DATE DUE

VOLUME 1

Principles AND Practice of SURGICAL PATHOLOGY AND CYTOPATHOLOGY

THIRD EDITION

VOLUME 1

PRINCIPLES AND PRACTICE OF SURGICAL PATHOLOGY AND CYTOPATHOLOGY

THIRD EDITION

EDITED BY

STEVEN G. SILVERBERG, M.D.

Professor of Pathology, and Director of Anatomic Pathology,
Department of Pathology, University of Maryland Medical System,
Baltimore, Maryland

ASSOCIATE EDITORS

RONALD A. DeLELLIS, M.D.

Professor, Department of Pathology,
Tufts University School of Medicine;
Department of Pathology, New England Medical Center,
Boston, Massachusetts

WILLIAM J. FRABLE, M.D.

Professor, Department of Pathology, Virginia Commonwealth University,
Medical College of Virginia; Director, Division of Surgical Pathology,
Medical College of Virginia Hospitals, Richmond, Virginia

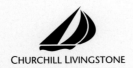

CHURCHILL LIVINGSTONE

New York, Edinburgh, London, Madrid, Melbourne, San Francisco, Tokyo

Library of Congress Cataloging-in-Publication Data

Principles and practice of surgical pathology and cytopathology / edited by
  Steven G. Silverberg, Ronald A. DeLellis, William J. Frable. — 3rd ed.
      p.   cm.
    Rev. ed. of: Principles and practice of surgical pathology. 2nd ed. 1990.
    Includes bibliographical references and index.
    ISBN 0-443-07541-7 (set : alk. paper)
    1. Pathology, Surgical. 2. Pathology, Cellular.   I. Silverberg,
Steven G., Date. II. DeLellis, Ronald A. III. Frable, William
J. IV. Title: Principles and practice of surgical pathology.
    [DNLM: 1. Pathology, Surgical.   WO 142 P9567 1997]
  RD57.P73   1997
  617′.07—dc21
  DNLM/DLC
  for Library of Congress   97-2455
                                                                   CIP

Distributed in the United Kingdom by Churchill Livingstone, Robert Stevenson House, 1–3 Baxter's Place, Leith Walk, Edinburgh EH1 3AF, and by associated companies, branches, and representatives throughout the world.

Medical knowledge is constantly changing. As new information becomes available, changes in treatment, procedures, equipment and the use of drugs become necessary. The editors/authors/contributors and the publishers have, as far as it is possible, taken care to ensure that the information given in this text is accurate and up to date. However, readers are strongly advised to confirm that the information, especially with regard to drug usage, complies with the latest legislation and standards of practice.

The Publishers have made every effort to trace the copyright holders for borrowed material. If they have inadvertently overlooked any, they will be pleased to make the necessary arrangements at the first opportunity.

Acquisitions Editor: *Marc Strauss*
Assistant Editor: *Vicky Stapf*
Production Editor: *Bridgett L. Dickinson*
Production Supervisor: *Laura Mosberg Cohen*
Cover Design: *Jeannette Jacobs*

Printed in Singapore

First published in 1997   7   6   5   4   3   2   1

To Kiyoe

Dolores, Renata, and Mark

Mary Ann, Deborrah, and Geraldine

Contributors

Jorge Albores-Saavedra, M.D.
Professor of Pathology, and Director, Division of Anatomic Pathology, Department of Pathology, University of Texas Southwestern Medical Center at Dallas, Dallas, Texas

Neil H. Anderson, M.D., M.R.C. Path.
Consultant Cytopathologist, Belfast Link Laboratories, Royal Hospitals Trust, The Belfast City Hospital Trust, Belfast, Ireland

Daniel A. Arber, M.D.
Staff Pathologist, Division of Pathology, City of Hope National Medical Center, Duarte, California

Paul L. Auclair, D.M.D., M.S.
Chairman, Department of Oral Pathology, Naval Dental School, Bethesda, Maryland

Alberto G. Ayala, M.D.
Professor, Division of Pathology, Department of Anatomic Pathology, The University of Texas M.D. Anderson Cancer Center, Houston, Texas

Leon Barnes, M.D.
Professor of Pathology and Otolaryngology, Department of Pathology and Laboratory Medicine, University of Pittsburgh School of Medicine; Chief, Division of Head and Neck Pathology, and Co-Director, Anatomic Pathology Services, Department of Pathology, Presbyterian University Hospital, Pittsburgh, Pennsylvania

Alan H. Beggs, Ph.D.
Assistant Professor, Department of Pediatrics, Harvard Medical School, Boston, Massachusetts; Research Associate, Department of Medicine, Children's Hospital, Boston, Massachusetts

Fred T. Bosman, M.D.
Professor and Director, Department of Pathology, Institut Universitaire de Pathologie, Lausanne, Switzerland

David G. Bostwick, M.D.
Professor, Department of Laboratory Medicine and Pathology, Mayo Medical School; Department of Laboratory Medicine, Mayo Clinic, Rochester, Minnesota

Peter G. Bullough, M.B., Ch.B.
Professor, Department of Pathology, Cornell University Medical College; Director, Department of Laboratory Medicine, Hospital of Special Surgery, New York, New York

Allen Burke, M.D
Adjunct Professor, Department of Pathology, Georgetown University School of Medicine; Associate Chair, Department of Cardiovascular Pathology, Armed Forces Institute of Pathology, Washington, D.C.

Karen L. Chang, M.D.
Staff Pathologist, Division of Pathology, City of Hope National Medical Center, Duarte, California

Alison D. Cluroe, B.Med.Sc, B.M., B.S., F.R.C.P.A.
Senior Lecturer, Department of Pathology, Auckland University School of Medicine; Consultant, Histopathology, Auckland Hospital, Auckland, New Zealand

Melissa J. Contos, M.D.
Assistant Professor, Department of Pathology, Virginia Commonwealth University, Medical College of Virginia, Richmond, Virginia

Bernard Czernobilsky, M.D.
Professor, Department of Pathology, Medical School of the Hebrew University and Hadassah, Jerusalem, Israel; Senior Consultant, Department of Pathology, Tel-Aviv Sourasky Medical Center, Tel-Aviv, Israel

Umberto De Girolami, M.D.
Associate Professor, Department of Pathology, Harvard Medical School; Director of Neuropathology, Department of Pathology, Brigham and Women's Hospital, Boston, Massachusetts

Ronald A. DeLellis, M.D.
Professor, Department of Pathology, Tufts University School of Medicine; Department of Pathology, New England Medical Center, Boston, Massachusetts

Ruby Delgado, M.D.
Assistant Professor and Co-Director, Immunohistochemistry Laboratory, Department of Pathology, University of Texas Southwestern Medical Center at Dallas, Dallas, Texas

Franco G. DeNardi, M.D.
Professor, Department of Pathology, McMaster University Faculty of Health Sciences; Staff Pathologist, Department of Laboratory Medicine, Hamilton Health Sciences Corporation, Henderson Division, Hamilton, Ontario, Canada

Ralph C. Eagle, Jr., M.D.
Professor, Departments of Ophthalmology and Pathology, Jefferson Medical College of Thomas Jefferson University; Director, Department of Pathology, Wills Eye Hospital, Philadelphia, Pennsylvania

Gary L. Ellis, D.D.S.
Assistant Chairman, Department of Oral and Maxillofacial Pathology, Armed Forces Institute of Pathology, Washington, D.C.

Robert A. Erlandson, Ph.D.
Associate Professor, Department of Pathology, Cornell University Medical College; Attending Electron Microscopist, Department of Pathology, Memorial Sloan-Kettering Cancer Center, New York, New York

Jose Esteban, M.D.
Professor, Department of Pathology, Georgetown University School of Medicine; Director of Cytopathology, Department of Pathology, Georgetown University Medical Center, Washington, D.C.

Garrey T. Faller, M.D.
Assistant Professor, Department of Pathology, Tufts University School of Medicine; Staff Pathologist, Department of Pathology, Carney Hospital, Boston, Massachusetts

Robert E. Fechner, M.D.
Professor, Department of Pathology, University of Virginia School of Medicine; Director of Anatomic and Surgical Pathology, Department of Pathology, University of Virginia Health Sciences Center, Charlottesville, Virginia

Cecilia M. Fenoglio-Preiser, M.D.
MacKenzie Professor and Director, Department of Pathology and Laboratory Medicine, University of Cincinnati College of Medicine, Cincinnati, Ohio

Linda D. Ferrell, M.D.
Professor, Department of Anatomic Pathology, University of California, San Francisco, School of Medicine, San Francisco, California

Mary Ann S. Frable, M.D.
Professor, Department of Otolaryngology, Virginia Commonwealth University, Medical College of Virginia, Richmond, Virginia

William J. Frable, M.D.
Professor, Department of Pathology, Virginia Commonwealth University, Medical College of Virginia; Director, Division of Surgical Pathology, Medical College of Virginia Hospitals, Richmond, Virginia

Henry F. Frierson, Jr., M.D.
Associate Professor, Department of Pathology, University of Virginia School of Medicine, Charlottesville, Virginia

Yao Shi Fu, M.D.
Senior Pathologist, Department of Pathology, St. Joseph Medical Center, Burbank, California

Parvin Ganjei, M.D.
Professor, Department of Pathology, University of Miami School of Medicine; Director of Surgical Pathology and Cytopathology, Department of Pathology, Jackson Memorial Medical Center, Miami, Florida

Mari Garcia-Moliner, M.D.
Assistant Professor, Department of Pathology, Tufts University School of Medicine; Attending Pathologist, New England Medical Center, Boston, Massachusetts

Kim R. Geisinger, M.D.
Professor, Department of Pathology, Bowman Gray School of Medicine of Wake Forest University; Director, Surgical Pathology and Cytopathology, North Carolina Baptist Hospitals, Winston-Salem, North Carolina

Loren E. Golitz, M.D.
Professor, Departments of Dermatology and Pathology, University of Colorado School of Medicine; Chief, Department of Dermatology, Denver General Hospital, Denver, Colorado

Zachary D. Goodman, M.D., Ph.D.
Chief, Department of Hepatic and Gastrointestinal Pathology, Armed Forces Institute of Pathology, Washington, D.C.

Robert O. Greer, Jr., D.D.S., Sc.D.
Professor, Department of Pathology, University of Colorado School of Medicine; Professor and Chairman, Division of Oral and Maxillofacial Pathology, University of Colorado School of Dentistry, Denver, Colorado

David J. Grignon, M.D.
Associate Professor, Department of Pathology, Wayne State University School of Medicine; Director of Anatomical Pathology, Department of Pathology, Harper Hospital, Detroit, Michigan

Prabodh Gupta, M.D.
Professor, Department of Pathology and Laboratory Medicine, University of Pennsylvania School of Medicine; Director, Department of Cytopathology and Cytometry, University of Pennsylvania Medical Center, Philadelphia, Pennsylvania

A. Marion Gurley, M.B., Ch.B
Anatomical Pathologist, Dr. Colin Laverty and Associates, Eastwood, N.S.W., Australia

Elizabeth H. Hammond, M.D.
Professor, Department of Pathology, University of Utah School of Medicine; Chairman, Department of Pathology, LDS Hospital, Intermountain Health Care, Salt Lake City, Utah

John M. Hardman, M.D.
Professor, Department of Pathology, University of Hawaii John A. Burns School of Medicine, Honolulu, Hawaii

Bruce C. Horten, M.D.
Attending Pathologist, Department of Pathology, Lenox Hill Hospital; Medical Director, Impath Laboratories, New York, New York

Eva Horvath, Ph.D.
Department of Pathology, St. Michael's Hospital, Toronto, Ontario, Canada

Christopher B. Hubbard, M.S.
Department of Pathology, Duke University School of Medicine; Manager, Pathology Informatics, Department of Pathology, Duke University Medical Center, Durham, North Carolina

Kamal G. Ishak, M.D., Ph.D.
Chairman, Department of Hepatic and Gastrointestinal Pathology, Armed Forces Institute of Pathology, Washington, D.C.

Edward C. Klatt, M.D.
Associate Professor, Department of Pathology, University of Utah School of Medicine; Medical Director of Autopsy, Department of Pathology, University Hospital, Salt Lake City, Utah

Michael J. Kornstein, M.D.
Associate Professor, Department of Pathology, Virginia Commonwealth University, Medical College of Virginia, Richmond, Virginia

Kalman Kovacs, M.D.
Professor, Department of Pathology, University of Toronto Faculty of Medicine; Staff Pathologist, Department of Pathology, St. Michael's Hospital, Toronto, Ontario, Canada

Ernest E. Lack, M.D.
Director of Anatomic Pathology and Professor, Department of Pathology, Georgetown University School of Medicine, Washington, D.C.

Ginette Lajoie, M.D.
Lecturer, Department of Pathology, University of Toronto Faculty of Medicine; Staff Pathologist, Department of Pathology, Toronto Hospital, Toronto, Ontario, Canada

Zoltan Laszik, M.D., Ph.D.
Renal Research Fellow, Department of Pathology, University of Oklahoma College of Medicine; Department of Pathology, University Hospitals, Oklahoma City, Oklahoma

Frederick D. Lee, M.D., F.R.C.P. (Glas.), F.R.C. Path.
Consultant and Honorary Professor, Department of Pathology, Glasgow Royal Infirmary and University NHS Trust, Glasgow, Scotland

Merle A. Legg, M.D.
Emeritus Chairman, Department of Pathology, New England Deaconess Hospital, Boston, Massachusetts

Beatriz Lifschitz-Mercer, M.D.
Senior Lecturer, Department of Pathology, Tel Aviv University, Sackler School of Medicine; Chief, Department of Pathology, Tel Aviv Sourasky Medical Center, Tel Aviv, Israel

James Linder, M.D.
Professor, Department of Pathology and Microbiology, University of Nebraska College of Medicine, Omaha, Nebraska

Massimo Loda, M.D.
Assistant Professor, Department of Pathology, Harvard Medical School; Director of Molecular Pathology, Department of Pathology, New England Deaconess Hospital, Boston, Massachusetts

Trevor A. Macpherson, M.B., Ch.B., M.S.
Professor, Department of Pathology, University of Pittsburgh School of Medicine; Chief, Department of Pathology, Magee-Womens Hospital, Pittsburgh, Pennsylvania

John Maksem, M.D.
Chief, Department of Pathology, Mercy Hospital, Des Moines, Iowa

Shahla Masood, M.D.
Professor and Associate Chair, Department of Pathology, University of Florida Health Science Center; Chief of Pathology, University Medical Center, Gainesville, Florida

Maria J. Merino, M.D.
Chief, Surgical Pathology, Laboratory of Pathology, National Cancer Institute, National Institutes of Health, Bethesda, Maryland

Nabila E. Metwalli, M.D.
Professor, Department of Pathology, University of Alexandria Medical School, Alexandria, Egypt

Roberta R. Miller, M.D.*
Clinical Professor, Department of Pathology and Laboratory Medicine, University of British Columbia Faculty of Medicine; Pathologist, Department of Pathology and Laboratory Medicine, Vancouver Hospital and Health Sciences Centre, Vancouver, British Columbia, Canada

A. Scott Mills, M.D.
Associate Professor, Department of Pathology, Virginia Commonwealth University, Medical College of Virginia, Richmond, Virginia

Joan M. Mones, M.D.
Clinical Assistant Professor, Department of Pathology, University of Miami School of Medicine, Miami, Florida; Attending Pathologist, Parkway Regional Medical Center, Boston, Massachusetts

Azorides R. Morales, M.D.
Professor and Chairman, Department of Pathology, University of Miami School of Medicine; Chief, Laboratory Services, Jackson Memorial Medical Center, Miami, Florida

Nestor L. Müller, M.D.
Professor, Department of Radiology, University of British Columbia Faculty of Medicine; Associate Head for Academic Affairs, Department of Radiology, Vancouver Hospital and Health Sciences Centre, Vancouver, British Columbia, Canada

Diane L. Mullins, M.D.
Assistant Professor, Department of Pathology and Laboratory Medicine, University of Florida College of Medicine, Gainesville, Florida

George F. Murphy, M.D.
Professor, Department of Pathology, and Director of Medical Education, Jefferson Medical College of Thomas Jefferson University, Philadelphia, Pennsylvania

Tibor Nadasdy, M.D., Ph.D.
Assistant Professor, Department of Pathology, Johns Hopkins University School of Medicine, Baltimore, Maryland

Mehrdad Nadji, M.D.
Professor, Department of Pathology, University of Miami School of Medicine; Director of Anatomic Pathology, Department of Pathology, Jackson Memorial Medical Center, Miami, Florida

Hideo Namiki, M.D.
Clinical Professor, Department of Pathology, University of Hawaii John A. Burns School of Medicine, Honolulu, Hawaii

Guy E. Nichols, M.D.
Assistant Professor, Department of Pathology, University of Virginia School of Medicine; Department of Pathology, University of Virginia Health Sciences Center, Charlottesville, Virginia

Lucien E. Nochomovitz, M.D.
Chief, Department of Anatomic Pathology, Winthrop-University Hospital, Mineola, New York

*Deceased.

Amy E. Noffsinger, M.D.
Assistant Professor, Department of Pathology and
Laboratory Medicine, University of Cincinnati College of
Medicine, Cincinnati, Ohio

Jan M. Orenstein, M.D.
Professor, Department of Pathology, George Washington
University School of Medicine and Health Sciences,
Washington, D.C.

Robert R. Pascal, M.D.
Professor, Department of Pathology and Laboratory
Medicine, Emory University School of Medicine; Surgical
Pathologist, Division of Anatomic Pathology, Department
of Pathology, Emory University Hospital, Atlanta, Georgia

Karl H. Perzin, M.D.
Professor, Division of Clinical Surgical Pathology,
Columbia University College of Physicians and Surgeons;
Attending Surgical Pathologist, Department of Pathology,
Presbyterian Hospital, New York, New York

Bruce D. Ragsdale, M.D.
Instructor, Department of Dermatology, University of
Alabama School of Medicine, Birmingham, Alabama;
Dermatopathologist, Central Coast Pathology Consultants,
San Luis Obispo, California

Robert R. Rickert, M.D.
Clinical Professor, Department of Pathology and Laboratory
Medicine, UMDNJ-New Jersey Medical School, Newark,
New Jersey; Co-chairman, Department of Pathology, Saint
Barnabas Medical Center, Livingston, New Jersey

Robert H. Riddell, M.D.
Professor, Department of Pathology, McMaster University
Faculty of Health Sciences; Chief of Service, Anatomical
Pathology, Department of Laboratory Medicine, Hamilton
Health Sciences Corporation, Hamilton, Ontario,
Canada

Jae Y. Ro, M.D.
Professor, Division of Pathology, Department of Anatomic
Pathology, The University of Texas M.D. Anderson
Cancer Center, Houston, Texas

Stanley J. Robboy, M.D.
Professor, Departments of Pathology, and Obstetrics and
Gynecology, Duke University School of Medicine;
Director, Gynecologic and Obstetric Pathology,
Departments of Pathology, and Obstetrics and Gynecology,
Duke University Medical Center, Durham, North Carolina

Elizabeth C. Roberts, M.B., Ch.B.
Resident Physician, Department of Pathology, Oregon
Health Sciences University School of Medicine, Portland,
Oregon

Lawrence M. Roth, M.D.
Professor, Department of Pathology, Indiana University
School of Medicine; Director of Surgical Pathology,
Department of Pathology, Indiana University Hospital,
Indianapolis, Indiana

Sanford I. Roth, M.D.
Professor, Department of Pathology, Northwestern
University Medical School; Attending Pathologist,
Department of Pathology, Northwestern Memorial
Hospital, Chicago, Illinois

Frank R. Rudy, M.D.
Clinical Assistant Professor, Department of Pathology,
Pennsylvania State University College of Medicine, Hershey,
Pennsylvania; Chairman, Department of Laboratories,
Pinnacle Health Hospitals, Harrisburg, Pennsylvania

Joseph D. Sabella, M.D.
Chief (retired), Brookside Hospital Laboratory, San Pablo,
California; Chairman and Chief Executive Officer
(retired), The Doctors' Company, Napa, California

Mario J. Saldana, M.D.
Professor (Emeritus/Active), Department of Pathology,
University of Miami School of Medicine; Attending
Pathologist, Cedars Medical Center, Miami, Florida;
Consulting Pathologist, Mount Sinai Medical Center,
Miami Beach, Florida,

Khalil Sheibani, M.D.
Clinical Professor, Department of Pathology, University
of Southern California School of Medicine, Los Angeles,
California; Pathologist, Department of Pathology, Western
Medical Center, Santa Ana, California

Mark E. Sherman, M.D.
Associate Professor, Division of Cytopathology and
Gynecologic Pathology, Department of Pathology, Johns
Hopkins Medical Institutions, Baltimore, Maryland

Maria Shevchuk, M.D.
Associate Professor of Clinical Pathology, Department of
Pathology, New York University School of Medicine;
Department of Pathology, Lenox Hill Hospital, New York,
New York

Mary K. Sidawy, M.D.
Associate Professor, Department of Pathology, George
Washington University School of Medicine and Health
Sciences; Director of Cytopathology, Department of
Pathology, George Washington Medical Center,
Washington, D.C.

Fred G. Silva, M.D.
Lloyd E. Rader Professor and Chairman, Department
of Pathology, University of Oklahoma College of
Medicine; Director, Renal Pathology Laboratory,
Department of Pathology, and Chief, Pathology
Services, University Hospitals, Oklahoma City,
Oklahoma

Steven G. Silverberg, M.D.
Professor of Pathology, and Director of Anatomic
Pathology, Department of Pathology, University of
Maryland Medical System, Baltimore, Maryland

Jan F. Silverman, M.D.
Professor and Vice Chairman, Director of Cytology,
Department of Pathology and Laboratory Medicine,
East Carolina University School of Medicine,
Greenville, North Carolina

Harlan J. Spjut, M.D.
Professor, Department of Pathology, Baylor College of
Medicine, Houston, Texas

Gregg A. Staerkel, M.D.
Assistant Professor, Division of Pathology, Department of
Anatomic Pathology, University of Texas M.D. Anderson
Cancer Center, Houston, Texas

Michael W. Stanley, M.D.
Professor, Department of Pathology, University of Arkansas
College of Medicine, Little Rock, Arkansas

Timothy T. Stenzel, M.D., Ph.D.
Resident, Department of Pathology, Duke University
Medical Center, Durham, North Carolina

Nora C. J. Sun, M.D.
Professor, Department of Pathology, University of
California, Los Angeles, UCLA School of Medicine, Los
Angeles, California; Head, Hematopathology, Department
of Pathology, Harbor-UCLA Medical Center, Torrance,
California

Aron E. Szulman, M.B., Ch.B.
Emeritus Professor, Department of Pathology, University
of Pittsburgh School of Medicine; Pathologist,
Department of Pathology, Magee-Womens Hospital,
Pittsburgh, Pennsylvania

Sana O. Tabbara, M.D.
Associate Professor, Department of Pathology, George
Washington University School of Medicine and Health
Sciences, Washington, D.C.

Myron Tannenbaum, M.D., Ph.D.
Professor, Departments of Pathology and Surgery,
University of South Florida College of Medicine, Tampa,
Florida; Department of Veterans Affairs Medical Center,
Bay Pines, Florida

Lisa A. Teot, M.D.
Assistant Professor, Department of Pathology and
Laboratory Medicine, University of Rochester School of
Medicine and Dentistry, Rochester, New York

Kamal Thapar, M.D., Ph.D.
Fellow, Divsion of Neurosurgery, Department of Surgery,
University of Toronto Faculty of Medicine; Division of
Neurosurgery, St. Michael's Hospital, Toronto, Ontario,
Canada

William M. Thurlbeck, M.D.
Emeritus Professor, Department of Pathology and
Laboratory Medicine, University of British Columbia
Faculty of Medicine; Consultant Pathologist, Department
of Pathology and Laboratory Medicine, Vancouver
Hospital and Health Sciences Centre, Vancouver,
British Columbia, Canada

Peter G. Toner, D.S.C., F.R.C.P., F.R.C. Path.
Musgrave Professor, Department of Pathology, School
of Clinical Medicine, The Queen's University of Belfast;
Director of Laboratory Medicine, Belfast Link
Laboratories, Royal Hospitals Trust, The Belfast City
Hospital Trust, Belfast, Ireland

Renu Virmani, M.D.
Research Professor, Department of Pathology,
Vanderbilt University School of Medicine, Nashville,
Tennessee; Chair, Department of Cardiovascular
Pathology, Armed Forces Institute of Pathology,
Washington, D.C.

Frank Vuitch, M.D.
Associate Professor and Co-Director, Department of
Pathology, University of Texas Southwestern Medical
Center at Dallas, Dallas, Texas

Lawrence M. Weiss, M.D.
Director of Surgical Pathology, Department of Anatomic
Pathology, City of Hope National Medical Center,
Duarte, California

James E. Wheeler, M.D.
Professor, Department of Anatomic Pathology, Hospital
of the University of Pennsylvania, Philadelphia,
Pennsylvania

Edward J. Wilkinson, M.D.
Professor and Interim Chairman, Department of
Pathology, Immunology, and Laboratory Medicine,
University of Florida College of Medicine, Gainesville,
Florida

Washington C. Winn, Jr., M.D.
Department of Pathology and Laboratory Medicine,
University of Vermont College of Medicine; Microbiology
Laboratory, Medical Center Hospital of Vermont,
Burlington, Vermont

James M. Woodruff, M.D.
Professor, Department of Pathology, Cornell University
Medical College; Attending Pathologist, Department of
Pathology, Memorial Sloan-Kettering Cancer Center, New
York, New York

Hong-Yi Yang, M.D., Ph.D.
Professor, Department of Pathology, University of Hawaii
John A. Burns School of Medicine, Honolulu, Hawaii

Richard J. Zarbo, M.D., D.M.D.
Professor, Department of Pathology, Case Western Reserve
University School of Medicine, Cleveland, Ohio; Head,
Division of Surgical Pathology, Henry Ford Health System,
Detroit, Michigan

Preface

The genesis of the first edition of this work dates back more than 15 years, at which time it became apparent that the field of surgical pathology had become so complex that there was a need for a text authored by an international group of experts, most of whom had already written monographs or major review articles in their specific areas. The stated goals of that edition were to provide a thorough and authoritative survey of the field of surgical pathology and to present the information needed in a practical format that would be useful to the pathologist in training or practice. Another new concept at that time was for the chapters to be at least in part specimen-oriented rather than disease-oriented, so that lesions likely to be encountered as medical biopsy specimens were sometimes discussed in separate chapters from those seen primarily in surgical resection specimens of the same organs. Several chapters at the beginning of the first volume were provided as introductory material, and included discussions of subjects considered not unique to any one organ or organ system, but rather applicable to many of the specific site chapters.

These concepts have weathered the subsequent years well, but it also became clear that there was still room for improvement. For many years, my colleagues and I have emphasized the intimate relationship between the disciplines of surgical pathology and cytopathology, demanding not only that both cytologic and tissue specimens be correlated in individual cases (a more and more frequent situation with the increasing popularity of fine needle aspiration biopsy), but also that each pathologist be capable of applying the lessons of one discipline to the problems of the other. In order to aid the reader in fully realizing these goals, the decision was made to convert the current edition into a text of both surgical and cytopathology. In most instances, both the surgical and cytopathology of a single organ or system are integrated in a single chapter, while in others the scope of the subject made it easier and (we hope) more effective to use adjacent chapters. As has been the case since the first edition of this text, we have been fortunate to be able to persuade some of the preeminent experts in cytopathology to contribute the pertinent chapters or chapter sections.

Equally apparent is the fact that techniques considered to be of research interest only at the time of our first edition are now an integral part of the practice of surgical and cytopathology. Additionally, new economic and regulatory imperatives have created new pitfalls as well as opportunities for the pathologist. Both new biotechnological advances and new applications of quality improvement are not only covered where appropriate in each organ-based chapter, but have also contributed to an expansion of the introductory section (the "Principles" of "Principles and Practice") from 7 chapters in the first edition to 10 in the current one.

I have been extremely fortunate in the introduction of these major changes to have been aided by two new Associate Editors without whose advice and assistance this task might well have been impossible to accomplish. Drs. DeLellis and Frable not only supervised the molecular and technical and cytopathologic sections, respectively, but were active partners at every stage of the development of the entire project. They deserve a major share of the credit for the success of the book, and certainly a great deal of my own gratitude.

Equally deserving are the numerous talented authors who contributed the 62 individual chapters. Some of these authors have been with us from the beginning, while more than half represent new contributors. The latter are yet another vehicle for keeping the final product as fresh and exciting as the field of surgical and cytopathology itself, and we are indeed fortunate to have so many gifted physicians enter our specialty each year.

We are all, of course, surrounded by relatives, friends, and colleagues who are a constant source of inspiration to us. In addition, our mentors over the years have instilled in us the ability and the desire to reach our goals. For my own part, these have included the late Drs. Abou Pollack, Harry Greene, Averill Liebow, Fred Stewart, and Frank Foote, as well as the happily still active Drs. Claude Gompel, Leopold G. Koss, and Saul Kay. My colleagues and students at the University of Colorado, George Washington University, and now the University of Maryland have all played a major role in the development of this work through its three editions. Dr. DeLellis gratefully acknowledges the help and support of his many colleagues in the Department of Pathology at Tufts University School of Medicine and the New England Medical Center. Dr. Frable would also like to acknowledge the assistance of the faculty and staff of the Division of Surgical and Cytopathology of the Virginia Commonwealth University, Medical College of Virginia. The editorial and production staff at Churchill Livingstone have been very helpful to us all, with particular thanks to Marc Strauss, Victoria Stapf, and Bridgett Dickinson. Finally, my parents, Esther and the late Bertram Silverberg, were instrumental in the early development of my career, and my wife, Kiyoe, has been a constant source of support over the past 30 years.

Steven G. Silverberg, M.D.

Contents

General Philosophy and Principles of Surgical Pathology and Cytopathology

Steven G. Silverberg

What is surgical pathology? Probably the best definition is that surgical pathology is the discipline that deals with the anatomic pathology of tissues removed from living patients. Many surgical pathologists expand this definition to include smears, aspirates, and body fluids as well, so cytopathology is usually considered within the domain of surgical pathology. Indeed, it has been my philosophy for many years that it is difficult to be an excellent surgical pathologist without also practicing cytopathology, and virtually impossible to be an excellent cytopathologist—especially in the era of fine needle aspiration of almost every organ—without also obtaining and retaining expertise in general surgical pathology.

By the above definition, surgical pathology differs from autopsy pathology in (1) the nature of the specimens seen most frequently, and (2) the usual immediacy of the decisions to be made and their relation to the subsequent management of an individual patient. The latter distinction is perhaps more immediately apparent. The diagnosis made by the surgical pathologist or cytopathologist often precedes the treatment of the patient and, in fact, in such instances usually influences or even determines what such treatment will be. On the other hand, the role of the autopsy pathologist, or morbid anatomist, invariably begins after treatment has ended and includes an assessment of the appropriateness and adequacy of the therapeutic regimens employed.

The first difference listed above between surgical and autopsy pathology is also an important one to remember, however. As an example, diagnostic material from the heart forms a fairly small (but currently increasing) portion of the workload of the surgical pathologist, whereas it is a major (if not the major) consideration in the practice of autopsy pathology. By contrast, the skin and the female genital tract are usually not studied extensively at autopsy, yet together they comprise more than one-half the specimens seen in most practices of surgical pathology. Thus, it is apparent that the reading and continuing education that must be undertaken to keep up to date in the two fields is quite different, almost justifying their characterization as entirely separate disciplines. By contrast, the basic skills essential to the practice of surgical pathology are the same as those learned in the performance of autopsies, and there are few

practicing surgical pathologists who do not continue their involvement with autopsy pathology as well.

PRACTICE OF SURGICAL PATHOLOGY

Whether working in an academic medical center or a small community hospital, the surgical pathologist always functions as a teacher and often as a researcher. The main role of the surgical pathologist, however, is still essentially the practice of medicine, which is sometimes easy to forget, particularly for the pathologist who does not regularly see living patients. The results of such distance may be disastrous for both the pathologist and the patient. The role of the surgical pathologist should be that of a consultant to the clinician for the ultimate benefit of the patient, and this role must be remembered even when the pathologist is in the laboratory, far from direct contact with either the clinician or the patient.

Furthermore, despite the traditional name of the field (surgical pathology), the practitioner soon learns that service to, and contact with, general and specialty surgeons comprises only a small part of the total practice. Because the workload of the modern surgical pathologist also includes specimens from dermatologists, gynecologists, gastroenterologists, pediatricians, nephrologists, and physicians in many other specialties, the pathologist must have some familiarity with each of these fields and the clinical problems encountered therein. Thus the formative and continuing education must consist of training not only in morphologic interpretation but also in the clinical practice of medicine. The most effective surgical pathologists are often those who have had some advanced clinical training after their undergraduate medical education and thus are best able to place the specimens they receive into the proper clinical context.

This need for clinical competence is even more apparent for cytopathologists who perform their own fine needle aspiration biopsies (FNABs). We have found that sometimes interventional cytopathologists can localize and aspirate small masses after repeated failures by even very experienced clinicians. As pointed out in Chapter 10, exact knowledge by the cytopathologist of the clinical context of the aspirated mass can be extremely useful in making the correct diagnosis, as well as in knowing whether a paucicellular aspirate is representative of the lesion and diagnosable as benign or is truly insufficient for diagnosis. Cytopathologists who perform FNABs are also well aware of the clinical effort involved in obtaining pertinent historic data, in reassuring the patient, and in dealing with the fortunately rare complications of the procedure.

Consultative Role of the Surgical Pathologist

By recalling the relationship between the surgical pathologist and the clinician and patient, the general principles of the approach to a specimen are greatly simplified. Surgical pathologists should deal with each specimen as if they were the clinician—or, better yet, the patient—awaiting the surgical pathology report. Questions such as whether to photograph a gross specimen, how many sections to submit of a particular lesion, how carefully to search for lymph nodes in a radical procedure, whether to order recuts or special stains, whether to write or dictate a microscopic description, and so forth all become answerable in terms of the single basic question, "Were I either the clinician or the patient in this case, what information would I need about this specimen, and how can that information best be supplied?"

Given this approach, the answers to different but similar questions about the same specimen may initially appear to be at odds; this apparent contradiction is easily resolved, however, when the ultimate benefit to the patient is considered. For example, the question of whether to perform radiography on a breast resection specimen is usually answered in the affirmative, since the information obtained from this procedure will assist the surgical pathologist in guaranteeing that the clinically suspicious lesion has been removed and that no other grossly inapparent but clinically important lesions are present in the same specimen.[1] On the other hand, the question of whether to perform laborious fat-clearing procedures for the axillary contents received as part of a mastectomy specimen is usually resolved negatively, since the information that may be obtained from this procedure (detection of additional small lymph nodes and perhaps even additional micrometastases) does not appear to influence either the prognosis or the treatment significantly.[2]

Thus, the approach to any specimen received in the surgical pathology laboratory obviously depends on the specific clinical problem to be resolved by the interpretation of that specimen. Therefore, it is essential that each specimen be accompanied by an adequate description of what it represents, as well as an appropriate clinical history. The surgical pathologist should design the request form so the clinician filling out the form is sure to appreciate the need for supplying this information. Recent progress toward some degree of standardization of the surgical pathology report may aid in making the information more universally available.[3] If adequate clinical information is not received with a particular specimen, the surgical pathologist is completely justified in not processing that specimen until the appropriate information is obtained. The telephone should also

be an important part of the surgical pathologist's equipment. Submitting physicians should be called promptly if any question exists about a specimen submitted.

Similarly, the responsibility of the surgical pathologist does not end when a diagnosis has been made and recorded on the surgical pathology report. If the diagnosis differs significantly from what was clinically suspected, or if it requires any immediate response by the clinician, the clinician should be contacted promptly rather than waiting for the report by the usual route of distribution. If the diagnosis made is an uncommon one, the significance of which is not likely to be understood by the clinician, the surgical pathologist should be sure that the meaning of the term is explained and a pertinent reference provided, either verbally or in the body of the surgical pathology report (preferably by both means).

The importance of communication between the clinician and the pathologist is often underestimated by both parties. This is particularly true of surgical pathologists, who perhaps become too familiar with the "What do you think of this slide without any history?" type of quiz they often receive during residency. It is essential to remember, however, that the practice of surgical pathology is not an intellectual game, but rather a serious facet of the practice of medicine, often with life or death implications. Thus, when dealing with any living patient, all the available clinical information should be presented to the surgical pathologist responsible for the case. This is obviously of less importance in some cases than in others, but it is easier to invoke it as a general rule to which occasional exceptions will be made than to face a constant struggle in obtaining clinical information when it is urgently needed.

These comments pertaining to communication between the clinician and the surgical pathologist are indicative of the role of the surgical pathologist as a clinical consultant. The clinician would certainly not think of calling in a gynecologist as a consultant to evaluate a possible pelvic mass without providing both adequate clinical data and the reason for the consultation; similarly, the clinician should not obtain a consultation from the surgical pathologist without the same courtesy. To continue the same analogy, just as the clinician would not demand that the gynecologic consultant perform a specific diagnostic or therapeutic procedure, the surgical pathologist should not be required to perform a particular stain, a frozen section, or any other procedure on the tissues submitted. The other side of the coin is that it then becomes the role of the surgical pathologist to decide what special stains or other studies to perform based on an interpretation of all the clinical and pathologic data available in a given case, and it is the surgical pathologist's responsibility to be sure that all this information has indeed been supplied.

In cytopathology as well, the issue of communication is extremely important and (as mentioned above in association with the performance of FNAB) may involve the patient directly as well as through the medium of the clinician. The problem of communicating the result of a suspicious Papanicolaou (Pap) smear to the submitting clinician and ultimately to the patient, and of ensuring timely and appropriate follow-up, is one that becomes even more obvious when it results in malpractice litigation.[4] If the cytopathologist does not also personally see the tissue specimen accompanying or following a Pap smear, a bronchial wash, an FNAB, or some other cytologic specimen, communication with the surgical pathologist who receives that tissue specimen also becomes crucial in the process of quality assurance (see Ch. 2). This process is obviously a two-way street, and the surgical pathologist equally needs to compare the tissue diagnosis with cytopathologic material from the same patient.

Interpathologist Consultation in Surgical Pathology

The question of consultations in surgical pathology is frequently puzzling for the novice. It is always difficult to find the proper middle ground between the hesitancy to ever ask for a consultation and the temptation to seek consultation on virtually every case that is not entirely routine. We who practice surgical pathology are fortunate that it is far easier to transport slides to an expert consultant than to transport the patient; therefore, there is never really an excuse for not obtaining a consultation in situations in which it is indicated, and thus we are safer in erring on the side of overutilization rather than underutilization of this service.

Internal consultation should always be used in questionable cases. Thus, if three members of a group at a particular institution practice surgical pathology, all three should review such a case, and the final report should express the consensus diagnosis. If such a consensus is unobtainable, or if doubt remains, outside consultation is then sought. A good general rule to follow is that one outside consultant should be used for each case. Nothing is more disturbing to the practicing pathologist than to send slides from a case to three different eminent consultants and get three different answers. The consultant should be chosen for expertise in a particular field of surgical pathology or because the referring pathologist has had previous favorable experience with that consultant—not because the consultant is located at a famous institution, although the person chosen may lack the credentials of an expert consultant in the particular case to be referred.

Having chosen the consultant, it is essential to provide that individual with the same courtesies that we expect our clinicians to provide to us.[5] Thus, the name, age, and sex of the patient, the hospital and/or surgical pathology number, and the pertinent clinical history should be submitted, as well as a copy of the surgical pathology report in which the gross pathologic features of the case are described. The slides submitted should be adequate in both quantity and quality, since the function of a consultant is not to overcome someone else's inadequate histotechnique. Specially stained slides, if pertinent, should also be submitted, or at least unstained slides or paraffin blocks on which consultants may perform the stains they deem necessary. Referring pathologists should always include their own diagnoses, or the differential if a final diagnosis has not been reached. If questions about the clinical management of the case exist, these should be asked directly in the referring letter. Unless there is some compelling reason for wanting these slides returned (such as the lesion being seen on only one slide or the block being unavailable), the consultant should be permitted to retain the submitted slides. When the report of the consultant is received by the referring pathologist, it should always be made available to the clinician, even (or especially) if it is at variance with the referring pathologist's original diagnosis.

The surgical pathologist should always be willing to send a case for consultation if so requested by the clinician, but certainly the surgical pathologist is free to state that a consultation is not really necessary if such is the case. If the clinician requests a specific consultant, and the pathologist believes that that individual is inappropriate for the case in question, the clinician should be so informed. If the clinician still insists on that consultant, the pathologist should probably acquiesce but is certainly entitled to send the case to another consultant as well. This is one of the few acceptable reasons for violating the "one consultant per case" rule mentioned earlier.

Consultant pathologists are entitled to adequate clinical information and histologic material and in most instances should be able to retain the slides (especially if the patient is being treated in their institution). If these slides or the clinical data submitted are in any way inadequate, consultant pathologists should feel free to make the same demands of the referring pathologist that they would make of their clinicians or of their laboratory, and they should not make a diagnosis on the basis of inadequate clinical or pathologic data. They may need to request the paraffin blocks or fixed tissues for processing in their own laboratory; the fear of insulting the referring pathologist by asking for this material should not outweigh the responsibility to the patient of rendering a diagnosis only on optimal preparations.

Consultations on cytopathologic material sent to pathologists outside one's own institution are more problematic, since no paraffin block exists (except in the case of material processed as a cell block) from which to cut additional slides, and the referring pathologist may therefore hesitate to risk loss or breakage of the only glass slide showing a worrisome finding. Photomicrographs may be useful in this situation, and even more immediacy is provided by the rapidly developing field of telepathology, by which high quality photographic images can be transferred virtually instantaneously to the consultant.[6,7] This technology is clearly available—but perhaps less necessary —for tissue consultations as well, and may be of particular value in obtaining rapid help with a difficult frozen section interpretation.[8]

Intraoperative Consultation in Surgical Pathology

The question of false positive diagnoses is particularly relevant with respect to frozen section examinations. Older reports of frozen section results in breast lesions, for example, have generally indicated that the frequency of false positive diagnoses (something being called cancer that in reality is benign) should be zero, that false negative diagnoses comprise about 1 percent of cases, and that diagnosis must be deferred to permanent sections in 1 to 2 percent of the cases.[9–11] Several points should be emphasized with reference to these figures. First, authors who publish results of frozen section examination (or, for that matter, of anything) are invariably those who have a great deal of experience with the technique; the surgical pathologist who performs 100 frozen section examinations a year is likely to have considerably poorer results than one who performs 1,000 a year. Second, the frequency of false positive diagnoses is inversely related to that of deferred diagnoses, so the attempt to "force" a diagnosis in a difficult situation is likely to lead to the feared result of a false positive interpretation. Thus, there should be no shame in equivocating in such a situation, and sometimes (e.g., for intralobular and intraductal mammary lesions, questionable lymphomas), discretion is usually the better part of valor. Third, most false negative interpretations are probably due to sampling error and are thus unavoidable. Despite our competence in gross pathology, when one or two sections are taken from a 10 cm specimen, we will invariably encounter situations in which the definitive diagnosis is not made until many more sections are examined the following day.

Finally, my colleagues and I[12–15] as well as others[16,17] have commented on recent changes in both the indications for frozen section examination and the specimens most frequently encountered. In almost one-half of our cases, the examination is performed not primarily for a diagnosis, but rather to comment on the adequacy of the specimen for subsequent diagnosis, to select tissue for special studies (e.g., hormone receptors, lymphoid cell markers, flow cytometry), or to demonstrate gross pathology and thus ensure better communications. Thus, the proportion of cases with a deferred diagnosis has increased considerably since the early reports. Similarly, the proportion of breast cases (still the most frequent organ site involved) with occult or "minimal" cancer has also increased markedly, contributing as well to an elevated proportion of both deferred and false negative diagnoses.

In actuality, "frozen section" examination is a poor term, since many intraoperative consultations (the preferred term) do not result in performance of frozen section examinations. It is the responsibility of the surgical pathologist, as the consultant in this situation, to decide exactly what needs to be done; if the gross appearance of the specimen is characteristic, or if the diagnosis can be made by the imprint or smear technique alone, the performance of a frozen section examination may be unnecessary. Similarly, freezing of tissues may not only be unnecessary but may actually be contraindicated in certain situations. For example, if the specimen submitted is so small that frozen section examination would be likely to exhaust the tissue completely, and if the frozen section diagnosis is likely to be either difficult to make or unnecessary for the immediate management of the patient, then certainly this procedure should not be performed. This has become particularly notable in recent years in the intraoperative management of mamographically directed breast biopsies.[18,19]

The role of the frozen section examination in providing instant gratification for the surgeon should be commented on further at this point. Since most departments of pathology charge the patient an additional fee for these examinations, both the clinician and the pathologist should understand that frozen sections should be performed only when they will provide information of immediate or ultimate value in patient management. Thus, a breast biopsy specimen should certainly be frozen if immediate mastectomy is contemplated (a rare event today in most hospitals), but the tissue should probably not be frozen if the surgeon plans to delay definitive surgery by several days even if the results of the biopsy are positive for carcinoma. However, intraoperative consultation may still be indicated to obtain fresh tumor tissue for estrogen and progesterone receptor assays or flow cytometric analysis, or for both. Even this need has diminished, however, with the development of technology to perform these studies on routinely fixed and embedded tissues. As another example, in a case of suspected malignant lymphoma, intraoperative consultation may be requested to determine whether diagnostic tissue has indeed been removed before the incision is closed but such consultation should not be requested to provide a definitive diagnosis unless the physician plans to institute therapy immediately (e.g., in a case of spinal cord compression or superior vena cava syndrome).

Special mention should be made of the surgical practice of requesting frozen section examination to determine the adequacy of margins in a resection for cancer. This is done most frequently in the head and neck area: such tissues are often difficult to freeze and section because of the high fat content. In addition, it is apparent that in a large resection specimen, only a limited number of frozen section examinations can be performed perpendicular to the tumor and its resection margins while the patient is still waiting under anesthesia. Thus, a report of a positive margin is of great value, but a negative report does not by any means guarantee that tumor will not be found when permanent sections of the adjacent tissues are examined. Thus, I usually remind our surgeons that frozen section examinations in this situation are analogous to the old bumper sticker in that, if you need this, "you are too darn close."

Margins on tumor resections, incidentally, are one of those situations in which cytologic preparations do not add significantly to the information obtained by performing a classic frozen section examination. Unless massive amounts of tumor are present at a resection margin (usually enough to be visible grossly), the results of the imprint will probably still be negative for tumor cells. By contrast, we have found these preparations of considerable assistance as a complement to frozen section examination in many situations; in some cases, they even supplant the frozen section examination itself.[13–15,20,21] For example, false negative results on a lymph node containing a small volume of metastatic cancer are more likely to be obtained from a frozen section examination than from a smear or imprint preparation of that lymph node. The main reason is that multiple cut surfaces of the node can be processed on one slide using the cytologic technique, as opposed to the multiple frozen sections that would be necessary to examine the node as thoroughly without the use of imprints. Also, since freezing artifact is not a factor in the imprint preparation, a few cancer cells are more easily distinguished from the surrounding population of lymphocytes and histiocytes than they are in the artifactually distorted frozen section. Imprints or smears also are often of more value than the classic frozen section in the case of a tumor that is largely necrotic, in which a few malignant cells can be lost in the sea of necrosis on the frozen section but are usually easily visible on the cytologic preparation.

There are relatively few other situations in which the imprint is of more value than the frozen section examination, but many situations exist in which it is of equal (or at least complementary) value. When only a small tissue sample is provided and the possibility exists that a frozen section examination would exhaust the specimen and leave none available for permanent sections, a positive imprint can preclude the necessity of performing the frozen section examination and can thus preserve the tissue in its entirety. Since imprints are also quicker to perform, time (an essential consideration) is saved in the operating room. Toward this end, I have used imprints extensively in the intraoperative evaluation of cases of hyperparathyroidism and have found that they are at least as accurate as the frozen section examination in distinguishing parathyroid tissue from thyroid, lymph node, thymus, or adipose tissue.[22] Indeed, we can also distinguish normal or atrophic from hyperfunctioning parathyroid glands in almost all cases.[23] In other non-neoplastic situations as well, the cytologic technique has been helpful; for example, I have been able to identify ganglion cells in smears from sympathetic ganglia that were submitted for intraoperative evaluation. A more complete summary of the technique and our experience with it is available elsewhere.[15]

Before leaving the topic of intraoperative cytology entirely, it is worth mentioning that this technique can prepare the surgical pathologist for the interpretation of fine needle aspiration specimens. An excellent way for surgical pathologists to prepare for reading specimens of this sort is to perform touch preparations or smears on all tumors received fresh in the operating room, and for that matter even to perform needle aspirations of these tissues themselves before beginning to accept in vivo specimens from their clinicians. As in the case of frozen section examinations, discretion is often the better part of valor, and the results of an aspiration should never be reported as positive without absolute certainty that tumor is indeed present. As in other cytologic techniques, the emphasis should be on reporting in terms of the anticipated histopathologic diagnosis, rather than using a "negative-suspicious-positive" or numeric grading system (see Ch. 10 for a more complete discussion of this general topic).

The Surgical Pathology Report

The subject of special stains and their uses and abuses is obviously important in surgical pathology. The question of which (if any) special stains to use in a particular case is best resolved by a consideration of the clinical significance of the report in that case. Since special stains are performed most frequently in the search for and interpretation of either infectious or neoplastic disease, their use in these two situations is covered in more detail in Chapters 3 and 7, respectively. General principles of histochemistry and immunohistochemistry are discussed respectively in Chapters 4 and 5. Similarly, questions of how many sections to submit from a particular gross specimen, how these sections should be taken and labeled, whether multiple or serial sections are required, and similar considerations are best decided with reference to an individual case. Thus, such questions are dealt with in the individual chapters of this text relating to specific organs and organ systems. In general terms, however, perhaps the most important single consideration is that of consistency in the practice of surgical pathology within a given laboratory. Thus, if one surgical pathologist in the laboratory does not use the letter "I" as a designation for tissue sections be-

cause of its possible confusion with the Roman numeral "I" none of the pathologists submitting tissue in that laboratory should use that designation. If one pathologist uses a particular designation for resection margins, then all colleagues should use the same designation. Only in this manner can submitting clinicians be guaranteed that the terms of a surgical pathology report they receive on a Monday will mean the same as the terms of the report they receive on Tuesday. Similarly, when all the surgical pathologists in that laboratory have gone elsewhere, their successor or successors will be able to review old slides and old reports and be aware of exactly what they signify.

This brings us to the topic of the correct way to prepare a surgical pathology report; the best statement that can be made is that there is no single best way. The most important aspect to remember is that the report should be prepared with the best interests of the clinician and the patient in mind. Thus, the most important features are clarity, brevity, and careful attention to those details that may influence the management of the patient. In general terms, those portions of the clinical history that are relevant to the specimen should always be included in the final report, as should the exact source of the specimen and the condition in which it is received (e.g., in formalin, fresh, unfixed and poorly preserved, intact, or previously opened). All necessary measurements should be performed before the specimen is dissected, and these measurements (including weight) should be recorded. The description of the gross pathology encountered should proceed from the general to the specific; for example, the presence of a tumor must be noted before its characteristics are described in detail. In general terms, the portion of a specimen (or multiple specimens) described first should be that in which the clinician is most interested, although there may be exceptions to this rule (e.g., when peripheral specimens are received first for frozen section examination and thus are described first in the gross description). If anything has been done to the specimen before its gross examination and sectioning, this should be mentioned in the surgical pathology report. Thus, if a frozen section examination has been performed, the final report should mention this fact, should contain the exact (i.e., word-for-word) frozen section report rendered to the clinician, and should indicate who performed the frozen section examination and rendered the report (in many instances, the pathologist who performed the frozen section examination may not be the same one who cuts, examines, and eventually signs out the case). Similarly, if portions of tissue have been removed for electron microscopic examination, hormone receptor analysis, virologic or other cultures, or any study other than histologic examination, this should also be noted in the final report.

If the gross specimen is a complex one, a photograph may add immeasurably to the dictated or written gross description. Photographs should be taken before the specimen is extensively dissected and may be repeated if necessary during and after the process of dissection as well. Important gross details should be adequately labeled in the photograph; a Polaroid or other instant photographic technique may be extremely valuable for this purpose. Finally, the gross dictation should always include the eventual disposition of the specimen, since this is the only way that future reviewers of the case will have of knowing what each slide represents. This rule should be followed whether the specimen is a single, small piece of tissue that is submitted in toto or a radical resection for cancer, in which 100 or more sections may be submitted, with the relationship of the label for each section to its exact source duly recorded in a "slide key" accompanying the gross description.

In addition to the possible benefit mentioned earlier for future reviewers, the advantage of a careful recording of the disposition of the gross specimen may be more immediate. Thus, in the unfortunate event that a specimen is lost or confused with another specimen, the gross dictation and slide key may resolve the possible serious confusion resulting in this situation. Similarly, if the gross description indicates that four pieces of tissue were submitted from a particular biopsy, and only three appear on the slide produced by the histotechnologist, the pathologist knows instantly that the block should be inspected and sections of deeper levels ordered.

The same rules of reason that pertain to gross descriptions and dictations apply equally to both the microscopic description and the final diagnosis. In both sections of the report, the clinically most significant lesions should precede the incidental findings, even if the portion of the specimen containing the latter was processed grossly before the former. As a general rule, what is visible with the scanning lens of the microscope should be described before what is visible with the high-power objective. For example, the pushing versus infiltrating character of the margin of a tumor should always be described before its degree of nuclear pleomorphism or mitotic activity. The microscopic description should be just that, rather than a diagnosis or prognostic commentary. Thus, a phrase such as "a tumor that appears to be of low grade malignancy" should never appear in the microscopic description but should be reserved for a comment appended to the final diagnosis. Information included in the microscopic description should be as specific as possible; thus "vascular invasion" should be replaced by an exact characterization of the type of vessel (e.g., artery, vein, capillary, lymphatic) invaded, and "chronic inflammation" should yield to an enumeration of the specific cells (lymphocytes, histiocytes, plasma cells) comprising the infiltrate.

Similarly, the final diagnosis should be as specific as possible, should list diagnoses in their order of clinical importance, and should be inclusive of all the specimens received (not forgetting, for example, the unremarkable appendix received with the hysterectomy specimen for cervical cancer). Terminology will vary with the individual laboratory, but again some attempt should be made at standardization. For example, tumors may be subdivided as well, moderately, or poorly differentiated or as grade I, II, or III, but not as both on different days or by different pathologists. The diagnosis should also be clinically relevant, so for a squamous cell carcinoma of the cervix, possibly neither of the above grading systems would be used, but perhaps an indication as to whether the tumor is keratinizing, large cell nonkeratinizing, or small cell.[24] If terminology used is likely to be confusing to the clinician, it should be clearly defined in an appended comment, perhaps with a suitable bibliographic reference. Better yet, clinicians should also be contacted in person or by telephone to be sure they fully understand the information the pathologist is seeking to convey.

Although the essentials of a microscopic description have been detailed above, it should be noted that there has been a great deal of debate in recent years over the necessity for any microscopic description at all in a surgical pathology report. In our laboratory, my colleagues and I have adopted the middle ground between those who demand a microscopic description on every specimen and those who consider it totally unnecessary. Normal appendices, cervical biopsy specimens showing only chronic cervicitis, unremarkable hernia sacs, and the like are described grossly and given a diagnosis, with the microscopic features omitted; the time thus saved is put to good use in ensuring that the microscopic descriptions for diagnostic biopsy specimens, tumor resections, and other "nonroutine" specimens are complete to the point of containing all the pertinent observations.

As mentioned previously, a current trend exists toward standardization of the surgical pathology report, not just within each institution but between different institutions as well.[3] One such useful technique is use of computerized checklists to ensure that the clinically relevant information (e.g., tumor size, histologic type, grade, status of resection margins, involvement of lymphatic and blood vessels, and so forth) is always included in the same format in every report. An extensive discussion of computerized reports and checklists is presented in Chapter 8.

Standardization of cytopathology reports is also rapidly becoming the rule rather than the exception. The Bethesda System for reporting Pap smears has already become the standard in the United States. In this system (discussed in greater detail in Ch. 49), not only are diagnostic impressions recorded in a checklist fashion, but statements concerning the adequacy of the specimen are standardized as well. Similar systems are being worked out for the reporting of breast and thyroid FNAB results, as well as other types of cases.[25,26]

NEW ADJUNCTS TO THE PRACTICE OF SURGICAL AND CYTOPATHOLOGY

The history of the field of surgical pathology contains innumerable techniques that were initially developed as basic research tools and subsequently became adapted to the diagnostic armamentarium. Many of the techniques we now consider as routine (e.g., cryostat procedures for frozen section preparation, electron microscopy, immunohistochemistry, and fine needle aspiration cytology) were at one time a novelty—to our antecedents, or even to us. In the previous edition of this book, this section briefly discussed a few of the new adjuncts already in place in some surgical pathology laboratories and some that were anticipated to become commonplace while that volume was still in use. The main subjects discussed were flow cytometry, various molecular biologic techniques, morphometry, computeriztion, and telepathology. With the exception of morphometry, which, because it is still both expensive for start-up equipment and time and labor intensive, has remained largely a research tool, the other fields have become so much a part of the routine practice of surgical and cytopathology that they are now covered in detail elsewhere in the current edition. The reader is referred to Chapters 7 to 9 for more complete discussions.

QUALITY ASSURANCE

Quality assurance has become an important facet of surgical and cytopathology in the modern era of accountability. The relation of quality assurance to malpractice liability is discussed in Chapter 2, but a few words are in order on general principles. We do not believe that quality assurance is meaningful if quality is absent, and much of what has already been discussed above—communication with the clinician, the role of internal and external consultation, correlation of intraoperative with final diagnoses, preparation of the surgical pathology report, the use of new techniques, and so forth—provides the framework of quality. The essence of quality assurance, then, is the documentation that these activities are actually taking place. Complete and up-to-date procedure manuals (containing procedures that are really being followed), written recording of consultations and communications, and careful review of reports in general and diagnoses in particular form the essence of a quality assurance program. Ways of achieving these goals are too numerous to detail here, but attention to the items discussed in this chapter and in more detail in Chapter 2 and 3, as well as material available from local and national pathology societies, should provide a framework on which to build.

TRAINING IN SURGICAL AND CYTOPATHOLOGY

It is difficult to be specific about training without first defining the ultimate goal of the individual to be trained. For example, the resident who desires to become an academic surgical/cytopathologist should spend a minimum of 3 years of training in anatomic pathology, with at least 2 of those years devoted to surgical pathology and cytology. Ideally, at least 1 more year is advisable, as is training in more than one institution (both because of the variety of specimens seen in different institutions and because of the exposure to several different philosophies). A prolonged period of exposure to specialized techniques (such as electron microscopy, immunohistochemistry, FNAB) and/or fields of study (dermatopathology, hematopathology, gynecologic pathology) is also advisable. The neophyte academic surgical pathologist is also well advised to undertake and complete some research project or projects during training and to experience the difficulties and triumphs resulting from the presentation and publication of the results thereof.

On the other hand, the training program in surgical pathology for the resident who spends a total of 2 years (or less) each in anatomic and clinical pathology before taking the board examinations and entering clinical practice must, by virtue of the length of time on surgical and cytopathology rotations, be considerably different. At institutions in which training is received in several different hospital laboratories, many residents follow the latter path. Although the nature of the workload differs both quantitatively and qualitatively from one laboratory to the next within such training programs, the directors of these laboratories should believe that the principles to be learned by the trainee are similar in each laboratory. Thus, we at The George Washington University formulated the following list of fundamentals that residents are expected to master during their training:

1. Cognizance of their own role in the clinical situation in relation to both the clinician and the patient. Residents are responsible for the surgical specimen from the time it is obtained from the patient until the final report is received by the clinician. They should ensure that the specimen is received in time and in proper condition for processing, that the slides are prepared to their satisfaction, and that the diagnosis is received and understood as early as possible by the clinician.
2. Ability to perform in a reasonable time a technically adequate frozen section examination and to deliver an appropriate interpretation. In this situation, residents should be able to communicate with the surgeon to obtain and deliver pertinent information. Residents should also be aware of the limitations of frozen section technique, should know when a diagnosis must be deferred, and should be able to apply special techniques such as imprints, which complement or supplant the frozen section examination.
3. Ability to identify, describe, and submit appropriate sections from specimens commonly encountered in surgical pathology practice. Trainees should establish which cases need to be processed first in a day's workload. They should be able to dictate the gross descriptions of the great majority of cases in final form at the cutting table; to identify the specimens received, how they are processed, and what each section submitted represents, in clear enough fashion that this information is immediately evident to anyone subsequently reading the report; and to recognize the importance of maintaining the specimen for subsequent diagnostic workup and for teaching.
4. Cooperation with investigators studying human tissues, to the extent that patient care is not compromised.
5. Ability to determine whether slides received are adequate in number and quality and to take appropriate remedial steps if they are not. Residents should be aware of uses and abuses of special stains, recuts, and similar techniques; should be able to assign priorities for the earlier and more extensive investigation of more important cases; and should be able to write a clinically relevant, concise but complete, organized, and intelligible microscopic description on every case for which such a description is required.
6. Ability to diagnose correctly the great majority of commonly encountered lesions, awareness of the existence of other lesions, and knowledge of when and how to seek consultation. Trainees should develop a systematic approach to slide examination, to ensure that lesions, even if they are not always correctly interpreted, will at least not be overlooked. They should also be able to relate the histologic findings to the clinical and gross features of the case.
7. Cognizance of new and specialized techniques in such fields as histochemistry, electron microscopy, immunopathology, molecular biology, and specimen radiography and their applications to diagnostic surgical pathology. It is important to have knowledge of when it is appropriate to submit tissues for

these and other studies, and in what form the tissue must be submitted for the studies to be successful.

8. Understanding the clinical manifestations and natural history of lesions encountered. This demands independent reading, beginning with standard textbooks (especially, we hope, this one) and progressing to familiarity with and critical reading of current clinical and pathologic literature.

9. Familiarity with the technical aspects of histopathology as related to surgical pathology. This includes techniques of sectioning, embedding, and staining, comparative values of different fixatives, operation and servicing of microtomes and cryostats, and similar problems.

Although this list of goals might easily be modified in different institutions that train residents in surgical pathology, we believe that goals should be established by each institution for its own training program. Both trainees and those who are responsible for their training should be aware of these goals and should monitor the program carefully to be sure they are being met. Similarly, the wording should be changed somewhat to apply to training in cytopathology, but very similar goals will still apply. For example, the reference to frozen sections will be altered to rapid interpretation of FNAB specimens, and the emphasis on gross pathology will change to clinical localization of masses for FNAB. Nevertheless, training overall should emphasize the similarities rather than the differences between the two disciplines, and opportunities to compare cytologic and tissue pathologic manifestations of the same lesions should always be provided.

A word should also be said about training in surgical pathology for nonpathologists. Although it is our strong conviction that surgical pathology should be practiced by pathologists, we also believe that, just as the pathologist with advanced clinical experience is often a better pathologist, the general surgeon, gynecologist, dermatologist, or other clinical specialist who has been exposed to a rotation in surgical pathology during training is often the better for this experience as well. These rotations by clinical trainees through the surgical pathology service will often be limited to one or a few months, and the goals of the training in this situation should be as follows: (1) to instill an appreciation of the role of the surgical pathologist as a consultant in the appropriate clinical field; (2) to develop a recognition of the importance of adequate communication (including the provision by the clinician of appropriate clinical histories and specimen descriptions) in the performance of this consultative role of the surgical pathologist; (3) to develop a respect for the specimen as the primary vehicle for this communication, together with an appropriate appreciation of proper techniques of fixation and submission of specimens; (4) to develop a realization of what surgical pathologists cannot do, so as to expect fewer miracles from them in subsequent clinical practice; (5) to develop some concept of basic principles of gross pathology, so that inflammatory, neoplastic, traumatic, and other processes can be distinguished in the operating room or the clinic; and (6) to develop the same sort of familiarity with microscopic interpretation, and with the clinical and pathologic significance of the main entities encountered in the individual field of clinical practice, so that a surgical pathology report may

be interpreted and slides reviewed with the surgical pathologist with more confidence in the future.

RESEARCH IN SURGICAL AND CYTOPATHOLOGY

According to the Random House Dictionary of the English Language, research is defined as "diligent and systematic inquiry or investigation into a subject in order to discover or revise facts, theories, applications, etc." We have emphasized that most surgical pathologists do indeed perform research as defined in this manner.[27] We have classified the types of research performed by the surgical pathologist and directly related to surgical pathology as (1) observational; (2) manipulative with human tissues; (3) experimental with nonhuman models; and (4) technical, instructional, and delivery. A few comments are offered below on each of these categories of research in surgical pathology; the same comments are equally applicable to cytopathology.

Observational Research

The first of these, designated observational research, is probably the most common, and certainly the most common outside the university or academic setting. The role of the surgical pathologist in this form of research is the observation of the results of an experiment of nature. The subject chosen depends on the material available in one's own institution, although collaborative relationships with other pathologists or other institutions (or both) may add to the volume of material observed. The results of this form of research may range from the report of a single case to a major clinical-pathologic-epidemiologic review.

Although this type of project—particularly the case report—has often been denigrated, it is worth noting that many new and important entities in the surgical pathology literature were originally described in the form of a single case report, and many new and important observations on previously described entities have been made in the same format. This does not mean that every case report is equally valuable, and certainly many have added nothing but verbiage and paper to the world's resources. (The same statement, of course, can equally be made of many other research projects, including many that have been well funded by tax dollars).

Manipulative Research with Human Tissues

In the second category of research in surgical pathology are those studies that involve some degree of manipulation with human tissues. The importance of the role of the surgical pathologist in making such tissues available for study has been commented on briefly earlier and should be emphasized again at this time. It is equally important for surgical pathologists to remember, however, that their primary role is that of a diagnostician: they must be careful not to give away so much tissue for research that the amount retained is inadequate for the provision of the diagnostic and prognostic information for which it was originally sent.

In this kind of research, the surgical pathologist may serve merely as the collector of tissues for others, or may be the primary researcher. Human tissues obtained from living patients may be used for organ or cell culture, transplantation into animals, study by DNA spectrophotometry or flow microfluorimetry, immunohistochemistry, transmission or scanning electron microscopy, genotyping, or other studies.[28] If any of these techniques is found to be of diagnostic importance for the patient, this sort of research may not only provide interesting biologic data but may also add new tools to the diagnostic armamentarium of the surgical pathologist.

This type of research is currently under pressure from several different sources. The first is the managed care mentality and the emphasis on cost-cutting, often at the expense of quality, that it engenders. Thus any time or effort expended by the surgical or cytopathologist in research may be deemed to be nonproductive and wasteful unless it is supported by grant or contract revenue. Even more worrisome are current attempts by usually well meaning legislators, attorneys, and ethicists to limit access to patient-derived pathologic material and pertinent clinical and epidemiologic data in the name of privacy and confidentiality of genetic data. Obviously, any cellular or tissue specimen can now be used to obtain genetic information about the patient from whom it was obtained. It thus becomes even more important than before for the pathologist to become the guardian of these specimens, ensuring that they will be released only for legitimate research purposes and that appropriate confidentiality will be maintained.[29,30]

Experimental Research with Nonhuman Models

In the category of experimental research with nonhuman models, I refer to those studies that are carried out in vitro or in animals but are related directly to human disease. Again, the surgical pathologist may personally perform this research or may function as a consultant to, or collaborator with, a basic scientist. The morphologic skills of surgical pathologists are often invaluable to basic scientists who are working in this sort of system and cannot by themselves transpose these histologic observations to the appropriate human disease.

Technical, Instructional, and Delivery Research

Finally, research in the technical, instructional, and delivery aspects of surgical pathology is a rapidly expanding field. This includes such projects as developing and perfecting new techniques that can be applied to the diagnosis of human disease, developing new models for training in surgical and cytopathology, and developing new techniques for providing better service in surgical and cytopathology to clinicians and referring pathologists alike. Many of the currently accepted standard techniques in the field arose from someone's pioneering research of this sort in the past.

Summary

One of the most attractive aspects of the field of pathology in general, and surgical and cytopathology in particular, is that this wide diversity of research models enables interesting and satisfying research to be performed outside the traditional academic setting. Thus, many pathologists in community hospital practice situations perform significant research, and this trend may be magnified in the future. The image of research in surgical pathology as being somehow unable to compete for academic stature with more basic experimental research is fortunately being supplanted by an appreciation of the fact that both good and bad research are performed in both fields, and that the quality and significance of research in surgical pathology are often equal to those of more "fundamental" studies.

Funding has often been a problem for research in surgical pathology in the past, but my colleagues and I firmly believe that good research in surgical pathology should be as fundable by the grant mechanism as good research in any other field. The emphasis in this statement, however, should be placed on the word "good" and surgical pathologists must be sure that the scientific reasoning and methodology applied to their research can stand up to criticism by full-time scientists as well as by other surgical pathologists. Time and physical facilities are also important to the performance of research in surgical pathology, and those who are responsible for providing these must be made aware of the importance of research to both the practice and teaching of surgical pathology.

CAVEATS AND OPPORTUNITIES FOR THE FUTURE

As discussed above and elsewhere in this volume, this is both an exciting and a dangerous time in the field of surgical and cytopathology. The excitement comes from the application of new technologies to the diagnosis of human tissue and cellular material, but the danger is inherent in the cost-cutting and legalistic climate in which, just as we are able to make more accurate diagnoses and investigate more fully the underlying mechanisms of the diseases we diagnose, we may be strongly discouraged or even forbidden to do so by nonmedical personnel who do not begin to understand the issues involved. Pathologists must familiarize themselves with these issues and become ardent advocates for both their patients of today and their yet unborn patients of the 21st century.

REFERENCES

1. Schwartz GF, Feig SA, Patchefsky AS: Clinicopathologic correlations and significance of clinically occult mammary lesions. Cancer 41:1147, 1978

2. Morrow M, Evans J, Rosen PP, Kinne DW: Does clearing of axillary lymph nodes contribute to accurate staging of breast cancer? Cancer 53:1329, 1984

3. Association of Directors of Anatomic and Surgical Pathology: Standardization of the surgical pathology report. Am J Surg Pathol 16:84–86, 1992

4. Greening SE, Somrak TM: Medicolegal issues in cytology: legal principles and liability outlook. pp. 65–81. In: Cytopathology Annual 1994. ASCP Press, Chicago, 1994

5. Association of Directors of Anatomic and Surgical Pathology: Consultations in surgical pathology. Am J Surg Pathol 17:743–745, 1993

6. O'Brien MJ, Sotnikov AV: Digital imaging in anatomic pathology. Am J Clin Pathol, suppl. 1, 106:S25–S32, 1996

7. Black-Schaffer S, Flotte TJ: Current issues in telepathology. Telemed J 1:95–105, 1995

8. Oberholzerm M, Fischer HR, Christen H, et al: Telepathology: frozen section diagnosis at a distance. Virchows Arch 426:3–9, 1995

9. Ackerman LV, Ramirez GA: The indications for and limitations of frozen section diagnosis. Br J Surg 46:336–350, 1959

10. Holaday WJ, Assor D: Ten thousand consecutive frozen sections. Am J Clin Pathol 61:769–777, 1974

11. Nakazawa H, Rosen P, Lane N, Lattes R: The frozen section experience in 3000 cases. Am J Clin Pathol 49:41–51, 1968

12. Silverberg SG: The role of the pathologist in oncology. pp. 174–188. In McKenna RJ, Murphy GP (eds): Fundamentals of Surgical Oncology. Macmillan, New York, 1986

13. Esteban JM, Zaloudek C, Silverberg SG: Intraoperative diagnosis of breast lesions. Am J Clin Pathol 88:681–688, 1987

14. Oneson RH, Minke JA, Silverberg SG: Intraoperative pathologic consultation: an audit of 1,000 recent consecutive cases. Am J Surg Pathol 13:237–243, 1989

15. Nochomovitz L, Sidawy M, Silverberg SG, et al: Intraoperative Consultation. A Guide to Smears, Imprints, and Frozen Sections. ASCP Press, Chicago, 1989

16. Agnantis NJ, Apostolikas N, Christodoulou I, et al: The reliability of frozen section diagnosis in various breast lesions: a study based on 3452 biopsies. Recent Results Cancer Res 90:205–210, 1984

17. Fessia L, Ghiringhello B, Arisio R, et al: Accuracy of frozen section diagnosis of breast cancer detection. A review of 4436 biopsies and comparison with cytodiagnosis. Pathol Res Pract 179:61–66, 1984

18. Silverberg SG, Association of Directors of Anatomic and Surgical Pathology, Fechner RE: Current controversy: frozen section examination of nonpalpable or small palpable breast lesions. Pathol Case Rev 1:2–5, 1996

19. Oberman HA: A modest proposal. Am J Surg Pathol 16:69–70, 1992

20. Sidawy MK, Silverberg SG: Intraoperative cytology: back to the future? Am J Clin Pathol 96:1–3, 1991

21. Mair S, Lash RH, Suskin D, Mendelsohn G: Intraoperative surgical specimen evaluation: frozen section analysis, cytologic examination, or both? A comparative study of 206 cases. Am J Clin Pathol 96:8–14, 1991

22. Geelhoed GW, Silverberg SG: Intraoperative imprints for the identification of parathyroid tissue. Surgery 96:1124–1130, 1984

23. Sasano H, Geelhoed GW, Silverberg SG: Intraoperative cytologic evaluation of lipid in the diagnosis of parathyroid adenoma. Am J Surg Pathol 12:282–286, 1988

24. National Cancer Institute Workshop: The revised Bethesda System for reporting cervical/vaginal diagnoses: report of the 1991 Bethesda workshop. JAMA 267:1892, 1992

25. Sneige N, Staerkel GA, Caraway NP, et al: A plea for uniform terminology and reporting of breast fine needle aspirates. Acta Cytol 38:971–972, 1994

26. The Papanicolaou Society of Cytopathology Task Force on Standards of Practice: Guidelines of the Papanicolaou Society of Cytopathology for the examination of fine needle aspiration specimens from thyroid nodules. Mod Pathol 9:710–715, 1996

27. Silverberg SG: The surgical pathologist as researcher. Am J Clin Pathol 75:452, 1981

28. Trump BF, Harris CC: Human tissues in biomedical research. Hum Pathol 10:245, 1979

29. Grody WW: Molecular pathology, informed consent, and the paraffin block. Diagn Mol Pathol 4:155–157, 1995

30. Association of Directors of Anatomic and Surgical Pathology: Use of human tissue blocks for research. Hum Pathol 27:519–520, 1996

2

Quality Control, Assurance, and Improvement in Anatomic Pathology

Richard J. Zarbo
Robert R. Rickert

During the past two decades increasing attention has been focused on the quality of diagnostic performance in anatomic pathology. Although such attention is certainly related in part to an accelerating interest in this area on the part of government, accrediting agencies, third party payers, health care consumers, and the media, historic review suggests that most of the impetus has been provided by the specialty of pathology itself.

Quality control measures were well established in the various sections of the clinical laboratory long before formal implementation in anatomic pathology. In the mid-1940s interlaboratory comparison programs were under development, beginning with the seminal work of Sunderman[1] and colleagues in Philadelphia. The first comprehensive reports addressing what we would now regard as quality control and quality assurance issues in anatomic pathology began to appear in the late 1960s and early 1970s.[2–6] Dorsey[7] has recently provided an excellent historic review of the evolution of laboratory quality assurance.

In this chapter, we present an overview of quality assurance in anatomic pathology and, with appropriate historic considerations, attempt to frame in broad perspective the topic of quality assurance as it pertains to the various sections of anatomic pathology. Definitions are presented, general principles discussed, and components to be considered in a comprehensive quality assurance program enumerated. Our purpose is to provide the reader with sufficient background, understanding, and specific information to develop a quality assurance program that will meet patient care needs as well as satisfy the necessary accreditation and regulatory requirements.

QUALITY ASSURANCE OBJECTIVES

It is important to consider the main objective of quality assessment and assurance, which is not only to pacify the accreditation surveyor or laboratory inspector or satisfy the often burdensome regulatory requirements. The fundamental objective of quality assessment in all areas of anatomic pathology is to ensure that we provide the referring physician with a quality diagnostic report based on the interpretation of optimal technical preparations.

Anatomic pathology is a profession that can be likened to a service industry providing one essential component in the assembly process of a complex service, namely, patient care. Without the anatomic pathologist's product, the process often grinds to a halt, for this is a component on which other critical professional decisions and further medical services are often predicated. However, as recently observed by Dr. John Batsakis,[8] "Pathology does not make ball-bearings; it deals with biologic systems, incompletely understood, and imperfectly measured or subjectively assessed." As an oversimplification then, the product of the pathologist is a diagnosis made from the examination of tissue specimens. However, to examine the quality of this product is to consider the following characteristics culminating from numerous sequential technical and professional steps in the testing process: accuracy, completeness and medical relevance of information content, timeliness, consistency, availability, and cost effectiveness. How to best ensure or improve the quality of this medical service product, especially in the present cost-conscious environment, is the current focus of pathologists, administrators, professional societies, and accrediting agencies.

DEFINITIONS OF QUALITY CONTROL AND ASSURANCE

A significant cause of confusion in understanding the various issues concerned with implementing quality assurance programs in all areas of medicine is the often imprecise use of terminology. In the past, the terms *quality control* and *quality assurance* were often used interchangeably and without definition. Add to this the lack of a generally accepted definition of the word *quality*, and confusion is not surprising but expected. *Quality* of patient care is currently defined by the Joint Commission on Accreditation of Healthcare Organization's (JCAHO) *Accreditation Manual for Hospitals, 1992* as "the degree to which patient care services increase the probability of desired patient outcomes and reduce the probability of undesired outcomes, given the current state of knowledge." The JCAHO defines *quality control* as a "scientific and technical process that is implemented on a daily basis by the non-medical staff of the laboratory and which is supervised by the pathologist." *Quality assurance* "adds the application of medical judgment to the responsibilities of the pathologist."

The College of American Pathologists (CAP) in the glossary section of the *Standards for Laboratory Accreditation* defines *quality control* in the following manner: "Quality control is an integral component of quality assurance and is the aggregate of processes and techniques so derived to detect, reduce and correct deficiencies in an analytic process."[24] A complementary definition of quality control that has served the CAP Laboratory Accreditation Program very well for many years is attributed to Dr. Raymond Bartlett[9] and states that "quality control is a surveillance process in which the actions of people and performance of equipment and materials are observed in some systematic, periodic way which provides a record of consistency of performance and action taken when performance does not conform to standards which have been established in the laboratory." Perhaps the most succinct and certainly most pungent definition is that offered by the late Dr. Israel Diamond, who regarded quality control as "man's feeble attempt to repeal Murphy's Law." *Quality assurance* is defined by CAP as follows: "Quality assurance in laboratory medicine is the process of assuring that all pathology services involved in the delivery of patient care have been accomplished in a manner appropriate to maintain excellence in medical care."

From the above discussion, it is clear that current definitions of quality control focus mainly on technical, procedural, and process issues, whereas the broader concept of quality assurance deals with outcome.

QUALITY IMPROVEMENT

Recently, the United States Federal Government, through the Clinical Laboratory Improvement Amendments of 1988 (CLIA '88),[10] has broadly defined quality assurance as "an ongoing process for monitoring and evaluating every step of the laboratory's testing operation including preanalytic, analytic and postanalytic processes." This definition places a different and distinct emphasis on the focus of those seeking to ensure or improve pathology and laboratory medicine services. An example of these steps in the total test cycle is illustrated for surgical pathology in Figure 2-1.[11]

The approaches to assuring quality in pathology have matured throughout the 1990s, beginning with quality control of laboratory testing, progressing to quality assessment and assurance activities that often address regulatory requirements, and finally incorporating total quality management or continuous quality improvement principles for improvement of quality. Each concept has built on previous ones, assessing intralaboratory analytic quality, laboratory quality, and customer and data-driven scientific models for the creation of protocols, practices, and system designs that include quality as a patient outcome. Because of the manual and interpretive nature of the anatomic pathology service, formal assessments of laboratory practice have been inconsistently documented, whereas in the clinical laboratory, the analytic component of the testing cycle has been well addressed by the emphasis on daily laboratory quality control practices and external quality assessment (proficiency testing). Quality assurance is a broader perspective, incorporating evaluation and documentation of the preanalytical (mainly prelaboratory) and postanalytical (mainly postlaboratory) aspects of the test cycle, in the quest to assure quality of service.

We believe that many future quality improvements will be seen in the preanalytic and postanalytic stages of the testing process, which have not benefited from as much attention by pathologists and laboratory professionals. The current management focus, not only in business but also in medicine, is an adoption of a continuous quality improvement model to im-

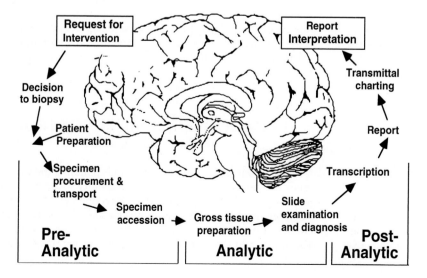

Fig. 2-1. Surgical pathology total test cycle.

prove the level of service continuously through measurement and comparison with a performance standard or benchmark before implementing process changes. This is a scientific approach to making changes, predicated on the collection of meaningful data, identification of root causes of problems, and development of appropriate solutions. This assessment is continuous, incorporating a sequence of steps referred to as "plan; do; check; and act," thereby resulting in incremental and continuous improvement. The functional linkage of this continuous quality improvement process with quality assurance is the systematic capture of information from clinicians and other health care "customers" as it relates to improving quality of services and satisfaction of regulatory and accreditation requirements.

The concept of continuous quality improvement is founded on the precepts that (1) sources of defects in quality are often built into the system and are not usually caused by deficiencies in people; (2) identifying problems (by data collection) is to recognize opportunities for improvement (inspection should not instill fear of punitive actions and bias in data collection); and (3) appropriate measurements can be used as a basis of understanding and revising processes to effect improvement. Specific points that are directly applicable to development of a functional Quality Assurance Plan in Anatomic Pathology are as follows: "(1) improving quality may, in the long run, be the best way to control costs; (2) an effort to develop better system designs is a more efficient way to control quality than is mass inspection of the final product; (3) quality assurance should have as its major goal continual improvement, not finding 'flaws'; (4) quality control requires the constant attention and support of the highest status individuals in organizations; (5) quality control requires statistical sophistication; and (6) quality improvement is unlikely to occur in an atmosphere of fear."[12]

subscription quality improvement program termed *Q-Probes*, offered since 1989 by the CAP.[13] Presently over 1,450 laboratories in the United States, Canada, Australia, New Zealand, Hong Kong, Belgium, Brazil, Scotland, Saudi Arabia, and Singapore participate through anatomic and clinical pathology modules of large and small hospital programs. These predesigned quality improvement studies enable laboratory personnel to assess quality of services objectively by comparison of individual laboratory performance with that of overall and peer group data collected in a uniform manner over the same defined time intervals.

To date, 82 Q-Probes studies have examined attributes of pathology and laboratory medicine practices and performance with generation of reference data for the purpose of benchmarking to effect quality improvement. These reference databases have been used by laboratories as target values to direct specific changes in laboratory practice in a systematic quality improvement process. Individualized participant reports allow benchmarking not only from percentile rank from the aggregate data, but also from differences stratified by peer group parameters. Using this quality improvement tool, laboratories have been able to benchmark various aspects of the preanalytic, analytic, and postanalytic stages of the test cycle in pathology and laboratory medicine. Many of these Q-Probes studies, conducted in all aspects of anatomic pathology, have been published in the peer-reviewed literature and the performance benchmarks described in a 1995 chapter added to the CAP's *Quality Improvement Manual in Anatomic Pathology*.[14] It is anticipated that the establishment of reference databases or benchmarks of quality practice based on this kind of aggregate database will provide baseline measurements or target values to direct specific changes in practice through a systematic quality improvement process.

REFERENCE DATABASES AND BENCHMARKING

Many laboratories throughout the world evaluate and document their own performance in many activities as components of quality assurance programs. However, in general, these data are viewed without a frame of reference to assess relative performance and upon which to base process improvements, since many steps of the laboratory testing process have not been examined formally. We believe that the availability of comparative data, in these times of diminishing resources, would be extremely helpful in defining the optimal performance expectations of specific laboratory services. Individual laboratories would further benefit by comparison of their organization's performance with that of other organizations with defined system designs and processes, so-called benchmarking. The JCAHO has also recommended that quality improvement activities designed to study and improve processes that affect patient outcomes would benefit by such external comparisons. This benchmarking process of measuring performance against and adopting key system processes of the best performers implies the use of a large database.[11]

An example of benchmarking in pathology is the voluntary

QUALITY ASSURANCE PARAMETERS

Numerous Anatomic Pathology activities, composing the total test cycle illustrated in Figure 2-1 would benefit from assessment and improvement, and several ways of examining these processes exist. These activities can be classified into procedural, technical, diagnostic, and professional components.[15] They include not only many aspects of laboratory processes such as tissue transportation, handling, accession, dissection, labeling, embedding, sectioning, and staining, but also the professional components of diagnostic accuracy, medical usefulness of report content, and timeliness of communication.

Possible targets of measurement can also be viewed under the general evaluation categories of structure, process, and outcome. Components of *structure* pertain to availability of institutional resources or system aspects of care such as diagnostic protocols. This would include hospital and laboratory administration policies, physical facilities, equipment, staff allocation, and qualifications. *Process* evaluation focuses on policy, procedure, and individual steps in the delivery of care or provision of a service. For anatomic pathology this would include aspects of laboratory management, policy, and procedures covering those activities leading up to and directly involved in the making of a diagnosis. For example, measurement could focus on accuracy, timeliness, and technical skill in applying diagnostic protocols.

Obviously, the most difficult parameter to measure in pathology is the effect on clinical patient *outcome*. The end products of technical activities and value judgments in anatomic pathology are diagnosis oriented. These are reflected in the numerous components of the anatomic pathology consultation, including the accuracy of the pathologic diagnosis. These can be considered interim outcomes in the assessment of quality rather than clinical end points related to immediate change in patient health status. Therefore, issues that relate to *diagnosis*, information content provided, and pathologist performance rather than the impact on patient management and treatment are more readily addressed in pathology. It is recognized that the distinctions made among structure, process, and outcome can be quite arbitrary, that they do not stand alone, and that they have meaning only in the context of the others and are therefore interdependent aspects of quality of care. However, these distinctions do have organizational, educational, and conceptual value in the assessment of the many factors that may potentially influence quality care.[16]

SPECIAL ASPECTS OF ANATOMIC PATHOLOGY

The development of both quality control and quality assurance systems in the various sections of anatomic pathology presents special challenges. These relate mainly to the nature of the test result and the cognitive processes that lead to that result. In surgical pathology, autopsy pathology, and cytopathology, we are not dealing with a quantitative value generated by a sophisticated analytic instrument (i.e., an objective "result" that may be subjected to a variety of statistical evaluations to document its accuracy and precision) rather, we are concerned with a consultative medical opinion developed by the pathologist through subjective evaluation and interpretation of the gross and microscopic attributes of the tissue examined. The subjective nature of the diagnostic process and its outcome not only challenge the pathologist's ingenuity in developing quality control and quality assurance programs but also call attention to distinctions between the two entities in anatomic pathology that are more blurred than in clinical pathology. Whereas the technical and procedural events that prepare the specimen and produce the analyte (slide) are surely quality control issues, the diagnostic opinion offered is a patient management activity oriented to outcome and therefore concerned with quality assurance. Assessing the quality of the report itself combines elements of both quality control and quality assurance. For example, review of a diagnostic report for typographic errors is a quality control activity; evaluating the content of the report in a case of colorectal cancer is clearly quality assurance.

As we approach the design and development of a quality assurance program for anatomic pathology, it is important to recall that the kinds of activities fundamental to this process are not new, rather, they represent commonplace and traditional practices of our specialty that have existed for generations.

Quality assurance in anatomic pathology did not begin with the early reports published in the late 1960s; it did not begin with the accreditation efforts of CAP; it did not begin with the JC-AHO and its Agenda for Change; and it surely did not begin with government regulation or the media. Quality assurance in anatomic pathology, in our view, was initiated when some pathologist long ago shared a diagnostic problem with a colleague. Unfortunately, the quality assurance significance of many activities that are part of our daily professional lives is sometimes overlooked. We do not need to invent new techniques as much as we need to develop systems of organization and documentation of our current and often routine activities. By doing so, even with the limits inherent in monitoring subjective opinions, programs can be developed that both contribute to and help document the quality of our diagnostic activities.

GENERAL PRINCIPLES AND ESSENTIAL ELEMENTS OF A QUALITY ASSURANCE PROGRAM

A comprehensive quality assurance program must incorporate a variety of elements that include procedural and technical activities (process or quality control), considerations related to the professional role of the pathologist in arriving at a diagnostic conclusion (quality assurance), and an evaluation of the quality of the diagnostic report (features of both quality control and quality assurance). These general features are applicable to all disciplines and services within anatomic pathology (surgical pathology, the autopsy, and cytopathology), and the process elements must include all the laboratories that support these services, including general histology, electron microscopy, immunohistochemistry, and molecular pathology. A number of publications address these general principles as well as provide specific suggestions and formats for program design and data collection.[15,17–28] An important resource for the development and implementation of a quality assurance program in anatomic pathology is the CAP *Quality Improvement Manual in Anatomic Pathology*.[29]

As we review the essential features to include in a comprehensive program, it is important to understand that individual programs will vary in the specific mechanisms and operational details that accomplish these goals. Programs must be tailored to the individual practice setting, and specific design will depend on variables such as the volume and type of case material, number of pathologists, representation of subspecialty interests, and existence of undergraduate and postgraduate teaching responsibilities. A program designed and implemented in a large teaching facility with 10 or more pathologists, subspecialty expertise, and a residency program may be inappropriate and unworkable in a small hospital with one or two pathologists. Nonetheless, the general principles must apply in all practice settings.

Penner[20] has divided the components of quality assurance in anatomic pathology into internal and external components, as outlined in Table 2-1. Cowan[23] has recently defined an information system approach to quality assurance in anatomic pathology. Recognizing that the pathologist's product is infor-

Table 2-1. Components of Anatomic
Pathology Quality Assurance

I. Internal components
   A. Personnel
      1. Staff qualifications
      2. Continuing education
   B. Specimens
      1. Acquisitions
      2. Handling and preparation
   C. Reports
   D. Performance evaluation
II. External components
   A. Procedures
      1. Source and type of material
      2. Standards for evaluation of diagnosis
   B. Types of programs
      1. Education
      2. Evaluation

(From Penner,[20] with permission.)

mation, Cowan[23] emphasizes that the practice of anatomic pathology should be evaluated as a system for producing and effectively communicating information. He has identified these important issues in quality assurance, illustrated in Table 2-2.

As noted in the introductory paragraph, we view quality assurance in anatomic pathology as comprising three interrelated levels of activity, which are outlined in Table 2-3.[19] Included are the various elements presented in Penner's[20] and Cowan's[23] formulations, but they are expressed in a slightly different manner. Each component is described and discussed below. Obviously, individual pathologists will conceptualize these elements in their own way. Hopefully, the text that follows provides a framework within which quality assurance indicators can be identified and individual programs developed and implemented to achieve our stated objective.

Table 2-2. Issues in Quality Assurance

Definitions of standards
Monitors
Professional performance/peer review
   Accuracy in diagnosis
   Communication
   Timeliness
   Efficiency
System operation
   Turnaround time
   Control and processing
   Technical proficiency
   Efficiency
Use of quality assurance information
   Department management
   Performance-based credentialing
   Accreditation

(From Cowan,[23] with permission.)

Table 2-3. Principle Elements of a Comprehensive
Quality Assurance Program in Anatomic Pathology

I. Technical and procedural elements (quality control)
   A. Specimen identification/audit trail/acceptance
   B. Specimen handling and processing
   C. Procedure manuals
   D. Instrument maintenance
   E. Record keeping
II. Professional role of the pathologist (quality assurance)
   A. Review of previous material
   B. Cytologic/histologic correlation
   C. Intraoperative consultation (frozen section)
   D. Personal consultation and peer review
   E. Institutional consultation
   F. Teaching conference/committee review
   G. Continuing education, performance improvement, and self-assessment activities
III. Quality of the diagnostic report (quality control and quality assurance)
   A. Clinical information
   B. Transcription/typographic accuracy
   C. Timeliness
   D. Quality/adequacy of descriptions
   E. Adequacy of diagnostic information

Technical and Procedural Elements

Included here are activities that are basically quality (process) control in type and do not differ significantly from those in the various sections of clinical pathology. In anatomic pathology they deal mainly with the procurement of the specimen, maintenance of the integrity of its identity, and assurance of the quality of specimen handling and processing to achieve an optimal technical preparation for diagnostic interpretation. As in all other quality control and quality assurance activities, written description and documentation are essential.

Specimen Identification/Audit Trail/Acceptance

Fastidious patient/specimen identification is obviously essential. Procedures should provide stepwise tracking that permits precise identification at each point at which the specimen changes hands. In surgical pathology and cytopathology, this auditing process must begin at the specimen source in the operating room, clinic, or doctor's office. Personnel at these sites should be provided with written instructions for proper collection, labeling, preservation, and submission of tissues and specimens. Written specimen receipt and acceptance policies should also be established and available. Current practices and benchmarks related to laboratory-identified deficiencies in specimen accessioning and patient identification have been defined in a 1994 Q-Probes study conducted in 417 institutions and comprising 1,004,115 surgical pathology specimens.[30]

Specimen Handling

Written procedures for the proper handling and dissection of various types of specimens are very useful. The extent and complexity of this type of document may vary depending on variables such as department size, volume and type of specimens, and existence of a training program. In some practice settings, simple guidelines may suffice, whereas in a large practice with a high volume of complex specimens, a comprehensive manual may be required. In departments with postgraduate trainees, a comprehensive manual defining the proper description, dissection, and histologic sampling of all types of tissues and specimens is especially important. Not only is the manual an excellent teaching adjunct, but it promotes consistency in the handling of complicated specimens. Some pathology services prefer to develop their own internal manuals, while others choose one of those currently published. Whichever type of document is used, it is important that the procedures described are those being followed. The procedures outlined for a given department will also provide a basis for evaluation of the adequacy of the descriptions and information contained within the diagnostic report (see below).

Tissue Processing and Procedure Manuals

Technical manuals in the various sections of anatomic pathology are just as essential as in clinical pathology. In general histology, electron microscopy, immunohistochemistry, and cytology laboratories, procedure manuals should be available that describe accurately the technical activities of the laboratory. They should contain basic information concerning tissue and specimen processing and define the staining methods in use and their source. Just as in clinical pathology, the technical manual should accurately represent the procedures in place. They are also subject to the same annual review process applicable in the various sections of clinical pathology. Data from a 1994 Q-Probes study documenting the rate, source, and type of extraneous tissue present on surgical pathology slides define the current state of quality of surgical pathology slide production.[31]

Instrument Maintenance

A schedule should be developed for the monitoring and servicing of all instruments in use in anatomic pathology. Intervals for the changing of solutions in tissue processors should be defined and records kept. The acceptable ranges of temperature should be determined for all temperature-dependent equipment, including paraffin baths and dispensers, water baths, tissue processors, refrigerators, ovens, and cryostats. Records of periodic checks should be maintained. Microtomes should be clean, well maintained, and properly lubricated and the knives kept sharp and free of nicks. Maintenance and service records should be available to the technical staff responsible for operating the equipment.

Record Keeping

Systematic maintenance of written records and documents is important in providing consistent and high quality technical preparations in anatomic pathology. In addition to those described in the previous sections, the laboratories should keep accurate records of specimens processed, slides prepared, and special stains made. The various technical and procedural elements of quality assurance just described are concerned with

the production of optimal preparations for diagnostic interpretation by the pathologist. To evaluate the laboratory's success and consistency in achieving this goal, records addressing each of the elements should be maintained. Examples of forms used to monitor such diverse items as requisition form adequacy, specimen rejection, tissue fixation, and stain quality may be found in the publication of Travers[22] and in the CAP *Quality Improvement Manual In Anatomic Pathology*.[29]

Professional Role of the Pathologist

The pathologist's professional responsibility in achieving a diagnosis is clearly an issue concerned with quality assurance. It is also the most difficult area of quality assurance to evaluate, mainly because of the subjective, consultative nature of the pathologist's medical responsibility. It is important to emphasize again that pathologists have traditionally been involved in these quality assurance procedures. What is needed is a comprehensive program that organizes and documents these activities. The specific combinations of activities included and the systems employed to document this area of quality assurance will vary somewhat depending on the size of the staff, the volume and variety of case material, and other departmental resources.

Review of Previous Material

Examination of the patient's previous records and materials often contributes to the quality of a diagnostic consultation on a current specimen. For example, recognition of an adenocarcinoma in the lung as metastatic may depend on the availability of an adequate history and review of previous material from the patient's rectal cancer. An individual department should develop a systematic process to identify, retrieve, and review relevant previous material in its files. Capturing information about previous pathologic examinations in other institutions is often a more vexing problem, requiring the cooperation of the submitting physician and often the ingenuity of the pathologist. This review process is an integral and important part of quality assurance in all areas of anatomic pathology.

Cytologic-Histologic Correlation

Correlative review of all relevant pathologic material enhances the consultative process in anatomic pathology. This is an essential area of quality assurance in both surgical pathology and cytopathology and serves an important educational role as well. Multi-institutional reference databases of cytologic-histologic correlation for comparative performance assessment have been derived from Q-Probes studies of breast and lung fine needle aspiration biopsies and cervical biopsies.[32–34]

Intraoperative Consultation

Diagnoses rendered during surgery should be directly communicated to the operating surgeon. The frozen section slide should be properly labeled and retained with the rest of the case, and the report should be made part of the permanent written record.[29] Correlation and comparison of frozen section and

Table 2-4. Frozen Section Consultation: Comparison of Literature Experience With Q-Probes Data

Parameter	Literature	Q-Probes 1989	1990	1994
No. institutions	19	297	461	233
No. aggregate FS cases	42,891	52,464	90,538	13,364
No. aggregate FS diagnoses	NA	79,647	121,668	18,532
FS diagnosis deferral rate (%)	0.2–6.1	4.2	3.2	4.6
FS error rate (median %)[a]	1.9	1.7	1.4	1.8
FS error range (10th–90th)[a]	1–3.7	0–5	0–4.2	0–7.5

[a] FS error is the discordance based on frozen section (FS) diagnoses corrected for deferred diagnoses.

final diagnoses is one of the most traditional quality assurance practices in anatomic pathology. When significant disparities are identified, they should be reconciled in writing. As with other areas of quality assurance in anatomic pathology, until recently very few objective data have been available against which performance could be evaluated.[35] The Q-Probes program has established multi-institutional reference databases of numerous intraoperative consultation quality attributes defining ordering indications, diagnostic accuracy, deferral rates, causes of error, effect of error on patient management, and immediate intraoperative outcomes.[36–39] Three Q-Probes studies of frozen section-permanent section correlation conducted in 1989, 1990, and 1994 have collectively examined diagnostic accuracy in more than 156,000 frozen section cases from 991 institutions.[36–38,40,41] The benchmarks derived from these multi-institutional studies compared with the literature experience are presented in Table 2-4, as are unique data related to the specific reasons for frozen section discordances[38] (Table 2-5). In addition to the Q-Probes data collection devices, examples of data collection documents addressing intraoperative (frozen section) consultations may be found in the CAP *Quality Improvement Manual In Anatomic Pathology*.[29]

Table 2-5. Reasons for Frozen Section Discordance

Reason	%
Misinterpretation of original frozen section	31.8
Microscopic discrepancy between frozen section (negative) and permanent section (positive) from frozen block	30.0
Gross sampling error	31.4
Technical problem in preparing frozen section	3.1
Specimen labeling error	0.1
Lack of clinical data	1.2
Other	2.5

(Data from Gephardt and Zarbo.[37])

Personal Consultation and Peer Review

In all areas of anatomic pathology the assessment of diagnostic "accuracy" or "correctness" is essentially a matter of peer consensus. Whereas the comparison of resection specimens for cancer with the biopsies on which the therapeutic decision to resect was made provides an opportunity for "outcome" review, this involves only a minority of cases processed in most laboratories. Consultation and peer review have therefore been traditional cornerstones of the quality assurance process in anatomic pathology. Although pathologists have traditionally shared difficult and otherwise interesting cases with colleagues, the quality assurance significance of this exercise has sometimes been overlooked.

It is important that consultations, both intra-and extra-departmental, be documented. The mechanism for case selection chosen by a specific department may vary considerably depending on the staff size, case material, and subspecialty interests of the pathologists. In large departments with training programs and active internal consultation, documentation of peer review may be quite simple. In other practice settings more elaborate case selection techniques may be required, with review criteria based on diagnostic categories or percentage of cases. Some of the more common mechanisms include (1) routine examination of every case by a second pathologist, (2) documentation of cases reviewed for presentation at tumor boards and other clinical-pathologic conferences, (3) routine review of all malignant diagnoses, (4) routine review of a predetermined percentage of cases, (5) routine review of report copies only, and (6) extradepartmental review of cases. Some reports have documented the efficacy of detecting and correcting diagnostic errors, but none have noted the cost effectiveness of these procedures.[25,27,28,42–46]

Regardless of the case selection methods used, peer review consultations will generally fall into either of two categories, prospective and retrospective.[22] In the *prospective* approach, case review takes place prior to release of the diagnostic report.[47] Advantages include simplicity, use of consultative patterns already in existence in the laboratory, and application of quality assurance review before the final diagnosis is rendered. The latter point permits resolution of diagnostic differences and decisions to seek additional consultation prior to final diagnosis. Disadvantages include the potential for some case categories to escape scrutiny altogether and an assumption that the peer reviewer has concurred in the diagnostic formulation of an entire case when only selected slides were seen. In our opinion, this latter issue is potentially the most significant drawback and is especially likely when unofficial or "curbside" consultations are solicited from colleagues. *Retrospective* techniques incorporate case review after diagnoses are reported. The major advantages of this approach are the scope of review, which often incorporates broad categories of cases, integration of this professional peer review with review of the report format itself, and generally easier identification of quality issues. The major disadvantage, of course, is the identification of problems after they have occurred. In our experience many departments utilize combinations of these two approaches, together with other peer review activities. The CAP *Quality Improvement Manual In Anatomic Pathology*[29] and the recent report of Travers,[22] present sample formats for documenting quality assurance review and defining discrepancies.

Extradepartmental consultations are another important and traditional quality assurance technique. Although outside consultation is usually sought for difficult diagnostic problems, routine cases are also often sent to other institutions when a patient is referred for an additional opinion or treatment, or both. The maintenance of the written report of these consultations is an important part of quality assurance.

The ease with which internal peer consultation is implemented depends to some extent on the size of the staff. Intradepartmental review is not difficult to organize in a large department. However, this kind of review is difficult to accomplish for the solo practitioner. Pathologists in these practice settings may establish a cooperative review arrangement with a colleague in a similar setting, may do "blind" review of their own previously reported cases, may take advantage of the consultative services available through some pathology societies, and may participate in the various self-assessment programs to be described.

The level of diagnostic consensus in surgical pathology has been addressed in several studies from a variety of institutions. In an experimental project of the CAP, a peer panel reached a diagnostic consensus in 77 percent of 250 slides.[6] Owen and Tighe[48] demonstrated greater than 90 percent consensus. These authors found a discordance rate of 2 percent for "major" differences and 5 percent for "minor" differences among senior pathologists and 8 percent for "major" and 11 percent for "minor" differences among junior pathologists. A prospective peer review of 3,000 consecutive cases from a military hospital revealed 7.8 percent of cases in which at least one reviewer disagreed with the preliminary diagnosis (92.2 percent concordance). In 2.2 percent of cases, disagreement was sufficient to modify the final diagnosis.[47] In a recent report from Southampton University Hospitals in England based on a random review of 2 percent of surgical pathology cases, 20 of 518 (3.9 percent) of the reports were considered "unsatisfactory." In six of these, the unsatisfactory report could have affected patient management.[27] Another report from the same institution has described a "clinicopathologic meeting" format as a means of auditing diagnostic performance.[28] This review of 416 cases resulted in an altered diagnosis in 9 percent, a refined diagnosis in 10 percent, and no change in 81 percent. Amended diagnoses resulted in major management changes in 3.8 percent, minor management changes in 2.9 percent, and no management change in 93.3 percent. This meeting approach also incorporated input from the submitting clinical services and demonstrated that gastroenterology (endoscopic biopsy specimens) had the largest number of cases with clinically significant diagnostic changes.

Institutional Consultation

In many institutions, institutional consultation is a required formal review of pathologic materials, resulting from the transfer of a patient from a different hospital or clinic. This policy is meant to ensure that clinical interventions, such as major surgery, radiotherapy, or chemotherapy, are performed for appropriate conditions. A recent review by Abt and colleagues[49] of pathology slides from outside institutions on 777 patients referred to a university hospital documented an overall discrepant diagnosis rate of 9.1 percent, with discrepancies higher (21 percent) for cytologic than surgical pathology (7.8 percent) cases reviewed. This appears to be a cost-effective quality assurance exercise with medicolegal implications, reflected in the finding that discrepant diagnoses resulted in 5.8 percent of cases in which diagnostic and therapeutic procedures were changed.

Teaching Conference and Committee Review

Conference and committee reviews are largely hospital-based activities that offer additional opportunities for pathology case review and documentation of diagnostic accuracy, terminology, and report content adequacy. Examples are tumor boards and clinical specialty conferences, clinicopathologic conferences, and surgical case review (tissue committee). With appropriate documentation of the re-examination of these cases, quality assurance interests are served. Furthermore, these types of review are easily incorporated into the quality assurance program of the institution.

Continuing Education and Performance Improvement Activities

Organized programs of continuing education and self-assessment may contribute significantly to the department's quality assurance program. Most pathologists attend local, state, regional, and/or national professional educational meetings. These provide exposure to recognized authorities on a variety of topics in anatomic pathology. Sharing the material at a later date with departmental colleagues enhances the value of these exercises. Several professional societies also offer teleconference programs that provide similar continuing education programs without the need to leave the laboratory.

A number of excellent self-improvement/self-assessment programs are available through national pathology organizations. For many years the American Society of Clinical Pathologists has sponsored the Check Sample Program, which exposes the subscriber to interesting case material followed by a critique prepared by a recognized authority on the subject presented. The more recently developed Check Path program provides results that permit peer group comparison. The Armed Forces Institute of Pathology offers Histopathology Quality Assessment Surveys to all pathologists in Military and Veterans Affairs Treatment Facilities. The surveys are sent four times a year and are designed to present challenging unknown cases to the pathologist. Feedback is provided after completion of each survey. The CAP developed the Performance Improvement Program in Diagnostic Surgical Pathology and Cytopathology to provide a self-assessment and performance improvement activity based on "expert" consensus diagnosis.[50] The program approximates practice conditions and uses original patient slides chosen from cases submitted by participants.

These types of external quality assurance programs are often viewed as "proficiency" testing exercises. In our judgment they are important educational activities but as presently configured are not an appropriate model for accreditation, licensure, or performance standard setting purposes.[15] Cramer and colleagues[51] have recently and very thoughtfully addressed the potential pitfalls in the design of proficiency tests in anatomic pathology. These authors note appropriately that variability in diagnostic classification does not necessarily indicate that a mistake has been made. The range of interobserver variability, even among "experts," has been amply demonstrated in recent reports addressing borderline lesions of the breast.[52,53] The report by Schnitt and associates[53] did demonstrate that enhanced interobserver concordance may be obtained with the use of standardized criteria.

QUALITY OF THE DIAGNOSTIC REPORT

The most important end point of our professional responsibility in anatomic pathology is the generation of an accurate and timely diagnostic report. Evaluation of the quality of the report should take place at several levels and should involve elements of both quality control and quality assurance. The principles of review are applicable to all disciplines within anatomic pathology, although specific details and requirements will vary among them.

Clinical Information

Because diagnostic evaluation of specimens in anatomic pathology is a medical consultation, the availability of adequate and relevant clinical information is essential to fulfill our patient care responsibilities. Virtually all pathologists have had to deal with requisition forms devoid of the clinical information necessary to provide proper diagnostic consultation. Although provision of clinical information by the clinician is a requirement of accrediting organizations, this deficiency on the specimen requisition form was the most common, acounting for roughly 40 percent of all deficiencies in a recent Q-Probes study of over one million specimens.[30] Varying degrees of success in solving this problem have been achieved. Pathologists must be industrious in their efforts to obtain the necessary clinical information to serve the needs of the patient. The adequacy of the information furnished in the requisition form should be part of the quality assurance review process. This is an area in which involvement of the institution's quality assurance apparatus can be used to provide additional leverage.

Transcription/Typographic Accuracy

Transcription and typographic accuracy, a largely quality control activity, is the primary responsibility of the "sign-out" pathologist. However, the effectiveness of the proofreading process may be enhanced by the use of additional "sets of eyes." Typographic accuracy may benefit from review by responsible clerical staff at the time the report is prepared and from review of the completed report by residents or additional pathologists, or by both. This review process may be formalized on a rotational basis. Although many errors of this type are insignificant, the unintended inclusion or exclusion of words such as "no,"

"present," or "absent" may have profound consequences. Furthermore, a report containing spelling, grammatical, and other typographic errors reflects negatively on the professionalism of the department.

Timeliness

The clinical usefulness of our consultative reports in anatomic pathology requires that they be available to referring physicians in a timely fashion. For surgical pathology the Laboratory Accreditation Program of the CAP requires that most routine case reports be available within two working days.[54,55] More complex specimens requiring prior fixation, complicated dissection, special studies, or additional consultation will understandably require more time for complete processing and reporting. The Association of Directors of Anatomic and Surgical Pathology recommends that the verbal report be available within two working days from time of specimen accessioning in the laboratory and within three working days until the final report is signed. This recommendation also allows additional time for special procedures.[25] CAP Q-Probes studies of 1992 and 1993 have developed reference databases of intralaboratory timeliness for surgical pathology routine biopsies and complex specimens, examining the influence of laboratory characteristics and practices on turnaround time.[56] The actual performance of most laboratories in these studies meets or exceeds the proposed standards.

Provisions for more rapid reporting of certain specimens are commonly available in the form of provisional or interim reports. The department should have a mechanism to keep the referring physician informed when a reporting delay is anticipated. The referring physician should be immediately notified when delays result from unexpected findings of clinical or therapeutic significance.

Quality and Adequacy of Descriptions

The "sign-out" pathologist is ultimately responsible for the precision, uniformity, consistency, and accuracy of the descriptive information recorded in the diagnostic report. The format and content should reflect the reporting requirements developed for the individual department. The descriptions provided should be clear and concise and contain adequate information regarding anatomic source, organ or tissue type, laterality, size and/or weight, measurements, and extent of any gross lesions. They should be free of typographic, spelling, and grammatical errors. Whether microscopic descriptions are included is a decision to be made by the specific pathology department, often with the advice and consent of the medical staff. If included in the report, the microscopic findings should be consistent with and support the final diagnosis. The use of dissection guidelines/manuals is important in establishing a reporting standard for the department against which compliance can be evaluated. Systematic review of completed diagnostic reports provides an ongoing evaluation of the quality and completeness of the descriptions provided.

Reporting documents in both surgical and autopsy pathology should provide adequate information about tissue block and slide identification. Inclusion of this information in the report provides necessary identification of special sections, such as those from resection margins, deepest penetration of tumor, and lymph node levels, and also greatly facilitates later consultative review. The frustration experienced when attempting to review undesignated slide material from a complicated case is well known to most pathologists. The provision of an appropriate key or summary of sections with each report not only enhances the quality of the document but also provides an inventory report of blocks prepared.

Adequacy of Diagnostic Information

The primary goal of our efforts in anatomic pathology is to provide a report that is not only accurate and timely but also contains clinically relevant information that contributes to patient care. Evaluation of the diagnostic information provided is clearly a quality assurance exercise. Findings described and diagnoses rendered in a pathology report may be entirely factually correct but may fail to address important patient management questions specifically asked or implied in the requisition. For example, evaluation of a series of mucosal biopsies in a patient with inflammatory bowel disease may correctly identify the diagnostic features of long-standing ulcerative colitis, but the value of the consultation is limited if the presence or absence of dysplasia is not noted when this was the primary indication for the biopsy procedure. Similar types of deficiencies in achieving the full potential of our consultations may occur in all areas of anatomic pathology.

For neoplasms, the diagnostic report should not only communicate the correct diagnosis but also provide sufficient information regarding grade of tumor and extent of disease for use in standard systems of grading and staging of tumors. An international system of staging is now available. The fourth edition of the *Manual for Staging of Cancer* of the American Joint Committee on Cancer[57] and the publications of the Union International Contre le Cancer in 1987 provide identical recommendations. An important adjunct for the diagnostic reporting of neoplasms is the series of guidelines that have been developed by the CAP. These address the data to be included in consultation reports on various types of cancer including breast cancer, bladder cancer, and Hodgkin's disease.[58] Additional guidelines for prostate, colorectal, lung, and ovarian cancer have recently been published.[59–62] Several CAP Q-Probes multi-institutional studies have addressed the adequacy of surgical pathology reports including those for colorectal carcinoma, breast carcinoma, lung carcinoma, and bladder carcinoma.[63–66]

A standard terminology should be established for the department and the institution and physicians that it serves, using a standardized glossary such as Systematized Nomenclature of Human and Veterinary Medicine (SNOMED). Specific classifications that may be chosen include the World Health Organization's *Histologic Typing of Tumors* and the Armed Forces Institute of Pathology's *Atlas of Tumor Pathology*. Recent reports directed toward the development of standardized diagnostic terminology for cytopathology have resulted in the Bethesda system[67] and its subsequent revision.[68]

The important point to be emphasized is the need for the individual pathology service to establish reporting criteria and to adopt a uniform diagnostic nomenclature for the department. Once established and defined, the guidelines will serve as a benchmark for quality assurance review to help ensure that appropriate and complete information is contained in each report.

The Association of Directors of Anatomic and Surgical Pathology has recently proposed standardization of surgical pathology reports.[69] Their recommendations address both the format and content of the report and provide specific suggestions concerning demographic and specimen information, gross description, microscopic description and comment section, intraoperative consultation, and final diagnosis. The value of a standardized reporting format or checklists, or both, has been amply demonstrated in a recent report by Zarbo.[63] This report was based on a Q-Probes study of the adequacy of surgical pathology reports of resected colorectal carcinomas. The one practice significantly associated with increased likelihood of providing complete diagnostic information was the use of a standardized report form or checklist. The recent literature contains examples of standardized surgical pathology forms or checklists to facilitate production of synoptic reports for common cancers.[70–72] See Chapter 8 for a more complete discussion of this subject.

ORGANIZATION AND DOCUMENTATION OF QUALITY ASSURANCE

In the preceding sections we have described various components that may be included in a comprehensive quality assurance program for anatomic pathology. It is important that the program be organized and described in a written document. Documentation of compliance with the elements selected for the program must also be maintained. In the planning process it is often helpful to develop an inventory of those activities of the department that, in the broadest sense, have quality assurance implications. As previously emphasized, these will include both quality control (process) and quality assurance (outcome) activities. Since the number of possible activities that can be included far exceeds those that can be reasonably accomplished, the individual department must select the activities that in its judgment are most likely to enhance the quality of its patient care services. These should involve all areas of anatomic pathology providing services and include activities concerned with the quality of the technical preparations, the role of the pathologist, and the quality of the completed diagnostic report. It is appropriate to remind the reader of the admonition regarding documentation, which has long guided the Laboratory Accreditation Program of the CAP: "If it isn't written, it didn't happen."

IMPLEMENTATION OF THE QUALITY ASSURANCE PLAN

Regardless of institution size, it is the pathologist's role to implement the quality assurance plan. This would include responsibility to organize and guide projects, develop indicators and standards, and, based on analysis of the data, diagnose causes. These activities should be overseen by a pathologist who is strongly supported or in a position to effect change. Because quality assurance should be an ongoing concern of all the laboratory employees, the plan is most efficiently implemented with the formal input of pathologists, laboratory supervisors, and key technologist/technicians.

This is most readily accomplished by formation of an Anatomic Pathology Quality Assurance Committee, which meets at regularly designated intervals (e.g., monthly). The quality assurance plan should be described in a written document identifying how it is to be carried out e.g., the mission, key players, their responsibilities, what is being done, how, and over what time frame. The committee should function to oversee and coordinate quality assurance monitoring and evaluation activities and in doing so provide a measure of assurance in the delivery of continually improved quality care in anatomic pathology.

Quality assurance activities should focus on *prospective*, continuous monitoring and evaluation of high volume and/or high risk service activities. The prospective collection of data rather than retrospective audits reflects the influence of the proactive rather than reactive approach to quality management. The starting point should be the committee's development of appropriate indicators (measurable variables) or monitors to audit the most important aspects of care provided. Each monitor, with defined methodology of actual data organization and collection, should then be delegated to a committee member to oversee. The data are then analyzed and interpreted by the committee to clarify potential or actual problems identified by this monitoring process. Information from these monitoring and evaluation activities may result in committee recommendations for corrective action. Documentation of the findings and recommendations from the completed monitor should be submitted quarterly to the Pathology Departmental Quality Assurance Committee and the Hospital Quality Assurance Department.

The documentation format should consist of pertinent, interpreted monitor findings or minutes of committee meetings specifically addressing the monitor. Any corrective actions taken are assessed by remonitoring to document the effectiveness of these actions on performance improvement. Again, relevant information is communicated and integrated into Departmental and Hospital Quality Assurance Programs. A departmental newsletter is also an excellent opportunity to communicate selected findings of good performance, opportunities for improvement, and changes in the policies or procedural aspects (process) of interacting with the laboratory.

ROLE OF SPECIALTY SOCIETIES AND ACCREDITING AND REGULATORY AGENCIES

A number of voluntary accrediting agencies and other national organizations have had important roles in the development and promotion of quality assurance activities in the hos-

pital in general and in pathology in particular. Some of these such as the American Society of Clinical Pathologists, the CAP, the United States and Canadian Academy of Pathology, the International Academy of Pathology, state pathology societies, and various subspecialty pathology organizations have made major contributions to quality assurance through the development and presentation of numerous educational programs for our specialty. The American Society of Cytopathology sponsors educational programs and offers a voluntary accreditation program for cytology laboratories.

The Laboratory Accreditation Program of the CAP was initiated in 1961 with the primary objective of improving the quality of laboratory services through voluntary participation, professional peer review, education, and compliance with established performance standards. The essential criteria by which laboratories are judged are defined in the CAP *Standards for Laboratory Accreditation*, 1996 Edition.[24] The Laboratory Accreditation Program conducts on-site inspections on a biennial schedule with a self-inspection conducted by the laboratory in the interim year. Inspections are conducted by peer professionals trained in the accreditation process, and team leaders are always pathologists. Currently, more than 5,000 laboratories in the United States and a number of foreign countries participate in this program. Compliance with the Standards is evaluated using a series of checklists that address all aspects of laboratory operation. In anatomic pathology the accreditation process thoroughly examines broad issues of quality control/quality assurance including specimen handling procedures, equipment, safety, personnel, reports, and the overall management principles that comprise quality in all areas of anatomic pathology. All the essential components of quality control/quality assurance that have been described in this chapter are addressed in the checklist. Specific mechanisms and operational details are not mandated. Laboratory directors are encouraged, within the basic framework, to develop their own programs to meet individual requirements. The various quality assurance programs, educational activities, and written materials provided by the professional organizations noted earlier may assist in meeting accreditation requirements.

The CAP Laboratory Accreditation Program has and will continue to be a voluntary laboratory improvement activity based on education and peer review. Nonetheless, since shortly after its inception, the Program has acquired a quasi-regulatory role through its relationship with other organizations and agencies.[73] For more than 20 years, the Laboratory Accreditation Program of CAP was "deemed" an equivalent program for interstate licensure requirements under the Clinical Laboratory Improvement Act (CLIA) of 1967. Following the passage of CLIA 1988 amendments and the promulgation of regulations, the CAP Laboratory Accreditation Program sought deemed status from the Health Care Financing Administration. In June of 1994 the CAP was notified that its Laboratory Accreditation Program was approved by the latter group. The CAP Laboratory Accreditation Program, because of its deeming authority, may now be used by laboratories to meet federal licensure requirements. The Laboratory Accreditation Program also meets licensure requirements in approximately 25 states. Since 1978, the JCAHO, with the agreement of the Health Care Financing Administration, has accepted the CAP Laboratory Accreditation Program in lieu of its own inspection of hospital laboratories. The JCAHO now has a formal written agreement with the CAP. When the laboratory elects the CAP program for accreditation, the JCAHO will not conduct the laboratory portion of its survey process. However, the JCAHO will review the entire quality improvement program of the institution including that of the pathology and medical laboratory services.

The JCAHO (formerly JCAH) is a private, not-for-profit organization that has been responsible since 1951 for a voluntary survey program of standardization, inspection, and accreditation. Presently this program includes 5,400 acute care and general hospitals and 3,200 other health care organizations. The latter include mental health centers, outpatient clinics, nursing homes, substance abuse and rehabilitation programs, and hospices. The JCAHO is composed of five member organizations (the American College of Surgeons, American College of Physicians, American Hospital Association, American Medical Association, and American Dental Association) that appoint its 21 member Board of Commissioners. The JCAHO plays a key role in the development of standards and survey procedures and also confers accreditation on organizations that meet its standards. The federal government ties hospital accreditation to Medicare and Medicaid certification. In addition, 43 states tie JCAHO accreditation to licensure.

The JCAHO *Accreditation Manual for Hospitals* contains quality assurance standards and required characteristics that apply to the organization and that apply specifically to the laboratory.[74] In its Monitoring and Evaluation Series the JCAHO discusses its approach to evaluation of quality assurance of pathology and medical laboratory services.[75] The JCAHO poses the following questions to "help pathology and medical laboratory personnel assess the adequacy of their monitoring and evolution activities." These coincide with their 10 Step Monitoring and Evaluation Model, a form of quality assurance implementing continuous quality improvement principles:

1. Has responsibility for the department's or service's monitoring and evaluation been assigned?
2. Has the scope of service been delineated?
3. Have the important aspects of service been identified?
4. Have indicators of quality and appropriateness of care been identified?
5. Have thresholds for evaluation been established?
6. Have relevant data been collected?
7. When thresholds for evaluation are reached, has evaluation been initiated?
8. Have actions been taken to resolve identified problems or to improve patient care services?
9. Has service improved, has monitoring continued, and is there documentation?
10. Has the information from monitoring and evaluation activities been communicated to the organization-wide quality assurance program?

Although specific clinical indicators have not been developed by JCAHO for pathology, pathology-related issues are presently covered within other specialty- and organization-wide indicators. For example, surgical pathology report adequacy for resected lung, colorectal, and female breast cancers are among the oncology clinical indicators currently undergoing beta field testing.[75]

It is clear that regulatory agencies of government have identified and will continue to focus on quality assurance issues in the medical laboratory, including anatomic pathology. Nowhere is this more apparent than in cytopathology. Up to this time, the voluntary accrediting agencies have had major roles in pathology quality assurance and, through relationships with government agencies, have assisted laboratories in meeting regulatory requirements.

DISCOVERABILITY AND CONFIDENTIALITY

In discussions of quality assurance activities in health care, concern in often expressed about the protection of quality assurance information. In some states laws protect information collected for quality assurance purposes from subpoena.[76] To be protected, documents must be specifically identified as quality assurance documents. Care should be taken to protect the identities of patients and health care providers in all quality assurance reports. In some states where quality assurance records are not specifically protected by statute, the courts have protected these documents in specific cases. In these cases, public policy interests served by the existence of quality assurance activities have been held to exceed the interest of the specific litigant. It is very important that laboratory directors be aware of legal issues pertaining to quality assurance documents in the jurisdiction where they practice.

REFERENCES

1. Sunderman FW: The origin of proficiency testing for clinical laboratories in the United States. pp. 6–7. In: Proceedings of the Second National Conference on Proficiency Testing. National Council of Health Laboratory Services, Bethesda, MD, 1975
2. Nakazawa H, Rosen P, Lane N: Frozen section experience in 3,000 cases. Am J Clin Pathol 49:41–51, 1968
3. Feinstein AR, Gelfman NA, Yesner R: Observer variability in the histopathologic diagnosis of lung cancer. Am Rev Respi Dis 101:671–684, 1970
4. American Society of Cytology, 18th Scientific Meeting; Honolulu (Nov. 8, 1970). Forum on criteria for certification, licensure and quality control of cytology laboratories. Acta Cytol 15:562–576, 1971
5. Royal College of Pathologists of Australia, Board of Education, Sydney: Reports of Surveys: 1969, 1970, 1971. The College of Sydney, Sydney, Australia. 1971
6. Penner DW: Quality control and quality evaluation in histopathology and cytology. pp. 1–19. In Sommers SC (ed): Pathology Annual. Appleton-Century-Crofts, E. Norwalk, CT, 1973
7. Dorsey DB: Evolving concepts of quality in laboratory practice: a historical overview of quality assurance in clinical laboratories. Arch Pathol Lab Med 113:1329–1334, 1989
8. Batsakis JG: Quality assurance: sisyphean or sibylline. Arch Pathol Lab Med 114:1173–1174, 1990
9. Bartlett R: Quality Control in Clinical Microbiology. American Society of Clinical Pathologists (CCE), Chicago, 1988

10. U.S. Department of Health and Human Services: Medicare, Medicaid and CLIA Programs: clinical laboratory improvement amendments of 1988 (CLIA, '88) final rules. Federal Registry, Washington, DC, 57:7183–7184, 1992

11. Zarbo RJ: Improving quality in pathology and laboratory medicine. Am J Clin Pathol 102:563–564, 1994

12. Berwick DM: Continuous improvement as an ideal in health care. N Engl J Med 320:53–56, 1989

13. Howanitz PJ: Quality assurance measurements in departments of pathology and laboratory medicine. Arch Pathol Lab Med 114:1131–1135, 1990

14. QAS-Quality Assurance Committee: Benchmarking with multi-institutional reference databases for quality improvement (1995). pp. 127–183. In Travers H (ed): Quality Improvement Manual in Anatomic Pathology. College of American Pathologists, Northfield, IL, 1993

15. Rickert RR: Quality assurance goals in surgical pathology. Arch Pathol Lab Med 114:1157–1162, 1990

16. Bachner P: Quality assurance: an accreditation perspective. Lab Med 20:159–162, 1989

17. Langley FA: Quality control in histopathology and diagnostic cytology. Histopathology 2:3–18, 1978

18. Murthy MSN, Derman H: Quality assurance in surgical pathology — personal and peer assessment. Am J Clin Pathol 75:462–466, 1981

19. Rickert RR: Quality assurance in anatomic pathology. Clini Lab Med 6:697–706, 1986

20. Penner DW: Quality assurance in anatomic pathology. p. 297. In Howanitz PJ, Howanitz JH (eds): Laboratory Quality Assurance. McGraw-Hill, New York, 1987

21. Rickert RR, Maliniak RM: Intralaboratory quality assurance of immunohistochemical procedures: recommended practices for daily application. Arch Pathol Lab Med 113:673–679, 1989

22. Travers H: Quality assurance in anatomic pathology. Lab Med 20:85–92, 1989

23. Cowan DF: Quality assurance in anatomic pathology: an information system approach. Arch Pathol Lab Med 114:129–134, 1990

24. Standards for Laboratory Accreditation. College of American Pathologists, Northfield, IL, 1996

25. Association of Directors of Anatomic and Surgical Pathology: Recommendations on quality control and quality assurance in anatomic pathology. Am J Surg Pathol 15:1007–1009, 1991

26. Ramsay AD: Locally organized medical audit in histopathology. J Clin Pathol 44:353–357, 1991

27. Ramsay AD, Gallagher PJ: Local audit of surgical pathology: 18 months' experience of peer review based quality assessment in an English teaching hospital. Am J Surg Pathol 16:476–482, 1992

28. McBroom HM, Ramsay AD: The clinicopathologic meeting: a means of auditing diagnostic performance. Am J Surg Pathol 17:75–80, 1993

29. Travers H (ed): Quality Improvement Manual in Anatomic Pathology. College of American Pathologists, Northfield, IL, 1993

30. Nakhleh RE, Zarbo RJ: Surgical pathology specimen identification and accessioning. Arch Pathol Lab Med 120:227–233, 1996

31. Gephardt GN, Zarbo RJ: Q-Probe 94–03: Extraneous Tissue in Surgical Pathology Slides: Data Analysis and Critique. College of American Pathologists, Northfield, IL, 1995

32. Zarbo RJ, Howanitz PJ, Bachner P: Interinstitutional comparison of performance in breast fine-needle aspiration cytology: a Q-Probe quality indicator study. Arch Pathol Lab Med 115:743–750, 1991

33. Zarbo RJ, Fenoglio-Preiser CM: Interinstitutional database for comparison of performance in lung fine-needle aspiration cytology. A College of American Pathologists Q-Probe study of 5264 cases with histologic correlation. Arch Pathol Lab Med 116:463–470, 1992

34. Jones BA, Novis DA: Cervical biopsy-cytology correlation. A College of American Pathologists Q-Probes study of 22,439 correlations in 348 laboratories. Arch Pathol Lab Med 120:523–531, 1996

35. Dankwa EK, Davies JD: Frozen section diagnosis: an audit. J Clin Pathol 38:1235–1240, 1985

36. Zarbo RJ, Hoffman GG, Howanitz PJ: Interinstitutional comparison of frozen section consultation. A College of American Pathologists Q-Probe study of 79,647 consultations in 297 North American institutions. Arch Pathol Lab Med 115:1187–1194, 1991

37. Gephardt GN, Zarbo RJ: Interinstitutional comparison of frozen section consultations. A College of American Pathologists Q-Probes study of 90,538 cases in 461 institutions. Arch Pathol Lab Med 120:804–809, 1996

38. Novis DA, Gephardt G, Zarbo RJ: Interinstitutional comparison of frozen section consultation in small hospitals: a College of American Pathologists Q-Probes study of 18,532 frozen section consultation diagnoses in 233 small hospitals. Arch Pathol Lab Med 1996 (in press)

39. Zarbo RJ, Schmidt WA, Bachner P, et al: Indications and immediate patient outcomes of pathology intraoperative consultations: a College of American Pathologists/Centers for Disease Control and Prevention outcomes working group study. Arch Pathol Lab Med 120:19–25, 1996

40. Hoffman GG: Q-Probe 89-01A: Surgical Pathology Frozen Section Consultations: Data Analysis and Critique. College of American Pathologists Northfield, IL, 1990

41. Gephardt G, Zarbo RJ: Q-Probe 90–20A: Surgical Pathology Frozen Section Consultation: Data Analysis and Critique. College of American Pathologists, Northfield, IL, 1991

42. Henson DE: Editorial: opportunities unexplored. Arch Pathol Lab Med 114:565, 1990

43. Henson DE, Frelick RW, Ford LG, et al: Results of a national survey of characteristics of hospital tumor conferences. Surg Gynecol Obstet 170:1–6, 1990

44. Safrin RE, Bark CJ: Surgical pathology signout. Routine review of every case by a second pathologist. Am J Surg Pathol 17:1190–1192, 1993

45. Association of Directors of Anatomic and Surgical Pathology: Consultations in surgical pathology. Am J Surg Pathol 17:743–745, 1993

46. Lind AC, Bewtra C, Healy JC, et al: Prospective peer review in surgical pathology. Am J Clin Pathol 104:560–566, 1995

47. Whitehead ME, Fitzwater JE, Lindley SK, et al: Quality assurance of histopathologic diagnoses: a prospective audit of three thousand cases. Am J Clin Pathol 81:487–491, 1984

48. Owen DA, Tighe JR: Quality evaluation in histopathology. BMJ 1:149–150, 1975

49. Abt AB, Abt LG, Olt GJ: The effect of interinstitution anatomic pathology consultation on patient care. Arch Pathol lab Med 119:514–517, 1995

50. Penner DW, Bradford S, Hyman MP: Taking a quantum leap in histopathology and cytopathology. Pathologist 11:777–779, 1983

51. Cramer SF, Roth LM, Ulbright TM: The mystique of the mistake: with proposed standards for validating proficiency tests in anatomic pathology. Am J Clin Pathol 96:774–777, 1991

52. Rosai J: Borderline epithelial lesions of the breast. Am J Surg Pathol 15:209–221, 1991

53. Schnitt SS, Connolly JL, Tavassoli FA: Interobserver reproducibility in the diagnosis of ductal proliferative breast lesions using standardized criteria. Am J Surg Pathol 16:1133–1143, 1992

54. College of American Pathologists Committee on Laboratory Accreditation: Inspection Checklist I, Laboratory General. College of American Pathologists, Northfield, IL, 1994

55. College of American Pathologists Commission on Laboratory Accreditation: Inspection Checklist VIII, Anatomic Pathology and Cytopathology. College of American Pathologists, Northfield, IL, 1994

56. Zarbo RJ, Gephardt GN, Howanitz PJ: Intralaboratory timeliness of surgical pathology reports: results of two College of American Pathologists Q-Probes studies of biopsies and complex specimens. Arch Pathol Lab Med 120:234–244, 1996

57. Beahrs OH, Henson DE, Hutter RVP, et al: Manual for Staging of Cancer. 4th Ed. American Joint Committee on Cancer. Lippincott-Raven, Philadelphia, 1992

58. Hutter RVP: Guidelines for data to be included in consultation reports on breast cancer, bladder cancer and Hodgkin's disease. Pathologist 40:18–23, 1986

59. Henson DE, Hutter RVP, Sobin LH, et al: Protocol for the examination of specimens removed from patients with colorectal carcinoma. A basis for checklists. Arch Pathol Lab Med 118:122–125, 1994

60. Henson DE, Hutter RVP, Farrow G: Practice protocol for the examination of specimens removed from patients with carcinoma of the prostate gland. Arch Pathol Lab Med 118:779–783, 1994

61. Nash G, Hutter RVP, Henson DE: Practice protocol for the examination of specimens from patients with lung cancer. Arch Pathol Lab Med 119:695–700, 1995

62. Scully RE, Henson DE, Nielsen ML, et al: Practice protocol for the examination of specimens removed from patients with ovarian tumors: a basis for checklists. Arch Pathol Lab Med 119:1012–1022, 1995

63. Zarbo RJ: Interinstitutional assessment of colorectal carcinoma surgical pathology report adequacy: a College of American Pathologists Q-Probes study of practice patterns from 532 laboratories and 15,940 reports. Arch Pathol Lab Med 116:1113–1119, 1992

64. Fenoglio-Preiser CM, Zarbo RJ: Q-Probe 90-14A: Breast Carcinoma Surgical Pathology Report Adequacy. Data Analysis and Critique. College of American Pathologists, Northfield, IL, 1990

65. Gephardt GN, Baker PB: Interinstitutional comparison of bladder carcinoma surgical pathology report adequacy. A College of American Pathologists Q-Probes study of 7234 bladder biopsies and curettings in 268 institutions. Arch Pathol Lab Med 119:681–685, 1995

66. Gephardt GN, Baker PB: Q-Probe 91–06A: Lung Carcinoma Surgical Pathology Report Adequacy: Data Analysis and Critique. College of American Pathologists, Northfield, IL, 1992

67. National Cancer Institute Workshop: The 1988 Bethesda System for reporting cervical/vaginal cytological diagnoses. JAMA 262:931–934, 1989

68. The revised Bethesda System for reporting cervical/vaginal cytologic diagnoses: report of the 1991 Bethesda Workshop. Anal Quant Cytol Histol 14:11–163, 1992

69. Association of Directors of Anatomic and Surgical Pathology: Standardization of the surgical pathology report. Am J Surg Pathol 16:84–86, 1992

70. Rosai J: Standardized reporting of surgical pathology diagnosis for the major tumor types: a proposal. Am J Clin Pathol 100:240–255, 1993

71. Robboy SJ, Bentley RC, Krigman H, et al: Synoptic reports in gynecologic pathology. Int J Gynecol Pathol 13:161–174, 1994

72. Markel SF, Hirsch SD: Synoptic surgical pathology reporting. Hum Pathol 22:807–810, 1991

73. Duckworth JK: Laboratory licensure and accreditation pp. 334–353. In Howanitz PJ, Howanitz JH (eds): Laboratory Quality Assurance. McGraw-Hill, New York, 1987

74. Joint Commission on Accreditation of Health Care Organizations: Accreditation Manual for Hospitals. JCAHO, Chicago, IL, 1992

75. Joint Commission on Accreditation of Health Care Organizations: Monitoring and Evaluation in Pathology and Medical Laboratory Services. JCAHO, Chicago, IL, 1989

76. Butch SH: The role of the clinical laboratory in quality assurance and risk management. In: American Society of Clinical Pathologists, Fall 1989 Teleconference Series, University of Michigan, Ann Arbor, MI, 1989

3

Medicolegal Principles and Problems

Joseph D. Sabella

A malpractice claim against a pathologist is a demand for compensation by a patient or a patient's family for an alleged injury that the claimant believes was caused by a negligent error by the pathologist. The claim may be made without the filing of a lawsuit, simultaneously with the filing of a lawsuit, or a lawsuit may follow. The great majority of claims are accompanied or followed by lawsuits. A claim can also result from a negligent error by persons supervised by the pathologist; under the legal doctrine of *respondeat superiore*, the master is responsible for the servant. This type of claim can be made even when subordinates are not direct employees of the pathologist if the facts indicate that the pathologist had a duty to supervise their work.

The liability experience of pathologists and the accompanying loss data presented in this chapter are derived mainly from the experience of a large, doctor-owned, medical malpractice insurer that insures over 2,000 pathologists, about 1,800 of whom are insured under a program endorsed by the College of American Pathologists The College program has been continuously with the company from January 1, 1986 to the time of this writing, a period of 10 years. Added to this experience is that of the approximately 200 pathologists who are separately insured, some of whose experience dates back to 1976. The aggregate of this experience represents the most comprehensive information available regarding the malpractice liability and loss experience of pathologists. Quantitative information presented in this chapter is derived from the experience of the pathologists in the College program; qualitative attributes of claims are from the combined experience[1,2] (personal communication, The Doctors' Company).

Most of the conclusions presented here are the result of reviews of claims by panelists who individually reviewed slides and reports independently before joining together with claims representatives and defense lawyers to discuss the cases and give guidance in their management. Unfortunately, when pathologists review slides through the "retrospectoscope," whether for the defense or for the plaintiff, hindsight tends to be 20/20. It is impossible for the reviewer to relive the experience of the original pathologist, which may have been influenced by such factors as the urgency and time demand of a frozen section, the pressure from the clinician for a decision, the absence of the wisdom of experts yet to be consulted, and the lack of insight provided by the natural history of a disease as it unfolds over time. Nevertheless, in conducting these review panels, an attempt was made to create maximal "prospectoscopic" objectiv-

ity. Only the minimal historic information available to the original pathologist and a brief gross description of the tissue were made available to the panelists before they reviewed slides. Only after they had made their own diagnoses were they given additional information, such as follow-up history, slides and reports of any subsequent biopsies, and the reports of consulting pathologists.

OVERVIEW OF PATHOLOGISTS' LIABILITY

Claims against pathologists have risen in recent years,[1,2] (personal communication, The Doctors' Company). Figure 3-1 shows the frequency of claims nationwide, from 1988 through June 30, 1995. Claim frequency is expressed as claims/100 insured, with pathologists shown on the lower-line and the average frequency for all specialties combined on the upper.

Figure 3-1 shows a sharp rise in pathologists' claim frequency in the early years, but this is more apparent than real and occurs because the pathologists had been insured under a claims-made policy, which covers claims that are made in a current policy year, arising from incidents in that year or from incidents that occurred in prior years covered by the policy. Because the pathologists were part of an endorsed program that was started in 1986 and that did not cover incidents (occurrences) prior to that year, the early years reflect an immature experience. Thus the increase in claims against pathologists from 1988 through 1991 from slightly over 3 claims/100 to 6 claims/100 pathologists cannot be interpreted as including an underlying increase in frequency because of the confounding factor of the maturation of the liability experience itself. However, the increase after 1991 from six claims to nine by mid-1995, a 38.5 percent increase, is indicative of a real and substantial rise in frequency.

It should be noted that in 1988 the average frequency for all specialties was over 19/100 insured, but by 1991, when the pathology experience had matured, the all-insured frequency had fallen to slightly over 15, 2.3 times that of pathologists. By mid-1995, the average frequency of all insured had risen to nearly 19, and that of pathologists to 9, a ratio of 2.1. This indicates that the claim frequency of pathologists has risen in tandem with that of all physicians.

Further discussion of the insurance aspects of pathologists' liability requires that some technical insurance terms be ex-

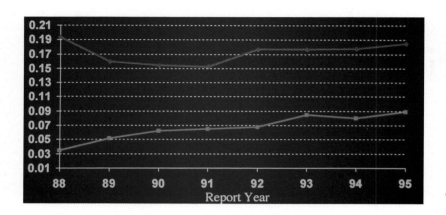

Fig. 3-1. Claim frequency. Pathologists versus the average among all specialties nationwide 1986 through June 1995. Red, all specialities; blue, pathology.

plained. *Reserves* are funds set aside by the insurer in expectation of future payment. *Indemnity* is defined as monies actually paid to claimants or reserved for such payment in the future. *Allocated loss expense* includes all expenses paid or reserved that are allocable to specific claims. These include such items as fees of defense attorneys (the largest), expert testimony and review of cases, record copying, and so on. *Earned premium* is the total of all premiums collected by the insurer that are applicable to separate, specific years of coverage. *Loss ratio* is indemnity payments and reserves plus allocated loss expenses and reserves divided by earned premium. The loss ratio does not include in the numerator the general expenses of operating a company's claims department (*unallocated loss expense*), nor does it include the other general administrative expenses. *Investment income* is an important factor in the economics of insurance and is earned from investing the company's case reserves and *surplus* funds (*capital and surplus* when speaking of commercial insurers). Surplus (or capital and surplus) consists of uncommitted funds that support the taking of risk by an insurer and serves as a source of funds in the event that reserves prove inadequate to cover future losses.

Figure 3-2 shows that in the years 1987 and 1988, when the loss experience was very immature, the losses were less than the premium, but from 1989 through mid-1995, losses exceeded premium by substantial margins, reaching a peak in 1993 of over 180 percent. If one adds to this the insurer's other operating expenses, losses in 1993 were more than twice the premium.

The reductions in the loss ratios in 1994 and the first half of 1995 do not reflect an improving loss experience, but instead are the result of large increases in premiums in those years. Despite the improvement in the loss ratios of 1994 and the first half of 1995, the losses exceeded not only the premiums, but also the total of the addition of the investment income allocable to the premium. In short, despite substantial increases in premiums, pathologists have not paid their way from 1989 through mid-1995.

While pathologists experience only about half as many claims as all specialities combined, their claims have two important characteristics. The first is that the ultimate development of the claims experience for a given year of coverage (the coverage year) lags behind that of the average of all specialties by about 1 year. In other words, the interval between the end of a given year of coverage and the time when substantially all the claims arising from incidents occurring in that year are reported is 1 year longer than the average interval for all specialties. This lag in the reporting of pathology claims is not the result of a disinclination by pathologists to report, but is caused instead by the nature of the great majority of the errors committed by pathologists that lead to claims against them, such as missed cancers and, with Papanicolaou (Pap) smears, missed premalignant dysplasias as well. When such false negative errors occur, the usual course of events starts with a lack of appropriate treatment In many cases, months may elapse before persistent complaints or findings or new signs and symptoms lead to a re-eval-

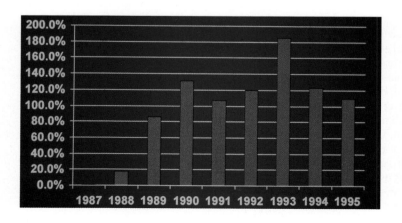

Fig. 3-2. CAP program loss ratios, 1987 through June 1995 by report year (case basis).

uation of the patient. In cases of missed cervical intraepithelial neoplasia (CIN), the delay in definitive diagnosis and therapy can be much longer, occasionally up to several years, a problem that is compounded because many women do not have yearly Pap smears.

Ultimately, due to persistence or development of symptoms or findings, further workup of the patient leads to the correct diagnosis, at which time disease may be advanced. At this point, the previous slides are reviewed and the error is detected. Appropriate treatment then follows, often including protracted radiotherapy or chemotherapy. When treatment is completed, the attention of the patient and family, which up to that time has been focused on the immediate problems of the illness and its treatment, now turns to the original error by the pathologist. The patient may conclude that the error has compromised the chance for cure, a lawyer is consulted who agrees, and a claim is made. When the patient dies of the disease before the claim is made or the claim is unresolved at the time of death, the dependents will make the claim.

The second important characteristic of claims against pathologists is that they are of high severity, that is, they are for larger than average damages. As of September 30, 1995, the average case reserve of the insurer for all specialties combined was $97,388, but for the most recent 289 pathology claims it was $150,511, 54.5 percent higher because a missed diagnosis of cancer often leads to severe injury including death, with high damages and proportionately high demands for compensation (personal communication, The Doctors' Company).

Because this combination of frequency, severity, and late claims development has produced large losses and a worsening loss experience for pathologists, it is important that they become familiar with (1) the basics of the law of medical malpractice, (2) the causes of claims against them, and (3) the steps that can be taken to manage their risk.

ANATOMY OF A CLAIM: DUTY + NEGLIGENCE + INJURY + ANGER = CLAIM

Duty

A clinician does not owe a duty to render care to a person unless that person has been accepted as a patient. While the choice to accept or reject a patient applies unambiguously to a clinician in private office practice, it is absent in certain situations wherein such duty is implied. Examples are emergency room physicians, clinicians covering an emergency roster, or physicians under contract or employed by hospitals, clinics, or managed care organizations.

The question of the pathologist's duty is a more complex one. When a patient is referred by a clinician for a procedure such as fine needle aspiration biopsy or a bone marrow examination, in theory the pathologist has the choice to accept or not accept the patient. However, in nearly all instances, the pathologist's relationship to a hospital, private laboratory, or medical group

carries with it an implied duty to accept such patients. Similarly, when an anatomic pathology specimen or laboratory specimen is accepted, or if the pathologist agrees to perform a postmortem examination, the pathologist owes a direct duty to the referring physician to analyze or examine the specimen or deceased, to obtain correct answers and diagnoses to the extent possible, and to report the results in a timely manner to the physician.

In addition to the pathologist's direct duty to the referring clinician, there is an indirect duty to the patient, and, in the case of an autopsy, to the family. Although this duty can be characterized as secondary to that owed to the referring clinician, it is nonetheless real. This point is raised because in several recent cases the clinician has been remiss in following up after a worrisome pathology or cytology report or laboratory abnormality, and the plaintiff's attorney has attempted to show that the pathologist had a direct duty to the patient to ensure proper follow-up and treatment, either by making sure the clinician followed up appropriately or by reporting the abnormality directly to the patient. Such claims have been strenuously resisted, because establishment of such a duty in case law would profoundly disrupt relationships and communications among pathologists, clinicians, and patients. One can imagine the nightmare of both the clinician and the pathologist communicating to the patient every abnormal clinical laboratory test, or surgical pathology or cytopathology diagnosis, or communicating autopsy findings directly to families or other persons legally entitled to them.

The above notwithstanding, it is becoming more common for the patient or members of the family to wish to speak directly to the pathologist regarding biopsy, cytology, or autopsy findings. The motivation for such direct consultation may range from simple curiosity to reasons as serious as suspicion of a serious error by the clinician or pathologist. This point is explored later in this chapter

Negligence

Negligence is defined as not performing professionally at the expected standard of care. In pathology the standard of care is defined legally as using such care as a reasonably prudent pathologist would use in similar circumstances. The standard of care in any given case is established by the testimony of expert witnesses. In some states the so-called locality rule prevails, which defines standard of care as that of a reasonably prudent pathologist in the same geographic locale. In many states, however, this is not the case, and highly specialized academic pathologists can testify as to the standard of care to be imposed on nonacademic, private practitioners, and even on solo practitioners in rural areas This problem is further complicated by the existence of national specialty certification, which implies uniform national standards of competence.

Implicit in the definition of negligence is the concept that because the practice of medicine is an inexact science, no liability exists if a pathologist (or any physician) makes an error in judgment that is not negligent. While this is correct as an abstract concept of law, the reality is that if a case goes to trial before a jury, the standard of care will be established by which expert witnesses the jury chooses to believe: those for the defense or those for the plaintiff. It is important to keep in mind that whereas pathologists, who are educated in the sciences and highly trained and knowledgeable in statistics, have a well grounded concept of what is scientifically true, "truth" to a plaintiff's lawyer is what he or she can convince a jury to believe. This conundrum notwithstanding, the concept of allowable, non-negligent errors of judgment that do not create liability is important in the give and take of managing claims and negotiating their closure short of trial.

Injury and Causation

Assuming that the elements of duty and negligence have been demonstrated, the plaintiff must also prove that the negligent error caused an *injury*. In legal parlance this is called *causation*. In theory, even if an error can be shown to be negligent, if it did not injure the patient there should be no liability. While these are well established principles of law, the everyday practice of law is not always so abstract. Many of the claims against pathologists involve the discovery of a missed diagnosis of cancer that has delayed treatment for a short time, frequently only a few months. Subsequent diagnosis followed by appropriate treatment may then show a locally advanced lesion or extensive metastases that the plaintiff attributes to this short delay in treatment. It would be the exceedingly rare case in which this was true, but again, the problem is not what is medically true, but what a jury can be induced to believe. It appears to be fixed firmly in the minds of the public that cancer is virtually always curable if treated early, strongly implying the converse, that any delay at all can result in advanced disease with lost chance of cure.

The problem of causation is further complicated because the legal definition of injury is not restricted to physical injury. Three decades ago, case law was such that psychological injury unaccompanied by physical injury was not compensable. This principle was adhered to because it was understood that the demonstration, evaluation, and proof of pure psychological injury was fraught with great difficulty and that the adoption of such a broad definition of injury would allow claims that could not be properly adjudicated and would increase the likelihood of spurious and even fraudulent claims. However, under relentless pressure over the past 30 years from an aggressive and burgeoning plaintiff bar to expand liability and plaintiffs' rights, the definition of injury has evolved to include pure psychological injury.

This is not an abstract problem for pathologists because, although most claims against pathologists are for missed cancer, there is a smaller but significant number of claims for false positive cancer diagnoses. In some cases in which the error is not immediately discovered, unnecessary and possibly disfiguring surgery or extensive radiotherapy or chemotherapy may be administered, resulting in an actual immediate injury or the justifiable fear of future injury. However, even in cases in which the error is discovered early enough to prevent inappropriate treatment or to abort it after only a few treatment sessions, plaintiffs nevertheless may now claim purely psychological injury such as fear of cancer.

Anger

In civil claims and lawsuits, especially those involving individuals, the element of anger is nearly always present. The only exceptions in medical liability are cases of catastrophic injury such as severely damaged newborns or severe paralysis causing total disability of a breadwinner, situations in which the family and patient face economic catastrophe. Faced with ruinous present and future expenses, these patients or their families may make a claim and sue, even when no great anger is felt toward the doctor, if they believe their problems were caused by the doctor's error.

Anger, of course, requires a target. When directed at a clinician, anger is often engendered by a poor outcome or serious complication following a diagnostic procedure or treatment, or when the clinician has missed a diagnosis that the patient or the family believes has resulted in an injury. In such instances, the patient or family may conclude, rightly or wrongly, that the doctor has not been open in discussing the situation and may even believe that they are the victims of a cover-up. From that point it is a short distance to a lawyer's office.

As to pathologists as targets of anger, it was not very long ago that pathologists were relatively anonymous to patients, in large part because of the way in which they were compensated, often a percentage of income from the entire laboratory operation or by salary. However, now that most pathologists bill patients directly for anatomic pathology services and for other personally performed services such as fine needle aspiration biopsies, they have lost their anonymity and have become identifiable to patients as caregivers. As a result, if the patient or family believes that an error in histopathologic or cytopathologic diagnosis has occurred that has harmed the patient, the pathologist is now a more readily identifiable target of anger.

When a clinician communicates with a patient or family concerning an adverse outcome, whether or not an actual error has been committed by anyone involved in the patient's care, the clinician is in a position to ensure that the communication is accurate and reasonable, and if any miscommunication with the patient or family or misunderstanding by them has occurred, the clinician is in a position to correct it. However, the communication problem faced by the pathologist who has made an error, or is believed to have made an error, is considerably more difficult, because any initial discussion with the patient or family rarely takes place directly with the pathologist. Instead such critically important communication often involves an intermediary, the clinician, and sometimes multiple clinicians. Thus, the pathologist is frequently not able to ensure appropriate, coordinated communication with the patient or family regarding a perception of error. This can be an especially serious problem if the clinician is unsympathetic or has poor rapport with the pathologist or with the patient or family, or because the clinician has developed severe anxiety over a possible legal action, and in a misguided attempt at self-exoneration tries to lay blame ("dumps") on others, including the pathologist. The anxiety felt by physicians when concerned over a possible malpractice action, coupled with the stress of dealing with a severely injured patient, can induce counterproductive behavior that in itself can increase the chance that they or others involved in the patient's care will face litigation.

Now that pathologists have become identified to patients as caregivers, it is becoming more common for patients to ask to speak directly to them about surgical and cytopathology diagnoses and autopsy findings. The pathologist should welcome these opportunities to deal directly with patients, and more is said on this point in the section on risk management below.

Another source of claims against physicians is the allegation that the patient did not give an *informed consent* to a diagnostic or therapeutic procedure that entails risk. Patients or parents of minors who are injured by the procedure can later claim that they would not have consented to the procedure if the risk of adverse outcome or complications had been explained beforehand. To date, the issue of informed consent has not been a problem for pathologists, but in view of the increasing number of diagnostic procedures being personally performed by them, a reminder that they need to obtain informed consent is in order.

GENESIS OF CLAIMS AGAINST PATHOLOGISTS

Nearly all claims against pathologists are the result of errors in surgical pathology and cytopathology, and all but a small number of these claims arise from failure to diagnose cancer or premalignant dysplasia[1,2] (personal communication, The Doctors' Company).

In the following discussion, further insurance terms are defined as follows. *Losses* are funds already paid or reserved (set aside) to be paid in the future for claims. Claims for which payment has been made are called *paid losses*, and those for which no payment has as yet been paid but for which funds have been reserved for future payment are called *unpaid losses*. Funds held in reserve are called *loss reserves*. Both payments and loss reserves are for payment of *indemnity* and *allocated loss expenses*. Indemnity is defined as payment to a claimant for compensation of injuries. As previously defined, allocated loss expenses are those expenses allocable to specific claims.

As an aside, with respect to indemnity payments it should be remembered that when the fee of the claimant's lawyer's is to be paid on a contingency basis (the most common arrangement), a substantial portion of the sums paid to claimants (usually at least a third and often more of the settlement or award)

will in turn be paid to their lawyers. Moreover, payment of the high expenses entailed in pursuing a contested malpractice claim are also the responsibility of the claimant rather than of the lawyer and therefore are paid by the claimant in addition to the contingency fee. When protracted litigation has resulted in a modest indemnity payment, the major portion of the award goes not to compensate the injured patient, but is consumed instead in paying the plaintiff's lawyer and the expenses attendant on the litigation. Because there are no public records of amounts paid by plaintiffs to their lawyers as fees and for litigation expenses, the proportion of indemnity payments that are actually retained by plaintiffs is unknown.

The amounts shown in Figure 3-3 as paid include (1) payments of indemnity and allocated claims expense for those claims closed with indemnity, (2) payments of only allocated claims expense for those claims closed without indemnity, and (3) payments only of allocated claims expense for those claims that are still open and are under active management.

As shown in Figure 3-3, clinical pathology claims account for only 2.9 percent of loss reserves and 3.1 percent of paid losses. The paucity of claims in clinical pathology is, at first glance, surprising, when one considers the many millions of laboratory tests that are performed daily, the varying conditions of urgency and time demand, both for ordering and reporting, and the many ways in which errors can occur, such as technical errors, misidentification of specimens, and results going astray, to name just a few. Errors in the transfusion service have been a particularly source of concern to pathologists because of the potential for serious injury and death, but they too have been uncommon.

Further analysis suggests a number of reasons for this surprisingly good record. The actual number of errors in comparison with the workload is small. Refined techniques and reagents, automated analyzers that reduce the chance for human error, stringent quality control, computerization with automated specimen identification, carefully written procedure manuals, close supervision of the clinical laboratory by pathologists who are well trained in clinical pathology, and better trained technologists have all contributed to this favorable experience. Moreover, errors in clinical pathology rarely cause patient injury. Clinicians will usually be skeptical of anomalous test results and before acting on them will have them repeated. Also, patients are usually unaware of laboratory errors unless, as is

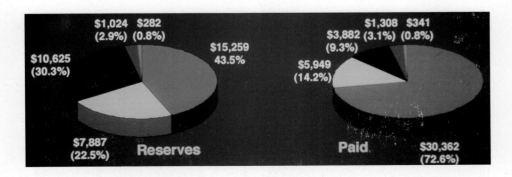

Fig. 3-3. Pathology claims. Aggregate paid and reserved, 1986 through June 1995 (to the nearest thousand). Unpaid losses = $35,077 (45.6 percent); paid losses = $41,842 (54.4 percent); total incurred = $76,919 (100 percent). Green, surgical pathology; yellow, cervicovaginal smears; black, cytopathology–other; red, clinical pathology; light blue, autopsies.

$1,024 $282
(2.9%) (0.8%)
$15,259 43.5%
$10,625 (30.3%)
$7,887 (22.5%) Reserves

$1,308 $341
(3.1%) (0.8%)
$3,882 (9.3%)
$5,949 (14.2%)
Paid $30,362 (72.6%)

rarely the case, the error has led to inappropriate diagnostic procedures or treatment that has resulted in substantial economic, physical, or psychological injury. Thus, even though a clinical laboratory error might actually be negligent, the additional elements of a claim (injury and anger) are absent.

Of great interest in Figure 3-3 is that, of total aggregate incurred losses of $76,919,000, $42,842,000 (54.4 percent) has actually been paid. When one considers the characteristics of pathology claims mentioned earlier, that the claims-made liability experience had not matured until 1991, and that a 1 year lag exists in the development of pathology claims, the payment of this large proportion of the losses is a remarkable record. It is also an effective counterpoint to the oft-repeated statements by plaintiff lawyers that malpractice losses are an illusion created by the idiosyncratic accounting practices of insurance companies.

ANALYSIS OF ANATOMIC PATHOLOGY CLAIMS

Autopsies

Claims arising from autopsies have been very uncommon, accounting for less than 1 percent of both unpaid and paid losses. All were for autopsies in which proper consent had not been obtained or that were on performed on the wrong body.

Surgical and Cytopathology

As mentioned above, claims in surgical and cytopathology accounted for nearly all the losses. Unpaid losses (loss reserves) for these claims were $33,771,000 (96.3 percent) of the total loss reserves of $35,077,000, and paid losses were $40,193,000 (96.1 percent) of the total paid of $41,842,000.

Figure 3-4 shows a breakdown of the most recently reported 200 claims. Figure 3-4A shows the frequency of the various claims as a percentage of the total, and Figure 3-4B shows the claims as a percentage of the total dollar losses incurred. It should be noted that since these claims are recent, most of the incurred losses are in loss reserves rather than having been paid. Thus, the final costs and their distribution among the various claims will not be known with certainty for a number of years. Nonetheless, the comparison of the aggregate data in Figure 3-3 with that of the more recent data in Figure 3-4 is useful in demonstrating loss trends.

Figure 3-3 shows that in the aggregate experience, surgical pathology accounted for 59.3 percent of the incurred losses. (This number is derived by adding surgical pathology reserves, $15,259,000, to surgical pathology payouts, $30,362,000, giving a total incurred for surgical pathology, $45,621,000, and dividing this number by the total incurred losses for all claims, $76,919,000, times 100.)

In comparison, Figure 3-4B shows that of the more recent claims, incurred losses in surgical pathology stayed the same, 60 percent of the total incurred losses, but there was a large de-

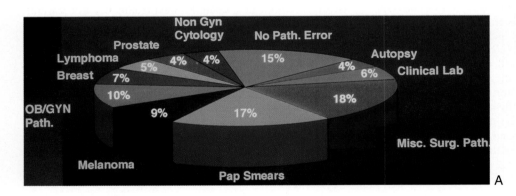

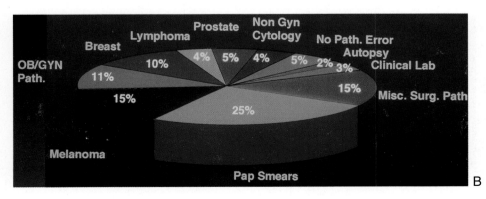

Fig. 3-4. **(A)** Relative frequency of the 200 most recent claims. **(B)** Relative cost of the 200 most recent claims.

crease in the proportion of nongynecologic cytology losses from the 18.9 percent of total aggregate incurred losses shown in Figure 3-3 to 4 percent of the more recent losses depicted in Figure 3-4B. The reasons for this decrease are not apparent, but in my colloquies with colleagues in different parts of the country about pathologists' liability, a suggestion has been made that in some areas, the number of fine needle aspiration biopsies is decreasing as they are being supplanted by biopsies using thin cutting needles.

Most of the errors in surgical and cytopathology were judged by reviewers to be below the standard of care. A few cases were considered to be undiagnosable with techniques available at the time of the error. As more sophisticated methods of analysis such as immunohistochemistry come into more widespread use, the small number of such undiagnosable cases should become even smaller in the future. Even though most of the errors were judged to be negligent, some of these claims lacked one or more of the other elements of a claim: injury or causation. As pointed out above, however, defending claims on the basis that the delay in diagnosis did not cause an injury is difficult if a case goes to trial before a jury. This is especially true in anatomic pathology where the evidence of error is, in a sense, more *concrete* than is often the case in claims against clinicians.

An important factor in the genesis of claims was poor communication from clinician to pathologist or pathologist to clinician. Another was poor communication within pathology groups (i.e., the absence of intragroup consultation or its documentation). These factors are addressed below.

As shown in Figure 3-4A, 53 percent of the most recent 200 cases arose from alleged errors in surgical pathology, and 21 percent were from cytopathology. The 15 percent of claims in which no error by the pathologist could be demonstrated included a mixture of surgical and cytopathology cases. The absence of error did not, however, preclude the occurrence of these claims and that they were so numerous is a comment on the lax legal standards that exist in our civil justice system.

Gynecologic Pathology

As shown in Figure 3-4, the most common claims in surgical pathology were in gynecologic pathology, accounting for 10 percent of the most recent 200 claims and 11 percent of the total incurred losses. The high incidence of gynecologic pathology claims does not signify that they are disproportionately more common, but instead reflects that gynecologic specimens are the most common tissues dealt with by the pathologist. These claims involved a variety of errors, many of which were judged to be negligent, but no discernible pattern occurred from which useful recommendations toward claim prevention can be made.

Melanoma

Figure 3-4 shows that missed melanomas gave rise to the second most common claims, accounting for 9 percent of the most recent 200 claims, but for a disproportionate 15 percent of the incurred losses[1,2] (personal communication, the Doctors' Company). Analysis of prior claims also showed a substantial number of missed melanomas.[1] The errors were made by both general pathologists and dermatologists certified in dermatopathology. A frequent contributor to the problem was the use of the shave biopsy technique by the clinician, which resulted in small samples of lesional tissue and also made it impossible to measure tumor thickness, assess depth of invasion, and evaluate margins.

An illustrative case is that that of a young man on whom a shave biopsy of a pigmented lesion of the arm was performed. The section contained scanty lesional tissue in both the dermoepidermal junction and the small amount of dermis that was present. The pathologist diagnosed compound nevus. He had not inked the tissue, because he did not believe that margins would be an issue in a shave (incisional) biopsy. The patient returned to his physician nearly 1 year later with a recurrence at the biopsy site, and workup at that time confirmed that the recurrence was frankly malignant and also revealed advanced metastatic disease. For the review by the insurer's panel, the pathologist submitted the original slide plus multiple recuts that were requested so as to allow simultaneous review by the members of the review panel. When the reviewers examined the original slide, they were unanimously concerned about cytologic atypia that they considered borderline in nature, and a tiny, inconspicuous focus, was seen near one end of the section that was frankly malignant. Examination of the deeper levels in the recuts showed extensive, easily diagnosable melanoma. The pathologist had overlooked the very small malignant focus in the original slide and therefore had not ordered deeper sections, which would have made the melanoma readily diagnosable. The panel concluded that four negligent errors had been committed: failing to note the cytologic atypia, missing the small malignant focus in the original slide, failing to ink for margins, and not cutting deeper levels. This case illustrates the need to ink all small biopsies even when margins are not expected to be an issue, to ensure that sections are full-face. Suggestions for handling small biopsies are presented below in the risk management section.

In most of the cases of missed melanoma, the diagnosis was readily apparent and the reviewers judged the error to be negligent. In some of these cases, because the melanoma was missed, no second, more extensive resection had been done, as is usual after minimal resections of apparently benign lesions that turn out to be malignant on pathologic examination. Nevertheless, in many of these cases the primary lesion had in fact been completely excised, as shown by inked margins that were free of tumor and by the absence of subsequent recurrence at the biopsy site. Moreover, some of these lesions were thin and superficial and thus had a good prognosis; no further treatment would have been indicated. Unfortunately, in the cases reviewed, the patients developed metastatic disease despite the previous complete excision of the primary lesion and the good prognosis of those lesions that were thin and superficial. Therefore these misses are examples of negligent errors that did not cause an injury. However, as previously mentioned, such cases are difficult to defend on the basis of causation when the error by the pathologist is frankly below the standard of care, and the evidence sits on a slide for anyone to see. Moreover, a causation defense is made doubly difficult by plaintiffs' experts who will testify, contrary to accepted medical opinion, that had the correct diagnosis been made, regional lymphadenectomy would have been carried out and would have increased the chance for cure.

The surgical pathology literature contains few data on errors, not just regarding melanoma, but other diagnoses as well. One study reported on variability in the pathologic diagnosis of melanoma by three recognized experts.[3] The paper did not deal with the *benign versus malignant* issue since all the cases in the study were known melanomas. It did, however, demonstrate that while excellent agreement existed among the three regarding lesion thickness, correlation regarding histologic type was poor. The kappa value for the latter was 0.48. The kappa value is a measure of agreement between or among observers that exceeds the probability that different observers would have agreed purely by chance. A kappa of 0 indicates that any apparent agreement has been entirely by chance, and a kappa of 1 reflects perfect agreement beyond chance.[4]

Recommendations

The shave biopsy technique should be avoided when excising pigmented lesions (excluding such trivial lesions as pigmented seborrheic keratoses). This recommendation is made fully realizing that indications for shave biopsy may exist in special situations such as when excisional biopsy of a lesion that is almost certainly benign would cause unacceptable scarring. Nonetheless, this technique should be used very sparingly, and when the pathologist is called on to examine these biopsies, special care should be taken, including inking the specimen, not to assess margins but to ensure that the sections examined represent full-face cuts.

Lymphoma

Figure 3-4 shows that lymphoma was the third most common cause of claims among the most recent 200 claims, comprising 5 percent of the total and 4 percent of the incurred losses. Lymphoma was also a prominent cause of claims in the prior aggregate experience. Most of the errors were judged by the insurer's review panels to be below the standard of care, but a small number of cases were judged to be difficult, with disagreement among the reviewers as to whether the diagnosis was or was not lymphoma. An important difference, however, between the defendant pathologists and the review panel members was that the reviewers would have sought expert consultation in these difficult cases.

Among the lymphoma claims, extranodal lymphoma was a more common problem than its incidence relative to nodal lymphoma would suggest. As is commonly appreciated, it can be difficult to differentiate extranodal lymphomas from exuberant lymphoid hyperplasias or intense chronic inflammatory reactions or, as is not uncommonly the case, a mixture of the two. An illustrative case is one in which a 43-year-old man presented with a left otitis media; examination revealed a swelling in the nasopharynx on the same side. This was biopsied and diagnosed as lymphoid hyperplasia by the pathologist. The patient was treated conservatively but did not respond to the therapy. Three months later, he was rebiopsied and small cleaved cell lymphoma was diagnosed by a pathologist at another institution. Workup at that time revealed widespread disease.

The reviewers found the first biopsy to consist almost entirely of lymphoid hyperplasia and chronic inflammation, but they were able to identify several small foci that showed lymphoma. Apparently the pathologist zeroed in on the extensive, exuberant inflammation and overlooked these few small foci. The diagnosis of small cleaved cell lymphoma in the slides submitted from the rebiopsy was readily apparent. However, the 3 month delay in the diagnosis of a low grade lymphoma was certainly not the cause of the patient's advanced disease at the time of the second biopsy. The difficulty of the causation defense is reiterated.

This case teaches a number of lessons. The first is that the pathologist should have been aware that otitis media in an adult should always raise the possibility of neoplastic obstruction of the eustachian tube by a nasopharyngeal lesion. The second is that extranodal lymphoma, especially when it is associated with ulceration and secondary infection, can present a mixture of inflammation, hyperplasia, and lymphoma; depending on the vagaries of sampling by the clinician, the inflammatory/hyperplastic reaction can overshadow the neoplastic change, rendering it inconspicuous. The differentiation of lymphoma from inflammation or lymphoid hyperplasia is frequently further complicated because the clinician often submits a small amount of tissue from extranodal sites, frequently as multiple small fragments with obscuring crush artifact. Whenever the pathologist is faced with this kind of biopsy material, special care should be taken to avoid being distracted by the predominant reactive changes.

Some of the problems in the pathologic diagnosis of lymphoma should be overcome by the greater availability of immunohistochemical techniques and by new kinds of DNA and other testing that will become available in the future. Currently, however, pathology of the lymphomas is difficult and will remain so, at least in the near future, especially for pathologists who have limited experience with these relatively uncommon lesions. Considering the frequency of cases in which the panel reviewers concluded they would have sought consultation, it would be wise for pathologists with limited exposure to these disease to consider seeking consultation more frequently.

Breast

Figure 3-4 shows that errors in the diagnosis of breast lesions were the fourth most common cause of claims, constituting 7 percent of the most recent 200, and a disproportionate 10 percent of the incurred losses. This frequency is not surprising considering that breast disorders themselves are very common, and that the pathologist is frequently called on to diagnose them. These claims demonstrated a variety of errors including poor communication between clinician and pathologist, insufficient correlation with the clinical facts and with the results of special tests such as mammography and ultrasonography, poor technique in examining submitted tissue, and inadequate histologic examination and characterization of the neoplasms. The claims revealed few cases of simple missed cancer, which is in accord with a report indicating excellent agreement among experts as to benign versus malignant breast lesions. Areas of disagreements were found in borderline cases and in judging the degree of tumor differentiation.[5] Nearly all the errors in the reviewed cases were judged by the review panelists to be below the standard of care.

In some of the lumpectomy cases, the specimens were not inked for margins, and these patients had recurrences that were discovered many months later, at which time they had axillary node or distant metastases. All such claims alleged loss of chance of cure. In some of the cases, the delay was only a few months, and the patients presented with extensive node metastases that could not have been caused by the relatively short delay. Once again, however, the difficulty of defending negligent errors in pathology on the basis of causation must be stressed.

One illustrative case combines a number of the errors that were encountered in these breast cases (although not all in such a combination). A lumpectomy and axillary node dissection were performed for an obvious invasive ductal carcinoma correctly diagnosed by the pathologist. The lumpectomy specimen was not inked for margins. The pathologist noted that noninfiltrating carcinoma was also present but did not stress that it was extensive, both intermixed with the invasive tumor and at considerable distance from it. He also failed to note that foci of noninvasive cancer were present at the edge of some of the sections, which, despite the absence of inking, probably represented involvement of the resection margin. The stromal lymphatics were extensively involved which the pathologist did describe. Seven lymph nodes were examined and said to be free of tumor. No postoperative radiotherapy or chemotherapy was given. This fact calls the judgment of the clinician into question, because, even though the nodes were termed negative, the report of lymphatic invasion was an indication for considering additional treatment.

One year later the breast lesion recurred at the site of the previous biopsy, and a second lumpectomy showed a recurrent invasive ductal carcinoma identical in histologic appearance to the first tumor. Persistence of extensive noninfiltrating cancer was also found. Three additional lymph nodes were excised, one of which showed a metastatic focus. Review of the original slides showed that three of the seven nodes previously diagnosed as free of tumor actually contained single micrometastases, which, although inconspicuous, were judged as diagnosable by the reviewers. A modified radical mastectomy was then performed.

Recommendations

A number of lessons may be learned from the breast claims. (1) Lumpectomy specimens should always be inked to ascertain and report the adequacy of excision (this really should go without saying!). (2) Lymph nodes should be scanned and then examined at 100 power so as not to miss micrometastases. (3) The presence and degree of noninvasive cancer and other findings such as lymphatic invasion should be described and their implications for postoperative treatment and possible recurrence noted in the report. (4) The pathologist should always be aware of the physical findings and of special tests such as mammography and unltrasonography.

Prostate

Figure 3-4 shows that errors in prostate biopsies accounted for 4 percent of the most recent 200 claims and 5 percent of the in-

curred losses. Unlike most of the claims against pathologist, which were false negative cancer diagnoses, the most common claims arising from the prostate were for false positive cancer diagnoses made on thin cutting needle biopsies, which led to radical prostatectomy. The claims alleged impotence due to unnecessary surgery. The most common error was over-reading microglandular atrophy as carcinoma. The histology failed to show nuclear enlargement or atypia and nucleoli were not prominent.

Recommendations

Although nuclear and nucleolar changes are not always found in prostate cancer, the pathologist should nevertheless be wary of diagnosing such cancer in very small biopsies on the basis of a microglandular pattern alone without nuclear and nucleolar changes.

Nongynecologic Cytopathology

These claims involved specimens of many kinds and from multiple sites, but fine needle aspiration biopsies (FNABs) of the breast were the most common, reflecting the relatively high incidence of breast pathology and the popularity of this technique in assessing breast disease.

Figure 3-3 gives the aggregate experience from 1986 through June 30, 1995; nongynecologic cytopathology accounted for 30.3 percent of all claims reserves and 9.3 percent of all payments. Of the 200 most recent claims, the incidence of nongynecologic claims has fallen sharply to 4 percent, and such claims account for only 4 percent of the incurred losses (Fig. 3-4). One possible reason for this reduction is that pathologists are becoming more skilled at interpreting FNABs. Another is that fewer FNABs are being performed, as biopsies by thin cutting needle are becoming more common, not only to sample breast and other masses, but also to perform stereotactically directed incisional and even excisional biopsies of very small, mammographically detected breast lesions (mammogramomas).

In some of the claims in which the clinician had performed the FNAB, slides were of poor quality, mainly due to air drying. In others, smears were hypocellular. FNABs of any site can miss the lesion, and unless the pathologist has personally performed the procedure, it is not possible to assess the adequacy of the specimen. Clinicians vary in their ability to perform FNABs, and accepting the clinician's word that the needle was in the specimen is akin to believing "the check is in the mail." Even though certain specimens demonstrated these deficiencies, the pathologist sometimes went ahead and signed out the case as benign, after commenting on the hypocellularity or drying artifact.

Recommendations

Slides from whatever source, fluids or FNABs, that are of poor quality or are *unexpectedly* hypocellular should never be definitively signed out. Instead, the problem should be described and a pathologic diagnosis such as *insufficient for diagnosis* should be rendered. If the pathologists believe that FNABs should be repeated or that open biopsy or other examination is indicated, they should not hesitate to make that suggestion in the report.

This applies to any biopsy done by whatever means, but the problem of attempting to read poor slides was an especially prominent one in FNABs. Obviously hypocellularity would be of no concern in slides prepared from serous exudates or other lesions known to be hypocellular, such as non-neoplastic cysts.

In a few cases the pathologist used Pap smear terminology, suggesting that the error was due to application of inappropriate criteria to these nongynecologic smears. Diagnostic criteria vary with the source of the specimen, and the pathologist who reads nongynecologic smears should be aware of and pay attention to these differences.

In all the claims arising from false negative reports, patients were subsequently found to have cancer; when diagnosed later, most showed metastatic disease, resulting in the usual allegation of loss of chance of cure.

A few breast cases of false positive diagnoses started a chain of events that led to unnecessary surgery such as disfiguring modified radical mastectomy. The fault in these cases was as much that of the clinician, who proceeded with treatment without confirming the diagnosis, as it was that of the pathologist who made the error. That is, however, cold comfort. These claims were for unnecessary treatment with disfigurement, the attendant pain and suffering, and emotional stress including the fear of cancer.

One large cooperative study of breast FNAB results from 10 centers that assessed the accuracy of 23,063 breast FNABs reported inadequate smears in 6.5 percent of malignant lesions and 23.2 percent of benign lesions.[6] Sensitivity was 92.2 percent (7.8 percent false negatives) and specificity was 95.3 percent (4.7 percent false positives). This false positive rate was higher than is generally believed to be the case for this procedure. Inspection of the data from each of the institutions revealed that one center had a specificity of only 77.4 percent, whereas the other institutions' specificity ranged from a high of 98.0 percent to a low of 93.4 percent, essentially in accord with what is generally believed to be correct. Despite the improvement in the data by excluding this one statistical outlier, a degree of inaccuracy persists that raises the question of qualifying breast FNAB reports, and especially negative reports, with a warning to the clinician regarding the examination's rate of error.

With respect to false positive reports, if one were to judge from the relative infrequency of such claims, one could conclude that they are not an important liability problem. This relatively favorable experience may not be due to the lower incidence of false positive diagnoses, but rather may occur because in these instances only lumpectomy is performed (not disfiguring), the correct benign diagnosis is then made, and treatment such as mastectomy or intensive radiotherapy or chemotherapy is avoided. Thus the injury, unnecessary lumpectomy, is insufficient to cause the anger that precipitates a claim.

Gynecologic Cytology

Figure 3-3 shows that of all aggregate claims from 1986 through June 30, 1995, Pap smears accounted for 22 percent of all reserves and 14.2 percent of all payments. The paid amount, which is lower in proportion to the reserves, does not indicate a favorable payment experience, but rather an increasing number of these claims, which, because of their immaturity, remain open and reserved. This is borne out by the data in Figure 3-4A, showing that of the 200 most recent claims, Pap smears are the most frequent, with this single test accounting for 17 percent of claims. Figure 3-4B shows they comprise 25 percent of the incurred losses, an increase of 39 percent over the aggregate incurred losses of 18 percent (paid plus reserved) shown in Figure 3-3.

Nearly all these claims were for false negative findings that were *significant* misses, with significant defined as errors that resulted in the absence of appropriate follow-up in diagnosis and treatment. In these cases, the misses were retrospectively discovered after the patients had developed invasive cervical carcinomas, most of which were squamous and a few of which were adenocarcinomas. Most of the cases involved a single smear, but a few involved two consecutive smears, 1 or more years apart. The interval between the last missed smear and the diagnosis of carcinoma ranged from a few months to up to 3 years. This problem was compounded because many of these patients did not have annual Pap smears, and in many cases the interval between smears was long. Because the natural history of dysplasia or in situ carcinoma that goes on to become invasive cancer is usually one of slow progression, most of these cases of invasive carcinoma would probably have been avoided if the patients had been screened annually. The effect of the frequency of Pap smear examination on the risk of subsequently developing invasive squamous carcinoma is strong. It has been reported that no difference exists between annual and biennial examinations, but the relative risk of smears taken at 3 year intervals is 3.9 and that of never having had the examination is 12.3.[7]

In some cases the subsequent diagnosis of invasive cancer was made relatively soon after the missed smear, sometimes after only a few months. Thus, one must conclude that these tumors were invasive at the time the smear was missed. That these smears often contained few abnormal cells, consistent with the finding that invasive carcinoma of the cervix often sheds few abnormal cells and often none at all, provides corroboration. Moreover, when small numbers of abnormal cells were later discovered on retrospective review of the previous smears, their morphology was usually that of invasive rather than in situ carcinoma. Therefore, in many of these cases, despite misses that could be characterizeable by plaintiffs' experts as negligent, the elements of injury and causation were absent. However, the reader is again reminded of the difficulty inherent in defending negligent errors before a jury on the basis of absence of injury or causation.

As stated, a minority of these claims involved smears that contained very small numbers of abnormal cells dispersed among the many non-neoplastic epithelial and inflammatory cells, which together can number up to 300,000 on a single slide.[8] In such cases it is understandable that the abnormality could be missed, even by diligent observers. Unfortunately, however, most of the claims involved smears that were judged by reviewers to have contained sufficient numbers of abnormal cells to be diagnosable.

As noted earlier, an inevitable bias exists when slides are screened as special cases rather than as part of routine processing. It has been reported that many missed smears from patients with proven invasive carcinoma containing very few abnormal cells are repeatedly missed when inserted blindly into the routine screening process, but are recognized when reviewed as special cases even without the knowledge that the patient has invasive carcinoma.[9] A plaintiff's expert who is aware that the patient has invasive cancer has an even greater advantage and therefore an even stronger bias. Unfortunately, when a plaintiff's expert is given a slide to review that contains very few abnormal cells, the expert then embarks on a *treasure hunt* and, having found the rare cells that were missed in routine screening, testifies that the error was negligent Clearly, the *objective* standard of care in cervicovaginal cytology allows at least a 4 percent rate of laboratory false negatives, but experts, often with excellent credentials, can be found who set an unrealistically high standard of care.[9,10]

A significant number of cases showed abnormal cells that were not diagnosable as premalignant or malignant and were representative of cells identified in the Bethesda classification as *abnormal squamous cells of unknown significance* (ASCUS). The uncertainty of the significance of ASCUS (as well as abnormal glandular cells of unknown significance [AGUS]) is now well recognized. One study reported that when these cells are found, subsequent biopsies range from benign to dysplastic.[11] The same study assessed the reproducibility of readings using the Bethesda System by circulating 20 Pap smears, 4 of which were judged by the authors to be typical of their category, among five recognized experts in cytopathology. The experts unanimously agreed in 3 of the 4 "typical" smears, with unanimous agreement in only 7 of the 20 cases (35 percent). Among the other 13 cases a wide range of disagreement was found. In 2 cases diagnoses ranged from BCC (benign cellular changes) to ASCUS; in 3, from ASCUS to low grade intraepithelial squamous lesion (LSIL); in 2, from LSIL to HSIL (high grade); in 2, from BCC to LSIL; in 3, from ASCUS to HSIL; and in 1, from BCC to HSIL. The authors stated that qualifying comments were frequently used by the reviewers and that these diminished the significance of these discrepancies. However, a reading of the examples of the qualifying comments included in the report showed them to be quite diverse, and that the reviewers felt compelled to use them with such great frequency confirms the lack of precision and reproducibility of the Bethesda System categories BCC and ASCUS, even in expert hands.

Despite the wide recognition of this problem, or perhaps *because* of it, expert witnesses for the plaintiff (sometimes quite prestigious ones) can be found who will testify that the presence of these cells (sometimes called *litigation cells*) calls for a comment by the pathologist that the smear should be repeated or that other follow-up steps should be taken, and that not doing so is negligence on the part of the pathologist.[11]

In some of the claims, the pathologist did identify these cells properly but appended the word *benign* to the diagnosis or used it in a comment. Judging from the lack of timely clinical follow-up, even when the pathologist suggested repeat examination, this association of the word *benign* with ASCUS apparently falsely reassured the clinician.

Recommendation 1

Whenever ASCUS or AGUS are noted in a Pap smear report, the observation should usually be qualified by a comment, but the simple use of the descriptive adjective *benign* should be avoided.

When ASCUS or AGUS are found in a smear, the pathologist will frequently ask for a repeat smear. However, the actual value of a smear taken soon after a suspicious smear has been called into question. It has been reported that 60 percent of second smears will show no abnormality, even when the patient has disease.[8] The medical implications of this in terms of appropriate follow-up care are of serious concern. From a medicolegal standpoint, however, should there be a later claim involving a false negative smear, the request by the pathologist for a repeat smear improves defensibility (clearly an example of defensive medicine, unfortunately).

As was the case in nongynecologic cytopathology, a common error by the cytotechnologist or pathologist was to diagnose slides definitively that contained too few cells or that showed serious artifacts such as air drying. It has been estimated that 10 to 20 percent of all smears submitted to the laboratory are unsatisfactory.[8] Rendering a definitive diagnosis on defective smears is a trap that cytotechnologists and pathologists should avoid.

Recommendation 2

Whenever slides are deficient for any reason, diagnosis should not be attempted. Instead, the report should reflect the deficiency and suggest that the smear be repeated.

The only claim resulting from a false positive Pap smear was one in which a pathologist who interpreted previously screened slides for a large laboratory reviewed a slide taken from a postmenopausal woman and noted the presence of small cells *consistent with adenocarcinoma*; in his comment he asked that the smear be repeated. The final report was generated by a computer from a preset menu in a different city and was issued as *adenocarcinoma* without qualification and without review by the pathologist. Although the pathologist had communicated personally with the gynecologist regarding his uncertainty and was assured by him that the endometrium would be biopsied before any further treatment was carried out, the patient unfortunately did not return to the same gynecologist but saw a different one instead. The second gynecologist noted the unqualified cytology report of adenocarcinoma and without performing a confirmatory biopsy did a hysterectomy that showed only atrophic postmenopausal endometrium. The major error in this case was that of the gynecologist, but defense of the claim against the pathologist was complicated by the disparity between his qualified handwritten diagnosis and the unqualified, computer-generated diagnosis of adenocarcinoma.

Recommendation 3

When computer-generated reports are used (1) the array of possible "canned" diagnoses should reflect all the possible diagnoses that might be made by the pathologist, and the computer program should allow for exceptional diagnoses that are not on the menu to be recorded; (2) the report should faithfully include any qualifying comments; and (3) all abnormal cytology reports should be reviewed and signed by the pathologist who checks the final report against the original worksheets.

False Positive and False Negative Pap Smears

The reason why there are so few claims involving false positive reports is not that these errors do not occur, they are at least as common as false negatives. The paucity of such claims, even when the false positive diagnosis could be judged to be negligent, is due to the absence of the other two elements of a claim: (1) no serious injury beyond the expense of the unnecessary follow-up studies, perhaps coupled with the temporary stress of worrying about having cancer; and (2) no anger. Indeed, follow-up examination that fails to demonstrate the presence of a suspected premalignant or malignant lesion results instead in a sense of great relief in the patient.

As shown in Figures 3-3 and 3-4, the problem of liability for missed Pap smears is a serious and growing one. Plaintiff lawyers have become aware of the Pap smear's false negative rate, and whenever they are consulted by a woman who has invasive cervical carcinoma, they routinely ask for reports of previous smears; if any were reported as negative, they have them reviewed.

Numerous reports confirm a high rate of both false negative and false positive Pap smears. Since it is the false negatives that concern us, the following discussion is mainly confined to these. False negatives are variously defined as follows:

1. True false negatives, in which previous smears from patients subsequently proved by biopsy to have a premalignant or malignant lesion do not contain abnormal cells, even on retrospective review. True false negatives are more common in invasive lesions and have been reported to be as high as 75 percent.[12] These negative examinations can be the result of two possible causes: the lesion did not shed abnormal cells or the clinician used poor sampling technique.
2. Laboratory false negatives in which a smear or smears were called negative, a subsequent smear is positive, and retrospective review of the previous smear or smears reveals abnormal cells that were missed. A large range of error has been reported; this point is discussed below.
3. Laboratory false negatives in which subsequent biopsy shows a premalignant or malignant lesion.

The laboratory false negative rate for cervical intraepithelial neoplasia has been reported to range from 5 to 20 percent, and for invasive cancer up to 50 percent. Laboratory false negatives are defined as including both screening errors by cytotechnologists and interpretive errors by pathologists.

The most comprehensive report on Pap smear errors is that of the College of American Pathologists Interlaboratory Comparison Program.[13] False negatives and positives were based on consensus diagnoses by an expert committee, and the results showed a laboratory false negative rate of 4 percent for the years 1989 through 1993, and a laboratory false positive rate of 5 percent for 1993. It is questionable if this error rate can be superimposed on the "average" laboratory since participants in this program enrolled voluntarily and are presumed to have a spe-

cial interest in quality assurance. That performance of individual laboratories improved over time and that the group was composed of a preponderance of "seasoned" participants in all but the earliest years support the probability that these results are better than "average." These concerns notwithstanding, the results of this program would seem to describe a minimum of 4 percent for false negatives under favorable conditions of continuing training and close attention to quality assurance

A report that is probably more representative of "average" performance is one in which a group of women with negative smears had repeat smears three months later.[14] This study showed that true false negative results were 11.1 percent with a laboratory false negative rate of 7.4 percent, and a total false negative rate of 18.5 percent.

While the true false negative rate does not pertain directly to this discussion of pathologists' liability, the large number of aggregate false negatives resulting from the combination of nonshedding tumors, clinician sampling error, and laboratory error is of great concern as it pertains to quality of care. When one adds to this the overlapping effects of a high rate of patient noncompliance in obtaining annual examinations, not seeking care even when symptomatic, and unwillingness to undergo further diagnostic testing in the face of an abnormal smear, the reason why only about 7 in 10 cases of cervical carcinoma have been prevented becomes explainable.[9]

The advent of automated computerized screening may hold some promise for reducing the *laboratory* false negative Pap smear.[15,16] This equipment has been recently approved for rescreening smears that have been diagnosed as negative by the cytotechnologist (see Ch. 49). Since rescreening of only 10 percent of negative smears as currently required by law, whether done manually or by automation, is virtually useless in improving the accuracy of the Pap smear,[17] manufacturers of this equipment are urging that *all* negative smears be rescreened. However, since these instruments will display up to 25 fields for review on a monitor screen (or can be adjusted to show even more), and this in turn will lead to an indeterminate number of actual manual rescreens by a cytotechnologist and increased interpretations by a pathologist, their use may not significantly decrease the Pap smear workload at a time when the legal limits imposed on the number of cases that can be screened by a cytotechnologist have already created a shortage of these personnel. Moreover, the considerable additional expense entailed in the use of these instruments is in conflict with mounting pressures to decrease health care costs. Nevertheless, it is likely that automated rescreening of all negative smears would greatly improve Pap smear accuracy.

The major problem inherent in Pap smear liability is that both the public and the media do not understand that the Pap smear is not a definitive diagnostic test with 100 percent accuracy.[12,18,19] It is instead only a screening procedure with a combined sampling and laboratory false negative rate estimated to be as high as 20 percent and in the best laboratories a minimum laboratory false negative rate of 4 percent. Therefore, it has been suggested that Pap smear reports, like all clinical screening tests, be qualified as to their irreducible level of insensitivity[20]; this would serve as a reminder to clinicians to stress the need for yearly examinations.

In practice environments where the pathologist and the clinical staff have a close professional association, the pathologist is in a better position to make clinicians aware of the Pap smear's shortcomings. Even in these favorable environments, however, some question exists of the degree to which clinicians are imparting this information to their patients, are stressing to them the need for annual examination, and are taking the necessary steps to ensure patient notification and compliance. In practice situations in which the pathologist and clinicians do not have a close professional relationship (such as in large, geographically remote laboratories with Pap smear workloads in the tens or hundreds of thousands), the problem of communicating the Pap smear's imperfections is compounded. Moreover, the increasing centralization and depersonalization inherent in managed care, combined with its pressure and that of current public policy for lower costs, are in direct conflict with the increasing demands of quality assurance mandated by government regulation and reinforced by rapidly expanding liability.

MANAGING THE PATHOLOGIST'S RISK

Risk management is an insurance term that, in the context of medical malpractice, includes (1) preventing negligent errors that cause patient injury; (2) preventing, whenever possible, claims arising from injuries, whether negligent or not, (3) increasing defensibility when a claim is unavoidable; and (4) controlling the cost of claims in which a negligent error has actually occurred and has caused an injury. The second through fourth points do not imply any attempt to deprive deserving patients or their families of appropriate compensation. Instead, point two, preventing claims, attempts to assist physicians in dealing with adverse outcomes and complications to avoid the anger and resentment that may lead to claims. The aim of point three, increasing defensibility, is to ensure that physicians do not take actions that would increase liability or create liability for themselves or for others where actual malpractice has not occurred. The goal of point four, controlling the cost of claims in which there is negligence and injury, is to manage them in such a way as to ensure that compensation will be fair to both the plaintiff and the insured, that compensation will be proportional to the injury, and that, ultimately, insurance costs and their substantial contribution to health care costs will be controlled.

It must be stressed that suggestions offered in this section and elsewhere in this chapter for managing the pathologist's risk of professional liability should not be construed as standards of practice. The author recognizes that practices differ and that actions taken by pathologists to reduce their liability risk will need to be adapted to the geographic, professional, and administrative attributes of their practices.

Since very few claims were filed due to technical errors in the histopathology or cytopathology laboratory, this discussion does not deal with this aspect of quality control and assurance. Instead, it is confined to suggestions applying to actions that can be taken personally by the pathologist to reduce the risk of malpractice claims. The reader is referred to the literature and to Chapter 2 of this text for the strictly technical aspects of laboratory quality control and assurance.[21,22]

The suggestions for improving quality and reducing liability offered in this section are generally applicable to both the private and the academic practice of pathology. In some instances they may need to be modified to fit particular needs; the special needs of academic institutions in training and supervising residents, fellows, and technologists in training are not addressed here. The reader is referred to the literature applicable to academic institutions.[22,23]

Communication

The need for adequate and clear communication in surgical and cytopathology is twofold: from the clinician to pathologist and from the pathologist to the clinician. Most specimens can be correctly diagnosed by the pathologist even when little or no clinical information is supplied by the clinician. However, in many instances an accurate, clinically useful pathologic diagnosis is not possible without knowledge of the clinical context. Indeed, instances exist in which a lack of clinical data could result in a diagnosis by the pathologist that could harm the patient, for instance, when the pathologist was not informed as to whether a specimen consisting of multiple small fragments obtained by endoscopy represented an incisional biopsy of a malignant lesion solely for diagnosis, or was an attempt to excise a small lesion completely. Such knowledge would be essential before the pathologist could make any meaningful comment about the adequacy of excision (i.e., the presence of uninvolved tissue). If the pathologist merely rendered the correct diagnosis without apprising the clinician that little or no uninvolved tissue was present, and the clinician believed the lesion had been completely excised, the stage would be set for persistence of tumor that could later become advanced, resulting in an injury and possibly a malpractice claim.

The problem of getting clinicians to supply minimal essential clinical information on the requisition slip that accompanies the specimen is a perennial one, and it will most likely get worse as managed care expands the centralization of laboratory and pathology services and creates a gulf between the pathologist and the clinician. In most cases, no more than a few words of history are needed, but even such minimal information is often difficult to obtain. The pathologist must work hard at educating referring clinicians as to the importance of supplying clinical data, but convincing a small, recalcitrant minority to do this is a truly Sisyphean labor.

Although many cooperative clinicians supply this information and will discuss the pathologic findings with the pathologist in important cases, a few must always be phoned when information is needed. In the course of the pathologist's busy day, it can prove irksome to track down a clinician who may be operating at another hospital, may be gone for the afternoon, may reside far away in a different time zone, or may have just left for a 2 week vacation. Nevertheless, I have discovered, in many colloquies with pathologists on liability and risk management, that virtually all pathologists take the lead in securing essential clinical information when it has not been supplied with the specimen.

Much of the discussion in this chapter about errors by the pathologist may have given the reader the impression that errors are simply a matter of the wrong choice in a dichotomy of *positive* and *negative*, or *benign* and *malignant*. While this was true in many of the claims, it was not the case in all. The reality of the histopathologic and cytopathologic diagnosis of neoplasia is that the pathologist is often faced not with a choice between two distinct alternatives but among multiple morphologic patterns that represent a continuum from benign to inflammatory atypia to malignant. In addition, a further choice must be made from among the many subtle shadings of tumor differentiation and cytologic atypia and an evaluation performed of associated abnormalities such as the mitotic rate, abnormal mitoses, lymphatic invasion, depth of tumor penetration, and adequacy of resection margins. Moreover, the pathologist must be satisfied that the examined sections are full face and that no tissue critical to the diagnosis has been left behind in the paraffin blocks or cut through and lost. In addition, the pathologist must discount the many artifacts that could mislead and must also consider the adequacy (or inadequacy) of the submitted tissue or smears to answer the questions being asked, explicitly or implicitly, by the clinician or, if not being asked, should be. Pathologists must also walk a fine line, in good part intuitive, between being too decisive and making diagnoses that are beyond their skills, and being indecisive and qualifying too many opinions with or without seeking consultation. In the former case the danger exists of harmful error and in the latter the danger of being irrelevant to the care of the patient. The *art* of pathology is not just to do all of these things, demanding though they are. It also includes the need to be skilled in the *semantics* of reporting—conveying meaning to the clinician of such clarity that the best possible care of the patient will result.[1,23]

If the pathologist phones the clinician regarding an important surgical pathology or cytopathology diagnosis, the call should be recorded and should include the date and the name of the person contacted. If it is necessary to give the report to a staff person, the pathologist must take special care that the recipient is accurately transcribing it and should always insist that the message be read back. It is surprising how often the report becomes distorted, for example, the "no" being left out of the sentence: "there is *no* evidence of malignancy." If the final report has not been typed at the time the call is made, the notation of the call can become an integral part of the report. If the report has already gone out, the call can be noted in the laboratory's electronic or paper file copy or in a separate electronic or paper log. It is presumed that the pathologist will be familiar with state requirements regarding electronic versus paper files.

The Small or Multiple, Small-Fragment Specimen

Earlier, allusion was made to the problems inherent in processing small specimens or those that consist of multiple, very small fragments. Over the years, a marked change has occurred in the kinds of biopsies and other surgical specimens that come to the pathologist. Not very long ago specimens were often large, and the pathologist could easily orient them in space, identify surgical margins, and thus ensure a thorough examination. With the advent of the fiberoptic endoscope, however, biopsies have become not only small, but often in multiple tiny fragments that cannot be oriented and in which surgical margins cannot be identified. In addition to endoscopic biopsies, small specimens such as small skin ellipses have always existed. When preparing these biopsies, it is customary to apportion multiple fragments in one or among multiple cassettes in such a manner that the paraffin blocks will contain more than one fragment. When embedded in this way, individual fragments invariably come to lie at slightly different levels within the block; in the case of thin slices such as those from an ellipse of skin, the fragments may not be oriented perfectly in the horizontal plane. Thus, when the block is sectioned, some of the fragments may not be reached by the knife, others can be lost in the waste sections that are cut to obtain a full-face of the block, and parts of thin tissue slices that lie at slightly different angles within the block may not be present on the slide because they have been cut through and lost or because the level of cut did not reach them.

A consensus existed among the review panelists that the remedy for these problems is to avoid overfilling cassettes and to section all small biopsies at three step-section levels at the first cutting.[1] When deeper sections are ordered after the first cuts are reviewed, the need to create a new full-face cut of the block, in which very small fragments have already been made even smaller, often results in cutting through and losing some of the tissue, resulting in an inadequate examination of which the pathologist may not be aware. Conversely, a disadvantage in obtaining three levels at the first cutting is that often very little tissue remains available in the block for special studies. However, this can be overcome by mounting some of the intermediate sections on slides and saving them unstained for a period of time that will ensure their availability if needed later. When cutting three step sections, the number of slides can be minimized by mounting all three levels on one slide when size permits.

The panelists also recommended inking all small specimens other than those that consist of multiple very small fragments. Although it is customary for pathologists to ink tissue when surgical margins are an issue, this is usually not done when a biopsy is incisional and margins are not expected to be of concern. However, even when margins are not an issue, all small fragments should be inked to ensure that the fragments are examined in their entirety. The example of the melanoma case described earlier, in which deeper sections of a shave biopsy prepared for the review panelists made a difficult diagnosis an easy one, is a case in point.

Intragroup Consultation

In some cases intragroup consultation would almost certainly have avoided the error and subsequent claim. The review panelists recommended that such consultation be done without fail when even the slightest question about the diagnosis exists. Unfortunately, nearly all these claims involved diagnoses that although erroneous, raised no questions in the mind of the pathologist who signed out the case. This last point resulted in a number of suggestions by the review panelists, and these have been supplemented by suggestions from the many pathologists throughout the country who have attended programs in risk management that I have conducted or in which I have participated.

The following cases should have intragroup consultation with one or more colleagues, and the results of such consultation should be recorded either in the report itself or in a separate record: (1) cases in which the slightest doubt exists about the diagnosis; (2) all malignant diagnoses (basal cell carcinomas of the skin excepted); (3) diagnoses that are a surprise to the clinician or to the pathologist; (4) diagnoses that carry with them the need for further, potentially harmful diagnostic procedures or protracted or potentially harmful therapy; (5) cases in which correlation with the clinical data raises serious contradictions or questions; and (6) all diagnoses of special interest. Although the adoption of these recommendations would go a long way toward ensuring appropriate intragroup consultation, it would not avoid the irreducible number of errors where the diagnosis is *obviously benign*—but wrong.

The solo practitioner cannot carry out intragroup consultation, but it might be possible, depending on distances, for these pathologists to arrange timely review of critical diagnoses with a nearby pathologist and to review the less urgent diagnoses at regular intervals. Telepathology may also be an option in the future.

Lawyers have raised the question of exposing more than one pathologist to litigation if the surgical or cytology report records the intragroup consultation with one or more colleagues or with a nearby pathologist, and the diagnosis later turns out to be in error and precipitates a claim. This is unfortunately true. However, that one or more additional opinions were requested by the pathologist would increase defensibility against the allegation of negligence. Moreover, intuition tells us that the number of claims avoided by such consultation would more than counterbalance any increased liability arising from what should be a much smaller number of errors. However, little experience exists to date in this regard, and only time and further experience will tell us if intuition will be supported by empiricism. Liability questions aside, however, such consultation is advisable for optimal patient care.

The Inadequate Specimen

The earlier admonition not to make a definitive diagnosis on a specimen that is inadequate is repeated here. This problem had been mainly confined to gynecologic and nongynecologic cytopathology, especially in FNABs and Pap smears. The diagnosis should reflect the specimen's inadequacy, and the pathologist should feel no hesitation in recommending in the report that the examination be repeated or that other indicated tests be done. Such recommendation takes on heightened significance in those practice situations in which a heavy workload is largely composed of referrals from distant clinicians with whom the pathologist has no close professional relationship.

Some clinicians object to such written recommendations by the pathologist on the basis that the pathologist does not fully understand the clinical context and the possible reasons why such recommendations might not be followed. Their concern is that if they do not comply with the recommendation and future litigation ensures, their liability would be ensured. This is a specious objection, because when the clinician has reason not to follow the pathologist's recommendation, this can be stated in a simple, brief entry in the patient's record. Moreover, although

this chapter is concerned mainly with professional liability, we must remember that the basic goal of both the pathologist and the clinician is the best possible care of the patient; if this is accomplished through cooperation, and the rate of injury goes down, liability will also subside.

Direct Communication Between the Pathologist and the Patient

As stated earlier, now that pathologists bill patients directly and are personally performing more diagnostic procedures, they have become identified to patients as caregivers. In discussions with pathologist throughout the country, I have discovered that requests by patients or their families to communicate directly with the pathologist are becoming more common. In myriad situations such direct personal contact with patients could occur; it is beyond the scope of this chapter to provide detailed guidelines for every one of them. Nevertheless, a brief discussion is in order. In the following, whenever the word *patient* is used, a *member or members of the family* is also implied.

A patient may wish to speak to the pathologist in situations ranging in import from simple curiosity about the pathologic findings to a demand for an explanation of what is perceived to be an error by the pathologist or the clinician. Obviously, different approaches by the pathologist would be required depending on the context of the discussion, but regardless of the reasons for the patient's request to speak to the pathologist, prior discussion with the clinician is imperative so that the pathologist may fully understand the clinical issues and the clinician comprehend all the implications of the pathologic diagnosis. In some instances the patient will be misinformed, and a reasonable explanation that addresses the patient's concerns could turn aside any anger or resentment that might be building. In other instances, the patient will be concerned about an unavoidable adverse outcome or complication when no one is at fault, and a straightforward explanation coupled with the assurance that everything possible is being done to remedy the situation could suffice to put the patient's mind at rest. In other instances, the problem might simply be one of poor communication by the clinician regarding an adverse outcome or the patient's status, and cooperation between the pathologist and clinician in clarifying the situation might suffice to abort any problem.

The most serious situation would be one in which the patient has been seriously injured due to an apparently negligent error by the clinician or by the pathologist. Any discussion with the patient in this context is best carried out jointly with the clinician whenever possible; such discussion requires frankness and honesty, coupled with a sincere wish (conveyed to the patient) to repair the situation to the greatest extent possible. In the event of pathologist error, the pathologist may be at a disadvantage in communication because the initial discussion of the pathologist's error with the patient has often been carried out by the clinician. If the clinician has poor rapport with the patient or with the pathologist, the situation can become even more complicated. Whenever the possibility of future litigation exists, it is imperative that the clinician and the pathologist contact their professional liability carriers for advice and assistance.

Consultants and Differences of Opinion

A consultant must be chosen carefully, because a pathologist can be held liable for the consultant's error under the legal doctrine of *vicarious liability*. Simply stated, this means that since the pathologist was responsible for choosing the consultant, if the consultant makes an error that leads to litigation, the referring pathologist can also become a target.[1]

In those instances in which the pathologist defers a diagnosis pending consultation, the report should state clearly that the diagnosis has been deferred. Any speculation as to diagnostic possibilities should be included only as a comment, which should also state that a final report will be issued after the consultant's opinion has been received. A special file, computerized or otherwise, should be created to ensure that the reply is in fact received and transmitted to the patient's record, the clinician, and the pathology files.

If the referring pathologist agrees with the consultant, this should be stated on the final pathology report. If the pathologist disagrees with the consultant, and the issue is not settled through direct communication with the consultant, a second interim report should be issued stating the disagreement and that additional consultation is being sought. Ultimately a final report must be made that summarizes the various opinions and is distributed as above.

Another situation that recurred in the claims was one in which the pathologist made a diagnosis of a malignant tumor, radical disfiguring surgery such as amputation was carried out, and the patient was then referred to another institution for postoperative radiotherapy or chemotherapy. Routine review of the original slides at the second institution before the initiation of treatment showed the lesion to be benign and the patient then made a claim alleging unnecessary surgery and disfigurement. As in the above situation, the pathologist is obliged either to agree or disagree with the reviewing pathologist; disagreement means that the issue must be resolved through further consultation, and the final diagnosis or other resolution of the problem must be reported and appropriately distributed.

Substantial disagreement in diagnosis between the original pathologist and the reviewing pathologist at the referral institution has been reported. In one recent report, among 777 referrals, the rate of error in cytology including FNABs, was 21 percent and in surgical pathology 7.8 percent. A change in patient evaluation or therapy occured in 5.8 percent of the cases.[24,25]

In the event that the pathologist has made a significant error that is discovered later, an obligation to issue and distribute an amended report exists; such a report would state and correct the error. The pathologist should avoid defensiveness and should merely state the facts. In such a situation it is advisable for the pathologist to phone the clinicians involved in the patient's care and to inform the professional liability insurer.

WHAT TO DO WHEN SLIDES, BLOCKS, OR REPORTS ARE REQUESTED

Most requests for slides and other materials are for medical purposes; in the interest of good medical care, all pathologists comply immediately.[26] It is useful if the patient has given prior consent for transfer of data; if not, such consent should be secured. Although materials are often sent without such consent in urgent situations, to date no claims have alleged invasion of privacy. When possible, original slides should not be sent, and representative recuts should be sent instead. If comparable recuts cannot be prepared or the request is for cytology slides, original slides must be sent. Since it often proves difficult to ensure the return of original slides and blocks, a suspense system should be in place to make sure they are returned: if litigation ensues at some future time, only the original slides and the blocks from which they were prepared would be considered legal evidence. If the request is from a lawyer, or otherwise carries any hint of possible litigation either against the pathologist or others, the pathologist should be careful not to send the original slides or blocks. For surgical pathology slides, recuts certified by the pathologist to be representative should be sent if they are acceptable to the requester. If recuts are not acceptable or impossible, as is the case with cytology slides, the pathologist should offer to have a reviewing pathologist examine the slides on the original pathologist's premises. Of course, a lawyer may be able to secure a court order compelling the pathologist to turn over the original slides and blocks, but in such an instance, the pathologist would have the protection of the court if the slides or blocks were lost or damaged. The technical legal term for damage or loss is *spoliation of evidence*. If the pathologist is obliged to turn over original surgical pathology slides, with or without the blocks, recuts should first be made whenever possible to ensure their availability if the originals are lost or damaged.

Cytology slides may be donated to quality assurance programs, provided they can be retrieved if needed for review for medical or legal reasons. In fact, concurrence by the program's reviewers would be beneficial in corroborating the original diagnosis.

CONCLUSIONS

Surgical Pathology

Surprisingly little literature exists concerning errors in surgical pathology. One study referred to above reported the results of reviews of known melanomas and showed poor agreement regarding the thickness of the lesions.[3] Two other studies, one of breast carcinoma[5] and a second of rectal carcinoma[27] indicated that when slides were circulated among experts, significant errors such as benign vs. malignant were uncommon. Instead, discrepancies were in the assessment of tumor grade, an attribute that appeared to be highly subjective. A third, similar study showed the same wide variation in assessing the degree of atypia in cervical intraepithelial neoplasia.[28]

The errors discussed here, discovered as a result of litigation, are nearly all for missed diagnosis of cancer with claims alleging loss of chance of cure. A much smaller number of false positive diagnoses were found with claims of injury ranging from the purely psychological—fear of cancer—to unnecessary, disfiguring surgery or harmful radiotherapy or chemotherapy that was not indicated. Special areas of concern were melanomas, lymphomas, and prostate needle biopsies.

Suggestions for reducing the risk in these areas have been made. In addition, general suggestions for handling biopsy material and improving communication among pathologists, clinicians, and patients have been presented.

Cytopathology

The major problems in nongynecologic cytopathology were in FNABs, in which breast aspirates were especially common. Interestingly, the number of claims involving FNABs appears to have decreased recently. It is possible that this is a reflection of improved skill and performance, but some anecdotal evidence suggests that the decrease may partly have occurred because fewer FNABs are being performed as biopsy by thin cutting needle becomes more prevalent.

A good deal of this chapter has been devoted to the liability of the Pap smear. I have referred to it in the past as a "legal growth industry" because of the burgeoning liability of this single test. A number of suggestions have been made regarding this problem, including honest expert testimony regarding the actual standard of care, which must take into account the irreducible level of false negatives (a long uphill battle), the possible impact of automated rescreening, the contradiction between cost control and quality control, the need to educate clinicians and the public about the test's imperfections, and the possibility that all negative Pap smear diagnoses should be qualified as to the irreducible insensitivity of the examination. However, the most effective measure in preventing injury and liability from the false negative Pap smear, whether it results from a sampling or laboratory error, is to impress on patients the need for annual examination. Because the natural history of those cases of cervical intraepithelial neoplasia that do not regress spontaneously usually is one of slow progression, annual examination would virtually eliminate the injury of invasive cervical cancer and with it the liability for claims alleging loss of chance of cure.[8]

It will not be possible to eliminate completely the liability faced by pathologists, especially in a legal climate of ever expanding plaintiffs' rights, but I believe that if pathologists adapt the measures suggested here to their practices and remain receptive to further remedies that will become evident in the future through the ongoing study of claims against them, much can be done to contain the problem.

That the problem can be contained is as much a hope as it is a certainty, but in the words of Pindar, it is "Hope, which most of all, guides the changeful mind of mortals."

REFERENCES

1. A report of claims review panels (pathology) pp. 1–28. In: Risk Management Manual. The Doctors' Company. Napa, CA, 1993
2. Troxel D, Sabella JD: Problem areas in pathology practice. Am J Surg Pathol 18:821–831, 1994
3. Krieger N, Hiatt RA, Sagebiel RW, et al: Interobserver Variability among pathologists' evaluation of malignant melanoma: effects upon an analytical study. J Clin Epidemiol 47:897–902, 1994
4. Silcox P: Editorial: some issues in observer error studies in pathology. J Pathol 168:255–256, 1992
5. Beck JS Members of the Medical Research Council Breast Tumor Pathology Panel Associated With the United Kingdom Trial of Early Detection Of Breast Cancer: J Clin Pathol 38:1358–1365, 1985
6. Stefano C, Bonardi R, Cariaggi MP: Performance of fine needle aspiration cytology of the breast—multicenter study of 23,063 aspirates in ten Italian laboratories. Tumori 81:13–17, 1995
7. Kirk S, Chu Jo, Mandelson M, et al: Papanicolaou smear screening interval and risk of cervical cancer. Obstet Gynecol 74:838–843, 1989
8. Koss LG: The Papanicolaou test for cervical cancer detection, a triumph and a tragedy. JAMA 261:737–743, 1989
9. Austin RM: In search of a "reasonable person standard" for gynecologic cytologists. Diagn Cytopathol 11:216–218, 1994
10. Kline TJ: Cytopathology: negligence and a lawyer's opinion. Diagn Cytopathol 11:219, 1994
11. Young NA, Naryshkin So, Atkinson BF, et al: Interobserver variability of cervical smears with squamous abnormalities. Diagn Cytopathol 11:352–357, 1994
12. Wall Street Journal Jan 25:24, 1988
13. Davey DD, Nielsen ML, Frable WJ, et al: Improving accuracy in gynecologic cytology. Arch Pathol Lab Med 117:1193–1198, 1993
14. Beilby JOW, Bourne R, Guillebaud J, Steele ST: Paired cervical smears—a method of reducing the false negative rate in population screening. Obstet Gynecol 60:46–48, 1982
15. Koss LG: Reducing the error rate in Papanicolaou smears. One laboratory's experience with the PAPNET system. Physician Assistant Dec:548–552, 1954
16. Check WA: Pap devices seek to star in clinical galaxy. CAP Today 9:24–30, 1995
17. Melamed, MR: Presidential Address, 20th Annual Scientific Session Meeting, American Society of Cytology. Acta Cytol 17:285–288, 1973
18. Wall Street Journal Nov 2:1, 1987
19. Wall Street Journal Dec 29:17, 1987
20. Robb J: Editorial: the Pap smear is a cancer screening test: why not put the screening error rate in the report? Diagn Cytopathol 9:485–486, 1993
21. Brehaut D: Applied principles of quality assurance and quality control in the histopathology laboratory. Can J Med Technol 52:18–22, 1990
22. Rosai J, Bonfiglio TA, Corson JM, et al: Recommendations on quality control and quality assurance in surgical pathology and autopsy pathology. Mod Pathol 5:567–568, 1992
23. Cowan DF: Quality assurance in anatomic pathology. Arch Pathol Lab Med 114:129–134, 1990
24. Abt AB, Abt LG, Olt GJ: The effect of interinstitutional anatomic pathology consultation on patient care. Arch Pathol Lab Med 119:514–517, 1995
25. Silverberg SG: Editorial: the institutional pathology consultation; documentation of its importance in patient management. Arch Pathol Lab Med 119:493, 1995
26. Sabella JD: What to do when slides, blocks or tissues are requested. CAP Today Oct:26–28, 1992
27. Thomas GDH, Dixon MF, Smeeton NC, Williams NS: Observer variation in the histological grading of rectal carcinoma. J Clin Pathol 36:385–391, 1983
28. Robertson AJ, Anderson JM, Beck J: Observer variability in histopathological reporting of cervical biopsy specimens. J Clin Pathol 42:231–238, 1989

4

Cell and Tissue Staining Methods

Ronald A. DeLellis
Garrey T. Faller

Histochemistry is a hybrid science that bridges the gap between cytology/histology and analytical chemistry or biochemistry. Simply stated, the goal of the histochemist is to provide detailed chemical information in the context of cell and tissue structure. According to Lison, in fact, histochemistry is a science as old as histology itself. Francois-Vincent Raspail (1794–1878), a botanist by training, is generally regarded as the founder of histochemistry, and most of the early work in this field was devoted to the use of chemical methods for the elucidation of plant structure.[1] Over the past century, however, histochemistry has evolved from a largely empiric discipline to a highly sophisticated science that now includes immunohistochemistry and hybridization histochemistry (in situ hybridization). Both of these topics are covered in separate chapters in this volume. The purpose of this chapter is to provide an overview of general staining methods for the cytologist and histopathologist.

FIXATION

Tissue Fixation

A prerequisite to all cell and tissue staining methods is adequate fixation. The purposes of fixation are to inhibit autolysis and bacterial overgrowth, to prevent solubility of the components of interest, to preserve their localization at the sites in which they normally occur in living cells, and to provide appropriate conditions that will permit their coloration with specific dyes and dye mixtures.[2] Additionally, fixation is required to produce sufficient tissue rigidity to facilitate sectioning and slide preparation. The ability of various fixatives to achieve these goals depends on numerous variables, including the nature of the specific fixative, its rate of tissue penetration, the osmolality and pH of the fixative solution, the temperature, the length of fixation, and the size of the sample.

The components of various fixatives differ remarkably with respect to their effects on cells and tissues. While some of the components (e.g, ethanol) cause considerable cell shrinkage, others may result in unacceptable degrees of cell swelling. Accordingly mixtures of fixatives have been developed to mini-

mize some of these deleterious effects. Additional components, such as detergents, are also added to fixative solutions to facilitate tissue penetration. Adequate fixation can be achieved only when tissues are adequately prepared. Thus, tissue must be placed in fixative solutions as soon as they are obtained, and they must be thin enough to permit thorough penetration of the fixative. In most instances, tissue blocks must not exceed 2 to 3 mm in thickness. As a general rule, tissues should be fixed in at least 20 times their own volumes of fixative solutions.

In addition to standard liquid fixatives, vapor fixation following freeze-drying has also been used to preserve certain highly diffusible cell constituents such as catecholamines and very small peptide hormones.[3] Most recently, microwave fixation has been advocated for very rapid fixation of tissue samples; this subject is covered in detail in several reviews and monographs.[4,5]

Fixatives have been classified as cross-linking or precipitating types.[2,6–9] The most commonly used fixative in pathology practice is formaldehyde, a prototypic cross-linking fixative. Formaldehyde is a gas that is available as solution containing 37 to 40 percent by weight of the gas dissolved in water. It is also available as a solid polymer (paraformaldehyde).[7] Formaldehyde is used primarily as 10 percent neutral buffered solution (formalin), which is equivalent to 4 percent formaldehyde. The use of a buffer in formalin solutions is critical because of the formation of formic acid with prolonged storage. As noted by Pearse,[2] the reactions of formaldehyde with proteins are numerous and complex, since it can react with a number of functional end groups to form methylene bridges. The groups with which formaldehyde reacts include amino, imino and amido, peptide, guanyl, hydroxyl, carboxyl, sulfhydryl, and aromatic rings. Much of the fixation results from methylene bridge formation involving the epsilon amino groups of lysine and peptide links of another chain. The extent of cross-link formation is dependent on many factors, most importantly the duration of fixation. Although formalin penetrates tissues fairly rapidly, complete fixation requires relatively long periods of time. Tissues fixed in formalin for short periods (<4 hours) become completely fixed only as a result of their subsequent exposure to alcohols during dehydration procedures. The addition of zinc sulfate to formalin provides a combination cross-linking and precipitating fixative. Both glutaraldehyde and acrolein also represent cross-linking fixatives.

Generally, tissues fixed in glutaraldehyde are more extensively cross-linked than those fixed in formaldehyde. However, glutaraldehyde penetrates tissues poorly, and blocks must be very thin for complete fixation to occur.

Ethanol and methanol represent examples of precipitating (coagulating) fixatives, which have the ability to denature proteins.[2,6–9] Both of these reagents rupture the hydrogen bonds, which are responsible for maintaining the tertiary structure of proteins. Ethanol is rarely used alone as a tissue fixative. It may be combined with formalin (alcoholic formalin), which penetrates tissues more rapidly than formalin alone, or with a variety of other constituents. Carnoy's fluid, which is composed of a mixture of ethanol, chloroform, and acetic acid, basically serves as a precipitating fixative. By itself, acetic acid does not fix proteins, but it does coagulate nuclear chromatin and is useful for the preservation of chromosomes.[7] Carnoy's fluid fixation typically results in lysis of red blood cells and is also associated with considerable tissue shrinkage. It penetrates tissues rapidly but extracts lipids during the process of fixation. However, it provides an excellent fixative for the demonstration of glycogen. Picric acid, a major component of Bouin's fluid (picric acid, formalin, glacial acetic acid), is also classified as a precipitating fixative. It forms salts (picrates) with the basic groups of proteins.

Mercuric chloride is also a commonly used fixative, particularly in the form of formol sublimate (B5). It combines with the hydroxyl and carboxyl groups of proteins and with the phosphoric acid of nucleoproteins. In addition, mercury has a selective affinity for thiol groups. Since formol sublimate penetrates tissues very slowly, samples must be sectioned very thinly prior to fixation. Overfixation will result in excessive hardness of the tissues.[9] Zenker's fixative includes a combination of potassium dichromate, mercuric chloride, and glacial acetic acid. Chromium-containing fixatives have both cross-linking and precipitating effects. Because of their oxidizing effects, chromate fixatives convert adrenalin and noradrenalin into adrenochrome and noradrenochrome pigments (chromaffin reaction). Osmium tetroxide, which was formerly used as a lipid stain, is now employed primarily as a fixative for electron microscopy. The mechanism of fixation is not well understood, although some cross-linking appears to be involved. This fixative penetrates tissues slowly, and its use is limited to very small blocks.

Fixation and Processing of Cytologic Material

Fixation is crucial in maintaining cytologic detail in smears prepared from different body sites. Since chromatin is well preserved with alcoholic fixatives, wet fixation with 95 percent ethanol is generally recommended for most cytologic studies.[10] In wet fixation, a freshly prepared slide is submerged immediately into fixative for 15 to 30 minutes prior to staining. Other fixatives that have been used include methanol and isopropanol. Ten percent formalin had also been recommended in the past, but considerable loss of chromatin detail is usually seen. In some instances, air-dried preparations are used for subsequent Romanovsky type staining procedures.

Coating fixatives containing ethanol or its substitute and polyethylene glycol are also used frequently, particularly with cervicovaginal smears.[11] Coating fixatives are commercially available as spray fixatives, or they may be prepared directly in the laboratory. Polyethylene glycol is a wax-like substance that coats and protects the cells on the slide. Before staining, however, this coat must be dissolved by placing the slide in ethanol.

Transport of sputum, urine, cerebrospinal fluid, cyst fluid, effusions, and brushing and washing specimens to the laboratory should be immediate to prevent autolytic changes and bacterial overgrowth. If a delay in transporting or processing occurs, specimens should be refrigerated; alternatively, 50 to 70 percent ethanol may be added to the specimen in a 1:1 ratio.[11] It is important to note that when fixatives are added to fluid specimens, cells may have a decreased adherence to the glass slide.

Body fluids are usually centrifuged prior to subsequent preparative procedures.[11] After centrifugation, direct smears may be made from the cell pellet. One method is to use a pipette to aspirate and expel several drops of the cell button onto a slide; smears are then prepared by placing a second glass slide on top and gently pulling them apart.[12] This procedure effectively disperses the cells. If the specimen is clear or scanty, or both, and does not produce a pellet, cytocentrifugation or filter preparations may be the methods of choice.

Filter preparations are designed to produce a thin uniform dispersion of cells on a slide with minimal cell overlapping. Either a cellulose membrane filter or a polycarbonate filter may be used; both have slightly different characteristics. The ThinPrep process is one of the newest technologies and first requires transfer of cells into a preservative solution (Cytolyte or PreserveCyte). The cells are then automatically collected on a polycarbonate filter and transferred to a glass slide. Interestingly, recent studies have suggested that the false negative rate may be reduced when ThinPrep is used compared with conventional cervical cancer screening methods.[13–15]

Technical problems may exist with sputum, urine, and bloody specimens. Sputum produced by a deep cough is extremely viscous and difficult to concentrate by centrifugation. Commercially available mucolytic agents or 8 percent hydrochloric acid may be added to dissolve the mucus and facilitate centrifugation. Others, however, prefer to make direct smears without mucolytic agents based on the belief that tumor cells are concentrated in the mucus. Blood and white-tinged areas are usually sampled selectively. A second problematic specimen is voided urine, which is a hostile environment with a low pH, high osmolality, and the potential for bacterial contamination and overgrowth. Because the first voided morning specimen usually has the most degenerative changes, the second urine specimen of the day preceded by hydration and vitamin C ingestion is recommended.[16–18] Bloody specimens cause diagnostic problems when red cells overlap and obscure cells of interest. To eliminate or diminish this problem, a variety of lysing agents may be used.[11] One technique involves placing the glass slide into 50 to 70 percent ethanol or into modified Carnoy's fixative followed by 95 percent ethanol. Alternatively, after fixation in 95 percent ethanol, the slide may be placed into a urea solution or acid alcohol followed by 95 percent ethanol.

Fine needle aspiration smears may be wet fixed in alcohol-based fixatives or may be air-dried for Diff-Quik type stains.[12]

Any residual material in the needle may be collected in a cell wash medium (e.g., Cytolyte). Adjunctive preparations such as cell blocks or filter preparations may be made from this wash, if needed.

Cell blocks are often diagnostically useful and may provide architectural information not readily apparent from cell smears. They also offer the possibility of providing material for histochemical, immunohistochemical, or in situ hybridization studies. The cell block is prepared by centrifuging the specimen, pouring off the supernatant, fixing the cell pellet, and submitting it for paraffin embedding and sectioning. Ten percent buffered formalin is used most commonly, although other fixatives may also be employed for specific indications.[11] Alcohol is not generally recommended, since it hardens the cell pellet, which may cause it to crumble on sectioning.

Imprint preparations, made by touching a slide to the cut surface of a tissue, provide important cytologic detail that may not be readily apparent on frozen section or even permanent sections. In addition, a rapid diagnosis may be rendered by a touch preparation without having to prepare a frozen section.

MECHANISMS OF STAINING

Despite their continuous use for more than a century in pathology laboratories throughout the world, the specific mechanisms underlying most of the commonly used staining methods are poorly understood. Staining occurs as a result of interactions of cell and tissue components with single dyes or complex mixtures of dyes. Differing affinities between the dye and tissue binding sites result in selective staining of certain constituents. Reaction conditions may be adjusted to emphasize these selective affinities, thereby providing maximal contrast between intensely stained and less stained (or negative) components. For example, varying the pH and electrolyte concentrations of certain cationic dyes will permit the distinction of certain classes of acidic mucosubstances. Patterns of staining can be futher modified by tissue fixation, selective blocking or extraction procedures, and poststaining differentiation procedures.[10,19]

Dyes can potentially bind to cell and tissue structures by a variety of mechanisms, including electrostatic (coulombic) forces, hydrogen bonding, van der Waals forces, covalent binding, and hydrophobic interactions, an example of the latter being the preferential solubility of oil red O in lipid droplets.[10,19] Staining may occur through the action of an intermediary binding agent, which is referred to as a *mordant*. This term usually refers to metal ions that bind covalently to dye molecules to form dye-metal complexes. For example, aluminum potassium sulfate serves as a mordant for hematoxylin in Mayer's hematoxylin procedure. In fact, the oxidation product of hematoxylin, which is known as hematein, has a very low affinity for nuclei without the addition of the metal mordant. Alternatively, certain cellular and tissue components may have a direct affinity for metal salts. The Gordon-Sweet reticulin stain, for example, takes advantage of this phenomenon. Staining of a specific cellular compartment may also result from the formation of a colored compound in situ, as in the case of enzyme histochemical procedures.

Basic (cationic) dyes carry a net positive charge, which permits them to react with a variety of tissue-bound anionic sites, including phosphate groups of nucleic acids, sulfate groups of glycosaminoglycans, and carboxyl groups of proteins. The reaction of basic dyes with anionic sites is a pH-dependent phenomenon. At high pH, phosphate, carboxyl, and sulfate groups will stain positively. At acidic pH, only sulfate groups will be reactive. Thus, staining at controlled pH can provide important information on the chemical composition of the cell.

When some basic dyes react with tissue components, a color shift in the dye is produced. This phenomenon, termed *metachromasia*, reflects the presence of polyanions that are sufficiently close to form dimeric and polymeric aggregates of dye molecules (Fig. 4-1). Absorption properties of aggregated dye molecules differ from those of nonaggregated dye, resulting in the characteristic color shift.

Acidic (anionic) dyes, by contrast carry a net negative charge, which enables them to react with tissue-bound cationic moieties. In addition to electrostatic factors, additional factors

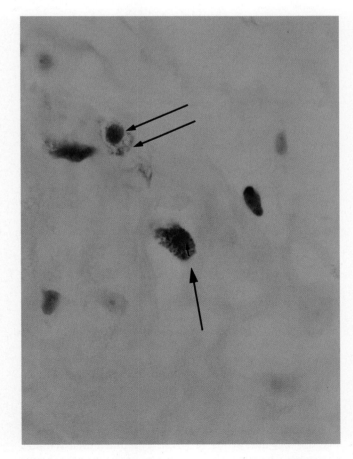

Fig. 4-1. Giemsa stain. Mast cell in this bladder biopsy is stained purple (single arrow). Degranulated mast cell is indicated by double arrows.

that are important in the reactions of acidic dyes include size and aggregation of the dye molecules and the permeability or texture of the tissue components stained.[19] Acidophilic components include cytoplasmic filaments, intracellular membranous components, and extracellular fibers.

The Papanicolaou stain consists of a mixture of cationic and anionic dyes.[11] Nuclei are stained first with hematoxylin. Slides are then rinsed in water and dehydrated with ethanol for cytoplasmic staining with orange G (OG) and EA solutions. Orange G contains a monochromatic dye and stains keratin orange. EA is a label given by Papanicolaou and contains eosin, light green, and the diazo dye Bismarck brown. Eosin stains the cytoplasm of mature squamous cells and nucleoli pink, and light green stains the more immature squamous cells and columnar cells green to blue. The role of Bismarck brown is poorly understood and it is often omitted from staining protocols. It is important to remember that the pink and green colors are not reliable in predicting the superficial versus the more immature nature of the squamous cells. Poorly understood factors such as fixation and pH may affect the colors, and superficial cells should be recognized as those with a low nuclear/cytoplasmic ratio and a pyknotic nucleus irrespective of the cytoplasmic coloration.

Nucleic Acids

The Feulgen reaction has been used extensively for the demonstration of DNA, particularly for cytophotometric applications.[20] When this technique is used for quantitative DNA analysis, it is imperative that all conditions be rigorously controlled. This procedure depends on the reaction of aldehyde or ketone groups with Schiff's reagent (fuchsin-sulfuric acid). In this method, treatment of DNA with hydrochloric acid results in the breakage of purine-deoxyribose bonds and the formation of aldehyde groups.[21] The reaction of aldehyde groups with Schiff's reagent results in a red-purple color. Prolonged treatment of sections with hydrochloric acid results in the depolymerization of DNA and a negative Feulgen reaction. RNA is completely hydrolyzed by the hydrochloric acid and does not stain. Fluorescent dyes, including acridine orange and auramine O, have also been used in place of Schiff's reagent.

Methyl green and pyronin Y are basic dyes that have been used for many years for the demonstration of DNA and RNA, respectively.[20] In properly stained sections, nuclei are green, and the cytoplasm is red to magenta. Specific and quantitative staining of DNA can be obtained by prolonged reaction with methyl green. It has been suggested that the specificity of the reaction is due to the presence of two tertiary amine groups on methyl green that become linked to the phosphate moieties in DNA. Pyronin Y, on the other hand, has an affinity for RNA. Prior to the advent of immunohistochemistry, pyronin Y was commonly used for the demonstration of plasma cells, which contain abundant cytoplasmic RNA.

The selective staining of nuclei by methyl green is related to dye size and the texture of DNA. The differential staining, therefore, is based on the competition of the dyes for anionic sites of differing accessibilities. Because of the extensive contamination of methyl green dye lots by methyl violet, the methyl

green must be extracted in chloroform extensively before use. Granules of eosinophilic leukocytes, some mucins, and osteoid also stain positively with pyronin Y under these conditions. Proof of the presence of specific nucleic acids can be obtained by treatment of sections with DNAse or RNAse before staining.

Acridine orange is a basic dye that has been used for the demonstration of DNA and RNA.[20] With this technique, RNA exhibits a red fluorescence and DNA appears green. This type of staining pattern is referred to as fluorescence metachromasia. The orthochromatic form of the dye fluoresces green, and the metachromatic form has a red fluorescence. Because of the overlap between the green and red fluorescence, treatment of sections with RNAse improves the coefficient of variation between the fluorescence readings of acridine orange-stained nuclei.

Considerable interest has recently arisen in quantitating the nucleolar organizing regions as a reflection of the proliferative activity of tumor cells. The nucleolar organizing regions are loops of DNA that transcribe RNA and that are related to the formation of the nucleolus. They can be demonstrated with aqueous silver nitrate, and the resultant nucleolar organizing regions (AgNORs) are stained black.[22] It is important that sections be sufficiently thin to permit quantitation of the AgNORs, since there is a relationship between the number of AgNORs and proliferative activity.

Proteins and Connective Tissue Elements

Methods for proteins include those that have been developed for the demonstration of specific amino acids and those that depend on the physical interaction of dyes with complex fibrous protein molecules. Staining for amino acids is based on reactions of dyes with specific end groups that can be demonstrated histochemically on the basis of characteristic color reactions. The most frequently encountered amino groups are those in the epsilon position on the side chain of lysine.[23] Accordingly, cross-linking fixatives such as formaldehyde should not be used for the demonstration of amino groups in tissue, since methylene bridges form between them. Examples of specific end groups demonstrable by histochemical methods include amino, guanido, indolyl, and sulfhydryl (thiol) groups.[23]

The ninhydrin (triketo-hydrindene-hydrate)-Schiff reaction occurs because ninhydrin oxidizes alpha-amino acids to form carbon dioxide, ammonia, and the next lower aldehyde.[23] The aldehydes produced then react with Schiff's reagent to produce a purple product. Blocking reactions can be used concurrently to establish the specificity of the reaction. Tyrosine-containing proteins can be demonstrated on the basis of the reaction of constituent phenyl groups with a mixture of mercuric sulfate, sulfuric acid, and sodium nitrite (Millon reaction). The indole groups of tryptophan and tryptamine can be demonstrated on the basis of their reactions with p-dimethylaminobenzaldehyde (DMAB). Indole groups react with DMAB to form beta-carboline, which is then oxidized by sodium nitrite to produce a blue pigment. Numerous other methods are available for the demonstration of amino acid end groups, and they are covered in detail in standard histochemistry texts.

Although methods for amino acids are rarely used in practice, methods for fibrous proteins are among the most com-

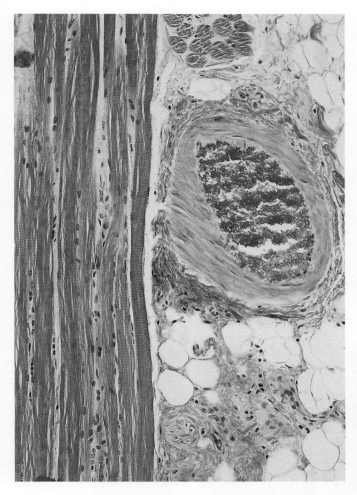

Fig. 4-2. Gomori's trichrome stain. Collagen is stained blue, and skeletal muscle fibers are stained red.

methods employ two or more anionic dyes in combination with phosphomolybdic acid or phosphotungstic acids. In the Mallory technique, which employs acid fuchsin, orange G, aniline blue, and phosphomolybdic acid, muscle and fibrin are stained red, whereas collagen and reticulin are stained blue. The Masson method employs Ponceau acid fuchsin, phosphomolybdic acid, and aniline blue or light green. With this method, muscle, red blood cells, and fibrin are red and collagen and reticulin are blue (aniline blue) or green (light green). The Gomori method employs chromotrope 2R, fast green or aniline blue, and phosphotungstic acid. This is a one-step procedure resulting in green or blue staining of collagen and red staining of muscle, red blood cells, and fibrin (Fig. 4-2).

Reticulin fibers, which consist primarily of type III collagen in a glycoprotein matrix, can be demonstrated by a variety of techniques, including the periodic acid-Schiff (PAS) reaction.[24] The Gordon-Sweet technique, however, is the most selective and most widely used method for the demonstration of reticulin fibers (Fig. 4-3). Hydroxyl groups of adjacent hexose sugars are oxidized to aldehydes by potassium permanganate. The aldehydes subsequently reduce silver diamine ion to metal-

monly used procedures in pathology.[24] The major fibrous proteins of connective tissue include collagen, reticulin, and elastin. These substances have differing physicochemical characteristics that permit them to be stained selectively in histologic preparations. Methods based on the use of mixtures of anionic dyes color different tissue components selectively. It has been suggested that the differential staining observed with these methods is based on the size of the dye, the numbers of cationic sites in the tissues, and the textures of the various components. Smaller dyes, according to this hypothesis, quickly penetrate structures composed of tightly and loosely woven proteinaceous units and react with cationic sites.[24] Upon washing, the dye molecules would be eluted first from the loosely woven units, and the liberated cationic sites should be free to react with a second (or third) anionic dye. Whether this explanation is correct, however, remains to be determined.

In the van Gieson procedure, which employs acid fuchsin and picric acid, collagen stains red, whereas muscle and red cells stain yellow. The trichrome methods are valuable for providing additional discrimination of tissue components. These

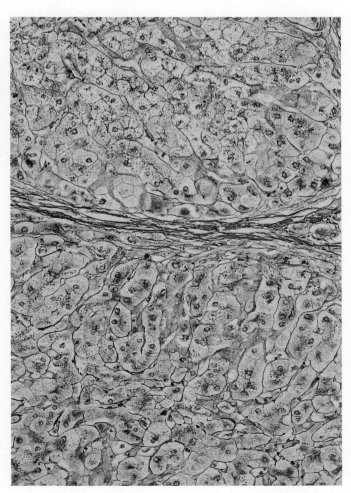

Fig. 4-3. Gomori's reticulin stain. Reticulin fibers surrounding cords of liver cells are stained black.

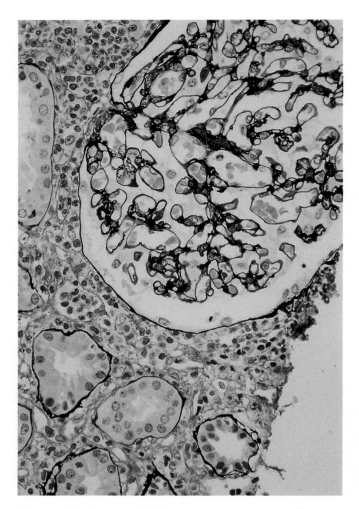

Fig. 4-4. The Jones modified hexamine silver technique. The renal glomerular capillary basement membranes and the tubular basement membranes are stained black.

lic silver, and the reaction may be further modified by the use of a toner such as gold chloride.

Basement membranes are complex structures that are resolvable at the ultrastructural level into three major zones: (1) the lamina rara, which is composed of complex carbohydrates; (2) the lamina densa, which is composed primarily of type IV collagen together with a variety of glycoproteins; and (3) the lamina reticularis, which is composed of fibrous proteins that are continuous with the surrounding fibrous tissue elements.[24] Carbohydrate constituents are responsible for the PAS positivity of basement membranes. The hexamine silver method (the Jones technique) is particularly useful for the demonstration of the thin basement membranes present within glomeruli and at the junction of epithelia with underlying stroma (Fig. 4-4). The basis of this method is that periodate-generated aldehydes selectively reduce an alkaline hexamine silver salt solution. The collagenous components of basement membranes are demonstrable with trichrome methods.

Elastic tissue, which consists of elastin and glycoprotein, can be demonstrated by many different techniques. Both hydrogen bonding and van der Waals forces are most likely involved in the staining of elastic tissues by different dyes.[24] The Verhoeff method utilizes a mixture of iodine, ferric chloride, and hematoxylin followed by ferric chloride differentiation. Elastic fibers stain black with this method as a result of the formation of a metallic (iron)-dye (hematein)-lake (Fig. 4-5). Weigert's resorcin fuchsin has also been used extensively for the demonstration of elastic fibers, which appear blue to black in appropriately stained sections. Aldehyde fuchsin, although popular at one time, is less selective for elastic fibers than other staining procedures. Elastic fibers appear purple with this method. Orcein is a naturally occurring vegetable dye, which has been used since 1890 for the demonstration of elastic fibers. With this stain, elastic fibers are stained dark brown; however, some variability in staining color and intensity is related to differences in dye lots. A modification of the orcein staining technique that involves preoxidation of tissue sections with potassium permanganate is effective for the demonstration of cells that have been infected with hepatitis B virus[25] (Fig. 4-6).

Amyloid appears as a pink amorphous intercellular material in hematoxylin and eosin-stained sections. Grossly, amyloid

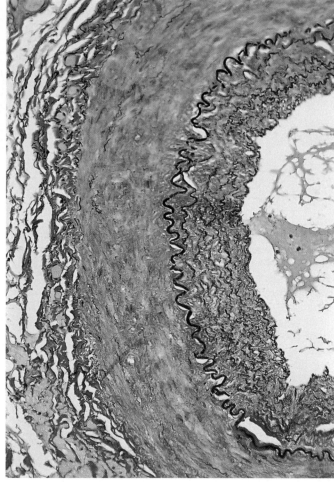

Fig. 4-5. Verhoeff's elastic fiber stain. The elastic fibers in the arterial wall are stained black.

Pretreatment of sections with potassium permanganate has been used to distinguish amyloid type AA (sensitive to effect of pretreatment) from non-type AA amyloids, which are resistant to the effects of potassium permanganate.[28] The underlying mechanisms for these differences are unknown. Recently, however, the specificity of potassium permanganate for this differentiation has been called into question. Both thioflavine T and S have been used for the demonstration of amyloid.[29] Although these dyes have high levels of sensitivity, their specificity is less than that of Congo red.[30]

Fibrin is a fibrillar substance that is deeply eosinophilic because of its high concentration of basic amino acids.[24] Fibrin also stains positively with Mallory's phosphotungstic acid hematoxylin (PTAH) and exhibits a positive reaction with DMAB due to its high tryptophan content. Fibrinoid is variably metachromatic with toluidine blue. In contrast to the uniform blue stain of fibrin with PTAH, fibrinoid stains orange-yellow to blue.

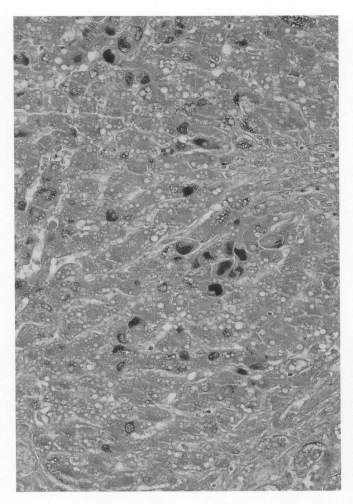

Fig. 4-6. Modified orcein stain for the demonstration of hepatitis B virus-infected cells. Positive cells are stained red-brown. Copper-associated protein also stains positively with this method.

can be demonstrated by treating tissues with Gram's iodine. Amyloid-rich tissues develop a deep brown coloration that can be converted to blue violet following treatment with sulfuric acid. The positive iodine stain is most likely related to the spatial configuration rather than the chemical composition of the beta-pleated sheet.[26] Amyloid deposits are variably PAS positive and stain pale blue or green with trichome methods. Moreover, amyloid deposits exhibit metachromasia following treatment with crystal violet.

The most specific method for the demonstration of amyloid is the alkaline Congo red method developed by Puchtler et al.[27] In this technique, alcoholic Congo red is combined with sodium chloride at alkaline pH (Fig. 4-7). The combination of high pH and saturated salt inhibits ionic binding of Congo red to tissue sections and serves to increase the specificity of the reaction. Congo red-stained amyloid deposits exhibit a green birefringence in polarized light. Other congophilic tissue components such as elastic fibers and the granules of eosinophilic leukocytes, on the other hand, are nonbirefringent.

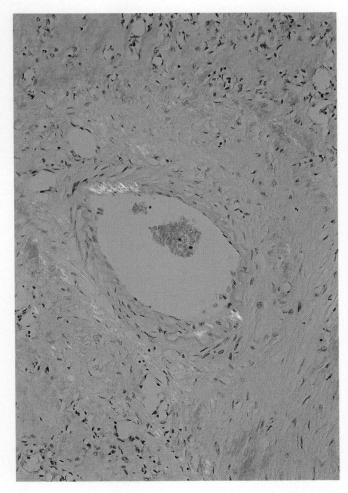

Fig. 4-7. Congo red stain photographed in partially polarized light. The amyloid deposits exhibit green birefringence.

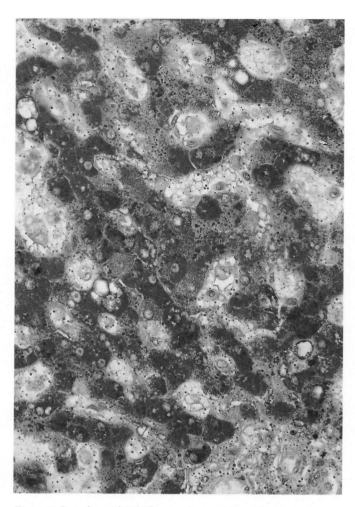

Fig. 4-8. Periodic acid-Schiff stain of normal liver. The hepatocytes contain abundant glycogen, which is stained magenta with this stain.

Carbohydrates

The carbohydrates and mucosubstances (complex carbohydrates) are ubiquitously distributed constituents that subsume major metabolic and structural roles.[31] They may occur in free or bound forms within cells and in a variety of extracellular compartments. A simple carbohydrate is a monosaccharide such as glucose, whereas glycogen represents a complex carbohydrate or polysaccharide, the major storage form of glucose. Free monosaccharides cannot be demonstrated by standard histochemical staining methods, but glycogen can be visualized by the PAS method.

The histochemical classification of the mucosubstances is both complex and confusing, partly because the mucosubstances are heterogeneous and are often composed of admixtures of different sugar-containing residues.[31] The *glycosaminoglycans* are strongly anionic substances that form a major constituent of the connective tissue mucins. They consist of unbranched long chain polysaccharides containing aminated monosaccharides or amino sugars. The glycosaminoglycans in-

clude keratan sulfate, sialoglycans (neuraminic acid), dermatan sulfate, chondroitin 4 and 6 sulfates, heparan sulfate, and hyaluronic acid. The *proteoglycans* include complexes of glycosaminoglycans and protein. They are large complexes with an average molecular weight of approximately 10^5 K. *Glycoconjugates* include *glycoproteins*, *glycolipids*, and *proteoglycans*. The glycoproteins include a complex family of carbohydrates linked with protein. The molecules of glycoproteins are generally smaller than those of proteoglycans, and their carbohydrate moieties contain fewer sugars. The oligosaccharide chains of glycoproteins are often branched, whereas the polysaccharides of proteoglycans tend to be unbranched. The glycoprotein oligosaccharides are characterized by wide variability in the types and order of individual sugars; polysaccharides of proteoglycans are much less diverse. Glycosaminoglycans always contain the carboxyls of uronic acids or carboxyls and sulfates. Some glycoproteins contain the carboxyls of sialic acid or carboxyls and sulfates. Some glycoconjugates are devoid of anionic groups and are classified as neutral mucosubstances.

Numerous staining techniques are available for the demonstration of mucosubstances in tissue sections.[31] Some of them depend on the selective affinity of cationic dyes for anionic sites in the carbohydrates, and others depend on the demonstration of the vicinal glycols in the molecules. An additional approach for the characterization of carbohydrate constituents involves the use of lectins that have affinities for specific external or internal sugar molecules. The use of lectins for this purpose is described in detail elsewhere.[32]

One of the most useful procedures for the demonstration of carbohydrate derivatives in tissue sections is the PAS reaction.[31] This reaction is based on the principle that products with vicinal glycol groups or their amino or alkylamine derivatives are oxidized by periodic acid to form dialdehydes that react with Schiff's reagent to produce a magenta color. A variety of cell and tissue products will stain positively with PAS, including glycogen, glycoproteins, and glycolipids (Fig. 4-8). Glycogen can be distinguished from other PAS-positive elements on the basis of its susceptibility to digestion with diastase (Fig. 4-9).

The PAS stain has been used extensively in pathology laboratories for the demonstration of neutral *mucins*. It also reacts with certain acidic mucins containing sialic acid but not with sulfated acidic mucins. The PAS stain can be used in conjunction with Alcian blue (AB), which stains sialylated and sulfated mucins, to provide a "pan"-mucin stain (Fig. 4-10). AB is a cationic dye that has a high affinity for acidic mucosubstances containing sulfate esters or carboxyl groups of uronic acid. At pH 2.5, all acidic glycoproteins and glycosaminoglycans exhibit positive staining with AB. The combination of PAS and AB is also useful for studying inflammatory and metaplastic conditions of the gastrointestinal tract. For example, in cases of gastric intestinal metaplasia, differential staining of goblet cells and gastric mucous cells can be achieved with this combined stain (Fig. 4-10). Further distinction of the acidic mucins can be achieved by varying the pH and electrolyte concentration of the staining solution. At pH 1.0, both weakly and strongly sulfated acid mucosubstances will be positively stained with AB, while at pH 0.2 only strongly sulfated mucosubstances will be reactive. The critical electrolyte concentration method, in

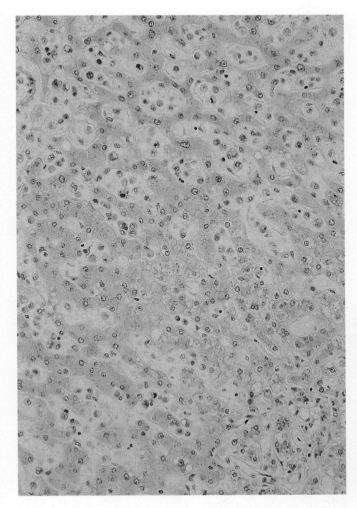

Fig. 4-9. Diastase-digested periodic acid-Schiff stain (same tissue sample as in Fig. 4-8). The glycogen deposits have been digested as a result of the diastase treatment.

conjunction with AB, is an important approach for the differentiation of acidic mucosubstances.[33] The basis of this method is that both sulfated mucosubstances and glycosaminoglycans containing carboxyl groups bind AB in the presence of low concentrations (<0.3 M) of electrolytes. At molarities in excess of 0.8 M, only sulfated mucosubstances stain positively.

Sulfated mucins can also be demonstrated by the high iron diamine method.[34] In this procedure, a mixture of diamine salts is oxidized by ferric chloride to produce a black cationic chromogen that stains sulfate ester groups black/brown. When sections are counterstained with AB, sulfated mucins will stain black/brown, and carboxylated mucins will stain blue.

Treatment of sections with hyaluronidase prior to staining with AB is a useful approach to establish the identity of an acidic mucosubstance. It should be remembered, however, that testicular hyaluronidase will digest hyaluronosulphate and chondroitin sulfates A and C in addition to hyaluronic acid.[31] The finding of enzyme-labile AB-positive material in a biopsy

of a pleural tumor, for example, supports the diagnosis of mesothelioma, since these tumors are rich in hyaluronic acid. Treatment of sections with sialidase is a useful approach to confirm the identify of a sialic acid-rich mucosubstance.

The mucicarmine stain is a widely used empiric method for the demonstration of mucosubstances (Fig. 4-11). With this procedure, neutral mucins are negative or weakly positive, whereas strongly sulfated mucosubstances are variably positive. Other acidic mucins, including hyaluronic acid, are strongly mucicarminophilic.

Lipids

The lipids comprise a complex group of substances that include both unconjugated (free fatty acids and free cholesterol) and conjugated lipids (ester lipids, phospholipids, and sphingosine-based substances, including sphingomyelins, cerebrosides, sulfatides, and gangliosides). Since lipids are extracted by the

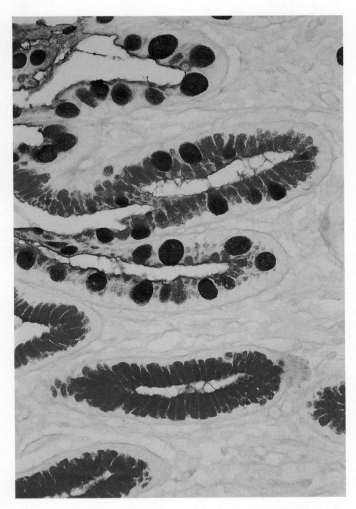

Fig. 4-10. Alcian blue/periodic acid-Schiff stain (pH 2.5) of stomach with complete intestinal metaplasia. The mucous cells are magenta (periodic acid-Schiff positive), and the goblet cells are purple, indicating a mixture of acidic and neutral mucins.

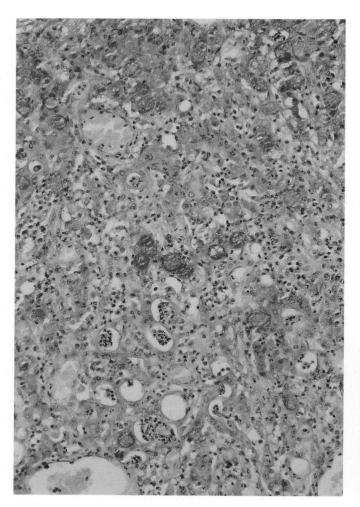

Fig. 4-11. Southgate's mucicarmine stain of poorly differentiated adenocarcinoma. Mucin deposits are stained red.

organic solvents used in paraffin tissue processors, studies of lipids should be performed on unfixed or formalin-fixed frozen sections.

The oil-soluble dyes, including the various members of the Sudan family, are invaluable reagents for the demonstration of lipids in tissue sections, since they are more soluble in lipid than in the alcoholic solutions in which they are usually prepared. The standard Sudan black technique selectively stains unsaturated lipids, cholesterol esters, triglycerides, and some phospholipids. With a bromination step prior to staining, lecithin, free fatty acids, and free cholesterol will be stained positively in addition to the moieties stained by unmodified Sudan black.

Oil red O is one of the most popular methods for staining lipids in the surgical pathology laboratory[35] (Fig. 4-12). With this technique, unsaturated hydrophobic lipids, triglycerides, and cholesterol stain orange-red, whereas phospholipids stain pink. Cholesterol can be distinguished from cholesterol esters with the digitonin reaction using an oil red O counterstain. Digitonin forms a birefringent complex with cholesterol, and cholesterol esters stain positively with oil red O.

Methodologies for the demonstration of sphingomyelins, cerebrosides, gangliosides, and sulfatides are discussed in detail in several monographs.[36] In most neuropathology laboratories, luxol fast blue is used for the demonstration of myelin, which appears blue to green (Fig. 4-13). Degenerating myelin can be demonstrated with the Marchi technique, which employs osmium tetroxide. Degenerated myelin is stained black, and normal myelin has a light brown coloration.

Pigments and Minerals

Pigments of various types are commonly found in many types of cells and tissues.[37] Some pigments are related to fixation, and others are naturally occurring. One of the most commonly encountered pigments is acid formaldehyde hematin (*formalin pigment*). This pigment occurs most commonly in bloody tissues that have been fixed in unbuffered formalin. Formalin pigment appears most often as a yellow-brown to black microcrystalline substance that is iron negative. Typically, formalin pigment, in contrast to most naturally occurring pigments, is birefringent.

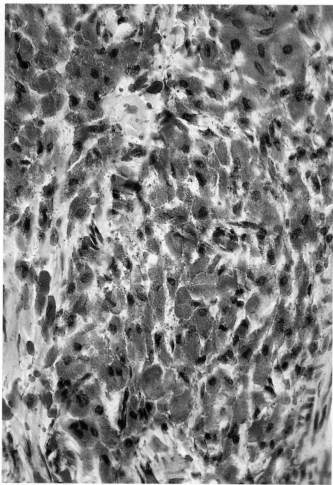

Fig. 4-12. Oil red O stain of skin biopsy from a patient with hyperlipoproteinemia. Lipid deposits are stained red.

lipofuscin is Sudan black B positive and will also reduce ferricyanide to ferrocyanide (the Schmorl reaction). Ceroid represents a form of lipofuscin at an early stage of oxidation.

Pseudomelanosis (*melanosis coli*) pigment has many similarities to lipofuscin.[37] It is typically yellow to brown and granular. Pseudomelanin is nonbirefringent but exhibits a yellow to orange autofluorescence. It is usually acid-fast negative, but it may in some instances exhibit only faint staining. Iron stains are generally negative, although a few iron-positive granules may be admixed with the pigment.

Melanin pigment appears as yellow, brown, or brown to black granules in a variety of normal and pathologic tissues. This pigment is nonbirefringent and does not exhibit the typical autofluorescence of lipofuscin. In contrast to other pigments, melanin can be bleached with hydrogen peroxide, chlorine water, chromic acid, or potassium permanganate. Bleaching of melanin is sometimes required to confirm its identify and to facilitate interpretation of cytologic features of heavily pigmented cells. Melanin deposits are negative for iron using the Prussian blue reaction and are usually PAS negative. The Fontana-

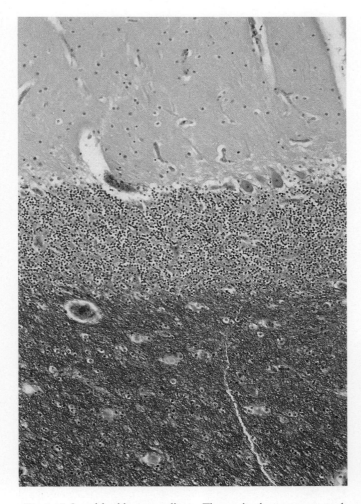

Fig. 4-13. Luxol fast blue stain of brain. The myelin deposits are stained blue.

The pigment usually occurs in extracellular sites in areas of recent hemorrhage, but it may also occur within cells. Formalin pigment can be removed with alcoholic picric acid. The appearance and chemical composition of formalin pigment is similar to malaria pigment, which is also birefringent. In sections fixed in formol sublimate, mercury pigment appears as a large yellow-brown birefringent crystalline material. This pigment may be removed by treating sections with Lugol's iodine. Chromic oxide pigment, which also appears in extracellular sites, can be removed by treatment of sections with acid alcohol.

The lipofuscins (lipochrome pigments) are among the most commonly encountered naturally occurring pigments.[37] They are derived in part by the oxidation of unsaturated tissue lipids or lipoproteins. Lipofuscin most often appears as a golden-brown intracellular pigment that is nonbirefringent and iron negative. Its histochemical characteristics partly depend on the state of oxidation of its component lipids. It is autofluorescent, PAS positive, and variably acid fast (Fig. 4-14). In addition,

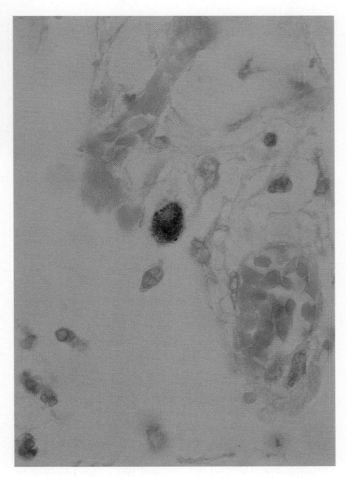

Fig. 4-14. Ziehl-Neelsen stain of lipofuscin deposits in a pulmonary macrophage. The lipofuscin deposits are weakly acid fast and stain red-purple.

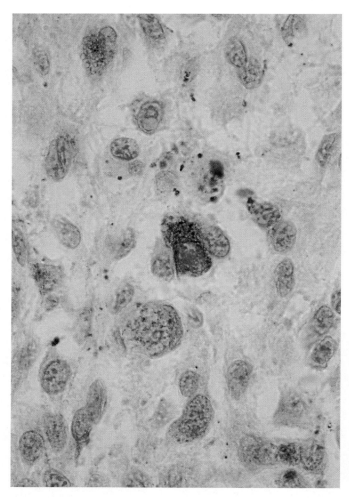

Fig. 4-15. Fontana-Masson stain of malignant melanoma. The melanin deposits within the cytoplasm are stained black.

Masson argentaffin technique stains melanin granules black (Fig. 4-15); however, it should be remembered that argentaffin granules in enteroendocrine cells and chromaffin cells will also give a positive reaction. Moreover, lipofuscin deposits are variably positive with the Fontana-Masson method. The ferric ferricyanide reduction technique (Schmorl's stain) has also been used for the demonstration of melanins, but the specificity of this method is low, since many reducing substances, including lipofuscins, argentaffin granules, and keratohyaline, will give a positive result.

Hemosiderin pigment, which represents ferric iron complexed to protein, also appears as a yellow-brown pigment but is not autofluorescent. Perls' Prussian blue reaction is typically positive, but acid-fast and PAS stains are negative (Fig. 4-16). In the Prussian blue reaction, ferric iron reacts with potassium ferrocyanide to produce an insoluble blue product (ferric ferrocyanide). The Turnbull blue method can be used to demonstrate ferrous iron and ferric iron that has been reduced to the ferrous state.

Bile pigment (bilirubin) and hematoidin crystals are identical substances. Bilirubin is derived as an iron-free pigment from biliverdin, which is an intermediary in the breakdown of hemoglobin by cells of the reticuloendothelial system. The crystalline forms of bilirubin or hematoidin are birefringent but not autofluorescent. Specific identification of bile pigment can be accomplished by treatment of sections with concentrated nitric acid, which oxidizes the pigment progressively to red, purple, and blue-green products (Gmelin reaction). In the Stein technique, bilirubin is oxidized by iodine to form a green biliverdin pigment.

Porphyrin pigments rarely occur in tissues in sufficient concentrations to be visible by light microscopy.[37] When they are present, they may appear as yellow to brown/black granular deposits. The most valuable approach for their identification depends on a characteristic orange-red autofluorescence in ultraviolet light. Since the fluorescence fades rapidly, sections must be examined immediately after they are prepared.

Copper is present in many normal tissues; however, its concentration is too low to permit detection by histochemical

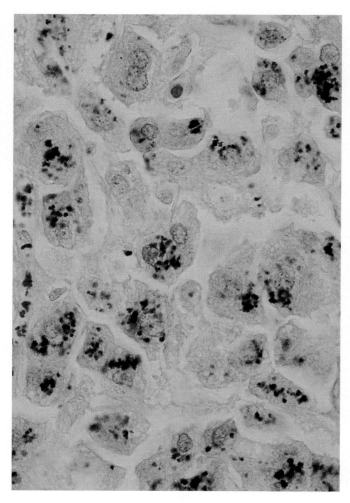

Fig. 4-16. Perls' stain of liver with increased iron stores. Sites of ferric iron deposition are stained blue.

mine silver method is also a useful approach for the demonstration of urate deposits.

Amines and Peptide-Containing Cells

The biogenic amine-containing cells of the adrenal medulla, paraganglia, and gastrointestinal tract can be demonstrated selectively by a variety of staining methods. In the classic chromaffin reaction, tissues are fixed in a potassium dichromate-containing fixative. The amine products are subsequently oxidized to colored quinone products, which polymerize to form adrenochrome and noradrenochrome pigments. The iodate ion will also oxidize biogenic amines with the formation of similar pigments. Biogenic amines also have the ability to reduce silver directly (argentaffin positivity). The chromaffin reaction has a low level of sensitivity and has been replaced in most laboratories by the formaldehyde and glyoxylic acid methods. In the formaldehyde-induced fluorescence method, freeze-dried tissue samples or air-dried touch preparations are exposed to formal-

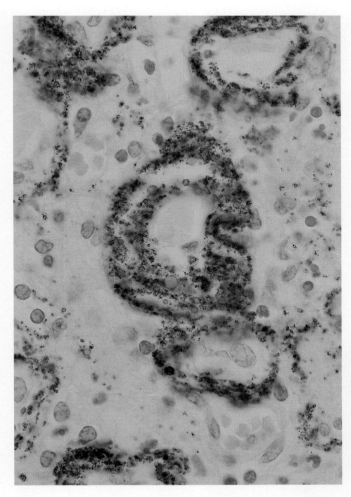

Fig. 4-17. von Kossa's stain of kidney with nephrocalcinosis. Phosphate and carbonate deposits are stained black.

methods. Copper concentration is typically increased in the livers of patients with Wilson's disease and in patients with primary biliary cirrhosis. In the method developed by Uzman, copper forms a green-black complex with rubeanic acid. Copper-associated protein can be demonstrated by a modified orcein technique, which also demonstrates cells containing hepatitis B surface antigen. Rhodamine is an additional stain for the demonstration of copper.

Calcium has been demonstrated traditionally in tissue sections with the von Kossa stain; however, this silver-based method demonstrates phosphates and carbonates rather than calcium (Fig. 4-17). Since phosphates and carbonates are invariably complexed to calcium in human tissues, a positive von Kossa reaction is indicative of the presence of calcium. Alizarin red S, a synthetic anthraquinone dye, is particularly useful for the detection of small amounts of calcium (Fig. 4-18).

Urate deposits can be identified most accurately in unstained fresh tissues or in scrapings with polarized light. Since the urate crystals are soluble in aqueous solutions, alcohol is the fixative of choice. Urates may be demonstrated with the Schultz reaction or by the DeGalantha procedure. The Gomori methena-

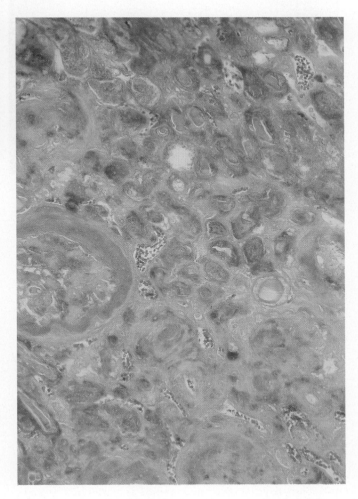

Fig. 4-18. Alizarin red stain of kidney with nephrocalcinosis. Calcium deposits are stained orange-red.

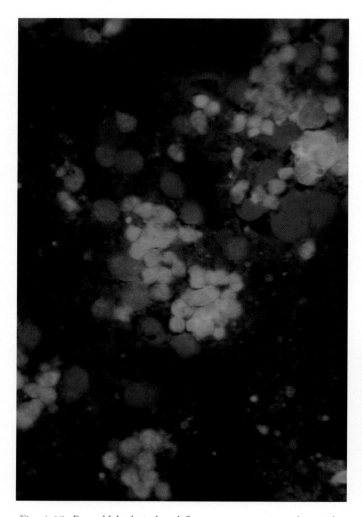

Fig. 4-19. Formaldehyde-induced fluorescence reaction of a touch preparation of a neuroblastoma. The presence of green fluorescence indicates the presence of catecholamines.

dehyde vapor and form isoquinoline (norepinephrine, epinephrine) or beta-carboline (serotonin) derivatives[38] (Fig. 4-19). These products can be distinguished because of their characteristic emission maxima in ultraviolet light. The principle of the glyoxylic acid method is essentially the same as the formaldehyde-induced fluorescence method.[39] A major advantage of the glyoxylic acid method is that fresh frozen samples may be used in place of freeze-dried samples.

Other methods that have been used for the demonstration of biogenic amine-containing cells include the Masson-Hamperl argentaffin method, the argyrophil techniques, the alkaline diazo method, and the Schmorl ferricyanide method. Cells that are rich in biogenic amines or other reducing substances have the capacity to reduce silver directly and are termed *argentaffin positive* (Fig. 4-20). Those cells that are stained positively by previously reduced silver are classified as argyrophilic (Fig. 4-21). It should be remembered that only a small proportion of argyrophil-positive cells is argentaffinic.

Several methods are available for the demonstration of histamine. The most sensitive is a fluorescent method that employs O-phthaldialdehyde (OPT) in freeze-dried samples.[40] Tissues fixed in Carnoy's fluid have also been used for the demonstration of histamine with OPT.

The protein constituents of endocrine secretory granules can be demonstrated by a variety of techniques. One of the most useful is the Grimelius argyrophil method[41] (Fig. 4-21 and 4-22). An excellent correlation exists between argyrophilia, as seen with this method, and the distribution of chromogranin, as demonstrated by immunohistochemistry. Two additional stains that have been used for the demonstration of endocrine secretory granules are lead hematoxylin[42] and toluidine blue following acid hydrolysis (masked metachromasia).[43]

Several stains are also available for the differentiation of cell types within the adenohypophysis (e.g., PAS-orange G) and pancreatic islets (protargol-aldehyde fuchsin), but they have been largely supplanted by immunohistochemical methods.

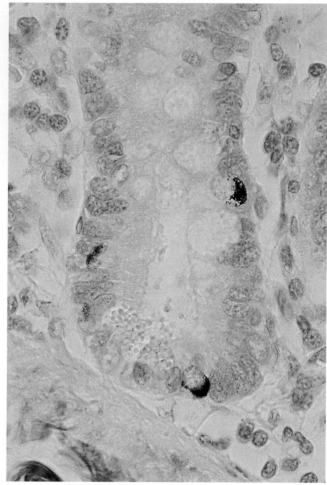

Fig. 4-20. Masson-Fontana stain for the demonstration of argentaffin cells in the terminal ileum. The argentaffin cells are stained black.

mogenic indicator is added after hydrolysis of the substrate is completed.

With very few exceptions, enzyme histochemical procedures must be performed on fresh frozen tissue samples or on tissue samples that have been briefly fixed before cryostat sectioning. Chloroacetate esterase is one clinically useful enzyme that can be demonstrated in formalin-fixed paraffin-embedded samples in cells of granulocytic lineage and mast cells (Fig. 4-23).

Enzyme histochemical methods have relatively limited applications in diagnostic pathology laboratories.[45-47] Currently, this approach is used primarily for evaluation of muscle biopsies and for the subclassification of leukemias. For example, the myofibrillar ATPase reaction is the most reliable method for the distinction of muscle fiber types (Fig. 4-24). At alkaline pH, for example, type 1 muscle fibers stain lightly for ATPase, and type 2 fibers stain darkly. At acid pH, type 1 fibers stain darkly, type 2A fibers stain lightly, and type 2B fibers stain with intermediate intensity. Oxidative enzymes such as NADH are present in high concentrations in type 1 fibers, but are present in low to intermediate concentrations in type 2 fibers. Phosphorylase ac-

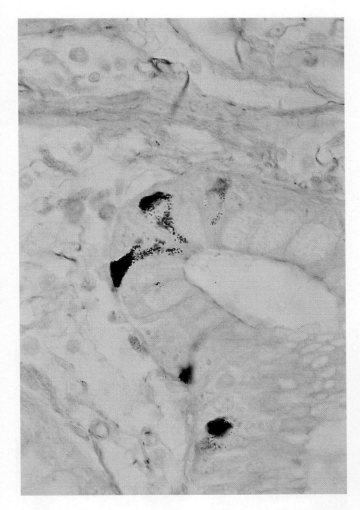

Fig. 4-21. Grimelius' stain for the demonstration of argyrophil cells in the colon. The argyrophil cells are stained black.

Enzyme Histochemistry

Histochemistry has provided a successful approach for the demonstration of a wide variety of oxidative and hydrolytic enzymes.[44] A positive staining reaction results from the formation of a colored product in situ. Numerous approaches have been developed for the demonstration of enzymes in tissue sections. These include metal precipitation reactions, simultaneous coupling procedures, and postincubation staining methods. The phosphatase enzymes may be demonstrated by the incubation of sections with a phosphate substrate. Hydrolysis of the substrate leads to the liberation of phosphate groups, which are free to react with a metallic cation such as lead. The sections are then incubated with ammonium sulfide, with the formation of lead sulfide, which appears as a black precipitate. In simultaneous coupling reactions, the enzyme hydrolyzes a substrate with the formation of a colorless intermediary product that is free to react with a chromogenic indicator incorporated into the incubating solution. In postincubation coupling methods, the chro-

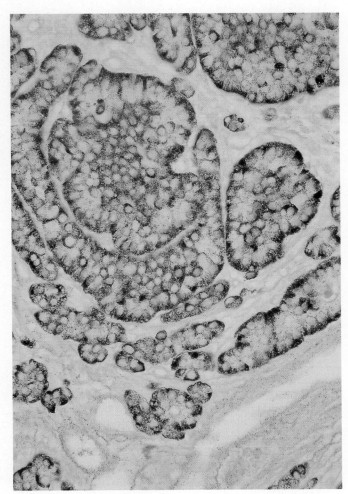

Fig. 4-22. Grimelius' stain of mid-gut carcinoid tumor. A positive stain is indicated by the presence of brown/black intracytoplasmic granules.

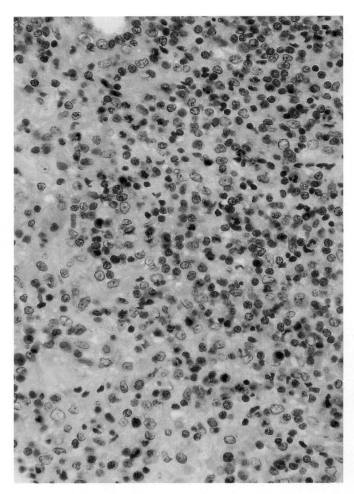

Fig. 4-23. Choroacetate esterase stain (Leder's stain) using hexazonium pararosaniline as the chromogen. Cells of granulocytic lineage are stained red.

The acid-fast stain was developed in 1881 by Ziehl and Neelson, who used carbol-fuchsin, a mixture of fuchsin and phenol, to stain mycobacteria. Mycobacteria have a high lipid content in their cell walls and resist conventional Gram staining. Phenol reportedly depresses surface tension and facilitates the entry of dye ions, which bind to mycolic acid present in the bacterial cell wall.[48] Additionally, either heat (the Ziehl-Neelson method) or a stronger solution of the dye (the Kinyoun method) are required to allow this stain to penetrate the organism. Mycobacteria resist a subsequent decolorization step with strong acid alcohols and stain red (Fig. 4-26). A modified acid-fast stain using Fite's method is recommended for nocardia and certain strains of the leprosy bacilli, which are both partially acid fast. In this method, a mixture of vegetable oil and xylene is used both to preserve and protect the lipid capsule, and a weaker 1 percent aqueous solution of sulfuric acid is the decolorizer rather than 3 percent hydrochloric acid in alcohol.[48] Methylene blue is the counterstain for both procedures.

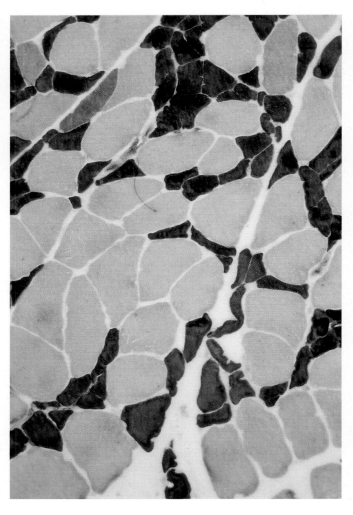

Fig. 4-24. ATPase reaction in muscle biopsy with evidence of type 2 fiber atrophy. The type 2 fibers are stained black.

tivity, on the other hand, is high in type 2 fibers but low in type 1 fibers.

Microorganisms

Most bacteria are divided into either Gram-positive or Gram-negative groups based on the color of the organisms after staining with crystal violet and iodine. A decolorizing solution of ethanol and acetone is added, followed by counterstaining with safranin.[48] Gram-positive bacteria resist decolorization and stain blue-black (Fig. 4-25). Gram-negative bacteria decolorize and stain red after counterstaining. The exact mechanism through which certain bacteria are Gram positive and others Gram negative is poorly understood. One hypothesis is that crystal violet and iodine are both ion association reagents.[49] Several modifications exist of the Gram stain for paraffin-embedded tissue.[48,50]

shown a range of 22 to 50 percent correlation.[55–57] False positive smears also exist, with rates reported from 3 to 50 percent; these may be due to death of organisms by drug therapy, by severe decontamination procedures, or by tap water contaminants. It is important to note that conventional stains have a reduced affinity for dead mycobacteria; however, the dead bacteria fluoresce just as well as viable ones. Also, numerous reports exist of *Mycobacterium gordone*, a common tap water contaminant, causing false positives. Filtration of all solutions is recommended for mycobacterial specimens to prevent this contamination problem.

PAS and methenamine silver are the two most popular stains used to demonstrate the carbohydrate components of fungi. Whichever stain is used is a matter of preference because both stain fungi equally well. The PAS stain tends to give more background staining but also provides more information on the cellular reaction. The Gridley modified PAS technique for fungi combines the chromic acid-Schiff (Bauer) and aldehyde

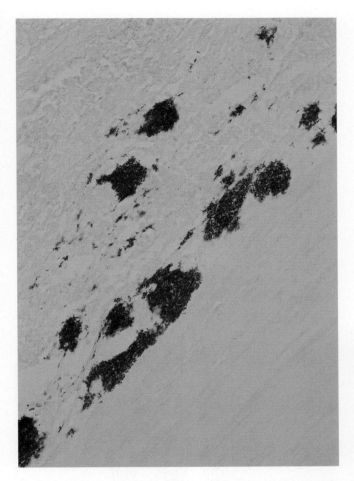

Fig. 4-25. Gram stain. Gram-positive organisms in this brain abscess are stained blue.

A fluorescent stain with the basic dyes auramine O and rhodamine B is an alternative to the traditional acid-fast stain and may be superior.[48] Acid-fast organisms fluoresce red-yellow on a dark background. The advantage of this stain is that it is more sensitive and much less tedious than traditional acid-fast stains because screening can be accomplished at low power.[51] Also, the tubercle bacilli may have a higher affinity for this dye than carbol fuchsin. One study showed that 15 to 18 percent of culture-positive specimens had positive fluorescent stains with negative conventional acid-fast stains.[52] The Centers for Disease Control and Prevention (CDC) recommends that the auramine-rhodamine stain be decolorized and restained with the conventional stains for confirmation of a positive result.

It should be recognized that the microscopic detection of acid-fast organisms irrespective of the stain used has a low sensitivity, because approximately 10,000 mycobacterial organisms/ml of fluid are required for detection.[53,54] Thus all specimens should be submitted for culture. Studies that have examined culture-positive specimens for smear positivity have

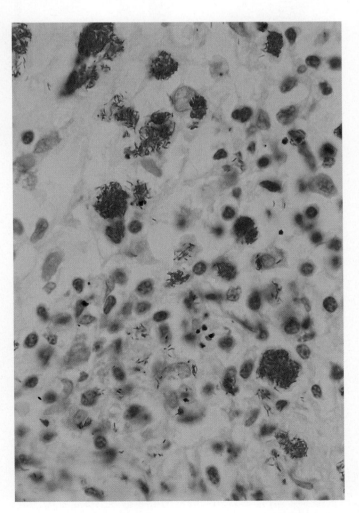

Fig. 4-26. Acid-fast stain of lymph node with *Mycobacterium avium-intracellulare* infection. Organisms are stained red.

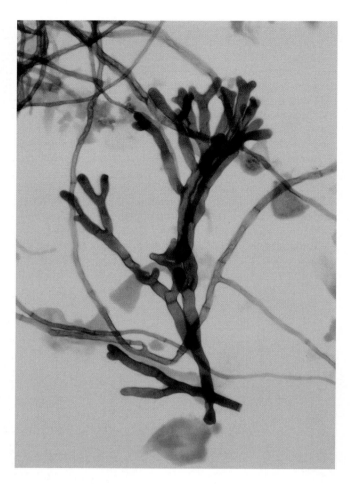

Fig. 4-27. Methenamine silver stain of bronchoalveolar lavage specimen. Hyphae of *Aspergillus* organisms are positively stained.

fuchsin techniques. Chromic acid oxidizes tissue and fungal polysaccharides to aldehydes, which then combine with the Schiff reagent. Because chromic acid is a weaker oxidizer than periodic acid, less background staining is seen. It is important to note that nocardia and actinomycetes are not stained with the Gridley method.

The Grocott methenamine silver technique is a modification of Gomori's methenamine silver stain. Like the PAS reaction, aldehydes are produced in the fungal cell wall by oxidation of 1:2 glycol groups. However, as in the Gridley modified PAS technique, 5 percent chromium trioxide (chromic acid) is the oxidizer rather than periodic acid. A methenamine silver (hexamine) mixture is then reduced by the aldehydes to metallic silver, which is black (Fig. 4-27). It should be remembered that many other tissue constituents, including mucins, glycogen, and other carbohydrates will also be stained by this method.

The methenamine silver stain is also commonly used for the

demonstration of the cyst walls of *Pneumocystis carinii* (Fig. 4-28), whereas the Giemsa or modified Giemsa (Diff-Quik) stains are trophozoite stains. In addition, the Giemsa stain also demonstrates numerous other organisms including *Helicobacter pylori*, amebae, giardia, and cryptosporidia. Air-dried smears as well as sections from paraffin-embedded tissue may be used.

Both the mucicarmine stains and India ink preparations are commonly utilized to detect cryptococci. The mucicarmine stain uses the dye carmine and aluminum as a mordant to stain the mucopolysaccharide capsule of the organism deep rose to red. Hematoxylin is used for nuclear staining and metanil yellow for counterstaining. The India ink technique, on the other hand, provides a negative image of the organisms. It involves mixing a drop of India ink with a drop of specimen and looking for the negative images of encapsulated budding yeast. The background appears black, and the organisms are unstained.

The Warthin-Starry and the Dieterle stains are silver-based methods used to identify bacteria not readily identified by the Gram stain. The Warthin-Starry stain is commonly used to

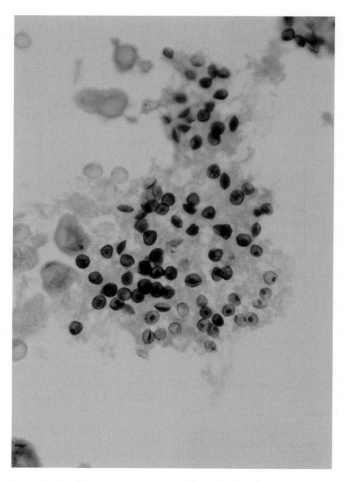

Fig. 4-28. Methenamine silver stain of bronchoalveolar lavage specimen. Cystic forms typical of *Pneumocystis carinii* are stained black.

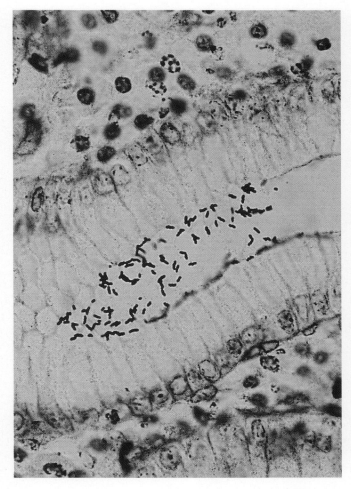

Fig. 4-29. Warthin-Starry stain of gastric biopsy with numerous *Helicobacter pylori* organisms, which are stained black.

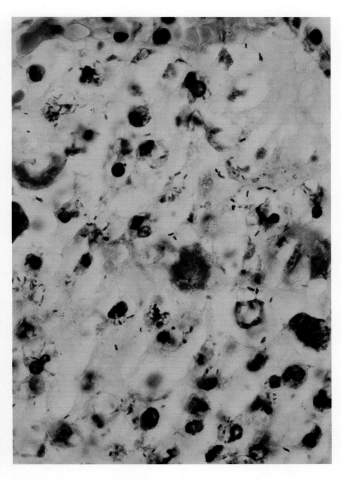

Fig. 4-30. Dieterle's stain for *Legionella pneumophila*. The coccobacillary forms are stained black.

identify *H. pylori* (Fig. 4-29), spirochetes, and the organism of cat-scratch disease; the Dieterle stain is recommended for identification of *Legionella*[48] (Fig. 4-30). These organisms are argyrophilic, that is, they absorb silver from solution and require a reducing agent to make them visible. The Dieterle stain uses hydroquinone to reduce the silver nitrate, uranyl nitrate to decrease background staining, and a gum mastic alcohol solution for even impregnation. As in other silver stains, positively staining organisms are visible because bound silver nitrate when reduced to metallic silver becomes black. A careful hematoxylin and eosin examination usually reveals *H. pylori* on the mucosal surface if it is present. However, if the clinical suspicion is high and organisms are not identified, the Warthin-Starry silver stain is recommended. A combination of the Steiner stain, hematoxylin and eosin, and Alcian blue at pH 2.5 (Genta stain) provides simultaneous visualization of organisms and tissue morphology.[58] *Treponema pallidum* and *Borrelia burgdorferi*, the etiologic agents of syphilis and Lyme disease, respectively, as well as the Donovan bodies of granuloma inguinale, are also visualized.[59,60]

REFERENCES

1. Pearse AGE: Historical introduction. pp. 1–14. In: Histochemistry. Theoretical and Applied. 4th Ed. Vol. 1. Churchill Livingstone, Edinburgh, 1980
2. Pearse AGE: The chemistry and practice of fixation. pp. 97–158. In: Histochemistry. Theoretical and Applied. 4th Ed. Vol. 1. Churchill Livingstone, Edinburgh, 1980
3. Pearse AGE: Freeze drying of biological tissues. In: Histochemistry. Theoretical and Applied. 4th Ed. Vol. 1. Churchill Livingstone, Edinburgh, 1980
4. Leong ASY, Daymon ME, Milios J: Microwave irradiation as a form of fixation for light and electron microscopy. J Pathol 146:313–332, 1985
5. Hopwood D: Cell and tissue fixation, 1972–1982. Histochem J 17:389–442, 1985
6. Hopwood D: Fixation and fixatives. pp. 21–42. In Bancroft JD, Stevens A (eds): Theory and Practice of Histological Techniques. Churchill Livingstone, Edinburgh, 1990
7. Kiernan JA: Histological and Histochemical Methods. Theory and Practice. Pergamon, Oxford, 1981
8. Baker JR: Introduction to fixation. pp. 14–30. In: Cytological

Technique: the Principles Underlying Routine Methods. 5th Ed. Science Paperbacks and Methuen, London, 1966

9. Banks PM: Technical aspects of specimen preparation and introduction to special studies. pp. 1–21. In Jaffe ES (ed): Surgical Pathology of the Lymph Nodes and Related Organs. WB Saunders, Philadelphia, 1995

10. Bancroft JD, Cook HC: Manual of Histochemical Techniques and their Diagnostic Application. Churchill Livingstone, Edinburgh, 1994

11. Keebler CM, Somrak TM: Cytopreparative techniques. pp. 412–447. In: The Manual of Cytotechnology. 7th Ed. ASCP, Chicago, 1993

12. Woronzoff-Dashkoff KP: The Ehrlick-Chenzinsky-Plehn-Malachowski-Romanowsky-Nocht-Jenner-May-Grünwald-Leishman-Reuter-Wright-Giemsa-Lillie-Roe, Wilcox stain. The mystery unfolds. Clin Lab Med 13:759–771, 1993

13. Wilbur DC, Cibas ES, Meritt S, et al: ThinPrep processor. Clinical trials demonstrate an increased detection rate of abnormal cervical cytologic specimens. Am J Clin Pathol 101:209–214, 1994

14. Hutchinson ML, Agarwal P, Denault T: A new look at cervical cytology: ThinPrep multicenter trial results. Acta Cytol 36:499–504, 1992

15. Hutchinson ML, Isenstein LM, Goodman AK, et al: Homogeneous sampling accounts for the increased diagnostic accuracy using the ThinPrep processor. Am J Clin Pathol 101:215–219, 1994

16. Ro JY, Staerkel GA, Ayala AG: Cytologic and histologic features of superficial bladder cancer. Urol Clin North Am 19:435–453, 1992

17. Hossein M, Yazdi MB: Genitourinary cytology. Clin Lab Med 11:369–377, 1991

18. Koss LG: Diagnostic Cytology and its Histopathologic Bases. 4th Ed. Lippincott-Raven, Philadelphia, 1992

19. Horobin, RW: An overview of the theory of staining. pp. 93–105. In Bancroft JD, Stevens A (eds): Theory and Practice of Histopathological Techniques. Churchill Livingstone, Edinburgh, 1990

20. Stevens A, Bancroft JD: Proteins and nucleic acids. pp. 143–153. In Bancroft JD, Stevens A (eds): Theory and Practice of Histological Techniques. Churchill Livingstone, Edinburgh, 1990

21. Pearse AGE: Nucleic acids and nucleoproteins. pp. 248–293. Histochemistry. Theoretical and Applied. 3rd Ed. Vol. 1. Little, Brown, Boston, 1968

22. Ploton D, Menager M, Jeannesson P, et al: Improvement in the staining and in the visualization of the argyrophilic proteins of the nucleolar organizing regions at the optical level. Histochem J 18:5–14, 1986

23. Pearse AGE: Proteins and amino acids. pp. 106–179. Histochemistry. Theoretical and Applied. 3rd Ed. Vol. 1. Little, Brown, Boston, 1968

24. Bradbury P, Gordon KC: Connective tissues and stains. pp. 119–142. In Bancroft JD, Stevens A (eds): Theory and Practice of Histological Techniques. Churchill Livingstone, Edinburgh, 1990

25. Shikata T, Uzawa T, Yoshiwara N, et al: Staining methods for Australia antigen in paraffin sections—detection of cytoplasmic inclusion bodies. Jpn J Exp Med 44:25, 1974

26. Cooper JH: Selective amyloid staining as a function of amyloid composition and structure. Lab Invest 31:232, 1974

27. Puchtler H, Sweat F, Levine M: On the binding of Congo red by amyloid. J Histochem Cytochem 10:355, 1962

28. Wright JR, Calkins E, Humphrey RL: Potassium permanganate reaction in amyloidosis. Lab Invest 36:274, 1977

29. Vassar PS, Culling FA: Fluorescent stains with special reference to amyloid and connective tissue. Arch Pathol 68:487, 1959

30. McKinney B, Grubb C: Nonspecificity of thioflavine T as amyloid stain. Nature 205:1023, 1965

31. Cook HC: Carbohydrates. pp. 177–213. In Bancroft JD, Stevens A (eds): Theory and Practice of Histological Techniques. Churchill Livingstone, Edinburgh, 1990

32. Goldstein IJ, Hayes CE: The lectins: carbohydrate binding proteins of plants and animals. Adv Carbohydr Chem Biochem 35:127–340, 1978

33. Scott JE, Dorling J: Differential staining of acid glycosaminoglycans (mucopolysaccharides) by Alcian blue in salt solutions. Histochemie 5:221–233, 1965

34. Sorvari TE: Histochemical observations on the role of ferric chloride in the high iron diamine technique for localizing sulphated mucosubstances. Histochem J 4:193–204, 1972

35. Bayliss-High OB: Lipids. pp. 215–244. In Bancroft JD, Stevens A (eds): Theory and Practice of Histological Techniques. Churchill Livingstone, Edinburgh, 1990

36. Adams CWM: Neurohistochemistry. Elsevier Science, Amsterdam, 1965

37. Stevens A: Pigments and minerals. pp. 245–267. In Bancroft JD, Stevens A (eds): Theory and Practice of Histological Techniques. Churchill Livingstone, Edinburgh, 1990

38. Falck B, Owman CA: A detailed methodological description of the fluorescence method for the cellular distribution of biogenic monoamines. Acta Univ Lund 7:5–23, 1965

39. DeLaTorre JC, Surgeon JW: A methodological approach to rapid and sensitive monoamine histofluorescence using a modified glyoxylic acid technique: the SPG method. Histochemistry 49:81, 1976

40. Shelley WB, Öhman S, Parnes HM: Mast cell stain for histamine on freeze-dried embedded tissue. J Histochem Cytochem 16:433–439, 1968

41. Grimelius LA: A silver nitrate stain for A_2 cells of human pancreatic islets. Acta Soc Med Upsal 73:243–270, 1968

42. Solcia E, Capella C, Vasallo G: Lead hematoxylin as a stain for endocrine cells. Significance of staining and comparison with other selective methods. Histochemistry 20:116, 1969

43. Solcia E, Vasallo G, Capella C: Selective staining of endocrine cells by basic dyes after acid hydrolysis. Stain Technol 43:257–263, 1968

44. Bancroft JD, Cook HC: Enzyme histochemistry. pp. 289–322. Manual of Histological Techniques and Their Diagnostic Application. Churchill Livingstone, Edinburgh, 1994

45. Dubowitz V: Muscle Biopsy: A Practical Approach. Bailliere Tindall, London, 1985

46. Leder LD: Uber die selektive fermentcytochemische Darstellung von neutrophilen myeloischen Zellen Gewebsmastzellen in Paraffinschnit. Kurze wissenschaftliche Mitteilungen 42:11, 1964

47. Stevens A: Enzyme histochemistry. Diagnostic applications. pp. 401–412. In Bancroft JD, Stevens A (eds): Theory and Practice of Histological Techniques. Churchill Livingstone, Edinburgh, 1990

48. Stevens A: Micro-organisms. pp. 289–308. In Bancroft JD, Stevens A (eds): Theory and Practice of Histological Techniques. Churchill Livingstone, Edinburgh, 1990

49. Noda Y, Toei K: A new bacterial staining method involving gram stain with theoretical considerations of the staining mechanism. Microbios 70:49–55, 1992

50. Glynn JH: The application of the Gram stain to paraffin sections. Arch Pathol 20:896–899, 1935

51. Niejadlik DC: Clinical Diagnosis and Management by Laboratory Methods. pp. 510, 1079. 18th Ed. WB Saunders, Philadelphia, 1991

52. Eisenstadt J, Hall GS, Gibson SM, Dunbar D: Mycobacteria. pp. 703–755. In Mahon CR, Manuchs T (eds): Textbook of Diagnostic Microbiology. WB Saunders, Philadelphia, 1995

53. Kox LF: Tests for detection and identification of mycobacteria. How should they be used? Respir Med 89:339–408, 1995

54. Koneman EW: Mycobacterium tuberculosis. pp. 635–676. Diagnostic Microbiology. 4th Ed. Lippincott-Raven, Philadelphia, 1992

55. Boyd JC, Marr JJ: Decreasing reliability of acid-fast smear techniques for the detection of tuberculosis. Ann Intern Med 82:489–492, 1975

56. Pollock HM, Wieman EJ: Smear results in the diagnosis of mycobacterioses using blue light fluorescence microscopy. J Clin Microbiol 5:329–331, 1977

57. Rickman TW, Moyer NP: Increased sensitivity of acid fast smears. J Clin Microbiol 11:618, 1980

58. Genta RM, Robason GO, Graham DY: Simultaneous visualization of Helicobacter pylori and gastric morphology. A new stain. Hum Pathol 25:221–226, 1994

59. Van der Sluis JJ: Laboratory techniques in the diagnosis of syphilis: a review. Genitourin Med 68:413–419, 1992

60. Pfister HW, Wilske B, Weber K: Lyme borreliosis: basic science and clinical aspects. Lancet 343:1013–1016, 1994

5

Immunohistochemical Techniques

Mehrdad Nadji
Azorides R. Morales

Labeled antibodies that permit visualization of specific substances in tissue sections have been in use for more then 50 years. Fluorescein isothiocyanate and other fluorescent compounds were the first substances to be bound to antibodies.[1] Colloidal metals such as ferritin and mercury were next to be conjugated with antibodies.[2,3] It was only after the introduction of enzyme-labeled antibodies that immunohistochemical techniques were accepted as simple, versatile, and practical tools in diagnostic histopathology.[4,5] Today, great advances have been made in the development and refinement of various immunohistologic methods.[6–10] The introduction of monoclonal antibodies into the realm of immunohistochemistry has ensured the availability of an unlimited source of highly specific reagents for histologic demonstration of various cell and tissue antigens.[9,11] Many commercial sources now offer good quality antibodies, detection systems, and immunohistochemical staining kits. Automated immunohistochemical machines have become viable alternatives to the manual procedures. Consequently, diagnostic immunohistochemistry has become an integral part of a pathology laboratory, and one can safely predict that it will continue to remain valuable for many years to come.

This chapter first examines the technical aspects of the immunohistochemical methods, including brief notes related to the specimen, fixation, staining procedure, reagents, and controls, as well as potential pitfalls and means to avoid them. Second, analytical aspects of this technique are reviewed and selection of markers, interpretation of results, and potential analytical pitfalls are discussed. Details concerning the use of markers in specific diagnostic situations are discussed in chapters devoted to pathologic lesions of each organ.

DIFFERENT TECHNIQUES

Immunohistochemical techniques are a group of immunolabeling procedures that are capable of demonstrating various substances in cells and tissues. These techniques are based on the ability of specific antibodies to localize and bind to corresponding antigens. The binding reaction is not visible unless the antibody is tagged with a label that either absorbs or emits light and thus produces a contrast or a color.

Fluorescein compounds, when excited by ultraviolet light, emit light within the visible wavelengths. The color of the emitted light depends on the nature of the compound. Fluorescein isothiocyanate, for example, emits green light, whereas rhodamine produces red fluorescence. Other fluorescent substances have been introduced in recent years that emit light of other colors.[12] As a group, immunofluorescence methods require the use of fresh or fresh frozen tissue. The reaction results are visualized on a dark background. The requirement for fresh tissue, together with the lack of morphologic detail and permanency of stains, has limited the use of immunofluorescence methods to evaluation of immunologic disorders, particularly in kidney and skin.

Various metals, such as iron, gold, and mercury, have been used as labels for immunohistochemical methods.[2,3,13] All produce sufficient electron opacity for visualization by light and electron microscopy. The poor penetration of metal conjugates and their nonspecific deposition in the background are the major drawbacks of immunometal methods. Immunogold methods are the most popular of these techniques and are used predominantly for ultrastructural localization of substances such as hormones. The immunogold-silver staining technique is one of the highly sensitive immunohistochemical procedures.[13,14]

Enzymes are currently the most widely used labels in immunohistochemistry.[15,16] The enzyme-antibody complexes retain their immunologic and enzymatic properties and are therefore able both to bind to specific antigens in tissue and to change the color of a suitable chromogen. Peroxidase and alkaline phosphatase are the commonly used enzymes, with peroxidase being the label of choice for most diagnostic immunohistochemical assays.

In immunohistochemistry, the labels are either directly bound to the primary, secondary, or tertiary antibodies, or they are indirectly introduced into the reaction by the use of other substances such as haptens, biotin, polymers, or protein A. Currently available immunohistochemical techniques are a large, heterogeneous group of procedures that differ from one another by the type of label, the number of antibodies, and the type of nonimmunologic substances used. Major categories of immunohistochemical methods are listed in Table 5-1. Only those immunoperoxidase procedures with widespread routine usage in diagnostic histopathology are discussed in more detail.

Table 5-1. Different Immunohistochemical
Methods

Labeled antibody methods[17,18]
   Direct
   Indirect
Unlabeled antibody procedures[17-19]
   Hybrid antibody[20]
   Immunoglobulin bridge[21,22]
   Enzyme-antienzyme[23]
   Labeled antigen[24]
   Protein A label[25]
   Hapten-labeled antibody[26]
   Biotin-avidin[27]
   Avidin-biotin conjugate[28]
   Labeled avidin D[29]

Peroxidase-Antiperoxidase Method

Application of the primary antibody in the peroxidase-antiperoxidase (PAP) method is followed sequentially by a second antibody and a PAP complex. The second antibody acts as a bridge between the first antibody and the PAP-soluble complex. This technique that was introduced by Sternberger's group[23] in 1970 has been until recently one of the most popular immunoperoxidase procedures. The apparent decline in popularity of the PAP technique was partly due to the difficulties in producing murine PAP complexes for use with monoclonal antibodies. Although this problem has been overcome by production of monoclonal PAP complexes, its relatively lower sensitivity has led to wider use of newer methods.[30]

Avidin-Biotin-Peroxidase Complex Method

Biotin, an egg-white protein, has an intense affinity for a low molecular weight vitamin, avidin. This interaction, with an association constant that is several million times greater than antigen-antibody binding, is practically irreversible. In the avidin-biotin-peroxidase complex (ABC) method, the secondary biotinylated antibody is followed by a preformed complex of avidin-biotin-peroxidase.[28] The resulting large latticework complexes can deliver many active peroxidase molecules and hence the ABC techniques have one of the highest sensitivities of all immunohistochemical methods.

Streptavidin-Biotin Procedure

The streptavidin-biotin procedure is a modification of the ABC method in which streptavidin has replaced avidin. Isolated from *Streptomyces avidinii*, streptavidin has the same high affinity for biotin.[31] Immunohistochemical systems based on the peroxidase-labeled or alkaline phosphatase-labeled streptavidin-biotin complexes have a sensitivity comparable to the conventional ABC techniques, although an ABC kit with increased load of peroxidase complexes has proved to be the most

sensitive commercially available detection system for routine immunohistochemistry.[32]

TECHNICAL ASPECTS

This section examines the various factors that are involved in the performance of immunostaining techniques. Since most immunohistochemical procedures currently used in anatomic pathology are immunoperoxidase methods, we have limited our discussion primarily to the application of these techniques to histologic and cytologic specimens.

The Histologic Specimen

Frozen Section

Because routine fixation and processing reduce the amount of immunohistochemically detectable antigens, cryostat sections were preferred for immunohistochemistry of low copy antigens when monoclonal antibodies were first introduced.[6-10] However, with increasing availability of highly sensitive detection systems and the advent of antigen retrieval technologies, routine use of frozen sections for immunohistochemistry has been drastically reduced.

When immunohistochemistry of frozen samples is anticipated, one should note that cell and tissue antigens are best preserved when the specimen is immediately and rapidly frozen. This can be accomplished by prompt immersion of a block of tissue, no larger than $1.0 \times 1.0 \times 0.3$ cm, in liquid nitrogen (snap freezing). A mixture of isopentane and liquid nitrogen will result in a more uniform freezing of tissue and hence the best preservation of histomorphology.[8] Slow freezing of the specimens by placing them in a freezer will result in considerable antigen loss and poor morphologic detail. Thawing and refreezing the specimens also have a negative impact on histologic detail and preservation of tissue antigens.

Embedding compounds will facilitate preparation of good quality frozen sections, but because evidence exists that embedded frozen tissues gradually lose their cellular antigens, prolonged storage of histologic material in embedding medium is not recommended. Snap-frozen fresh tissues without supporting media, however, can be stored at −70°C for long periods of time without appreciable antigen loss.

Plastic-Embedded Tissue

Thin sections from tissues embedded in different types of plastics, such as araldite, epoxy resin, and methacrylate, demonstrate excellent morphologic detail. For immunohistochemistry, however, it is necessary to remove the resin with sodium ethoxide and to re-expose the antigens by protease digestion or heat-induced retrieval techniques.[33,34] Nevertheless, even with these additional steps, immunohistochemical reactions in plastic-embedded tissue yield unpredictable results. Therefore plastic sections are not recommended for routine immunohistochemistry in diagnostic pathology. A number of pre- and postembedding methods have been described for immunoelectron microscopy; however, a discussion of those procedures is beyond the scope of this chapter.

Paraffin-Embedded Specimens

The applicability of immunohistochemical procedures to paraffin-embedded tissue is the most important factor responsible for their popularity and widespread use in diagnostic pathology. Every pathology file is now a potential source for numerous retrospective studies. No conclusive evidence shows the degree of deleterious effect that different types of commercially available paraffin may have on various antigens. However, when fixed and processed tissue is embedded in paraffin, immunohistochemically detectable tissue antigens remain intact in the block for many years and will not decrease by prolonged storage.

Fixatives

It is safe to say that no ideal fixative for immunohistochemistry currently exists. All fixatives, in one way or another, adversely affect the immunohistochemically detectable cell and tissue antigens.[35] Among the factors that influence the choice of fixative are its availability, price, safety, and suitability for one or more antigens. Cell and tissue substances differ in their susceptibility to various fixatives. An optimal fixative for intermediate filaments, for example, may cause deterioration of plasma proteins. In prospective immunohistochemical studies, therefore, the choice of fixative depends on the type of antigens that are to be detected. This section briefly examines the advantages and limitations of some of the more commonly used fixatives.

Formalin

Although 10 percent neutral formalin is the most widely available and economical fixative, it is not the best for immunohistochemistry.[36,37] The deteriorating effect of formalin is more evident with certain plasma proteins, such as light and heavy chain immunoglobulins. Most other cytoplasmic antigens, however, withstand formalin fixation and can be demonstrated adequately either directly or by retrieval techniques. Formalin is also the best available fixative for preservation of nucleic acids in archival tissues used for molecular biologic studies.

Alcohol-Containing Fixatives

Alcohols and alcohol-based fixatives, such as Carnoy's and methacarn, have the advantage of penetrating tissue rapidly. They are the fixatives of choice for a few cell markers, including intermediate filaments.[38,39] Most other tissue antigens, however, are not adequately preserved in alcohol-containing fixatives. Also, the tissues fixed in alcoholic solutions shrink and harden quickly and may exhibit poor morphology.

Picric Acid-Containing Fixatives

Bouin's and Zamboni's are the two most commonly used fixatives in this group.[40] With the exception of intermediate filaments and immunoglobulins, most other cytoplasmic antigens can be demonstrated successfully in tissue fixed in Bouin's solution.[41] Bouin's fixation is particularly advantageous in preserving viral antigens and peptide hormones. Zamboni's solution (picric acid-paraformaldehyde) is also suitable for electron microscopy.[40]

Mercuric Fixatives

B5 and other mercuric chloride-containing fixatives, such as Zenker's and Susa's, are better than formalin in preserving histologic detail, particularly nuclear morphology. These fixatives are also the best for immunohistochemical demonstration of immunoglobulins as well as most lymphoid cell markers in paraffin-embedded tissues.[42,43] Mercuric fixatives, however, are not recommended for most other cellular antigens. These fixatives produce undesirable background staining and may result in erroneous interpretation of staining reactions.

Other Fixatives

In recent years a number of fixatives have been commercially introduced as potential nontoxic alternatives to neutral buffered formalin.[44] Most of these solutions are alcohol based and contain additional substances such as acetic acid, sodium chloride, zinc sulfate, ethylene glycol, and others.[39] In our experience, and that of others, none of these reagents performs as well as formalin in preserving the morphology and antigenicity of histologic material.[44] Most of these alternative fixatives also cost considerably more than buffered formalin.

Fixatives for Frozen Section

A number of fixatives have been recommended for frozen sections. Cell surface antigens are best preserved in sections fixed briefly in cold acetone (5 minutes at 4°C). Good results are also obtained in frozen sections fixed for a few minutes in ethanol, formalin, and picric acid-paraformaldehyde. Sections should be fixed immediately for best morphologic preservation. If fixation is apt to mask or denature the antigen under study, it can be delayed until after the primary antibody has been applied. Immunohistochemistry of unfixed frozen tissue will result in diffusion of the antigens, increased background staining, and poor morphologic results.[8]

Fixation Process

To achieve the highest quality immunohistochemical results, the tissue should be fixed promptly, thoroughly, and adequately.[7,45] Delay in fixation, inadequate fixation, and overfixation are all equally detrimental to good immunohistochemistry and may cause analytic errors. Adequate penetration of the fixative can be achieved only by trimming the histologic specimen properly before fixation. Optimal formalin fixation time for a $1.0 \times 1.0 \times 0.3$ cm block of tissue is between 12 and 18 hours. For fixatives containing alcohol, picric acid, and mercuric chloride, the optimal fixation time is 2 to 5 hours, provided that the tissue block is not larger than 0.5 × 0.5 × 0.2 cm.[8] Prolonged fixation results in a progressive loss in immunohistochemically detectable antigens. This is particularly true of overfixation in formalin, which often necessitates pretreatment of tissue to unmask susceptible proteins.[46]

Rapid fixation of tissue can be achieved by using a conventional microwave oven. Fixation time in formalin, for example, can be reduced to a few seconds, preserving both morphology and stainable tissue antigens.[47] Rapid microwave fixation will also obviate the need for protease digestion or heat-induced antigen retrieval.

Decalcification

Different decalcifying solutions, such as EDTA, formic acid, and nitric acid, do not significantly alter the antigenicity of various cell and tissue substances.[48] However, tissues should not be left in decalcifying solutions any longer than necessary. If antigen loss is anticipated during decalcification, the specimen should be fixed first and then placed in decalcifying solution.

Processing and Embedding

Processing and embedding appear to have little effect on immunostaining of fixed tissue. Some low copy cellular antigens, however, may be lost during routine processing and embedding. In recent years, alternative tissue processing and paraffin-embedding techniques have been described that result in an improved preservation of cellular antigens for immunostaining.[49,50] For example, a procedure in which the tissue is freeze-dried and then embedded directly in paraffin is reported to produce staining results with an intensity equal to, or greater than, that observed in frozen sections.[50]

Histologic Sections

Four micrometer thick sections of paraffin-embedded tissue provide the best preparations for immunostaining. Thicker sections, folded sections, and sections with tears or nicks from the microtome are undesirable for immunohistochemistry.[41,45] Histologic sections such as these are easily washed off during the procedure. Furthermore, thick or folded sections absorb immunologic reagents nonspecifically and cause false positive results.

There is evidence that prolonged storage of paraffin sections may result in the loss of certain tissue antigens.[51] It is advisable therefore, to utilize freshly cut histologic sections to circumvent the possible adverse effects of storage on immunohistochemistry.

Adhesion of Section to the Slide

Loss of frozen or paraffin sections from the slide during immunohistochemical staining is not uncommon. This problem is even more pronounced when sections are subjected to protease digestion or heat-induced antigen retrieval using a microwave oven. Various adhesives (including albumin, gelatin, silane, chrome alum, and even regular paper glue) have all been applied to slides to prevent this loss. The most efficient method to minimize cell and tissue loss during immunostaining is the use of slides that either are poly-L-lysine coated or electrostatically charged.[52,53] The latter option is more convenient and effective but also more expensive.

Melanin Bleaching

The peroxidase label is usually visualized using diaminobenzidine (DAB) as chromogen, with the formation of dark brown granules. Pigments of similar color, such as melanin, when present in excessive amounts may interfere with correct interpretation of immunoperoxidase results. Treatment of the sections with potassium permanganate and oxalic acid before beginning the staining procedure appears to be the least damaging to stainable antigens and tissue morphology.[54] Alternatively, one could use a chromogen that produces a different color, or convert the color of melanin into blue by treating the section with Azure B.

Use of Previously Stained Slides

The consideration for performance of immunohistochemistry usually comes about after examination of routinely fixed and stained histologic or cytologic slides. If additional material is not available for immunohistochemistry (e.g., no tumor left in the paraffin block of a small biopsy), one can utilize the previously stained slides. Most cellular antigens can be detected in hematoxylin and eosin- or Papanicolaou-stained samples. Destaining of slides is not necessary. Protease digestion or heat-induced antigen retrieval should not be attempted unless the original slide was coated with proper adhesives. Immunohistochemistry can also be repeated on samples that have reacted negatively for other antigens.

Staining Procedure

Although immunoperoxidase staining is simple enough for any qualified technician to perform, it may harbor a potential pitfall in each step of the procedure. The following recommendations are intended for the improvement of staining results and prevention of technical mishaps during the procedure.

Clearing and Rehydration

These steps are for removal of the paraffin by a clearing agent such as xylene and rehydration of tissue sections by their immersion in decreasing grades of ethanol. Shortcuts in these steps will result in poor morphologic resolution of the final products. Clearing reagents are now on the market that can be used as alternatives to xylene. Their performance is comparable to xylene; their prices, however, are considerably higher.

Inhibition of Endogenous Peroxidase Activity

Endogenous peroxidase and peroxidase-like activity can be inhibited by several means. The technique most commonly used is immersion of the slides in a freshly prepared 1 : 4 solution of

3 percent hydrogen peroxidase in absolute methanol.[55] If it is not inhibited, the peroxidase and peroxidase-like activity of various cells may interfere with interpretation of stains, particularly in frozen sections. Some workers, however, choose not to block endogenous peroxidase and to use its activity as an internal control for evaluation of the chromogen reaction. When a heat-induced antigen retrieval procedure is used, the endogenous peroxidase activity will also be reduced.

Reduction of Nonspecific Background Staining

Nonspecific background staining of tissues, such as collagen, smooth and skeletal muscle, and certain mitochondrion-rich cells like hepatocytes and oncocytes, is a common nuisance of immunoperoxidase techniques.[41,45] These nonspecific background stains are more common when conventional polyclonal antisera are used. Some monoclonal antibodies, particularly those of mouse ascites origin, may also produce similar results. Preincubation of histologic sections with high concentrations of a protein solution, such as nonimmune serum or albumin, may reduce undesirable background staining, although ordinarily it cannot be avoided completely.[55] Use of the primary antibody in its highest possible dilution may also help reduce this unwanted reaction. Because of the increased sensitivity of the immunoperoxidase techniques in recent years as well as refinement of reagents and detection systems, background staining is no longer a major problem in most laboratories.

Antigen Retrieval

Aldehyde fixatives cause protein cross-linkages that may result in masking of many tissue antigens. Removal of these cross-linkages by various techniques have been shown to improve drastically immunohistochemistry of formalin-fixed histologic sections. Two common methodologies for unmasking tissue antigens are protease digestion and retrieval of antigens by heat.

Protease Digestion

Trypsin and other proteolytic enzymes have been used to enhance immunohistochemical reactions by unmasking antigens and increasing the contrast between the specific reaction and nonspecific background staining.[56] In addition to trypsin, pepsin, pronase, ficin, protease types VII, VIII, and XIV, collagenase, and DNase have all been used in immunohistochemistry.[57,58] Although antigen retrieval by heat is rapidly replacing protease digestion, a number of antibodies still perform best on predigested tissues. Before it is utilized in immunohistochemistry, several facts should be known about proteolytic digestion. First, enzymatic predigestion is not for all antigens; it may enhance detection of a few markers, but no enhancement or false negative staining may occur with a number of others.[59] Second, there is no universal optimal proteolytic enzyme. The choice of enzyme depends on the type of antigen (e.g., intermediate filaments), its location (cytoplasm, nucleus), and the type of fixative and embedding medium used. Trypsin, for example, is a good enzyme to enhance the immunohistochemistry of cytokeratins in formalin-fixed, paraffin-embedded tissues. It may, however, have an adverse effect on the demonstration of cytokeratins in ethanol-fixed tissues.[46] Third, different tissue antigens require different protease concentrations, temperatures, and incubation times for optimal performance. Finally, the length of the enzymatic digestion period should be adjusted to the extent of tissue exposure to the fixative. Tissue that has been fixed in formalin for several weeks requires a longer digestion period than those fixed for one or two days.[46]

Heat-Induced Antigen Retrieval

Although the underlying mechanisms are not completely understood, heating histologic sections in a buffer solution helps to recover the masked antigens for immunohistochemistry. There are three types of heating devices currently used for this purpose: microwave ovens, autoclaves, and pressure cookers.

Microwave Oven

Microwaves have been in use in histology laboratories for many years. They have primarily been utilized to facilitate, or accelerate, various histologic procedures including tissue fixation, impregnation, processing, and embedding, as well as to expedite different histochemical stains.[60] Shi and colleagues[61] were the first to report the use of the microwave oven in immunohistochemistry, demonstrating its remarkable contribution to localization of many tissue antigens. Their original buffer, lead isothiocyanate, has now been replaced by 0.01 M citrate buffer (pH 6).[62–64] In most cases, acceptable antigen retrieval can be obtained by irradiating the histologic sections in a citrate buffer for 4 to 10 minutes.[62–66] Considerable variation, exists, however, in the energy level of different microwave ovens. Furthermore, microwave ovens heat unevenly, resulting in cold and hot spots. The use of rotating trays and larger buffer volumes will reduce the uneven heating effect of conventional microwave ovens. Microwave ovens have now been designed specifically for histology laboratories. They heat more evenly, but their prices are much higher.

Autoclave and Pressure Cooker

Autoclaves and pressure cookers, alternative methods of heating, were introduced recently to circumvent some of the problems associated with microwave ovens.[67,68] They produce an evenly distributed heat with no violent boiling of buffer solutions. Pressure cooking, in particular, is relatively simple to perform and has the advantage of producing temperatures of up to 120°C without a significant loss of the buffer solution.

Incubation with the Primary Antibody

The optimal incubation time for most primary antibodies is 20 to 30 minutes at room temperature (20° to 22°C). Overnight (18 hour) incubation of sections at 4°C will increase the sensitivity of the procedure with some monoclonal antibodies. With the use of antigen retrieval systems, overnight incubations are no longer necessary.

Antibody Titration and Shelf Life

The optimal concentration of a primary antibody should be determined by applying serial dilutions of that antibody to several sections of a known positive tissue.[7] The slide with the best specific reaction and the least background staining reflects the optimal dilution for that antibody. Prediluted antibodies, such as those in commercial staining kits, are usually titrated for a tissue with an average amount of antigen and may not be suitable for tissues containing either more or less than that amount.

The stability and shelf life of most immunologic reagents used in immunohistochemistry are ordinarily indicated by the supplier. Although many antibodies perform well for many months or years beyond their suggested expiration dates, they ultimately lose their reactivities if stored at 4°C. Most frequently used reagents may be frozen in small portions and used after thawing. Frozen reagents have an indefinite shelf life, but repeated thawing and freezing diminishes their reactivity.[41,45]

Reagents

Monoclonal Antibodies

The use of conventional polyclonal antisera in immunohistochemistry has been drastically reduced in recent years in favor of utilization of monoclonal antibodies. Monoclonal antibodies are relatively easy to produce; they are also specific, with little batch-to-batch variation.[9] By contrast, because their reactivity is usually against an epitope rather than the whole antigen, they may result in lesser sensitivity of antigen detection in histologic sections. Today, however, because of the usage of various antigen unmasking techniques in immunohistochemistry, the sensitivity of most monoclonal antibodies is comparable to that of polyclonal antibodies. Since different types of antigens may share common epitopes, monoclonal antibodies may recognize and bind to a number of unrelated antigens. This specific pattern of cross-reactivity is best demonstrated by the apparent reactivity of certain monoclonal antibodies developed against lymphocyte antigens with cells of other lineages, such as epithelial cells. It should be remembered therefore, that monoclonal antibodies are generally epitope specific, and their use does not guarantee antigen specificity. Finally, occasional unexpected reactivities have been reported with some monoclonal antibodies that are prepared from mouse ascites fluid.[69] These nonspecificities are not observed, however, when supernatant from hybridomas of the same clone are used.

Detection Systems

Prepackaged combinations of various linking antibodies and peroxidase (or alkaline phosphatase) complexes are now commercially available. Many of these ready-to-use detection systems are of good quality and obviate the need for frequent titrations of secondary antibodies and peroxidase conjugates. The optimal incubation time for most of these detection complexes (such as ABC and streptavidin) is 30 to 60 minutes at room temperature.

Chromogenic Substrates

Chromogens are another important group of reagents in immunohistochemistry. DAB is the most widely used chromogen for the immunoperoxidase technique. It produces brown granules at the reaction site that are not soluble in organic solvents. The intensity of the reaction, therefore, remains unchanged for years in storage. Because of the suspected carcinogenicity of DAB, other chromogens for peroxidase have been introduced.[70] One of the most popular of these alternative chromogens is aminoethylcarbazole (AEC). It produces a cherry-red color that, unlike DAB, is soluble in alcohol and clearing reagents. Therefore, it requires special aqueous mounting media to coverslip the slides, which reduces the morphologic resolution of histologic sections. In addition, AEC-stained slides gradually lose their reaction intensity in storage. Since AEC is also a suspected carcinogen, there is no valid reason for its use as an alternative to DAB. Stable mixed solutions of DAB and hydrogen peroxide that can be reused during the course of several days are now being marketed in large volume containers. These relatively safe preparations reduce the risk of daily contact with DAB powder that may occur during weighing and solution preparation. Other chromogens for peroxidase are less popular because of technical difficulties that complicate their use.[71] Furthermore, many have the same disadvantages as AEC. All chromogens for peroxidase should be disposed of according to the supplier's instructions.

Signal Amplification

In an attempt to increase the sensitivity of immunohistochemical procedures, a variety of techniques have been described. In some of these methods, the steps of a given procedure are repeated two times or more, whereas in others a combination of two different techniques is recommended.[72,73] These combination techniques are generally more time consuming and may cause increased nonspecific background staining. More recently, a signal amplification method was introduced that is based on the peroxidase-catalyzed deposition of a biotinylated compound at the site of antigen-antibody reaction.[74,75] The precipitated compound provides many more biotin molecules for binding to the subsequent avidin-peroxidase complexes.

Color Enhancement

A number of metallic solutions can be used to enhance the color of DAB in positive cells.[76] We use a 1 percent cupric sulfate solution for 5 minutes. Others have used osmium tetroxide (toxic), nickel, or cobalt salts. Color enhancement is particularly useful for black-and-white photography.

Counterstaining

Hematoxylin is the most popular nuclear counterstain for immunoperoxidase-stained tissues. The choice of the type of hematoxylin depends on the type of chromogen used. Since AEC is soluble in organic solvents, it should be used with Mayer's hematoxylin, which is not alcohol based.[8] Also, when intranuclear antigens are being studied, the counterstain should be cytoplasmic. For localization of steroid receptors and p53 and Ki-67 proteins, for example, we first use cupric sulfate color enhancement and then counterstain the cytoplasm with fast green.

Staining for Two or More Antigens

Different immunohistochemical methods for concurrent localization of more than one antigen in the same tissue section have been described.[8] They result in the production of two or more colors, each of which signals the presence of a different substance. Although most of these techniques are relatively simple to perform, their routine use in diagnostic pathology has little practical value. Furthermore, the color of one chromogen may overshadow the other, and the recognition of double or triple staining in one cell or area could become difficult.

CYTOPATHOLOGIC SPECIMENS

In recent years, cytology has played an increasingly important role in the diagnosis of human diseases, particularly those of a neoplastic nature. In fact, cytologic specimens may be the only diagnostic samples available from a patient with cancer.[77] Many ancillary tests traditionally carried out on histologic material are, therefore, being performed on cytologic specimens. One such technique, immunocytochemistry, has already proved to be important in diagnostic cytopathology.[78–82]

Specimen Types

Immunocytochemistry can be performed on most cytologic samples, including exfoliated cells, effusions, and fine needle aspirations.[78] Filter preparations are not suitable, however, because filters absorb immunologic reagents and cause unacceptable background staining.[80]

Cytologic samples easily demonstrate cytoplasmic antigens. Localization of certain intranuclear antigens, however, may require additional steps to enhance the membrane permeability in imprints, smears, and centrifuged specimens. Pretreatment of slides with a 0.10 percent solution of Triton X-100 for 5 to 10 minutes will increase the permeability of the membranes, thus enhancing the sensitivity of the technique. Cytocentrifugation of cellular specimens with a high content of protein may produce a precipitated film over cellular material and decrease penetration of reagents into the cells. To prevent this effect, gentle washing of the cells before cytocentrifugation with a solution of phosphate-buffered saline is recommended. To reduce the detachment of cells during the immunoperoxidase procedure, we coat the slides with poly-L-lysine or use electrostatically charged slides. Cell block preparations are particularly well suited for immunohistochemistry.

Fixation

In cytology, the duration of fixation is more important than the type of fixative used. Good immunostaining results can be obtained by fixing cytologic samples briefly (2 to 5 minutes) in common fixatives such as alcohol or buffered formalin. Brief fixation is preferred, because longer exposure to fixatives (days or weeks) may decrease the sensitivity in detecting certain cellular antigens, such as plasma proteins and intermediate filaments.

As we discussed before, immunocytochemistry can detect most cellular antigens in previously fixed and Papanicolaou-stained samples. Destaining of slides is not necessary.

Immunocytochemical Procedure

Immunocytochemical methods for cytologic specimens are identical to those used in histology.[77,80] Cytologic samples, for example, could be included in a batch with histologic sections; no technical modifications are needed. We do not, however, recommend protease digestion for cytologic specimens, primarily because the process detaches cells from the slide. In fact, because fixation time is short, protease digestion is usually not needed to unmask antigens in cytologic samples. On the other hand, use of microwave or other heat-induced antigen retrieval techniques are quite acceptable and useful in cytologic specimens.[83]

AUTOMATED IMMUNOHISTOCHEMISTRY

Automation is an expected development for an analytic procedure such as immunohistochemistry which is composed of well defined steps and standardized variables such as volume, time, and temperature. The limiting factor for automated immunohistochemistry has always been the requirement for reagent volume control. Recent innovations have solved this important problem by using either capillary action or pipettes to deliver immunologic reagents to the glass slides.[84,85] The entire process is controlled by a computer.

The greatest advantage of automated immunohistochemistry is improved intra- and interlaboratory reproducibility of assays. The cost of automation includes initial instrument purchase price plus the higher cost of prepackaged reagents. If one opts for automated immunohistochemistry, the following questions should be answered. Is the instrument versatile enough to be used for other techniques (e.g., in situ hybridization)? Is the system closed (works only with its own prepackaged reagents), or open (can use other reagents)? Are all required steps performed by the machine, or must steps such as heating, antigen retrieval, and so forth be done before loading slides on the instrument? How user-friendly is the software? Finally, how much space will the machine occupy? Although cost saving is not usually significant when automated techniques are compared with the manual methods, the former are capable of completing significantly larger workloads in considerably shorter times.

CONTROLS

As with other immunologic techniques, the results of immunohistochemical reactions are not valid unless proper controls are used and evaluated in each procedure. For standard immunoperoxidase procedures, two important control slides should be included: a positive control and an antibody (negative) control.[41]

Positive Control

A positive control is a histologic section that is known to contain the antigen under study. For a negative reaction to be considered truly negative, the known positive slide must be positive. The use of positive controls of intermediate intensity is preferable, because they become negative if the sensitivity of the reaction is reduced. A strongly positive control may still be positive and thus cause a false negative interpretation of the case under study.

Antibody (Negative) Control

An antibody control should also be included in every immunoperoxidase procedure. Its negativity validates positive results. Replacement of the primary antibody on an adjacent slide by the same antibody preabsorbed with the antigen under study is the most reliable antibody control. In most instances, however, a more practical antibody control is used by replacing the primary antibody with either nonimmune serum or another antibody with a different specificity. The use of a buffer solution as a replacement for primary antibody is not acceptable.

Probably the most reliable controls in immunohistochemistry are internal (built-in) positive and negative controls.[45] These represent different components of the tissue under study that are expected to react either positively or negatively with the antibody used. The use of the intermediate filament vimentin has also been advocated as an internal control for the assessment of antigen damage in immunohistochemistry.[86] Since it is present in practically every tissue, absence of vimentin reactivity may indicate poor fixation quality.

Controls for linking antibodies, peroxidase complexes, and avidin-biotin reagents are not ordinarily included in routine immunoperoxidase staining. Similarly, sections of tissues known to be negative for the antigen under study are not required to be included in every procedure provided that the specificity of the antibody is predetermined. Panels of known negative and positive tissues, however, are an integral part of evaluation of the specificity of every newly acquired antibody. The specificity of antibodies can be conveniently and economically tested on multiple tissue samples embedded in a single paraffin block.[87,88] The multitissue approach simplifies the screening of newly developed monoclonal antibodies to a considerable degree. These methods also consume smaller amounts of antibody and other reagents compared with the conventional practice of using several different tissue sections.

For all cytologic samples, both the known positive and antibody controls should consist of cytologic specimens.[80] One can ensure the availability of known positive cytologic slides by organizing a file of imprints from normal and neoplastic tissues known to contain various antigens. For antibody controls, however, duplicate slides of the case under study may not be available. In that situation, two separate circles can be etched with a diamond pen in the same cytologic slide. The primary antibody is added to one circle, whereas the other is covered with the control reagent.

ANALYTICAL ASPECTS

Selection of Markers

Immunocytochemistry can be used both to classify and to prognosticate tumors. Choice of markers depends entirely on their purpose. For example, selection of appropriate immunostains for classifying tumors depends on several factors, including clinical findings, morphologic appearance of the lesion, the differential diagnosis, and, most importantly, the availability of markers for the entities within that differential diagnosis.

A reasonable differential diagnosis is based on the morphology of the tumor, the clinical information, and the probability of a certain neoplasm occurring in the patient's age group in that anatomic location. Using this information, two or more markers should be selected because most immunohistochemical markers are nonspecific and are found in more than one type of cell. When used in panels, however, these markers help in general categorization of tumors (e.g., epithelial, lymphoid). The number of antibodies used in a panel depends entirely on the breadth of differential diagnosis and preference of the pathologist. Generally, one or two antibodies are used as the main reagents, whereas additional antibodies play a confirmatory role.

Similarly, a wide choice of markers is now available for evaluating the biologic behavior of tumors. These include markers reflecting cell kinetics, markers of tumor invasion and metastasis, and those markers that are important for treatment, such as steroid receptors and products of drug-resistance genes.

Evaluation of Results

From the moment of examination of the routine stains to the time of interpretation of immunohistochemical reactions, the skill and experience of the pathologist are the most important factors determining the diagnostic value of the technique. The importance of these factors becomes even more evident when the results are evaluated and incorporated into the final diagnosis. An experienced observer is familiar not only with the characteristics of a true positive reaction but also with the possibility of variability of results and potential sources of technical and analytical errors.

True Positive Reaction

When DAB is used as a chromogen, a true positive immunoperoxidase reaction not only stains cells brown but has several characteristics as well, familiarity with which will help the observer avoid false positive interpretations. The most important quality of a true positive reaction is its heterogeneity in distribution within single cells, among a group of cells, or throughout a neoplasm. In individual cells, the crisp brown granules of DAB may occupy all of the cytoplasm, the perinuclear area alone, or simply one of the poles of a cell. Diffuse, pale brown, or a single-tone yellow staining of neoplastic cells is, in all likelihood, nonspecific.

The site of positive reaction within a cell is another clue to the specificity of the staining. Most immunohistochemical markers are localized in either intracytoplasmic or intranuclear locations. Simultaneous cytoplasmic and nuclear staining of variable proportions are seen with some viral antigens, neuronal enolase, and S-100 protein. In fact, in the absence of nuclear staining, one should question the validity of a positive reaction for S-100 protein. Distinctive patterns of the localization of antigens in certain normal and neoplastic cells will also help verify a true positive reaction. For example, familiarity with the characteristic perinuclear or punctate staining of small cell carcinoma for cytokeratins aids in separating it from a potential neospecific reaction.

Negative Reaction

True negative reactions are difficult to verify in immunohistochemistry, even when appropriate controls are used.[89] When faced with a negative immunohistochemical reaction, two explanations are possible: cells elaborate the antigen under study but we are unable to demonstrate it, or cells do not express the antigen.

When cells express an antigen and we are unable to demonstrate it by immunohistochemistry, we are dealing with a false negative result. A false negative reaction may occur because of a technical problem related to the specimen, fixation, processing, the procedure, or the reagents used, or because the sensitivity of the method is lower than the threshold necessary to detect trace amounts of an antigen. Technical problems leading to false negative results can be identified and corrected if appropriate positive controls, both built-in and external, are used and evaluated in each procedure. True negative reactions, however, are more difficult to prove, even when positive controls are positive; consequently, negative results in immunohistochemistry are not usually as meaningful as positive reactions.

Problems in Interpretation

The potential pitfalls of immunoperoxidase procedures can be divided into technical problems and errors in interpretation of results. The two, however, are closely related because any technical mishap will show up under the microscope eventually and may lead to problems in interpretation.[41] With refinement of methods and availability of high quality reagents, the technical problems of immunohistochemistry have decreased drastically in recent years. Problems associated with the technique's analytical aspects have shown a relative increase, however. These problems are particularly evident in smaller laboratories, where the test volume is insufficient for the observer to gain adequate experience in all aspects of the procedure.[44] Many of the potential technical problems of the immunoperoxidase technique were addressed before. Here, we briefly review some of the common causes of false positive and false negative interpretations.

False Positive Stains

Crushed cells, degenerated and necrotic cells, and histiocytes and macrophages all absorb reagents nonspecifically and may therefore lead to erroneous interpretation. This phenomenon is particularly common when conventional polyclonal antisera are used. Similarly, cells in mitosis, tumor giant cells, and neoplastic cells with active phagocytosis and cannibalism stain nonspecifically for a variety of antigens, particularly for circulating substances. Nonspecific staining is also seen in intermediate and superficial cells of keratinizing and nonkeratinizing squamous epithelia.

The free edges of histologic sections at times exhibit nonspecific positive reactions. Also, cells that float in fluids, such as body cavity effusions or the contents of vesicles or cysts, may show nonspecific membrane staining for antigens present in that fluid. Undissolved granules of DAB or other chromogens produce spots of nonspecific positive reaction in histologic sections. Passive diffusion of an antigen from tissues containing large amounts of that substance to adjacent negative cells is another source of false positive results.

Failure to block the activity of endogenous peroxidase may lead to nonimmunologic positivity of cells that possess peroxidase or peroxidase-like activity. False positive immunohistochemical results may also be seen when cells contain endogenous biotin. A vivid example of this phenomenon is reported in gestational endometrial glands in which peroxidase-labeled avidin compounds bind to the biotin present in their optically clear nuclei.[90]

False Negative Stains

It is not unusual to observe complete lack of staining for different antigens in tissues known to contain them in a condensed or consolidated form. For example, the keratin layer of skin, Russell bodies in plasma cells, and colloid in thyroid follicles may not stain for cytokeratin, immunoglobulins, or thyroglobulin, respectively. The inability of reagents to penetrate these solidified structures is the explanation for this phenomenon. This view is supported by the presence of a rim of positivity in their more penetrable peripheries and by enhancement of staining after protease digestion. Another cause of false negative staining in tissues known to contain the substance under study is the prozone effect. This occurs when the tissue contains unusually large concentrations of antigen to the extent that the antigen-antibody reaction does not take place unless the antibody is substantially diluted. A plasmacytoma, for example, may not stain for the expected immunoglobulin with usual concentrations of the antibody, whereas a lower concentration of the same antibody will produce satisfactory results. This phenomenon is more likely to be seen when polyclonal antisera are used.

Diagnostic Sensitivity and Specifity

The sensitivity of an immunohistochemical method is the smallest amount of an antigen that it can detect. This is usually represented by the lowest staining intensity that will distinguish the antigen from the background. Although current immunohistochemical techniques are sensitive enough to provide useful information about a variety of diagnostic problems, even the most sensitive methods have limits below which the reaction cannot be detected. On the other hand, supersensitive immunohistochemical methods may not be desirable for routine diagnostic use, simply because they increase the frequency of uncommon aberrant results (e.g., cytokeratin positivity in nonepithelial cells).

Although closely related, diagnostic sensitivity and technical sensitivity for detection of an antigen are not the same. No matter how sensitive a technique might be, one cannot achieve the highest diagnostic sensitivity if the target antigen is not uniformly expressed by all the cells or tissues that are expected to contain it. Therefore, in addition to the technical sensitivity, the diagnostic sensitivity is dependent on the pattern of distribution and the frequency of expression of an antigen.

The specificity of a diagnosis derived from the immunohistochemical staining for an antigen depends not only on the technical specificity but also on the specificity of that antigen for the suspected diagnosis. Therefore, no matter how specific the method and the antibody might be, one cannot achieve acceptable diagnostic specificity if the antigen is not specific for that diagnosis.

Technical specificity may also be discussed in terms of specificity of the method as well as of the antibody. Testing for the nonspecificity of the method is relatively simple; it is accomplished by omitting each reagent, one at a time, to pinpoint the source of the nonspecific staining. Although various methods exist for evaluating the specificity of an antibody, it must be recognized that in routine diagnostic pathology these additional tests are both cumbersome and impractical. In such instances, one relies not only on information provided by the commercial source of the reagents but also on other facts such as clinical history, histomorphology, histochemistry, and electron microscopy to validate the specificity of the results.

QUALITY ASSURANCE

Immunohistochemical methods are now an essential part of diagnostic anatomic pathology. By themselves, however, immunohistochemical tests do not have independent diagnostic significance and are regarded as ancillary techniques complementing clinical and morphologic observations.[44,91–93] Therefore, one cannot overemphasize the importance of the pathologist for recognizing the indication for performance of such assays and also including the results as elements of final diagnostic opinions.

Quality assurance in anatomic pathology is the process of ensuring that excellence is maintained in all components of care delivery to a patient. Since anatomic pathology tests do not produce quantitative values, development of a comprehensive quality assurance program in this discipline is challenging.[92] Nevertheless, quality assurance in anatomic pathology should address the control of the quality of a procedure such as immunohistochemistry, as well as the issues related to the pathologist's activities in utilizing the test results as a component of overall patient care.

Quality Control

Most quality control measures for immunohistochemistry are similar to those used in a conventional histology laboratory. They are, however, supplemented by specific methods required to control the quality of immunologic methods. Quality control standards in immunohistochemistry should therefore address every aspect of the procedure, from the moment tissue is obtained to the time the results are interpreted.

Maintenance of an acceptable turnaround time for immunohistochemical tests is of utmost importance in the overall patient management. Ordinarily, a laboratory should be able to complete most immunohistochemical stains within 24 to 48 hours. Long delays in performance of the stains and, hence, their late incorporation in the final report is contrary to the fundamental goal of providing physicians with accurate, timely, and clinically relevant diagnoses.

Finally, details of all technical and interpretational activities of an immunohistochemistry laboratory should be carefully recorded and maintained. Every change or modification in methodology or reagents must be clearly documented in the laboratory manual. Occurrence of any technical or analytical mishap and the means of its correction should also be adequately described and made available for future reference.

Reproduciblity of Results and Governmental Regulation

The need for improvement in standardization and reproducibility of immunohistochemistry has attracted the attention of pathology organizations and governmental agencies. A number of surveys on interlaboratory reproducibility of immunohistochemical stains have been conducted. The results of the first such study, by the College of American Pathologists, have shown more than 80 percent concordance between participating and reference laboratories.[94] Also, a number of pathology groups, along with the Biologic Stain Commission and the Food and Drug Administration, have been involved in the regulation of immunohistochemical reagents.[93–96] In fact, at the time of this writing, the Food and Drug Administration intends to classify most immunohistochemical reagents as class I medical devices, which require only proper labeling and vendors' adherence to good manufacturing practices.[97] Pathologists thus can use these reagents for clinical purposes according to their best medical judgment. A few "stand-alone" diagnostic immunohistochemical tests will, however, be categorized as either class II or III medical devices, requiring more rigorous documentation of their accuracy and precision.[97]

Role of the Pathologist

Pathologists are responsible for all aspects of the operation of efficient and reliable immunohistochemistry laboratories. It is advisable, even in smaller laboratories, that a single pathologist be placed in charge of daily operations, to monitor the technical performance consistently and ensure the quality of the results.[44] The director of an immunohistochemistry laboratory should also have hands-on experience at the bench level to be able to identify and correct potential technical problems that may occur. Furthermore, the pathologist should continuously evaluate the staining procedures and experiment with new reagents and techniques as they become available. The director of an immunohistochemistry laboratory must be completely familiar with the relevant literature on the applications of the technique and commit time to participate in the continuing educational activities devoted to this specialty.

Another important component of a comprehensive quality assurance program in immunohistochemistry is validation of results by the pathologist in charge. This can be accomplished internally by correlating the staining results with the patient's clinical history, prior histologic or cytologic findings, and the clinical follow-up. Although they are less practical, positive immunohistochemical stains could also be confirmed by electron microscopy or by molecular pathologic studies such as detection of mRNA expression or DNA amplification relevant to the protein product under study. Additionally, consultant immunohistochemistry laboratories could be utilized periodically to verify some of the diagnostic conclusions derived from immunostaining. This is particularly suitable for less experienced laboratories, since it helps them to gain experience and confidence.[44]

Finally, for the purpose of communication with the clinician and documentation of incurred charges, the result of all immunohistochemical stains should be included in every pathology report (either original or supplemental). It is the responsibility of the pathologist to incorporate *all* positive and negative staining results in the final report irrespective of their diagnostic significance.[98] This is particularly important for the exchange of information among pathology laboratories and for the accumulation of data on the predictive value of various immunohistochemical markers.

REFERENCES

1. Coons AH, Creech HJ, Jones RN: Immunological properties of an antibody containing a fluorescent group. Proc Soc Exp Biol Med 47:200–202, 1941
2. Singer SJ: Preparation of an electron-dense antibody conjugate. Nature 183:1523–1524, 1959
3. Zhdanoff VM, Azdova NB, Kulberg AY: The use of antibody labeled with an organic mercury compound in electron microscopy. J Histochem Cytochem 13:684–687, 1965
4. Avrameas S, Uriel J: Methode de marquage d'antigenes et d'anticorps avec des enzymes et son application en immunodiffusion. CR Acad Sci 262:2543–2545, 1966
5. Nakane PK, Pierce GB Jr: Enzyme-labeled antibodies: preparation and application for the localization of antigens. J Histochem Cytochem 14:929–931, 1966
6. DeLellis RA: Diagnostic Immunohistochemistry. Masson, New York, 1981
7. Nadji M, Morales AR: Immunoperoxidase Techniques. A Practical Approach to Tumor Diagnosis. American Society of Clinical Pathologists Press, Chicago, 1986
8. Taylor CR, Cote RJ: Immunomicroscopy: A Diagnostic Tool for the Surgical Pathologists. WB Saunders, Philadelphia, 1994
9. Wick MR, Siegal GP (eds): Monoclonal Antibodies in Diagnostic Immunohistochemistry. Marcel Dekker, New York, 1988
10. Elias JM: Immunohistopathology. A Practical Approach to Diagnosis. American Society of Clinical Pathologists Press, Chicago, 1990
11. Kohler G, Milstein C: Continuous culture of fused cells secreting antibody of predefined origin. Nature 256:495–497, 1975
12. Mullins JM: Overview of fluorophores. Methods Mol Biol 34:107–116, 1994
13. Holgate CS, Jackson P, Cowen PN, Bird CC: Immunogold-silver staining: new method of immunostaining with enhanced sensitivity. J Histochem Cytochem 31:938–944, 1983
14. Roth J, Saremaslani P, Warhol MJ, Heitz PU: Improved accuracy in diagnostic immunohistochemistry, lectin histochemistry and in situ hybridization using a gold-labeled horseradish peroxidase antibody and silver intensification. Lab Invest 67:263–269, 1992
15. Mason DY, Sammons R: Alkaline phosphatase and peroxidase for double immunoenzymatic labeling of cellular constituents. J Clin Pathol 31:454–460, 1978
16. Suffin SC, Muck KB, Young JC: Improvement of the glucose oxidase immunoenzyme technique. Use of tetrazolium whose formazan is stable without heavy metal chelation. Am J Clin Pathol 71:492–496, 1979
17. Taylor CR: Immunoperoxidase techniques. Practical and theoretical aspects. Arch Pathol Lab Med 102:113–121, 1978
18. Heyderman E: Immunoperoxidase techniques in histopathology: application, methods and controls. J Clin Pathol 32:971–978, 1979
19. Falini B, Taylor CR: New developments in immunoperoxidase techniques and their application. Arch Pathol Lab Med 107:105–117, 1983
20. Hammerling U, Aoki T, Wood HA, et al: New visual markers of antibody for electron microscopy. Nature 223:1158–1159, 1969
21. Sternberger LA: Some new developments in immunocytochemistry. Microskopie 25:346–361, 1969
22. Mason TE, Phifer RF, Spicer SS, et al: An immunoglobulin-enzyme bridge method for localizing tissue antigens. J Histochem Cytochem 17:563–569, 1969
23. Sternberger LA, Hardy PH Jr, Cuculis JJ, Mayer HG: The unlabeled antibody-enzyme method of immunohistochemistry. Preparation and properties of soluble antigen-antibody complex (horseradish peroxidase-antihorseradish peroxidase) and its use in identification of spirochetes. J Histochem Cytochem 18:315–333, 1970
24. Mason DY, Sammons RE: The labeled antigen method of immunoenzymatic staining. J Histochem Cytochem 27:832–840, 1979
25. Goding JW: Use of staphylococcal protein A as an immunological reagent. J Immunol Methods 20:241–253, 1978
26. Jasani B, Thomas DW, Williams ED: Use of monoclonal antihapten antibodies for immunolocalization of tissue antigens. J Clin Pathol 34:1000–1002, 1981
27. Warnke R, Levy R: Detection of T and B cell antigens with hybridoma monoclonal antibodies: a biotin-horseradish peroxidase method. J Histochem Cytochem 28:771–776, 1980
28. Hsu SM, Raine L, Fanger H: Use of avidin-biotin peroxidase complex (ABC) in immunoperoxidase techniques: a comparison between ABC and unlabeled antibody (PAP) procedures. J Histochem Cytochem 29:577–580, 1981
29. Sharma HM, Kauffmann EM, Conrad CM: An improved immunoperoxidase technique using horseradish peroxidase avidin D. Lab Med 20:109–112, 1989
30. Mason DY, Cordell JL, Abdulaziz Z, et al: Preparation of peroxidase:antiperoxidase (PAP) complexes for immunohistologic labelling of monoclonal antibodies. J Histochem Cytochem 30:1114–1122, 1982
31. Chaiet L, Wolf FJ: The properties of streptavidin, a biotin-binding protein produced by Streptomycetes Arch Biochem Biophys 106:1–5, 1964

32. Swanson PE, Wick MR: Commercial avidin-biotin-peroxidase complex kits. Am J Clin Pathol 91:S43–S44, 1989

33. Pedraza MA, Mason D, Doslu FA, et al: Immunoperoxidase methods with plastic-embedded materials. Lab Med 15:113–115, 1984

34. Suurmeijer AJ, Boon ME: Notes on the application of microwaves for antigen retrieval in paraffin and plastic tissue sections. Eur J Morphol 31:144–150, 1993

35. Dapson RW: Fixation for the 1990's: a review of needs and accomplishments. Biotech Histochem 68:75–82,1993

36. Miller HRP: Fixation and tissue preservation for antibody studies: a review. Histochem J 4:305–320, 1972

37. Puchtler H, Meloan SN: On the chemistry of formaldehyde fixation and its effect on immunohistochemical reactions. Histochemistry 82:201–204, 1985

38. Gown AM, Vogel AM: Monoclonal antibodies to human intermediate filament proteins. II. Distribution of filament proteins in normal human tissues. Am J Pathol 114:309–321, 1984

39. Bostwick DG, Al Annouf N, Choi C: Establishment of the formalin-free surgical pathology laboratory. Utility of an alcohol-based fixative. Arch Pathol Lab Med 118:298–302, 1994

40. Somogyi P, Takagi H: A note on the use of picric acid-paraformaldehyde-glutaraldehyde fixative for correlated light and electron microscopic immunocytochemistry. Neuroscience 7:1779–1783, 1982

41. Nadji M, Morales AR: Immunoperoxidase. Part I. The technique and its pitfalls. Lab Med 14:767–771, 1983

42. Bosman FT, Lindeman J, Kuiper G, et al: The influence of fixation on immunoperoxidase staining of plasma cells in paraffin sections of intestinal biopsy specimens. Histochemistry 53:57–62, 1977

43. Leathem A, Atkins N: Fixation and immunohistochemistry of lymphoid tissue. J Clin Pathol 33:1010–1012, 1980

44. Miller RT: Immunohistochemistry in the community practice of pathology. Part 1. General considerations, technical factors, and quality assurance. Lab Med 22:457–464, 1991

45. Nadji M: Immunoperoxidase techniques. Facts and artifacts. Am J Dermatopathol 8:32–36, 1986

46. Battifora H, Kopinski M: The influence of protease digestion and duration of fixation on the immunostaining of keratins. A comparison of formalin and ethanol fixation. J Histochem Cytochem 34:1095–1100, 1986

47. Login GR, Schmitt SJ, Dvorak AM: Rapid microwave fixation of human tissues for light microscopic immunoperoxidase identification of diagnostically useful antigens. Lab Invest 57:585–591, 1987

48. Mukai K, Yoshimura S, Anzai M: Effects of decalcification on immunoperoxidase staining. Am J Surg Pathol 10:413–419, 1986

49. Sato Y, Mukai K, Watanabe S, Goto M, Shimosato Y: The AMeX method. A simplified technique of tissue processing and paraffin embedding with improved preservation of antigens for immunostaining. Am J Pathol 125:431–425, 1986

50. Stein H, Gatter K, Asbahr H, Mason DY: Use of freeze-dried, paraffin-embedded sections for immunohistologic staining with monoclonal antibodies. Lab Invest 52:676–683, 1985

51. Prioleau J, Schnitt SJ: p53 antigen loss in stored paraffin slides. N Engl J Med 332:1521–1522, 1995

52. Mazia D, Schatten G, Sale W: Adhesion of cells to surfaces coated with poly-L-lysine. J Cell Biol 66:198–200, 1975

53. Huang WM, Gibson SJ, Facer P, et al: Improved section adhesion for immunocytochemistry using high molecular weight polymers of L lysine as a slide coating. Histochemistry. 77:275–279, 1983

54. Alexander RA, Hiscott PS, Hart RL, Grierson I: Effect of melanin bleaching on immunoperoxidase, with reference to ocular tissues and lesions. Med Lab Sci 43:121–127, 1986

55. Burns J: Immunohistochemical methods and their application in the routine laboratory. p.337. In Anthony PP, Woolf N (eds): Recent Advances in Histopathology. Churchill Livingstone, London, 1978

56. Curran RC, Gregory J: The unmasking of antigens in paraffin sections of tissue by trypsin. Experientia 33:1400–1401, 1977

57. Taschini PA, MacDonald DM: Protease digestion step in immunohistochemical procedures: ficin as a substitute for trypsin. Lab Med 18:532–636, 1987

58. Mauro A, Bertolotto I, Germano I, et al: Collagenase in immunohistochemical demonstration of laminin, fibronectin and factor VIII/RAg in nervous tissue after fixation. Histochemistry 80:157–163, 1984

59. Ordonez NG, Manning JT, Brooks TE: Effect of trypsinization on the immunostaining of formalin-fixed, paraffin-embedded tissues. Am J Surg Pathol 12:121–129, 1988

60. Boon ME, Kok LP, Ouwerkerk-Noordam E: Microwave-stimulated diffusion for fast processing of tissue: reduced dehydrating, clearing, and impregnating times. Histopathology 10:303–309, 1986

61. Shi SR, Key ME, Kalra KL: Antigen retrieval in formalin-fixed paraffin-embedded tissues: an enhancement method for immunohistochemical staining based on microwave heating of tissue sections. J Histochem Cytochem 39:741–748, 1991

62. Gown AM, de Wever N, Battifora H: Microwave-based antigenic unmasking. A revolutionary technique for routine immuno-histochemistry. Appl Immunohistochem 1:256–266, 1993

63. Leong ASY, Milios J: An assessment of the efficacy of the microwave antigen retrieval procedure on a range of tissue antigens. Appl Immunohistochem 1:267–274, 1993

64. Beckstead, JH: Improved antigen retrieval in formalin-fixed, paraffin-embedded tissue. Appl Immunohistochem 2:274–281, 1994

65. Cattoretta G, Suurmeijer AJH: Antigen unmasking on formalin-fixed paraffin-embedded tissues using microwaves: a review. Adv Anat Pathol 2:2–9, 1995

66. Taylor CR, Shi SR, Chaiwun B, et al: Strategies for improving the immunohistochemical staining of various intranuclear prognostic markers in formalin-paraffin sections: androgen receptor, estrogen receptor, progesterone receptor, p53 protein, proliferating cell nuclear antigen, and Ki-67 antigen revealed by the antigen retrieval technique. Hum Pathol 25:263–270, 1994

67. Bankflalvi A, Navabi H, Bier B, et al: Wet autoclave pretreatment for antigen retrieval in diagnostic immunohischemistry. J Pathol 174:223–228, 1994

68. Miller K, Auld J, Jessup E, et al: Antigen unmasking in formalin-fixed routinely-processed paraffin wax-embedded sections by pressure cooking: a comparison with microwave oven heating and traditional methods. Adv Anat Pathol 2:60–64,1995

69. Bonetti F, Pea M, Martignoni G, et al: False positive immunostaining of normal epithelia and carcinomas with ascites fluid preparations of antimelanoma monoclonal antibody HMB45. Am J. Clin Pathol 95:454–459, 1991

70. Sheibani K, Tubbs RR: Enzyme immunohistochemistry: technical aspects. Semin Diagn Pathol 1:235–250, 1984

71. Sheibani K, Lucas FV, Tubbs RR, et al: Alternitive chromogens as substitutes for benzidine for myeloperoxidase cytochemistry. Am J Clin Pathol 75:367–372, 1981

72. Lansdorp PM, Van der Kwast TH, DeBoer M, Zeijlemaker WP: Stepwise amplified immunoperoxide staining. I. Celluar morphology in relation to membrane markers. J Histochem Cytochem 32:172–178, 1984

73. Swanson PE, Hagen KA, Wick MR: Advin-biotin-antiperoxdase (ABPAP) complex. An immunocytochemical method with enhanced sensitivity. Am J Clin Pathol 88:162–176, 1987

74. Bobrow MN, Harris TD, Shaughnessy KS, Litt GJ: Catalized reporter deposition, a novel method of signal amplification: application to immunoassays. J Immunol Meth 125:279–285, 1989

75. Merz H, Malisuis R, Mannweiler S, et al: ImmunoMax. A maximized immunohistochemical method for the retrieval and enhancement of hidden antigens. Lab Invest 73:149–156, 1995

76. Hsu S-M, Soben E: Color modification of diaminobenzidine (DAB) precipitation by metallic ions and its application for double immunohistochemistry. J Histochem Cytochem 30:1079–1082, 1982

77. Nadji M, Ganjei P, Morales AR: Immunohistochemistry in contemporary cytology. The technique and its application. Lab Med 25:502–508, 1994

78. Nadji M: The potential value of immunoperoxidase techniques in diagnostic cytology. Acta Cytol 24:442–447, 1980

79. Li Cy, Lazcano-Villareal O, Pierre RU, Yam LT: Immunocytochemical identification of cells in serous effusions. Technical considerations. Am J Clin Pathol 88:696–706, 1987

80 Nadji M, Ganjei P: Immunocytochemistry in diagnostic cytology. A 12-year perspective. Am J Clin Pathol 94:470–475, 1990

81. Lidang Jensen M, Johansen P: Immunocytochemical staining of serous effusions: an additional method in routine cytology practice? Cytopathology 5:93–103, 1994

82. Masood S: Prognostic and diagnostic implications of estrogen and progesterone receptor assays in cytology. Diagn. Cytopathol 10:263–267, 1994

83. Reynolds GM, Young FI, Young JA, et al: Microwave oven antigen retrieval applied to the immunostaining of cytopathology specimens. Cytopathol 5:345–358, 1994

84. Tubbs RR, Bauer TW: Automation of immunohistology. Arch Pathol Lab Med 113:653–657, 1989

85. Grogan TM: Automated immunohistochemical analysis. Am J Clin Pathol 98:S35–S38, 1992

86. Battifora H: Assessment of antigen damage in immunohistochemistry. The vimentin internal control. Am J Clin Pathol 96:669–671, 1991

87. Battifora H: The multitumor (sausage) tissue block: novel method for immunohistochemical antibody testing. Lab Invest 55:244–248, 1986

88. Miller RT: Multitumor "sandwich" blocks in immunohistochemistry. Simplified method of preparation and practical uses. Appl Immunohistochem 1:156–159, 1993

89. Nadji M: The negative immunocytochemical result: what does it mean? Diagn Cytopathol 2:81–82, 1986

90. Yokoyama S, Kashima K, Inoue S, et al: Biotin-containing intranuclear inclusions in endometrial glands during gestation and puerperium. Am J Clin Pathol 99:13–17, 1993

91. Heyderman E, Warren PJ, Haines AMR: Immunohistochemistry today: problems and practice. Histopathology 15:653–658, 1989

92. Rickert RR, Maliniak RM: Intralaboratory quality assurance of immunohistochemical procedures. Recommended practices for daily application. Arch Pathol Lab Med 113:673–679, 1989

93. Elias JM, Gown A, Jaffe E, et al: Quality control in immunohistochemistry: report on a workshop sponsored by the Biological Stain Commission. Am J Clin Pathol 92:836–843, 1989

94. Wold LE, Corwin DJ, Rickert RR, et al: Interlaboratory variability of immunohistochemical stains. Results of cell marker survey of the College of American pathologists. Arch Pathol Lab Med 113:680–683,1989

95. Taylor CR: Quality assurance and standardization in immunohistochemistry. A proposal for the annual meeting of the Biological Stain Commission, June, 1991. Biotech Histotech 67:110–117, 1992

96. Taylor CR: Report of the Immunohistochemistry Steering Committee of the Biological Stain Commission. "Proposed format: package insert for immunohistochemistry products." Biotech Histotech 67:323–328,1992

97. CAP Today, Volume 10, March 1996

98. Banks PM: Incorporation of immunostaining data in anatomic pathology reports. Am J Surg Pathol 16:808, 1992

6

Molecular Diagnostic Techniques

Massimo Loda
Ronald A. DeLellis

Decoding the instructions carried by the linear arrangements of the four nucleotides of DNA has been a daunting task since the discovery of DNA structure in 1953.[1] Akin to the discovery of microorganisms at the beginning of the century, advances in molecular biology and genetics have had a profound impact on the elucidation of several human diseases that had thus far eluded understanding. The precise definitions of the structural and functional defects that lie at the basis of human diseases are radically changing the approach to the diagnosis, prevention, and therapy of most of these ailments.

The development of increasingly more sophisticated instrumentation, such as DNA synthetizers and sequencers that are amenable to automation, and the global endeavor of the Human Genome Project, are providing detailed chromosomal maps so that sequences and markers from every region of all chromosomes are being made available for use.[2] The use of these nucleic acid probes to study disease processes defines molecular pathology. Molecular diagnostics is thus the application of this concept to all areas of pathology.

The technologic application of molecular biology spans all fields of anatomic, surgical, and cytopathology. Specific applications include microbiology, infectious diseases, transplantation and transfusion medicine, and inherited genetic disorders, including single gene defects, chromosomal disorders, and multifactorial diseases such as atherosclerosis, diabetes, or cancer. Molecular diagnostics is intimately associated with traditional genetics, particularly cytogenetics. This is especially true in the field of oncology, where, for instance, acquired chromosomal abnormalities such as translocations have led to the discovery of several oncogenes associated with distinct clinicopathologic entities.

This chapter deals with the aspects of molecular diagnostics that have direct applicability in surgical and cytopathology and includes (1) a brief overview of the fundamentals of molecular biology; (2) the genes implicated in pathogenetic mechanisms of cancer, infectious disease, inherited disorders, and transplantation; and (3) the diagnostic applications of molecular biology in experimental and diagnostic pathology.

BACKGROUND

DNA-RNA-Protein

DNA encodes the genetic information in all organisms. DNA is made up of two complementary, antiparallel strands of nucleotide bases aligned on a deoxyribose phosphate backbone; these strands run opposite to one another and exhibit molecular complementarity (Fig. 6-1). This means that the nucleoside adenosine (A) always pairs with thymidine (T), whereas guanosine (G) does so with cytosine (C). The molecular complementarity of the base pairs represents the cornerstone of recombinant DNA technology. Coding DNA, which is ultimately translated into proteins, represents less than 5 percent of the 3 billion nucleotides that comprise the human genome. It is arranged in the chromosomes as genes interspersed by noncoding regions of DNA. An estimated 100,000 genes are present in human DNA, organized and distributed among the 46 chromosomes.

Genomic coding DNA is translated into the 20 amino acids, a process that is mediated via the transcription of the relatively unstable intermediate single-stranded messenger RNA (mRNA). This differs from DNA by a uracil (U) residue in place of thymidine. RNA transcription is capable of significant amplification of the signal it encodes. The final product of a gene is the assembly of the amino acids into functional proteins.

Most of the variability among individuals occurs in noncoding eukaryotic DNA. This variability, known as genetic polymorphism, can be ascribed to length variation of repetitive sequences present in multiple copies throughout the genome. Simple sequences are present in tandem arrays called satellites or microsatellites according to their lengths.[3] The length of a set of satellites is unique to each individual. DNA fingerprinting used in forensic pathology utilizes probes to these regions or amplification of these sequences with polymerase chain reaction (PCR) to genotype and match specimens. Microsatellites

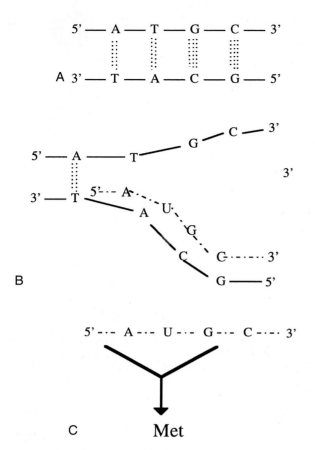

Fig. 6-1. Transcription and translation of DNA. **(A)** Double-stranded (ds) DNA. **(B)** Transcription. **(C)** Translation. Sense and antisense, antiparallel strands of DNA (double-stranded DNA) show complementarity between cytosine (C) and guanine (G) as well as between thymine (T) and adenine (A) bases. Dotted lines show hydrogen bonds. RNA is transcribed off the antisense DNA strand. The unique base of RNA, uracil (U), is chemically very similar to thymine (T) in that it specifically base pairs with adenine. In the process of translation, the RNA molecule serves as template for the amino acids that will form proteins.

constitute one of the most abundant classes of repetitive DNA in the human genome. Alleles at these sites are stably inherited and are now one of the most useful classes of genetic polymorphic sequences used in linkage analysis.[4] In addition, several tumor types display alterations in microsatellite sequences, a phenomenon known as microsatellite instability.[5–10] This is often due to malfunctioning of DNA repair enzymes (see below).

Another class of repeated DNA sequences is that of short interspersed elements, which are present in thousands of copies in each genome but do not differ significantly from individual to individual. The most abundant short interspersed element is that of the Alu repeats.

Recombinant DNA Technology

The basis of the ability to manipulate nucleic acids in vitro is molecular hybridization, or the complementary base pairing between two nucleic acid strands. Key to this ability is the use of enzymes that modify nucleic acids by cutting DNA at predetermined loci (restriction endonucleases), reattach loose ends (ligases), or synthetize identical copies to the template (DNA and RNA polymerases). Since RNA is unstable, another important enzyme, reverse transcriptase, allows the generation of a copy of an RNA molecule into complementary DNA (cDNA). These fragments of isolated DNA can then be inserted into highly replicating units of other organisms such as bacterial plasmids, amplified, and expressed. Recombinant DNA technology allows the isolation and subsequent indefinite amplification of a single gene from a background of "contaminating" DNA. The subsequent study of gene function and regulation is thereby greatly simplified.

Molecular Hybridization

Hybridization is defined as the process of duplex (double-stranded) molecule formation that occurs between the target DNA or RNA and its complementary nucleic acid probe. Hybridization can be accomplished in solution (e.g., PCR), on solid support such as nitrocellulose or nylon membranes (e.g., Southern blots), or at the cellular and subcellular levels (in situ hybridization). Fundamental to the correct performance and interpretation of hybridization assays is the concept of stringency, which is defined as the number of mismatched nucleotides tolerated in the probe-target hybrid. The higher the stringency, the lower the number of tolerated mismatches. The principal physical and chemical components that increase the stringency of a hybridization reaction include high temperature, high concentration of organic solvents such as formamide, and low salt concentration.

Probes

Nucleic acid probes are segments of DNA or RNA of variable length that may be labelled either radioisotopically or with a variety of nonisotopic reporter molecules and revealed with a color reaction. In addition, photon-emitting, chemiluminescent molecules may be utilized. The isotopes most frequently used are ^{32}P for filter hybridization and ^{35}S or, more recently, ^{33}P for in situ hybridization.[11] In routine molecular diagnostics nonisotopic probes are rapidly replacing radiolabeled probes, particularly in commercially available kits, because they are generally easier to manipulate, have a long shelf life and low cost, and do not require radioisotopic containment facilities.

The types of probes that can be utilized range from short (up to 50 bp) single-stranded, synthetic oligonucleotides, to complementary RNA probes of intermediate size (commonly ranging from 200 to 800 bp in length), to long (one to several thousand bases in length) double-stranded DNA probes.

Single-stranded DNA oligonucleotide probes are primarily used in PCR reactions, in allele-specific filter hybridization assays for the detection of point mutations, and in in situ hybridization.[12] They can be custom synthetized if the target sequence is known without the need of obtaining a cloned fragment of the gene of interest. Moreover, their cost is relatively low. If appropriately stringent conditions are used, oligonucleotides can detect even single base pair mismatches either in the PCR assay[13,14] or in filter hybridization,[15] making these probes ideal for screening assays. Disadvantages include the limited number of reporter molecules that can be tagged onto them, resulting in a low signal/noise ratio, and the narrow window between specific signal and loss of it.

RNA probes (riboprobes) are synthetized in vitro with RNA polymerase from cloned DNA templates inserted in transcription-efficient plasmids (Fig. 6-2). Riboprobes, particularly suited for use in in situ hybridization, are used in RNAse protection assays that detect mismatches and are sometimes used in Northern hybridization. The advantages of riboprobes, particularly in in situ hybridization assays, include the elevated incorporation of reporter molecules in a longer stretch of nucleotides, the greater stability of target RNA-riboprobe hybrids compared with DNA-RNA hybrids, and the ability to digest with ribonuclease (RNAse) unhybridized, single-stranded, labeled probe fragments. This results in a significant decrease in background. In addition, when riboprobes are compared with oligonucleotide probes in in situ detection, their intermediate length, while not inhibiting entrance into cells, affords a greater likelihood of hybridization to stretches of RNA that remain available for binding after tissue processing. Disadvantages of riboprobes include RNA instability (diminished shelf life) and the extreme susceptibility to ubiquitous RNAses, requiring special measures when handling slides and glassware.

Finally, DNA probes are longer (typically 1 to 3 kb), and are labeled by either random priming or nick-translation methodologies.[16] They are particularly suitable for use in solid support hybridization assays as well as in fluorescent in situ hybridization (FISH).

Filter Hybridization

Filter hybridization entails the detection by a specific probe of target DNA or RNA sequences previously bound in an irreversible fashion to a solid substrate. Genomic DNA can be irreversibly bound to a nitrocellulose or a nylon filter and hybridized with a labeled probe directed toward the gene of interest. With this technique, called dot-blot hybridization, one can assess the number of copies of a given gene, when the intensity of the hybridization signal at various dilutions is compared with that of a known standard.

Another technique used in the assessment of gene copy number is Southern blot hybridization, in which DNA is cut at specific sites by restriction endonucleases prior to gel elec-

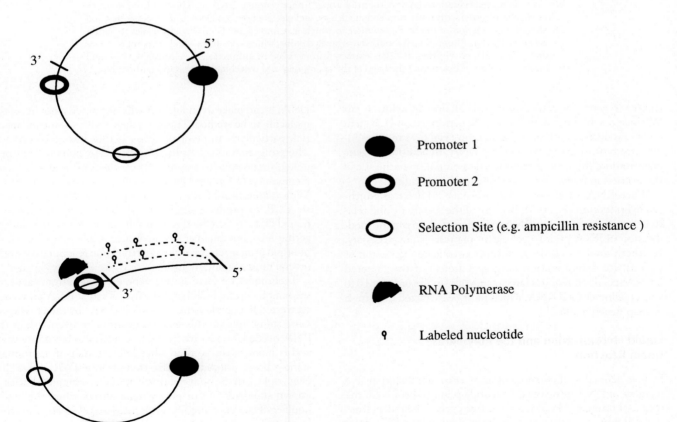

Fig. 6-2. Generation of riboprobes. The recombinant DNA of interest to be used as probe is inserted into a bacterial plasmid and flanked by promoters of RNA polymerase. The bacterial DNA has a selection site to allow preferential growth of the recombinant plasmid. To generate the riboprobe, the plasmid is first linearized, i.e., cut on the opposite end of the promotor to be used and then a labeled complementary copy of the insert is generated by RNA polymerase. The antisense (3′ to 5′) riboprobe synthetized is then able to hybridize to the sense (5′ to 3′) native target.

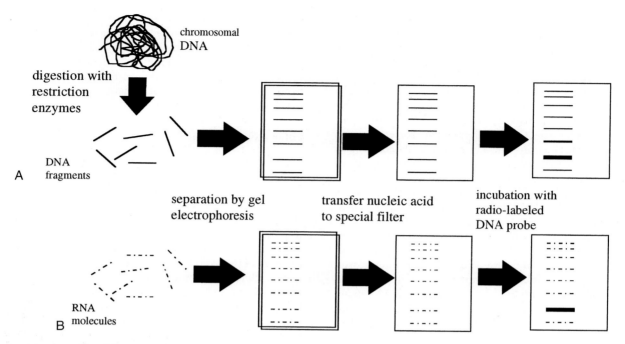

Fig. 6-3. Filter hybridization. (A) Southern blotting. Intact genomic DNA is extracted from tissue or cultured cells, digested with restriction endonucleases, and electrophoresed. DNA is then denatured and transferred onto a nylon or nitrocellulose filter to which it is irreversibly bound by ultraviolet radiation ("cross-linked"). The filter is then hybridized to a labeled probe, which reveals the band of appropriate size (arrow). (B) Northern blotting. RNA is extracted from tissue or cultured cells, electrophoresed, and transferred to a filter. Detection of the band of the appropriate size is accomplished as in Southern blot.

trophoresis and transferred onto nitrocellulose or nylon filters. Whereas dot-blot hybridization can be performed on PCR-generated products, Southern hybridization (Fig. 6-3) requires intact (fresh or snap-frozen) genomic DNA. In addition to gene quantitation, this assay permits the determination of the size of the restriction fragment to which the probe hybridizes.

When RNA is the target, the technique is known as Northern hybridization (Fig. 6-3). Because of the specificity and relatively small size of each mRNA to be detected, enzymatic modification of RNA prior to gel electrophoresis is not necessary. Northern analysis allows quantitation of gene expression as well as size determination (i.e., specificity) of the targeted mRNA species. It requires large quantities (in the order of 10 to 15 μg) of intact total RNA, which must be extracted from fresh or snap-frozen material.

Liquid Hybridization and the Polymerase Chain Reaction

PCR is defined as the exponential in vitro amplification of a segment of DNA using oligonucleotide primers specific for the region of interest.[17] PCR is a repetitive cycle of heat denaturation of DNA, annealing of the primers flanking the DNA fragment to be amplified, and extension of the annealed primers by thermostable DNA polymerase to synthetize an identical molecule (Fig. 6-4). The reaction results in the exponential amplification of the target fragment. By allowing preferential synthesis of a single segment of DNA on the background of extraneous

DNA, it can make available virtually unlimited amounts of the molecule to be studied. The scant availability of starting material, particularly in cytopathology, is thus less of an obstacle when this technique is utilized for diagnostic purposes. Furthermore, it is possible to amplify short segments of genomic, complementary, or foreign DNA extracted from archival material. Many Variants of PCR suit specific needs, including asymmetric PCR to produce single-stranded DNA for sequencing, nested PCR to increase the sensitivity of the reaction when targeting low copy number genes,[14] or multiplex PCR in which multiple primer sets are utilized in the same reaction to amplify several targets simultaneously.[18]

Techniques for quantitating gene expression from small tissue samples utilize PCR amplification of target RNA previously converted to complementary DNA (cDNA) by the enzyme reverse transcriptase. This method utilizes one-twentieth of the RNA needed for a Northern blot, is much less labor intensive, and is more sensitive than filter hybridization if appropriate standards are utilized. Reverse-transcriptase-PCR (RT-PCR) (Fig. 6-4) can be semiquantitative (i.e., compared with a known standard[19,20]) or purely quantitative when the actual number of copies of amplificant is measured.[21,22] The standards or controls used in semiquantitative RT-PCR can either be internal to the reaction (competitive PCR) or run side by side.[22] The nucleic acid molecules used as standards in the reaction should ideally be of approximately the same size and have the same primer-binding sequence to minimize preferential amplification of either the target or the control as a function of dif-

Generation of first strand cDNA (RT)

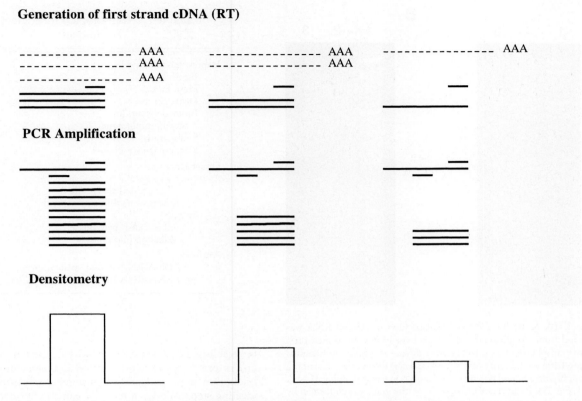

PCR Amplification

Densitometry

Fig. 6-4. Polymerase chain reaction PCR and quantitative PCR. Total RNA (dotted lines) is extracted from either tissue or cells, utilizing oligo-dT, random primers, or, as in this cartoon, specific antisense primer complementary to the gene of interest. A thermostable DNA copy (solid line) of the mRNA is synthetized using the enzyme reverse transcriptase. The specific upstream primer is added and the segment is amplified by PCR. Semiquantitation or pure quantitation (depicted by the histogram) of the gene of interest is then accomplished by one of several techniques. One such method is shown here: using serial dilutions of starting RNA, results are compared with RT-PCR of a housekeeping gene such as alpha-tubulin. Alternatively, an internal control (e.g., a plasmid containing a similar sequence) can compete in the PCR reaction with the target sequence, and the results are expressed as a ratio of the two PCR products.[23] Finally, liquid hybridization of the amplified product with a tagged internal probe can be quantified by electrochemiluminescence, which can detect targets at the attomole (10–12) level.[21]

ferent stringencies. An additional control can be a gene expressed constitutively by the cells or tissue to be tested to serve as an internal control reflecting sample integrity.[22] RT-PCR can also be applied to paraffin-embedded tissue.

Quantitative PCR has a variety of diagnostic applications, including assessing expression of oncogenes,[20,23] tumor suppressor genes, neuroendocrine peptide hormones, cytokines,[23] and RNA viruses such as the human immunodeficiency virus,[24,25] as well as hepatitis C virus and cytomegalovirus in transplant patients specifically to monitor efficacy of therapy[14,26–29] (Fig. 6-5).

In Situ Detection

In situ hybridization (ISH) is used to localize DNA and RNA at the cellular level. The method involves the localization on tissue sections or cytologic preparation of labeled RNA or DNA molecules that hybridize with complementary target DNA or RNA sequences in the cell.[30] The technique was originally developed by two independent groups in 1969.[31,32]

Oligonucleotides, cDNAs, or riboprobes may be labeled with ³H, ³²P, ³⁵S, or ³³P and detected by autoradiography. ³³P permits markedly reduced film or emulsion exposure without apparent loss of resolution. The use of ISH techniques to study gene expression has grown in the last few years with the development of nonisotopic detection methods. Nonradioactive hybridization methods require that the probe contain a reporter molecule (Table 6-1) introduced chemically or enzymatically to render it detectable by affinity cytochemistry. Nonisotopic methods offer significant advantages including high probe stability, safety, essentially no waste disposal problems, and a level of sensitivity approaching isotopically labeled probes in some instances. A number of different types of nucleic acid probes can be prepared for use in ISH: double-stranded DNA, single-stranded DNA, oligonucleotides, and single-stranded antisense (complementary) RNA types. In general, DNA probes are less

A.

B.

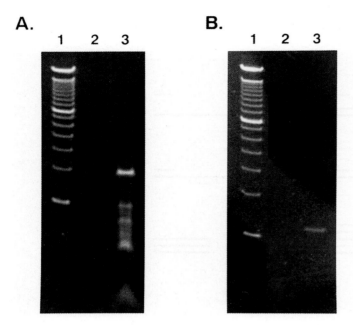

Table 6-1. Nonisotopic Probe Labeling Techniques

Hapten modified probes
Biotin
Photobiotin
Digoxigenin
Bromodeoxyuridine
Acetylaminofluorene
Sulfonation
Mercury trinitrophenyl
Direct labeling
Fluorochromes
Tetramethylrhodamine
Fluorescein thiosemicarbozide
Enzymes
Horseradish peroxidase
Alkaline phosphatase
Antibodies
Anti DNA-RNA hybrid antibodies
Anti RNA-RNA hybrid antibodies

Fig. 6-5. **(A & B)** RT-PCR of hepatitis C virus (HCV) RNA was extracted from paraffin-embedded core liver biopsy performed on a patient transplanted for end-stage liver disease secondary to hepatitis C-related disease. Integrity of RNA was assessed by reverse transcribing and amplifying a housekeeping gene (G protein subunit alpha, 205 bp, lane 3, Fig. A). Recurrence of hepatitis in the graft was confirmed by RT-PCR with specific primers to the 5′ noncoding region of the HCV RNA virus (115 bp, lane 3, Fig. B).[14] One hundred base pair molecular weight markers are run in lane 1 (Figs. A and B). The no reverse transcriptase negative controls are run simultaneously (lane 2, Figs. A and B).

sensitive than RNA probes and are used in high copy number target systems, for example, viral DNA, or when a high labeling efficiency is required to visualize single targets as in FISH. RNA probes are preferentially used in applications in which the target is in low copy numbers and is thus particularly suitable for mRNA detection. The FISH technique allows localization of chromosomal sequences, including genes (Fig. 6-6). It is a recent development of conventional cytogenetics that allows identification of translocations, deletions, loss of heterozygosities, assessment of gene amplification, and assignment of genetic loci to newly cloned genes.[33–36] FISH is especially effective when performed on touch imprints.[35] Numerous probe types are available for FISH analyses. These include tandem repeat (centromeric or a satellite) probes, which are useful for assessing chromosome copy number. Regional or locus-specific probes are useful for identification of translocations, amplifications, and deletions, while whole chromosome probes (painting probes) are useful for identifying structural rearrangements. FISH is particularly valuable in the assessment of chromosomal alterations in solid tumors, which are less amenable to conventional cytogenetic analysis.[37] FISH forms the basis of a new discipline of cytogenetics defined as molecular cytogenetics.

Important conditions to obtain optimal in situ labeling may

be established experimentally by varying the type and length of probes, pretreatment steps, duration and temperature of the hybridization step, stringency, and number of posthybridization washing steps. We have recently gained considerable experience with the use of a new, computerized, barcode-controlled instrument, the Ventana Gen II, which performs fully automated ISH including FISH, immunohistochemistry, or a dual-staining combination of ISH and immunohistochemistry on up to 40 slides simultaneously. With the use of this instrument all the variables outlined above can be tightly controlled, with resultant increased reproducibility, reduced hybridization time, and diminished labor.[38]

ISH techniques have been used successfully to localize oncogenes such as N-*myc*, c-*myc*, or c-*erb*-B2 in tumor cells.[39] In addition, messenger RNAs for hormones have been localized in endocrine tumor cells in the absence of the protein product of the same gene as assessed by immunohistochemistry. For example, most null cell adenomas of the pituitary gland have been shown to express the alpha chain of glycoprotein hormones.[40] Hormone receptors can also be demonstrated effectively by ISH. Moreover, this technique is useful to distinguish nonspecific uptake of hormones from hormone synthesis. The relationship between nucleic acid targets and submicroscopic cellular structures can be studied when ISH is applied at the ultrastructural level.[41]

The level of sensitivity of ISH when conditions and tissue preparation are optimal is about 20 copies per cell.[42] In recent years strategies to improve the threshold of detectable copy number for each cell has resulted in the development of a technique known as in situ PCR, which entails amplification via the PCR of target sequences (DNA or RNA) at the cellular level prior to ISH (indirect in situ PCR).[42–51] Prior to PCR amplification cells need to be permeabilized to allow reagent entry. Amplification can then be performed on either cells in suspension or glass slides. In the direct, less specific method,

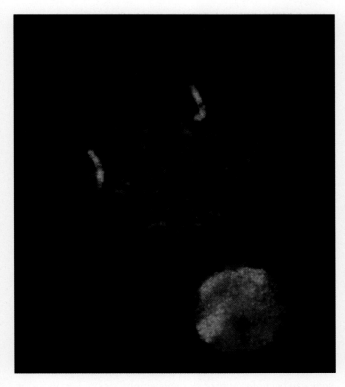

Fig. 6-6. Fluorescent in situ hybridization (FISH). Human peripheral leukocytes were separated over a Ficoll gradient and the white cells cultured to maximize the number of mitotic figures. Hybridization was performed in an automated instument (Ventana Medical Systems, Tucson, AZ) with Spectrum Green-labeled chromosome 1 whole chromosome paint. (Courtesy of Maria Pallavicini and Maija Wessman, University of California, San Francisco, CA and Ron Zeheb, Ventana Medical Systems, Tucson, AZ.)

labeled nucleotides are directly incorporated in the amplified product. In the preferable indirect method, ISH with a labeled probe is performed after amplification of the target is completed. Applications of this technique include detection of microorganisms, especially viruses, single copy genes, and chromosomal translocations. The methodology is not perfect to date. It is of paramount importance to have rigorous controls to interpret results correctly because of the ease with which false positive results are obtained. Mispriming by both endogenous fragmented DNA acting as PCR probes or repair of fragmented DNA in archival tissues can give rise to nonspecific signals. Results obtained on cells in suspension are still superior to those in paraffin-embedded tissue. A RT in situ PCR has also been described. Routine clinical application still awaits resolution of the obstacles mentioned above.

Tissues

As a result of more effective screening and sophisticated diagnostic techniques (e.g., mammography or prostate-specific antigen serum levels for breast and prostate carcinoma, respec-

tively) cancers are being detected at an earlier stage, and tumor size at primary diagnosis is constantly diminishing (as many as 30 percent of breast cancers seen in our institution are <1 cm in diameter), while tumor tissue is used for an increasing number of markers for prognostic assessment. It follows that the amount of tissue available for molecular studies is ever so much smaller.

To circumvent this problem, archival tissue can be utilized for molecular analyses. DNA and RNA can both be successfully extracted from paraffin-embedded tissue utilizing sequential steps of deparaffinization, protein digestion, and removal of non-nucleic acid material by organic extraction.[13,52–54] RNA obtained from archival material is amenable to RT to generate cDNA (Fig. 6-5). Genomic DNA, cDNA, or foreign (e.g., viral) DNA can then be amplified by PCR, provided the target fragments are kept small (optimally up to 400 bp in length). This is necessary because of nucleic acid fragmentation in tissue processing.[12,13] Less stringent conditions are also required for the DNA polymerase to synthetize an intact complementary strand from the discontinuous template nucleic acid fragments of the target.

Animal Models

Animal models of human disease form the basis of experimental pathology and provide the best paradigm for the assessment of molecular findings in routine pathology practice. Two models for the study of gene function as it relates to human diseases are transgenic and knockout animals.

Transgenic animals are defined as those in which foreign DNA (usually a human gene) is introduced into fertilized cells and is subsequently inherited in the progeny of the host. They provide the means to explore complex biologic functions of a given gene in vivo.[55] The inserted gene can become integrated in the host genome at several chromosomal sites. By virtue of the way in which the construct is designed, it can be overexpressed in all tissues when transcription is driven by a strong constitutive promoter (e.g., cytomegalovirus promoter), or its expression can be restricted by tissue-specific or developmentally regulated promoters.[56,57]

Knockout mice provide the ideal experimental setting when it is important to assess the consequences of loss of function of a gene. Standard knockout mice are made by specifically inactivating the gene of choice in embryonic stem cells. These are then injected into the mouse embryo, where they have the potential to develop into the different cell types. As in transgenic mice, the inactivated gene is carried in the germline and passed to the progeny. A major problem is death in utero, when, as is often the case, the gene turns out to be essential for normal development. To overcome this problem genes may be selectively knocked out using cell type-specific gene targeting.[58]

Models of several human diseases have been produced by such gene targeting, including Gaucher's disease, cystic fibrosis, Huntington's disease, and fragile X syndrome.[59–63] In addition, gene targeting has been extended to overexpression of mutated oncogenes,[64,65] mismatch repair genes,[66,67] and complex genetic diseases in which environmental and genetic influences both play a pathogenetic role, such as atherosclerosis.[68]

MOLECULAR PATHOLOGY OF CANCER

The role of molecular pathology in cancer diagnosis is focused on assessing mutations in oncogenes and tumor suppressor genes (both somatic and germline), determining overexpression of oncogenes or loss of function for suppressor genes, assessing clonality, and determining susceptibility to cancer by tracing genes or chromosomal regions closely linked (in recombination) to yet unidentified genes by means of linkage analysis.

Clonality

Assessment of clonality is especially useful when evaluating borderline lesions such as atypical lymphoid proliferations, atypical hyperplasias of breast and endometrium, or thyroid follicular nodules. In these settings a polyclonal population of cells would be indicative of benign polyclonal hyperplasia while a clonal one would point to a neoplastic process.

Many methods have been used to demonstrate clonality in tissues, including analysis of karyotypic abnormalities, gene rearrangements or translocations, point mutations in oncogenes and tumor suppressor genes, viral sequences such as the terminal repeat episomal sequence of the Epstein-Barr virus, microsatellite instability, loss of heterozygosity, and, most importantly, dosage compensation. Dosage compensation is the process whereby the level of X-linked gene expression is equalized between sexes by methylation of either the maternal or paternal allele.[69] X-chromosome inactivation assays (which can be utilized only in females) have utilized methylation-dependent restriction fragment length polymorphisms, as well as a variety of probes, including glucose-6-phosphate dehydrogenase, phosphoglycerate kinase 1, and the androgen receptor genes, all of which are located on the X chromosome.[70–73] The choice of the gene in the assessment of clonality, to be clinically useful, must take into account the degree of polymorphism of the locus in the population. The proportion of clonal cells in the tissue to be examined should be at least 20 percent. To apply this principle to tissue sections or cytologic preparations in which the pathologist is able to select dysplastic cells or areas of broderline malignancy, the simple technique of selective ultraviolet radiation fractionation can be applied.[52] This method consists of protection of pathologic areas of interest from ultraviolet radiation, which nicks and inactivates nucleic acids, on a histologic or cytologic slide, and subsequent extraction of DNA from the selected and relatively pure population of cells for PCR amplification and analysis.

A different approach used in the assessment of clonality is the concomitant use of multiple molecular techniques. This approach has recently been utilized in establishing the monotypic nature of Reed-Sternberg cells, which, because of their relative rarity, have escaped isolation in sufficient quantities.[74] In the study by Inghirami et al,[74] a combination of immunohistochemistry, interphase cytogenetics, static cytometry, and mutation analysis of the p53 gene contributed to defining unique and individualized DNA profiles of Reed-Sternberg cells, which remain constant over time.

Oncogenes and Tumor Suppressor Genes

In 1970 Rous sarcoma virus was shown to carry a gene able to transform a normal cell into a cancer cell. Shortly thereafter this gene, called src, was shown to be present in normal cells.[75,76] This finding definitively implicated genes in the pathogenesis of cancer. It also suggested that other retroviruses might derive their transforming properties from the acquisition of cellular genes involved in the normal regulation of growth: the proto-oncogenes. Since then over 70 oncogenes with transforming properties and 12 tumor suppressor genes have been identified to date.

Proto-oncogenes are highly conserved and are important in cellular pathways involved in growth and differentiation. They acquire the ability to transform normal cells as a result of a mutational event occuring in a critical portion of the gene. Only one of the two alleles needs to be mutated to confer (dominant) oncogenic properties to that gene. Many oncogenes, including src, have been found to be tyrosine kinases, enzymes that phosphorylate proteins on tyrosine residues, and thus act as regulatory proteins. Most oncogenes identified thus far are part of the cell's growth regulatory pathways and range from growth factors to their receptors, intracellular signal transducers, and nuclear transcription factors.

The activation of oncogenes is associated with increased expression of their protein products. Overexpression of an oncogene can occur because of genomic amplification, juxtaposition to strong viral or tissue-specific promoters controlling its transcription (e.g., following a translocation event), or by constitutive (deregulated) expression that follows a mutational event.

The assessment of oncogene mutations or overexpression may have both diagnostic and prognostic utility. For instance, assessing copy number of the N-myc oncogene, whether by ISH, dot-blot hybridization, or FISH, helps in staging childhood neuroblastoma.[33,77] Overexpression of c-erb-B2, or neu, is correlated with poor prognosis in breast carcinoma.[77–81]

Since many proto-oncogenes are tyrosine kinases, it follows that the function of such proteins involved in pathways of growth and differentiation can be modulated by reversible phosphorylation.[82,83] Several oncogenes, including c-erb-B2 and epidermal growth factor receptor, commonly amplified in breast and bladder cancers, transmit signals through the proto-oncogene ras, leading to the activation by phosphorylation of one or a pair of 42 to 44 kd mitogen-activated protein (MAP) kinases.[78–81,84] ras itself is constitutively activated by point mutations in as many as 30 percent of human cancers.[85] MAP kinase activation is thus a central step in tumor growth stimulation by the most widely expressed and activated human oncogenes. Among the targets of MAP kinases are other kinases, nuclear transcription factors, and other proteins with roles in cell cycle activation, which ultimately relay the information to the nucleus.[86]

Phosphatases are enzymes whose function is the dephosphorylation of other proteins including proto-oncogenes. Since their action opposes that of kinases, they are crucial proteins in the maintenance of an equilibrium in processes of cellular growth, differentiation, and death.[83] A novel family of phosphatases has been identified that inactivates MAP kinase by dephosphorylating both threonine and tyrosine residues.[87]

These enzymes have a similarity to cdc25, a protein that controls cell entry into mitosis, and are called *MAP kinase phosphatases* (MKP).[88] Homologues from yeast to humans have been isolated, a testimony of their conservation and importance through evolution.[89–92] The human prototype of MKPs, MKP-1, is the product of immediate early genes induced by the same agents that regulate MAP kinase activity.[93] We recently showed by ISH that MKP-1 was overexpressed early in the carcinogenic pathway in prostate, colon, breast, bladder, and lung tumors (Fig. 6-7), with progressive loss of expression with higher grade and stage. Aggressive tumors with poor prognosis (hepatocellular and pancreatic) express little or none of this phosphatase. MKP-1 may thus be a regulatory checkpoint in cancers that are activated by oncogenes encoding upstream components along the MAP kinase cascade, such as *ras*, as well as an early marker for a wide range of human epithelial tumors. MKP-1 may thus have both diagnostic and prognostic significance.[94] Furthermore, we found that the human homologue of another dual-specificity phosphatase, the cell cycle regulator cdc 25, is overexpressed at the mRNA level in breast carcinomas with poor prognosis[95] (Fig. 6-8). This ISH finding complemented the in vitro data pointing to the oncogenic role of this gene in tumors.

Tumor suppressor genes code for proteins whose loss of function results in transformation. For this to occur both alleles must be inactivated. When one allele is inactivated in the germline, such a genotype is transmitted to all somatic cells, rendering them more susceptible to a second mutational event on the remaining functional allele. This results in a greater predisposition to cancers in families carrying such germline mutations.[96–100] Since germline mutations are present in all cells, comparison with DNA extracted from normal tissue is important in the assessment of the inactivation of the second allele in tumor DNA. Germline inactivation of a tumor suppressor gene is often the result of gross rearrangements occurring in the region where the gene is located. Studies determining loss of heterozygosity play an important role in the discovery of such genes as well as in genetic linkage analysis.[101] Two of the most intensely studied tumor suppressor genes are the retinoblastoma (*Rb*) and the p53 genes. Hereditary retinoblastoma serves as a prototype of hereditary human cancer.[98] Retinoblastoma develops in about 90 percent of those who harbor an inactivating mutation at this locus. In addition, *Rb* hereditary inactivating mutations have been implicated in the development of other types of tumors, including osteosarcomas, soft tissue tumors, small cell carcinoma of the lung, and breast and bladder cancers.[102] DNA polymorphisms within the retinoblastoma gene can be used to determine the risk of cancer in affected kindreds.[98]

Sporadic mutations in the p53 tumor suppressor gene, most often occurring late in carcinogenesis, are the single most common genetic alteration observed in human cancer.[103,104] In addition, germline p53 mutations confer predisposition to cancer.[99,100] Finally, cancers tend to develop over three to six month periods in p53 knockout mice.[105–107]

Rearrangement of chromosomes resulting in translocations, insertions, or deletions may result in oncogene activation or inactivation of suppressor genes. Microinsertion/deletions of DNA, or single base-pair changes represented by transitions or transversions (point mutations), may also cause oncogene activation or render a suppressor gene inoperative. This occurs as a result of amino acid substitution (missense mutations), premature truncation of message and protein (nonsense mutations), altered reading frame due to frameshift mutations with altered amino acid sequence downstream of the mutation, or aberrantly spliced RNA due to mutations in sequences at intron-exon junctions important for RNA splicing. As a result of these events, the biologic properties of the gene product may be altered.

Since mutations play such an important role in cancer and inherited genetic diseases, it follows that highly conserved mechanisms whose role is to maintain genetic integrity should be in place in normal cells. The molecular machinery responsible for the maintenance of genetic integrity was discovered in *Escherichia coli* in 1976.[108] Yeast and human homologues of these enzymes have recently been demonstrated; their fundamental role in human cancer is underscored by two findings.[109,110] Microsatellite instability is frequently demonstrated in several human cancers of diverse tissue origin, and, more importantly, inherited cancer syndromes such as the autosomal

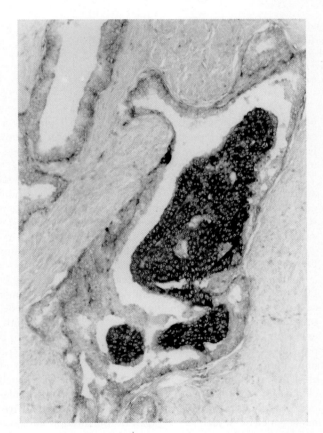

Fig. 6-7. Ribroprobe in situ hybridization for MKP-1 in prostate carcinoma. A paraffin section of an invasive cribriform carcinoma of the prostate was hybridized with a digoxigenin-labeled antisense riboprobe for MKP-1. Detection of the signal was accomplished by nitroblue tetrazolium (NBT). Note intense cytoplasmic positivity of tumor cells growing within a normal duct that expresses the gene only in basal cells.

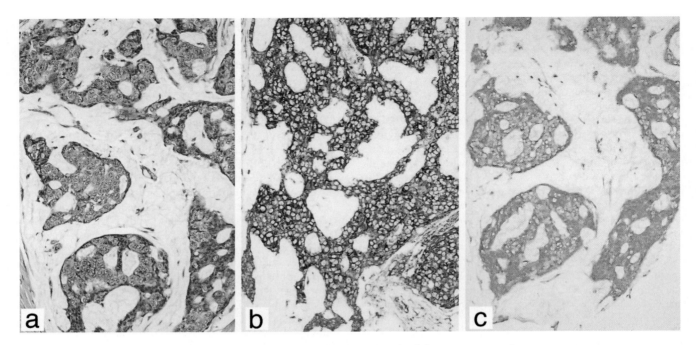

Fig. 6-8. (a–c) Riboprobe in situ hybridization for cdc 25 A and B in breast carcinoma. Invasive, mucin-producing breast carcinoma probed on an automated in situ hybridization instrument (Ventana ES, Ventana Medical Systems, Tucson, AZ) with antisense RNA probes to cdc25 A (overexpressed, Fig. b) and cdc25 B (no expression, Fig. c). In spite of high homology (60 percent) between isoforms A and B, with appropriate stringencies the hybridization reaction is specific. (Fig. a, hematoxylin and eosin.)

dominant hereditary nonpolyposis colon cancer syndrome have been found to harbor defects in mismatch repair genes.[9,109–111] These genes, *hMsh*1 and -2 and *hPMS*1 and -2, seem to be inherited as recessive genes in that normal cells in patients who inherit an altered allele show low mutability, whereas when both copies are inactivated in tumors, the result is hypermutability.[9,108,109] Mouse models with targeted disruption of the *Msh*2 gene display an increased predisposition to cancer, particularly lymphomas.[67]

Gene Rearrangements

Hematopathology has undoubtedly contributed the most significant advances in the understanding of oncogenesis. This is a consequence of important discoveries by molecular biologists that contributed to elucidation of the development and function of the immune system and also because pure populations of neoplastic hemopoietic cells became available.

Diagnostic molecular hematopathology takes advantage of two events that take place in hematopoietic oncogenesis: gene rearrangements and chromosomal translocations. The former has been used as a marker of clonality, whereas the latter result in activations of proto-oncogenes with the production of chimeric oncoproteins. Techniques aimed at identifying these genetic events provide additional clinically relevant data for the diagnosis and classification of lymphoid neoplasms beyond the knowledge that can be obtained with immunophenotyping. Immunoglobulin and T cell receptor genes are frequently in-

volved in chromosomal aberrations since they are physiologically rearranged to generate active antigen-receptor proteins. Furthermore, they may be utilized diagnostically in the assessment of clonality of lymphoid lesions.

The immunoglobulin or T cell receptor genes, or both, rearrange at the DNA level prior to clonal expansion in lymphoid cells. Exons encoding the variable (V), diversity (D), constant (C), and joining (J) regions of these molecules are linearly located on a stretch of genomic DNA. One of each of these regions randomly recombines after the intervening noncoding DNA is spliced out. Since a given rearrangement is unique to a committed cell and its derivative clone, Southern blotting or PCR techniques (able to detect as little as 0.8 percent of tumor cells in a background of normal/reactive cells[112]) are used to detect clonal populations in either fresh or archival tissues, otherwise undetectable by immunohistochemical methods. This is particularly useful for the analysis of T cell neoplasms, since no immunophenotypic markers are available for assessment of clonality. It is important to bear in mind that even though clonality is most often correlated with cancer, clonal populations of lymphoid cells can be detected in patients with immune deficiencies such as postorgan transplantation immunosuppression or the acquired immunodeficiency syndrome in the absence of overt malignancy.[113] When interpreting results of gene rearrangement studies, it is therefore very important to analyze the results in the context of morphologic, immunophenotypic, and clinical data.

Aside from assessing clonality, gene rearrangement studies can be useful in assigning lineage derivation of neoplasms of uncertain classification. For instance, gene rearrangement studies have shown that certain lymphomas failing to express immunophenotypic markers of either B or T cell lineage (so-called null cell lymphomas) are of B cell lineage.[114]

Translocations

Translocations and inversions have long been recognized by cytogeneticists. Distinct translocations in both hematologic and solid tumors result either in the activation of proto-oncogene products or, more frequently, in the translation of novel tumor-specific fusion proteins.[115] These proteins are often transcriptional factors. Since these fusion proteins are specific markers for individual subtypes of neoplasias, they are both potential targets for therapy design and ideal markers for the detection of minimal residual disease.

The Philadelphia chromosome in chronic myelogenous leukemia led to the discovery of the $210^{bcr/abl}$ tyrosine kinase oncogene. The retrovirally encoded *bcr/abl* gene has subsequently been shown to induce chronic myelogenous leukemia in irradiated experimental animals, thus establishing a firm pathogenetic role for this protein in the genesis of this disease.[116,117]

The translocation t(11;14)(q13;q32) results in overexpression of the putative oncogene cyclin D1 (*bcl*-1) in 30 to 50 percent of intermediate (mantle cell) lymphocytic lymphomas[118,119] as detected by Southern hybridization and, more recently, in up to 94 percent of these neoplasms when PCR-based methods are used.[120] The presence of this translocation has resulted in reclassification of some cases of small lymphocytic lymphomas as intermediate lymphomas.

Over 90 percent of follicular lymphomas have a t(14;18)(q32;q21) translocation in which the *bcl*-2 gene is moved under the control of the IgH promoter during the early stages of pre-B development.[121] The *bcl*-2 proto-oncogene codes for a protein that localizes to the inner mitochondrial membrane and whose major function is inhibition of apoptosis.[122,123] Since the *bcl*/JH breakpoints on the chromosome are tightly clustered, the chimeric sequence is easily amenable to amplification with PCR. This technique has been used to detect minimal residual disease in bone marrow before autologous transplantation.[124]

Another classic translocation in lymphoid malignant tumors is the t(8;14)(q24;q32) of Burkitt's lymphomas, in which the c-*myc* oncogene is juxtaposed to the immunoglobulin gene, resulting in its constitutive activation.[115] The importance of c-*myc* overexpression in the pathogenesis of B cell lymphomas is underscored by the similar molecular findings in Burkitt's lymphoma in acquired immunodeficiency syndrome (AIDS) patients.[125] and by the development of B cell lymphomas in transgenic mice that carry DNA sequences from a breakpoint junction of an 8;14 translocation in their germline.[126]

The t(2;5) translocation is typical of anaplastic large cell (Ki-1-positive) lymphomas. The resultant chimeric protein consists of the N-terminal portion of nucleophosmin fused to the kinase domain of a novel transmembrane tyrosine kinase named ALK.[127–129] Hodgkin's lymphomas, by contrast, do not harbor this translocation.[129] PCR amplification of the nucleophosmin/ALK locus may thus be of value in distinguishing cases in which borderline morphology between the two entities occurs. In addition, Downing et al[130] found that neither anaplastic morphology nor Ki-1 expression predicted the presence of this molecular lesion in a series of 21 high grade lymphomas including immunoblastic and diffuse large cell types. These results suggest that the t(2;5) translocation may define a distinct genetic subgroup of high grade lymphomas with variable histology and immunophenotype.

The presence of a t(15;17) is diagnostic of acute promyelocytic leukemia (PML). It results from the chimeric fusion of two genes, the retinoic acid receptor alpha and the PML gene.[131] Since responsiveness to trans retinoic acids depends on the presence of this translocation, its detection by RT-PCR is of paramount importance in routine clinical practice. The assay is also used in the detection of minimal residual disease.[132] Long-term survival seems to be associated with eradication of PML/retinoic acid receptor alpha as detected by RT-PCR.[133–134]

INFECTIOUS DISEASES

Diagnostic molecular microbiology applies the principles of nucleic acid hybridization to the detection and characterization of pathogenic microorganisms associated with infectious disease. PCR-based methods are replacing media-based biologic amplification. Fastidious organisms or viruses such as hepatitis C virus (HCV), which cannot be cultured, are now targets of molecular techniques. Finally, new organisms are being identified by molecular methods and their association with human diseases elucidated.

Molecular identification of microorganisms is especially useful (1) to avoid misinterpretation of false positive serology due to the presence of cross-reacting antibodies to host antigens or to antigens of related organisms, (2) to identify pathogenic organisms prior to seroconversion, (3) to follow therapeutic response to therapy (4) to identify mutations responsible for drug resistance, (5) to subtype different strains in related members of a genus, and (6) for the rapid and accurate identification of organisms that require elaborate and long media-based cultures.

Mycobacterial infections have recently resurfaced as diseases with significant clinical impact; they have a mortality of 60 percent if left untreated.[135] The diagnosis of tuberculosis has been complicated by an increase in the frequency of mycobacterial infections in immunocompromised patients. Inadequate treatment of many patients has led to an increase in the proportion of patients with drug-resistant strains of *Mycobacterium tuberculosis*.[136] Microscopic diagnosis of acid-fast bacilli is time consuming, non-species-specific, and insensitive, especially in treated patients.[137] Culture of such organisms requires weeks, resulting in delays in therapy or inappropriate treatment of unaffected individuals. Molecular diagnostics can thus play an important role in adequate and timely treatment as well as in patient follow-up. Species-specific PCR for mycobacteria can be performed on a variety of samples including sputum and paraffin-embedded tissue.[138–139] PCR is both very sensitive and specific when results are compared with bacteriologic and clinical data.[137]

Human papillomavirus has been strongly implicated in the pathogenesis of cervical, vulvar, anal, and penile cancer by several cytologic, epidemiologic, and molecular biology studies.[140–143] The methodology of choice in the detection of the carcinogenic subtypes is, however, still controversial.[143,144] Subtype-specific ISH probes are commercially available. With appropriate stringencies, carcinogenic subtypes such as human papillomavirus 16 may be detected in paraffin-embedded tissue specimens[145] (Fig. 6-9).

Epstein-Barr virus (EBV) is a double-stranded DNA herpesvirus that can persist in latent form in both epithelial cells and B lymphocytes. In most cases, EBV infection results in a self-limiting, transient lymphoproliferative disorder. In immunosuppressed states, however, such as human immunodeficiency virus (HIV) infection or in therapeutic immunosuppression following organ transplantation, reactivation of latent infection may contribute to the development of full-blown cancers. Initially EBV drives the cell to become activated. The virus then blocks further differntiation, committing the cell to indefinite T cell independent proliferation. EBV has thus been implicated in the pathogenesis of several neoplasms, including

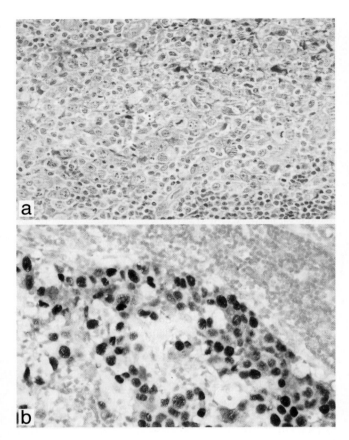

Fig. 6-10. Oligonucleotide probe in situ hybridization of Epstein-Barr early RNA (EBER) in Ki-1 lymphoma. **(a)** Hematoxylin and eosin stain of anaplastic, large cell (Ki-1-positive) lymphoma. **(b)** Automated in situ hybridization for EBER using digoxigenin-labeled oligonucleotides (cocktail of two probes). Note intense nuclear staining of tumor cells.

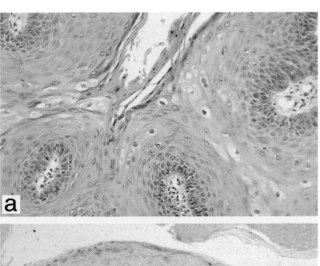

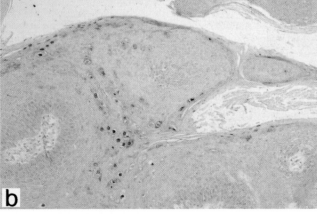

Fig. 6-9. DNA probe in situ hybridization of human papillomavirus HPV 16 in penile condyloma. **(a)** Hematoxylin and eosin stain of penile lesion showing koilocytotic change and parakeratosis. **(b)** Automated in situ hybridization with HPV 16 digoxigenin-labeled DNA probe. Note nuclear localization of viral DNA in nuclei of koilocytotic cells.

Burkitt's lymphoma, undifferentiated nasopharyngeal carcinoma, Hodgkin's disease, and post-transplantation lymphomas. As is the case for most microorganisms, a variety of techniques, including ISH and PCR, can be utilized to assess the presence of the actively replicating virus. EBV has been found in a subset (40 to 50 percent) of AIDS-related lymphomas and in most primary lymphomas of the central nervous system.[146,147] EBV DNA detection in cerebrospinal fluid by PCR is 100 percent sensitive and 99 percent specific in the diagnosis of central nervous system lymphomas.[148] The terminal repeat regions of the virus have been used as markers of clonality in angiocentric immunoproliferative lesions.[149] Nonisotopic ISH for Epstein-Barr early RNA can be easily accomplished in paraffin-embedded tissues using oligonucleotide primers (Fig. 6-10). Molecular detection of the EBV genome in lymphomas arising in immunocompromised patients may alter therapeutic strategies.

HCV is a small, positive-stranded RNA virus, approximately 10 kb long, considered to be the major causative agent of non-A, non-B hepatitis.[150] Several antibody tests of increasing specificity have been developed to diagnose infection or immunity or both to the disease. Patients who are infected with HCV may take as long as five months to seroconvert.[151] Antibody-based tests have, therefore, a limited utility in the diagnosis of acutely infected patients as well as in the follow-up of seropositive patients transplanted for hepatitis C. Although immunohistochemical and molecular tissue localizations of HCV have occasionally been reported, the viral titer in most tissue specimens available is quite inferior to the sensitivity of antibody-based assays or molecular hybridization assays without prior amplification.[152,153] We recently found that 27 percent of anti-HCV antibody-positive patients were negative by RT-PCR, whereas less than one percent of seronegative patients were PCR positive.[14] End-stage liver disease caused by HCV is the reason for as many as 30 percent of orthotopic liver transplantations (OLT) in some centers, including our own. We recently assessed HCV recurrence after OLT by nested RT-PCR in serum and liver of 41 patients with OLT, 32 of whom were transplanted for HCV or hepatitis B virus-related disease or for both. Results were compared with liver function tests, liver histology, and antibody status. Recurrent HCV (60 percent overall) was associated with mild to moderate hepatitis.[14] These results demonstrated that molecular techniques are mandatory to determine graft reinfection after liver transplantation and showed that HCV recurrence is usually associated with only mild to moderate hepatitic changes compatible with graft survival.

HIV is a retrovirus that causes a chronic and fatal disease in humans. One of the theories put forth to explain how HIV evades the immune system is the extremely low levels of gene expression in the circulating mononuclear cells it infects, even during "clinical latency."[154] Detection and precise quantitation of viral load by quantitative PCR techniques is extremely important in following antiviral therapeutic regimens in these patients. In fact, a positive correlation exists between clinical stage and absolute level of viral replication.[155] The sensitivity of quantitative PCR techniques for detecting HIV can be as high as one proviral molecule in 80,000 cells.[23] PCR techniques are also used to detect the virus prior to seroconversion or in newborns of seropositive mothers in whom maternal circulating anti-HIV antibodies interfere with serologic diagnosis.[156]

GENETIC DISEASES

A genetic variation that has no clinically relevant phenotypic effect is known as a polymorphism. The analysis of DNA polymorphism in the context of a population forms the basis of the study of genes causing inherited diseases. During meiosis, pairs of homologous chromosomes exchange equivalent segments. It follows that alleles close together on the same chromosome are more likely to be transmitted together during meiosis. When polymorphic loci are linked to mutant alleles or to as yet unidentified genes, they may be used in tracing families by means of linkage analysis and eventually mapping, identifying, and cloning the gene of interest (positional cloning). A prime example has been the linkage of the early-onset type of familial breast cancer to chromosome 17q21,[155] which resulted in cloning of the breast and ovarian cancer susceptibility gene BRCA 1, inherited mutations of which have been identified in five of eight kindreds studied.[156–158]

The role of genetics in clinical practice resides in its impact in the etiology of an ever increasing number of diseases. Genetic disorders can be broadly subdivided into three categories: (1) single gene defects such as cystic fibrosis, Huntington's disease, or muscular dystrophies; (2) chromosomal abnormalities such as aneuploidy, resulting in Down's syndrome; and (3) complex diseases such as atherosclerosis, diabetes, and cancer, which recur in families with patterns that are not strictly mendelian, in which environmental factors variably affect multifactorial genetic traits.

Cystic fibrosis is an autosomal recessive disorder that results from mutations in the CFTR gene. It is characterized by abnormal mucus production, which results in recurrent pulmonary infection and pancreatic insufficiency. Whereas inheritance of the diseased gene can be traced by polymorphic markers, molecular testing usually by PCR and allele-specific hybridization (ASO) of the over 200 disease-associated mutations has become a significant challenge.

Unstable trinucleotide repeats, which are highly polymorphic in the normal population, are responsible for Huntington's disease, fragile X syndrome, and myotonic dystrophy, among others.[159] Expansion of these repeats to a critical length results in full expression of the disease phenotype. PCR or Southern blots may be utilized in their detection. For Huntington's disease, knockout models have provided clues to suggest that the human disease involves a gain of function of the encoded *Hdh* gene.[60,61]

Because of the consequences that molecular test results have on affected patients and their progeny, molecular genetic testing has great influence on ethical issues that go beyond the mere ability to apply the technology.

TRANSPLANTATION

Transplantation of organs such as liver, which is rich in leukocytes of bone marrow origin and precursor dendritic cells, results in the ubiquitous and long-term persistence of these cells in recipient tissues. Persistence of multilineage leukocyte chimerism has been associated with long-term acceptance of transplanted organs.[160] In addition, the ratio of polymorphic DNA markers between donor and recipient plays a major role in the assessment of donor cell engraftment after bone marrow transplantation.[21,161,162] Molecular methods used in the detection of host cells include flow cytometry, FISH for the Y chromosome in female recipients, immunostaining for HLA markers, and PCR amplification of either Y chromosome or HLA sequences.

Typing by HLA methods using molecular techniques achieves a more precise donor-recipient match with subsequent increased potential for graft survival. Molecular HLA matching also provides a research tool to investigate MHC disparity and transplant complications. Molecular typing methods include sequence-specific amplification, hybridization with oligonucleotide probes, heteroduplex formation, and direct nucleotide sequencing. Data thus far available suggest that some HLA disparities may be tolerated, whereas others are highly immunogenic in bone marrow transplant patients.[163–166]

GENE THERAPY

Gene therapy aims to induce the expression of new proteins in the host by introducing their functional coding genes in target cells.[167,168] These proteins are then used either for therapeutic purposes or to gain understanding in the biology of the disease.[169,170] One hundred six gene therapy clinical trials are currently ongoing, half of which involve cancer patients. The remainder deal with inherited genetic diseases such as adenosine deaminase deficiency, cystic fibrosis, hemophilia, or hemoglobinopathies, as well as with HIV. Perhaps the most interesting type of gene therapy from a diagnostic standpoint is the induction of expression of a given protein to tag specific cells (gene marking).[171] This has permitted us to ascertain that relapse after autologous bone marrow transplant is the result of reinfusion of surviving tumor cells in the marrow.[172] The first authorized human gene therapy was performed in 1990, to correct an inherited genetic disease; the adenosine deaminase gene was successfully replaced in an 8-year-old boy. Two independent clinical trials have recently established that adenosine deaminase gene therapy has contributed to therapeutic improvement of severe combined immune deficiency.[173,174]

The strategy frequently utilized in cancer patients is to insert into tumor cells genes expressing molecules (e.g., interleukin-2) that will induce a natural immune attack against the transfected neoplastic cells. Alternatively, cells can be driven to express thymidine kinase, a herpesvirus protein. Patients can then be treated with antiviral agents such as gancyclovir, which will result in tumor cell death. The fate of cells subjected to gene therapy can potentially also be traced by radiologic methods or in routine surgical pathology or cytopathology specimens. In a mouse model, radiolabeled antisense oligonucleotides against the c-myc oncogene have been used in vivo to detect mammary tumor uptake by noninvasive imaging.[175]

Delivery systems for therapeutic genes include viral vectors (retroviruses, adenoviruses, adeno-associated viruses, and herpesviruses) and cationic liposomes. However, since somatic-cell gene therapy has moved so rapidly from the laboratory to clinical investigation, some obstacles, such as efficient targeting of cells and adequate expression of the transgene, remain to be overcome. Some viral vectors (adenoviruses) provoke immunologic reactions while others (retroviruses) carry potential replication risks. Since these are not insurmountable problems, the therapeutic use of human genes whose structure, function, and regulation are being elucidated by molecular biologists is bound to have an enormous impact on the practice of medicine and pathology in the years to come.

CONCLUSIONS AND FUTURE PROSPECTS

Understanding the molecular events that underlie the pathogenesis of disease is bringing about a fundamental change in the way in which we must approach disease. The path to a complete elucidation of the molecular basis of disease, however, is still far from complete. Only a fraction of the estimated number of human genes has been identified and sequenced, while the function of only a few is currently known. Molecular pathology will play an essential role in elucidating the patient care applications of discoveries at the molecular and biochemical level.

REFERENCES

1. Watson JD, Crick FHC: Genetical implications of the structure of deoxyribosenucleic acid. Nature 171:737, 1953
2. McKusick V: Mapping and sequencing the human genome. N Engl J Med 320:908–15, 1989
3. Jeffreys AJ, Wilson V, Thein SL: Hypervariable "minisatellite" regions in human DNA. Nature 314:67–73, 1985
4. Weissenbach J, Greenpay G, Dilo C: A second-generation linkage map of the human genome. Nature 359:794–801, 1992
5. Liu B, Nicolaides NC, Markowitz S, et al: Mismatch rapair gene defects in sporadic colorectal cancers with microsatellite instability. Nature Genet 9:48–55, 1995
6. Uchida T, White JJ Jr, Neuwirth H: DNA minisatellites demonstrate somatic DNA changes in most human bladder cancers. Cytogenet Cell Genet 53:61–63, 1990
7. Thein SL, Jeffreys AJ, Gooi HC, et al: Detection of somatic changes in human cancer DNA by DNA fingerprint analysis. Br J Cancer 55:353–356, 1987
8. Thibodeau SN, Bren G, Schaid D: Microsatellite instability in cancer of the proximal colon. Science 260:816–819, 1993
9. Aaltonen LA, Peltomäki P, Leach FS, et al: Clues to the pathogenesis of familial colorectal cancer. Science 260:812–816, 1993
10. Wooster R, Cleton-Jansen AM, Collins N, et al: Instability of short tandem repeats (microsatellites) in human cancers. Nature Genet 6:152–156, 1994
11. Baskin DG, Stahl WL: Fundamentals of quantitative autoradiography by computer densitometry for in situ hybridization, with emphasis on ^{33}P. J Histochem Cytochem 41:1767–1776, 1993
12. Loda M: Polymerase chain reaction-based methods for the detection of point mutations in oncogenes and tumor suppressor genes. Hum Pathol 25:564–571, 1994
13. Stork P, Loda M, Bosari S, et al: Detection of K-ras mutations in pancreatic and hepatic neoplasms by non-isotopic mismatched polymerase chain reaction. Oncogene 6:857–862, 1991
14. Loda M, Fiorentino M, Meckler J, et al: Hepatitis C virus reinfection in orthotopic liver transplant patients with or without concomitant hepatitis B infection. Diagn Mol Pathol 5:81–87, 1996
15. Verlaan-de Vries M, Bogaard ME, van den Elst H, et al: A dot-blot screening procedure for mutated ras oncogenes using synthetic oligodeoxynucleotides. Gene 50:313–320, 1986
16. Ausubel FM, Brent R, Kingston RE, et al (eds): Current Protocols in Molecular Biology. John Wiley & Sons, New York, 1994
17. Saiki RK, Scharf S, Faloona F, et al: Enzymatic amplification of β-globin genomic sequences and restriction site analysis for diagnosis of sickle cell anemia. Science 230:1350–1354, 1985
18. Manam S, Nichols WW: Multiplex polymerase chain reaction amplification and direct sequencing of homologous sequences: point mutation analysis of the ras genes. Anal Biochem 199:106–111, 1991
19. Columbyova L, Loda M, Scadden DT: Thrombopoietin receptor expression in human cancer cell lines and primary tissues. Cancer Res 55:3509–3512, 1995
20. Loda M, Giangaspero F, Badiali M, et al: p53 gene expression in medulloblastoma by quantitative polymerase chain reaction. Diagn Mol Pathol 1:36, 1992
21. Wang A, Doyle M, Mark DF: Quantitation of mRNA by the polymerase chain reaction. Proc Natl Acad Sci USA 86:9717–9721, 1989

22. Crotty PL, Staggs RA, Porter PT: Quantitative analysis in molecular diagnostics. Hum Pathol 25:572–579, 1994

23. Neubauer A, Neubauer B, He M, et al: Analysis of gene amplification in archival tissue by differential polymerase chain reaction. Oncogene 7:1019–1025, 1992

24. Simmonds P, Balfe P, Peutherer JF, et al: Human immunodeficiency virus-infected individuals contain provirus in small numbers of peripheral mononuclear cells and at low copy numbers. J Virol 64:864–872, 1990

25. Bagnarelli P, Menzo S, Valenza A, et al: Quantitative molecular monitoring of human immunodeficiency virus type 1 activity during therapy with specific antiretroviral compounds. J Clin Microbiol 33:16–23, 1995

26. Nakagawa H, Shimomura H, Hasui T, et al: Quantitative detection of hepatitis C virus genome in liver tissue and circulation by competitive reverse transcription-polymerase chain reaction. Dig Dis Sci 39:225–233, 1994

27. Gretch D, Corey L, Wilson J, et al: Assessment of hepatitis C virus RNA levels by quantitative competitive RNA polymerase chain reaction: high-titer viremia correlates with advanced stage of disease. J Infect Dis 169:1219–1225, 1994

28. Wright TL, Combs C, Kim M, et al: Interferon-alpha therapy for hepatitis C virus infection after liver transplantation. Hepatology 20:773–779, 1994

29. Weber B, Nestler U, Ernst W, et al: Low correlation of human cytomegalovirus DNA amplification by polymerase chain reaction with cytomegalovirus disease in organ transplant recipients. J Med Virol 43:187–193, 1994

30. Wilcox JN: Fundamental principles of in situ hybridization. J Histochem Cytol 41:1725–1733, 1993

31. Pardue M, Gall JG: Molecular hybridization of radioactive DNA to the DNA of cytological preparations. Proc Natl Acad Sci USA 64:600–604, 1969

32. John HL, Birnstiel ML, Jones KW: RNA: DNA hybrids at the cytological level. Nature 223:582–587, 1969

33. Misra DN, Dickman PS, Yunis EJ: Fluorescence in situ hybridization (FISH) detection of MYCN oncogene amplification in neuroblastoma using paraffin-embedded tissue. Diagn Mol Pathol 4:128–135, 1995

34. Persons DL, Hartmann LC, Herath JF, et al: Interphase molecular cytogenetic analysis of epithelial ovarian carcinomas. Am J Pathol 142:733–741, 1993

35. McManus AP, Gusterson BA, Pinkerton CR, et al: Diagnosis of Ewing's sarcoma and related tumours by detection of chromosome 22q12 translocations using fluorescence in situ hybridization on tumour touch imprints. J Pathol 176:137–142, 1995

36. Beck JLM, Hopman AHN, Feitz WFJ, et al: Numerical aberrations of chromosomes 1 and 7 in renal cell carcinomas as detected by interphase cytogenetics. J Pathol 176:123–135, 1995

37. Wolman SR: Fluorescence in situ hybridization: a new tool for the pathologist. Hum Pathol 25:586–590, 1994

38. Grogan TM, Rangel C, Rimsza L, et al: Kinetic-mode, automated double-labeled immunohistochemistry and in situ hybridization in diagnostic pathology. p. 79–100 In: Advances in Pathology and Laboratory Medicine. Mosby–Year Book, St. Louis, 1995

39. DeLellis RA: In situ hybridization techniques for the analysis of gene expression: applications in tumor pathology. Hum Pathol 25: 580–585, 1994

40. Lloyd RV, Jin L, Fields K, et al: Analysis of pituitary hormones and chromogranin A mRNAs in null cell adenomas, oncocytomas and gonadotroph adenomas by in situ hybridization. Am J Pathol 139: 553–564, 1991

41. Morey AL: Non-isotopic in situ hybridization at the ultrastructural level. J Pathol 176:113–121, 1995

42. Komminoth P, Long AA: In situ polymerase chain reaction and its applications to the study of endocrine diseases. Endocrinol Pathol (in press)

43. Komminoth P, Long AA, Ray R, et al: In situ polymerase chain reaction detection of viral DNA, single-copy genes, and gene rearrangements in cell suspension and cytospins. Diagn Mol Pathol 1:85–97, 1992

44. Long AA, Komminoth P, Lee E: Comparison of indirect and direct in situ polymerase chain reaction in cell preparations and tissue sections. Detection of viral DNA, gene rearrangements and chromosomal translocations. Histochemistry 99:151–162, 1993

45. Nuovo GJ: PCR In Situ Hybridization. Protocols and Applications. 2nd Ed. Lippincott-Raven, Philadelphia, 1992

46. Yap EPH, McGee JOD: Slide PCR: DNA amplification from cell samples on microscopic glass slides. Nucleic Acids Res 19:4294, 1991

47. Nuovo GJ, Margiotta M, MacConnell P, et al: Rapid in situ detection of PCR-amplified HIV-1 DNA. Diagn Mol Pathol 1:98–102, 1992

48. Bagasra O, Hauptman S, Lischner HW, et al: Detection of human immunodeficiency virus type I provirus in mononuclear cells by in situ polymerase chain reaction. N Engl J Med 326:1385–1391, 1992

49. Pestaner JP, Bibbo M, Bobroski T, et al: Potential of in situ polymerase chain reaction in diagnostic cytology. Acta Cytol 38:676–680, 1994

50. Patel VG, Shum-Siu BW, Heniford TJ, et al: Detection of epidermal growth factor receptor mRNA in tissue sections from biopsy specimens using in situ polymerase chain reaction. Am J Pathol 144:7–14, 1994

51. Patterson BK, Till M, Otto P, et al: Detection of HIV-I DNA and messenger RNA in individual cells by PCR-driven in situ hybridization and flow cytometry. Science 260:976–979, 1993

52. Shibata D: Extraction of DNA from paraffin-embedded tissue for analysis by polymerase chain reaction: new tricks from an old friend. Hum Pathol 25:561–563, 1994

53. Mies CM: Molecular biological analysis of paraffin-embedded tissues. Hum Pathol 25:555–560, 1994

54. Stanta G, Schneider C: RNA extracted from paraffin-embedded human tissues is amenable to analysis by PCR amplification. Biotechniques 11:304–308, 1991

55. Cuthbertson RA, Klintworth GK: Transgenic mice—gold mine for furthering knowledge in pathobiology. Lab Invest 58:484–502, 1988

56. Greenberg NM, DeMayo F, Finegold MJ, et al: Prostate cancer in a transgenic mouse. Proc Natl Acad Sci USA 92:3439–3443, 1995

57. Morgan BA, Izpisúa-Belmonte JC, Duboule D: Targeted misexpression of Hox-4.6 in the avian limb bud causes apparent homeotic transformation. Nature 358:236–239, 1992

58. Gu H, Marth JD, Orban PC, et al: Deletion of a DNA polymerase β gene segment in T cells using cell type-specific gene targeting. Science 265:103–106, 1994

59. Tybulewics VL, Tremblay ML, Lamarca ME, et al: Animal model of Gaucher's disease from targeted disruption of mouse glucocerebrosidase gene. Nature 357:407–410, 1992

60. Nassir J, Floresco SB, O'Kusky JR, et al: Targeted disruption of the Huntington's disease gene results in embryonic lethality and behavioral and morphologic changes in heterozygotes. Cell 81:811–823, 1995

61. Duyao MP, Auerbach AB, Ryan A, et al: Inactivation of the mouse Huntington's disease gene homolog Hdh. Science 269:407–410, 1995

62. Clarke LL, Grubb BR, Gabriel SE, et al: Defective epithelial chloride transport in a gene-targeted mouse model of cystic fibrosis. Science 257:1125–1128, 1992

63. Snouwaert JN, Brigman KK, Latour AM, et al: An animal model for cystic fibrosis made by gene targeting. Science 257:1083–1088, 1992

64. Muller WJ, Sinn E, Pattengale PK, et al: Single-step induction of mammary adenocarcinoma in transgenic mice bearing the activated c-neu oncogene. Cell 54:105–115, 1988

65. Lavigueur A, Maltby V, Mock D, et al: High incidence of lung, bone, and lymphoid tumors in transgenic mice overexpressing mutant alleles of the p53 oncogene. Mol Cell Biol 9:3982–3991, 1989

66. Baker SM, Bronner CE, Zhang L, et al: Male mice defective in the

DNA mismatch repair gene *PMS2* exhibit abnormal chromosome synapsis in meiosis. Cell 82:309–319, 1995

67. de Wind N, Dekker M, Berns A, et al: Inactivation of the mouse *Msh 2* gene results in mismatch repair deficiency, methylation tolerance, hyperrecombination, and predisposition to cancer. Cell 82:321–330, 1995

68. Smithies O, Maeda N: Gene targeting approaches to complex genetic diseases: atherosclerosis and essential hypertension. Proc Natl Acad Sci USA 92:5266–5272, 1995

69. Ryner LC, Swain A: Sex in the '90s. Cell 81:483, 1995

70. Vogelstein B, Fearon ER, Hamilton SR, et al: Use of restriction fragment length polymorphisms to determine the clonal origin of human tumors. Science 227:642–645, 1985

71. Apel RL, Ezzat S, Bapat BV, et al: Clonality of thyroid nodules in sporadic goiter. Diagn Mol Pathol 4:113, 1995

72. Mutter GL, Chaponot ML, Fletcher JA: A polymerase chain reaction assay for non-random X chromosome inactivation identifies monoclonal endometrial cancers and precancers. Am J Pathol 146: 501–508, 1995

73. Shroyer KR, Gudlaugsson EG: Analysis of clonality in archival tissues by polymerase chain reaction amplification of PGK-1: Hum Pathol 25:287–292, 1994

74. Inghirami G, Macri L, Rosati S, et al: The Reed-Sternberg cells of Hodgkin disease are clonal. Proc Natl Acad Sci USA 91:9842–9846, 1994

75. Martin GS: Rous sarcoma virus: a function required for the maintenance of the transformed state. Nature 227:1021–1023, 1970

76. Varmus HE: The molecular genetics of cellular oncogenes. Annu Rev Genet 18:553–612, 1984

77. Fabbretti G, Valenti C, Loda M, et al: N-MYC gene amplification/expression in localized stroma-rich neuroblastoma. Hum Pathol 24:294–297, 1993

78. Slamon DJ, Clak GM, Wong SG, et al: Human breast cancer: correlation of release and survival with amplification of the HER-2/neu oncogene. Science 235:177–182, 1987

79. Slamon DJ, Godolphin W, Jones LA, et al: Studies of the HER-2neu proto-oncogene in human breast and ovarian cancer. Science 244:707–712, 1989

80. Lee AK, Wiley B, Loda M, et al: DNA ploidy, proliferation and *neu*-oncogene overexpression in breast carcinoma. Mod Pathol 5:61–67, 1992

81. Gusterson BA, Gelber RD, Goldhirsch A, et al: The international (Ludwig) breast cancer study group. Prognostic importance of c-erb B-2 expression in breast cancer. J Clin Oncol 10:1049–1056, 1992

82. Bishop JM: The molecular genetics of cancer. Science 235:305–311, 1987

83. Charbonneau H: 1002 protein phosphatases? Annu Rev Cell Biol 8:463–493, 1992

84. Sidransky D, Messing E: Molecular genetics and biochemical mechanisms in bladder cancer. Oncogenes, tumor suppressor genes, and growth factors, review. Urol Clin North Am 19:629–639, 1992

85. Bos JL: Ras oncogenes in human cancer: a review. Cancer Res 49:4682–4689, 1989

86. Ruderman JV: MAP kinase and the activation of quiescent cells. Curr Opion Cell Biol 5:207–213, 1993

87. Alessi DR, Smythe C, Keyse SM: The human CL100 gene encodes a Tyr/Thr-protein phosphatase which potently and specifically inactivates MAP kinase and suppresses its activation by oncogenic ras in *Xenopus* oocyte extracts. Oncogene 8:2015–2020, 1993

88. Kumagai A, Dunphy WG: Regulation of the cdc25 protein during the cell cycle in *Xenopus* extracts. Cell 70:139–151, 1992

89. Guan K, Hakes DJ, Wang Y, et al: A yeast protein phosphatase related to the vaccina virus VH1 phosphatase is induced by nitrogen starvation. Proc Natl Acad Sci USA 89:12175–12179, 1992

90. Keyse SM, Emslie EA: Oxidative stress and heat shock induce a human gene encoding a protein-tyrosine phosphatase. Nature 359:644–647, 1992

91. Kwak SP, Hakes DJ, Mastell KJ, Dixon JE: Isolation and characterization of a human dual specificity protein tyrosine phosphatase gene. J Biol Chem 5:3596–3604, 1994

92. Rohan PJ, Davis P, Moskaluk CA, et al: PAC-1, a mitogen-induced nuclear protein tyrosine phosphatase. Science 259:1763–1766, 1993

93. Sun H: MKP-1 (3CH134), an immediate early gene product, is a dual specific phosphatase that dephosphorylates MAP kinase in vivo. Cell 75:487–493, 1993

94. Loda M, Capodieci P, Mishza R, et al: Expression of MAP kinase phosphatase-1 (MKP-1) in the early phases of human epithelial carcinogenesis. Am J Pathol (in press)

95. Galaktionov K, Lee AK, Eckstein J, et al: Cdc25 phosphatases as potential human oncogenes. Science 269:1575–1577, 1995

96. Horowitz JM, Yandell DW, Park SH, et al: Point mutational inactivation of the retinoblastoma antioncogene. Science 243:937, 1989

97. Malkin D, Li FP, Strong LC, et al: Germ line p53 mutations in a familial syndrome of breast cancer, sarcomas, and other neoplasms. Science 250:1233, 1990

98. Wiggs J, Nordenskjöld M, Yandell D, et al: Prediction of the risk of hereditary retinoblastoma, using DNA polymorphism within the retinoblastoma gene. N Engl J Med 318:151–157, 1988

99. Birch JM, Hartley AL, Blair V, et al: Cancer in the families of children with soft tissue sarcoma. Cancer 66:2239–2248, 1990

100. Garber JE, Goldstein AM, Kantor AF, et al: Follow-up study of twenty-four families with Li-Fraumeni syndrome. Cancer Res 51:6094–6097, 1991

101. Housman D: Human DNA polymorphism. N Engl J Med 332:318–320, 1995

102. Yandell DW, Campbell TA, Dayton SH, et al: Oncogenic point mutations in the human retinoblasoma gene: their application to genetic counselling. N Engl J Med 321: 1689–1695, 1989

103. Levine AJ, Momand J, Finlay CA: The p53 tumour suppressor gene. Nature 351:453, 1991

104. Kastrinakis WV, Ramchurren N, Rieger KM et al: Increased incidence of p53 mutations is associated with hepatic metastases in colorectal neoplastic progression. Oncogene 11:647–652, 1995

105. Sands A, Donehower LA, Bradley A: Gene-targeting and the p53 tumor-suppressor gene, review. Mutat Re 307:557–572, 1994

106. Harvey M, McArthur MJ, Montgomery CA, et al: Spontaneous and carcinogen-induced tumorigenesis in p53-deficient mice. Nature Genet 5:225–229, 1993

107. Donehower LA, Harvey M, Slagle BL: Mice deficient for p53 are developmentally normal but susceptible to spontaneous tumours. Nature 356:215–221, 1992

108. Cox EC: Bacterial mutator genes and the control of spontaneous mutations. Annu Rev Genet 10:135, 1976

109. Fishel R, Lescoe MK, Rao MRS, et al: The human mutator gene homolog *MSH2* and its association with hereditary nonpolyposis colon cancer. Cell 75:1027, 1993

110. Leach FS, Nicolaides NC, Papadopoulos N, et al: Mutations of a *mutS* homolog in hereditary nonpolyposis colon cancer. Cell 75:1215, 1993

111. Nicolaides NC, Papadopoulos N, Liu B, et al: Mutations of two *PMS* homologues in hereditary nonpolyposis colon cancer. Nature 371:75–80, 1994

112. Benhattar J, Delacretaz F, Martin P, et al: Improved polymerase chain reaction detection of clonal T-cell lymphoid neoplasms. Diagn Mol Pathol 4:108–112, 1995

113. Cossman J, Uppenkamp M, Sundeen J, et al: Molecular genetics and the diagnosis of lymphoma. Arch Pathol Lab Med 112:117–127, 1988

114. Cleary ML, Trela MJ, Weiss LM: Most null cell lymphomas are B lineage neoplasms. Lab Invest 53:521–525, 1985

115. Rabbitts TH: Chromosomal translocations in human cancer. Nature 372:143–149, 1994

116. Nowell PC, Hungerford DA: A minute chromosome in human chronic granulocytic leukemia. Science 132:1197, 1960

117. Daley GO, Van Etten RA, Baltimore D: Induction of chronic myelogenous leukemia in mice by the 210[bcr/abl] gene of the Philadelphia chromosome. Science 247: 824–830, 1990

118. Medeiros LJ, Van Krieken JH, Jaffe ES: Association of bcl-1 rearrangements with lymphocytic lymphomas of intermediate differentiation. Blood 76:2086–2090, 1990

119. Williams ME, Westermann CD, Swerdlow SH: Genotypic characterization of centrocytic lymphoma: frequent rearrangement of the chromosome 11 bcl-1 locus. Blood 76:1387–1391, 1990

120. Rimokh R, Berger F, Delsol G, et al: Detection of the chromosomal translocation t(11;14) by polymerase chain reaction in mantle cell lymphomas. Blood 83:1871–1875, 1994

121. Bakhshi A, Jensen JP, Goldman P, et al: Cloning the chromosomal breakpoint of t(14;18) human lymphomas: clustering around J$_H$ on chromosome 14 and near a transcriptional unit on 18. Cell 41: 899–906, 1985

122. Wagner AJ, Small MB, Hay N: Myc-mediated apoptosis is blocked by ectopic expression of Bcl-2. Mol Cell Biol 13:2432–2440, 1993

123. Baffy G, Miyashita T, Williamson JR, et al: Apoptosis induced by withdrawal of interleukin-3 (IL-3) from an IL-3-dependent hematopoietic cell line is associated with repartitioning of intracellular calcium and is blocked by enforced Bcl-2 oncoprotein. J Biol Chem 268:6511–6519, 1993

124. Gribben JG, Freedman AS, Neuberg D, et al: Immunologic purging of marrow assessed by PCR before autologous bone marrow transplantation for B-cell lymphoma. N Engl J Med 325:1525–1533, 1991

125. Neri A, Barrige F, Knowles DM, et al: Different regions of the immunoglobulin heavy-chain locus are involved in chromosomal translocations in distinct pathogenetic forms of Burkitt lymphoma. Proc Natl Acad Sci USA 85:2748–2752, 1988

126. Adams JM, Harris AW, Pinkert CA, et al: The c-myc oncogene driven by immunoglobulin enhancers induces lymphoid malignancy in transgenic mice. Nature 318:533–538, 1985

127. Herbst H, Anagnostopoulos J, Heinze B, et al: ALK gene product in anaplastic large cell lymphomas and Hodgkin's disease. Blood 86:1694–1700, 1995

128. Shiota M, Nakamura S, Ichinohasama R, et al: Anaplastic large cell lymphomas expressing the novel chimeric protein p80[NPM/ALK]: a distinct clinicopathologic entity. Blood 86:1954–1960, 1995

129. Ladanyi M, Cavalchire G, Morris SW, et al: Reverse transcriptase polymerase chain reaction for the Ki-1 anaplastic large cell lymphoma-associated t(2;5) translocation in Hodgkin's disease. Am J Pathol 145:1296–1300, 1994

130. Downing J, Weisenburger D, Kossakowska A: Molecular detection of t(2;5) of non-Hodgkin's lymphoma by RT-PCR, abstracted. In Proceedings of the Molecular Pathology 1994 Meeting, Rockville, MD, November 1994

131. Pandolfi PP, Alcalay M, Fagioli M, et al: Genomic variability and alternative splicing generate multiple PML/RARα transcripts that encode aberrant PML proteins and PML/RARα isoforms in acute promyelocytic leukemia. EMBO J 11:1397–1407, 1992

132. Miller WH Jr, Levine K, DeBlasio A, et al: Detection of minimal residual disease in acute promyelocytic leukemia by a RT-PCR assay for the PML/RARa fusion mRNA. Blood 82:1689–1694, 1993

133. Diverio D, Pandolfi PP, Biondi A, et al: Absence of reverse transcription-polymerase chain reaction detectable residual disease in patients with acute promyelocytic leukemia in long-term remission. Blood 82:3556–3559, 1993

134. Laczika K, Mitterbauer G, Korninger L, et al: Rapid achievement of PML-RARα polymerase chain reaction (PCR)-negativity by combined treatment with all-trans-retinoic acid and chemotherapy in acute promyelocytic leukemia: a pilot study. Leukemia 8:1–5, 1994

135. Brudney K, Dobkin J: Resurgent tuberculosis in New York City: human immunodeficiency virus, homelessness, and the decline of tuberculosis control programs. Am Rev Respir Dis 144:745–749, 1991

136. Frieden TR, Fujiwara PI, Washko RM, et al: Tuberculosis in New York City—turning the tide. N Engl J Med 333:229–233, 1995

137. Eisenach KD, Cave MD, Crawford JT: PCR detection of Mycobacterium tuberculosis. pp. 191–196. Persing DH, Smith TF, Tenover FC, White TJ (eds): Diagnostic Molecular Microbiology. Principles and Applications. American Society for Microbiology Press, Washington, DC, 1993

138. Tötsch M, Werner Schmid K, Brömmelkamp E, et al: Rapid detection of mycobacterial DNA in clinical samples by multiplex PCR. Diagn Mol Pathol 3:260–264, 1994

139. Ghossein RA, Ross DG, Salomon RN, et al: Rapid detection and species identification of mycobacteria in paraffin-embedded tissues by polymerase chain reaction. Diagn Mol Pathol 1:185–191, 1992

140. Barrasso R, De Brux J, Croissant O, Orth G: High prevalence of papillomavirus-associated penile intraepithelial neoplasia in sexual partners of women with cervical intraepithelial neoplasia. N Engl J Med 317:916–923, 1987

141. zur Hausen H: Papillomaviruses in anogenital cancer as a model to understand the role of viruses in human cancers. Cancer Res 49: 4677–4681, 1989

142. Pfister H: Human papilloma viruses and genital cancers. Adv Cancer Res 48:113–147, 1987

143. Monk BJ, Cook N, Ahn C: Comparison of the polymerase chain reaction and Southern blot analysis in detecting and typing human papilloma virus deoxyribonucleic acid in tumors of the lower female genital tract. Diagn Mol Pathol 3:283–291, 1994

144. Schiffman MH: Validation of hybridization assays: correlation of filter, in situ, dot-blot and PCR with Southern blot. pp. 169–179. In: The Epidemiology of Cervical Cancer and Human Papilloma Virus. International Agency for Cancer Research, Lyon, 1992

145. Clavel C, Binninger I, Boutterin MC, et al: Comparison of four non-radioactive and ³⁵S based methods for the detection of human papillomavirus DNA by in situ hybridization. J Virol Methods 33:253–266, 1991

146. Hamilton-Duitot S, Pallensen G, Franzman MB, et al: AIDS-related lymphoma. Histopathology, immunophenotype, and association with Epstein-Barr virus as demonstrated by in situ nucleic acid hybridization. Am J Pathol 138:149–163, 1991

147. MacMahon EME, Glass JD, Hayward SD, et al: Epstein-Barr virus in AIDS-related primary central nervous system lymphoma. Lancet 338:969–973, 1991

148. Cinque P, Brytting M, Vago L, et al: Epstein-Barr virus DNA in cerebrospinal fluid from patients with AIDS-related primary lymphoma of the central nervous system. Lancet 342:398–401, 1993

149. Medeiros LJ, Peiper SC, Elwood L, et al: Angiocentric immunoproliferative lesions: a molecular analysis of 8 cases. Hum Pathol 22:1150–1157, 1991

150. Choo Q, Kuo G, Weiner AJ, et al: Isolation of a cDNA clone derived from a blood borne non-A non-B viral hepatitis genome. Science 244:359–364, 1989

151. Alter HJ, Purcell RH, Shih JW, et al: Detection of antibody to hepatitis C virus in prospectively followed transfusion recipients with acute and chronic non-A non-B hepatitis. N Engl J Med 321: 1494–1500, 1989

152. Blight K, Rowland R, de la Hall P, et al: Immunohistochemical detection of the NS4 antigen of hepatitis C virus and its relation to histopathology. Am J Pathol 142:1568–1573, 1993

153. Hiramatsu N, Hayashi N, Haruna Y, et al: Immunohistochemical detection of hepatitis C virus-infected hepatocytes in chronic liver disease with monoclonal antibodies to core, envelope and NS3 regions of the hepatitis C virus genome. Hepatology 16:306–311, 1992

154. McCune JM: Viral latency in HIV disease. Cell 82:183–188, 1995

155. Piatak M, Saag MS, Yang LC, et al: High levels of HIV-1 in plasma during all stages of infection determined by competitive PCR. Science 259:1749–1754, 1993

156. Peckham C, Gibb D: Mother to child transmission of the human immunodeficiency virus. N Engl J Med 333:298–302, 1995

157. Hall JM, Lee MK, Newman B, et al: Linkage of early-onset familial breast cancer to chromosome 17q21. Science 250:1684–1689, 1990.

158. Miki Y, Swensen J, Shattuck-Eidens D, et al: A strong candidate for the breast and ovarian cancer susceptibility gene BRCA 1. Science 266:66–71, 1994

159. Huntington's Disease Collaborative Research Group: A novel gene containing a trinucleotide repeat that is expanded and unstable on Huntington's disease chromosomes. Cell 72:971–983, 1993

160. Starzl TE, Demetris AJ, Rao AS, et al: Migratory nonparenchymal cells after organ allotransplantation with particular reference to chimerism and the liver, review. Prog Liver Dis 12:191–213, 1994

161. Blazar BR, Orr HT, Arthur DC, et al: Restriction fragment length polymorphisms as markers of engraftment in allogeneic marrow transplantation. Blood 66:1436–1444, 1985

162. Nakao S, Nakatsumi T, Chuhjo T: Analysis of late graft failure after allogeneic bone marrow transplantation: detection of residual host cells using amplification of variable number of tandem repeats loci. Bone Marrow Transplant 9:107–111, 1992

163. Baxter-Lowe LA: Molecular techniques for typing unrelated marrow donors: potential impact of molecular typing disparity on donor selection, review. Bone Marrow Transplant, suppl. 4, 14:S42–50, 1994

164. Ugozzoli L, Wallace RB: Application of an allele-specific polymerase chain reaction to the direct determination of ABO blood group phenotype. Genomics 12:670–674, 1992

165. Santamaria P, Boyce-Jacino MT, Lindstrom AL: HLA class II "typing": direct sequencing of DRB, DQB, and DQA genes. Hum Immunol 33:69–81, 1992

166. Lo YM, Patel P, Newton CR, et al: Direct haplotype determination by double ARMS: specificity, sensitivity and genetic applications. Nucleic Acids Res 19:3561–3567, 1991

167. Blau HM, Springer ML: Gene therapy—a novel form of drug delivery. N Engl J Med 333:1204–1207, 1995

168. Whartenby KA, Abboud CN, Marrogi AJ, et al: The biology of cancer gene therapy. Lab Invest 72:131–145, 1995

169. Kessler DA, Siegel JP, Noguchi PD, et al: Regulation of somatic cell gene therapy by the food and drug administration. N Engl J Med 329:1169–1173, 1993

170. Crystal RG: Transfer of genes to humans: early lessons and obstacles to success. Science 270:404–410, 1995

171. Morgan RA, Cornetta K, Anderson WF: Applications of the polymerase chain reaction in retroviral-mediated gene transfer and the analysis of gene-marked human TIL cells. Hum Gen Ther 1:135–149, 1990

172. Brenner MK, Rill DR, Moen RC, et al: Gene-marking to trace origin of relapse after autologous bone marrow transplantation. Lancet 341:85–86, 1993

173. Bordignon C, Notarangelo LD, Nobili N, et al: Gene therapy in peripheral blood lymphocytes and bone marrow for ADA⁻ immunodeficient patients. Science 270:470–475, 1995

174. Blease RM, Culver KW, Miller AD, et al: T lymphocyte-directed gene therapy for ADA–SCID: initial trial results after four years. Science 270:475–480, 1995

175. Dewanjee MK, Ghafouripour AK, Kapadvanjwala M, et al: Noninvasive imaging of c-myc oncogene messenger RNA with indium-111-antisense probes in a mammary tumor-bearing mouse model. J Nucl Med 35:1054–1063, 1994

7

Flow and Image Cytometry

Henry F. Frierson, Jr.
James Linder

For more than a decade flow cytometry (FCM) and image cytometry have been used in the clinical laboratory as techniques for the analysis of cellular antigens and DNA content in cells from histologic and cytologic specimens. These cytometric techniques have clear value in selected applications, but improvements in instrumentation, cell preparation and analysis, and computer software continue. The utility of cytometric analysis in assisting diagnosis or determining prognosis in some applications is unsettled and requires further investigation. This introductory chapter summarizes FCM and image cytometry as they apply to surgical pathology and cytopathology. The chapter is devoted chiefly to methodologic aspects of specimen preparation, staining, cytometric analysis, data handling and interpretation, and quality control. Sources of variation, many of which lead to poor intra-and interlaboratory reproducibility, are highlighted. Particular diagnostic or prognostic applications are not addressed but can be found, when appropriate, in the chapters covering specific organ systems.

FLOW CYTOMETRY

FCM is a rapid and objective measurement of the intensity of fluorescence emitted by dyes that have been excited, most commonly by an argon-ion laser, to emit light at a higher wavelength. Its greatest clinical application is the enumeration of B and T cells as labeled by monoclonal antibodies coupled with a fluorescent tag. FCM has great value in the immunophenotyping of lymphoid proliferations present in peripheral blood, bone marrow, lymph nodes, and effusion specimens. It has important diagnostic utility in the examination of lymphoid proliferations sampled by fine needle aspiration. Because immunophenotyping of lymphoid proliferations, surface marker analysis of lymphocytes in immunodeficiency diseases, enumeration of reticulocytes, and detection of antiplatelet antibodies among other cytometric tasks fall within the domain of the clinical hematology and immunology laboratories, they are not discussed in this chapter, which is limited to methodologic considerations in the analysis of ploidy and proliferative fraction of solid tumors.

FCM allows the detection of gross changes in ploidy of interphase cells. It is able to resolve DNA content abnormalities when an excess or deficiency of at least two of the largest chromosomes exists. Because the finding of DNA aneuploidy is suggestive but not specific for the presence of malignant cells, DNA analysis has been investigated primarily for its potential prognostic impact. The value of ploidy and S-phase fraction (SPF) as prognostic factors for patients with solid tumors is currently limited, however, and reflects the discordant results recorded in hundreds of articles in the literature. Sources for the disparate data are numerous and include variations in patient selection, specimen type and number, use of fresh vs. archival material, methods of tumor disaggregation and staining, criteria for histogram interpretation, data analysis, and therapy. Most of these sources relate to the lack of standardization in FCM methodology. For the assessment of potential prognostic value, data from FCM analysis must be compared with the results of known, time-tested clinically important prognostic parameters. For instance, when examining the value of ploidy and proliferative fraction for invasive mammary carcinomas, FCM results must be analyzed in comparison with tumor size, axillary lymph node status, histologic grade, and histologic type in multivariate statistical analysis.[1]

As an important step in providing guidelines for the implementation of clinical DNA cytometry, a Consensus Conference was held in 1992 to evaluate the state of knowledge of the clinical utility of DNA analysis and to formulate recommendations regarding its methodology.[2–8] The 32 flow cytometrists who participated in the conference formulated a framework for the development of standards for DNA analysis. The participants also reviewed the literature to determine whether FCM had clinical value for patients with neoplasms of the breast,[4] bladder,[6] colon or rectum,[7] prostate,[5] or hematopoietic system.[8] Unfortunately, the conference, consisting largely of a highly selected group of cytometrists, had few or no representatives from surgical pathology, surgical or medical oncology, or other disciplines whose members routinely participate in the diagnosis or management of patients with cancer. Ultimately, the evaluation of DNA analysis by FCM as an important clinical tool requires prospective studies of large numbers of patients who are uniformly diagnosed, staged, and treated, and who are evaluated after long-term follow-up intervals. At this time, the more traditional prognostic parameters must be given the strongest consideration in the management of patients with cancer.

Basic Principles and Instrumentation

A flow cytometer measures the fluorescence from particles (labeled whole cells or nuclei) as they pass single file in a fluid sheath through a light beam, the source of which is most often an argon-ion laser. Thousands of particles may be analyzed in a few seconds or minutes, depending on the flow rate. A series of optical filters and mirrors separates and reflects the wavelengths of light. The light then falls on detectors that produce analogue signals that are digitized and displayed at specific channels in the histogram. The numbers generated relate to the amount of fluorescence emitted or light scattered by individual particles. In a single parameter histogram, the amount of fluorescence (channel numbers) is plotted on the x axis, and the number of particle counts per channel is plotted on the y axis.

The critical requirement of a single cell suspension is achieved by a conical nozzle and a laminar flow, in which sample fluid is introduced at a higher pressure into the sheath fluid. The procedure centers the monodispersed sample within the sheath fluid. A proper alignment of the laser beam with the stream containing the particles to be analyzed is necessary for accurate measurement. Forward-angle light scatter of a sample particle is proportional to its size, whereas 90 degree light scatter is indicative of cell granularity.

Argon-ion lasers produce a strong light at a wavelength of 488 nm. Fluorescent dyes absorb the laser light and emit light at a longer wavelength. If more than one fluorochrome is used, the emission spectra of each must have no or very minimal overlap. For surface marker analysis of lymphocytes, two-color analysis has become a standard procedure, and even three or more color analysis is being performed in clinical laboratories. The collection of labeled particles of interest in a histogram is accomplished by placing gates (windows). Data gathered for light scatter and fluorescence intensity are stored in a computer for subsequent analysis. The sorting of cells by the instrument after they pass through the laser beam is currently difficult and time consuming and has been little used in the routine clinical setting. Future improvements in reagents, electronics, and computer software will permit even more rapid and accurate assessment of multiple cellular parameters.

Specimen Disaggregation and Preanalytic Preparation

Both tissue (biopsy and excision specimens) and cytologic samples are suitable for FCM analysis (Fig. 7-1). Results obtained for specimens that are submitted fresh are superior to those for samples that have been fixed and embedded in paraffin. Fresh samples can be analyzed immediately, stored frozen as small tissue blocks or as disaggregated cells in a cryoprotective agent, or fixed in ethanol for subsequent analysis. We have obtained high quality DNA histograms for cells that have been frozen in a dimethylsulfoxide-citrate buffer for more than five years.[9] Fixation of cells in ethanol allows easy specimen transport and facilitates the interlaboratory comparison of results.[10,11]

Specimens that contain numerous cell clumps, abundant de-

bris, or a scarcity of neoplastic cells lead to histograms that are difficult or even impossible to analyze. When sheets or clusters of cells are present in a sample, disaggregation can be accomplished by adding a detergent, exposing the cells to an enzyme such as pepsin or trypsin, using a vortex, or passing the sample through a syringe equipped with a thin needle. Fresh samples typically have less debris, show increased fluorescence intensity, and lead to lower coefficients of variation compared with fixed, paraffin-embedded samples. Cytologic specimens suitable for DNA content analysis include effusion, washing, brushing, cerebrospinal fluid, and fine needle aspiration samples.[12] Bladder barbotage specimens are preferred over voided urine samples, as the latter typically show cell degeneration and have a poor cell yield. Bladder irrigation specimens may be refrigerated for up to 12 hours without serious degradation, but for later analysis, they should be stored frozen or fixed.[6]

Fresh tissue samples for FCM analysis should be submitted soon after procurement. False DNA aneuploidy has been observed in normal tissues that have undergone autolysis.[13] In autopsy specimens, false peaks are usually seen in samples procured more than 20 hours after death, but they may be seen in pancreatic specimens removed as soon as three hours postmortem.[13] If necessary, fresh tissue specimens can be transported to the laboratory in a suitable medium such as RPMI-1640 culture medium, 5 percent fetal calf serum, and 1 percent penicillin-streptomycin.[14] Samples may remain in such medium at 4°C for 2 to 3 days without adversely affecting results.

A variety of mechanical and enzymatic methods of dissociation have been used to disaggregate tissue samples. It is possible that no single method is superior for every type of tissue specimen. Mechanical procurement of single cells from solid tissues is usually preferred over enzymatic methods and may be accomplished by mincing, scraping, or ex vivo fine needle aspiration.[14-20] Both scraping and ex vivo needle aspiration allow the conservation of small specimens for histologic analysis.[16] In a study comparing mincing breast cancer tissue specimens in culture medium with scraping their surface using a scalpel blade and rinsing the blade in culture medium, no differences in histogram quality were observed.[14] Heterogeneity of ploidy and SPF occur within solid tumors, but their extent differs according to the particular study, tumor type, and specimen type.[21] This is reflected, in part, in the range for DNA aneuploidy reported for various solid tumors. As an extreme example, many studies have found that approximately 60 to 65 percent of invasive breast carcinomas are DNA aneuploid and that 5 to 20 percent are DNA multiploid; in a controversial study, one group, however, reported that with multiple sampling, 89 percent of their breast cancers showed DNA aneuploidy and 61 percent were DNA multiploid.[22-24] These authors reported that four samples of tumor were required for the highest sensitivity. In a study of fresh colon carcinoma specimens, it was recommended that at least three samples of tumor be analyzed for accurate ploidy analysis, since the authors found that analysis of only a single specimen would have resulted in the lack of detection of DNA aneuploidy in approximately one-third of the cases.[25] In regard to heterogeneity of SPF, a 45 percent disagreement rate was found when each of four samples of mam-

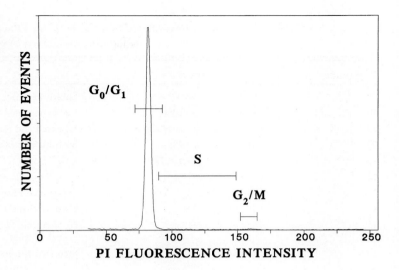

Fig. 7-1. Flow cytometric analysis allows the determination of ploidy (DNA diploidy in this histogram) and the number of cells in G0/G1 S, and G2/M phases of the cell cycle (propidium iodide stain). Half-peak CV of G0/G1 peak 2.5 percent.

mary carcinoma was analyzed.[26] These authors concluded that the intratumor variation in ploidy and SPF was due more to uncertainty in histogram interpretation and proliferative fraction analysis than to true intratumoral heterogeneity.[26] It seems clear, however, that multiple samples are preferable to a single specimen for FCM analysis and that the likelihood of finding DNA aneuploidy and an elevated SPF increases as the number of sites analyzed in a neoplasm increases. It is recommended that multiple samples of a neoplasm be pooled and thoroughly mixed prior to FCM analysis. Although some degree of intratumoral heterogeneity certainly exists in breast, colon and rectum, lung, bladder, and prostate carcinomas, among others, the clinical importance of this finding is largely unknown.[3] The ploidy status of a primary tumor, however, is largely reflective of that for its metastasis.[15]

Although the use of fresh samples usually leads to superior FCM results, hundreds of retrospective studies have utilized archival formalin-fixed, paraffin-embedded tissue specimens. A good correlation is often seen between the ploidy results for fresh and fixed specimens, although fixed specimens typically have much more debris, leading to poorer resolution of peaks (and hence a lower frequency of detection of DNA aneuploidy) and higher values for SPF[10,21 27-30] (Fig. 7-2). In one large study, approximately 90 percent of 1,400 paraffin-embedded tumors were evaluable for ploidy and approximately 70 percent for SPF.[21] The quality of histograms for paraffin-embedded samples is affected by tissue damage prior to fixation, amount of debris, and section thickness.[10,31] Poorly fixed tissue specimens lead to poor quality histograms. For paraffin-embedded tissues, formalin has been shown to be the most suitable fixative for FCM analysis, since increased debris and high coefficients of variation are seen for samples fixed in Zenker's, B-5, AZF, Bouin's, and Omnifix (Omni, Xenetics Biomed, Irvine, CA) fixatives.[32,33] False DNA aneuploidy has been noted for Carnoy's fixed specimens prior to fixation in formalin and embedding in paraffin.[34] Although it has been little studied as a fixative for FCM analysis, glutaraldehyde has been noted to enhance the relative fluorescence intensity compared with cells

Fig. 7-2. Histogram from a formalin-fixed, paraffin-embedded invasive breast carcinoma shows DNA diploidy and also abundant debris to the left of the G0/ G1 peak (peak A). Half-peak CV of peak A 5.1 percent.

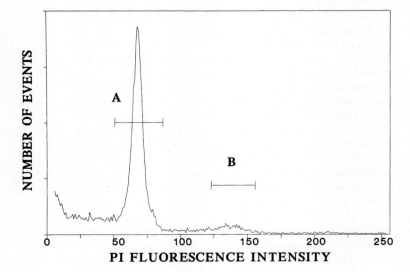

Table 7-1. Modifications of Hedley's Method[a] for Flow Cytometric Analysis of Formalin-Fixed, Paraffin-Embedded Specimens

Reference	Authors	Procedure
29	Schutte et al, 1985	Substituted trypsin for pepsin
38	Stephenson et al, 1986	Recommended >50 μm sections
39	Sickle-Santanello et al, 1988	Dewaxed and rehydrated sections in cassettes in specially designed container
40	Amberson et al, 1988	Sections in cassettes dewaxed and rehydrated in automatic tissue processor
41	Babiak and Poppema, 1991	
42	Heiden et al, 1991	
31	Hedley, 1989	Substituted Histoclear (National Diagnostics, Somerville, NJ) for xylene
42	Heiden et al, 1991	Used subtilisin Carlsberg and then stained without washing and centrifugation
43	Wang et al, 1993	For keratinized squamous cell carcinomas, pretreatment with 85% formic acid/0.3% H_2O_2 followed by subtilisin Carlsberg
20	Crissman et al, 1988	Increased pepsin incubation time
44	Pollack et al, 1993	
45	Ciancio et al, 1993	
46	Zalupski et al, 1993	Substituted trypsin or pronase for pepsin for sarcomas
47	Albro et al, 1993	Substituted proteinase K and heat for pepsin for liver tissue

[a] For Hedley's method, see Hedley et al.[27]

fixed in formalin.[35] The best results for formalin-fixed tissues occur with fixation times between 8 and 24 hours, as deterioration in histogram quality occurs with more prolonged fixation.[33] Formalin interferes with the intercalation of the fluorescent dye into DNA, causing a lowering of fluorescence intensity and a shift of the G0/G1 peak to the left in the histogram. It has been noted that resuspending formalin-fixed (not paraffin-embedded) cells in phosphate-buffered saline and heating them to 75°C for at least one hour prior to staining with propidium iodide enhances the fluorescence intensity to levels similar to that for fresh cells.[36] For simultaneous staining of DNA, intracellular proteins, and cell surface antigens, paraformaldehyde has been found to be a suitable fixative.[37]

The initial procedure for FCM analysis of formalin-fixed, paraffin-embedded specimens was published by Hedley and colleagues in 1983.[27] With this method, 30 μm thick sections are dewaxed in xylene, rehydrated in decreasing concentrations of ethanol, washed in distilled water, and incubated with 0.5 percent pepsin, pH 1.5, at 37°C for 30 minutes. Paraffin blocks that contain well preserved cells with little necrosis should be selected for analysis. Normal cells must also be present in the blocks to serve as an internal DNA diploid standard. Numerous modifications of Hedley's original technique have been described[20,29,31,38–47] (Table 7-1). In one of the most important modifications, paraffin sections 50 μm thick or greater were found to yield better histograms, as decreased section thickness resulted in an increase in debris and a decrease in relative height of the DNA aneuploid peak.[38] Other modifications in Hedley's original method concern the enzymatic digestion of tissue.[29,42–49] It is possible that the optimal enzyme and its length of incubation varies according to the type of tissue to be disaggregated from the paraffin block. No standardized methodology for FCM analysis of formalin-fixed, paraffin-embedded specimens currently exists.

Isolation of Nuclei or Whole Cells and Staining

In addition to mechanical methods, enzymatic (collagenase, pepsin, pronase, trypsin, and so forth), detergent (Triton X-100, NP-40), and chemical (EDTA, EGTA) treatments have been used for the dissociation of cells from fresh or frozen tissue specimens.[3] As discussed above, mechanical methods are, in general, preferable to enzymatic means of liberating cells from tissue samples. Depending on the method, however, differences may be found in cell recovery, viability, and histogram quality.[50] Loss of DNA aneuploid cells in squamous cell carcinomas has been reported for mechanically dissociated cells, whereas reduction in DNA aneuploid cells has been observed in enzymatic preparations of colonic adenocarcinomas.[51] Collagenase has been found to be useful for the enzymatic release of cells from soft tissue neoplasms, but it is unsatisfactory for prostate tissue specimens.[52,53]

Quite often a combination of mechanical, enzymatic, and detergent treatments is used to produce a single cell suspension. A popular method for preparing bare nuclei for FCM analysis was described in 1983 by Vindelov and colleagues,[9,54–57] who exposed mechanically dissociated cells in suspension to a detergent-trypsin digestion. This method can be used for both fresh and formalin-fixed, paraffin-embedded samples, but it precludes the simultaneous measurement of DNA content and labeling of surface or cytoplasmic antigens by fluorescein isothiocyanate (FITC)-conjugated antibodies, however.

Multiparameter (especially multicolor) FCM analysis assists in improving the detection of neoplastic cells in heterogeneous populations present in clinical samples. Reagents that preserve membranes and cytoplasm for multicolor analysis include buffered formaldehyde acetone,[58] paraformaldehyde and ethanol,[59] lysolecithin,[60] and saponin.[61] With two-color DNA analysis, whole cells are released from tissue mechanically, fixed in 50 percent ethanol, stained with propidium iodide, and labeled with either FITC-cytokeratin or FITC-leukocyte common antigen (CD45) antibodies[62–66] (Fig. 7-3). For analyzing epithelial cells in specimens that also contain inflammatory and stromal cells, this dual labeling with a DNA binding dye and an FITC-conjugated antibody to cytokeratin assists in de-

tecting small DNA aneuploid peaks and also renders a more accurate assessment of SPF[62–67] (Table 7-2). In a two-color analysis of mammary adenocarcinomas, the range for cytokeratin-positive cells was 25 to 41 percent.[62] Dual labeling is particularly helpful for SPF determination in DNA diploid neoplasms, because both neoplastic and non-neoplastic cells fall in the same G0/G1, S, and G2/M peaks in the histogram. The DNA content of lymphoid cells is easily assessed when the DNA dye is used along with an FITC-conjugated antibody to CD45. CD45-conjugated magnetic microspheres have also been used to deplete tumor-infiltrating lymphocytes, enhancing the assessment of ploidy and SPF.[68] Others recently reported that it was possible to dual label specimens that had

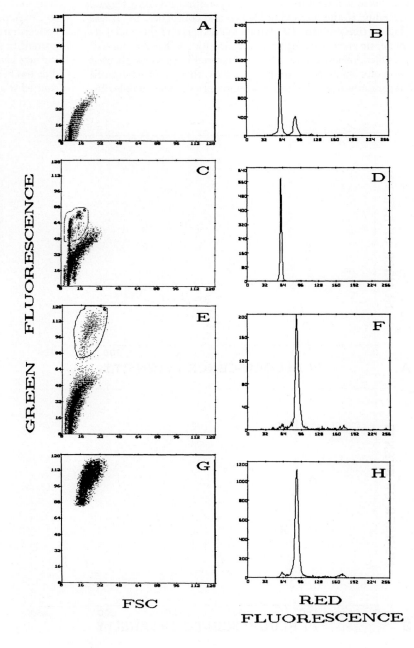

Fig. 7-3. This DNA aneuploid breast carcinoma was stained with the ONESHOT two-color method. Left column, forward angle light scatter versus log green fluorescence dot-plots show binding of FITC-bound monoclonal antibody. Right column, the DNA content of the specific tumor subpopulations. (A) Nonspecific FITC fluorescence is seen using staining with non-immune mouse IgG-FITC propidium iodide (PI). (B) The corresponding ungated histogram shows two distinct G0/G1 peaks. (C) The CD45+ cells are indicated in the CD45-FITC/PI-stained aliquot. (D) The histogram of the CD45+ cells defines the DNA diploid population as the lower of the two peaks in the ungated histogram. (E) The cytokeratin (CK)-positive cells are indicated in the CK-FITC/PI-stained sample. (F) The cytokeratin-positive cells show the DNA aneuploid cells as a single peak. (G) "Live" gating of the CK-FITC/PI-stained sample allows the acquisition of only those cells that are CK positive. (H) The corresponding histogram is composed of 20,000 CK-positive events. (From Zarbo et al,[66] with permission.)

Table 7-2. Advantages of Two-Color Flow
Cytometric Analysis

Identification of DNA diploid peak

Enhanced detection of small DNA aneuploid peaks

Limits S-phase fraction determination to epithelial cells

Assists in classifying DNA tetraploid and near tetraploid populations

Allows deconvolution of overlapping peaks by gating

(Adapted from Zarbo et al,[62] with permission.)

been fixed in formalin, embedded in paraffin, and disaggregated according to the method of Hedley and colleagues.[69,70] It was claimed that enough cytoplasm remained around the nuclei after pepsin treatment such that staining for cytokeratin was still possible. Although only a few laboratories have routinely used two-color analysis for fresh specimens, the use of whole-cell preparations instead of bare nuclei from fresh tissue samples has

been recommended by participants in the 1992 Consensus Conference.[3] Hence, results from the literature regarding ploidy and SPF for solid tumors that were based on single parameter analysis must be repeated using the two-color method. Future multiparametric measurements of solid tumors will also likely include assessments of proliferation-associated antigens, oncoproteins, and surface antigen determinants.

Several fluorochromes that bind to DNA have been found useful in FCM analysis.[3,71] These include propidium iodide, ethidium bromide, acridine orange, DAPI, and Hoechst 33342 and 33358. DAPI and the Hoechst dyes are DNA base pair affinity-specific stains, whereas the others intercalate into double-stranded nucleic acids. Since propidium iodide, ethidium bromide, and acridine orange bind to double-stranded RNA, cells must be pretreated with RNAse. Stoichiometric binding to DNA may be affected by several variables including acid concentration and enzymatic treatments. For all dyes it is important to use a saturating concentration, because understaining may cause inaccurate DNA content results.[3] Propidium iodide has been by far the most popular dye in clinical FCM. It is excited at a 488 nm wavelength and emits at 610 nm. Acridine

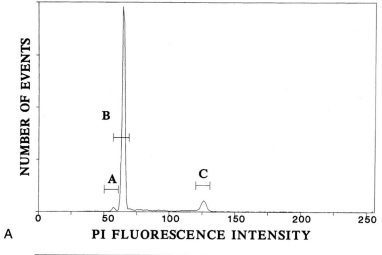

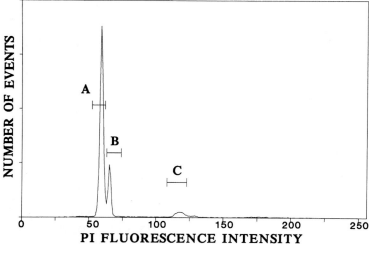

Fig. 7-4. (A) In this sample containing cells from an adrenal neuroblastoma only 1.8 percent of the cells were in G0/G1 peak A. (B) With the addition of normal human peripheral blood lymphocytes, peak A is determined to represent the G0/G1 peak of DNA diploid cells, whereas peak B represents neoplastic G0/G1 cells with a DNA index of 1.13. Half-peak CV of peak A, 2.0 percent and peak B, 1.7 percent.

orange has been used for the assessment of RNA content.[72] In one study, significant differences in double-stranded RNA excess were noted between neoplastic and non-neoplastic tissues, whereas no differences were seen in single-stranded RNA content.[73]

For the assessment of ploidy and calculation of the DNA index, the DNA diploid standard is quite important. The most appropriate DNA diploid standard consists of internal nonneoplastic cells present in the clinical specimen that contains the neoplastic cells. At times, it is useful to add biologic standards (chiefly normal human peripheral blood lymphocytes) to fresh specimens as a control to identify the DNA diploid peak (Fig. 7-4). It is critical that such control cells be prepared in the same manner as the sample cells and that they be added prior to staining, because variations in dye binding occur when stained control cells are added to stained sample cells.[74,75] For formalin-fixed, paraffin-embedded specimens, no control cells of any kind should be mixed with the sample.

Cell Quantity and Analysis

The measurement of DNA content is affected by numerous conditions that include laser power, fluorochrome binding, salt concentration of the cell suspension, instrument sensitivity, and amplification of signal.[36] Poorly controlled processing or instrument/analytic variables may lead to differences in channel location for peaks.[76] Beads of varying fluorescence intensity are typically used to provide instrument linearity.[3] Just before FCM analysis, cells must be monodispersed, which can be accomplished by vortexing the suspension, syringing through small (27 gauge) needles, or sonication.[77] The number of particle aggregates (doublets, triplets, and so forth) must be minimized. When the cell sample is sparse, the flow rate can be reduced to as low as 5 to 10 cells/sec.[57] It is recommended that at least 10,000 events be collected during analysis, but DNA aneuploid peaks may be clearly visible during analysis of fewer cells.[3] A sufficient quantity of debris should be collected so that software programs can be used for its subtraction. The lowest G0/G1 peak should probably be placed at a channel number no lower than 50 (in a 256 channel histogram).[3] Samples should contain at least 20 percent tumor cells, but DNA aneuploidy can be observed in specimens that contain less than this.[3] Obviously, a high percentage of tumor cells leads to a more accurate SPF determination.

Ploidy Assessment and Histogram Interpretation

As a percentage of total autosomal DNA, the DNA content of chromosomes ranges from 4.3 (chromosome 1) to 0.8 percent (chromosome 21).[55] The DNA content of female cells is 1.5 percent higher than that of male cells.[55] The minimal difference in DNA content required for the appearance of a bimodal peak is twice the coefficient of variation.[55] Hence, for the detection of a DNA content difference of 4 percent, each of the two resolved peaks would need to have a coefficient of variation of approximately 2 percent. In clinical samples, most cells are present in the G0/G1 peak, while fewer cells are in S-phase or in the postsynthetic (G2) or mitotic phase (M).

Visual inspection of the histogram is an important indication of its quality. In addition, inspection of the fluorescence/light scatter dot-plot may provide assistance in its evaluation.[57] Some histograms are inadequate for assessment, because there is too much debris or a high coefficient of variation of the G0/G1 peak. DNA aneuploidy (abnormal DNA stemline) should be reported only when two separate G0/G1 peaks are present (with the corresponding additional S-phase and G2/M peak).[74] The DNA index is calculated by dividing the mean relative DNA content (channel number) of diploid G0/G1 cells into the mean relative DNA content (channel number) of DNA aneuploid G0/G1 cells.[74] Hence, the DNA index for a DNA diploid peak is 1.0, whereas that for an abnormal stemline is less or more than 1.0. By convention, the first G0/G1 peak for paraffin-embedded samples is considered DNA diploid; with this guideline, DNA hypodiploidy cannot be determined for formalin-fixed, paraffin-embedded specimens (DNA hypodiploidy, however, occurs in only approximately 2 percent of neoplasms). In addition to the coefficient of variation, the proportion of cells in each peak is important for peak separation.[78] In general, 2 to 5 percent of all cells must be present in a particular channel location before a small peak becomes manifest. Peridiploid DNA aneuploid peaks may be difficult to resolve, particularly when abundant debris is seen in formalin-fixed, paraffin-embedded specimens.[30] Problematic G0/G1 peaks are broad or asymmetric. Such peaks may harbor unresolvable peridiploid DNA aneuploid peaks. A skewing to the right of the DNA diploid peak simulating an abnormal stemline, however, occurs in bladder barbotage specimens that contain numerous polymorphonuclear leukocytes. False DNA aneuploidy may occur from autolyzed normal tissue.[13] For autolyzed specimens, a shoulder to the right of the DNA diploid G0/G1 peak, a false DNA aneuploid peak with a small coefficient of variation (CV), or a broad peak with a high coefficient of variation may be seen. False peaks appear after short postmortem intervals in autolyzed tissues that contain digestive enzymes such as the pancreas.[13] Such peaks usually have a low DNA index and appear at least partially fused with the DNA diploid peak. False peaks are rarely seen in poorly fixed surgical material that has been embedded in paraffin.[79]

The definition of DNA tetraploidy has not been uniform.[80] As presently defined, DNA tetraploid cells have a DNA index ranging from 1.9 to 2.1 (Fig. 7-5). A DNA tetraploid population is present when a larger number of cells appears in the DNA diploid G2/M peak than the G2/M cells of the normal tissue counterpart.[3] Previous authors have defined DNA tetraploidy using arbitrary cutoff values for the number of cells in G2/M such as at least 15 or 20 percent of all events, or they have used a statistical approach of more than 2 or 3 standard deviations above the G2/M mean for the cells of the normal tissue counterpart.[3] It is possible that the definition of DNA tetraploidy should be established for neoplasms according to their anatomic site of origin.[3]

Accurate determination of DNA tetraploidy is difficult when cell aggregates are numerous. When doublets are suspected, triplets are also typically observed in the histogram. If a DNA tetraploid peak is truly present, then a G2/M peak at 8N should

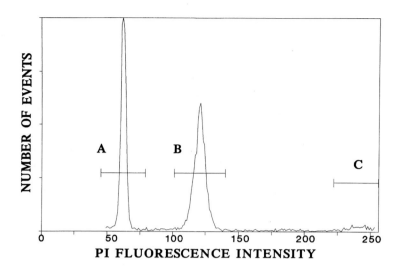

Fig. 7-5. Invasive breast carcinoma histogram. Peak B contains DNA tetraploid cells (DNA index, 1.95), whereas peak C represents the corresponding G2/M peak. Half-peak CV of peak A, 2.8 percent and peak B, 3.0 percent.

be apparent, and corresponding cells should appear in the SPF. Some software programs assist in eliminating cell aggregates from analysis. Two-color FCM analysis may be especially useful when histograms show increased numbers of cells in G2/M.[62,65]

The definition of DNA multiploidy has also varied, which is part of the reason for the differences in multiploidy frequency reported for particular neoplasms. DNA multiploidy has usually been defined as the presence of multiple DNA aneuploid G0/G1 peaks (Fig. 7-6). Differences of 10 percent or more in the DNA index (what constitutes a real difference in DNA index?) for peaks found in histograms from separate samples of a neoplasm may not always represent DNA multiploidy but may only reflect methodologic variability. DNA multiploidy is probably best defined as the presence of two or more DNA aneuploid G0/G1 peaks in the same histogram.[22,24] Neoplasms show heterogeneity of DNA content not only when they are multiploid but also when DNA aneuploidy is observed in one sample of a particular neoplasm and only DNA diploidy detected in another area of the same tumor.

It is clear that histograms may be difficult to classify and that

classification is to some extent subjective (Table 7-3). Lack of agreement in histogram interpretation was shown by Joensuu and Kallioniemi,[81] who circulated histograms from paraffin-embedded samples among six investigators. In this study designed to contain many different and sometimes difficult types of histograms, in only 44 percent of histograms was ploidy agreed on by all; in 85 percent concordance was reached by five of the six participants. The difficulty inherent in histogram interpretation is just one of the many reasons for disparities in the frequency of DNA aneuploidy reported for particular solid neoplasms.

Coefficient of Variation

The CV of the G0/G1 peak is the single most important parameter of histogram quality.[57] It is affected by differences in sample (inherent properties and fixation), preparation and staining, and instrument performance. It is quite important for studies to report the mean and range of CV values for controls

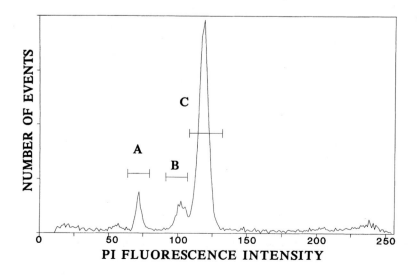

Fig. 7-6. DNA multiploidy is determined when multiple DNA aneuploid G0/G1 peaks are present. This histogram from an invasive breast carcinoma shows two DNA aneuploid peaks (DNA index of peak B, 1.40; DNA index of peak C 1.64). Half-peak CV of peak A, 2.6 percent, peak B, 12.1 percent, and peak C, 2.7 percent.

Table 7-3. Difficulties in Histogram Interpretation of Ploidy

Asymmetric peaks
Broad (high CV) peaks
Small peaks
Hypodiploid debris
Tetraploidy vs. increased G2/M

Abbreviation: CV, coefficient of variation.

Table 7-4. Complicated Histograms for Analysis of S-Phase Fraction

Skewed DNA diploid peak or peridiploid peaks
Multiple DNA aneuploid peaks
Overlapping peaks
High CVs
Small peaks

Abbreviation: CV, coefficient of variation.

and tumor samples and the method of CV calculation in order that the quality of results can be ascertained.[74] The half-peak CV is a measure of the peak width at half its height, and the full-peak CV is based on the width at the base of the peak. The half-peak CV is used more commonly. For fresh tissue samples, the goal for the CV for the DNA diploid G0/G1 peak should be less than 5 percent, whereas for formalin-fixed, paraffin-embedded samples the goal for diploid CVs should be no higher than 8 percent. In the consensus review for colorectal carcinoma, the authors recommended a goal of less than 6 percent for full peak CV.[7] CVs for DNA aneuploid peaks may be higher, however. Neoplasms with CVs less than 8 percent are recommended for useful SPF determination.[3] Higher CVs may render SPF determination inaccurate.

S-Phase Fraction

The number of cells in S (synthetic) phase has been recommended for the reporting of the proliferative component, although the number of cells in S+ G2/M is also reflective of the proliferative fraction.[3] In DNA aneuploid tumors, the SPF for the DNA aneuploid peak should be reported. When it is impossible to resolve completely the proliferating DNA aneuploid cells from the DNA diploid population, either the weighted average value for SPF of both peaks can be reported or it can be assumed that all cells in S-phase are neoplastic cells. It is the consensus opinion that the former approach is preferable to the latter.[3]

In comparing SPF with other methods of identifying proliferating cells such as tritiated thymidine labeling or bromodeoxyuridine labeling, SPF typically results in higher values. An important reason for this finding concerns the major source of error in SPF determination, debris, which results from necrosis, mechanical disaggregation, or enzymatic dissociation, and is nearly always a more severe problem for paraffin-embedded material than for fresh specimens.[82] The correlation of SPF with the thymidine-labeling index is better for DNA aneuploid than for DNA diploid neoplasms, because non-neoplastic diploid cells contaminate the DNA diploid peak.[83] The correlation between SPF and in vitro bromodeoxyuridine labeling has been reported to be poor.[84]

Types of histograms that result in difficult or impossible SPF determination are listed in Table 7-4. Table 7-5 lists the numerous sources of variation in SPF analysis. Higher values for

SPF are typically seen for paraffin-embedded specimens compared with fresh samples. Specimens in which tumor cells comprise less than 15 to 20 percent of the total population are unsatisfactory for SPF, while histograms that contain greater than 20 percent aggregates and debris are also unsatisfactory.[3] Background aggregates and debris is an important software calculation in the accurate assessment of SPF. It is the ratio of the estimated number of aggregates and debris to the total number of particle events over the region from the lowest G0/G1 mean to the highest G2/M mean.[3] A paucity of neoplastic DNA diploid cells leads to a particularly inaccurate assessment of SPF. Two-color multiparametric analysis is helpful for the calculation of SPF for DNA diploid neoplasms, since keratin-positive epithelial cells may be analyzed separately. Using this two-color approach, however, neoplastic epithelial cells cannot be distinguished from those epithelial cells that are non-neoplastic.

Aggregates can be reduced either by hardware pulse gating or by software modeling. The issue of whether to use hardware gating or software methods for aggregate correction is controversial.[3] Hardware gating depends on instrumentation, particle shape, and operator selection of gate regions.[3] With gating to minimize aggregates, peak vs. integral or pulse width vs. integral signals is used.[85] Software methods of excluding aggregates and debris should be restricted to events collected without hardware gating.[3]

Algorithms for debris compensation have evolved from single models to more complex nuclear cutting models. A good correlation in SPF for frozen and paraffin-embedded tissues is

Table 7-5. Sources of Variation in S-Phase Fraction Determination by Flow Cytometry

Fresh vs. paraffin-embedded samples
Debris
Particle aggregates
Debris subtraction methods
No. of neoplastic cells
Analytic techniques
Software algorithms for modeling
Single parameter vs. two-color analysis
Intratumoral heterogeneity
Coefficient of variation of G0/G1 peak

seen when debris is subtracted with multicut or single cut algorithms.[86] Debris compensation models allow more accurate SPF estimates than uncompensated histograms. In one study in which a sliced nuclear debris subtraction method was used for paraffin-embedded breast carcinomas, the median uncorrected SPF was 7.6 percent, and the median corrected value was 5.7 percent.[87] It is probable that debris compensation should be performed for histograms from all types of specimens including those having only 5 percent or less debris.[88] A standard exponential debris subtraction algorithm often results in oversubtraction, however.[85,88] The calculation of SPF depends greatly on the particular methodology employed[89] (Table 7-6). Sophisticated mathematical modeling software programs such as Multicycle (Phoenix Flow Systems, San Diego, CA)[90] and Modfit (Verity Software House, Topsham, ME)[91] are currently recommended for SPF analysis[3] (Fig. 7-7). They include nuclear cutting and exponential debris compensation algorithms. In a study of frozen breast carcinomas, SPF values were highest with the polynomial model without background subtraction and the histogram-dependent exponential function, intermediate with the rectangle model, and lowest with the model with classic exponential background subtraction.[89,92–94] These models produced markedly different estimates; a median variability of about 50 percent was observed for SPF for the same neoplasm. For three of the four models, however, variability was reduced to 15 to 20 percent. An algorithm has recently been reported for fully automated SPF determination.[95] Although this automated analysis does not replace human supervision, it does serve as a guideline for less experienced users, facilitates interlaboratory comparisons, and assists in extensive recalculations of large datasets.

Studies comparing SPF with prognosis have generally divided SPF values into two or three groups. The establishment of cutoff values is to some degree artificial, since SPF is a continuous variable. For each particular type of neoplasm, individual laboratories must set their own range of SPF values, establishing the cutoff points for low, intermediate, and high SPF. Values set by one laboratory should not be adopted by another, because interlaboratory differences in type of specimen, data analysis, and methodology usually exist. Most studies evaluating SPF and prognosis have used rather primitive cell cycle models without debris and aggregate subtraction.[4] Hence, studies using the most sophisticated modeling techniques along

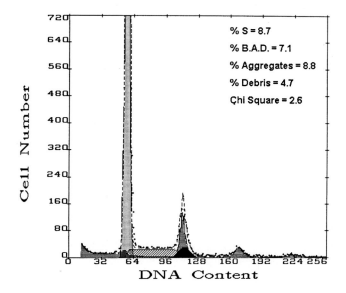

Fig. 7-7. Using Multicycle (Phoenix Flow Systems, San Diego, CA), an accurate assessment of S-phase and the amount of background aggregates and debris can be made. (Courtesy of Richard J. Zarbo, M.D., D.M.D., Detroit, MI.)

with multiparametric analysis are needed to evaluate the prognostic importance of SPF fully. In one such study of 168 cytokeratin-stained fresh colorectal carcinomas, Zarbo and colleagues[96] used state of the art software and found no consistent association between SPF and survival for patients with any tumor stage.

In lieu of mathematical calculation of SPF by FCM, other methods for determining the percentage of cells in S-phase can be employed. SPF can be measured by FCM for cells labeled with antibodies bromodeoxyuridine and idoxuridine.[97,98] Cells can incorporate the thymidine analogue into DNA either in vitro or in vivo. In vivo double labeling with idoxuridine and bromodeoxyuridine allows for more accurate estimation of potential doubling time. Non-neoplastic cells in the sample, however, cannot be excluded from analysis.[97] Fluorescent antibodies to Ki-67, proliferating cell nuclear antigen, or the various cyclins can be used to determine the percentage of nonquies-

Table 7-6. Algorithms Used for Calculation of S-Phase Fraction by Flow Cytometry

Reference	Mathematical Model	Algorithm
91	Model of Baisch et al	Simple rectangle without functions for debris subtraction
92	Polynomial (Dean-Jett model)	Series of rectangles without background subtraction
89, 90	Histogram-dependent exponential function (Multicycle[a]; Modfit[b])	Nonlinear least-squares fitting with background subtraction
93	Classic exponential function (Lampariello model)	Maximum likelihood as parameter estimation with background subtraction

[a] Phoenix Flow Systems, San Diego, CA.
[b] Verity Software House, Topsham, ME.

cent cells, but these antibodies have been used sparingly in FCM analysis.

Quality Control

Lack of standardization of FCM procedures for DNA analysis has largely been responsible for nonuniformity of results among laboratories. Variations in methodology and measurement of ploidy and SPF by FCM are numerous and include type of specimen analyzed, specimen disaggregation and staining, instrument calibration, data analysis and interpretation, and quality control. Wheeless and colleagues[99] identified three sources of variation affecting FCM in general and its transportability: (1) interlaboratory variation that is constant across time (generally reflecting stable differences in instrument set-up and laboratory techniques); (2) differences that are not constant across time (inconsistencies in preparation of samples, staining, and analysis); and (3) measurement variability (affecting sensitivity of technique). These important sources of variation were discovered in studies from the Bladder Cancer Flow Cytometry Network established by the National Cancer Institute, in which replicate samples were analyzed in five different laboratories.[99–102] Several groups of other investigators have also examined issues of reproducibility for FCM analysis.[103,104] In a study of 43 Italian laboratories each of which used their own staining and measurement protocols, good intralaboratory reproducibility was found for ploidy, but statistically significant differences were noted among laboratories for DNA index and CV.[104] In 1988, the College of American Pathologists introduced a proficiency testing program for DNA content analysis for clinical laboratories.[105] In a report published in 1994, results of ploidy analysis obtained from a mean of 241 participating laboratories on 19 unknowns from 1990 to 1992 showed a mean correct response rate of 86 percent (range, 58 to 97 percent) for modal number of DNA aneuploid peaks.[106] Incorrect responses were most commonly associated with near DNA diploid and DNA tetraploid unknowns, while some laboratories demonstrated consistent deviations from the mean of DNA index determination, which probably indicates problems in instrument linearity. SPF results for five specimens revealed wide interlaboratory variation, although the means were close to reference values. The largest range for SPF was 0 to 97 percent. These results clearly reveal the severity of differences for obtaining reproducible results for SPF among clinical laboratories. Reproducibility for SPF can be improved if laboratories use the same mathematical model for calculation.[89] The optimal and most reproducible mathematical approach for calculating SPF needs to be defined and agreed on.

The 1992 Consensus Conference served to establish a framework for the standardization of DNA analysis by FCM. The published guidelines addressed the standardization of specimen sampling, processing, instrument performance, and data and histogram analysis. Although important recommendations were made, several other issues remain to be addressed before all clinical laboratories process, stain, and analyze clinical material in a uniform manner. The need for methodologic improvement and standardization continues. The value of DNA analysis of ploidy and SPF as prognostic determinants will be clarified when the most highly developed FCM methods are employed in large prospective studies of fresh specimens from uniformly treated patients.[107] In addition, the impact of FCM analysis can only be assessed when each of the most important time-tested prognostic parameters has been incorporated into the multivariate statistical model. It is anticipated that in addition to ploidy and SPF determination, FCM will be used to study the clinical importance of a myriad of oncogene products. Multiparameter analysis by FCM will permit the study of surface membrane components, cytoplasmic proteins, receptors, and nuclear factors that may ultimately be shown to impart useful clinical information. An FCM method to measure estrogen receptor on cytokeratin-stained breast cancer cells has been described using the biotinylated antibody 1D5.[108]

LASER SCANNING CYTOMETRY

DNA analysis of ethanol-fixed, propidium iodide-stained imprints or smears can be performed by a recently developed microscope slide-based automatic laser scanning cytometer (CompuCyte Corporation, Cambridge, MA).[109] In a comparison with FCM and image cytometry, the laser scanning cytometer showed concordance for ploidy in over 90 percent of 53 cancers.[109] Good correlation in SPF was also seen between the laser scanning cytometer and the flow cytometer. Like the flow cytometer, the laser scanning instrument is automated and leads to rapid and reliable SPF determination. Like image cytometry, it has a minimal tissue requirement and the potential for visual selection of cells to be measured. Although this technology is still in the developmental stage, the instrument has the potential to measure multiple cellular parameters rapidly for thousands of cells. In addition to DNA content analysis, the applications include the quantitation of cell receptors and oncoproteins, immunophenotyping of hematolymphoid cells, and determining chromosome copy number by fluorescence in situ hybridization.

IMAGE CYTOMETRY

Image cytometry, also termed *image analysis*, has similarities to and differences from flow cytometry.[110] Image cytometry has relative strengths and weaknesses compared with flow cytometry, depending on the particular application or the specimen type being analyzed. Image cytometry broadly refers to the quantitative measurement of morphologic features in histologic tissue sections or cytologic preparations. Measurements may be made on individual cells or noncellular tissue components, or on the relationships between cells. A variety of parameters can be measured using different physical techniques (e.g., laser-induced fluorescence, stoichiometric binding of dyes, enzymatic reduction of chromogens). The most common application of image cytometry is the quantitation of DNA content. Image cytometry has real or perceived diagnostic utility in some clinical settings and is a powerful research tool.

Comments cited earlier in this chapter relating to the determination of ploidy by flow cytometry also apply to image cytometry. The most critical issues relate to the lack of standardization in both specimen processing analysis and interpretation of data.[111] Efforts continue to improve standardization, particularly through committees of the International Academy of Cytology.

Basic Principles and Instrumentation

Computers and video technology are central to all applications of image cytometry.[112] The technique depends on the initial capture of an image in digital format, which can then be subjected to mathematical analysis.[113] Image capture is usually performed with a video camera mounted on a light or fluorescent microscope. The analogue signal from this camera is converted to digital form through an analog-to-digital conversion process. The resulting digital data can reside in the computer memory or on other memory media. In this format it can be displayed on a computer monitor, or manipulated or analyzed by computer software.

A concept central to image cytometry is the notion of a *pixel* or picture element. This is represented by a discrete digital value in the computer memory. The number of pixels that comprise an image is determined by the quality of the video camera and the rate that the video signal from the camera is sampled by the analog-to-digital converter. Depending on the camera and the software configuration, images may be captured in black and white or in color. In black-and-white images individual pixels are assigned a numeric value ranging from 0 to 255 (so-called gray levels). The latter represents the highest level of transmitted light. Numeric values can also be assigned to the light intensity that a camera simultaneously captures in red, green, and blue wavelengths, so-called RGB color. Color-sensitive cameras are useful for the analysis of DNA ploidy as well as quantitative immunohistochemistry, which relies on colored chromogens.

Preanalytic Preparation

The specimens suitable for image cytometry include thin tissue sections or cytologic preparations (cell smears or cytocentrifuge or monolayer preparations). Most of the sample preparation techniques previously cited for preparing cell suspensions for flow cytometric analysis work equally well for image cytometry. The primary goal of cytopreparation is the depositing of cells onto a glass slide with a minimum of cell overlap. This greatly facilitates the measurement of morphologic features of individual cells.

Cell and Tissue Staining

For the measurement of DNA content, image cytometry can be performed on nuclei stained with fluorochromes or dyes. With the exception of laser scanning microscopy, a hybrid between image and flow cytometry, fluorochromes are rarely used. The major reagent used for DNA quantitation is the Feulgen stain, which binds to DNA in a stoichiometric fashion. Quantitative immunohistochemistry, the other major clinical application of image cytometry, may utilize the entire gamut of monoclonal antibodies that mark antigens expressed within, or on the surface of cells, or to other tissue components.

Image Analysis

The digital image can be subjected to a variety of measurements by various software tools. Fundamentally, image analysis is achieved by the assessment of the mathematical values of individual pixels that comprise the image. These measurements might include the pixel intensity, the relationship of the pixels to each other, or the number of pixels. Through such measurements it is possible to describe morphometric features of cells, such as nuclear shape, size, texture, or the relationship between cells (so-called contextual karyometry). It is also possible to sum the optical density of specific regions of the cell, such as the nucleus, that has been stained by a specific chromogen. DNA content is determined in this fashion. The Feulgen staining intensities of cells under examination are compared with normal human diploid cells (that are known to have a mass of 7.14 picograms of DNA per nucleus). Through the use of a standard curve, cells with unknown DNA content can be identified. When image cytometry is performed on histologic tissue sections of neoplasms, normal cell nuclei are often included in the same tissue section. These normal nuclei have been subjected to the same fixation, sectioning, and staining as the neoplasm being measured and can serve as internal controls.

Ploidy Assessment

The measurement of the optical density of the population of cells allows the preparation of a DNA histogram plotting the DNA mass in picograms on the horizontal axis relative to the number of cells on the vertical axis. In a normal human sample, most cells will have a mass of 7.14 pg/cell nucleus, reflecting the G0/G1 peak. A smaller number of cells will be G2 or mitotic phase, so-called G2/M peak. The intervening distance between the G0/G1 peak and the G2/M peak corresponds to the SPF. This is analogous to flow cytometry; however, the number of cells in S-phase are usually too few to measure by image cytometry, unless monoclonal antibodies are used that specifically mark cells in the DNA synthetic phase. Many of the same factors that effect the shape of the flow cytometry histogram can also complicate the assessment of image cytometry DNA histograms. Thus, debris, inflammatory cells, or specimen autolysis can affect the shape of and the ability to interpret the histogram.

Despite technical differences between flow and image cytometry, a high concordance elists between ploidy measurements obtained by the two techniques.[114–119] Depending on the source of the sample and methodology used in analysis, concordance exceeds 90 percent.[120,121] Thus, the choice of technique for clinical applications is often a matter of personal preference. Conceptually, flow cytometry is the preferred analytic tool for fluid samples, such as blood and body fluids. Flow cytometric methods allow the measurement of large numbers of cells, thus achieving high statistical reliability in a relatively short time. However, cells that are infrequent in the population may be undetectable.[122] Image cytometry typically involves the measurement of a few hundred cells. While this is slower, and potentially more labor intensive, it allows the morphologic visualization of cells so that individual cells with specific attributes can be selected for measurement. In some instances, this affords image cytometry greater sensitivity (and clinical utility) over flow cytometry for ploidy determination.[114,123] As discussed elsewhere, DNA ploidy may be prognostically significant or useful in planning therapy.[123–125]

Quantitative Immunohistochemistry

The number of cells that are usually analyzed by image cytometry is too few for accurate assessment of cell proliferation. S-phase determination is one example in which immunohistochemical stains can be combined with the quantitative power of image cytometry.[126] Several monoclonal antibodies specifically bind to nuclear antigens expressed on cells in the proliferating phase of the cell cycle.[127] These include MIB-1, Ki-67, antibodies to DNA polymerase alpha, and proliferating cell nuclear antigen.[128,129] Individual cells, or tissue sections stained by the immunohistochemical technique, can be examined by image cytometry to determine the proportion of cells in a sample that mark with the antibody. These antibodies provide an alternative to the counting of mitoses, which is classically performed in surgical pathology. Tissue sections that have been treated with these monoclonal antibodies may be examined to determine the relative proportion of cells that are in the proliferative phase of the cell cycle. Thus, a proliferating cell fraction is determined that is comparable to the SPF of the DNA histogram obtained by flow cytometry. Depending on the software program, the percent of positive nuclei may be determined, or a percentage of the total nuclear area present in the tissue section. These determinations may require the simultaneous assessment of DNA content in the tissue section.

A more common application of quantitative immunohistochemistry is the measurement of estrogen or progesterone receptor expression in carcinomas of the breast or other organs.[130–132] Depending on antibodies used in the analysis, immunohistochemical staining can either be performed on fresh frozen, imprint, or formalin-fixed materials. By using standard curves, the mass of receptor protein in nuclei can be determined (usually expressed as femtomoles). A good correlation elists between the immunohistochemical determination of receptors and standard biochemical methods of analysis. The immunohistochemical method has distinct advantages, notably that it requires far less tissue than the biochemical method, and it is possible to visualize the tumor cells. This latter point can be particularly useful in an sample having a relatively small proportion of tumor, in which erroneous results may be obtained from normal breast tissue that either does or does not express receptors.

Although not in broad clinical use, quantitative immunohistochemistry has been used to measure the protein product of oncogenes such as HER-2/neu and p53. The expression of such oncoproteins from various tumors as well as its prognostic significance is currently under evaluation.[133] The potential of measuring resistance of tumors to chemotherapy by quantitating P-glycoprotein has been demonstrated.[134]

Morphology

Classic morphometric measurement is not widely used in the daily practice of pathology. The measurement of muscle or nerve fiber size and shape is used as an adjunct by some neuropathologists.[135] Likewise, some investigators advocate the determination of nuclear contour in some T cell lymphomas.[128]

Cytology Automation

Efforts to automate the examination of the cervical vaginal Papaniclaou smear have fueled many of the advances in image cytometry.[136,137] Since the introduction of the Papaniclaou smear in the 1950s, research efforts have been focused on application of image cytometry for screening and also for diagnostic interpretation of cytologic materials. After many years of frustration, recent improvements in computer technology, software design, and slide preparation techniques have made automated cytology feasible. Several commercial instruments measure various cell parameters to classify cells as normal or abnormal. Approaches include the classic measurement of nuclear size, shape, and texture, as well as the use of nonalgorithmic neural networks. Preliminary studies of these technologies show that they give favorable results in the identification of classification of abnormal cells. Automated instruments have been produced that have been proposed to have a role in quality assurance activities in cytology, as comprehensively reviewed in *Acta Cytologica*.[138]

REFERENCES

1. Frierson HF Jr: Ploidy analysis and S-phase fraction determination by flow cytometry of invasive adenocarcinoma of the breast. Am J Surg Pathol 15:358–367, 1991
2. Hedley DW, Shankey TV, Wheeless LL: DNA cytometry consensus conference. Cytometry 14:471, 1993
3. Shankey TV, Rabinovitch PS, Bagwell B, et al: Guidelines for implementation of clinical DNA cytometry. Cytometry 14:472–477, 1993
4. Hedley DW, Clark GM, Cornelisse CJ, et al: Consensus review of the clinical utility of DNA cytometry in carcinoma of the breast. Cytometry 14:482–485, 1993
5. Shankey TV, Kallioniemi O-P, Koslowski JM, et al: Consensus review of the clinical utility of DNA content cytometry in prostate cancer. Cytometry 14:457–500, 1993
6. Wheeless LL, Badalament RA, deVere White RW, et al: Consensus review of the clinical utility of DNA cytometry in bladder cancer. Cytometry 14:478–481, 1993
7. Bauer KD, Bagwell CB, Giaretti W, et al: Consensus review of the clinical utility of DNA flow cytometry in colorectal cancer. Cytometry 14:486–491, 1993
8. Duque RE, Andreeff M, Braylan RC, et al: Consensus review of the

clinical utility of DNA flow cytometry in neoplastic hematopathology. Cytometry 14:492–496, 1993

9. Vindelov LL, Christensen IJ, Keiding N, et al: Long-term storage of samples for flow cytometric DNA analysis. Cytometry 3:317–322, 1983

10. Alanen KA, Klemi PJ, Joensuu H, et al: Comparison of fresh, ethanol-preserved, and paraffin-embedded samples in DNA flow cytometry. Cytometry 10:81–85, 1989

11. Alanen KA, Klemi PJ, Taimela S, Joensuu H: A simple preservative for flow cytometric DNA analysis. Cytometry 10:86–89, 1989

12. Frierson HF Jr: Ploidy and proliferative fraction analysis of cytologic specimens. pp. 596–613. In Keren DF, Hanson CA, Hurtubise P (eds): Flow Cytometry and Clinical Diagnosis. ASCP Press, Chicago, 1994

13. Alanen KA, Joensuu H, Klemi PJ: Autolysis is a potential source of false aneuploid peaks in flow cytometric DNA histograms. Cytometry 10:417–425, 1989

14. Torres FX, Mackowiak PG, Brown RD, et al: Comparison of two methods of mechanical disaggregation of scirrhous breast adenocarcinomas for DNA flow cytometric analysis of whole cells. Am J Clin Pathol 103:8–13, 1995

15. Frankfurt OS, Slocum HK, Rustum YM, et al: Flow cytometric analysis of DNA aneuploidy in primary and metastatic human solid tumors. Cytometry 5:71–80, 1984

16. Eliasen CA, Opitz LM, Vamvakas EC, et al: Flow cytometric analysis of DNA ploidy and S-phase fraction in breast cancer using cells obtained by ex vivo fine-needle aspiration: an optimal method for sample collection. Mod Pathol 4:196–200, 1991

17. Bach BA, Knape WA, Edinger MG, Tubbs RR: Improved sensitivity and resolution in the flow cytometric DNA analysis of human solid tumor specimens. Use of in vitro fine-needle aspiration: and uniform staining reagents. Am J Clin Pathol 96:615–627, 1991

18. Cornacchiari A, Grigolato PG, Facchetti F, et al: Usefulness of the scraping method for DNA flow cytometry in breast tumors. Cytometry 19:263–266, 1995

19. Lee TK, Wiley AL Jr, Esinhart JD, et al: Variations associated with disaggregation methods in DNA flow cytometry. Anal Quant Cytol Histol 15:195–200, 1993

20. Crissman JD, Zarbo RJ, Niebylski CD, et al: Flow cytometric DNA analysis of colon adenocarcinomas. A comparative study of preparatory techniques. Mod Pathol 1:198–204, 1988

21. Kallioniemi O-P: Comparison of fresh and paraffin-embedded tissue as starting material for DNA flow cytometry and evaluation of intratumor heterogeneity. Cytometry 9:164–169, 1988

22. Beerman H, Smit VTHBM, Kluin PM, et al: Flow cytometric analysis of DNA stemline heterogeneity in primary and metastatic breast cancer. Cytometry 12:147–154, 1991

23. Kute T: Response to Beerman et al: flow cytometric analysis of DNA stemline heterogeneity in primary and metastatic breast cancer, letter. Cytometry 12:155, 1991

24. Beerman H, Cornelisse CT: Response to Dr. Kute's letter to the editor, letter. Cytometry 12:156, 1991

25. Wersto RP, Liblit RL, Deitch D, Koss LG: Variability in DNA measurements in multiple tumor samples of human colonic carcinoma. Cancer 67:106–115, 1991

26. Ferno M, Baldetorp B, Ewers S-B, et al: One or multiple samplings for flow cytometric DNA analyses in breast cancer—prognostic implications? Cytometry 13:241–249, 1992

27. Hedley DW, Friedlander ML, Taylor IW, et al: Method for analysis of cellular DNA content of paraffin-embedded pathological material using flow cytometry. J Histochem Cytochem 31:1333–1335, 1983

28. Klemi PJ, Joensuu H: Comparison of DNA ploidy in routine fine needle aspiration biopsy samples and paraffin-embedded tissue samples. Anal Quant Cytol Histol 10:195–199, 1988

29. Schutte B, Reynders MMJ, Bosman FT, Blijham GH: Flow cytometric determination of DNA ploidy level in nuclei isolated from paraffin-embedded tissue. Cytometry 6:26–30, 1985

30. Frierson HF Jr: Flow cytometric analysis of ploidy in solid neoplasms: comparison of fresh tissues with formalin-fixed paraffin-embedded specimens. Hum Pathol 19:290–294, 1988

31. Hedley DW: Flow cytometry using paraffin-embedded tissue: five years on. Cytometry 10:229–241, 1989

32. Herbert DJ, Nishiyama RH, Bagwell CB, et al: Effects of several commonly used fixatives on DNA and total nuclear protein analysis by flow cytometry. Am J Clin Pathol 91:535–541, 1989

33. Esteban JM, Sheibani K, Owens M, et al: Effects of various fixatives and fixation conditions on DNA ploidy analysis. A need for strict internal DNA standards. Am J Clin Pathol 95:460–466, 1991

34. Carr, RF, Abaza AM: False aneuploidy in flow cytometric DNA analysis of paraffin embedded tissue: effects of Carnoy's fixation. Cytometry 14:668–672, 1993

35. Kute TE, Gregory B, Galleshaw J, et al: How reproducible are flow cytometry data from paraffin-embedded blocks? Cytometry 9:494–498, 1988

36. Overton WR, McCoy JP Jr: Reversing the effect of formalin on the binding of propidium iodide to DNA. Cytometry 16:351–356, 1994

37. Schmid I, Uittenbogaart CH, Giorgi JV: A gentle fixation and permeabilization method for combined cell surface and intracellular staining with improved precision in DNA quantification. Cytometry 12:279–285, 1991

38. Stephenson RA, Gay H, Fair WR, Melamed MR: Effect of section thickness on quality of flow cytometric DNA content determinations in paraffin-embedded tissues. Cytometry 7:41–44, 1986

39. Sickle-Santanello BJ, Farrar MB, DeCenzo JF, et al: Technical and statistical improvements for flow cytometric DNA analysis of paraffin-embedded tissue. Cytometry 9:594–599, 1988

40. Amberson JB, Wersto RP, Agarwal V, et al: Preparation of paraffin-embedded tissue for flow and image cytometric analysis: an improved and more efficient procedure, abstracted. Cytometry, suppl. 2:34, 1988

41. Babiak J, Poppema S: Automated procedure for dewaxing and rehydration of paraffin-embedded tissue sections for DNA flow cytometric analysis of breast tumors. Am J Clin Pathol 96:64–69, 1991

42. Heiden T, Wang N, Tribukait B: An improved Hedley method for preparation of paraffin-embedded tissues for flow cytometric analysis of ploidy and S-phase. Cytometry 12:614–621, 1991

43. Wang N, Pan Y, Heiden T, Tribukait B: Improved method for release of cell nuclei from paraffin-embedded cell material of squamous cell carcinomas. Cytometry 14:931–935, 1993

44. Pollack A, Ciancio G, Terry NHA, Block NL: Recognition and reduction of artifacts from autolysis in paraffin-embedded tissue using DNA/nuclear protein flow cytometry. Cytometry 14:565–568, 1993

45. Ciancio G, Pollack A, Block NL: Flow cytometric analysis of DNA and nuclear protein in paraffin-embedded tissue. Cytometry 14:205–209, 1993

46. Zalupski MM, Maciorowski Z, Ryan JR: DNA content parameters of paraffin-embedded soft tissue sarcomas: optimization of retrieval technique and comparison to fresh tissue. Cytometry 14:327–333, 1993

47. Albro S, Bauer KD, Hitchcock CL, Wittwer CT: Improved DNA content histograms from formalin-fixed, paraffin-embedded liver tissue by proteinase K digestion. Cytometry 14:673–678, 1993

48. Schultz DS, Zarbo RJ: Comparison of eight modifications of Hedley's method for flow cytometric DNA ploidy analysis of paraffin-embedded tissue. Am J Clin Pathol 98:291–295, 1992

49. Tagawa Y, Nakazaki T, Yasutake T, et al: Comparison of pepsin and trypsin digestion on paraffin-embedded tissue preparation for DNA flow cytometry. Cytometry 14:541–549, 1993

50. Chassevent A, Daver A, Bertrand G, et al: Comparative flow DNA

analysis of different cell suspensions in breast carcinoma. Cytometry 5:263–267, 1984

51. Ensley JF, Maciorowski, Z, Hassan M, et al: Variations in DNA aneuploid cell content during tumor dissociation in human colon and head and neck cancers analyzed by flow cytometry. Cytometry 14:550–558, 1993

52. Zalupski MM, Ryan JR, Ensley JF, et al: Development and optimization of tissue preparative methodology for DNA content analysis of soft tissue neoplasms. Cytometry 14:922–930, 1993

53. Konig JJ, van Dongen JW, Schroder FH: Preferential loss of abnormal prostate carcinoma cells by collagenase treatment. Cytometry 14:805–810, 1993

54. Vindelov LL, Christensen IJ, Nissen NI: A detergent-trypsin method for the preparation of nuclei for flow cytometric DNA analysis. Cytometry 3:323–327, 1983

55. Vindelov LL, Christensen IJ, Jensen G, Nissen NI: Limits of detection of nuclear DNA abnormalities by flow cytometric DNA analysis. Results obtained by a set of methods for sample-storage, staining and internal standardization. Cytology 3:332–339, 1983

56. Vindelov LL, Christensen IJ, Nissen NI: Standardization of high-resolution flow cytometric DNA analysis by the simultaneous use of chicken and trout red blood cells as internal reference standards. Cytometry 3:328–331, 1983

57. Vindelov LL, Christensen IJ: A review of techniques and results obtained in one laboratory by an integrated system of methods designed for routine clinical flow cytometric DNA analysis. Cytometry 11:753–770, 1990

58. Slaper-Cortenbach ICM, Admiraal LG, Kerr JM, et al: Flow cytometric detection of terminal deoxynucleotidyl transferase and other intracellular antigens in combination with membrane antigens in acute lymphatic leukemias. Blood 72:1639–1644, 1988

59. Lakhanpal S, Gonchoroff NJ, Kazmann JA, et al: A flow cytofluorometric double staining technique for simultaneous determination of human mononuclear cell surface phenotype and cell cycle phase. J Immunol Methods 96:35–40, 1987

60. Schroff RW, Bucana CD, Klein RA, et al: Detection of intracytoplasmic antigens by flow cytometry. J Immunol Methods 70:167–177, 1984

61. Jacob MC, Favre M, Bensa J-C: Membrane cell permeabilization with saponin and multiparametric analysis by flow cytometry. Cytometry 12:550–558, 1991

62. Zarbo RJ, Visscher DW, Crissman JD: Two-color multiparametric method for flow cytometric DNA analysis of carcinomas using staining for cytokeratin and leukocyte-common antigen. Anal Quant Cytol Histol 11:391–402, 1989

63. Zarbo RJ: Quality control issues and technical considerations in flow cytometric DNA and cell cycle analysis of solid tumors. pp. 425–469. In Keren DF, Hanson CA, Hurtubise P (eds): Flow Cytometry and Clinical Diagnosis. ASCP Press, Chicago, 1994

64. Brown RD, Zarbo RJ, Linden MD, et al: Two-color multiparametric method for flow cytometric DNA analysis. Standardization of spectral compensation. Am J Clin Pathol 101:630–637, 1994

65. Van der Linden JC, Herman CJ, Boenders JGC, et al: Flow cytometric DNA content of fresh tumor specimens using keratin-antibody as second stain for two-parameter analysis. Cytometry 13:163–168, 1992

66. Zarbo RJ, Brown RD, Linden MD, et al: Rapid (one-shot) staining method for two-color multiparametric DNA flow cytometric analysis of carcinomas using staining for cytokeratin and leukocyte common antigen. Am J Clin Pathol 101:638–642, 1994

67. Ramaekers FCS, Beck HLM, Fritz WFJ, et al: Application of antibodies to intermediate filament proteins as tissue-specific probes in the flow cytometric analysis of complex tumors. Anal Quant Cytol Histol 8:271–280, 1986

68. Kenyon NS, Schmittling RJ, Siiman O, et al: Enhanced assessment of DNA/proliferative index by depletion of tumor infiltrating leukocytes prior to monoclonal antibody gated analysis of tumor cell DNA. Cytometry 16:175–183, 1994

69. Frei JV, Martinez VJ: DNA flow cytometry of fresh and paraffin-embedded tissue using cytokeratin staining. Mod Pathol 6:599–605, 1993

70. Frei JV, Rizkalla K, Martinez VJ: Proliferative cell indices measured by DNA flow cytometry in node-negative adenocarcinomas of breast: accuracy and significance in cytokeratin-stained archival specimens. Mod Pathol 7:925–929, 1994

71. Myc A, Traganos F, Lara J, et al: DNA stainability in aneuploid breast tumors: comparison of four DNA fluorochromes differing in binding properties. Cytometry 13:389–394, 1992

72. Darzynkiewicz Z, Traganos F, Sharpless T, Melamed MR: Conformation of RNA in-situ as studied by acridine orange staining and automated cytofluorometry. Exp Cell Res 95:143–153, 1975

73. el-Naggar AK, Batsakis JG, Teague K, et al: Single- and double-stranded RNA measurements by flow cytometry in solid neoplasms. Cytometry 12:330–335, 1991

74. Heidemann W, Schumann J, Andreeff M, et al: Convention on nomenclature for DNA cytometry. Cytometry 5:445–446, 1984

75. Iverson OE, Laerum OD: Trout and salmon erythrocytes and human leukocytes as internal standards for ploidy control in flow cytometry. Cytometry 8:190–196, 1987

76. Price J, Herman CJ: Reproducibility of FCM DNA content from replicate paraffin block samples. Cytometry 11:845–847, 1990

77. Gonchoroff NJ, Ryan JJ, Kimlinger TK, et al: Effect of sonication on paraffin-embedded tissue preparation for DNA flow cytometry. Cytometry 11:642–646, 1990

78. Benson, NA, Braylan RC: Evaluation of sensitivity in DNA aneuploidy detection using a mathematical model. Cytometry 15:53–58, 1994

79. Joensuu H, Alanen KA, Klemi PJ, Aine R: Evidence for false aneuploid peaks in flow cytometric analysis of paraffin-embedded tissue. Cytometry 11:431–437, 1990

80. Joensuu H, Alanen K, Falkmer UG, et al: Effect of DNA ploidy classification on prognosis in breast cancer. Int J Cancer 52: 701–706, 1992

81. Joensuu H, Kallioniemi O-P: Different opinions on classification of DNA histograms produced from paraffin-embedded tissue: Cytometry 10:711–717, 1989

82. Haag D, Feichter G, Goerttler K, Kaufmann M: Influence of systematic errors on the evaluation of the S phase portions from DNA distributions of solid tumors as shown for 328 breast carcinomas. Cytometry 8:377–385, 1987

83. Meyer JS, Coplin MD: Thymidine labeling index, flow cytometric S-phase measurement, and DNA index in human tumors. Am J Clin Pathol 89:586–595, 1988

84. Lloveras B, Garin-Chesa P, Myc A, Melamed M: In vitro bromodeoxyuridine labeling of malignant neoplasms. A comparative study with flow cytometry cell-cycle analysis. Am J Clin Pathol 101:703–707, 1994

85. Bagwell CB, Mayo SW, Whetstone SD, et al: DNA histogram debris theory and compensation. Cytometry 12:107–118, 1991

86. Weaver DL, Bagwell CB, Hitchcox SA, et al: Improved flow cytometric determination of proliferative activity (S-phase fraction) from paraffin-embedded tissue. Am J Clin Pathol 94:576–584, 1990

87. Kallioniemi O-P, Visakorpi T, Holli K, et al: Improved prognostic impact of S-phase values from paraffin-embedded breast and prostate carcinomas after correcting for nuclear slicing. Cytometry 12:413–421, 1991

88. Wersto RP, Stetler-Stevenson M: Debris compensation of DNA histograms and its effect on S-phase analysis. Cytometry 20:43–52, 1995

89. Silvestrini R: Quality control for evaluation of the S-phase fraction by flow cytometry: a multicentric study. The SICCAB Group for Quality Control of Cell Kinetic Determinations. Cytometry 18:11–16, 1994

90. Rabinovitch PS: Practical considerations for DNA content and cell cycle analysis. pp. 117–142. In Bauer KD, Duque RE, Shankey TV (eds): Clinical Flow Cytometry: Principles and Applications. Williams & Wilkins, Baltimore, 1993

91. Bagwell CB: Theoretical aspects of flow cytometry data analysis. pp. 41–61. In Bauer KD, Duque RE, Shankey TV (eds): Clinical Flow Cytometry: Principles and Applications. Williams & Wilkins, Baltimore, 1993

92. Baisch H, Goehde W, Linden W: Analysis of PCP-data to determine the fraction of cells in the various phases of the cycle. Radiat Environ Biophys 12:31–37, 1975

93. Dean P, Jett J: Mathematical analysis of DNA distributions derived from flow microfluorometry. J Cell Biol 60:523–527, 1974

94. Lampariello F, Del Bino G: Automatic parameter estimation of flow cytometric DNA distributions in the study of cell kinetics. In Int Fed Autom Cont. Pergamon Press, New York, 1988

95. Kallioniemi O-P, Visakorpi T, Holli K, et al: Automated peak detection and cell cycle analysis of flow cytometric DNA histograms. Cytometry 16:250–255, 1994

96. Zarbo RJ, Nakhleh RE, Brown R, et al: Prognostic significance of flow cytometry (FCM) synthetic phase fraction (SPF) in 168 cytokeratin (CK) stained colorectal carcinomas, abstracted. Mod Pathol 8:71A, 1995

97. Going JJ, Stanton PD, Cooke TG: Influences on measurement of cellular proliferation by histology and flow cytometry in mammary carcinomas labeled in vivo with bromodeoxyuridine. Am J Clin Pathol 100:218–222, 1993

98. Pollack A, Terry HA, Wu CS, et al: Specific staining of iododeoxyuridine and bromodeoxyuridine in tumors double labelled in vivo: a cell kinetic analysis. Cytometry 20:53–61, 1995

99. Wheeless LL, Coon JS, Cox C, et al: Measurement variability in DNA flow cytometry of replicate samples. Cytometry 10:731–738, 1989

100. Coon JS, Deitch AD, de Vere White RW, et al: Interinstiutional variability in DNA flow cytometric analysis of tumors. The National Cancer Institute's Flow Cytometry Network experience. Cancer 61:126–130, 1988

101. Coon JS, Deitch AD, de Vere White RW, et al: Check samples for laboratory self-assessment in DNA flow cytometry. The National Cancer Institute's Flow Cytometry Network experience. Cancer 63:1592–1599, 1989

102. Wheeless LL, Coon JS, Cox C, et al: Precision of DNA flow cytometry in interinstitutional analyses. Cytometry 12:405–412, 1991

103. Kallioniemi O-P, Joensuu H, Klemi P, Koivula T: Inter-laboratory comparison of DNA flow cytometric results from paraffin-embedded breast carcinomas. Breast Cancer Res Treat 17:59–61, 1990

104. Danesi DT, Spano M, Altavista P: Quality control study of the Italian Group of Cytometry on flow cytometry cellular DNA content measurements. Cytometry 14:576–583, 1993

105. Homburger HA, McCarthy R, Deodhar S: Assessment of interlaboratory variability in analytical cytology. Results of College of American Pathologists flow cytometry study. Arch Pathol Lab Med 113:667–672, 1989

106. Coon JS, Paxton H, Lucy L, Homburger H: Interlaboratory variation in DNA flow cytometry. Results of the College of American Pathologists' survey. Arch Pathol Lab Med 118:681–685, 1994

107. Frierson HF Jr: The need for improvement in flow cytometric analysis of ploidy and S-phase fraction, editorial. Am J Clin Pathol 95:439–441, 1991

108. Brotherick I, Lennard TWJ, Cook S, et al: Use of the biotinylated antibody DAKO-ER ID5 to measure oestrogen receptor and cytokeratin positive cells obtained from primary breast cancer cells. Cytometry 20:74–80, 1995

109. Martin-Reay DG, Kamentsky LA, Weinberg DS, et al: Evaluation of a new slide-based laser scanning cytometer for DNA analysis of tumors. Comparison with flow cytometry and image analysis. Am J Clin Pathol 102:432–438, 1994

110. Weinberg DW: Relative applicability of image analysis and flow cytometry in clinical medicine. pp. 359–371. In Bauer KD, Duque RE, Sharkey TV (eds): Flow Cytometry: Principles and Applications. Williams & Wilkins, Baltimore, 1993

111. Gill J: Image analysis in pathology: what are the issues? Hum Pathol 20:203–204, 1989

112. Inoue S: Video Microscopy. Plenum, New York, 1986

113. Wells WA, Rainer RO, Memoli VA: Basic principles of image processing. Am J Clin Pathol 98:493–501, 1992

114. Bauer TW, Tubbs RR, Edinger MG, et al: A prospective comparison of DNA quantitation by image and flow cytometry. Am J Clin Pathol 93:322–326, 1990

115. Chabanas A, Rambeaud JJ, Seigneurin D, et al: Flow and image cytometry for DNA analysis in bladder washings: improved concordance by using internal reference for flow. Cytometry 14:943–950, 1993

116. Claud RD, Weinstein RS, Howeedy A, et al: Comparison of image analysis of imprints with flow cytometry for DNA analysis of solid tumors. Mod Pathol 2:463–467, 1989

117. Colombel MC, Pous MF, Abbou CC et al: Computer assisted image analysis of bladder tumour nuclei for morphonuclear and ploidy assessment. Anal Cell Pathol 6:137–147, 1994

118. Wilbur DC, Zakowski MF, Kosciol CM, et al: DNA ploidy in breast lesions: a comparative study using two commercial image analysis systems and flow cytometry. Anal Quant Cytol Histol 12:28–34, 1990

119. Wojcik EM, Katz RL, Johnston DA, et al: Comparative analysis of DNA ploidy and proliferative index in fine needle aspirates of non-Hodgkin's lymphomas by image analysis and flow cytometry. Anal Quant Cytol Histol 15:151–157, 1993

120. Danque PO, Chen HB, Patil J, et al: Image analysis versus flow cytometry for DNA ploidy quantitation of solid tumors: a comparison of six methods of sample preparation. Mod Pathol 6:270–275, 1993

121. Dawson AE, Norton JA, Weinberg DS: Comparative assessment of proliferation and DNA content in breast carcinoma by image analysis and flow cytometry. Am J Pathol 136:1115–1124, 1990

122. Taylor SR, Zachariah S, Chakraborty S, et al: Ploidy studies by image analysis on fine needle aspirates of the breast. Acta Cytol 37:923–928, 1993

123. Pindur A, Chakraborty S, Walch, Wheeler TM: DNA ploidy measurements in prostate cancer: differences between image analysis and flow cytometry and clinical implications. Prostate 25:189–198, 1994

124. Bauer KD, Merkel DE, Winter JN, et al: Prognostic implications of ploidy and proliferative activity in diffuse large cell lymphomas. Cancer Res 46:3173–3178, 1986

125. Michie BA, Black C, Reid RP, et al: Image analysis derived ploidy and proliferation indices in soft tissue sarcomas: comparison with clinical outcome. J Clin Pathol 47:443–447, 1994

126. Weinberg DS: Proliferation indices in solid tumors. Adv Pathol Lab Med 5:163, 1992

127. Bravo R: Synthesis of the nuclear protein cyclin (PCNA) and its relationship with DNA replication. Exp Cell Res 163:287–293, 1986

128. Schwartz BR, Pinkus G, Bacus S, et al: Cell proliferation in non-Hodgkin's lymphomas: digital image analysis of Ki-67 staining. Am J Pathol 134:327–336, 1989

129. Pesce CM: Defining and interpreting diseases through morphometry. Lab Invest 56:568–575, 1987

130. Allred DC, Bustamante M, Daniel CO, et al: Immunocytochemical analysis of estrogen receptors in human breast carcinomas: evaluation of 130 cases and a review of the literature regarding concordance with the biochemical assay and clinical relevance. Arch Surg 125:107–113, 1990

131. Auger M, Katz RL, Johnston DA, et al: Quantitation of immuno-cytochemical estrogen and progesterone receptor content in the fine needle aspirates of breast carcinoma using the SAMBA 4000 image analysis system. Anal Quant Cytol Histol 15:274–280, 1993

132. Bacus S. Flowers JL, Press MF, et al: The evaluation of estrogen receptor in primary breast carcinoma by computer-assisted image analysis. Am J Clin Pathol 90:233–239, 1988

133. Bacus SS, Chin D, Stern RK, et al: HER-2/neu oncogene expression, DNA ploidy and proliferation index in breast cancers. Anal Quant Cytol Histol 14:433–445, 1992

134. Grogan T, Dalton W, Rybski J, et al: Optimization of immuno-cytochemical P-glycoprotein assessment in multidrug-resistant plasma cell myeloma using three antibodies. Lab Invest 63:815–824, 1991

135. Castleman KR, Chui LA, Martin TP, et al: Quantitative muscle biopsy analysis. Monogr Clin Cytol 9:101, 1984

136. Wied GL, Bartels PH, Bahr GF, et al: Taxonomic intracellular system (TICAS) for cell identification. Acta Cytol 12:180–204, 1968

137. Wied GL, Bartels PH, Bibbo M, et al: Image analysis in quantitative cytopathology and histopathology. Hum Pathol 20:549–571, 1989

138. Bibbo M, Wied GL (eds): New industrial developments in automated cytology. Acta Cytol 40:1–72, 1996

8

Computers in Surgical and Cytopathology

Stanley J. Robboy
Timothy T. Stenzel
Christopher B. Hubbard
Steven G. Silverberg

Once a luxury, hospital computers have become a necessity for the delivery of quality patient care. Used primarily for financial bookkeeping many years ago, they now assist in all aspects of daily patient care. Systems for anatomic pathology (AP), initially focusing on the production of the AP report, now aim at comprehensive reporting, encoding of diagnoses, management, quality control, infinite archiving of reports, and scientific uses. The demands placed on any AP system become ever more complex and demanding, due to the rapidly changing world of pathology buffeted by managed care, consolidation of laboratories point of service considerations for both acquisition of specimens and delivery of reports, regulations,* and ever present risk management, as well as because the pathology report must add value to that already available through the more central hospital information system.[1] This chapter briefly describes the goals of an AP computerized system, highlights problems encountered in departmental computerization, covers the types of current systems in use, which are largely character based, and emphasizes the need for the systems now entering into use that are graphic in nature. Considerations in choosing systems are discussed elsewhere.[2,3]

In the new world of managed care, in which "optimal" care translates into hospital stays that are rather short, rapid turnaround time from receipt of the specimen until a report is in the clinician's hands is of paramount import. The desired goal is to have most of each daily load reported within 24 hours and all but the largest specimens or those requiring special handling, consultations, additional stains and so forth completed within 48 hours. All of this must be done without increased frenzy.

Rather than taxing the laboratory personnel, AP computer systems must resolve impediments and streamline everyone's efforts. This chapter discusses issues germane to all pathology departments, but emphasizes trends in which laboratories are becoming larger, the number of pathologists in a practice are multiple, interlinked technical work centers transcend multiple locations, and an entrepreneurial spirit is important to growth.

THE REPORT

The pathology report, the culmination of the pathologist's work effort, has evolved over recent years into a highly complex document reflecting both the conjoint work product of multiple specialists and increased information. As such, it reflects issues revolving around accession, interactions occurring during specimen workup, and concepts about design and interaction; the aim is to produce and, if need be, amend the final report later.

Issues of Accession

Patient Registration, Demographics, and Linkages

Every specimen accessioned requires linkage to a particular patient. This assumes that the system maintains a patient master index, which can continuously upgrade all pertinent demographic data such as change of last name in case of marriage and calculate current age from date of birth. The system should automatically link all the patient's specimens, whether inpatient, outpatient, from a doctor's office or free-standing clinic, or outside slides from another institution. Master indices are needed, which include information about the pathology staff, the technical staff, and submitting physicians, with information about whether they are staff or resident, within or outside the institution, telephone and fascimile numbers, and other pertinent demographics.

---

* In the United States, the agencies/acts most commonly involved are the Joint Commission on Accreditation of Healthcare Organizations (JCAHO), Clinical Laboratory and Improvement Act (CLIA), Food & Drug Administration (FDA), and College of American Pathologists (CAP). In the United Kingdom, the agencies/acts include the Medicines Control Agency MCA, Clinical Pathology Accreditation (CAP) and Royal College of Pathologists (RCP).

Log-in, Accession Number Assignment, Check Digits/Letters and Specimen Routing

Log-in is typically performed at the surgical pathology laboratory, although in the multioffice department all remote sites may serve this function, even if simply to acknowledge receipt of the specimen. The accession (case) number assigned is unique for each specimen received from a single surgical episode. It also commonly incorporates a check digit or letter as an internal control to ensure that an entered number is correct. Modern systems, in various permutations, have unique specimen accession numbers composed of identifiers for site, case type, year, and numeric sequence order. The ordering site is usually suppressed (identifier indicating that the specimen coming to the central laboratory from the hospital, 1; freestanding center, 2; and so forth. The case type is commonly two letters. The first describes whether the specimen is surgical, cytologic, or of autopsy origin ("S," "C," or "A"), and the second indicates the subtype of specimen (e.g., "SF," specimen entry as after *frozen* section consultation; "SL," surgical specimen, *large* type). These are followed by the year, and the next available number is computer assigned. Thus, SF-95-00080 is the eightieth surgical specimen received in 1995. The "F" indicates that a frozen section examination was performed on it prior to accessioning. Usually the bucket number is sequential for all surgical specimens regardless of the type of surgical specimen (e.g., SL-95-00081 might follow SF-95-00080). In such instances, the second letter can serve a double purpose as an internal check letter (see Robboy et al,[4] for a detailed description of a check letter/digit).

Additional information entered at log-in can have multiple practical uses. Inclusion of tissue type helps route cases to the appropriate subspecialist pathologist in those departments where multiple pathologists work simultaneously. It also aids the production of individual work logs for each person who subsequently will be involved in any of the various specimens.

Components of a Specimen: Identification

A major advance in the past decade has been development of systems that uniquely identify and trace each part of the specimen received. Usually a unique identifier is sequentially assigned within a case number for each specimen container (e.g., SF-95-00080A, -00080B, -00080C, or 1, 2, 3, or I, II, III, and so forth). Within each code, a unique number is then assigned to each resulting paraffin block (e.g., A1, A2, A3, and so forth). This is key in workload assessment, billing, tracking, retrieval, and, as a major timesaver, automatic cassette labeling with an imprinting device.

Anticipation of Workup

The evolving subspecialties in surgical pathology and changing notions of what is considered an optimal workup, which vary among institutions, require automated accommodation at the time of accession if specimens are to be examined in the most productive and efficient manner. As examples, at some institutions, liver biopsy specimens are routinely processed to include hematoxylin and eosin H&E stained slides at multiple levels, as well as special stains with aldehyde fuchsin and Masson trichrome; gastric biopsies include 2 H&E-stained slides, one with periodic acid-Schiff/alcian blue and an immunostain for *Heliobacter*. Some specimens routinely have slides prepared at two levels, whereas others, such as cervical and skin biopsies, routinely have three. Systems that automatically identify a specimen as a liver biopsy without further human intervention will automatically order the appropriate number of levels and special stains so that each work group will know promptly what is to be received shortly for processing. Turnaround time is therefore greatly shortened.

Interaction With the Specimen

Once accessioned, every specimen will have many interactions with numerous persons as well as transaction recording devices.

Initial Interactions: Production of Labels, Cassettes, Worksheets and Logs

As a general philosophy of system design, information captured at accession or later during the work flow should eliminate or minimize steps that in the past required human effort. The initial such by-products of today's computer systems are labels and log lists. Current regulations require that specimen containers and requisition forms be tagged with appropriate identifying information. Current systems automate this function by printing adhesive labels that generally exhibit the accession number, container number, patient name, and hospital unit number and can be attached to the container itself and the request forms. Similarly, cassette labeling/imprinting devices have semiautomated the labeling of the tissue cassettes anticipated to be needed. Finally, most systems should automatically produce adhesive labels for the coverslipped slide, usually to include accession number, patient name, hospital unit number, container number, block number, and level number (e.g., SF-95-00080 D3-L2 [container D, block 3, level 2 in the block]; sometimes the label is also bar coded.

Larger laboratories are often organized so that multiple grossing bays are in operation simultaneously. Once the specimen is accessioned, the system requires the ability to direct each specimen to its appropriate grossing bay or, if the specimen consists only of slides referred in for consultation, to the responsible pathology specialist.

As a by-product of this initial human interaction, the system needs to produce multiple logs. In addition to a master log listing all cases accessioned, specialty logs are often desirable. These may list the cases by individual grossing bay (e.g., large specimens, small specimens, skins), or may alert laboratories about special procedures requested (e.g., immunocytochemistry, electron microscopy, or flow cytometry). These logs should be either automatically produced daily or available on demand as desired. In systems on a network, the printed log should be directed for printing at any printer desired.

Gross Examination

Gross examination of the specimen often requires many interactions with the system. Photographs and radiographs are taken, portions of tissues sent to/from tissue banks, estrogen/progesterone receptor levels noted, electron microscopy and immunopathology performed, and so forth, all of which must be recorded. Since each portion of tissue selected for microscopic examination is placed in a unique user-specified cassette (A1, A2, A3 ..., or B, C..., and so on), it is common for additional cassettes to be required beyond the prelabeled number or, conversely, excess prelabeled cassettes must be discarded. The laboratory must reconcile the expected and actual workload. Also, because complex specimens are often received in pieces over the course of a day, it is important that computer systems show the last cassette number used to prevent duplicate cassette numbers from being issued.

Histologic Processing

Processing of specimens for microscopic examination is an art. In today's world of cost management, histology technologists must know before their work begins which tissues are expected and the appropriate handling of each. The system must permit the technologist to reconcile daily the anticipated versus actual workload. Systems that automate slide etching are enormous help, so as to provide permanent labeling of the slide itself. Similarly, much time is saved and accuracy achieved when the computer has prepared slide labels, as described earlier.

Review of Prior History, Including Image Retention

Knowledge of a patient's prior history and the ability to review the slides from prior operations dramatically impact on the pathologist's ability to render an insightful diagnosis on current material. This goal requires that the older style card catalogues be absorbed into the computer history files and that the pathology system maintain forever the information about the historic and current findings. At a minimum, any current system should maintain indefinitely a cross-index of the patient's name, hospital unit number, pathology accession number, and final diagnoses and be capable of easily producing a historic log. The entire report, including all gross and microscopic descriptions, should be maintained on-line for extended periods and preferably indefinitely. Three months of retention on-line is an absolute minimum; a year is a more realistic practical minimum. Current JCAHO standards require the final pathology report to be available in paper or a retrievable form for at least 20 years (CLIA requires 10 years). Many departments already keep them indefinitely.

As imaging systems become integrated into common use, it would be desirable to retain selected digitized images on-line for user-defined periods, with a period of 5 to 10 years as the realistic minimum if such images are to be useful for historic comparison with current materials. Newly introduced digital cameras produce pictures of acceptable quality that require only about 25 kb of storage (or 40,000 images/GB of storage). It is anticipated that all images will be maintained for the time that the report itself is maintained electronically.

Transcription and Editing

Transcription is a thorny and complicated issue. Virtually all departments have at least two to a sizable pool of transcriptionists whose major contribution is typing. Any number of transcriptionists will be involved during various periods while the report is being synthesized.

Several major advances have greatly streamlined transcriptionist efforts or even eliminated this function. One such advance is a central dictation system, apart from the computer system. Any member of the pathology staff, assistant, resident, or pathologist can dictate any aspect of the report, such as gross or microscopic sections, the final report, or any addition into the system. The secretarial professional then directly transcribes it into the AP computer system. The advantage to this system is that all telephones in the hospital or country are transformed into virtual dictation stations, thus freeing pathologists from dictating in confined areas or the need to use or transport special media (dictabelts) from one area to another. Some systems also offer hardwired stations that feature push-button identification of the dictating pathologist, the type of specimen being reported, and, with bar coding, the pathology number. These enhancements save precious time and promote enhanced accuracy.

A second major advance, the integrated voice interpreter, enables the pathologist to dictate directly into the computer, which translates the spoken words into words composed of characters. Such software add-ons are now showing sufficient reliability, speed, and accuracy to make them cost-efficient and thus enhance the automated report by removing one time-consuming and expensive step.

Finally, computer systems with user-friendly text editors ("word processors") enable residents and pathologists to edit their report directly once the draft has been entered. This can eliminate the need for the pathologist to return the draft with changes that the transcriptionist must reenter into the computer, which again saves time and drastically shortens turnaround times. In general, sufficient numbers of terminals strategically located, including a terminal in the pathologist's home when linked to the hospital via modem, greatly shorten the turnaround time to the point at which the final report is available to the clinicians.

Images

Pathologists frequently make drawings of specimens to highlight anatomic findings and to document economically where the labeled tissue sections are located with respect to the entire specimen. The modern system should permit the images to be scanned and incorporated into the report. Photographs are also commonly taken of gross specimens and increasingly of microscopic fields. Such images have required photographic media, and the prints and films with images have traditionally been stored separately from the pathology report. Now an increased ability exists to both capture and store the images digitally in the computer.[4] As image capture systems become easier to use and more inexpensively priced, and as laser printers are better able to reproduce the images with sufficient quality, images will very likely be included as an important and expected part of the final pathology report.

Prospective Quality Assurance

Today's computing systems are capable of a quality assurance level that is truly of benefit to the patient. For example, since 1991, the Duke AP computer system has listed at the beginning of each work day all cases for which cytologic and biopsy specimens are to be examined for the same patient.[5] After the component portions are independently reviewed in the respective divisions of Cytology or Gynecologic Pathology, but before any results are released to the clinicians, the diagnoses are compared for discrepant findings. When discordance exists, the specimens are reviewed; if the discordance persists, the case is rereviewed to identify the cause. Interpretative errors are sometimes found, although rarely. Usually the discordance reflects differences in sampling. When warranted, the surgical pathologist and cytologist conjointly issue a note, which has sometimes aided clinicians in recognizing that the highly abnormal cells in the smear (the usual case) may have come from an area (usually higher in the endocervical canal) that has not been biopsied. The clinician, confident that the discordant findings are valid, will often proceed immediately with further workup, which has led to the early identification of a tumor. The entire procedure, from accession to the release of the final diagnosis, usually occurs within 24 hours.

Interaction to Produce/Revise the Final Report

Verification of the pathology report is the final step; the pathologist reviews the entire report to ensure that it accurately portrays the findings. The discussion below describes the events immediately preceding and during verification and the demands placed on computer sophistication.

Authentication by Specialty Pathologists

When a portion of tissue is examined in a subspecialty laboratory by a pathologist other than the one responsible for the case as a whole, it has become increasingly important for the subspecialist to produce an independent report (as a subsection of the report as a whole) and to verify the findings; then lockout procedures can prevent anyone else from changing it in any way, even though the primary pathologist incorporates the findings into the overall diagnosis for the case as a whole. Error correction procedures with appropriate audit trails are also needed, as discussed below.

Diagnostic Coding and Charge Capture

Diagnostically coded surgical pathology reports facilitate both statistical evaluation and access to cases at later times. Several coding systems of choice exist, which largely reflect the country where the pathologist resides. The modern computer system must be capable of handling all systems. The SNOMED International Coding Scheme (CAP)[†] predominates in the United States; elsewhere alternate coding schemes are common (e.g., the READ Code in the United Kingdom). If SNOMED International is the nomenclature of choice, the system should crosswalk to SNOMED II, its forerunner. For many systems it is necessary that both coding schemes function simultaneously so that older cases coded with SNOMED II can be retrieved while new cases are coded with current versions. Finally, systems require translation crosswalks to codes such as the International Classification of Disease (ICD)-9 CM, now commonly required when submitting claims for payment.

CAP regulations mandate that all CLIA-approved surgical pathology laboratories have a diagnostic coding system in use. Manual coding by an experienced coder is superior for accuracy, brevity, and inclusion of minimal extraneous noise (superfluous or incorrect diagnoses). Unfortunately, highly experienced coders are rare, expensive, and a luxury virtually no department will enjoy in the future. Furthermore, manual coding systems are almost never current with case production. Current computer systems are now available that code the natural English text at the time of diagnosis. Such systems contain substantial noise, but they can be highly accurate, especially when they permit the pathologist, in the process of verifying the report, to edit, correct, or add codes.

The subject of billing systems for surgical pathology is enormously complex, even ignoring little appreciated aspects such as major management and scientific tools for examining productivity and resource consumption. At a minimum, and regardless of whether the pathologist wishes to bill through the pathology computer system or through secondary systems that are hospital or independently based, it is mandatory that the systems capture all charge information and tag each unit of work to the pathologist who actually performed the service. Since the Health Care Finance Administration (HCFA) has mandated that Current Procedural Terminology (CPT)-4, a specific charging code, be used for Medicare patients and numerous other insurers have followed suit, it is also important that the AP billing system be capable of identifying the appropriate primary CPT-4 code, the name of the pathologist associated with each code representing a unit of work (e.g., who performed the operating room consultation, which often differs from the person rendering the final diagnostic report or the electron microscopic analysis), and the corresponding ICD-9 CM clinical code. With focused regulatory reviews becoming more prevalent, it is also important that systems require the pathologist to verify the billing information captured and not

---

† SNOMED is a highly structured hierarchical coding scheme that uniquely specifies location (topography), appearance (morphology), physiologic changes (function), pathogens and animal vectors (living organisms), products (chemicals, drugs and biologic products), devices and activities commonly associated with disease and trauma (physical agents, activities, and forces), list of occupations (occupations), social conditions and relationships of importance in medicine (social context), entities comprising all of the above (diseases/diagnoses), and treatment (procedure).[6]

permit the case to be completed until the billing information has been certified correct and complete. At a minimum, the system should permit not only the capture of the primary code (e.g., 88305 for a diagnostic biopsy), but the ability to modify it (e.g., the second and subsequent unit of work might incorporate CPT modifiers for reduced work, such as 88305–52 for each subsequent independent biopsy performed during the same session). System capabilities should also permit the manual capture of additional charges for procedures done such as special stains.

The system must allow capture of any of these data at multiple points in the workflow and not simply at completion of the report. Also, the system must permit the pathologist to tag individual components of work done for purposes other than patient care (research or teaching) and thus allow alternate accounts to be charged. Finally, the system must allow for the possibility that some newer coding system will be used, which at this time is under consideration by certain U.S. governmental agencies.

Report Authentication by Consulting Pathologists

Risk management concerns, which are increasingly common, have led consulting pathologists to submit their opinions in writing to the pathologist of record, or to co-sign the final pathology report. In the event of co-signature, the computer system must be able to cue reports for the consultants' signatures in addition to, but before the pathologist of record. Reports should not be released for general inquiry until all co-signers have authenticated the report.

Report Review and Authentication by Pathologist of Record

As a final step prior to release of a case for external publication, either as hard copy or for transmission on-line, the pathologist of record must review the record and authenticate it as correct. The pathologist must have the freedom to review and modify any aspects of the report, except for those subsections previously verified by the subspecialist who performed and has taken responsibility for that particular segment, such as electron microscopy.

Report verification, a necessity for all systems, depends on system security ensuring that only pathologists can verify the case. Systems with a hierarchic granting of privileges can permit only pathologists to verify reports and, when desired, allow proxy privileges whereby another pathologist can substitute and authenticate (but also accept legal responsibility) for the pathologist of record. Also, systems incorporating electronic signature by the authenticating pathologist greatly reduce the time to verification since the pathologist may authenticate the case from the office or the surgical pathology area, or by modem from home or even when traveling.

Correction/Revision of Authenticated Reports

A small percentage of cases will always require the addition of supplemental information after the "final report" is authenticated (e.g., new results received after the case is completed, such as estrogen/progesterone findings on a breast lumpectomy specimen). Revisions are more difficult when portions of the original text are supplanted and superseded by the revised report. Whereas the original report should be unavailable to general inquiry once the report is superseded, regulations require that it nonetheless be retained in the system (see the section on quality assurance below for system-automated flagging of such reports).

The Final Report with Distribution and Management Uses

Construction of the final report involves both functional and technical aspects. Functionality, the subject of the second part of this chapter (the standardized [synoptic] report), addresses which findings should be included in the report and which formats help the clinician to grasp the report's content. More technical aspects of the report revolve around inclusion of critical nondiagnostic information with emphasis on cogent presentation. Among more successful reports, key demographic information (patient's name, hospital unit number, date of birth/age) is clustered, often in the upper right-hand corner, with the hospital or laboratory name and telephone number in the upper left. Near the pathology number is both the collection (operative) date and accession date. This is important to note, as commonly the turnaround time for the pathology department will be superb, but the overall time from when the office procedure was performed to the time the diagnosis was rendered may be poor, especially when, for example, an extra day was consumed before the specimen even reached the pathology department. Listing of the date allows praise or blame where due. Departments vary as to where the diagnosis block is placed. Regardless, highlighting the area (either by enlarging and putting in bold face the word *diagnosis* or shading/coloring the region) renders it prominent. If the specimen consists of slides received in referral from another institution, for the first line of the diagnosis block it is useful to list the name of the referral institution, the accession number of that institution, and the original operative date (Fig. 8-1). Finally, in all reports, it is important that the system identify each person who has worked on each section.

Report Printing and Distribution

The use of both laser printers and hospital information networks has profoundly changed how final pathology reports can be distributed. In the past, the use of multiple carbon forms necessitated that the reports all be printed at the pathology office

---

FINAL DIAGNOSES

Outside referral S95-2065, Nearby Hosp, Operative date 5/15/95

Endometrium, Pipelle biopsy: Adenocarcinoma, FIGO grade 3.

Fig. 8-1. Diagnoses section of report for slides referred from an outside institution.

and there separated, after which the individual copies could be manually sorted, segregated, and distributed to the patient chart on the hospital floor, the record room if appropriate, the various treating physicians, the pathology department, and other interested parties. Modern systems now can tailor this process somewhat more effectively. The copy for the patient's chart can be batch printed, but grouped in some more logical order (e.g., by nursing center). Copies for each requesting physician and for each consulting physician can be batch printed together by physician name, which both saves secretarial labor in the pathology department and more likely ensures that the reports will reach the desired physicians. Additional reports can be distributed as needed to other clinical and administrative departments such as the Tumor Committee, Billing Office, and Utilization Review. As more robust printer languages are developed, it is likely that printing may become distributed to network printers (i.e., directly by the printer at each nursing station, or in the physicians' offices). Possibly the report distribution may even become centralized, such that one major hospital computer/printer will receive all reports (pathology, radiology, electrocardiogram), regroup them, and distribute them in batch by each patient.

Quality Assurance, Care Mapping, and Outcome Management

Quality assurance (QA), also called TQM (total quality management) and CQI (continuous quality improvement), is an integral part of both departmental and hospital overall quality management programs. Common types of reports that measure aspects of the department as a whole include turnaround time analysis, specimen quality analysis, correlations between intraoperative and final diagnosis, and interlaboratory consultation diagnoses. Others are more specific for individual patients or individual pathologists. The former is exemplified by the prospective cytology-pathology correlation programs described above. The latter includes notification to pathologists of cases pending (report for each pathologist of cases not verified within 3 days). This latter program in particular has been shown to reduce tardiness in reports by 90 percent (unpublished data). Newer forms of quality assessment such as "care mapping" and "outcome management" are new terms to the hospital lexicon. These assessments cross department lines, focus on multiple interactions, and can affect patient outcome. AP systems should be designed with flexible retrieval systems such that any and all data items within the total pathology database can be accessed and selected items forwarded to other systems for amalgamation into the greater analytic process.

Management Reporting

Management reporting, an exhaustive subject, covers virtually every aspect of the pathology department. Examples have been given throughout this chapter that list various reports in use. In general, most reports tend to be daily logs of pending work, workload statistics, billing statistics, warning lists, and crisis lists.

INFORMATION RETRIEVAL AND APPLICATIONS

The ability to retrieve information in the format desired and on a timely basis continues to be a critical aspect of any system, and can have a great impact on a pathologist's performance, whether in terms of numbers of specimens completed, intellectual input on a case, or scientific review of cases. In a perverse sense, the well designed system does not improve the pathologist. Rather, it vastly reduces the effort ("scut time" or "exhaustion factor") required to obtain the information needed to complete any given task. Examples are discussed in the three categorical sections below.

General Inquiry

General inquiry functions are those modules that are in general use and that easily permit all facets of the surgical pathology system to be recalled in a complete fashion, and in an easy to use manner. Common inquiries include status of report, historic diagnoses for a patient, and work outstanding for a given individual or processing area. Access must be available by patient history number, patient name, accession number, specimen description (e.g., frozen section, small biopsy, outside slides, and so on), requesting physician, consulting physician, responsible resident, responsible pathologist, diagnosis, specimen (organ) type, general work area, and specific work area.

Presentation Format

One of the most difficult tasks in any system is a design to permit the user (whether clinician, pathologist, technician, or quality control officer) to view only the information desired in a format that is complete while pleasing to the eye and economical in space and time. For example, the clinician wishes to review all operations that clinician has performed over the past two days. The report presentation module in this case would build a queue of cases delimited (filtered) by clinician and time. Most anatomic pathology systems used in hospitals today are linked to a Hospital Information System, which the clinician would use to review the report. Because each individual pathology report is in actuality composed of component sections (i.e., diagnosis, gross examination, clinical history), the AP systems should be able to reorder the report and, for the Hospital Information System, store first those sections of most import to care workers (i.e., the diagnosis), and show in an inset box whether any part was revised since the original report was finalized.

Scientific-Historic Information Retrieval

A well designed computer system should not be an impenetrable black box, but rather a shell in which the data collected can be freely accessed, manipulated, and retrieved for any form of analysis desired. The system, using either internal or external instructions (which pull raw data into a secondary data man-

BONE LESIONS

DESIRED SNOMED DIAGNOSES FOR SEARCH:
CODE: (T1*)
  AND CODE: (M8*-9* AND NOT M8***0 AND NOT M9***0)

OR ANY LESION WITH
  SNOMED CODE: (M904*) OR (M918*-934*)

BOOLEAN CODE
((T1*) AND (M8*-9* AND NOT M8***0 AND NOT M9***0))
  OR
((M904*) OR (M918*-934*))

EXPLANATION
Where *=wild card, any combination of bone (T1) and tumor that is not benign (M8-9, but 5th digit not "0"); or any tumor of synovium (M904 series); or any tumor with osteoid (M918-20 series), chondromatous change (M921-924 series), giant cell tumor (M925), miscellaneous bone tumor (M926 series), or odontogenic tumor (M927-934 series).

Fig. 8-2. Complex Boolean algorithm for SNOMED computer search on bone lesions. (Modified from Robboy et al,[7] with permission.)

agement system where they can be further analyzed), should be able to generate a list of specimens with a particular diagnosis and then, for example, further select the list by age, sex, year, or other factors collected by the system. It should be able to retrieve cases involving electron microscopy, photographs, or deep-frozen tissue and to generate lists of patients whose diagnoses or case histories are unusual and merit further study. It should be capable of preparing daily, on an ongoing basis, lists of patients in the hospital with specific diseases so that the pathologist with special interests can rapidly identify and monitor those cases. Figure 8-2 portrays an example of a reasonably simple retrieval algorithm that uses nested Boolean logic to search daily for all bone cancers plus other specific diseases for the staff pathologist interested in orthopedic disease.

Applications

Quality assurance takes many forms. The cytology-biopsy correlations discussed above are an example of prospective quality assurance. While some quality assurance programs will be designed to satisfy regulatory agency promulgations, some can also be designed to have a major impact on self-teaching. As an example, in one system,[8] every specimen authenticated by pathology is computer examined against the radiology diagnostic computer system as to whether the patient had a radiographic examination of the relevant region: did the patient with gastric biopsy have an upper gastrointestinal series? On an ongoing basis, the pathologic diagnosis is sent to the responsible radiologist, giving immediate follow-up on the preoperative studies. This form of self-evaluation undoubtedly sharpens diagnostic skills, which in turn clearly benefits the patient.

American medicine devotes great effort to the care of pa-

tients with cancer. That care includes hospital tumor registries established to monitor the course of patients and increase understanding of the natural history of malignant disease. In one system,[9] the hospital's main tumor registry and a subsidiary registry maintained by the gynecology service saved considerable time and effort required to obtain and pursue all pathology reports once the pathology computer system routinely began to send these registries a listing of all new patients with applicable diagnoses. As an extra benefit, specimens with non-neoplastic diagnoses, such as negative lymph node biopsies, can be identified and transmitted, thereby indicating the patient that was alive at that moment, and pushing back by 1 year the time when the registry would next have to obtain follow-up information. The savings in terms of registry personnel was substantial.

Most hospitals devote substantial efforts to conferences, both for patient care and for the general education of students, residents, and staff. Use of the computer system to prepare complete lists of patient materials has saved the pathologist several hours in preparation time for each conference.

THE BACK OFFICE

Regulatory Compliance

The JCAHO, CLIA, and CAP have promulgated explicit and detailed standards for operation of anatomic pathology services. These cover a wide range of activities, from security, to documented quality control in all aspects of specimen flow, to monitoring of equipment and testing together with record maintenance. This subject is beyond the scope of this chapter, but newer models of computer systems should incorporate modules that will collect, store, and report all these regulatory items, a formidable undertaking.

ON THE HORIZON

Bar Codes Incorporated

Spurred on by both rules of regulatory agencies and outcomes of judicial proceedings, hospital personnel have recognized the need for systems that track the movement and location of a wide variety of surgical pathology acquisitions in a far more complex manner than that practiced in prior years. Incorporation of bar-code technology may help provide a portion of the answer. Two immediate applications involve slide inventory and the tracking of material to be disposed of or permanently archived. A major problem for nearly every pathology laboratory is found in the slide file room, where materials have been removed for study only to become permanently lost. A subsidiary issue is the acquisition of slides referred from an outside institution prior to the time the patient is examined in the hospital and the question of their subsequent location. Are they in the department, the central slide file room, or an individual pathologist's office, or have they been returned to the initial referring hospital? Bar codes on individual slides should greatly facilitate a solution. Similarly, the portion of the specimen received in formalin and not used for microscopic examination is generally discarded after several weeks to months. Bar-coded specimen containers should help permit the individual pathologist who wishes a particular specimen to be saved indefinitely to note this through the computer system at the pathologist's own sign-out desk, which would prevent the technologist from discarding the material when the specimen is checked before disposal. This could apply not only to formalin-fixed tissues but also to foreign bodies such as breast prostheses or other hardware or tissues for which retention is desired for any purpose. The retained material is often critical as proof that the standard of care was breached neither by the hardware manufacturer nor by the surgeon who installed the equipment.

On-Line References

In recent years many types of interactive information systems have been developed. The most widespread is Medline, a product of the National Library of Medicine; it is available in various networked versions, including local CD-ROM. Newly released image-based systems on video disk or CD-ROM are interactive atlas references[10-12] and expert systems[13] to aid in the diagnosis of the difficult specimen.

The Extended Laboratory

Merger mania has rapidly changed the landscape of the practice of pathology. Many independent hospital departments operated by a single group of pathologists may wish to utilize the same system simultaneously, which requires the systems to be capable of supporting and using interactively multiple independent hospital record numbering systems, but also partitioning the various databases to prevent co-mingling of data. Where outreach programs are used, the systems must be capable of allowing searches across databases. With managed care and prospects of distributed regional services becoming more likely, the AP system will also have to identify a patient's records that are found in various health care facilities; a universally adopted form of a unique patient identifier, such as social security number, may foster the linkages. As covered above, systems must already track specimen movement to and from outlying facilities.

Telepathology

Transmission of images is an area of much need and promise. One immediate use is transmission from the frozen section suite in the pathology laboratory into the operating room, which would permit the pathologist to show the surgeon exactly what the findings are in the specimen submitted while their import is under discussion. Transmission of images in real time or in slightly less than real time is becoming necessary for consultation among colleagues separated by significant physical distance. Electronic mail has been suggested as a low cost mechanism for transmission of an initial set of images to determine whether a diagnosis can be confidently achieved or whether ad-

ditional material is needed. Each individual participating in the consultation should be able to annotate the image displayed. Remote control of a distant microscope has been shown to be functional for frozen section consultation over long distances, whereby the consultant is able to move the slide on the stage and focus through the image in multiple planes.[14,15] Other uses have also been described.[16]

Instrument Interfaces

Relatively few automated instruments are used in surgical pathology, a situation that is rapidly changing. The major instruments that transmit results are the flow cytometer and image analysis systems. Systems already in use that require interfaces include dictation and voice recognition systems. Slide and cassette labelers as well as image transfer systems also require interfaces.

The Computer and the GUI Interface

This chapter has specifically ignored hardware considerations inasmuch as the success of the system lies largely with software specifications and the functionalities built into it, and to a smaller extent on the hardware and brand name of the maker. This is not to minimize the exponentially greater changes that have occurred over the past 25 years in equipment used and capabilities.

With the recent improvements and advances in capability and reliability in both personal computers and servers, as well as the ability to network with more traditional forms of computing hardware, we expect coming generations of systems to be graphic, with input and output screens that have windows, pop-up boxes, and the full range of mouse features seen today. In addition, insets will display pictures in the form of diagrams and images of gross and microscopic findings.

STANDARDIZED (SYNOPTIC) REPORTS

Enormous strides in medical knowledge have required that substantially new types of information be included in the surgical pathology report for it to be accurate, thorough, and useful. Some changes reflect the enlarged scope of testing (immunocytochemistry, nucleic acid probes, electron microscopy, and so forth). Another set of changes reflects the increasing use of standardized protocols in the treatment of cancers or other diseases, which demand that details be evaluated and reported. Rather than simply noting the presence or absence of cancer, the pathologist must now identify completely (sometimes exhaustively) the gross, histologic, and chemical particulars that may be necessary to select treatment, evaluate outcome, and estimate prognosis.

In general, the concept of what constitutes the report reflects two very different issues. One is the content of the information that is important to be reported. The other is the organization and presentation of the data in a form that is easy to display

Fig. 8-3. Endometrial tumor. Synoptic organization of items of diagnostic import that affect the behavior of tumor and that should be considered for inclusion in the final report. (From Robboy et al,[17] with permission.)

electronically, intuitively easy to understand, and appropriately formatted for the many current and potential uses.

The basis of any report is first and foremost knowledge of those findings that are important to evaluate. The example given in Figure 8-3 is for the uterine corpus.[17] Many of the items enumerated help the clinician to stage the disease. Others are known to influence the biologic behavior of disease or are currently being investigated for potential biologic import in the treatment of patients. It is axiomatic that this inventory, being dynamic, will be updated periodically to incorporate new advances in medical science. Such checklists should not be adopted slavishly; fixation with "pigeonholing" according to the checklist may hinder rather than foster open-mindedness as specimens are examined.

Once agreement exists as to the features deemed important, decisions must be made as to optimal formats of presentation. Within the past 5 years, many pathologists[18–23] and larger pathology organizations[24–30] have vigorously undertaken assessment of requirements for greater clarity and formats that will standardize data and provide ease of comprehension. This section addresses the issue of presentation in general, with specific examples. Each chapter in this book describes the appropriate information to present for the organs described.

The CAP is currently developing formatted checklists, or practice protocols[26]; these have been a major multidisciplinary cooperative effort of pathologists, surgeons, medical oncologists, radiotherapists, and others knowledgeable about the pathology and treatment of specific cancers. Practice protocols for several organs have already been completed.[29,30] Every organ of the body will eventually be described. Below is the pending CAP recommendation for uterine specimens removed for either treatment or staging (Fig. 8-4).

The design for presenting the diagnostic findings has been and continues to be one of the more controversial aspects of the report. Complexity often obscures and leads to unreadable or less than intelligent reports. Simplicity, by contrast, often leads to reports with insufficient information. Checklists, while convenient, especially for computer statistical analysis, require myriads of forms even for the same organ, are sometimes conceptually difficult to grasp, and are usually awkward when linking the multiple containers for each portion of the specimen that requires its own appropriate diagnosis. Examples of various formats are given below.

Figures 8-5 and 8-6 present the diagnostic findings in two formats in conformity with CAP guidelines. The first method groups diagnoses into blocks and presents the final diagnostic impressions *in order of descending importance* (Fig. 8-5). This is particularly significant so that important diagnoses are not inadvertently missed if they are placed in some other area of the final report (e.g., if the diagnoses are numbered according to the illogical and random order in which the specimen parts

---

APPENDIX 4: ENDOMETRIAL CANCER
(EXCLUDES STROMAL TUMORS)
(FIGO STAGING INCORPORATES PATHOLOGICAL FINDINGS)

Operative procedure: _____   Case: _____
Diagnosis:
Uterus: _____ (histology) (__% each major cell type)
    FIGO grade __, measuring __ × __ × __ cm
    with extension into _____
    and metastases to _____ lymph nodes
    and _____ (other sites).
Tumor penetrates _____ mm into _____ thick myometrium.

1 Architectural grade:
    (% solid growth) G1- Well-differentiated (5% or less solid growth)
                      G2- Moderately differentiated (6–50% solid growth)
                      G3- Poorly differentiated (over 50% solid growth)
    • Solid excludes squamous growth
    • Notable nuclear atypia, inappropriate for architectural grade, raises the nuclear grade by 1.
    • Nuclear grade takes precedence for clear cell, squamous & serous CA.

2 Special_Attributes
    Nuclear grade: 1 (Uniform nuclei, small nucleoli, rare mitoses)
    (glandular)   2 (More variability, larger nucleoli, more mitoses)
    (controversial)   3 (Pleomorphic, many mitoses)
    Squamous
    differentiation   __ % total neoplasm

3 Size of uterus: Weight _____ g; __ × __ × __ cm
    Size of tumor   __ × __ cm (length/width)
    Thickness of
    myometrium: __ mm
    Deepest invasion: None __ mm Serosa_involved

4 Location: Unifocal Multifocal
                           Ant Post Cornua
                           Fundus Body Lower_uterine_segment
                           Polyp (involves limited_to)

5 Extrauterine tumor
    Ovary   No Left Right Histology: _____
                               Synchronous v metastasis
    Fallopian tube   No Left Right
    Broad ligament   No Left Right
    Cervix   No Yes Supfl/glands Wall/stroma
                               Endocervix Exocervix
    If endocervix curetted No Tumor_only_(No_stroma) EC_with_implant
                               EC_with_invasion_into_stroma
    Parauterine   No Yes Left Right
    Vagina   No Yes
    Pelvic Peritoneum   No Yes
    Cul-de-sac   No Yes
    Omentum   No Yes
    Large Intestine   No Yes
    Other   No _____ (where)

6 Vascular involvement   No Yes_type_Uncertain
                               Lymphatics Blood_vessel Both

7 Tissues adjacent to cancer
    Nonhyperplastic   Prolif Secretory Atrophy Disordered_prolif
    Hyperplasia   Simple Complex Atypical

8 Ascites (>100 cc)   Absent Neg Pos
    Pelvic washing   Neg Pos

9 Special studies
    DNA ploidy   Euploid Tetraploid Aneuploid
    Estrogen-receptor   Neg Pos
    Progesterone-receptor Neg Pos
    S-Phase fraction
    Other   Yes, _____ Specify

10 Non-neoplastic endometrium/uterine
    Metaplasia   Squamous Mucinous Ciliary Clear_cell
                           Eosinophilic_cell Surface_syncytial
                           Papillary Other, Specify
    Adenomyosis   No Yes W_tumor
    Arias-Stella   No Yes
    Other   Yes, _____ Specify

	Left	Right
11 Lymph nodes: NOS	None ____ of _____ contain metastases	
Parauterine	None __/__ w Mets	None __/__ w Mets
Internal Iliac (hypogastric)		
Obturator (med ext iliac)	None __/__ w Mets	None __/__ w Mets
External iliac	None __/__ w Mets	None __/__ w Mets
Common iliac	None __/__ w Mets	None __/__ w Mets
Pelvic, NOS	None __/__ w Mets	None __/__ w Mets
Aortic, NOS	None __/__ w Mets	None __/__ w Mets
Inguinal, NOS	None __/__ w Mets	None __/__ w Mets

12 Serum blood levels
    CA-125

RESECTION/STAGING OF UTERUS
(Guidelines of College of American Pathologists)

Relevant clinical information
Patient identification (name, age/birthdate, unique ID)
Pertinent history & Type of procedure
Anatomic site (organs resected) & Orientation of the specimen
Physician/source of specimen & Date of procedure

Macroscopic (gross) examination
Fresh or in fixative (specify type)
External aspect (document extent of resection)
  Size (three dimensions) & Weight of uterus
  Constituent organs/tissues
  Documentation of areas marked by surgeon
Uterine corpus; For mass, give:
  Location & Size (3 dimensions)
  Description (exophytic, endophytic, consistency, etc.)
  Anatomic extent (invasion into myometrium, serosa, parametria,
    extension into cervix, attachment to or invasion of adjacent
    structures/organs)
  Relation to margins (parametrial, lower cervical, attached organs)
  Additional tumors
    Describe each possible primary cancer as above
    Multiple tumor nodules not regarded as primaries--
      Indicate size (range), number, location
    Other lesions (leiomyomas, adenomyosis, leiomyomas, polyps, etc)
Other organ(s)/tissue(s) (cervix, ovaries, tubes, others resected)
  General description
  If mass: Location, Size, Description, Anatomic extent, Margins
  Other macroscopic features
Lymph nodes submitted as part of resection specimen
  Location & Number
  Description (size, evidence of metastasis, other pertinent features)
Separately submitted lymph nodes
  Location (as specified by surgeon) & Number
  Description (size, evidence of metastasis, other pertinent features)
Other separately submitted tissues (e.g., staging biopsies, omentectomy)
  Location (as specified by surgeon)
  Description
Sections to be submitted for microscopic evaluation
  Primary tumor: demonstrate deepest myometrial invasion, distance
    from serosa, and isthmic/cervical or parametrial involvement.
  Show interface with adjacent benign endomyometrial junction.
  Other endometrial lesions--at least one section each
    Section(s) of grossly uninvolved endometrium

Ovaries, fallopian tubes and peritoneal & lymph node biopsies
Omentum, Vaginal cuff, & Other organs/tissues, as appropriate
Tissue submitted for special studies if done--specify

Microscopic evaluation and diagnosis
Uterine corpus
  If neoplasm
    Histologic type & Histologic grade
    Site (specify fundus, cornu, corpus, isthmus)
    Size (if different from gross measurement)
    Anatomic extent
    Presence/absence of vascular/lymphatic invasion.
    Margins (serosa/parametrium, cervical, others as indicated.
    Status of area(s) marked by surgeon
    Other findings--specify (e.g., endometrial hyperplasia, adenomyosis, etc.)
Other organ(s)/tissue(s) [for lymph nodes, see below]
  If neoplasm
    Histologic type & Histologic grade
    Site (e.g., ovary, fallopian tube, cervix, etc.)
    Designate whether metastatic, direct extension, or separate primary
    Size, Anatomic extent & Margins (if pertinent)
    Status of areas(s) marked by surgeon
    Other pathologic findings--specify (e.g., endometriosis, etc.)
Lymph nodes
  Site(s)
  Number with Total number examined & Number positive for tumor
  Other features (including benign glandular inclusions)
Other separately submitted tissue (e.g., staging biopsies, omentum)
  If neoplasm, type & Metastatic vs possible separate primary
  Benign inclusions
  Other findings

Results/status of special studies, if done, specify
Comments as relevant;
  Correlate with other specimens.
Correlate with clinical information;
  Explain discordance.
Provide sufficient information for staging.

Fig. 8-4. Endometrial tumor. Guidelines for formatted practice protocol developed by the College of American Pathologists. (Modified from Silverberg et al,[27] with permission.)

FINAL DIAGNOSES

E. Uterus, endometrium:

    Endometrioid adenocarcinoma, FIGO gr 3,
       3x3x2 cm, arising in anterior lower uterine segment
       Invasive 9 mm into wall 1.2 cm thick
       Involving wall of cervix
       With metastases to:

C.   Right external iliac lymph nodes: 1 of 6 nodes.
F.   Left common iliac lymph nodes: 2 of 5 nodes.

E. Myometrium: Leiomyomas, multiple, 2 cm maximum
E. Right ovary: Brenner tumor (4 mm)

The following tissues are free of tumor:
A. Vulva, biopsy: Lichen sclerosus
B. Omentum: Fibroadipose tissue.
D. Aortic lymph node, one node.
E. Fallopian tubes, bilateral, and left ovary
G. Left external iliac lymph nodes, 7 nodes.
H. Right common iliac lymph nodes, 2 nodes.
I. Right obturator lymph nodes, 3 nodes.
J. Left obturator lymph nodes: Fat only.

Fig. 8-5. Example of diagnoses for operative specimen for endometrial tumor. Formatted report listing diagnoses in order of importance and use of grouping to distinguish positive from negative findings.

FINAL DIAGNOSES

E. Uterus
    Endometrium: Endometrioid adenocarcinoma, FIGO grade 3,
       3x3x2 cm, arising in anterior lower uterine segment
       Invasive 9 mm into wall 1.2 cm thick
       Involving wall of cervix
    Myometrium: Leiomyomas, multiple, 2 cm maximum
    Right ovary: Brenner tumor (4 mm)
    Fallopian tubes, bilateral, & left ovary: No pathologic diagnosis

C. Right external iliac lymph nodes:
    Metastatic endometrioid adenocarcinoma in 1 of 6 nodes.

F. Left common iliac lymph nodes:
    Metastatic endometrioid adenocarcinoma in 2 of 5 nodes.

A. Vulva, biopsy:
    Squamous epithelium with hyperkeratosis.

B. Omentum:
    Fibroadipose tissue.

D. Aortic lymph node:
    No tumor in one node.

G. Left external iliac lymph nodes:
    No tumor in 7 nodes.

H. Right common iliac lymph nodes:
    No tumor in 2 nodes.

I. Right obturator lymph nodes:
    No tumor in 3 nodes.

J. Left obturator lymph nodes:
    Fat only.

Fig. 8-6. Second example of diagnoses for operative specimen for endometrial tumor. The information is identical to that in Fig. 8-5 but is organized both by descending order of importance and by the separate listing of each specimen container received.

UTERINE CORPUS- HYSTERECTOMY
FOR ENDOMETRIAL CARCINOMA

SPECIMEN:

SP # _____

_____

Pt. Name _____

_____[procedure]

Fellow/Att _____

Date _____

DIAGNOSIS:

V1   No residual endometrial carcinoma

Tumor Type
V2   Adenocarcinoma of endometrium
V3   Endometrioid type, NOS
V4   Endometrioid with squamous metaplasia
                (adenoacanthoma)
V5   Endometrioid, adenosquamous subtype
V6   Endometrioid, villoglandular subtype
V7   Clear cell type
V8   Papillary serous type
V9   Mixed type, composed of the following
                patterns: _____
(-)
              _____

V10   Malignant mixed mullerian tumor of endometrium
V11   With heterologous elements
V12   Without heterologous elements
(-)
              _____

Histologic Grade (For Endometrioid Types only)
V13   FIGO grade I (≤ 6% solid growth)
V14   FIGO grade II (6-50% solid growth)
V15   FIGO grade III (> 50% solid growth)
V16   FIGO grade not applicable
(-)
              _____

Nuclear Grade (For Endometrioid Types only)
V17   Nuclear grade 1
V18   Nuclear grade 2
V19   Nuclear grade 3
(-)
              _____

Depth of Invasion
V20   The tumor is limited to the endometrium
V21   The tumor invades to ≤ half of myometrium
V22   The tumor invades to > half of myometrium
V23   The maximal thickness of myometrial invasion
            is _____ *mm* [Important!]
V24   The thickness of the myometrium in the area
            of maximal tumor invasion is _____ *mm*
            [Important!]
(-)
              _____

Endocervical Invasion
V25   No endocervical invasion is identified
V26   Endocervical invasion is present in the mucosa only
V27   Endocervical invasion is present in the stroma only
V28   Endocervical invasion is present both in the mucosa
            and the stroma
(-)
              _____

Vascular Invasion
V29   No vascular invasion is identified
V30   Vascular invasion is present
(-)   _____

Endometrium
V31   The endometrium is unremarkable
V32   The endometrium shows the following abnormality(ies):
V33   Atrophy
V34   Simple hyperplasia without atypia
V35   Simple hyperplasia with atypia
V36   Complex hyperplasia without atypia
V37   Complex hyperplasia with atypia
V38   Polyp(s)
V39   Radiation changes
(-)   _____

Myometrium
V40   The myometrium is unremarkable
V41   The myometrium shows the following abnormality(ies):
V42   Adenomyosis
V43   Leiomyoma(s)
(-)   _____

Adnexae
V44   All adnexae are unremarkable
V45   The right fallopian tube shows _____
V46   The right ovary shows _____
V47   The left fallopian tube shows _____
V48   The left ovary shows _____
V49   All other adnexae are unremarkable
(-)
              _____

Lymph Nodes
V50   The lymph node status is as follows (expressed
            as the number of metastatic nodes in relation to
            the total number of nodes examined):
V51   Right obturator: _____
V52   Right pelvic: _____
V53   Right external iliac: _____
V54   Right internal iliac: _____
V55   Right periaortic: _____

V57   Left obturator: _____
V58   Left pelvic: _____
V59   Left external iliac: _____
V60   Left internal iliac: _____
V61   Left periaortic: _____
(-)   _____

**For Synchronous Ovarian and Endometrial
Carcinomas of Similar Histology (if applicable):**

V62   Note: The superficial character of the endometrial
            carcinoma suggests that it represents an independent
            primary rather than a metastasis from the ovarian
            carcinoma

Fig. 8-7. Synoptic form for hysterectomies done for endometrial cancer useful for computer coding. (Modified from Rusai,[25] with permission.)

FINAL DIAGNOSES

Pseudomyxoma peritonei:
   Arising in
      B. Appendix: as mucinous cystadenoma
Metastasis, resembling mucinous cystadenoma, to
      A. Right ovary, 980 grams unilocular cyst
Implants with both mucinous columnar epithelium & mucin to
      H. Umbilicus
Extensive mucinous deposition without tumor cells involving,
      C. Right diaphragm
      D. Omentum
      E. Bladder flap
      F6 Serosa of fallopian tubes
      F7 Serosa of left ovary
      G. Posterior cul de sac

Uterus (F):
   Endometrium: Proliferative phase.
   Myometrium: Leiomyomata, multiple, 8 mm maximum
   Cervix: No pathologic diagnosis
   Serosa: See above

Fig. 8-8. Example of formatted diagnoses in a complex case with multiple organ involvement

were received in the pathology laboratory). Lymph nodes and diagnostic biopsies without tumor are also grouped together in one section, thus aiding the clinician who reads the report and must utilize its findings. The second method also lists diagnoses by order of importance, but describes each specimen container individually (Fig. 8-6). This method is longer and can be more difficult to read when the overall case is complex. In both examples, the diagnoses are labeled with the appropriate container number in which the gross specimens were received in the pathology laboratory (and which correspond to the microscopic slides).

Two final formats are presented. One, a check-box type of final report, is designed for computer coding (Fig. 8-7). The other exemplifies a complex case with multiple organ involvement in which formatting can greatly foster comprehension of the total report (Fig. 8-8).

ACKNOWLEDGMENTS

We wish to thank Mr. Neal Patterson, President, Cerner Corporation (Kansas City, MO) and Ms. Jean Fitzpatrick, Product Manager for Anatomical Pathology, Cerner Corporation, for their many insights into the philosophy and practical applications of present and future anatomic pathology systems. Both have graciously spent many hours in discussing these matters over the past decade. We wish also to thank Mrs. Beverly Oxford, System Manager for the Duke AP computer system, and Mr. Joe Pietrantoni, Program Analyst for the Duke AP computer system, for their continual help.

REFERENCES

1. Friedman BA, Mitchell W: Integrating information from decentralized laboratory testing sites. The creation of a value-added network. Am J Clin Pathol 99:637–642, 1993
2. Elevitch F, Treling C, Spackman K, et al: A clinical laboratory information systems survey. A challenge for the decade. Arch Pathol Lab Med 117:12–21, 1993
3. Friedman BA, Mitchell W, Singh K: Differentiating between marketing-driven and technology-driven vendors of medical information systems. Arch Pathol Lab Med 118:784–788, 1994
4. Schubert E, Gross W, Siderits RH, et al: A pathologist-designed imaging system for anatomic pathology sign-out, teaching, and research. Semin Diagn Pathol 11:263–273, 1994
5. Ibrahim SN, Coogan AC, Wax TD, et al: Prospective correlation of cytologic/histologic cervical specimens. Am J Clin Pathol 106:319–324, 1996
6. Cote R, Rothwell DJ, Beckett RS, Palotay JL: The Systematized Nomenclature of Human and Veterinary Medicine (SNOMed). Ed 3.1. College of American Pathologists Press, Northfield, IL, 1995
7. Robboy SJ, Altshuler BA, Chen HS: Retrieval in a computer-assisted pathology encoding and reporting system (CAPER). Am J Clin Pathol 75:654–661, 1981
8. Greenes RA, Bauman RA, Robboy SJ, et al: Immediate pathologic confirmation of radiologic interpretation by computer feedback. Radiology 127:381–383, 1978
9. Aller RD, Robboy SJ, Poitras JW, et al: Computer assisted pathology encoding and reporting system (CAPER): an on-line computer system developed at the Massachusetts General Hospital. Am J Clin Pathol 68:715–720, 1977
10. Morawietz G, Rittinghausen S, Mohr U: Visual documentation of neoplasms as part of the REGISTRY Nomenclature Information System. Zentralbl Pathol 138:431–434, 1992
11. Heller DS: Gynecologic Pathology (CD-ROM). Blackwell Science, Boston, 1995
12. Robboy SJ, Norris HJ: Cervical Pathology (CD-ROM). Chapman Hall, New York, 1996
13. Robboy SJ, Norris HJ: Cervical Pathology. An Interactive Videodisc and Expert System. Intellipath, Santa Monica, CA, 1995
14. Oberholzer M, Fischer HR, Christen H, et al: Telepathology: frozen section diagnosis at a distance. Virchows Arch 426:3–9, 1995
15. Weinstein RS, Bloom KJ, Krupinski EA, Rozek LS: Human performance studies of the video microscopy component of a dynamic telepathology system. Zentralbl Pathol 138:399–403, 1992
16. Shimosato Y, Yagi Y, Yamagishi K, et al: Experience and present status of telepathology in the National Cancer Center Hospital, Tokyo. Zentralbl Pathol 138:413–417, 1992
17. Robboy SJ, Bentley RC, Krigman H, et al: Synoptic reports in gynecologic pathology. Int J Gynecol Pathol 13:161–174, 1994
18. Kempson R: Checklists for surgical pathology reports. An important step forward, editorial. Am J Clin Pathol 100:196–197, 1992
19. Kempson RL: The time is now: checklists for surgical pathology reports. Arch Pathol Lab Med 116:1107–1108, 1992
20. Leslie KO, Rosai J: Standardization of the surgical pathology report: formats, templates and synoptic reports. Semin Diagn Pathol 11:253–257, 1994
21. Markel SF, Hirsch SD: Synoptic surgical pathology reporting. Hum Pathol 22:807–810, 1991
22. Ngadiman S, Hoda SA: Checklists for surgical pathology reports. Arch Pathol Lab Med 117:569, 1992
23. Scurry J, Patel K, Wells M: Gross examination of uterine specimens. J Clin Pathol 46:388–393, 1993

24. Association of Directors of Anatomic and Surgical Pathology: Standardization of the surgical pathology report. Am J Surg Pathol 16:84–86, 1992
25. Rosai J: Standardized reporting of surgical pathology diagnoses for the major tumor types. Am J Clin Pathol 100:240–255, 1993
26. Ruby SG, Henson DE: Practice protocols for surgical pathology. Arch Pathol Lab Med 118:120–125, 1994
27. Silverberg SG, Hutter RVP, Henson DE: Practice protocol for the examination of specimens from patients with uterine cancer. Arch Pathol Lab Med (in press)
28. Henson DE, Hutter RVP, Sobin LH, Bowman HE: Protocol for the examination of specimens removed from patients with colorectal carcinoma. A basis for checklists. Arch Pathol Lab Med 118:122–125, 1994
29. Henson DE, Hutter RVP, Farrow G: Practice protocol for the examination of specimens removed from patients with carcinoma of the prostate gland. Arch Pathol Lab Med 118:779–783, 1994
30. Nash G, Hutter RVP, Henson DE: Practice protocol for the examination of specimens from patients with lung cancer. Arch Pathol Lab Med 119:695–700, 1995

9

Electron Microscopy

A. Marion Gurley
Alison D. Cluroe
Elizabeth C. Roberts

*What we must decide is perhaps how we are
valuable, rather than how valuable we are.*
Edgar Z. Friedenberg
"The Impact of the School"
The Vanishing Adolescent, 1959

Despite the advent and expansion of immunohistochemical techniques in the field of surgical pathology, and thus perhaps a more constricted role for the ultrastructural examination of tissue samples, areas of pathology both neoplastic and non-neoplastic remain in which electron microscopy is still an invaluable tool. When dealing with a muscle biopsy or a poorly differentiated sarcoma, for example, identification of specific fine structural detail may sometimes be the only means of providing a definite answer. The pathology literature reveals that for a variety of lesions the correlation of clinical information, light microscopy, immunohistochemistry, and electron microscopy is the only way to provide a real understanding of the true nature and pathogenesis of a particular lesion.[1] In the minds of some pathologists electron microscopy has become relegated to the domain of the researchers and perhaps teachers within our discipline. Often cost is misguidedly cited as a reason for not pursuing electron microscopy, and immunohistochemistry is seen by some as the modern day pathologist's answer to all ills. We should be cautious, however, about putting all our proverbial eggs into one basket. Most main centers already have electron microscopes in service and, used selectively, electron microscopy can still prove a cost-effective ancillary technique.[2]

SPECIMEN HANDLING

Many standard electron microscopy texts include chapters outlining in detail the theory and practice of tissue selection, fixation, processing, and staining, and interested readers should consult these for more information.[3–6] These subjects are summarized briefly here. They are also covered in more detail in Chapter 15 of this text.

Tissue for electron microscopy is best received fresh and should be placed in fixative as soon as possible after removal from the body. If tissue cannot be fixed immediately it is best kept at 4°C, but never frozen or allowed to air dry. For adequate fixation tissue should be submitted in 1 mm³ blocks, having been cut with a sharp knife while immersed in a few drops of fixative. Some specimens require special handling procedures, including renal and muscle biopsies. Tissue fragments from both ends of a needle biopsy of kidney are taken to ensure that cortex is sampled. Muscle biopsies are best fixed while in isometric clamps or, alternatively, fastened to an applicator stick to prevent contraction artifact.[7]

Glutaraldehyde is the fixative of choice for electron microscopy, with osmium tetroxide as the postfixative. Osmium acts both as a fixative and an electron-dense stain. Glutaraldehyde causes cross-linkage of proteins, and osmium fixes by combining with lipid. It is convenient to have individual small vials of glutaraldehyde stored in the laboratory refrigerator. Once in fixative, tissue should remain at 4°C and can be stored for several days. A minimum period of 1 hour is required for adequate fixation; prolonged fixation is not recommended. Formalin-fixed tissue may be used for electron microscopy but marked disruption of intracellular architecture often ensues. Methods of retrieval of paraffin-embedded tissue exist, but ultrastructural preservation is usually poor.[6]

Tissue for ultrastructural examination is embedded in plastic or resin and then semithin (thick) sections are cut using a glass knife and stained with a metachromatic dye (usually toluidine blue). Semithin sections are required to confirm the presence of the desired cells and to select the best tissue block for thin sectioning. In the case of renal biopsies semithin sections are used to locate glomeruli and in muscle biopsies to select the most longitudinal fibers. Final thin sections are cut on a diamond knife.

Routine staining in our laboratory is performed with uranyl acetate followed by lead citrate. Special staining protocols exist for various tissues to highlight specific components. For instance, demonstration of glycogen with potassium ferricyanide or ferrocyanide and osmium tetroxide is useful.[8,9] The addition of tannic acid will highlight collagen in skin biopsies that may be submitted for confirmation of epidermolysis bullosa; however, some authors stain these biopsies with uranyl acetate and lead citrate.[10] Biopsies for ciliary dysfunction can also be stained with lead citrate and uranyl acetate, but tannic acid may be added to improve the contrast of the dynein arms.[11]

It is possible to process material from fine needle aspiration biopsies for electron microscopy.[12–14] Negative staining techniques are used to study particulate specimens and are especially used to identify viruses.[6]

ELECTRON MICROSCOPY IN NON-NEOPLASTIC DISORDERS

The main areas of nontumor pathology referred to our unit are renal biopsies for assessment of glomerular disease, muscle biopsies and then in decreasing order of frequency, biopsies for ciliary dysfunction or for potential metabolic storage disorders, skin biopsy for assessment of epidermolysis bullosa, occasional tissue for the identification of microorganisms, endomyocardial biopsies, and peripheral nerve biopsies.

Renal Biopsy in Glomerular Disease

Glomerular basement membrane thickening seen by light microscopy can be resolved by electron microscopy into electron-dense deposits. These may be located either within the basement membrane or on the epithelial or endothelial side thereof. Thus, assessment of the ultrastructural detail of the glomerulus for the presence, absence, or location of membrane deposits in the glomerulonephritides aids in the classification of disease type. Evaluation of renal biopsy specimens involves use of the complementary procedures of light microscopy, electron microscopy, and immunofluorescence. However, some diagnoses can only be achieved by ultrastructural study of basement membrane changes. A good example is *minimal change nephrotic syndrome*, in which ultrastructural examination shows diffuse loss of foot processes in visceral epithelial cells.[15] This change cannot be appreciated on light microscopy. Another example is *systemic lupus erythematosus* (SLE), a condition in which the location and extent of glomerular involvement at an ultrastructural level provides an indication of the likely prognosis. The abundant subendothelial deposits seen rarely in other glomerulonephritides are almost characteristic of SLE, and when extensive these deposits appear as the characteristic wire-loop lesions that can then be seen on light microscopy. Another valuable ultrastructural feature of SLE is the presence within the renal biopsy of aggregates of microtubular structures or undulating tubules within endothelial cells.[16]

Skeletal Muscle Biopsy

Within our unit ultrastructural examination of skeletal muscle biopsy specimens has proved valuable not only in adding to nonspecific light microscopic findings, but also in providing a diagnosis after the tissue appeared essentially normal under light microscopy. Many muscle disorders produce only nonspecific myopathic changes on electron microscopy. Ultrastructurally, these commonly seen features include myofiber loss or disarray, Z-band streaming, and external lamina reduplication. However, some disorders have quite specific ultrastructural features that allow a definitive diagnosis. For example, in the appropriate clinical setting, structurally abnormal mitochondria

(crystalloids, increased mitochondrial size or number) (Fig. 9-1), when combined with the presence of ragged red fibers on a modified trichrome stain, may be regarded as constituting a *mitochondrial myopathy*.

Myopathy with tubular aggregates is a condition clinically associated with pain on exercise. The most prominent pathologic finding is the presence of large numbers of tubular aggregates located within the subsarcolemmal region.[17] Some *inflammatory myopathies* have helpful electron microscopic features; for example, in dermatomyositis, in addition to nonspecific myofibrillar changes, undulating tubules within the endothelial cells are present in most cases. Exocytosis of dark bodies is another feature seen in *dermatomyositis* but is more common in *polymyositis*. The presence of plasma cells beneath the basement membrane of muscle fibers, invasion of muscle fibers by mononuclear inflammatory cells, reduplication of basal lamina (often with multiple layers), and exocytosis of dark bodies are all features that point to a diagnosis of *polymyositis*. Ultrastructural confirmation of the presence of the characteristic abnormal filaments of *inclusion body myositis* is required for diagnosis of this disorder. The 15 to 18 nm diameter filaments may be found within the nuclei or, more commonly, within the cytoplasm of muscle fibers. In *Nemaline rod myopathy*, the presence of Nemaline bodies is the hallmark of both the infantile and adult forms. The rods show continuity within myofilaments and appear to originate from the Z discs.[18]

Ciliary Abnormalities (Distinction Between Acquired and Congenital Conditions)

Electron microscopy is the only means of establishing the presence of ciliary dysmorphology. It also allows distinction between a variety of acquired and congenital ciliary defects that result in impaired mucociliary transport.[19] Acquired changes are seen in the vast majority of the specimens passing through our unit. The presence of a morphologically recognized congenital ciliary abnormality is, in our experience, extremely rare, and the label should be used with caution at all times. Acquired ciliary changes are a common finding in patients with a history of recurrent respiratory tract infection. These, of course, by the very nature of their condition, are also the patients in whom the suspicion of a congenital ciliary abnormality is raised. Care must be taken not to overinterpret the acquired ciliary changes as the very much rarer congenital variety. When interpreting ciliary ultrastructure, the following three points should be kept constantly in mind:

1. Genetic ciliary abnormality should affect *all* cilia at *all* sites and at *all* times
2. Acquired ciliary abnormalities are usually focal and temporary
3. Some genetic ciliary disorders probably have no structurally recognizable abnormality

A variety of specific ciliary defects are genetic in origin. Examples include complete lack of dynein arms, defective ciliary spokes, and outer dynein arm defect. It must be noted, however, that dynein arms and radial spokes are often difficult to visualize ultrastructurally, even under the best conditions. The interpre-

Fig. 9-1. Mitochondrial myopathy in a 45-year-old woman with muscle weakness. "Ragged red" fibres seen on immunohistochemical staining. Electron microscopy revealed increased numbers of abnormal mitochondria with crystalline inclusions. (× 14,480.)

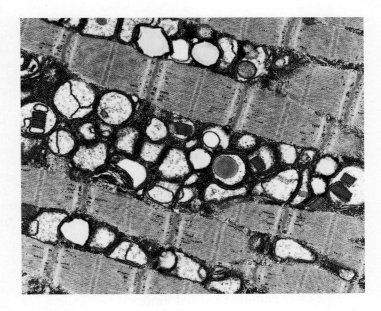

tation should therefore be guarded and the previously discussed points borne in mind. Examples of the more common acquired nonspecific ciliary defects are compound cilia, in which multiple axonemes are present within a common cell membrane, disorganized axonemes, and internalized or shed cilia (i.e. cilia projecting into the cytoplasm of the cell). An excellent article on the evaluation of ciliary dysfunction by Mierau et al[20] covers most of the important facts relating to the handling and interpretation of ciliary biopsies and presents a good cilial biopsy protocol. Because genetic error affects all cilia, at all sites, at least two sites must be sampled to establish a generalized rather than a local abnormality. The defects observed in both sites should be identical. Genetic error is permanent, and, if the above criteria have been satisfied, evaluation of an additional biopsy taken at a later date should be carried out before a definite diagnosis of a congenital cilial abnormality may be made.

Metabolic Storage Diseases

When a metabolic storage disorder is suspected, the samples collected and subsequently submitted for electron microscopy generally consist of liver and/or muscle and occasionally nerve. Electron microscopy may have a significant role to play in the final diagnosis in this area.[21] Once again, the combination of light microscopy, immunohistochemistry, and electron microscopy may provide a suitably distinctive picture to guide biochemical analysis in the correct direction for a definite diagnosis. In general, in suspected cases of storage disorder, one is looking for the accumulation of an abnormal product, excess of a normal constituent, or abnormal location of that constituent within cells. Examples of such conditions include *glycogen storage disorders*, in which depending on the type of disorder, excess free cytoplasmic or membrane-bound glycogen may be identified within cells. The different variants of the *neural ceroid lipofuscinoses* have ultrastructurally distinct inclusions for example, the late infantile form has dense curvilinear lamellar inclusions,

whereas the juvenile form has typical finger print profiles. The fibrogranular and lamellar inclusions of the different types of *mucopolysaccharidoses* are yet another example. Whenever a metabolic storage disorder is suspected, small tissue samples should be preserved in glutaraldehyde for possible ultrastructural examination.

Skin Biopsy for the Assessment of Epidermolysis Bullosa

Ultrastructural examination of skin biopsy specimens in epidermolysis bullosa is extremely useful in the classification of the different types. Overlap exists between the clinical and histopathologic features of the different forms. Electron microscopy, however, permits determination of the level of blister formation and hence the level of cleavage within the skin upon which the classification is based.[22]

Diagnostic Microbiology

The role of the electron microscope in the identification of various organisms lies mostly within the field of virology. However, in certain limited circumstances electron microscopy has a role to play in the diagnosis of bacterial disease (see below). Rapid diagnosis of some viral diseases, from a variety of body fluids or tissue samples, can often be achieved by ultrastructural analysis provided that a relatively high concentration of viral particles ($>10^5$ to 10^6/ml) is present to allow for visualization. The advantages of electron microscopy are that tissue culture of the virus is not necessary. The use of rapid embedding procedures followed by negative staining permits electron microscopy to be performed within 20 to 60 minutes and avoids the need for virus-specific reagents.[23] The use of immunoelectron microscopy allows for visualization of a virus when particle numbers are too small for direct detection.

Although virology laboratories now regularly utilize molecular techniques, including polymerase chain reaction and specific nucleic acid viral probes, direct ultrastructural visualization still offers the most rapid method of documenting the presence and type of viral particle. We have found ultrastructural examination useful in the identification of *Orf virus* particles in skin biopsy samples (Fig. 9-2). Ultrastructural examination is also useful when the location, not just the presence of an organism, is diagnostically important. For example, spirochetes are normally found within the human gastrointestinal tract, but in patients presenting with diarrhea and inflammatory bowel lesions spirochetes have been identified invading the lamina propria and within macrophages. Electron microscopy of bowel samples in our case of suspected intestinal spirochetosis was able to identify the spirochete organisms invading the bowel wall. Other organisms infecting the intestinal tract, particularly in human immunodeficieny virus-infected patients, have also been characterized with the use of electron microscopy.[24]

Endomyocardial Biopsy

Electron microscopy of endomyocardial biopsies has proved to be of some importance in evaluating the effects of drug toxicity or uncovering disease etiology in cardiac muscle specimens. Examples include assessment of the cardiotoxic effects of the antineoplastic anthracyclin derivatives Adriamycin and Daunomycin. Both of these agents have been associated with the development of cardiomyopathy.[25,26] The clinical course is characterized by progressive cardiac enlargement and dilation and with the development of congestive cardiac failure. The ultrastructural findings are not specific for anthracyclin-related cardiomyopathy; however, monitoring possible cardiotoxicity by the means of the ultrastructural changes in sequential endomyocardial biopsies in patients receiving anthracycline is of

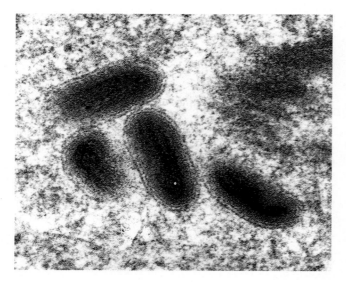

Fig. 9-2. Orf virus, in a 29-year-old man with nonhealing ulcer of the right small finger. Electron microscopy revealed viral particles in epidermal keratinocytes. (× 125,260.)

value. Two types of cell damage have been identified on electron microscopic examination. These are *vacuolar degeneration* and *myofibrillar loss*. Vacuolar degeneration occurs where the sarcoplasmic reticulum and T-tubule system are dilated with formation of large swollen vacuoles that coalesce to form membrane-bound spaces. This may be associated with loss of mitochondrial membranes and cristae and disorganization of nuclear chromatin. *Myofibrillar loss* may occur at the same time as vacuolar degeneration and may be partial or complete.[27] Ultrastructural analysis of endomyocardial biopsies has also proved to be of use in the identification of some specific heart muscle diseases. Examples include the identification of the randomly arranged, rigid, nonbranching rods characteristic of amyloid fibrils in amyloidosis or excess glycogen deposits in the various types of glycogen storage disorder.

Peripheral Nerve Biopsy

Infrequently within our unit we receive a length of sural nerve for assessment in cases of suspected neuropathy. Electron microscopy can be useful in identifying a variety of different nerve lesions.

For example, *axonal degeneration or atrophy* is characterized by the formation of columns of Schwann cells with their processes enclosed by basal lamina, the so-called bands of Büngner.

Segmental demyelination is characterized by "onion bulb" formation. This may be prominent enough to be identified by light microscopy but occasionally may require ultrastructural study to distinguish the process from clusters of degenerating axons. The onion bulbs are composed of concentric layers of Schwann cells, basal lamina, and longitudinally orientated bundles of collagen fibrils surrounding demyelinated or remyelinated axonal processes.

Ultrastructural examination of Schwann cells or endoneural, perineural, and epineural cells may demonstrate altered cellular organelles, or intra-and/or extracytoplasmic deposits, which can allow for a specific diagnosis to be made in some cases and which may not be appreciated at the light microscope level. Examples can be seen in patients with *Krabbe's disease*, in which Schwann cells and endoneural macrophages are seen to contain pleomorphic electron-lucent lipid deposits.[28] In addition, the highly characteristic cerebroside deposits, with an angulated and twisted tubular appearance, may be seen within endoneural macrophages. Early or small deposits of amyloid fibrils may be detected on ultrastructural examination of the supporting cells at a stage before they are visible under the light microscope.

NEOPLASTIC DISORDERS

It is not within the scope of this chapter to cover the ultrastructural features of all common neoplasms. Reference should be made to individual tumor sections, to Chapter 15, and to electron microscopy texts.[4,5,29] This next section concentrates on highlighting those areas of tumor pathology in which the discriminating pathologist will find electron microscopic examination of most value. Most cases referred to our unit would fall into the first two or three categories within this list.

Poorly Differentiated and Undifferentiated Neoplasms

Sometimes the tumor is so poorly differentiated as to provide few clues as to the nature of the lesion. This is particularly the case in the poorly differentiated, small, round, blue cell tumors of children and adolescents, including rhabdomyosarcoma, Ewing's sarcoma, primitive neuroectodermal tumors, neuroblastoma, and non-Hodgkin's lymphoma. The presence of a few microtubules, synapses, and neurosecretory granules may allow for the differentiation of neuroblastoma from the occasional thick and thin filaments or myosin-ribosome complexes of a poorly differentiated rhabdomyosarcoma.[30] Erlandson[30] states that myosin-ribosome complexes, in his experience, constitute the minimum criterion for diagnosis of rhabdomyosacroma. These complexes consist of a few rigid 15 nm filaments associated with numerous free ribosomes (Fig. 9-3).

In adults, when dealing with a poorly differentiated round or spindle cell tumor, the differential diagnosis can include rhabdomyosarcoma, leiomyosarcoma (Fig. 9-4), angiosarcoma, monophasic synovial sarcoma, amelanotic melanoma, undifferentiated small cell carcinoma, malignant peripheral nerve sheath tumor, and myofibroblastic lesions. Many of these tumors have characteristic electron microscopic findings. For example, the identification of stage II melanosomes at the ultrastructural level allows for a diagnosis of amelanotic melanoma (Fig. 9-5), whereas the ultrastructural diagnosis of malignant vascular lesions (Fig. 9-6) requires the demonstration of one or more of the following features[31]:

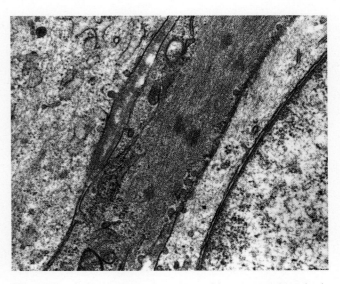

Fig. 9-4. Leiomyosarcoma in a 59-year-old woman with multiple subcutaneous nodules and no known primary tumor. Light microscopy revealed a poorly differentiated sarcoma. Electron microscopy revealed occasional cells containing thin filaments with focal densities, micropinocytotic vesicles, and the presence of external lamina. (× 35,000.)

1. Weibel-Palade bodies
2. Lumens lined by plump cells with atypical nuclei and long bipolar cytoplasmic processes joined by tight junctions
3. Pinocytotic vesicles
4. Partial investment of the nonluminal cell membrane by basement membrane
5. Arrays of disorganized cytoplasmic vimentin filaments

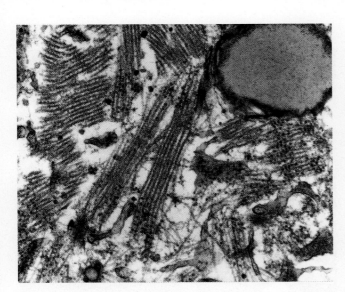

Fig. 9-3. Rhabdomyosarcoma in a 46-year-old man. Peroneal mass attached to bulbar urethra showing poorly differentiated sarcoma on light microscopy. Electron microscopy revealed the minimal criteria for diagnosis of a rhabdomyosarcoma, myosin-ribosome complexes. (× 44,330.)

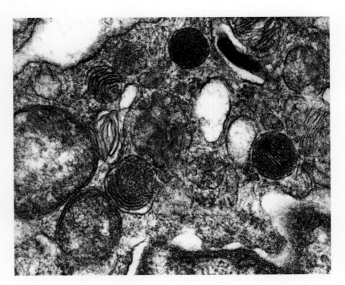

Fig. 9-5. Malignant melanoma in a 42-year-old man with poorly differentiated malignant spindle cell lesion of the left shoulder. Electron microscopy revealed numerous pleomorphic melanosomes. (× 61,900.)

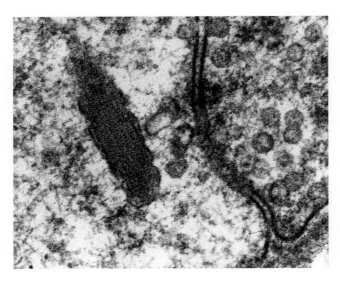

Fig. 9-6. Angiosarcoma in a 60-year-old woman with a solitary adrenal mass thought to be an adrenal cortical carcinoma. Electron microscopy revealed numerous pinocytotic vesicles and infrequent Weibel-Palade bodies (shown here). Occasional slit-like channels consistent with lumina and thin wisps of basal lamina were seen in other areas. (× 20,820.)

To make this diagnosis in a very poorly differentiated lesion the minimal criteria would be the presence of Weibel-Palade bodies in the cytoplasm of the malignant cells and/or lumen formation with associated pinocytotic vesicles[32] (Fig. 9-6).

Diagnosis of Mesothelioma

The diagnosis of mesothelioma is of obvious importance both medically and legally; it is based on appropriate clinical history, radiologic findings, morphology, and, increasingly, immunochemistry. However, the morphology, which is classically biphasic, can present a variety of patterns, including dominance of either the epithelial or spindle cell component. Furthermore, the spindle cell component, when dominant, may manifest a variety of patterns simulating various soft tissue neoplasms.[33] The propensity of this neoplasm to involve biopsy tracks means that large tissue biopsies and even biopsy cores are avoided in favor of the smaller needles required to procure pleural fluid for cytologic examination. The distinction between epithelial malignant mesothelioma and adenocarcinoma can often be difficult. When examining pleural fluid even a classic biphasic tumor may only exfoliate cells from the epithelial component. The demonstration of neutral mucins within the cytoplasm or glandular structures of the tumor will clinch the diagnosis of adenocarcinoma. However, the absence of appropriate staining does not necessary imply a mesothelioma. The literature contains large numbers of papers attesting to the utility of immunocytochemistry in the diagnosis of mesothelioma.[34–39] Essentially, mesotheliomas are usually epithelial membrane antigen (EMA) positive and negative for carcinoembryonic antigen (CEA), Leu-M1, B72.3, and BerEP4. Pulmonary adenocarcinomas are also positive for EMA, but will usually express positivity for at least two of the other antibodies. In a female patient, however, the most likely cause of a malignant pleural effusion is metastatic carcinoma of the breast, not metastatic pulmonary adenocarcinoma.[40] In this instance immunocytochemical studies may not be helpful because of the overlap in staining patterns between carcinoma of the breast and mesothelioma.[41] Although this distinction can usually be made on clinical, radiologic, or morphologic grounds alone, ultrastructural examination may be more rewarding than immunocytochemical examination in difficult cases. Most studies examining the utility of immunocytochemistry have used electron microscopic examination of mesothelioma as the gold standard.[39] The most important ultrastructural finding is the presence of long, slender, branching microvillous processes (Fig. 9-7) in the malignant mesothelial cells. Furthermore, these microvilli are distributed circumferentially around the cell. Interestingly, some early studies in which immunogold localization of EMA has been performed show that this antigen is distributed in relation to the microvilli.[35]

In practice in making a diagnosis of malignant mesothelioma we correlate the clinical, radiologic, morphologic (cytologic and/or histopathologic), and immunochemical results. If all features of the case are in keeping with malignant mesothelioma, we accept this diagnosis. However, if one or more of the preceding factors is conflicting or equivocal, we proceed with an ultrastructural examination of pleural fluid or pleural biopsies to confirm the diagnosis.

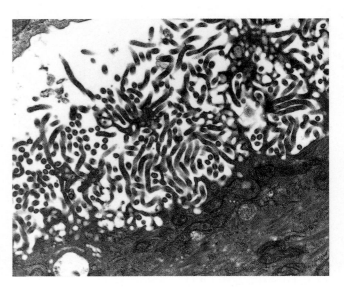

Fig. 9-7. Mesothelioma in a 80-year-old with malignant pleural effusion. Electron microscopy revealed large cells with long slender microvilli and prominent bundles of tonofilaments. (× 19,340.)

Confusing, Aberrant, or Unexpected Immunohistochemical Staining Patterns

Cases in which the immunohistochemistry fails to provide a definite diagnosis are not uncommon, for the following reasons: intrinsic properties of the tumor, technical processing problems, nonspecific immunostaining (i.e., cytokeratins in melanoma), false positive or false negative staining, or simply selection of an inappropriate antibody panel because of misleading or lack of helpful histologic features at the light microscopic level. Examples of this instance would include small cell or poorly differentiated neuroendocrine carcinomas in which the number of neurosecretory granules present within the lesion are insufficient to allow for positive immunostaining. Ultrastructural study of a suspected gastrointestinal stromal tumor (gastrointestinal autonomic nerve tumor) is still necessary before this diagnosis can be made. A highly characteristic ultrastructural feature of these tumors in the numerous synaptic structures containing dense-core neurosecretory granules of variable diameter and/or empty vesicles. These are often joined by rudimentary cell junctions to other cell processes. In addition, curved collagen fibrils known as skeinoid fibers are also seen in some cases (Fig. 9-8).

Not all tumors have a distinctive immunohistochemical staining pattern.[42] Examples include malignant peripheral nerve sheath tumors, monophasic synovial sarcoms, poorly differentiated leiomyosarcoma, hemangiopericytoma, and malignant fibrous histiocytoma. Primitive neuroectodermal tumors are classic examples of neoplasms that, because of their wide degree of differentiation, may stain positively for different antigens in different cases.[43] These tumors frequently show immunohistochemical evidence of neuroblastic or neuronal differentiation; however, glial, epithelial, melanocytic, and rhabdomyoblastic differentiation have also been detected.[44–47]

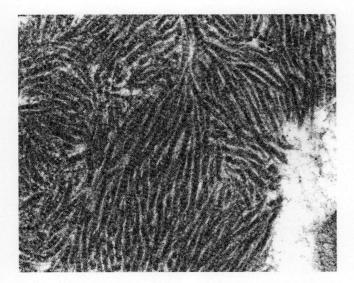

Fig. 9-8. Gastrointestinal autonomic nerve tumour. Skeinoid fibers from a fine needle aspirate. (× 37,330.)

The literature is reporting an increasing number of cases of anomalous immunostaining. For example, the nonspecific staining for cytokeratins in leiomyosarcoma,[48] rhabdomyosarcoma,[49] and lymphoma[50] may result in an incorrect diagnosis.

Fine Needle Aspiration

Because of the cost effectiveness of fine needle aspiration, this technique has become increasingly popular in the workup of mass lesions. Pressure has been increasing to provide specific tumor diagnoses, which has been reflected in the increasing proportion of fine needle aspiration material seen in electron microscopy laboratories.[51] Electron microscopic examination frequently has an advantage over immunocytochemical stains because of the vagaries of cell block preparation and the amount of material required to perform a panel of immunoperoxidase stains. As has been pointed out, the very nature of immunoperoxidase is that it can only test a particular hypothesis. Usually multiple stains are needed to test the different hypotheses included within the differential diagnosis.[52] Conversely, a good quality ultrastructural examination of only a very small number of tumor cells can potentially exclude multiple diagnoses and confirm a specific diagnosis. It may do so even when the correct diagnosis was not originally considered. The literature contains many semiquantitative studies of the efficacy of electron microscopy of fine needle aspiration specimens. Various studies quote figures between 44.5 and 79.6 percent for the proportion of cases in which ultrastructural examination either confirmed the original cytologic diagnosis or provided a more specific diagnosis.[53–59] Some of the studies go on to quantitate the number of cases in which the ultrastructural examination gave a more precise diagnosis than the cytologic diagnosis.[53,54,56,58,59] These figures range from 11 to 47.4 percent. When an attempt was made to identify cases in which the ultrastructural examination permitted a more specific diagnosis that was of clinical significance the figures ranged from 27.1 to 55.5 percent.[55,56,58,59]

The large variation in the foregoing figures probably represents not only differences in the efficacy of ultrastructural examination in the various institutions, but also differences in study design. The figures are also influenced by a large variation in the percentage of cases in which an adequate ultrastructural examination could be carried out. These figures range from 20.4 to 36 percent.[54,56–59] It has been suggested, and it is certainly our experience, that filtration procedures to concentrate the cell sample and remove blood from fine needle aspiration samples are useful in improving the material available for ultrastructural examination.[12–14] It has also been our practice to perform a rapid examination of Diff-Quik-stained material at the time the fine needle aspiration is performed. This allows assessment of adequacy of the material. A request can then be made for repeat passes. It also allows the cytopathologist to formulate a differential diagnosis and select cases appropriately in which it is anticipated that ultrastructural examination may be of use.[60] For example, it has been our experience that ultrastructural examination can almost always contribute to the workup of small round cell neoplasms identified in fine needle aspirates

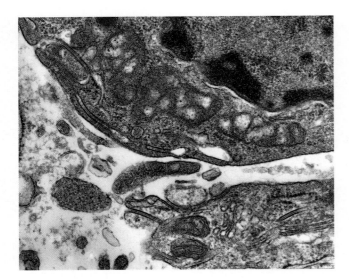

Fig. 9-9. Langerhans cell histiocytosis in a 11-year-old boy. Fine needle aspirate of T5 vertebral body mass. Electron microscopy revealed classic Birbeck's granules. (× 35,000)

from pediatric patients. Other authors have also found ultrastructural examination to be extremely useful in this group of tumors.[52]

Tumors That Require Electron Microscopic Examination for Their Accurate Diagnosis

In some tumors specific fine structural details must be identified for the correct diagnosis to be achieved. The identification of the classic tubular structure with a striated core consistent with a Birbeck's granule within histiocytic-appearing cells is one means of making a definitive diagnosis of a Langerhans cell histiocytosis (Fig. 9-9), and its presence may be useful in excluding those rare cases of true histiocytic lymphoma that can superficially mimic Langerhans cell histiocytosis. The diagnosis of chromophobe renal cell carcinoma is achieved by identifying the presence of numerous cytoplasmic vesicles throughout the tumor cells.[61] Alveolar soft part sarcoma is thought by many to be of muscle origin. However, the reports of immunohistochemical staining in the literature are confusing.[62] Ultrastructural identification is easy if the membrane-bound rhomboid crystals are found. These are formed by the crystallization of the larger secretory granules, which are often associated with small dense granules adjacent to the Golgi apparatus. Myoepithelial lesions are identified by their unique combination of actin filaments with fusiform densities orientated to the long axis of the cells and the presence of perinuclear tonofilaments and desmosomes.

Typical Classic Neoplasm

In addition to unusual neoplasms, classic neoplasms should be submitted to electron microscopy. This allows accumulation of a bank of ultrastructural data that may have definite value in the solution of more difficult diagnostic problems. Familiarity with the fine structural characteristics of these tumors may well aid in evaluation of a lesion consisting of only poorly differentiated cells. For example, our databank has proved useful in aiding diagnosis of very poorly differentiated angiosarcoma and poorly differentiated rhabdomyosarcoma.

In addition, our electron microscopy unit is based in a teaching and research facility, and thus we undoubtedly have a responsibility to accumulate useful material that may continue to contribute to our knowledge of tumor pathogenesis at an ultrastructural level.

REFERENCES

1. Mackay B: Editorial. Ultrastructural Pathol 19:iii, 1995
2. Erlandson RA, Rosai J: A realistic approach to the use of electron microscopy and other ancillary diagnostic techniques in surgical pathology. Am J Surg Pathol 19:247–250, 1995
3. McKay B: Diagnostic Electron Microscopy. Appleton-Century-Crofts, E. Norwalk, CT, 1981
4. Ghadially FN: Diagnostic Electron Microscopy of Tumours. 2nd Ed. Butterworths, London, 1985
5. Erlandson RA: Diagnostic Transmission Electron Microscopy of Tumours. Lippincott-Raven, Philadelphia, 1994
6. Hayat MA: Principles and Techniques of Electron Microscopy. 3rd Ed. MacMillan, Press New York, 1989
7. Carpenter S Karpati G: Pathology of Skeletal Muscle. Churchill Livingstone, New York, 1984
8. De Bruijn WC, den Breejen P: Selective glycogen contrast by hexavalent osmium oxide compounds. Histochem J 6:61, 1974
9. White DL, Mazurkiewicz JE, Barnett RJ: A chemical mechanism for tissue staining by osmium tetroxide-ferrocyanide mixtures. J Histochem Cytochem 27:1084–1091, 1979
10. Tidman MJ, Eady AJ: Evaluation of anchoring fibrils and other components of the epidermal junction in dystrophic epidermolysis bullosa by a quantitative ultrastructural technique. J Invest Dermatol 84:374–377, 1985
11. Pysher TJ, Neustein HB: Ciliary dysmorphology. Perspect Pediatr Pathol 8:101–131, 1984
12. Akhtar M, Ali MA, Owen EW: Application of electron microscopy in the interpretation of fine needle aspiration biopsies. Cancer 48:2458–2463, 1981
13. Akhtar M, Bakry M, Nash EJ: An improved technique for processing aspiration biopsy for electron microscopy. Am J Clin Pathol 85:57–60, 1986
14. Akhtar M, Bakry M, Al-Jeaid AS, McClintock JA: Electron microscopy of fine needle aspiration biopsy specimens: a brief review. Diagn Cytopathol 8:278–282, 1992
15. Arakawa M: A scanning electron microscopic study of the human glomerulus. Am J Pathol 64:457–466, 1971
16. Balow JE: Lupus nephritis (NIH Conference). Ann Intern Med 106:79–94, 1987
17. Lewis PD: "Myopathy" with tubular aggregates. J Neurol Sci 13:381–388, 1971
18. Engel WK, Oberc MA: Abundant nuclear rods in adult-onset rod disease. J Neuropathol Exp Neurol 34:119–132, 1975
19. Pysher TJ, Neustein HB: Ciliary dysmorphology. Perspect Pediatric Pathol 8:101–131, 1984
20. Mierau GW, Agostini R, Beals TF, et al: The role of electron microscopy in evaluating ciliary dysfunction: report of a workshop. Ultrastruct Pathol 16:245–254, 1992
21. Dustin P, Tondeur M, Libert J: Ultrastructural changes in metabolic

disease. p. 159. In Johannassen JV (ed): Electron Microscopy in Human Medicine. Vol. 2. Cellular Pathology: Metabolic and Storage Diseases. McGraw-Hill, New York, 1978

22. Eady RAJ, Tidman MJ: Diagnosing epidermolysis bullosa. Br J Dermatol 108:621–626, 1983.

23. Miller SE: Electron microscopy in rapid viral diagnosis. EMSA Bull 19:53–59 1989.

24. Orenstein JM: The role of electron microscopy in infectious disease diagnosis. J Histotechnol 18:211–224, 1995

25. Bristow MR, Mason JW, Billingham ME, Daniels JR: Doxorubicin cardiomyopathy: evaluation of phonocardiography, endomyocardial biopsy and cardiac catheterisation. Ann Intern Med 88:168–175, 1978

26. Lefrak EA, Pitha J, Rosenheim S, Gottlieb JA: A clinicopathologic analysis of Adriamycin cardiotoxity. Cancer 32:302–314, 1973

27. Billingham ME, Mason JW, Bristow MR, Daniels JR: Anthracycline cardiomyopathy monitored by morphological changes. Cancer Treat Rep 62:865–872, 1978

28. Schocet SS, McCormick WF, Powell GF: Krabbes' disease: a light and electron microscopic study. Acta Neuropathol (Berl) 36:153–160, 1976

29. Henderson DW, Papadimitriou JM, Coleman M: Ultrastructural appearances of tumours. Diagnosis and Classification of Human Neoplasia by Electron Microscopy. 2nd Ed. Churchill Livingstone, London, 1986

30. Erlandson RA: The ultrastructural distinction between rhabdomyosarcoma and other undifferentiated "sarcomas." Ultrastructural Pathol 11:83–101, 1987

31. Erlandson RA: Ultrastructural diagnosis of amelanotic malignant melanoma: aberrant melanosomes, myelin figures or lysosomes? Ultrastruct Pathol 11:191–208, 1987

32. MacKay B, Ordóñez NG, Huang WL: Ultrastructural and immunocytochemical observations on angiosarcomas. Ultrastruct Pathol 13:97–110, 1989

33. Moran CA, Suster S, Koss MN: The spectrum of histologic growth patterns in benign and malignant fibrous tumours of the pleura. Semin Diagn Pathol 9:169–180, 1992

34. Leong AS, Stevens MW, Mukherjee TM: Malignant mesothelioma: cytologic diagnosis with histologic, innumohistochemisal and ultrastructural correlation. Semin Diagn Pathol 9:141–50, 1992

35. van der Kwast TH, Versnel MA, Delahaye M, et al: Expression of epithelial membrane antigen on malignant mesothelioma cells. An immunocytochemical and immunoelectron microscopic study. Acta cytol 32:169–174, 1988

36. Sheibani K, Shin SS, Kezirian J, Weiss LM: Ber-EPA antibody as a discriminant in the differential diagnosis of malignant mesothelioma versus adenocarcinoma. Am J Surg Pathol 15:779–784, 1991

37. Nance KV, Silverman JF: The utility of ancillary techniques in effusion cytology. Diagn Cytopathol 8:185–189, 1992

38. Bedrossian CW, Bonib S, Moran C: Differential diagnosis between mesothelioma and adenocarcinoma: a multimodal approach based on ultrastructure and immunocytochemistry. Semin Diagn Pathol 9:124–140, 1992

39. Wick MR, Loy T, Mills SE, et al: Malignant epithelial pleural mesothelioma versus peripheral pulmonary adenocarcinoma: a histochemical, ultrastructural and immunohistologic study of 103 cases. Hum Pathol 21:759–766, 1990

40. Johnston WW: Cytologic correlations. p. 1070. In Dail DH, Hammar SP (eds): Pulmonary Pathology. Springer-Verlag, New York, 1987

41. Bedrossian WM, Mashood S: Immunocytochemistry applied to cytologic specimens. pp. 351–352. In Leong A S-Y (ed): Applied Immunohistochemistry for the Surgical Pathologist. Edward Arnold London, 1993

42. Miettinen M: Immunohistochemistry of solid tumours. Brief view of selected problems, review. Acta Pathol Microbiol Immunol Scand 98:191–199, 1990

43. Llombart-Bosch A, Lacombe MJ, Peydro-Olaya A, et al: Malignant peripheral neuro-ectodermal tumours of bone other than Askin's neoplasm: characterisation of 14 new cases with immunohistochemistry and electron microscopy. Virchows Arch [A] 412:421–430, 1988

44. Cavazzana AO, Ninfo V, Roberts J, Triche TJ: Peripheral neuroepithelioma: a light microscopic, immunocytochemical and ultrastructural study. Mod Pathol 5:71–78, 1992

45. Hachitanda Y, Tsuneyoshi M, Enjoji M, et al: Congenital primitive neuroectodermal tumour with epithelial and glial differentiation. An ultrastructural and immunohistochemical study. Arch Pathol Lab Med 114:101–105, 1990

46. Jimenez CL, Carpenter BF, Robb IA: Melanotic cerebellar tumour. Ultrastruct Pathol 11:751–759, 1987

47. Dickinson DW, Hart MN, Menezes A, Cancilla PA: Medulloblastoma with glial and rhabdomyoblastic differentiation. J Neuropathol Exp Neurol 42:639–647, 1983

48. Brown DC, Theaker JM, Banks PM, et al: Cytokeratin expression in smooth muscle tumours. Histopathology 11:477–486, 1987

49. Coindre JM, de Mascarel A, Trojani M, et al: Immunohistochemical study of rhabdomyosarcoma. Unexpected staining with S-100 protein and cytokeratin. J Pathol 155:127–132, 1988

50. de Mascarel A, Merlio J-P, Coindre J-M, et al: Gastric large cell lymphoma expressing cytokeratin, but no leukocyte common antigen. A diagnostic dilemma. Am J Clin Pathol 91:478–481, 1989

51. Strausbauch P, Neil J, Debbs DJ, Silverman JF: The impact of fine needle aspiration biopsy on a diagnostic electron microscopy laboratory. Arch Pathol Lab Med 113:1354–1356, 1989

52. Mierau GW, Berry PJ, Orsini EN: Small and round cell neoplasms; can electron microscopy and immunohistochemical studies accurately classify them? Ultrastruct Pathol 9:99–111, 1985

53. Willis EJ, Carr S, Philips J: Electron microscopy in the diagnosis of percutaneous fine needle aspiration specimens. Ultrastruct Pathol 11:361–387, 1987

54. Sehested M, Francis D, Hainau B: Electron microscopy of trans-thoracic fine needle aspiration biopsies. Acta Pathol Microbiol Immunol Scand [A] 91:457–461, 1983

55. Ravinsky E, Quinouez GE, Paraskevas M et al: Processing fine needle aspiration biopsies for electron microscopy examination. Experience implementing a procedure. Acta Cytol 37:661–666, 1993

56. Dardick I, Yazdi HM, Brosko C et al: A quantative comparison of light and electron microscopic diagnoses in specimens obtained by fine needle aspiration biopsy. Ultrastruct Pathol 15:105–129, 1991

57. Gurley AM, Silverman JF, Lasaletta MM, et al: The utility of ancillary studies in paediatric FNA cytology. Diagn Cytopathol 8:137–146, 1992

58. O'Reilly PE, Brueckner J, Silverman JF: Value of ancillary studies in fine needel aspiration cytology of the lung. Actol Cytol 38:144–150, 1994

59. Sehested M, Juul N, Hainau B, Torp-Pederson S: Electron microscopy of ultrasound guided fine needle biopsy specimens. Br J Radiol 60:351–353, 1987

60. Dabbs DJ, Silverman JF: Selective use of electron microscopy in fine needle aspiration cytology. Acta Cytol 32:880–884, 1988

61. Bonsib SM, Lager DJ: Chromophobe cell carcinoma: analysis of five cases. Am J Surg Pathol 14:260–267, 1990

62. Erlandson RA: Ultrastructural features of specific human neoplasms with clinicopathologic, immunohistochemical and cytogenetic correlations. p. 272. In Diagnostic Transmission Electron Microscopy of Tumours. Lippincott-Raven, Philadelphia, 1994

10

Fine Needle Aspiration

William J. Frable

Aspiration biopsy, aspiration cytology, or fine needle aspiration biopsy (FNAB) has enjoyed a rebirth in the United States in the past 15 years.[1] It is contributing substantially to timely diagnosis of neoplastic and non-neoplastic disease, thus reducing the necessity for an open surgical biopsy. Common clinical sites for FNAB are breast, thyroid, and lymph nodes.[2] Sophisticated radiologic imaging has detected many clinically silent lesions that can be sampled by FNAB within the chest, abdomen, and pelvis.[3] High resolution mammography and stereotactic needle placement have allowed sampling of nonpalpable breast lesions, while transrectal ultrasound of the prostate can uncover target lesions for directed sampling.[4,5] By current definition, FNAB is performed with needles of external diameter 1.0 mm or less, typically 22, 23, or 25 gauge needles.[6] These fine needles for sampling tumors cause minimal trauma and carry virtually no risk of complications, except for transthoracic sampling and (rarely) transabdominal aspiration.[7]

HISTORY

Martin and Ellis[8] were the first to report on the sampling of tumors by means of small gauge needles in 1930. This method became quite popular at Memorial Sloan-Kettering Cancer Center, with the publication of a number of successful clinical studies through the late 1950s. However, the procedure failed to be adapted in other major medical centers throughout the United States. Led by a group of experienced Swedish clinicians who were specialists in hematology and oncology, aspiration biopsy cytology had a resurgence in post-World War II Europe.[9–13] Both clinicians and pathologists from the United States studied in Sweden in the early 1970s and with their help FNAB again came to be recognized as a useful biopsy method for diagnosing tumors.[14]

Although very few comprehensive studies of technology assessment of FNAB have been reported, this procedure seems to be quite cost effective.[15] Cytopathologists who are well trained in this technique are still in short supply, but FNAB and general cytology have received increased attention and training time in most pathology residency programs. An increasing number of fellowships also provide in-depth training in FNAB specifically. A variety of radiologic imaging methods, computed tomography, ultrasonography, and image-intensified fluoroscopy have stimulated radiologists to perform FNA.[3,16] It is important for surgical and cytopathologists to work closely with these new interventional radiologists to maximize the effectiveness of FNAB for deep lesions.[17]

PLANNING FOR IMPLEMENTATION OF FNA IN PRACTICE

Either a surgeon, clinician, or cytopathologist may perform the aspiration biopsy. If surgeons or clinicians wish to perform the aspiration, then it is very important to work closely with the pathologist who will process the smears and interpret them. Stewart's[18] comment of 60 years ago still holds today: "Aspiration biopsy is as good as the combined intelligence of the clinician and pathologist makes it."[18]

A pathology department may decide to embark on development of an aspiration biopsy service. Abele and Miller[19] have detailed from their extensive experience the evolution from a hospital-based service to a free-standing clinic. For success in the clinic setting, dedicated personnel must be familiar with the needs of patients. The utility of FNA must initially be proved to clinicians. This is best accomplished by providing on-demand service that includes hospitalized patients, outpatient clinics, and travel to attending physicians' offices. With growth of the FNAB service, it will become necessary to perform aspirations within specified hours.

Suitable space to examine patients is required. Within a hospital clinic this space should be close to the pathology department but a separately designated area that is both quiet and comfortable for patients. Staff must be sufficient to assist the pathologists and provide clerical support.[19]

As described by Abele and Miller,[19] physicians may next request that the aspiration be performed in their office in preference to some location in the pathology laboratory. FNA lends itself to a traveling biopsy situation, because the equipment that must be transported is minimal. The major disadvantage is the traveling from office to office for single biopsies in even a modest-sized metropolitan area. However, this does promote the use of aspiration biopsy, which, if successful, leads to the formation of a free-standing clinic. A presentation to clinicians is also a useful marketing strategy. The experience of Abele and miller[19] should be reviewed carefully before undertaking the development of a free-standing FNAB clinic.

EXAMINATION OF THE PATIENT AND INFORMED CONSENT

Before starting the FNAB the patient is informed about what to expect. I have used the analogy of an ordinary venipuncture, that is, the procedure will take no longer to perform nor be more uncomfortable than drawing a blood sample. The pathologist may wish to develop a patient brochure that reviews the FNAB procedure (see Appendix 10-1). This can be given to the patient before the initial visit. The information of importance includes the general indications for FNAB, what it is intended to accomplish, and a summary of the few potential complications. Use of a standard consent form is optional in my view, but certainly verbal consent is important and it is probably a good idea to have a witness present, for example, a nurse or office assistant. In the case of FNAB performed on children it is recommended that a consent be obtained either verbally or in writing from parents. Informed written consent should be obtained for any deep aspiration biopsy, with or without imaging, particularly in the case of biopsy of the chest, abdomen, or pelvis.[20]

Where FNAB is being performed by clinicians and surgeons, success will only be obtained by a close working relationship between the responsible clinician and the cytopathologist. This is absolutely essential if the cytopathologist has no opportunity to examine the patient and must rely on information about the patient and the target being sampled which in transmitted from the clinician taking the biopsy. It is of great importance that a detailed description of the location of the mass for biopsy, its consistency upon aspiration, the clinical history of the patient, and the clinician's differential diagnosis be either clearly recorded on the report form by the aspirator or personally communicated to the cytopathologist.[21]

The cytopathologist's responsibility is to render a report meaningful to the clinician. The final diagnostic report must make sense within the framework of the patient's clinical presentation. The quality of the aspirate should be reported. It is important that no attempt be made to develop a definitive interpretation from an inadequate aspirate or even from a good aspirate when important clinical information is not provided. When the initial cytologic diagnosis does not fit the clinical situation, caution is advised. No major therapeutic decisions should be made on the basis of the cytologic findings alone.[6,22]

Equipment Needed

The following equipment is needed for a rapid and efficient performance of FNAB:

1. Cameco Syringe Pistol (Precision Dynamics, San Fernando, CA), Aspir-Gun (Everst, Linden, NJ), or other type of aspiration handle
2. 10 or 20 ml disposable plastic syringe with straight or Leur-Lock Tip (Becton Dickinson, Rutherford, NJ), depending on aspiration gun handle size
3. 22 to 25 gauge, 0.6 to 1.0 mm external diameter disposable needles, 3.8, 8.8, 15 and 20 cm long, with or without stylus

4. Alcohol sponges; Betadene sponges for deeper aspirations of transabdominal, transthoracic, bone, or deep soft tissue
5. Sterile gauze pads
6. Microscopic glass slides with frosted ends
7. Small vial of balanced salt solution or RPMI tissue culture transport media, or both
8. Vial of 50 percent alcohol for sample of aspirate for flow cytometry if needed
9. Suitable alcohol spray fixative for immediate fixation of wet smears
10. Vial of local anesthesia, 1 to 2 percent lidocaine (optional); topical spray anesthesia for aspirates in children or intraoral aspirations
11. Small vial of buffered glutaraldehyde for fixing aspirate for electron microscopy if required

A small plastic tray will conveniently hold all the equipment. Some pathologists who have set up free-standing FNAB clinics prefer to inject local anesthesia for all patients undergoing aspiration biopsy. They employ the equipment used by dentists and available from dental supply houses: 30 gauge disposable needles, 2.0 ml disposable cylinders of 2 percent lidocaine hydrochloride, with or without epinephrine, and a reusable metallic injection handle. Local anesthesia is then very precisely dispensed along the planned needle tract without tissue distortion that might affect palpation of the aspiration biopsy target. This method generally avoids the anesthetic burn.[19] Anesthetic guns are also available that dispense a short burst to deaden the skin surface only. These have been advocated when performing aspiration biopsy on masses encountered in children.

Preliminary Steps

FNAB may usually be repeated enough times to procure suitable amounts of aspirate for both diagnostic purposes and special tests, such as flow cytometry, immunohistochemistry, electron microscopy, or even molecular diagnosis, unless the patient is apprehensive.[23–39] It is not apparent that using local anesthesia ameliorates patient apprehension. It is important to take time to explain the procedure to the patient completely, since this is more likely to allay the fear of needles or any medical procedure. Taking time to gain the patient's confidence is most important. Under no circumstances should an uncooperative patient undergo aspiration biopsy. There may be exceptions to this rule in children, with parental permission, if the child can be restrained adequately.

The following preliminary steps should be followed for successful aspiration biopsy[2]:

1. Review the medical history of the patient and determine the clinical problem with relation to the lesion to be biopsied.
2. Decide whether the biopsy is indicated.
3. Attempt to determine by palpation the location of the target mass to be biopsied in relationship to surrounding structures. Estimate the depth of the lesion. Determine the optimal approach to accomplish the aspiration biopsy. A deeply located mass is usually best approached directly and

perpendicularly to the skin surface. Very superficially located tumors and those that are very small are best approached by penetrating the skin at a nearly horizontal plane, and then subsequently feeling for the lesion when advancing the tip of the needle.

4. The patient should be placed in a comfortable position for the FNAB but with the mass readily palpable and easily stabilized during the biopsy. This is very important in head and neck lesions, where the prominence of an enlarged lymph node, or lump, may be dependent on whether the patient is lying down or sitting up (Fig. 10-1). The prominence of the sternocleidomastoid muscle and its relationship to cervical lymph nodes require that the patient be positioned so that a minimum of soft tissue is traversed before reaching the target. It is helpful to place a small pillow under the patient's upper back when aspirating thyroid lesions. This will extend the neck, making the nodule appear more prominently. Aspirate thyroid nodules only within a perpendicular plane to the transverse vertebral process, and within a groove bounded medially by the trachea and laterally by the medial border of the sternocleidomastoid muscle (Fig. 10-2). The transverse process of the vertebra acts as a reference point for deep-lying thyroid nodules.

   Aspirating within the groove described and in a perpendicular plane avoids puncturing the carotid artery laterally and the trachea medially. If the carotid artery should be punctured, blood will begin to flow freely into the syringe. Withdraw the needle and place pressure on the artery at the site of the puncture for a full 10 minutes. If the trachea is inadvertently punctured, this is of no consequence. It will be apparent when suction is applied to the syringe, since only air will be withdrawn. Remove the needle and repeat the aspiration. The patient may cough at the time the trachea is punctured.

5. Take time to examine the patient's lesion thoroughly while describing the technique and what is to be accomplished with it.

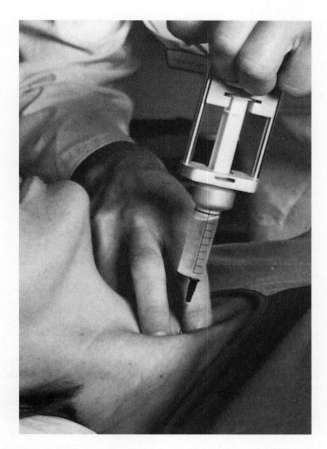

Fig. 10-2. Aspiration biopsy of thyroid mass. Thyroid nodule is immobilized between two fingers within a groove bounded laterally by the sternocleidomastoid muscle and medially by the larynx. A perpendicular plane for the position of the aspiration needle is utilized with the transverse vertebral process acting as a deep reference point if necessary.

Performing the Aspiration

The aspiration is performed as follows[20]:

1. Grasp the lesion with one hand, usually between two fingers, or push it into a position where it seems fixed and stable.
2. Prepare the skin with an alcohol sponge as for venipuncture.
3. Lay the syringe pistol with attached needle against the skin at the determined puncture site and angle.
4. With a quick motion insert the needle through the skin.
5. Advance the needle into the mass.
6. Puncture of the target may be tested by differences in resistance, by feeling that a capsule was penetrated, or by moving the syringe pistol very slightly laterally and detecting a corresponding movement of the mass beneath the fingers.
7. Apply suction to the aspirating syringe, usually about one-third the length of the syringe barrel.
8. Move the needle back and forth within the tumor with short, quick strokes and in slightly different directions.
9. Note at all times the junction of the needle and the hub of the syringe for the appearance of any specimen.

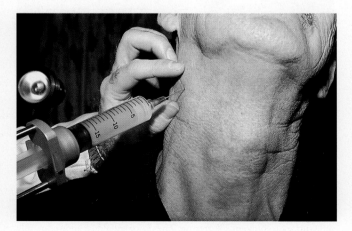

Fig. 10-1. Position for aspiration biopsy of an enlarged cervical lymph node. Examining chair with a headrest should be used for stability.

10. At the first appearance of any sample at the junction of the syringe and the needle, release the trigger of the syringe pistol and let the vacuum in the syringe equate to normal.
11. With air pressure in the syringe equalized, withdraw the needle from the mass.
12. Apply gentle pressure to the puncture site with a sterile gauze pad. The patient, a nurse, or an assistant may apply pressure to the puncture site while the aspirator turns to smear preparation and appropriate fixation.

Never withdraw the needle from the mass with any vacuum in the syringe pistol. With residual vacuum the small aspiration sample will be drawn into the syringe. It is quite difficult to recover the aspirate from the barrel of the syringe and the sample also begins to dry immediately. It could be irretrievably lost. If a cyst is encountered, it should be evacuated as completely as possible. After aspiration of any cyst, it is essential that the patient be re-examined for any residual mass, and if one is detected a repeat FNAB should be attempted on that mass.

The basic aspiration technique described is the same for deep lesions following the administration of local anesthesia through the chest or abdominal wall to the pleura or peritoneum. Many radiologists prefer to place a guide needle, usually 18 gauge, to the surface of the target, check its position by imaging, and then place the actual aspiration needle through the guide needle, again checking the position of the aspirating needle within the target by imaging.[40]

The amount of suction should be modified in accordance with the type of target. For example, in the thyroid, minimal or no suction is often sufficient to obtain a biopsy, since the thyroid is generally quite vascular, exceptions being some tumors and chronic forms of thyroiditis.[41,42] Reactive lymph nodes and some cases of chronic sialoadenitis also produce excessive blood if too much suction is applied. The needle-only technique may prove quite useful for FNAB of the thyroid and lymph nodes, and in very small lesions.[43]

Aspiration is usually most effective when one describes with the needle a small cone, with the apex at the point where the needle penetrates the skin. If the target is large, multiple separate aspirates are indicated, describing overlapping cones. It is critical to successful aspiration to keep the material within the needle and not to aspirate excessive blood or fluid, which dilutes the cellular composition of the specimen. Therefore, the aspiration itself should be of very short duration in most cases. Excellent instructional videos are now available that emphasize the points above, and others in addition, for achieving successful aspiration biopsy.[44,45]

Developing expertise at performing FNAB takes practice. This is possible using both cadavers and surgical specimens. A collection of biopsies from both normal tissue and tumors may be procured. Good technique with FNAB is appreciated by the patient.

SMEAR PREPARATION

The following steps should be followed in the preparation of FNAB smears[2]:

1. Immediately after completing the aspiration biopsy, detach the needle from the syringe; then pull back on the syringe pistol, filling the syringe with air.
2. Reattach the needle and place the tip of the needle in the center of a plain glass slide, touching the surface (Fig. 10-3).
3. Advance the plunger of the syringe to express a small drop of the sample, approximately 2 to 3 mm in diameter, onto the slide.
4. Quickly continue this procedure over a series of slides.
5. Invert a second plain glass slide over the drop; as it spreads, pull the two slides apart horizontally in a single gentle motion (Fig. 10-4).
6. An alternative smear method, when the drop spreads, is to pull the two slides apart vertically (compression smears).
7. Repeat the above procedure for all slides; fix some of the slides immediately in 95 percent ethyl alcohol, or other suitable fixative depending on stain preference.
8. Allow unfixed smears to air dry.

It is quite important to place the bevel of the needle against the slide as the sample is expressed so that no air gap exists between the end of the needle and the surface of the slide. Splattering the biopsy over the surface of the slide is prevented, as is excessive air drying of the aspirate prior to fixation in alcohol. By practicing the smear-making methods, it is possible to place nearly all the aspirated material, normally 4 or 5 drops, in a 3.8 cm (1½ in.) needle, over a series of slides and then begin actual smear preparation. With the rapid Papanicolaou method of

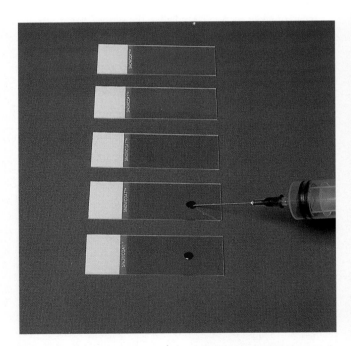

Fig. 10-3. Placing the aspirate on the slide. Drops of aspiration sample are expressed from the needle onto a series of slides by advancing the plunger of the syringe. The bevel of the needle should be touching the slide surface to prevent splattering. The drops should be approximately 2.0 mm in diameter, but their size will vary depending on the consistency of the aspirate.

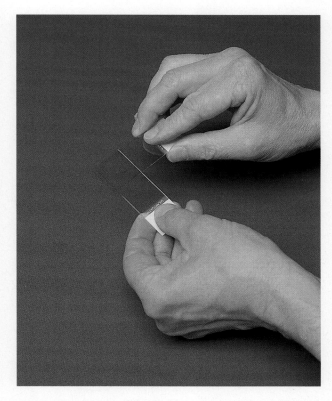

Fig. 10-4. Smears are made by quickly inverting another slide over the drop of sample. The aspirate sample will spread in a circular fashion, and the smears may be made by pulling the slides apart vertically or, as illustrated, pulling the slides apart horizontally in the same manner in which a smear of bone marrow is prepared.

Yang and Alvarez[46] all smears may be air dried. The most important point is to have the smear occupy only a small area of the slide. With good smear technique a tissue-like pattern is created. The area of the smear that must be reviewed by the cytopathologist is reduced, enhancing potentially important diagnostic features (Fig. 10-5).

Bloody or Fluid-diluted Aspirates

Some aspiration biopsies are diluted by excessive blood or fluid. Most aspirates from non-neoplastic goiter of the thyroid are largely composed of blood or colloid, or both, with relatively few follicular cells. Inexperienced interventional radiologists often provide samples that are excessively diluted by blood. For aspiration biopsy, more sample volume whether it is blood or fluid, is not better. It is quite difficult to make good smears from largely blood specimens. The liquid nature of these aspirates results in smears that occupy large areas of the slide. Diagnostic cells that may be present are usually found at the edges of the smears, and they consist mostly of single cells. When bloody or diluted aspirates are encountered the following steps may help in concentrating whatever cellular material might be present [40] (Fig. 10-6):

1. Place the drop of biopsy on the slide as described above; because of the liquid nature of the aspirate this will be 5 to 10 mm in diameter.
2. The slide with the drop of biopsy is held in the left hand.
3. Next take a second slide with the right hand bringing the edge of that slide up to the drop.
4. Note that the drop of biopsy sample spreads along the edge of the slide. As it does, begin to push the edge of the slide in the right hand toward the end farthest from the drop, but only about halfway toward the end of the slide in the left hand. This maneuver is in effect the same as making a blood smear.
5. Reaching the halfway point as described above, lift the spreader slide (in the right hand) straight up off the slide in the left hand.
6. Immediately tilt the smear slide that is in the left hand away from the leading edge of the smear; note that the blood runs back toward the point where the drop of sample was placed originally.
7. Next begin smear preparation with the lateral clean edge of the slide in the right hand (spreader slide) but only from the leading edge of the smear slide in the left hand.
8. Tissue particles that may be present will be concentrated in that part of the smear that was prepared from the leading edge of the slide in the left hand.

The method of smear preparation outlined above is difficult to perform. It requires practice and dexterity. If a specimen is largely fluid, then it is appropriate to use standard cytologic techniques, as one would for handling any other fluid submitted to the laboratory. I prefer cytospin preparations because they recover sufficient cells, and immunohistochemical staining can be performed on them if needed. Use of filters has largely disappeared as have cell spreads of buttons of material obtained from some fluids after centrifugation.

When deep aspirations or intraoperative aspiration biopsies consist mostly of blood, all the blood pulled into the syringe is best processed as a cell block (see below). Only the aspiration sample left within the needle should be used to prepare smears. Even a few milliliters of blood drawn up into the syringe can result in the rapid formation of a clot. Clotting of blood will greatly interfere with good smear preparation. Cells and small tissue fragments obtained become entrapped within the clotted blood (Fig. 10-7). The aspirate cannot be spread evenly on the slide, distorting any useful diagnostic pattern to the smear. The presence of the blood with entrapped cells also results in heavy and uneven staining.[21]

Cell Block Preparation

Samples for cell blocks may be handled by one of several techniques; simple centrifugation and the addition of 10 percent neutral buffered formalin to the resulting cell button, addition of thromboplastin or bacterial agar to the cell button, or use of the commercially available cytoblock system.[47] The cytoblock system has been found to be most satisfactory.[21] With any cell block method or very small biopsy fragments, it is important to work closely with the histotechnologist so that blocks are trimmed carefully to preserve ribbons of thin sections

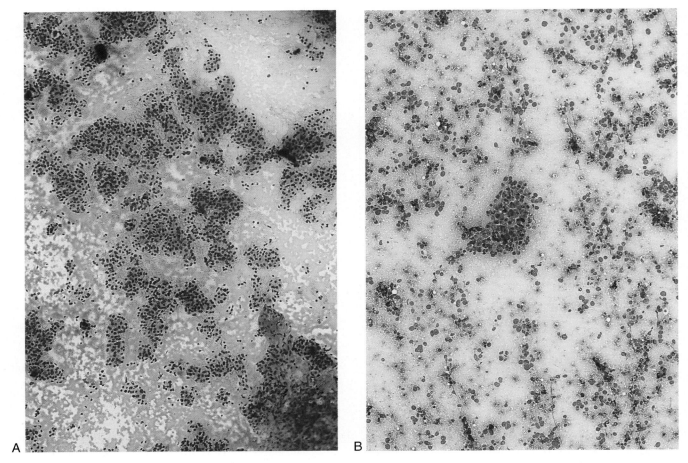

Fig. 10-5. Pattern diagnosis in fine needle aspiration biopsy smear. **(A)** Follicular neoplasm of the thyroid. Cellular smear with clustering of follicular cells illustrating a scalloped pattern at the edges of the large fragments. This pattern is created from the multiple proliferation of closely packed follicles seen histologically in follicular neoplasms. (Diff-Quik, × 100.) **(B)** Infiltrating duct carcinoma of the breast with a pattern of sheets, loose clusters, and single tumor cells comprising a cellular aspirate. A finely granular necrosis is in the background of the smear. This pattern recapitulates the histology of poorly differentiated infiltrating duct carcinoma of the breast. (Diff-Quik, × 100.)

of the biopsy. Some of these cell block slides should be stained initially, for example, those that are odd numbered, while saving others for special stains if needed. Cell block sections are usually more consistent for the application of immunohistochemistry, with the exception of lymphoproliferative diseases, in which cytospins provide good preparations if enough cells are obtained from the FNA[48] (Fig. 10-8).

Tissue Microcores

The tip design of the Franseen style needle, used principally in transthoracic and transabdominal FNAB, seems to result in procuring microcores from the aspiration procedure. These small cores must be dislodged by inserting the stylus into the needle and pushing them out onto a plain glass slide. These cores should not be smeared. That will only result in distortion of the cells, resulting in poor diagnostic material.[2,20] To prepare

some smears, at least in an effort to provide a provisional diagnosis, gently roll the microcore over a small area of the slide. Then the core should be placed very quickly in suitable fixative and processed as a small biopsy. As these tissue cores may be quite slender, it is imperative to work closely with a knowledgable histotechnologist to obtain good tissue sections and not destroy much of the tissue when trimming the paraffin block. These microcores require even more skill in histology than handling core needle biopsies of liver or kidney.

Specimen Problems (Including Cysts)

FNAB may obtain fluid that is clear and yellow in color, usually from breast cysts. This fluid does not need to be examined cytologically and can be discarded. Cyst fluid that is cloudy or aspirated should be sent for cytologic examination. Following evacuation of a cyst by FNAB, re-examination for any residual

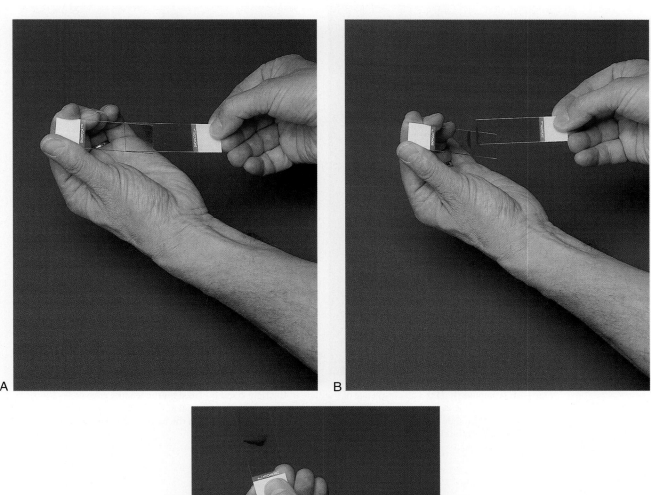

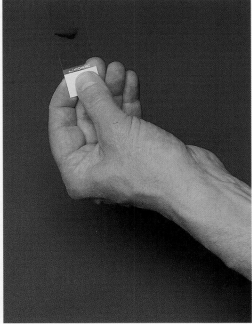

Fig. 10-6. Technique for making smears from aspirates diluted by blood. **(A)** A drop of aspiration sample is placed near the frosted end of a slide held in the left hand. The edge of a second slide held in the right hand is placed on the drop, which will spread along the edge of the slide. The slide in the left hand is pulled about halfway down the surface of the slide in the right hand in the manner of making a blood smear. **(B)** The slide in the left hand is then lifted vertically and **(C)** the slide in the right hand is held vertically so that the liquid blood runs back toward the original site of the drop of sample. (*Figure continues.*)

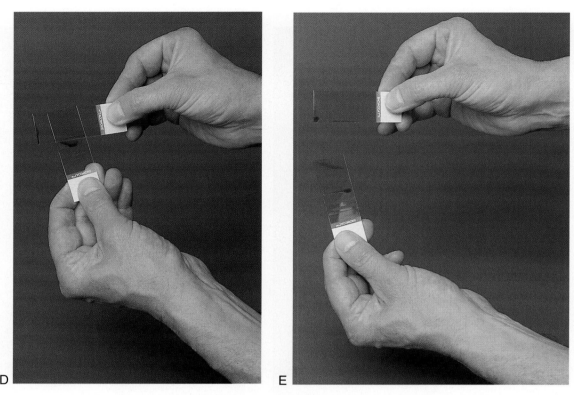

Fig. 10-6 (*Continued*). (**D**) The clean edge of the slide in the right hand is placed on the leading edge of the smear on the slide in the left hand. (**E**) A smear is then made from the material at the leading edge toward the end of the slide held in the left hand. An additional smear is made from the material on the edge of the slide held in the right hand, the spreader slide.

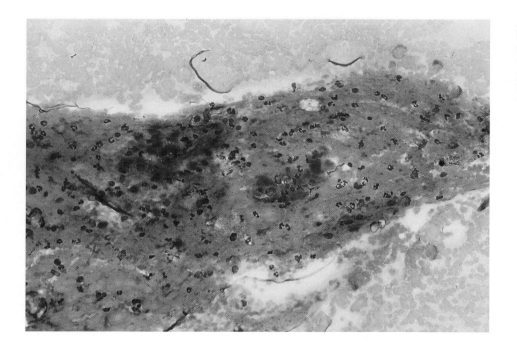

Fig. 10-7. Effects of prior clotting of blood on preparation of smears from an aspiration biopsy. Blood that has partially clotted traps cells, disrupting the pattern of the smear and obscuring details of individual and groups of cells. (Diff-Quik, × 250.)

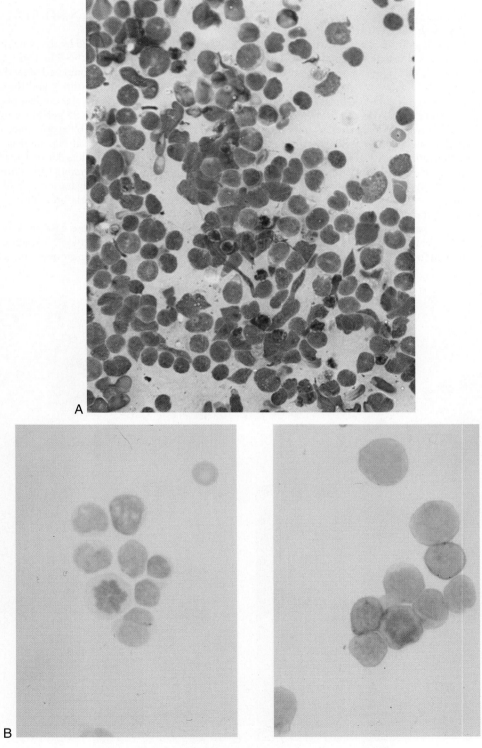

Fig. 10-8. **(A)** FNA smear and **(B)** cytospin of FNA of an enlarged supraclavicular mass in a nine-year-old patient. Interpretation of the smears indicated acute lymphoblastic lymphoma (Fig. A). Pan B cell marker is negative (left) while CD1a, a T cell marker, is strongly positive (Fig. B), (right). With the use of cytospins for immunohistochemistry, the smear background is quite clean. (Fig. A, Diff-Quik, Fig. B, peroxidase-antiperoxidase.)

mass is much more important than submitting the clear yellow fluid for cytologic examination. When aspirating masses in and around the thyroid, a cyst with water-clear fluid may be encountered. This is essentially diagnostic of a parathyroid cyst.[49] All that clear fluid or a portion of it may be submitted for determination of parathormone levels. They are usually quite elevated.

A rare and difficult to recognize lesion is cystic papillary carcinoma of the thyroid. Clinical clues to this condition are fresh blood in a thyroid cyst fluid, a residual mass after aspiration of a thyroid cyst, or a cyst that immediately refills after aspiration.[50] In my experience the vast majority of thyroid cysts that do reaccumulate fluid are cystic non-neoplastic goiters. The reaccumulation takes place slowly over weeks, months, or even years. Use of thyroid suppression may keep this process in check. A good policy is to aspirate the cyst two to three times. If on suppression therapy the cyst refills again, surgical excision should be considered. Occasionally such a case will be cystic degeneration of a follicular adenoma.

FIXATIVES AND STAINS

Air-dried smears are stained by the Romanowsky method or one of a number of variations.[2,21] The Diff-Quik stain is used in my laboratory. This stain is composed of methyl alcohol, which is the fixative, followed by eosin Y and then azure A. Smears that are spray fixed with one of a number of commercial products available or wet fixed in 95 percent ethyl, methyl, or isopropyl alcohol are stained with Papanicolaou (Pap) stain or one of its modifications. The rapid Pap stain is very useful, as all smears may be air dried. Cell loss during fixation and staining is markedly reduced with the rapid Pap staining developed by Yang and Alvarez.[46] The rehydration step also lyses red blood cells, eliminating their effects on staining and clearing the background of the smears.[46]

It has been helpful in some cases to have the rapid Pap-stained smears to compare cytologic features with air-dried Diff-Quik-stained smears. Nuclear grooves and intranuclear inclu-

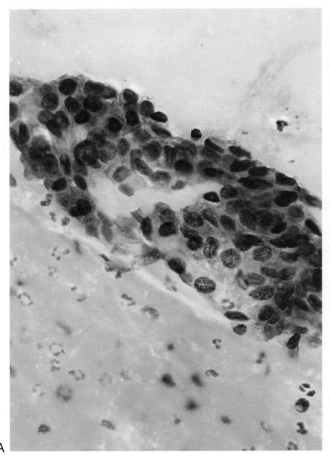
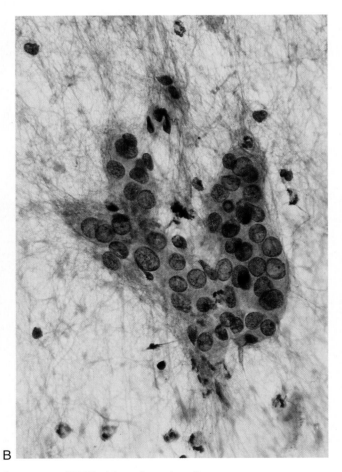

Fig. 10-9. Comparison of Diff-Quik and rapid Papanicolaou stains in FNAB of thyroid mass (papillary carcinoma of the thyroid). **(A)** Diff-Quik-stained smear reveals clusters of cells with elongated nuclei. The pattern suggests papillary carcinoma, but the nuclear features, either grooves or intranuclear inclusions, are not convincing. (Diff-Quik, × 600.) **(B)** Rapid Papanicolaou stain shows the same pattern of cell clusters, but the nuclear features, both grooves and inclusions, are much more obvious. (Rapid Papanicolaou, × 600.)

Table 10-1. Comparison of Air-Dried and Wet-Fixed Smears

	Air-Dried Smear, Romanowsky Stain	Wet-Fixed Smear, Papanicolaou Stain
Dependence on smear technique	Strong	Moderate
Dry smear	Good fixation	Drying artifacts common
Wet smear	Artifacts common	Good fixation
Tissue fragments	Cells poorly seen, heavy ground substance staining	Individual cells clearly seen
Cell and nuclear area	Exaggerated, differences enhanced	Comparable to tissue sections
Cytoplasmic detail	Well demonstrated	Poorly demonstrated
Nuclear detail	Different pattern from Papanicolaou stain	Excellently demonstrated
Nucleoli	Not always discernible	Well demonstrated
Stromal components	Well demonstrated and often differentially stained	Poorly demonstrated
Partially necrotic tissue	Poor definition of cell detail	Good definition of single intact cells

(From Orell et al,[54] with permission.)

sions may be easier to observe in some cases of papillary carcinoma of the thyroid (Fig. 10-9). An added advantage is that clinicians performing their own aspiration biopsies do not have to consider the details of fixation of smears; rather, the laboratory can decide which smears should be stained by this rapid Pap method and which can be optimally prepared by the use of other stains.

If smears are fixed with spray fixative it is important to allow them to dry for at least 1 hour prior to staining. When using aerosol-spray fixatives, do not hold the can closer than 1 ft from the slide. The propellant in the spray fixative may freeze the cells, which creates an artifact indistinguishable from a typical air-drying artifact.[51]

Before staining smears with any rapid hematoxylin and eosin method, fix them by immersion for a few seconds in equal parts of 50 percent ethyl alcohol and 10 percent neutral buffered formalin. When staining with a quick hematoxylin and eosin method, in the rinsing steps use hot (tap, not boiling) water. This will also improve the overall quality of staining and sharpen cell detail.[21]

Samples for immunohistochemistry are prepared by rinsing either a separate aspirate from the lesion or a portion of the aspiration biopsy into balanced salt solution. Cytospins are made from the needle rinse and may be either air dried or fixed in 95 percent ethyl alcohol. I prefer air drying. Direct smears or cytospins, either air dried or fixed to be used for immunohistochemistry, may be preserved in a deep freezer for up to four weeks. Either fixed or deep-frozen aspirate samples are also suitable for molecular diagnostic methods. Recent studies have identified several additional methods that may be helpful in improving immunostaining of cytologic specimens, including the use of microwave methods for antigen retrieval.[48,52]

Both personal preference and experience often dictate which stain or stains will be used on aspiration biopsy smears. Cytopathologists with an orientation toward surgical pathology may prefer a rapid hematoxylin and eosin stain.[53] Those with a major experience in cytopathology most often prefer the Pap stain.[17] Individuals influenced by a hematologic background or trained in the aspiration biopsy clinic at the Karolinska Institute in Stockholm like the Romanowsky, May-Grünwald-Giemsa, straight Giemsa, or Wright's stains, or, in the United States, Diff-Quik.[4,6,9–11,54] The Romanowsky stain and its variations result in a metachromasia of any stromal elements, with epithelial or other types of cells viewed in contrast to that stroma. The major advantage of this stain is its rapidity, which can lead to an immediate diagnosis following the aspiration biopsy. The quality of the aspirate can also be checked. Depending on the initial evaluation, repeat aspiration biopsies may be obtained for both diagnosis and special studies.

Table 10-1 compares the properties of air-dried versus wet-

Table 10-2. Comparison of Features Emphasized in Romanowsky Stains and Conventional Papanicolaou Stain

Tissue Type	Romanowsky	Papanicolaou
Epithelial	Mucin, intracellular or extracellular; colloid (thyroid); secretory granules (prostate); lipofuscin granules (seminal vesicles); lipid vacuoles; fire flares (thyroid); bare bipolar nuclei (benign breast); bile plugs; basement membrane globules (adenoid cystic carcinoma); amyloid	Squamous differentiation/keratinization; oncocytes (salivary gland tumors); psammoma bodies
Lymphoid	Cytoplasmic basophilia; lymphoglandular bodies; hematopoietic cells; lipid vacuoles	Nuclear outline; nuclear chromatin pattern; nucleoli

(From Orell et at,[54] with permission.)

fixed smears.[54] Table 10-2 lists the features emphasized by the Romanowsky stains compared with the conventional Pap stain as outlined originally by Orell and colleagues.[54]

ANCILLARY TECHNIQUES AND APPLICATIONS

Several special techniques may improve the diagnostic results of aspiration biopsies.[23,25,27] Immunohistochemical staining may be performed directly on smears, on microcore biopsy or any cell block samples, and on cytospin preparations of aspirates, as described above. Immunohistochemistry applied to direct smears may result in significant background staining.[55] If the cells in question are stained intensely, this represents a positive reaction for the antibody in question. The positive detection of a terminally differentiated protein, such as gastrin or prostate-specific antigen, is quite reliable on direct smears because of the highly intense staining. Any background positivity can be ignored. The basic differential between lymphoma and undifferentiated carcinoma is also quite reliable on direct smears. To obtain a clean background and in cases of lymphoproliferative disease, cytospin preparations provide good differentiation between positive and negative staining for various types of lymphoid cells and may be used to determine clonality.[56] Flow cytometry of aspirates may be utilized in the same manner to segregate various population of lymphoid cells[26] (Fig. 10-10). Fluorescent in situ hybridization can be used on FNAs to detect numeric chromosome abnormalities. The method described by Cajulis and Frias-Hidvegi[38] has good sensitivity and specificity. This technique has application when only a few tumor cells are present in a given specimen or in aspirations in which it is difficult to distinguish benign from malignant cells.[38]

INTERPRETATION OF THE REPORT

A number of important components should be included in a completed FNAB report.[21] Demographics, history, and the precise procedure performed are compiled by the aspirator, either clinician or cytopathologist. The microscopic features and diagnosis are the responsibility of the cytopathologist. The final diagnosis should include the site as well as the morphology as observed, for example, "benign mixed tumor of right parotid salivary gland." The cytologic diagnoses are formatted in the same way as standard surgical pathology diagnoses. They are complete diagnoses.[6] If a definite diagnosis cannot be made, this needs to be stated. Such reports are much less specific. Examples would be "atypical cells of undetermined type or significance, from aspirate of left cervical lymph node" or "nondiagnostic aspirate of right breast mass."

Recommendations for appropriate additional studies are an important part of the report and may include a request for repeat aspiration biopsy, a recommendation for an open biopsy, or another management plan.[20] These various recommendations are dependent on the degree of certainty of the cytopathologist in the reporting of the aspiration biopsy coupled with a synthesis of the clinical information and results of the physical examination of the lesion, including how it felt during the FNAB. An intraoperative frozen section should be specifically suggested if after aspiration biopsy the cytopathologist cannot make a definitive malignant diagnosis and major surgery is planned. With respect to the current medical malpractice climate in the United States, it may be advisable to confirm a malignant aspiration biopsy diagnosis by frozen section, particularly if the contemplated surgery is extensive. Even with this caveat, the aspiration biopsy is still quite useful because, among patients with suspected malignant tumors, it distinguishes between those definitely requiring immediate surgery and those who do not.

COMPLICATIONS AND LIABILITY

Most "lumps and bumps" in patients who present for FNAB are superficially located and not in direct relationship to anatomic structures hazardous for biopsy. Complications from properly performed FNAB of superficial masses are few and of little consequence.[17] They include some minor discomfort in the region of the aspiration, usually of no more than a few hours' duration, some minimal ecchymosis of the aspiration site, and (rarely) small hematomas.[21] Complications are directly related to needle size. They have been less than 0.03 percent in a review of published series when needles of finer gauge than 20 have been used.[7] Tumor cells seeding the needle tract have been reported only rarely with this size needle. Most reported cases of that complication are poorly documented. I have observed no cases of needle tract seeding in over 13,000 superficial and deep aspirations performed since 1972.

Reports have documented tissue damage or the displacement of tumor cells causing confusion in the interpretation of subsequent surgical biopsies or inability to make a diagnosis on the surgical specimen. Careful examination of these cases indicates the use of larger needles than 22 gauge or thin needles with tip design that ensures damage to tissue in comparison with the conventional straight beveled needle used to draw a blood sample. Other reports suggest that an ill-trained or inexperienced clinician performing FNAB accounts for most or all of the cases in a given series.[7,57,58]

While taking a superficial FNAB, particularly in the area of the head and neck, some patients may experience lightheadedness or actual syncope.[59] Most of these patients have a past history of vasovagal responses to needle puncture. This informa-

---

Fig. 10-10. **(A)** Smear and **(B)** flow cytometry for lymphoid markers of fine needle aspiration biopsy of a lumbar mass, soft tissue large cell lymphoma. Cells from aspirate of the tumor were labeled for lymphoid markers and scanned. A monoclonal population of lymphoid cells is demonstrated, supporting a diagnosis of lymphoma. (Fig. A, Diff-Quik, × 400.)

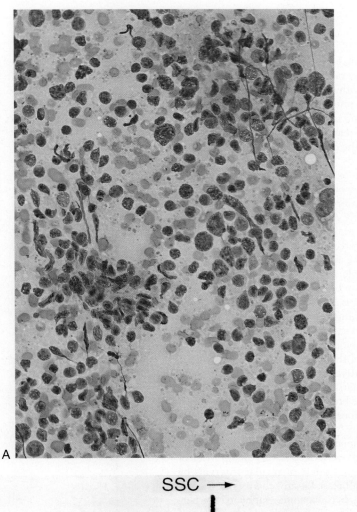

A

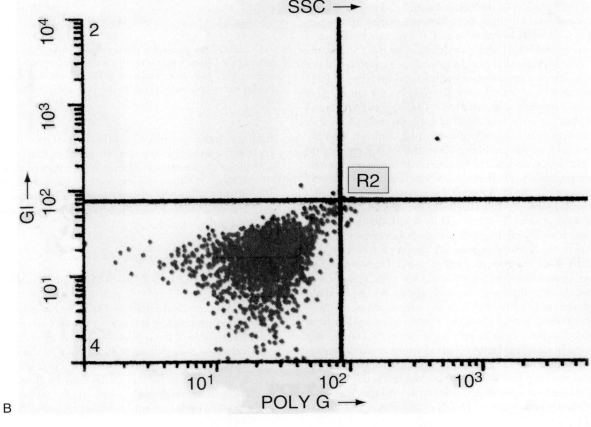

B

tion can be uncovered prior to biopsy, allowing appropriate precautions to be taken. A very rare complication with breast aspiration, and occasionally with sampling of a supraclavicular or high axillary lymph node, is pneumothorax.[7] When performing FNAB of the mammary gland in patients with small breasts, or a mass deeply placed at the margin of the breast, direct the aspiration needle away from the chest wall to avoid this complication.

In addition to complications of the procedure, FNAB is vulnerable to legal action in two other areas. These are a false positive diagnosis of malignancy or false negative diagnosis when a malignant tumor is present.[6] A false negative diagnosis may arise in several ways: failure to recognize or find malignant cells that are present; poorly prepared or inadequate samples; not actually sampling the tumor by aspiration; and intrinsic features of some tumors, for example marked sclerosis, which make them unsuitable for aspiration biopsy. The first problem, failure to recognize malignant cells, is entirely the responsibility of the cytopathologist. The remaining problems are those of the aspirator and focus on the importance of attention to details in every part of the aspiration biopsy method.[20]

FNAB of the breast more than other sites presents the potential problem of false negative results.[17,40] Patients may be referred or aspirated by clinicians for vague "thickenings" of the breast. These changes in the breast do not constitute a defined mass and are rarely suspicious for malignancy.[21] The entire breast is found to be "lumpy." Following a benign aspiration biopsy report, and a benign appearance of the mammogram, the risk of a breast cancer being overlooked is very small. Most of these patients can be followed safely at regular intervals by physical examination of the breast for any changes or the development of a definite mass. Serial mammography may be performed as well, as an added safeguard. If a documented plan of follow-up is established and is understood by the patient, the rare small carcinoma that may be missed for a time should not cause any change in prognosis once the diagnosis is established. Emphasis should be placed on a defined plan for follow-up of this group of patients with negative FNAB to avoid a potential adverse effect of an unrealistically long-term sense of security from a false negative result. Ultimately, the clinician must decide for each case the likelihood that an FNAB is representative of the lesion and, with the degree of confidence in the FNA interpretation, whether to accept a diagnosis of negative for malignancy as the final step in the patient's evaluation.[20]

Invariably, false positive diagnoses are the result of overreading atypical cells. They are usually few in number for any given case. If an FNAB diagnosis of malignancy does not fit the clinical picture, the clinician must ask for a review of the slides, specifically with that information in mind. Even with good sampling, masses that consistently yield few cells, regardless of the suspicion of malignancy, are nearly always benign. One notable exception is with FNAB of the breast, where both fibroadenomas and benign phyllodes tumors often exhibit large numbers of atypical cells in aspiration biopsy.[60] Tumor cells from fibroadenoma and benign phyllodes tumors may even appear to infiltrate fat that is found in smears, thus simulating a pattern of invasive breast carcinoma. Myoepithelial cells are usually present in these cases, frequently in large numbers. When they are present in an FNAB of the breast, this always

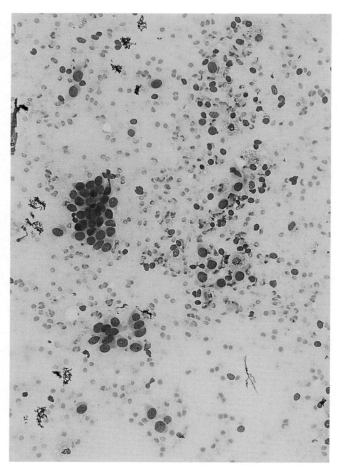

Fig. 10-11. False positive aspiration biopsy from cystosarcoma phyllodes of the breast. Smear is cellular with clusters and loose sheets and single tumor cells. Note variation in nuclear size and shape. In other fields, oval naked nuclei were present. (Diff-Quik, × 250.)

indicates either a benign mass or at least one in which the pathologist should not report anything more than a suspicion of a malignant breast tumor. They may be few in number and easily overlooked by the cytopathologist in some challenging cases (Fig. 10-11). When the typical patterns of breast cancer are not easily recognized on FNAB, it is important to be careful with the final interpretation.

PROBLEMS FOR THE CLINICIAN

The most common pitfall for the clinician is failure to procure a good specimen.[20] It is not appropriate to judge this from the total volume of the aspirate but rather from the number of cells found and their pattern of distribution on the slide. A large volume of sample is not better when most of it is only blood or cyst fluid. The target for the FNAB must be clearly identified. A clinical differential diagnosis should be transmitted to the pathologist. The important questions are as follows: what are the indications for this aspiration biopsy, and what do I wish to learn to influence my management of this patient?

PROBLEMS FOR THE PATHOLOGIST

The pathologist's most common difficulty is trying to read too much into a limited FNAB, particularly with insufficient clinical information. Listed below are seven golden rules of aspiration biopsy. They should be kept in mind at all times.[61]

1. Be aware of the limitations of FNAB for the body site being sampled.
2. Obtain cellular samples that are adequate and well prepared.
3. Be aware of the diagnostic pitfalls for each body site sampled.
4. Correlate cytologic impressions with the patient's history and physical findings.
5. Live within your experience and limitations.
6. Compare the cytology of FNA with tissue samples whenever they are available.
7. Maintain good lines of communication among the clinician, cytopathologist, and patient.

REFERENCES

1. Frable WJ: Needle aspiration biopsy: past, present, and future. Hum Pathol 20:504–517, 1989
2. Frable WJ: Aspiration cytology. pp. 239–251. In Keebler CM, Somrak TM (eds): The Manual of Cytotechnology. 7th Ed. ASCP Press, Chicago, 1993
3. Salzman AJ: Imaging techniques in aspiration biopsy. pp. 17–38. In Linsk JA, Franzen S (eds): Clinical Aspiration Cytology. 2nd Ed. Lippincott-Raven, Philadelphia, 1989
4. Linsk JA, Franzen S: Clinical Aspiration Cytology. p. 35. 2nd Ed. Lippincott-Raven, Philadelphia, 1989
5. Masood S: Fine needle aspiration biopsy of non palpable breast lesions. pp. 33–63. In Schmidt W (ed): Cytopathology Annual 1994. ASCP Press, Chicago, 1994
6. Stanley MW, Lowhagen T: Fine Needle Aspiration of Palpable Masses. pp. 3–5. Butterworth-Heinemann, Boston, 1993
7. Powers CN: Fine needle aspiration biopsy: perspectives on complications. The reality behind the myths. pp. 71–98. In Schmidt W (ed): Cytopathology Annual 1996. ASCP Press, Chicago, 1996
8. Martin HE, Ellis, EB: Biopsy by needle puncture and aspiration. Ann Surg 92:169–181, 1930
9. Lopes Cardozo P: Clinical Cytology. Stafleu, Leiden, 1954
10. Zajicek J: Aspiration Biopsy Cytology. Part I. Cytology of Supradiaphragmatic Organs. Vol. 4. pp. 1–15, 20–26. Monographs in Clinical Cytology. S. Karger, New York, 1974
11. Soderstrom N: Fine Needle Aspiration Biopsy. pp. 13–18. Almqvist & Wiksell, Stockholm, 1966
12. Webb AJ: Through a glass darkly (the development of needle aspiration biopsy). Bristol Med Chir J 89:59–68, 1974
13. Dahlgren SE, Nordenstrom B: Transthoracic Needle Biopsy. Almqvist & Wiksell, Stockholm, 1966
14. Frable WJ: The history of fine needle aspiration biopsy: the American experience. pp. 91–100. In Schmidt W (ed): Cytopathology Annual 1994. ASCP Press, Chicago, 1994
15. Raab SS, Bottles K, Cohen MB: Technology assessment in anatomic pathology. An illustration of test evaluation using fine-needle aspiration biopsy. Arch Pathol Lab Med 118:1173–1180, 1994
16. Hopper KD, Abendroth CS, Sturtz KW, et al: Fine-needle aspiration biopsy for cytopathologic analysis: utility for syringe handles, automated guns, and the nonsuction method. Radiology 185:819–824, 1992
17. Frable WJ: Thin-Needle Aspiration Biopsy. pp. 184, 185, 231, 232. Vol. 14. In Bennington JL (ed): Major Problems in Pathology. WB Saunders, Philadelphia, 1983
18. Stewart FW: The diagnosis of tumors by aspiration biopsy. Am J Pathol 9:801–812, 1933
19. Abele JS, Miller TR: Implementation of an outpatient needle aspiration biopsy service and clinic: a personal perspective. pp. 43–71. In Schmidt W (ed): Cytopathology Annual, 1993. Williams & Wilkins, Baltimore, 1993
20. Frable WJ: Fine needle aspiration biopsy. pp. 33–45. In Banks P, Kraybill WG (eds): Pathology for the Surgeon. WB Saunders, Philadelphia, 1996
21. Frable WJ: Fine needle aspiration biopsy. pp. 625–642. In Bibbo M (ed): Comprehensive Cytopathology. 2nd Ed. WB Saunders, Philadelphia, 1996
22. Orell SR: The two faces of fine-needle biopsy: its role in the teaching hospital and in the community. Diagn Cytopathol 8:557–558, 1992
23. Mazhar R, Kovatich A, Ehya H: Utility of polyclonal and monoclonal antibodies against carcinoembryonic antigen in hepatic fine-needle aspirates. Diagn Cytopathol 11:358–362, 1994
24. Ostrowski ML, Brown RW, Wheeler TM, et al: Leu-7 immunoreactivity in cytologic specimens of thyroid lesions, with emphasis on follicular neoplasms. Diagn Cytopathol 12:297–302, 1995
25. Nizzoli R, Bozzetti C, Savoldi L, et al: Immunocytochemical assay of estrogen and progesterone receptors in fine needle aspirates from breast cancer patients. Acta Cytol 38:933–938, 1994
26. Wojcik EM, Katz RL, Johnston DA, et al: Comparative analysis of DNA ploidy and proliferative index in fine needle aspirates of non-Hodgkin's lymphoma by image analysis and flow cytometry. Anal Quant Cytol Histol 15:151–157, 1993
27. Johnson DE, Powers CN, Rupp GN, et al: Immunocytochemical staining of fine-needle aspiration biopsies of the liver as a diagnostic tool for hepatocellular carcinoma. Mod Pathol 5:117–123, 1991
28. Katz RL, Hirsch-Ginsberg C, Childs C, et al: The role of gene rearrangements for antigen receptors in the diagnosis of lymphoma obtained by fine-needle aspiration: a study of 63 cases with concomitant immunophenotyping. Am J Clin Pathol 96:479–490, 1991
29. Katz RL, Patel S, Brooks T: Immunocytochemistry of lymphoproliferative disorders using the Ficoll-hypaque technique on cytologic specimens. pp. 265–272. In Schmidt W (ed): Cytopathology Annual 1993. Williams & Wilkins, Baltimore, 1993
30. Sneige N, Dekmezian RH, Katz RL, et al: Morphologic and immunocytochemical evaluation of 220 fine needle aspirates of malignant lymphoma and lymphoid hyperplasia. Acta Cytol 34:311–322, 1990
31. Dabbs DJ, Silverman JF: Selective use of electron microscopy in fine needle aspiration cytology. Acta Cytol 32:880–884, 1988
32. Brooke PK, Wakely PE Jr, Frable WJ: Utility of electron microscopy as an adjunct in aspiration cytology diagnosis, abstracted. Lab Invest 4:22A, 1991
33. Boon ME, Schut JJ, Suurmeijer AJH, et al: Confocal microscopy of false-negative breast aspirates. Diagn Cytopathol 12:42–50, 1995
34. Corkill ME, Katz R: Immunocytochemical staining of c-erbB-2 oncogene in fine-needle aspirates of breast carcinoma: a comparison with tissue sections and other breast cancer prognostic factors. Diagn Cytopathol 11:250–254, 1994
35. Kube MJ, McDonald DA, Quin JW, et al: Use of archival and fresh cytologic material for the polymerase chain reaction. Analyt Quant Cytol Histol 16:174–182, 1994
36. Martin AW, Davey DD: Comparison of immunoreactivity of neu oncoprotein in fine-needle aspirates and paraffin-embedded materials. Diagn Cytopathol 12:142–147, 1995

37. Cartagena N, Katz RL, Hirsch-Ginsberg C, et al: Accuracy of diagnosis of malignant lymphoma by combining fine-needle aspiration cytomorphology with immunocytochemistry and in selected cases, Southern blotting of aspiration cells: a tissue-controlled study of 86 patients. Diagn Cytopathol 8:456–464, 1992

38. Cajulis RS, Frias-Hidvegi D: Detection of numerical chromosomal abnormalities in malignant cells in fine needle aspirates by fluorescence in situ hybridization of interphase cell nuclei with chromosome-specific probes. Acta Cytol 37:391–396, 1993

39. Heinrichs M, Striepecke E, Bocking A: Quantitative analysis of the neu oncogene in normal and transformed epithelial breast cells by fluorescence in situ hybridization and laser scanning microscopy. Anal Quant Cytol Histol 16:233–239, 1994

40. Koss LG, Woyke S, Olszewski W: Aspiration Biopsy. Cytologic Interpretation and Histologic Bases. 2nd Ed. pp. 21–23, 43, 193–196. Igaku Shoin, New York, 1993

41. Zajdela A, Zillhardt P, Voillemot N: Cytological diagnosis by fine needle sampling without aspiration. Cancer 59:1201–205, 1987

42. Kinney TB, Lee MJ, Filomena CA, et al: Fine-needle biopsy: prospective comparison of aspiration versus non aspiration techniques in the abdomen. Radiology 186:549–552, 1993

43. Zajdela A, Zillhardt P, Voillemot N: Cytological diagnosis by fine needle sampling without aspiration. Cancer 59:1201–1205, 1987

44. Ljung B: Thin Needle Aspiration Biopsy: An Instructional Video. Department of Cytopathology, University of California, San Francisco, San Francisco, CA, 1992

45. Grohs HK: Fine Needle Aspiration and Smear Making Techniques: An Instructional Video. International Institute for Applied Cyto Science. Manchester, MA, 1992

46. Yang GCH, Alvarez II: Ultra-fast Papanicolaou stain: an alternative preparation for fine-needle aspiration cytology. Acta Cytol 39:55–60, 1995

47. Harris MJ: Cell block preparation. Three-percent bacterial agar and plasma-thrombin clot methods. Cytotech Bull 11:6–7, 1974

48. Shield PW, Perkins G, Wright RG: Immunocytochemical staining of cytologic specimens. How helpful is it? Am J Clin Pathol 105:157–162, 1996

49. Silverman JF, Khazanic PG, Norris HT et al: Parathyroid hormone (PTH) assay of parathyroid cysts examined by fine-needle aspiration biopsy. Am J Clin Pathol 86:776–780, 1986

50. Davidson HG, Campora RG: Thyroid. pp. 660–662. In Bibbo M (ed): Comprehensive Cytopathology. WB Saunders, Philadelphia, 1991

51. Holmquist MD: The effect of distance in aerosol fixative of cytologic specimens. Cytotech Bull 15:25–27, 1979

52. Osborn M, Domogala W: Immunocytochemistry. pp. 1011–1051. In Bibbo M (ed): Comprehensive Cytopathology. WB Saunders, Philadelphia, 1991

53. Hadju SI. The value and limitations of aspiration cytology in the diagnosis of primary tumors Acta Cytol 33:741–790, 1989

54. Orell SR, Sterrett GF, Walters Max N-I, et al: Manual and Atlas of Fine Needle Aspiration Cytology. pp. 8–33. 2nd Ed. Churchill Livingstone, New York, 1992

55. Abendroth CS, Dabbs DJ: Immunocytochemical staining of unstained versus previously stained cytologic preparations. Acta Cytol 39:379–386, 1995

56. Skoog L, Tani E, Svedmyr E, et al: Growth fraction in non-Hodgkin's lymphomas and reactive lymphadenitis determined by Ki-67 monoclonal antibody in fine needle aspirates. Diagn Cytopathol 12:234–239, 1995

57. Lee KC, Chan JKC, Ho LC: Histologic changes in the breast after fine-needle aspiration. Am J Surg Pathol 18:1039–1047, 1994

58. LiVolsi VA, Merino MJ: Worrisome histologic alterations following fine needle aspiration of thyroid. Mod Pathol 3:59A, 1990

59. Powers CN, Frable WJ: Fine Needle Aspiration Biopsy of the Head and Neck. Butterworth-Heinemann, Boston, 1996

60. Dusenbery D, Frable WJ: Fine needle aspiration cytology of phyllodes tumor. Potential diagnostic pitfalls. Acta Cytol 36:215–221, 1992

61. Feldman, PS, Covell JL, Kardos TF: Fine Needle Aspiration Cytology. Lymph Node, Thyroid, Salivary Gland. pp. 9–10. ASCP Press, Chicago, 1989

Appendix 10-1
Fine Needle Aspiration Biopsy

Your Appointment for an Aspiration Biopsy

Your doctor has recently found that you have a lump and has scheduled you for or requested a fine needle aspiration biopsy (FNAB). This procedure is a good way to find out what this lump might be because it is fast, safe and reliable and will cause you only minimal discomfort. FNAB is not new, having been invented in the United States over 60 years ago. FNAB has been in continuous use at this institution for over 20 years. FNAB is also a procedure quite useful for determining the nature of lumps found in children. This pamphlet will explain what FNAB is and will answer some of your questions. Please read it carefully. If you have other questions write them down in the space on the back of this pamphlet or ask the doctors who will perform the aspiration biopsy (when you come for your appointment). All your questions will be answered before the biopsy is done.

Why Do I Need a Biopsy?

A lump may result from several different causes, including infection, excessive tissue growth or fluid collection, a benign tumor, or a malignancy (cancer). Most lumps are not malignant but your doctor's treatment of the lump will depend on its exact nature. FNAB is a simple test that often tells the doctor how to proceed with your treatment.

Are There Alternatives?

Until recently, the usual method of obtaining a tissue diagnosis was a minor operation called a surgical biopsy. Surgical biopsy is highly reliable, but can involve some discomfort, is usually more expensive, and has several risks, such as bleeding, infection, and scar tissue formation. FNAB can, in most cases, accurately determine the nature of the lump more safely and comfortably than surgical biopsy.

How Is the Aspiration Biopsy Performed?

After cleansing the skin overlying the lump, a very small needle is passed through the skin and into the mass. The needle is less than 1 mm in diameter. It is smaller than the needles used in most laboratories to draw blood from your arm. During the procedure you may briefly feel some discomfort like that encountered when a laboratory technician draws blood from your arm. The FNAB takes only a few seconds to perform. One to three separate biopsies of the lump are taken during your visit.

After the aspiration biopsy, you will be able to drive, return to work, or perform any other activity that you normally do. Continue taking any medicine your doctor has given you as directed, since the biopsy does not affect medication schedules.

What Are the Risks Associated with Fine Needle Aspiration Biopsy?

FNAB poses no significant risk to you. Some patients report a mild, dull, throbbing sensation in the area of the biopsy, which usually subsides within 30 to 60 minutes. This minor discomfort does not bother most patients and requires no medication. A small bruise or tenderness may occur at the aspiration site. If you experience any unusual discomfort or swelling, please call your doctor. Some patients have experienced light-headedness as may also occur with the giving of a sample of blood. This is quite rare with FNAB. Please inform your doctor if you have experienced this problem in the past when a blood sample was taken.

Some patients have expressed concern that passage of the needle through a tumor might cause the tumor to spread. This concern has been examined by scientists at several universities and is considered highly unlikely.

Finally, the risk of infection exists at any time the skin is penetrated. However several thousand biopsies have been done by the aspiration service without a single case of infection having been reported to date.

What Result Can I Expect from this Biopsy?

About 85 to 90 percent of the time, the biopsy result can tell the doctor the exact nature of the lump so that correct treatment can be determined. About 5 percent of the time the biopsy can tell something about the lump, but will not give the doctor all of the information that may be needed to determine your treatment. In the remaining 5 to 10 percent of cases, it is not possible to obtain enough tissue from a particular lump for an accurate diagnosis on which to begin treatment. When this happens, the doctor will often order a surgical biopsy or other tests. It is important to find out exactly what the lump is.

How Long Does It Take to Obtain the Results of the Fine Needle Aspiration Biopsy?

The material obtained by aspiration biopsy is immediately examined under the microscope by a physician experienced in cytopathology to make a preliminary diagnosis of your problem and to ensure that a sufficient amount of tissue is present for final study and special tests if they are indicated. We will notify your doctor of preliminary findings, who will make them known to you on request. If you have been referred by a physician outside of this institution, the physicians directing the aspiration biopsy service may make the preliminary results of your biopsy known to you on request.

Your doctor is notified of the final results of your biopsy only after all the tissue obtained is thoroughly examined. In most cases this process takes 24 to 48 hours. However, you may have to wait an extra day or two if special tests are required on your aspiration biopsy sample.

Any More Questions?

Please write them down below.

_____

_____

_____

_____

_____

The Aspiration Biopsy Service is available to answer questions from 8:00 AM to 4:30 PM weekdays at the following numbers:

11

Infectious Diseases

Washington C. Winn, Jr.
William J. Frable

The microbial world is vast, and the portion that impinges on human activities is a minute part of the universe. Bacteria are an integral part of the world around us, and we could not live without them. They are even an integral part of our bodies, colonizing our digestive tube from start to finish. Many human diseases are actually the result of chance encounters with infectious agents that have another, more productive role in nature. For instance, most filamentous fungi exist in nature to process decaying vegetation, not to infect immunocompromised humans. In fact, from the microbe's point of view, infection of an "accidental host" such as a human is truly a dead end. The equine encephalitis viruses or the borrelial spirochete of Lyme disease perpetuate their species within an enzootic cycle. If they were limited to infection of humans, they would soon be on the endangered species list.

Of the small number of contacts between pathogenic microbes and humans, only occasionally is a physician called to participate in the resultant illness, still less commonly is a specimen taken for analysis, and least likely of all is the submission of tissue for pathologic study. The view of infectious disease from the surgical pathology suite, or even from the cytopathology laboratory is, therefore, a very constricted and narrowly defined prospect. The cytopathologist is much more likely to receive a sputum sample for detection of malignant cells than for infectious organisms. The surgical pathologist is more likely to dissect a pulmonary segment that was resected for cancer than for infection. What then is the importance of infectious disease for a surgical pathologist? First, the surgical cutting room may be the first place that a fully treatable disease is defined, with the ability to define the therapeutic approach hanging on the correct handling of the tissue or smears. Second and equally important, the examination of tissue specimens is often the court of last resort for unraveling a serious, but puzzling disease of a possibly infectious nature. If the specimen is not handled correctly, the last opportunity may have been lost, or a second invasive procedure may be required.

The subset of infectious diseases that require the anatomic pathologist's attention includes infections that produce significant morbidity, elude detection or definition by less invasive diagnostic means, cause localized lesions or at least dysfunction of specific organs that can be aspirated or biopsied, or elicit a host response that suggests clinically and/or pathologically a noninfectious process. Most serious systemic viral and bacterial infections are diagnosed by sampling blood or body fluids without the necessity for aspiration or biopsy of organs. Although morphologic study is important for some viral and bacterial infections, fungal and parasitic disease requires far greater emphasis

than would be predicted from their frequency in outpatients, in whom viral infections predominate, or in hospitalized patients, in whom bacterial infections present the greatest challenges.

The goal of this chapter is to discuss the host reactions to common pathogens encountered by surgical pathologists and cytopathologists and to review the differential diagnosis of microbes that can be detected and possibly identified in tissue. The discussion emphasizes infections that are likely to be encountered in the United States and Canada, but it is important to recognize that the greatest challenges are presented by unusual presentations of common diseases or common presentations of unusual diseases. The microbiologist or surgical pathologist in the Middle East or Central America would have little difficulty recognizing the presence of *Leishmania* spp. in tissue or imprint smears, but leishmaniasis may be a difficult challenge for a pathologist in the United States. We have observed significant delays in therapy and unnecessary morbidity for the patient because a leishmanial infection was not recognized in the initial biopsy. Certain infections, such as viral hepatitis, some gastrointestinal infections, and Whipple's disease, are covered in the chapters devoted to the relevant organ system.

APPROACHES TO ETIOLOGIC DIAGNOSIS

The diagnosis of infectious diseases is a cooperative endeavor among the anatomic pathologist (here, the surgical pathologist or cytologist with a team of histotechnologists and pathologist assistants), the clinical microbiologist (the pathologist or other doctoral scientist with a team of medical technologists), and the clinician (especially the infectious disease physician). A clinician faced with classic chickenpox in an immunocompetent patient does not require laboratory support for the diagnosis. The microbiologist who isolates *Mycobacterium tuberculosis* knows that the etiology of a disease has been established. Similarly, the surgical pathologist who views the diagnostic spherules of *Coccidioides immitis* can define the etiologic agent as well as describe the host response and extent of disease. Far more often, however, the activities of the three principal players are complementary. In pharmacologic terms they are always additive, but are often synergistic. The special contribution that the broadly trained pathologist can bring to the challenge is the integration of clinical knowledge, microbiology, and morphologic pathology. Such an individual is in the perfect position to be the linchpin of the operation, coordinating the activities of the various specialists in a referral facility or serving

Table 11-1. Approaches to the Etiologic Diagnosis of Infectious Diseases

Diagnostic Method	Technique	Specimen Required	Advantages	Disadvantages	Comments
Clinical diagnosis	Clinical history Travel history Occupational history Other data	None	Provides clues to exposure or risk factors	Rarely provides etiologic diagnosis	
Morphologic diagnosis	Histologic sections: H&E	Fresh or fixed tissue	Essential information on host response and other disease processes	Usually not etiologically specific	
Morphologic diagnosis	Histologic sections or smears: histochemistry	Fresh or fixed tissue or smears	Defines morphology of some agents and relation of agent to host response	Often provides only a presumptive diagnosis	Nonspecificity an advantage if the likely agent is not known
Immunologic diagnosis	Histologic sections or smears: immunofluorescence or immunoenzyme assay	Fresh or fixed tissue or smears	Definitive identification of some agents	Must know target antigens; limited library of commercial reagents	Some antigens altered by fixation, especially with fluorescence, requiring pretreatment
Molecular diagnosis	Histologic sections or smears: in situ hybridization	Fresh or fixed tissue or smears	Definitive identification of some agents	Limited availability or commercial reagents	Still in the realm of research for most agents
Molecular diagnosis	Amplification techniques (e.g., PCR)	Fresh tissue or paraffin blocks	Definitive identification		Research status

Abbreviations: H&E, hematoxylin and eosin; PCR, polymerase chain reaction.

multiple roles in a smaller institution. To achieve the goal of producing such broadly trained pathologists it is essential that residency programs encourage (or preferably require) pathologists-in-training to cross divisional lines, to provide optimal solutions to clinical problems. It is equally essential that residents recognize the unique challenges of integrated pathology and treat them as opportunities rather than administrative burdens.

Approaches to the establishment of an etiology for an infectious process are summarized in Table 11-1. The clinical impression leads to the formulation of an initial hypothesis. To the extent that the working hypothesis is correct and is communicated to the other participants, the likelihood increases that the correct diagnostic steps are taken in an expeditious manner. Once a specimen has been collected, an early dichotomous pathway should develop.

Macroscopic Examination

Inspection, selection, and possibly dissection are required for specimens that are too large to be processed in toto or are inhomogeneous (or both). This process is familiar to the surgical pathologist, but it also occurs in the microbiology laboratory.

Cytologic Examination

The utility of cytologic examination of imprint smears in the surgical pathology laboratory is becoming increasingly appar-

ent. A cytologic specimen may be the first indication of an infectious disease. Imprints may be stained by a variety of methods, as discussed below. It is essential, however, that an adequate number of imprint smears be made before the specimen is placed in fixative solution. It is almost always easier to examine a thin smear for infectious agents than to search through the planes of a 5 μm thick specimen with a histochemical stain that has been adapted for use on fixed, embedded tissue. The preparation of smears allows the parallel use of sections when the imprints may not be effective. The surgical pathologist who places everything into formalin solution without making smears is like the fighter who ties one hand behind his back. The surgeon who places the tissue in formalin solution before submitting it to the laboratory is tying the hands of all participants behind their backs. It should be noted that the microbiologist is also performing cytologic analysis with the traditional Gram smear: the details of many infectious agents and the cellular inflammatory response may be observed. The only difference between Gram and Papanicolaou stains is that the details of the bacteria are observed more effectively in the first and the details of the tissue cells are seen more clearly in the second.

Direct Detection with Histochemical Stains

A variety of histochemical stains has been developed over the years for evaluation of infectious agents. None is specific, but in combination with the morphology of the microbe, the host response, and the clinical history a presumptive etiologic diagnosis may often be rendered with a certainty that approaches microbiologic, immunologic, or genetic identification. Despite all the advantages of modern science, Gram stain remains the most useful rapid diagnostic technique in the microbiology laboratory. Similarly, the hematoxylin and eosin (H&E) stain remains the mainstay of the histology laboratory. The most common histochemical stains used for detection of infectious agents in smears and tissues are summarized in Table 11-2. The subject has been reviewed extensively in the microbiology literature.[1] The classic manual of staining procedures prepared at the Armed Forces Institute of Pathology[2] has been updated recently.[3] Many of these stains appear deceptively simple on paper, but are devilishly difficult to perform reliably and consistently. When options exist, it is best to pick the single technique that the local histology laboratory finds most congenial. A histology laboratory that consistently turns out a good tissue Gram stain or silver impregnation stain should be complimented frequently and vocally.

Bacteria

The premier method for histochemical detection of bacteria in smears and tissues remains the Gram stain, described over 100 years ago by a Danish microbiologist, Hans Christian Gram. The advantages of this method include simplicity and differentiation of bacteria into those that retain crystal violet after treatment with iodine and decolorization with alcohol, acetone, or a mixture of the two (Gram positive) and those that lose the blue dye after decolorization (Gram negative). A counterstain, usually saffranin, is applied to color the cellular material and the Gram-negative bacteria. Addition of 0.05 percent acid fuchsin to the counterstain enhances the staining of pale, fastidious Gram-negative bacteria without overstaining the cells.

Several modifications of Gram stains have been developed for histologic sections. The Brown and Brenn method and the Brown-Hopps technique are the most widely employed.[4] In general, the Brown and Brenn method works better for Gram-positive organisms, whereas the Gram-negative species are better displayed by the Brown-Hopps stain. Other adaptations of Gram stain, such as the MacCallum-Goodpasture method, are less successful at differentiating bacteria from background material (despite the eminence of the two pathologists who originated this technique).

The best approach to identifying bacteria in tissue is to have prepared imprint smears that can be stained by the Gram method. Once the material is embedded and sectioned, the Brown-Hopps method is the best single stain for bacteria. It must be recognized that several versions of the Brown-Hopps procedure are extant, and they are decidedly not equally good at coloring Gram-negative bacteria. A variation of the procedure that was developed at the Armed Forces Institute of Pathology is most satisfactory for demonstration of fastidious and pale-staining bacteria.[3] (Note that this procedure is *not* the same as the Brown-Hopps stain in the *Manual of Histologic Techniques* published by that organization.[2]) Despite the apparent simplicity of the protocols, there is sufficient art in producing a tissue Gram stain that the goal can be frustratingly elusive. One of the authors evaluated a case of *Yersinia enterocolitica* ap-

pendicitis, in which the bacilli were demonstrated clearly by the Dieterle stain (a silver impregnation method) but not at all by the recommended version of the Brown-Hopps stain. However, adjacent sections stained at the Armed Forces Institute of Pathology displayed the Gram-negative bacilli as well as the silver stain—and with the additional information of Gram reactivity. A good test of the adequacy of a tissue Gram stain is adequacy to color pale-staining organisms such as *Bordetella pertussis*, *Brucella* spp., *Legionella* spp., or a variety of anaerobic bacteria. Do not assume that the stain is adequate because Gram-negative bacilli can be seen in a section of colonic tissue.

The second important group of bacterial stains comprises the silver impregnation stains, originally designed for spirochetes that do not stain by the Gram method. The Warthin-Starry, Levaditi, Dieterle, and Steiner methods provide essentially similar results, the choice depending on the abilities of the individual laboratory. Although these stains were developed for the demonstration of *Treponema pallidum*, they have taken on new importance as highly sensitive stains for all bacterial species. We owe our knowledge of the etiologic agents of cat-scratch disease[5] (*Bartonella henselae* and possibly *Afipia felis*) and chronic gastritis with lymphoid aggregates (*Helicobacter pylori*)[6] to the sensitivity of these stains, which demonstrated conclusively the presence of—at the time—unknown bacteria that were intimately associated with the pathologic process. Cat-scratch disease had long been thought to be infectious in nature, but chronic gastritis was considered a chemical disease until the observation of the curved bacilli in gastric tissue set investigators on the correct path. *Legionella pneumophila* was first demonstrated by inoculation of experimental animals and staining of the infected tissues with the Gimenez stain, but the bacteria were first demonstrated in human tissue with a modification of the Dieterle spirochete stain.[7] (Once again, it is likely that the bacteria were not seen originally in sections stained by the Brown-Hopps and Brown and Brenn methods because of technical problems or the variation of the stain that was used. In retrospect, the bacteria were stained weakly by these methods.[8] If the Brown-Hopps stain is working correctly, it will color *L. pneumophila* distinctly.)

The silver impregnation stains are entirely nonspecific, a feature that is a virtue when the characteristics of an infectious agent are not known. Drawbacks of these stains are the absence of information about Gram reactivity, the distortion of bacterial morphology by deposition of silver salts, and the greater propensity toward detecting contaminating environmental bacteria picked up in processing (an unwanted byproduct of the great sensitivity of the stains).

Other stains, not primarily associated with detection of bacteria, will also stain these prokaryotic organisms. The Gimenez stain, which was designed for the rickettsiae, depends on carbol fuchsin for staining and, as such, is essentially the final component of the Gram stain with a sensitive counterstain. The Gimenez technique was designed for smears but was adapted to frozen sections for staining of *L. pneumophila*.[8] Methylene blue and acridine orange are sometimes used on smears but have not been used commonly to detect bacteria in sections. Other stains that are not intended primarily for detection of bacteria will demonstrate them on occasion, especially if large numbers of bacteria are present: Giemsa, periodic

Table 11-2. Histochemical Stains for Demonstrating Infectious Organisms

Stain	Cytologic (C) or Histologic (H)	Intended Organisms	Other Possible Organisms	Artifacts	Comments
Gram stain	C	Bacteria	Some yeasts and molds; rarely *Pneumocystis* organisms	Stain debris (Gram-positive); fibrin (Gram-negative)	First choice for demonstration of bacteria
Gimenez stain	C, H (frozen sections)	Bacteria, rickettsiae			Uncommonly used
Brown and Brenn	H	Bacteria	Some yeasts and molds	Mast cell granules; nuclear debris (Gram-positive); fibrin, cell membranes (Gram-negative)	Best for Gram-positive bacteria
Brown-Hopps	H	Bacteria	Some yeasts and molds	See Brown and Brenn	Best for Gram-negative bacteria
MacCallum-Goodpasture	H	Bacteria	Some yeasts and molds	See Brown and Brenn	Uncommonly used
Silver impregnation stains (Warthin-Starry, Dieterle, Levaditi, Steiner)	C, H	*Treponema* spp., *Leptospira* spp., *Borrelia* spp.	Bacteria, especially *Bartonella* spp., *Helicobacter* spp.	Carbon, tissue debris	Very sensitive, but nonspecific general bacterial stain
Ziehl-Neelsen, Kinyoun	C, H	Mycobacteria	Schistosomal eggs; some partially acid-fast organisms may stain	Lipofuscin; other acid-fast debris	Cytologic and histologic preparations may be complementary
Modified Ziehl-Neelsen or Kinyoun (Putt, Fite, Fite-Farraco)	C, H	*Nocardia* spp.	Mycobacteria (especially *M. leprae*, rapidly growing mycobacteria), schistosomal eggs, *Legionella micdadei*, *Rhodococcus* spp.	See Ziehl-Neelsen	The Putt stain is reportedly less specific than the Fite stain on tissue
Periodic acid-Schiff	C, H	Fungi	Bacteria (e.g., *Tropheryma whippeliae*), foamy exudate of *Pneumocystis* organisms	Glycogen; Russell bodies	
Gomori methenamine silver	C, H	Fungi (including *Pneumocystis*)	Bacteria, including *Nocardia* spp., *Actinomyces* spp.	Fibrin, elastin, collagen, erythrocytes, capillaries	Preferred stain for fungi
Gridley stain	S	Fungi	See periodic acid-Schiff	See periodic acid-Schiff	Counterstain provides better contrast than periodic acid-Schiff
Hematoxylin and eosin		Some parasites, molds, and dimorphic yeast; viral inclusions			General histologic stain; screening for infectious agents
Papanicolaou stain	C	Some parasites, yeasts, viral inclusions	Bacteria, molds		General cytologic stain; screening for infectious agents
Giemsa stain	C, H	Some parasites, dimorphic fungi	Bacteria	Phagocytized material	

acid-Schiff (PAS), and Gomori methenamine silver (GMS) (especially if stained too darkly) stains, some counterstains for acid-fast procedures (such as methylene blue), and even H&E.

Mycobacteria

The principle of the acid-fast stain is that the wall of the my-cobacteria, which has a high content of fatty acids, retains dyes that are not subsequently leached by acid or acid-alcohol solu-tions. The traditional stain is the Ziehl-Neelsen stain, which incorporates carbol fuchsin, and has been adapted for histologic sections. An alternative approach is use of a fluorochrome dye, such as auramine, rhodamine, or a combination of the two. Acid-fast organisms appear red when sections stained with car-bol fuchsin are viewed with the light microscope; they appear yellow (auramine), red (rhodamine), or orange (auramine-rho-damine) when viewed with a fluorescence microscope. In ei-ther case the reaction is a chemical reaction based on acid fast-ness, not an immunologic reaction. The fluorochrome dyes are best detected with an epifluorescence microscope and a halo-gen light source. It is not necessary to use a mercury vapor lamp for this purpose.

Most microbiology laboratories find the fluorochrome method most convenient, because it is possible to screen many smears at low power (10 to 25 × objective). Most surgical pathologists have found the light microscopic approach more congenial. In large series of cases, consisting mostly of sputum smears, the fluorochrome stain has been slightly more sensitive than the Ziehl-Neelsen method, but slightly less specific.[9,10] Ei-ther approach can be used, depending on the comfort of the ex-aminer and the availability of a fluorescence microscope of good quality. Both the fluorochrome and carbol fuchsin slides retain their characteristics well in storage.

Reports in the microbiology literature show that some my-cobacteria, particularly the rapid growers *Mycobacterium fortui-tum* and *M. chelonae* do not stain reliably with the traditional acid-fast stains.[11] For the demonstration of these species, as well as other partially acid-fast bacteria, it is necessary to use a mod-ified decolorization method, such as use of sulfuric acid instead of hydrochloric acid in the Ziehl-Neelsen stain for smears. The modified acid-fast stains have also been adapted for histologic sections. The most commonly used procedure is the Fite stain, which incorporates a xylene-peanut oil solution for gentle de-colorization. The modified acid-fast stains are tricky to perform, because insufficient decolorization may cause a falsely positive reaction. It has been reported that the Putt stain may color the filaments of *Actinomyces israelii* (a non-acid-fast bacterium) red.[12,13]

Mycobacteria may be visualized occasionally with other stains. They are weakly Gram positive, and some bacterial cells may stain clearly blue with the Gram stain if large numbers of organisms are present. In smears the mycobacteria may appear as nonstaining ghosts against a proteinaceous background. The GMS stain may color these organisms, particularly if the stain is dark.

Fungi

Two major groups of stains are in use for detection of fungi: stains for the chitin in the cell walls of fungi and analine dyes that emphasize the cellular detail of the organisms. The two most commonly used procedures for staining cell walls are the GMS stain for fungi and the PAS procedure. Both of these stains may be applied successfully to either smears or histologic sections. The fungal cells appear black with the silver stain and red with the PAS technique. The material in the cell walls is not glycogen, and the reaction is thus resistant to diastase. A modification of the PAS method by Gridley makes most fungi stand out clearly against a yellow background, in contrast to the less differentiated red-blue background of the traditional PAS method. A more recent addition to the armamentarium is Cal-cofluor, a dye used in the textile industry as a whitener. Calco-fluor binds to the chitin of fungal cell walls and fluoresces blue-white when exposed to ultraviolet light.[14,15] The calcofluor stain is usually applied to smears but may also be used on histo-logic sections.

Stains that reveal cellular detail may also stain the cell walls of fungi. A Romanovsky stain, such as one of the variations of the Giemsa stain, is often used for demonstration of the cellu-lar structure of dimorphic yeasts, particularly *Histoplasma capsu-latum*. The Giemsa (or Wright) stain is routinely used on smears. It has also been applied to histologic sections, but in our experience the Giemsa stain is more often done than done well on tissue. A poorly performed Giemsa stain may be misleading if it defines some detail of human cells without coloring the fungal cells adequately. The H&E and Papanicolau stains are also useful for visualizing the cellular details of fungi and are more often helpful than the Giemsa stain because they are used for initial staining and evaluation of histologic and cytologic preparations, respectively. In addition, the Gram stain will color—either partially or completely—the cell walls and nu-clear details of some fungi, particularly yeast cells and their pseudohyphae. The cytoplasm of some yeast may appear vari-ably acid fast, but the cell walls do not stain.[16]

Other histochemical procedures are important for highly se-lective indications. Stains for the mucopolysaccharide capsules of certain fungi, especially *Cryptococcus neoformans*, are useful. The mucicarmine stain is used most frequently, but Alcian blue may also be employed. The melanin pigment in the walls of de-matiacious molds and in *C. neoformans* can be demonstrated with the Fontana-Masson stain.[17]

Pneumocystis carinii cysts may also be detected with the tolu-idine O stain in smears[18,19] and the Gram-Weigert stain in smears or tissue.[19,20] The Calcofluor stain has also been used for detection of cysts in smears.[18,21] For most pathology laborato-ries, the GMS stain is most familiar and is probably the single best stain for cysts. Trophozoites are not colored by the cyst stains. To detect this important stage of the organism it is nec-essary to use a Romanovsky stain, such as the Giemsa or Diff-Quik stains.

Viruses and Parasites

The most important stains for recognition of viral inclusions and parasites are the first-line ones: H&E for tissue sections and the Papanicolaou stain for cytologic preparations. In addition, the Giemsa stain is useful for observing the fine details of some protozoa in both smears and histologic sections. Special stains for viral inclusions have been described, but they offer no ad-vantages over the H&E stain.

Quality Control

Selection of appropriate material for quality control of histochemical stains is critical for assurance that results are correct. The ideal controls have the following characteristics:

1. The source of the controls matches the source of the test material (e.g., bronchoalveolar lavage and histologic sections containing *P. carinii* are both available for use with corresponding clinical specimens)

2. The control organism matches the organism sought in the test material, if there are differences in the staining characteristic of organisms that might be used as controls (e.g., *P. carinii* and *Aspergillus* spp. as controls for the GMS stain or use of *Nocardia* spp. for the modified acid-fast stain); if the test section contains mucin-secreting epithelium, staining of cellular mucin may serve as an additional positive control for the mucicarmine stain

3. Use of a control organism that presents a challenge for the histochemical stain in addition to the normal control, if appropriate (e.g., *L. pneumophila* in addition to *Escherichia coli*)

4. The positive control slide should contain enough organisms to be found without an extended time-consuming search, but should not have masses of organisms. An acid-fast control in which the mycobacteria can be seen as a red cloud at low magnification is little assurance that small numbers of mycobacteria will be detected. It is difficult to develop broad guidelines, but in general there should be

   a. A concentration of large organisms, such as fungal hyphae or dimorphic yeast, that requires scanning of at least half of the slide at low power (10 × objective lens)

   b. A concentration of small organisms, such as bacteria and mycobacteria, that requires evaluation of relevant areas of the section with a 40 × objective by an experienced observer or with a 100 × objective by an average observer

5. Use of a negative control only if it provides additional information. The normal tissue of histologic sections can serve as a negative control in most situations, including tissue Gram stains and GMS, PAS, and mucicarmine stains. It is important to recognize that having a separate negative control does not substitute for experience in evaluating and recognizing artifacts and staining irregularities, because no single block of tissue will contain all possible distractors. It is essential, however, to include a negative control slide for the silver impregnation stains, such as the Warthin-Starry stain, because of their propensity to detect small numbers of contaminating bacteria, probably introduced in tap water used to float paraffin-embedded sections in water baths. Although contamination with environmental mycobacteria in water is uncommon, it is probably judicious to include a negative control slide for mycobacteria

Several schemes have been described for "manufacturing" control slides in vitro.[22–24] The traditional approach of using purchased or home-made clinical material works best if sufficient time and attention are devoted to the task. This process must have commitment from the leaders of the histology laboratory and cannot be shunted off as an afterthought. Sharing of resources among laboratories may be necessary to accumulate the necessary material. A modest amount of tissue will last for many years if very small blocks are prepared. The only means of obtaining cytologic material with which to evaluate *P. carinii* are to prepare a stock of smears from a positive bronchoalveolar lavage or imprints from lung tissue or to make imprints from rats in which *Pneumocystis* infection has been induced by treatment with corticosteroids. If the positive control material for *Pneumocystis* organisms is also to be used for immunofluorescence with monoclonal antibodies that react with human organisms, the rat material will not be acceptable.

Suggested infectious processes for quality control material are listed in Table 11-3. When more than one organism is suggested, the tissue may be mounted in the same block for ease of processing. It is acceptable to store unstained paraffinized sections for positive controls, but the negative control slides should be prepared fresh each time, at least from the point of sectioning the paraffin block. If parallel preparation of slides is not done, it will not be possible to assess the possibility of environmental contamination, the most likely source being the water bath.

Immunologic Detection

Direct detection of infectious agents in smears and tissues using in situ (solid phase) assays has great potential for adding both specificity and sensitivity to the histochemical approach. The two techniques that have been used most commonly are immunofluorescence, either direct or indirect, and enzyme immunochemistry, usually employing horseradish peroxidase or alkaline phosphatase as detection systems. Biotin-avidin amplification techniques have also been applied. Many antigens are altered by formalin fixation, so that the antigenic sites are no longer available for reactivity, especially with fluorescein-conjugated antibodies. If fixed tissue sections are to be examined, pretreatment of the sections with trypsin or ammonium chloride may be necessary. Commercial reagents are available for immunologic detection of some viruses, such as herpes simplex virus, cytomegalovirus, and adenovirus; for bacteria, such as *Legionella* spp. and *T. pallidum*; and for parasites, such as *Toxoplasma gondii*.

In some cases, such as toxoplasmosis, immunoenzyme techniques increase the sensitivity with which sporozoites can be detected in an inflammatory reaction.[25,26] In other cases, such as the viral and bacterial pathogens, the molecular approaches do not appear to add sensitivity to that provided by histochemical stains. Monoclonal antibodies may still provide value by providing definitive identification of agents, such as viruses, that have been demonstrated with histochemical stains, but that have atypical morphology. In addition, immunologic techniques may allow definitive identification of bacterial agents that cannot be differentiated by histochemical means. The specificity of commercial agents must be scrutinized carefully, however. The available reagents for herpes simplex virus are not type specific. Although the antibodies are labeled as to the immunizing serotype, cross-reactions between types 1 and 2 prevent an identification that is more specific than herpes simplex virus. Nonspecific staining of optically clear nuclei in gestational endometrium has been described after use of peroxidase-conjugated antisera to herpes simplex virus.[27]

Table 11-3. Quality Control for Histochemical Stains

Type of Organism	Type of Stain	Positive Control	Negative Control
Bacteria	Gram	1. Staphylococcal or pneumococcal infection 2. Enteric Gram-negative bacillus infection 3. *Legionella* pneumonia	Optional
	Silver impregnation	1. Cat-scratch disease 2. *Legionella* pneumonia	Uninfected tissue
Spirochetes	Silver impregnation	*Treponema pallidum*	Uninfected tissue
Fungi	Gomori methenamine Silver Periodic acid-Schiff Gridley	*Aspergillus* or Zygomycetes Infection	Optional
	Mucicarmine	*Cryptococcus neoformans*	Mucin-negative *Blastomyces dermatitidis*
	Fontana-Masson	*Cryptococcus neoformans* or dematiacious fungus infection	*Aspergillus* spp. or Zygomycetes
Pneumocystis carinii	Gomori methenamine silver; Gram-Weigert	*Pneumocystis carinii* infection	Uninfected lavage; tissue optional
Various	Giemsa	*Pneumocystis carinii* or *Toxoplasma gondii* tachyzoites or *Leishmania* spp. infection	Optional

In certain situations, the specificity of the reactions may be compromised not only by immunologic cross-reactions, but also by environmental contamination, much as are histochemical stains. We have observed cases in which an erroneous diagnosis of *L. pneumophila* infection was rendered, based on detection of environmental bacteria that had been picked up in the course of processing the sections. Errors can often be avoided—whether the technique is histochemical, immunologic, or molecular—by careful correlation of the special studies with the clinical history and the host response to the putative pathogens.

Molecular Detection in Tissue

Molecular detection of infectious agents in tissue is a promising technique for the future. Several approaches have been taken. In situ demonstration of genetic material has been accomplished by DNA hybridization and by the polymerase chain reaction. An alternative approach is to retrieve archival tissue from paraffin blocks and perform molecular analysis on extracted tissue. The techniques have been applied to many infectious agents, but most remain in the province of the research laboratory. Nucleic acids are degraded to varying extents by formalin fixation, so fresh or frozen tissue is preferred. When the suitability of fixation has been formally investigated, as for detection of human papillomavirus, formalin appears to be an adequate or even preferred fixative.[28] In situ hybridization kits for some viral antigens are commercially available.

Use of the Microbiology Laboratory

Maximal information for the clinician will be obtained when data from the surgical pathology and microbiology laboratories are combined. In order for that to happen someone at the front end of the process must think to submit part of the specimen for culture. The role of the microbiology laboratory is to provide an etiologic diagnosis when the cytopathologic and histopathologic findings are nonspecific and to produce isolates for molecular characterization and antibiotic susceptibility studies. Morphologic studies are important for agents that have not yet been cultured successfully or reliably. In addition, pathologic analysis is important for documenting the role of an infectious agent in a clinical infection. It is good practice for the surgical pathologist or the clinical microbiologist (or both) to freeze unused tissue from a potentially infectious case, because subsequent morphologic analysis may suggest an etiologic agent that was not considered when the cultures were ordered. If frozen sections suggest an infectious agent, it is worth culturing the specimen even if its microbiologic integrity may have been compromised. For instance, recovery of M. *tuberculosis* provides important information under any circumstances.

TISSUE RESPONSE TO INFECTIOUS AGENTS

The body has a limited repertory of responses to injury. A particular injury elicits a response that is determined by the nature of the injury (in the case of infectious diseases, the nature of the infecting organism) and the characteristics of the host. Certain generalizations are possible, and they form the basis for discussion to provide an organizational framework that will facilitate comprehension of an extensive and complex list of infections. Not surprisingly, the complexity of microbes and the hosts they infect are so great that numerous exceptions exist. The exceptions can sometimes be understood once the biology is elucidated, but often one must be content with phenomenology.

Several major types of histologic response can be delineated: acute inflammation and abscess formation; granulomas with or without necrosis; lymphohistiocytic reactions, vascular infection, hemorrhage, and infarction; and combinations of acute and chronic inflammation. The detection and differentiation of classes of infectious agents in tissue is discussed along with the tissue response most closely associated with that class of agents. Major exceptions to the typical association of the type of microbe and the histologic response are also discussed.

The status of host immunologic and cellular defenses can also have significant influences on the cellular response to infectious agents. Some of these influences are considered where appropriate.

It should also be noted that some infections are not associated with a recognizable cellular reaction in the affected tissue. The most common explanation for serious infections without an inflammatory response is that the pathogenic mechanism of the infection is production of a toxin that exerts its effects biochemically. Two examples are cholera, which is a disease of intestinal fluid secretion, and botulism, which is a disorder of neuromuscular transmission. Such infections, however serious, are not likely to result in the submission of tissue for morphologic study, and they are not considered.

Acute Inflammatory Response and Abscess Formation: Bacterial Pathogens and Their Mimics

The acute inflammatory response, represented at the cellular level by the polymorphonuclear neutrophil, is the basis of the body's reaction to almost any injury. An acute thermal injury is differentiated from an accompanying bacterial infection by the intensity of that inflammatory response, rather than the quality of that reaction. The difference can be understood if the thermal injury is viewed as a one-time event, however intense, whereas the bacterial infection presents the body with a self-replicating antigen and consequently an intense and prolonged inpouring of acute inflammatory cells. The major clinical and pathologic presentations of acute bacterial infection are cellulitis, formation of abscesses or (in a preformed cavity) empyemas, gas formation, and undifferentiated acute inflammation.

Major Presentations

Cellulitis

Cellulitis is a spreading infection of soft tissue usually associated with an acute inflammatory response (Fig. 11-1). The classic pathogens that cause cellulitis are *Staphylococcus aureus* and *Streptococcus pyogenes* (group A beta-hemolytic streptococcus). The lesion is an undifferentiated acute inflammatory response that dissects through fascial planes.

Classic streptococcal cellulitis does not produce necrosis of tissue. In the 1980s we witnessed the reappearance of severe, life-threatening forms of *S. pyogenes* infection, which were caused by certain serotypes and included necrotizing cellulitis/fasciitis, sometimes associated with myonecrosis and myositis.

Necrotizing cellulitis/fasciitis with or without myositis are also produced by mixtures of anaerobic bacteria or mixtures of aerobic and anaerobic bacteria, which may result in synergistic gangrene. Particularly in persons who are afflicted with diabetes mellitus or severe peripheral vascular disease, many bacterial species not usually associated with cellulitis, such as members of the Enterobacteriaceae, may produce this lesion. Clostridial cellulitis is considered under gas-forming infections.

Cellulitis and fasciitis may take on special characteristics and ominous implications when they occur in certain anatomic locations. The two most dramatic are Ludwig's angina and Fournier's gangrene (perineal phlegmon). In both conditions polymicrobial infection that includes anaerobic bacteria dissects rapidly through tissue planes and may cause uncontrollable, life-threatening infection. Ludwig's angina is caused by a mixture of oral bacteria and begins in the floor of the mouth or retropharyngeal space. The infection may end fatally, with compromise of the airway. Fournier's gangrene is a variant of synergistic infection that is caused by a mixture of perineal bacteria of fecal origin. Spread of the disease through the pelvis into the peritoneum may occur so rapidly that even aggressive antimicrobial therapy and surgical debridement cannot keep up.

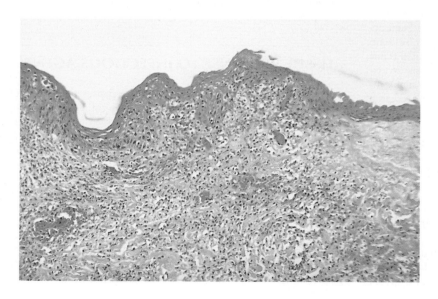

Fig. 11-1. Streptococcal dermatitis and cellulitis. An acute inflammatory response with polymorphonuclear neutrophils and edema disrupts the basal layer of the epidermis, the dermis, and the subcutaneous tissue. (H&E stain, original magnification × 50; *Streptococcus pyogenes* isolated in pure culture from the tissue.)

Fig. 11-2. *Clostridium* necrotizing infection of the colon. Scant inflammation and edema disrupt the wall of the colon and coat the serosal surface. The most prominent feature of the infection is the large amount of gas that has accumulated in the tissue. It might be dismissed as fat, except that the clear spaces occur in sites where fat does not exist. (H&E stain, original magnification × 5; *Clostridium septicum* isolated in pure culture from the patient.) (Courtesy of Stephen Allen, M.D.)

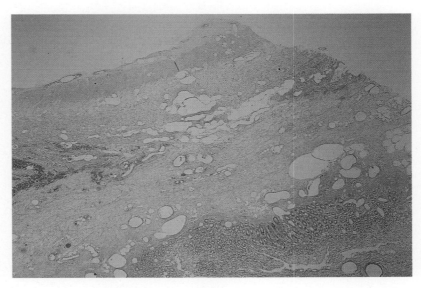

Gas-Forming Infections

Gas-forming infections are most commonly caused by clostridial species, of which the most common are *Clostridium perfringens* and *C. septicum*.[29–31] Clostridal cellulitis and particularly myonecrosis are often characterized by minimal cellular inflammation, being associated with tissue necrosis, a proteinaceous exudate, and bubbles of gas in the tissues. *C. septicum* causes necrotizing infection in the gastrointestinal tract (Fig. 11-2). Distant foci of myonecrosis caused by this pathogen should prompt a search for neoplastic disease in the gastrointestinal tract, which provides a portal of entry for the bacilli. Rarely hemolytic exotoxins produced by *C. perfringens* produce a syndrome of fatal, massive intravascular hemolysis, particularly after gallbladder surgery.

Diffuse Acute Inflammation

Diffuse acute inflammation is the hallmark of pyogenic bacterial infection. The most common infectious agents are the major Gram-positive agents: staphylococci; streptococci, including *Streptococcus pneumoniae* and *Enterococcus* spp.; the Gram-negative bacilli, including *Haemophilus* spp., the enteric bacilli, and nonfermenting bacilli, such as pseudomonads and *Acinetobacter* spp.; and a variety of anaerobic bacteria. *Clostridium* spp. are often participants in mixed bacterial infections that are not associated with gas formation.

Abscess and Empyema Formation and Necrotizing Infection

Necrotizing infection and formation of abscesses or empyema are features of pyogenic bacterial pathogens except for *Haemophilus* spp. and *S. pneumoniae*. The classic abscess-forming pathogen is *S. aureus*, but a variety of Gram-negative facultatively anaerobic and strictly anaerobic bacilli must also be considered. The cytology of abscesses is usually directed toward the bacterial pathogen with a Gram smear, rather than toward the host cell, but fine needle aspiration (FNA) is performed occasionally on pyogenic lesions when the nature of the process has not been clear to the clinician (Fig. 11-3).

Fig. 11-3. Staphylococcal abscess, lymph node aspirate. Erythrocytes and polymorphonuclear neutrophils are seen on an edematous background. Some of the neutrophils contain ingested cocci and show the vacuolated degeneration produced by bacterial products. The Gram reaction of the cocci cannot be determined, nor can their alignment (clusters or chains) be accurately assessed in their intracellular location. (Giemsa stain, original magnification × 1,000; *Staphylococcus aureus* isolated in pure culture from the lymph node.)

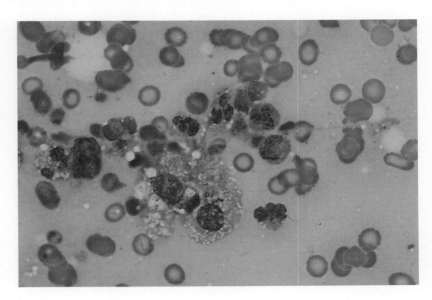

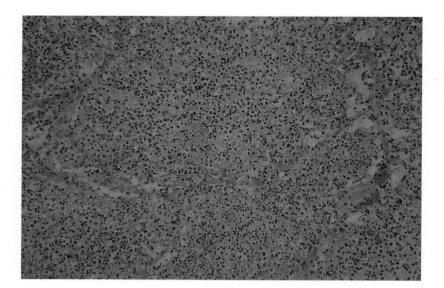

Fig. 11-4. *Legionella pneumophila* pneumonia. The cellular exudate in the airspaces consists of edema, fibrin, and polymorphonuclear neutrophils, many of which have undergone leukocytoclasis, producing a dusty appearance. (H&E stain, original magnification × 100; *Legionella pneumophila*, serogroup 1 isolated in pure culture from the lung.)

Specific Pathogens

Legionella Species

Legionella spp., particularly *L. pneumophila*, causes an acute lobular pneumonia that is more common and more severe in patients who have compromised immunologic or pulmonary defense mechanisms (legionnaire's disease). A second clinical syndrome, Pontiac fever, is self-limited and will not be seen by surgical pathologists. The airspaces in legionnaire's disease are choked with fibrin and acute inflammatory cells, but paradoxically a productive cough develops in only approximately 50 percent of patients. Leukocytoclasis of the airspace exudate is characteristic, but not diagnostic (Fig. 11-4). The bacteria, which are both extracellular and intracellular within macrophages, can be demonstrated with the Warthin-Starry or equivalent stain (Fig. 11-5) or by direct immunofluorescence. Fixation of the tissue in formalin is not detrimental to the rele-

vant antigens. Abscesses are demonstrable in as many as 20 percent of autopsied lungs, but are not usually evident antemortem.[32]

Vibrio Species

Vibrio cholerae causes a toxin-mediated, noninflammatory infection that is limited to the intestinal epithelium. Other *Vibrio* spp., particularly *V. vulnificus*, cause necrotizing infection of the skin and soft tissues (Fig. 11-6) after introduction of the bacteria into the skin or gastrointestinal tract by salt water or shellfish that have been harvested from contaminated water.[33,34] The infections have occurred most commonly in Gulf Coast states but have also been described in patients who have been exposed to brackish water in the interior of the United States.[35] *Aeromonas* spp. cause similar infections after exposure to fresh water.[36] Disseminated infection, which may be fatal, occurs in some cases.

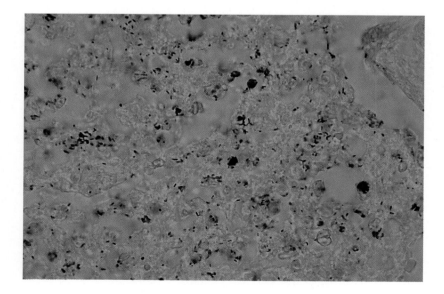

Fig. 11-5. *Legionella pneumophila* pneumonia. Numerous bacteria are demonstrated by silver impregnation, which distorts and enlarges the outlines of the bacilli. Clusters of bacteria reflect their position within the cytoplasm of monocyte/macrophages. The Gram reaction cannot be determined in this preparation. (Dieterle stain, original magnification × 1,000; *Legionella pneumophila*, serogroup 1 isolated in pure culture from the lung.)

Fig. 11-6. *Vibrio* necrotizing inflammation in soft tissue. An intense acute inflammatory response destroys the subcutaneous tissue. Involvement of a small artery can be seen. (H&E stain, original magnification × 45; *Vibrio vulnificus* isolated in pure culture from the tissue.) (Courtesy of David Walker, M.D.)

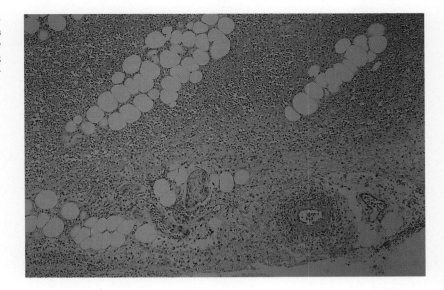

Nocardia Asteroides

Nocardia asteroides is an aerobic actinomycete that produces mycetoma (as discussed later) and acute infection of the lung, particularly in immunocompromised patients.[37,38] Dissemination from the lung, especially to the brain, may result. The inflammatory respose is usually purulent, and abscesses may result (Fig. 11-7), but nocardial pneumonia may also be chronic, in which case fibrosis and granulomas may be found (Fig. 11-8). *N. asteroides* is readily demonstrable as branching, filamentous Gram-positive bacilli (Fig. 11-9), which also stain well with the methenamine silver technique. The documentation of filaments and branching is important, because other Gram-positive bacilli may be filamentous or may display rudimentary branching, or both. Differentiation of *Nocardia* from *Actinomyces* can be made by evaluation of the clinical presentation, the absence of sulfur granules in systemic infection, and the demonstration of partial acid fastness in the bacilli. Modified acid-fast stains such as the Fite stain must be employed and interpreted carefully, as discussed later.

Smears and Tissue Sections

The interpretation of Gram-stained smears and sections is decidedly more difficult than the technical performance of the staining procedure. The myth that interpretation of the Gram stain is a simple task probably derives from the memory of administrative physicians whose only contact with the challenge came in a medical school microbiology course. Certain coccal organisms, such as some streptococci, have a tendency to elongate, producing confusion with Gram-positive bacilli. Conversely, some Gram-negative bacilli, such as *Haemophilus influenzae* and particularly *Acinetobacter* spp., can be quite coccal. *Clostridium* spp., including *C. perfringens*, have a distressing propensity for easy decolorization, and these important

Fig. 11-7. *Nocardia* pneumonia in an immunosuppressed patient. Necrotizing infection with formation of abscesses has destroyed the pulmonary parenchyma. The exudate consists of masses of polymorphonuclear neutrophils. (H&E stain, original magnification × 45; *Nocardia asteroides* isolated in pure culture from the lung.)

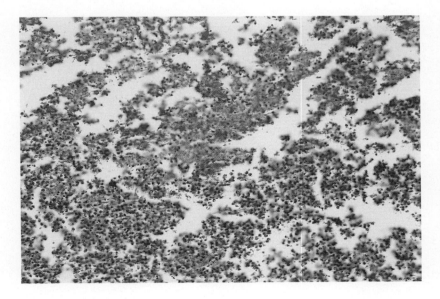

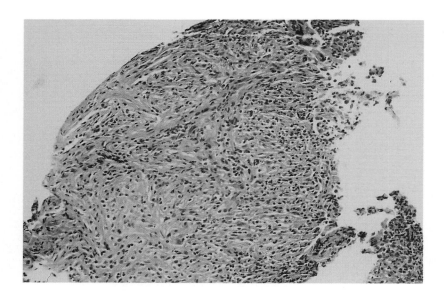

Fig. 11-8. *Nocardia* pneumonia. A well organized, noncaseating granuloma of macrophages is present in the interstitium. Transbronchial biopsy. (H&E stain, original magnification × 200; *Nocardia asteroides* isolated in pure culture from the specimen.)

pathogens may present as Gram-negative bacilli. By contrast, some Gram-negative bacteria regularly and stubbornly retain some of the crystal violet, appearing magenta or even blue. The legitimacy of these challenges is well illustrated by the fact that one clostridial species, *Clostridium clostridiiforme*, was classified for many years as a *Bacteroides* sp. (a Gram-negative genus). Additionally, *Gardnerella vaginalis*, a participant in mixed infections of the female genital tract, has been classified at various times as *Haemophilus vaginalis* (Gram-negative) and *Corynebacterium vaginale* (Gram-positive). Gram-positive bacteria that have been damaged by antimicrobial therapy or the inflammatory response may stain Gram-negative. When bacteria are within phagocytes, it is usually impossible to determine whether they are in chains (e.g., streptococci) or in clusters (e.g., staphylococci), because they are conforming to the structure of the phagosome. In all these situations the clues to the correct identification include the type of infection, careful analysis of the morphology of the bacteria, and assessment of

most of the population. As in most areas of pathology, it is dangerous to make a determination based on a single cell or small group of cells, whether eukaryotic or prokaryotic.

The problems of interpretation of the Gram stain are compounded in tissue sections, where organisms may be in multiple planes of focus or may be sectioned obliquely. The tissue versions of the Gram stain also tend to stain the bacteria less crisply. In particular, Gram-negative species may come out looking magenta or rose colored rather than a definitive red or pink.

Bacterial Mimics

If extensive cellular or tissue necrosis is present, a variety of organisms may elicit a neutrophilic inflammatory response. Examples may be found among the fungi (*Candida* spp.), the parasites (*T. gondii* and *Leishmania* spp.), and the viruses (herpes simplex virus and adenovirus).

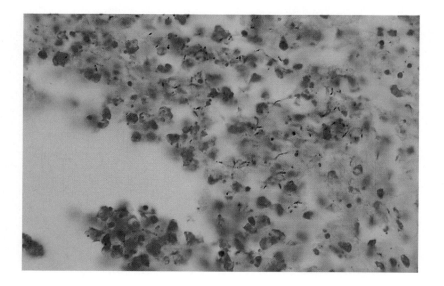

Fig. 11-9. *Nocardia* pneumonia. Thin, branching, irregularly staining Gram-positive bacilli course through necrotic pulmonary tissue. Same case as Fig. 11-7. (Brown and Hopps stain, original magnification × 1,000.)

Macrophage-Associated Infections and Granulomas: Mycobacteria, Fungi, Parasites, and Their Mimics

Acid-Fast Bacteria: Smears and Tissue Sections

The first step in detection of acid-fast bacteria is recognition that an appropriate stain should be performed, based on clinical suspicion or suggestive cellular response in H&E-stained sections. Granulomas or disorganized collections of macrophages are the usual clues, but a low index of suspicion should be maintained when the etiologic agent of the inflammatory process is not evident. Granulomas are organized collections of macrophages that have been activated by specific cellular immune responses. Macrophages may take the form of epithelioid histiocytes—so-called because they line up in a fashion that may resemble epithelium—and Langhans giant cells, which typically have nuclei marginated at the cell membrane. Granulomas may be intact or may display several types of central necrosis. Caseation consists of an eosinophilic material in which the ghosts of cells may still be visible. The necrotic material in some infectious granulomas stains intensely eosinophilic, resembling the fibrinoid necrosis seen in rheumatoid granulomas. Finally, the necrotic center consists of degenerating (but not ghost) inflammatory cells. These granulomas are often large and irregular, producing an appearance called stellate necrosis. Certain infectious agents are associated with particular types of necrosis, but the overlap is sufficient that an etiologic diagnosis should not be assumed. For instance, tuberculosis commonly elicits a caseating granulomatous response, but some infections may be characterized by noncaseating granulomas that are indistinguishable from those seen in sarcoidosis (Fig. 11-10).

Chronic inflammation with necrosis or acute inflammation (or with both) but without well formed granulomas characterizes some mycobacterial infections, particularly those caused by M. fortuitum, M. chelonae, and M. abscessus (Fig. 11-11), and are typical of nocardial infections.

Several other bacterial species, primarily Rhodococcus equi and Legionella micdadei, which elicit a response of macrophages or polymorphonuclear neutrophils, or both, may be partially or completely acid fast. Rhodococcus organisms produce chronic and granulomatous inflammation, including caseating granulomas and malacoplakia[39–41] (Fig. 11-12). L. micdadei causes an inflammatory exudate that consists of polymorphonuclear neutrophils or macrophages, or both, but granulomas are not seen.[32] In the case of L. micdadei the bacteria lose the property of acid fastness after they have been isolated in culture. Rhodococcus is only occasionally acid fast. The lesions of leprosy may be either granulomatous (Fig. 11-13) in patients with active cell-mediated immune responses or may consist of aggregates of poorly organized macrophages when cellular immunity is less aggressive. The numbers of mycobacteria also reflect the efficacy of the host response. In tuberculoid (granulomatous) leprosy, organisms may be difficult to find, whereas the macrophages (Lepra cells) of lepromatous leprosy are packed with acid-fast bacteria. A similar lesion is caused by the Mycobacterium avium complex in immunosuppressed patients, predominantly those who are infected with the human immunodeficiency virus (HIV). Large collections of macrophages distort and replace normal tissue (Fig. 11-14), and the cells are stuffed with mycobacteria[42,43] (Fig. 11-15). Because M. avium complex bacteria are stained with the PAS procedure, these nongranulomatous lesions may resemble Whipple's disease, particularly in the gastrointestinal tract and in lymphoid tissue.[44] An even greater challenge for the surgical pathologist is presented by the spindle cell pseudotumor that is caused by M. avium complex in HIV-infected patients[45] (Fig. 11-16). These lesions may be found in skin, lymphoid tissue, or bone. The cells resemble smooth muscle or fibroblasts but are histiocytes by immunohistochemical staining. They contain large numbers of mycobacteria (Fig. 11-17).

Sections should be scanned with a 40 × objective, concentrating on areas of granulomatous inflammation, necrosis, or acute inflammation. If acid-fast organisms are not seen and the

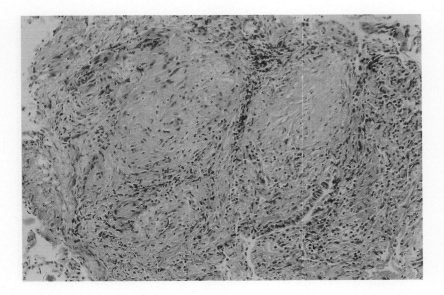

Fig. 11-10. Mycobacterium tuberculosis. Noncaseating granulomas with multinucleated giant cells in the submucosa of a bronchus. Transbronchial biopsy. (H&E stain, original magnification × 100; Mycobacterium tuberculosis isolated in pure culture from specimen.)

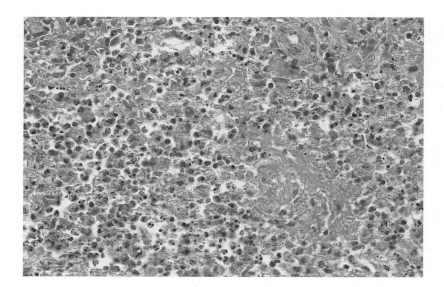

Fig. 11-11. Rapid grower mycobacterial infection of soft tissue. Necrotizing inflammation consisting of macrophages and a minor component of polymorphonuclear neutrophils. (H&E stain, original magnification × 400; *Mycobacterium abscessus* isolated in pure culture from specimen.)

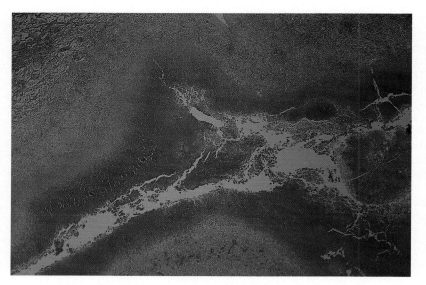

Fig. 11-12. *Rhodococcus* pneumonia. A large caseating granuloma is present. Other areas of the specimen were infiltrated by masses of unorganized macrophages. (H&E stain, original magnification × 5; *Rhodococcus equi* isolated in pure culture from the specimen.) (Courtesy of David Walker, M.D.)

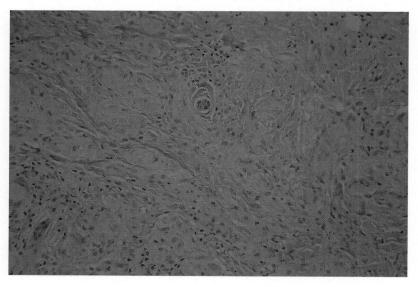

Fig. 11-13. Cutaneous leprosy. The dermis is infiltrated with epithelioid macrophages organized into confluent granulomas. Small numbers of acid-fast bacilli were present. (H&E stain, original magnification × 200.)

Fig. 11-14. Disseminated infection in the spleen of a patient infected with the human immunodeficiency virus. Masses of macrophages with abundant cytoplasm replace the splenic tissue and resemble the lesion of Whipple's disease. (H&E stain, original magnification × 200; *Mycobacterium avium* complex isolated in pure culture from tissue.) (Courtesy of David Walker, M.D.)

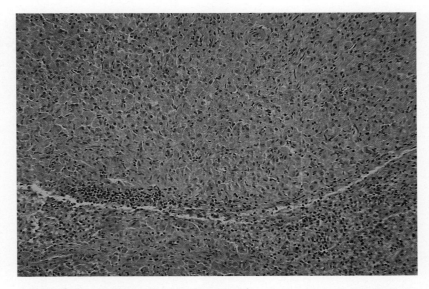

Fig. 11-15. Acid-fast stain of the tissue shown in Fig. 11-14. The cells are packed with mycobacteria. (Original magnification × 1,000.)

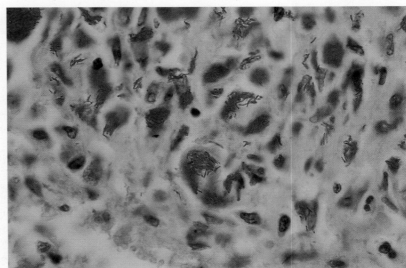

Fig. 11-16. Spindle cell tumor of soft tissue in a patient infected with the human immunodeficiency virus. Despite the elongated appearance of the cells, suggesting an origin from myofibroblasts, immunohistochemical stains documented their origin from macrophages. (H&E stain, original magnification × 500.) (Courtesy of Ann-Marie Nelson, M.D.)

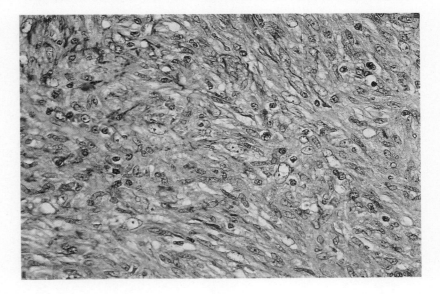

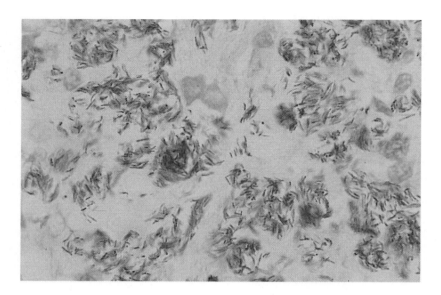

Fig. 11-17. Acid-fast stain of the tissue shown in Fig. 11-16. The cells are packed with acid-fast bacilli, compatible with *Mycobacterium avium* complex. (Ziehl-Neelsen stain, original magnification × 1,000.) (Courtesy of Ann-Marie Nelson, M.D.)

histologic response strongly suggests mycobacterial disease, the sections should be examined with a 100 × oil immersion lens. Attention should be focused on areas of necrosis and on macrophages, including giant cells. If acute, necrotizing inflammation is present, these areas should be examined closely. Morphologic differences have been described among mycobacteria, such as the cording produced by M. *tuberculosis*; large, banded bacilli of M. *kansasii*; long, broad, sometimes banded bacilli of M. *marinum*; and pleomorphic, occasionally coccobacillary cells of M. *avium* complex.[11] It is safest, however, to wait for help from the microbiology laboratory. Bacilli of the M. *avium* complex can be demonstrated with the PAS technique. Mycobacteria are Gram-positive bacilli and may be weakly Gram positive after staining, especially in smears. The mycobacteria may also appear as ghosts against an inflammatory background.[46]

If the conventional acid-fast stain fails to demonstrate bacilli in lesions with morphology suggestive of mycobacterial or no-

cardial disease, a modified stain should be employed. The modified stains should not be used as the first-line approach unless nocardial disease is suspected, because the modified decolorization is tricky. False positive acid fastness has been described in cases of actinomycosis when the Putt method was employed.[12,13] The Fite method is preferred in tissue sections. Partial acid fastness indicates that a portion of the bacterial population will be stained or, in the case of *Nocardia* spp., that portions of individual organisms will stain positively.

Cytologic Diagnosis of Mycobacterial Infections

Tuberculosis, still a predominant infection in third world countries, is making a resurgence in the United States with the recent identification of drug-resistant strains.[47] This infection may be encountered and diagnosed or at least suspected from the interpretation of cytologic samples principally obtained by FNA biopsy.[48] Several examples have been seen in FNA of en-

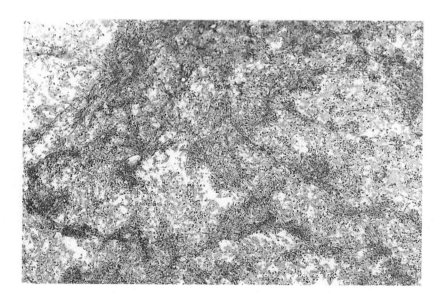

Fig. 11-18. Tuberculosis infection in cervical lymph node. Fine needle aspiration demonstrates acute inflammatory cells in a necrotic granular-appearing background. No actual granulomas are seen, but the background suggests tuberculosis. (Diff-Quik stain, original magnification × 50.)

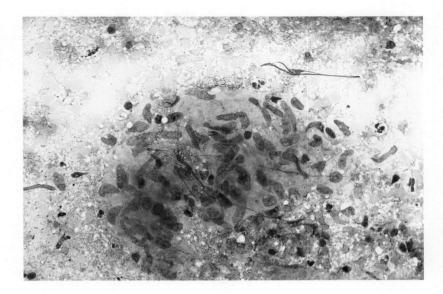

Fig. 11-19. Tuberculosis of the lung. Fine needle aspiration of a lung mass demonstrates epithelioid granuloma in a granular necrotic background. The same type of granuloma, most often in a clear smear background, can be seen in sarcoid. (Diff-Quik stain, original magnification × 400.)

larged cervical lymph nodes, particularly in children. Figure 11-18 illustrates a typical picture of necrosis and relatively acute inflammation but without well formed granulomas. The background of relatively homogeneous necrosis in the absence of any atypical cells suggesting a neoplasm is the morphologic clue that leads to performance of special stains to identify the organisms. Careful search of additional smears is often necessary to find them. The same picture may appear in an aspiration biopsy of the lung, but more intact granulomas may also be found within the necrotic background (Fig. 11-19).

With infection by atypical mycobacteria in patients with the acquired immunodeficiency syndrome (AIDS), the cytologic and histologic picture is quite different. In both bronchial lavage and FNA samples of the lung or lymph nodes or even cutaneous or soft tissue masses, many histiocytes are seen that in air-dried smears stained with Romanowsky methods appear like Gaucher cells. They have been termed pseudo-Gaucher cells

and were described in bone marrow smears and originally in an aspirate of an inguinal lymph node from a patient who had been injected with bacille Calmette-Guérin to treat superficial carcinoma of the bladder.[46,49] Few to many clear, thin, slightly curved areas appear in these smears both in the background and within the histiocytic cells, so-called negative images[46] (Fig. 11-20). These areas that do not stain with water-based stains represent the atypical mycobacteria that are easily stained with acid-fast stains and that usually occur in profusion in such smears (Fig. 11-21). Infection with *Nocardia*, usually in respiratory cytologic samples (Fig. 11-22) produces a similar finding, although the organisms are larger and tend to branch. More specific identification is required by culture or other methods as the morphology is not specific. Because it is the waxy cell wall of these organisms that prevents penetration by water-based stains, smears that are fixed in alcohol (e.g., the Papanicolaou stain) will not demonstrate this feature.

Fig. 11-20. Atypical mycobacterial infection in mediastinal lymph nodes. Fine needle aspiration of enlarged mediastinal lymph nodes demonstrates homogeneous metachromatic material with only a few inflammatory cells. Note the curved short clear spaces seen throughout the smear, "negative images" that represent the large number of organisms. Patient suffered from the acquired immunodeficiency syndrome. (Diff-Quik stain, original magnification × 400.)

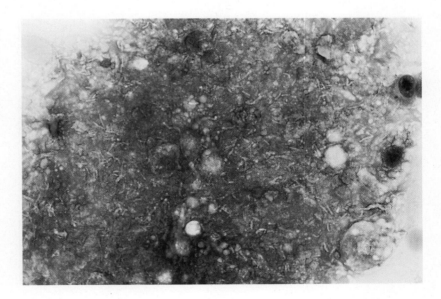

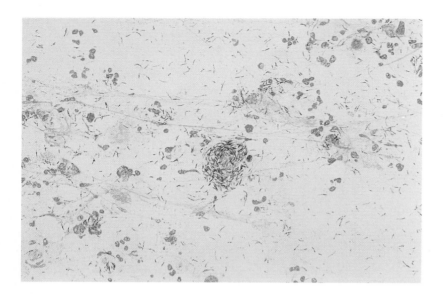

Fig. 11-21. Similar case as is illustrated in Figure 11-20; from fine needle aspiration of a cervical lymph node. The organisms stain acid fast. (Ziehl-Neelsen stain, original magnification × 600.)

Fungi: Smears and Tissue Sections

Fungi take two distinctive morphologic forms: yeasts and filamentous molds. Some species may produce both forms, concurrently or depending on temperature of incubation. Most molds, referred to as hyaline, have colorless or lightly colored hyphae, whereas a minority of species, known as dermatiacious fungi, contain pigments such as melanin in their cells. An excellent reference for morphologic identification of fungi in tissue is the atlas assembled by Chandler and Watts.[50]

Yeasts

Yeasts or blastoconidia are single-celled organisms that reproduce by a process called budding. The systemic dimorphic fungi include *Histoplasma capsulatum*, *Blastomyces dermatitidis*, *Coc-cidioides immitis*, *Sporothrix schenckii*, *Penicillium marneffii*, and some dematiacious fungi. When grown at 37°C in the laboratory or in the body of an infected host, the form is a budding yeast (*Histoplasma*, *Blastomyces*, or *Sporothrix*), a yeast-like form (*P. marneffii* and some dematiacious fungi), or a spherule (sporangium) with endospores (*C. immitis*).

The best overall stain for yeast in tissue is the routine H&E procedure. Even if a special stain is needed to detect fungi, the H&E stain may provide needed cytologic clues as to the identification. Several additional clues can be used to facilitate the identification of yeast in tissue (Table 11-4). The size of the yeast provides an important clue for identification. Approximate sizes may be inferred by comparison with adjacent cells. Greater accuracy can be achieved by use of an ocular micrometer. Clinical history, the organ(s) infected, and the tissue re-

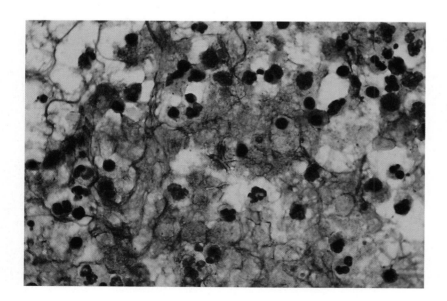

Fig. 11-22. *Nocardia* species. Bronchial washing from patient with lung infiltrate radiographically suggestive of carcinoma. Note the few curved negative images in the center of the field, which are larger than those seen in mycobacterial infection. Special stain and proof by culture or other methods are necessary. (Diff-Quik stain, original magnification × 1,000.)

Table 11-4. Identification of Yeasts in Smears and Tissue

Yeast	Size (μm)	Cellular Detail	Staining	Histologic Response	Location in Tissue	Hyphal Forms	Comments
Histoplasma capsulatum	3–5	Thin wall; budding ±; single nucleus; large distorted forms in old granulomas	H&E+, GMS+, PAS+, mucin−, FM−	Macrophage, granuloma with or without necrosis	Intracellular macrophage, extracellular in necrosis	No	Must be differentiated from small *Candida*, *Torulopsis*, small-form *Blastomyces*
Histoplasma duboisii	8–15		H&E+, GMS+, PAS+, mucin−, FM−		Intracellular macrophage, giant cells	No	Predominantly found in Africa
Blastomyces dermatitidis	8–15	Thick wall; budding +; multiple nuclei	H&E+, GMS+, PAS+, mucin±, FM−	Macrophage, granuloma, microabscess	Intracellular macrophages and giant cells; extracellular in microabscesses	No	Must be differentiated from *Cryptococcus*, developing spherules of *Coccidioides*
Coccidioides immitis	5–30	Thin wall; budding −; endospore formation; hyphae may be found in pulmonary cavities	H&E+, GMS+, PAS+, mucin−, FM−	Macrophage, granuloma	Intracellular macrophages and giant cells	Rare	Developing spherule must be differentiated from *Blastomyces*
Sporothrix schenckii	2–6	Thin wall; elongated (cigar-shaped); budding +	H&E+, GMS+, PAS+, mucin−, FM−	Macrophage, granuloma	Intracellular macrophages and giant cells	No	Rarely seen; Splendore-Hoeppli phenomenon may occur
Candida spp.	3–6	Thin wall; budding pseudohyphae	H&E+, GMS+, PAS+, mucin−, FM−	PMNL with or without abscesses; macrophage, granuloma	Extracellular in pus; intracellular in macrophage	Yes	Differentiate from *Torulopsis*, *Histoplasma*, filamentous molds
Torulopsis spp.	2–5	Thin wall; budding	H&E+, GMS+, PAS+, mucin−, FM−	PMNL	Extracellular	No	Rare pathogen
Cryptococcus neoformans	2–20	Thin wall; budding; variable size; round but may have distorted forms	H&E+, GMS+, PAS+, mucin+, FM+	Macrophage, giant cells, granuloma; scant reaction	Intracellular in macrophage and giant cell; extracellular without tissue reaction	Very Rare	Differentiate from *Blastomyces*
Malassezia furfur	2–5	Thin wall; septa between daughter cells	H&E+, GMS+, PAS+, mucin−, FM−			No	Rare; primarily in infants with lipid infusions
Penicillium mameffi	2–5	Thin wall; division by septation					
Chromoblasto-mycosis	5–12	Division by septation					

Abbreviations: H&E, hematoxylin and eosin; GMS, Gomori methenamine silver; PAS, periodic acid-Schiff; FM, Fontana-Masson; PMNL, polymorphonuclear leukocyte.

sponse to the yeast may be useful clues. Finally, in some instances histochemical stains may be useful for differentiation of certain yeasts.

Histoplasma Capsulatum. *H. capsulatum* is a small yeast that measures 3 to 5 μm. It is important to note that yeast cells in old caseous lesion may be moderately to very large and quite distorted. *H. capsulatum* has a close association with macrophages and is usually found intracellularly in active infections. Macrophages in which the cytoplasm is packed with small oval structures suggested to early investigators that the organism was a protozoan parasite similar to *Leishmania*, hence the name *Histoplasma* (tissue plasmodium). The clear spaces

that may be seen around the yeast are artifacts of fixation that yielded the species name (Fig. 11-23). The cadaver of this intracellular association may be seen in old healed lesions, because clusters of extracellular yeast may be tightly bound, reflecting their former location in a viable cell. *H. capsulatum* is typically oval, has a single nucleus in H&E-stained sections, and buds via a narrow base. Both viable and nonviable yeast cells stain well with methenamine silver (Fig. 11-24) and the PAS technique after diastase digestion. In active lesions with intracellular yeast the morphology can be delineated best with Giemsa or H&E stains.

Histoplasmosis occurs in a variety of forms, depending on the immune status of the host.[51] The most common clinical mani-

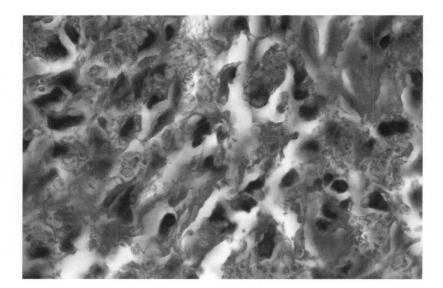

Fig. 11-23. Mucosal histoplasmosis. An infiltrate in the tongue consists of macrophages that are packed full of small, oval yeasts. The clear space around the nuclear material is not a capsule. A single nuclear mass can be seen in some yeast cells. (H&E stain, original magnification × 1,000; *Histoplasma capsulatum* isolated from tissue.)

festation is asymptomatic or minimally symptomatic infection. In the hyperendemic areas of the country—roughly the Ohio and Mississipi River valleys and the central Appalachian mountains—as many as 90 percent of the population may show immunologic evidence of prior infection. Immunocompetent patients may experience an acute self-limited pneumonia, in which granulomas may not be prominent initially.[52] The tissue response may be noncaseating granulomas, caseating granulomas with an organization that varies from quite loose to very tight (Fig. 11-25) or unorganized collections of macrophages. A continuum exists from the macrophage collections to the loosely organized granulomas. As in leprosy, the histologic response appears to correspond to the extent to which cellular immunity is operative.

Dissemination of yeast throughout the reticuloendothelial system often follows the pulmonary infection. The end result of the primary encounter is usually a healed granuloma in the lung, lymph nodes, liver, or spleen. Concentric rings of calcification in a solitary lung nodule, which may be demonstrable in chest radiographs, are highly suggestive of histoplasmosis. Disseminated infection occurs in immunosuppressed patients, classically the elderly but now predominantly patients infected with HIV.[53–55] Lesions are most common in organs of the reticuloendothelial system and the gastrointestinal tract. Unimpeded growth of yeast in HIV-infected patients may produce gastrointestinal lesions that resemble neoplasms macroscopically (Fig. 11-26).

The organ systems in which *H. capsulatum* will be seen most commonly are therefore the lung, the gastrointestinal tract, and the reticuloendothelial organs, whereas the skin and the musculoskeletal system are much less commonly involved.[56] In active infection the macrophage is the key cell (Figs. 11-23 and 11-24). Chronic pulmonary disease, which occurs primarily in men with chronic obstructive lung disease, resembles cavitary

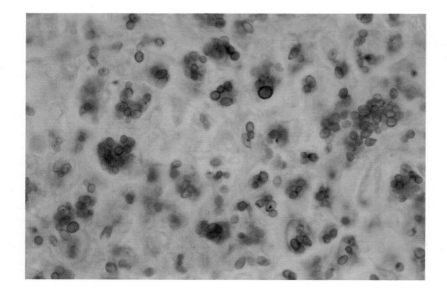

Fig. 11-24. The small uniform yeasts shown in Fig. 11-23 are well demonstrated by a silver stain. Although the cellular elements are not well stained, the intracellular location of the yeast is betrayed by the clustering. (Gomori methenamine silver stain, original magnification × 1,000.)

Fig. 11-25. Miliary histoplasmosis of the lung. A well formed interstitial granuloma with slight central fibrinoid necrosis is surrounded by an abundant mantle of lymphocytes. (H&E stain, original magnification × 25; *Histoplasma capsulatum* genes demonstrated in tissue by polymerase chain reaction.) (Courtesy of James Smith, M.D.).

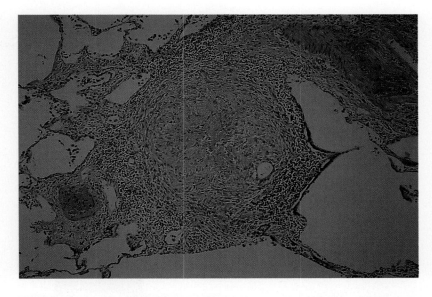

tuberculosis[57] (Fig. 11-27). Lesions may consist entirely of infected macrophages when infection disseminates in immunosuppressed individuals. Infected circulating mononuclear cells may be demonstrated, particularly in HIV-infected individuals. As immunologic reactivity increases, formation of increasingly well organized granulomas, which may be either caseating or noncaseating, results in focal lesions. Whenever tuberculosis enters the differential diagnosis, histoplasmosis should be close behind. Neutrophilic inflammation and microabscesses are not seen. Fibrosing mediastinitis is frequently attributed to *H. capsulatum*, but the yeasts are not usually demonstrable in sections.[58,59]

The differential diagnosis of *Histoplasma* in tissues and smears includes protozoan parasites, a rare small form of *B. dermatitidis*, *P. carinii*, and other small yeasts. The protozoa may be differentiated because they do not stain with methenamine silver. The small forms of *B. dermatitidis* retain their broad-based budding and have multiple nuclei if examined closely. *Candida* spp. usually produce a neutrophilic inflammatory response with or without granulomas, are often accompanied by hyphae or pseudohyphae, and are most commonly extracellular. *Torulopsis (Candida) glabrata* overlaps *Histoplasma* in size but is a rare cause of tissue infection. Particularly in older or florid lesions, in which the yeast cells of *H. capsulatum* demonstrate greater variation in size and morphology, confusion with the cysts of *P. carinii* may result. We have seen a case that was variously diagnosed as histoplasmosis or granulomatous pneumocystosis by experienced pathologists. Molecular amplification studies eventually established the etiology of the infection as *H. capsulatum*.

Blastomyces Dermatitidis. *B. dermatitidis* is a medium-sized yeast that measures 8 to 15 μm. It is roughly spherical or subspherical in shape and has a distinctive thick cellular wall that may almost appear refractile in H&E-stained sections, and a single broad-based bud. *B. dermatitidis* has multiple nuclei and

Fig. 11-26. Colonic mass in disseminated histoplasmosis in patient infected with the human immunodeficiency virus. The inflammatory mass resembles an annular, constricting carcinoma. (*Histoplasma capsulatum* isolated from patient.) (Courtesy of David Walker, M.D.)

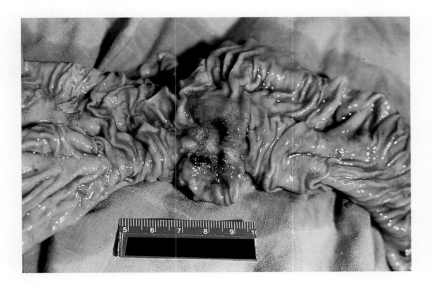

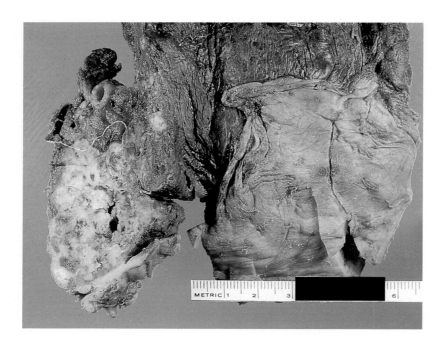

Fig. 11-27. Chronic pulmonary histoplasmosis. A lobectomy specimen, obtained because of the suspicion of neoplastic disease, demonstrates dense parenchymal granulomatous inflammation with fibrosis, a cavitary lesion, and overlying dense pleural fibrosis. Postoperatively, a sputum specimen obtained 6 weeks previously yielded *Histoplasma capsulatum*.

is usually demonstrated well with H&E stains (Fig. 11-28). The yeasts are also stained well with methenamine silver and the PAS technique. Some strains are weakly or moderately well colored with the mucicarmine stain, a point to remember when depending on this technique for documentation of *C. neoformans* (Fig. 11-29).

The endemic zone for blastomycosis covers much of the eastern United States and overlaps that of histoplasmosis. This infection is much less common than histoplasmosis and almost always occurs as single, sporadic cases, whereas histoplasmosis more commonly causes epidemic disease. Infection is almost always contracted through the respiratory system, resulting in asymptomatic infection, self-limited pneumonia, or localized infection, which may be mistaken for neoplastic disease.[60,61]

Disseminated infection usually results in cutaneous and skeletal disease. Chronic, ulcerating, hyperkeratotic skin lesions may suggest the possibility of squamous cell carcinoma (Fig. 11-30). Aggressive, systemic infection has been observed in immunosuppressed patients.[62]

The histologic response in blastomycosis is granulomatous, often with a characteristic mixture of acute inflammation including microabscesses. In the skin a pronounced overlying pseudoepitheliomatous hyperplasia is frequently seen (Fig. 11-30). Yeast cells are usually found in macrophages or multinucleated giant cells and in the microabscesses (Figs. 11-28 and 11-30). *B. dermatitidis* must be differentiated from *C. neoformans*, from developing spherules of *C. immitis*, and in parts of Africa from *Histoplasma duboisii*. The yeast cells of *Cryptococcus*

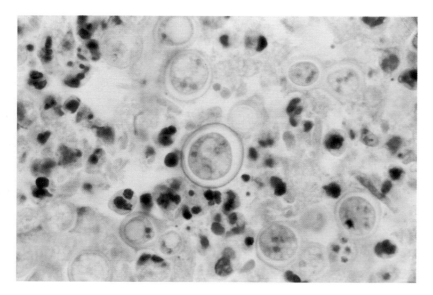

Fig. 11-28. Localized blastomycosis was an incidental finding in an autopsy. Yeast cells of *Blastomyces dermatitidis* demonstrate multiple nuclei, thick cell walls, broad-based budding, and an artifactual separation of the cytoplasm from the cell wall. (H&E stain, original magnification × 1,000.)

Fig. 11-29. Yeast cells of *Blastomyces dermatitidis* in a granulomatous lesion are colored by the mucicarmine stain. The correct diagnosis must be made by careful morphologic study of the yeast or by fungal culture, or by both. (Mucicarmine stain, original magnification × 250.)

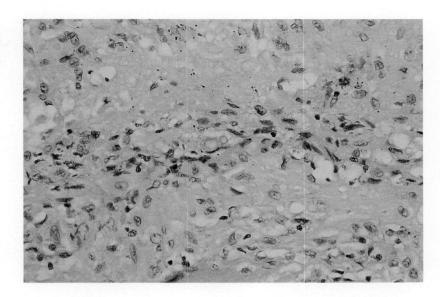

are more uniformly round and more variable in size, have a thin wall, and bud with a narrow base. The capsule of *C. neoformans* is always stained by the mucicarmine and Fontana-Masson methods, whereas *Blastomyces* organisms are usually negative with the former and always with the latter (although we have seen a case in which a false positive Fontana-Masson stain led to an incorrect diagnosis). *Coccidioides* can be eliminated if budding yeast cells are demonstrated; in their absence the differentiation can be accomplished by evaluation of the thick cell wall and the search for more completely developed spherules.

Extremely rarely hyphal forms of *B. dermatitidis* have been reported in lung tissue and sputum obtained from immunosuppressed patients.[63] The unusual small form of *B. dermatitidis* (Fig. 11-31) must be differentiated from *H. capsulatum*.[64]

Cryptococcus Neoformans. *C. neoformans* is a variably sized yeast that ranges from 2 to 20 μm in diameter, with a prepon-

derance of cells measuring 4 to 8 μm. The sexual form of the fungus, *Filobasidiella neoformans*, which is not found in human tissue or demonstrated in clinical laboratories, is a basidiomycete—the closest thing we have to an infectious mushroom. Other species of *Cryptococcus* are only rarely, if ever, human pathogens.

C. neoformans has a thin wall and a narrow-based bud. The great variability in size and the uniformity in shape of the spherical cells are useful clues to the diagnosis. The yeasts are moderately well stained by the H&E stain and are well displayed with the methenamine silver and PAS techniques. Staining of the often abundant polysaccharide capsule with the mucicarmine stain (Fig. 11-32) and demonstration of a melanin pigment with the Fontana-Masson stain are useful histochemical clues to the correct etiology. Most strains of *C. neoformans* are heavily encapsulated in tissue, although they may lose much of the polysaccharide after isolation in the clinical laboratory.

Fig. 11-30. Cutaneous blastomycosis is characterized by pseudoepitheliomatous hyperplasia, granulomatous inflammation, and microabscesses composed of polymorphonuclear neutrophils. (H&E stain, original magnification × 45.)

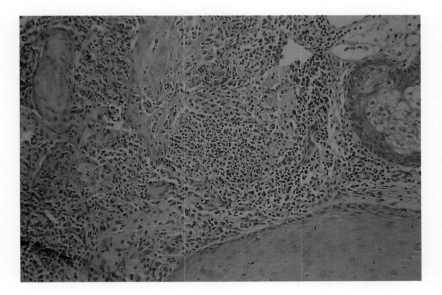

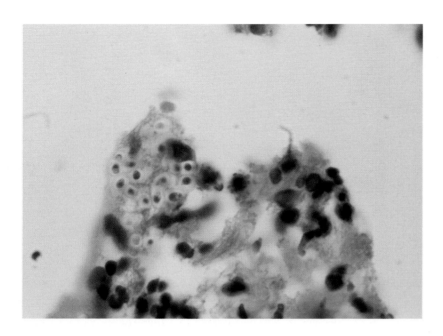

Fig. 11-31. *Blastomyces dermatitidis*, small form in a macrophage, resembling the yeast cells of *Histoplasma capsulatum*. The correct identification can be made by careful observation of multiple nuclei and broad-based budding or most definitively by culture. (H&E stain, original magnification × 1,000.)

The large capsule, which does not stain with H&E, often produces a clear zone around the yeast cell, the in vivo equivalent of the India ink preparation in the clinical laboratory. The mucicarmine stain usually colors the area of the capsule directly around the cell wall, leaving the mass of capsule comparatively unstained (Fig. 11-32). Some strains of *C. neoformans* are poorly encapsulated, both in vivo and in vitro. In these cells the mucicarmine stain produces a thin rim of staining at the cell wall. Very rarely, pseudohyphae of *C. neoformans* may be demonstrated in tissue[65] (Fig. 11-32).

Cryptococcosis is a worldwide cosmopolitan infection, which is primarily acquired through the respiratory tract. The pulmonary-lymph node complex is demonstrated only rarely.[66,67] Active pulmonary infection may result, but the clinical manifestations are dominated by disseminated infection, especially to the central nervous system.[68] Much less commonly, primary inoculation into the skin may produce localized cutaneous infection, which resembles the chronic, crusted lesions of blastomycosis or may present as cellulitis.[69] Cryptococcal infections are frequently seen in HIV-infected patients.[70] The histologic response appears to depend on the degree of encapsulation of the yeast cells. Most often the fully encapsulated cells produce a relatively noninflammatory process in which the encapsulated yeasts produce a gelatinous mass. It is easy to miss the fungal nature of the infection if poorly staining yeast are missed in an H&E-stained section (Fig. 11-33). Minimally encapsulated strains elicit a granulomatous inflammatory response with multinucleated giant cells[71] (Fig. 11-33). The yeasts are located intracellularly in macrophages and giant cells.

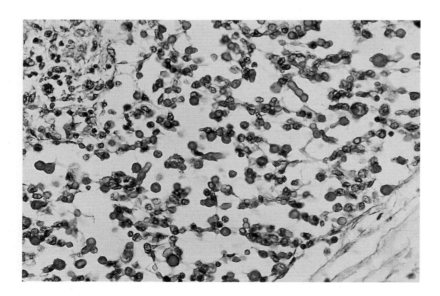

Fig. 11-32. The mucopolysaccharide capsules of *Cryptococcus neoformans* in a mediastinal lymph node are well demonstrated. There is minimal inflammatory reaction, the lymphocytic architecture being disrupted by clear spaces and the yeast cells. The yeast cells are round and vary in size. The capsule closest to the cell wall is stained. A few short pseudohyphae can be seen. (Mucicarmine stain, original magnification × 400.)

The primary differential diagnosis of cryptococcosis is with blastomycosis and coccidioidomycosis. The inflammatory response, the relatively uniform shape, and the greatly variable size of the yeast cells should suggest the correct diagnosis. Histochemical stains are useful, particularly the mucicarmine and Fontana-Masson stains.[72] Combination of these two stains has been described.[73] The possibility that B. dermatitidis may stain with the mucicarmine stain must be remembered.

Sporothrix Schenckii. S. schenckii is a small, round to oval yeast that measures 2 to 6 μm in size. The yeasts are rarely seen in histologic sections, both because they are sparse and because they stain poorly with H&E. Likewise, the characteristic elongated, "cigar-shaped" cells are not commonly encountered. A characteristic, but not diagnostic feature of sporotrichosis is the asteroid body, an eosinophilic structure measuring up to 100 μm. The asteroid body is produced by accretion of proteinaceous material around a yeast cell, the Splendore-Hoeppli phenomenon.[74] Unfortunately, the asteroid bodies, which were frequently reported in early cases from South African miners, are not commonly seen in the United States. S. schenckii stains well with the methenamine silver and PAS techniques. A potential pitfall is the presence of cigar-shaped structures in sarcoid-like granulomas in lymph nodes, known as Hamazaki-Wesenberg bodies.[50] These nonbiologic structures can be differentiated from yeast cells by their inherent yellow-brown pigmentation.

The distribution of Sporothrix is worldwide. Epidemics in the United States have been associated particularly with agricultural products, particularly sphagnum moss.[75,76] The classic description of the patient as an alcoholic rose gardener is not often accurate, but a modern analogy was contributed by a group of beer-guzzling fraternity brothers who acquired their infection when they were passing straw-packed bricks along a chain line as they constructed a masonry wall.[77] The portal of entry is usually the skin, resulting in a local lesion that may be followed by lymphangitis and proximal lesions in skin or lymph nodes, or both. Disseminated infection occurs uncommonly, primarily to the skeletal system and the lung. The occasional entry of S. schenckii into the respiratory tract results in a primary granulomatous pneumonia that must be differentiated from other fungal and mycobacterial processes.[78]

Histologically, the process is granulomatous, with both caseating and noncaseating lesions. A component of acute inflammation and microabscesses may be present. The differential diagnosis of sporotrichosis clinically and pathologically includes swimming pool granuloma caused by Mycobacterium marinum, tularemia caused by Francisella tularensis (which may also result in lymphangitis and proximal lesions), blastomycosis, and neoplastic disease. Because the causative microbes are rarely demonstrated in tissue, the etiology must often be resolved by culture.

Candida Species. Candida spp. are the most common causes of fungal infection in hospitalized patients and those who are immunosuppressed.[79] Candida albicans is by far the most common pathogen, but in some locations C. tropicalis has been equally or more frequent as a nosocomial pathogen.[80] Other species that may be encountered with some frequency are C. guilliermondii, C. parapsilosis,[81] and C. krusei,[82] which is especially important because of its intrinsic resistance to the imidazole class of antifungal agents. T. (Candida) glabrata is a small yeast that produces urinary tract infections, fungemia, and endocarditis; it is not often encountered in tissue specimens.

Candida spp. are small elliptical yeasts that measure 3 to 6 μm in size. They commonly produce pseudohyphae both in vivo and in vitro, which differentiates them from most of the other commonly encountered yeasts. The yeast cells stain well with H&E, Gram stain, methenamine silver, and PAS techniques. The psuedohyphae consist of budding yeast cells that have not separated, producing elongated structures that have nonparallel walls at the cellular junctions (Fig. 11-34). True hyphae, which are also produced by C. albicans, have parallel cell walls.

Candida spp. produce a variety of clinical infections, most commonly of the skin, nails, vagina, and mucocutaneous areas.

Fig. 11-33. Cryptococcal osteomyelitis. A poorly encapsulated strain of Cryptococcus neoformans has elicited a granulomatous reaction. Variably sized, round yeast cells are present in macrophages and multinucleated giant cells. (H&E stain, original magnification × 400; Cryptococcus neoformans isolated in pure culture from the lesion.)

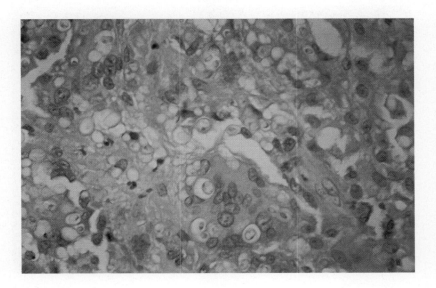

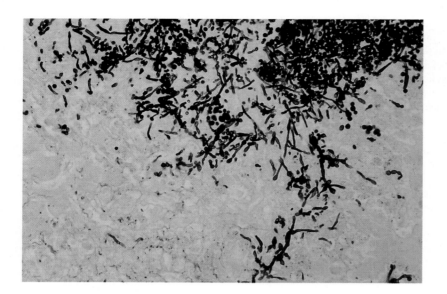

Fig. 11-34. *Candida* liver abscess. A combination of budding yeast and pseudohyphae makes the most likely etiologic diagnosis candidiasis. (Gomori methenamine silver stain, original magnification × 45; *Candida albicans* isolated in pure culture from the patient.)

More serious infections include oral candidiasis (thrush); disease of the gastrointestinal tract (Fig. 11-35), especially the lower esophagus; endocarditis; and disseminated infection that may involve any organ.[83] Infection of the central nervous system and primary infection of the lungs are uncommon.[84,85] The portals of entry are usually the skin or the gastrointestinal tract. The histologic response is usually pyogenic (Fig. 11-35), but granulomatous lesions or mixed acute and chronic inflammation may result.

The differential diagnosis on initial analysis usually includes bacterial pathogens (which may also be present). Once the presence of yeasts and pseudohyphae are recognized, the diagnosis is usually obvious (Fig. 11-34). If yeasts alone are present, they must be differentiated from dimorphic yeasts, which usually have different clinical and pathologic presentations. The pseudohyphae must be differentiated from hyaline molds, such as *Aspergillus* spp.

Yeast-Like Fungi

Coccidioides Immitis. *C. immitis* is a dimorphic fungus that reproduces in vivo and at 37°C by endosporulation rather than by budding. A mature spherule contains many endospores (Fig. 11-36), which are released when the spherule ruptures. Each of the endospores enlarges and develops into a new spherule. The smallest endospores measure 5 μm, whereas the mature spherules range from 30 to 100 mm in size, occasionally reaching 200 mm. Spherules and their endospores are stained well by H&E. Spherules that are developing from released endospores may also be visible but are more reliably seen after staining by the methenamine silver or PAS techniques (Fig. 11-37). The endospores also stain with the special stains, but the wall of the spherule is not stained by the PAS technique and is only variably stained with methenamine silver. In pulmonary cavitary disease oxygenation of the cavity may lead to the development of the filamentous phase of the fungus. A more unusual occur-

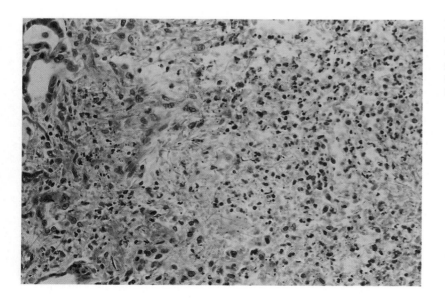

Fig. 11-35. *Candida* gastrointestinal infection. A necrotizing mucosal infection includes a neutrophilic and mononuclear inflammatory response. Pseudohyphae, which can be seen coursing through the tissue, are too large to be bacteria. (H&E stain, original magnification × 45.)

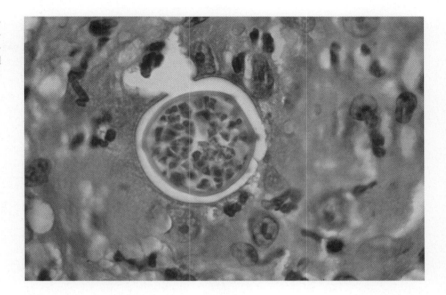

Fig. 11-36. *Coccidioides immitis* spherule in a multinu-cleated giant cell. The thick wall of the spherule en-closes many endospores. Among commonly seen fun-gal infections the spherule is distinctive and diagnostic. (H&E stain, original magnification × 1,000.) (Courtesy of Louis Rosati, M.D.)

rence was the presence of spherules and arthroconidia in the nervous system of a patient with a cerebrospinal fluid reser-voir.[86] The arthroconidia of the mold phase are the infective form. Thus certain surgical specimens are at least theoretically infectious, whereas the yeast phase of dimorphic fungi is infec-tious only if inoculated directly into tissue.

The distribution of *C. immitis* is limited to the southwestern United States, but the disease is increasingly seen throughout the country because of increasing travel.[87] The arthroconidia are so infectious that a brief sojourn in an endemic area may re-sult in infection. Recent increases in the frequency of infection in California may be related to more favorable conditions for dissemination of the arthroconidia during periods of drought.[88] Infection, which is acquired through the respiratory tract, is usually asymptomatic or minimally symptomatic. Acute or chronic pneumonia may result, and progressive, disseminated disease may occur, particularly in immunocompromised pa-

tients.[89,90] The organs most commonly involved are the skin, bones, and central nervous system.[91] The inflammatory process in coccidioidomycosis is granulomatous, but acute inflamma-tion and microabscesses may also be seen. Granulomas may be either caseating or noncaseating.

As the endospores of *C. immitis* develop, they overlap *Histo-plasma*, *Cryptococcus*, and *Blastomyces* in size. The lesions most closely resemble those of blastomycosis, and, as has been men-tioned, the developing spherules may resemble the yeast cells of *Blastomyces*. Developing spherules may be found in macrophages, in multinucleated giant cells, or extracellularly. Endosporulation documents *Coccidioides*, whereas demonstra-tion of budding yeast eliminates the possibility of this fungus. The differential diagnosis may be very difficult when few non-diagnostic forms are present. Immunofluorescence has been used successfully to arbitrate difficult cases, but the reagents are unfortunately not widely available. Of course, if the clinician or

Fig. 11-37. Coccidioidomycosis. A developing spherule of *Coccidioides immitis* is located in a multinu-cleated giant cell. The primary differential diagnosis at this stage of development is with *Cryptococcus neofor-mans* and *Blastomyces dermititidis*. (Periodic acid-Schiff stain, original magnification × 250.)

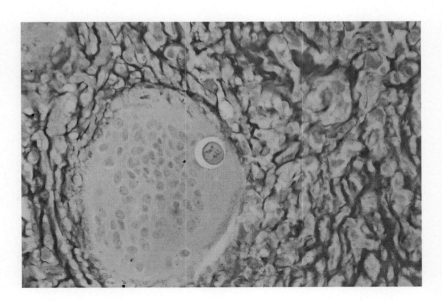

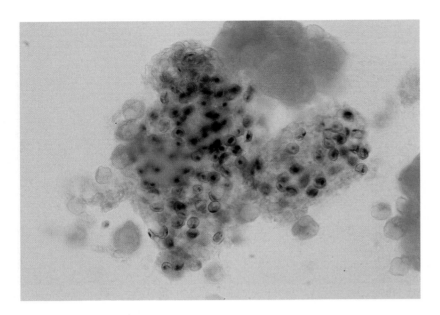

Fig. 11-38. *Pneumocystis* pneumonia. Clusters of cysts are present in the foamy alveolar exudate. Collapsed cysts produce the helmet shape. The focal thickening of the cyst wall can be seen as black marks. (Gomori methenamine silver stain, original magnification × 450.)

pathologist had the forethought to culture the specimen, the answer should be forthcoming from the microbiology laboratory.

Pneumocystis Carinii. *P. carinii* is often considered a parasite, but molecular genetic analysis has established its place among the fungi.[92] Similar organisms, which are found in other animal species such as rodents, probably represent other species.[93] *P. carinii* contains a cyst stage in which internal spores, referred to as trophozoites, develop. It is thought that the trophozoites are released from the mature cysts. The organism has not been cultured for more than a few passages in vitro, and the life cycle is not known definitively. The mature trophozoites measure 2 to 4 μm in size and can be stained by Romanovsky stains, such as the Giemsa or Diff-Quik stain. They are difficult to visualize in small numbers because of their small size. The cysts measure 5 to 8 *mm* and are roughly spherical but frequently appear par-

tially collapsed, producing the so-called helmet-shaped form (Fig. 11-38). A thickening of the cyst wall often produces a darker comma-shaped area of staining with the methenamine silver technique.

The cysts stain poorly or not at all with H&E or Giemsa stains, but occasionally the cysts may be outlined as ghosts by these stains or by Gram stain, and internal trophozoites may sometimes be visualized.[94] The PAS technique does not color the cysts but does stain the "foamy exudate" in which the cysts are often enmeshed and that is thought to be elaborated by the organism. The cysts are well stained by the methenamine silver procedure, but the optimal staining times are slightly different from those used for other fungi. The histology laboratory should be apprised, therefore, that *Pneumocystis* is being considered. The cysts are also stained by the Gram-Weigert technique (Fig. 11-39) as well as by Calcofluor white and toluidine blue in smears, as discussed earlier. *Pneumocystis* cysts fluoresce when

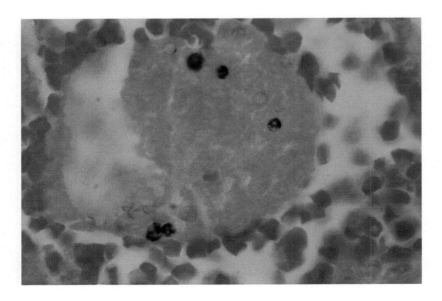

Fig. 11-39. *Pneumocystis* pneumonia. Cysts are demonstrated on the background of the foamy alveolar exudate. (Gram-Weigert stain, original magnification × 1,000.)

smears are stained by the Papanicolau technique and examined in a fluorescence microscope.[95] For most pathologists the Diff-Quik, Giemsa, and/or rapid methenamine silver stains are the choices for immediate study. Fluoresceinated monoclonal antibodies to *P. carinii*, which are commercially available, have proved equivalent to or more sensitive than other methods for detection of both trophozoites and cysts in most studies.[96–98] Screening of specimens is facilitated by use of fluorescence microscopy, but the comparative sensitivity of the techniques in a particular institution will depend heavily on the skill and diligence of the observers. Immunofluorescence has not been applied extensively to tissue sections, and some of the monoclonal reagents do not react with organisms that have been fixed in formalin.

Pneumocystosis is distributed worldwide and usually occurs as sporadic infection, but small outbreaks have been described.[99] The portal of entry is believed to be the respiratory tract, and the predominant organ affected is the lung. Subclinical infection is not commonly recognized but is probably a frequent occurrence as judged by the prevalence of antibody[100] and occasional demonstration of the organisms in lung tissue of patients without symptoms referable to the lower respiratory tract.[101] Symptomatic infection occurs almost invariably in immunosuppressed individuals. The infection was first described in malnourished infants in Europe, but steroid therapy and neoplastic disease, particularly of the hematopoietic system, were the most important risk factors before the appearance of HIV infection.[102] Pneumocystosis was the infection that initially defined AIDS, and most infections now occur in HIV-infected individuals.[103,104] Coinfecting organisms, particularly cytomegalovirus, are commonly present.[105] The institution of prophylactic therapy with trimethoprim-sulfamethoxazole has significantly reduced the incidence of this infection.[106] Disseminated infection was rare in the pre-AIDS era, but infection of virtually every organ system has been reported in HIV-infected patients.[107]

The histologic response to *P. carinii* is quite varied. An interstitial pneumonia rich in plasma cells was described in malnourished children (Fig. 11-40) but is not often seen in its pure form. The most typical reaction is a modest mononuclear infiltrate in the interstitium accompanied by a prominent intra-alveolar accumulation of foamy material that is colored by the PAS technique (Fig. 11-39). This exudate may calcify.[108] The other common inflammatory response is diffuse alveolar damage (Fig. 11-41) with mononuclear interstitial inflammation, proliferation of pneumocytes, and accumulation of fibrin with hyaline membranes in the airspaces.[109] Less common histologic responses include granulomatous inflammation,[110] vascular invasion, vasculitis, and cavitary lesions, especially in patients infected with HIV.[111] Most cases of disseminated infection are characterized by pools of "foamy exudate" that disrupt the normal architecture of the organ and in which large numbers of cysts are present. The efficacy of bronchoalveolar lavage and cytologic examination has resulted in fewer biopsy samples being submitted for evaluation.[112]

If the classic foamy exudate is present, there is little difficulty in establishing the correct diagnosis. Diffuse alveolar damage calls into play a large differential of infectious and noninfectious etiologies. The cysts must be differentiated from small yeasts, such as *Candida* spp. or *H. capsulatum*. Erythrocytes that have been overstained with the methenamine silver method also provide a challenge for the unwary observer.

Cytologic Diagnosis. The most common infection of the respiratory tract seen both in patients with AIDS and in other immunocompromised patients is *P. carinii*.[113] This organism is tightly bound within the alveolar framework of the lung, produces little or no inflammatory reaction, and can be difficult to detect in respiratory tract specimens unless direct sampling is used (i.e., bronchial lavage, brushings, washings, and FNA biopsies). In air-dried smears stained by Romanowsky methods (Wright's stain, May-Grünwald, Giemsa, and the most popular of these stains, Diff-Quik), the morphology is a metachromatic tangled mass of fibrin-like material containing the dark small trophozoites. (Fig. 11-42). At high magnification there is a suggestion of separate cyst walls surrounding the trophozoites, the whole mass of material reproducing a cast of the alveolus. In the Papanicolaou stain (Fig. 11-43) the individual trophozoites do

Fig. 11-40. *Pneumocystis* plasma cell pneumonia. The original presentation of this infection. An interstitial mononuclear infiltrate including many plasma cells is not accompanied by a significant inflammatory response in the airspaces. (H&E stain, original magnification × 250.)

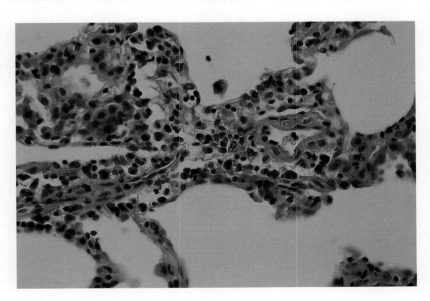

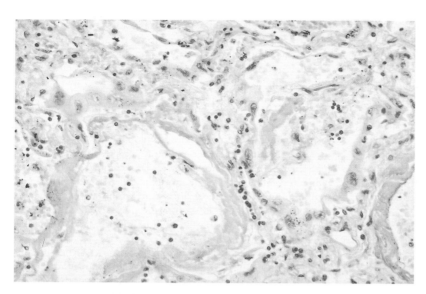

Fig. 11-41. *Pneumocystis* pneumonia. The histologic response is characterized by diffuse alveolar damage, including mononuclear interstitial inflammation and exudation of fibrin into the airspaces with hyaline membranes. (H&E stain, original magnification × 200.)

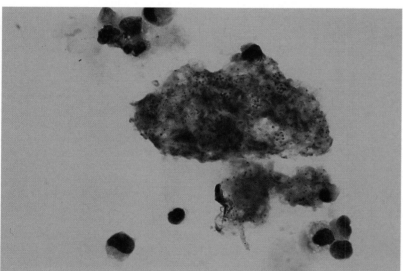

Fig. 11-42. *Pneumocystis* pneumonia. The smear of a bronchoalveolar lavage contains clusters of trophozoites and cysts in a clump of foamy alveolar exudate. The intracystic trophozoites are visible. (Giemsa stain, original magnification × 1,000.)

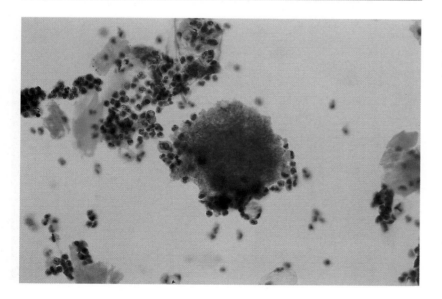

Fig. 11-43. *Pneumocystis carinii* in bronchial washing. Cluster of organisms enmeshed in fibrin and surrounded by a few inflammatory cells. There is a vague outline of small cysts, but the trophozoites are not seen with the Papanicolaou stain. (Papanicolaou stain, original magnification × 1,000.)

not stain, but the cyst walls of multiple cysts embedded in the fibrin matrix are more apparent. The inflammatory reaction to *Pneumocystis* organisms is usually minimal unless, as often happens, another pathogen is present. Figure 11-44 demonstrates both *Pneumocystis* and herpes inclusions in material obtained by bronchial washing from an area of infiltrate detected radiographically in the lung. This patient suffered from AIDS, in which multiple infections are not uncommon.

Penicillium Marneffii. *P. marneffii* is a recently recognized opportunistic fungal infection that appears to be endemic in Asia.[114,115] Immunocompetent patients have been infected, but most patients have been immunocompromised. In the United States most patients have been HIV-infected individuals who have traveled to Asia. The portal of entry is thought to be the lung, resulting in a chronic pneumonia and on occasion dissemination to peripheral organs, particularly the liver. Accumulations of macrophages, which may undergo necrosis, form the basic histopathologic response. Numerous intracellular yeast-like cells that measure 2 to 5 μm in size resemble *H. capsulatum* most closely. If budding yeast cells are identified, the possibility of *Penicillium* infection can be eliminated. The yeast-like cells of *P. marneffii* divide by septation. Occasionally, elongated, sausage-shaped cells with septa can be demonstrated, establishing the diagnosis in conjunction with the clinical presentation and histologic response.

Chromoblastomycosis. Chromoblastomycosis is a chronic infection of skin and subcutaneous tissue that is caused by several genera of dematiacious (pigmented) fungi, particularly *Fonsecaea pedrosoi*.[50] The infection is most prevalent in tropical and subtropical regions. In the United States it is uncommon but is most often documented in the southern states. As the name implies, the clinical and histologic appearance of the lesions resembles blastomycosis most closely. The chronic lesions are caused by direct inoculation of the fungi, so they are most often seen on exposed parts of the lower extremities. The histologic response is granulomatous, with the inclusion of microabscesses and a profound pseudoepitheliomatous hyperplasia that accounts for the verrucous, tumor-like skin masses. The hallmark of the infection is the presence of dark brown, thick-walled muriform cells that measure 5 to 12 μm (Fig. 11-45). These structures, which are diagnostic of the infection, are referred to as sclerotic bodies. Special stains are not necessary because of the intrinsic pigmentation. As is true in blastomycosis, the yeast-like cells are found in the microabscesses surrounded by polymorphonuclear neutrophils. The sclerotic bodies divide by septation, which may be visualized in the brown cells.

Prototheca Species. *Prototheca* spp. are achlorophyllous algae that occasionally cause infection of the skin and subcutaneous tissue and often infect bursae, especially that of the olecrenon.[116-118] They are considered with the fungi because of their morphologic and cultural similarities. The diagnostic form is a sporangium that contains up to 20 endospores (Fig. 11-46). The sporangia of the two most common species, *P. wickerhamii* and *P. zopfii*, measure 2 to 12 μm and 10 to 25 mm in diameter, respectively. Crowding of the endospores, each of which has a single nucleus and its own cell wall, causes molding of the endospores that may resemble septation. The sporangia of *P. wickerhamii* may assume the form of a morula— a central endospore surrounded by peripheral endospores. The sporangia and endospores are stained well with H&E, although in some cases only the walls of the individual endospores are colored. The structures are also demonstrated well with the methenamine silver and PAS techniques.

The histologic response in cutaneous lesions is a scant mononuclear infiltrate with focal necrosis and many interspersed sporangia. Inflammation of the bursa may include granulomas with or without necrosis (Fig. 11-47). The differential diagnosis is not difficult if the observer is familiar with this organism. Other organisms that form sporangia, such as *C. immitis*, are considerably larger. In H&E-stained sections the sporangia may be mistaken for strange multinucleated host cells.

Fig. 11-44. *Pneumocystis carinii* and herpesvirus infection in bronchial wash. Small fibrin masses of *Pneumocystis* organisms are seen mixed with enlarged ground-glass nuclei of herpesvirus in bronchial cells. Note the acute inflammatory background, which is highly unusual with the presence of *Pneumocystis* organisms alone. The patient suffered from the acquired immunodeficiency syndrome. (Diff-Quik stain, original magnification × 250.)

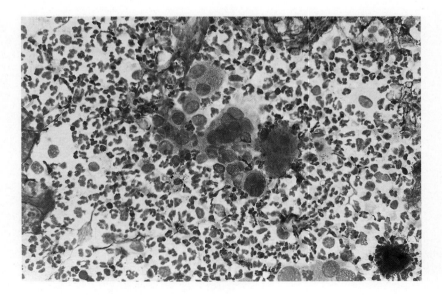

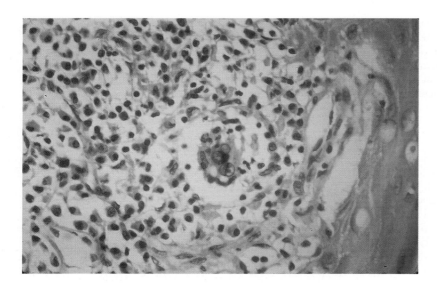

Fig. 11-45. Chromoblastomycosis. Yellow-brown yeast-like cells are present in a mononuclear inflammatory exudate in the upper dermis. The yeast-like cells, some of which have septa, are referred to as sclerotic bodies. They are produced by several species of dematiacious fungi. (H&E stain, original magnification × 450.)

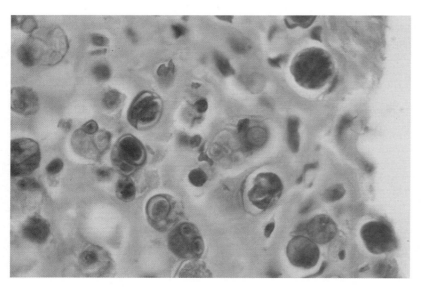

Fig. 11-46. Protothecosis. The inflammatory lesion contains numerous sporangia with internal spores. The cells of these achlorophyllous algae can be misinterpreted as multinucleated cells with inclusions. (H&E stain, original magnification × 1,000; *Prototheca wickerhamii* isolated from specimen in pure culture.)

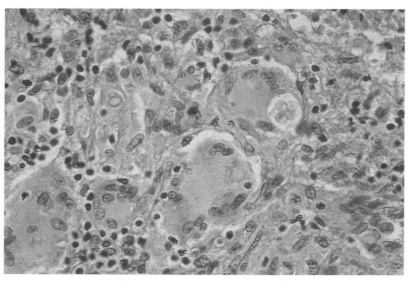

Fig. 11-47. Protothecosis. After resection of the lesion shown in Fig. 11-46, recurrent disease was characterized by few organisms and a granulomatous inflammatory response. The algae are present in the cytoplasm of multinucleated giant cells. (H&E stain, original magnification × 500; *Prototheca wickerhamii* isolated in pure culture from tissue.)

Fig. 11-48. Blastomycosis of the lung. Fine needle aspiration of a lung mass clinically suspected to be carcinoma demonstrates organisms with broad-based budding in a background of inflammation. (Diff-Quik stain, original magnification × 1,000.)

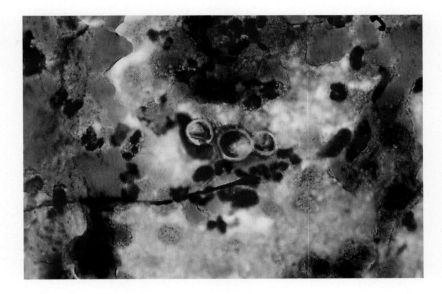

Cytologic Diagnosis of Dimorphic Fungal Infections

Primary mycotic infections may occur in the respiratory tract and initially be mistaken clinically and radiographically for a lung neoplasm. The budding organisms of blastomycosis found in the FNA biopsy of a lung mass are seen in Figures 11-48 and 11-49, stained with Diff-Quik and Papanicolaou reagents, respectively. The organisms of blastomycosis have an internal structure that resembles a nucleus, at least in its staining characteristics, and is called a nuclear body. This is in contrast to the cytomorphology of *Cryptococcus* (Fig. 11-50), which has a narrow-based, teardrop-shaped budding and an opaque or homogeneous center bounded by a thick capsule. *Cryptococcus* organisms may show a flattened surface and a crystalline-like center, which is actually an artifact of coverslipping Papanicolaou-stained slides. Most of these yeast-like organisms are rigid, and the irregularly flattened side of *Cryptococcus* may trap a very small air bubble, which when viewed in the microscope will refract light, giving the appearance of a small crystal in the center of the organism (Fig. 11-51). An interesting case of the use of FNA biopsy is illustrated in Figures 11-52 to 11-54. This patient was suffering from Addison's disease and was found to have bilateral adrenal masses (Fig. 11-52). Aspiration demonstrated organisms of *Cryptococcus* (Fig. 11-53) stained with mucicarmine to demonstrate the capsule and with GMS (Fig. 11-54) to illustrate the size range and narrow-based budding of these organisms.

An example of coccidiomycosis is seen in a sputum sample in a patient who had AIDS but who was also from the dusty desert area of the Southwestern United States, where the organism is commonly found. The irregularity of the spherules of this organism may appear as debris contaminating the sample (Fig. 11-55). Figure 11-56 shows a single small early spherule with a thin but distinct capsule. Such a structure may be ignored as plant material or some other contaminant in the sample. When these organisms are seen in a background of granuloma formation, more distinctly in a FNA biopsy, the diagnosis is much easier.

Fig. 11-49. Blastomycosis of the lung. Bronchial washing in patient suspected of having carcinoma of the lung demonstrates organism with broad-based budding in a background of inflammation. (Papanicolaou stain, original magnification × 1,000.)

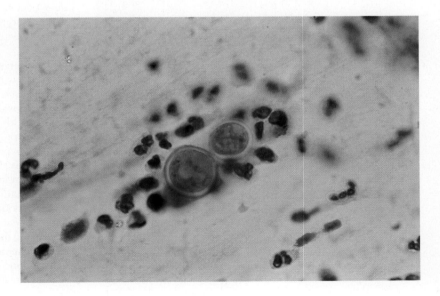

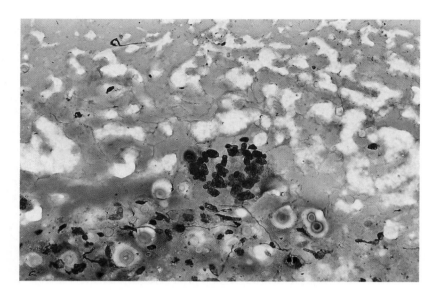

Fig. 11-50. *Cryptococcus neoformans* infection of lung. Patient with the acquired immunodeficiency syndrome with pulmonary infiltrate. Many round yeasts are present with thick capsules and narrow-based budding. (Diff-Quik stain, original magnification × 600.)

H. capsulatum is rarely identified in sputum, bronchial washing, or brushing specimens as the organism is either not present or is present in very small numbers when only a single or several granulomas are present. In children, who may acquire a very disseminated form in the lung, the organisms may be found within multiple histiocytes.[119] An example of the aspiration of a solitary lung mass demonstrates these small organisms in a large multinucleated giant cell as small symmetrical clear round spaces with very small central darker dot-like structures (Fig. 11-57). Special stains, such as the methenamine silver or PAS

with light green techniques, are usually required to identify or confirm the presence of this small organism. The cell block from this lung aspirate (Fig. 11-58) demonstrates a small granuloma with a multinucleated giant cell. On close examination very small round clear areas are seen in the cytoplasm of some cells making up the granuloma. A barely detectable small slightly darker dot is present in some of these clear areas. These two features together characterize the yeast cells of *H. capsulatum*.

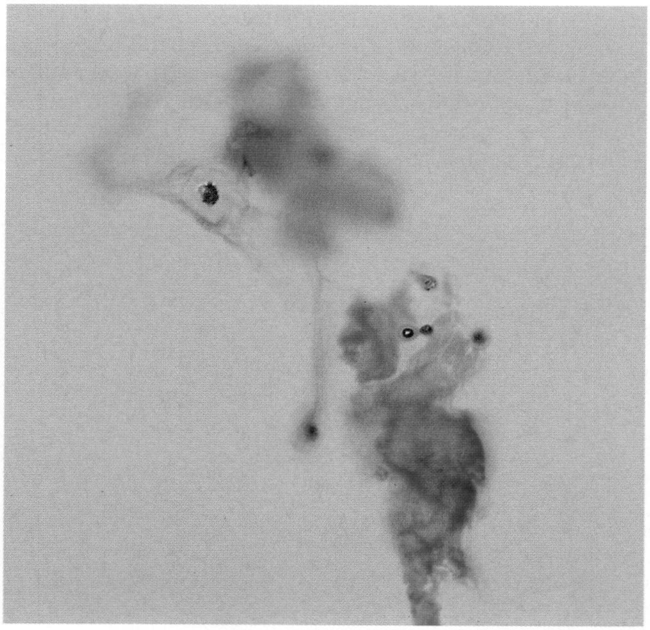

Molds

Filamentous fungi can be characterized by size, pigmentation, and septation. The largest group of human pathogens are the hyaline molds, which have hyphae without intrinsic pigmentation. Hyaline molds include the zygomycetes and the hyphomycetes. The various members of either group cannot be distinguished morphologically from each other except in the rare event that diagnostic asexual reproductive structures are present. The second, less common group of pathogens are the dematiacious fungi that have hyphae with intrinsic pigmentation of varying degrees. The morphologic features of filamentous fungi are summarized in Table 11-5.

Zygomycetes. Zygomycetes (formerly phycomycetes) are hyaline fungi with broad, sparsely septate hyphae that branch haphazardly, often at right angles (Fig. 11-59). They measure 5 to 20 μm in width. The most common human pathogen is *Rhizopus* spp. Other members of the group include *Mucor* spp., *Rhizomucor* spp., *Absidia* spp., and *Cunninghamella* spp. The Zygomycetes produce two major forms of clinical disease.[120,121] The first is rhinocerebral zygomycosis (formerly called, incorrectly in most instances, mucormycosis), in which infection in the nose and paranasal sinuses extends into the orbit or cerebrum, or both. The second form is pulmonary infection with or without disseminated disease. Risk factors for either type of infection are diabetic ketoacidosis and malignancies, particularly of the hematopoietic system. Less common infections are primary cutaneous and gastrointestinal infection, usually at the site of a break in host defenses (such as cutaneous burns or gas-

Fig. 11-51. *Cryptococcus neoformans* infection of the meninges. Morphology of *Cryptococcus* organisms demonstrating crystalline-like center, which is an artifact due to the flattened shape of some of the organisms. (Papanicolaou stain, original magnification × 200.)

Fig. 11-52. *Cryptococcus neoformans* infection of the adrenal glands in a patient with Addison's disease. Fine needle aspiration was performed to determine the cause of Addison's disease in a patient with enlargement of both adrenal glands. Metastatic carcinoma was suspected. Computed tomography-guided needle aspiration demonstrates needle in plate.

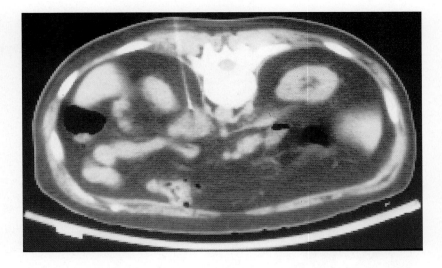

Fig. 11-53. *Cryptococcus neoformans* infection of the adrenal glands. Organisms seen on smears of aspiration stained with mucicarmine to demonstrate the capsule. (Mucicarmine stain, original magnification × 1,000.)

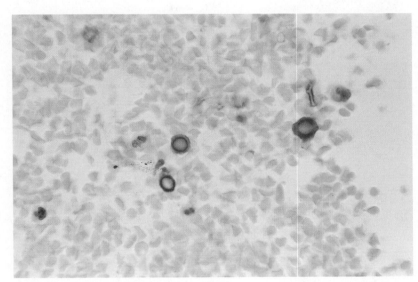

Fig. 11-54. *Cryptococcus neoformans* infection of the adrenal glands. Multiple round yeasts have narrow-based, tear-drop budding. (Gomori methenamine silver stain, original magnification × 1,000.)

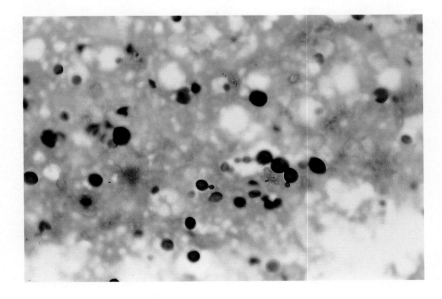

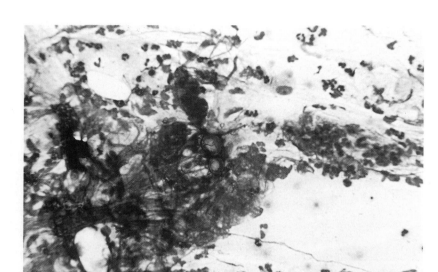

Fig. 11-55. *Coccidiodes immitis* in sputum. A patient suffering from the acquired immunodeficiency syndrome and residing in the desert area of the Southwest developed pulmonary infiltrate. Two rounded blue-staining spherules are seen in a background of marked acute inflammation. (Diff-Quik stain, original magnification × 400.)

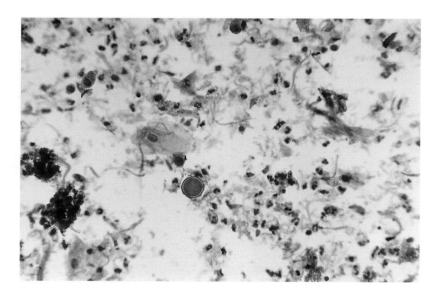

Fig. 11-56. *Coccidioides immitis* in sputum. Same case as Fig. 11-55 with larger orange-staining spherule in a background of inflammation. (Papanicolaou stain, original magnification × 400.)

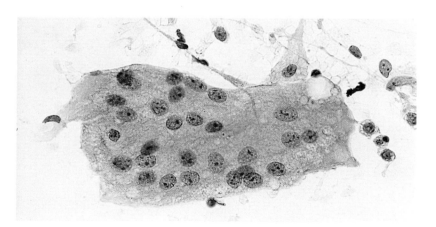

Fig. 11-57. Histoplasmosis of lung. Fine needle aspiration of a lung nodule demonstrated the pattern of granulomatous inflammation. Large multinucleated giant cell in this figure has small round clear areas (some with a very faint central dot) that represent the organism. (Papanicolaou stain, original magnification × 600.)

Fig. 11-58. Histoplasmosis infection of lung. Cell block from case illustrated in Fig. 11-57. Small granuloma is present with multinucleated giant cell. Organisms of histoplasmosis were demonstrated with special stains. (H&E stain, original magnification × 400.)

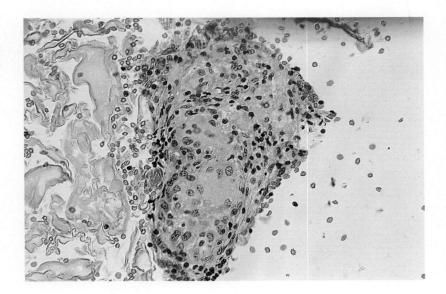

Table 11-5. Morphologic Characteristics of Filamentous Molds in Smears and Tissue

Mould	Size (μm)	Cellular Detail	Staining	Histologic Response	Vascular Invasion	Yeast Forms	Comments
Zygomycetes	5–20	Broad, ribbon-like hyphae; rarely septate; right angle branching	H&E±; BH±; GMS±; PAS±; FM −	PMNLs with or without abscesses; hemorrhage; necrosis	Yes	No; cross-sections may resemble large, distorted yeast cells	*Rhizopus* most common; cannot differentiate species
Aspergillus spp.	3–6	Thin hyphae of variable size; septate; acute angle branching	H&E±; BH±; GMS+; PAS+; FM −	PMNLs with or without abscesses; macrophages, granulomas; hemorrhage; necrosis	Yes	No; cross-sections may resemble distorted yeast cells	Cannot be differentiated from other hyaline molds; A. *niger* mycetomas may have calcium oxalate crystals
Other hyaline molds	2–8	Thin hyphae of variable size; septate; acute angle branching	H&E±; BH±; GMS+; PAS+; FM −	PMNLs with or without abscesses; macrophages, granulomas; hemorrhage; necrosis	Yes	No; cross-sections may resemble distorted yeast cells	Most common are *Scedosporium apiospermum* (*Pseudallescheria boydii*) and *Fusarium* spp.
Candida spp.	3–5	Thin hyphae and pseudohyphae; septate or connected blastoconidia; acute angle branching	H&E±; BH±; GMS+; PAS+; FM −	PMNLs with or without abscesses; macrophages, granulomas	Uncommon	Yes	Cannot differentiate species
Dematiacious molds	2–6	Thin hyphae	Unstained +; H&E±; BH±; GMS+; PAS+; FM +	PMNLs with or without abscesses; necrosis; macrophages, granulomas	No	Yeast-like cells in chromoblastomycosis (sclerotic bodies)	Tissue response varies with species and type of disease

Abbreviations: H&E, hematoxylin and eosin; BH, Brown-Hopps; GMS, Gomori methenamine silver; PAS, periodic acid-Schiff; FM, Fontana-Masson; PMNL, polymorphonuclear leukocyte.

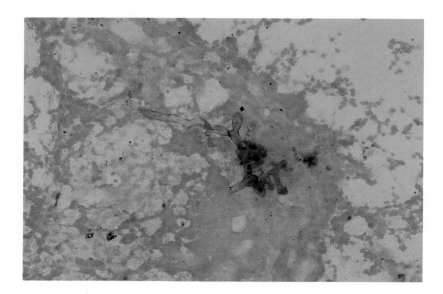

Fig. 11-59. Zygomycetes in a fine needle aspirate of an hepatic abscess. Large, somewhat crumpled, ribbon-like hyphae branch at right angles and do not have septae. Notice that folding of the hyphae produces transverse densities that may resemble septae. This group of fungi often stains as well or better with H&E than with special stains. (Gomori methenamine silver, original magnification × 400.)

trointestinal ulcers) or after application of occlusive bandages that were contaminated with fungal spores.[122]

A characteristic feature of zygomycosis is invasion of the hyphae into the walls of blood vessels, producing thrombosis and infarction. The infections are, therefore, usually necrotizing and hemorrhagic. The thin walls of the hyphae result in distortion and collapse of the structures. Sparse septae may be seen, and collapsed hyphae, folded on themselves, may mistakenly be taken for septae. The Zygomycetes must be differentiated from hyphomycetes, such as *Aspergillus* spp., in which the width of the hyphae is at the lower end of the range. Swollen hyphae or hyphae cut in cross-section can be mistaken for yeast. The Zygomycetes usually stain as well with H&E as they do with methenamine silver or PAS methods. Little is to be gained, therefore, from performing the special stains.

Aspergillus Species. *Aspergillus* spp. are hyaline, septate hyphae that branch dichotomously. The most common human pathogens are *A. fumigatus*, *A. flavus*, and *A. niger*. The hyphae measure 3 to 6 μm in width. They stain moderately well with H&E and are well demonstrated by methenamine silver and PAS techniques.

Aspergillosis comes in three forms: allergic bronchopulmonary disease, mycetoma, and invasive disease. Allergic bronchopulmonary aspergillosis has several manifestations.[123,124] Chronic eosinophilic pneumonia is characterized by macrophages and eosinophils in the interstitium and airspaces, sometimes Charcot-Leyden crystals, and aggregation of the eosinophils into microabscesses. In the distal airways impaction of mucus and endobronchial inflammation may be present. If hyphae are not demonstrated, the lesion cannot be differentiated from other causes of eosinophilic pneumonia. Mucoid impaction is characterized by inspissated plugs of mucus with eosinophils and Charcot-Leyden crystals in the lumens of large bronchi. Fungal hyphae may be difficult to demonstrate. A similar pathologic process has been described in the paranasal sinuses.[125] Allergic bronchocentric granulomatosis is a chronic granulomatous process that partially or completely destroys the

walls of bronchi and bronchioles. The inflammation commonly involves adjacent arterioles and arteries but is clearly centered on the bronchial tree. Hyphal fragments are present in the bronchial lumens but do not invade the parenchyma. In the nonasthmatic patient other causes of granulomatous inflammation, such as mycobacteria, *H. capsulatum*, and *B. dermatitidis*, should be considered.[126]

Mycetomas (aspergillomas) occupy pre-existing cavities in the lung, usually produced by tuberculosis, or the cavities of the paranasal sinuses (Fig. 11-60). Masses of hyphae, many of which are distorted, stain poorly and are presumably dead; they occupy the cavity but do not invade tissue. Cavities are also produced in the course of invasive aspergillosis, but they have a much more sinister implication in this setting (Fig. 11-61). A form of minimally invasive disease that is somewhere between pure mycetoma and invasive aspergillosis does occur. The major complication is erosion of the infiltrating hyphae, surrounding chronic inflammation, or superimposed acute inflammation into adjacent blood vessels. The mycetoma cavities are usually exposed to the air, which allows the development of fruiting heads, asexual reproductive structures that are ordinarily seen only in the microbiology laboratory. The presence of conidiophores with swollen vesicles, phialides, and chains of conidia confirms the genus and may even allow identification of the infecting species (Fig. 11-62). Calcium oxalate crystals may be seen in the tissue adjacent to mycetomas caused by *A. niger*. They are well demonstrated with polarized light and provide strong presumptive evidence as to the etiology (Fig. 11-63).

Invasive aspergillosis, the most serious clinical form, occurs primarily in patients who are immunocompromised, especially those who are neutropenic. The portal of entry is usually the lung, but it may be through compromised skin or gastrointestinal epithelium. *Aspergillus* spp. are angioinvasive and produce destructive, necrotizing lesions analogous to those produced by the zygomycetes. Cavitary lesions in the lung may be produced by infarction and then overgrown by the invading fungi (Fig. 11-61).

The histopathology of invasive aspergillosis is dominated by

Fig. 11-60. *Aspergillus niger* mycetoma of lung. A large, thick-walled cavity contains brown grumous material that consists of masses of hyphae.

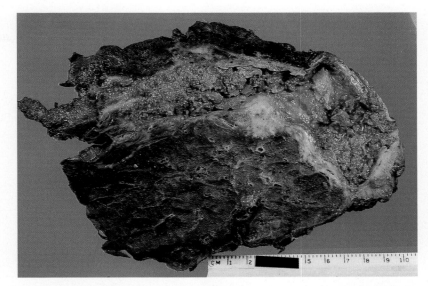

Fig. 11-61. *Aspergillus fumigatus* invasive disease with cavitation. The necrotizing infection has produced cavities in which masses of white mold are growing. The clinical implications of these "mycetomas" is that of the underlying invasive infection.

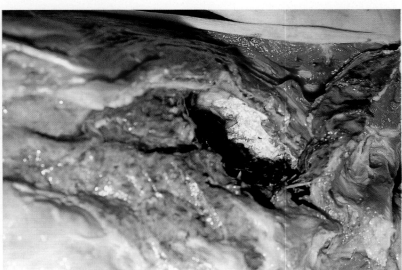

Fig. 11-62. *Aspergillus niger* fruiting head in a mycetoma. A conidiophore supports elongated phialides. Small dark spores and pieces of other phialides are present in the surrounding tissue. Although the spores and fruiting heads are colored, the hyphae of *Aspergillus*, a hyphomycete, are not pigmented. These asexual structures occur when the mold grows in air, indicating that the cavity of the mycetoma communicated with the bronchial tree. (H&E stain, original magnification × 400.)

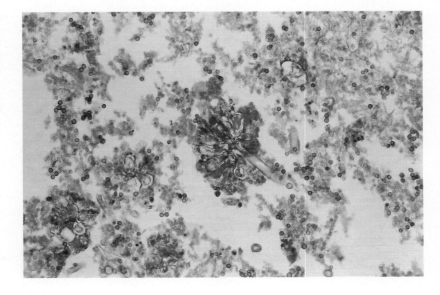

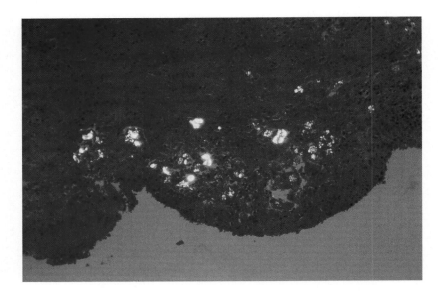

Fig. 11-63. Calcium oxalate crystals in an *Aspergillus niger* mycetoma of the lung. The presence of these crystals provides a presumptive diagnosis of the infecting fungal species. (H&E stain with polarized light, original magnification × 40.)

hemorrhage and necrosis, and acute inflammation is common if the patient has adequate circulating neutrophils. Less commonly, the inflammatory response in smoldering infection is granulomatous. The diagnosis of hyphomycete infection can be made by recognition of thin, septate, dichotomously brancing hyphae (Fig. 11-64). The differential diagnosis includes thin hyphae of zygomycetes and pseudohyphae of *Candida* spp. The presence of numerous septae, which may be best seen with special stains, differentiates these hyphae from those of the zygomycetes. Differentiation of *Candida* pseudohyphae from irregular mold hyphae is usually not difficult, and the presence of budding yeast cells establishes the diagnosis. *Aspergillus* spp. cannot be differentiated in tissue from other hyphomycetes that are less common, but sufficiently common to warrant circumspection in the report (Fig. 11-65). A firm diagnosis of aspergillosis is not possible. A report of "hyphomycete (or mold) such as *Aspergillus* spp." is more accurate.

Other Hyphomycetes. Other hyphomycetes that produce serious infection are numerous. The most commonly identified agents are *Scedosporium (Pseudoallescheria) boydii*[127] and *Fusarium* spp.[128–130] These fungi produce invasive infection; mycetomas, especially of the paranasal sinuses; ulcerative keratitis; and rarely dermatomycosis. Virtually any fungus can be pathogenic in a host with the requisite risk factors, emphasizing the importance of culturing all specimens when an infectious etiology is a possibility. In lesions that are chronic or of unknown etiology and are of clinical consequence it is entirely appropriate to obtain a fungus culture if an invasive procedure for procurement of tissue has been performed. A recent case of *Paecilomyces lilacinus* bursitis would have been hopeless to diagnose without supporting mycologic data.[131]

Phaeohyphomycosis. *Phaeohyphomycosis* is a term used to describe cutaneous or systemic infections caused by dematiacious

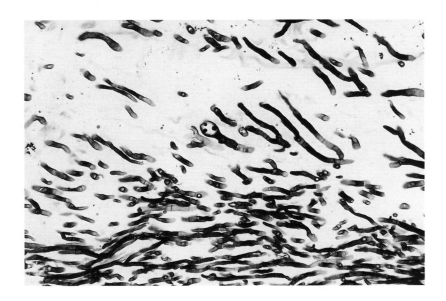

Fig. 11-64. *Aspergillus* morphology. The thin, regular hyphae are septate and branch at acute angles (dichotomously). A single swollen hyphal segment is present. On the basis of this morphology *Aspergillus* cannot be differentiated from other hyphomycetes. (Gomori methenamine silver stain, original magnification × 400.)

Fig. 11-65. *Pseudallescheria boydii* (*Scedosporium apiospermum*) myocarditis. The thin, septate hyphae with dichotomous branching cannot be differentiated reliably from *Aspergillus*. (Methenamine silver stain, original magnification × 400.) (Courtesy of David H. Walker, M.D.)

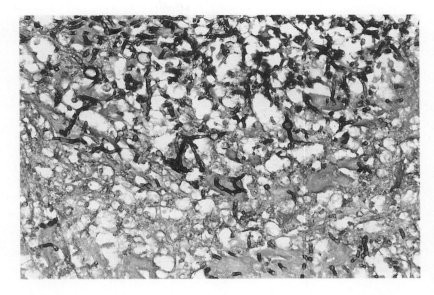

(naturally pigmented) molds.[50] The most common lesions are localized subcutaneous infections that result from direct entry of the fungus through the skin (Fig. 11-66). Many of these molds are commonly found in nature, associated with vegetation. Occasionally, the vehicle for entry—usually a splinter or thorn—may be seen in the lesion. Granulomatous inflammation in the subcutaneous tissue is the hallmark of the infection, and the epidermis is usually uninvolved. As a result the clinical presentation is ordinarily a firm of fluctuant nodule. The fluctuance results from the formation of cystic spaces in the granulomas, producing a phaeomycotic cyst. The infecting fungus cannot be identified specifically without culture. *Exophiala* spp. and *Phialophora* spp. are the most common causes of phaeomycotic cyst, and diffuse granulomatous inflammation is commonly caused by *Bipolaris* spp., *Wangiella* spp., and *Alternaria* spp.[50] The therapy is simple excision of the lesion.

Systemic infection, which is very uncommon, usually affects the central nervous system and is caused by *Cladosporium (Xy-lohypha) bantianum*. The portal of entry is probably the lung, but pulmonary infection is not evident. A destructive infection with tissue necrosis is the result, and the inflammatory response may include either granulomas or purulent inflammation. The remarkable trophism for the brain is unexplained. Septate hyphae, some with bizarre swollen forms, and occasionally yeast-like cells are found in the necrotic material or abscesses (Fig. 11-67).

The diagnosis of phaeohyphomycosis is established by demonstration of yellow-brown, septated hyphae in the lesions. Special stains are not usually necessary because of the naturally occurring pigment, but methenamine silver and PAS techniques do stain the fungi well. In fact, an unstained section is sometimes useful for demonstration of the hyphae unobscured by histochemical staining. The dematiacious fungi contain melanin. If the pigmentation of the hyphae is slight and the identification is in doubt, the Fontana-Masson stain may be used to document the nature of the organisms (Fig. 11-67).

Fig. 11-66. Phaeohyphomycosis. An inoculation lesion of the subcutaneous tissue includes a granuloma with multinucleated giant cells. A mass of brown pigmented hyphae is contained in the granuloma. The fungus is identified by the pigment as dematiacious, but the specific identification cannot be made from the morphology. (H&E stain, original magnification × 400.)

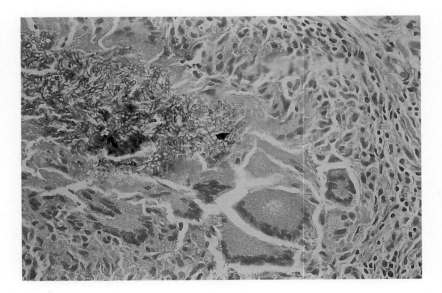

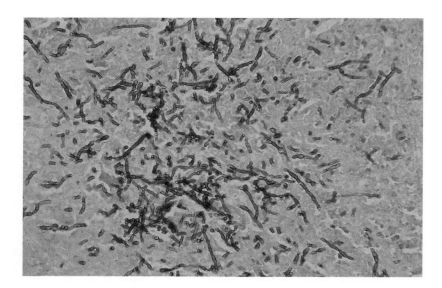

Fig. 11-67. Phaeohyphomycosis of the brain. Septate, branching hyphae in a necrotic lesion. The hyphae are colored by demonstration of melanin in their walls. (Fontana-Masson method, original magnification × 400; *Cladosporium (Xylohypha) bantianum* isolated from specimen.)

Cytologic Diagnosis of Mold Infections. Among saprophytic fungi, the respiratory tract is also a common site of infection. The most frequently encountered organism is *Aspergillus* (Fig. 11-68). Organisms with their typical tree-branching pattern can be found in sputum, bronchial washings and brushings, and fine needle aspirates. The target in the respiratory tract is often a mass lesion, a mycetoma, that clinically and radiographically may look quite like a lung neoplasm. It should be remembered that this and other saprophytes may grow within necrotic areas of malignant tumors. It is therefore prudent that when these organisms are identified in cytologic samples, particularly from the respiratory tract, care is taken to screen for the presence of malignant tumor cells.

Parasites: Smears and Tissue Sections

Parasites can be broadly divided into protozoa, nematodes, cestodes, and trematodes. Although they are of major importance on a global scale, parasitic infection is not commonly encountered in most surgical pathology laboratories. The discussion is, therefore, limited to infections that might be reasonably encountered. A superb photographic atlas of parasites in tissues[132] and a scholarly treatise on the pathology of parasitic disease[133] have been published recently. Protozoa are unicellular organisms, most of which are free living in the environment. Most of the important human pathogens are parasitic, and many have life cycles that involve insect vectors or nonhuman reservoirs, or both. Nematodes, cestodes, and trematodes are round worms, flat worms, and flukes, respectively.

Protozoa

Entamoeba Histolytica. *Entamoeba histolytica* is a protozoan parasite that is transmitted by the fecal-oral route.[134,135] The pathologic tissue form is the trophozoite, which measures from 10 to 60 μm in size. Trophozoites in tissue are usually 20 mm or greater in diameter. The most common disease is acute infec-

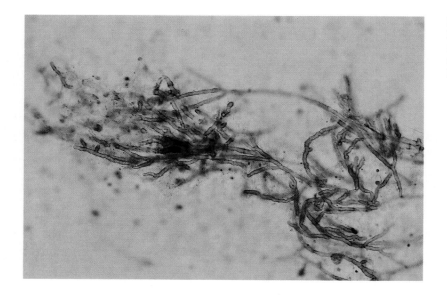

Fig. 11-68. *Aspergillus* species infection in the lung. Patient with large lung mass clinically suspected to be carcinoma. Multiple branching hyphae are seen in the aspiration smears in a necrotic background. (Papanicolaou stain, original magnification × 400.)

tion of the gastrointestinal tract, known as amebic dysentery. Systemic infection usually results in infection of the liver, but other organs may be involved. Active gastrointestinal disease is often not present in patients with hepatic amebic abscesses. The frequent occurrence of amebae in asymptomatic homosexual men has concentrated attention toward the varying pathogenicity of intestinal amebae.[136] A small form of *Entamoeba*, *Entamoeba hartmanni*, resembles *E. histolytica* but measures less than 10 mm in size and is not pathogenic. A proposal has been put forward to place avirulent strains that resemble *E. histolytica* morphologically in a separate species.[137]

The tissue response to *E. histolytica* is necrotizing and hemorrhagic, but without appreciable acute inflammation (Fig. 11-69). The designation of the destructive liver lesions as amebic abscess is, therefore, something of a misnomer. Trophozoites are usually demonstrated in the necrotic lesions without difficulty if the possibility is considered. The amebae are irregular in shape, reflecting their motility by formation of pseudopods. Trophozoites are often positioned in clear lacunae that are produced by pulling away of the adjacent inflammatory exudate, calling attention to the protozoa (Fig. 11-69). The amebic nucleus measures 3 to 4 μm in size with a punctate central karyosome (nucleolus), whereas the cytoplasm has a vacuolated appearance and may contain ingested erythrocytes. If trophozoites are not clearly visualized in H&E-stained sections, the PAS technique may be applied to make the amebae stand out against the necrotic background. Amebae must be differentiated from macrophages, which are also stained by the PAS technique, by close examination of the cellular morphology, and by analysis of the nuclear detail in the H&E-stained sections.

Free Living Amebae. Free living amebae include *Acanthmoeba* spp., which cause destructive infections of the skin, cornea, and central nervous system, and *Naegleri fowleri*, which causes an acute destructive meningoencephalitis.[138,139] Recently, a new genus, *Balamuthia*, has been defined; this organism is believed to be responsible for some infections previously attributed to

Acanthamoeba.[140] Both genera occur in warm fresh and brackish water and in soil, from which sources they enter the human host directly. The path to the central nervous system is believed to be through the nasal cavity for *Naegleria*, whereas *Acanthameba* reaches the brain through the bloodstream after entry into the respiratory tract.

Morphologically, the two genera overlap sufficiently that definitive diagnosis of trophozoites is impossible without culture or immunochemical stains. *Acanthamoeba* spp., but not *Naegleria* spp., however, produce cysts in tissue. The trophozoites of *Acanthamoeba* measure 15 to 35 μm in size. Actively motile trophozoites of *Naegleria* measure 15 to 30 μm by 6 to 9 μm, whereas rounded trophozoites measure 9 to 15 μm in diameter. The amebae contain a single nucleus with a prominent central karyosome (Fig. 11-70). The cysts of *Acanthamoeba* measure 15 to 20 μm in diameter, but they may measure up to 30 μm. Cysts have a thick double wall, which varies in morphology by species. Nuclear morphology is difficult to discern, but cytoplasmic globules can often be seen in histologic sections. The trophozoites must be differentiated from macrophages on the basis of nuclear morphology. If the nucleus is not present in the plane of section, differentiation is not possible.

The histologic response to *Acanthamoeba* is granulomatous with multinucleated giant cells. *Naegleria* encephalitis is an acute infection, and the meninges are infiltrated with polymorphonuclear neutrophils and macrophages intermixed with amebae, which may be difficult to distinguish without careful study (Fig. 11-70).

Toxoplasma Gondii. *T. gondii* is a coccidian parasite that undergoes sexual replication in the gastrointestinal tract of cats. After the oocysts develop in the environment, humans may ingest the resulting sporozoites, which disseminate throughout the body. Rapidly multiplying parasitic forms are referred to as tachyzoites. *T. gondii* is an intracellular pathogen, but a very nondiscriminating one, as virtually any nucleated cell in the body may be infected. The dividing tachyzoites fill the infected cell, eventually producing a pseudocyst. Within this pseudocyst

Fig. 11-69. *Entamoeba histolytica* liver abscess. Multiple amebae with fine cytoplasm are present in a hemorrhagic, necrotic exudate. The nuclei are small with a small karyosome (nucleolus) and fine nuclear chromatin. (H&E stain, original magnification × 1,000.)

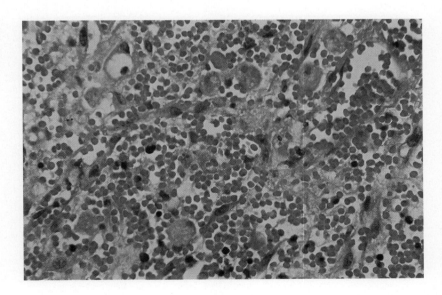

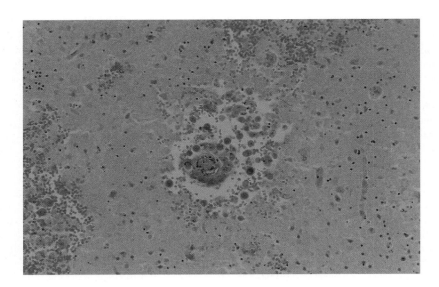

Fig. 11-70. *Acanthamoeba* encephalitis. Multiple amebae are present in a Virchow-Robin space. At higher magnification the amebic nuclei contain a large karyosome and coarse chromatin. There is necrosis and hemorrhage in the surrounding brain. (H&E stain, original magnification × 50.)

the more slowly developing forms are referred to as bradyzoites. Individual tachyzoites are crescent shaped and measure approximately 2 by 6 μm (Fig. 11-71). Tissue cysts are round to subspherical and measure from 5 to 100 μm in size and are packed with hundreds of bradyzoites. All the forms stain with H&E or Giemsa, but careful search may be required to detect them. Bradyzoites stain well with the PAS technique, but tachyzoites stain less well. The cyst wall stains weakly by the PAS technique but is intensely colored with the methenamine silver technique. The tachyzoites and bradyzoites, by contrast, do not stain with silver impregnation techniques. As previously noted, use of immunofluorescence or immunoenzyme techniques facilitates detection of parasites in necrotic lesions.[25,26]

Acute infection is most often manifested by a syndrome that resembles Epstein-Barr virus disease. The characteristic pathology in the affected lymph nodes (see Ch. 20) includes follicular hyperplasia with tingible bodies and small, noncaseating, ep-

ithelioid granulomas in follicular centers and in interfollicular areas. Peripheral sinuses are crowded with macrophages, and plasma cells are common. *Toxoplasma* cysts are found in lymph nodes only with great rarity.[141] Parasites were not detected in a group of serologically documented cases even when molecular techniques were employed.[142] A more serious result of acute infection is chorioretinitis, which is usually diagnosed by serology and clinical presentation. In pregnant women transplacental migration of the protozoa to the fetus may produce severe or fatal intrauterine infection.

In immunosuppressed patients severe disease may be produced by accelerated multiplication in many organs, most importantly the brain and the lung.[143] The cyst forms do not elicit a pathologic reaction, but their rupture to release tachyzoites produces an acutely necrotizing and hemorrhagic inflammatory process. The inflammatory response and the degree to which cerebral lesions are encapsulated are determined, however, by

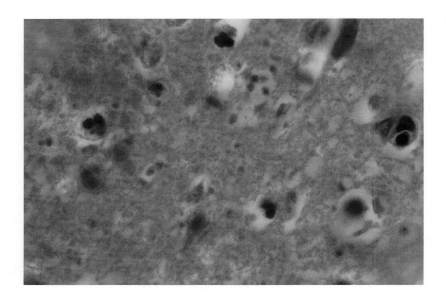

Fig. 11-71. Cerebral toxoplasmosis. Multiple oval *Toxoplasma gondii* tachyzoites are present in a necrotic lesion. The nuclei and cytoplasm are demonstrated, but the kinetoplast cannot be appreciated in this preparation. (H&E stain, original magnification × 1,000.)

the immunologic status of the host.[144] In the lung an interstitial pneumonitis and diffuse alveolar damage may precede the necrotizing phase.[145]

The pseudocysts of *Toxoplasma* must be differentiated from other coccidian and microsporidian parasites, which produce larger cysts, predominantly in the heart and skeletal muscle. Macrophages infected with *H. capsulatum* must not be mistaken for *Toxoplasma*. If doubt exists, demonstration of the yeast cells with methenamine silver will resolve the issue.

Trypanosoma Cruzi. *Trypanosoma cruzi* is a protozoan parasite of the New World that produces both acute and chronic infection, known as Chagas' disease. It is unusual in the United States but may be seen particularly in the states that border Mexico. The parasite has both flagellated (trypomastigotes) and nonflagellated (amastigotes) forms. In tissue the amastigote is usually encountered. The most serious consequences of acute infection are myocarditis and encephalitis, which may be more frequent in immunosuppressed patients.[146] Amastigotes, which are round to oval and measure 1.5 to 4 μm, accumulate in myofibers or in glial cells, evoking an intense acute inflammatory response. In chronic Chagas' disease, the amastigotes multiply in the autonomic ganglia of the gastrointestinal tract, resulting in megaesophagus and megacolon.

The amastigotes of *T. cruzi* are differentiated from *T. gondii* and the yeast cells of *H. capsulatum* by the presence of a cellular kinetoplast in addition to a nucleus, although this structure may be difficult to visualize in histologic sections. Staining of the yeast cells of *H. capsulatum* with the methenamine silver technique provides an additional clue to that pathogen. The amastigotes of *Leishmania* spp. are similar to those of *Toxoplasma*, but the former predominantly infect cells of the skin, mucous membranes, liver, and spleen, whereas the latter predominantly affect the brain, myocardium, and smooth muscle.

Leishmania Species. *Leishmania* spp. are protozoan parasites that are distributed widely throughout the Old and New Worlds. Travel to Mexico and Central and South America is responsible for most cases seen in the United States.[147] Leishmaniasis, including visceral disease, was one of the infectious diseases most commonly noted in veterans of the recent Gulf War.[148]

Leishmaniasis occurs as relatively benign, but unsightly cutaneous disease; potentially disfiguring mucocutaneous infection; and disseminated, potentially fatal infection, known as kala-azar. The type of infection is roughly associated with the country of origin, but molecular techniques are now available for definitive characterization of the risks if the protozoan can be isolated in culture. Disseminated infection may occur more frequently in severely immunosuppressed patients.[149,150]

Leishmania spp. are intracellular parasites that are associated prominently with macrophages as amastigotes. There is no flagellated form in tissue. The histologic response in cutaneous and mucocutaneous disease consists of accumulations of macrophages; noncaseating granulomas with giant cells may also be present. It is not uncommon to find an intermixed acute inflammatory response with microabscesses. Pseudoepitheliomatous hyperplasia of the overlying dermis may be present. The differential diagnosis of the skin lesions includes other mixed inflammatory infections, such as blastomycosis or chromoblastomycosis. Once the amastigotes are recognized they must be differentiated from other parasites and from *H. capsulatum*, as discussed already. Demonstration of the kinetoplast in the amastigotes narrows the differential diagnosis to *T. cruzi* (Fig. 11-72).

Flagellates. The most common infections found in routine cervical vaginal smears are *Trichomonas vaginalis*[151] (Fig. 11-73), a flagellate parasite, or an increased mixed bacterial flora, covering and tightly adherent to the surface of squamous cells, currently designated bacterial vaginosis.[152] The squamous cells covered with bacteria were formerly believed to represent *Gardnerella* (*Haemophilus*) organisms, and the cells were named *clue cells*[153] (Fig. 11-74). These peculiar cells were felt to be a rather specific finding, but that is no longer considered true, as any bacterial overgrowth (probably the result of change in vaginal

Fig. 11-72. Cutaneous leishmaniasis. Numerous amastigote forms of *Leishmania* are contained in macrophages. Other areas of the biopsy contained a neutrophilic inflammatory response to necrotic tissue or secondary irritants. Despite the numerous organisms, the etiology was not recognized at the time of initial interpretation. (H&E stain, original magnification × 500.)

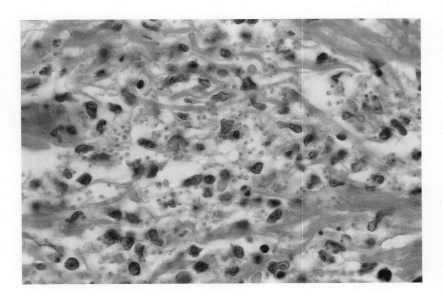

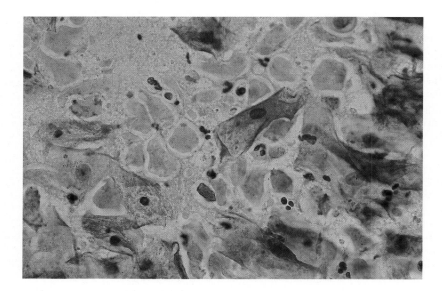

Fig. 11-73. *Trichomonas vaginalis* in a cervical vaginal smear. Many gray-green vaguely outlined organisms are seen between scattered superficial squamous cells. (Papanicolaou stain, original magnification × 600.)

pH or hormonal status, or both) may lead to overgrowth of bacteria, normally present in small numbers, which will coat the surface of superficial squamous cells from the cervix or vagina.

Other Protozoa. *Cryptosporidium parvum, Isospora belli, Cyanospora* spp., and several genera of microsporidia infect the gastrointestinal tract and occasionally other organs. They are discussed in Chapter 38.

Nematodes

A variety of roundworms infect humans, but few reside sufficiently long in tissue to be seen in surgical specimens. In general morphology many common characteristics are seen, but also many individual variations. Some features permit characterization of the roundworms in histologic sections, but identification of the infecting parasite requires considerable experience. The nematodes are worm-like, nonsegmented, bilaterally symmetric, and pseudocoelomate. The cuticle consists of three distinct layers, which may be exaggerated in degenerating worms. A thin superficial epicuticle may also be present. The cuticle of most nematodes contains transverse striae or annulations, which may impart the appearance of segmentation. Longitudinal ridges, called alae, ranging from one to three in number, are termed cervical, longitudinal, or caudal depending on their location. The presence, number, and morphology of the alae are useful clues to the nature of the worm. Nematodes also contain a hypodermis, muscles, digestive system, reproductive system, and nervous system.

Visceral Larva Migrans. Visceral larva mirgans is caused by the migrating larvae of nonhuman nematodes, most commonly *Toxocara* canis and *T. cati*. After a human host ingests eggs, larvae of the human roundworm *Ascaris lumbricoides* migrate through the wall of the gastrointestinal tract, to the liver, through the lungs, and back into the gastrointestinal tract, where they develop into mature worms. The tissue phase of the

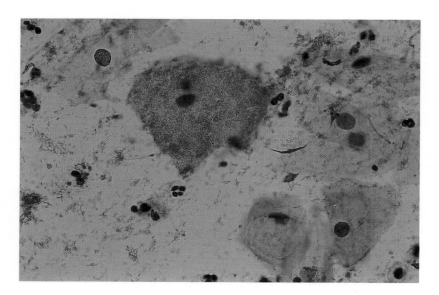

Fig. 11-74. Bacterial vaginosis, cervical vaginal smear. Squamous cell covered with small coccobacillary organisms with many additional organisms in the background. These cells are referred to as clue cells, indicating a bacterial overgrowth of mixed type in the vagina. (Papanicolaou stain, original magnification × 600.)

Fig. 11-75. Visceral larva migrans. A degenerating nematode larva is trapped in a lymph node. The worm is surrounded by a granuloma, and frequent eosinophils are present in the adjacent node. (H&E stain, original magnification × 16.) (Courtesy of Sandy Dorman, M.D.)

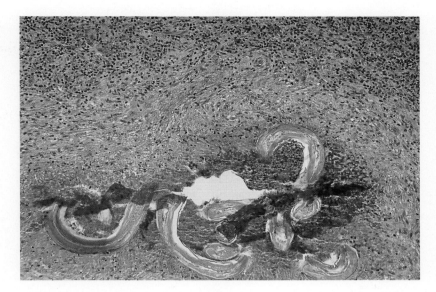

life cycle is transient, and, although symptoms may be provoked, only rarely is tissue damage seen. The larvae of nonhuman ascarid worms, however, wander through the tissues of the body until they come to rest in an organ, where they die and produce an inflammatory response. The tissue response consists of chronic, granulomatous inflammation with many eosinophils. The dying larva is present in the center of the lesion, but serial sections may be necessary to demonstrate it (Fig. 11-75). Excision of the lesion is curative.

Enterobius Vermicularis. The pin worm causes its clinical symptoms as ova hatch and migrate into the perianal area. The mature worms live in the cecal area and may migrate into the appendix, where they are occasionally seen incidentally in the lumen of appendectomy specimens. The cuticle with its transverse striations and lateral alae suggests that the specimen is a nematode (Fig. 11-76). If the section happens to include an ovary with eggs, a definitive identification is easy.

Dirofilaria Species. *Dirofilaria* spp. are common parasites of a variety of animal species and are transmitted to new hosts by the bite of a mosquito. When the filaria enter a human host, localized nodules are produced, most commonly in the skin (typically *Dirofilaria tenuis* from raccoons) or in the lungs (typically *Dirofilaria immitis* from dogs). The histologic response is granulomatous, with a component of acute inflammation in the early lesions. In pulmonary coin lesions, which are often resected because of the possibility of neoplastic disease,[154,155] the association of the process with a pulmonary artery may be detectable. The species of *Dirofilaria* can be differentiated (at least by experts) in histologic sections.[156]

Strongyloides Stecoralis. *Strongyloides stercoralis* differs from hookworm in that it can produce autoinfection of humans, because the eggs do not require a stage of development in the environment before infective larvae hatch. Chronic *Strongyloides* infection may occur in immunocompetent individuals, but se-

Fig. 11-76. *Enterobius vermicularis* in the lumen of an appendix is an incidental finding. Symptoms occur when the gravid female migrates to the perianal area to lay her eggs. The worm is identified as a nematode by the characteristic morphology, including the prominent lateral alae. In this case a specific identification can be made, because the section has serendipitously revealed the characteristic pinworm eggs in the gonad. (H&E stain, original magnification × 250.)

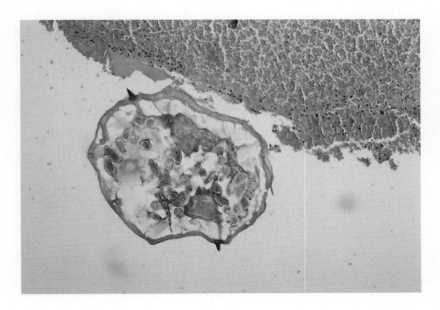

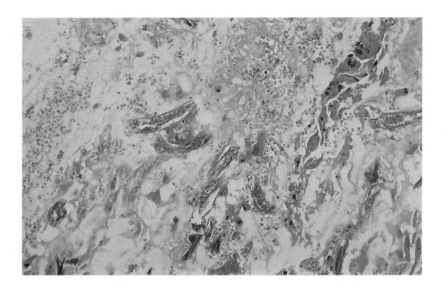

Fig. 11-77. *Strongyloides stercoralis* hyperinfection in the small intestine. Many sections of larvae are present in the necrotic mucosa, intermixed with large numbers of yeast cells. The worms can be identified as nematodes but not characterized more specifically from this section; however, it is unlikely that any other parasite would produce this picture. Careful study of sections or visualization of whole worms in feces can establish the diagnosis definitively. (H&E stain, original magnification × 100.)

vere disease is found primarily in immunosuppressed individuals, who may have been infected many years earlier.[157] As the infective rhabditiform larvae migrate from the gastrointestinal tract through the lungs, they may produce large accumulations of larvae in the gastrointestinal tract. Systemic symptoms result, and ulceration of the gastrointestinal tract may occur (Fig. 11-77).

Trichinella Spiralis. *Trichinella spiralis* naturally infects swine, rats, and a variety of wild animals, such as bears and cougars. The larvae of *T. spiralis* infect only striated muscle, where they mature and are encapsulated by the host. They may remain viable for many years, but eventually die and calcify. The symptoms of the infection include muscle aches and tenderness, myocardial dysfunction, and periorbital edema from involvement of ocular muscle.[158] An acute inflammatory response may be demonstrated in muscle early in the disease (Fig. 11-78). Later the larvae calcify, and the infection becomes quiescent. The in-

fection is transmitted only when one carnivorous animal eats the flesh of the other, releasing the larvae, which then burrow into the intestinal epithelium of the new host. Trichinosis elicited such paranoia in 19th century Europe that it is said there were more meat inspectors than soldiers in Bismarck's Germany. The infection has been virtually eliminated in the United States by stopping the practice of feeding offal to swine. Most infections are now associated with consumption of inadequately cooked game. The larvae can be identified specifically by their morphologic characteristics, but the typical clinical presentation and cellular location are virtually diagnostic.

Cestodes

Cestodes include the fish tapeworm, *Diphyllobothrium latum*; the pork tapeworm, *Taenia solium*; the beef tapeworm, *Taenia saginata*; and the dog tapeworm, *Echinococcus granulosus*. The adult tapeworm consists of a "head" (scolex) that contains a groove (*Diphyllobothrium*), suckers (*T. saginata*), or suckers and hook-

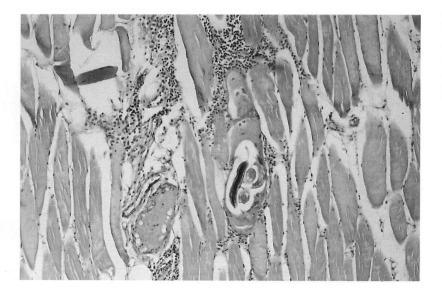

Fig. 11-78. *Trichinella spiralis* myositis. A nematode larva has encysted in a skeletal muscle fiber. The diagnosis can be made from the characteristic location of the worm. Intense focal inflammation reflects the acuteness of the infection with reaction to encysting or dying larvae. Eventually the larvae will calcify. (H&E stain, original magnification × 200.)

lets (*T. solium* and *Echinococcus granulosus*). A short undifferentiated "neck" connects the scolex to a long series of segments, also called proglottids. Each proglottid contains male and female genital systems. The genital systems become increasingly mature as the proglottids progress caudally. Microscopically, the proglottids of cestodes contain an acellular, homogeneous tegument beneath which is a layer of nuclei and thin bands of longitudinal and circular muscle. Most of the segment is composed of a loose network of fluid and cells. Distinctive round to oval calcareous bodies that contain calcium carbonate identify the worm as a cestode.

When an embryonated egg of *T. solium* or *E. granulosus* is ingested by a human intermediate host, the larval form penetrates the intestinal wall and migrates to a variety of organs, depending on the species. Larvae of the pork tapeworm develop into a cysticercus, which consists of the larva in a fluid-filled space that is referred to as a bladder. The most common site for development of cysticerci is the skin and subcutaneous tissue, where the larvae become encapsulated, die, and eventually calcify. Next in frequency is the retina and the central nervous system, where the cysticerci are not encapsulated and cause significant morbidity and mortality, sometimes years after the primary infection. *T. solium* infection is common in Mexico, so cases of cysticercosis are most likely to be seen in states along the southern border.[159] Fully developed cysticerci are round or oval and measure from 5 to 15 mm in length by 4 to 12 mm in diameter. The "bladder worms," therefore, form a space-occupying lesion that may cause symptoms by pressure on adjacent brain. If the larva dies, an intense inflammatory response may be produced, causing an acute exacerbation of symptoms. The larva can be seen in the clear fluid of the cysticercus and can be identified, at least to being a cestode, by general morphology including calcareous bodies. If a larva is not found, documentation of the nature of the lesion is difficult.

When humans ingest an egg of the dog tapeworm, *E. granulosus*, the larval form migrates to an organ, usually the liver or lung, where it develops into a hydatid cyst. A germinal layer of the hydatid cyst gives rise to brood capsules that eventually re-

sult in new cysts, called daughter cysts, producing an enlarging mass of increasingly complicated cysts. The final result resembles a giant balloon that is filled with myriads of tiny balloons (Fig. 11-79). Within each daughter cyst are numerous protoscoleces, which have an invaginated head complete with hooklets. Degenerated brood capsules, scoleces, and hooklets floating in the cyst fluid are referred to as hydatid sand. Large hydatid cysts may measure 20 cm or more in size and may take years to develop.

In histologic sections the germinal epithelium of the cyst wall and the protoscoleces can be demonstrated, complete with hooklets and calcareous corpuscles typical of cestodes (Fig. 11-80). As long as the cyst is intact, the symptoms relate primarily to the effects of a large space-occupying lesion. When a cyst ruptures, an anaphylactic reaction may occur, and, if the patient survives, new cysts may form from the scoleces released from the ruptured cysts.

The most common natural cycle of *E. granulosus* includes development of hydatid cysts in herbivores, such as sheep, and mature worms in the intestinal tract of carnivores, such as dogs. Humans function as incidental, "dead end" intermediate hosts. Many human infections in the United States are seen in patients who were infected years previously in sheep-raising areas of the Old World. Basque sheep herders brought the infection to the Western United States, however, and indigenous foci remain well established.

Trematodes

Schistosomes. The most important flukes in the United States are the schistosomes, which have a complex life cycle. Human species are endemic throughout the world, but none exists in the continental United States. The final developmental stage of schistosomes, the fork-tailed cercariae, swim freely in water and penetrate the skin of human hosts. Avian schistosomes, which are found in the continental United States, proceed no further than the skin, where they produce a disease known as swimmer's itch. The clinical disease and pathology produced by schistosomes depends on the species and the stage of dis-

Fig. 11-79. Echinococcal cyst of the liver. Eight liters of cysts and daughter cysts were present in a cyst that had slowly enlarged over a period of 10 to 20 years. Hydatid sand can be seen as granular material in the clear cyst fluid.

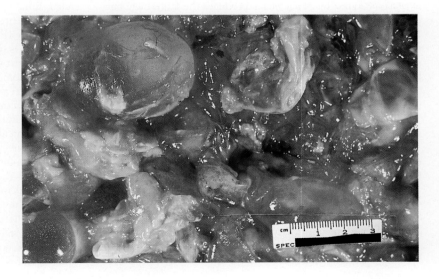

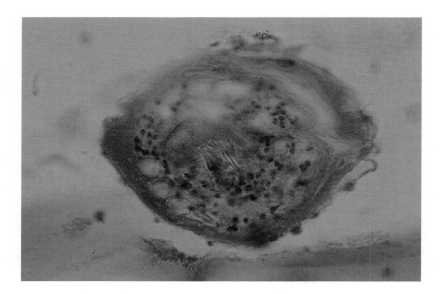

Fig. 11-80. A protoscolex of *Echinococcus granulosus*, including the refractile hooklets, is demonstrated. (H&E stain, original magnification × 250.)

ease.[160,161] *Schistosoma mansoni* migrates through the body, eventually lodging in the hemorrhoidal venous plexus. Eggs migrate into the intestinal tract and are excreted.

Gastrointestinal symptoms including diarrhea and even dysentery may result. The most serious manifestations of infection result from migration of eggs to the liver and spleen. *S. mansoni* occurs in Africa, the Arabian peninsula, Brazil, and the Caribbean, including Puerto Rico. *S. japonicum*, the oriental blood fluke, migrates to the superior mesenteric or portal veins. Eggs are deposited in the gastrointestinal tract, especially the small bowel, and the liver. *S. haematobium*, which is endemic in Africa, southern Europe, the Middle East, and parts of India, localizes in the vesicle and pelvic venous plexuses. Eggs migrate through the wall of the bladder and are excreted in the urine.

Mature worms are only rarely identified in histologic specimens. The chronic infection is dominated by the tissue reaction to the eggs. A cellular infiltrate of neutrophils and eosinophils is followed by a granulomatous reaction including multinucleated giant cells. Fibrosis eventually results. Eggs in the intestine, liver, and spleen are most likely to be *S. mansoni* or *S. japonicum*. Typically *S. japonicum* produces the largest egg burden, and the eggs are most likely to calcify. Many of the eggs are difficult to identify, because of distortion, collapse, or calcification. The classic lateral spines of *S. mansoni* or the terminal spines of *S. haematobium* may be demonstrated in some eggs, however. The end result of extensive fibrotic response to deposited eggs in the intrahepatic biliary system is referred to as pipestem cirrhosis. Eggs in the bladder represent infection with *S. haematobium*. Visualization of the eggs in tissue with acid-fast stains has been described.

Granulomatous Infections Caused by Other Microbes

Syphilis

Syphilis is an age-old disease caused by *T. pallidum* subsp. *pallidum*. The lesions of primary and secondary syphilis are characterized by prominent endothelial cells in proliferating small blood vessels and by a mononuclear inflammatory infiltrate

that is rich in plasma cells (Fig. 11-81). In the placenta there is also often relative villous immaturity.[162] The lesions of primary and secondary syphilis are less commonly granulomatous.[163] Fully formed granulomas, known as gummas, are a feature of late syphilis. In an age that has witnessed an unfortunate resurgence in syphilis, it is important to think of this possibility in unusual granulomatous lesions or inflamed foci that have a high proportion of plasma cells or vascular proliferation. The spirochetes can be demonstrated by silver impregnation techniques, such as the Warthin-Starry or related techniques (Fig. 11-82) or by staining with fluoresceinated antibodies.[164]

Cat-Scratch Fever

Cat-scratch fever is caused by *Bartonella (Rochalimaea) henselae* and perhaps by *Afipia felis*. A primary lesion at the site of the scratch, usually of a kitten, is often not visible, and the disease is dominated by regional lymphadenitis.[165–167] The basic lesion is a necrotizing granuloma that often has an irregular outline, referred to as stellate necrosis. The interior of the granuloma is composed of degenerating mononuclear and polymorphonuclear inflammatory cells. Palisading epithelioid histiocytes and multinucleated giant cells and surrounding fibrosis complete the picture (Fig. 11-83). The intense inflammatory reaction often extends through the capsule of the lymph nodes and into the adjacent soft tissue. The differential diagnosis of necrotizing granulomas with stellate necrosis includes tularemia (*F. tularensis*), *Yersinia* infection, and lymphogranuloma venereum (*Chlamydia trachomatis*). The causative organism is usually not visualized in these infections, so the diagnosis may be suggested by the clinical presentation and the organ system involved, but the definitive diagnosis must be made by culture or serology, or both. Granulomas with caseous necrosis may also be present, expanding the differential diagnosis to include mycobacterial and fungal infection. Severe, prolonged disease and systemic infection have been reported.[168]

Bartonella organisms are not demonstrated by tissue Gram stains but may be visualized by the Warthin-Starry or related silver impregnation techniques.[5,169] Short, fat bacilli, the morphology of which is distorted by the silver salts, are present in

Fig. 11-81. Secondary syphilis of the anus. Pseudoepitheliomatous hyperplasia, proliferation, and arborization of capillaries are seen, as well as a mononuclear infiltrate that includes many plasma cells. (H&E stain, original magnification × 50.)

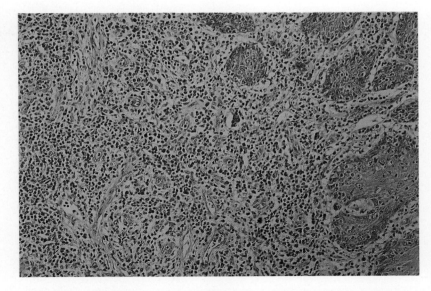

Fig. 11-82. Congenital syphilis. Tightly coiled spirochetes in the placenta establish the diagnosis. Fluoresceinated antibodies are also available for an immunologically specific diagnosis. (Warthin-Starry stain, original magnification × 1,000.)

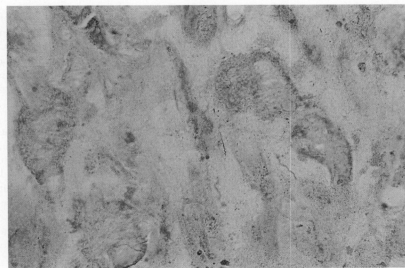

Fig. 11-83. Cat-scratch disease caused by *Bartonella henselae*. A large geographic granuloma with central necrosis is present in a lymph node that drained the site of a cat scratch. The patient had elevated levels of IgM and IgG antibody to *Bartonella henselae*, but not to *Afipia felis*. (H&E stain, original magnification × 20.)

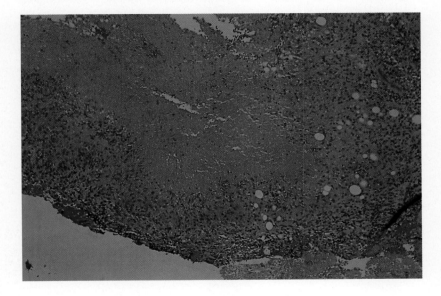

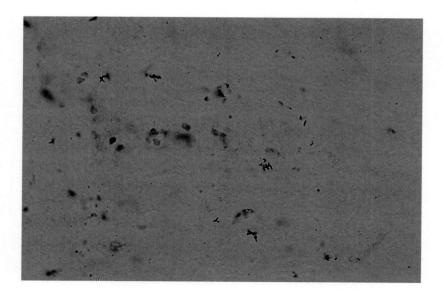

Fig. 11-84. Short plump bacilli were identified in the lymph node pictured in Fig. 11-83. The morphology of the bacilli is obscured by the silver deposition. (Warthin-Starry stain, original magnification × 1,000.)

early lesions, particularly in vascular areas (Fig. 11-84). In our experience the bacilli are more often photographed than seen, so the diagnosis rests at the moment on demonstration of a serologic response to the bacteria. The etiologic agents can be recovered in culture, but the necessary procedures are difficult, tedious, and not often accomplished in microbiology laboratories.

Cytologic Diagnosis of Lymph Node Cat-Scratch Infections.
Enlarged lymph nodes are a frequent target for aspiration biopsy. Historically aspiration of lymph nodes was used to diagnosis sleeping sickness in the early 1900s.[170] Today a variety of infections may be encountered in such samples, and certain aspiration patterns, while not specific, may suggest an infectious etiology in the appropriate clinical setting. The most frequently encountered of these is cat-scratch disease. Smear patterns are of three types: an early phase with a hyperplastic reactive pattern and few granulomas (Fig. 11-85); a middle phase with many granulomas of stellate shape and suppuration (Fig. 11-86); and a late phase that is largely a necrotic smear pattern obscuring many granulomas.[171] It has not been possible to identify the organisms with special stains on smears, and identification of the organisms with special stains on section is quite problematic.

Tularemia

Tularemia, a zoonotic infection that is caused by *F. tularensis*, is widely distributed through the United States.[172–176] Infection is acquired from direct contact with infected animals, particularly rabbits (rabbit fever), but ticks may also transmit the infection. Several clinical forms of the infection may result. Most common is ulceroglandular tularemia, which resembles sporotrichosis clinically. An inflammatory lesion at the site of injury is followed by lymphangitic spread and involvement of

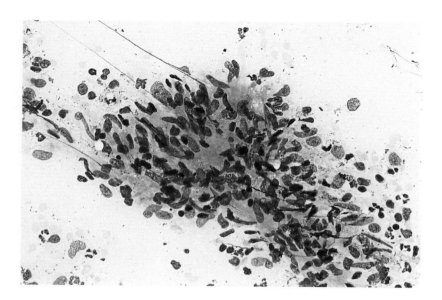

Fig. 11-85. Cat-scratch disease. Fine needle aspiration of an enlarged cervical lymph node with a reactive pattern of mixed lymphoid cells. Clinical correlation is required as the aspiration pattern is nonspecific. (Diff-Quik stain, original magnification × 400.)

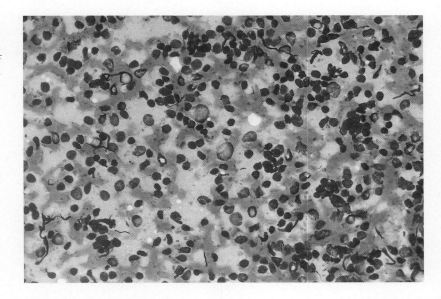

Fig. 11-86. Cat-scratch disease. Fine needle aspiration of an enlarged cervical lymph node with a stellate granuloma and some acute inflammatory cells. Clinical correlation is required, as even with the presence of granulomas and suppuration the aspiration pattern is nonspecific. (Diff-Quik stain, original magnification × 600.)

regional lymph nodes. The basic inflammatory lesion is a necrotizing granuloma that resembles the lesion of cat-scratch disease and must be differentiated from the same alternative diagnoses (Fig. 11-87). Less common forms of infection include oculoglandular tularemia, a typhoidal form without an obvious portal of entry, and primary tularemia pneumonia.

Yersinia Species

Yersinia spp. produce varied clinical disease depending on the species. Yersinia pestis, which is the most venerable and most virulent pathogen, causes human plague, which in many respects resembles tularemia.[177,178] The infection is transmitted by fleas from infected rodents to humans who come in close contact. Historically, rats have been the primary host, but indigenous infection in the southwestern United States is associated with contact with infected prairie dogs. The most common type is ulceroglandular, which is dominated by enlarged, fluc-

tuant lymph nodes draining the primary inoculation site. Primary lesions and lymphangitic spread are not prominent. Histologically, the lymph nodes, which are more likely to be aspirated than surgically resected, are replaced by necrotizing granulomas and acute inflammation. The bacteria can be demonstrated in the lesions with methelene blue or Gram stain, and they are easily cultured. Direct immunofluorescence is available in some public health laboratories for rapid, specific identification of the pathogen. Primary plague pneumonia, which can result in human to human spread, has a high mortality and is the most feared form of the disease.

Two other species, Y. enterocolitica and Y. pseudotuberculosis, produce acute disease in the gastrointestinal tract and the draining mesenteric lymph nodes.[179–182] Necrotizing granulomas may cause ulceration in the mucosa of the ileum or appendix (Fig. 11-88). Alternatively, a syndrome of granulomatous mesenteric lymphadenitis may occur without primary lesions in

Fig. 11-87. Oculoglandular tularemia. A large geographic granuloma with prominent palisading of epithelioid histiocytes and central necrosis occupies a cervical lymph node. The patient had inoculated her eye when she squashed an engorged tick, after which she developed conjunctivitis followed by lymphadenopathy. She developed a serologic response to Francisella tularensis and responded to treatment with tetracycline. (H&E stain, original magnification × 15.)

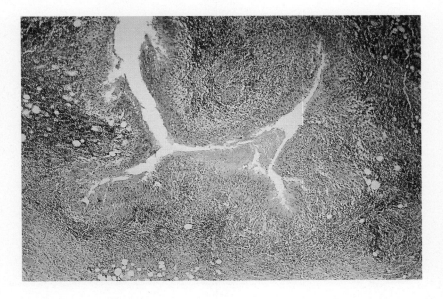

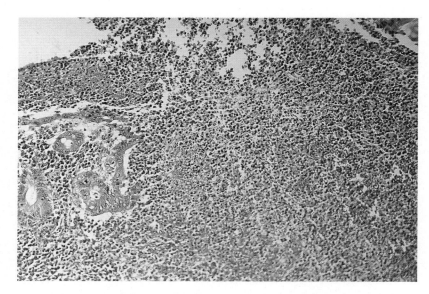

Fig. 11-88. *Yersinia* appendicitis. An ulcerated lesion is populated by mononuclear cells and polymorphonuclear neutrophils. The surface lesion communicated with a large submucosal stellate granuloma. (H&E stain, original magnification × 30; *Yersinia enterocolitica* isolated from feces.)

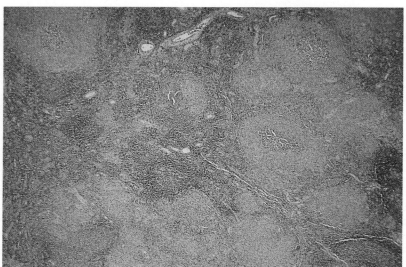

Fig. 11-89. *Yersinia* mesenteric lymphadenitis. Multiple stellate, necrotizing granulomas replace a mesenteric lymph node. The inflammation extended into the surrounding fat. The preoperative diagnosis was acute suppurative appendicitis, but the appendix was macroscopically and microscopically normal. (H&E stain, original magnification × 5; *Yersinia pseudotuberculosis* isolated from lymph nodes.)

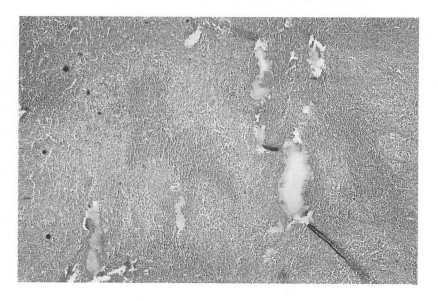

Fig. 11-90. Lymphogranuloma venereum. A large portion of an inguinal lymph node is replaced by a suppurative granuloma that contains necrotic macrophages and polymorphonuclear neutrophils. Such lymph nodes appear fluctuant on physical examination. (H&E stain, original magnification × 5.)

the gastrointestinal tract (Fig. 11-89). Clinically, mesenteric lymphadenitis resembles acute appendicitis, but the surgeon finds fluctuant, matted mesenteric nodes and a normal appendix. Y. enterocolitica is more often associated with primary gastroenteritis and ulcerating intestinal lesions, whereas Y. pseudotuberculosis is associated more closely with mesenteric lymphadenitis. Multinucleated giant cells are said to be more common in Y. pseudotuberculosis infection. Both species can cause septicemia in immunosuppressed patients and in individuals with iron overload syndromes.

Lymphogranuloma Venereum

Lymphogranuloma venereum, which is caused by the L1 to L3 serotypes of Chlamydia trachomatis, is a sexually transmitted infection that results in enlarged inguinal lymph nodes.[183] The lymph nodes are fluctuant because of extensive necrotizing granulomas with stellate necrosis (Fig. 11-90). Extension of the chronic inflammation into the perirectal tissues can result in fibrosis and strictures. Lymphogranuloma venerum serotypes can also cause granulomatous proctitis, most often described in homosexual men.[184,185] Other serotypes produce genital infection in men and women. In the infants of infected mothers inclusion conjunctivitis or a distinctive neonatal pneumonia may result.[186] Chlamydia psittaci causes a chronic interstitial pneumonia and endocarditis, and a newly recognized species, Chamydia pneumoniae, is the etiologic agent of an interstitial pneumonia that has not been characterized histologically.[187] Lymphogranuloma venereum is the only infection that is likely to be seen by a surgical pathologist.

Cytologic Diagnosis of Chlamydial Genital Infections. It was believed in the past that relatively specific cytologic changes occurred in squamous cells found in Chlamydia infection in the female genital tract (Fig. 11-91). This has not proved to be the case when compared with cultures taken at the time of the cervical smear.[151,188,189] These cytologic findings are now considered to be nonspecific, in other words, related to inflammation and tissue repair.

Coxiella Burnetii

Coxiella burnetii is a rickettsia-like bacterium that causes pneumonia (Q fever) and endocarditis. It is associated with dairy products and body fluids of a variety of animals.[190,191] Laboratory workers have developed Q fever after exposure to infected sheep.[192] Hepatitis with noncaseating granulomas may be encountered by the surgical pathologist in liver biopsies.[193,194] So-called fibrin ring granulomas consist of macrophages and lymphocytes around a central hole. They are distinctive findings in Q fever but may be seen in several other infections.[195,196]

Brucella Species

Brucella spp. produce disseminated infection after exposure to infected milk products or animal parts of goats (Brucella melitensis), cattle (B. abortus), or swine (B. suis).[197,198] The reticuloendothelial system is a particular target of these bacteria, which usually produce multiple, small, noncaseating granulomas[199–201] (Fig. 11-92). Larger granulomas with necrosis may occasionally result. Calcified healed granulomas in the spleen have been described in patients who have been infected with B. suis.

Infections Associated with Acute Inflammation, Granulomas, and Chronic Inflammation

Many of the infections already discussed may be associated with predominantly acute or granulomatous inflammation admixed with a minor component of the other inflammatory response. Examples of such infections include blastomycosis, coccidioidomycosis, chromoblastomycosis, and nocardiosis. A few infections are, however, typically characterized by a balanced mixture of acute and chronic inflammation.

Actinomycosis

Actinomycosis is caused by one of several species of Actinomyces, most commonly Actinomyces israelii. These bacteria are

Fig. 11-91. Chlamydia infection in cervical/vaginal smear. Large vacuole in endocervical cells with very small pink elementary bodies. These changes are suggestive but have not demonstrated acceptable sensitivity and specificity when compared with cultures to detect Chlamydia. (Papanicolaou stain, original magnification × 1,000.)

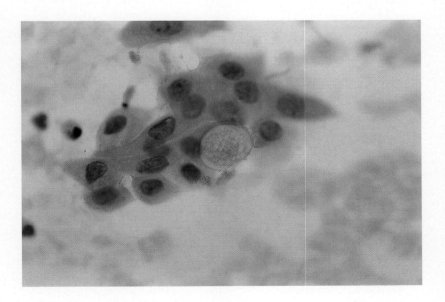

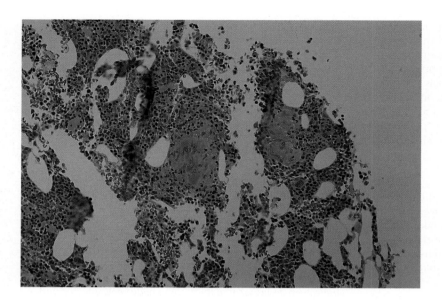

Fig. 11-92. Brucellosis. Several small noncaseating granulomas are present in the bone marrow of a patient with an undifferentiated febrile disease. He had not been exposed to brucella since he worked in an abattoir 30 years previously. (H&E stain, original magnification × 40; *Brucella suis* isolated from blood in pure culture.)

normal inhabitants of the upper respiratory tract, gastrointestinal tract, and female genital tract. The associated infections occur in organs or soft tissue adjacent to these structures: cervicofacial, thoracic, abdominal, and pelvic actinomycosis.[202] The infection was first described in cattle as lumpy jaw, caused by *A. bovis*. Similar human disease was later shown to be caused by *A. israelii*. *Rothia dentocariosa* and other species of *Actinomyces* may also produce the infection.

The hallmarks of the infection are extensive chronic inflammation and fibrosis that produces firm, tumor-like nodules. Intermixed in the chronic inflammatory masses are islands of neutrophilic inflammation that result in draining sinuses. The characteristic actinomycotic sulfur granules, named for their macroscopic appearance, are found in the middle of the neutrophilic pools (Fig. 11-93). Sulfur granules consist of a mass of filmentous, branching Gram-positive bacteria enmeshed in an eosinophilic matrix of uncertain composition. At the edge of the granules are eosinophilic club-shaped structures, an example of the Splendore-Hoeppli phenomenon. Polymorphonuclear neutrophils often cling to the edge of the granules, which may measure several millimeters in size and be visible to the naked eye. The sulfur granules are well demonstrated by H&E stains, but the bacteria cannot be seen without special stains. Tissue Gram stain, particularly the Brown and Brenn stain, or the methenamine silver technique reveal tangled bacterial filaments coursing throughout the granule (Fig. 11-93). The actinomycetes are not colored by the PAS or Gridley techniques. Sulfur granules are distinct from colonies of various bacteria, without the proteinaceous matrix or peripheral clubs, that may be seen in a variety of infections or as colonizing flora in the crypts of the tonsils. Pelvic actinomycosis has been associated with the use of intrauterine contraceptive devices and suggests a more chronic, recalcitrant course than similar infections lacking actinomycetes.[203,204]

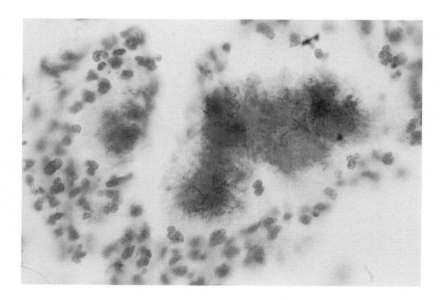

Fig. 11-93. Pleuropulmonary actinomycosis. Thin, branching Gram-positive bacilli are demonstrated in a sulfur granule. Most of the substance of the granule consists of an amorphous ground substance. (Brown-Hopps stain, original magnification × 1,000; *Actinomyces israelii* isolated from specimen.)

Botryomycosis

Botryomycosis is an uncommon disease process that resembles actinomycosis clinically and pathologically but is caused by bacteria other than *Actinomyces*.[205,206] The most common bacterial pathogen is *S. aureus*, but several Gram-negative bacteria and other Gram-positive bacteria may be the etiologic agents. Grains of bacterial colonies may be present, or the structures may appear identical to actinomycotic sulfur granules. Diagnosis is made by culture or by demonstration of cocci or bacilli in the granules instead of filamentous Gram-positive bacilli.

Cytologic Diagnosis

Actinomycosis may also be recognized on aspiration biopsies and has been seen frequently in the past in cervical/vaginal smears in patients who have intrauterine contraceptive devices (IUDs).[151,207] The appearance of the organisms is similar in both situations: a relatively amorphous mass of material with some filamentous club-like structures on the surface surrounded by polymorphonuclear leukocytes (Fig. 11-94) within a background of heavy acute inflammation. The organisms may be few in number, requiring a thorough search of the smears whenever a very heavy inflammatory exudate is present. Clinically enlarged nodes or masses in the neck may be very indurated and suggest an advanced head and neck carcinoma. In patients with IUDs a large pelvic mass with induration of the vagina may stimulate an advanced ovarian or uterine carcinoma. Since IUDs have largely been abandoned, these cases are now quite rare, as is the identification of this organism in cervicovaginal smears.

Mycetoma

Mycetoma is a chronic, tumorous infection of the skin and subcutaneous tissue, usually of the lower extremities.[50] The pathogens are introduced directly into the host through the skin by trauma. Histologically, a mixture of acute and chronic inflammation with grains of varying morphology is seen, depending on the etiologic agent. Mycetoma may be caused by aerobic actinomycetes, particularly *Actinomadura* spp. (causing the designation Madura foot), *Nocardia* spp. (including *N. asteroides*), *Nocardiopsis* spp., and *Streptomyces somaliensis*. Eumycotic mycetomas are caused by a variety of hyphomycetes (white grain mycetoma) and dematiacious fungi (black grain mycetoma). The differentiation is made by demonstration of bacteria or fungi in the grains with appropriate special stains.

Infections Associated with Lymphohistiocytic Inflammation: Viruses and Their Mimics

Viruses are obligate intracellular pathogens of enormous variety and vigor, despite their limited genetic resources. Virus infections are among the most common in the world but will be encountered by surgical pathologists less frequently than bacterial, fungal, and parasitic infections for several reasons. Viral infections do not often result in invasive diagnostic procedures because the diagnosis can be made by culturing accessible secretions or by testing serum for antibodies. The list of viruses that infect hospitalized or immunocompromised patients is relatively short. Some of the most lethal viruses that produce all too abundant pathologic material, such as the arenaviruses (e.g., Lassa virus) and filoviruses (e.g., Ebola virus) occur in remote parts of the world, and are unlikely to be encountered in the United States.

A single viral agent, HIV, is responsible for an explosion of interest in and concern about many of the infectious agents discussed in this chapter. HIV does cause disease other than destruction of the immune system, but it is the secondary infectious agents, rather than HIV itself that results in the submission of a surgical specimen. Viruses exert their effects at the cellular level, and the cellular reaction is a response to damage done to individual cells. Although some important exceptions are seen, the primary lesion is individual cell death and the tissue response is mononuclear.

Viruses are too small to be seen with the light microscope.

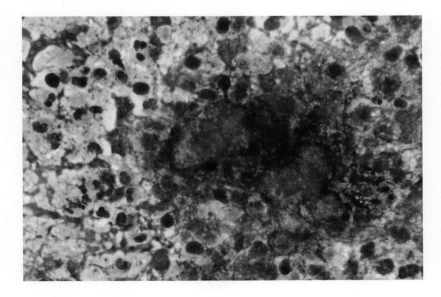

Fig. 11-94. Actinomycosis. Fine needle aspiration of enlarged and partially fixed neck mass thought clinically to be metastatic carcinoma from an intraoral primary. Large ball-like cluster of organisms with filaments and clubs on the surface seen in a background of marked acute inflammation. (Diff-Quik stain, original magnification × 400.)

The surgical pathologist is able to contribute diagnostic information primarily in those infections in which masses of viral particles (inclusions) are sufficiently large to be seen with the light microscope. Viral inclusions are formed by masses of developing or complete viral particles as they are assembled in the infected cell. Viruses contain either RNA or DNA, but, with a rare exception, not both. As a general rule the inclusions of DNA-containing viruses are found in the nucleus, whereas RNA-containing viruses are assembled in the cytoplasm (Table 11-6). Several treatises on the cellular morphology of viral infections are available.[1,208,209]

Viruses: Smears and Tissue Sections

Influenza Virus

Influenza virus is an RNA-containing myxovirus that causes sporadic and epidemic respiratory disease. Influenza viruses types A and B are the primary causes of epidemic respiratory infection, and influenza A virus is the only agent that produces pandemic disease. The most common manifestation is a syndrome of fever, nonproductive cough, and intense myalgias known as "the flu." Secondary bacterial pneumonia is a feared complication that is caused most commonly by S. aureus, Streptococcus pneumoniae, and H. influenzae. In epidemics, primary influenza virus pneumonia is a cause of fatal infection. The hallmark of influenza infection of the lower respiratory tract is diffuse alveolar damage, a host response that is shared by most other viral respiratory pathogens. Mononuclear interstitial inflammation is accompanied by proliferation of pneumocytes and accumulation of fibrin with hyaline membranes in the airspaces (Fig. 11-95). Inclusions are not found, and the diagnosis must be made by demonstration of viral antigen or by culture.

Rarely, influenza virus may cause myositis (sometimes with myoglobinuria) and myocarditis.[210]

Parainfluenza Viruses

Parainfluenza viruses are of four serotypes. They usually cause upper respiratory tract infection or croup (laryngotracheobronchitis) but may produce bronchiolitis and pneumonia, which are especially common in infections caused by serotype 3 strains. Diffuse alveolar damage may be accompanied by multinucleated syncytial giant cells in type 2 and type 3 infection (Fig. 11-96). Inclusions are not usually seen. The histologic appearance of lung tissue infected with parainfluenza viruses that produce giant cells and inclusions is identical to the host reaction to respiratory syncytial virus.

Respiratory Syncytial Virus

Respiratory syncytial virus is the most common cause of bronchiolitis and pneumonia in infants and young children but may also produce serious infection and epidemic disease in adults.[211,212] Peribronchiolar inflammation and diffuse alveolar damage are accompanied by syncytial giant cells, which may contain eosinophilic intranuclear inclusions (Fig. 11-97).

Measles Virus

Measles virus enters the body through the upper respiratory tract, after which it disseminates through the body. The maculopapular skin rash is the most familiar manifestation of infection. The most serious complications are pneumonia and encephalitis. In the lung, diffuse alveolar damage is accompanied by syncytial giant cells (the original giant cell pneumonia). The giant cells contain intranuclear inclusions and occasionally cytoplasmic inclusions (Fig. 11-98). Warthin-Finkeldey giant

Table 11-6. Viral Inclusions

Virus	Nucleic Acid	Location	Staining	Comments
Herpes simplex virus	DNA	Intranuclear	Eosinophilic	Multinucleated giant cells; cannot be differentiated from varicella-zoster virus
Varicella-zoster virus	DNA	Intranuclear	Eosinophilic	Multinucleated giant cells; cannot be differentiated from herpes simplex virus
Cytomegalovirus	DNA	Intranuclear and intracytoplasmic	Amphophilic to basophilic	Cytomegaly; cytoplasmic inclusions are variably present
Epstein-Barr virus	DNA	Intranuclear	Eosinophilic	Only rarely present
Smallpox virus	DNA	Intracytoplasmic	Eosinophilic	Guarneri bodies
Parvovirus B19	DNA	Intranuclear	Basophilic	Erythroid precursors
JC virus	DNA	Intranuclear	Basophilic	Present in oligendroglia
Measles virus	RNA	Intranuclear and intracytoplasmic	Eosinophilic	Inclusions present in epithelioid giant cells; not present in Warthin-Finkeldey giant cells
Respiratory syncytial virus	RNA	Intracytoplasmic	Eosinophilic	Syncytial giant cells
Parainfluenza virus	RNA	Intracytoplasmic	Eosinophilic	Irregularly present in type 2 and type 3 strains; syncytial giant cells
Rabies virus	RNA	Intracytoplasmic	Eosinophilic	Negri bodies; irregular staining may be caused by included cellular material

Fig. 11-95. Influenza virus pneumonia. The histologic reaction is manifested by acute alveolar damage with mononuclear interstitial inflammation and exudation of fibrin with hyaline membranes in the airspaces. Inclusions are not produced by influenza viruses. The diagnosis can be suspected from the clinical history but must be confirmed by serology or most definitively by culture. (H&E stain, original magnification × 50.)

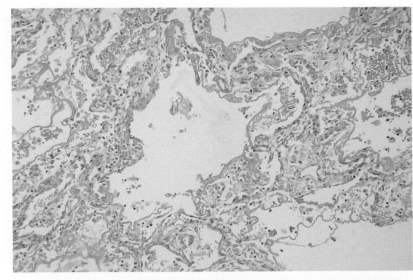

Fig. 11-96. Giant cell pneumonia caused by parainfluenza virus 3. There is a mononuclear interstitial infiltrate. The virus has produced numerous multinucleated syncytial giant cells in the pulmonary membrane. Inclusions were not demonstrated. (H&E stain, original magnification × 200; parainfluenza virus type 3 isolated from lung.)

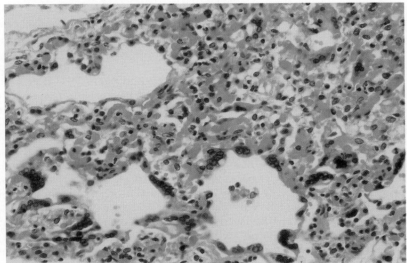

Fig. 11-97. Giant cell pneumonia caused by respiratory syncytial virus. The histologic response resembles that seen in parainfluenza virus infection. A multinucleated syncytial giant cell in an airspace contains an eosinophilic intracytoplasmic inclusion, which is difficult to distinguish at this magnification. (H&E stain, original magnification × 200; respiratory syncytial virus isolated from lung.)

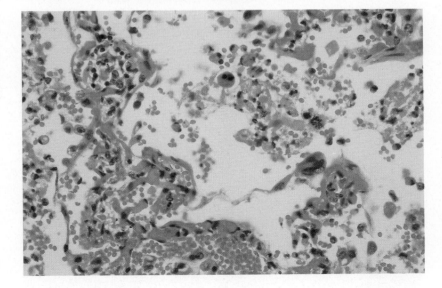

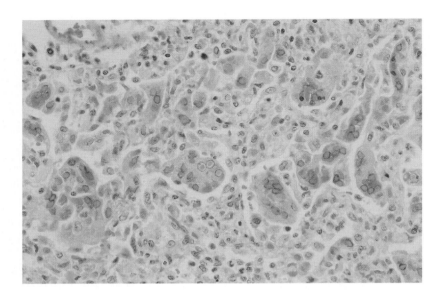

Fig. 11-98. Giant cell pneumonia caused by measles virus. There is a mononuclear infiltrate in the interstitium and the airspaces. Numerous multinucleated syncytial giant cells contain eosinophilic intranuclear and intracytoplasmic inclusions. (H&E stain, original magnification × 400.)

cells in lymphoid tissue may have a different pathogenesis and do not contain inclusions.

Herpes Simplex Virus

Herpes simplex virus is ubiquitous and extremely versatile in its ability to cause human disease. Type 1 strains, which predominantly infect the upper half of the body, are found in people of all ages, beginning in early childhood. Sexually transmitted type 2 strains make their appearance in adolescence and almost exclusively infect the genitourinary systems and skin of the lower body. Pathologists are most likely to encounter herpes simplex virus in cytologic preparations of genital lesions (type 2) or skin (either type). The primary lesions on the skin or mucosa are maculopapules followed quickly by vesicles, caused by infection of squamous epithelium and subsequent disruption of the keratinocytes. Keratinolysis produces intraepidermal bullae, and multinucleated giant cells are present in the adjoining intact epithelium. Mucosal lesions ulcerate so quickly that the

vesicles are less commonly seen (Fig. 11-99). Cytologic preparations are obtained by scraping the base of an ulcer or unroofed vesicle. Smears may be air dried and stained with a Romanovsky or H&E stain (Fig. 11-100), a procedure known as a Tsanck preparation. Alternatively, the smear may be fixed and stained by the Papanicolau technique. The inclusions of herpes simplex virus are homogeneous and often fill the nucleus, pushing the normal nucleoprotein to the periphery of the nuclear envelope. In formalin-fixed H&E-stained sections, artifactual shrinkage of the inclusion produces a halo between the eosinophilic inclusion and the more basophilic peripheralized chromatin. It is easy to miss inclusions that do not have a halo. In cytologic preparations inclusions are often difficult to discern, but molding of the nuclei in multinucleated cells assists in differentiating the virally infected cell from its normal neighbors.

The sensitivity of cytologic diagnosis is very high in skin lesions, but unfortunately not so high in infections of the female

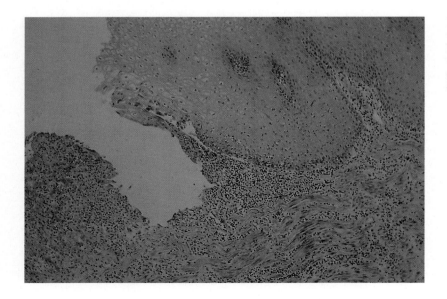

Fig. 11-99. Herpes simplex esophagitis. There is intense mixed inflammation beneath ulcerated epithelium. Several epithelial cells at the edge of the ulcer (identifiable at this magnification by their condensed eosinophilic appearance) contain intranuclear viral inclusions. (H&E stain, original magnification × 50.)

Fig. 11-100. Tsanck preparation. A multinucleated giant cell is demonstrated in this scraping from the base of a vesicular lesion. Intranuclear inclusions are not seen, but the molding of the nuclei is clearly demonstrated. It is not possible to distinguish between herpes simplex and varicella-zoster viruses with this technique. (Diff-Quik stain, original magnification × 1,000.)

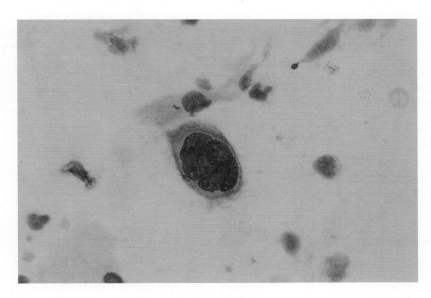

genital tract. The specificity of cytologic diagnosis by experienced investigators is also high, but atypical, reactive cells have been misinterpreted as herpes-infected cells in cytologic preparations.[213] Herpes simplex and varicella-zoster viruses produce inclusions that cannot be differentiated by morphologic criteria. Use of dual antibodies with different fluorescent labels has been successfully evaluated as a means of diagnosing vesicular skin lesions.[214] Anomalous immunostaining with antisera to herpes simplex virus has been described in optically clear nuclei in gestational endometrium, leading to an erroneous diagnosis of intrauterine herpes infection.[27]

Type 1 herpes simplex virus is the most common cause of sporadic viral encephalitis, and type 2 virus also causes serious life-threatening systemic infection in neonates whose mothers have active genital infections at the time of vaginal delivery and in patients whose host defenses are compromised. Diagnosis of herpes simplex infection in brain biopsies was once a prerequisite for therapy, but the advent of effective, nontoxic drugs has reduced the necessity of obtaining brain tissue. In a large study of diagnostic methods for herpes encephalitis, histologic examination was only 56 percent sensitive and 86 percent specific.[215] Both sensitivity and specificity were improved by use of immunofluorescence.

Disseminated infection may cause destructive disease in many organs, particularly the liver (Fig. 11-101), if the patient is immunocompromised. Necrotizing infection in the liver, adrenal glands, or other organs is typically seen in severely immunosuppressed patients, such as recipients of organ transplants and in neonates who have disseminated gestational infection (Fig. 11-101). Herpetic esophagitis is characterized by ulcerating lesions that may be coinfected with *Candida* spp. In other situations compromise of physical defenses may increase the risk of herpes simplex virus infection. Cutaneous disease is associated with damage to the normal epidermis by physical

Fig. 11-101. Herpes hepatitis in disseminated neonatal infection. Extensive necrosis and hemorrhage are seen in the hepatic cords. Most of the intact cells shown here at the edge of necrotic lesions contain eosinophilic intranuclear inclusions. The inclusions vary from homogeneous masses that fill the nucleus to condensed aggregates on viral nucleoprotein that are separated from marginated nuclear chromatin by an artifactual clear halo. Multinucleated giant cells are present. It is not possible to differentiate herpes simplex and varicella-zoster viruses cytopathologically, but the clinical presentation suggests type 2 herpes simplex virus as the culprit. (H&E stain, original magnification × 500; herpes simplex virus type 2 isolated from tissue.)

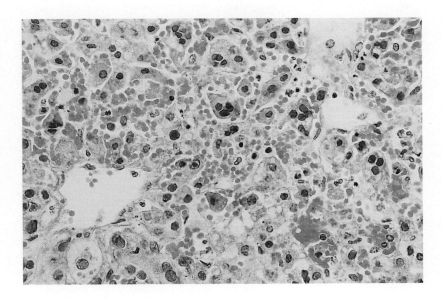

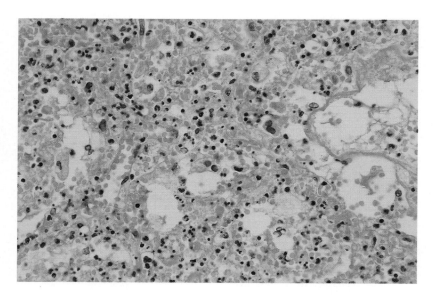

Fig. 11-102. Herpes simplex virus pneumonia. Extensive necrosis and leukocytoclasis are seen in the airspace infiltrate, which includes polymorphonuclear neutrophils. The intense reaction suggests a bacterial etiology at first glance, but the correct etiology is revealed by eosinophilic intranuclear inclusions in a few cells. (H&E stain, original magnification × 200; herpes simplex virus type 1 isolated in pure culture from specimen.)

abrasions in wrestling matches ("herpes gladiatorum") or by thermal burns. Similarly, destructive corneal infection results from direct inoculation of herpes simplex virus into the eye. Patients who are intubated and at risk of aspiration have a higher than normal incidence of herpetic infection in the lower respiratory tract. The virus is usually type 1 and probably enters the lungs from the where it may be shed asymptomatically. The distribution of inflammation in the lungs is patchy. By contrast, viremic type 2 infection in neonates or type 1 infection in immunosuppressed adults usually results in multifocal, punctate pulmonary lesions.

The unitary lesion in herpetic infections is the accumulation of damaged cells, which may result in extensive necrosis as the cells rupture. The inflammatory response includes mononuclear cells, and a pattern of diffuse alveolar damage is often found. In addition, however, an intense polymorphonuclear neutrophilic response is elicited by the extensive necrosis (Fig.

11-102). The exuberance of the acute inflammatory response may mislead the observer into assuming that the etiology is bacterial. If, as often happens, all mental processes of the surgical pathologist cease at the determination of a bacterial etiology, the nature of the infection may be missed completely.[216] Careful observation of the section will reveal the presence of inclusions in epithelium. Multinucleated giant cells are often present but are not as dramatic as in some other viral infections.

Cytologic Diagnosis. Infection of the female genital tract by the herpes virus is quite symptomatic on the external genitalia but clinically silent when involving the cervix. Characteristic ground-glass changes or cells with definite inclusion bodies (or both) may be seen in cervicovaginal smears stained by the Papanicolaou method[216a] (Fig. 11-103). Whereas the incidence of this infection in the female genital tract seemed rather common from even causal observations in the 1960s and 1970s, it is

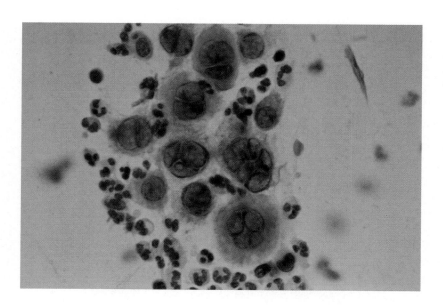

Fig. 11-103. Herpes virus in cervical/vaginal smear. Multinucleated cells with a ground-glass appearance to the nuclei, the so-called seeds in pomegranate appearance typical of herpes virus infection. (Papanicolaou stain, original magnification × 600.)

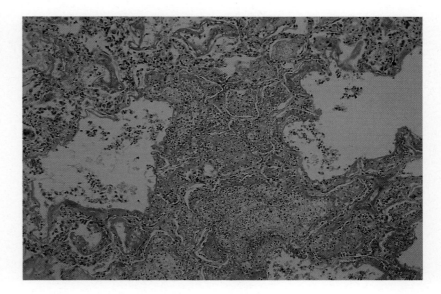

Fig. 11-104. Varicella-zoster pneumonia. A portion of a focal lesion, suggesting intravascular dissemination of virus, is pictured. Interstitial inflammation and an intense inflammatory exudate are seen in the airspaces, consisting of leukocytes and fibrin with hyaline membranes. (H&E stain, original magnification × 50.)

much less often seen today, at least in cytologic samples from the cervix. Detection of herpes virus inclusions in the cervical smear can be important in the pregnant patient near term, as a vaginal delivery may result in increased risk of infection of the newborn, with devastating results.[217]

Varicella-Zoster Virus

Varicella-zoster virus causes chickenpox on initial contact and shingles when the virus in spinal ganglia is reactivated. The diagnosis is usually obvious clinically, and difficult cases can be resolved without recourse to biopsy. In immunosuppressed patients and in pregnant women varicella-zoster virus can produce severe pneumonia and disseminated infection. The lesions and the viral inclusions closely resemble those of herpes simplex (Fig. 11-104), so the etiology must be determined by culture or by detection of specific viral antigens or nucleic acids.

Epstein-Barr Virus

Epstein-Barr virus is important as a cause of both infectious mononucleosis and certain neoplasms. Mononucleosis is usually diagnosed serologically, and the participation of the virus in neoplasms must be evaluated with molecular techniques. Occasionally a liver biopsy will be obtained if hepatitis occurs in a patient who does not have other classic findings of mononucleosis. A nonspecific mononuclear infiltrate is present in the parenchyma, and extensive hepatocellular necrosis is not seen (Fig. 11-105). Rarely, inclusions that resemble those of herpes simplex have been reported.

Cytomegalovirus

Cytomegalovirus is the virus most often seen by surgical pathologists, because of its ubiquity and its prominence in infections of immunocompromised patients. Infection of virtually any organ may occur. Interstitial pneumonitis, myocarditis, and he-

Fig. 11-105. Epstein-Barr virus hepatitis. A focus of hepatocellular necrosis and mononuclear cell inflammation is seen in the parenchyma. Mild hepatitis is common in infectious mononucleosis, but clinical illness that leads to a biopsy is distinctly unusual. (H&E stain, original magnification × 400.)

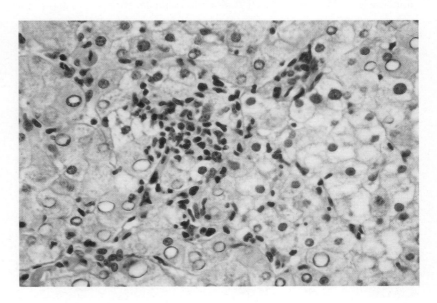

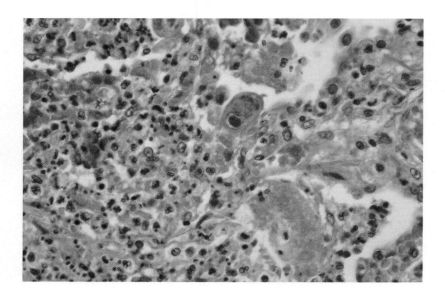

Fig. 11-106. Cytomegalovirus pneumonia. Mononuclear interstitial inflammation and mixed inflammation with nuclear fragmentation are seen in the airspaces. A large cytomegalic cell with an amphophilic intranuclear inclusion surrounded by a halo and irregular, granular, basophilic cytoplasmic inclusions is present. In addition, several clumps of eosinophilic exudate indicate an accompanying infection with *Pneumocystis carinii.* (H&E stain, original magnification × 500.)

patitis have classically presented the most common clinical problems.[218–221] The pneumonia is usually diffuse, but focal and even miliary lesions have been described.[222]

The dilemma with cytomegalovirus is less to document the presence of infection in an individual patient than to establish that this virus, which persists for many years in tissues, has caused the clinical disease. Multiple cells that have been infected with this virus may be demonstrated in tissues that display no inflammatory reaction. For decades many pathologists believed that cytomegalovirus did not cause gastrointestinal disease, but that infected macrophages or endothelial cells populated ulcerating lesions previously caused by other agents. Experience with HIV-infected patients has convinced all observers that cytomegalovirus does cause ulcerative disease in the gastrointestinal tract from the esophagus through the colon.

The histologic response to cytomegalovirus is principally mononuclear. The infected cell is globally enlarged, with a large, amphophilic to basophilic intranuclear inclusion (Fig. 11-106). Granular basophilic inclusions are present in the cytoplasm of many infected cells. Multinucleated giant cells are not produced by cytomegalovirus.

Cytologic Diagnosis. Cytomegalovirus infection any also be identified in cytologic smears from the cervix, although rarely (Fig. 11-107). The characteristic very large intranuclear inclusion bodies can be found in endocervical or endometrial gland cells. In female patients with AIDS, this organism can be widely disseminated but may first be detected in the cervical smear; such a finding is quite rare in the patient with an intact immune system.[223]

Adenovirus

Adenovirus causes disease of virtually every organ system. Specific serotypes are associated with some adenovirus infections, most of which cause morbidity but not mortality. Lower respi-

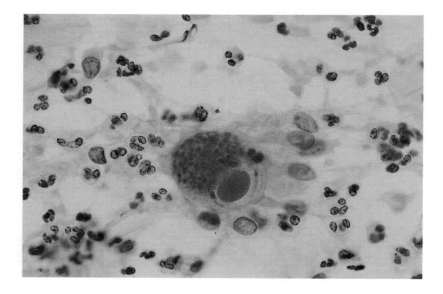

Fig. 11-107. Cytomegalovirus inclusion in a cervical/vaginal smear. There is a single probable endocervical cell with a large intranuclear inclusion and many smaller intracytoplasmic inclusions. (Papanicolaou stain, original magnification × 1,000.)

Fig. 11-108. Adenovirus hepatitis. Extensive hepatocellular necrosis and many cells with intranuclear viral inclusions are seen. Some of the eosinophilic inclusions are separated by an artifactual halo from the peripheralized nuclear chromatin, similar to the cytopathology produced by herpes simplex virus. Other inclusions are more basophilic and completely fill the nuclei, producing "smudge" cells. Compare these inclusions with those of herpes simplex in Fig. 11-101. The herpetic inclusions do not obliterate the nuclear membrane, and multinucleated giant cells are not found in adenovirus infections. (H&E stain, original magnification × 250.)

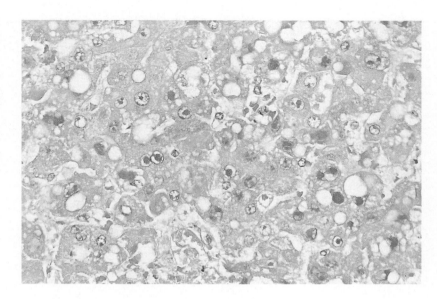

ratory infection occurs rarely in immunocompetent individuals, primarily military recruits who are under considerable stress. Disseminated infection and severe hepatitis have been documented in recipients of organ transplants. Cells infected with adenovirus contain intranuclear inclusions that initially resemble the eosinophilic inclusions of herpes viruses. As the inclusion matures it becomes more basophilic and increasingly fills the nucleus (Fig. 11-108). Eventually the inclusion may obscure the outline of the nuclear membrane, producing a "smudge cell." The early adenovirus inclusions must be differentiated from herpes simplex and varicella-zoster viruses. The late inclusions can resemble those of cytomegalovirus and must also be differentiated from degenerated cells.

Papoviruses

Papoviruses consist of papillomaviruses, which cause human warts, papillomas, and epithelial neoplasia (see Ch. 49); poly-

omaviruses, which cause disease in immunosuppressed patients; and vacuolating agents, which do not cause human disease. The most important polyomaviruses, SV40 and JC virus, cause progressive multifocal leukoencephalopathy, a disease that is more likely to be seen by the autopsy pathologist than the surgical pathologist. Multiple foci of demyelination without inflammation are produced in the subcortical white matter. Oligodendroglia are the target cells, in which accumulation of virions produce a basophilic intranuclear inclusion (Fig. 11-109).

Human Parvovirus 19

Human parvovirus 19 produces erythema infectiosum (fifth disease) in children, nonimmune hydrops in pregnant women, and acute arthritis in adults. Parvovirus infections are most likely to be seen by surgical pathologists in bone marrow biopsies from patients with hemoglobinopathies and chronic he-

Fig. 11-109. Progressive multifocal leukoencephalopathy. An infected oligodendroglial cell contains a basophilic inclusion that fills the nucleus. The loose neuropil reflects accompanying demyelination. The polyomaviruses (most commonly JC virus and SV40 virus) are very difficult to culture, but the etiology can be confirmed by documenting the characteristic virions ultrastructurally. (H&E stain, original magnification × 1,000.)

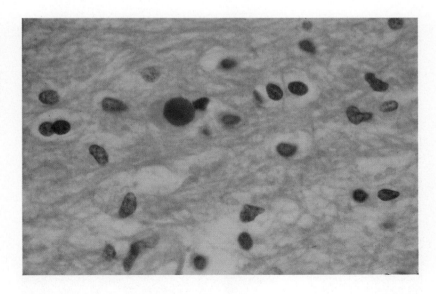

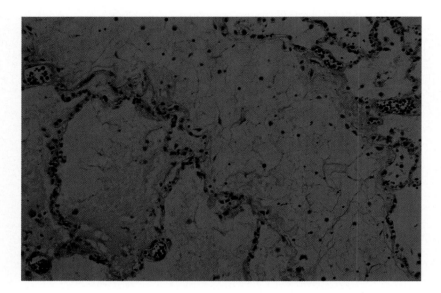

Fig. 11-110. Hantavirus pulmonary syndrome. The histopathologic reaction is relatively noninflammatory, consisting of edema in the interstitium and airspaces as a result of viral infection of the vascular endothelium. Large immunoblastic cells are often present. (H&E stain, original magnification × 20; Sin Nombre virus demonstrated in tissue.) (Courtesy of Sherif Zaki, M.D.)

molytic anemia. Parvovirus B19 may cause aplastic crisis in these patients, and basophilic intranuclear inclusions can be demonstrated in erythroid precursors.

Molluscum Contagiosum

Molluscum contagiosum is the only poxvirus that is likely to be encountered in the surgical pathology laboratory. A distinctive raised, umbilicated skin lesion(s) provides little diagnostic challenge and is not usually biopsied unless the nodules are atypical. The elevated mass consists of enlarged, proliferated keratinocytes that contain large masses of eosinophilic cytoplasmic inclusions.

Hantaviruses

Hantaviruses classically produced hemorrhagic fever, such as Korean hemorrhagic fever, and a milder infection called nephropathia endemica. The spectrum of disease expanded considerably in the 1990s when acute respiratory disease in the Four Corners area of the American Southwest was attributed to

a new hantavirus, now known as Sin Nombre virus. Other related viruses have been discovered in the eastern United States, but very few infections have so far been attributed to these agents. The infection presents as acute respiratory failure, and the pulmonary pathology includes prominent pulmonary edema and enlarged immunoblastic lymphoid cells[224,225] (Fig. 11-110). The capillary leakage is produced by viral infection of the endothelium.

Other Viral Infections

Other viral infections that are unlikely to be seen by the surgical pathologist include rabies with intracytoplasmic inclusions (Negri bodies), enteroviral infections, and a variety of hemorrhagic fever viruses in several taxonomic groups.

Viral Mimics

The most important infection in the mimic group is pertussis, which will rarely be seen by the surgical pathologist. *Bordetella*

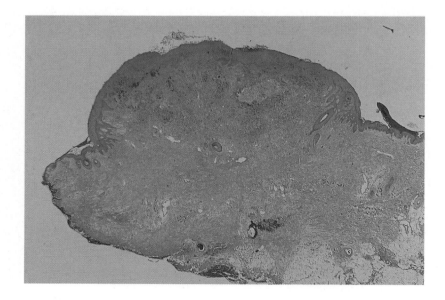

Fig. 11-111. Bacillary angiomatosis. A nodular cutaneous lesion consists of inflammatory cells and proliferating small blood vessels. The lesion resembles a pyogenic granuloma. (H&E stain, original magnification × 5.) (Courtesy of Ann-Marie Nelson, M.D.)

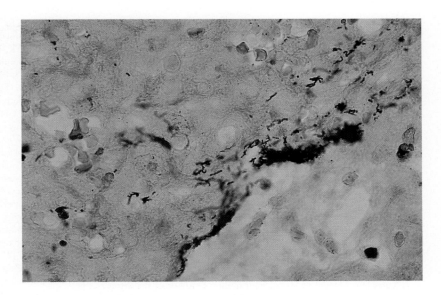

Fig. 11-112. Bacillary angiomatosis. Multiple bacilli are demonstrated in the vascular lesion. The morphology of the Gram-negative bacilli is distorted by the silver impregnation. (Warthin-Starry stain, original magnification × 1,000.) (Courtesy of Ann-Marie Nelson, M.D.)

pertussis elicits a lymphocytic response in the epithelium of the respiratory tract from the larynx to the lower airways. Rare fatal cases are characterized by lymphocytic infiltrates in the peribronchial and peribronchiolar mucosa.

Infections of the Cardiovascular System and Vascular Endothelial Cells

The vascular system is involved primarily or secondarily in many infectious diseases. Bacterial intravascular infections occur as secondary infections of damaged endothelium—bacterial endocarditis and mycotic aneurysm. The neutrophilic inflammatory response is differentiated from thrombus by the intensity of the neutrophilic response and the demonstration of bacteria in the lesions. The endothelium is the primary target for *Rickettsia rickettsii*, the causative agent of Rocky Mountain spotted fever. Vasculitis may also be seen in meningococcemia,

which may be associated with disseminated intravascular coagulation. *Pseudomonas aeruginosa* occasionally produces a "vasculitis" in which bacterial colonies obliterate the walls of blood vessels and may contribute to the necrotizing character of the infections.

Bartonella (Rochalimaea) quintana is the historic agent of trench fever.[226] This bacterium was first demonstrated by molecular techniques to be the etiologic agent of two non-neoplastic diseases of vascular proliferation that occur in HIV-infected individuals.[227] Bacillary angiomatosis consists of capillary proliferation, leudocytoclastic debris, and amorphous material that represents colonies of bacteria.[228] The lesion resembles pyogenic granuloma histologically (Fig. 11-111). The bacteria can be demonstrated with the Warthin-Starry stain or related silver impregnation procedures (Fig. 11-112). The lesions of bacillary angiomatosis have also been demonstrated in lymph nodes.[228] Similar lesions in the viscera, especially the liver, are known as peliosis[228] (Fig. 11-113).

Fig. 11-113. Peliosis hepatis. A noninflammatory vascular lesion in the liver of a patient infected with the human immunodeficiency virus is caused by *Bartonella henselae*. (H&E stain, original magnification × 33.) (Courtesy of Ann-Marie Nelson, M.D.)

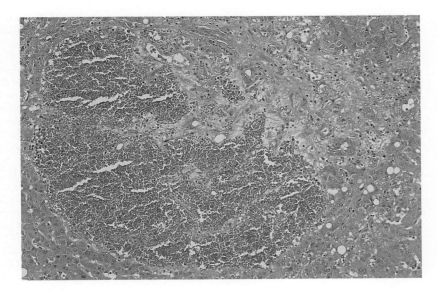

Vascular invasion is an important component of fungal infections caused by the zygomycetes and certain hyphomycetes, such as *Aspergillus* spp., as discussed previously. Certain viruses also have an attraction for the vasculature, in this case endothelial cells. The most important of these viruses for surgical pathologists is the new group of respiratory hantaviruses. Other hemorrhagic fever viruses that are not indigenous to the United States also affect the endothelium. Cytomegalovirus and varicella-zoster virus are common viral agents that infect the endothelium, and the histopathology may be influenced by this tropism.

REFERENCES

1. Woods GL, Walker DH: Detection of infection or infectious agents by use of cytologic and histologic stains. Clin Microbiol Rev 9:382, 1996

2. Luna LG: Manual of Histologic Staining Methods of the Armed Forces Institute of Pathology. 3rd Ed. McGraw-Hill, New York, 1968

3. Prophet EB, Mills B, Arrington JB, et al (eds): Laboratory Methods in Histotechnology. American Registry of Pathology, Washington, 1992

4. Brown RC, Hopps HC: Staining of bacteria in tissue sections: a reliable gram stain method. Am J Clin Pathol 60:234, 1973

5. Wear DJ, Margileth AM, Hadfield TL, et al: Cat scratch disease: a bacterial infection. Science 221:1403, 1983

6. Marshall BJ: Unidentified curved bacilli on gastric epithelium in active chronic gastritis. Lancet 2:1273, 1983

7. Chandler FW, Hicklin MD, Blackmon JA: Demonstration of the agent of Legionnaires' disease in tissue. N Engl J Med 297:1218, 1977

8. Greer PW, Chandler FW, Hicklin MD: Rapid demonstration of *Legionella pneumophila* in unembedded tissue. An adaptation of the Gimenez stain. Am J Clin Pathol 73:788, 1980

9. Needham GM: Comparative efficacy of direct microscopy (two methods) and cultures in the diagnosis of tuberculosis. Mayo Clin Proc 32:1, 1957

10. Hertz C, Pawlicki SA, Green RA: Fluorescent staining and microscopy for detection of acid-fast bacilli. Univ Mich Med Center J 32:196–199, 1966

11. Woods GL, Meyers WM: Mycobacterial diseases. pp. 843–865. In Damjanov I, Linder J (eds): Anderson's Pathology. 10th Ed. CV Mosby, St. Louis, 1996

12. Robboy SJ, Vickery AL Jr: Tinctorial and morphologic properties distinguishing actinomycosis and nocardiosis. N Engl J Med 282:593, 1970

13. Lowe RN, Azimi PH, McQuitty J: Acid-fast *Actinomyces* in a child with pulmonary actinomycosis. J Clin Microbiol 12:124, 1980

14. Monheit JE, Brown G, Kott MM, et al: Calcofluor white detection of fungi in cytopathology. Am J Clin Pathol 85:222, 1986

15. Monheit JE, Cowan DF, Moore DG: Rapid detection of fungi in tissues using calcofluor white and fluorescence microscopy. Arch Pathol Lab Med 108:616, 1984

16. Wages DS, Wear DJ: Acid-fastness of fungi in blastomycosis and histoplasmosis. Arch Pathol Lab Med 106:440, 1982

17. Wood C, Russel-Bell B: Characterization of pigmented fungi by melanin staining. Am J Dermatopathol 5:77, 1983

18. Baselski VS, Robison MK, Pifer LW, Woods DR: Rapid detection of *Pneumocystis carinii* in bronchoalveolar lavage samples by using Cellufluor staining. J Clin Microbiol 28:393, 1990

19. Gosey LL, Howard RM, Witebsky FG, et al: Advantages of a modified toluidine blue O stain and bronchoalveolar lavage for the diagnosis of *Pneumocystis carinii* pneumonia. J Clin Microbiol 22:803, 1985

20. Rosen PP, Martini N, Armstrong D: *Pneumocystis carinii* pneumonia. Diagnosis by lung biopsy. Am J Med 58:794, 1975

21. Kim YK, Parulekar S, Yu PK, et al: Evaluation of calcofluor white stain for detection of *Pneumocystis carinii*. Diagn Microbiol Infect Dis 13:307, 1990

22. Elston HR: Synthetic controls for microbiological stains in histopathology. Lab Med 17:750, 1986

23. Tseng CH, Tseng C: Laboratory method for producing tissue controls for fungal stains. Lab Med 22:637, 1991

24. Jung WK: In vitro positive controls for histochemical stains of bacteria and fungi. Am J Clin Pathol 84:342, 1985

25. Sun T, Greenspan J, Tenenbaum M, et al: Diagnosis of cerebral toxoplasmosis using fluorescein-labeled antitoxoplasma monoclonal antibodies. Am J Surg Pathol 10:312, 1986

26. Conley FK, Jenkins KA, Remington JS: *Toxoplasma gondii* infection of the central nervous system. Use of the peroxidase-antiperoxidase method to demonstrate toxoplasma in formalin fixed, paraffin embedded tissue sections. Hum Pathol 12:690, 1981

27. Sickel JZ, di Sant'Agnese PA: Anomalous immunostaining of 'optically clear' nuclei in gestational endometrium. A potential pitfall in the diagnosis of pregnancy-related herpesvirus infection. Arch Pathol Lab Med 118:831, 1994

28. Nuovo GJ, Silverstein SJ: Comparison of formalin, buffered formalin, and Bouin's fixation on the detection of human papillomavirus deoxyribonucleic acid from genital lesions. Lab Invest 59:720, 1988

29. Stevens DL, Musher DM, Watson DA, et al: Spontaneous, nontraumatic gangrene due to *Clostridium septicum*. Rev Infect Dis 12:286, 1990

30. Kaiser CW, Milgrom ML, Lynch JA: Distant nontraumatic clostridial myonecrosis and malignancy. Cancer 57:885, 1986

31. Narula A, Khatib R: Characteristic manifestations of clostridium induced spontaneous gangrenous myositis. Scand J Infect Dis 17:291, 1985

32. Winn WC Jr, Myerowitz RL: The pathology of the *Legionella* pneumonias. A review of 74 cases and the literature. Hum Pathol 12:401, 1981

33. Beckman EN, Leonard GL, Castillo LE, et al: Histopathology of marine vibrio wound infections. Am J Clin Pathol 76:765, 1981

34. Woo ML, Patrick WG, Simon MT, French GL: Necrotising fasciitis caused by *Vibrio vulnificus*. J Clin Pathol 37:1301, 1984

35. Tacket CO, Barrett TJ, Mann JM, et al: Wound infections caused by *Vibrio vulnificus*, a marine vibrio, in inland areas of the United States. J Clin Microbiol 19:197, 1984

36. Joseph SW, Daily OP, Hunt WS, et al: *Aeromonas* primary wound infection of a diver in polluted waters. J Clin Microbiol 10:46, 1979

37. Simpson GL, Stinson EB, Egger MJ, Remington JS: Nocardial infections in the immunocompromised host: a detailed study in a defined population. Rev Infect Dis 3:492, 1981

38. Javaly K, Horowitz HW, Wormser GP: Nocardiosis in patients with human immunodeficiency virus infection. Report of 2 cases and review of the literature. Medicine 71:128, 1992

39. Emmons W, Reichwein B, Winslow DL: *Rhodococcus equi* infection in the patient with AIDS: literature review and report of an unusual case. Rev Infect Dis 13:91, 1991

40. van Etta LL, Filice GA, Ferguson RM, Gerding DN: *Corynebacterium equi*: a review of 12 cases of human infection. Rev Infect Dis 5:1012, 1983

41. Lasky JA, Pulkingham N, Powers MA, Durack DT: *Rhodococcus equi* causing human pulmonary infection: review of 29 cases. South Med J 84:1217, 1991

42. Horsburgh CR Jr: *Mycobacterium avium* complex infection in the acquired immunodeficiency syndrome. N Engl J Med 324:1332, 1991

43. Klatt EC, Jensen DF, Meyer PR: Pathology of *Mycobacterium avium-intracellulare* infection in acquired immunodeficiency syndrome. Hum Pathol 18:709, 1987

44. Gillin JS, Urmacher C, West R, Shike M: Disseminated *Mycobacterium avium-intracellulare* infection in acquired immunodeficiency syndrome mimicking Whipple's disease. Gastroenterology 85:1187, 1983

45. Umlas J, Federman M, Crawford C, et al: Spindle cell pseudotumor due to *Mycobacterium avium-intracellulare* in patients with acquired immunodeficiency syndrome (AIDS). Positive staining of mycobacteria for cytoskeleton filaments. Am J Surg Pathol 15:1181, 1991

46. Maygarden SJ, Flanders EL: Mycobacteria can be seen as "negative images" in cytology smears from patients with acquired immunodeficiency syndrome. Mod Pathol 2:239, 1989

47. Wassersug JD: Tuberculosis epidemic: forgotten rules for its control. Pharos 57:32, 1994

48. Metre MS, Jayaram G: Acid-fast bacilli in aspiration smears from tuberculous lymph nodes: an analysis of 255 cases. Acta Cytol 31:17, 1987

49. Lopes Cordozo P: Atlas of Clinical Cytology. Hertogenbosch, Targa b.v., 1979

50. Chandler FW, Watts JC: Pathologic Diagnosis of Fungal Infections. ASCP Press, Chicago, 1987

51. Goodwin RA, Des Prez RM: Pathogenesis and clinical spectrum of histoplasmosis. South Med J 66:13, 1973

52. Reynolds RJ III, Penn RL, Grafton WD, George RB: Tissue morphology of *Histoplasma capsulatum* in acute histoplasmosis. Am Rev Respir Dis 130:317, 1984

53. Johnson PC, Khardori N, Najjar AF, et al: Progressive disseminated histoplasmosis in patients with acquired immunodeficiency syndrome. Am J Med 85:152, 1988

54. Reddy P, Gorelick DF, Brasher CA, Larsh H: Progressive disseminated histoplasmosis as seen in adults. Am J Med 48:629, 1970

55. Wheat LJ, Connolly-Stringfield PA, Baker RL, et al: Disseminated histoplasmosis in the acquired immune deficiency syndrome: clinical findings, diagnosis and treatment, and review of the literature. Medicine (Baltimore) 69:361, 1990

56. Studdard J, Sneed WF, Taylor MR Jr, Campbell GD: Cutaneous histoplasmosis. Am Rev Respir Dis 113:689, 1976

57. Goodwin RA, Owens FT, Snell JD, et al: Chronic pulmonary histoplasmosis. Medicine (Baltimore) 55:413, 1995

58. Loyd JE, Tillman BF, Atkinson JB, Des Prez RM: Mediastinal fibrosis complicating histoplasmosis. Medicine (Baltimore) 67:295, 1988

59. Goodwin RA, Nickell JA, Des Prez RM: Mediastinal fibrosis complicating healed primary histoplasmosis and tuberculosis. Medicine (Baltimore) 51:227, 1972

60. Sarosi GA, Hammerman KJ, Tosh FE, Kronenberg RS: Clinical features of acute pulmonary blastomycosis. N Engl J Med 290:540, 1974

61. Witorsch P, Utz JP: North American blastomycosis: a study of 40 patients. Medicine (Baltimore) 47:169, 1968

62. Pappas PG, Threlkeld MG, Bedsole GD, et al: Blastomycosis in immunocompromised patients. Medicine (Baltimore) 72:311, 1993

63. Atkinson JB, McCurley TL: Pulmonary blastomycosis: filamentous forms in an immunocompromised patient with fulminating respiratory failure. Hum Pathol 14:186, 1983

64. Case Records of the Massachusetts General Hospital. Case 49-1988: *Histoplasma capsulatum* or *Blastomyces dermatitidis?* N Engl J Med 320:1699, 1989

65. Freed ER, Duma RJ, Shadomy HJ, Utz JP: Meningoencephalitis due to hyphae-forming *Cryptococcus neoformans*. Am J Clin Pathol 55:30, 1971

66. Salyer WR, Salyer DC, Baker RD: Primary complex of *Cryptococcus* and pulmonary lymph nodes. J Infect Dis 130:74, 1974

67. Baker RD: The primary pulmonary lymph node complex of cryptococcosis. Am J Clin Pathol 65:83, 1976

68. McDonnell JM, Hutchins GM: Pulmonary cryptococcosis. Hum Pathol 16:121, 1985

69. Anderson DJ, Schmidt C, Goodman J, Pomeroy C: Cryptococcal disease presenting as cellulitis. Clin Infect Dis 14:666, 1992

70. Chuck SL, Sande MA: Infections with *Cryptococcus neoformans* in the acquired immunodeficiency syndrome. N Engl J Med 321:794, 1989

71. Farmer SG, Komorowski RA: Histologic response to capsule-deficient *Cryptococcus neoformans*. Arch Pathol 96:383, 1973

72. Ro JY, Lee SS, Ayala AG: Advantage of Fontana-Masson stain in capsule-deficient cryptococcal infection. Arch Pathol Lab Med 111:53, 1987

73. Lazcano O, Speights VO Jr, Bilbao J, et al: Combined Fontana-Masson-Mucin staining of *Cryptococcus neoformans*. Arch Pathol Lab Med 115:1145, 1991

74. Lurie HI: Histopathology of sporotrichosis. Notes on the nature of the asteroid body. Arch Pathol 75:421, 1963

75. Grotte M, Younger B: Sporotrichosis associated with sphagnum moss exposure. Arch Pathol Lab Med 105:50, 1981

76. Coles FB, Schuchat A, Hibbs JR, et al: A multistate outbreak of sporotrichosis associated with sphagnum moss. Am J Epidemiol 136:475, 1992

77. Sanders E: Cutaneous sporotrichosis. Beer, bricks, and bumps. Arch Intern Med 127:482, 1971

78. England DM, Hochholzer L: Primary pulmonary sporotrichosis. Report of eight cases with clinicopathologic review. Am J Surg Pathol 9:193, 1985

79. Saral R: *Candida* and *Aspergillus* infections in immunocompromised patients: an overview. Rev Infect Dis 13:487, 1991

80. Wingard JR, Merz WG, Saral R: *Candida tropicalis*: a major pathogen in immunocompromised patients. Ann Intern Med 91:539, 1979

81. Weems JJ Jr: *Candida parapsilosis*: epidemiology, pathogenicity, clinical manifestations, and antimicrobial susceptibility. Clin Infect Dis 14:756, 1992

82. Goldman M, Pottage JC Jr, Weaver DC: *Candida krusei* fungemia. Report of 4 cases and review of the literature. Medicine (Baltimore) 72:143, 1993

83. Johnson TL, Barnett JL, Appelman HD, Nostrant T: *Candida* hepatitis. Histopathologic diagnosis. Am J Surg Pathol 12:716, 1988

84. Haron E, Vartivarian S, Anaissie E, et al: Primary *Candida* pneumonia. Experience at a large cancer center and review of the literature. Medicine (Baltimore) 72:137, 1993

85. Parker JC Jr, McCloskey JJ, Lee RS: Human cerebral candidosis—a postmortem evaluation of 19 patients. Hum Pathol 12:23, 1981

86. Meyer PR, Hui AN, Biddle M: *Coccidioides immitis* meningitis with arthroconidia in cerebrospinal fluid: report of the first case and review of the arthroconidia literature. Hum Pathol 13:1136, 1982

87. Stevens DA: Coccidioidomycosis. N Engl J Med 332:1077, 1995

88. Pappagianis D: Marked increase in cases of coccidioidomycosis in California: 1991, 1992, and 1993. Clin Infect Dis, suppl. 1, 19:S14, 1994

89. Galgani JN, Ampel NM: Coccidioidomycosis in human immunodeficiency virus-infected patients. J Infect Dis 162:1165, 1990

90. Fish DG, Ampel NM, Galgiani JN, et al: Coccidioidomycosis during human immunodeficiency virus infection. A review of 77 patients. Medicine (Baltimore) 69:384, 1990

91. Vincent T, Galgiani JN, Huppert M, Salkin D: The natural history of coccidioidal meningitis: VA-Armed Forces cooperative studies, 1955–1958. Clin Infect Dis 16:247, 1993

92. Edman JC, Kovacs JA, Masur H, et al: Ribosomal RNA sequence shows *Pneumocystis carinii* to be a member of the fungi. Nature 334:519, 1988

93. Walzer PD, Linke MJ: A comparison of the antigenic characteristics of rat and human *Pneumocystis carinii* by immunoblotting. J Immunol 138:2257, 1987

94. Macher AM, Shelhamer J, MacLowry J, et al: *Pneumocystis carinii* identified by gram stain of lung imprints. Ann Intern Med 99:484, 1983

95. Ghali VS, Garcia RL, Skolom J: Fluorescence of *Pneumocystis carinii* in Papanicolaou smears. Hum Pathol 15:907, 1984

96. Wolfson JS, Waldron MA, Sierra LS: Blinded comparison of a direct immunofluorescent monoclonal antibody staining method and a Giemsa staining method for identification of *Pneumocystis carinii* in induced sputum and bronchoalveolar lavage specimens of patients infected with human immunodeficiency virus. J Clin Microbiol 28:2136, 1990

97. Midgley J, Parsons PA, Shanson DC, et al: Monoclonal immunofluorescence compared with silver stain for investigating *Pneumocystis carinii* pneumonia. J Clin Pathol 44:75, 1991

98. Kovacs JA, Gill V, Swan JC, et al: Prospective evaluation of a monoclonal antibody in diagnosis of *Pneumocystis carinii* pneumonia. Lancet 2:1, 1986

99. Singer C, Armstrong D, Rosen PP, Schottenfeld D: *Pneumocystis carinii* pneumonia: a cluster of eleven cases. Ann Intern Med 82:772, 1975

100. Pifer LL, Hughes WT, Stagno S, Woods D: *Pneumocystis carinii* infection: evidence for high prevalence in normal and immunosuppressed children. Pediatrics 61:35, 1978

101. Sheldon WH: Subclinical *Pneumocystis* pneumonitis. AMA J Dis Child 97:287, 1959

102. Walzer PD, Perl DP, Krogstad DJ, et al: *Pneumocystis carinii* pneumonia in the United States. Epidemiologic, diagnostic, and clinical features. Ann Intern Med 80:83, 1974

103. Gottlieb MS, Schroff R, Schanker HM, et al: *Pneumocystis carinii* pneumonia and mucosal candidiasis in previously healthy homosexual men. Evidence for a new acquired cellular immunodeficiency. N Engl J Med 305:1425, 1981

104. Masur H, Michelis MA, Greene JB, et al: An outbreak of community-acquired *Pneumocystis carinii* pneumonia. Initial manifestation of cellular immune dysfunction. N Engl J Med 305:1431, 1981

105. Wang NS, Huang SN, Thurlbeck WM: Combined *Pneumocystis carinii* and cytomegalovirus infection. Arch Pathol 90:529, 1970

106. Schneider MME, Hoepelman AIM, Schattenkerk JKME, et al: A controlled trial of aerosolized pentamidine or trimethoprim-sulfamethoxazole as primary prophylaxis against *Pneumocystis carinii* pneumonia in patients with human immunodeficiency virus infection. N Engl J Med 327:1836, 1992

107. Telzak EE, Cote RJ, Gold JW, et al: Extrapulmonary *Pneumocystis carinii* infections. Rev Infect Dis 12:380, 1990

108. Lee MM, Schinella RA: Pulmonary calcification caused by *Pneumocystis carinii* pneumonia. A clinicopathological study of 13 cases in acquired immune deficiency syndrome patients. Am J Surg Pathol 15:376, 1991

109. Askin FB, Katzenstein AL: *Pneumocystis* infection masquerading as diffuse alveolar damage: a potential source of diagnostic error. Chest 79:420, 1981

110. Cupples JB, Blackie SP, Road JD: Granulomatous *Pneumocystis carinii* pneumonia mimicking tuberculosis. Arch Pathol Lab Med 113:1281, 1989

111. Travis WD, Pittaluga S, Lipschik GY, et al: Atypical pathologic manifestations of *Pneumocystis carinii* pneumonia in the acquired immune deficiency syndrome. Review of 123 lung biopsies from 76 patients with emphasis on cysts, vascular invasion, vasculitis, and granulomas. Am J Surg Pathol 14:615, 1990

112. Golden JA, Hollander H, Stulbarg MS, Gamsu G: Bronchoalveolar lavage as the exclusive diagnostic modality for *Pneumocystis carinii* pneumonia. A prospective study among patients with acquired immunodeficiency syndrome. Chest 90:18, 1986

113. Johnson WW, Elson CE: Respiratory tract. pp. 340–352. In Bibbo M (ed): Comprehensive Cytopathology. WB Saunders, Philadelphia, 1991

114. Jones PD, See J: *Penicillium marneffei* infection in patients infected with human immunodeficiency virus: late presentation in an area of nonendemicity. Clin Infect Dis 15:744, 1992

115. Deng ZL, Connor DH: Progressive disseminated penicilliosis caused by *Penicillium marneffei*. Report of eight cases and differentiation of the causative organism from *Histoplasma capsulatum*. Am J Clin Pathol 84:323, 1985

116. Nosanchuk JS, Greenberg RD: Protothecosis of the olecranon bursa caused by achloric algae. Am J Clin Pathol 59:567, 1973

117. Chandler FW, Kaplan W, Callaway CS: Differentiation between *Prototheca* and morphologically similar green algae in tissue. Arch Pathol Lab Med 102:353, 1978

118. Holcomb HS 3d, Behrens F, Winn WC Jr, et al: *Prototheca wickerhamii*—an alga infecting the hand. J Hand Surg [Am] 6:595, 1981

119. Butler JC, Heller R, Wright PF: Histoplasmosis during childhood. South Med J 87:476, 1994

120. Sugar AM: Mucormycosis. Clin Infect Dis, suppl. 1, 14:S126, 1992

121. Marchevsky AM, Bottone EJ, Geller SA, Giger DK: The changing spectrum of disease, etiology, and diagnosis of mucormycosis. Hum Pathol 11:457, 1980

122. Gartenberg G, Bottone EJ, Keusch GT, Weitzman I: Hospital-acquired mucormycosis (*Rhizopus rhizopodiformis*) of skin and subcutaneous tissue: epidemiology, mycology and treatment. N Engl J Med 299:1115, 1978

123. Bosken CH, Myers JL, Greenberger PA, Katzenstein AL: Pathologic features of allergic bronchopulmonary aspergillosis. Am J Surg Pathol 12:216, 1988

124. Katzenstein AL, Liebow AA, Friedman PJ: Bronchocentric granulomatosis, mucoid impaction, and hypersensitivity reactions to fungi. Am Rev Respir Dis 111:497, 1975

125. Katzenstein AL, Sale SR, Greenberger PA: Pathologic findings in allergic aspergillus sinusitis. A newly recognized form of sinusitis. Am J Surg Pathol 7:439, 1983

126. Myers JL, Katzenstein AL: Granulomatous infection mimicking bronchocentric granulomatosis. Am J Surg Pathol 10:317, 1986

127. Scherr GR, Evans SG, Kiyabu MT, Klatt EC: *Pseudallescheria boydii* infection in the acquired immunodeficiency syndrome. Arch Pathol Lab Med 116:535, 1992

128. Wheeler MS, McGinnis MR, Schell WA, Walker DH: *Fusarium* infection in burned patients. Am J Clin Pathol 75:304, 1981

129. Louie T, el Baba F, Shulman M, Jimenez-Lucho V: Endogenous endophthalmitis due to *Fusarium*: case report and review. Clin Infect Dis 18:585, 1994

130. Gamis AS, Gudnason T, Giebink GS, Ramsay NK: Disseminated infection with *Fusarium* in recipients of bone marrow transplants. Rev Infect Dis 13:1077, 1991

131. Westenfeld F, Alston WK, Winn WC: Complicated soft tissue infection with prepatellar bursitis caused by *Paecilomyces lilacinus* in an immunocompetent host: case report and review. J Clin Microbiol 34:1559, 1996

132. Orihel TC, Ash LR: Parasites in Human Tissues. ASCP Press, Chicago, 1994

133. Gutierrez Y: Diagnostic Pathology of Parasitic Infections with Clinical Correlations. Lea & Febiger, Philadelphia, 1990

134. Adams EB, MacLeod IN: Invasive amebiasis—amebic dysentery and its complications. Medicine (Baltimore) 56:315–324, 1977

135. Adams EB, MacLeod IN: Invasive amebiasis—amebic liver abscess and its complications. Medicine (Baltimore) 56:325–334, 1977

136. Sorvillo FJ, Strassburg MA, Seidel J, et al: Amebic infections in asymptomatic homosexual men, lack of evidence of invasive disease. Am J Publ Health 76:1137, 1986

137. Diamond LS, Clark CG: A redescription of *Entamoeba histolytica* (Schaudinn, 1903; emended Walker, 1911) separating it from *Entamoeba dispar* (Brumpt, 1925). J Euk Microbiol 40:340, 1993

138. Ma P, Visvesvara GS, Martinez AJ, et al: *Naegleria* and *Acanthamoeba* infections: a review. Rev Infect Dis 12:490, 1990

139. Tan B, Weldon-Linne CM, Rhone DP, et al: *Acanthamoeba* infection presenting as skin lesions in patients with the acquired immunodeficiency syndrome. Arch Pathol Lab Med 117:1043, 1993

140. Visvesvara GS, Martinez AJ, Schuster FL, et al: Leptomyxid ameba: a new agent of amebic meningoencephalitis in humans and animals. J Clin Microbiol 28:2750, 1990

141. Cohen C, Trapuckd S: *Toxoplasma* cyst with toxoplasmic lymphadenitis. Hum Pathol 15:396, 1984

142. Weiss LM, Chen YY, Berry GJ, et al: Infrequent detection of *Toxoplasma gondii* genome in toxoplasmic lymphadenitis: a polymerase chain reaction study. Hum Pathol 23:154, 1992

143. Oksenhendler E, Cadranel J, Sarfati C, et al: *Toxoplasma gondii* pneumonia in patients with the acquired immunodeficiency syndrome. Am J Med 88:5–18N, 1990

144. Falangola MF, Reichler BS, Petito CK: Histopathology of cerebral toxoplasmosis in human immunodeficiency virus infection: a comparison between patients with early-onset and late-onset acquired immunodeficiency syndrome. Hum Pathol 25:1091, 1994

145. Nash G, Kerschmann RL, Herndier B, Dubey JP: The pathological manifestations of pulmonary toxoplasmosis in the acquired immunodeficiency syndrome. Hum Pathol 25:652, 1994

146. Oddo D, Casanova M, Acuna G, et al: Acute Chagas' disease (*Trypanosomiasis americana*) in acquired immunodeficiency syndrome: report of two cases. Hum Pathol 23:41, 1992

147. Melby PC, Kreutzer RD, McMahon-Pratt D, et al: Cutaneous leishmaniasis: review of 59 cases seen at the National Institutes of Health. Clin Infect Dis 15:924, 1992

148. Magill AJ, Grögl M, Gasser RA Jr, et al: Visceral infection caused by *Leishmania tropica* in veterans of operation desert storm. N Engl J Med 328:1383, 1993

149. Fernandez-Guerrero ML, Aguado JM, Buzon L, et al: Visceral leishmaniasis in immunocompromised hosts. Am J Med 83:1098, 1987

150. Berenguer J, Moreno S, Cercenado E, et al: Visceral leishmaniasis in patients infected with human immunodeficiency virus (HIV). Ann Intern Med 111:129, 1989

151. Gupta PK, Frost JK: Human urogenital trichomoniasis: epidemiology, clinical and pathological manifestations. pp. 399–410. In Kulda J, Cerkasov J (eds): Proceedings of the Symposium on Trichomonads and Trichomoniasis. Acta Univ Carol, 1988

152. Kurman RJ, Solomon D: The Bethesda System for Reporting Cervical/Vaginal Cytologic Diagnosis. Springer-Verlag, New York, 1994

153. Schnadig VJ, Davie KD, Shafer SK, et al: The cytologist and bacterioses of the vaginal-ectocervical area: clues, commas and confusion. Acta Cytol 33:287, 1988

154. Mizrachi HH, Lieberman PH, Tolui SS, Sun T: Pulmonary dirofilariasis: mimicry of well-differentiated squamous carcinoma. Hum Pathol 20:818, 1989

155. Ro JY, Tsakalakis PJ, White VA, et al: Pulmonary dirofilariasis: the great imitator of primary or metastatic lung tumor. A clinicopathologic analysis of seven cases and a review of the literature. Hum Pathol 20:69, 1989

156. Gutierrez Y: Diagnostic features of zoonotic filariae in tissue sections. Hum Pathol 15:514, 1984

157. Kaye D: The spectrum of Strongyloidiasis. Hosp Pract (Off Ed) 23:111–126, 1988

158. Pinals RS: Fever, eosinophilia, and periorbital edema. Hosp Pract (Off Ed) 23:55–74, 1988

159. Shandera WX, White AC Jr, Chen JC: Neurocysticercosis in Houston, Texas: a report of 112 cases. Medicine (Baltimore) 73:37, 1994

160. King CH: Acute and chronic schistosomiasis. Hosp Pract (Off Ed) 26:117–130, 1991

161. Smith JH, Christie JD: The pathobiology of *Schistosoma haematobium* infection in humans. Hum Pathol 17:333, 1986

162. Qureshi F, Jacques SM, Reyes MP: Placental histopathology in syphilis. Hum Pathol 24:779, 1993

163. Murray FE, O'Loughlin S, Dervan P, et al: Granulomatous hepatitis in secondary syphilis. Ir J Med Sci 159:53, 1990

164. Ito F, Hunter EF, George RW, et al: Specific immunofluorescence staining of *Treponema pallidum* in smears and tissues. J Clin Microbiol 29:444, 1991

165. Margileth AM, Hayden GF: Cat scratch disease. N Engl J Med 329:53, 1993

166. Schwartzman WA: Infections due to *Rochalimaea*: the expanding clinical spectrum. Clin Infect Dis 15:893, 1992

167. Carithers HA: Cat-scratch disease. An overview based on a study of 1,200 patients. Am J Dis Child 139:1124, 1985

168. Margileth AM, Wear DJ, English CK: Systemic cat scratch disease: report of 23 patients with prolonged or recurrent severe bacterial infection. J Infect Dis 155:390, 1987

169. Miller Catchpole R, Variakojis D, Vardiman JW, et al: Cat scratch disease. Identification of bacteria in seven cases of lymphadenitis. Am J Surg Pathol 10:276, 1986

170. Cohen MB, Miller TR, Bottles K: Classics in cytology; note on fine needle aspiration of the lymphatic glands in sleeping sickness. Acta Cytol 30:451, 1986

171. Stastny JF, Wakely PE Jr, Frable WJ: Cytologic features of necrotizing granulomatous inflammation consistent with cat-scratch disease. Diagn Cytopathol 15:108, 1996

172. Pullen RL, Stuart BM: Tularemia analysis of 225 cases. JAMA 129:495, 1945

173. Stuart BM, Pullen RL: Tularemic pneumonia. Review of American literature and report of 15 additional cases. Am J Med Sci 210:223, 1945

174. Mille RP, Bates JH: Pleuropulmonary tularemia. A review of 29 patients. Am Rev Respir Dis 99:31, 1969

175. Brooks GF, Buchanan TM: Tularemia in the United States—epidemiologic aspects in the 1960's and follow-up of the outbreak of tularemia in Vermont. J Infect Dis 121:357, 1970

176. Evans ME, Gregory DW, Schaffner W, McGee ZA: Tularemia: a 30-year experience with 88 cases. Medicine (Baltimore) 64:251, 1985

177. Reed W, Palmer D, Williams RC Jr, Kisch AL: Plague in the Southwestern United States—a review of recent experience. Medicine (Baltimore) 19:465, 1970

178. Reilly CG, Kates ED: The clinical spectrum of plague in Vietnam. Arch Intern Med 126:990, 1970

179. Sternby NH: Morphologic findings in appendix in human *Yersinia enterocolitica* infection. Contrib Microbiol Immunol 2:141, 1973

180. Gleason TH, Patterson SD: The pathology of *Yersinia enterocolitica* ileocolitis. Am J Surg Pathol 6:347, 1982

181. Finlayson NB, Fagundes B: *Pasteurella pseudotuberculosis* infection: three cases in the United States. Am J Clin Pathol 55:24, 1971

182. Hubbert WT, Peteny CW, Glasgow LA: *Yersinia pseudotuberculosis* infection in the United States: septicemia, appendicitis, and mesenteric lymphadenitis. Am J Trop Med Hyg 20:679, 1971

183. Scieux C, Barnes R, Bianchi A, et al: Lymphogranuloma venereum: 27 cases in Paris. J Infect Dis 160:662, 1989

184. Klotz SA, Drutz DJ, Tam MR, Reed KH: Hemorrhagic proctitis due to lymphogranuloma venereum serogroup L2—diagnosis by fluorescent monoclonal antibody. N Engl J Med 308:1563, 1983

185. Quinn TC, Goodell SE, Mkrtichian E, et al: *Chlamydia trachomatis* proctitis. N Engl J Med 305:195, 1981

186. Beem MO, Saxon EM: Respiratory-tract colonization and a distinctive pneumonia syndrome in infants infected with *Chlamydia trachomatis*. N Engl J Med 296:306, 1977

187. Grayston JT: Infections caused by *Chlamydia pneumoniae* strain TWAR. Clin Infect Dis 15:757, 1992

188. Bernal JN, Martinez MA, Dabancens A: Evaluation of proposed cytomorphologic criteria for the diagnosis of *Chlamydia trachomatis* in Papanicolaou smears. Acta Cytol 33:309, 1989

189. Geerling S, Nettum JA, Linder LE, et al: Sensitivity and specificity of the Papanicolaou-stained cervical smear in the diagnosis of *Chlamydia trachomatis* infection. Acta Cytol 29:671, 1985

190. Reimer LG: Q fever. Clin Microbiol Rev 6:193, 1993

191. Spelman DW: Q fever. A study of 111 consecutive cases. Med J Aust 1:547, 1982

192. Hall CJ, Richmond SJ, Caul EO, et al: Laboratory outbreak of Q fever acquired from sheep. Lancet 1:1004, 1982

193. Srigley JR, Vellend H, Palmer N, et al: Q-fever. The liver and bone marrow pathology. Am J Surg Pathol 9:752, 1985

194. Pellegrin M, Delsol G, Auvergnant JC, et al: Granulomatous hepatitis in Q fever. Hum Pathol 11:51, 1980

195. Lobdell DH: 'Ring' granulomas in cytomegalovirus hepatitis. Arch Pathol Lab Med 111:881, 1987

196. Ruel M, Sevestre H, Henry-Biabaud E, et al: Fibrin ring granulomas in hepatitis A. Dig Dis Sci 37:1915, 1992

197. Pfischner WCE, Tshak KG, Neptune EM: Brucellosis in Egypt. A review of experience with 228 patients. Am J Med 22:915, 1957

198. Buchanan TM, Faber LC, Feldman RA: Brucellosis in the United States 1960–1972. An abbatoir-associated disease. Part 1. Clinical features and therapy. Medicine (Baltimore) 53:403, 1974

199. Hunt AC, Bothwell PW: Histological findings in human brucellosis. J Clin Pathol 20:267, 1967

200. Simpson WM: Undulant fever (brucellosis)—a clinicopathologic study of ninety cases occurring in and about Dayton, Ohio. Ann Intern Med 4:238, 1930

201. Spink WW, Hoffbauer FW, Walker WW, Green RA: Histopathology of the liver in human brucellosis. J Lab Clin Med 34:40, 1949

202. Brown JR: Human actinomycosis: a study of 181 subjects. Hum Pathol 4:319, 1973

203. Schmidt WA: IUDs, inflammation, and infection: assessment after two decades of IUD use. Hum Pathol 13:878, 1982

204. Bhagavan BS, Gupta PK: Genital actinomycosis and intrauterine contraceptive devices. Cytopathologic diagnosis and clinical significance. Hum Pathol 9:567, 1978

205. Wilson DJ: Botryomycosis. Am J Pathol 35:153, 1959

206. Greenblatt M, Heredia R, Rubenstein L, Alpert S: Bacterial pseudomycosis ("botryomycosis"). Am J Clin Pathol 41:188, 1964

207. Burkman RT, Schlesselman S, McCaffrey L, et al: The relationship of genital tract *Actinomyces* and the development of pelvic inflammatory disease. Am J Obstet Gynecol 143:585, 1982

208. Strano AJ: Light microscopy of selected viral diseases (morphology of viral inclusion bodies). Pathol Annu 11:53, 1976

209. Cheville NF: Cytopathology in Viral Diseases. S Karger, Basel, 1975

210. Engblom E, Ekfors TO, Meurman OH, et al: Fatal influenza A myocarditis with isolation of virus from the myocardium. Acta Med Scand 213:75, 1983

211. Englund JA, Sullivan CJ, Jordan MC, et al: Respiratory syncytial virus infection in immunocompromised adults. Ann Intern Med 109:203, 1988

212. Takimoto CH, Cram DL, Root RK: Respiratory syncytial virus infections on an adult medical ward. Arch Intern Med 151:706, 1991

213. Stowell SB, Wiley CM, Powers CN: Herpesvirus mimics. A potential pitfall in endocervical brush specimens. Acta Cytol 38:43, 1994

214. Brumback BG, Farthing PG, Castellino SN: Simultaneous detection of and differentiation between herpes simplex and varicella-zoster viruses with two fluorescent probes in the same test system. J Clin Microbiol 31:3260, 1993

215. Nahmias AJ, Whitley RJ, Visintine AN, et al: Herpes simplex virus encephalitis: laboratory evaluations and their diagnostic significance. J Infect Dis 145:829, 1982

216. Foley FD, Greenawald KA, Nash G, Pruitt BAJ: Herpesvirus infection in burned patients. N Engl J Med 282:652, 1970

216a.Coleman DV: Cytological diagnosis of virus-infected cells in cervical smears. Diagn Gynecol Obstet 4:363–373, 1982

217. DeMay RM: The Art & Science of Cytopathology. ASCP Press, Chicago, 1995

218. Fend F, Prior C, Margreiter R, Mikuz G: Cytomegalovirus pneumonitis in heart-lung transplant recipients: histopathology and clinicopathologic considerations. Hum Pathol 21:918, 1990

219. Craighead JE: Cytomegalovirus pulmonary disease. Pathobiol Annu 5:197, 1975

220. Myers JD, Spencer HCJ, Watts JC, et al: Cytomegalovirus pneumonia after human marrow transplantation. Ann Intern Med 82:181, 1975

221. Heurlin N, Brattstrom C, Tyden G, et al: Cytomegalovirus the predominant cause of pneumonia in renal transplant patients. A two-year study of pneumonia in renal transplant recipients with evaluation of fiberoptic bronchoscopy. Scand J Infect Dis 21:245, 1989

222. Beschorner WE, Hutchins GM, Burns WH, et al: Cytomegalovirus pneumonia in bone marrow transplant recipients: miliary and diffuse patterns. Am Rev Respir Dis 122:107, 1980

223. Sickel JZ, Rutkowski MA, Bonfiglio TA: Cytomegalovirus inclusions in routine cervical Papanicolaou smears: a clinicopathologic study of three cases, abstract ed. Acta Cytol 35:646, 1991

224. Nolte KB, Feddersen RM, Foucar K, et al: Hantavirus pulmonary syndrome in the United States: a pathological description of a disease caused by a new agent. Hum Pathol 26:110, 1995

225. Zaki SR, Khan AS, Goodman RA, et al: Retrospective diagnosis of hantavirus pulmonary syndrome, 1978–1993: implications for emerging infectious diseases. Arch Pathol Lab Med 120:134, 1996

226. Maurin M, Raoult D: *Bartonella (Rochalimaea) quintana* infections. Clin Microbiol Rev 9:273, 1996

227. Relman DA, Loutit JS, Schmidt TM, et al: The agent of bacillary angiomatosis. An approach to the identification of uncultured pathogens. N Engl J Med 323:1573, 1990

228. LeBoit PE, Berger TG, Egbert BM, et al: Bacillary angiomatosis. The histopathology and differential diagnosis of a pseudoneoplastic infection in patients with human immunodeficiency virus disease. Am J Surg Pathol 13:909, 1989

12

Immunologically Mediated Diseases

Edward C. Klatt
Elizabeth H. Hammond

IMMUNE MECHANISMS OF TISSUE INJURY

Immunologic tissue injury results from a variety of pathologic mechanisms involving antigens and antibodies. Antigens may be exogenous to the host, such as microbiologic agents, plant materials, pharmacologic agents, or chemical compounds, while endogenous antigens from body tissues may be involved in pathogenesis of autoimmune diseases. The reactions can be localized or systemic, subclinical or life threatening. The nature of the tissue injury depends on the nature of the antigen, the location of the antigen, and the type, avidity, and amount of antibody. Interaction of antigen and antibody with inflammatory cells producing cytokines, as well as with a variety of chemical mediators of inflammation, also determines the type and degree of tissue injury. Based on antigen-antibody interactions, four major hypersensitivity reactions have been defined.[1]

Type I Hypersensitivity

Pathogenesis

Sensitization to an antigen leads to production of preformed antibody, either at the site of entrance of antigen—often the mucosa of the respiratory or gastrointestinal tract—or in lymph nodes that drain the site of antigen entrance, by B lymphocytes assisted by CD4 lymphocytes. The high affinity antibody, mainly IgE, is bound to mast cells and peripheral blood basophils.[2,3] Further antigen contact in previously sensitized persons leads to an anaphylactic response because the antigen cross-links the Fc receptors of IgE molecules attached to mast cells and basophils, causing release of stored chemical mediators including biogenic amines (principally histamine) in the process of degranulation.[4,5]

Anaphylaxis occuring within 5 to 60 minutes of antigen contact leads to histamine release, with vasodilation and exudation of fluid from venules, submucosal gland secretion, and bronchial smooth muscle contraction. Mast cells are often localized around blood vessels, enhancing histaminic effects. This immediate response produces little tissue damage. Grossly, af-

fected tissues are edematous, and lumens of bronchi are filled with mucoid secretions.[2] If the inflammatory response continues, even in the absence of additional antigen, secondary mediators are released that recruit additional inflammatory cells including eosinophils, neutrophils, and macrophages (Fig. 12-1). This can occur hours after initial exposure to antigen. The granulocytes can release proteases and hydrolases to enhance inflammation and increase tissue destruction. However, necrosis and ulceration of mucosal surfaces are uncommon.[6]

Clinical and Pathologic Features

Examples of localized anaphylaxis include localized skin swelling (hives) with urticaria, allergic rhinitis (hay fever from plant pollens), allergic conjunctivitis (watery eyes), and allergic gastroenteritis with diarrhea (food allergy from allergens in fish, wheat, or milk products). Approximately 10 percent of persons experience some degree of atopy, as evidenced by a propensity for allergic reactions. Systemic anaphylaxis can be life threatening, as illustrated by administration of penicillin or bee sting suffered by a sensitized individual. Consequences include laryngeal edema and extensive bronchoconstriction, both of which contribute to severe respiratory distress. Extensive vasodilation with exudation leads to hypotension with shock.[2]

Type II Hypersensitivity

Type II reactions are quite diverse. The common immunologic mechanism uniting them is the attachment of an antibody to a specific tissue antigen fixed at a specified site. Thus, these are antibody-dependent hypersensitivity reactions.

Complement-Mediated Cytotoxicity

Circulating antibody can be directed against antigens on red blood cell (RBC) membranes. With a major transfusion reaction from ABO incompatibility, the naturally occurring anti-A and/or anti-B antibody in patient serum will attach to donor RBCs, and hemolysis will ensue in minutes. In hemolytic disease of the newborn, most often due to Rh incompatibility be-

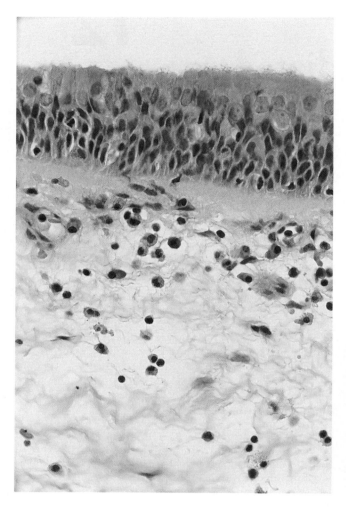

Fig. 12-1. Type I hypersensitivity reaction. Beneath the nasal mucosa is marked stromal edema with scattered eosinophils.

tween mother and fetus, maternal IgG crosses the placenta and attaches to fetal RBCs, with ensuing hemolysis, fetal anemia, organomegaly, and jaundice. Autoimmune diseases with a hemolytic anemia component typically involve a warm IgG autoantibody directed against the patient's own RBCs, and extravascular hemolysis over weeks to months occurs, mainly in spleen. With ongoing hemolysis, extramedullary hematopoiesis may occur in liver and spleen; bone marrow shows erythroid hyperplasia.[7]

Goodpasture's Syndrome

Goodpasture's syndrome, which has an incidence of 0.3 in 100,000, represents a special case of complement-mediated cytotoxicity in which an autoantibody is directed against the noncollagenous domain of the alpha 3 collagen chain of type 4 collagen in glomerular and pulmonary capillary basement membranes. The attachment of antibody triggers the complement cascade, with resultant basement membrane destruction and pulmonary or glomerular hemorrhage. Immunofluores-

cence with antibody to IgG and/or IgA will demonstrate a linear staining pattern in glomerular capillaries on renal biopsy (Fig. 12-2). This immunologic injury leads to a rapidly progressive (crescentic) glomerulonephritis.[8]

Antibody-Dependent Cell-Mediated Cytotoxicity

Antibody dependent cell-mediated cytotoxicity (ADCC) involves immunoglobulin, mostly IgG, which attaches to fixed tissue antigens. The bound immunoglobulins present their Fc receptors to a variety of inflammatory cells that can attach to these receptors, including neutrophils, eosinophils, macrophages, and natural killer (NK) cells. Attachment of IgG to Fc receptor triggers membrane perturbations in the inflammatory cells, leading to release of proteases and destruction of cells that have the attached antibody.[4,9] ADCC is a naturally occurring immune response useful in defense against parasites invading tissues. It is an important mechanism of allograft rejection, particularly in renal transplants.[10]

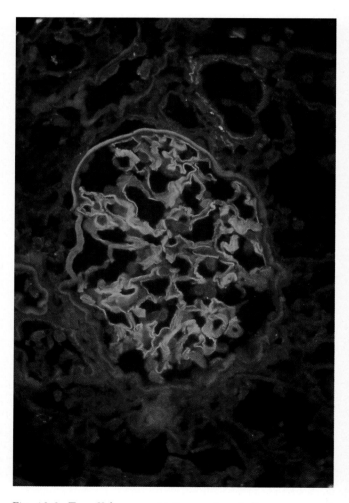

Fig. 12-2. Type II hypersensitivity reaction. A linear pattern of immunoglobulin deposition with antibody to IgG is seen in the glomerulus with Goodpasture's syndrome.

Antireceptor Antibody-Mediated Cellular Dysfunction

A reaction occurs when an autoantibody is produced against specific cell surface receptors. The autoantibodies block the receptors, producing cellular dysfunction. Autoimmune thyroid diseases, including Graves' disease and Hashimoto's thyroiditis, develop when receptor autoantibodies have functional activity with attachment to thyroid-stimulating hormone receptors on thyroid follicular epithelial cells. Serologic testing may reveal antithyroglobulin and antimicrosomal antibodies. Lymphocytic infiltrates and lymphoid follicles can appear in both conditions.[11] Autoantibody directed against acetylcholine receptors on striated muscle leads to muscular weakness with myasthenia gravis.[12]

Type III Hypersensitivity

Pathogenesis

Immune complexes formed of antigen and antibody, principally IgG, IgM, and IgA, may be localized and formed in situ, or they may be systemic circulating complexes that become deposited at specific locations. Larger complexes bind more avidly and are more easily phagocytized by cells of the mononuclear phagocyte system. Complexes not removed by phagocytosis are available for deposition elsewhere. Complexes formed of antibody with higher avidity or antigens with specific tissue affinity will also determine the pattern of distribution.[13,14]

Circulating immune complexes tend to deposit at tissue interfaces with basement membranes, where they become trapped (Fig. 12-3). Sites include small arteries, arterioles, and capillaries of the vascular system, particularly in kidney and lung, where a vasculitis results. Body cavities lined by mesothelium such as pleura, pericardium, peritoneum, and synovium may have serositis. Epidermal basement membrane can be involved. Complement activation occurs and yields biologically active fragments that increase neutrophilic infiltration, promote phagocytosis, increase vascular permeability, and damage cell membranes. Proteases released by attracted neutrophils lead to further tissue damage. Vascular damage leads to activation of platelets to produce microthrombi and activation of Hageman factor to promote vasodilation with edema.[15]

Clinical Findings

The autoimmune collagen vascular diseases are in large part mediated via immune complex deposition. The serum antinuclear antibody (ANA) test is invariably positive, and a higher ANA titer generally correlates with more active disease. Serum assays for total hemolytic complement, C3, and C4 are often low. Pancytopenia can occur, and anemia of chronic disease is common. Immune responses with infections from viral, bacterial, and parasitic agents may also be implicated in immune complex disease.

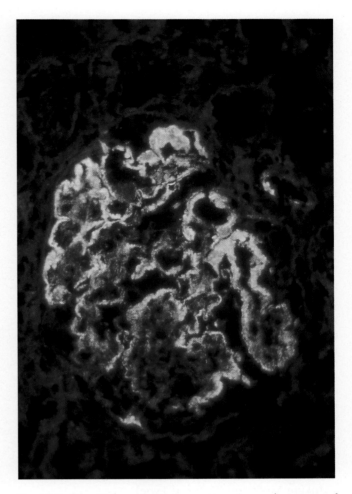

Fig. 12-3. Type III hypersensitivity reaction. A granular pattern of immunoglobulin distribution with antibody to C3 is seen in a glomerulus in this case of systemic lupus erythematosus.

Pathologic Findings

Nonspecific changes of edema with tissue swelling may be seen grossly. Inflammation may lead to effusions with fibrinous exudates on serosal surfaces. Skin rashes are common. Endocarditis may appear, with bland platelet fibrin vegetations. The microscopic pathologic findings include vasculitis (sometimes with fibrinoid necrosis) with arteritis or capillaritis, endocarditis, serositis (pericarditis, pleuritis, peritonitis), synovitis, dermatitis, and glomerulonephritis. Vascular microthrombi may appear, sometimes in association with localized ischemia and infarction. Immunosuppressive therapy may diminish the inflammatory response seen in biopsied tissues.

Serum Sickness

Serum sickness is a generalized immune complex disease that occurs on administration of a foreign protein. Once common with passive immunization utilizing large amounts of foreign (animal) serum, it is now seen with the use of antithymocyte globulin, hepatitis serum immunoglobulin, anti-CD3 mouse monoclonal antibody (OKT3), and vaccines (tetanus antiserum). The foreign protein stimulates a primary immune response approximately 5 days after administration. If the original antigen has not been cleared from circulation, then immune complexes begin to form. Increased vascular permeability aids immune complex deposition. Clinical findings of fever, lymphadenopathy, cutaneous eruptions, and arthralgias occur 8 to 12 days after injection. Circulating immune complexes can be found along with decreased serum C3 and C4 complement. Pathologic findings in skin eruptions consist of perivascular edema with collections of lymphocytes and macrophages but few neutrophils and no necrosis of vessels, although immune complexes can be demonstrated in vessel walls by immunofluorescence.[16]

Arthus Reaction

The Arthus reaction, a local immune complex disease following injection of a foreign protein into the dermis of a previously sensitized person, will create a localized excess of antigen that forms complexes with preformed antibody precipitating at the site of injection. IgG Fc receptors may contribute to inflammation by activating macrophages, neutrophils, NK cells, and mast cell responses. The complexes incite an intense vasculitis with fibrinoid necrosis and thrombosis. This can be accompanied by vascular leakage with localized hemorrhage or by focal ischemic necrosis.[17]

Type IV Hypersensitivity

Cytokine-Mediated (Delayed Type) Hypersensitivity

Previous sensitization with an antigen may produce long-lived CD4 lymphocytes that can recognize the antigen on a further encounter, in association with HLA class II molecules on antigen-presenting cells, which then release a variety of cytokines, including interleukin-1 (IL-1), interferon-gamma, and tumor necrosis factor-alpha. The cytokines attract blood monocytes, which become tissue macrophages. Cytokines recruit additional lymphocytes and macrophages. Tissue injury is mediated by macrophages and endothelial cell cytokines and chemical mediators released by this reaction. This is the mechanism for many granulomatous diseases.[18]

Clinically, the earliest inflammation takes about 12 to 48 hours to appear, and reaches a peak at 2 to 3 days. It is the basis for contact dermatitis (e.g., poison ivy), and for defense against persistent intracellular infectious agents (particularly mycobacteria and fungi. It is thus the basis for the tuberculin skin test as well as skin testing with *Candida* and mumps antigens to assess cell-mediated immune function. Microscopically, inflammation begins with localized collections of lymphocytes and macrophages associated with swollen capillary endothelial cells. Over time, as cell numbers increase, a granuloma forms that is a localized, firm, tan-white nodule that can range in size from a few millimeters to a centimeter or more. Larger granulo-

mas tend to have central caseation, although noninfectious sarcoid granulomas are typically noncaseating (Fig. 12-4). Delayed type hypersensitivity may also play a role in tumor immunity and in cellular allograft rejection.[19]

T Cell-Mediated Cytotoxicity

Cells to which T cell-mediated cytotoxicity is directed have HLA class I molecules that aid in antigen presentation; specific target cell surface antigen is recognized by cytotoxic CD8 lymphocytes. This process produces focal cell necrosis without widespread, grossly apparent, tissue injury.[20] Clinically, conditions resulting from this immune mechanism are diverse, including viral infections such as hepatitis and inflammatory responses to neoplasms. Allografts used in transplantation in which HLA matching is not exact are also subject to a cytotoxic lymphocytic response. The cytotoxic response leads to target cell membrane injury and release of specific cytotoxic substances such as perforin by the CD8 cells.[21]

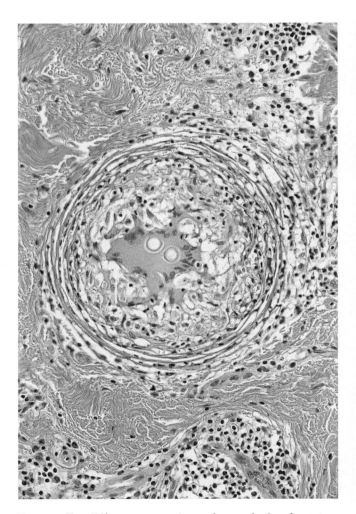

Fig. 12-4. Type IV hypersensivity. A granuloma with a Langhans giant cell contains two spherules of *Coccidioides immitis*.

VASCULITIS

Vasculitis is a feature of many immunologic diseases, infections, and drug reactions. Patient presentations are protean and include fever, weight loss, malaise, arthralgia, and myalgia. One or more immunologic hypersensitivity reactions may contribute to the inflammation. The pattern of vascular involvement and the nature of the inflammatory response help to characterize different patterns of vasculitis.[22,23] Tissue diagnosis with biopsy can be aided by clinical laboratory testing for antineutrophil cytoplasmic autoantibodies (ANCA). By immunofluorescence microscopy, ANCAs can be divided into a cytoplasmic staining pattern (cANCA), which correlates with antiproteinase 3 antibody, and a perinuclear pattern (pANCA) of staining, which correlates with antimyeloperoxidase antibody. The presence of cANCA (antiproteinase 3) is more indicative of Wegener's granulomatosis, whereas the presence of pANCA (antimyeloperoxidase antibody) more strongly suggests a vasculitis typical of microscopic polyarteritis or idiopathic crescentic glomerulonephritis. A positive ANA test, particularly if high titered, suggests a systemic autoimmune disease.[24]

Type III Hypersensitivity

Type III hypersensitivity plays a role in many vasculitides. An acute hypersensitivity vasculitis affecting small arteries and arterioles with predominantly neutrophilic inflammation and leukocytoclasis may be seen in association with many infections and drugs and with serum sickness. A chronic hypersensitivity vasculitis in any size artery with mainly lymphocytic inflammation is typical of vasculitis with autoimmune diseases Fig. 12-5. The skin is often affected, but almost any organ can be involved.

Polyarteritis Nodosa

By contrast, type III hypersensitivity with polyarteritis nodosa affects medium to small arteries in skin and many visceral organ sites, waxing and waning at different times, so the clinical manifestations are numerous and confusing. Vascular involvement is focal and segmental, with mixed inflammatory cell infiltrates that can be acutely necrotizing, although healed chronic lesions show mainly fibrosis. Microaneurysms can be found, and pANCA is often present. A "microscopic" polyarteritis nodosa variant occurs with segmental necrotizing glomerulonephritis.

Wegener's Granulomatosis

Wegner's granulomatosis typically affects small arteries and veins of the upper and lower respiratory tract and kidney; other organs are less commonly involved. Types II, III, and IV hypersensitivity reactions all contribute, and cANCA is often present. Capillaritis is common, but not fibrinoid vascular necrosis. Mixed inflammatory cell infiltrates, but with few

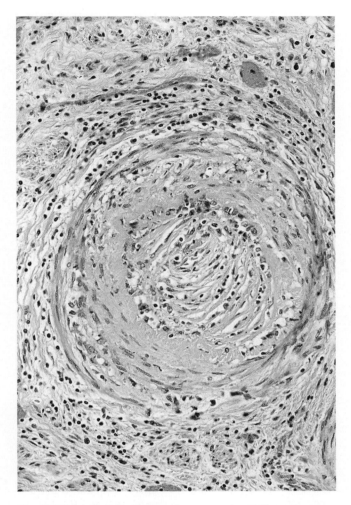

Fig. 12-5. Vasculitis. Predominantly mononuclear infiltrates are seen in this mesenteric artery in a case of systemic lupus erythematosus.

eosinophils, accompany necrotizing and non-necrotizing granulomatous inflammation to produce areas of geographic necrosis surrounded by palisading epithelioid macrophages and giant cells. Fibrosis occurs with chronic lesions.

Allergic Granulomatous Vasculitis

Allergic granulomatous vasculitis, also known as Churg-Strauss vasculitis, has a broad pattern of involvement including both small arteries and arterioles as well as veins and venules, with contributions from types I, III, and IV hypersensitivity. Affected persons often have a history of atopy with bronchial asthma. Peripheral eosinophilia, often marked, and cANCA are present. Upper and lower respiratory tract, viscera (particularly heart), and skin can all be involved. There are mainly extravascular mixed inflammatory cell infiltrates, often including a prominent component of eosinophils, with necrotizing granulomas. Eosinophilic vasculitis can appear in either arteries or veins. Tissue necrosis with a granulomatous reaction including giant cells can also be seen.

Giant Cell and Takayasu's Arteritides

Arteritides resulting mostly from type IV hypersensitivity include giant cell arteritis and Takayasu's arteritis. In the former, the typical pattern of involvement includes the temporal artery and branches of carotid arteries. One-sixth of cases may have involvement of the aorta and its major branches. It can be quite focal, requiring serial sections even of a small biopsy. The inflammation is mixed with scattered giant cells. If it is chronic, only fibrosis may be seen. Takayasu's arteritis involves the aorta, particularly the arch, and pulmonary, coronary, and renal arteries can be involved. The inflammation, which early on appears granulomatous, can produce aneurysms and predispose to dissection. If chronic, fibrosis is present.

AUTOIMMUNE DISEASES

Pathogenesis

Loss of self-tolerance and activation of the immune system can lead to a variety of autoimmune conditions. MHC expression by many cells plays an important role in this process, along with T lymphocytes. Many pathologic lesions seen with autoimmune diseases are a consequence of immune hypersensitivity reactions, particularly immune complex-mediated disease.

Systemic Lupus Erythematosus

Systemic lupus erythematosus (SLE) represents the classic systemic immune complex disease. Serum ANA testing often reveals a "rim" pattern, and anti-double-stranded DNA and anti-Smith autoantibodies can be present that are quite specific for SLE. Antiphospholipid antibodies are frequent and are associated with endothelial damage to produce thromboses. Histologic patterns of vasculitis range from leukocytoclastic to lymphocytic and may occur in any organ, although treatment may dampen the inflammatory response. Skin lesions demonstrate hydropic degeneration of the basal layer, upper dermal edema, purpura, vasculitis, and edema. Immune complexes can be identified by immunofluoresence with staining for IgG, C1q, and C3. Serositis, with or without fibrinous exudates, is common in body cavities. Arthritis is nonerosive. Libman-Sacks endocarditis can occur. The spleen demonstrates concentric periarteriolar fibrosis ("onion-skinning"). Glomerulonephritis is common and can result in end-stage renal disease. *Discoid lupus erythematosus* differs from SLE mainly because the skin and not the visceral organs are involved. Drug-induced SLE is unlikely to display severe vasculitis or extensive organ involvement.[25]

Progressive Systemic Sclerosis (Scleroderma)

Patients with anti-DNA topoisomerase I antibody are more likely to have diffuse disease, whereas the presence of anticentromere antibody suggests a more limited CREST syndrome (calcinosis, Raynaud's phenomenon, esophageal dysfunction, sclerodactyly, and telangiectasia). Even though the condition is immunologically mediated, minimal inflammation is present, and the major histologic finding is fibrosis, best seen with a trichrome stain. The skin shows extensive dermal fibrosis. The submucosa and mucosa of the gastrointestinal tract, and the lower esophagus in particular, can show extensive fibrosis, leading to strictures and dysmotility. An alveolitis may precede restrictive lung disease, with interstitial fibrosis that may progress to honeycomb change. A patchy myocardial fibrosis can occur, and arrhythmias are common. In some cases primary biliary cirrhosis can be present, or a myositis similar to polymyositis. Sjögren's syndrome can occur concurrently. Renal hyperplastic arteriolosclerosis with concentric intimal endothelial proliferation in small arcuate and interlobular arteries can lead to severe hypertension and arteriolar fibrinoid necrosis with cortical microinfarcts.[26]

Rheumatoid Arthritis

A proliferative synovitis with pannus formation, articular cartilage erosion, and joint destruction with deformity is common in rheumatoid arthritis. Symmetric involvement of small joints of the hands and feet occurs. Microscopically, the pannus demonstrates marked chronic inflammation containing lymphoid follicles with many CD4 lymphocytes and numerous plasma cells. Rheumatoid nodules, which are localized areas of fibrinoid necrosis surrounded by palisading epithelioid macrophages, lymphocytes, and plasma cells, can appear in soft tissues at pressure points such as the elbow or in visceral locations. Most patients have rheumatoid factor, which is an autoantibody (mostly IgM) formed against the Fc portion of autologous IgG. A very high titer of rheumatoid factor can be associated with concomitant vasculitis similar to polyarteritis nodosa but involving mainly small peripheral arteries.[27]

Other Autoimmune Diseases

Polymyositis results in an inflammatory myopathy, sometimes in association with other autoimmune diseases, and the presence of a skin rash with histologic features similar to the skin changes of SLE suggests a diagnosis of dermatomyositis. *Mixed connective tissue disease* overlaps with other autoimmune diseases and has features of SLE, polymyositis, and systemic sclerosis, but generally without serious organ involvement leading to renal or pulmonary failure. *Sjögren's syndrome* primarily involves salivary and lacrimal glands with chronic inflammation and atrophy, but a predilection exists for coexistence of other autoimmune diseases and for development of malignant lymphomas.[28,29]

Miscellaneous Endocrine Autoimmune Diseases

Type 1 diabetes mellitus is thought to result from alteration of beta cells in islets of Langerhans by viral or chemical factors followed by abnormal MHC expression and autoimmune destruction mediated via T lymphocytes and cytokine release. Histologically, lymphocytic insulitis with edema and loss of islet cells is seen, culminating in loss of islets.[30] *Addison's disease* is most commonly the result of autoimmune destruction of adrenal cortex; initially lymphocytic infiltrates cause cortical destruction, followed by fibrosis and atrophy.[31] *Lymphocytic hypophysitis* is a rare postpartum disorder that can account for pituitary failure.[32]

PRIMARY IMMUNODEFICIENCY DISEASES

X-Linked Agammaglobulinemia

Pathogenesis

Congenital agammaglobulinemia (Bruton's disease) results from a genetic defect on the long arm of the X chromosome, so that males are primarily affected. The mutations affect production of a tyrosine kinase active in early B cells that diminishes their maturation and leads to virtual absence of all immunoglobulin classes.[33]

Clinical Features

Less than 100 mg/dl of serum IgG is present and no detectable IgA or IgM. When protective maternal antibody begins to disappear late in infancy, bacterial infections become more numerous, particularly respiratory tract infections, otitis media, and skin infections. *Haemophilus influenzae* and *Streptococcus pneumoniae* are more common than *Staphylococcus aureus* and *Streptococcus pyogenes*. Viral and fungal infections are not increased, although a propensity exists for development of vaccine-associated poliomyelitis and echovirus meningoencephalitis. Chronic diarrhea with giardiasis may occur. Arthritis of large joints may result from *Ureaplasma urealyticum* infection. With time, about 20 percent of affected persons will develop an autoimmune disease such as rheumatoid arthritis, SLE, or dermatomyositis.[34]

Pathologic Findings

Grossly, lymph nodes and tonsils appear atrophic, but the thymus is normal in size. Microscopically, lymphoid tissues have only rare follicles that lack germinal centers, inconspicuous sinuses, and capsular fibrosis. Plasma cells are absent from lymph nodes, spleen, bone marrow, and gut-associated lymphoid tissues, and circulating B cells are virtually absent, although T cells are normal in number. Pre-B cells are present.

DiGeorge's Syndrome

Pathogenesis

DiGeorge's syndrome (or sequence) is a field defect of third and fourth pharyngeal pouch development in utero during organogenesis in the first trimester of pregnancy. A specific deletion on the long arm of chromosome 22 has been implicated.[35]

Structures that may be aplastic or hypoplastic include thymus, parathyroid glands, great vessels, and esophagus. As with all syndromes involving congenital anomalies, the presence of one anomaly makes other anomalies more likely. DiGeorge's syndrome may be further subclassified as complete, in which thymic tissue is almost totally absent or partial, in which such tissue is only decreased.[36,37]

Clinical Features

Children with complete DiGeorge's syndrome have normal levels of circulating immunoglobulin, although in some cases serum IgE is increased and IgA is decreased. They have markedly decreased numbers of circulating T lymphocytes, making them susceptible to fungal and viral infections. Children with partial DiGeorge's syndrome have only a slight decrease in peripheral T lymphocytes and have increased infections, but with less frequency and less severity than children who have the complete form. Accompanying aplasia of the parathyroid glands can lead to life-threatening hypocalcemia that may appear soon after birth.[36]

Pathologic Findings

In complete DiGeorge's syndrome the thymus, normally a prominent prepubertal anterior mediastinal structure, is difficult to distinguish from adipose tissue; in the partial variant the thymus is recognizable but is smaller than normal. Microscopically, the complete variant demonstrates a lack of normal cortex and medulla, with only scattered Hassall's corpuscles and a few lymphocytes. Lymph nodes have follicles but decreased numbers of T cells in paracortical and mantle zones, and the periarteriolar cuffs of lymphocytes in spleen are virtually absent. Plasma cells and immunoblasts, however, are present. The partial variant shows decreased numbers of lymphocytes in the thymus and other lymphoid structures.[36,37]

Severe Combined Immunodeficiency

Pathogenesis

Variants of severe combined immunodeficiency (SCID) result from different defects with different inheritance patterns, but all demonstrate some degree of failure in development of both humoral and cell-mediated immunity. Over half of the cases are an X-linked form due to a mutation on the long arm of the X chromosome, which produces a defective gamma chain of the IL-2 receptor. Lack of an intact IL receptor renders early lymphocytes incapable of normal differentiation and development into functional T and B cells in response to growth factors.[38] Other SCID cases will demonstrate autosomal recessive inheritance linked to a lack of the enzyme adenosine deaminase. This enzyme is involved in purine metabolism, and its deficiency results in production of metabolites toxic to lymphocytes.[39]

Clinical Findings

Affected infants have markedly decreased circulating lymphocytes (<1000/μl), although NK cell levels may be normal or high. A greater decrease tends to be present in cell-mediated immunity than in humoral immunity. Normal or increased numbers of B lymphocytes may be present with the X-linked form, but these cells still do not function properly. Very little serum IgG is found and virtually no IgM or IgA. Infants develop *Candida* skin rashes and thrush, persistent diarrhea, severe respiratory tract infections with *Pneumocystis carinii* and *Pseudomonas* soon after birth, and failure to thrive after 3 months of age. Severe viral infection can occur. Maternal T lymphocytes crossing the placenta may produce graft-versus-host disease.[34,40]

Pathologic Findings

The thymus in SCID is not developed beyond initial embryogenesis, does not descend to the anterior mediastinum, and displays virtual absence of lymphocytes and Hassall's corpuscles. Lymphoid tissues throughout the body are hypoplastic, with severe depletion of lymphocytes.

Selective (Isolated) IgA Deficiency

Pathogenesis

About 1 in 500 persons of European descent has a virtual lack of circulating IgA as well as secretory IgA, which in most cases results from failure of the IgA type of B lymphocytes to transform into plasma cells capable of producing IgA or from impaired survival of IgA-producing plasma cells. Some patients may have deficiencies in IgG subclasses 2 or 4 (or both), with increased IgG subclasses 1 and 3. Some patients go on to develop common variable immunodeficiency, suggesting a similar defect in B cell maturation and function.[41–43]

Clinical Features

Selective IgA deficiency is defined by a serum IgA less than 50 mg/dl; a partial IgA deficiency is diagnosed when serum IgA is more than 50 mg/dl but less than 2 standard deviations below normal. Because IgA functions to protect mucosal surfaces, some affected patients are at increased risk of respiratory, gastrointestinal, and urinary tract infections, most often bacterial, and diarrhea is common. More severely affected persons may even have a sprue-like illness with malabsorption. Atopy, as demonstrated by asthma, can be present. Concomitant autoimmune diseases, particularly SLE and rheumatoid arthritis, can be present. About one-half of IgA-deficient persons develop anti-IgA antibodies of the IgE type, so that transfusion of blood products containing serum with normal IgA levels leads to severe systemic anaphylaxis.[42,44,45]

Pathologic Findings

The gross and microscopic architecture of lymphoid organs appears normal. Plasma cells containing IgA are absent.

Common Variable Immunodeficiency

Pathogenesis

Common variable immunodeficiency (CVID) comprises a heterogenous group of disorders (incidence of 1 in 100,000) that can involve both humoral and cell-mediated immunity. Although numbers of circulating B lymphocytes are normal, impaired secretion of one or more immunoglobulin isotypes exists, usually IgG or IgA. A selective abnormality of T cell activation, as demonstrated by decreased synthesis of interleukins (IL-2, -4, and -5) has been identified. Patients may have impaired gastrointestinal mucosal immunity. Another variant results from either a decrease in CD4 cells or an increase in CD8 cells. Also occurring is a variant resulting from the presence of T and B lymphocyte autoantibodies.[34,46,47]

Clinical Findings

One-half of CVID cases are diagnosed before age 21, but in some cases complications do not develop until adolescence or adulthood. At least two of the three main serum immunoglobulin isotypes are decreased. Persons with CVID are prone to recurrent bacterial infections, particularly sinusitis, bronchitis, pneumonia, bronchiectasis, and otitis. *Bordetella pertussis* infections occur in childhood. Viral infections are uncommon, although recurrent herpes simplex with eventual herpes zoster is an exception. Giardiasis is common. The incidence of autoimmune diseases is increased, particulary hemolytic anemia, thrombocytopenia, and pernicious anemia. In about two-thirds of cases, normal numbers of circulating B lymphocytes are present. A decrease in immunoglobulins is found, generally in all classes but more often IgG and IgA and sometimes only IgG.[34,46,48]

Pathologic Findings

Lymphadenopathy, gastrointestinal lymphoid hyperplasia, and splenomegaly are often present. Grossly, both thymic and lymphoid tissues develop normally. Microscopically, germinal centers of lymphoid follicles can appear hyperplastic with increased B lymphocytes. Both nodal and extranodal lymphoid proliferations may be present that range from reactive to atypical lymphoid hyperplasia. An increased tendency exists for nonspecific noncaseating sarcoid-like granulomas to be present in liver, spleen, lymph nodes, and bone marrow. Both Hodgkin's disease and non-Hodgkin's lymphomas are more frequent. Inflammatory bowel diseases are more common, and an increased risk exists for gastric carcinoma. Some affected persons develop amyloidosis.[34,46,49]

Wiskott-Aldrich Syndrome

Pathogenesis

Inheritance of Wiskott-Aldrich syndrome occurs in an X-linked recessive pattern because of a defective gene on the short arm of the X chromosome. The immunodeficiency is accompanied by thrombocytopenia and eczema. Circulating platelets are markedly decreased. T lymphocytes exhibit cytoskeletal disorganization and loss of microvilli by electron microscopy, and they express little CD43 by immunohistochemical staining.[34,50]

Clinical Findings

The level of serum IgG is usually normal, along with a decrease in IgM, but often an increase in both IgA and IgE. The initial onset of disease in early childhood is accompanied by recurrent bacterial infections, particularly to encapsulated bacteria such as S. pneumoniae, with development of pneumonia, meningitis, and septicemia. Later, failure of T lymphocyte function may predispose to recurrent herpetic infections and to P. carinii pneumonia. Thrombocytopenia may be severe enough to result in a bleeding diathesis.[34]

Pathologic Findings

Grossly, thymus and lymph nodes appear normal. Microscopically, T lymphocytes can be depleted in paracortical areas of lymphoid tissues and T lymphocytes decreased in peripheral blood. Numbers of megakaryocytes in bone marrow are normal.

Ataxia-Telangiectasia

Pathogenesis

Ataxia-telangiectasia, a very rare autosomal recessive disease, results from a genetic defect on the long arm of chromosome 11 that predisposes to chromosome breakage and rearrangement, particularly on chromosomes 7 and 14, leading to a high risk of neoplasia and a marked sensitivity to radiation.[51]

Clinical Findings

The symptoms usually begin between 9 months and 2 years of age as a triad of progressive cerebellar ataxia, mucocutaneous telangiectasias, and recurrent respiratory tract infections with a variety of bacterial and fungal organisms. Immunoglobulin deficiencies, particularly IgA and/or IgE, may be present, although serum IgM is usually elevated.[52]

Pathologic Findings

Thymic atrophy is found with lymphocyte depletion and absence of Hassall's corpuscles. Lymph nodes demonstrate T cell depletion in paracortical areas and mantle zones and eventually become atrophic. Recurrent pulmonary infections lead to bronchiectasis and fibrosis. The neoplasms that occur are often lymphomas (usually B cell) and leukemias, but an increased risk of solid tumors also exists.[51]

Other Primary Immunodeficiency Disorders

Deficiencies of complement components are uncommon but can be associated with syndromes resembling SLE. Chédiak-Higashi syndrome is a rare autosomal recessive disorder in which peripheral blood neutrophils, monocytes, and lymphocytes contain giant cytoplasmic granules and patients have leukopenia, making them susceptible to bacterial and fungal infections of skin, mucous membranes, and respiratory tract. In chronic granulomatous disease, neutrophils and monocytes lack the enzyme NADPH oxidase, which is needed to generate intracellular oxidants that destroy phagocytosed infectious organisms, particularly catalase-positive agents such as S. aureus, Candida, and Aspergillus, so that chronic infections are common.[53]

ACQUIRED IMMUNODEFICIENCY SYNDROME

Pathogenesis and Clinical Features

The human immunodeficiency virus (HIV), a retrovirus of the lentivirus family, causes the acquired immunodeficiency syndrome (AIDS). HIV infection leads to relentless destruction of the immune system that puts all HIV-infected persons at risk of illness and death from opportunistic infectious and neoplastic complications. The great majority of AIDS cases are caused by HIV-1.[54] HIV primarily infects cells with CD4 cell surface receptor molecules, including cells of the mononuclear phagocyte system, principally CD4 lymphocytes, blood monocytes, tissue macrophages, dendritic cells, and microglial cells. HIV has the additional ability to mutate easily because its reverse transcriptase enzyme introduces a mutation approximately once every 2,000 incorporated nucleotides. The rapid turnover of HIV and CD4 lymphocytes promotes an origin of new strains of HIV that can resist immune attack, are more cytotoxic, can generate syncytia more readily, can resist drug therapy, or result in variability of pathologic lesions as different cell types are targeted or different cytopathic effects are elicited during the course of infection. The biologic properties of HIV can vary even within an individual HIV-infected person.[55,56]

A second HIV designated HIV-2 has appeared in West Africa but only sporadically elsewhere. The transmission of HIV-2 is similar to that for HIV-1, but perinatal transmission is much less frequent, there is a longer latent period before the appearance of AIDS, a less aggressive course of AIDS, and a lower viral load, with higher CD4 lymphocyte counts. This may explain the limited spread of HIV-2 (less efficient transmission, particularly via heterosexual and perinatal modes). The mortality rate from HIV-2 infection is only two-thirds that for HIV-1.[57-59]

Replication of HIV may first occur within inflammatory cells at the site of infection or within peripheral blood mononuclear cells, but replication quickly shifts to lymphoid tissues of the body, including lymph nodes, spleen, liver, and bone marrow. Besides nodes, the gut-associated lymphoid tissue provides a substantial reservoir for HIV. Macrophages and Langerhans cells in epithelia such as the genital tract are important both as reservoirs and vectors for spread of HIV because they can be HIV infected but are not destroyed. Within lymph nodes, HIV virions are trapped in the processes of follicular dendritic cells where they may infect CD4 lymphocytes that are percolating through the node. The follicular dendritic cells themselves become infected, but are not destroyed.[54]

Presence of HIV in genital secretions and blood, and to a lesser extent breast milk, is significant for spread of HIV, but transmission via saliva, urine, tears, and sweat does not routinely occur because of the low concentration of HIV in these fluids.[54,60] HIV is mainly spread as a sexually transmissible disease.[61] Transmission through parenteral exposure with injected drug use, however, is highly efficient because many more peripheral blood mononuclear cells capable of either harboring or becoming infected by HIV are in blood than are present in other body fluids. Mothers with HIV infection can pass the virus transplacentally, at the time of delivery through the birth canal, or through breast milk. Congenital AIDS occurs, on average, in about 25 to 30 percent of babies born to HIV-1-infected mothers.[62]

Acute HIV infection may produce a mild disease resembling infectious mononucleosis that diminishes over 1 to 2 months. Fever, lymphadenopathy, pharyngitis, diffuse erythematous rash, arthralgia/myalgia, diarrhea, and headache are the commonest symptoms. Biopsied lymph nodes reveal reactive changes.[54,63,64] Generally, within 3 weeks to 3 months an immune response is accompanied by a simultaneous decline in HIV viremia and presence of positive serologic HIV tests. The CD4 lymphocytes rebound in number, but not to preinfection levels.[65]

A clinically latent period of HIV infection lasts on average from 8 to 10 years, during which time enough of the immune system remains intact to prevent most infections, but viral replication actively continues in lymphoid tissues.[66] A decrease in the total CD4 count below $500/\mu l$ presages the development of clinical AIDS, and a drop below $200/\mu l$ not only defines AIDS, but also indicates a high probability for the development of AIDS-related opportunistic infections and/or neoplasms, or death.[67,68] Plasma HIV-1 RNA increases as plasma viremia becomes more marked. For perinatally acquired HIV infection, latency before clinical AIDS may be shorter than in adults.[69]

HIV-Related Lymphadenopathy

Lymphadenopathy with HIV infection can be seen in the absence of opportunistic infections and neoplasms and is termed *HIV-related lymphadenopathy* (HIVL). It can occur with primary HIV infection or at any time during progression through AIDS. Loss of normal nodal architecture as the immune system fails is marked by development of generalized lymphadenopathy with large nodes that vary in size over time but usually do not exceed 3 cm. This condition is called *persistent generalized lymphadenopathy*. At least 25 percent of persons with AIDS have lymphadenopathy at some time.[70] HIVL can be grouped into four major patterns that follow in sequence and parallel the decline in CD4 lymphocytes. With the exception of the follicular hyperplasia pattern with follicular fragmentation, which is seen most frequently in inguinal and axillary lymph nodes, these patterns appear in lymph nodes throughout the body, regardless of the presence or absence of gross lymph node enlargement, and they indicate that a single node biopsy will yield valid findings.[70,71]

Hyperplasia dominates early HIVL lesions, and the initial pattern, *follicular hyperplasia without follicular fragmentation*, demonstrates reactive follicular centers that vary widely in size and shape. The follicles may represent more than two-thirds of the cross-sectional area of the lymph node. Within the follicles are tingible body macrophages, mitoses, large lymphocytes, plasma cells, foci of hemorrhage, cytolysis, and scattered small lymphocytes singly or in clusters. The second pattern, *follicular hyperplasia with fragmentation* (Fig. 12-6), has follicles that encompass less than two-thirds of the cross-sectional area of the lymph node, and the interfollicular area contains large numbers of plasma cells, perisinus cells, sinus histiocytes, and immunoblasts. The network of dendritic reticulum cells is disrupted. Foci of hemorrhage appear in germinal centers, with necrosis and follicular infiltration by small lymphocytes as the process progresses. Mantle zones are reduced or absent. Warthin-Finkeldey type giant cells, or polykaryocytes that represent syncytia of HIV-infected lymphocytes, can be demonstrated.

With progression of HIV infection, regressive changes appear (Fig. 12-7), and the third pattern, *follicular involution*, shows more pronounced overall hypocellularity than the pre-

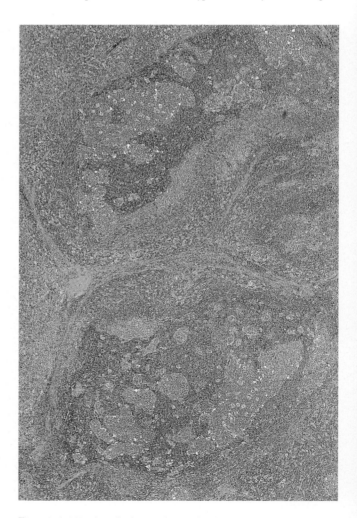

Fig. 12-6. HIV lymphadenopathy, early phase. Hyperplastic follicles are undergoing fragmentation. Hemorrhage and many tingible body macrophages are also present.

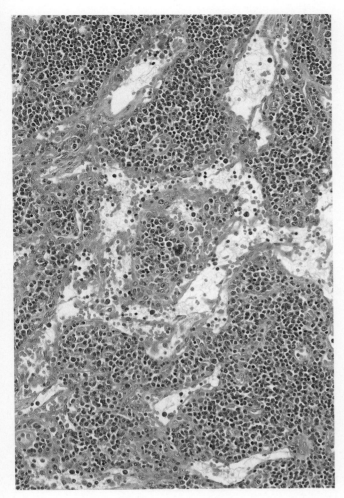

Fig. 12-7. HIV lymphadenopathy, late phase. Involution and loss of germinal centers with prominent sinuses may be seen. A multinucleated giant cell is seen in the center. (Courtesy of Glenn Segal D.O.)

ceding patterns. Follicles are present but are small and lack tingible body macrophages and mantle zones and are often hyalinized (scarred). Arborizing postcapillary venules with high endothelia are prominent. The final pattern, *follicular depletion*, has absent follicles. The lymph node cortex is narrow or undefined, and the medulla occupies two-thirds or more of the cross-sectional area. Small blood vessels appear prominent, and scattered histiocytes appear in sinuses. Immunoblasts and/or plasma cells may be seen throughout the node.[70,71]

Prior to the onset of AIDS, most nodes will have follicular hyperplasia, with or without follicular fragmentation, while almost 90 percent of AIDS patients have follicular atrophy or depletion patterns. Although nodes in AIDS can be small, they are routinely enlarged to 1 to 2 cm. During the hyperplastic phase, germinal centers contain mostly CD19+ B lymphocytes, which may account for hypergrammaglobulinemia. However, CD4 lymphocytes continue to decrease as a patient moves from follicular hyperplasia to depletion.[70,71] At least 10% of HIV-1-infected persons are long survivors, who show no marked progressive decline in immune function. In addition, their nodal

architecture is maintained, with neither the hyperplasia nor the lymphocyte depletion common with progression to AIDS. Although peripheral blood mononuclear cells contain detectable HIV-1 and viral replication continues, their viral burden is low.[72]

Opportunistic Infections

Infections seen in association with AIDS are characterized by more extensive organ involvement, dissemination to multiple organs, poor inflammatory response, decreased sensitivity of serologic testing, and diminished response to antimicrobial agents when compared with patients who do not have AIDS. The most common organ sites biopsied are lung, gastrointestinal tract, liver, lymph node, and bone marrow. Stereotaxic brain biopsy is occasionally performed. Most acute life-threatening infections will involve the lungs. For light microscopy, special stains including Gomori methenamine silver, periodic-acid Schiff, and acid-fast stain are very helpful for identifying most opportunistic infections.

Immunohistochemical staining for specific infectious agents can be helpful when the classic patterns of inflammation are lacking, when scant tissue is available, when organisms are not numerous, or when histologic appearances are ambiguous.[73]

The most common opportunistic infection is *P. carinii*, which produces an extensive pneumonia in nearly all cases and is not commonly disseminated. Bronchoalveolar lavage and/or transbronchial biopsy provide the best diagnostic yield. Atypical features are frequent and include scant intra-alveolar foamy exudate, intersititial mononuclear infiltrates, interstitial fibrosis, granuloma formation, diffuse alveolar damage, and bronchiolitis.[74] Cytomegalovirus (CMV) is frequent and can appear in any organ, but the most commonly biopsied sites are lung and gastrointestinal tract. No gross or microscopic findings are specific for CMV, although foci of inflammation, hemorrhage, and/or necrosis at any site should be searched for to show the characteristic cytomegalic cells containing intranuclear inclusions and basophilic cytoplasmic inclusions.[75]

Fungal infections are common. Candidiasis usually appears as oral thrush and sometimes produces a tracheobronchial or esophageal infection, but it is rarely disseminated. Crytococcosis often involves lung and meninges, but it can become disseminated. Histologically, the organisms often lack capsules, and inflammation is scant. Histoplasmosis and coccidioidomycosis are infrequent infections but can be widely disseminated, particularly to lung and lymphoreticular organs. Aspergillosis is not frequent but is more likely to appear with bone marrow suppression or corticosteroid therapy.[76,77]

Mycobacterial infections occur in two patterns. Infection with *Mycobacterium tuberculosis* resembles that in non-AIDS patients and is predominantly a pulmonary infection, but with more extensive and disseminated disease. The granulomas are poorly formed but show some epithelioid macrophages, Langhans giant cells, and lymphocytes. Infection with *Mycobacterium avium* complex is more disseminated but usually involves lymphorecticular organs, typically lymph nodes, spleen, and liver. Organomegaly is common, but grossly visible miliary granulomas appear infrequently, and microscopically diffuse sheets or nodular collections of large macrophages stuffed with mycobacteria are seen. Acid-fast and auramine fluorescent stains reveal many organisms, and blood or tissue cultures are helpful for diagnosis.[78,79]

Other infections include toxoplasmosis, which produces multiple acute and chronic abscesses in the brain but is less common in other organs, where mixed inflammatory infiltrates may be seen. Finding the characteristic pseudocysts can be difficult, and immunohistochemical staining can aid in recognizing tachyzoites. Herpes simplex infections appear as single or grouped vesicles on the skin or in the oral cavity, esophagus, or perianal region. Histologically, multinucleated cells with mauve to gray, ground-glass inclusions are present. Dissemination is uncommon.[80,81] Bacterial pneumonias and septicemias are common with AIDS and are best diagnosed with microbiologic culture.

Lymphoid Interstitial Pneumonitis

Lymphoid interstitial pneumonitis (LIP) is a diagnostic criterion for AIDS in childhood but is not frequently seen in adults. It must be differentiated from other infiltrative and interstitial pulmonary diseases. LIP cannot be distinguished grossly. Tissue diagnosis is made by open lung biopsy because bronchoscopic biopsies are frequently nondiagnostic. Peripheral blood may show plasmacytosis and eosinophilia.[82]

The earliest microscopic finding is hyperplasia of bronchus-associated lymphoid tissue with aggregates of lymphocytes and plasma cells in a bronchovascular distribution and minimal interstitial inflammation. In more advanced lesions, all lung fields demonstrate a diffuse interstitial infiltrate of lymphocytes, plasma cells, and histiocytes (Fig. 12-8). Additional features can include lymphoid aggregates with germinal centers, intraluminal fibrosis, increased alveolar macrophages, and type II pneumonocyte hyperplasia. Advanced cases may demonstrate confluent pulmonary nodules several centimeters in size. Rarely, poorly formed granulomas may be present, but progressive pulmonary interstitial fibrosis is rare. Unlike chronic or nonspecific interstitial pneumonitis, LIP is more florid and extensive and has a tendency to infiltrate alveolar septa. In LIP, unlike malignant lymphomas, small lymphocytes predominate, Immunohistochemical staining of questionable infiltrates will demonstrate a polyclonal cellular proliferation with LIP.[83]

A pattern of pulmonary lymphoid hyperplasia is characterized by lymphoid follicles with or without germinal centers that often surround bronchioles. The most florid form of lymphoid hyperplasia involving the lung in HIV-infected children is known as polyclonal B cell lymphoproliferative disorder (PBLD). With PBLD nodular infiltrates of polyclonal B lymphocytes and CD8 cells are seen. Other organs may be involved by PBLD.[84]

Brain Findings with AIDS

The differential diagnosis of cerebral mass lesions in AIDS includes non-Hodgkin's lymphoma, toxoplasmosis, and progressive multifocal leukoencephalopathy (PML). Lymphomas tend to be large single masses but may be infiltrative and ill defined.

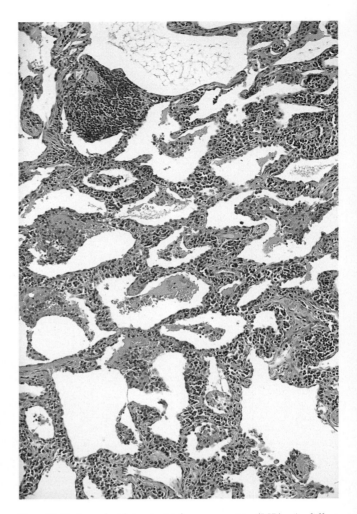

Fig. 12-8. Lymphoid interstitial pneumonitis (LIP). A diffuse interstitial infiltrate of lymphocytes, plasma cells, and histiocytes is seen, along with a small lymphoid aggregate. (Courtesy of Donald G. Guinee, Jr., M.D.)

Toxoplasmosis often produces smaller multiple masses that are ring enhancing on radiographic scans. Opportunistic infections with CMV and cryptococcosis usually do not produce mass lesions. Cryptococcosis most often produces a meningitis, but without marked inflammation. Biopsy may help to distinguish these lesions, but sampling error is often a problem.[73]

HIV infection of microglia and macrophages residing in the brain leads to a variety of changes and specific pathologic findings seen on brain biopsy, particularly in patients with dementia. Microscopic examination often reveals *HIV encephalitis*, a subacute encephalitis consisting of multiple foci with mononuclear cells typical of small macrophages, microglia, and multinucleated giant cells (Fig. 12-9). These are often seen near small blood vessels. They appear less commonly scattered in the gray matter or leptomeninges. The multinucleated giant cells, often numerous, are the hallmark of HIV infection involving the central nervous system, and HIV can be demonstrated in their cytoplasm by immunocytochemistry with antibody to gp41 or

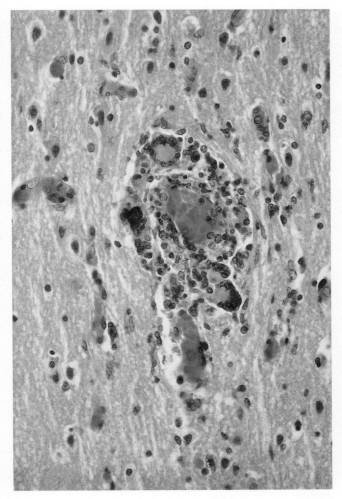

Fig. 12-9. HIV encephalitis. The cerebral cortex has perivascular inflammatory infiltrates containing prominent multinucleated cells. (Courtesy of Jeannette J. Townsend, M.D.)

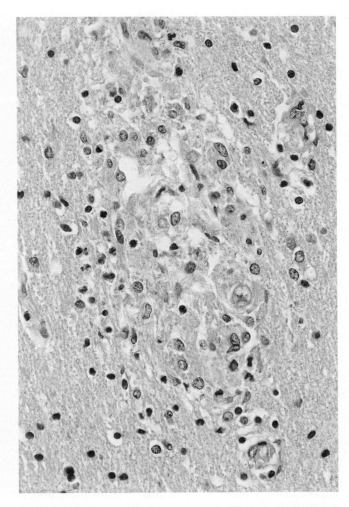

Fig. 12-10. HIV encephalitis. A microglial nodule is present containing plump reactive astrocytes and inflammatory cells, including macrophages.

by polymerase chain reaction methods utilizing antibodies to gp41 or p24.[85–87]

HIV leukoencephalopathy, which overlaps with HIV encephalitis, produces diffuse bilateral damage to cerebral and cerebellar white matter. Grossly the lesions are similar to multiple sclerosis plaques. Microscopically, the predominantly perivascular lesions demonstrate myelin debris in macrophages, reactive astrocytosis, hemosiderin in macrophages, multinucleated giant cells, and little or no inflammation. Vacuolar myelin swellings can appear, as well as axonal damage. Oligodendroglial cells appear normal. Without the presence of multinucleated giant cells, the diagnosis depends on finding of HIV antigen in macrophages.[88]

Microglial nodules in both gray and white matter are collections of plump reactive astrocytes and inflammatory cells, including macrophages (Fig. 12-10). They are often located near small capillaries that may have plump endothelial cells with nearby hemosiderin-laden macrophages. Sometimes the macrophages can give rise to multinucleated cells. Small foci of necrosis may be seen in or near these nodules. Microglial nodules are not specific for HIV infection and may be present with neoplasia, traumatic focal necrosis, or infection by viral, protozoal, or bacterial organisms. Specific etiologic agents in microglial nodules may not be present, but fungi, CMV inclusions, and *Toxoplasma gondii* can sometimes be identified. Some microglial nodules contain HIV by immunohistochemical staining.[86,88]

PML results from human papovavirus infection (designated JC virus, from the polyoma subgroup) affecting primarily white matter. PML can occur in any immunocompromised patient. Cerebrospinal fluid analysis is typically normal, although some patients may have mild protein elevations along with mononuclear cell pleocytosis. Oligoclonal bands may be found as well.[89] Myelin-producing oligodendrocytes are targeted in PML, leading to focal areas of white matter granularity a few millimeters in size that may coalesce. Abnormalities of white matter range

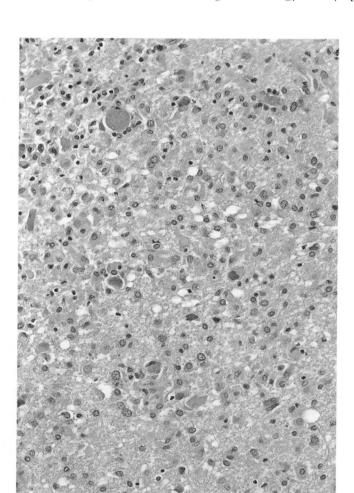

Fig. 12-11. Progressive multifocal leukoencephalopathy (PML). Astrocytosis with bizarre astrocytes, macrophages, and several large oligodendrocytes with ground glass nuclei.

from pallor to demyelination to necrosis. The gray-white matter junction is typically involved along with adjacent cortical gray matter. The lesions are usually centered around capillaries and demonstrate demyelination with perivascular monocytes, T cells, astrocytosis with bizarre or enlarged astrocytes (with occasional mitotic figures), and central lipid-laden macrophages. At the periphery are large "ballooned" oligodendrocytes infected with JC virus which have enlarged ground-glass nuclei containing viral antigen (Fig. 12-11). Immunohistochemical staining or in situ hybridization methods can help identify the JC virus. Multinucleated giant cells containing HIV may also be present.[90]

Neoplasms with AIDS

Non-Hodgkin's Lymphomas

AIDS-related lymphomas arise in polyclonal B cell proliferations from diminished immunosurveillance with decreasing CD4 lymphocyte counts, destruction of follicular dendritic cells allowing B cell clonal proliferation, chronic antigen stimulation marked by polyclonal hypergammaglobulinemia, Epstein-Barr virus (EBV) infection, and cytokine deregulation. These B cell proliferations are best characterized clinically as persistent generalized lymphadenopathy. A monoclonal proliferation eventually arises from a single clone that has accumulated sufficient genetic abnormalities. That AIDS-related lymphomas are almost always high grade helps in diagnosis, which can be difficult because tissues obtained by stereotaxic brain biopsy, bronchoscopic lung biopsy, or endoscopic gastrointestinal biopsy may be scant. Immunohistochemical staining may aid in defining a monoclonal cell population consistent with a neoplastic proliferation or in identifying the nature of lymphomatous infiltrates when necrosis is extensive.[91,92]

Grossly, non-Hodgkin's lymphomas with AIDS may appear as small infiltrates, focal nodular lesions, multicentric nodules, or larger tumor masses. Smaller lymphomatous lesions appear white to tan with irregular borders; larger masses with definable margins are accompanied by necrosis and hemorrhage, producing a variegated cut surface. Gastrointestinal tract, liver, lungs, and brain are most often affected, and lymph node and bone marrow involvement are much less frequent.[73]

Microscopically, systemic non-Hodgkin's lymphomas seen with AIDS fall into two broad categories, both of B cell origin. About one-third are classified as small noncleaved cell lymphomas (Burkitt or Burkitt-like lymphomas) in the Working Formulation classification. These lymphomas demonstrate c-myc activation in all cases, p53 mutation in some cases, and EBV infection in a minority of cases. The cells have round nuclei with one or more prominent nucleoli and scant cytoplasm arranged in diffuse sheets that form a discrete mass or intersect irregularly and infiltrate normal tissues without significant necrosis (Fig. 12-12). Uniformly distributed macrophages containing phagocytosed debris are present, and occasional mitoses are seen. Plasmablastic features including eccentric nuclei and a well defined Golgi zone may occur.[93]

The second broad category, comprising virtually all primary central nervous system lymphomas seen with AIDS and about two-thirds of systemic lymphomas, is best termed diffuse large cell lymphoma. These can be either large cell immunoblastic lymphomas or large noncleaved cell lymphomas in Working Formulation classification. They often demonstrate EBV infection and occur when the CD4 cell count is lower. These lymphomas are essentially an expansion of EBV-infected B lymphocytes.[91] The immunoblastic type consists of cells having moderate to large amounts of cytoplasm with or without plasmacytic features of eccentric nuclei and basophilic cytoplasm, large round to oval nuclei, and prominent single nucleoli. The large cell type has less cytoplasm and one or more peripheral nucleoli in a nucleus with finely dispersed chromatin. Necrosis is often a prominent feature, and mitoses are frequent.[93]

Kaposi's Sarcoma

A human herpesvirus-like agent (human herpesvirus 8) has been identified in skin lesions of Kaposi's sarcoma in both classic and AIDS-associated forms as well as in the Kaposi's sarcoma of HIV-negative homosexual men. This agent appears to be sexually transmitted independently of HIV. Although the skin is involved in over 75 percent of cases and is often the site of initial clinical presentation, visceral Kaposi's sarcoma mainly

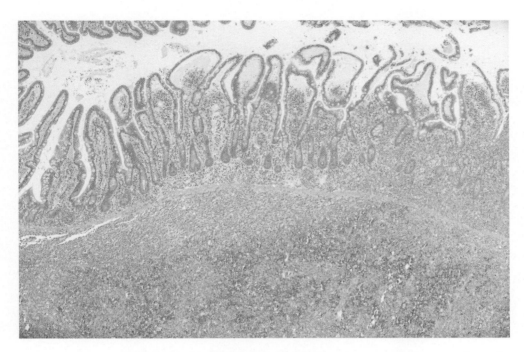

Fig. 12-12. Small noncleaved cell lymphoma in AIDS. The lymphomatous infiltrates involve the small intestinal mucosa and submucosa.

involving the lungs, lymph nodes, and gastrointestinal tract is also present in 75 percent of cases.[94–96]

Diagnosis is best made by skin biopsy. Bronchoscopic and gastrointestinal endoscopic biopsy may yield a diagnosis of Kaposi's sarcoma but these methods are hampered by sampling error because of the focal nature of the lesions. Although it is common for Kaposi's sarcoma to become widely disseminated, some patients may have only one site or focus of involvement, not necessarily skin. This sarcoma has a propensity to infiltrate around large vascular structures, near epithelial or mesothelial surfaces, or near the capsules of organs. The natural history, however, is progression over time to involve multiple sites in multiple organs.[73]

Gross and Microscopic Features

Three gross pathologic patterns of skin involvement are seen: patch, plaque, and tumor (Figs. 12-13 to 12-15). The early lesions of the *patch stage* are clinically as well as microscopically quite inconspicuous. These flat or macular blue to red-purple lesions often resemble bruises. Cutaneous lesions may occur anywhere on the trunk and extremities, but a propensity for facial involvement is seen. Lesions on the neck, upper trunk, and arms may follow the skin cleavage lines in a dermatomal distribution pattern similar to lesions of pityriasis rosea.[95]

The patch stage shows a superficial and perivascular proliferation of spindle cells arranged in parallel arrays around the vessels or beneath the epidermis. The involved vessels often appear straighter than usual and seem to cut through the dermis. The Kaposi's sarcoma cells may be fusiform to epithelioid, with eosinophilic cytoplasm and prominent round, oval, or fusiform nuclei. Nuclear pleomorphism and hyperchromatism may not be pronounced, and RBCs may not be seen. Helpful findings include individually necrotic cells, a mononuclear cell infiltrate, presence of epithelioid cells, dilated irregular vascular spaces, and perivascular distribution. Over time the perivascular spindle cell proliferation becomes more prominent and can be observed around skin appendages. RBCs are present in the slit-like spaces in association with occasional deposits of golden-brown hemosiderin granules either free or within macrophages.[97]

Stasis dermatitis of the lower legs can appear similar but has newly formed capillaries located close to the epidermis surrounded by an edematous to fibrotic dermis, often accompanied by hemosiderin granules. The patch and the *plaque stages* of Kaposi's sarcoma also show chronic inflammatory infiltrates that may be perivascular or diffuse or both and of varying severity. These infiltrates consist of lymphoid cells, plasma cells, and some histiocytes. As a result, they may resemble granulation tissue, but the presence of atypical spindle cells, large protruding endothelial cells, extravasated erythrocytes, hyaline globules, and hemosiderin pigment should suggest a diagnosis of Kaposi's sarcoma.

Grossly visible red-purple nodules varying in size from a few millimeters to several centimeters represent the *tumor stage*. A solitary nodule may be present, but multiple nodules that in severe cases may become confluent over a wide area are common. Microscopically, spindle cells are numerous, RBC extravasation is pronounced, and hemosiderin pigment is abundant. Phagocytosis of erythrocytes leads to intracytoplasmic slits and formation of erythrophagosomes that are the hyaline globules seen by hematoylin and eosin staining.[98] The entire lesion appears as a mass, although it rarely has discrete borders. Infiltration around adjacent adnexal structures or into underlying adipose tissue is common. Overlying epidermis is usually intact.

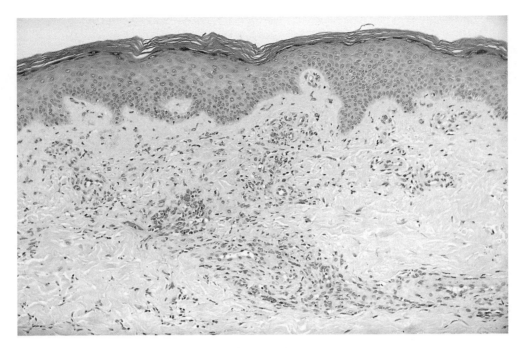

Fig. 12-13. Kaposi's sarcoma of skin. Upper dermal ill-defined vascular spaces with red blood cell extravasation are seen.

The spindle cells of Kaposi's sarcoma have features of both endothelium and smooth muscle. Immunohistochemical staining for endothelium-associated CD34 or CD31 may be helpful, since lymphatic endothelium does not contain CD34. Factor VIII-related antigen will be found in some, but not all, of the vascular portions and rarely in spindle cell components. All Kaposi's sarcoma lesions demonstrate positivity for vimentin. Radiation or chemotherapeutic effect may produce involutional changes including loss of atypical spindle cells, absence of vascular spaces, fibrosis, and extensive hemosiderin deposition. More often, treatment leads only to partial regression, with decreased numbers of atypical cells. The diagnosis is suggested at low power by the presence of a localized nodule or infiltrate.[99] Other lesions that may partially mimic Kaposi's sarcoma include bacillary (epithelioid) angiomatosis, capillary hemangioma, sclerosing hemangioma, pyogenic granuloma, papular angioplasia, amelanotic melanoma, and spindle cell squamous carcinoma.[100,101]

Miscellaneous Finding with AIDS

Hepatic steatosis is frequently identified. Lymph nodes may demonstrate deposition of amorphous pink hyaline material that is not amyloid. Hemosiderosis in spleen and liver is common. An HIV nephropathy with features similar to focal segmental glomerulosclerosis may occasionally be seen during the course of HIV infection in patients with renal failure.[102] A dilated cardiomyopathy may develop in some AIDS patients. Cervical squamous dysplasias and carcinomas are more frequently seen in women with HIV infection, whereas males having sex with other males are more likely to have anal squamous dysplasias and carcinomas. Both are also related to human pa-

pillomavirus infection.[103,104] Leiomyosarcomas have also rarely been reported in adolescent and adult AIDS patients and may be associated with EBV infection of smooth muscle cells.[105]

OTHER SECONDARY IMMUNODEFICIENCY CONDITIONS

Idiopathic CD4+ T Lymphocytopenia

Markedly decreased CD4 lymphocyte counts can appear in some persons manifesting signs and symptoms of immunodeficiency in the absence of HIV infection and are classified as having idiopathic CD4+ T lymphocytopenia. Persons with this condition may have a risk factor for HIV infection or even an opportunistic infection, but the CD4 lymphocyte count does not progressively decrease over time as with AIDS, and serum immunoglobulin levels are normal. This disorder appears to be rare and is generally associated with transient illness.[106]

Iatrogenic Immunologic Disorders

Immunosuppressive therapy with chemotherapeutic agents, corticosteroids, and cyclosporine will produce varying degrees of immune dysfunction. T lymphocytes are predominantly affected, with varying loss of humoral immunity. Patients receiving immunosuppressive therapy can develop one or more bacterial, fungal, viral, and protozoal opportunistic infections. The degree of immunosuppression in general correlates with the risk for infection. Extreme debilitation accompanying malnutrition

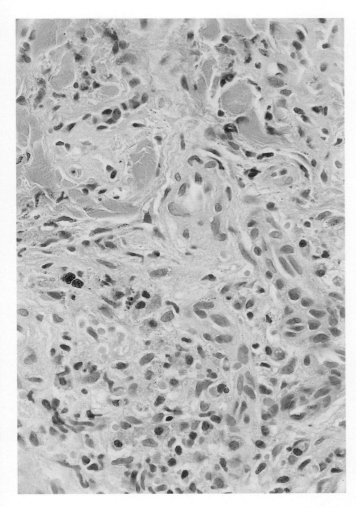

Fig. 12-14. Kaposi's sarcoma of skin. Atypical cells, hyaline globules, and hemosiderin deposition are present.

associated with poverty, dementia, and wasting with malignancies can eventually diminish immune responses enough to increase the risk of opportunistic infections.[107,108]

Post-transplantation lymphoproliferative disorder (PTLD) may occur in transplant recipients. PTLD occurs in less than 1 percent of allogeneic bone marrow recipients, in 1 to 5 percent of renal allograft recipients, and in up to 20 percent of cardiac transplant patients. Patients treated with cyclosporine or OKT3 can have onset of PTLD as early as 1 month following transplantation. A PTLD is typically an extranodal B cell proliferation of host origin associated with EBV infection that does not respond to chemotherapy or radiation. Several morphologic patterns are seen, none of which should be labeled malignant lymphoma. One pattern of PTLD is a simple reactive lymphoid hyperplasia that usually resolves spontaneously. A polymorphic PTLD pattern demonstrates cellular atypia and even invasion, but frequently responds to a reduction in immunosuppressive therapy. A monomorphic PTLD, however, less frequently responds to reduced immunosuppression and is more aggressive.[109]

Patients receiving organ transplants who require long-term

immunosuppressive therapy have an increasing risk for each year of survival of development of cancers, including lymphoproliferative disorders (leukemias, non-Hodgkin's lymphomas, and Hodgkin's disease), Kaposi's sarcoma, and carcinomas, particularly cutaneous carcinomas. Lymphomas are often extranodal, and the cutaneous carcinomas can be multifocal.[110] Patients who receive therapy with interferon or IL-2 may develop manifestations of autoimmune disease.[18]

AMYLOIDOSIS

Clinical Findings

Immunologic mechanisms may play a role in the deposition of amyloid, an abnormal proteinaceous substance that is defined by histopathologic criteria. Amyloid deposition is associated with a number of conditions including chronic infections, autoimmune diseases, aging, inherited disorders, and plasma cell dyscrasias. The most common clinical findings are weight

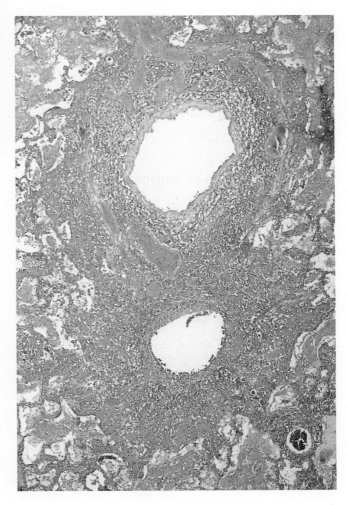

Fig. 12-15. Kaposi's sarcoma of lung. The neoplasm appears in a perivascular and peribronchial distribution.

loss, fatigue, renal failure, congestive heart failure, carpal tunnel syndrome, and peripheral neuropathy. The most commonly affected organs are heart, liver, and kidney. The gastrointestinal tract and lung are also commonly involved but generally their involvement does not lead to clinical manifestations.[111]

Nature of Amyloid

Regardless of underlying disease, amyloid appears with hematoylin and eosin stains as a homogeneous eosinophilic material between the cells of tissues and is distinguished from other pink amorphous "hyaline" deposits by its staining with alkaline Congo red (Figs. 12-16 to 12-18). In routine histologic sections from formalin-fixed and paraffin-embedded tissues, the Congo red dye will line the amyloid fibrils so that they not only appear red-orange by light microscopy, but also will have an apple-green birefringence under polarized light. By electron microscopy, amyloid appears as a beta-pleated sheet composed of fibrils ranging from 7.5 to 10 nm in width that are nonbranching and of indefinite length and associated with a P component (similar to serum C-reactive protein) that is doughnut shaped and pentagonal. Staining with thioflavin T will demonstrate amyloid by fluorescence microscopy in the blue-violet range.[111,112]

Tissue Diagnosis

Diagnosis of amyloidosis is made by tissue biopsy. Sites with a high ($\geq$ 75 percent) yield include heart, liver, skin, kidney, small intestine, sural nerve, rectum, and tongue. In addition, aspiration of the abdominal fat pad can be performed.[111] Immunohistochemical staining can be done to subclassify the amyloid proteins present.[113]

Types of Amyloidosis

Amyloidosis is subclassified based on the nature of the proteinaceous material forming the amyloid fibrils and the disease states that coexist with it. Amyloidosis can also be classified as systemic or localized. The amyloid is deposited extracellularly and interferes with organ function because it occupies space and displaces normal cellular constituents. Amyloid is often deposited in vascular walls.[112]

Immunologic Amyloidosis

The the most common type of amyloidosis seen in the United States is immunologic. The light chains (Bence Jones proteins) secreted by plasma cells with multiple myeloma contribute to amyloid formation. The fibrils are of the amyloid light chain type, and they can be deposited in any tissue, although liver, spleen, adrenal, and kidney are the most common sites of deposition.[111]

Reactive Systemic Amyloidosis

Amyloidosis can be secondary to chronic inflammatory conditions such as an autoimmune disease, tuberculosis, osteomyelitis, bronchiectasis, ulcerative colitis, or chronic skin

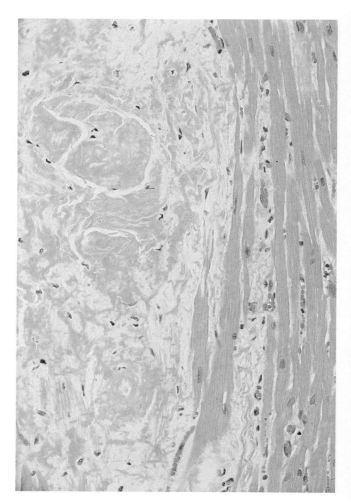

Fig. 12-16. Amyloid. Amorphous pink deposits of amyloid are seen in the heart.

infections. Malignant tumors such as Hodgkin's disease and renal cell carcinoma may also give rise to this form of amyloidosis. The fibrils are of the amyloid-associated type and are composed of a precursor serum protein known as serum amyloid-associated protein. The amyloid can be deposited in any tissue.[114]

Heredofamilial Amyloidosis

The best characterized form is *familial Mediterranean fever*, inherited as an autosomal recessive trait associated with recurrent inflammation of joints and serosal surfaces. The amyloid fibrils are composed of amyloid-associated protein derived from serum amyloid-associated protein in serum. The distribution of amyloid is widespread in tissues.[112] A variety of familial autosomal dominant conditions lead to amyloidosis, and most have as a precursor protein the serum prealbumin transthyretin. Some are associated with progressive peripheral neuropathy, whereas other forms affect the kidney, eye, and heart.[115]

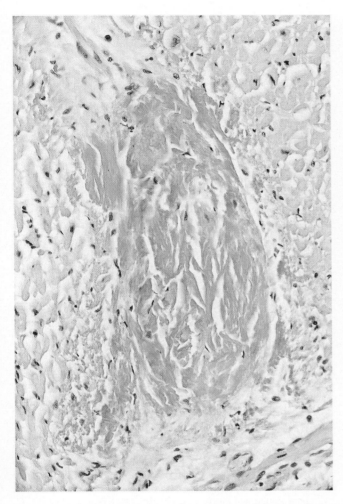

Fig. 12-17. Amyloid. An orange-red appearance with Congo red stain is seen in cardiac muscle.

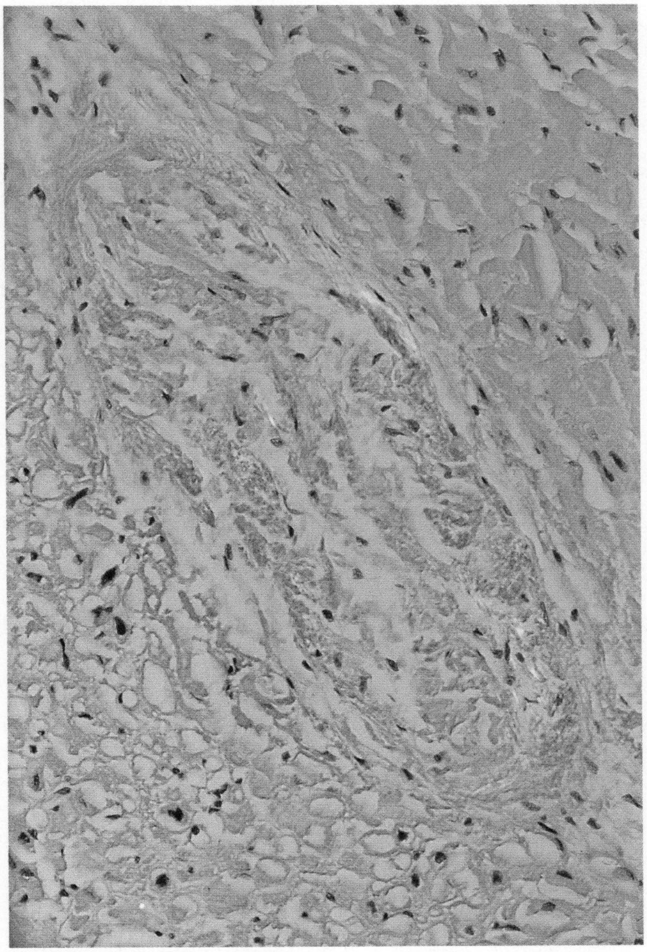

Fig. 12-18. Amyloid. When stained with Congo red and viewed under polarized light, the amyloid deposits in cardiac muscle demonstrate an apple-green birefringence

Hemodialysis-Associated Amyloidosis

Persons on long-term hemodialysis can have amyloidosis due to the retention in serum of beta-2-microglobulin, which forms the amyloid fibrils. Amyloid is mainly deposited in joint tissues.[116]

Localized Amyloidosis

Only a single organ is involved in the localized form, with nodular amyloid deposits. The lung, larynx, skin, urinary bladder, or tongue may be involved. In some of these cases, infiltrates of plasma cells may be found, and the amyloid is of the light chain type. In some endocrine neoplasms, particularly medullary carcinomas of the thyroid gland, the amyloid deposited is derived from polypeptide hormones secreted by the neoplasms. Amyloid may also be identified in the islets of Langerhans of persons with type II diabetes mellitus.[112]

Cardiac Amyloidosis

Cardiac amyloid mainly occurs in association with immunologic light chain amyloid. However, a *senile cardiac amyloidosis* involving the atria, with fibrils derived from atrial natriuretic peptide, is quite common in the elderly but is usually asymptomatic. A more significant variant results in atrial and ventricular amyloid deposition in adults and is derived from serum transthyretin protein. This latter form of amyloidosis can produce an infiltrative (restrictive) cardiomyopathy.[117]

Cerebral Amyloidosis

An amyloid angiopathy may be present in the brain either as a rare inherited condition or in association with Alzheimer's disease and with Down's syndrome. Amyloid derived from beta-amyloid (A4) protein can be present in the cores of the senile plaques or in small arteries with Alzheimer's disease and does not appear to contribute to the pathogenesis of the dementia.

Familial cerebral amyloid angiopathy can lead to significant intracerebral and subarachnoid hemorrhage caused by loss of vascular integrity.[112,118]

REFERENCES

1. Virella G: Hypersensitivity reactions. Immunol Ser 58:329–341, 1993
2. Bochner BS, Lichtenstein LM: Anaphylaxis. N Engl J Med 324:1785–1790, 1991
3. O'Hehir RE, Garman RD, Greenstein JL, Lamb JR: The specificity and regulations of T-cell responsiveness to allergens. Annu Rev Immunol 9:67–95, 1991
4. Ravetch JV, Kinet JP: Fc receptors. Annu Rev Immunol 9:457–492, 1991
5. Tan HP, Lebeck LK, Nehlsen-Cannarella SL: Regulatory role of cytokines in IgE-mediated allergy. J Leuk Biol 52:115–118, 1992
6. Borish L, Joseph BZ: Inflammation and allergic response. Med Clin North Am 76:765–787, 1992
7. Izui S: Autoimmune hemolytic anemia. Curr Opin Immunol 6:926–930, 1994
8. Kelly PT, Haponik EF: Goodpasture's syndrome: molecular and clinical advances. Medicine 73:171–185, 1994
9. Fanger MW, Erbe DV: Fc gamma receptors in cancer and infectious disease. Immunol Res 11:203–216, 1992
10. Sung MW, Yasumura S, Johnson JT, et al: Natural killer (NK) cells as effectors of antibody-dependent cytotoxicity with chimeric antibodies reactive with human squamous-cell carcinomas of the head and neck. Int J Cancer 61:864–872, 1995
11. LiVolsi VA: The pathology of autoimmune thyroid disease: a review. Thyroid 4:333–339, 1994
12. Berrih-Aknin S: Myasthenia gravis: a model of organ-specific autoimmune disease. J Autoimmun 8:139–143, 1995
13. O'Meara YM, Feehally J, Salant DJ: The nephritogenic immune response. Curr Opin Nephrol Hyperten 3:318–328, 1994
14. Tagami H: The role of complement-derived mediators in inflammatory skin diseases. Arch Dermatol Res, suppl. 1, 284:S2–S9, 1992
15. Sams WM Jr: Human hypersensitivity angiitis. Immunol Ser 46:585–604, 1989
16. Lawley TJ, Bielory L, Gascon P, et al: A prospective clinical and immunologic analysis of patients with serum sickness. N Engl J Med 311:1407–1413, 1984
17. Sylvestre DL, Ravetch JV: Fc receptors initiate the Arthus reaction: redefining the inflammatory cascade. Science 265:1095–1098, 1994
18. Schattner A: Lymphokines in autoimmunity–a critical review. Clin Immunol Immunopathol 70:177–189, 1994
19. Beck JS: Skin changes in the tuberculin skin test. Tubercle 72:81–87, 1991
20. Blanchard D, van Els C, Borst J, et al: The role of the T cell receptor, CD8, and LFA-1 in different stages of the cytolytic reaction mediated by alloreactive T lymphocyte clones. J Immunol 138:2417–2421, 1987
21. Trautwein G: Immune mechanisms in the pathogenesis of viral diseases: a review. Vet Microbiol 33:19–34, 1992
22. Parums DV: The arteritides. Histopathology 25:1–20, 1994
23. Mandell BF, Hoffman GS: Differentiating the vasculitides. Rheum Dis Clin North Am 20:409–442, 1994
24. Li PK, Leung JC, Lai FM, et al: Use of antineutrophil cytoplasmic autoantibodies in diagnosing vasculitis in a Chinese population. Am J Nephrol 14:99–105, 1994
25. Boumpas DT, Austin HA 3rd, Fessler BJ, et al: Systemic lupus erythematosus: emerging concepts. Part I. Ann Intern Med 122:940–950, 1995
26. Perez MI, Kohn SR: Systemic sclerosis. J Am Acad Dermatol 28:525–547, 1993
27. Panayi GS: The pathogenesis of rheumatoid arthritis and the development of therapeutic strategies for the clinical investigation of biologics. Agents Actions, suppl. 47:1–21, 1995
28. Lynch JP III, Hunninghake GW: Pulmonary complications of collagen vascular disease. Annu Rev Med 43:17–35, 1992
29. Kalovidouris AE: Immune aspects of myositis. Curr Opin Rheumatol 4:809–814, 1992
30. Campbell IL, Harrison LC: Molecular pathology of type 1 diabetes. Mol Biol Med 7:299–309, 1990
31. Kong MF, Jeffcoate W: Eighty-six cases of Addison's disease. Clin Endocrinol 41:757–761, 1994
32. Koshiyama H, Sato H, Yorita S, et al: Lymphocytic hypophysitis presenting with diabetes insipidus: case report and literature review. Endocrinol J 41:93–97, 1994
33. Conley ME, Fitch-Hilgenberg ME, Cleveland JL, et al: Screening of genomic DNA to identify mutations in the gene for Bruton's tyrosine kinase. Hum Mol Genet 3:1751–1756, 1994
34. Rosen FS, Cooper MD, Wedgwood RJ: The primary immunodeficiencies. N Engl J Med 333:431–440, 1995
35. Kurahashi H, Akagi K, Inazawa J, et al: Isolation and characterization of a novel gene deleted in DiGeorge syndrome. Hum Mol Gen 4:541–549, 1995
36. Levy-Mozziconacci A, Wernert F, Scambler P, et al: Clinical and molecular study of DiGeorge sequence. Eur J Pediatr 153:813–820, 1994
37. Junker AK, Driscoll DA: Humoral immunity in DiGeorge syndrome. J Pediatr 127:231–237, 1995
38. Noguchi M, Yi H, Rosenblatt HM, et al: Interleukin-2 receptor gamma chain mutation results in X-linked severe combined immunodeficiency in humans. Cell 73:147–157, 1993
39. Santisteban I, Arredondo-Vega FX, Kelly S, et al: Four new adenosine deaminase mutations, altering a zinc-binding histidine, two conserved alanines, and a 5' splice site. Hum Mutat 5:243–250, 1995
40. Stephan JL, Vlekova V, LeDeist F, et al: Severe combined immunodeficiency: a retrospective single-center study of clinical presentation and outcome in 117 patients. J Pediatr 123:564–572, 1993
41. Islam KB, Baskin B, Nilsson L, et al: Molecular analysis of IgA deficiency. Evidence for impaired switching to IgA. J Immunol 152:1442–1452, 1994
42. French MA, Denis KA, Dawkins R, Peter JB: Severity of infections in IgA deficiency: correlation with decreased serum antibodies to pneumococcal polysaccharides and decreased serum IgG2 and/or IgG4. Clin Exp Immunol 100:47–53, 1995
43. Liblau RS, Bach JF: Selective IgA deficiency and autoimmunity. Int Arch Allergy Immunol 99:16–27, 1992
44. Koskinen S, Tolo H, Hirvonen M, Koistinen J: Long-term persistence of selective IgA deficiency in healthy adults. J Clin Immunol 14:116–119, 1994
45. Sandler SG, Mallory D, Malamut D, Eckrich R: IgA anaphylactic transfusion reactions. Transfus Med Rev 9:1–8, 1995
46. Eisenstein EM, Sneller MC: Common variable immunodeficiency: diagnosis and management. Ann Allergy 73:285–292, 1994
47. Herbst EW, Armbruster M, Rump JA, et al: Intestinal B cell defects in common variable immunodeficiency. Clin Exp Immunol 95:215–221, 1994
48. Cunningham-Rundles C: Clinical and immunologic studies of common variable immunodeficiency. Curr Opin Pediatr 6:676–681, 1994
49. Sander CA, Medeiros LJ, Weiss LM, et al: Lymphoproliferative lesions in patients with common variable immunodeficiency syndrome. Am J Surg Pathol 16:1170–1182, 1992

50. Kenney D, Cairns L, Remold-O'Donnell E, et al: Morphological abnormalities in the lymphocytes of patients with Wiskott-Aldrich syndrome. Blood 68:1329–1332, 1986

51. Savitsky K, Bar-Shira A, Gilad S, et al: A single ataxia telangiectasia gene with a product similar to PI-3 kinase. Science 268:1749–1753, 1995

52. Gatti RA: Ataxia-telangiectasia. Dermatol Clin 13:1–6, 1995

53. Warren JS: Immunodeficiency diseases pp. 1580–1584. In McClatchey KD (ed): Clinical Laboratory Medicine. Williams & Wilkins, Baltimore, 1994

54. Levy JA: Pathogenesis of HIV infection. Microbiol Rev 57:183–289, 1993

55. Coffin JM: HIV population dynamics in vivo: implications for genetic variation, pathogenesis, and therapy. Science 267:483–489, 1995

56. Saag MS, Hammer SM, Lange JM: Pathogenicity and diversity of HIV and implications for clinical management: a review. J Acquir Immune Defic Syndr, suppl. 2, 7:S2–S11, 1994

57. Markovitz DM: Infection with the human immunodeficiency virus type 2. Ann Intern Med 118:211–218, 1993

58. Adjorlolo-Johnson G, DeCock KM, Ekpini E, et al: Prospective comparison of mother-to-child transmission of HIV-1 and HIV-2 in Abidjan, Ivory Coast. JAMA 272:462–466, 1994

59. Whittle H, Morris J, Todd J, et al: HIV-2 infected patients survive longer than HIV-1 infected patients. AIDS 8:1617–1620, 1994

60. Centers for Disease Control and Prevention: First 500,000 AIDS cases—United States, 1994. MMWR 44:849–853, 1995

61. Clemetson DB, Moss GB, Willerford DM, et al: Detection of HIV DNA in cervical and vaginal secretions. JAMA 269:2860–2864, 1993

62. St. Louis ME, Kamenga M, Brown C, et al: Risk for perinatal HIV-1 transmission according to maternal immunologic, virologic, and placental factors. JAMA 269:2853–2859, 1993

63. Sinicco A, Palestro G, Caramello P, et al: Acute HIV-1 infection: clinical and biological study of 12 patients. J Acquir Immune Defic Syndr 3:260–265, 1990

64. Henrard DR, Daar E, Farzadegan H, et al: Virologic and immunologic characterization of symptomatic and asymptomatic primary HIV-1 infection. J Acquir Immune Defic Syndr Hum Retrovirol 9:305–310, 1995

65. Coutlee F, Olivier C, Cassol S, et al: Absence of prolonged immunosilent infection with human immunodeficiency virus in individuals with high-risk behaviors. Am J Med 96:42–48, 1994

66. Pantaleo G, Graziosi C, Demarest JF, et al: HIV infection is active and progressive in lymphoid tissue during the clinically latent stage of disease. Nature 362:355–358, 1993

67. Centers for Disease Control and Prevention: Revised classification system for HIV infection and expanded surveillance case definition for AIDS among adolescents and adults. MMWR 41:1–19, 1992

68. Centers for Disease Control and Prevention: 1994 revised classification system for human immunodeficiency virus infection in children less than 13 years of age. MMWR 43:1–10, 1994

69. Tovo PA, deMartino M, Gabiano C, et al: Prognostic factors and survival in children with perinatal HIV-1 infection. Lancet 339:1249–1253, 1992

70. Baroni CD, Uccini S: The lymphadenopathy of HIV infection. Am J Clin Pathol 99:397–401, 1993

71. Ost A, Baroni CD, Biberfeld P, et al: Lymphadenopathy in HIV infection: histological classification and staging. Acta Pathol Microbiol Immunol Scand [Suppl] 8:7–15, 1989

72. Pantaleo G, Menzo S, Vaccarezza M, et al: Studies in subjects with long-term nonprogressive human immunodeficiency virus infection. N Engl J Med 332:209–216, 1995

73. Klatt EC, Nichols L, Noguchi TT: Evolving trends revealed by autopsies of patients with AIDS. Arch Pathol Lab Med 118:884–890, 1994

74. Saldana MJ, Mones JM: Pulmonary pathology in AIDS: atypical Pneumocystis carinii infection and lymphoid interstitial pneumonitis. Thorax, suppl. 49:S46–S55, 1994

75. Smith MA, Brennessel DJ: Cytomegalovirus. Infect Dis Clin North Am 8:427–438, 1994

76. Stansell JD: Pulmonary fungal infections in HIV-infected persons. Semin Respir Infect 8:116–123, 1993

77. Wheat LJ: Histoplasmosis and coccidioidomycosis in individuals with AIDS. A clinical review. Infect Dis Clin North Am 8:467–482, 1994

78. Barnes PF, Bloch AB, Davidson PT, Snider DE Jr: Tuberculosis in patients with human immunodeficiency virus infection. N Engl J Med 324:1644–1650, 1991

79. Klatt EC, Jensen DF, Meyer PR: Pathology of Mycobacterium avium-intracellulare infection in patients with AIDS. Hum Pathol 18:709–14, 1987

80. Tschirhart DL, Klatt EC: Disseminated toxoplasmosis in the acquired immunodeficiency syndrome. Arch Pathol Lab Med 112:1237–1241, 1988

81. Quinnan GV Jr, Masur H, Rook AH, et al: Herpesvirus infections in the acquired immune deficiency syndrome. JAMA 252:72–77, 1984

82. Moran CA, Suster S, Pavlova Z, et al: The spectrum of pathological changes in the lung in children with the acquired immunodeficiency syndrome. Hum Pathol 25:877–882, 1994

83. Travis WD, Fox CH, Devaney KO, et al: Lymphoid pneumonitis in 50 adult patients infected with the human immunodeficiency virus: lymphocytic interstitial pneumonitis versus nonspecific interstitial pneumonitis. Hum Pathol 23:529–541, 1992

84. Joshi VV, Kauffman S, Oleske JM, et al: Polyclonal polymorphic B-cell lymphoproliferative disorder with prominent pulmonary involvement in children with acquired immunodeficiency syndrome. Cancer 59:1455–1462, 1987

85. Gray F, Lescs MC: HIV-related demyelinating disease. Eur J Med 2:89–96, 1993

86. DeGirolami U, Smith TW, Hénin D, Hauw JJ: Neuropathology of the acquired immunodeficiency syndrome. Arch Pathol Lab Med 114:643–655, 1990

87. Achim CL, Wang R, Miners DK, Wiley CA: Brain viral burden in HIV infection. J Neuropathol Exp Neurol 53:284–294, 1994

88. Gray F, Gherardi R, Scaravilli F: The neuropathology of the acquired immunodeficiency syndrome (AIDS). Brain 111:245–266, 1988

89. von Einsiedel RW, Fife TD, Aksamit AJ, et al: Progressive multifocal leukoencephalopathy in AIDS: a clinicopathologic study and review of the literature. J Neurol 240:391–406, 1993

90. Hair LS, Nuovo G, Powers JM, et al: Progressive multifocal leuko-encephalopathy in patients with human immunodeficiency virus. Hum Pathol 23:663–667, 1992

91. Herndier BG, Kaplan LD, McGrath MS: Pathogenesis of AIDS lymphomas. AIDS 8:1025–1049, 1994

92. Gaidano G, Pastore C, Lanza C, et al: Molecular pathology of AIDS-related lymphomas: biologic aspects and clinicopathologic heterogeneity. Ann Hematol 69:281–290, 1994

93. Raphael, M, Gentilhomme O, Tulliez M, et al: Histopathologic features of high-grade non-Hodgkin's lymphomas in acquired immunodeficiency syndrome. Arch Pathol Lab Med 115:15–20, 1991

94. Moore PS, Chang Y: Detection of herpesvirus-like DNA sequences in Kaposi's sarcoma in patients with and those without HIV infection. N Engl J Med 332:1181–1185, 1995

95. Tappero JW, Conant MA, Wolfe SF, Berger TG: Kaposi's sarcoma: epidemiology, pathogenesis, histology, clinical spectrum, staging criteria and therapy. J Am Acad Dermatol 28:371–395, 1993

96. Serraino D, Zaccarelli M, Franceschi S, Greco D: The epidemiology of AIDS-associated Kaposi's sarcoma in Italy. AIDS 6:1015–1019, 1992

97. Niedt GW, Myskowski PL, Urmacher C, et al: Histology of early lesions of AIDS-associated Kaposi's sarcoma. Mod Pathol 3:64–70, 1990

98. Kao GF, Johnson FB, Sulica VI: The nature of hyaline (eosinophilic) globules and vascular slits of Kaposi's sarcoma. Am J Dermatopathol 12:256–267, 1990

99. Ioachim HL, Adsay V, Giancotti FR, et al: Kaposi's sarcoma of internal organs. Cancer 75:1376–1385, 1995

100. Blumenfeld W, Egbert BM, Sagebiel RW: Differential diagnosis of Kaposi's sarcoma. Arch Pathol Lab Med 109:123–127, 1985

101. LeBoit PE, Berger TG, Egbert BM, et al: Bacillary angiomatosis: the histopathology and differential diagnosis of a pseudoneoplastic infection in patients with human immunodeficiency virus disease. Am J Surg Pathol 13:909–920, 1989

102. Stone HD, Appel RG: Human immunodeficiency virus-associated nephropathy: current concepts. Am J Med Sci 307:212–217, 1994

103. Vermund SH, Kelley KF, Klein RS, et al: High risk of human papillomavirus infection and cervical squamous intraepithelial lesions among women with symptomatic human immunodeficiency virus infection. Am J Obstet Gynecol 165:392–400, 1991

104. Kiviat NB, Critchlow CW, Holmes KK, et al: Association of anal dysplasia and human papillomavirus with immunosuppression and HIV infection among homosexual men. AIDS 7:43–49, 1993

105. Zetler PJ, Filipenko D, Bilbey JH, Schmidt N: Primary adrenal leiomyosarcoma in a man with acquired immunodeficiency syndrome (AIDS). Arch Pathol Lab Med 119:1164–1167, 1995

106. Smith DK, Neal JJ, Holmberg SD: Unexplained opportunistic infections and CD4+ T-lymphocytopenia without HIV infection. N Engl J Med 328:373–379, 1993

107. Frey FJ, Speck RF: Glukokortidoide und Infekt. Schweiz Med Wochenschr 122:137–146, 1992

108. Jerrells TR: Immunodeficiency associated with ethanol abuse. Adv Exp Med Biol 288:229–236, 1991

109. Craig FE, Gulley ML, Banks PM: Posttransplantation lymphoproliferative disorder. Am J Clin Pathol 99:265–276,1993

110. Penn I: Tumors after renal and cardiac transplantation. Hematol Oncol Clin North Am 7:431–445, 1993

111. Kyle RA, Gertz MA: Primary systemic amyloidosis: clinical and laboratory features in 474 cases. Semin Hematol 32:45–59, 1995

112. Stone MJ: Amyloidosis: a final common pathway for protein deposition in tissues. Blood 75:531–545, 1990

113. Hoshii Y, Takahashi M, Ishihara T, Uchino F: Immunohistochemical classification of 140 autopsy cases with systemic amyloidosis. Pathol Int 44:352–358, 1994

114. Liepnieks JJ, Kluve-Beckerman B, Benson MD: Characterization of amyloid A protein in human secondary amyloidosis: the predominant deposition of serum amyloid A1. Biochim Biophys Acta 1270:81–86, 1995

115. Varga J, Wohlgethan JR: The clinical and biochemical spectrum of hereditary amyloidosis. Semin Arthritis Rheum 18:14–28, 1988

116. Drueke T, Touam M, Zingraff J: Dialysis-associated amyloidosis. Adv Ren Replace Ther 2:24–39, 1995

117. Hesse A, Altland K, Linke RP, et al: Cardiac amyloidosis: a review and report of a new transthyretin (prealbumin) variant. Br Heart J 70:111–115, 1993

118. Maury CP: Molecular pathogenesis of beta-amyloidosis in Alzheimer's disease and other cerebral amyloidoses. Lab Invest 72:4–16, 1995

13

Transplant Pathology

Elizabeth H. Hammond

MECHANISMS OF HUMAN ALLOGRAFT REJECTION

Although our understanding of mammalian immune regulation has been much more clearly defined in the last few years, the precise importance of various mechanisms underlying human allograft rejection is still open to considerable speculation. Allograft rejection in animals does not exactly parallel that in humans; human leukocyte antigens (HLA) important in transplantation have a different spectrum of tissue localization, and organ-specific transplantation antigens that must be playing a role in allograft rejection have not been defined.[1–3] The following discussion summarizes the current state of our knowledge concerning alograft rejection with the above caveats in mind.

When an allograft is introduced, specific T lymphocyte responses against the foreign histocompatibility (HLA) antigens of the donor are initiated.[2] T cells recognize foreign HLA class II antigens and are activated to proliferate, differentiate, and secrete a panel of soluble growth differentiation factors called cytokines. These cytokines induce further expression of HLA class II antigens on grafted tissue, stimulate B lymphocytes to produce antibodies against determinants on the transplant, and facilitate the development of specific effector functions, including cytotoxicity and cytokine-mediated effector functions (similar to delayed hypersensitivity responses) mediated by CD4+ lymphocytes and macrophages. Damage to the allograft occurs by direct parenchymal injury or indirectly by vascular damage in the allograft leading to ischemic changes.[2] Figure 13-1 depicts these interactions.

HLA Molecules and Antigen Recognition

Transplants from genetically different persons are rejected because of the barrier imposed by alloantigens and coded by the major histocompatibility complex (MHC).[4] The human MHC, called the HLA complex, encompasses about 4,000 kb on the short arm of chromosome 6 and contains multiple genes.[5] It encodes the polymorphic cell-associated glycoproteins, class I molecules (HLA-A, -B, and -C), and class II molecules (HLA-DP, -DQ, and -DR), which determine the recognition of antigen by T lymphocytes. Class I molecules are constitutively expressed by most cells and tissues, most strongly by the vascular endothelium and lymphoid cells.[6] Class II molecules are con-

stitutively expressed only by a small number of cell types, including B lymphocytes, monocytes, follicular dendritic cells, and capillary endothelial cells. However, class II antigen expression can be induced on a variety of cells by cytokines such as interferon-gamma (IFN-gamma) and tumor necrosis factor-alpha (TNF-alpha).[2,3,7] Cells whose class II molecules are up-regulated under such circumstances include activated T lymphocytes, endothelial cells, renal tubular epithelial cells, liver bile duct epithelial cells, and pancreatic beta cells. MHC expression by the graft is very important because T cell recognition of foreign antigen requires the participation of MHC molecules.[8] The antigen receptors of T lymphocytes interact specifically with the composite ligand, made up of a peptide fragment of a foreign protein bound in the peptide binding groove of an MHC molecule. The physiologic function of the MHC molecules is thus to present antigens to the receptors of T cells.[4] The interaction between T cell receptors and HLA peptide complexes presumably evolved to allow the recognition of foreign peptides in the context of the host HLA, to destroy infected cells. In transplant rejection, however, foreign HLA is recognized in association with host peptides or foreign peptides, or both. Thus, the surfaces presented by foreign HLA peptide complexes to host T cell receptors will be different in both the HLA molecules and the bound peptide. This property, coupled with the diversity of bound peptides, probably accounts for the high number of T lymphocytes that are stimulated by foreign HLA antigens.[9]

The great polymorphism of MHC molecules provides a mechanism for increasing the number of peptides that can be presented. Increasing the number of different MHC molecules expressed by a person expands the range of peptides that can be bound and broadens T cell responsiveness. Class I and class II loci are highly polymorphic; most humans express six different molecules of each class. Thus it is likely that unrelated humans will have different HLA types. The phenomenon of transplant rejection is a direct consequence of the advantage to the species of having more HLA types so that the likelihood of encountering a pathogen against which all members of a population have a poor response generally decreases.[8,10]

Antigen-Presenting Cells

Antigen-presenting cells, present in the graft, are critical to the process of T cell activation. Such cells consist of dendritic reticulum cells, macrophages, and endothelial cells of the graft

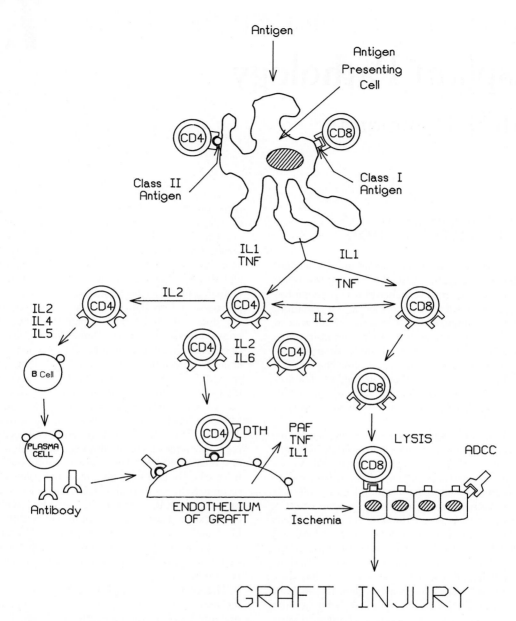

Fig. 13-1. Allograft rejection. Diagram illustrating the interaction of recipient cells with solid organ allograft tissue. (Figure drawn by Thomas H. Hammond.)

venules and capillaries.[11,12] By virtue of their capacity to express MHC II antigens, these cells are able to activate CD4-expressing lymphocytes, which then produce interleukin-2 (IL-2), leading to proliferation of CD4- and CD8-expressing cells.[2,3]

T Cell Activation

The initiation of an immune response depends on the antigen-specific interaction of the T cell receptor with alloantigen and leads to T cell activation. Within seconds to minutes of their addition to T cells, alloantigens induce a variety of bio-

chemical events that induce T cells to produce cytokines, proliferate, and differentiate. The initial event is the rise in cytoplasmic free calcium, which is thought to result from the action of the inositoltriphosphate on a specific receptor, leading to calcium release.[13] Other messengers are certainly involved, including protein kinase C, phosphoryl lipase C, and tyrosine kinase. After these complex biochemical changes, the early consequences of T cell activation include the expression of cytokines that act on a variety of cells, starting with (IL-2).[14] A little later, IL-3 is produced and stimulates the proliferation of stem cells, which can in turn differentiate into granulocytes and macrophages. IFN-gamma is also produced, inducing the expression of MHC class II molecules on endothelial cells and monocytes and triggering other macrophage functions. B cell growth and the differentiation factors IL-4, IL-5, and IL-6 induce clonal expansion of B cells that have been stimulated by specific antigen, leading to the production of specific antibodies. After this burst of cytokine production, T cells divide under the influence of IL-2 and IL-4 and begin to assume different effector functions such as cytotoxicity. Finally, a group of very late activation molecules is produced 7 to 14 days after stimulation.

Accessory Molecules

Associated with the T cell receptor on the cell surface is the CD3 molecular complex. These CD3 polypeptides assemble with the T cell receptor intracellularly; the complex is then transported to the cell surface. The relative contribution of these CD3 peptides to receptor conformation and signal transduction is still unknown.[15] The interaction of host lymphocytes with donor antigens is not limited to the antigen-specific complexes of T cell receptors with HLA molecules and CD3. At least five additional pairs of accessory molecules can contribute to this interaction. These antigen-independent receptor-ligand pairs are involved to various degrees in cell adhesion, activation (signal transduction), and specific effector function. It is now known that the CD4 molecule binds MHC class II molecules and that the CD8 molecule binds MHC class I molecules. Thus, the CD4 subset of peripheral blood lymphocytes reacts preferentially with MHC class II molecules, whereas CD8 cells react preferentially with MHC class I molecules. These receptor-ligand pairs increase the avidity of interaction between the T cells and targets. Other lymphocyte receptor-ligand pairs are shown in Table 13-1.[1,16–18]

Mechanisms of Effector Function in Allograft Rejection

Specific and Nonspecific Cytotoxicity

CD8+ cells can differentiate into cytotoxic cells that are specific for single cell surface antigens (cytotoxic T lymphocytes [CTL]). The mechanism by which such CTLs develop from CD8+ T lymphocytes is complex and incompletely understood. However, this process is triggered by recognition of MHC class I specificities in concert with the T cell receptor.[1–3,19–21] Such mature CTLs then specifically bind to their target tissue and deliver a lethal hit. Three potential mechanisms of this cytotoxicity are under investigation: pore formation in target cells produced by pore-forming proteins (perforins, cytolysins); release of cytokines such as TNF-beta that may injure the cell membrane directly; or release of proteolytic enzymes such as serine esterases that may damage the cell membrane directly or activate cytotoxic precursors.[2,3,19]

Nonspecific cytotoxic cells such as macrophages and natural killer cells may bind to target parenchymal cells in the allograft via Fc receptor binding of specific IgG bound to such cells. Macrophages are capable of causing cytocidal activity via secretion of proteases. They also accelerate inflammation and repair. This mechanism, known as antibody-dependent cell-mediated cytotoxicity, may be activated with or without participation of complement.[20,21]

Cytokine-Mediated Effector Function (Delayed Type Hypersensitivity)

Cytokine production is initiated by CD4+ sensitized cells that have recognized the antigen on antigen-presenting cells or vascular endothelium in association with MHC class II molecules. Such specifically sensitized CD4 cells then secrete cytokines (IL-1, IL-2), which recruit other CD4+ cells and recruit and activate macrophages.[22,23] Graft destruction is then instigated by microvascular injury, ischemia, and macrophage cytotoxicity. Such mononuclear phagocytes are an essential component of graft inflammatory responses. They act as antigen-presenting cells in grafts and, by virtue of their activation in the context of antigen recognition, produce a variety of cytokines that amplify the immune response. IFN-gamma, produced by such cells, is capable of transforming blood-borne monocytes into mature tissue macrophages. IL-1, secreted primarily by such cells, mobilizes polymorphonuclear leukocytes (particularly eosinophils) and acts as a potent fibroblast-activating factor.[24,25] IFN-gamma and IL-1 are also produced by activated endothelial cells, which in addition produce platelet activating factor (PAF) and amplify the inflammatory consequences of cytokine-mediated reactions.[22–24] Several studies have looked at expression of cytokines in human tissues undergoing rejection using in situ hybridization or polymerase chain reaction techniques. IL-1, IL-2, IL-4, IL-5, IL-6, IFN-gamma, and TNF have all been found in rejection allografts as opposed to non-rejection allografts. The expression of these factors in infection as opposed to rejection has not been described.[25–27] IL-2 and IL-2 receptor also appear in the blood and urine during acute rejection. Studies have evaluated the diagnostic utility using serum enzyme-linked immunosorbent assays and found no significant value because levels are similarly elevated in the presence of infection of the allograft.[28,29] Table 13-2 catalogues the cytokines important in allograft rejection.

Table 13-1. Receptor-Ligand Pairs in the Interaction Between T Lymphocytes and Targets

Receptor	Ligand
T cell receptor	HLA and peptide
CD4	HLA-DR (MHC class II)
CD8	HLA-A, -B, -C (MHC class I)
CD11a, -18 (LFA-1; integrin)	ICAM-1, ICAM-2
CD2 (LFA-2; erythrocyte rosette receptor)	LFA-3
CD44 (receptor for hyaluronic acid)	Addressin

Abbreviations: LFA, leukocyte function-associated antigen; ICAM, intercellular adhesion molecule.

Table 13-2. Cytokines That Mediate Allograft Rejection

Cytokine	Source	Target Cells and Biologic Properties
IL-1	Virtually any cell, including monocytes, macrophages, endothelial cells, keratinocytes, and glial cells	Activates resting T cells; is a cofactor for other hematopoietic growth factors; induces sleep, fever, corticotropin release, and other systemic acute-phase responses; stimulates synthesis of other lymphokines (IL-2, IFN-gamma); stimulates production of collagenases; increases bone resorption by osteoclasts; activates macrophages; renders endothelial cells more adhesive for leukocytes
TNF-alpha	Macrophages, activated T cells, NK cells	Mimics many actions of IL-1 on T cells, B cells, macrophages, and endothelial cells; induces acute phase reactions; inhibits lipoprotein lipase in fat cells; inhibits hematopoietic stem cells; cytotoxic to parenchymal cells by triggering apoptosis
TNF-beta (lymphotoxin)	Activated T cells	Produces parenchymal cell lysis without contact by triggering apoptosis
IL-2	Activated T cells	Stimulates growth of activated T and B cells; activates and promotes growth of NK cells; activates monocytes
IL-4	Activated T cells	Growth and differentiation factor for activated B and T cells; growth factor for mast cells; increases expression of HLA class II antigens on B cells
IL-5	Activated T cells	Induces differentiation of activated B cells into antibody-producing plasma cells
IL-6	Activated T cells, fibroblasts, monocytes	Enhances maturation of activated T and B cells; stimulates growth of hematopoietic progenitor cells; inhibits growth of fibroblasts
IFN-gamma	Activated T cells, NK cells	Activates macrophages and induces expression of HLA class II molecules on macrophages and many other cells; suppresses hematopoietic progenitor cells; activates endothelial cells; antiviral activity

Abbreviations: IL, interleukin; TNF, tumor necrosis factor; IFN, interferon; NK, natural killer.

Antibody-Mediated Effector Function

Specific sensitization of CD4+ cells and generation of IL-2, IL-4, and IL-5 promote B cell differentiation and generation of antigraft antibodies, which can promote graft destruction via antibody-dependent cell-mediated cytotoxicity or complement-mediated cytotoxicity, or both mechanisms. Activation of mononuclear phagocytes leads to activation of the arachidonic acid pathway, leading to thrombocyte aggregation and accumulation. Finally, such activation also leads to activation of the extrinsic coagulation pathway via tissue factor. These effects ultimately lead to vascular endothelial injury, fibroblast proliferation, and occlusive vasculopathy with tissue ischemia. The contribution of these factors to chronic rejection is therefore very important.[20,21,30,31]

PATHOLOGIC MANIFESTATIONS OF ACUTE ALLOGRAFT REJECTION

Acute Cellular Rejection of Allografts

Lymphoid and Macrophage Infiltrates

The most common manifestation of allograft rejection is the infiltration of the allograft by lymphocytes, which presumably are

there to destroy the parenchyma of the graft. Pathologically, this process is recognized by finding large numbers of activated lymphocytes (accompanied by macrophages) infiltrating parenchymal structures of the allograft, such as the kidney tubules, the cardiac myocytes, the bronchioles, or the bile ducts.[32–35] The lymphoid infiltrate may be accompanied by small numbers of other inflammatory cells such as neutrophils or eosinophils. The process of acute cellular rejection in bone marrow is not often appreciated pathologically; destruction of the bone marrow takes place without observation and is manifested by lack of adequate numbers of leukocytes in the circulation and of precursor cells in the marrow.[36] The pathologic features of allograft rejection are illustrated in Figures 13-2 to 13-4.

Vascular Infiltration of Lymphocytes (Endothelialitis)

Since the infiltrating cells arrive in the allograft via the blood, adherence and penetration of the capillaries, arterioles, and venules by lymphoid cells is often considered a part of the rejection process.[37–39] The notable exception to this involvement of the microvasculature in descriptions of the rejection process is the heart, in which involvement of the microvasculature is ignored.[40] In other solid organ allografts, endothelialitis (endothilitis) is a well recognized part of acute rejection, making the diagnosis of significant allograft rejection more certain. In the kidney, for example, the involvement of arteries or

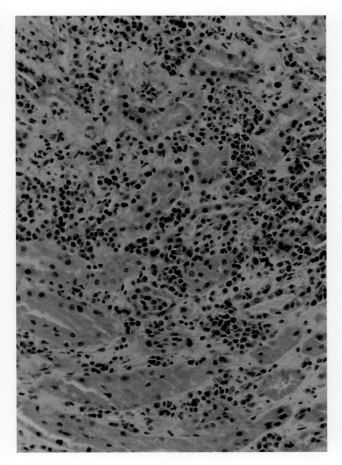

Fig. 13-2. Lymphoid cells are generally invading the renal tubules in this photograph of a kidney biopsy with acute cellular rejection.

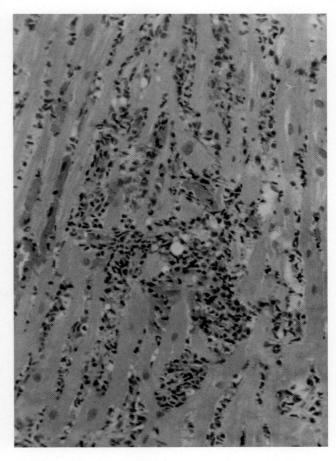

Fig. 13-3. Cardiac biopsy illustrating the architectural distortion of myocytes by invading lymphoid cells. Macrophages as part of the infiltrate are difficult to appreciate. Myocyte damage can be assumed because of the distorted arrangement of myocytes. This biopsy is thus an example of moderate cellular rejection, International Society for Heart and Lung Transplantation (ISHLT) grade 3A.

Table 13-3. Acute Cellular Rejection Features

Organ	Primary Target	Endothelial Target	Differential Diagnosis
Kidney	Tubular epithelial cells	Microvasculature, arterioles (50% of acute rejection involves arterioles)	Infection, ischemia, cyclosporine toxicity, acute tubular damage, interstitial nephritis
Heart	Myocytes	None specified as part of process; arteriolitis rare	Ischemia, biopsy site artifact, Quilty lesion, infection
Liver	Bile duct epithelium	Venulitis of portal and central veins; endothelialitis secures diagnosis of rejection	Hepatitis, drug toxicity, bile duct obstruction, sepsis, ischemia, hyperalimentation toxicity
Lung	Bronchioles, alveolar lining cells	Arteriolitis/venulitis necessary for diagnosis of moderate rejection	Infection, BALT, biopsy site, ischemia
Bone marrow (GVHD)	Keratinocytes, intestinal lining cells, bile duct epithelium, salivary glands	None known	Chemotherapy, radiation effects

Abbreviations: GVHD, graft-versus-host disease; BALT, bronchus-associated lymphoid tissue.

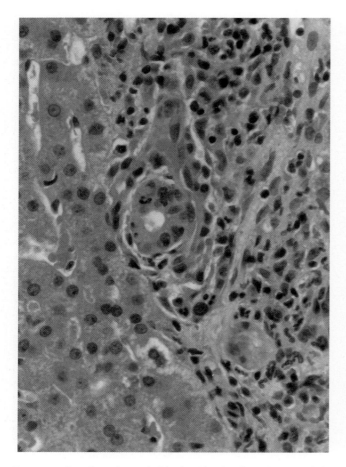

Fig. 13-4. Portal triad invaded by lymphoid cells and eosinophils. Vascular changes are inapparent. Since endothelialitis and a mixed infiltrate was seen in more than 50 percent of portal triads, the process was considered moderate cellular rejection. The liver parenchyma shown at lower left is unaffected.

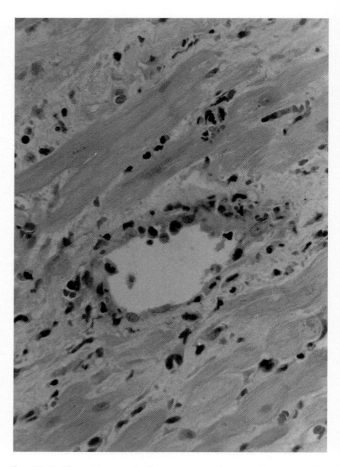

Fig. 13-5. Photomicrograph illustrating venulitis involving a cardiac biopsy. Lymphoid cells obviously invade this venule. No appreciable cellular rejection was apparent, but interstitial edema was obvious. Biopsy showed moderate vascular rejection. (From Hammond et al,[61] with permission.)

arterioles is found in 50 percent of acute cellular rejection, is designated as a pathognomonic feature, and is considered a poor prognostic feature.[37] In the liver, the endothelialitis involving venules is necessary to exclude other causes of inflammation of portal regions.[41] Table 13-3 illustrates the differences in the rejection findings in various solid organ allografts. Figures 13-5 and 13-6 illustrate the pathologic features in heart and liver allografts.

Differential Diagnosis of Acute Cellular Rejection

The major differential diagnosis of this process is infiltration of the allograft by lymphocytes for other reasons. In the kidney, infection may also cause an infiltrate that appears to invade tubular epithelium.[42] In the heart, lymphocytes are very uncommon, and are only found, associated with scarring, at the sites of pre-

Table 13-4. Grading Schema for Acute Rejection of Kidney Allografts

Grade	Banff Designation	Description
No rejection	g0, l0, t0, v0	No infiltrates or minimal ones; no tubulitis
Mild rejection	g0–1, l1, t1, v0–1	Infiltrate of lymphocytes occupying <50% of cortex; tubulitis
Moderate rejection	g0–2, l2, t2, v1–2	Infiltrate of lymphocytes occupying 50–100% of cortex; tubulitis and endothelialitis of arteries in 50%
Severe rejection	g1–3, l3, t3, v3	Mixed infiltrate of lymphocytes, eosinophils, and neutrophils; tubulitis and endothelialitis; vasculitis with/without thrombosis

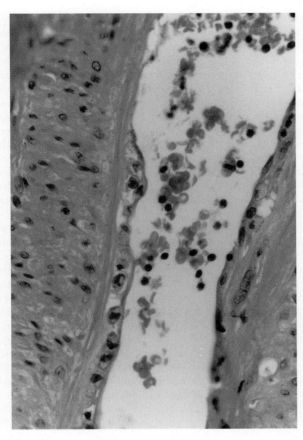

Fig. 13-6. This artery from a liver biopsy contains lymphoid cells infiltrating under the vascular endothelium. Such arteries are rarely found in biopsy specimens. Endothelialitis is much more commonly appreciated when it involves veins and arterioles.

vious biopsy or associated with ischemic damage related to transplantation.[43] In the lung, inflammation of bronchioles and interstitial spaces is also associated with infection of the lung, such as pneumonia.[44] In liver allografts, the portal regions often contain a few inflammatory cells such as lymphocytes, so that finding a portal infiltrate of lymphocytes is nonspecific.[45]

Grading the Severity of the Rejection Process

In each of these allografts, the severity of the process is considered and reported if the diagnosis of allograft rejection is established. The rules for each site are somewhat different, but all depend on an evaluation of the extensiveness of the infiltration process and the aggressiveness of the infiltration, that is, the amount of associated parenchymal damage. Grading schemes for the various allografts are given in Tables 13-4 to 13-7, and the reader is referred to the references for further information.[38–46]

Immunologic Mechanisms Related to Tissue Immunocytochemistry

With the advent of more sophisticated immunocytochemical techniques, it has become possible to evaluate the types of cells involved in the acute rejection process. Numerous CD4+ and CD8+ lymphocytes can be seen. Since the characteristics of the infiltrating cells may be altered by immunosuppression, the importance of these observations is doubtful. No opportunities exist to look at the composition of infiltrates in untreated human recipients. Therefore, studies of infiltrate composition cannot be reliably related to effector mechanisms. Since both CD4+ and CD8+ cells are found, it is likely that both cytokine-mediated and cytotoxic lymphocyte-mediated effector mechanisms are operative. Macrophage markers have also been evaluated. It is known that at least half of the infiltrating cells in most allografts are macrophages. Furthermore, the macrophages commonly express activation markers, suggesting that they are playing a role in antigen recognition as well as in nonspecific cytotoxicity.[47–50] Looking for macrophage activation markers is difficult except in frozen sections; therefore, we have little reliable information in human allograft systems. The same difficulty exists when looking for expression of vascular adhesion molecules such as intercelluler adhesion molecule or vascular cell adhesion molecule or cytokines like IL-2. The information is largely anecdotal. Studies evaluating amounts of production of these factors are also inconclusive, since it is rare for serial studies of allografts to be done in controlled settings. Evidence of cytokine-mediated allograft rejection is difficult to assess pathologically. Cytokine messenger (m)RNA can only be sought from fresh or frozen tissue or sections, and cytokine ex-

Table 13-5. Grading Schema for Acute Rejection of Heart Allografts

Grade	ISHLT Designation	Description
No rejection	0	No rejection
Focal mild	1A	One focus of interstitial lymphocytes
Diffuse mild	1B	Diffuse infiltrate of lymphocytes in one or more pieces
Focal moderate	2	One focus of space-occupying lymphoid infiltrate with myocyte damage
Multifocal moderate	3A	Multiple foci of space-occupying infiltrates of lymphocytes
Borderline severe	3B	Diffuse space-occupying infiltrates of lymphocytes in >75% of area
Severe	4	Polymorphic infiltrate of lymphocytes and neutrophils associated with edema, hemorrhage, and vasculitis

Abbreviation: ISHLT, International Society for Heart and Lung Transplantation.

Table 13-6. Grading Schema for Acute Cellular Rejection of Liver Allografts

Grade	Description
No rejection	No significant mixed infiltrates in portal triads
Consistent with/suggestive of rejection	Mixed infiltrate of lymphocytes and eosinophils in <50% portal regions; bile duct damage minimal
Mild rejection	Mixed infiltrate of lymphocytes and eosinophils in <50% of portal triads; bile duct damage, endothelialitis of venules and central veins
Moderate rejection	Mixed infiltrate involving >50% of triads with/without endothelialitis of venules
Severe rejection	Central balloon cell degeneration of hepatocytes with giant cells and/or vanishing bile ducts (manifestations of arteriopathy)

pression is relatively nonspecific, being also associated with inflammation and vascular ischemic damage.[51–54]

Acute Antibody-Mediated Rejection of Allografts

Hyperacute Rejection

In virtually all allografts, processes of rejection are described in which the allograft is lost due to deposition of preformed alloantibody directed against the graft in the newly ingrafted organ. Such rejection responses are usually rapid and occur in situations in which the recipient has circulating alloantibodies at the time of transplantation, typically against HLA antigens of the donor.[55,56] Since the advent of more sophisticated tissue typing methods, most donors and recipients are HLA typed prior to allografting, and cross-matches are performed to detect reactivity of recipients' serum antibodies directed against donor peripheral blood cells as antigens. Allografting across such barriers is rare for kidney tranplants. Cardiac and lung transplant recipients are often transplanted before cross-match results are available because of the short length of time that hearts and lungs can be perfused prior to tranplantation. Patients with circulating levels of panel-reactive antibodies greater than 20 percent are very likely to have positive cross-matches to many donors and are therefore prospectively cross-matched to prevent hyperacute rejection.[57] This makes the availability of organs much more limited for these patients. Liver transplant recipients rarely experience hyperacute rejection even in the presence of a positive cross-match, although hyperacute rejection has been reported. The cause of this resistence to hyperacute rejection is unknown, but it may relate to the availability of Kupffer cells to process the antigen-antibody complexes.[41,58]

Pathology of Hyperacute Rejection

The pathology of hyperacute rejection is nonspecific and depends on the time after transplant at which a biopsy is performed and how it is examined. Often, the organ is not biopsied and is received by the surgical pathologist as an explanted organ or is examined only at postmortem examination. Gross descriptions of the events by the surgeon may provide important clues to the correct diagnosis. Often, in such cases, the organ immediately appears well perfused and pink, after which it suddenly blanches and ceases to function. Attempts to improve the graft perfusion are usually unsuccessful, and the organ is removed in the case of kidney allografts. In liver, lung, or cardiac allografts, circulatory support for the allograft is often undertaken because the consequence of removal is a need for immediate retransplantation.

Microscopically, allografts lost to hyperacute humorally mediated rejection show a paucity of findings. Interstitial edema and hemorrhage are seen, and perhaps margination of neutrophils in capillaries and venules. If the process is prolonged, the allograft will show evidence of ischemia with parenchymal necrosis. Occasionally, thrombosis is also seen. If frozen tissue is available, the allograft may be examined immunocytochemically to detect antibody. In such cases, the antibody is detected attached to capillaries, venules, and arterioles.[57,58] Associated complement components are also found. Fibrin may or may not be present in the vessels and interstitium, depending on the duration of the post-transplant period. The mechanism of such responses is well characterized in animal models. Antibody is deposited on the vascular endothelium, which is rich in the HLA antigen(s) to which the antibody is directed. This de-

Table 13-7. Grading Schema for Acute Cellular Rejection of Lung Allografts

Grade	ISHLT Designation	Description
Minimal rejection	A1	Perivenular lymphoid infiltrates
Mild rejection	A2	Perivascular infiltrates of lymphocytes and eosinophils with endothelialitis and bronchiolitis
Moderate rejection	A3	Perivascular and alveolar infiltrates including neutrophils, endothelialitis, endothelial hyperplasia
Severe	A4	Confluent diffuse infiltrates with vasculitis and alveolar damage, necrosis, and hemorrhage
Lymphoid bronchitis	B1[a]	Lymphocytic infiltration of bronchi
Lymphoid bronchiolitis	B2[a]	Lymphocytic infiltration of terminal and respiratory bronchioles

[a] B lesions are not part of acute rejection; these lesions may be precursors to chronic rejection.

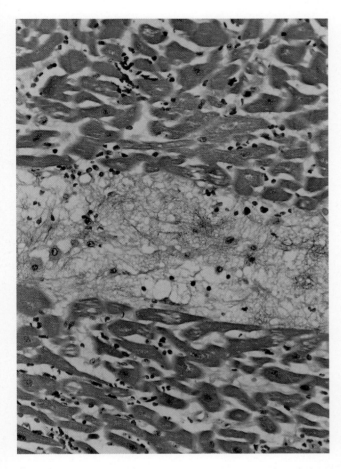

Fig. 13-7. Significant fibrillar edema seen in the interstitium of a heart that was rejected hyperacutely. Myocytes were focally hypereosinophilic and neutrophils are seen strewn around myocytes, suggesting ischemic damage.

posited antibody fixes complement components that attract neutrophils and promote tissue damage and destruction of the vessel walls. Such antibody and complement deposition also leads to elaboration of cytokines by the vascular endothelium, which aggravates the damage by increased inflammatory responses. The result of this reaction is the destruction of the microcirculation of the allograft, leading to ischemic damage and allograft loss.[37,41,44,59,60] An example of hyperacute rejection is shown in Figure 13-7.

Accelerated Antibody-Mediated Rejection

The antibody-mediated (humoral) reactions that take place in allografts are fortunately uncommon. Recipients may lack high levels of circulating antibodies at the time of transplantation, but develop them later in response to the massive antigen shedding that takes place shortly after transplantation. These antibodies may accumulate slowly and may damage the allograft in a more subtle fashion.

Microscopically, such rejection reactions resemble vasculitis or capillaritis, because they are manifested by adherence to and penetration of vascular walls by inflammatory cells (neutro-

phils, eosinophils, macrophages, and lymphocytes) and are associated with endothelial injury and fibrinoid necrosis of vascular walls.[37,41,40,58] Immunocytochemically, one can demonstrate that the process is humorally mediated. The allograft vasculature displays immunogobulin and complement components.[59,61] Figures 13-8 and 13-9 illustrate the pathologic features of accelerated cardiac rejection.

In kidney transplants, these deposits are localized to the arterioles and arteries; in cardiac vessels, deposits are found in the microvasculature. They can be detected by immunocytochemical evaluation of frozen sections of the allograft.

CHRONIC ALLOGRAFT VASCULOPATHY (CHRONIC REJECTION)

The long-term survival of solid organ allografts is compromised by the development of chronic vasculopathy, a form of chronic rejection.[62–64] Large arteries supplying the allografted organ with blood are slowly narrowed by concentric intraluminal fibrosis. This process develops slowly over time and eventually results in allograft loss due to vascular compromise. In cardiac trans-

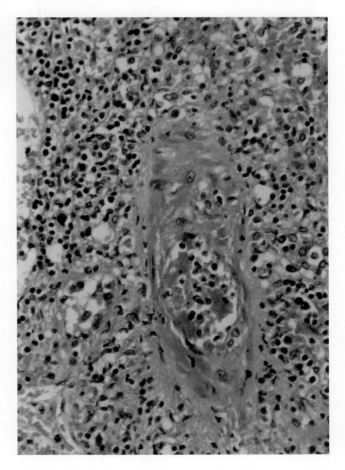

Fig. 13-8. A kidney biopsy with severe accelerated rejection contains a vessel with fibrinoid necrosis of the arterial wall (center).

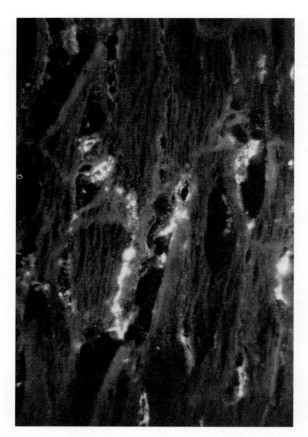

Fig. 13-9. Photomicrograph illustrating the accumulation of IgG in the capillaries of a cardiac biopsy with humoral rejection. Positive staining is seen as bright linear profiles. Areas staining also showed staining with antibody directed against HLA-DR, highlighting the distribution as vascular. No cellular infiltrates were seen histologically, and the patient responded to plasmapheresis. Slide incubated with fluorescein isothiocyanate labeled anti-human IgG. (× 250.) (From Hammond et al,[61] with permission)

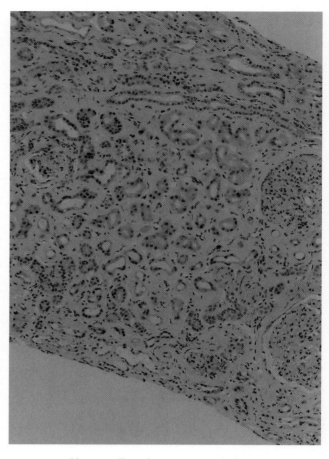

Fig. 13-10. Chronic allograft rejection in kidneys manifests by interstitial fibrosis and tubular atrophy. Biopsy contained a large artery with subintimal fibrous proliferation. No acute tubular damage is associated with the fibrosis and atrophy, making the differential diagnostic choice of cyclosporine nephrotoxicity unlikely.

plantation, up to 10 percent of patients develop allograft vasculopathy each year after transplantation. Ultimately, it is this process that causes allograft loss in most long-surviving transplant recipients.

Pathologic Manifestations of Vasculopathy

In each allograft the consequences of allograft vasculopathy are those of chronic ischemic damage, although the pathologic manifestations are organ specific (Table 13-8).

Table 13-8. Chronic Vasculopathy

Organ	Obliterative Vasculopathy	Parenchymal Manifestations	Differential Diagnosis
Kidney	Yes, with allograft loss	Tubular loss, interstitial fibrosis, periglomerular fibrosis	Cyclosporine or FK506 toxicity, chronic infection or obstruction, recurrent primary renal disease
Heart	Yes, with allograft loss	Myocardial infarction, global ischemic damage with heart failure, arrythmia	Atherosclerosis from donor, coronary artery embolus, persistent rejection
Liver	Yes, with allograft loss; loss can occur from vanishing bile duct syndrome	Central liver cell loss; bile duct loss	Primary biliary cirrhosis, chronic arterial injury, chronic obstruction
Lung	Yes, but not cause of allograft loss	Obliterative bronchiolitis leads to graft loss	Infection with repair

Kidney Allografts

In kidney allografts, this process is known as chronic vascular nephropathy or chronic rejection. This type of rejection is characterized by proliferative vasculopathy which involves the arteries and arterioles of the kidney.[63,64] Arteries have subintimal fibrosis without reduplication of the elastic lamina, a pattern reminiscent of malignant hypertensive vascular changes. The kidney parenchyma shows ischemic damage with patchy interstitial fibrosis, tubular damage and atrophy, and periglomerular fibrosis, in descending order of frequency. Figure 13-10 illustrates these features. Glomeruli commonly show collapse of tufts and may display a prominent glomerulopathy with marked reduplication of capillary membranes and slight increase in mesangial matrix, which is nonspecific. The extent of reduplication of capillary basement membranes is usually greater in allograft vasculopathy than in recurrent glomerulonephritis. The principal differential diagnosis is between chronic rejection and cyclosporine nephrotoxicity, which may produce a similar vasculopathic lesion that can occur earlier after transplant and is

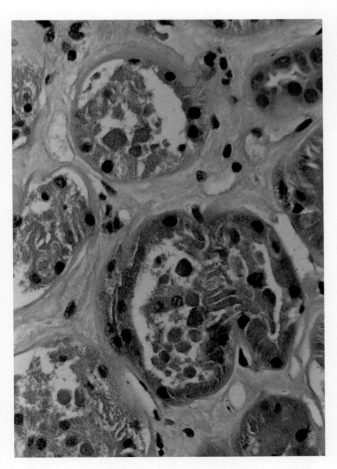

Fig. 13-11. Acute tubular damage associated with acute cyclosporine nephrotoxicity. The tubular epithelial cells are missing and desquamated. The photomicrograph was taken several months after transplant, a time at which such acute tubular damage is unlikely from perfusion-related acute tubular necroses.

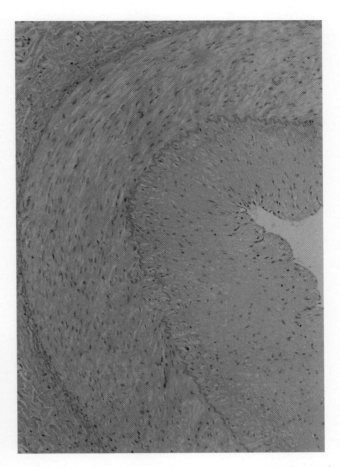

Fig. 13-12. A coronary artery with prominent concentric subintimal fibrosis. Patient died of an acute myocardial infarction 10 months after transplant.

associated with significantly more acute tubular damage. The type of tubular damage produced by cyclosporine nephrotoxicity is illustrated in Figure 13-11. FK506, another macrolide immunosuppressive agent, can also produce vasculopathy.[65–67]

Heart Allografts

As in other allografts, chronic allograft rejection results in ischemic injury to the allograft and its eventual loss.[68–70] The process involves the coronary vasculature generally and produces uniform concentric narrowing of coronary vessels that is progressive. Patients with this process eventually develop heart failure and allograft loss or die of acute painless myocardial infarction or arrythmia. Pathologically, the process is similar to that in other allografts. The grafts show concentric subintimal fibrosis (Fig. 13-12) associated with infiltration of the arterial wall by lymphocytes and macrophages. Accumulation of fatty macrophages is not a feature. On endomyocardial biopsy, the features of ischemic damage are irregular hypertrophy, interstitial scarring, and myocyte vacuolization. These features are not specific but are highly suggestive.[61]

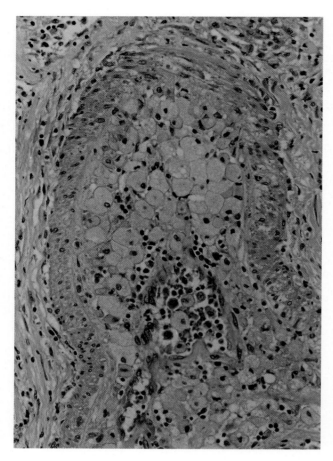

Fig. 13-13. Central artery from a chronically rejected liver showing subintimal fibrosis and fat-laden macrophages within the wall of the vessel.

Liver Allografts

Chronic rejection or vasculopathy is evidenced by clinical findings of progressive liver failure. The vasculopathic lesions are known as obliterative endarteritis, are seen only in the larger arteries of the liver, and are not found in needle biopsies. Histologically, lipid-laden macrophages or fibrosis accumulate in the subendothelial area of the vessel, with subsequent narrowing and occlusion. Grossly the vessel may be yellow because of the accumulated lipid. A vessel affected by this change is illustrated in Figure 13-13. As a result of the obliterative endarteritis, central ischemic changes occur in the hepatic parenchyma. This is characterized by ballooning degeneration and eventual confluent dropout of hepatic cells (Fig. 13-14). Multinucleated giant hepatic cells indicate regenerative activity. Lipochrome is prominent. Central fibrosis and collapse may be seen; only rarely does micronodular cirrhosis occur. Another rare type of chronic ischemic damage to the allograft is known as vanishing bile duct syndrome, which is characterized by complete absence of bile ducts in the portal triads. The portal triads appear fibrous, and no inflammatory infiltrate is present. This condition is thought to follow episodes of acute cellular rejection. Van-

ishing bile duct syndrome is occasionally reversible if not accompanied by vascular insufficiency.[71–73]

Lung Allografts

In lung allografts, chronic rejection chiefly manifests by chronic interstitial fibrosis and obliterative bronchiolitis. These are the pathologic lesions resulting from the ischemic damage produced by the vasculopathy of the larger vessels. Although chronic vascular changes occur that are similar in all respects to those in other solid organ transplants, the progressive obliteration of bronchioles assumes the greatest clinical importance.[74–79] This process appears to develop through a sequence of epithelial injury leading to submucosal scarring and finally total obliteration of bronchioles. This fibrotic scarring process involves both membranous and respiratory bronchioles and may be eccentric or concentric, with a residual lumen in the early stages.[78] Ultimately the airway lumen is totally obliterated by fibrous tissue. The smooth muscle layers of the bronchioles may be destroyed by extension of the fibrous tissue into the peribronchiolar interstitium, associated with mononuclear cell infiltration of all layers of the bronchiolar wall in the active phase. Epithelial damage with lymphocytic infiltration may be

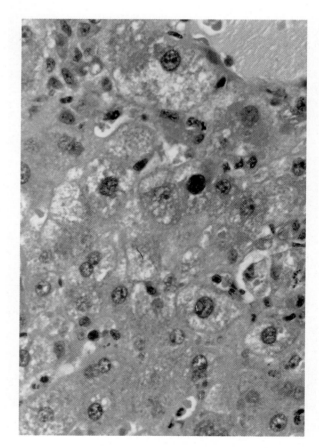

Fig. 13-14. Central balloon cell degeneration of liver cells that accompanied the vascular findings shown in Fig. 13-13. Upper right, a central vein.

present, in addition to the fibrosis.[79] Alternatively, the epithelium may be ulcerated, with subepithelial granulation tissue growing into the lumen in a polyploid fashion prior to scarring. During the active phase of obliterative bronchiolitis, perivascular infiltrates are noted in the adjacent parenchyma. In lung biopsies, bronchiolar scarring may only be evident on elastic stains demonstrating proximity of the fibrosed structure to the pulmonary arterioles and delineating the extent of luminal narrowing by submucosal fibrosis.[44,78] Extensive peribronchiolar fibrosis associated with destruction of the smooth muscle may result in extrinsic compression of the lumen in a constrictive form of obliterative bronchiolitis. The distribution of obliterative bronchiolitis is often patchy. Further evidence that obliterative bronchiolitis is a manifestation of chronic rejection is its frequent occurrence in nontransplant patients with immunologic lung disease. Obliterative bronchiolitis is well described in the collagen vascular diseases and has also been reported in bone marrow transplant recipients who have experienced graft-versus-host disease (GVHD).[74–79]

Mechanisms of Allograft Vasculopathy

It is strongly suspected on the basis of pathologic and experimental evidence that allograft vasculopathy is immunologically mediated, although the precise mechanisms are still in doubt. Experimentally, vasculopathy does not occur in autografts, lending support to this theory. The vasculature possesses endothelium that expresses HLA and other alloantigens and could serve as the target of both antigen recognition and antigen presenting cells.[80] Effector mechanisms are probably of both cellular and humoral types. The process is certainly aggravated by the inflammatory potential of the endothelial cells themselves, which serve to amplify any cycle of injury and repair incited by the chronic antigenic stimulation of the allografted organ. Other factors that might contribute to the process are still being sought and include diet and immunosuppressive agents such as cyclosporine and FK506, which are capable of producing vasculopathic changes. This field is under intense investigation.[62–70]

GRAFT-VERSUS-HOST DISEASE IN BONE MARROW TRANSPLANT RECIPIENTS

Another manifestation of chronic allostimulation is GVHD, a syndrome of dermatitis, panenteritis, hepatitis, scleroderma, and immunodeficiency occurring in bone marrow transplant recipients. It results from the transplantation of allogeneic lymphoid cells, which attack recipient epidermis, bowel epithelium, and liver cells. The precise immunologic mechanisms are poorly understood, but the severity of the process is clearly linked to the degree of HLA mismatch between donor and recipient. Direct damage to recipient lymphocytes in sites such as the thymus results in immunodeficiency.[81,82] Apoptosis of skin, gut, and bile duct epithelium results from direct cytotoxicity or indirectly through cytokine-mediated damage. Recent studies suggest that IL-1 and TNF play an important role in this process.[83,84]

Acute Form

Acute GVHD is a triad of dermatitis, enteritis, and hepatitis occurring within the first several weeks after transplantation in bone marrow transplant recipients. Pathologically, the lesions are composed of individual or groups of apoptotic parenchymal cells accompanied by minimal to moderate lymphocytic infiltrates. In the skin, bulla formation occurs in moderately severe cases and progresses to total epidermal loss. Without serial biopsies, the lesions are difficult to distinguish from erythema multiforme, early herpetic skin infections, direct acute toxicity of chemotherapy or radiation, and lichen planus. In the gut, the lesions consist of apoptotic crypt cells with associated lymphoid infiltration. Eventually, crypt abscesses develop associated with edema of the lamina propria. Total loss of gut epithelium can occur, with fatal bleeding. In the liver, apoptotic bile duct epithelial cells are the site of the immunologic injury, leading to cholestatic hepatitis, with eventual hepatocellular and cholangiolar cholestasis and hepatocytolysis. Endothelialitis can be seen but is not common, leading to diagnostic difficulties in distinguishing GVHD of the liver from chronic active hepatitis, Cytomegalovirus hepatitis, and veno-occlusive disease occurring as a result of chemotherapy or radiation toxicity. Oral mucositis caused by chemotherapy or radiotherapy, or both, clouds interpretation of mucositis for up to about 30 days after transplant.[85–89]

Chronic Form

Chronic GVHD occurrs 80 to 100 days after transplant. It is probably an autoimmune process superimposed on allogeneically initiated GVHD. The skin is the most frequently involved organ and resembles lichen planus and hypertrophic lupus erythematosus. Fibrous remodeling of the dermis occurs within weeks to months, leading to widening of the papillary dermis and ultimately scleroderma-like changes in the gross and microscopic appearance of the skin. Because of the serious sequelae of chronic GVHD, patients undergo screening skin biopsy 90 to 100 days after transplant to evaluate the need to maintain immunosuppression if chronic GVHD is present. Skin biopsy of a rash or the forearm has a sensitivity of 68 percent and a specificity of 91 percent. If a lichen planus pattern is seen, the patient has a significantly increased death hazard ratio. The surgical pathologic evaluation of these biopsies is thus very important. Biopsies should be taken from areas of rash or from the forearm and be full thickness so that intradermal changes can be evaluated. Active GVHD is diagnosed based on findings of epithelial cell necrosis (basal layer vacuolar degeneration or rare eosinophilic bodies even without inflammatory cells) around appendages or in the epidermis.[90–91]

The sicca syndrome (dry gland) is another major manifestation of chronic GVHD, affecting 80 percent of patients with the condition. Organs involved include mouth, eyes, nose, vagina, and urethra. Oral chronic GVHD is more difficult to diagnose histologically because the findings are somewhat nonspecific and range from pronounced lichenoid reaction to mucosal atrophy. A negative biopsy does not exclude the possibility of GVHD. To be considered truly negative, the

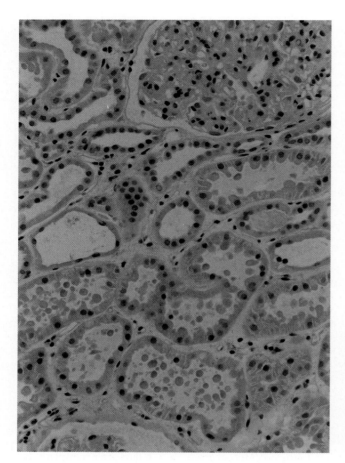

Fig. 13-15. Perfusion injury. Kidney tubules show desquamation and dilation. The glomerulus contains rare neutrophils. The cadaveric kidney was perfused for 24 hours prior to transplantation.

biopsy must contain both lip mucosa and salivary gland. By contrast, a positive lip biopsy in conjunction with other evidence of chronic GVHD constitutes extensive chronic GVHD, which prompts specific immunosuppressive therapy. Keratoconjunctivitis, another common manifestation of sicca syndrome, is best diagnosed clinically using slit lamp examination and decreased tear production (Schirmer's test). Other manifestations of chronic GVHD include difficulty in swallowing, reminiscent of scleroderma. Histologically, the lesions are composed of mucosal ulcerations with submucosal fibrosis and destruction of submucosal glands. Patients can also develop renal vasculopathy and bronchiolitis obliterans, indistinguishable from the chronic rejection of allografts of these organs.[90–95]

The pathogenesis of chronic GVHD involves autoimmunity superimposed on immunodeficiency. Patients develop immunodeficiency due to the thymic damage as a result of acute GVHD. Immunodeficiency of normal mechanisms for inducing self-tolerance could then lead to autoimmunity. Autoreactive T cells would then be postulated to produce cytokines in response to self-antigens, leading to chronic GVHD.[96–97]

OTHER PATHOLOGIC PROCESSES THAT INVOLVE ALLOGRAFTED ORGANS

Perfusion Injury

Allografts must be kept in a perfusing solution for variable lengths of time prior to transplantation for purposes of transport and logistics. The perfusing solutions vary with each allograft type, as do the time limits tolerated by the particular organ.

Kidney allografts can be kept successfully for 12 to 24 hours, livers can be kept for 36 hours, and heart and lung allografts must be used within 4 hours. Organs kept for prolonged periods in cold perfusing solutions show a variety of pathologic features related to the relatively ischemic state and the length of time of perfusion. In most cases, the histologic features resolve within 1 to 3 weeks after transplantation. Rarely, the graft is incapable of recovering from this ischemic insult, and primary graft failure results.

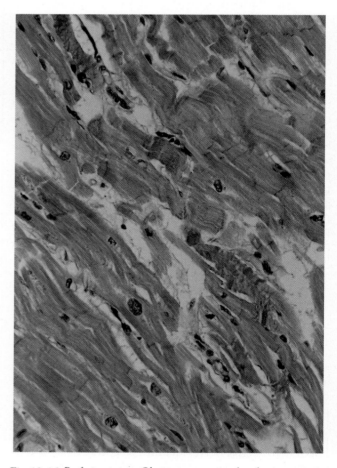

Fig. 13-16. Perfusion injury. Obvious contraction band necrosis is seen in this view of a cardiac biopsy taken from a patient several weeks after transplant. The process resolved spontaneously without sequelae. If such changes are seen after the initial month after transplant, they suggest humoral rejection or allograft vasculopathy causing ischemia.

Kidney Allografts

In kidney allografts, this perfusion effect manifests by acute tubular damage. Tubules are dilated and renal tubular epithelial cells slough, giving the luminal border a ragged appearance (Fig. 13-15). This process must be distinguished from cyclosporine nephrotoxicity, which can produce similar tubular damage. A glomerulitis may also occur, manifested by infiltration of glomeruli by neutrophils.[37]

Heart Allografts

Heart allografts may show focal areas of myocytolysis or contraction band necrosis (or both) as a manifestation of early ischemic damage induced by storage in perfusion solutions before transplantation. Figure 13-16 illustrates such contraction band necrosis. Hearts undergoing prolonged perfusion can also require heightened amounts of catecholamines early after transplantation. Catecholamine effects on the heart are seen in the form of punctate ischemic myocytes surrounded by neutrophils.[38]

Liver Allografts

Liver allografts often have widespread perfusion effects. Histologically this process is manifested by balloon cell degeneration

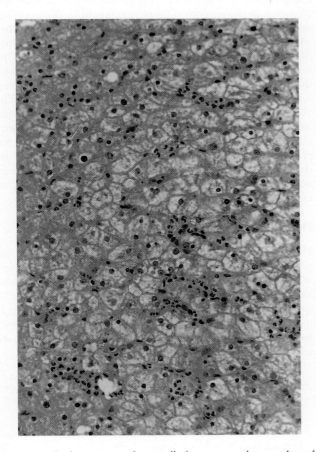

Fig. 13-17. Perfusion injury. Liver cells from a recently transplanted allograft show ballon cell degeneration and an infiltrate of neutrophils, an entity known as surgical hepatitis.

of hepatocytes, especially in central areas. Infiltrations of neutrophils may also be seen in liver lobules, a condition known as surgical hepatitis. Figure 13-17 shows balloon cell degeneration associated with perfusion.[41]

Lung Allografts

Lung allografts show diffuse alveolar damage as a manifestation of perfusion injury. Neutrophils may be associated with the damage, and desquamation of the alveolar lining cells associated with interstitial edema and hemorrhage occurs if the process is severe.[44]

Inflammation and Repair

Although the inciting events in allograft rejection are almost certainly immunologic, these responses are certainly amplified in various ways by inflammatory stimuli. All the cells, plasma proteins, and vascular constituents of inflammation are present in the allograft.[98–100] Many of the vascular and cellular responses of inflammation are mediated by chemical factors derived from the action of the inflammatory stimulus.[98–102] Figure 13-18 illustrates the Quilty phenomenon, an endocardial inflammatory process seen in cardiac allografts. The change occurs in biopsies with and without acute rejection.

Early after transplantation, a potent inflammatory stimulus is always present—ischemia, induced by the necessary removal from the donor, the delay, and the reimplantation. Such ischemia is of variable extent depending on circumstances; however, some parenchymal cell necrosis always exists, which triggers elaboration of inflammatory mediators.[101] In all solid organ allografts in the early post-transplant period, hallmarks of acute inflammation can be seen; vasodilation and vascular permeability, slowing of the circulation, and leukocyte margination, adhesion, and emigration are frequently present. These changes are protean in the first few biopsies and are not seen as manifestations of allograft rejection, but rather as manifestations of the perfusion injury that all allografts sustain.

Role of the Vascular Endothelium

The vascular endothelium assumes a central role in immune mechanisms as both stimulator and target cell and also has a central effector function in inflammatory responses, including production of adhesion molecules and inflammatory mediators such as IL-1, TNF, and PAF.[102–105] The endothelium also promotes amplification and prolongation of the inflammatory response by facilitating adhesion and emigration by neutrophils and macrophages. These cells, especially the long-lived macrophage, have the potential to secrete additional mediators into the extracellular spaces of the allograft, including neutral proteases, chemotactic factors for other leukocytes, reactive oxygen metabolites, products of arachidonic acid metabolism (especially prostaglandins and leukotrienes), complement components, coagulation factors, growth-promoting factors, PAF, IFN, and cytokines such as IL-1 and TNF.[47,48,106–108] These substances are potent amplifiers of tissue damage in the

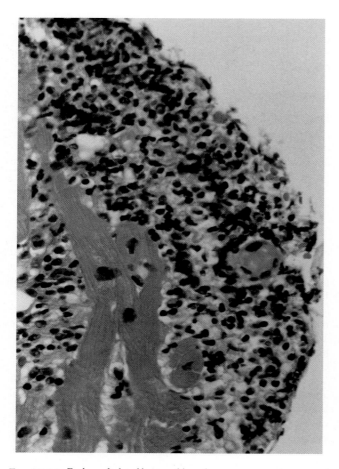

Fig. 13-18. Endocardial infiltrate of lymphocytes, macrophages, and other cells termed the *Quilty phenomenon*, after the first patient with the finding. The relationship of this inflammatory process to rejection is controversial.

allograft, and their effects are regulated by the interaction of the macrophage with its environment.

Role of the Coagulation, Kinin, and Complement Systems

The other important compartment active in inflammation is the blood plasma, with its complement, kinin, and coagulation systems. The complement system functions in inflammation by mediating biologic events that lead to chemotaxis of inflammatory cells (C5a, C5a des Arg), increased vascular permeability (C3a), opsonization (C3b, C3bi), and cell lysis (C5b-9).[47–50] Complement activation can be triggered by antigen-antibody complexes or by aggregated IgG, plasmin, endotoxin, or activation by necrotic cells such as myocytes. The kinin and clotting systems can be triggered by activation of Hageman factor (factor XII) due to interaction with collagen or basement membrane, a situation potentiated by ischemic necrosis. Activation of Hageman factor leads to release of bradykinin, a potent mediator of vascular permeability, which amplifies inflammation. Activated Hageman factor also initiates the clotting and fibrinolytic sys-

tems, which can lead to further chemotaxis of inflammatory cells, activation of complement components, and recurrent Hageman factor activation, leading to further cyclic inflammatory stimuli.[3,18,109–113] The coagulation and fibrinolysis systems are tightly regulated by endothelial cell anticoagulant and procoagulant activities. The natural expression of these regulatory substances and their alteration by allograft rejection is the subject of intense investigation in heart and kidney allografts. Alteration of the coagulation and fibrinolytic systems provides a common pathway for both acute and chronic tissue damage regardless of whether the response is initiated by immunologic or inflammatory stimuli.[114–116]

Role of Immunosuppressive Drug Toxicity

Cyclosporine Toxicity

The principal effect of cyclosporine is related to nephrotoxicity. In all solid allograft patients, nephrotoxicity can occur with cyclosporine use. Pathologically, it manifests by acute tubular damage with isometric vacuolization of tubules and dystrophic calcification. Cyclosporine is also toxic to endothelial cells and can produce a thrombotic process involving arteries and glomeruli in rare patients. This process resembles the hemolytic uremic syndrome. When much higher doses of cyclosporine were routinely used, a vasculopathy was describe in which medial hyalinosis of arteries and arterioles was prominent. Currently, this is a rare phenomenon. With chronic cyclosporine use, a chronic form of nephropathy results, expressed pathologically by persistent tubular damage and interstitial fibrosis. This process is difficult to distinguish from chronic allograft rejection in kidney transplant recipients and may coexist with chronic vasculopathy or may exacerbate it. In cardiac transplant recipients, no specific cardiac toxicity is seen, although the Quilty phenomenon is more frequent in patients treated with cyclosporine and was originally attributed to a drug effect.[37]

FK506 Toxicity

FK506, another macrolide immunosuppressive drug, can also result in nephrotoxicity, although the extent of the problem and the frequency are less than with cyclosporine. Patients with kidney allografts develop an acute and chronic form of toxicity similar to that of cyclosporine. Isometric vacuolization of tubules is more prominent with this agent. No specific drug effects of FK506 on heart, lung, or liver allografts have been described.[37]

REFERENCES

1. Krensky AM, Weiss A, Crabtree G, et al: T-lymphocyte-antigen interactions in transplant rejection. N Engl J Med 322:510–517, 1990
2. Mason DW, Morris PJ: Effector mechanisms in allograft rejection. Annu Rev Immunol 4:119–145, 1986
3. Dinarello CA, Mier JW: Lymphokines. N Engl J Med 317:940–945, 1987

4. Sachs DH, Hansen TH: The major histocompatibility complex. pp. 445–488. In Paul, WE (ed): Fundamental Immunology. Lippincott-Raven, Philadelphia, 1989

5. Campbell RD, Trowsdale J: Map of the human major histocompatibility complex. Immunol Today 14:349–352, 1993

6. Daar AS, Fuggle SV, Fabre JW, et al: The detailed distribution of HLA A B C antigens in normal human organs. Transplantation 38:287–292, 1984

7. Daar AS, Fuggle SV, Fabre JW, et al: The detailed distribution of MHC class II antigens in normal human organs. Transplantation 38:293–298, 1984

8. Robinson MA, Kindt TJ: Major histocompatibility complex antigens and genes. pp. 489–539. In Paul WE (ed): Fundamental Immunology. 2nd Ed. Lippincott-Raven, Philadelphia, 1989

9. Hughes AL, Nei M: Pattern of nucleotide substitution at major histocompatibility complex class I loci reveals overdominant selection. Nature 33:167–170, 1988

10. Gregersen PK: HLA class II polymorphism: implications for genetic susceptibility to autoimmune disease. Lab Invest 61:5–10, 1989

11. Wagner CR, Vetto RM, Burger DR: Subcultured human endothelial cells can function independently as fully competent antigen-presenting cells. Hum Immunol 13:33–47, 1985

12. Johnston RG Jr: Monocytes and macrophages. N Engl J Med 318:747–752, 1988

13. Weiss A, Imboden JB: Cell surface molecules and early events involved in human T lymphocytic activation. Adv Immunol 41:1–38, 1987

14. Smith KA: Interleukin-2: inception, impact and implication. Science 240:1169–1176, 1988

15. Davis MM, Bjorkman PJ: T-cell receptor genes and T-cell recognition. Nature 334:395–401, 1988

16. Parnes JR: Molecular biology and function of CD4 and CD8. Adv Immunol 44:265–311, 1989

17. Springer TA, Dustin ML, Kishimoto TK, Marlin SD: The lymphocyte function-associated LFA-1, CD2, and LFA-3 molecules: cell adhesion receptors of the immune system. Annu Rev Immunol 5:223–252, 1987

18. Berg EL, Goldstein LA, Jutila MA, et al: Homing receptors and vascular addressins: cell adhesion molecules that direct lymphocyte traffic. Immunol Rev 108:5–18, 1989

19. Royer HD, Reinherz EL: T-lymphocytes: ontogeny function and relevance to clinical disorders. N Engl J Med 317:1136, 1987

20. Miltenburg AM, Meijer-Paape ME, Weening II, et al: Induction of antibody-dependent cellular cytotoxicity against endothelial cells by renal transplantation. Transplantation 48:681–688, 1989

21. Hayry P: Generation and breakdown of a vicious cycle in context of acute allograft rejection. Transplant Proc 18:52–62, 1986

22. Cotran RS: New roles for the endothelium in inflammation and immunity. Am J Pathol 129:407–410, 1987

23. Pober JS: Cytokine-mediated activation of vascular endothelium. Am J Pathol 133:426–429, 1988

24. Dvorak HF, Galli SM, Drorak AM, et al: Cellular and vascular manifestations of cell-mediated immunity. Hum Pathol 17:122–127, 1986

25. Martinez OM, Krams SM, Sterneck M, et al: Intragraft cytokine profile during human liver allograft rejection. Transplantation 53:449–456, 1992

26. Hoffman MW, Wonigeit K, Steinhoff G, et al: Production of cytokines (TNF-alpha, IL-1-beta) and endothelial cell activation in human liver allograft rejection. Transplantation 55:329–335, 1993

27. Ruan XM, Quiao JH, Trento A, et al: Cytokine expression and endothelial cell and lymphocyte activation in human cardiac allograft rejection: an immunohistochemical study of endomyo-cardial biopsy samples. J Heart Lung Transplant 11:1110–1115, 1992

28. Colvin RB, Preffer FI, Fuller TC, et al: A critical analysis of serum and urine interleukin-2 receptor assays in renal allograft recipients. Transplantation 48:800–805, 1989

29. Chatenoud L, Ferran C, Legendre C, et al: In vivo cell activation following OKT3 administration. Systemic cytokine release and modulation by corticosteroids. Transplantation 49:697–702, 1990

30. Mannik M: Mechanisms of tissue deposition of immune complexes. J Rheumatol 13:35–38, 1987

31. Strom TB: The cellular and molecular basis of allograft rejection: fact and fancy. Transplant Proc 18:801–805, 1985

32. Hall BM, Cellular infiltrates in allografts. Transplant Proc 19:50–56, 1987

33. Billingham ME: Diagnosis of cardiac rejection by endomyocardial biopsy. Heart Transplant 1:25–30, 1982

34. Higgenbottam T, Stewart S, Penketh A, et al: Transbronchial lung biopsy for the diagnosis of rejection in heart-lung transpant patients. Transplant 46:532–539, 1988

35. Snover DC: Orthotopic liver transplantation: a pathological study of 63 serial liver biopsies from 17 patients with special reference to the diagnostic features and natural history of rejection. Hepatology 4:1212–1222, 1984

36. Sale GE, Buckner CD: Pathology of bone marrow in transplant recipients. Hematol Oncol Clin North Am 2:738–756, 1988

37. Colvin RB: Kidney transplantation. pp. 329–366. In Colvin RB, Bhan AT, McCluskey RT (eds): In Diagnostic Immunopathology. Lippincott-Raven, Philadelphia, 1995

38. Hammond EH: Cardiac transplantation. p. 367. In Colvin RB, Bhan AT, McCluskey RT (eds): Diagnostic Immunopathology. Lippincott-Raven, Philadelphia, 1995

39. Demetris AJ, Lasky S, Van Thiel DH, et al: Pathology of hepatic transplantation: a review of 62 adult allograft recipients immuno-suppressed with a cyclosporine/steroid regimen. Am J Pathol 118: 151–161, 1985

40. Hammond EH: Microvascular cardiac rejection. pp. 92–110. In Hammond EH (ed): Solid Organ Transplantation Pathology. WB Saunders, Philadelphia, 1994

41. Flinner RL, Hammond EH: Liver transplantation pathology. pp. 186–214. In Hammond EH (ed): Solid Organ Transplantation Pathology. WB Saunders, Philadelphia, 1994

42. Solez K, McGraw DJ, Beschorner WE, et al: Reflections on use of the renal biopsy as the "gold standard" in distinguishing transplant rejection from cyclosporine nephrotoxicity. Transplant Proc, 4 suppl. 1, 17:123–133, 1985

43. Billingham ME, Cary NR, Hammond EH, et al: A Working Formulation for the standardization of nomenclature in the diagnosis of heart and lung rejection: Heart Rejection Study Group. J Heart Transplant 9:587–592, 1990

44. Yousem SA, Berry GJ, Brunt EM, et al: A Working Formulation for the standardization of nomenclature in the diagnosis of heart and lung rejection: Lung Rejection Study Group. J Heart Transplant 9:593–601, 1990

45. Snover DC, Freese DK, Sharp HL, et al: Liver allograft rejection: an analysis of the use of biopsy in determining outcome of rejection. Am J Surg Pathol 11:1–10, 1987

46. Sibley RK, Payne W: Morphologic findings in the renal allograft biopsy. Semin Nephrol 5:294–306, 1985

47. Bogman MJ, Dopper IM, van de Winkel JG, et al: Diagnosis of renal allograft rejection by macrophage immunostaining with a CD14 monoclonal antibody, WT14. Lancet 2:235–238, 1989

48. Steinhoff G, Wonigeit K, Sorg C, et al: Patterns of macrophage immigration and differentiation in human liver grafts. Transplant Proc 21:398–400, 1989

49. Gassel AM, Hansmann ML, Radzun HJ, Weyland M: Human cardiac allograft rejection: correlation of grading with expression of different monocyte/macrophage markers. Am J Clin Pathol 94:274–279, 1990

50. Mues B, Brisse B, Zwadlo G, et al: Phenotyping of macrophages with monoclonal antibodies in endomyocardial biopsies as a new approach to diagnosis of myocarditis. Eur Heart J 11:1–18, 1990

51. Colvin RB: Diagnostic use in transplantation. Clinical applications of

monoclonal antibodies in renal allograft biopsies. Am J Kidney Dis 11:126–130, 1988

52. Nickeleit V, Miller M, Cosimi AB, Colvin RB: Adhesion molecules in human renal allograft rejection: immunohistochemical analysis of ICAM-1, ICAM-2, ICAM-3, VCAM-1, and ELAM-1. pp. 380–387. In Lipsky PE, Rothlein R, Kishimoto TK, et al (eds): Structure, Function, and Regulation of Molecules involved in Leukocyte Adhesion. Springer-Verlag, New York, 1993

53. Noronha, IL, Eberlein GM, Hartley B, et al: In situ expression of tumor necrosis factor-alpha, interferon-gamma, and interleukin-2 receptors in renal allograft biopsies. Transplantation 54:1017–1024, 1992

54. Noronha IL, Weis H, Hartley B, et al: Expression of cytokines, growth factors, and their receptors in renal allograft biopsies. Transplant Proc 25:891–894, 1993

55. Myburgh JA, Cohen I, Gecelter L, et al: Hyperacute rejection in human-kidney allografts. Shwartzman or Arthus reaction? N Engl J Med 281:131–135, 1969

56. Matas AJ, Scheinman JI, Rattazzi LC, et al: Immunopathological studies of the ruptured human renal allograft. Surgery 98:922–926, 1976

57. Carpenter CB, Milford EL: HLA matching in cadaveric renal transplantation. Immunol Allergy Clin North Am 9:45–60, 1989

58. Demetris AJ, Juffe R, Tzakis A, et al: Antibody-mediated rejection of human orthotopic liver allografts/a study of liver transplantation across ABO blood group barriers. Am J Pathol 132:489–502, 1988

59. Hammond EH, Yowell RL, Nunoda S, et al: Vascular (humoral) rejection in heart transplantation: pathologic observations and clinical implications. J Heart Transplant 8:430–443, 1989

60. Barr ML, Cohen DJ, Benvenisty Al, et al: Effect of anti-HLA antibodies on the long-term survival of heart and kidney allografts. Transplant Proc 25:262–264, 1993

61. Hammond EH, Hansen J, Spencer LS, et al: Vascular rejection in cardiac transplantation: histologic, immunopathologic and ultrastructural features. Cardiovasc Pathol 2:21–34, 1993

62. Salomon RN, Hughes CCW, Schoen FJ, et al: Human coronary transplantation-associated arteriosclerosis: evidence of a chronic immune reaction to activated graft endothelial cells. Am J Pathol 138:791–798, 1991

63. Wynn JJ, Pfaff WW, Patton PR, et al: Late results of renal transplantation. Transplantation 45:329–333, 1988 1988

64. Häyry P, Mennander A, Räisänen-Sokolowski A, et al: Pathophysiology of vascular wall changes in chronic allograft rejection. Transplant Rev 7:1–12, 1993

65. Myers BD, Ross J, Newton L, et al: The long-term course of cyclosporine-associated chronic nephropathy. Kidney Int 33:590–600, 1988

66. Coffman T, Carr DR, Yarger W, Klotman P: Evidence that renal prostaglandin and thromboxane production is stimulated in chronic cyclosporine nephrotoxicity. Transplantation 43:282–285, 1987

67. First MR, Smith RD, Weiss MA, et al: Cyclosporine-associated glomerular and arteriolar thrombosis following renal trans-plantation. Transplant Proc 21:1567–1570, 1989

68. Clinton SK, Libby P: Cytokines and growth factors in atherogenesis. Arch Pathol Lab Med 116:1292–1300, 1992

69. Gordon D, Reidy MA, Benditt EP, Scharwtz SM: Cell proliferation in human coronary arteries. Proc Natl Acad Sci USA 12:4600–46004, 1990

70. Reed E, Cohen DJ, Barr ML, et al: Effect of anti-HLA and anti-idiotypic antibodies on the long-term survival of heart and kidney allografts. Transplant Proc 24:2494, 1992

71. Grond J, Gouw ASH, Poppema S, et al: Chronic rejection in liver transplants: a histopathologic analysis of failed grafts and antecedent serial biopsies. Transplant Proc 18:128–135, 1988

72. Ludwig J, Weisner RH, Butts KP, et al: The acute vanishing bile duct syndrome (acute irreversible rejection) after orthotopic liver transplantation. Hepatology 7:476–83, 1987

73. Vierling JM, Fennell RH Jr: Histopathology of early and late human hepatic allograft rejection: evidence of progressive destruction of interlobular bile ducts. Hepatology 5:1076–1082, 1985

74. Kramer MR, Stoehr C, Whang JL, et al: The diagnosis of obliterative bronchiolitis following heart-lung transplantation: low yield of transbronchial biopsy. J Heart Lung Transplant 12:675–681, 1993

75. Yousem, SA, Burke C, Billingham ME: Pathologic pulmonary alterations in long-term human heart-lung transplantation. Hum Pathol 16:911–923, 1985

76. Scott JP, Higgenbottam TW, Clelland CA: Natural history of chronic rejection in heart-lung transplant recipients J Heart Transplant 9:510–515, 1990

77. Sibley RK, Berry GJ, Tazelaar HD, et al: The role of transbronchial biopsies in the management of lung transplant recipients. J Heart Lung Transplant 12:308–324, 1993

78. Stewart S: Pathology of lung transplantation. Semin Diagn Pathol 9:210–219, 1992

79. Milne DS, Gascoigne A, Wilkes J, et al: The immunohistopathology of obliterative bronchiolitis following lung transplantation. Transplantation 54:748–750, 1992

80. Gouw ASH, Huitema S, Grand J, Sluot MJ: Early induction of MHC antigens in human liver grafts. Am J Pathol 133:81–94, 1988

81. Dilly SA, Sloane JP, Psalti ISM: The cellular composition of human lymph nodes after allogenic bone marrow transplantation: an immunohistological study. J Pathol 150:213–221, 1986

82. Muller-Hermelink HK, Sale GE, Borisch B, Storb R: Pathology of the thymus after allogenic bone marrow transplantation in man. A histologic immunohistochemical study of 36 patients. Am J Pathol 129:242–256, 1986

83. Burakoff SJ, Degg HJ, Ferrara J, Atkinson K, (eds): Graft-vs.-Host Disease: Immunology, Pathophysiology, and Treatment. Marcel Dekker, New York, 1990

84. van Bekkem DW, deVries JM, van der Waaij D: Lesions characteristic of secondary disease in germ free heterologous radiation chimeras. J Natl Cancer Inst 38:223–231, 1967

85. Sale GE, Lerner KG, Barker EA, et al: The skin biopsy in the diagnosis of acute graft-versus-host disease in man. Am J Pathol 89:621–635, 1977.

86. Epstein RJ, McDonald GB, Sale GE, et al: The diagnostic accuracy of the rectal biospy in acute graft-versus-host disease: a prospective study of thirteen patients. Gastroenterology 78:764–771, 1980

87. Parkman R, Champagne J, DeClerck Y, et al: Cellular interactions in graft-versus-host disease. Transplant Proc 19:53–54, 1987

88. McDonald GB, Shulman HM, Sullivan KM, Spencer GD: Complications of marrow transplantation. I. Intestinal and hepatic complications of human bone marrow transplantation. Gastro-enterology 90:460–477, 1986

89. Shulman HM, Sharma P, Amos D, et al: A coded histologic study of hepatic graft-versus-host disease after human bone marrow transplantation. Hepatology 8:463–470, 1988

90. Snover DC, Weisdorf SA, Ramsey NK, et al: Hepatic graft-versus-host disease: a study of the predictive value of liver biopsy in diagnosis. Hepatology 4:123–130, 1984

91. Nakhleh R, Miller W, Snover D: The significance of mucosal versus salivary gland changes in lip biopsies in the diagnosis of chronic graft-versus-host disease. Arch Pathol Lab Med 113:932–934, 1989

92. Jack MK, Jack GM, Sale GM, et al: Ocular manifestations of graft-versus-host disease. Arch Opthalmol 101:1080–1084, 1983

93. Janin-Mercer A, Saurat JH, Bourges M, et al: The lichen planus-like and sclerotic phases of graft-versus-host disease in man: an ultrastructural study of six cases. Acta Derm Venereol (stockh) 61:187–193, 1981

94. Wingard JR, Piantadosi S, Vogelsang G, et al: Predictors of death from chronic graft-versus-host disease after bone marrow transplantation. Blood 74:1428–1435, 1989

95. Graze PR, Gale RP: Chronic graft-versus-host disease: a syndrome of disordered immunity. Am J Med 66:611–620, 1979

96. Beschorner WE, Saral R, Hutchins GM, et al: Lymphocytic bronchitis associated with graft-versus-host disease in recipients of bone marrow transplants. N Engl J Med 299:1030–1034, 1978

97. Beschorner WE, DiGennaro KA, Hess AD, Santos GW. Cyclosporine and the thymus: influence on irradiation and age on thymic immunopathology and recovery. Cell Immunol 110:350–364, 1987

98. Ryan G, Majno G: Acute inflammation, a review. Am J Pathol 86:185–194, 1977

99. Harlan JM: Consequences of leukocyte vessel wall interactions in inflammatory and immune reactions. Semin Thromb Hemost 13:434–444, 1987

100. Gallin JI (ed): Inflammation: Basic Principles and Clinical Correlates. Lippincott-Raven, Philadelphia, 1992

101. Cochrane CG. Gimbrone MA (eds): Biological Oxidants: Generation and Injurious Consequences. Academic Press, San Diego, 1992

102. Cotran RS: New roles for the endothelium in inflammation and immunity. Am J Pathol 129:407–413, 1987

103. McManus LM: Pathobiology of platelet activating factor. Pathol Immunopathol Res 5:104–117, 1986

104. Braquet P, Hosford D, Braquet M, et al: Role of cytokines and platelet activating factor in microvascular immune injury. Int Arch Allergy Immunol 88:88–93, 1989

105. Le J, Vilcek J: TNF and IL 1: cytokines with multiple overlapping biological activities. Lab Invest 56:234–248, 1987

106. Unanue, ER, Allen PM: The basis for the immunoregulatory role of macrophages and other accessory cells. Science 236:551–557, 1987

107. Nathan CF: Secretory products of macrophages. J Clin Invest 79:319–326, 1987

108. Johnston RB: Monocytes and macrophages. N Engl J Med 318:747–752, 1988

109. Ross GD (ed): Immunobiology of the Complement System. Lippincott-Raven, Philadelphia, 1988

110. Muller-Eberhard HJ: Molecular organization and function of the complement system. Annu Rev Biochem 57:321–347, 1988

111. Samuelsson B, Dahlen SE, Lindgren JA, et al: Leukotrienes and lipotoxins: structure, biosynthesis and biologic effects. Science 237:1171–1176, 1987

112. Schafer H, Mathey D, Hugo F, Bhakdi, S: Deposition of the terminal C5b-C9 complex in infarcted areas of human myocardium. J Immunol 137:1945–1949, 1986

113. Roth GJ: Platelets and blood vessels: the adhesion vent. Immunol, Today 13:100–105, 1992

114. Cines DB: Disorders associated with antibodies to endothelial cells. Rev Infect Dis, suppl. 4, 11:705–711, 1989

115. Shaddy RE, Prescott SM, McIntyre TM, Zimmerman GA: Role of endothelial cells in transplant rejection. pp. 35–48. In Hammond EH (ed): Solid Organ Transplantation Pathology. WB Saunders, Philadelphia, 1994

116. Faulk WP, Labarrerre CA: Fibrinolytic and anticoagulant control of hemostasis in human cardiac and renal allografts. PP. 49–66. In Hammond EH (ed): Solid Organ Transplantation Pathology. WB Saunders, Philadelphia, 1994

14

Iatrogenic Lesions

Robert E. Fechner
Guy E. Nichols

The clinical application of hundreds of new therapeutic and diagnostic agents in the past few decades has added iatrogenic problems as a new dimension to the practice of medicine. Iatrogenic changes occur in diverse situations ranging from hyperplastic endometrium in women taking estrogen to life-threatening radiation-induced malignant tumors. The pathologist may be involved in the diagnosis of adverse drug reactions. In most cases of suspected adverse drug reaction, the diagnosis is made on clinical grounds, but sometimes a biopsy is done in an effort to distinguish a drug-induced reaction from some other cause. A detailed discussion of the morphologic effects of drug therapy is beyond the scope of this chapter. We will largely limit the discussion to drug effects that cause or mimic neoplasia.

REACTION TO DIAGNOSTIC PROCEDURES

Trauma of Biopsy

Distortion of tissue due to the physical trauma at the moment of biopsy can alter the architectural pattern or the cytologic detail, or both. When a small piece of benign glandular mucosa is twisted or compressed, the evenly spaced distribution of normal glands is lost, and the irregular pattern may be worrisome. The problem is compounded if cytologic atypia is present, as in atrophic gastritis. Perhaps the most common mechanical distortion of glandular epithelium is seen in endometrial curettings where telescoping of the epithelium may be mistaken for adenomatous hyperplasia. The loss of stroma between glands also gives a false impression of hyperplastic crowding (Fig. 14-1).

Mechanical compression and disruption of nuclei are especially common in small biopsy specimens along the edge of the tissue where cup forceps have severed the fragment from the parent organ. Lymphocytes and neutrophils are susceptible to this alteration, as well as epithelium. The cells of oat cell carcinoma of the lung are particularly prone to this type of damage. Nonetheless, even when much of the biopsy specimen is distorted, it is usually possible to identify a few intact cells and to make a cytologic diagnosis.

Tissue removed by surgical resection after a recent biopsy can have many alterations in the normal parenchyma and stroma at the biopsy site. The site is usually readily identified by the necrosis and hemorrhage along the edges of the incised tissue or needle track. In addition, changes may be present several millimeters away due to disruption of the blood supply beyond the area of direct trauma. Completely necrotic parenchyma is easily recognized, but epithelium that is still viable can have enlarged nuclei, and when these cells are set in a degenerating collapsing stroma, the normal architecture may be severely altered. Reactive fibroblasts and endothelial cells further complicate the picture. The latter form small solid buds or cords of cells lacking a lumen or having an irregularly shaped lumen. The individual cells often have large vesicular nuclei with huge nucleoli and frequent mitoses. By cytologic criteria, the reactive cells raise the possibility of malignancy. Small aggregates of atypical cells in foci of hemorrhage or necrosis must not be diagnosed as epithelial unless unequivocal evidence exists of specialized functions such as keratin formation or mucin secretion. Even when they are recognized as epithelial, cells in these foci must be interpreted with extreme caution, since regenerative and degenerative changes of normal epithelium are often prominent.

Necrosis of fat after an incisional or needle biopsy may be confusing, especially in the breast. The nuclei of degenerating fat cells or reactive histiocytes range from hyperchromatic to vesicular but usually are small and lack the large nucleoli seen in reactive fibroblasts and endothelial cells. Occasionally, they are arranged in small nests or in a circular configuration that mimics adenocarcinoma. Cytologic smears of fat necrosis obtained by breast fine needle aspiration (FNA) demonstrate numerous finely vacuolated macrophages in a hypocellular background of lymphocytes, multinucleated giant cells, and acellular debris.[1,2] Scarcity of branched epithelial groups distinguishes fat necrosis from intraductal papilloma of the breast, which also exhibits numerous foam cells in FNA specimens.[1]

Necrosis of parenchymal elements after a biopsy is often accompanied by vigorous repair. Re-epithelialization of the endometrium or endocervix after curettage is characterized by cells of variable size having nuclei that are dense and angulated and lack polarity (Fig. 14-2). These changes are most marked on the surface but may be seen in the underlying glands as well. The surface location of most of the atypical cells is the most helpful feature distinguishing them from adenocarcinoma. If the glands are involved, their even distribution with intervening stroma helps separate them from neoplastic glands, which are crowded, lack a regular pattern of distribution, and have little or no normal stroma between the glands.

Cytologic smears obtained after recent cervical biopsy or

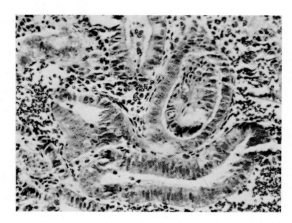

Fig. 14-1. Mechanical distortion of normal proliferative endometrium due to curettage. Note telescoping of epithelium within glandular lumens and loss of stroma between glands. No cytologic atypia is seen, nor is this the pattern of true architectural abnormality of hyperplasia.

conization demonstrate reactive changes similar to those seen in histologic sections, but a lack of tissue architecture makes distinction from malignancy more problematic in smears. Reactive changes, generally referred to as reparative or regenerative in nature, are seen for up to 6 weeks after biopsy and consist of large sheets of glandular or metaplastic squamous cells with variably enlarged nuclei and enlarged, often multiple nucleoli.[3] In contrast to invasive cancers, reparative cells demonstrate fine, evenly distributed chromatin, only rare atypical single cells, and a lack of nuclear hyperchromasia. Because distinction of reparative change from malignant tumors can be difficult, cytologic follow up should not be performed until 6 weeks after biopsy or conization.

In some cases, endocervical cytologic specimens can yield suspicious glandular cells for years after conization. In these cases, atypical groups and single glandular cells demonstrate hyperchromatic, irregular nuclear membranes and increased nuclear/cytoplasmic ratios that are easily confused with adenocarcinoma in situ. These atypical glandular cells can be distinguished from cells of adenocarcinoma in situ by a lack of nuclear enlargement and lack of nuclear crowding as well as pathologist awareness of conization history.[4] Their long-term persistence in endocervical smears appears to result from post-conization shortening of the endocervical canal that leads to sampling of low endometrial and high endocervical epithelium.[5] Conization can also shift the squamocolumnar transformation zone superiorly, so that routine cotton swab sampling no longer adequately samples endocervical epithelium. Endocervical brush sampling is more efficacious in these cases.[6]

Surgical specimens of mucosa from the oral cavity obtained after a biopsy may contain reactive changes in the minor salivary glands. The trauma of the original biopsy produces degeneration of the salivary gland lobules, which then undergo squamous metaplasia (Fig. 14-3). The squamous cells distend acini and ducts, forming complex branching arrangements that simulate either squamous or mucoepidermoid carcinoma. The cytologic blandness of the squamous cells coupled with the surrounding remnants of degenerated acini permit recognition of these changes as reactive rather than malignant. The appearance is identical to that described in the spontaneously occurring entity of necrotizing sialometaplasia of the palate.[7] Squamous metaplasia of acini has also been described in the major salivary glands after biopsy[8] and in the larynx.[9]

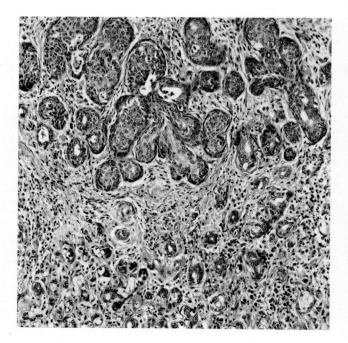

Fig. 14-3. Tissue from resection of palate showing squamous metaplasia in minor salivary gland tissue 8 days after incisional biopsy specimen detected squamous carcinoma. Degeneration of acini with loss of lobular pattern is seen in lower half of field, while squamous epithelium fills acini and ducts in upper half of field. The epithelium is cytologically bland.

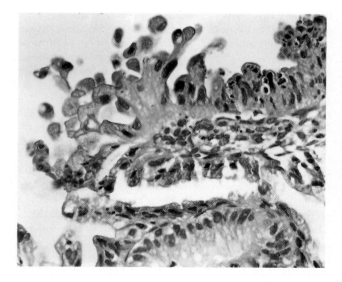

Fig. 14-2. Endocervical epithelium 12 days after endometrial curettage. Surface is lined by elongated cells with pleomorphic dense nuclei intermixed with neutrophils. Normal endocervical gland is at bottom.

Hambrick[10] described the fate of colonoscopic polypectomy sites. Initially, there is acute inflammation in the submucosa, and over a period of 2 weeks granulation tissue covers the defect as the inflammation subsides. By the end of 3 weeks, the site is completely resurfaced by normal colonic mucosa. Atypical epithelial changes are not mentioned.

Granulomas with a central necrobiotic zone surrounded by palisading histiocytes occur in the prostate, kidney, cervix, salpinx, and ovaries of patients who have had previous surgical procedures.[11–15] Electrocautery has been used in many of the operations, but the pathogenesis of these granulomas is unknown. The granulomas have been found from 1 week to 3 years after surgery. Electrocautery has been used in many of the operations, and various metals have been identified in the granulomas.[16] These metals are derived from the cutting loops. This is sometimes referred to as *diathermy pigment*.[17] Aluminum oxide, apparently derived from laser housings, has been identified in the granulomas of one case.[18]

Thermal Artifact

Thermal artifacts are found in a variety of cauterized specimens obtained by electrocautery or laser.[19] The changes are most severe at the edges but can reach the central portion of thin tissue fragments. It is sometimes possible to reach unaffected tissue by deeper sectioning beyond the peripheral thermal changes. The line of demarcation between the damaged area and normal tissue is quite abrupt. In one illustration of a high power field of perineural invasion by prostatic carcinoma, one-half the circumference of the nerve was uninterpretable due to thermal damage, whereas the other half had completely intact cells with good nuclear detail that allowed a firm diagnosis of carcinoma.[20] Tissue removed by laser will have a thin rim of thermal change identical to thermal changes from electrocautery.

Loop electrosurgical excision procedure (LEEP) is being used more frequently to excise cervical squamous intraepithelial lesions, sometimes following cytologic diagnosis without confirming tissue biopsy. Thermal artifact from LEEP is identical to laser-induced thermal damage, consisting of a variably thick zone of densely eosinophilic coagulation-desiccation (approximately 0.1 to 0.5 mm) underlying a thin, superficial zone of carbonization (approximately 0.02 mm).[21,22] In the hands of experienced operators, LEEP thermal artifact does not limit accurate histologic evaluation of resection margins.[21–25] In our experience, the usual LEEP artifact actually facilitates margin evaluation in fragmented specimens that can not be oriented and inked following excision. Occasionally LEEP causes excessive tissue fragmentation and thermal damage that limits histologic evaluation of margins, presumably due to loop size or operator inexperience.[26,27]

A signet ring configuration of lymphocytes and stromal cells in transurethral resections may be mistaken for carcinoma. This artifact is probably thermal.[28]

Implantation of Normal Epithelium

Symptomatic intradural extramedullary squamous-cell-lined cysts measuring up to 2 cm in size have occurred at the site of lumbar punctures carried out 1 to 23 years previously. It appears that the pathogenesis is the use of needles with improperly fitting stylets that carry skin into the spinal canal.[29] Squamous epithelium has also been implanted in the meniscus of a joint.[30]

Implantation of Abnormal Epithelium

Clumps of adenomatous cells from tubular adenomas can be found in the submucosa two to 21 days after removal by forceps biopsy or polypectomy. If resection is carried out in this time span, it is possible to mistake this for adenocarcinoma. The cells eventually disappear, but mucous pools are persistent.[31]

A surgical breast biopsy has often been subjected to one or more needling procedures such as FNA core needle biopsy, needle localization, or infiltration with local anesthetic.[32–34] Irregular nests of epithelium dislodged into the interductal stroma from ductal carcinoma in situ can mimic invasive carcinoma. Fragments of epithelium from ductal carcinoma in situ have also been seen in the subcapsular sinus of lymph nodes and in lymphovascular spaces within the breast.[34] Whether or not this has any potential for disseminated metastasis has not been determined. "Pseudoinvasion" of vascular spaces has been attributed to needle injection of local anesthetic in the cervix.[35]

Fine Needle Aspiration Changes in Subsequently Excised Tissue

Previous lymph node FNA can produce hemorrhage, focal fibroblastic organization, and occasional nodal infarction but rarely limits subsequent histologic evaluation[36,37] FNA of kidney, thyroid, and salivary gland solid tumors rarely leads to extensive tumor necrosis.[38,39] After FNA, nearly 10 percent of breast biopsies have changes attributable to the procedure. These include infarction of fibroadenomas and papillomas as well as displaced epithelium[40] (Fig. 14-4). Six days after an FNA, a 3 cm mesenteric mass with reactive fibroblasts was attributed to the FNA. It mimicked sarcoma at the time of frozen section.[41] Worrisome histologic alterations following FNA of the thyroid are seen in resected thyroid glands that have been previously aspirated. Acute changes such as inflammation, hemorrhage, and infarction are easily recognized. Chronic changes are potentially misleading and include pseudoinvasive tracking of epithelium through the capsule, atypical metaplasia, and nuclear clearing.[42]

Needle Track Seeding

Ever since the introduction of needle aspiration, critics have claimed that it carries significant risk for dissemination of malignant tumors by needle track seeding. Experiments in animals, early clinical experience with large bore needles, and sporadic case reports continue to fuel these concerns.[43] However, an extensive survey of recent intra-abdominal FNA experience using fine bore needles, usually 22 gauge but up to 19 gauge, indicates that needle track seeding of malignant cells is a rare complication. It occurs in less than 0.01 percent of total cases,

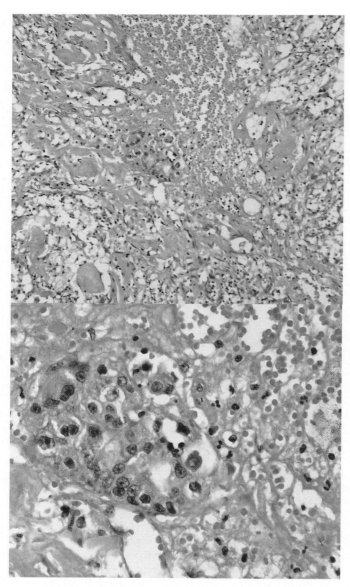

Fig. 14-4. Lumpectomy specimen has cytologically atypical epithelium associated with extravasated erythrocytes and neutrophils. Patient had fine needle aspiration 2 days before with diagnosis of "malignant cells." The biopsy showed cytologically identical ductal carcinoma in situ (DCIS). The cells illustrated here are thought to be displaced cells from DCIS and not infiltrating carcinoma. (Low and high power of same cluster of cells.)

although in a higher percentage of pancreatic cancers.[43] Risk of seeding appears to be related to the number of needle passes.[43,44] Peritoneal seeding is an even rarer complication of intra-abdominal FNA.[45] Some authors continue to warn against needle aspiration of ovarian cysts based not on statistically significant data but on sporadic case reports of intra-abdominal spread.[46] These concerns are also based in large part on separate, controversial reports of malignant peritoneal implantation following surgical ovarian cyst rupture. The overall complication rate for ovarian cyst FNA of 1 to 2 percent is mostly

due to pain, bleeding, and infection[47] and only rarely to tumor seeding. Cutaneous seeding may rarely occur following FNA of the thyroid.[48]

Radiographic Media

Barium sulfate is seen on the enteric mucosa as chalky white strands. Microscopically it consists of fine, fairly uniform golden granules. They are not doubly refractile. Barium elicits little inflammatory reaction when it reaches an extraluminal location through a perforated diverticulum or fistula. It lies free or is found in histiocytes. Rarely, foreign body giant cells are seen, but without well formed granulomas. When barium is found in areas of severe inflammatory and fibrous reaction, the response is due to concomitant fecal contamination rather than to barium per se. In one case, reaction was sufficient to cause ureteral obstruction.[49] Occasionally, barium is forced into the rectal mucosa at the time of barium enema and produces a polypoid mass.[50] In another report, barium entered the peritoneal cavity through a perforated duodenal ulcer and was still visible on radiographs 4 years later.[51]

The media used in hysterosalpingograms are oil-based iodine-containing compounds. The dye may be retained, and in one patient was visualized in a salpinx 25 years after the salpingogram.[52] In another patient, foreign body granulomas of the peritoneum were found that were attributed to extravasted medium.[53] The condition referred to as xanthomatous or lipoid salpingitis is characterized by a submucosal accumulation of foam cells; occasionally a history of a salpingogram will be obtained.

REACTION TO PHYSICAL AND CHEMICAL AGENTS

Starch, Cotton Lint, Cellulose, Gelfoam, and Talc

Rubber surgical gloves were introduced by Halsted to protect the hands of his scrub nurse from irritating disinfectants used in the operating room and later were found to protect the patient from infection as well.[54] Talcum powder was used to facilitate the donning of the gloves. By the 1940s, it was clear that the powder caused intestinal adhesions, fecal fistulas, and delayed wound healing and occasionally led to death. Since the 1950s, cornstarch mixed with 2 percent magnesium oxide (Bio-sorb) has become the most widely used agent, but rice starch is also available, and both can produce a granulomatous reaction.[55] Most symptomatic cases are due to peritonitis. Starch may be introduced into the abdomen by vaginal examination[56] and paracentesis,[57] as well as at laparotomy. Granulomatous reactions have also occurred in the pleura, middle ear, oral cavity, and brain.[58]

Symptoms of starch peritonitis usually begin in the second or third week after an otherwise uneventful recovery from surgery. Low grade fever and signs of peritonitis are often present; these gradually resolve after several days. If an exploratory laparo-

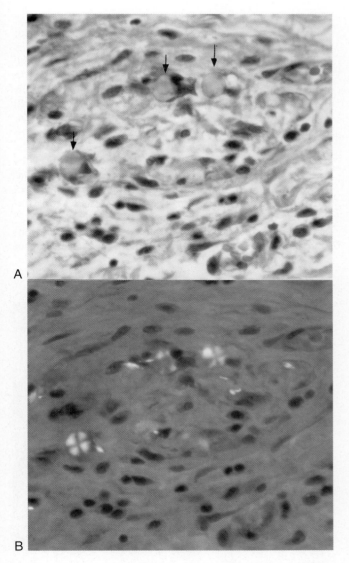

Fig. 14-5. Spherical particles of Bio-sorb (arrows) in subserosal fibrous tissue. **(A)** Specimen was obtained at time of closure of colostomy 5 weeks after previous surgery. Identical field under polarized light shows Maltese-cross configuration of Bio-sorb. **(B)** The small irregular shreds of doubly refractile material probably represent cotton lint from gauze sponges or packs.

nosis can be made by examination with polarized light.[59] FNA of talc and starch granulomas demonstrate characteristic birefringent silicate crystals ranging in size from 2 to 100 µm[60] and Maltese cross-shaped birefringent crystals,[61] respectively, within epithelioid histiocytes and multinucleated giant cells. Birefringent starch granules have also been detected extracellularly and intracellularly in cerebrospinal fluid filter preparations.[62]

In one patient, who underwent exploratory laparotomy because of starch peritonitis and then underwent surgery 18 months later, starch granules were found in calcified foreign body granulomas.[63]

Lint from cotton gauze sponges also produces a granulomatous or fibrous reaction.[64] Initially, the fragments of lint are up to 50 mm in width and are several times longer. They are ragged, irregularly shaped particles that are pale pink or violaceous in H&E sections and are shown to better advantage with polarized light. Over time, they disintegrate and exist as tiny particles that require polarized light to be seen. At this stage, the distinction from starch granules is based on the formation of Maltese crosses in the latter, whereas the cotton lint lacks this property (Fig. 14-5).

Fibrous adhesions from patients who have had previous surgery almost invariably contain foreign material, whether it be glove powder or cotton lint.[64] Absorbable hemostatics and the vehicles of antimicrobial agents are other potential irritants that may enhance adhesion formation.[65]

Cellulose fibers are the major component of disposable surgical gowns and drapes. The fibers have produced symptomatic granulomatous peritonitis, as well as other complications.[66] They are 5 to 15 mm in width and up to several hundred microns in length with twists at many levels that result in obliquely transverse folds. On cross-section, they are doughnut shaped, with a central empty space surrounded by the fiber wall. The material is faintly pink in H&E sections, PAS positive,

tomy is done, the peritoneum is found to be focally or diffusely studded with granulomas ranging from 1 mm to more than 1 cm in size. Omental necrosis or matting of the fat into discrete masses may be found.

The histologic response to the starch ranges from scattered histiocytes, lymphocytes, and neutrophils to well formed granulomas containing foreign body giant cells. The larger granulomas may have central necrosis.[57] The starch particles are seen on hematoxylin and eosin (H&E) sections as faintly eosinophilic particles averaging 3 to 10 mm in size. They stain deeply with periodic acid-Schiff (PAS) reagent and under polarized light have a Maltese-cross birefringence (Fig. 14-5). Peritoneal or pleural fluid contains the granules, and the diag-

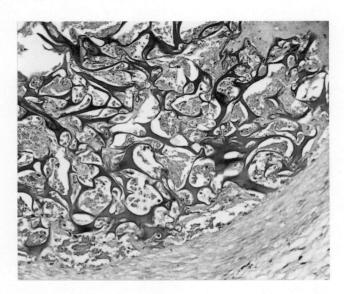

Fig. 14-6. Gelfoam has an irregular spiculated appearance. The material is in an artery injected before resection of a hemangioma in this region.

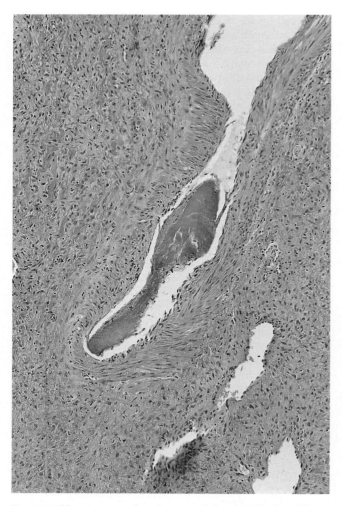

Fig. 14-7. Homogeneous, densely eosinophilic microfibrillar collagen (Avitene) embolus in a nasopharyngeal angiofibroma. Endothelialization and recanalization occur within days of embolization.

doubly refractile, and is found inside multinucleated giant cells or embedded in fibrous tissue.

Embolizing Agents

Surgical pathologists encounter arterial embolization materials in resected vascular lesions of the central nervous system (CNS) and tumors that are preoperatively embolized to optimize hemostasis. Therapeutic arterial embolization of intractable epistaxis or hemoptysis is less likely to be detected in histologic sections.[67] A number of chemical embolization materials are used, sometimes in combination.[68,69] These include Gelfoam, an absorbable gelatin that appears microscopically as basophilic, spiculated masses (Fig. 14-6). It may produce a severe foreign body reaction in the brain.[70] Avitene is a resorbable, microfibrillar collagen that forms intensely eosinophilic emboli that become rapidly endothelialized and

recanalized and incite a minimal tissue reaction[69] (Fig. 14-7). Nonresorbable polyvinyl alcohol particles form irregular, intravascular emboli that are admixed with blood elements (Fig. 14-8). Polyvinyl alcohol particles are poorly stained by H&E but appear densely black on elastic stain.[71] They may induce an acute vasculitis and foreign body reaction[72] but are essentially chemically inert, producing long-term vascular occlusion with recanalization and calcification.[73] The liquid embolization material, bucrylate (isobutyl 2-cyanoacrylate), is partially dissolved during xylene tissue processing and is translucent by H&E staining. It is best demonstrated in tissue sections by ether-based oil red O staining.[74] Of the commonly used embolization materials, bucrylate appears to induce the most severe tissue reaction in the form of vasculitis, vessel necrosis, foreign body reaction, and occasional extravascular extrusion.[69] Lipiodol-mediated delivery of cytotoxic drugs can be demonstrated in resected hepatocellular carcinoma by Sudan stain but not by H&E.[75]

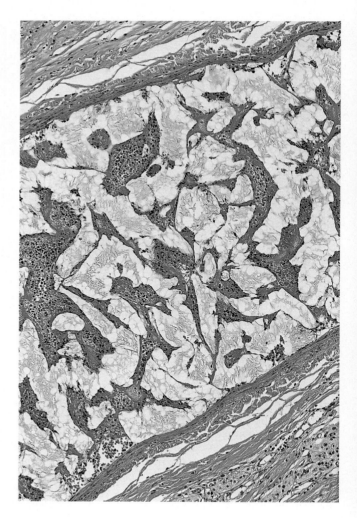

Fig. 14-8. Section from an intracranial meningioma following preoprative embolization and resection. Irregular, intravascular polyvinyl alcohol particles admixed with normal blood elements appear weakly basophilic by H&E staining.

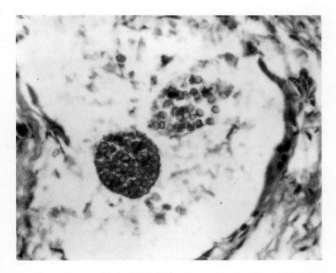

Fig. 14-9. Myospherulosis consists of an aggregate of altered red cells surrounded by a membrane. A fibrous and histiocytic inflammatory change is seen at the periphery. Patient had previous surgery for sinusitis that included packing with petroleum-impregnated gauze. (Courtesy of Thomas M. Wheeler, M.D., Methodist Hospital, Houston, TX.)

Myospherulosis

In 1977 Kyriakos[76] reported that tissue removed from paranasal sinuses or the middle ear had small sacs containing spherules about the size of erythrocytes (Fig. 14-9). The name myospherulosis was chosen because of the identification of the findings with previously described cases from Africa, which occurred in muscle. All the patients of Kyriakos had had previous operations that included packing with gauze impregnated with antibiotic ointment. Rosai[77] and Travis et al[78] proved that the spherules are erythrocytes that become enveloped in a sac. Wheeler et al[79] demonstrated that erythrocytes undergo the same change in vitro when incubated with human fat. This finding accounts for myospherulosis in soft tissues at injection sites.[80] Myospherulosis has also been demonstrated in the brain.[81] In cytologic smears, myospherulosis is essentially identical to its histologic image, isolated or sac-like aggregates of 4 to 7 μm spherules that presumably represent erythrocytes altered by previous lipid exposure. In addition to petroleum-based intramuscular injections, FNA detection of myospherulosis has been associated with previous breast biopsy, fat necrosis, and invasive breast cancer.[82] Therefore, cytologic detection of myospherulosis indicates erythrocyte exposure to either endogenous or exogenous lipids and is a potential, albeit unusual, harbinger of underlying carcinoma.

Steroid Injection

A granulomatous reaction resembling rheumatoid nodules develops in the nasal mucosa after injection with steroids. The central amorphous area is apparently the injected substance itself.[83] A similar reaction occurs in keloids injected with steroids.[84] Rupture of tendons sometimes follows steroid injection, but histologic findings are not specific.[85] Connective tissue steroid injection sites demonstrate similar deposits of amorphous, acellular material, but often no surrounding inflammatory reaction is present.[86]

Oleogranuloma

Oleogranulomas (lipid granulomas, oleomas, paraffinomas) are reactive masses that occur as a reaction to a variety of oils that have been injected, topically applied, or used as a lubricant during dilation of the cervix. The histiocytic response may not produce a clinically detectable mass until years later, at which time rapid enlargement is possible.[87] Lesions have been reported in the rectum, parametrium, and pleural space.[88,89]

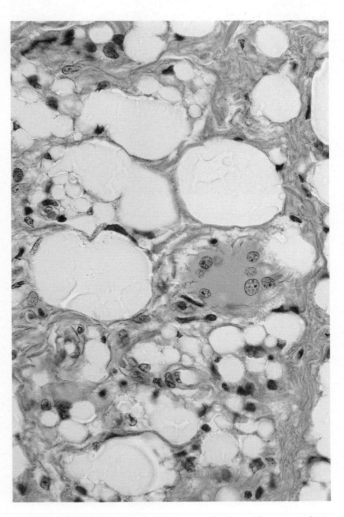

Fig. 14-10. Silicone in capsule of patient with silicone breast prosthesis removed because of contracture of fibrous capsule. Silicone-gel is seen as variously sized droplets.

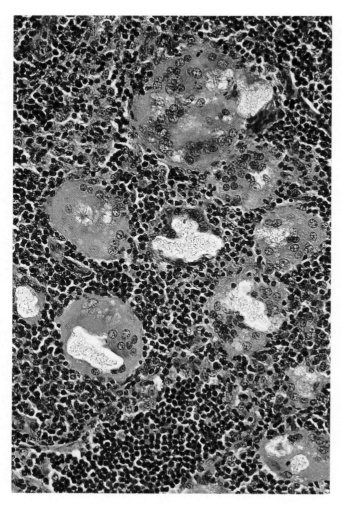

Fig. 14-11. Inguinal lymph node from patient with silicone prosthesis of hip joint. The translucent strands and globules of silicone are found within giant cells.

Lubricating Jellies and Contraceptive Creams

Lubricating jellies should not be used prior to obtaining cervicovaginal smears, since these can obscure cytologic detail and limit interpretation.[90] In addition, plant cellular materials found in some commercial lubricants may resemble neoplastic cells in cervicovaginal smears.[91]

Silicone

Silicone injections of the breast are no longer used, but many women still carry this substance and have symptoms that sometimes lead to biopsy. The reaction is fibrous and histiocytic. Many of the histiocytes have an irregular configuration, and the silicone produces a fine to coarse cytoplasmic vacuolization. Such cells may be mistaken for malignant lipoblasts.

More than 2 million silicone breast prostheses have been im-

planted in the United States alone since their introduction in the 1960s.[92] Dense fibrous capsule formation or prosthetic rupture often leads to removal. Many of the fibrous capsules are lined with a cellular membrane histologically, immunohistochemically, and ultrastructurally identical to synovium.[93,94] This synovial metaplasia has been described in sutured skin, after repeated subcutaneous injections of air, and at the bone-cement interface of loosened hip prostheses.[95] The capsules and soft tissue beyond the capsule contain a variety of foreign material including droplets of silicone (Fig. 14-10), fragments of the prosthetic bag envelope, polyurethane, and talc.[96] No evidence suggests an increase in "connective tissue" diseases in patients with silicone implants.[97]

Silicone can appear in giant cells in the axillary nodes. Cytologic smears of silicone lymphadenopathy demonstrate refractile silicone fragments, both intracellular and extracellular, as well as asteroid bodies. FNA offers a relatively noninvasive method for excluding malignant lymphadenopathy in these patients.[98] Cases of carcinoma have been reported in patients with prostheses, but no evidence thus far shows an increased incidence of cancer unless the patient had been irradiated.[99] Although needle aspiration in patients with silicone breast implants carries some risk of puncture radiographically guided and unguided FNA attempts can still be performed to rule out malignant tumors. Cytologic smears in these cases occasionally detect silicone granulomas that exhibit loose aggregates of epithelioid histiocytes with variably sized, clear cytoplasmic vacuoles and little epithelium.[100]

Symptomatic splenomegaly due to macrophages filled with silicone has been reported in a patient undergoing hemodialysis. The silicone was presumably from the roller pumps.[101] It may also be found in the liver and kidney.

Silicone lymphadenopathy is seen in nodes draining joints that have silicone prostheses[102] (Fig. 14-11). The adenopathy can occur in the absence of synovitis or malfunction of the prosthesis.[103–105] However, cytologic demonstration of silicone elastomer microshards in fluids that accumulate adjacent to silicone joint prostheses may be an indication for removal of prostheses.[106]

Intrauterine Devices

Intrauterine devices (IUDs) produce epithelial erosion and acute inflammation at the point of contact with the endometrium. Squamous metaplasia and foreign body granulomas are encountered rarely.[107] Secretory development is delayed by 3 days or more in about 30 percent of women wearing these devices.[108]

Serious complications include perforation of the uterus and extrauterine infection consisting usually of tubo-ovarian abscess. Inexplicably, the abscesses are nearly always unilateral, unlike "ordinary" pelvic inflammatory disease, which is almost always bilateral.[109] Disproportionate numbers of abscesses are secondary to actinomyces, with its characteristic inflammatory response of a purulent exudate mixed with foamy histiocytes.

A constellation of cytologic abnormalities can be seen in the cervicovaginal smears of women using IUDs. In the early weeks after IUD insertion, smears show a prominent macrophage response followed by nonspecific reparative and degenerative changes similar to those that follow biopsy procedures.[110] Subsequent cellular changes that are specific for IUDs are easily confused with adenocarcinoma. These include shedding of glandular cells and occasional metaplastic squamous cells with prominent cytoplasmic vacuolization and variable degrees of nuclear enlargement, hyperchromasia, nucleolar prominence, nuclear membrane irregularity, and neutrophilic infiltration.[111,112] Less commonly, bizarre cells with high nuclear/cytoplasmic ratios and cytoplasmic protrusions can also be confused with malignancy. Pathologist awareness of IUD history helps to avoid a false diagnosis of malignant tumor.

In cytologic preparations, IUD-associated actinomycoces typically appear as irregular dense masses with radiating, filamentous bacterial organisms recognizable only at the periphery. Less commonly they appear as loose colonies of branched filaments. Similar but distinct filamentous aggregates that are surrounded by a dense rim of inflammatory cells are often inappropriately termed "sulfur granules." These can represent actinomycoces but are not specific, since they are also seen in other infections.[112] Fragments of IUD material, polarizable sulfa crystals from topical ointments, contraceptive creams, hematoidin crystals, and uncharacterized radiate crystals associated with pregnancy can also be confused with actinomycoces.[112,113] IUD usage is occasionally associated with calcifications and psammoma bodies in cervicovaginal smears, findings that otherwise would suggest the possibility of ovarian or endometrial adenocarcinoma.[114]

Cryotherapy

The degree of damage to tissue by intense cold depends on the temperature and duration of application. In the uterine cervix, the epithelium becomes contracted and degenerates almost instantly. The sharp line of demarcation is only a few cells wide. Blood vessels regenerate a new endothelial lining after about 2 weeks. After a few months the only marker of previous cryosurgery is the hyalinized but patent blood vessels.[115]

In the immediate days following cervical and vaginal cryotherapy, smears contain a background of necrotic cellular debris and acute inflammation that should not be confused with malignant tumor diathesis. Early after cryotherapy cytoplasmic vacuolization is seen that remains for weeks and occasionally for months.[116] Reparative changes identical to those seen in postbiopsy smears are seen following cryotherapy as well as electrocautery, laser ablation, and radiotherapy. In contrast to radiotherapy, cryotherapy changes lack significant nuclear and cytoplasmic enlargement and nuclear irregularity. In contrast to laser therapy and electrocautery, cryotherapy does not produce prominent epithelial cell elongation.[117] The duration of cytologic abnormalities that follow cryotherapy, electrocautery, and laser ablation varies with the mode of therapy, individual technique, and anatomic extent of treatment but generally lasts for 6 weeks or longer.[118] Cervical cryotherapy, electrocautery, and laser ablation can shift the squamocolumnar transformation zone superiorly into the endocervical canal, similar to conization, necessitating endocervical brush instead of cotton swab sampling of endocervical epithelium.[6,119]

Postcryotherapy histologic changes in the prostate resemble those seen in the cervix. Early necrosis and inflammation is followed by granulation tissue, fibrosis, and focal re-epithelialization.[120] To minimize postcryotherapy complications, transrectal sonography is used to monitor hyperechoic periprostatic freeze damage as a signal for termination of therapy. Hyperechoic damage is not a good indicator of tumor destruction since prostatectomy specimens removed 3 to 10 months following ultrasound-proven "complete" freezing often contain viable carcinoma.[121]

Orthopedic Hardware

A variety of materials are used in prosthetic devices. The materials used and the tissue reactions are discussed in detail in Chapter 22. The carcinogenic effect of the various materials has been of concern, since the substances used in prostheses produce sarcomas in rodents. The relevance of these studies to humans remains to be determined. Thus far only three cases of sarcoma have developed at the site of a hip prosthesis. One patient was a 77-year-old woman who developed pain 2 years after arthroplasty; she had malignant fibrous histiocytoma.[122] Another patient had an osteosarcoma 5 years after surgery,[123] and one other patient had a malignant fibrous histiocytoma 4 years after insertion of a prosthesis.[124] Between 1956 and 1980, five sarcomas were reported in sites where metal plates had been inserted for traumatic fracture.[125,126] Even if no cause-and-effect relationship exists in some of these cases, they attest to the rarity of neoplasms associated with the 300,000 to 400,000 total joint replacements inserted each year worldwide.[127]

Metallic components from hip prostheses can evoke a florid histiocytic response in the pelvic lymph nodes.[128] This alteration has been found in patients having pelvic lymphadenectomy for urinary bladder or prostatic cancer.[129] It has been confused with carcinoma.[130]

Teflon Paste and Proplast

A paste containing the polymer polytetraflorethane (Teflon) is used to correct vocal cord paralysis and for treatment of urinary incontinence.[131] Microscopically, it consists of shiny yellow particles in a myriad of shapes and sizes ranging from 6 to 100 mm (Fig. 14-12). The injected bolus becomes surrounded by a fibrous rim with some penetration between the particles. Mononuclear and multinucleated histiocytes also display a histiocytic response. In several patients treated for vocal cord paralysis, the material has entered the neck, resulting in a mass. Teflon can be recognized on FNA.[132] The overlying epithelium of the vocal cord has not shown atypical changes nor have any other recognizable adverse reactions occurred despite the presence of small particles within the lymphatics or blood vessels.

Granulomatous foreign body reactions to Teflon can be demonstrated by FNA. In one case, periurethral injection resulted in a macroscopic Teflon cyst that yielded no giant cell or inflammatory infiltrate by FNA, only irregular, birefringent Teflon particles.[133]

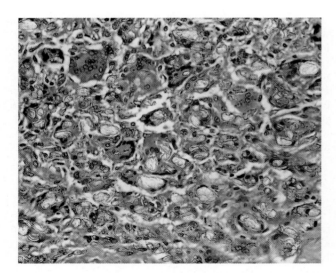

Fig. 14-12. Teflon paste within vocal cord. Irregular particles provoke a fibrous and histiocytic reaction.

Proplast is a polymer of Teflon and carbon used mainly in cosmetic surgery for filling soft tissue defects. Its porosity permits ingrowth of capillaries and connective tissue, which helps anchor the material in place. Occasionally the material may shift so the desired cosmetic effect is lost; the implant is then removed. The soft tissue around the prosthesis contains foreign body giant cells, some of which have small punctate particles of the carbon component.[134]

Suture Materials

The thoughtful pathologist always removes suture material before submitting a block of tissue for embedding. Nevertheless, small fragments of suture may be buried in the middle of the block or may be in a stage of disintegration and not grossly detectable. A surgeon occasionally asks whether suture is present in an excised focus of inflammation; if so the surgeon may wish to know the type of material.

Sutures are divided into two groups, absorbable and nonabsorbable. Absorbable sutures include catgut (derived from sheep or beef intestines), collagen, polyglycolic acid, and polyglactin 910, which is a copolymer of glycolic and lactic acids in a ratio of 9:1. The nonabsorbable sutures are nylon, cotton, polyester (Dacron), polypropylene, steel, and silk. Silk is generally placed in this category although it disintegrates and eventually disappears after a period of many months to years.[135]

All sutures provoke a tissue response. Catgut is destroyed by the proteolytic enzymes of neutrophils and, therefore, requires inflammation to be absorbed. The absorbable synthetic polymers are hydrolyzed by water and do not require enzymatic degradation, but nonetheless they evoke a histiocytic and fibrous reaction.[136] The response to silk and cotton includes neutrophils, lymphocytes, or macrophages and eventually ends with a fibrous reaction accompanied only by macrophages. All the other materials excite a histiocytic response with minimal

fibrosis.[137] Rarely, silk suture evokes a necrobiotic granuloma closely resembling rheumatoid nodules.[138]

On microscopic examination some sutures are always specifically identifiable (e.g., catgut), whereas others can only be placed in a general category (e.g., multifilamentous synthetic agents). Silk, Dacron, and cotton are always multifilamentous. Nylon and steel are produced in either a mono- or multifilamentous form. Polypropylene is manufactured only as a monofilament. Catgut, whether plain or chromic, is a homogeneous faintly eosinophilic or amphophilic substance (Fig. 14-13). The multiple filaments of silk are of similar size but are round, square, or triangular when seen in cross-section (Fig. 14-14). Each of the filaments in the multifilament synthetic sutures are round and of identical size (Fig. 14-15). Randomly scattered tiny black specks are seen both in Dacron and nylon. Polyglactin and polypropylene tend to have a glossy, transparent appearance.[137] Some sutures are covered on the surface with Teflon to decrease the abrasive effect, and minute fragments may be flaked off into the adjacent tissue.

On occasion, the inflammatory reaction to suture after resection of a portion of the gastrointestinal tract produces a mass sufficiently large to be seen as a filling defect on barium examination. A few patients have undergone re-exploration because the defect was believed to be a recurrence of neoplasm at the suture line or a new primary in another organ into which suture had migrated.[139,140]

In sites of previous surgery for neoplasia, reactive suture granulomas can be clinically worrisome for recurrent disease. Pathologic evaluation by needle aspiration typically demonstrates multinucleated giant cells with intracytoplasmic fragments of suture material, obviating the need for additional surgery. However, FNA smears of suture granulomas occasionally lack these diagnostic features and instead show a predominance of reactive spindle cells with mild nuclear pleomorphism. Depending on the histology of the original tumor, these findings can paradoxically augment suspicion for a malignant tumor and can necessitate rebiopsy.[141]

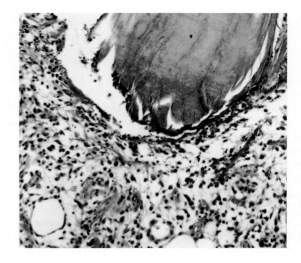

Fig. 14-13. Catgut suture is fairly homogeneous material with inflammatory response, including many neutrophils.

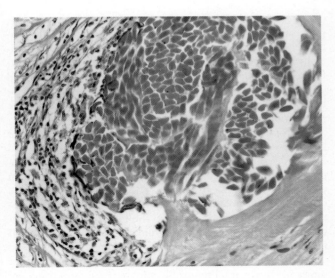

Fig. 14-14. Silk suture is always multifilamentous with irregularly shaped, dark filaments

Monsel's Solution

Monsel's solution (20 percent ferric subsulfate) is commonly used by dermatologists as a styptic or hemostatic after superficial skin biopsies. The compound may be in spindle cells with large vesicular nuclei[142] and may seep as deeply as skeletal muscle.[143] If the diagnosis on the biopsy specimen is melanoma and the area is subsequently excised, the interpretation of the depth of invasion is hampered by the distorted cells and pigment.

Vascular Prostheses

Three patients with sarcoma arising in the region of a Dacron or Teflon-Dacron graft have been reported. The strongest case for a cause-and-effect relationship is presented by Weinberg and Maini,[144] even though the tumor arose only 14 months after insertion of the graft.

UNTOWARD RESULTS OF SURGICAL PROCEDURES

Implantation of Normal Tissue

Normal colonic mucosa deep in the wall of the bowel was found when a colostomy was closed after 8 years. Presumably it was implanted at the original procedure.[145] Six of 19 patients with localized colitis cystica profunda of the rectum had a history of previous rectal surgery.[146] It is possible that the procedure implanted mucosa or altered the muscularis mucosae to permit downward extension of glands.

Thyroid tissue has been described in the lateral neck after prior surgery. The adjacent suture material suggests mechanical

implantation.[147] Omentum has been implanted in the endometrium following operative perforation of the uterus.[148]

The fallopian tube is sometimes caught in the incision at the time of vaginal hysterectomy and can produce a vaginal mass on subsequent examination. The biopsy speciment shows tubal architecture with its normal complement of cells; degenerative and regenerative cytologic alterations can be seen in the form of cells with enlarged or dense nuclei. Stratification of the cells can be prominent.

Alterations due to Cardiac Procedures

Fragments of tissue from suctioning of the pericardial cavity during surgery produces artifacts due to a mixture of adipose tissue, pericardial mesothelium, and foreign material.[149] Cardiac catheterization may also account for some of these mixtures of cells, and they may cause confusion with malignant neoplasm or endomyocardial biopsies.[150]

Ventriculoperitoneal Shunts

Ventriculoperitoneal shunts are occasionally occluded by overgrowths of reactive inflammatory tissue, peritoneal mesothelium, or CNS tissues including choroid plexus, glia, and meninges. Occluding tissues may be submitted for histologic examination to exclude recurrent neoplasia. Associated intraventricular inflammatory and foreign body reactions can be seen in cerebrospinal fluid.[151] Tissue from primary CNS tumors or, less commonly, benign choroid plexus may embolize through the shunt into the peritoneal cavity, where they appear cytologically positive or suggestive of malignant tumor, respectively.[152] Benign glial nodules as well as neoplasms have spread to the peritoneal cavity.[153,154]

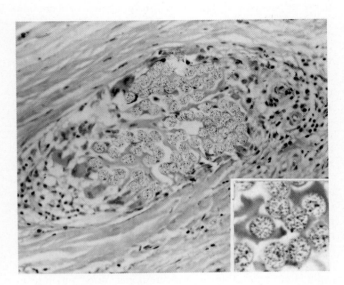

Fig. 14-15. Cross-section of Dacron, which had been in place for 2 years, showing foreign body giant cells between the individual filaments.

Alterations at the Site of Anastomoses

Numerous alterations, including roughly 50 adenocarcinomas, have been reported in the colon in the immediate area of ureterosigmoidostomies. Some are adenomatous polyps with prominent submucosal cysts resembling colitis cystica profunda. The carcinomas are weighted by undifferentiated and mucin-producing tumors. The neoplasms are closely related to the length of time that the patients have had the ureterosigmoidostomy (an average of about 20 years). One patient developed cancer at age 17.[155] This argues strongly in favor of a causal relationship: the urinary stream produces premalignant changes and ultimately a malignant neoplasm.[156,157] Carcinoma can occur even after early external diversion.[158]

Gastric polyps around gastroenterostomy stomas have included small discrete masses as well as completely circumferential proliferations, which on occasion have prolapsed into the lumen. Microscopically, dilated glands protrude through the muscularis and the term *gastritis cystica polyposa* has been proposed.[159]

Even in the absence of a gross polyp, sections from the gastric mucosa at the anastomotic site may display abnormalities, including dilated glands and a decrease in chief and parietal cells. If an erosion or ulcer is present, the adjacent epithelium can have regenerating, immature cells with a high nuclear/cytoplasmic ratio that line irregular glands of variable sizes.[160,161] An increased incidence of gastric cancer exists in patients with gastroenterostomies,[162] and the tumors may arise in the polyps.[163] Thirty-seven years after a Billroth II resection, a squamous carcinoma developed in the gastric stump.[164]

Postoperative Abdominal Cysts

Peritoneal cysts may develop several months to 5 years after surgery, particularly in patients who have had a postoperative course with signs of peritonitis or wound infection.[165] Most patients are women with a previous history of pelvic or abdominal surgery, endometriosis, or pelvic inflammatory disease.[166] The cysts may be free-floating, may be embedded in the retroperitoneum, or may be attached to any of the abdominal viscera. They are unilocular or multilocular and contain clear, yellow, or green-brown fluid. The cysts are lined by low cuboidal or flattened mesothelium-like cells, squamous epithelium, or no cells at all. The wall is fibrous with variable vascularity and inflammation. The pathogenesis is not clear but possibly relates to walled-off areas of inflammation. The rapid growth that sometimes occurs may be due to osmotic forces secondary to hemorrhage.

In histologic sections, the cystic configuration, previous operative history, prominent chronic inflammation, stromal reaction, and mild to moderate degree of nuclear atypia indicate a reactive process.[166] Malignant mesotheliomas are rarely prominently cystic.[167] FNA of peritoneal inclusion cysts can yield reactive, hypertrophic mesothelial cells with nuclear enlargment and prominent nucleoli that suggest malignant tumor, especially after previous surgery for carcinoma. Wide variation in mesothelial cell size, cytoplasmic vacuolation, and multinucleation may be seen, identical to reactive mesothelial changes in other serous fluids. Fine chromatin, regular nuclear membranes, prominent but regular nucleoli, ruffled plasma membrane contours, and characteristic intercellular spaces or "windows" generally allow distinction from recurrent malignant tumor. In difficult cases, immunohistochemical staining panels performed on cytologic fluids, including the mesothelium-specific antibody ME1, or standard paraffin-based panels on cell block preparations are useful.[168,169]

The formation of lymphocysts is a complication of pelvic or renal surgery. The cyst contains a clear slightly yellow fluid and is devoid of lining cells. Symptoms are related to a mass compressing the ureter, bladder, colon, or vessels, resulting in edema of the lower extremities. The origin from lymphatic channels is documented by numerous reports in which lymphangiography medium has filled the mass.[170] Meticulous attention to ligation of lymphatic trunks at the time of the original surgery minimizes cyst formation.[171]

Mesenteric cysts, usually lined by luteal cells, can follow surgery of the ovary. Presumably minute portions of ovary are dislodged and implant on the peritoneum, where they survive and enlarge.[172]

Reactions Resembling Neoplasms

Proppe et al[173] described a highly cellular spindle cell proliferation with numerous mitotic figures that occurred in the vagina after a variety of surgical procedures. The largest mass was 4 cm in diameter. A similar proliferation has occurred in the prostatic urethra and urinary bladder following transurethral resections and in the endocervix.[174] The lesions appear 2 weeks to 3 months after surgery. Clinical history is essential since postoperative spindle cell nodules (PSCN) of the bladder and prostate can be histologically identical to spontaneous spindle cell proliferations ("inflammatory pseudotumors"), which are sometimes associated with underlying carcinomas.[175] Focal immunohistochemical staining for cytokeratins in some PSCN may confound this differential. PSCN and spontaneous spindle cell proliferations also share histologic features with two primary genitourinary tract cancers spindle cell carcinoma and leiomyosarcoma. Accurate diagnosis frequently requires immunohistochemistry in addition to clinical history.[176] FNA smears of reparative mesenchymal proliferations, including PSCN and inflammatory pseudotumors, occasionally demonstrate sufficient spindle cell hypercellularity and pleomorphism to be confused with cancer. A prominent inflammatory background in these cases should alert the pathologist not to make a definitive cytologic diagnosis of sarcoma.[177]

A highly cellular fibrohistiocytic proliferation with nuclear atypia resembling liposarcoma has occurred in sites in which sclerosing agents were used for the repair of hernia. Silica has been identified in these foci. Although this material is no longer used, the interval between injection and lesion has ranged up to 40 years; therefore, this lesion may still be seen.[178] Broad aggregates of histiocytes with eosinophilic granular cytoplasm may accumulate at the site of surgical trauma and resemble granular cell tumor. The granular cytoplasm is lipofuscin, which is usually acid fast.[179]

Fig. 14-16. Entrapped mesothelial cells mimic adenocarcinoma. This is from the wall of a postoperative peritoneal inclusion cyst. (Courtesy of Philip B. Clement, M.D., Vancouver General Hospital, Vancouver, BC.)

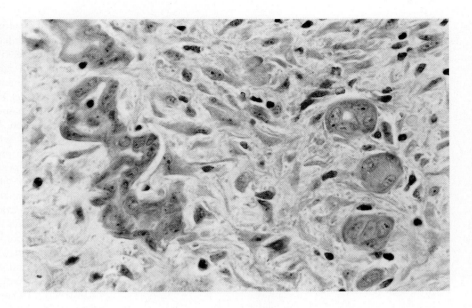

Unilocular or multilocular cysts that raise the possibility of malignant neoplasm have been found in women who have undergone previous surgery.[180] Entrapped, markedly atypical mesothelial cells with mitotic activity mimic adenocarcinoma (Fig. 14-16).

Malignant Neoplasms

A few malignant tumors have arisen at the site of previous surgery. One of the 200 malignant fibrous histiocytomas reported by Weiss and Enzinger[181] arose 8 years later at the excision site for a lipoma. Two additional cases, one at an amputation site and the other in a hernioplasty scar, have been reported.[182] Whether these are coincidental is arguable.

REACTIONS TO CYTOTOXIC DRUGS AND IMMUNOSUPPRESSION

Chemotherapy for cancer and some nonmalignant conditions involves potent agents that may have morphologic as well as physiologic effects on a variety of normal tissues. The toxicity of the various agents is diverse. Much of the morbidity consists of gastrointestinal symptoms, bone marrow suppression, cutaneous alterations, and hepatic or renal impairment. The surgical pathologist is uncommonly involved in these problems, with some notable exceptions. For example, perforation of the small intestine in patients with widespread lymphoma was a rare event prior to chemotherapy but now occurs due to drug-induced massive necrosis of tumor within the bowel wall.[183] Some tumors also display behavioral changes such as unusual sites of metastases[184–186] or a more widespread distribution.[187–189] Whether this reflects immune suppression that fa-

cilitates spread of the tumor or is due to an increased duration of survival is uncertain. Cavitation of pulmonary metastases can occur due to chemotherapy and can be confused with inflammatory lesions.[190] Hepar lobatum results from a chemotherapeutic effect on breast cancer metastatic to the liver.[191]

Changes in Normal Epithelium

Alkylating agents can induce epithelial abnormalities that mimic malignancy in many organs, notably lung, lower urinary tract, and cervix.[192–197] Multidrug chemotherapeutic regimens that include alkylating agents have produced marked epithelial atypia in diagnostic specimens from the breast[198,199] and esophagus.[200] Histologic effects of chemotherapy are usually seen in resected specimens following preoperative therapy.

Biopsies, FNAs, or cytologic smears of sputum, bronchoalveolar, urine, or cervicovaginal origin may contain identical abnormal cells, raising the possibility of metastases or a second primary neoplasm. Since alkylating agents can cause secondary solid tumors, this distinction is especially problematic. Cytologic changes due to alkylating agents mimic radiation-induced changes as well as cancers and include cytomegaly, increased nuclear size, increased nuclear/cytoplasmic ratio, bizarre shapes, cytoplasmic vacuolization, and occasionally hyperchromasia (Fig. 14-17). Morphometric image analysis of urine cytologies cannot clearly distinguish these toxic changes from malignancy.[201] A continuous spectrum of atypia from minimally enlarged, non-neoplastic cells to bizarre giant cells and the detection of cilia on atypical pulmonary cells indicate drug-induced change. However, in cases with extreme atypia, clinical history may be the most important discriminator.

Urine cytology is particularly affected by the alkylating agent cyclophosphamide,[202] which is concentrated in urine, and by

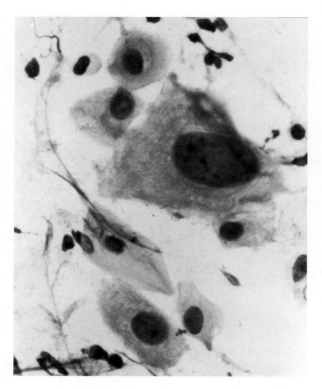

Fig. 14-17. Cells in sputum of a patient receiving busulfan for leukemia. He had pneumonia but no pulmonary neoplasm. The wide variation in size of qualitatively similar cells is the characteristic spectrum for this cytopathy.

intravesical cytotoxic therapy, although effects of the latter are less likely to resemble malignancy.[195,203] Nonalkylating agents such as bleomycin can cause changes similar to alkylating agents in the lung.[197]

Chemotherapy for mammary carcinoma may produce multilobated cells within otherwise normal ducts of the breast. These do not resemble the cells of carcinoma in situ and undoubtedly reflect chemotherapy effect.[199] Atrophy of lobules may be focally prominent. A teardrop appearance has been seen in some breasts treated with chemotherapy and may reflect hormonal (Tamoxifen) therapy. Rarely, no residual carcinoma is detectable. The tumor site has been replaced by a nodular fibrous reaction accompanied by histiocytes.[204]

Extensive cytoplasmic vacuolization is found in glands of normal or hyperplastic prostate.[205] Involutional changes and basal cell hyperplasia, may also be seen.

The effects of topical podophyllin therapy on condyloma acuminatum are frequently claimed to mimic high grade squamous intraepithelial neoplasia. Acute post-therapy changes of edema, increased mitotic activity, and single cell keratinocyte degeneration and necrosis are followed by hyperkeratosis and mixed inflammation, all of which resolve within 2 to 6 weeks. Persistence of orderly maturation and lack of diagnostic nuclear atypia allow distinction from high grade dysplasia.[206] By con-

trast, topical cytotoxic therapy with 5-fluorouracil can produce nonspecific chemical mucositis and nonhealing ulcers.[207]

Intravesical bacilles Calmette-Guérin immunotherapy for transitional cell carcinoma or high grade urothelial dysplasia induces a prominent granulomatous response in both the bladder and prostate. In addition to caseating and noncaseating granulomas, squamous metaplasia and a mixed inflammatory infiltrate are seen. Urine cytology demonstrates degenerating epithelial cell debris in a background of abundant mixed inflammation, but granulomatous features are not prominent. Prostatic FNA specimens taken after bacille Calmette-Guérin therapy contain similar features but also demonstrate histiocytes and multinucleated giant cells, similar to prostatic FNA smears following transurethral resections.[197]

Toxic pulmonary effects of the antiarrhythmic drug amiodarone are morphologically striking, although they do not resemble malignancy. A prominent alveolar infiltrate of foamy macrophages and occasional vacuolated parenchymal cells demonstrates characteristic cytoplasmic lamellar inclusions by ultrastructural examination.[208] These toxic changes can be monitored by bronchoalveolar lavage[209] and are rarely seen in pleural fluids.[210]

Changes in Neoplastic Epithelium

It is now common to give preoperative chemotherapy with or without radiotherapy prior to a surgical resection. The appearance of the treated cancer in the surgical specimen may have major implications for the type of additional therapy, as exemplified in the treatment of osteosarcoma. In this instance, the continuation of the preoperative chemotherapy regimen depends on the amount of viable tumor present in the resected tissue. Similarly, therapeutic judgments may be made based on the appearance of neoplasm in patients who have received preoperative chemotherapy for carcinoma of the breast. In one study, the appearance of the tumor and the ability to grade it histologically was identical to the prechemotherapy biopsy in many instances.[211]

Kennedy et al[199] illustrated an extraordinary vacuolization of neoplastic cells such that they resembled foamy histiocytes. Epithelial markers were identified by immunohistochemistry, indicating that these were persistent epithelial cells.

Chemotherapy-induced changes in malignant tumors do not necessarily indicate a lethal effect. Morphologic and kinetic monitoring of pulmonary small cell carcinomas during multidrug chemotherapy demonstrates drug-induced vacuolization and nuclear enlargement that do not inevitably lead to cell death.[212]

Histologic Maturation After Chemotherapy

Cytotoxic drug therapy may accentuate maturation of various elements in residual neoplasms. Testicular mixed germ cell tumors can have only benign-appearing elements in metastases after chemotherapy.[213] Many ovarian immature teratomas and a few adenocarcinomas have shown maturation after drug therapy.[214] A plausible explanation is based on the premise that neoplasms have heterogeneous subpopulations that react differently to the same therapeutic agent, with the less well differentiated component being more susceptible. This phenomenon has been reported frequently since the advent of chemotherapy, but it should be kept in mind that an identical maturation of metastatic germ cell tumors was reported prior to the chemotherapy era.[215]

Resected germ cell tumors that contain predominantly benign mature elements must be examined carefully, because they may also have small foci of malignancy. The malignancy can be present even when previously elevated serum markers have returned to normal.[213] Cytologic atypia, as opposed to obviously invasive cancer, does not seem to be an adverse prognostic factor in males.[216]

Residual rhabdomyosarcoma of childhood sometimes has a high proportion of rhabdomyoblasts and strap cells after chemotherapy. It occurs only when similar cells are focally present in the original tumor.[217,218] Other types of soft tissue sarcomas also have a lower histologic grade after chemotherapy (with or without concomitant radiotherapy).[219] This finding again suggests that high grade populations of cells are more susceptible to therapy than low grade clones.

Differentiation of neuroblastoma to ganglioneuroblastoma with a predominance of mature atypical ganglion cells and fewer immature malignant cells has been found after cytotoxic chemotherapy for neuroblastoma. Differentiation did not, however, correlate with prognosis.[220]

Hepatoblastomas may have small areas of osteoid in the original tumor, which may occupy large areas after chemotherapy. Such a predominance of "benign tissue" does not seem to be a favorable prognostic sign, although this point is arguable.[221]

An autopsy study of patients with choriocarcinoma disclosed that a few patients had residua consisting only of atypical cytotrophoblasts.[222] Similar trophoblasts can be seen in surgically resected choriocarcinomas after chemotherapy. These cells resemble intermediate trophoblasts and may reflect an insensitivity of this stage of trophoblastic differentiation to chemotherapy.

Patients with Wilms' tumor may receive preoperative chemotherapy. Up to 90 percent of the tumor mass may become necrotic, mainly in the replicating, undifferentiated elements.[223] Mature heterotopic elements such as cartilage, fat, and skeletal muscle persisted after therapy. A few tumors consisted almost entirely of skeletal muscle.[224] Favorable outcomes were associated with extensive tumor necrosis (>90 percent), low mitotic activity, and high degrees of differentiation of residual tumor.[224]

Persistent Non-Neoplastic Tumor Mass

A tumor mass can persist after chemotherapy, radiotherapy, or a combination of the two. It can be interpreted as a therapeutic failure and result in additional, unnecessary therapy. After an adequate course of therapy, persistent tumor masses that are resected often consist only of inflamed fibrous tissue with necrotic areas lacking any neoplasm. It has been reported in lymph nodes from patients with Hodgkin's disease,[225] large cell lymphoma,[226] and testicular embryonal carcinoma.[227,228] This phenomenon has also occurred in the spleen.[226]

Thymic Hyperplasia

The thymus may become hyperplastic after chemotherapy and may mimic a mediastinal neoplasm. The cause is unknown.[229,230]

Non-Neoplastic Lymphadenopathy

Enlarged lymph nodes following therapy for malignant neoplasm always raise the possibility of metastatic disease. In one instance, a man developed rapidly enlarging axillary nodes 1 month after completion of chemotherapy for lymphoma. The node consisted only of a narrow rim of lymphoid tissue surrounding normal mature fat.[231] Fatty replacement is commonly seen in nodes removed during axillary dissections for carcinoma of the breast, but rapid growth is not a feature of such nodes.[232]

Geis et al[233] reported five renal transplant recipients in whom gigantic systemic lymphadenopathy developed shortly after transplantation. It rapidly resolved with no evidence of residual disease from 6 to 15 months later. These patients had received antithymocyte globulin and presumably had a transient reaction to this agent. The biopsies were indistinguishable from diffuse large cell lymphoma. In another report, a similar reaction developed in the soft tissue at the site of antilymphocytic globulin injection.[234] These may represent variant forms of post-transplantation lymphoproliferative disorders.

Drug-Associated Neoplasms

Secondary malignant tumors are attributed to a number of cytotoxic drugs, most notably the alkylating agents.[235] Alkylating agent therapy is associated with aggressive, acute nonlymphocytic leukemias, which typically evolve through a myelodysplastic phase, occur 5 to 10 years following primary therapy, and demonstrate abnormalities of chromosomes 5 or 7.[236] Acute leukemia has also been reported after alkylating agents were used in the treatment of rheumatoid arthritis or multiple sclerosis.[237] In contrast to alkylating agents, topoisomerase inhibitors lead to secondary acute nonlymphocytic leukemias that do not evolve through a myelodysplastic phase, occur 2 to 3 years following primary therapy, and demonstrate abnormalities of chromosomes 11q23.[238,239]

Second primary cancers have followed successful chemotherapy for Hodgkin's disease, non-Hodgkin's lymphoma, multiple myeloma, pulmonary small cell undifferentiated carcinoma, ovarian and breast carcinoma, and polycythemia vera. Within 20 years of therapy for Hodgkin's disease, second neoplasms include a predominance of solid tumors, mostly gastric and pulmonary carcinomas, in addition to earlier occurring acute leukemias and non-Hodgkin's lymphoma.[240,241] Adjuvant radiotherapy appears to play a role in the development of secondary solid tumors. By contrast, non-Hodgkin's lymphoma therapy carries a negligibly increased relative risk of development of solid tumors but is clearly associated with secondary acute leukemia.[242] Leukemia developed 30 to 90 months after the onset of therapy in 0.3 percent of nearly 6,000 women treated for ovarian cancer.[243]

Carcinoma of the urinary bladder has occurred 1 to 10 years after chemotherapy. Most patients were being treated with cyclophosphamide for lymphoma. Dysplastic lesions, some interpreted as carcinoma in situ, were present in addition to invasive carcinoma. Some of the carcinomas were of unusual types, such as mucus-secreting carcinoma,[244] spindle cell carcinoma,[245] and a disproportionate number of squamous cancers.[246] A leiomyosarcoma of the bladder occurred in a 17-year-old boy treated at age 4 with cyclophosphamide.[247] A fibrosarcoma-like tumor has also been seen.[248]

Presumably drug-induced secondary malignant tumors arise by direct, mutagenic effects of cytotoxic therapy, as evidenced by characteristic chromosomal abnormalities, or by immunosuppressive mechanisms that result in decreased tumor surveillance.

Immunosuppressed patients at increased risk of neoplasms include recipients of bone marrow and solid organ transplants who are on prolonged immunosuppressive therapy. One uncommon hazard is to receive a donor organ containing carcinoma and then develop metastases from the transplanted neoplasm.[249] More importantly, the risk of developing a primary neoplasm is estimated to be 80 times greater than in the general population.[250] Neoplasms have been reported in more than 2,000 renal transplant recipients, occurring at a much younger age than in persons with similar tumors in the general population.[251] Malignant lymphoma, Kaposi's sarcoma, and squamous carcinoma of the cervix, lip, tongue, and anogenital region have been the main offenders. The squamous carcinomas, including the cutaneous tumors, are capable of widespread metastases. One sarcoma, malignant fibrous histiocytoma of bone, has been reported in a renal transplant patient.[252]

Post-transplantation lymphoproliferative disorders (PTLD) represent a heterogeneous spectrum of Epstein-Barr virus (EBV)-related lymphoid proliferations. Incidence varies with the intensity of cyclosporine or monoclonal anti-T lymphocyte therapy and with the organ being transplanted. The vast majority of PTLD are B cell proliferations arising in lymph nodes or extranodal sites, frequently the gastrointestinal tract or lung. Classification and prognostication are notoriously difficult due to wide variations in histomorphology, immunoglobulin light chain expression, and immunoglobulin gene rearrangements.[253,254] PTLD are best classified by a molecular modification of Frizzera's morphologic scheme.[255] *Plasmacytic hyperplasias* are paracortical expansions of cytologically normal plasmacytoid lymphocytes and plasma cells with preservation of normal nodal architecture. They are polyclonal and regress following reduction of immunosuppression. *Polymorphic PTLD* (formerly subdivided into polymorphic hyperplasia and polymorphic lymphoma) are polymorphous lymphocyte proliferations that efface normal nodal architecture and contain numerous immunoblasts. Further subclassification based on cytologic atypia or necrosis is not necessary. They are monoclonal, demonstrate clonal patterns of EBV infection, and often regress following reduction of immunosuppression. Like the hyperplasias, they do not exhibit molecular oncogene abnormalities. *Lymphomas/myelomas* are monomorphous, cytologically malignant proliferations that are histologically identical to their nontransplantation-associated counterparts. They are monoclonal, demonstrate clonal patterns of EBV infection, and

less frequently regress following immunosuppression reduction. In contrast to polymorphic PTLD, they demonstrate oncogene or tumor suppressor gene abnormalities, or both. T cell lymphomas represent a minor fraction of PTLD and exhibit more frequent cutaneous involvement, decreased response to immunosuppression reduction, and a lesser association with EBV.[256] Pediatric PTLD are uncommon. They are more often associated with primary EBV infection and involvement of Waldeyer's ring.[257]

Hormonal Effects

Early in utero exposure to diethylstilbestrol (DES) results in vaginal adenosis, predominantly of the endocervical type, in most exposed women. Vaginal smears contain increased numbers of metaplastic squamous cells and endocervical type columnar cells.[258] Approximately 1 percent of DES-exposed

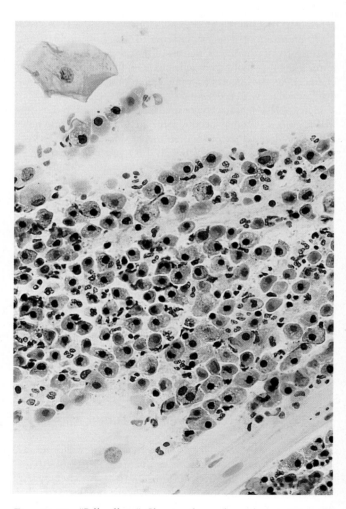

Fig. 14-18. "Pill effect." Sheets of pseudoparakeratotic, small, metaplastic-appearing squamous cells with dense, pyknotic nuclei and fine cytoplasmic vacuolization in a cervicovaginal smear from a woman using oral contraceptives. Note superficial squamous cell (upper left; Papanicolaou stain).

women develop vaginal or cervical clear cell adenocarcinoma.[259] Vaginal cytology has been used to follow patients for neoplasia, but its reliability depends on sampling technique.[258] DES-exposed males occasionally develop benign epididymal cysts, but they exhibit no cytologic abnormalities in urine or prostatic fluid.

Multiple forms of preoperative endocrine therapy for prostatic adenocarcinoma produce neoplastic gland shrinkage, cytoplasmic vacuolization, nuclear degeneration, and inflammation that can limit postprostatectomy tumor grading. In some instances, tumor cells have voluminous vacuolated cytoplasm mimicking histiocytes, as described above in mammary carcinoma. Benign prostrate glands exhibit atrophy, squamous and transitional cell metaplasia, vacuolization, and basal hyperplasia. Preoperative endocrine therapy does not completely ablate tumor but does appear to decrease involvement of surgical resection margins and extent of prostatic intraepithelial hyperplasia.[260–262]

Squamous metaplasia of normal prostatic glands occurs during estrogen therapy. In addition, several cases of adenocarcinoma with a malignant squamous element (adenosquamous carcinoma) have been diagnosed after two to nine years of estrogen therapy for pure adenocarcinoma in the original biopsy.[263,264]

Gonadotropin-releasing hormone agonists are used to shrink leiomyomas. Resected tumors often have marked cytoplasmic contraction with crowded nuclei, imparting a hypercellular appearance. This is not accompanied by nuclear atypia or mitotic activity.[265]

Oral Contraceptive ("Pill") Effect

Pseudoparakeratosis is an unusual, infrequently described cytologic drug effect seen in the cervicovaginal smears of a minority of women using oral contraceptives.[266] It consists of focal groups of very small, discohesive, metaplastic-appearing cells with pyknotic nuclei and dense orangeophilic or cyanophilic cytoplasm with fine vacuolization (Fig. 14-18). Small cell size and vacuolization help to distinguish pseudoparakeratosis from high grade dysplasia or parakeratosis.

Radiation Recall by Drugs

The ability of a cytotoxic drug to cause signs or symptoms localized to a previously irradiated area constitutes the radiation recall phenomenon. The changes produced by the drug are clinically and pathologically indistinguishable from radiation damage occurring in the absence of drug therapy. In most instances, the administration of the drug has produced erythema or necrosis in previously irradiated skin. In addition, recall has been seen in the small intestine,[267] esophagus,[268] and lung.[269]

IONIZING RADIATION

The pathologist receives irradiated tissue in four main clinical situations: (1) planned surgical resections in patients

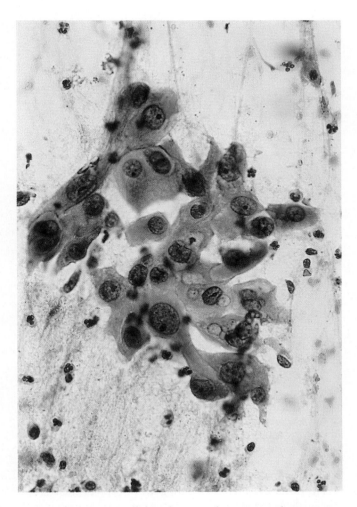

Fig. 14-19. Acute cellular changes of ionizing radiation in a cervicovaginal smear include nuclear and cytoplasmic enlargement and vacuolization, multinucleation, prominent nucleoli, amphophilic cytoplasmic staining, and irregular cell shapes (Papanicolaou stain.)

treated with preoperative radiation; (2) biopsy specimens from patients treated by radiation with the intent to cure but who have possible postirradiation persistent tumor; (3) non-neoplastic tissue resected because of late radiation damage; and (4) resection or biopsy specimens of postirradiation neoplasms.

High energy radiation capable of producing ionization within living cells is generated either in the form of x-rays from a vacuum tube external to the body or in the form of beta and gamma rays emitted from the nuclei of radioactive atoms that are placed into the organ containing the neoplasm. The physiologic and morphologic changes are identical regardless of the source.

Radiation in therapeutic doses injures every living tissue to some degree. The beneficial result in cancer therapy is based on the difference in the sensitivity and regenerative capacity of normal versus malignant cells. Indeed, it is the deleterious effect of radiation on non-neoplastic tissue that limits the radiation dose.

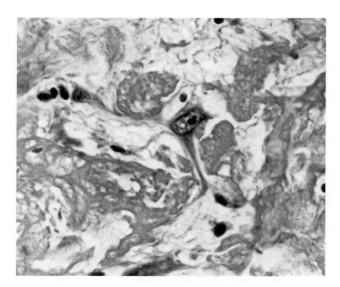

Fig. 14-20. Greatly enlarged fibroblasts with long cytoplasmic processes are typical, but not pathognomonic, of radiation damage. The stroma shows the splotchy, amorphous, hyalinized stroma characteristic of radiation effect.

The clinical effect of radiation on normal tissue can be divided into early and late phases. The temporal cutoff is arbitrary, but early is variably defined as any alteration occurring from eight weeks to six months after initiation of therapy, and late is any time thereafter. Late changes may follow continuously on early changes, or a symptom-free interval of weeks to many years may elapse before late changes declare themselves clinically.

The histologic alterations during the early phase include epithelial damage and connective tissue changes. Exquisitely sensitive cells such as those in the crypts of the small intestine show nuclear swelling and clumping of chromatin within minutes after receiving 50 to 100 cGy. Acute cellular changes include nuclear and cytoplasmic enlargement, cytoplasmic vacuolization, amphophilic cytoplasmic staining, nuclear membrane irregularity, multinucleation, prominent nucleoli, and occasional bizarre or "tadpole" shapes[270] (Fig. 14-19). Although both nuclear and cytoplasmic enlargement is seen, the N/C ratio may be slightly increased. Nuclear degeneration, including pyknosis and karyorrhexis is seen, but chromatin usually remains diffuse, fine, and normochromic. Occasional cells exhibit hyperchromasia. Acute radiation changes have been best described for cervical squamous epithelium, but similar changes are seen in endocervical cells.[271] These changes correlate ultrastructurally with swelling of mitochondria, dilation of the endoplasmic reticulum, the formation of vesicles, an accumulation of lipid, and an increase in lysosome-like bodies. In addition, disintegration of the Golgi apparatus, mitochondria, cytoplasmic filaments, and centrioles may occur. Late epithelial radiation effects, which can last for many years, include persistent nuclear and cytoplasmic enlargement but not vacuolization. In cervical smears, elongated parabasal-like cells resembling atrophy and enlarged endocervical cells may demonstrate nuclear hyperchromasia. Reparative changes also occur in

about one-third of patients. The constellation of radiation changes resembles cancer, as evidenced by higher false positive rates for malignant cytologic diagnoses in the postirradiation setting. Malignant cells are generally distinguished from benign radiation change by increased N/C ratios and coarse, hyperchromatic chromatin.

Stromal changes are probably triggered by damage to the endothelium of capillaries.[272] The endothelial cytoplasm becomes swollen and vacuolated, and nuclear enlargement is present. These damaged cells result in an alteration of the histohematic barrier manifest by edema and a fibrinous exudate. A patchy fibrous reaction ensues, and the combination of collagen and persisting fibrin produces eosinophilic hyalinized areas. Ultrastructurally, the hyalinized areas are a mixture of collagen bundles and cytoplasmic fragments that are cemented together by an amorphous finely granular protein substance. Large fibroblasts are often conspicuous, with proportionately enlarged nuclei that are either vesicular or hyperchromatic. Sometimes fibroblasts stand out due to basophilia secondary to abundant rough endoplasmic reticulum. Occasionally angulated tapering cytoplasmic projections are seen, which have been called swallowtail fibroblasts or radiation fibroblasts (Fig. 14-20). Fibroblasts with this appearance are not found exclusively in irradiated tissue, however. Areas of intense inflammation due to any cause may display bizarre fibroblasts, especially when infection is present; radiation damage is not pathognomonic for this appearance.[273]

Endothelial damage is also seen in arterioles and muscular arteries but apparently does not acutely affect their function because of the large lumen. Within several weeks, however, intimal and medial fibrosis or hyalinization may drastically alter the configuration of the muscular arteries, and rarely an intimal ac-

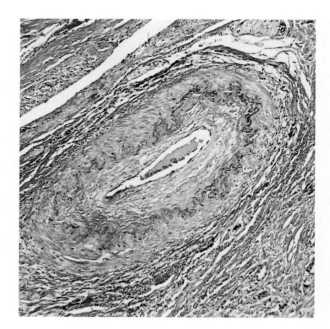

Fig. 14-21. Artery from soft tissue of neck 1 year after patient received 6,000 cGy. The internal elastica is discontinuous, intimal fibrous thickening is seen, and the adventitia is fibrotic.

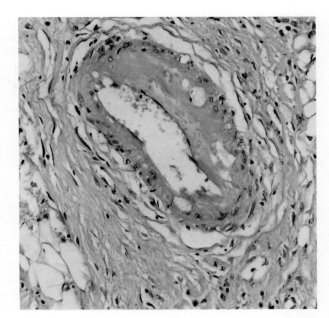

Fig. 14-22. Small artery with vacuolated and hyalinized media. This can be either an early or late radiation change.

cumulation of foam cells occurs, which compromises the lumen (Figs. 14-21 to 14-23). The changes along the course of a vessel may be spotty, so in any one tissue section relatively few sites of vascular damage are seen even though extensive connective tissue changes are evident. Arteries are affected far more often than veins, except for the unique sensitivity of hepatic veins.

Traditionally, late radiation damage has been attributed to

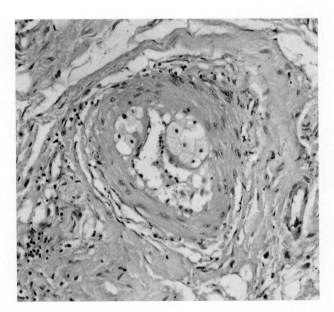

Fig. 14-23. Intimal foam cells are covered with endothelium. The change can be found at the completion of radiotherapy (as in this case) or can be seen many years later.

progressive arterial sclerosis accompanied by stromal fibrosis. Many epithelial changes such as ulceration of the rectum or skin are considered secondary to vascular insufficiency rather than a persisting direct effect on the epithelial cells per se. The compromised vasculature presumably makes an irradiated tissue permanently susceptible to devastating damage if it becomes infected or is traumatized.[274]

Effect on Neoplasms

The effect of radiation on the gross and microscopic appearance of a tumor is unpredictable. Attempts to predict tumor ra-

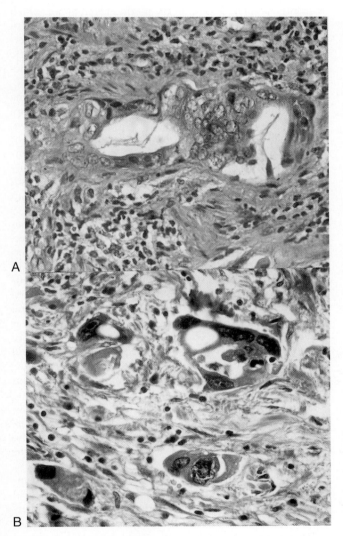

Fig. 14-24. (A) Well differentiated adenocarcinoma of prostate before irradiation (B) Immediately after the conclusion of 5,500 cGy, the tumor in the resected specimen showed bizarre nuclei and minimal formation of lumens. The postirradiation section came from the immediate area of the original biopsy, and none of the residual tumor resembled the preradiation pattern. We have seen this change in needle biopsies more than one year after radiation in patients with normal prostatic serum antibody.

diation response based on tumor differentiation (e.g., keratinizing vs. nonkeratinizing squamous cancers) or cytologic changes in adjacent benign epithelium[275–277] have been unsuccessful.[278] For example, if two laryngeal squamous cancers with the same histologic pattern and clinical stage of disease are given preoperative radiotherapy, one tumor may be completely absent in the resected specimen, whereas the other persists and is identical to the original biopsy. More often, the tumor is altered, with the most frequent change being necrosis. Many tumor cells undergo nuclear and cytoplasmic enlargement and vacuolization identical to that seen in normal epithelium. Sometimes the cells assume a gigantic size, with grotesquely shaped, densely hyperchromatic nuclei. The tumor pattern or degree of differentiation may be altered. Squamous carcinoma frequently has more keratin in the postirradiated tumor, which may or may not be associated with intact tumor cells.[279] This phenomenon probably reflects the sensitivity of poorly differentiated (immature) cells to radiation, whereas postmitotic cells are capable of maturing and carrying out specialized functions before dying. Increased pleomorphism and cytomegaly occur in the cells of undifferentiated nasopharyngeal carcinoma following radiotherapy. These are transient and usually disappear after 8 weeks.[280]

Generally, residual adenocarcinoma is histologically unchanged. This has been especially well documented for endometrial and prostatic carcinoma.[281,282] Occasionally, however, the malignant cells have grotesque cytologic features with gigantic nuclei and a degree of pleomorphism far greater than the original tumor (Fig. 14-24).

Squamous metaplasia has been described in adenocarcinomas of the breast and endometrium and in small cell undifferentiated carcinoma of the lung after irradiation.[283] However, squamous metaplasia can be seen in nonirradiated tumors of these types, and one must raise the question of sampling deficiencies in the small amounts of tissue available before irradiation. In an extensive study of irradiated uteri, Silverberg and DeGiorgi[281] found that squamous elements were first seen after irradiation in five cases, but in three others the squamous elements were noted in sections of the initial biopsy specimen and not in sections of the uterus after hysterectomy. They concluded that this was more likely a result of sampling variation than a direct effect of irradiation.

Transitional cell carcinomas of the urinary bladder tend to have more nuclear pleomorphism after irradiation, whereas carcinoma in situ is not altered. Squamous differentiation in the carcinoma has been described, but it raises the same questions as these described above.[284]

Residual carcinoma in a specimen resected as part of a combined radiotherapeutic and surgical approach is not unexpected because of the short interval between completion of radiotherapy and surgery. The prognostic significance of residual tumor in resected specimens is frequently raised, but few data answer this question. Residual carcinoma of the endometrium does not seem to affect the prognosis adversely if the tumor is in a favorable stage, namely, confined to the endometrium.[281] For laryngeal carcinoma, patients without residual tumor have a better survival, but this again probably correlates with a more favorable initial clinical stage.[285]

A far more perplexing problem arises when intact tumor cells are found in tissue biopsies or cytologic smears from a patient irradiated for cure and for whom surgery was not planned. What is the reproductive capacity of these cells? Intact tumor cells with normal staining characteristics must be sufficiently metabolically active to maintain their appearance. Nonetheless, this intactness does not ensure their ability to complete the next cell division or the one after that. Suit and Gallager[286] showed that irradiated tumor samples histologically identical to the original tumor failed to grow when transplanted into other animals, whereas nonirradiated samples of the tumor grew when transplanted. Viability as measured by histologically intact cells is not to be equated with further growth potential. This has been demonstrated in uteri removed after irradiation[281] and in serial biopsies of patients with prostatic carcinoma who have been radiated.[282] Thus, the pathologist should limit the interpretation of tumor cells to the observation that "morphologically intact tumor cells are present," because an accurate prediction of future growth cannot be made. The significance of malignant cells in postirradiation cervicovaginal smears may depend on the post-therapy interval and degree of radiation change. In early postirradiation smears, malignant cells may be difficult to distinguish from acute, benign radiation change. This may explain conflicting reports regarding the clinical significance of malignant cells in the early weeks after therapy. Malignant cells with marked acute radiation changes presumably have little or no potential for replication,[287] although some authors claim that any persistence is ominous.[288] Malignant cells exhibiting little to no radiation effect or those present greater than one to four months after therapy are an indication for aggressive clinical evaluation for residual disease.[270,287] Cervicovaginal cytology is only 50 percent sensitive in detecting cancer in those patients destined for recurrence, presumably because of limited sampling due to fibrosis.[270]

Postirradiation high grade dysplasia of the cervix is difficult to detect clinically and occurs with higher frequency than dysplasia in nonirradiated patients. Whether reported cases of postirradiation dysplasia include patients with unrecognized invasive disease is uncertain, but those who present within 3 years of completing therapy have a very high rate of recurrent invasive disease and poor survival.[270]

The problem of persistent tumor after irradiation for cure comes up most often in squamous cancers of the head and neck and cervix. Some carcinomas of the larynx undergo regression accompanied by mucosal healing, but edema continues to be present at the site of the tumor. The difficulty in finding carcinoma in biopsy specimens from the edematous area is frustrating. Goldman et al[289] found that tumor in postirradiation resected specimens often consisted only of scattered microscopic foci less than 0.5 mm in diameter. Furthermore, when the mucosa is intact, the tumor will not be reached, unless a deep biopsy is performed. Even in the absence of tumor in a biopsy, progressive edema 3 to 6 months after radiotherapy may be an indication for surgical resection. Tumor will be found in almost all these resection specimens.[290,291]

Paradoxically, cutaneous metastases may be sharply confined to the field of previous irradiation. This may be due to increased vasculature secondary to the radiation.[292] The effects on normal tissues that are commonly irradiated will now be considered.

Skin and Mucous Membranes

The early phase of radiation dermatitis is occasionally seen when skin is excised en bloc after preoperative radiotherapy. The epidermis and dermis are edematous, and the capillaries are dilated and lined by swollen endothelial cells. The cells of the pilosebaceous apparatus and sweat glands may be enlarged or focally necrotic.

In the late phase, the epidermis is atrophic in some areas and acanthotic in others. Hyperkeratosis is common. Atypical nuclei and individual cell keratinization are similar to those seen in solar keratosis. The dermal collagen bundles are swollen and often hyalinized, with variable staining. Fibrocytes associated with "new" collagen are irregularly distributed. The capillaries are usually ectatic and appear to be held rigidly open by the dense stroma about them. The pilosebaceous apparatus is usually absent altogether, but sweat glands may persist. Inflammation is negligible unless the skin is ulcerated.[293] Mucous membranes show the same changes as the skin except for damage to the minor salivary glands in place of the skin appendages.

Salivary Glands

The acute effect of radiation on salivary glands is manifest clinically by mucositis; microscopically distention of the ducts and acini, with secretions, is seen. By the end of a course of radiotherapy, however, the lobular architecture is destroyed because of a loss of acini and a chronic inflammatory infiltrate. Ducts and acini may contain cells with enlarged nuclei (two to three times normal size), which may be either vesicular or hyperchromatic (Fig. 14-25). Fibrous tissue is increased, particularly within the lobules, but the broad bands of fibrosis seen in cases of obstruction are not attained.[294] It was also found that intralobular fat persisted in irradiated glands, whereas it was ab-

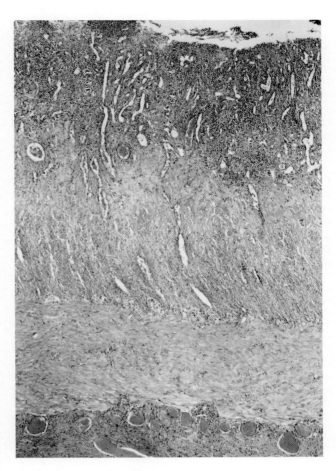

Fig. 14-26. Segment of obstructed small intestine removed 4 years after radiotherapy for carcinoma of cervix. The stenotic segment has ulcerated mucosa, greatly thickened and fibrotic submucosa, focal necrosis and fibrosis of the circular muscle layer, a normal longitudinal muscle layer, and serosal fibrosis with ectatic vessels.

sent in glands with obstructive disease. The epithelium of both ducts and acini may be partly replaced by squamous epithelium; occasionally, it irregularly distends the ducts and acini to a point where they may be confused with squamous carcinoma.[295] This may be particularly problematic if an enlarged, hard submandibular gland is removed because it is thought to be a lymph node with metastases.

Intestine

Either the small or large intestine may require surgical intervention for late radiation damage, which may appear within a few months after completion of therapy or may not be seen until more than 10 years later. Radiation enterocolitis manifests symptoms of obstruction due to a narrowed segment that ranges from 0.5 to 5 cm in length but is usually 1.5 to 2 cm long. Lesser degrees of edema and fibrosis extend away for 3 to 4 cm. The mucosa is usually ulcerated, but partial re-epithelialization may occur. Vascular damage is spotty but is invariably present both

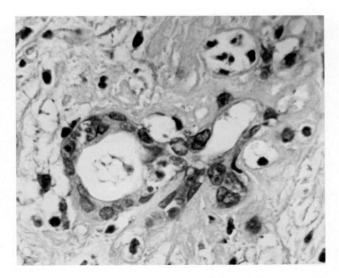

Fig. 14-25. Salivary gland at completion of 5,800 cGy of therapy for carcinoma of the oral cavity. Most acini are destroyed, and the remaining cells have pleomorphic nuclei.

within the bowel wall and the adjacent mesentery. The circular muscular layer is particularly susceptible to destruction and fibrous replacement, whereas the outer longitudinal layer is almost always spared (Fig. 14-26). Since radiation damage is a progressive, continuing process, edema and inflammation are also present.[296]

Colonic glands may be located in the muscularis as a late change. The epithelium of the glands is normal or atrophic, and its appearance is identical to that seen in colitis cystica profunda.[297]

Modest doses (2,000 to 2,500 cGy) of preoperative radiation produce marked atypia in non-neoplastic colonic mucosa. The changes are not permanent, since biopsy specimens from colostomy sites after 2 months do not show the change even though the line of resection had atypia at the time of the operation.[298] Similar cytologic changes plus villous atrophy occur in the small intestinal mucosa. Doses as low as 1,000 cGy produce severe but transient alterations.

Liver

Radiation damage to the liver is unique because the major site of vascular injury is to veins, namely, the small radicles of the hepatic venous system. Sclerosis of the portal vein is rare, and arterial lesions have not been reported.[299] The central veins and small sublobular hepatic veins undergo an intimal thickening that is unrelated to overt thrombosis.

Kidney

Radiation damage to the glomeruli, tubules, and vessels of the kidney is not accompanied by much inflammation; therefore the term *radiation nephropathy* is preferable to the more widely used term *radiation nephritis*. Luxton and Kunkler[300] followed 54 patients for up to 12 years and grouped them into five major clinical groups: (1) acute radiation nephropathy, (2) chronic radiation nephropathy, (3) asymptomatic proteinuria, (4) benign hypertension; and (5) malignant hypertension. From a morphologic viewpoint, Mostofi[301] divided radiation changes into four categories that serve to emphasize the different changes seen in the clinical groups. These categories are (1) mild sclerosing nephrosis, (2) severe sclerosing nephrosis with mild to severe nephrosclerosis, (3) mild to severe sclerosing nephrosis with hypertensive necrotizing vasculitis, and (4) nephroglomerulosis. Sclerosing nephrosis consists of small or collapsed tubules intermixed with interstitial fibrosis (Fig. 14-27). Nephroglomerulosis is predominantly a glomerular affliction; in contrast to most cases in the other groups, it begins within 3 to 12 months after irradiation. The dominant change is in the glomeruli, almost all of which have decreased lobulation and thickening of the capillary walls simulating membranous glomerulonephritis. By electron microscopy, disruption of hypertrophic endothelial and epithelial cells from the basement membrane is seen.[302] In a few instances, the affected zone has been sharply demarcated, and the remainder of the kidney was normal, presumably because only a portion of the kidney was lying in the field of radiation. This possibility must be kept

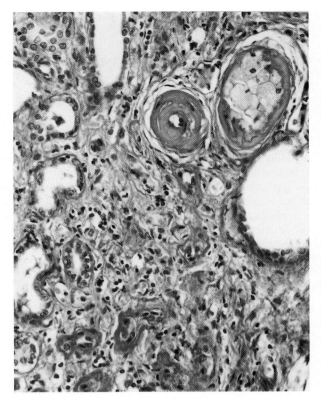

Fig. 14-27. Sclerosing nephrosis secondary to radiation consists of atrophic tubules separated by fibrous tissue. A markedly hyalinized arteriole is present, as well as an artery with intimal foam cells. The patient had been irradiated 10 years previously for testicular carcinoma.

in mind because of the potential for sampling error at the time of needle biopsy.

Urinary Bladder

Transitional epithelium is readily damaged by radiation, and almost all patients will exfoliate abnormal cells whether the therapy is directed to a primary cancer of the bladder or an adjacent pelvic organ. The cells and nuclei are enlarged and the cytoplasm is often vacuolated.[303] Nuclei are wrinkled, mildly hyperchromatic, enlarged more or less in proportion to the cytoplasm, and tend to be multiple. Radiation-induced changes, like postsurgical and cytotoxic drug effects, limit the accuracy of urine cytology.[304] This is especially true following low grade transitional cell carcinoma. In a small number of cases, definitive distinction of cancer from benign radiation effect may be impossible, requiring further cytologic or histologic evaluation.[305] Radiation-induced alterations generally disappear within a few months after completion of therapy.[306] Abnormal cells noted beyond that time can be evaluated using standard criteria, especially if intervening urine cytologies are free of atypical cells. Recurrent high grade transitional cell carcinomas demonstrate high N/C ratios, marked hyperchromasia, and coarse chromatin. The presence of malignant-appearing cells in transitional epithelium from a patient who has been irradiated for primary bladder carcinoma probably reflects radioresistant invasive carcinoma or carcinoma in situ. The latter is a likely source for the later development of invasive carcinoma.[306,307]

The rich vasculature of the bladder and its abundant submucosal connective tissue renders this organ susceptible to late complications of radiation. Approximately 1 to 3 percent of long-term survivors will develop chronic devastating damage to the bladder in the form of deep ulceration, fibrotic contraction, or fistula formation in the absence of tumor. Patients undergoing cyclophosphamide therapy experience more frequent and severe toxicity when it is combined with pelvic irradiation.[308]

Prostate

Radiation-induced atypia in benign prostatic epithelium and stroma is similar to that described for other organs. In carcinoma, decreased numbers of irregularly distributed neoplastic glands limit accurate Gleason scoring, and tumor cell N/C ratios may be decreased to the point of appearing anucleate. The significance of residual cancer in irradiated prostate gland biopsies is controversial but appears to indicate increased recurrence and spread of disease as well as decreased survival.[309]

Biopsies of men whose prostatic carcinoma has been radiated often show squamous metaplasia with marked cytologic atypia in the non-neoplastic glands, larger prostatic ducts, and prostatic urethra. In other glands, necrotic epithelium exposes corpora amylacea to the stroma, eliciting a giant cell reaction. The seminal vesicles become atrophic and fibrotic.[310]

Uterus

Intracavitary radiation for endometrial carcinoma produces changes in the cervix, endometrium, and myometrium. The squamous lining of the exocervix is often obliterated, and only a fibrinous exudate lies on the surface. The endocervical epithelium may be pleomorphic, with either hyperchromatic or vacuolated nuclei that frequently lie in the middle or luminal end of the cell. Mucin is diminished. The distinction from adenocarcinoma involving the endocervix is readily made because, despite their cytologic changes, the glands are normally spaced.

Nuclear and cytoplasmic alterations are especially common in the endometrium treated with intracavitary radium. Markedly abnormal cells are found not only in the endometrium but in foci of adenomyosis. The latter might be diagnosed incorrectly as invasive adenocarcinoma. Misinterpretation can be avoided by knowing that residual endometrial adenocarcinoma characteristically shows little change when compared with preoperative biopsy material, whereas the non-neoplastic endometrium is severely altered.[281] The epithelium forms an irregular layer one to four cells thick with some cells protruding above the surface and attached to the epithelial lining only by a thin strand of cytoplasm (Fig. 14-28). Most cells are greatly enlarged and have a polygonal, round, or extremely attenuated shape rather than the normal cuboidal or low columnar configuration. The cytoplasm ranges from a powdery ground-glass appearance through a finely or coarsely

eosinophilic granularity. Vacuolization is present in some cells as either tiny droplets or large vacuoles. Nuclei are occasionally normal, but most are enlarged and may be round, angulated, or have an irregular contour due to numerous folds and convolutions. Small nucleoli are frequent. The endometrial stromal cells do not undergo these cytologic changes although inflammation and edema are invariably present. Thus, the presence of bizarre endometrial cells adjacent to endometrial stromal cells is virtual proof that the epithelial cells are non-neoplastic. In rare cases, myometrial cells are enlarged and vacuolated after intracavitary radiation.[311]

Thyroid

Numerous changes are found in the thyroid, including colloid nodules with foci of hyperplasia identical to those seen in nonirradiated thyroid. Small foci of hyperplasia are also scattered throughout the parenchyma, with the columnar cells forming small tufts. Occasionally, a nodule is composed of small fingers of thyroid tissue forming tiny lumens. Large, dense nuclei may be found either in hyperplastic nodules or within individual follicles. Oxyphilic cells are frequent and are often associated with a lymphocytic infiltrate.[312]

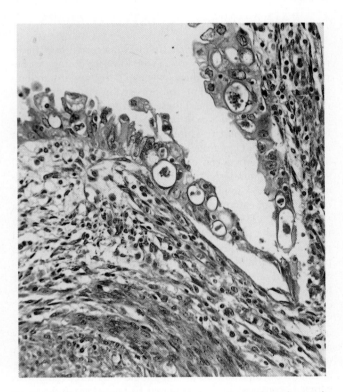

Fig. 14-28. Focus of adenomyosis after intracavitary radium therapy for endometrial carcinoma. The epithelium is stratified, and a few cells are attached only by a strand of cytoplasm. Many cells are vacuolated, and nuclear pleomorphism is present. The endometrial stroma beneath the epithelium is edematous and inflamed, but the stromal cells are not atypical. Normal myometrium is at the bottom of the field.

Many nodules have been classified as adenomas, since they have a trabecular pattern. When nuclear abnormalities are superimposed, the possibility of carcinoma is raised. In the absence of invasion, such nodules are probably best considered atypical adenomas.[313]

Breast

Patients treated for breast cancer with primary radiotherapy may subsequently develop clinical or mammographic abnormalities that are biopsied. In some instances, fat necrosis has mimicked a primary tumor on physical examination. It may be located near the biopsy site and may result in fixation of the skin.[314] The most characteristic radiation affect is the presence of atypical epithelial cells in the terminal duct/lobular unit, accompanied by atrophy and lobular fibrosis. Occasionally, epithelial atypia is seen in larger ducts.[315] FNA smears from irradiated breasts typically demonstrate nuclear atypia, epithelial hypocellularity, and fat necrosis. Radiation-induced benign nuclear enlargement and prominent nucleoli may be difficult to distinguish from carcinoma, but smears from recurrent cancer typically demonstrate abundant, discohesive malignant cells.[316]

RADIATION-ASSOCIATED TUMORS

Tumors associated with radiation have occurred in patients receiving high dose therapy for cancer, low dose therapy for benign conditions, multiple diagnostic exposures, and internal radiation due to deposition of isotopes used in diagnostic procedures (thorium dioxide) and therapeutic procedures (^{131}I).[317]

A threshold may not exist below which radiation has no effect, a concept summarized in the following manner by Rubin and Casarett[318]: (1) a finite probability exists that the smallest amount of radiation can cause a significant change in a cell such as gene mutation, (2) a finite probability exists that such a cell alteration may be an event in a complex multievent mechanism of carcinogenesis, (3) the probability that such a single event will complete the carcinogenic mechanism in an individual of a population depends on the size of the exposed population and on the number of individuals in it that are so predisposed, and (4) it is therefore reasonable to assume that no threshold dose exists in a population in which there is not at least one patient who requires merely this one cell change to complete a carcinogenic event.

The following principles must be kept in mind when assigning radiation as the probable cause of a neoplasm. The new tumor must have been in the field of radiation. The organ in which it arises must have been previously documented as being normal. A symptom-free period should pass after radiation, which is conventionally considered to be at least 5 years. In point of fact, however, strong arguments can be made for radiation-induced tumors arising within 2 or 3 years after irradiation.

Most tumors attributed to radiation are malignant, although a few benign osseous and neurogenic neoplasms appear to have been radiation induced.[319,320] Generally speaking, the gross and microscopic appearances of radiation-induced tumors are not distinctive, and their behavior parallels the course of disease that would be expected for the same histologic type of tumor arising in a nonirradiated organ. The few exceptions to these statements will be noted in the subsequent sections. Radiation damage to normal structures may or may not be found in the region of the tumor, and the presence of radiation damage in the surrounding non-neoplastic tissue is not a requisite for the diagnosis of a radiation-induced tumor.

Skin

Postirradiation basal or squamous cell carcinomas of the skin are most common on the face and usually manifest 20 or more years after irradiation for benign conditions.[321] The latency period varies from 3 to 64 years, however.[322] The role of radiation is securely established by the occurrence of cancers in unusual locations such as the antecubital fossa or forearm after irradiation of these areas for dermatitis.[323] Multiple lesions are the rule, both synchronously and metachronously. Their number far exceeds the multiple lesions that are also characteristic of cutaneous cancers in nonirradiated patients. The squamous carcinomas are more aggressive than those arising in actinic keratosis. Nonetheless, skin damaged by radiation need not inevitably develop cancer even when the injury is severe enough to produce necrosis.[322]

Atypical fibroxanthomas have arisen in skin that had been irradiated.[324] Most appeared more than 15 years after irradiation, but a few were seen in less than 5 years. Angiosarcoma of the skin of the breast has occurred after lumpectomy and radiation.[325]

Sinonasal Region

Sinonasal small cell neoplasm after retinoblastoma has been reported in a few cases. In one case, immunohistochemical evidence suggested a primitive neuroectodermal tumor.[326] Another case was completely devoid of differentiation.[327]

Salivary Gland

Low dose radiation to the head in childhood increases the incidence of mixed tumors. In one study, 2 of 971 persons who received radiation had mixed tumors, whereas the expected number was 0.04 cases.[328] Other tumors include Warthin's tumor, mucoepidermoid tumor, or unclassified carcinoma.[329–331] A few patients receiving high dose radiotherapy for carcinoma have later developed malignant tumors of the parotid gland.[332]

Intestine

About 35 colorectal carcinomas have been reported in patients who had previous irradiation, usually of the uterine cervix. Castro et al[333] analyzed 24 patients with colorectal carcinoma who were long-term survivors (5 to 28 years) of uterine cancer treated with radiotherapy. They found that in 13 cases the segment of bowel bearing the tumor had vascular and stromal changes consistent with radiation injury. Moreover, 13 patients had colloid carcinoma, which otherwise constitutes only about 10 percent of colon cancers. Qizilbash[334] described a treacherous combination wherein a papillary adenocarcinoma surrounded the margin of an ulcerated radiation-induced stricture. Colloid carcinoma has occurred in a child in the field of irradiation for Wilms' tumor.[335]

Angiosarcoma of the small intestine developed in a woman 8 years after postoperative irradiation for ovarian carcinoma.[336] We have seen one case of small intestinal angiosarcoma 12 years after radiation for squamous cancer of the cervix.

Uterus

Several hundred cases of endometrial cancer have been reported after irradiation of the uterus for endometrial bleeding from benign disease. It is uncertain how many of these are radiation induced, since many of the cases received radiation for abnormal endometrial bleeding and may have been predisposed to adenocarcinoma. Furthermore, many of the postirradiation lesions were diagnosed as adenocarcinoma in situ, and the almost universal lack of illustrations leaves the exact nature of the lesions in question. It is possible that some of the cases may have been postirradiation cytopathy of normal endometrium.

The frequency of bona fide endometrial cancer in patients receiving radiation for squamous cancer of the cervix was studied by Fehr and Prem,[337] who found 12 examples in 2,294 patients, which was more than double the expected number. The proportion of mixed müllerian sarcomas was striking. Looking at it from another direction, Norris and Taylor[338] found that 15 percent of 477 patients with uterine sarcomas had a history of irradiation. The tumors included mixed müllerian sarcomas, endometrial stromal sarcomas, and unclassified sarcomas. Leiomyosarcoma did not seem to be related. The behavior of postirradiation mixed müllerian sarcomas has been reported as more aggressive than spontaneous tumors in one study,[339] but not in another study.[340] Postirradiation endometrial adenocarcinoma has a dismal outlook.[341]

Bone

Approximately 200 sarcomas have been reported at the site of a benign bone lesion that was irradiated. About three-fourths of these patients received what would now be considered unacceptably high doses. Moreover, most of the irradiated lesions (such as giant cell tumors) would currently be treated with newer surgical techniques. Postirradiation tumors have included osteosarcomas, fibrosarcomas, chondrosarcomas, and malignant fibrous histiocytomas.[342] The latent period has varied from slightly less than 3 years to 30 years with an average of 6 years for tumors occurring in weight-bearing bones and 14 years in non-weight-bearing bones.[343]

A new complication appears to be emerging from the successful treatment of Ewing's sarcoma by local irradiation to the primary coupled with systemic chemotherapy. Four of 10 patients who had lived 5 or more years after the initial diagnosis of Ewing's sarcoma developed an osteosarcoma at the site of the original tumor.[344]

Postirradiation sarcoma in previously normal bone is a rare event. A review of about 6,000 patients treated for malignant disease disclosed 2 osteosarcomas arising in bone that had been normal at the time of treatment 5 and 11 years previously.[345] This is 0.03 percent of all patients treated or 0.1 percent of the 5 year survivors. In another study, Tountas et al[346] found 10 postradiation sarcomas, representing 0.035 percent of 5 year survivors. In children, genetic factors seem to play a role.[347]

Benign osseous tumors in the field of high dose radiotherapy have all been osteochondromas. They occur when the radiation is given in childhood.[319,348]

Soft Tissue

Most sarcomas in irradiated soft tissues are on the chest or shoulder 4 to 16 years after radiation for breast carcinoma.[349,350] Most have metastasized. The lesions have had the conventional histologic patterns of malignant fibrous histiocytoma, fibrosarcoma, chondrosarcoma, or a mixture of the latter two.[351,352] One fibrosarcoma had large, bizarre cells resembling so-called radiation fibroblasts interspersed among more typical foci of fibrosarcoma, a pattern that is occasionally seen even in the absence of prior radiation.[353] Postradiation sarcomas of the head and neck are rare. Malignant schwannomas have occurred in radiated soft tissues and have pursued a highly aggressive course. About one-half have been in patients with von Recklinghausen's disease.[354] Angiosarcoma is a rare postirradiation sarcoma.[355,356]

Breast

Cancer of the breast has been reported in women in their 20s who received radiation to the chest during the first two decades of life, either for metastatic tumor[357] or benign conditions[358] Adult women receiving radiation for mastitis or other benign breast disease have shown a twofold increase in frequency of breast cancer,[359] as have women undergoing repeated, prolonged fluoroscopic examination of the chest during therapy for tuberculosis.[360] Cancer of the breast appears to be slightly increased in patients treated with radiation for Hodgkin's disease.[361] Cancers in irradiated women tend to have less desmoplasia than cancers in controls.[362] Carcinoma of the male breast has been reported at age 46 after irradiation at puberty for gynecomastia[363] and at age 35 after low dose irradiation in infancy.[364] The possible tumorigenic effect of repeated mammograms remains to be determined.[365]

Central Nervous System

The most frequent radiation-induced tumor in the CNS is the so-called pituitary sarcoma, which is actually a fibrosarcoma with abundant collagen formation in some foci. Remnants of the irradiated adenoma are often scattered within the sarcoma. The latent period between irradiation and symptoms referable to the sarcoma ranges from 2.5 to 21 years, with an average of 7 years. The tumors do not metastasize, and death occurs from local growth.[366]

Donahue et al[367] described two patients with neurofibromas of the spinal cord 11 and 13 years after radiation to the mediastinum in childhood.

Meningiomas have been found in a few patients receiving either high dose or low dose irradiation. Watts[368] reported meningiomas 15 and 25 years after therapeutic irradiation for glioma. Three meningiomas occurred in a group of more than 5,000 patients receiving radiation to the scalp in childhood for tinea capitis, whereas none was present in the control group.[369] Radiation has been incriminated as a cause of malignant gliomas.[370] A spinal cord glioma arose in a region irradiated for Hodgkin's disease.[371]

Thyroid and Parathyroid

In 1950 Duffy and Fitzgerald[372] suggested an association between thyroid carcinoma in childhood and a prior history of irradiation to the thymus in infancy. The practice of using radiation to treat benign conditions such as acne or tonsillitis had largely ceased by 1960, but thyroid cancer continues to occur in these patients. As many as 7 percent of the persons who received radiation to the head or neck have been found to have thyroid carcinoma.[373] In one report, 40 percent of the adults operated on for thyroid cancer between 1968 and 1972 had a history of irradiation.[374]

Virtually all the cancers have been classified as papillary, follicular, or mixed.[375] In one patient, medullary carcinoma was found in a gland also containing papillary cancer.[376] There is one report of a case of anaplastic carcinoma in a 32-year-old man who was irradiated at age 7.[377]

The thyroid gland removed from a patient with a history of irradiation almost always contains multiple nodules. As often as not, the clinically palpable nodule is either an adenoma or colloid nodule, and the carcinoma is present elsewhere. The cancers may be small, and in one series nearly one-half of the tumors were not found at the time of frozen section examination. Extensive sampling was required to disclose foci of carcinoma, which were 2 to 3 mm in size.[313] Frozen section interpretation is also complicated when non-neoplastic follicles with nuclear atypia are trapped within inflammatory fibrous areas. Multifocal bilateral cancers are common.[378]

Nearly a dozen cases of thyroid cancer have been reported in patients receiving relatively high doses of[131] I for Graves' disease.[379] Nuclear pleomorphism, oncocytic change, and multiple small adenomas are also seen.[380]

Patients treated with radiation for medulloblastoma receive an estimated 200 to 3,000 cGy to the thyroid, and several carcinomas have been reported.[381] Doses in excess of this are probably not associated with a markedly increased risk of cancer, perhaps because more of the injured thyroid cells are rendered incapable of division.[382] Nonetheless, several cases of papillary cancer have occurred after high dose radiation for Hodgkin's disease.[383,384]

The possibility that low dose irradiation may produce adenomas or hyperplasia in parathyroid glands has been raised. Several investigators have obtained a history of low dose irradiation in 14 to 30 percent of patients with hyperparathyroidism.[385] The irradiated glands do not have special histologic features, except for a possible increase in the proportion of oncocytes.[386] The latter has not been the subject of an adequately controlled study. The association of thyroid carcinoma and hyperparathyroidism (excluding medullary carcinoma and patients with syndromes of multiple endocrine adenomas) may in part be explained by irradiation. Nonetheless, in one series of 40 patients with coexistent parathyroid adenoma and thyroid carcinoma, only one had a history of prior irradiation.[386]

Mesothelium

Approximately a dozen pleural or peritoneal mesotheliomas have been reported 7 to 31 years after medium to high dose radiation, often for breast carcinoma.[387] An especially convincing argument for radiation as a causative agent can be made in a woman in whom mesothelioma developed at age 28; she had had a lung lesion radiated when she was 4 years old.[388]

Thorium Dioxide

Thorotrast is the trade name for a radioactive suspension of thorium dioxide used between 1930 and 1950 as a contrast medium. More than 50,000 persons received the agent,[389] including at least 4,300 Americans.[390] More than 90 percent of the Thorotrast remains in the reticuloendothelial system for life, as brown, shiny, granules. In the liver, it is found in Kupffer cells or in histiocytes. At the site of arterial injection, a progressive fibrous reaction around extravasated dye can continue for years, and sarcomas have been reported.[391,392] More than 200 neoplasms have been reported overall.[393] More than one-half of the tumors are hepatic (approximately one-third angiosarcomas, one-third cholangiocarcinomas, and one-third hepatocellular carcinomas).[394] Rarely, all three types occur simultaneously.[395] The occurrence of tumors as long as 36 years after exposure indicates a lifelong risk.[396] Several osteosarcomas have been reported.[397] A detailed bibliography of Thorotrast-associated neoplasms has been published.[389]

Thermal Therapy

Numerous studies on the use of hyperthermia have shown that it enhances radiotherapy or chemotherapy, or both.[398] Hyperthermia alone damages small vessels and presumably contributes to cytotoxic effects.[399] Alterations in experimental and human tumors are not specific. The quantity of necrosis or the frequency of absent tumor in the resected specimen may be increased when compared with resected specimens from patients treated with either radiation or chemotherapy alone.[400–402]

REFERENCES

1. Maygarden SJ, Novotny DB, Johnson DE, et al: Subclassification of benign breast disease by fine needle aspiration cytology. Comparison of cytologic and histologic findings in 265 palpable breast masses. Acta Cytol 38:115–129, 1994

2. Feldman PS, Covell JL: Fine Needle Aspiration Cytology and its Clinical Applications: Breast and Lung. p 47. American Society of Clinical Pathologists Press, Chicago, 1985

3. Vooijs GP: Benign proliferative reactions, intraepithelial neoplasia and invasive cancer of the uterine cervix. pp. 153–230. In Bibbo M (ed): Comprehensive Cytopathology. WB Saunders, Philadelphia, 1991

4. Lee KR: Atypical glandular cells in cervical smears from women who have undergone cone biopsy. A potential diagnostic pitfall. Acta Cytol 37:705–709, 1993

5. Pacey F, Ayer B, Greenberg M: The cytologic diagnosis of adenocarcinoma in situ of the cervix uteri and related lesions. III. Pitfalls in diagnosis. Acta Cytol 32:325–303, 1988

6. Partoll LM, Javaheri G: Cervical cytology after cryosurgery, laser ablation and conization A comparison of the cotton swab and endocervical brush. Acta Cytol 37:876–878, 1993

7. Fechner RE: Necrotizing sialometaplasia. A source of confusion with carcinoma of the palate. Am J Clin Pathol 67:315, 1977

8. Batsakis JG, Sneige N, El-Naggar AK: Fine-needle aspiration of salivary glands: its utility and tissue effects. Ann Otol Rhinol Laryngol 101:185, 1992

9. Walker GK, Fechner RE, Johns ME, et al: Necrotizing sialometaplasia of larynx secondary to atheromatous embolization. Am J Clin Pathol 77:221, 1982

10. Hambrick E: The fate of colonoscopic polypectomy sites. Dis Colon Rectum 19:400, 1976

11. Evans SC, Goldman RL, Klein HZ, et al: Necrobiotic granulomas of the uterine cervix. Probable post-operative reaction. Am J Surg Pathol 8:841, 1984

12. Herbold DR, Frable WJ, Kraus FT: Isolated noninfectious granulomas of the ovary. Int J Gynecol Pathol 2:380, 1984

13. Balogh K: Palisading granuloma in the kidney after open biopsy, letter. Am J Surg Pathol 10:441, 1986

14. Spagnolo DV, Waring PM: Bladder granulomata after bladder surgery. Am J Clin Pathol 86:430, 1986

15. Epstein JI, Hutchins GM: Granulomatous prostatitis: distinction among allergic, nonspecific, and posttransurethral resection lesions. Hum Pathol 15:818, 1984

16. Henry L, Wagner B, Faulkner MK, et al: Metal deposition in post-surgical granulomas of the urinary tract. Histopathology 22:457–465, 1993

17. Agel NM: Necrobiotic granulomas of the urogenital system. J Clin Pathol 48:185, 1995

18. Thurrell W, Reid P, Kennedy A, Smith JHF: Necrotising granulomas of the peritoneum. Histopathology 18:190, 1991

19. Fechner RE, Mills SE: Breast Pathology. Benign Proliferations, Atypias, and In Situ Carcinomas. p. 9. ASCP Press, Chicago, 1990

20. Tannenbaum M: Differential diagnosis in uropathology. II. Urologic artifact and/or pathologist's dilemma. Urology 4:485, 1974.

21. Baggish MS, Barash F, Noel Y, et al: Comparison of thermal injury zones in loop electrical and laser cervical excisional conization. Am J Obstet Gynecol 166:545–548, 1992

22. Chen R-J, Lee EF, Shih J-C: Does the loop electrosurgical excision procedure adversely affect the histopathological interpretation of cervical conization specimens? Acta Obstet Gynecol Scand 73:726, 1994

23. Oyesanya OA, Amerasinghe CN, Manning EA: Outpatient excisional management of cervical intraepithelial neoplasia. A prospective, randomized comparison between loop diathermy excision and laser excisional conization. Am J Obstet Gynecol 168:485–488, 1993

24. Felix JC, Muderspach LI, Duggan BD, et al: The significance of positive margins in loop electrosurgical cone biopsies. Obstet Gynecol 84:996–1000, 1994

25. Wright TC Jr, Richard RM, Ferenczy A, Koulos J: Comparison of specimens removed by CO_2 laser conization and the loop electrosurgical excision procedure. Obstet Gynecol 79:147, 1992

26. Messing MJ, Otken L, King LA, et al: Large loop excision of the transformation zone (LLETZ): a pathologic evaluation. Gynecol Oncol 52:207–211, 1994

27. Montz FJ, Holschneider CH, Thompson LDR: Large-loop excision of the transformation zone: effect on the pathologic interpretation of resection margins. Obstet Gynecol 81:976, 1993

28. Alguacil-Garcia A: Artifactual changes mimicking signet ring cell carcinoma in transurethral prostatectomy specimens. Am J Surg Pathol 10:795, 1986

29. Batnitzky S, Keucher TR, Mealey J Jr, et al: Iatrogenic intraspinal epidermoid tumors. JAMA 237:148, 1977

30. Strauchen JA, Strefling AM: Epidermal inclusion cyst of the meniscus. J Bone Joint Surg [Am] 64A:290, 1982

31. Dirschmid K, Kiesler J, Mathis G, et al: Epithelial misplacement after biopsy of colorectal adenomas. Am J Surg Pathol 17:1262, 1993

32. Boppana S, May M, Hoda S: Does prior fine-needle-aspiration cause diagnostic difficulties in histologic evalution of breast carcinomas? Lab Invest 70:13A, 1994

33. Youngson BJ, Cranor M, Rosen PP: Epithelial displacement in surgical breast specimens following needling procedures. Am J Surg Pathol 18:896, 1994

34. Youngson BJ, Liberman L, Rosen PP: Displacement of carcinomatous epithelium in surgical breast specimens following stereotaxic core biopsy. Am J Clin Pathol 103:598, 1995

35. McLaughlin CM, Devine P, Muto M, Genest DR: Pseudo-invasion of vascular spaces: report of an artifact caused by cervical lidocaine injection prior to loop diathrmy. Hum Pathol 25:208, 1994

36. Tsang WYW, Chan JKC: Spectrum of morphologic changes in lymph nodes attributable to fine needle aspiration. Hum Pathol 23:562, 1992

37. Behm FG, O'Dowd GJ, Frable WJ: Fine-needle aspiration effects on benign lymph node histology. Am J Clin Pathol 1984; 82:195–8.

38. Kern SB: Necrosis of a Warthin's tumor following fine needle aspiration. Acta Cytol 32:207, 1988

39. Keyhani-Rofagha S, Kooner DS, Keyhani M, O'Toole RV: Necrosis of a Hürthle cell tumor of the thyroid following fine needle aspiration. Case report and literature review. Acta Cytol 43:805, 1990

40. Lee KC, Chan JKC, Ho LC: Histologic changes in the breast after fine-needle aspiration. Am J Surg Pathol 18:1039–1047, 1994

41. Tabbara SO, Frierson HF Jr, Fechner RE: Diagnostic problems in tissues previously sampled by fine needle aspiration. Am J Clin Pathol 96:76–80, 1991

42. Livolsi VA, Merino MJ: Worrisome histologic alterations following fine-needle aspiration of the thyroid (WHAFFT). Pathol Annu 29:99–120, 1994

43. Smith EH: Complications of percutaneous abdominal fine-needle biopsy. Review. Radiology 178:253–258, 1991

44. Shenoy PD, Lakhkar BN, Ghosh MK, et al: Cutaneous seeding of renal carcinoma by Chiba needle aspiration biopsy. Case report. Acta Radiol 32:50–52, 1991

45. Pasieka JL, Thompson NW: Fine-needle aspiration biopsy causing peritoneal seeding of a carcinoid tumor. Arch Surg 127:1248–1251, 1992

46. Trimbos JB, Hacker NF: The case against aspirating ovarian cysts. Cancer 72:828–831, 1993

47. Andersen WA, Nichols GE, Avery SR, Taylor PT: Cytologic diagnosis of ovarian tumors: factors influencing accuracy in previously undiagnosed cases. Am J Obstet Gynecol 173:457–464, 1995

48. Hales MS, Hsu FSF: Needle tract implantation of papillary carcinoma of the thyroid following aspiration biopsy. Acta Cytol 34:801, 1990

49. Elliot JS, Rosenberg ML: Ureteral occlusion by barium granulomata. J Urol 71:692, 1954

50. Lewis JW Jr, Kerstein MD, Koss N: Barium granuloma of the rectum: an uncommon complication of barium enema. Ann Surg 181:418, 1975

51. Hayden RS: Perforation of duodenal ulcer during fluoroscopy. Disposition of barium sulfate in the abdominal cavity. Radiology 57:214, 1951

52. Fox RM, Malter IJ: Prolonged oviduct retention of iodized contrast medium. Obstet Gynecol 40:221, 1972

53. Kantor HI, Kamholz JH, Smith AL: Foreign-body granulomas following the use of Salpix. Report of a case simulating intraabdominal tuberculosis. Obstet Gynecol 7:171, 1956

54. Coder DM, Olander GA: Granulomatous peritonitis caused by starch glove powder. Arch Surg 105:83, 1972

55. Taft DA, Lasersohn JT, Hill JD: Glove starch granulomatous peritonitis. Am J Surg 120:231, 1970

56. Paine CG, Smith P: Starch granulomata. J Clin Pathol 10:51, 1957

57. Davies JD, Neely J: The histopathology of peritoneal starch granulomas. J Pathol 107:265, 1972

58. Aarons J, Fitzgerald N: The persisting hazards of surgical glove powder. Surg Gynecol Obstet 138:385, 1974

59. Sobel HJ, Schiffman RJ, Schwarz R, et al: Granulomas and peritonitis due to starch glove powder. Arch Pathol Lab Med 91:558, 1971

60. Housini I, Dabbs DJ, Coyne L: Fine needle aspiration cytology of talc granulomatosis in a peripheral lymph node in a case of suspected intravenous drug abuse. Acta Cytol 34:342–344, 1990

61. Tao LC, Morgan RC, Donat EE: Cytologic diagnosis of intravenous talc granulomatosis by fine needle aspiration biopsy. A case report. Acta Cytol 28:737–739, 1984

62. Reinhartz T, Lijovetzky G, Levij IS: Intracellular starch granules in cytologic material. Acta Cytol 22:36–37, 1978

63. Holmes EC, Eggleston JC: Starch granulomatous peritonitis. Surgery 71:85, 1972

64. Sturdy JH, Baird RM, Gerein AN: Surgical sponges. A cause of granuloma and adhesion formation. Ann Surg 165:128, 1967

65. Saxen L, Myllarniemi H: Foreign material and postoperative adhesions. N Engl J Med 279:200, 1968

66. Dragan MJ: Wood fibers from disposable surgical gowns and drapes. JAMA 241:2297, 1979

67. Tomashefski J Jr, Cohen AM, Doershuk CF: Longterm histopathologic follow-up of bronchial arteries after therapeutic embolization with polyvinyl alcohol (Ivalon) in patients with cystic fibrosis. Hum Pathol 19:555–561, 1988

68. Novak D: Embolization materials. pp. 295–312. In Diondelinger RF, Rossi P, Kurdziel JC, Wallace S (eds): Interventional Radiology. Thieme, New York, 1990

69. Schweitzer JS, Chang BS, Madsen P, et al: The pathology of arteriovenous malformations of the brain treated by embolotherapy. II. Results of embolization with multiple agents. Neuroradiology 35:468–474, 1993

70. Knowlson GTG: Gel-foam granuloma in the brain. J Neurol Neurosurg Psychiatry 37:971, 1974

71. Kepes JJ, Yarde WL: Visualization of injected embolic material (polyvinyl alcohol) in paraffin sections with Verhoeff-van Gieson elastica stain. Am J Surg Pathol 19:709–711, 1995

72. Germano IM, Davis RL, Wilson CB, et al: Histopathological follow-up study of 66 cerebral arteriovenous malformations after therapeutic embolization with polyvinyl alcohol. J Neurosurg 76:607–614, 1992

73. Davidson GS, Terbrugge KG: Histologic long-term follow-up after embolization with polyvinyl alcohol particles. Am J Neuroradiol, suppl. 4, 6:843–846, 1995

74. Lundie MJ, Ellyatt D, Kaufmann MB, et al: Staining procedure to aid in assessment of bucrylate histotoxicity in tissue sections. Arch Pathol Lab Med 109:779–781, 1985

75. Jinno K, Moriwaki S, Tanada M, et al: Clinicopathological study on combination therapy consisting of arterial embolization for hepatocellular carcinoma. Cancer Chemother Pharmacol 31:S7–12, 1992

76. Kyriakos M: Myospherulosis of the paranasal sinuses, nose and middle ear. A possible iatrogenic disease. Am J Clin Pathol 67:118, 1977

77. Rosai J: The nature of myospherulosis of the upper respiratory tract. Am J Clin Pathol 69:475, 1978

78. Travis WD, Li C-Y, Weiland LH: Immunostaining for hemoglobin in two cases of myospherulosis. Arch Pathol Lab Med 110:763, 1986

79. Wheeler TM, Sessions RB, McGavran MH: "Myospherulosis": a preventable iatrogenic nasal and paranasal entity. Arch Otolaryngol 106:272, 1980

80. White JT: Myospherulosis. South Med J 72:485, 1979

81. Mills SE, Lininger JR: Intracranial myospherulosis. Hum Pathol 13:596, 1982

82. Shabb N, Sneige N, Dekmezian RH: Myospherulosis. Fine needle aspiration cytologic findings in 19 cases. Acta Cytol 35:225–228, 1991

83. Wolff M: Granulomas in nasal mucous membranes following local steroid injections. Am J Clin Pathol 62:775, 1974

84. Santa Cruz DJ, Ulbright TM: Mucin-like changes in keloids. Am J Clin Pathol 75:18, 1981

85. Ford LT, DeBender J: Tendon rupture after local steroid injection. South Med J 72:827, 1979

86. Balough K: The histologic appearance of corticosteroid injection sites. Arch Pathol Lab Med 110:1168–1172, 1986

87. Hutton L: Oleothorax: expanding pleural lesion. AJR 142:1107, 1984

88. Hoare AM, Alexander-Williams J: Oleogranuloma of the rectum produced by Lasonil ointment. BMJ 2:997, 1977

89. Ghosh A: Lipogranuloma of the uterine parametrium. Br J Obstet Gynecol 83:409, 1976

90. Keebler CM: Cytopreparatory techniques. pp. 881–906. In Bibbo M (ed): Comprehensive Cytopathology. WB Saunders, Philadelphia, 1991

91. Avrin E, Marquet E, Schwartz R, et al: Plant cells resembling tumor cells in routine cytology. Am J Clin Pathol 57:303–305, 1972

92. Emery JA, Spanier SS, Kasnic G Jr, Hardt NS: The synovial structure of breast-implant-associated bursae. Mod Pathol 7:728–733, 1994

93. Hameed MR, Erlandson R, Rosen PP: Capsular synovial-like hyperplasia around mammary implants similar to detritic synovitis. A morphologic and immunohistochemical study of 15 cases. Am J Surg Pathol 19:433–438, 1995

94. Raso DS, Crymes LW, Metcalf JS: Histological assessment of fifty breast capsules from smooth and textured augmentation and reconstruction mammoplasty prostheses with emphasis on the role of synovial metaplasia. Mod Pathol 7:310, 1994

95. Edwards JCW, Sedgwick AD, Willoughby DA: The formation of a structure with the features of synovial lining by subcutaneous injection of air: an in vivo tissue culture system. J Pathol 134:147, 1981

96. Kasper CS: Histologic features of breast capsules reflect surface configuration and composition of silicone bag implants. Am J Clin Pathol 102:655–659, 1994

97. Strom BL, Reidenberg MM, Freundlish B, Schinnar R: Breast silicone implants and the risk of systemic lupus erythematosus. J Clin Epidemiol 47:1211, 1994

98. Tabatowski K, Elson CE, Johnston WW: Silicone lymphadenopathy in a patient with a mammary prosthesis. Fine needle aspiration cytology, histology and analytical electron microscopy. Acta Cytol 34:10–41, 1990

99. Frantz P, Herbst CA Jr: Augmentation mammoplasty, irradiation, and breast cancer. A case report. Cancer 36:1147, 1975

100. Dodd LG, Sneige N, Reece GP, et al: Fine-needle aspiration cytology of silicone granulomas in the augmented breast. Diagn Cytopathol 9:498–502, 1993

101. Bommer J, Ritz E, Waldherr R: Silicone-induced splenomegaly. Treatment of pancytopenia by splenectomy in a patient on hemodialysis. N Eng J Med 305:1077, 1981

102. Tabatowski K, Sammarco GJ: Fine needle aspiration cytology of silicone lymphadenopathy in a patient with an artificial joint. A case report. Acta Cytol 36:529–532, 1992

103. Christie AJ, Weinberger KA, Dietrich M: Silicone lymphadenopathy and synovitis. Complications of silicone elastomer finger joint prostheses. JAMA 237:1463, 1977

104. Christie AJ, Weinberger KA, Dietrich M: Recurrence of silicone lymphadenopathy. JAMA 245:1314, 1981

105. Travis WD, Balogh K, Abraham JL: Silicone granulomas: report of three cases and review of the literature. Hum Pathol 16:19, 1985

106. Friedlander GN, Potter GK, Tucker RS, et al: Silicone elastomer microshards in fluid from a painful metatarsophalangeal implant site. A case report. Acta Cytol 39:586–588, 1995

107. Ober WB: Effects of oral and intrauterine administration of contraceptives on the uterus. Hum Pathol 8:513, 1977

108. Czernobilsky B, Rotenstreich L, Mass N, et al: Effect of intrauterine device on histology of endometrium. Obstet Gynecol 45:64, 1975

109. McCormick JF, Scorgie RDF: Unilateral tubo-ovarian actinomycosis in the presence of an intrauterine device. Am J Clin Pathol 68:622, 1977

110. Sagiroglu N Sagiroglu E: The cytology of intrauterine contraceptive devices. Acta Cytol 14:58–64, 1970

111. Fornari ML: Cellular changes in the glandular epithelium of patients using IUD's—a source of cytologic error. Acta Cytol 18:341–343, 1974

112. Gupta PK: Intrauterine contraceptive devices. Vaginal cytology, pathologic changes, and clinical implications. Acta Cytol 26:571–613, 1982

113. Zaharopoulos P, Wong JY, Edmonston G, et al: Crystaline bodies in cervicovaginal smears. Acta Cytol 29:1035–1042, 1985

114. Barter JF, Orr JW, Holloway RW, et al: Psammoma bodies in a cervicovaginal smear associated with an intrauterine device—a case report. J Reprod Med 32:147–148, 1987.

115. Ostergard DR, Townsend DE, Hirose FM: Treatment of chronic cervicitis by cryotherapy. Am J Obstet Gynecol 102:426, 1968

116. Gondos B, Smith LR, Townsend DE: Cytologic changes in cervical epithelium following cryosurgery. Acta Cytol 14:386–389, 1970

117. Holmquist ND, Bellina JH, Danos ML: Vaginal and cervical cytologic changes following laser treatment. Acta Cytol 20:290–294, 1976

118. Koss LG: Diagnostic Cytology and Its Histologic Basis. p. 665. Lippincott-Raven, Philadelphia, 1992

119. Hoffman MS, Gordy LW, Cavanagh D: Use of the Cytobrush for cervical sampling after cryotherapy. Acta Cytol 35:79–80, 1991

120. Petersen DS, Milleman LA, Rose EF, et al: Biopsy and clinical course after cryosurgery for prostatic cancer. J Urol 120:308–311, 1978

121. Grampsas SA, Miller GJ, Crawford ED: Salvage radical prostatectomy after failed transperineal cryotherapy: histologic findings from prostate whole-mount specimens correlated with intraoperative transrectal ultrasound images. Urology 45:936–941, 1995

122. Bago-Granell J, Aguirre-Canyadell M, Nardi J, et al: Malignant fibrous histiocytoma of bone at the site of a total hip arthroplasty. J Bone Joint Surg [Br] 66B:38, 1984

123. Penman HG, Ring PA: Osteosarcoma in association with total hip replacement. J Bone Joint Surg [Br] 66B:632, 1984

124. Swann M: Malignant soft-tissue tumour at the site of a total hip replacement. J Bone Joint Surg [Br] 66B:629, 1984

125. Fechner RE: Bone and joints. p. 79. In Riddell RH (ed): Pathology of Drug-Induced and Toxic Diseases. Churchill Livingstone, New York, 1982

126. Lee YS, Rho RWH, Nather A: Malignant fibrous histiocytoma at site of metal implant. Cancer 54:2286, 1984

127. Goldring SR, Schiller AL, Roelke M, et al: The synovial-like membrane at the bone-cement interface in loose total hip replacements and its proposed role in bone lysis. J Bone Joint Surg [Am] 65A:575, 1983

128. O'Connell JX, Rosenberg AE: Histiocytic lymphadenitis associated with a large joint prosthesis. Am J Clin Pathol 99:314–316, 1993

129. Albores-Saavedra J, Vuitch F, Delgado R, et al: Sinus histiocytosis of pelvic lymph nodes after hip replacement. A histiocytic proliferation induced by cobalt-chromium and titanium. Am J Surg Pathol 18:83–90, 1994

130. Bjornsson BL, Truong LD, Cartwright J Jr, et al: Pelvic lymph node histiocytosis mimicking metastatic prostatic adenocarcinoma: association with hip prostheses. J Urol 154:470, 1995

131. McKinney CD, Gaffey MJ, Gillenwater JY: Bladder outlet obstruction after multiple periurethral polytetrafluoroethylene injections. J Urol 153:149–151, 1995

132. Wenig BM, Heffner DK, Oertel YC, Johnson FB: Teflonomas of the larynx and neck. Hum Pathol 21:617, 1990

133. Hanau CA, Chancellor MB, Alexander A, et al: Fine-needle aspiration of a periurethral Teflon-filled cyst following radical prostatectomy. Diagn Cytopathol 8:614–616, 1992

134. Freeman BS: Proplast, a porous implant for contour restoration. Br J Plast Surg 29:158, 1976

135. Peacock EE Jr, Van Winkle W Jr: Wound Repair. 2nd Ed. WB Saunders, Philadelphia, 1976

136. Postelthwait RW: Tissue reaction to surgical sutures. p. 263. In Dunphy JE, Van Winkle W Jr (eds): Repair and Regeneration. The Scientific Basis for Surgical Practice. McGraw-Hill, New York, 1968

137. Salthouse TN, Matlaga BS, Wykoff MH: Comparative tissue response to six suture materials in rabbit cornea, sclera, and ocular muscle. Am J Opththalmol 84:224, 1977

138. Alguacil-Garcia A: Necrobiotic palisading suture granulomas simulating rheumatoid nodule. Am J Surg Pathol 17:920, 1993

139. Shauffer IA, Sequeira J: Suture granuloma simulating recurrent carcinoma. AJR 128:856, 1977

140. Belleza NA, Lowman RM: Suture granuloma of the stomach following total colectomy. Radiology 127:84, 1978

141. Maygarden SJ, Novotny DB, Johnson DE, et al: Fine-needle aspiration cytology of suture granulomas of the breast: a potential pitfall in the cytologic diagnosis of recurrent breast cancer. Diagn Cytopathol 10:175–179, 1994

142. Amazon K, Robinson MJ, Rywlin AM: Ferrugination caused by Monsel's solution. Clinical observations and experimentations. Am J Dermatopathol 2:197, 1980

143. Olmstead PM, Lund HZ, Leonard DD: Monsel's solution. A histologic nuisance. J Am Acad Dermatol 3:492, 1980

144. Weinberg DS, Maini BS: Primary sarcoma of the aorta associated with a vascular prosthesis: a case report. Cancer 46:398, 1980

145. Rosen Y, Vaillant JG, Yerkmakov V: Submucosal mucous cysts at a colostomy site: relationship to colitis cystica profunda and report of a case. Dis Colon Rectum 19:453, 1976

146. Wayte DM, Helwig EB: Colitis cystica profunda. Am J Clin Pathol 48:159, 1967

147. Rosai J: Ackerman's Surgical Pathology. 7th Ed. CV Mosby, St. Louis, 1989

148. Armin A-R, Moradi A, Winters G: Posttraumatic intrauterine omental implantation mimicking lipomatous lesion 16 years later. Int J Gynecol Pathol 6:89, 1987

149. Courtice RW, Stinson WA, Walley VM: Tissue fragments recovered at cardiac surgery masquerading as tumoral proliferations. Evidence suggesting iatrogenic or artefactual origin and common occurrence. Am J Surg Pathol 18:167–174, 1994

150. Veinot JP, Tazelaar HD, Edwards WD, Colby TV: Mesothelial/monocytic incidental cardiac excrescences (cardiac MICE). Mod Pathol 7:9, 1994

151. Bigner SH, Elmore PD, Dee AL, et al: Unusual presentations of inflammatory conditions in cerebrospinal fluid. Acta Cytol 29:291–296, 1985

152. Bigner SH, Elmore PD, Dee AL, et al: The cytopathology of reactions to ventricular shunts. Acta Cytol 29:391–396, 1985

153. Hoffman HJ, Duffner PK: Extraneural metastases of central nervous system tumors. Cancer 56:1778, 1985

154. Lovell MA, Ross GW, Cooper PH: Gliomatosis peritonei associated with a ventriculoperitoneal shunt. Am J Clin Pathol 91:485–487, 1989

155. Recht KA, Belis JA, Kandzari J, et al: Ureterosigmoidostomy followed by carcinoma of the colon. Cancer 44:1538, 1979

156. Harford FJ, Fazio VW, Epstein LM, et al: Rectosigmoid carcinoma occurring after ureterosigmoidostomy. Dis Colon Rectum 27:321, 1984

157. Iannoni C, Marcheggiano A, Pallone F, et al: Abnormal patterns of colorectal mucin secretion after urinary diversion of different types: histochemical and lectin binding studies. Hum Pathol 17:834, 1986

158. Schipper H, Deckter A: Carcinoma of the colon arising at uretero-implant sites despite early external diversion. Pathogenetic and clinical implications. Cancer 47:2062, 1981

159. Littler ER, Gleibermann E: Gastritis cystica polyposa. (Gastric mucosal prolapse at gastroenterostomy site, with cystic and infiltrative epithelial hyperplasia.) Cancer 29:205, 1972

160. Koga S, Watanabe H, Enjoji M: Stomal polypoid hypertrophic gastritis. A polypoid gastric lesion at gastroenterostomy site. Cancer 43:647, 1979

161. Stemmermann GN, Nayashi T: Hyperplastic polyps of the gastric mucosa adjacent to gastroenterostomy stomas. Am J Clin Pathol 71:341, 1979

162. Morgenstern L, Yamakawa T, Seltzer D: Carcinoma of the gastric stump. Am J Surg 125:29, 1973

163. Bogomoletz WV, Potet F, Barge J, et al: Pathological features and mucin histochemistry of primary gastric stump carcinoma associated with gastritis cystica polyposa. A study of six cases. Am J Surg Pathol 9:401, 1985

164. Ruck P, Wehrmann M, Campbell M, et al: Squamous cell carcinoma of the gastric stump. A case report and review of the literature. Am J Surg Pathol 13:317–324, 1989

165. Monafo W, Goldfarb W: Postoperative peritoneal cyst. Surgery 53:470, 1963

166. Ross MJ, Welch WR, Scully RE: Multilocular peritoneal inclusion cysts (so-called cystic mesotheliomas). Cancer 64:1336–1346, 1989

167. Weiss SW, Tavassoli FA: Multicystic mesothelioma. An analysis of pathologic findings and biologic behavior in 37 cases. Am J Surg Pathol 12:737–746, 1988

168. O'Hara CJ, Corson JM, Pinkus GS, et al: A monoclonal antibody that distinguishes epithelial-type malignant mesothelioma from pulmonary adenocarcinoma and extrapulmonary malignancies. Am J Pathol 136:421–428, 1990

169. Nance KV, Silverman JF: Immunocytochemical panel for the identification of malignant cells in serous effusions. Am J Clin Pathol 95:867–874, 1991

170. Steinberg AO, Madayag MA, Bosniak MA, et al: Demonstration of 2 unusually large pelvic lymphocysts by lymphangiography. J Urol 109:477, 1973

171. Basinger GT, Gittes RF: Lymphocyst: ultrasound diagnosis and urologic management. J Urol 114:740, 1975

172. Payan HM, Gilbert EF: Mesenteric cyst-ovarian implant syndrome. Arch Pathol Lab Med 111:282, 1987

173. Proppe KH, Scully RE, Rosai J: Postoperative spindle cell nodules of genitourinary tract resembling sarcomas. A report of eight cases. Am J Surg Pathol 8:101, 1984

174. Kay S, Schneider V: Reactive spindle cell nodule of the endocervix simulating uterine sarcoma. Int J Gynecol Pathol 4:255, 1985

175. Lundgren L, Aldenborg F, Angervall L, et al: Pseudomalignant spindle cell proliferations of the urinary bladder. Hum Pathol 25:181–191, 1994

176. Wick MR, Brown BA, Young RH, et al: Spindle-cell proliferations of the urinary tract. An immunohistochemical study. Am J Surg Pathol 12:379–389, 1988

177. Powers CN, Berardo MD, Frable WJ: Fine-needle aspiration biopsy: pitfalls in the diagnosis of spindle-cell lesions. Diagn Cytopathol 10:232–240, 1994

178. Weiss SW, Enzinger FM, Johnson FB: Silica reaction simulating fibrous histiocytoma. Cancer 42:2738, 1978

179. Sobel HJ, Avrin E, Marquet E, et al: Reactive granular cells in sites of trauma. A cytochemical and ultrastructural study. Am J Clin Pathol 61:223, 1974

180. McFadden DE, Clement PB: Peritoneal inclusion cysts with mural mesothelial proliferation. A clinicopathologic analysis of six cases. Am J Surg Pathol 10:844, 1986

181. Weiss SW, Enzinger FM: Malignant fibrous histiocytoma: an analysis of 200 cases. Cancer 41:2250, 1978

182. Inoshita T, Youngberg GA: Malignant fibrous histiocytoma arising in previous surgical sites. Report of two cases. Cancer 53:176, 1984

183. Sherlock P, Oropeza R: Jejunal perforations in lymphoma after chemotherapy. Arch Intern Med 110:102, 1962

184. Hartmann WH, Sherlock P: Gastroduodenal metastases from carcinoma of the breast. An adrenal steroid-induced phenomenon. Cancer 14:426, 1961

185. Mayer RJ, Berkowitz RS, Griffiths CT: Central nervous system involvement by ovarian carcinoma. A complication of prolonged survival with metastatic disease. Cancer 41:776, 1978

186. Gercovich FG, Luna MA, Gottlieb JA: Increased incidence of cerebral metastases in sarcoma patients with prolonged survival from chemotherapy. Report of cases of leiomyosarcoma and chondrosarcoma. Cancer 36:1843, 1975

187. Telles NC, Rabson AS, Pomeroy TC: Ewing's sarcoma: an autopsy study. Cancer 41:2321, 1978

188. Lockwood WB, Broghamer WL Jr: The changing prevalence of secondary cardiac neoplasms as related to cancer therapy. Cancer 45:2659, 1980

189. Espana P, Chang P, Wiernik PH: Increased incidence of brain metastases in sarcoma patients. Cancer 45:337, 1980

190. Thalinger AR, Rosenthal SN, Borg S, et al: Cavitation of pulmonary metastases as a response to chemotherapy. Cancer 46:1329, 1980

191. Qizilbash A, Kontozoglou T, Sianos J, et al: Hepar lobatum associated with chemotherapy and metastatic breast cancer. Arch Pathol Lab Med 111:58, 1987

192. Koss LG, Melamed MR, Mayer K: The effect of busulfan on human epithelia. Am J Clin Pathol 44:385, 1965

193. Nelson BM, Andrews GA: Breast cancer and cytologic dysplasia in many organs after busulfan (Myleran). Am J Clin Pathol 42:37, 1964

194. Koss LG: Diagnostic Cytology and Its Histologic Basis. pp. 753–757. Lippincott-Raven, Philadelphia, 1992

195. Koss LG: Diagnostic Cytology and Its Histologic Basis. pp. 920–926. Lippincott-Raven, Philadelphia, 1992

196. Koss LG: Diagnostic Cytology and Its Histologic Basis. pp. 675–681. Lippincott-Raven, Philadelphia, 1992

197. Walloch JL, Hong HY, Bibb LM: Effects of therapy on cytologic specimens. pp. 860–877. In Bibbo M (ed): Comprehensive Cytopathology. WB Saunders, Philadelphia, 1991

198. Pinedo F, Vargas J, de Agustin P, et al: Epithelial atypia in gynecomastia induced by chemotherapeutic drugs. A possible pitfall in fine needle aspiration biopsy. Acta Cytol 35:229–233, 1991

199. Kennedy S, Merino MJ, Swain SM, et al: The effects of hormonal and chemotherapy on tumoral and nonneoplastic breast tissue. Hum Pathol 21:192–198, 1990

200. O'Morchoe PJ, Lee DC, Kozak CA: Esophageal cytology in patients receiving cytoxic drug therapy. Acta Cytol 27:630–634, 1983
201. Stella F, Battistelli S, Marcheggiani F, et al: Urothelial toxicity following conditioning therapy in bone marrow transplantation and bladder cancer: morphologic and morphometric comparison by exfoliative urinary cytology. Diagn Cytopathol 8:216–221, 1992
202. Forni AM, Koss LG, Geller W: Cytologic study of the effect of cyclophosphamide on the epithelium of the urinary bladder in man. Cancer 17:1348–1355, 1964
203. Rasmussen K, Petersen BL, Jacobo E, et al: Cytologic effects of thiotepa and Adriamycin on normal canine urothelium. Acta Cytol 24:237–233, 1980
204. Tabbara SO, Fechner RE, Edge SB: Pathologic assessment of post-chemotherapy mastectomies. Mod Pathol 3:98A, 1990
205. Armas OA, Aprikian AG, Melamed J, et al: Clinical and pathobiological effects of neoadjuvant total androgen ablation therapy on clinically localized prostatic adenocarcinoma. Am J Surg Pathol 18:979–991, 1994
206. Wade TR, Ackerman AB: The effects of resin of podophyllin on condyloma acuminatum. Am J Dermatopathol 6:109–122, 1984
207. Krebs HB, Helmkamp BF: Chronic ulcerations following topical therapy with 5-fluorouracil for vaginal human papillomavirus-associated lesions. Obstet Gynecol 78:205–208, 1991
208. Colgan T, Simon GT, Kay JM, et al: Amiodarone pulmonary toxicity. Ultrastruct Pathol 6:199–207, 1984
209. Martin WJ, Osborn MJ, Douglass WW: Amiodarone pulmonary toxicity: assessment by bronchial lavage. Chest 88:630–631, 1985
210. Stein B, Zaatari GS, Pine JR: Amiodarone pulmonary toxicity. Acta Cytol 31:357–361, 1987
211. Frierson HF, Fechner RE: Histologic grade of locally advanced infiltrating ductal carcinoma after treatment with induction chemotherapy. Am J Clin Pathol 102:154, 1994
212. Kuo SH, Luh KT: Monitoring tumor cell kinetics in patients receiving chemotherapy for small cell lung cancer. Acta Cytol 37:353–357, 1993
213. Tiffany P, Morse MJ, Bosl G, et al: Sequential excision of residual thoracic and retroperitoneal masses after chemotherapy for stage III germ cell tumors. Cancer 57:978, 1986
214. Hong SJ, Lurain JR, Tsukada Y, et al: Cystadenocarcinoma of the ovary in a four-year old: benign transformation during therapy. Cancer 45:2227, 1980
215. Willis GW, Hajdu SI: Histologically benign teratoid metastasis of testicular embryonal carcinoma: report of five cases. Am J Clin Pathol 59:338, 1973
216. Davey DB, Ulbright TM, Loehrer PJ, et al: The significance of atypia within teratomatous metastases after chemotherapy for malignant germ cell tumors. Cancer 59:533, 1987
217. Molenaar WM, Oosterhuis JW, Kamps WA: Cytological "differentiation" in childhood rhabdomyosarcomas following polychemotherapy. Hum Pathol 15:973, 1984
218. Molenaar WM, Oosterhuis JW, Oosterhuis AM, et al: Mesenchymal and muscle-specific intermediate filaments (vimentin and desmin) in relation to differentiation in childhood rhabdomyosarcomas. Hum Pathol 16:838, 1985
219. Wilson RE, Antman KH, Brodsky G, et al: Tumor-cell heterogeneity in soft tissue sarcomas as defined by chemoradiotherapy. Cancer 53:1420, 1984
220. Ogita S, Tokiwa K, Arizono N, Takahishi T: Neuroblastoma: incomplete differentiation on the way to maturation or morphological alteration resembling maturity? Oncology 45:148, 1988
221. Saxena R, Leake JL, Shafford EA, et al: Chemotherapy effects on hepatoblastoma. A histological study. Am J Surg Pathol 17:1266–1270, 1993
222. Mazur MT, Lurain JR, Brewer JI: Fatal gestational choriocarcinoma. Clinicopathologic study of patients treated at a trophoblastic disease center. Cancer 50:1833, 1982
223. Brisigotti M, Cazzutto C, Fabbretti G, et al: Wilms' tumour after treatment. Pediatr Pathol 12:397–406, 1992
224. Zuppan CW, Beckwith JB, Weeks DA, et al: The effect of preoperative therapy on the histologic features of Wilms' tumour. Analysis of cases from the Third National Wilms' Tumour Study. Cancer 68:385–394, 1991
225. Durkin W, Durant J: Benign mass lesions after therapy for Hodgkin's disease. Arch Intern Med 139:333, 1979
226. Stewart FM, Williamson BR, Innes DJ, et al: Residual tumor masses following treatment for advanced histiocytic lymphoma. Diagnostic and therapeutic implications. Cancer 55:620, 1985
227. Einhorn LH, Donohue J: Cis-diamminedichloroplatinum, vinblastine and bleomycin combination chemotherapy in disseminated testicular cancer. Ann Intern Med 87:293, 1977
228. Lamm DL, Wepsic HT, Feldman P, et al: Importance of alpha-fetoprotein in patients with seminoma. Urology 10:233, 1977
229. Shin M, Hoo K: Diffuse thymic hyperplasia following chemotherapy for nodular sclerosing Hodgkin's disease. Cancer 51:30, 1983
230. Carmosino L, DiBenedetto A, Feffer S: Thymic hyperplasia following successful chemotherapy. A report of two cases and review of the literature. Cancer 56:1526, 1985
231. Smith T: Fatty replacement of lymph nodes mimicking lymphoma relapse. Cancer 58:2686, 1986
232. Werbin N: Fatty changes and metastases in axillary lymph nodes. J Surg Oncol 25:145, 1984
233. Geis WP, Iwatsuki S, Molnar Z, et al: Pseudolymphoma in renal allograft recipients. Arch Surg 113:461, 1978
234. Deodhar SD, Kuklinca AG, Vidt DG, et al: Development of reticulum-cell sarcoma at the site of antilymphocyte globulin injection in a patient with renal transplant. N Engl J Med 280:1104, 1969
235. Boffetta P, Kaldor JM: Secondary malignancies following cancer chemotherapy. Acta Oncol 33:591–598, 1994
236. Rubin CM, Arthur DC, Woods WG, et al: Therapy-related myelodysplastic syndrome and acute myeloid leukemia in children: correlation between chromosomal abnormalities and prior therapy. Blood 78:2982–2988, 1991
237. Tchernia G, Mielot F, Subtil E, et al: Acute myeloblastic leukemia after immunodepressive therapy for primary nonmalignant disease. Blood Cells 2:67, 1967
238. Cortes J, O'Brien S, Kantarjian H, et al: Abnormalities in the long arm of chromosome 11 (11q) in patients with de novo and secondary acute myelogenous leukemias and myelodysplastic syndromes. Leukemia 8:2174–2178, 1994
239. Sandoval C, Pui CH, Bowman LC, et al: Secondary acute myeloid leukemia in children previously treated with alkylating agents, intercalating topoisomerase II inhibitors, and irradiation. J Clin Oncol 11:1039–1045, 1993
240. Klastersky J, Leleux A: Secondary neoplasms following cancer treatment with a special emphasis on lung tumors. Neoplasma 38:253–256, 1991
241. Cimino G, Papa G, Tura S, et al: Second primary cancer following Hodgkin's disease: updated results of an Italian multicenter study. J Clin Oncol 9:432–437, 1991
242. Ellis M, Lishner M: Second malignancies following treatment in non-Hodgkin's lymphoma. Leuk Lymphoma 9:337–342, 1993
243. Reimer RR, Hoover R, Fraumeni JR Jr, et al: Acute leukemia after alkylating-agent therapy of ovarian cancer. N Engl J Med 297:177, 1977
244. Dale GA, Smith RB: Transitional cell carcinoma of the bladder associated with cyclophosphamide. J Urol 112:603, 1974
245. Casko SB, Keuhnelian JG, Gutowski III, et al: Spindle cell cancer of bladder during cyclophosphamide therapy for Wegener's granulomatosis. Am J Surg Pathol 4:191, 1980
246. Wall RL, Clausen KP: Carcinoma of the urinary bladder in patients receiving cyclophosphamide. N Engl J Med 293:271, 1975

247. Seo IS, Clark SA, McGovern FD, et al: Leiomyosarcoma of the urinary bladder thirteen years after cyclophosphamide therapy for Hodgkin's disease. Cancer 55:1597, 1985

248. Carney CN, Stevens PS, Fried FA, et al: Fibroblastic tumor of the urinary bladder after cyclophosphamide therapy. Arch Pathol Lab Med 106:247, 1982

249. Peters MS, Stuard DI: Metastatic malignant melanoma transplanted via a renal homograft. A case report. Cancer 41:2426, 1978

250. Penn I, Starzl TE: Malignant tumors arising de novo in immunosuppressed organ transplant recipients. Transplantation 14:407, 1972

251. Penn I: Cancers of the anogenital region in renal transplant recipients. Analysis of 65 cases. Cancer 58:611, 1986

252. Barenfange J, Mazur JM, Mody N, et al: Malignant fibrous histiocytoma of bone in a renal-transplant patient. J Bone Joint Surg [Am] 62A:297, 1980

253. Craig F, Gulley M, Banks P: Posttransplantation lymphoproliferative disorders. Am J Clin Pathol 99:265–276, 1993

254. Swerdlow S: Post-transplant lymphoproliferative disorders: a morphologic, phenotypic and genotypic spectrum of disease. Histopathology 20:373–385, 1992

255. Knowles D, Cesarman E, Chadburn A, et al: Correlative morphologic and molecular genetic analysis demonstrates three distinct categories of posttransplantation lymphoproliferative disorders. Blood 85:552–565, 1995

256. van Gorp J: Posttransplant T-cell lymphoma: a review. Adv Anat Pathol 2:132–134, 1995

257. Lones M, Mishalani S, Shintaku I, et al: Changes in tonsils and adenoids in children with posttransplant lymphoproliferative disorder: report of three cases with early involvement of Waldeyer's ring. Hum Pathol 26:525–530, 1995

258. Bibbo M, Ali I, Al-Nageeb M, et al: Cytologic findings in female and male offspring of DES treated mothers. Acta Cytol 19:568–575, 1975

259. Zaino RJ, Robboy SJ, Bentley R, et al: Diseases of the vagina. pp. 131–184. In Kurman RJ (ed): Blaustein's Pathology of the Female Genital Tract. Springer-Verlag, New York, 1994

260. Grignon DJ, Sakr WA: Histologic effects of radiation therapy and total androgen blockade on prostate cancer. Cancer 75:1837–1841, 1995

261. Civantos F, Marcial M, Banks E, et al: Pathology of androgen deprivation therapy in prostate carcinoma. Cancer 75:1634–1641, 1995

262. Van de Voorde W, Elgamal A, Poppel H, et al: Morphologic and immunohistochemical changes in prostate cancer after preoperative hormonal therapy. Cancer 74:3164–3175, 1994

263. Devaney DM, Dorman A, Leader M: Adenosquamous carcinoma of the prostate: a case report. Hum Pathol 22:1046–1050, 1992

264. Wernert N, Goebbels R, Bonkhoff H, et al: Squamous cell carcinoma of the prostate. Histopathology 17:339–344, 1990

265. Crow J, Gardner RL, McSweeney G, Shaw RW: Morphological changes in uterine leiomyomas treated by GnRH agonist goserelin. Int J Gynecol Pathol 14:235, 1995

266. Patten SF Jr: Diagnostic cytopathology of the uterine cervix. pp. 66–68. In Weid GL (ed): Monographs in Clinical Cytology. 2nd Ed. Vol. 3. S Karger, New York, 1978

267. Stein RS: Radiation-recall enteritis after actinomycin-D and Adriamycin therapy. South Med J 71:960, 1978

268. Greco FA, Brereton HD, Kent H, et al: Adriamycin and enhanced radiation reaction in normal esophagus and skin. Ann Intern Med 85:294, 1976

269. Cassady JR, Richter M, Piro AJ, et al: Radiation-Adriamycin interactions: preliminary observations. Cancer 36:946, 1975

270. Shield PW, Daunter B, Wright RG: Post-irradiation cytology of cervical cancer patients. Cytopathology 3:167–182, 1992

271. Frierson HF, Covell JL, Andersen WA: Radiation changes in endocervical cells in brush specimens. Diagn Cytopathol 6:243–247, 1990

272. Fajardo LF, Berthrong M: Vascular lesions following radiation. Pathol Annu 23:297–330, 1988

273. Fajardo LF, Berthrong M: Radiation injury in surgical pathology. Part I. Am J Surg Pathol 2:159, 1978

274. White DC: The histopathologic basis for functional decrements in late radiation injury in diverse organs. Cancer 37:1126, 1976

275. Graham RM, Graham JB: Cytologic prognosis in cancer of the uterine cervix. Cancer 8:59–70, 1955

276. Graham RM, Graham JB: Sensitization response in patients with cancer of the uterine cervix. Cancer 13:5–14, 1960

277. Zerne SRM, Morris JM: Prognostic significance of cytologic response in radiation of gynecologic cancer. Obstet Gynecol 19:145–155, 1962

278. Koss LG: Diagnostic Cytology and Its Histologic Basis. pp. 673–675. Lippincott-Raven, Philadelphia, 1992

279. Skolnik EM, Soboroff BJ, Tardy ME Jr, et al: Preoperative radiation of larynx. Analysis of serial sections. Ann Otol Rhinol Laryngol 79:1049, 1970

280. Nicholls JM, Sham J, Chan C-W, Choy D: Radiation therapy for nasopharyngeal carcinoma: histologic appearances and patterns of tumor regression. Hum Pathol 23:742, 1992

281. Silverberg SG, DiGiorgi LS: Histopathologic analysis of preoperative radiation therapy in endometrial carcinoma. Am J Obstet Gynecol 119:698, 1974

282. Cox JD, Stoffel TJ: The significance of needle biopsy after irradiation for stage C adenocarcinoma of the prostate. Cancer 40:156, 1977

283. Gray SR, Hahn IS, Cornog JL Jr: Short-term effect of radiation on human neoplasms. Arch Pathol Lab Med 97:74, 1974

284. Neumann MP, Limas C: Transitional cell carcinomas of the urinary bladder. Effects of preoperative irradiation on morphology. Cancer 58:2758, 1986

285. Weymuller ER Jr: Prognostic importance of the tumor-free laryngectomy specimen. Arch Otol 104:505, 1978

286. Suit HD, Gallager HS: Intact tumor cells in irradiated tissue. Arch Pathol 78:648, 1964

287. Koss LG: Diagnostic Cytology and Its Histologic Basis. pp. 666–673. Lippincott-Raven, Philadelphia, 1992

288. Campos J: Persistent tumor cells in the vaginal smears and prognosis of cancer. Acta Cytol 14:519–522, 1970

289. Goldman JL, Cheren RV, Zak FG, et al: Histopathology of larynges and radical neck specimens in a combined radiation and surgery program for advanced carcinoma of the larynx and laryngopharynx. Ann Otol Rhinol Laryngol 75:313, 1966

290. Flood LM, Brightwell AP: Clinical assessment of the irradiated larynx. Salvage laryngectomy in the absence of histological confirmation of residual or recurrent carcinoma. J Laryngol Otol 98:493, 1984

291. Calcaterra TC, Stern F, Ward PH: Dilemma of delayed radiation injury of the larynx. Ann Otol Rhinol Laryngol 81:501, 1972

292. Diehl LF, Hurwitz MA, Johnson SA, et al: Skin metastases confined to a field of previous irradiation. Report of two cases and review of the literature. Cancer 53:1864, 1984

293. Tessmer CF: Radiation effects in skin. p. 146. In Berdjis CC (ed): Pathology of Irradiation. Williams & Wilkins, Baltimore, 1971

294. Harwood TR, Staley CJ, Yokoo H: Histopathology of irradiated and obstructed submandibular salivary glands. Arch Pathol Lab Med 96:189, 1973

295. Kashima HK, Kirkham WR, Andrews JR: Postirradiation sialadenitis. A study of the clinical features, histopathologic changes and serum enzyme variations following irradiation of human salivary glands. AJR 94:271, 1965

296. Perkins DE, Spjut HJ: Intestinal stenosis following radiation therapy. AJR 88:953, 1962

297. Gardiner GW, McAuliffe N, Murray D: Colitis cystica profunda occurring in a radiation-induced colonic stricture. Hum Pathol 15:295, 1984

298. Weisbrot IM, Liber AF, Gordon BS: The effects of therapeutic radiation on colonic mucosa. Cancer 36:931, 1975

299. Lewin K, Millis RR: Human radiation hepatitis. A morphologic study with emphasis on the late changes. Arch Pathol Lab Med 96:21, 1973

300. Luxton RW, Kunkler PB: Radiation nephritis. Acta Radiol Ther Phys Biol 2:169, 1964

301. Mostofi FK: Radiation effects on the kidney. p. 338. In Mostofi FK, Smith DE (eds): The Kidney. Williams & Wilkins, Baltimore, 1966

302. Kapur S, Chandra R, Antonovych T: Acute radiation nephritis. Light and electron microscopic observations. Arch Pathol Lab Med 101:469, 1977

303. Loveless KJ: The effects of radiation upon the cytology of benign and malignant bladder epithelia. Acta Cytol (Baltimore) 17:355, 1973

304. Wiener HG, Vooijs GP, van't Hof-Grootenboer B: Accuracy of urinary cytology in the diagnosis of primary and recurrent bladder cancer. Acta Cytol 37:163–169, 1993

305. Cowen PN: False cytodiagnosis of bladder malignancy due to previous radiotherapy. Br J Urol 47:405–412, 1975

306. Eposti PL, Edsmyr F, Moberger G, et al: Cytologic diagnosis in bladder carcinoma treated by supervoltage irradiation. Scand J Urol Nephrol 3:201, 1969

307. Tweeddale DN: Urinary Cytology. Little, Brown, Boston, 1977

308. Jayalakshmamma B, Pinkel D: Urinary-bladder toxicity following pelvic irradiation and simultaneous cyclophosphamide therapy. Cancer 38:701–707, 1976

309. Grignon DJ, Sakr WA: Histologic effects of radiation therapy and total androgen blockade on prostate cancer. Cancer 75:1837–1841, 1995

310. Bostwick DG, Egbert BM, Fajardo LF: Radiation injury of the normal and neoplastic prostate. Am J Surg Pathol 6:541, 1982

311. Mazur MT, Kraus FT: Histogenesis of morphologic variations in tumors of the uterine wall. Am J Surg Pathol 4:59, 1980

312. Spitalnik PF, Straus FH: Patterns of human thyroid parenchymal reaction following low-dose childhood irradiation. Cancer 41:1098, 1978

313. Komorowski RA, Hanson GA: Morphologic changes in the thyroid following low-dose childhood radiation. Arch Pathol Lab Med 101:36, 1977

314. Clarke D, Curtis JL, Martinez A, et al: Fat necrosis of the breast simulating recurrent carcinoma after primary radiotherapy in the management of early stage breast carcinoma. Cancer 52:442, 1983

315. Schnitt SJ, Connolly JL, Harris JE, et al: Radiation-induced changes in the breast. Hum Pathol 15:545, 1984

316. Filomena CA, Jordan AG, Ehya H: Needle aspiration cytology of the irradiated breast. Diagn Cytopathol 8:327–332, 1992

317. Hutchison GB: Late neoplastic changes following medical irradiation. Cancer 37:1102, 1976

318. Rubin P, Casarett GW: Clinical Radiation Pathology. WB Saunders, Philadelphia, 1968

319. Katzman H, Waugh T, Berdon W: Skeletal changes following irradiation of childhood tumors. J Bone Joint Surg [Am] 51A:825, 1969

320. Schore-Freedman E, Abrahams C, Recant W, et al: Neurilemomas and salivary gland tumors of the head and neck following childhood irradiation. Cancer 51:2159, 1983

321. van Vloten WA, Hermans J, van Daal WAJ: Radiation-induced skin cancer and radiodermatitis of the head and neck. Cancer 59:411, 1987

322. Martin H, Strong E, Spiro RH: Radiation-induced skin cancer of the head and neck. Cancer 25:61, 1970

323. Lazar P, Cullen SI: Basal cell epithelioma and chronic radiodermatitis. Arch Dermatol 88:172, 1963

324. Hudson AW, Winkelmann RK: Atypical fibroxanthoma of the skin: a reappraisal of 19 cases in which the original diagnosis was spindle-cell squamous carcinoma. Cancer 29:413, 1972

325. Moskaluk CA, Merino MJ, Danforth DN, Medeiros LJ: Low-grade angiosarcoma of the skin of the breast: a complication of lumpectomy and radiation therapy for breast carcinoma. Hum Pathol 23:710–714, 1992

326. Saw D, Chan JKC, Jagirdar J, et al: Sinonasal small cell neoplasm developing after radiation therapy for retinoblastoma: an immunohistologic, ultrastructural, and cytogenetic study. Hum Pathol 23:896–899, 1992

327. Frierson HF Jr, Ross GW, Stewart FM, et al: Unusual sinonasal small-cell neoplasms following radiotherapy for bilateral retinoblastomas. Am J Surg Pathol 13:947, 1989

328. Harzen RW, Pifer JW, Toyooka ET, et al: Neoplasms following irradiation of the head. Cancer Res 26:305, 1966

329. Walker MJ, Chaudhuri PK, Wood DC, et al: Radiation-induced parotid cancer. Arch Surg 116:329, 1981

330. Smith DG, Levitt SH: Radiation carcinogenesis: an unusual familial occurrence of neoplasia following irradiation in childhood for benign disease. Cancer 34:2069, 1974

331. Little JW, Rickles NH: Malignant papillary cystadenoma lymphomatosum. Report of a case, with a review of the literature. Cancer 18:851, 1965

332. Mark RJ, Poen J, Tran LM, et al: Postirradiation sarcomas. A single-institution study and review of the literature. Cancer 73:2653–2662, 1994

333. Castro EB, Rosen PP, Quan SHQ: Carcinoma of large intestine in patients irradiated for carcinoma of cervix and uterus. Cancer 31:45, 1973

334. Qizilbash AH: Radiation-induced carcinoma of the rectum. A late complication of pelvic irradiation. Arch Pathol Lab Med 98:118, 1974

335. Sabio H, Teja K, Elkon D, et al: Adenocarcinoma of the colon following treatment of Wilms' tumor. J Pediatr 95:424, 1979

336. Chen KTK, Hoffman KD, Hendricks EJ: Angiosarcoma following therapeutic irradiation. Cancer 44:2044, 1979

337. Fehr PE, Prem KA: Malignancy of the uterine corpus following irradiation-therapy for squamous cell carcinoma of the cervix. Am J Obstet Gynecol 119:685, 1974

338. Norris HJ, Taylor HB: Postirradiation sarcomas of the uterus. Obstet Gynecol 26:689, 1965

339. Meredith RF, Eisert DR, Kaka Z, et al: An excess of uterine sarcomas after pelvic irradiation. Cancer 58:2003, 1986

340. Varella-Duran J, Nochomovitz LE, Prem KA, et al: Postirradiation mixed müllerian tumors of the uterus. A comparative clinicopathologic study. Cancer 45:1625, 1980

341. Kwon TH, Prempree T, Tang C-K, et al: Adenocarcinoma of the uterine corpus following irradiation for cervical cancer. Gynecol Oncol 11:102, 1981

342. Huvos AG, Woodard HQ, Heilweil M: Postradiation malignant fibrous histiocytoma of bone. A clinicopathologic study of 20 patients. Am J Surg Pathol 10:9, 1986

343. Weatherby RP, Dahlin DC, Ivins JC: Postradiation sarcoma of bone. Review of 78 Mayo Clinic cases. Mayo Clin Proc 56:294, 1981

344. Chan RC, Sutow WW, Lindberg RD, et al: Management and results of localized Ewing's sarcoma. Cancer 43:1001, 1979

345. Phillips TL, Sheline GE: Bone sarcomas following radiation therapy. Radiology 81:992, 1963

346. Tountas AA, Fornasier VL, Harwood AR, et al: Postirradiation sarcoma of bone. A perspective. Cancer 43:182, 1979

347. Meadows AT, Strong LC, Li FP, et al: Bone sarcoma as a second malignant neoplasm in children: influence of radiation and genetic predisposition. Cancer 46:2603, 1980

348. Rutherford H, Dodd GD: Complications of radiation therapy: growing bone. Semin Roentgenol 9:15, 1974

349. Oberman HA, Oneal RM: Fibrosarcoma of the chest wall following resection and irradiation of carcinoma of the breast. Am J Clin Pathol 53:407, 1970

350. Travis EL, Kreuther A, Young T, et al: Unusual postirradiation sarcoma of chest wall. Cancer 38:2269, 1976

351. Langham MR Jr, Mills AS, DeMay RM, et al: Malignant fibrous histiocytoma of the breast. A case report and review of the literature. Cancer 54:558, 1984

352. Bobin JY, Rivoire M, Delay E, et al: Radiation induced sarcomas following treatment for breast cancer: presentation of a series of 14 cases treated with an aggressive surgical approach. J Surg Oncol 57:171–177, 1994

353. Senyszyn JJ, Johnston AD, Jacox HW, et al: Radiation induced sarcoma after treatment of breast cancer. Cancer 26:394, 1970

354. Sordillo PP, Helson L, Hadju SI, et al: Malignant schwannoma—clinical characteristics, survival, and response to therapy. Cancer 47:2503, 1981

355. Goette DK, Detlefs RL: Postirradiation angiosarcoma. J Am Acad Dermatol 12:922, 1985

356. Ulbright TM, Clark SA, Einhorn LH: Angiosarcoma associated with germ cell tumors. Hum Pathol 16:268, 1985

357. Ivins JC, Taylor WF, Wold LE: Elective whole-lung irradiation in osteosarcoma treatment: appearance of bilateral breast cancer in two long-term survivors. Skeletal Radiol 16:133, 1987

358. Iknayan HF: Carcinoma associated with irradiation of the immature breast. Radiology 114:431, 1975

359. Baral E, Larsson LE, Mattsson B: Breast cancer following irradiation of the breast. Cancer 40:2905, 1977

360. Mackenzie I: Breast cancer following multiple fluoroscopies. Br J Cancer 19:1, 1965

361. Yahalom Y, Petrek JA, Biddinger PW, et al: Breast cancer in patients irradiated for Hodgkin's disease: a clinical and pathological analysis of 45 events in 37 patients. J Clin Oncol 10:1674–1681, 1992

362. Dvoretsky PM, Woodard E, Bonfiglio TA, et al: The pathology of breast cancer in women irradiated for acute postpartum mastitis. Cancer 46:2257, 1980

363. Lowell DM, Martineau RG, Luria SB: Carcinoma of the male breast following radiation. Report of case occurring 35 years after radiation therapy of unilateral prepubertal gynecomastia. Cancer 22:581, 1968

364. Curtin CT, McHeffy B, Kolarsick AJ: Thyroid and breast cancer following radiation. Cancer 40:2911, 1977

365. Bailer JC III: Screening for early breast cancer: pros and cons. Cancer 39:2783, 1977

366. Powell HC, Marshall LF, Ignelzi AR: Post-irradiation pituitary sarcoma. Acta Neuropathol (Berl) 39:165, 1977

367. Donahue WE, Jaffe FA, Newcastle NB: Radiation-induced neurofibromata. Cancer 20:589, 1967

368. Watts C: Meningioma following irradiation. Cancer 38:1939, 1976

369. Modan B, Baidatz D, Mart H, et al: Radiation-induced head and neck tumours. Lancet 1:277, 1974

370. Marus G, Levin CV, Rutherford GS: Malignant glioma following radiotherapy for unrelated primary tumors. Cancer 58:886, 1986

371. Clifton MD, Amromin GD, Perry MC, et al: Spinal cord glioma following irradiation for Hodgkin's disease. Cancer 45:2051, 1980

372. Duffy BJ Jr, Fitzgerald PJ: Thyroid cancer in children: a report of 28 cases. J Clin Endocrinol 10:1296, 1950

373. Refetoff S, Harrison J, Karanfilski BT, et al: Continuing occurrence of thyroid carcinoma after irradiation to the neck in infancy and childhood. N Engl J Med 292:171, 1975

374. DeGroot L, Paloyan E: Thyroid carcinoma and radiation. A Chicago endemic. JAMA 225:487, 1973

375. Greenspan FS: Radiation exposure and thyroid cancer. JAMA 237:2089, 1977

376. Cerletty JM, Guansing AR, Engbring NH, et al: Radiation-related thyroid carcinoma. Arch Surg 113:1072, 1978

377. Komorowski RA, Hanson GA, Garancis JC: Anaplastic thyroid carcinoma following low-dose irradiation. Am J Clin Pathol 70:303, 1978

378. Schneider AB, Pinsky S, Bekerman C, et al: Characteristics of 108 thyroid cancers detected by screening in a population with a history of head and neck irradiation. Cancer 46:1218, 1980

379. McDougall IR, Kennedy JS, Thomson JA: Thyroid carcinoma following iodine-131 therapy. Report of a case and review of literature. J Clin Endocrinol 33:287, 1971

380. Sheline GE, Lindsay S, McCormack KR, et al: Thyroid nodules occurring late after treatment of thyrotoxicosis with radioiodine. J Clin Endocrinol 22:8, 1962

381. Roggli VL, Estrada R, Fechner RE: Thyroid neoplasia following irradiation for medulloblastoma. Report of two cases. Cancer 43:2232, 1979

382. Maxon HR, Thomas SR, Saenger EL, et al: Ionizing irradiation and the induction of clinically significant disease in the human thyroid gland. Am J Med 63:967, 1977

383. McDougall IR, Coleman CN, Burke JS, et al: Thyroid carcinoma after high-dose external radiotherapy for Hodgkin's disease: report of three cases. Cancer 45:2056, 1980

384. McHenry C, Jarosz H, Calandra D, et al: Thyroid neoplasia following radiation therapy for Hodgkin's lymphoma. Arch Surg 122:684, 1987

385. Russ JE, Scanlon EF, Sener SF: Parathyroid adenomas following irradiation. Cancer 43:1078, 1979

386. LiVolsi VA, LoGerfo P, Feind CR: Coexistent parathyroid adenomas and thyroid carcinoma. Can radiation be blamed? Arch Surg 113:285, 1978

387. Shannon VR, Nesbitt JC, Libshitz HI: Malignant pleural mesothelioma after radiation therapy for breast cancer. Cancer 76:437–452, 1995

388. Austin MB, Fechner RE, Roggli VL: Pleural malignant mesothelioma following Wilms' tumor. Am J Clin Pathol 86:227, 1986

389. Grampa G: Radiation injury with particular reference to Thorotrast. Pathol Annu 6:147, 1971

390. Telles NC: Follow-up of thorium dioxide patients in the United States. Ann NY Acad Sci 145:674, 1967

391. Kamiho A, Okabe K, Hirose T: Thorium dioxide granuloma of the neck with resultant fatal hemorrhage. Arch Otol 105:45, 1979

392. Hasson J, Hartman KS, Milikow E, et al: Thorotrast-induced extraskeletal osteosarcoma of the cervical region. Report of a case. Cancer 36:1827, 1975

393. Levy DW, Rindsberg S, Friedman AC, et al: Thoratrast-induced hepatosplenic neoplasia: CT identification. AJR 146:997, 1986

394. Smoron GL, Battifora HA: Thorotrast-induced hepatoma. Cancer 30:1252, 1972

395. Kojiro M, Kawano Y, Kawasaki H, et al: Thoratrast-induced hepatic angiosarcoma, and combined hepatocellular and cholangiocarcinoma in a single patient. Cancer 49:2161, 1982

396. Underwood JCE, Huck P: Thorotrast associated hepatic angiosarcoma with 36 years latency. Cancer 42:2610, 1978

397. Sindelar WF, Costa J, Ketcham AS: Osteosarcoma associated with Thorotrast administration. Report of two cases and literature review. Cancer 42:2604, 1978

398. Stewart JR, Gibbs FA Jr: Hyperthermia in the therapy of cancer. Perspectives on its promise and its problems. Cancer 54:2823, 1984

399. Badylak SF, Babbs CF, Skojal TM, et al: Hyperthermia-induced vascular injury in normal and neoplastic tissue. Cancer 56:991, 1985

400. Sugimachi K, Kai H, Matsufuji H, et al: Histopathological evaluation of hyperthermo-chemo-radiotherapy for carcinoma of the esophagus. J Surg Oncol 32:82, 1986

401. Sugaar S, LeVeen HH: A histopathologic study on the effects of radiofrequency thermotherapy on malignant tumors of the lung. Cancer 43:767, 1979

402. Skibba JL, Quebbeman EJ: Tumoricidal effects and patient survival after hyperthermic liver perfusion. Arch Surg 121:1266, 1986

15

Differential Diagnosis of Metastatic Tumors

Mary K. Sidawy
Fred T. Bosman
Jan M. Orenstein
Steven G. Silverberg

The differential diagnosis of metastatic tumors is a problem that has long perplexed surgical pathologists. Although as morphologists we have always endeavored to be as specific as possible in characterizing a neoplasm, whether primary or metastatic, until recently the correct identification of the primary site of a metastasis has been of only minor clinical importance. Within the past few years, however, the development of chemotherapeutic regimens that are fairly specific for certain primary sites has made it imperative that the diagnostic pathologist provide this information if at all possible. Fortunately, some of our diagnostic techniques have also improved simultaneously, so, although many mysteries still remain after thorough investigation, we are indeed often able to provide more information commensurate with clinical expectations.

This chapter is divided into several sections, which are presented in the usual order in which the surgical and cytopathologist deal with these problems. The first section is concerned with a discussion of some of the most common clinicopathologic problems in this area, with general recommendations for preliminary resolution of these problems by the interpretation of clinical and routine histopathologic and cytopathologic data. The second section concerns the application of histochemical methods, including the so-called special stains, while the third reviews the use of the newer but still relatively inexpensive immunohistochemical methods. Finally, the fourth section presents what at present is the final technique applied for differential diagnosis—ultrastructural analysis.

Fine needle aspiration has emerged in the last two decades as a reliable modality to evaluate primary and metastatic tumors. More recently, cytologic preparations have also been validated as acceptable techniques for the examination of intraoperative pathologic specimens with a diagnostic accuracy comparable to that of frozen section analysis.[1-4] Consequently, the pathologist is increasingly called on to interpret or handle cytologic material. In this chapter, the characteristic features and the shared similarities among certain tumors are emphasized. In some cases, the primary site of metastatic disease may be established by distinctive or diagnostic cytologic features. For instance, colonic adenocarcinomas reveal tall columnar malignant epithelial cells with elongated nuclei forming a palisade-like arrangement. Tumor necrosis is a characteristic finding. Metastatic prostatic adenocarcinomas reveal acinar structures, with a moderate amount of cytoplasm and low grade nuclei with prominent nucleoli. Metastatic carcinoids display dispersed cells with the typical "salt and pepper" chromatin. Follicular carcinomas of thyroid are characterized by microfollicle formation with central inspissated colloid. The presence of bile pigment is diagnostic of metastatic hepatocellular carcinomas. Large cells with abundant clear cytoplasm and rich vascularity characterize metastatic renal cell carcinomas. It is important to stress that such distinctive cytologic features are not always present, and review of slides of any previous material is essential. Cytologic samples are also suitable for ancillary studies including cytochemistry, immunohistochemistry, and ultrastructural analysis. Although the cytologic appearance of tumors is not often pathognomonic, the morphologic features coupled with clinical data and ancillary studies should allow a specific diagnosis to be made in many cases.

THE CLINICOPATHOLOGIC PROBLEM

The exact proportion of malignant tumors presenting as distant metastases with an occult primary source is difficult to determine, with figures as divergent as 1.5 percent[5] and 6.5 percent[6] cited in the recent literature. For the surgical or cytopathologist, however, these cases must be added to those in which a primary site is known or clinically suspected but histologic material from the primary tumor is not available for review. In these latter cases as well, the pathologist must be able to state whether the appearance of the metastatic disease is consistent with the known or suspected primary site.

Sites

The most common site of a metastatic cancer with an unknown primary source is a lymph node, particularly a cervical lymph node, and occasionally bone.[5–9] The most common histologic type of tumor seen in the cervical lymph nodes is squamous cell carcinoma,[5] and in this situation the primary site, if it is discovered, usually is in the head and neck region.[9–11] Lindberg[10] illustrated the specific nodal groups most likely to be involved by tumors originating in different sites in this region. Thus, it is particularly helpful to know the exact site of the lymph node submitted. It is also worth remembering that approximately 40 percent of metastases to cervical lymph nodes will be from subclavicular primary sites such as lung, gastrointestinal tract, pancreas, prostate, and breast.[11]

Another important point worth noting about cervical lymph node metastases is that they can often show a lymphoepithelioma pattern, in which individual tumor cells are intimately admixed with lymphocytes, often giving the false impression of a primary malignant lymphoma.[12] Reed-Sternberg-like cells have been reported in these cases, particularly when the primary site was in the nasopharynx. It has been shown that patients with this primary tumor site are likely to have antibodies to Epstein-Barr virus-associated antigens in their sera, and this information can be applied to immunoperoxidase stains or in situ hybridization (see Ch. 6) of the lymph nodes as well.[13]

After the cervical lymph nodes, metastases from unknown primary sites are next most frequently seen in axillary,[14] inguinal,[15] and supraclavicular[16] lymph nodes. Each of these again has its own characteristic pattern for the most likely primary tumor sites. For example, metastatic carcinoma in axillary nodes in women is far and away most likely to be from the breast. Indeed, unless the histologic characteristics of the tumor are totally inconsistent with a primary breast tumor, ipsilateral mastectomy will usually be performed in these cases if an obvious primary lesion is not detectable. It should be remembered, however, that carcinomas arising in the axillary tail of the breast can occasionally be mistaken for axillary lymph node metastases, especially when they contain a marked lymphocytic infiltrate, as in the case of medullary carcinoma (Fig. 15-1). In this instance, what is originally thought to be a metastasis may really be the primary tumor, and, of course, no other primary lesion will be found even after careful study of the mastectomy specimen. This situation (primary tumor in an unusual site initially thought to be metastatic) has been commented on in other sites as well.[17] If the possibility of a mammary primary tumor can be eliminated, the other common sources of axillary lymph node metastases are lung carcinomas and melanomas.

In the case of inguinal lymph node metastases, the most common occult primary sites in women are the cervix, endometrium, and ovary. Vulvar carcinoma, although common, usually has a clinically evident primary tumor. In men, the most frequent sites are prostate, anus, and rectum.[11] Supraclavicular lymph nodes are unique in that they can attract metastases from almost anywhere in the body, ranging from head and neck to mammary, pulmonary, gastrointestinal, and genitourinary primary sites.

After lymph nodes, the second most common site of metastasis from an unknown primary source is not clear-cut. In most

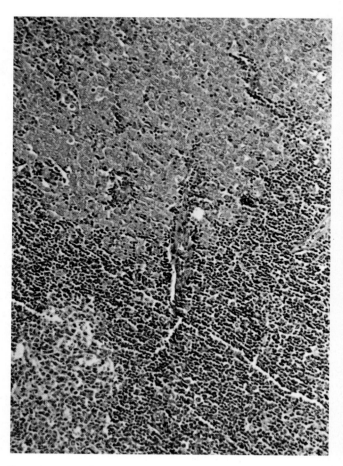

Fig. 15-1. Metastatic medullary carcinoma of breast in axillary lymph node. Sharp demarcation of tumor (above) from lymphoid tissue (below) suggests metastatic carcinoma rather than primary lymphoma. Germinal centers (below) and subcapsular sinus (not illustrated) indicated that this is a node rather than a lymphoid infiltrate in a primary carcinoma of the axillary tail of the breast.

series, however, the second most frequent anatomic location (and occasionally the most frequent) is bone.[5,18] Metastases to long bones and the vertebral column are about equally frequent, and are followed by those to ribs and the skull. The radiologist may be of help in establishing the primary site, since certain metastatic tumors, such as those from the prostate, kidney, thyroid, and neuroblastoma, are said to have distinctive radiologic features.[18] By contrast, the fact that these lesions often must be decalcified before sectioning may make histologic interpretation more difficult. It is always worthwhile to try to dissect out some uncalcified tissues for submission for histologic examination before decalcification of the major portion of the specimen.

After bone, the most frequent sites of metastases from occult primary lesions are (roughly in descending order) the lungs, liver, central nervous system, pleura, intestine, and skin.[5,6] Actually more frequent than several of these, but not listable as a single metastatic site, are those occult primary tumors manifesting as generalized or abdominopelvic peritoneal carcinomatosis.[19] Few rules are applicable for determining the primary source of metastases in these various sites, with the exception that common tumors (such as breast in women and lung in men) should obviously be thought of first. However, unusual metastatic patterns may often be demonstrated.

It can also not be overemphasized that malignant melanoma is the great clinical and pathologic mimic in this situation and should always be considered in the differential diagnosis of any metastatic tumor without a known primary source. Indeed, for unusual sites of metastatic disease (e.g., heart, gallbladder, prostate), melanoma is frequently the most common primary tumor found.

It should also be remembered that in most cases manifesting with metastases from an occult source, the primary site will never be found.[6,11,20] This is often true even after investigation at autopsy.[6] Thus, the question of how extensively to investigate these cases before treatment is instituted is still debatable and may eventually depend on a cost-benefit analysis.[6,20] In most series, metastatic squamous or undifferentiated carcinomas in cervical lymph nodes are associated with fairly good survival rates after radiotherapy,[5] and only 10 to 15 percent of other metastases from unknown primary sites turn out to be of a treatable type by currently available chemotherapeutic regimens.[6–8] Routine light microscopy is often not helpful in predicting favorable responses,[8] and the relative roles of immunohistochemistry[6] and electron microscopy[7,8,17] are still being evaluated.

Adenocarcinoma

Within the clinical spectrum of metastatic tumors from unknown primary sites, by far the most common histologic features are those of carcinoma, and if the cervical lymph node metastases are excluded, the overwhelmingly most common type is adenocarcinoma.[6–8,20,21] One of the main problems for the surgical pathologist in sites in which metastatic adenocarcinomas are frequently seen is the distinction of a metastasis from a primary tumor at that site.[17,22] The lung and liver are excellent examples of this problem. Needle biopsies, aspirations, or even resections often raise the question of metastatic carcinoma versus primary pulmonary or hepatic carcinoma. In the lung, a bronchioloalveolar histologic pattern or an admixture of squamous elements favors a primary lesion, whereas nodular circumscription of the tumor favors metastatic disease.

Distinctive cytologic features that allow a diagnosis of primary versus metastatic adenocarcinoma in the lung are often elusive. Certain features of bronchioloalveolar carcinoma may allow one to suggest this diagnosis based on cytologic material. Papillary fragments, and three-dimensional cell clusters with extreme depth of focus, have been emphasized.[23] The nuclei are bland and the cytoplasm is distended by single or multiple vacuoles. Nuclear pseudoinclusions and psammoma bodies may be observed.

In the liver, the appearance of primary hepatocellular carcinoma is often distinctive, particularly if bile or hyaline globules can be demonstrated. Cytologically, primary hepatocellular carcinoma displays, at least focally, some hepatocellular features. A trabecular pattern, macronucleoli, intranuclear inclusions, and bile pigment are characteristic features. Immuno-

logic markers such as alpha-fetoprotein may be demonstrable either in the serum or by immunoperoxidase study in the tumor. If these methods fail, ultrastructural examination may show characteristic hepatic morphologic features, with intercellular bile canaliculi and intracellular voluminous smooth endoplasmic reticulum. In the case of primary bile duct adenocarcinomas of the liver (cholangiocarcinomas), the tumor cells resemble bile duct epithelium and are easily recognizable as nonhepatocellular cytologically. The cells are individually dispersed or arranged in cohesive three-dimensional groups with gland formation. The cytoplasm may appear vacuolated, indicative of mucin secretion. However, distinction from a metastatic carcinoma is often impossible, particularly if the metastasis is of a ductal type (e.g., pancreas, common bile duct). Radiologic studies may be helpful, but often exploratory surgery will be necessary to make this distinction.

In other organs, the diagnostic problem may be that of distinguishing a metastatic adenocarcinoma from a histologically similar primary tumor that is not adenocarcinoma. Common problems here include mesotheliomas of the pleura, peritoneum, and pericardium, as well as papillary ependymomas and choroid plexus papillomas of the central nervous system. Another potential, but far less common, problem of a similar type involves the so-called adamantinoma of bone, most frequently seen in the tibia. The distinction in the case of both mesothelioma and the central nervous system tumors is best made on the basis of histochemical, immunohistochemical, and/or ultrastructural findings, which are discussed later in this chapter and in the appropriate organ-site chapters of this book.

A problem distinctive to the female genital tract concerns the differential diagnosis of endometrioid carcinoma of the ovary from a metastasis from a primary carcinoma of the endometrium. If the endometrium can be proved benign, the ovarian tumor can clearly be accepted as a primary endometrioid carcinoma. Similarly, if origin can be shown in a focus of endometriosis in the ovary, the tumor can also safely be considered primary. However, in many instances neither of these situations will pertain, and the primary or secondary nature of the ovarian tumor is then not clear. It is our impression that, although endometrial carcinoma does metastasize to the ovary, this situation is far less common than that of separate primary tumors in ovary and endometrium. A recent addition to the techniques used to make this distinction is flow cytometry; different ploidy levels in the two tumors strongly favor separate primaries. An even more recent addition is molecular analysis for loss of heterozygosity in the two tumors: different patterns suggest different primary tumors, while shared molecular features indicate that one tumor is primary and the other metastatic.[24] This subject is discussed in more detail in Chapters 51 and 52.

A similar situation exists with other metastatic tumors to the ovary, which may be mistaken for primary lesions and vice versa. Particularly difficult is the distinction between a primary ovarian mucinous carcinoma and a metastasis from the colon or rectum. Since the primary mucinous ovarian carcinomas are usually of the intestinal type, we know of no foolproof way at present to make this distinction. Bilaterality suggests metastatic disease but certainly does not rule out the possibility of bilateral primary ovarian tumors or a single ovarian primary lesion with metastasis to the contralateral ovary. Immuno-histochemical staining for HAM56 antibody (ovary positive, colon negative)[25] and for cytokeratins 7 and 20 (ovary, cytokeratin 7 positive and cytokeratin 20 negative; colon, cytokeratin 20 positive and cytokeratin 7 negative)[26,27] have recently proved useful in a few series. By contrast, if the tumor being considered is a carcinoid, bilaterality is virtually a guarantee of origin outside the ovary, whereas unilateral tumor is almost always primary and benign. Again, the reader is referred to Chapter 52 for a more complete discussion of these problems (see also discussion of tumor alkaline phosphatase below).

Another problem posed by the ovary, as well as other paired organs such as breast, lung, and kidney, is that of whether bilateral disease represents multiple primary foci or a single primary focus with contralateral metastasis. Again, this question is often impossible to answer with complete certainty, but both clinical and pathologic features of the individual case may help. For example, bilateral paired organ tumors without evidence of other dissemination suggest that both lesions are primary, whereas widespread disseminated disease suggests metastasis, or at least makes the problem a purely academic one. The presence of preneoplastic or preinvasive neoplastic changes associated with the tumor (e.g., in situ lobular or intraductal carcinoma associated with an infiltrating carcinoma of the breast) strongly suggests that the associated invasive tumor is primary at that site. Circumscription of most tumors suggests metastatic disease, whereas an infiltrating margin usually suggests a primary origin at that site. Strong histologic dissimilarity between the two tumors being considered suggests separate primary sources, whereas histologic identity suggests (but certainly does not prove) the possibility that one may be a metastasis from the other. Flow cytometry (identical versus different ploidy levels) may help here as well, as may molecular genetic studies.[28,29] Finally, in some organs, primary and metastatic lesions occupy somewhat different locations. For example, primary breast tumors occur within mammary tissue, whereas metastases to the breast may often be found in the subcutaneous fat. Similarly, although endobronchial metastases certainly exist, they are relatively uncommon, and thus this location might suggest a primary rather than a metastatic lung tumor.

Other Tumors

Although thus far we have considered the question of primary versus metastatic disease only in relation to adenocarcinomas, this differential diagnosis must often be considered in other types of malignant tumors as well. With respect to *squamous cell carcinomas*, the problem most frequently arises when a tumor is found in the lung of a patient who has previously been treated for squamous cell carcinoma of the head and neck region, esophagus, cervix, or other primary site. Again, in this instance, the clinical history will often be of primary importance. For example, late metastases from esophageal carcinomas are almost unknown, so a patient fortunate enough to survive for 5 or more years after treatment for this disease who then develops a squamous cell carcinoma in the lung can safely be assumed to have a new primary tumor. The precise location of the tumor is also helpful, in that primary squamous cell carcinoma of the

lung usually arises centrally from a major bronchus, whereas metastatic cancers to the lung tend to be more peripheral. As mentioned earlier, the circumscribed versus infiltrating character of the tumor margins also helps in the differential diagnosis. Finally, an admixture of other histologic types, such as oat cell or adenocarcinoma, also suggests a primary lung tumor. If doubt still persists after all these criteria are applied, and if disseminated disease is not present elsewhere, the patient is probably best treated for a new primary pulmonary carcinoma.

A fairly recent observation is that the same situation exists in the mediastinum and retroperitoneum of men when *malignant germ cell tumors* are found. As discussed in more detail in Chapter 34, the differential diagnosis between germ cell tumors and thymoma, lymphoma, and metastatic carcinoma in these sites may be a difficult one, and even when a malignant germ cell tumor is diagnosed with confidence, a primary lesion in the testis must be ruled out with care. In women, this is less of a problem, since primary mediastinal and retroperitoneal germ cell tumors are vanishingly rare.

The cytomorphology of extragonadal and metastatic germ cell tumors is sufficiently distinctive to allow specific diagnoses. The cytologic recognition of classic seminoma presents no difficulty.[30,31] The smears reveal a primarily dispersed population of large, round cells with scant to moderately abundant cytoplasm. The nuclear/cytoplasmic ratio is high. The nuclei are large, with prominent nucleoli and fine, evenly distributed chromatin. The tumor cells are very fragile, as evidenced by the numerous stripped nuclei and chromatin threads. The tigroid background seen in the Diff-Quik-stained preparations (Harelco, Gibbstown, NJ) is characteristic and is thought to result from disruption of the cytoplasm at the time of smearing. An admixture of lymphoid cells and occasional granulomas may be present. The cells of embryonal carcinoma are arranged in tightly cohesive clusters, in glandular or papillary formations. They show pronounced nuclear pleomorphism with coarse chromatin, and several prominent nucleoli.[31,32] Yolk sac or endodermal sinus tumors exhibit several patterns indicating their different morphologic expressions. The tumor cells occur singly, in tight or loose clusters, or reveal distinct papillary configuration. The cytoplasm is vacuolated. The nuclei are pleomorphic, with coarse chromatin clumping and prominent nucleoli.[31] Intra-and extracytoplasmic eosinophilic hyaline globules that are periodic acid-schiff (PAS) positive and diastase resistant are easily recognizable.[33] The recognition of hypervacuolated cells and pseudopapillary structures, and the demonstration of hyaline bodies help to distinguish this tumor. Choriocarcinoma reveals single and cohesive clusters of pleomorphic cells with bizarre hyperchromatic nuclei. The nuclei have irregular nuclear membranes and some have prominent nucleoli. The cytoplasm is dense and eosinophilic. Scattered multinucleated tumor giant cells with coarse chromatin and eosinophilic nucleoli are present.[31]

Immunoblastic lymphomas may be confused with seminomas owing to the dispersed population of cells with scant to moderate cytoplasm, round nuclei, and prominent central nucleoli. Thymomas are composed of a mixture of epithelial cells and lymphocytes in variable proportion depending on the histologic type. The epithelial cells occur in clusters and are bland, with little nuclear variability. The lymphoid cells in the background are generally small. In spindle cell thymomas, cohesive sheets of elongated epithelial cells are observed. The cytologic features of metastatic carcinomas depend on the histologic type and are discussed in more detail in the following sections.

The differentiation between germ cell tumors and lymphoma, thymoma, and metastatic carcinoma can be greatly facilitated by immunohistochemical methods. Carcinomas and most thymomas express cytokeratins, and lymphomas express leukocyte common antigen (LCA), as well as more cell type-specific antigens, whereas germ cell tumors often express alpha-fetoprotein or human chorionic gonadotropin. This is discussed in more detail in the section on immunohistochemistry and in Chapters 47 and 52.

The question of primary versus metastatic disease often arises when malignant *melanoma* is diagnosed as well, whether it be in the skin or in the much less common mucosal, meningeal, or ocular locations. The presence of either junctional activity (in skin or mucous membranes) or benign precursor cells (e.g., nevus cells) strongly suggests the primary origin of a melanoma at the site in question. The absence of these features on the initial sections—particularly if no history of a prior or concurrent primary melanoma elsewhere is available—mandates multiple sectioning of the tissue block in question. In all considerations of this problem, it should be remembered that melanomas frequently metastasize widely from occult primary sites, or as a delayed phenomenon many years after the primary source has been apparently successfully treated.

Since the suggestion of a primary site for a metastatic tumor depends in large measure on the histologic type of the tumor, the distinction between, for example, *squamous* and *adenocarcinoma* is an important but often difficult problem. The well differentiated squamous carcinoma showing keratin pearls and intercellular bridges does not pose this problem, nor does the well differentiated adenocarcinoma containing glands or ducts with lumina and obvious mucin production. By contrast, the metastatic tumor composed of solid nests or sheets of anaplastic cells without the above-mentioned attributes is often difficult to classify. Special stains may be of value, but in our experience if the tumor is so undifferentiated that mucin, for example, is not detected or at least suspected with the routine hematoxylin and eosin stain, it usually is not present in sufficient quantity to be detectable with a more specific stain.

Even in these poorly differentiated tumors, however, certain morphologic features may be of value. For example, a spindled appearance of some of the cells is more suggestive of squamous than adenocarcinoma, whereas extremely large solitary nucleoli are more frequently seen in adenocarcinomas. Cytologically, the presence of keratinization and a streaming arrangement of the nuclei are reliable features for classifying the tumor as squamous. The presence of tadpole cells, dense cytoplasm with well defined borders, nuclear pyknosis, and hyperchromasia also help in recognizing the squamous nature of the tumor. Metastatic adenocarcinoma shows three-dimensional groups with pleomorphic nuclei, vesicular chromatin, prominent nucleoli, and vacuolated cytoplasm. A potential difficulty may occur in the distinction of transitional cell carcinoma that has squamous or glandular differentiation from squamous cell carcinoma and adenocarcinoma. Metastatic transitional carcinoma reveals individual cells as well as papillary groups with or without fi-

brovascular cores. Tumor cells have dense granular cytoplasm, enlarged hyperchromatic nuclei, prominent nucleoli, and occasional intranuclear inclusions.[34] Emphasis has been placed on the presence of intracytoplasmic vacuoles and endoplasmic/ectoplasmic interfaces.[34] Cercariform transitional cells (defined as spindled, racquet-shaped malignant cells with long unipolar cytoplasmic processes) have been described as a distinct cytomorphologic clue that may be helpful in the diagnosis of metastatic transitional cell neoplasms of low grade.[35]

Electron microscopy can also be extremely helpful in these cases. It has been shown, for example, that so-called undifferentiated or poorly differentiated carcinomas of the cervix[36] and lung[37] can usually be identified as being of either squamous or glandular origin when examined with the electron microscope. More specific details of this differentiation are discussed later.

The differentiation between adenocarcinoma and squamous cell carcinoma can also be facilitated through the study of the expression of cell type-specific cytokeratins. Adenocarcinomas, for example, tend to express cytokeratin 18, which is usually absent in squamous cell carcinomas, which express cytokeratin 10. This approach is discussed in more detail in the section on immunohistochemistry.

Patterns of Growth

Spindle Cell Tumors

In many instances, metastatic or primary malignant tumors can be characterized by their pattern of growth, and a differential diagnosis can be formulated therefrom. Often the differential diagnosis includes not only different types of carcinoma, as discussed earlier, but noncarcinomatous neoplasms as well. For example, when the pattern of growth is that of a spindle cell tumor, the diagnostic possibilities include carcinoma, sarcoma, and melanoma. In the case of a primary tumor, the site involved may be the most important diagnostic criterion. For example, although both melanoma and various types of sarcoma have been reported in the larynx, a spindle cell tumor in that organ, particularly if it grows as a polypoid mass elevating the mucosa, is most likely to be a metaplastic squamous cell carcinoma ("pseudosarcoma"), and a careful search should be made for foci of in situ or invasive squamous cancer. In metastatic sites, of course, this sort of criterion is more difficult to apply, so a spindle cell tumor metastatic to the lung with no known primary site, for example, could equally be carcinoma, sarcoma, or melanoma. Although reticulin and trichrome stains are said to be of value in distinguishing spindle cell carcinomas from spindle cell sarcomas, we have rarely found this to be the case, and we prefer to rely on immunohistochemistry in combination with electron microscopy, if suitable tissue is available for study. Expression of cytokeratin practically rules out the possibility of sarcoma or melanoma, although in some sarcomas (e.g., epithelioid sarcoma and synovial sarcoma) cytokeratin expression has been reported. Melanomas almost without exception express S-100 protein, but this marker is by no means specific for melanoma. Various melanoma-specific monoclonal antibodies have been reported, but none of these appears to be entirely specific, although HMB 45 comes close and is extremely useful.

Lack of cohesiveness of the spindled tumor cells, a tendency for them to aggregate in nests, and, of course, the presence of stainable melanin also suggest that the spindle cell tumor in question is a malignant melanoma. Aspirates of melanomas reveal a variety of patterns including a pattern of relatively bland spindle or fusiform cells. The dispersed cell population, the presence of intranuclear cytoplasmic inclusions, bi- and multinucleation, and prominent nucleoli are helpful characteristic features. Melanin pigment may be present within the tumor cells or in the accompanying macrophages. The tumor cells in the spindle cell variant of squamous cell carcinomas are more cohesive, and the cytoplasm is tapered and bipolar. In contrast to melanomas, squamous carcinomas are positive for cytokeratin and negative for S-100 and HMB 45. Since sarcomas usually manifest as bulky primary tumors rather than as precocious metastases from occult primary sites, in practical terms they are far less likely than either carcinoma or melanoma to be the source of unexplained metastatic disease.

Large Round to Polygonal Cell Tumors

Another type of tumor cell morphologic pattern that is seen frequently, particularly in lymph nodes, is that of tumors composed of large round to polygonal cells (Table 15-1). This differential diagnosis is most common in adults, and the three most likely possibilities are carcinoma, lymphoma, and melanoma. As mentioned earlier in the discussion of spindle cell tumors, the presence of poor tumor cell cohesiveness, nesting, and/or stainable melanin is suggestive of melanoma, as is the presence of scattered multinucleate giant cells and of numerous intranuclear inclusions of cytoplasm. In a lymph node, tumor cells in the subcapsular sinus or sharply defined from normal lymphoid structures of the node (or displaying both patterns) suggest a metastatic carcinoma or melanoma. A diffuse infiltrate replacing and blending in with the surrounding lymphoid tissues (if any remain) is more suggestive of malignant lymphoma. Markedly convoluted or cleaved nuclei are likely to be seen in lymphoma cells as well. The presence of any glandular or squamous differentiation establishes the diagnosis of carcinoma. These three diagnostic possibilities, as well as the others listed in Table 15-1, are often better distinguished by histochemical or ultrastructural studies, as discussed later. Here again, immunohistochemistry may be helpful. In this differential diagnosis LCA, which will be expressed by all lymphoid cells, will assist in the identification of lymphoma, whereas the markers mentioned above may identify carcinoma or melanoma.

Small Round Cell Tumors

The problem of small round cell tumors (Table 15-2) is one that is encountered predominantly in the pediatric age group. Any tissue may be involved, but here bone is a particularly puzzling site, since both Ewing's sarcoma and malignant lymphoma may be primary tumors or metastatic lesions in bone. All the tumors listed in Table 15-2 can also be encountered in adults, with lymphomas, plasmacytomas, oat cell and lobular carcinomas, and carcinoid tumors being encountered more frequently in adults. The nuclei of plasmacytomas should be distinctive, as may those of some malignant lymphomas. Rosettes in neuroblastomas and brightly eosinophilic cytoplasm with or without cross-striations in embryonal rhabdomyosarcomas are, of course, also distinctive. Lobular carcinoma of the breast metastasizes in a sinus catarrh-like pattern in axillary lymph nodes (see Ch. 19) and may show a characteristic single file linear arrangement of tumor cells in other sites, such as the skin.

Cytologically, the appearance of noncohesive small cells generates the differential diagnosis listed in Table 15-2. Malignant lymphomas reveal a monotonous population of single cells with minimal cytoplasm. The presence of lymphoglandular bodies in the background suggests the lymphoid nature of the lesion. Ewing's sarcomas reveal small round cells arranged singly and in clusters with well defined scant granular cytoplasm. The presence of intracytoplasmic glycogen can be demonstrated with a PAS stain. The individual cells of neuroblastomas may resemble lymphomas; however, focal cellular cohesion and rosette formation help in distinguishing the two entities. Embryonal rhabdomyosarcomas also consist of small oval to round cells with eccentrically placed nuclei and scant granular cytoplasm arranged in loosely cohesive clusters. Plasmacytomas reveal a dispersed population of cells with features of plasma cells such as eccentric nuclei and chromatin arranged in a cartwheel pattern. The cytoplasm is sharply demarcated and demonstrates perinuclear clearing. Binucleate and multinucleate cells are frequent. Carcinoid tumors consist of dispersed or loosely cohesive aggregates of small uniform cells with round to oval nuclei and scanty cytoplasm. The stippled granular chromatin pattern and infrequent nucleoli are helpful features in recognizing the neuroendocrine nature of the tumor.[38] Small cell carcinomas consist of loosely cohesive medium-sized cells with round to oval hyperchromatic nuclei, scanty cyto-

Table 15-1. Large Round to Polygonal Cell Tumors

Carcinoma
Lymphoma
Melanoma
Plasmacytoma
Eosinophilic granuloma
Histiocytoma
Germinoma

Table 15-2. Small Round Cell Tumors

Lymphoma
Oat cell/carcinoid
Neuroblastoma
Ewing's sarcoma
Embryonal rhabdomyosarcoma
Plasmacytoma
Lobular carcinoma (breast)

plasm, salt and pepper chromatin, and inconspicuous nucleoli. The streaming arrangement of the cells, the nuclear molding, smearing of nuclear chromatin, and single cell and sheet-like necrosis are helpful diagnostic features.[38] Lobular carcinomas of the breast reveal relatively uniform small cells with irregular nuclei in a single cell pattern. Nucleoli may be indistinct or conspicuous. The presence of cytoplasmic lumina, which indent and push the nuclei to one end of the cells, indicates the glandular nature of the tumor. The single file arrangement of the cells and the presence of lumina with targetoid mucin are typical features of lobular carcinomas.[39]

In these small round cell tumors, special stains and immunohistochemical and ultrastructural studies may also provide the definitive answer. Immunohistochemical analysis here may include antibodies to cytokeratins, which will identify carcinomas; LCA, which will identify lymphoma; neurofilaments, which occur in neuroblastomas and occasionally also in carcinoids; neuron-specific enolase, chromogranin, and synaptophysin, which occur in neuroblastomas, oat cell carcinomas, and carcinoids; actin and desmin, which characterize myogenic differentiation; myoglobin, seen in rhabdomyosarcomas; and finally immunoglobulins, which characterize plasmacytomas.

Giant Cell Tumors

At the other end of the size spectrum, giant cell tumors (Table 15-3) may also pose diagnostic problems. For the most part, however, the tumors listed in Table 15-3 will manifest at clinically obvious primary sites rather than as distant metastases from an occult primary site. Giant cell carcinomas of the lung and pancreas, however, may represent an exception to this rule. Giant cell glioblastomas rarely metastasize but may be difficult to distinguish in their primary situation in the brain from metastatic giant cell carcinomas or sarcomas. The diagnosis of glioblastoma is generally inferred from its glial appearance. Cytologic preparations are well suited to demonstrate the characteristic fibrillary background of glioblastomas. This feature is only seen in neoplasms of glial or neuronal origin and is absent in metastatic carcinoma and lymphoma. In addition, smears of glioblastomas reveal bizarre, multinucleated giant cells, a wide range of nuclear and cytoplasmic abnormalities, and necrosis. Smears of giant cell carcinomas reveal pleomorphic multinucleate or mononucleate tumor giant cells with large, irregularly shaped nuclei, coarse, granular chromatin, and large prominent nucleoli. The cytoplasm is occasionally infiltrated by neutrophils. Pleomorphic sarcomas containing giant cells include fibrous histiocytomas, fibrosarcomas, and liposarcomas. Malignant fibrous histiocytomas produce cellular smears consisting of pleomorphic giant cells and mononuclear histiocytic round cells in addition to spindle cells.

Giant cell carcinomas, whether originating in lung, pancreas, thyroid, or other organs, frequently show a sarcomatoid histologic pattern; they may be identified as epithelial neoplasms only on immunohistochemical or ultrastructural examination, and even then often with difficulty. For this differential diagnosis, an immunohistochemical workup will include antibodies to cytokeratin, human chorionic genadotropin, and glial fibrillary acidic protein.

Clear Cell Tumors

A much more frequent diagnostic problem in the clinical situation of a metastasis from an occult primary site is that of tumors characterized by numerous clear cells (Table 15-4). Histochemical and ultrastructural studies have shown that the clear appearance of these cells by light microscopy may represent three different subcellular characteristics: (1) large amounts of intracytoplasmic glycogen, (2) organelle poor cytoplasm with little or no glycogen, and (3) fixation or other artifact.[40] Obviously, the determination of which of these three mechanisms is responsible for the clear cell morphologic features will influence the final diagnosis. Far and away the most common of the clear cell tumors—as well as the most likely to metastasize from an occult primary source—is primary clear cell carcinoma of the kidney. The cells of this tumor contain both glycogen and lipid and have a characteristic ultrastructural appearance. Clear cell sarcomas of tendon sheath may contain melanin and are generally considered to represent soft parts clear cell melanomas. Clear cell smooth muscle tumors infrequently metastasize; if they do, they should have an obvious primary tumor, usually in the gastrointestinal tract or the uterus. They should also show evidence of smooth muscle origin at the histochemical or ultrastructural level. Germinomas (seminoma in men, dysgerminoma in women) are a classic example of cells that appear clear because of a paucity of organelles. They contain little or no stainable glycogen (or, for that matter, anything else) and frequently show nucleoli with Chinese character-like nucleonemata. Immunohistochemical studies for the differenti-

Table 15-3. Giant Cell Tumors

Carcinoma
    Lung
    Pancreas
    Thyroid
Giant cell tumor of bone
Soft tissue sarcomas
Choriocarcinoma
Glioblastoma

Table 15-4. Clear Cell Tumors

Carcinoma
    Kidney
    Liver
    Adrenal
    Salivary gland
    Sweat gland
    Lung
    Thyroid
    Female genital tract
Clear cell sarcoma of tendon sheath
Leiomyoblastoma
Germinoma

ation between these tumor types will include antibodies to cytokeratins, cytokeratin subtypes (which may assist in characterizing the organ site of the primary carcinoma), desmin and actin (for leiomyoblastoma), and placental alkaline phosphatase (for germinoma).

Smears of metastatic renal clear cell carcinomas consist of dissociated or clusters of large cells with abundant foamy cytoplasm and a low nuclear/cytoplasmic ratio. The nuclei are bland, eccentric, and frequently contain single prominent nucleoli. The distinctive rich vascularity is a helpful feature. Papillary structures and psammoma bodies have been described.[41] Cytologically, clear cell sarcomas of tendon sheath show nests of epithelioid cells with clear cytoplasm, round vesicular nuclei, and prominent nucleoli. Epithelioid leiomyosarcomas are characterized by smears with many single polygonal cells having eccentric, atypical nuclei. The cytoplasm has a clear quality, with distinct cell borders.[42]

Although clear cell carcinomas are characteristically adenocarcinomas, squamous carcinomas may also show this appearance, either focally or diffusely. This has been pointed out in cases of so-called clear cell carcinomas of the lung, and it has been suggested that this is indeed not a distinct entity.[43] Smears demonstrate clusters of tumor cells with large, hyperchromatic nuclei and prominent nucleoli. The characteristic clear cytoplasm is not always well preserved in cytologic preparations.

Granular Cell Tumors

As in the case of clear cell tumors, an eosinophilic granular cell tumor may owe its light microscopic appearance to an increase in any one of several different organelles, including (1) mitochondria, (2) smooth endoplasmic reticulum, (3) dense lysosome-like bodies, (4) secretory granules, and (5) others.[44] Examples of each of these mechanisms can be found in the list of tumors in Table 15-5. For example, true oncocytomas of the

Table 15-5. Eosinophilic Granular
Cell Tumors

Carcinoma
  Kidney
  Liver
  Adrenal cortex
  Apocrine (breast, sweat gland)
  Hürthle cell (thyroid)
  Glassy cell (cervix)
Sarcoma
  Epithelioid
  Alveolar soft parts
Melanoma
Paraganglioma/pheochromocytoma
Oncocytomas
Granular cell tumor
Gemistocytic astrocytoma
Hilar/Leydig cell tumor
Luteoma
Decidua

salivary gland and other organs (which are rarely malignant) show marked mitochondrial hyperplasia demonstrable by phosphotungstic acid hematoxylin stain and by electron microscopy. Steroid hormone-secreting tumors, such as hepatic and adrenal cortical carcinomas and ovarian or testicular hilar or Leydig cell tumors and luteomas, characteristically demonstrate hyperplastic smooth endoplasmic reticulum.

Secretory granules are present in paragangliomas and pheochromocytomas, lysosome-like bodies in granular cell tumors, and rhomboid crystals in alveolar soft part sarcomas. Other tumors in this group may show a combination of these features. In any event, probably the single most common tumor listed in Table 15-5 that manifests initially with metastatic disease is malignant melanoma. Metastatic renal carcinomas are more frequently of the clear cell type, as described earlier, and the other entities listed either rarely manifest initially with metastatic disease or are benign (luteoma, decidual polyp) or so low grade malignant (oncocytomas, granular cell tumor, gemistocytic astrocytoma, hilar/Leydig cell tumors) that they rarely metastasize at all. The immunohistochemical distinction of melanoma from carcinoma has been discussed above.

Cytologically, hepatocellular carcinomas, adrenal cortical carcinomas, oncocytomas, renal cell carcinomas, and alveolar soft part sarcomas share certain features, but they also exhibit distinctive characteristics. The tumor cells of hepatocellular carcinomas resemble hepatocytes and display a trabecular arrangement characterized by three to four cell layers surrounded by spindled endothelial cells. The nuclei are overlapped and crowded, with loss of polarity. They are uniformly enlarged and have prominent nucleoli.[45] The cytologic appearance of adrenal cortical carcinomas ranges from well differentiated to highly anaplastic tumors. They all exhibit mitosis, loss of cohesion, cytologic atypia, hypercellularity, and preservation of cytoplasm. Well differentiated tumors have lipid-laden cells and enlarged hyperchromatic nuclei, and display a sinusoidal architectural pattern in cell block material. Poorly differentiated tumors show pleomorphism and bizarre forms. Renal oncocytomas reveal large uniform cells with abundant granular cytoplasm arranged singly or in loose aggregates. The nuclei are relatively small and lack nucleoli.[46] Alveolar soft part sarcomas show single and clustered atypical cells with ill-defined, abundant, vacuolated cytoplasm and oval nuclei containing prominent nucleoli. The cytoplasm stains negatively with oil red O and positively with PAS-diastase.[47,48]

HISTOCHEMISTRY

General Histochemical Methods

Histochemistry permits identification and histotopographic localization of substances in tissue sections. Its advantage over biochemical analysis of tissue homogenates is that the chemical composition of histologic structures can be studied in parallel with morphologic evaluation. Therefore, histochemical methods can provide parameters that are very valuable for the differential diagnosis of primary or metastatic tumors. Histochemical methods, however, have some inherent limitations. Special tissue processing may be required for optimal results, and, therefore, many techniques cannot be applied to routinely fixed and embedded specimens. Furthermore, many histochemical methods are not specific for one chemically defined substance but stain groups of more or less related molecules. Many of these components occur in more than one type of cell or tissue, and, therefore, very few histochemical methods are specific for a single cell type or tissue component.

Histochemistry includes special histologic staining methods, enzyme histochemical methods, and immunohistochemical methods, which are discussed in a separate section. Special stains often are not, but can be, quite specific, even though the chemical basis of many methods is still unclear. Enzyme histochemical methods generally are specific with regard to the interaction of a given enzyme with a given substrate. Most enzymes, however, are not cell or organ specific, and when organ-specific isoenzymes have been found, methods for their histologic detection have rarely been developed. Often the differences will be quantitative rather than qualitative. For this reason, semiquantitative assessment of patterns of staining of different enzymes in tumors usually gives more information than the reaction of a single enzyme. Consequently, thus far enzyme histochemistry has been of limited significance in the differential diagnosis of tumors. Nonetheless, in selected cases enzyme histochemistry can provide valuable information about the nature and origin of neoplastic tissue.

Existing staining methods and enzyme histochemical techniques are described in Chapter 4. Therefore, only a few general remarks are made here.

Tissue processing frequently affects the chemical composition of cells or intercellular structures. Fortunately, most of the special staining reactions can be successfully performed on routinely processed (i.e., formalin-fixed and paraffin-embedded) tissues. For some staining techniques special fixatives are recommended. In some cases, postfixation of a rehydrated section will be sufficient, but in others special tissue processing is essential. Lipid histochemical studies, for example, are practically impossible on paraffin sections because of the removal of most of the lipids by the organic solvents that are used in the embedding cycle. Formaldehyde-induced fluorescence of catecholamines can be performed on immersion-fixed tissues, but optimal results are obtained by freeze-drying of fresh frozen tissue and special paraffin embedding, because of the high solubility of these substances.[49]

With very few exceptions, routinely processed tissues are not suitable for enzyme histochemical studies. For almost all enzyme histochemical methods, cryostat sectioning of unfixed frozen tissue is the best processing method. The sections can subsequently be fixed according to the requirements for the enzyme of interest. Therefore, whenever differential diagnostic problems are anticipated and unfixed tissue is available, a representative sample should be snap frozen (preferably in isopentane quenched in liquid nitrogen) and stored at −70°C.

Selected special staining methods and enzyme histochemical methods that may be of use in studying metastatic tumors are listed in Tables 15-6 and 15-7, respectively.

Applications

A significant number of substances can be stained by means of a histochemical reaction. In many instances, positive staining indicates the presence of a category of substances rather than one chemically defined molecule (e.g., diastase-resistant PAS positivity indicates the presence of a macromolecule with

Table 15-6. Histochemical Staining Methods in Tumor Diagnosis

	Method	Substance	Diagnostic Application
Fibrillary proteins	Congo red; thioflavine van Gieson	Amyloid	Medullary thyroid carcinoma
		Collagen	Carcinoma, sarcoma, lymphoma
Carbohydrates	PAS, diastase degradable	Glycogen	Rhabdomyosarcoma, Ewing's sarcoma, renal adenocarcinoma
	PAS, diastase resistant	Neutral mucosubstances	Carcinomas, lymphomas of B cell type, hepatoma
	Alcian blue	Acid mucosubstances	Carcinomas, mesothelioma
Lipids	Oil red O	All lipid material	Liposarcoma, adrenal carcinoma, ovarian stromal cell tumors
	Perchloric acid-naphthoquinone	Cholesterol and derivatives	Adrenal carcinoma, ovarian stromal cell tumors
Nucleic acids	Methyl green-pyronine (MGP)	RNA and DNA	Lymphomas of B cell type
Pigments	Schmorl	Melanin	Melanoma
	Fouchet	Bile	Hepatoma
Neuroendocrine granules	Grimelius	Argyrophil granules	Neuroendocrine type carcinoid tumor
	Masson-Fontana	Argentaffin granules	Neuroendocrine type carcinoid tumor
	Formaldehyde-induced fluorescence	Catecholamines	Neuroendocrine type carcinoid tumor

Abbreviation: PAS, periodic acid-Schiff.

Table 15-7. Enzyme Histochemical Methods in Tumor Diagnosis

	Enzyme	Diagnostic Application
Phosphatases	Alkaline	Adenocarcinoma of lung, endometrium, kidney
	Acid	Prostatic carcinoma
		Carcinoid type tumors
		Monocytic leukemia
		Histiocytic sarcoma
		Convoluted lymphoma
	Acid, tartrate resistant	Hairy cell leukemia
	Adenosine triphosphatase (ATPase)	Rhabdomyosarcoma
Oxidases	Dihydroxyphenylalanine (DOPA) oxidase	Melanoma
Dehydrogenases	Nicotinamide adenine dinucleotide tetrazolium reductase (NADH-TR)	Rhabdomyosarcoma
Sulphatases	Arylsulphatase	Digestive tract adenocarcinoma
Esterases	Alpha-naphthyl (nonspecific) esterase	Carcinoid type tumors
		Monocytic leukemia
		Histiocytic sarcoma
Peptidases	Aminopeptidase	Adenocarcinoma of stomach, bile duct, urinary bladder, kidney

free hexose groups but is not specific for any single type of carbohydrate molecule). Therefore, at best, both staining techniques and enzyme histochemical reactions can give an indication of tissue type (e.g., epithelium vs. connective tissue) or differentiation (e.g., squamous vs. adenocarcinoma) rather than pointing toward an organ of origin. In modern practice, this is usually accomplished more easily with immunohistochemical techniques (see below).

Endocrine Tumors

Steroids in endocrine neoplasms, regardless of the tissue of origin, can be stained with general lipid staining methods such as oil red O. In addition, cholesterol and related substances can be stained by the perchloric acid-naphthoquinone reaction.[50] This reaction should be performed on fresh frozen sections and does not distinguish between different types of cholesterol esters.

Neuroendocrine tumors can be diagnosed and, to a certain extent, can also be differentiated according to the cell type of origin with different staining techniques.[51,52] In general, whenever a carcinoid type tumor consisting of solid nests or cords of monomorphic cells is encountered, the silver impregnation techniques serve as a method of screening. Argentaffin methods stain cells that can reduce ammoniacal silver solutions, resulting in a brown silver precipitate.[53] Argyrophil cells have to be treated with a reducing substance before they can react with the silver solution.[54] Absence of silver reactivity, however, does not preclude neuroendocrine origin. Although in the normal situation the neuroendocrine cells can be differentiated into different types according to their staining properties, these characteristics often are not valid for neoplastic cells because these may show abnormal patterns of reaction. For example, normal beta cells in pancreatic islets are not argyrophilic, but neoplastic beta cells often are.[55] In general, carcinoid type tumors in organs derived from the foregut tend to be argyrophilic, whereas mid- and hindgut carcinoids are argentaffin or areac-

tive.[51,52] In addition to the aforementioned silver staining methods, the aldehyde fuchsin, lead hematoxylin, and diazonium methods are useful for the visualization of neuroendocrine cells. Formaldehyde-induced fluorescence is an elegant method for the demonstration of biologic amine content.[49] Originally described for the demonstration of norepinephrine in the adrenal medulla, this method allows detection of many different related amines, which are converted into a fluorophore with a specific fluorescence emission spectrum through formaldehyde condensation.[56] Enzyme histochemistry of neuroendocrine tumors is not highly specific. Nonspecific esterases and acid phosphatases occur frequently but are also found in many other neoplasms.

Parafollicular or C cells of the thyroid also belong to the diffuse neuroendocrine system. The cells in parafollicular or medullary carcinoma of the thyroid frequently are argyrophilic. A rather characteristic feature of these tumors is the presence of amyloid. Unfortunately, this typical feature is often lost in metastases. The amyloid stains with Congo red or thioflavine. The dimethylaminobenzaldehyde method for tryptophan allows differentiation between the so-called amine precursor uptake and decarboxylation-amyloid in neuroendocrine tumors and immunoamyloid, because the former does not contain tryptophane.[57]

Melanocytes stain with many of the above-mentioned methods and are therefore regarded as of neural crest origin. As a result, in addition to the Schmorl method for melanin, argyrophil and argentaffin methods are also helpful for the diagnosis of melanoma, but only if melanin is present. Consequently, the diagnosis of amelanotic melanoma can be very difficult. Fortunately, the enzyme DOPA-oxidase is quite specific for melanocytes and can often be demonstrated even in the absence of melanin. The reaction, which has to be applied to cryostat sections of unfixed tissue, can be of great help in the diagnosis of melanoma. Immunohistochemistry and electron microscopy, however, are far more widely used.

Lymphomas

Histochemical methods are useful for the characterization of neoplastic cells in leukemia and lymphoma. In addition, several of these methods can be helpful in distinguishing lymphoma from nonlymphoid neoplasms.

Special stains of interest are the methyl green-pyronine (MGP) method and the PAS method. Pyronine in the MGP method stains the cytoplasm of immunoglobulin-synthesizing plasmacytoid and mature plasma cells. However, pyronine binds to RNA, and, therefore, all cells actively engaged in protein synthesis will be stained. Nevertheless, pyroninophilic cytoplasm of poorly differentiated diffusely growing cells in a tumor mass suggests plasmacytoid differentiation and therefore is supportive evidence for a lymphoma of the B cell type. PAS staining provides comparable information. Stored immunoglobulins in lymphoma cells can be found as globular or diffuse cytoplasmic PAS-positive diastase-resistant staining. This pattern of staining, therefore, also supports the diagnosis of lymphoma of the B cell type. Carcinoma cells, however, can also be PAS positive.

Several enzyme histochemical methods are helpful in the diagnosis of lymphoma and for further subtyping of lymphomas. Enzyme histochemical evaluation of lymphomas can be done on cryostat sections, but better results are obtained on imprint cytologic preparations of fresh specimens. The alpha-naphthyl (nonspecific) esterase method[58] shows diffuse cytoplasmic staining in monocytic and histiocytic cells but staining of one or more spot-like granules in the cytoplasm of T lymphocytes.[59] Diffuse cytoplasmic staining of this enzyme therefore will be found in monocytic leukemia, in true histiocytic lymphoma or sarcoma, and in Langerhans cell histiocytosis or malignant histiocytosis.

Acid phosphatase shows a pattern of staining similar to that of nonspecific esterase. Tartrate-resistant acid phosphatase positivity is highly suggestive of hairy cell leukemia.[60]

Carcinomas

In the differential diagnosis of metastatic carcinoma, histochemistry can contribute first to the differential diagnosis between carcinoma and other neoplasms, especially sarcoma, and second to the determination of the type of differentiation within a carcinoma and, if possible, the origin of the neoplasm. Unfortunately, with regard to the latter, the results are usually rather poor.

In distinguishing between anaplastic carcinoma and sarcoma or lymphoma, the arrangement of the tumor cells can be of help. With few exceptions, carcinoma cells tend to grow in solid nests and cords surrounded by connective tissue stroma, whereas sarcomas and lymphomas tend to grow diffusely. Reticulin and van Gieson stains will reveal the pattern of reticulin and collagen fibers and thereby accentuate the growth pattern of the neoplastic cells.

As mentioned earlier, MGP staining can be useful in the differentiation of undifferentiated large cell carcinoma from immunoblastic sarcoma of the B cell type, with the restriction that all cells actively engaged in protein synthesis will be pyroninophilic. For the differentiation of carcinoma from lesions derived from histiocytes, such as histiocytic sarcoma or Langerhans cell histiocytosis, enzyme histochemical staining for alpha-naphthyl (nonspecific) esterase and acid phosphatase can be helpful. These enzymes occur diffusely in the cytoplasm of cells of monocytic and histiocytic origin.

The production of mucopolysaccharides in an anaplastic carcinoma is an argument in favor of adenocarcinoma. In general, diastase-resistant PAS staining indicates the presence of neutral mucosubstances but—as in lymphomas—also of glycoproteins, whereas alcian blue staining indicates the presence of acid mucosubstances. More extensive histochemical differentiation of mucosubstances can be obtained by applying blocking procedures and enzyme digestion before staining. These methods, however, are of little help in the classification of neoplasms. An exception is the hyaluronidase-labile alcian blue staining of hyaluronic acid in mesothelioma. Although not entirely specific (chondroitin sulfate in cartilage is also degradable by hyaluronidase), this reaction can be useful for the diagnosis of mesothelioma.[61]

In very few cases, general histochemical methods will determine the final classification of carcinoma. Whenever hepatocellular carcinoma is suspected, the presence of diastase-resistant, PAS-positive hyaline intracytoplasmic globules is useful supportive evidence for this diagnosis.[62] In addition, in these tumors bile pigments can be stained with standard histochemical methods.

In some cases, enzyme histochemistry can help in establishing the origin of a metastatic carcinoma. Unfortunately, no enzymes have so far been found that are completely specific for a single cell or tissue type. This implies that, in addition to qualitative differences in enzyme content, quantitative differences have to be taken into account. Furthermore, the absence or presence of a given enzyme will usually be compatible with several different tissues of origin, and, therefore, staining for multiple enzymes will result in more specific information.

Acid phosphatase can be found in a wide variety of tumors. Extremely high activity of this enzyme in an adenocarcinoma, however, is almost diagnostic of prostatic origin. The presence of alkaline phosphatase in adenocarcinoma strongly favors pulmonary, endometrial, ovarian, or renal origin and virtually excludes the intestinal tract as the primary site. Determination of the activity of this enzyme in an ovarian neoplasm can therefore be helpful in distinguishing between a primary carcinoma of the ovary or metastatic endometrial carcinoma on the one hand and metastasis of breast or intestinal adenocarcinoma on the other.[63] Conversely, arylsulfatase activity in an adenocarcinoma strongly favors an intestinal origin.[64] Aminopeptidase is mostly found in adenocarcinoma of the stomach, bile ducts, urinary bladder, or kidney. Many other enzymes have been studied, but the lack of specificity and the enormous variability limit the diagnostic significance of these methods.

Mesenchymal Tumors

Special stains and histochemical methods have few useful applications in this area. Primary and metastatic localizations of soft tissue sarcomas not infrequently cause differential diagnostic problems, but in most cases, histochemical methods will be of little help. The same holds true for metastatic localizations of undifferentiated round cell neoplasms of bone (Ewing's sarcoma and malignant lymphoma), although the presence of glycogen in the former may be helpful. Nonetheless, in some differential diagnostic problems special stains can provide useful information and therefore deserve brief discussion.

In a localization of undifferentiated pleomorphic sarcoma, a differentiation will have to be made among malignant peripheral nerve sheath tumor, rhabdomyosarcoma, liposarcoma, and malignant fibrous histiocytoma. The presence of alpha-naphthyl esterase activity suggests histiocytic origin. Demonstration of intracytoplasmic lipid droplets with an oil red O stain will support the diagnosis of liposarcoma. One should, however, realize that reactive phagocytic cells, especially in tumors with necrosis, also contain lipid material. The rare cross-striated contractile elements in a rhabdomyosarcoma can be stained with the phosphotungstic acid hematoxylin method, as can the numerous mitochondria in oncocytes. In addition, quite often PAS-positive diastase-degradable glycogen deposits can be found in rhabdomyosarcoma cells. Enzyme histochemical techniques applied to fresh cryostat sections of tumor tissue can provide evidence of muscular origin in undifferentiated sarcomas. Although not entirely specific for muscular tissue, the presence of nicotinamide adenine dinucleotide tetrazolium reductase and adenosine triphosphatase strongly supports a diagnosis of rhabdomyosarcoma.[65] Immunohistochemical demonstration of myoglobin is, however, easier and more specific.

It should be stressed that among soft tissue tumors PAS staining is by no means unique for rhabdomyosarcoma. In alveolar soft part sarcoma the tumor cells usually show granular diastase-resistant PAS staining, whereas in synoviosarcoma the muco-substances in the slit-like spaces in the tumor are also PAS positive. For the differential diagnosis of these tumors, therefore, the PAS reaction is of little value. However, this method can be essential for the diagnosis of Ewing's sarcoma. In undifferentiated round cell neoplasms of bone, Ewing's sarcoma will have to be differentiated from malignant lymphoma and metastatic neuroblastoma. Of these, only Ewing's sarcoma always contains numerous PAS-stainable glycogen granules. In addition, both malignant lymphoma and neuroblastoma contain a fibrillar stroma, stainable with routine reticulin methods, which is not found in Ewing's sarcoma.

IMMUNOHISTOCHEMISTRY

Diagnostic pathology of neoplastic disease has benefitted tremendously from the development of immunohistochemical techniques and the availability of a wide range of specific (polyclonal and monoclonal) antibodies against diagnostically useful antigens. In oncologic research, considerable emphasis has been placed on the development of tumor-specific or tumor type-specific monoclonal antibodies. Tumor-specific antigens have not been detected, and even purportedly tumor type- or cell type-specific monoclonal antibodies frequently have limited specificity. Nonetheless, the hybridoma methodology for the development of monoclonal antibodies has resulted in a multitude of diagnostically useful reagents.[66]

Methodologic Considerations

The immunohistochemical methods and the principles of their application in surgical pathology are extensively reviewed in Chapter 5. It is of importance, however, to re-emphasize some essential considerations here because the reliability of diagnostic immunohistochemistry rests entirely on the quality of the applied immunohistochemical techniques and on the validity of the applied working hypotheses. In using immunoreactivity patterns for various antigens as a diagnostic tool, some general rules must be strenuously applied. These can be summarized in the following questions.

1. *Were the applied techniques valid?* In assessing the validity of the applied techniques, proper attention should be paid to tissue processing procedures and antibody specificity. Proper tissue processing is of paramount importance for reliable immunohistochemistry. In principle, for each antigen an appropriate tissue processing protocol has to be developed. Fortunately, however, for many antigens routine processing (including formalin fixation and paraffin embedding), if necessary in combination with enzyme pretreatment, is compatible with reliable immunohistochemistry. For each newly acquired antibody (especially for monoclonal antibodies) the compatibility with the local tissue processing conditions has to be ascertained.

   Antibody specificity is another crucial element in reliable immunohistochemistry. In most diagnostic histology laboratories, facilities for extensive immunochemical specificity testing are not available, making appropriate tissue controls absolutely essential, as outlined below.

2. *Were the controls adequate?* With all immunostaining procedures positive and negative controls should be utilized with material that has been processed similarly to the case material. Negative controls should include checks for nonspecific binding of the detection system (e.g., conjugates, peroxidase-antiperoxidase, avidin-biotin-peroxidas complex) as well as the primary antibody (nonimmune serum or absorbed antiserum).[67] Omission of controls may lead to serious misinterpretation of case material.

3. *Is the distribution of the antigen known in sufficient detail?* This aspect is of particular importance when monoclonal antibodies are used. The specificity of many monoclonal antibodies is largely defined on the basis of tissue reactivity tests, and therefore these can almost never be too exhaustive. This is demonstrated by the Leu-7 monoclonal antibody, which was originally claimed to react only with natural killer cells, but was subsequently found to react also with endocrine cells.[68] Also illustrating the importance of extensive testing is the CAM (cell adhesion molecule) 5.2 monoclonal anticytokeratin antibody, which occasionally also reacts with an epitope occurring in smooth muscle cells.[69] Similarly, some antigens were originally claimed to be specific for one organ or cell type but subsequently proved to be more widely distributed. Examples are neuron-specific enolase (NSE), which has been demonstrated in a variety of non-neural and non-neuroendocrine tissues,[70] and prostatic acid phosphatase, which occurs not only in the prostate but also in some normal and neoplastic endocrine cells.[71]

4. *Are markers of differentiation of normal cells also valid as markers of differentiation of neoplastic cells?* Marker-based classification relies on the assumption that neoplastic cells usually and perhaps always differentiate along the same lines as their normal counterparts and that markers of differentiation of normal cells will retain their differentiational specificity in neoplastic cells. Unfortunately, tumors tend to break rules. Many case reports illustrate the potential for aberrant differentiational behavior of neoplastic cells and call for cautious interpretation of marker patterns in the classification of tumors. Within this context, histogenetic concepts of tumor development have proved rather limited. The number of neoplasms of which the histogenesis has been conclusively established is restricted. Most histogenetic concepts have been inferred from circumstantial evidence.

Events such as the occurrence of endocrine cells in a considerable number of adenocarcinomas of various organs,[71] of vimentin immunoreactivity in certain carcinoma cells,[72] of keratin immunoreactivity in some smooth muscle tumors,[69] and of chorionic gonadotropin in a variety of carcinomas[73] are illustrations of the important basic notion that patterns of differentiation dominate the morphology and immunophenotype of neoplasms, rather than the ontogenetic derivation of the tissue in which the neoplasm developed.

Immunocytochemistry is commonly used and plays a significant role in the evaluation of cytologic samples.[74,75] For immunocytochemical studies, smears, cytospins, and 4 μm deparaffinized cell block sections may be used. Optimal fixatives for immunostaining of smears are alcohol and cold acetone.[76,77] Air-dried smears work best when they are postfixed in acetone.[78] For retrospective immunocytochemical stains, destained Papanicolaou smears are superior to air-dried, Diff-Quik-stained smears. It is important to emphasize that the type of fixation employed must be considered when evaluating immunocytochemical results. Variability of results secondary to fixation has been seen in a number of studies.[78,79] For instance, alcohol and paraformaldehyde fixatives aid the expression of intermediate filaments.[80] Variability in immunocytochemistry results is attributed to the unevenness of smears and superimposition of cells. Background staining in cytologic preparation is also a major problem and is due to the presence of protein-rich fluid and red blood cells.[81] When dealing with cytologic specimens, the antibody concentration and incubation time may need to be adjusted from what is generally used for formalin-fixed, paraffin-embedded tissue sections. Titering procedures for the primary antibodies using positive cytologic control specimens would allow for the development of optimal procedures.[78]

Applications

Diagnostic immunohistochemistry of malignant neoplasms calls for a systematic approach. It is absolutely essential to perform detailed morphologic studies before immunohistochemistry is applied. The morphologic analysis should lead to an exact identification of the diagnostic problem, preferentially phrased as a question to which marker immunohistochemistry

might provide an answer. The markers should be carefully chosen to allow an answer to the question, and the potential results of the marker studies should actually be anticipated in the decision as to which markers to choose. In reading the immunostained slides, the methodologic considerations should be taken into account before a final conclusion can be drawn.

One of the most difficult problems in surgical pathology is that of an undifferentiated metastatic tumor with an unknown primary. Careful and stepwise application of marker immunohistochemistry according to the following questions can be of tremendous help in this situation. The first question is whether or not the tumor expresses markers of carcinoma. If so, the tumor can either be a carcinoma or a biphasic neoplasm (e.g., epithelioid sarcoma, mesothelioma, or synovial sarcoma). If the lesion is a carcinoma, subsequently it must be decided which type of carcinoma it is and where the primary tumor might be located. If it is a biphasic neoplasm, further classification will have to be done. If the tumor does not express markers of carcinoma the second question will be whether the lesion might be a lymphoma, a melanoma, or a sarcoma. If it is a lymphoma, further morphologic and immunophenotypic classification is needed. If it is a sarcoma, the tumor will also have to be further classified. Markers for these different groups are listed in Table 15-8. Obviously, this approach is rather general. For specific situations more detailed or better tailored approaches might be envisaged.

Immunohistochemical Markers of Carcinoma

One of the most important developments with regard to the immunohistochemical classification of poorly differentiated or undifferentiated neoplasms has been the recognition of the tissue-specific expression of intermediate filaments. These filaments, which together with microfilaments, thick filaments, and microtubules constitute the cytoskeleton, consist of five different classes of proteins.[82] Cytokeratins occur almost exclusively in epithelial cells, vimentin predominantly in mesenchymal cells (but also under certain conditions in some epithelial cells), desmin and actin in muscle cells, neurofilament proteins in nerve cells, and glial fibrillary acidic protein in glial cells. Numerous studies have documented that this tissue-specific distribution is largely retained under neoplastic conditions.[82,83] Consequently, the typing of tumors by intermediate filament immunohistochemistry has become an important element in diagnostic pathology. More recently, the specific types of cytokeratins[84–86] have also been used to distinguish between carcinomas arising in different primary sites.[26,27,87]

For the recognition of the carcinomatous nature of a poorly differentiated metastatic lesion, immunohistochemical staining for cytokeratins is usually the first step. A variety of polyclonal or monoclonal antibodies are available that recognize a broad range of cytokeratins in routinely fixed and paraffin-embedded tissue, usually after trypsin digestion. Two other markers may be used to identify carcinomas, either singly or in combination with cytokeratins. These are epithelial membrane antigen (EMA) and desmosomal plaque protein. EMA was isolated from milk fat globule membranes and occurs almost exclusively in epithelial cells.[88,89] Desmosomal plaque protein is a major constituent of the cytoplasmic plaque of desmosomes and

Table 15-8. Markers for Classification of Undifferentiated Neoplasms

Diagnosis	Subtype	Initial Marker(s)	Additional Marker(s)
Carcinoma	Urothelial cell carcinoma	Cytokeratin, EMA, desmoplakin	Cytokeratin 7, vimentin
	Squamous cell carcinoma		Cytokeratin 10, vimentin
	Adenocarcinoma		Cytokeratins 8, 18, 19, vimentin
Biphasic	Synovial sarcoma	Cytokeratin, EMA, desmoplakin, vimentin	
	Epithelioid sarcoma	Cytokeratin, EMA, desmoplakin, vimentin	
	Mesothelioma	Cytokeratin, EMA, desmoplakin, vimentin	Cytokeratin 18
Lymphoma	B cell type	Leukocyte common antigen (CD45)	B cell antigens (CD19, CD20)
	T cell type	Immunoglobulins	T cell antigens (CD3, CD45RO)
	Histiocytic type	Lysozyme, alpha-1-AT, alpha-1-ACT, CD68	Ki-1 antigen (CD30)
Melanoma		S-100, NKI/C3	
Sarcoma	Basal lamina reactive	Vimentin	
	Myosarcoma	Laminin, type IV collagen	Desmin, actin, myoglobin
	Angiosarcoma		Factor VIII-related antigen,
	Liposarcoma		CD31, Ulex europaeus lectin
	Basal lamina nonreactive fibrosarcoma		
	Malignant fibrous histiocytoma		

Abbreviations: EMA, epithelial membrane antigen; alpha-1-AT, alpha-1 antitrypsin; alpha-1-ACT, alpha-1-antichymotrypsin; NK, natural killer.

consequently occurs exclusively in cells with desmosomes.[90] One of these markers may be sufficient to identify the epithelial nature of a poorly differentiated carcinoma. A negative immunostain, however, does not entirely exclude the possibility of a carcinoma, and therefore the use of more than one marker is recommended.

Among lesions positive for cytokeratin, EMA, and desmosomal plaque protein, synovial sarcoma, mesothelioma and epithelioid sarcoma form a special category. These neoplasms have characteristics of carcinoma as well as of sarcoma. Consequently, in addition to epithelial markers, sarcoma-associated vimentin immunoreactivity can also be found.[91] Coexpression of cytokeratin and vimentin, however, is not restricted to these tumors but has also been reported in (among others) renal adenocarcinomas, thyroid carcinomas, endometrial and ovarian carcinomas, mixed tumors of the salivary glands, and nephroblastomas.[91] Therefore, these tumors cannot be diagnosed on the basis of their pattern of expression of intermediate filaments alone. The diagnosis of a classic biphasic synovial sarcoma will usually be rather simple and will rarely require application of special techniques. If the tumor is monophasic, however, the diagnosis may require conventional histochemistry (alcian blue with hyaluronidase digestion) as well as immunohistochemistry and electron microscopy. The same holds true for epithelioid sarcoma, the diagnosis of which can be extremely difficult. For the tubular component of mesothelioma, the distinction from adenocarcinoma can often be made confidently by virtue of the absence of carcinoembryonic antigen (CEA) immunoreactivity in mesothelioma.[76,92] If the lesion is largely fibroblastic, the presence of cytokeratin immunoreactivity may be diagnostic. An additional parameter in the diagnosis of these neoplasms may be the pattern of immunoreactivity for the basal lamina proteins type IV collagen and laminin. These will not be expressed in a fibrosarcoma but will occur around individual spindle cells in mesothelioma or synovial sarcoma, around tubular configurations in mesothelioma or synovial sarcoma, and around cell nests in epithelioid sarcoma.[93]

If mesothelioma, synovial sarcoma, and epithelioid sarcoma can be excluded, a cytokeratin-positive lesion is most likely to be a carcinoma. The question then arises of which type of carcinoma is at hand. Occasionally, this will appear to be a question of academic interest, because further typing of the tumor will have no therapeutic implications. As some types of carcinoma can be rather successfully treated, however, further tumor typing may be required. The first step is to identify the carcinoma as of either squamous, transitional, or glandular (adenocarcinoma) differentiation. Here again intermediate filament typing may be extremely useful. Cytokeratin proteins comprise a family of more than 19 different polypeptides, which can be separated by two-dimensional gel electrophoresis on the basis of differences in charge and molecular weight. In the cytokeratin catalogue, cytokeratin 1 has a high isoelectric point and a high molecular weight, and cytokeratin 19 has a low isoelectric point and a low molecular weight. The important characteristic of cytokeratin peptides is that different epithelia exhibit expression of different combinations of cytokeratins.[84–86,94] Squamous epithelia contain the more basic and high molecular weight cytokeratins 1 to 6 as well as cytokeratins 9 to 14. Of these, cytokeratin 10 occurs only in keratinizing epithelia.[95] By contrast, cytokeratins 4 and 13 occur only in nonkeratinizing epithelia. Cytokeratins 8, 18, and 19 occur in "simple" epithelia, whereas cytokeratin 7 occurs exclusively in transitional epithelium. Monoclonal antibodies have been prepared that are reactive with a single or selected group of specific cytokeratins. Initially, with very few exceptions, these antibodies only reacted with the undenatured form of the polypeptide and therefore could not be applied to paraffin sections. More recently, versions applicable to archival tissues have become available, and these antibodies are now a powerful tool in the study of differentiation in neoplasma. Immunoreactivity for cytokeratin 10 only occurs in keratinizing squamous carcinomas. Immunoreactivity for cytokeratins 8, 18, and 19 occurs in many adenocarcinomas (excluding breast cancers), mesotheliomas, some transitional cell carcinomas, and neuroendocrine neoplasms. Immunoreactivity for cytokeratin 7 occurs in breast carcinomas and in many urogenital cancers.[26,27,84,87,96–98]

If, on the basis of the pattern of cytokeratin expression, a cancer has been tentatively identified as an adenocarcinoma, further analysis may be directed toward detection of the site of origin of the primary tumor. Specific markers exist for various organs (Table 15-9). Prostate-specific acid phosphatase and prostate-specific antigen (PSA) occur almost exclusively in prostate cancer,[99] although the former can also be detected in some endocrine tumors of the pancreas.[100] Estrogen receptor protein is a fairly reliable marker for breast carcinoma, although endometrial and ovarian adenocarcinomas, as well as occasional others, may also express this antigen, and poorly differentiated breast cancers are usually negative.[101] Thyroglobulin is a highly reliable marker of follicular and papillary thyroid carcinoma but unfortunately tends to be poorly expressed in anaplastic thyroid carcinoma.[102] CEA is still widely in use as a marker for adenocarcinomas, but it has a very wide distribution (which may in part be related to the tendency of anti-CEA antibodies to react also with many cross-reacting antigens) and also occurs in some squamous cell carcinomas and some neuroendocrine tumors.[103] Alpha-fetoprotein is associated with hepatocellular carcinomas but also occurs in germ cell tumors with yolk sac differentiation. Very few antigens, therefore, are absolutely specific for one organ site or tumor type.

Many different monoclonal antibodies have been reported with limited reactivity, allowing their use for tentative identification of the primary site of a metastatic carcinoma. The CA-125 antigen is suggestive but hardly specific for serous cystade-

nocarcinomas of the ovary.[104] Various monoclonal antibodies have been reported that react almost exclusively with renal cell adenocarcinoma.[105,106] Relatively specific monoclonal antibodies are also available for small cell carcinoma of the lung.[107] In some instances, monoclonal antibodies are useful because of predictable negativity in certain tumor types, for example CEA in mesothelioma[76] or HAM56 in colorectal carcinoma.[25] With hindsight, however, the optimistic expectations that hybridoma methodology would produce monoclonal antibodies to hitherto unknown tissue or cell type-specific antigens have not yet materialized.

A solid, nodular, or trabecular growth pattern in a carcinoma always raises the possibility of neuroendocrine differentiation. For neuroendocrine differentiation, the Grimelius argyrophil reaction is still a convenient screening procedure. A fairly wide variety of more or less specific immunohistochemical markers for endocrine differentiation, including enzymes, storage granule-related components, and peptides or amines, has been reported.

Of the enzymes investigated only the gamma-homodimeric form of the glycolytic enzyme enolase (NSE) has proved suitable as a universal marker for neuroendocrine differentiation. The enzyme occurs in neurons and in virtually all neuroendocrine cells and most of their neoplasms in the pancreas, gut, lung, and skin.[108] However, several studies have contested the specificity of NSE for neuroendocrine cells, showing that lymphocytes, some epithelial cells, smooth muscle cells, and a variety of neoplasms can also show NSE reactivity.[70] Nevertheless, NSE remains a useful marker, mostly because lack of NSE immunoreactivity makes neuroendocrine differentiation highly unlikely. Because its expression is not related to dense core granules, it is particularly useful in sparsely granulated tumors, such as small cell lung cancer. Final proof for the neuroendocrine nature of a neoplasm, however, requires the presence of additional markers, such as chromogranin, synaptophysin, or neurohormonal peptides.

Chromogranins are glycoproteins that occur in the dense core granules of chromaffin and other neuroendocrine cells. Three different chromogranins have been recognized: chromogranins A, B, and C (also called secretogranin II).[109,110] None of these shows a universal distribution, indicating that to avoid false negative results a search for chromogranin immunoreactivity should include antibodies against all three proteins. It should also be noted that in sparsely granulated tumors such as small cell lung carcinoma, chromogranin may not be detected at all. The main advantage of chromogranins as neuroendocrine markers lies in the fact that so far they have demonstrated absolute specificity for neuroendocrine cells. The same holds true for synaptophysin, a protein component of presynaptic vesicles.[111]

Endocrine tumors can be functionally classified according to the pattern of amine or peptide hormone production. An enormous variety of neurohormonal peptides has been discovered in recent years. Identification of the individual peptides requires a large collection of specific antibodies. For purely diagnostic purposes this will rarely be necessary. Although neuroendocrine tumors frequently produce the neurohormonal peptides that normally occur in the tissue of origin, ectopic hormones are often produced, thus limiting the predictability of the site of

Table 15-9. Markers for Subclassification of Carcinoma

Tumor	Markers
Follicular cell thyroid carcinoma	Thyroglobulin
Medullary thyroid carcinoma	Calcitonin
Prostatic adenocarcinoma	Prostatic acid phosphatase, prostate-specific antigen
Hepatocellular carcinoma	Alpha-fetoprotein
Embryonal carcinomas	
With yolk sac differentiation	Alpha-fetoprotein
With trophoblastic differentiation	Chorionic gonadotropin
Breast carcinoma	Estrogen receptor protein, alpha-lactalbumin, GCDFP-15
Ovarian serous carcinoma	CA-125
Gastrointestinal carcinomas (and others)	Carcinoembryonic antigen (CEA)
Neuroendocrine carcinomas	Neuron-specific enolase, chromogranins, synaptophysin, neurofilament, peptide hormones

the primary tumor on the basis of the pattern of hormone production. Furthermore, it is important to realize that a significant proportion of non-neuroendocrine carcinomas contains a subpopulation of tumor cells with neuroendocrine differentiation, including the production of peptide hormones. Therefore, the occurrence of neuroendocrine cells in a carcinoma does not provide sufficient evidence to classify the neoplasm as neuroendocrine. In an appropriate clinical and hematoxylin and eosin setting, however, a neuroendocrine classification is possible and will have important implications for specific chemotherapy.

Noncarcinomatous Tumors

If the tumor does not express markers of carcinoma, the question then arises of whether it is a lymphoma, a melanoma, or a sarcoma. For this categorization, vimentin has been advocated as a characteristic intermediate filament protein.[91,112] Indeed, these tumors usually show vimentin immunoreactivity. However, as has been indicated previously, vimentin expression can also be found in different types of carcinoma under various conditions. Furthermore, because vimentin expression does not differentiate between these different tumor types, vimentin is a marker with very limited potential. It can, however, serve as a marker of tissue immunoreactivity in a tumor in which all other immunostains are negative, since at least blood vessels and stromal cells should stain positively for vimentin in every specimen.[113]

Most lymphomas have fairly characteristic morphology, which permits their distinction from melanoma or soft tissue sarcoma fairly easily. In poorly differentiated neoplasms, however, this differential diagnosis can occasionally be extremely difficult. A good universal marker for normal and neoplastic lymphoid cells is LCA. Monoclonal antibodies are available against LCA that identify this antigen in routinely processed paraffin sections of almost all lymphomas.[114] Once a lesion has been identified as a lymphoma, further classification will be necessary. The immunophenotyping of lymphoma is extensively discussed in Chapter 20.

Melanomas can be extremely difficult to diagnose, especially when they are amelanotic, because their morphology may vary from rather carcinoma-like to purely sarcomatoid. S-100 protein has been widely advocated for the diagnosis of melanoma. This protein was initially isolated from glial and ependymal cells in the central nervous system but was subsequently also found in cells of the peripheral nervous system as well as in fat cells, chondrocytes, and melanocytes. Melanomas are almost always S-100 protein positive, but unfortunately this marker lacks sufficient specificity.[115,116] Its main use lies in the finding that when S-100 protein immunoreactivity is lacking, the lesion is unlikely to be a melanoma. For positive identification of melanoma a number of monoclonal antibodies have been developed. The most widely used and most specific at present (but lacking some of the sensitivity of S-100 protein) is HMB 45.[117]

The diagnosis of sarcoma is often reached by exclusion: if no morphologic or immunohistochemical characteristics of carcinoma, lymphoma, or melanoma are found, the lesion must be a sarcoma. This reasoning can be fortified significantly if the sar-

coma can be further classified. Since sarcomas infrequently present with metastatic disease from an occult primary site, their classification with and without immunohistochemical help is more appropriately discussed in detail in Chapter 18.

Finally, different markers also exist for neurogenic differentiation. The S-100 protein has already been discussed in connection with melanoma. It is also expressed in malignant peripheral nerve sheath tumors,[115,116] as is myelin basic protein, a component of the myelin sheath of Schwann cells.[118]

DIAGNOSTIC ELECTRON MICROSCOPY

The transmission electron microscope (TEM) is an established tool of the surgical pathologist.[119,120] Many pathology departments in teaching hospitals and in larger community hospitals have electron microscopes at their disposal for diagnostic purposes. In the surgical pathology service of The George Washington University Medical Center, approximately 2 percent of all nonrenal specimens are processed for TEM. In roughly one-third of these cases, the information revealed by the electron microscope proves necessary for arriving at a diagnosis and, thus, the patient is billed for the services. This often includes the evaluation of metastatic tumors with an unknown primary site. Immunohistochemistry is beginning to reduce the need for electron microscopic studies in this area, but we are still developing an understanding of its strengths and weaknesses. Meanwhile, TEM and immunohistochemistry are complementary and serve as mutual quality controls.[17,121,122] Undoubtedly, there will always be situations in which the electron microscope (e.g., surface specializations, organelle structure) and immunohistochemistry (e.g., detection of low molecular weight cytokeratin and surface antigens, identification of secretions and types of intermediate filaments) provides unique information.

Processing of Tissue for Ultrastructural Studies

Three factors are critical for the optimal ultrastructural study of tissue: speed, size, and sampling. Although neutral buffered glutaraldehyde is the preferred fixative, excellent results can be attained on tissue fixed with buffered formalin. Often more important than the fixative itself is the elapsed time between the dissociation of the tissue from its oxygen supply and when it finally is placed in the fixative. Degeneration begins the moment the blood supply is interrupted and is exaggerated by the degeneration and necrosis that often accompanies tumor growth. Prolonged surgical procedures, such as a Whipple's procedure, hysterectomy for uterine tumor, or cystectomy, regularly yield poorly preserved tissue. Ideally, tissue should be placed in glutaraldehyde in the frozen section room. However, the moment it is believed that ultrastructural evaluation may be needed on tissue already fixed in formalin, a thin piece of the tissue can be shaved off the well fixed exposed surface with a sharp scalpel or razor blade and transferred directly into glutaraldehyde for further fixation. For diagnostic purposes, the temperature of fixation is not critical; the glutaraldehyde should be stored in the refrigerator at 4°C for longevity (10 ml in scintillation vials), removed as needed (can come to room temperature while waiting), and returned to the refrigerator until processing. Size of the sample goes hand in hand with fixation speed, since the smaller the piece of tissue, the more rapidly it is thoroughly fixed. The electron microscopist speaks of 1 mm cubes or of no cell being more than 0.5 mm from a surface. Dicing the tissue with a sharp scalpel blade while it is submerged in a drop of fixative on, for example, a sheet of dental wax, is the optimal method. A simpler technique is to take a thin shaving of tissue from the cut surface of the fresh specimen and transfer it immediately to glutaraldehyde. This guarantees minimal handling and eliminates possible drying artifact. Sampling is especially important for the electron microscopist, considering the number of cells that can be reasonably examined. One should always sample areas of differing color and texture so as not to submit only necrotic or normal tissue, or only one facet of a complex tumor.

The most one can say about retrieving tissue from a paraffin block is that its efficacy is unpredictable. Because the patient is the one who may suffer from our lack of foresight, in our laboratory tissue is routinely retrieved from paraffin for ultrastructural studies. It is unclear exactly what determines potential success. Included are the nature of the tissue; its initial fixation, including fixative and speed; the actually processing into paraffin (heating, solvents, time scheme); how long it was in paraffin; and how it was handled after embedding, for example, during microtomy (freezing).[123] Paraffin embedding can be expected to disrupt and distort membranes, along with intercellular junctions and microvilli, as well as specific vacuoles such as mucin. On the positive side, intermediate filaments, including cytokeratin (tonofilaments/tonofibrils), and dense core granules are usually preserved. The paraffin block is matched with the last section cut for light microscopy, and the selected tissue is chipped out with a sharp razor blade or scalpel, diced into pieces of less than 1 mm,[3] and transferred to a scintillation vial containing 100 percent xylene. After rotating overnight at room temperature, the tissue is hydrated through alcohol containing increasing amounts of water, fixed for a few hours in glutaraldehyde, postfixed in osmium tetroxide, and processed into plastic in a routine fashion.

The surgical pathologists in our institution are taught to consider fixing portions of every specimen routinely for potential ultrastructural studies, in effect asking themselves, "Why should a sample of this specimen not be fixed in glutaraldehyde?" This applies equally to very small samples, such as transbronchial, mediastinal, and liver biopsies, because as long as the tissue can be seen by the electron microscopy technician, it can be processed and be quite adequate for TEM. Nothing is sacrificed by fixing a small fragment of tissue in glutaraldehyde, even if, in the rare case, lesional tissue is present only in the sample submitted for TEM. One possibility is to hold the piece of tissue set aside for TEM in buffered formalin until the hematoxylin and eosin-stained sections are reviewed. However, this could waste valuable time, especially when the tissue may be further held until special stains are reviewed. The light microscopic (LM) detail obtained in sections from plastic-embedded tissue is excellent; in fact, in some tissues (bone marrow, lymph node), 1 mm semithin sections are considered preferable because of the superior nuclear and cytoplasmic detail. The limitation of plastic-embedded tissue is in the area of special stains, especially using immunohistochemistry, but also routine cytochemistry. Our laboratory uses a combination of methylene blue and basic fuchsin-azure II for staining plastic sections. It stains collagen, glycogen, and mucin red (usually distinguished by location and pattern), and the nucleus and cytoplasm different shades and intensities of blue.

Electron microscopy is most efficiently and effectively employed when it is closely coordinated with LM, which, in turn, relies on clinical information. The electron microscopist may wait for the LM results before processing the tissue into plastic and, especially, before cutting thin sections. To conserve time, tissue is often processed into plastic before LM studies are complete.

The limitations of the electron microscope must be appreciated if it is to be optimally employed. First and foremost, the TEM is not used to distinguish benign from malignant, since that distinction is based on light microscopic criteria. Because of the nature of sampling in TEM, not finding a feature is not necessarily diagnostic. For example, finding intercellular junctions between otherwise undifferentiated cells excludes lymphopoietic cells. By contrast, absence of junctions suggests a lymphoma, but other features must also be consistent, such as the paucity of organelles, prominent ribosomes, and nuclear blebs.

The degree of differentiation of tumor cells is clearly appreciated at the ultrastructural level, and the findings are highly suggestive of the clinical behavior. Ultrastructural and immunohistochemical criteria are constantly being sought that predict behavior and response to therapy.

The determination of the type of epithelial tumor at the LM level depends on identifying features of the presumed tissue of origin, such as glandular organization and secretions for adenocarcinomas, or intercellular bridges and keratinization for squamous cell carcinomas. The prominence of these features forms a spectrum that extends from well to poorly differentiated. This spectrum, discerned at the LM level, is graphically demonstrated at the ultrastructural level; the electron microscope is capable of extending the spectrum to levels inaccessible to the LM. By LM, the tumor is noted to be undifferentiated, whereas at the TEM level, the spectrum is continued until eventually the tumor is also undifferentiated at the ultrastructural level. TEM also regularly reveals complexities not otherwise appreciated by LM, such as multidirectional differentiation (e.g., varying combinations of glandular, squamous, and neuroendocrine differentiation in a single tumor). The clinical significance of these observations is being evaluated.[124]

The use of TEM in evaluating tissue obtained by fine needle aspiration has great promise. Several studies have demonstrated the value of TEM in confirming or establishing a definite diagnosis.[75,125–127] When indicated by the clinical history or the preliminary assessment of a fine needle aspirate, it is useful to save a portion of the sample for possible electron microscopic evaluation. The aspirated material should be fixed in glutaraldehyde and the cell block embedded in epoxy resin.

TEM has also been employed with success in evaluating cells in effusions.[128,129] It has proved capable of distinguishing carcinomas from lymphomas, identifying reactive mesothelial cells, and assisting in ascertaining the origin of metastatic cells.

Applications

Small Round Cell Tumors

The small round or blue cell tumors of childhood include predominantly Ewing's sarcoma, neuroblastoma, rhabdomyosarcoma, and lymphoma.[130–136] Characteristically, neuroblastomas contain dense core neuroendocrine granules identical to those observed in small cell undifferentiated (oat cell) carcinomas of the lung and other locations. Similarly, the number of granules parallels the degree of differentiation. Such granules are typically located in broad, dendrite-like processes, where they may be associated with neurofilaments and microtubules, but they can also be found in the subplasmalemma. The key to distinguishing dense core granules from other dense granules, such as primary lysosomes, is their location and relative uniformity of size and shape. The diagnostic ultrastructural feature of a rhabdomyosarcoma is the combination of thick (15 nm) myosin and thin (7 nm) action filaments mimicking normal myogenesis (with or without Z-band formation). Ewing's sarcoma is a controversial tumor that may actually represent more than one lesion or a spectrum of lesions, possibly with neuroectodermal differentiation.[133–135] Depending on the mode of fixation, it characteristically has considerable amounts of glycogen at the LM level, which is more consistently seen by TEM. Glycogen is usually a nonspecific feature but, given the proper context, it can be highly suggestive. For both Ewing's sarcoma and lymphoma, no specific diagnostic ultrastructural features elist, and the pathologist must frequently exclude other small round cell tumors by LM, immunohistochemistry, and TEM.

Mesothelioma Vs. Adenocarcinoma

Distinguishing mesothelioma from primary or metastatic adenocarcinoma is often a difficult and not uncommon problem.[76,129,137,138] Ultrastructural criteria have been applied with some success, but the problem is best addressed by the combination of TEM, cytochemistry, and immunohistochemistry. Because the microvilli in epithelial mesotheliomas are characteristically so long, thin, and wavy or undulating, they are rarely seen entirely in the plane of a thin section. The microvilli lack a glycocalyx (a regular feature of adenocarcinomas of the lung), central microfilaments or core rootlets (a feature of alimentary tract tumors), or associated glycocalyceal bodies. The cells are joined near their bulging apical surface by tight junctions and laterally by prominent desmosomes and usually rest on a basal lamina. They contain variable amounts of glycogen, but no mucin, as well as bundles of tonofilaments or tonofibrils that are often perinuclear in location. Adenocarcinomas associated with the pleura have widely differing appearances depending on their origin. The first task is distinguishing an adenocarcinoma from a mesothelioma and then, as in any other possible metastatic site, determining the origin.

Mesotheliomas in effusion cytologic preparations are characterized by marked cellularity comprised of one cell population.

The mesothelial cells reveal a spectrum ranging from benign to reactive to malignant. The arrangement of the cells ranges from single cells to large fragments with scalloped borders. Papillary clusters with fibrovascular cores may be present. The presence of windows between the cells betrays the mesothelial origin. The cytoplasm is abundant, dense around the nucleus, and vacuolated at the periphery. Blebs on the cell surface may be noted. With the Papanicolaou stain, the two-tone appearance of the cytoplasm is appreciated. It is characterized by perinuclear eosinophilia and peripheral cyanophilia. The cytoplasm shows a concentric lamination around the nucleus that corresponds to perinuclear distribution of intermediate filaments. The nuclei are eccentric, with evenly dispersed chromatin. Binucleate and multinucleate cells are present. By contrast, effusions of adenocarcinoma contain tridimensional cell balls that appear as a second population distinct from the surrounding mesothelial cells. The cell balls have smooth borders shared by many cells. The cytoplasm is vacuolated, unlike the dense or concentrically laminated cytoplasm of mesothelial cells. The nuclear/cytoplasmic ratio is higher than in mesotheliomas.

Adenocarcinoma Vs. Squamous Cell Carcinoma Vs. Neuroendocrine Tumor

One of the most common requests made of a diagnostic electron microscopist is to assist in arriving at a more definitive diagnosis for a metastatic lesion that appears undifferentiated at the LM level. The distinction among adenocarcinoma, squamous cell carcinoma, and neuroendocrine carcinoma at the differentiated end of the spectrum is relatively easy, whereas at the other extreme it can be extremely difficult.[36,37,139] The basic criterion for an adenocarcinoma is the presence of lumina, defined as microvillus-lined spaces formed by cells joined by junctional complexes composed of desmosomes and tight junctions (modified terminal bar). These lumina will be more or less clearly formed, depending on the degree of differentiation; the cells may have other glandular features, such as mucinous granules in the periluminal cytoplasm and free mucin in the lumen. The basic criterion for the diagnosis of squamous cell carcinoma is cells joined by desmosomes associated with tails of cytokeratin (tonofilaments), which are also seen as bundles or tonofibrils free in the cytoplasm (Fig. 15-2). Keeping in mind that squamous cells are covered by pleomorphic villous processes that can be mistaken for microvilli and that small numbers of tonofibrils are regularly seen in adenocarcinomas will prevent confusion between poorly differentiated adenocarcinomas and squamous cell carcinomas. It will also prevent overdiagnosis of adenosquamous carcinomas. Neuroendocrine cell tumors are characterized by varying concentrations of dense core, neuroendocrine type, neurosecretory granules within processes or in the subplasmalemma (Fig. 15-3). Combinations of the three paths of differentiation are commonly encountered at the TEM level, especially in certain locations, such as the lung.[124,140]

Adenocarcinomas, whether clearly identified by LM or only at the electron microscopic level, often present initially or subsequently as metastases. The electron microscopist is regularly asked whether any ultrastructural features suggest the primary site.[141] Determining the source of a metastasis helps not only in honing the therapy but also in minimizing the time and extent

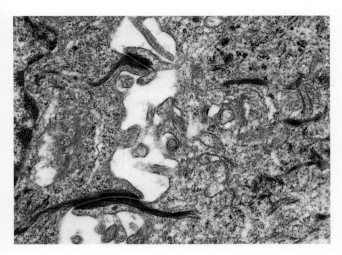

Fig. 15-2. Electron micrograph of a squamous cell carcinoma of the lung showing typical desmosomes with keratin tails (intercellular bridges) and bundles of tonofilaments. Villous processes between desmosomes can be mistaken for microvilli. (× 25,000.)

of the diagnostic workup. The distinction between primary and metastasis must always be considered in any lung lesion, whereas the lesion is clearly a metastasis in the brain, bones, or lymph nodes. In our experience, most adenocarcinomas of the lung, primary or metastatic, consist of cells resembling the nonciliated Clara cell, which is characterized by a bulging apical cytoplasm containing large, dense, often laminated granules, sometimes resembling surfactant granules, with varying amounts of apical glycogen, and relatively little mucin[142,143] (Fig. 15-4). Breast

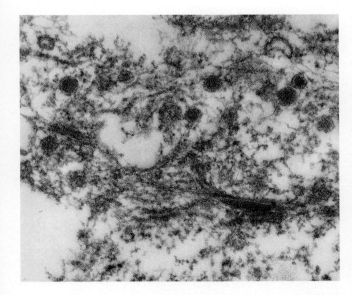

Fig. 15-3. Electron micrograph of a bronchial biopsy from a small cell carcinoma of the lung. Even though the tissue was fixed in formalin and embedded in paraffin and displays extremely poor general preservation, dense core granules measuring roughly 120 nm are still discernible. The structure in the lower right may represent a junction (× 51,000.)

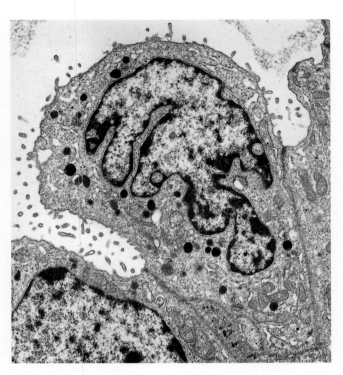

Fig. 15-4. Electron micrograph of a recurrent adenocarcinoma of the lung with a bronchioloalveolar growth pattern. Typical of Clara cells, there are relatively large dense bodies surrounding an irregular nucleus. The apical portion of the cell bulges into the lumen above the lateral junctions. (× 7,000.)

cancers typically have so-called intracytoplasmic microvillus-lined lumina surrounded by tonofilaments and dense secretory vacuoles that can be confused with dense core granules[144,145] (Fig. 15-5). The microvilli in each of these two common tumors are often described as nonspecific, irregular, pleomorphic, and

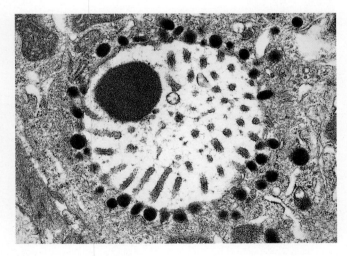

Fig. 15-5. Electron micrograph of a chest wall recurrence of an adenocarcinoma of the breast. The intracytoplasmic lumen is surrounded by small, dense secretory vacuoles and intermediate filaments. The lumen contains secretions, and the microvilli lack core rootlets. (× 24,000.)

lacking features characteristic of the alimentary tract, especially the colorectum. The latter include long core rootlets that extend deep into the apical cytoplasm and a prominent glycocalyx and abundant glycocalyceal bodies.[146] Although these features are especially common and prominent in tumors of the colorectal region, they can be seen in tumors from all portions of the alimentary tract, as well as in some mucinous tumors of the ovary and even in the lung (Fig. 15-6), where they resemble adenocarcinomas of the nasopharynx.[147] If the cells in a metastatic adenocarcinoma are dominated by glycogen and lipid, a renal primary should be considered.[148] Both features are nonspecific, even together, but their presence in relatively large amounts, in the proper setting, is highly suggestive. Lipid is a common sign of degeneration and is thus especially observed in association with necrosis in any tumor. Further subdivision of squamous cell carcinomas is presently not possible on the basis of TEM. Therefore, the location of the metastasis takes on special importance.

Anterior Mediastinal Tumors

Tumors of the anterior mediastinum can usually be distinguished by TEM.[149] Thymomas characteristically have well formed desmosomes and bundles of tonofilaments. Neuroendocrine tumors have characteristic dense core granules. Adenocarcinomas have glandular lumina; when no primary can be found, one should consider an extragonadal germ cell tumor, a lesion that responds well to therapy.[150] Identification of circulating or intratumoral alpha-fetoprotein or human chorionic gonadotropin, or both, will confirm this diagnosis. Lymphomas lack junctions, and this diagnosis can be supported by the absence of other findings. Germinoma is suggested by characteristic Chinese character-appearing nucleoli, although they are not unique to this lesion.

Soft Tissue Tumors

TEM plays a major role in the distinction of soft tissue sarcomas from one another and from other spindle cell tumors (squamous, renal cell, and other metaplastic carcinomas and malignant melanomas). Since soft tissue tumors rarely present as metastatic lesions, they are not discussed in detail here; the reader is referred to Chapter 18.

Diagnostic Features

Relatively few ultrastructural features are pathognomonic for a particular lesion. Electron microscopists have searched for such features as they have for clear histogenetic patterns. It has become appreciated that tumor cells are capable of differentiating along multiple pathways or combinations of pathways, regardless of their presumed cell of origin.[151,152] Tumors can vary in appearance due to time and therapy, and the phenotype of a lesion does not necessarily reflect a particular embryonal layer. Tumor cells share the same genetic information and, in parallel with the neoplastic state, distinctions recede and unusual combinations and patterns appear.

Within the proper context, the presence of premelanosomes and melanosomes is diagnostic of melanoma, but they can also be seen in other tumors derived from the neural crest, such as melanocytic schwannoma (Fig. 15-7) and soft tissue tumor of tendon sheath or clear cell sarcoma of soft parts (soft tissue melanoma). When dealing with melanosomes, in which the typical transversely oriented striations may be obscured by the pigment, one must always ascertain that the melanosomes are in the tumor cells and not in macrophages, especially in a lymph node.

Although in their normal cellular counterparts, the size, appearance, and even shape of secretory granules/vacuoles can tell something about their contents and thus the cell type, this

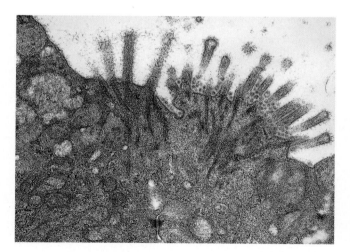

Fig. 15-6. Electron micrograph of a moderately differentiated mucinous adenocarcinoma of the right upper lobe of the lung (single lesion, 9 negative lymph nodes, no other primaries at 24 months). The "rigid" microvilli have prominent core rootlets, glycocalyx, and glycocalyceal bodies. Typical flocculent mucinous vacuoles are present (lower field). (× 32,000.)

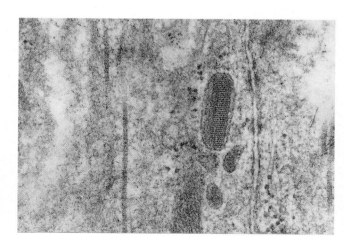

Fig. 15-7. Electron micrograph of malignant melanocytic nerve sheath tumor (malignant melanocytic schwannoma) apparently arising from the myenteric plexus of the stomach of a 24-year-old woman. Transversely striated premelanosomes are located in a long process joined to a second process by several small nonspecific junctions. (× 60,000.)

does not necessarily hold true for tumors. The crystalline appearance of insulin granules may be maintained, as well as the large halos with central or eccentric dense cores in epinephrine- and norepinephrine-containing pheochromocytomas, respectively. The Weibel-Palade body characteristic of endothelial cells is an elongated body with longitudinally oriented striated or tubular contents.[153] Unfortunately, these structures tend to be retained only in the more differentiated endothelial cell tumors. Characteristic crystalline inclusions are seen in certain rare tumors, such as alveolar soft parts sarcomas, juxtaglomerular or renin-secreting tumors, hilus cell tumors of the ovary, and interstitial or Leydig cell tumors of the testis. Birbeck or Langerhans bodies or granules are characteristic of variants of Langerhans cell histiocytosis, such as eosinophilic granuloma. Lamellar surfactant granules or myelinoid bodies are diagnostic for alveolar type II pneumocytes of the lung. Ribosome-lamellar complexes are especially common in hairy cell leukemia. Most of these lesions, however, rarely enter into the differential diagnosis of metastatic tumors.

At times the appearance of organelles can be helpful. Mitochondria of steroid-secreting cells and their tumorous counterparts (e.g., adrenocortical tumors) have tubulovesicular cristae. Plasma cells have stacks of rough endoplasmic reticulum that fill the cytoplasm to varying degrees, depending on the level of differentiation. The nucleus and nucleolus, which provide such critical information at the light microscopic level, are relatively uninformative at the ultrastructural level, although plasma cell neoplasms may maintain their cartwheel or clock-face pattern. The nuclear morphology is more helpful in mycosis fungoides/Sézary's syndrome, in which the nuclei are highly contorted and have a cerebriform appearance. However, complicated nuclei are not unique to this syndrome and must be considered in context.

REFERENCES

1. Esteban JM, Zaloudek C, Silverberg SG: Intraoperative diagnosis of breast lesions. Comparison of cytologic with frozen section technic. Am J Clin Pathol 88:681–688, 1987
2. Mair S, Lash RH, Suskin D, Mendelsohn G: Intraoperative surgical specimen evaluation: frozen section analysis, cytologic examination, or both? A comparative study of 206 cases. Am J Clin Pathol 96:8–14, 1991
3. Nochomovitz L, Sidawy M, Silverberg S, et al: Intraoperative Consultation. A Guide to Smears, Imprints, and Frozen Sections. ASCP Press, Chicago, 1989
4. Oneson RH, Minke JA, Silverberg SG: Intraoperative pathologic consultation. An audit of 1,000 recent consecutive cases. Am J Surg Pathol 13:237–243, 1989
5. Snee MP, Vyrnmuthu N: Metastatic carcinoma from unknown primary site: the experience of a large oncology centre. Br J Radiol 58:1091, 1985
6. Kirsten F, Chi CH, Leary JA, et al: Metastatic adeno- or undifferentiated carcinoma from an unknown primary site—natural history and guidelines for identification of treatable subsets. Q J Med 62:143, 1987
7. Hamilton CS, Langlands AO: ACUPS (adenocarcinoma of unknown primary site): a clinical and cost benefit analysis. Int J Radiat Oncol Biol Phys 13:1497, 1987
8. Maiche AG: Cancer of unknown primary. A retrospective study based on 109 patients. Am J Clin Oncol (CCT) 16:26–29, 1993
9. MacComb WS: Diagnosis and treatment of metastatic cervical cancerous nodes from an unknown primary site. Am J Surg 124:441, 1972
10. Lindberg R: Distribution of cervical lymph node metastases from squamous cell carcinoma of the upper respiratory and digestive tracts. Cancer 29:1446, 1972
11. Krementz ET, Cerise EJ: Metastatic lesions of undetermined source. Hosp Med 6:91, 1970
12. Giffler RF, Gillespie JJ, Ayala AG, et al: Lymphoepithelioma in cervical lymph nodes of children and young adults. Am J Surg Pathol 1:293, 1977
13. Pearson GR, Weiland LH, Neel HB III, et al: Application of Epstein-Barr virus (EBV) serology to the diagnosis of North American nasopharyngeal carcinoma. Cancer 51:260, 1983
14. Copeland EM, McBride CM: Axillary metastases from unknown primary sites. Ann Surg 178:25, 1973
15. Zaren HA, Copeland EM: Inguinal node metastases. Cancer 41:919, 1978
16. Agliozzo CM, Reingold IM: Scalene lymph nodes in necropsies of malignant tumors: analysis of one hundred sixty-six cases. Cancer 20:2148, 1967
17. Hammar S, Bockus D, Remington F: Metastatic tumors of unknown origin: an ultrastructural analysis of 265 cases. Ultrastruct Pathol 11:209–250, 1987
18. Papac RJ: Bone marrow metastases. A review. Cancer 74:2403–2413, 1994
19. Chu DZJ, Lang NP, Thompson C, et al: Peritoneal carcinomatosis in nongynecologic malignancy. A prospective study of prognostic factors. Cancer 63:364–367, 1989
20. Stewart JF, et al: Unknown primary adenocarcinoma: incidence of overinvestigation and natural history. BMJ 1:1530, 1979
21. Kambhu SA, Kelsen DP, Fiore J, et al: Metastatic adenocarcinomas of unknown primary site. Prognostic variables and treatment results. Am J Clin Oncol (CCT) 13:55–60, 1990
22. Viadana E, Au K-L: Patterns of metastases in adenocarcinomas of man. An autopsy study of 4,728 cases. J Med 6:1, 1975
23. Silverman JF, Finley JL, Park HK, et al: Fine needle aspiration cytology of bronchioloalveolar-cell carcinoma of the lung. Acta Cytol 29:887–894, 1985
24. Shenson DL, Gallion HH, Powell DE, Pieretti M: Loss of heterozygosity and genomic instability in synchronous endometrioid tumor of the ovary and endometrium. Cancer 76:650–657, 1995
25. Younes M, Katikaneni PR, Lechago LV, Lechago J: HAM56 antibody: a tool in the differential diagnosis between colorectal and gynecological malignancy. Mod Pathol 7:396–400, 1994
26. Berezowski K, Stastny JF, Kornstein MJ: Cytokeratins 7 and 20 and carcinoembryonic antigen in ovarian and colonic carcinoma. Mod Pathol 9:426–429, 1996
27. Wauters CCAP, Smedts F, Gerrits LGM, et al: Keratins 7 and 20 as diagnostic markers of carcinomas metastatic to the ovary. Hum Pathol 26:852–855, 1995
28. Tsao S-W, Mok C-H, Knapp RC, et al: Molecular genetic evidence of unifocal origin for human serous ovarian carcinomas. Gynecol Oncol 48:5–10, 1993
29. Li S, Han H, Resnik E, et al: Advanced ovarian carcinoma: molecular evidence of unifocal origin. Gynecol Oncol 51:21–25, 1993
30. Caraway NP, Fanning CV, Amato RJ, Sneige N: Fine-needle aspiration cytology of seminoma: a review of 16 cases. Diagn Cytopathol 12:327–333, 1995
31. Collins KA, Geisinger KR, Wakely PE Jr, et al: Extragonadal germ cell tumors: a fine-needle aspiration biopsy study. Diagn Cytopathol 12:223–229, 1995
32. Balsley E, Francis D, Jacobsen GK: Testicular germ cell tumors: classification based on fine needle aspiration biopsy. Acta Cytol 34:690–694, 1990

33. Mizrak B, Ekinci C: Cytologic diagnosis of yolk sac tumor. A report of seven cases. Acta Cytol 39:936–940, 1995

34. Johnson TL, Kini SR: Cytologic features of metastatic transitional cell carcinoma. Diagn Cytopathol 9:270–278, 1993

35. Powers CN, Elbadawi A: "Cercariform" cells: a clue to the cytodiagnosis of transitional cell origin of metastatic neoplasms? Diagn Cytopathol 13:15–21, 1995

36. Auersperg N, Erber H, Worth A: Histologic variation among poorly differentiated invasive carcinomas of the human uterine cervix. J Natl Cancer Inst 51:1461, 1973

37. Churg A: The fine structure of large cell undifferentiated carcinoma of the lung: evidence for its relation to squamous cell carcinomas and adenocarcinomas. Hum Pathol 9:143, 1978

38. Szyfelbein WM, Ross JR: Carcinoids, atypical carcinoids and small cell carcinomas of the lung: differential diagnosis of fine-needle aspiration biopsy specimens. Diagn Cytopathol 4:1–8, 1988

39. Robinson IA, McKee G, Jackson PA, et al: Lobular carcinoma of the breast: cytological features supporting the diagnosis of lobular cancer. Diagn Cytopathol 13:196–201, 1995

40. Batsakis JG, Regezi JA: Selected controversial lesions of salivary tissues. Otolaryngol Clin North Am 10:309, 1977

41. Dekmezian R, Sneige N, Shabb N: Papillary renal-cell carcinoma: fine-needle aspiration of 15 cases. Diagn Cytopathol 7:198–203, 1991

42. Smith MB, Silverman JF, Raab SS, et al: Fine-needle aspiration cytology of hepatic leiomyosarcoma. Diagn Cytopathol 11:321–327, 1994

43. Katzenstein A-LA, Prioleau PG, Askin FB: The histologic spectrum and significance of clear-cell change in lung carcinoma. Cancer 45:943, 1980

44. Askew JB Jr, Fechner RE, Bentinck DC, et al: Epithelial and myoepithelial oncocytes: ultrastructural study of a salivary gland oncocytoma. Arch Otolaryngol 93:46, 1971

45. Pisharodi LR, Lavoie R, Bedrossian CWM: Differential diagnostic dilemmas in malignant fine-needle aspirates of liver: a practical approach to final diagnosis. Diagn Cytopathol 12:364–371, 1995

46. Akhtar M, Ali AM: Aspiration cytology of chromophobe cell carcinoma of the kidney. Diagn Cytopathol 13:287–294, 1995

47. Husain M, Nguyen GK: Alveolar soft part sarcoma. Report of a case diagnosed by needle aspiration cytology and electron microscopy. Acta Cytol 39:951–954, 1995

48. Ordonez NG, Hickey RC, Brooks TE: Alveolar soft part sarcoma: a cytologic and immunohistochemical study. Cancer 61:325–331, 1988

49. Falck B, Hillarp NA, Thieme G, et al: Fluorescence of catecholamines and related compounds condensed with formaldehyde. J Histochem Cytochem 10:348, 1962

50. Adams CWM: A perchloric acid-naphthoquinone method for the histochemical localization of cholesterol. Nature 192:331, 1961

51. Jones RA, Dawson IMP: Morphology and staining patterns of endocrine cell tumours in the gut, pancreas and bronchus and their possible significance. Histopathology 1:137, 1977

52. Grimelius L, Wilander E: Silver impregnation and other non-immunocytochemical methods. p. 95. In Polak JM, Bloom SR (eds): Endocrine Tumours. Churchill Livingstone, Edinburgh, 1985

53. Singh I: A modification of the Masson-Hamperl method for staining of argentaffin cells. Anat Anz 115:81, 1964

54. Grimelius L: A silver nitrate stain for α2-cells in human pancreatic islets. Acta Soc Med Uppsal 73:243, 1968

55. Nieuwenhuijzen Kruseman AC, Knijnenburg G, Brutel de la Riviere G, et al: Morphology and immunohistochemically defined endocrine function of pancreatic islet cell tumors. Histopathology 2:389, 1978

56. Ewen SB, Rost FDW: The histochemical demonstration of catecholamines and tryptamines by acid and aldehyde-induced methods. Microspectrofluorimetric characterization of the fluorophores in models. Histochem J 4:59, 1972

57. Westermark P, Grimelius L, Polak JM, et al: Amyloid in peptide hormone-producing tumors. Lab Invest 37:212, 1977

58. Leder LD: Der Blutmonocyt. Springer-Verlag, Berlin, 1967

59. Grossi CE, Webb SR, Zicca A, et al: Morphological and histochemical analysis of 2 human T-cell subpopulations bearing receptors for IgM or IgG. J Exp Med 147:1405, 1978

60. Katayama I, Yang JPS: Reassessment of a cytochemical test for differential diagnosis of leukemic reticuloendotheliosis. Am J Clin Pathol 68:268, 1977

61. Roggli VL, Kolbeck J, Sanfilippo F, Shelburne JD: Pathology of human mesothelioma: etiologic and diagnostic considerations. Pathol Annu 22:91–131, 1987

62. Norken SA, Campagna-Pinto D: Cytoplasmic hyaline inclusions in hepatomas. Arch Pathol 86:25, 1968

63. Willighagen RGJ, Thiery M: Enzyme histochemistry of ovarian tumors. Am J Obstet Gynecol 100:393, 1968

64. Koudstaal J: The histochemical demonstration of arylsulphatase in human tumors. Eur J Cancer 11:809, 1975

65. Sarnat HB, de Millo DE, Siddiqui SY: Diagnostic value of histochemistry in embryonal rhabdomyosarcoma. Am J Surg Pathol 3:177, 1979

66. Kohler G, Milstein C: Continuous cultures of fused cells secreting antibodies of predefined specificity. Nature 256:495, 1975

67. Lee AK, DeLellis R: Immunohistochemical techniques and their applications to tissue diagnosis. p. 31. In Spicer SS (ed): Histochemistry in Pathological Diagnosis. Marcel Dekker, New York, 1987

68. Bunn PA Jr, Linnoila I, Minna JD, et al: Small cell lung cancer, endocrine cells of the fetal bronchus and other neuroendocrine cells express the leu-7 antigenic determinant present on natural killer cells. Blood 65:764, 1985

69. Norton AJ, Thomas JA, Isaacson PG: Cytokeratin-specific monoclonal antibodies are reactive with tumors of smooth muscle cells. An immunocytochemical and biochemical study using antibodies to intermediate filament cytoskeletal proteins. Histopathology 11:487, 1987

70. Schmechel DE: Gamma subunits of the glycolytic enzyme enolase: non-specific or neuron-specific. Lab Invest 52:239, 1985

71. Epstein JI: Prostate Biopsy Interpretation. 2nd Ed. Lippincott-Raven, Philadelphia, 1995, pp. 224–225

72. Roholl PJM, Ramaekers FCS, Bosman FT: Markers of carcinomas and sarcomas. Diagnostic implications. p. 227. In den Otter W, Ruitenberg EJ (eds): Tumor Immunology—Mechanisms, Diagnosis, Therapy. Elsevier, Amsterdam, 1987

73. Fukuyama M, Hayashi Y, Koike M, et al: Human chorionic gonadotrophin in lung and lung tumors. Immunohistochemical study on unbalanced distribution of subunits. Lab Invest 55:433, 1987

74. Domagala WM, Markiewski M, Tuziak T, et al: Immunocytochemistry on fine needle aspirates in paraffin miniblocks. Acta Cytol 34:291–296, 1990

75. Saleh H, Masood S: Value of ancillary studies in fine-needle aspiration biopsy. Diagn Cytopathol 13:310–315, 1995

76. Motoyama T, Watanabe T, Okazaki E, et al: Immunohistochemical properties of malignant mesothelioma cells in histologic and cytologic specimens. Acta Cytol 39:164–170, 1995

77. Shield PW, Perkins G, Wright RG: Immunocytochemical staining of cytologic specimens. How helpful is it? Am J Clin Pathol 105:157–162, 1996

78. Banks ER, Jansen JF, Oberle E, Davey DD: Cytokeratin positivity in fine-needle aspirates of melanomas and sarcomas. Diagn Cytopathol 12:230–233, 1995

79. Parham DM, Webber B, Holt H, et al: Immunohistochemical study of childhood rhabdomyosarcomas and related neoplasms. Results of an intergroup rhabdomyosarcoma study project. Cancer 67:3072–3080, 1991

80. Pettigrew NM: Techniques in immunocytochemistry. Application to diagnostic pathology. Arch Pathol Lab Med 113:641–644, 1989

81. Leong AS-Y: Immunostaining of cytologic specimens. Am J Clin Pathol 105:139–140, 1996

82. Wang E, Fishman D, Lieu RKH, Sun T-T (eds): Intermediate filaments. Ann NY Acad Sci 455, 1985

83. Battifora H: Clinical applications of the immunohistochemistry of filamentous proteins. Am J Surg Pathol, suppl. 1, 12:24–42, 1988

84. Miettinen M: Keratin immunohistochemistry: update of applications and pitfalls. Pathol Annu 28:113–143, 1993

85. Moll R, Franke WW, Schiller DL, et al: The catalog of human cytokeratins: patterns of expression in normal epithelia, tumors and cultured cells. Cell 31:11–24, 1982

86. Eichner R, Bonitz P, Sun TT: Classification of epidermal keratins according to their immunoreactivity, isoelectric point, and mode of expression. J Cell Biol 98:1388–1396, 1984

87. Loy TS, Calaluce RD: Utility of cytokeratin immunostaining in separating pulmonary adenocarcinomas from colonic adenocarcinomas. Am J Clin Pathol 102:764–767, 1994

88. Pinkus GS, Kurtin PJ: Epithelial membrane antigen—a diagnostic discriminant in surgical pathology: immunohistochemical profile in epithelial, mesenchymal and hematopoietic neoplasms using paraffin sections and monoclonal antibodies. Hum Pathol 16:929–940, 1985

89. True LD: Epithelial membrane antigens. pp. 5.1–5.28. In True LD (ed): Atlas of Diagnostic Immunohistopathology. Lippincott-Raven, Philadelphia, 1990

90. Moll R, Cowin P, Kapprell H-P, et al: Desmosomal proteins: new markers for identification and classification of tumors. Lab Invest 54:4, 1986

91. Azumi N, Battifora H: The distribution of vimentin and keratin in epithelial and nonepithelial neoplasms. A comprehensive immunohistochemical study on formalin- and alcohol-fixed tumors. Am J Clin Pathol 88:286–296, 1987

92. Gosh AK, Gatter KC, Dunnill MS, et al: Immunohistochemical staining of reactive mesothelium, mesothelioma and lung carcinoma with a panel of monoclonal antibodies. J Clin Pathol 40:19, 1987

93. Miettinen M, Foidart J-M, Ekblom P: Immunohistochemical demonstration of laminin, the major glycoprotein of basement membranes, as an aid in the diagnosis of soft tissue tumors. Am J Clin Pathol 79:306, 1983

94. Quinlan RA, Schiller DL, Hartfeld M, et al: Patterns of expression and organization in cytokeratin intermediate filaments. Ann NY Acad Sci 455:282, 1985

95. Debus E, Weber K, Osborn M: Monoclonal cytokeratin antibodies that distinguish simple from stratified squamous epithelia: characterization on human tissues. EMBO J 1:1641, 1982

96. Ramaekers FCS, Huijsmans A, Moesker O, et al: Monoclonal antibody to keratin filaments specific for glandular epithelia and their tumors: use in surgical pathology. Lab Invest 49:353, 1983

97. Debus E, Moll R, Franke WW, et al: Immunohistochemical distinction of human carcinomas by cytokeratin typing with monoclonal antibodies. Am J Pathol 114:121, 1984

98. van Muijen GNP, Ruiter DJ, Franke WW, et al: Cell type heterogeneity of cytokeratin expression in complex epithelia and carcinoma as demonstrated by monoclonal antibodies specific for cytokeratins 4 and 13. Exp Cell Res 162:97, 1986

99. Jobsis AC, De Vries GP, Anholt RRH, et al: Demonstration of the prostatic origin of metastasis: an immunohistochemical method for formalin-fixed embedded tissue. Cancer 41:1788, 1978

100. Kimura N, Sasano N: Prostate specific acid phosphatase in carcinoid tumours. Virchows Arch [A] 410:247, 1986

101. Veronese SM, Barbareschi M, Morelli L, et al: Predictive value of ER1D5 antibody immunostaining in breast cancer. A paraffin-based retrospective study of 257 cases. Appl Immunohistochem 3:85–90, 1995

102. Burt A, Goudie RB: Diagnosis of primary thyroid carcinoma by immunohistological demonstration of thyroglobulin. Histopathology 3:279, 1979

103. Muraro R, Wunderlich D, Thor A, et al: Definition by monoclonal antibodies of a repertoire of epitopes of carcinoembryonic antigen differentially expressed in human colon carcinomas versus normal adult tissues. Cancer Res 45:5769, 1985

104. Kawabat SE, Bast RC, Bhan AK, et al: Tissue distribution of a coelomic-epithelium-related antigen recognized by the monoclonal antibody OC 125. Int J Gynecol Pathol 2:275, 1983

105. Moon TD: A highly restricted antigen for renal cell carcinoma defined by a monoclonal antibody. Hybridoma 4:163, 1985

106. Oosterwijk E, Ruiter DJ, Wakka JC, et al: Immunohistochemical analysis of monoclonal antibodies to renal antigens: applications in the diagnosis of renal cancers. Am J Pathol 123:301, 1986

107. De Ley L, Broers R, Ramaekers FCS, et al: Monoclonal antibodies in clinical and experimental pathology of lung cancer. p. 191. In Ruiter DJ, Fleuren GJ, Warnaar SO (eds): Applications of Monoclonal Antibodies in Tumor Pathology. Martinus Nijhof, Dordrecht, 1987

108. Marangos PJ: Clinical utility of neuron-specific enolase as a neuroendocrine tumor marker. p. 181. In Polak JM, Bloom SR (eds): Endocrine Tumours. Churchill Livingstone, Edinburgh, 1985

109. Fischer-Colbrie R, Fischenschlager I: Immunological characterization of secretory proteins of chromaffin granules: chromogranins A, chromogranin B and enkephalin-containing peptides. J Neurochem 44:1854, 1985

110. Fischer-Colbrie R, Hagn C, Kilpatrick L, et al: Chromogranin C: a third component of the acidic proteins in chromaffin granules. J Neurochem 47:318, 1986

111. Wiedenmann B, Franke WW, Kuhn C, et al: Synaptophysin: a marker protein for neuroendocrine cells and neoplasms. Proc Natl Acad Sci USA 83:3500, 1987

112. Ramaekers FCS, Puts JJG, Moesker O, et al: Antibodies to intermediate filament proteins in the immunohistochemical identification of human tumours. An overview. Histochem J 15:691, 1983

113. Battifora H: Assessment of antigen damage in immunohistochemistry. The vimentin internal control. Am J Clin Pathol 96:669–671, 1991

114. Warnke RA, Gatter KC, Falini B, et al: Diagnosis of human lymphoma with monoclonal antileucocyte antibodies. N Engl J Med 309:1275, 1983

115. Nakajima T, Watanabe S, Sato Y, et al: An immunoperoxidase study of S-100 protein distribution in normal and neoplastic tissues. Am J Surg Pathol 6:715, 1982

116. Kahn HJ, Marks A, Thorn H, et al: Role of antibody to S-100 protein in diagnostic pathology. Am J Clin Pathol 79:341, 1983

117. Ordonez NG, Xiaolong J, Hickey RC: Comparison of HMB-45 monoclonal antibody and S-100 protein in the immunohistochemical diagnosis of melanoma. Am J Clin Pathol 90:385–390, 1988

118. Mogollon R, Penneys N, Albores-Saavedra J, et al: Malignant schwannoma presenting as a skin mass. Confirmation by the demonstration of myelin basic protein within tumor cells. Cancer 53:1190, 1984

119. Erlandson RA: Diagnostic Transmission Electron Microscopy of Tumors. Lippincott-Raven, Philadelphia 1994

120. Dickerson GR: Diagnostic Electron Microscopy: A Text/Atlas. Igaku-Shoin, New York, 1988

121. Erlandson RA, Rosai J: A realistic approach to the use of electron microscopy and other ancillary diagnostic techniques in surgical pathology. Am J Surg Pathol 19:247–250, 1995

122. Frost AR, Orenstein JM, Abraham AA, Silverberg SG: A comparison of the usefulness of electron microscopy and immunohistochemistry. One laboratory's experience. Arch Pathol Lab Med 118:922–926, 1994

123. Wang N-S, Minassian H: The formaldehyde-fixed and paraffin-em-

bedded tissues for diagnostic transmission electron microscopy. A retrospective study. Hum Pathol 18:715, 1987

124. Neal MH, Kosinski R, Cohen P, et al: Atypical endocrine tumors of the lung: histologic, ultrastructural, and clinical study of 19 cases. Hum Pathol 17:1264, 1986

125. Dabbs DJ, Silverman JF: Selective use of electron microscopy in fine needle aspiration cytology. Acta Cytol 32:880–884, 1988

126. Dardick I, Yazdi HM, Brosko C, Rippstein P: A quantitative comparison of light and electron microscopic diagnoses in specimens obtained by fine needle aspiration biopsy. Ultrastruct Pathol 15:105–129, 1991

127. Yazdi HM, Dardick I: What is the value of electron microscopy in fine needle aspiration biopsy? Diagn Cytopathol 4:177–182, 1988

128. Herrera GA, Wilkerson JA: Ultrastructural studies of malignant cells in fluids. Diagn Cytopathol 1:272, 1985

129. Bedrossian CWM: Malignant effusions: a multimodal approach to cytologic diagnosis. Igaku-Shoin, New York, 1994

130. Mawad JK, Mackay B, Raymond AK, Ayala AG: Electron microscopy in the diagnosis of small round cell tumors of bone. Ultrastruct Pathol 18:263–270, 1994

131. Mierau GW, Berry PJ, Orsini EN: Small round cell neoplasms: can electron microscopy and immunohistochemical studies accurately classify them? Ultrastruct Pathol 9:99, 1985

132. Mierau GW, Favara BE: Rhabdomyosarcoma in children: ultrastructural study of 31 cases. Cancer 46:2035, 1980

133. Cavazzana AO, Miser JS, Jefferson J, et al: Experimental evidence for a neural origin of Ewing's sarcoma of bone. Am J Pathol 127:507, 1987

134. Tsuneyoshi M, Yokoyama R, Hashimoto H, Enjoji M: Comparative study of neuroectodermal tumor and Ewing's sarcoma of the bone: histopathologic, immunohistochemical, and ultrastructural features. Acta Pathol Jpn 39:573–581, 1989

135. Ushigome S, Shimoda T, Takaki K, et al: Immunocytochemical and ultrastructural studies of the histogenesis of Ewing's sarcoma and putatively related tumors. Cancer 64:52–62, 1989

136. Pettit CK, Zukerberg LR, Gray MH, et al: Primary lymphoma of bone. A B-cell neoplasm with a high frequency of multilobated cells. Am J Surg Pathol 14:329–334, 1990

137. Warhol MJ, Corson JM: An ultrastructural comparison of mesotheliomas with adenocarcinomas of the lung and breast. Hum Pathol 16:50, 1985

138. Dardick I, Jabi M, Elliot M, et al: Diffuse epithelial mesothelioma: a review of the ultrastructural spectrum. Ultrastruct Pathol 11:503, 1987

139. Auerbach O, Frasca JM, Parks VR, et al: A comparison of World Health Organization (WHO) classification of lung tumors by light and electron microscopy. Cancer 50:2079, 1982

140. McDowell EM, Trump BF: Pulmonary small cell carcinoma showing tripartite differentiation in individual cells. Hum Pathol 12:286, 1981

141. Dvorak AM, Monahan RA: Metastatic adenocarcinoma of unknown primary site. Diagnostic electron microscopy to determine the site of tumor origin. Arch Pathol Lab Med 106:21, 1982

142. Kimura Y: A histochemical and ultrastructural study of adenocarcinoma of the lung. Am J Surg Pathol 2:253, 1978

143. Ogata T, Endo K: Clara cell granules of peripheral lung cancers. Cancer 54:1635, 1984

144. Sobrinho-Simoes M, Johannessen JV, Gould VE: The diagnostic significance of intracytoplasmic lumina in metastatic neoplasms. Ultrastruct Pathol 2:327, 1981

145. Nesland JM, Memoli VA, Holm R, et al: Breast carcinomas with neuroendocrine differentiation. Ultrastruct Pathol 8:225, 1985

146. Hickey WF, Seiler MW: Ultrastructural markers of colonic adenocarcinoma. Cancer 47:140, 1981

147. Weidner N: Pulmonary adenocarcinoma with intestinal-type differentiation. Ultrastruct Pathol 16:7–10, 1992

148. Mackay B, Ordonez NG, Khoursand J, et al: The ultrastructure and immunohistochemistry of renal cell carcinoma. Ultrastruct Pathol 11:483, 1987

149. Carlson G, Sibley RK: Anterior mediastinal neoplasms: an ultrastructural review. p. 253. In Russo J, Sommers SC (eds): Tumor Diagnosis by Electron Microscopy. Vol. 1. Field, Rich, New York, 1986

150. Richardson RL, Schoumacher RA, Fer MF, et al: The unrecognized extragonadal germ cell cancer syndrome. Ann Intern Med 94:181, 1981

151. Gould VE: Histogenesis and differentiation: a re-evaluation of these concepts as criteria for the classification of tumors. Hum Pathol 17:212, 1986

152. Silverberg SG: Histogenetic interpretation of immunohistochemical staining results. pp. 17–21. In Kindermann G, Lampe B (eds): Immunohistochemische Diagnostik gynäkologisher Tumoren. Thieme, New York, 1992

153. Carstens PHB: The Weibel-Palade body in the diagnosis of endothelial tumors. Ultrastruct Pathol 2:315, 1981

16

Inflammatory Diseases of the Skin

Loren E. Golitz

HANDLING AND PROCESSING OF SKIN BIOPSY SPECIMENS

It is important in the diagnosis of the inflammatory dermatoses to select the proper site for biopsy. In many diseases, such as lichen planus and psoriasis, biopsy of an older lesion may provide the most histologic information. Care should be taken, however, to avoid lesions that show excoriation and secondary infection. In the bullous dermatoses, it is preferable to biopsy an early vesicle because secondary changes in an older lesion may obscure the characteristic findings. In most cases of dermatitis, the inclusion of normal skin in the biopsy specimen is not necessary and may result in the oversight of important changes if the specimen is sectioned through the area of normal skin.

Types of Biopsies

Three types of skin biopsies are most often used in the diagnosis of the inflammatory dermatoses. The *excisional biopsy* obtains a generous amount of tissue and is the most desirable form of skin biopsy from the pathologist's point of view. A good excisional biopsy is elliptical and includes subcutaneous fat. This form of biopsy may be necessary for the interpretation of inflammatory changes in the subcutaneous fat such as erythema nodosum. The disadvantages of the excisional biopsy are the time required to perform the procedure and the necessity for sutures. A second form of skin biopsy is the *punch biopsy*. Most punch biopsy specimens are 4 mm in diameter; however, they vary from 2 to 8 mm in diameter. The punch biopsy obtains a round plug of skin, which frequently includes the superficial portion of the subcutaneous fat. In general, the punch biopsy is adequate for most inflammatory dermatoses with the exception of those that involve the fat and deep fascia. The punch biopsy is quick and easy to perform and does not require sterile technique or sutures; however, the resulting round scar is less desirable than the linear scar of an excisional biopsy. A third type of biopsy, the *shave biopsy*, may be preferable for those disorders that involve predominantly the epidermis and superficial dermis. The shave biopsy usually obtains a larger piece of epidermis than the 4 mm punch biopsy and is ideal for diseases such as psoriasis and lichen planus that do not involve the fat. The shave biopsy is performed quickly without the use of sterile technique or sutures. A fourth type of biopsy, the *curette biopsy*, is used for a variety of tumors by some clinicians but is generally unacceptable for the inflammatory dermatoses because it may provide an inadequate specimen or excessively traumatize the tissue. In all forms of skin biopsies, but particularly with the punch biopsy, care should be taken not to compress the tissue with the forceps because this tends to distort the histologic changes.

Fixation and Processing

The ideal fixative for skin biopsy specimens is 10 percent phosphate-buffered neutral formalin. A minimum of 8 hours should be allowed for fixation, although 24 hours is ideal. Large specimens should be sectioned to 4 mm or less in thickness to allow adequate fixation. In cold climates where tissue is sent through the mail, a fixative solution containing alcohol may be desirable to prevent the formation of ice crystals in the tissue.

When processing biopsy specimens of the inflammatory dermatoses, the epidermal surface should be inspected grossly, and the tissue should be bisected through the area of greatest alteration. For disorders with focal changes such as scabies, this may mean the difference between an accurate diagnosis and a nonspecific one. Most punch biopsy and shave biopsy specimens should be bisected and embedded with the cut surfaces down. Two millimeter punch biopsy specimens are small and should be embedded intact. Although excisional biopsy specimens of tumors are usually bisected through the narrow axis, more information may be obtained in the inflammatory dermatoses if they are bisected longitudinally. Hair shafts that protrude from the surface of the skin should be trimmed before embedding to avoid dulling the microtome blade and scratching the surface of the sections. Excessive fat should be trimmed from the specimen if the inflammatory process does not involve the subcutaneous fat.

HISTOLOGY OF NORMAL SKIN

Epidermis

The outer layer of the epidermis is known as the stratum corneum, keratin layer, or horny layer. This layer often shows a loose basketweave pattern, but on the palms and soles it is thick and compact. Skin from acral portions of the body may show a clear zone or stratum lucidum immediately beneath the keratin layer. Deep to the stratum lucidum is the granular cell layer, which is formed by partially flattened cells that contain deeply basophilic keratohyaline granules. The thickness of the granular cell layer varies from 1 to 10 cells and is usually proportional to the thickness of the stratum corneum. Beneath the granular cell layer is the stratum malpighii, also known as the squamous cell layer or prickle cell layer. The cells in this layer are polygonal and contain round to oval nuclei. The malpighian cells are attached to each other by modifications of their cell membranes known as prickles or desmosomes. The deepest layer of the epidermis is the basal cell layer. The basal cell layer contains two types of cells, epidermal basal cells and melanocytes. The basal cells are columnar and are attached to the underlying basement membrane by hemidesmosomes. Basal cells divide and daughter cells become the cells of the stratum malpighii. Almost all mitotic activity occurs in the basal cell layer; however, mitoses occur rarely one or two layers above the basal cell layer. About 28 to 30 days are required for a cell to move from the basal cell layer to the outer portion of the keratin layer where it is shed off. Approximately every tenth cell in the basal cell layer is a melanocyte, which produces a granular pigment known as melanin. Melanocytes have elongated dendritic processes that extend into the malpighian layer. Melanin pigment moves through the dendrites and is eventually found in the cytoplasm of the malpighian cells where it functions to screen the nucleus of these cells from ultraviolet radiation. A second type of dendritic cell, the Langerhans cell, occurs within the malpighian layer. This cell, which is not obvious in routinely stained sections, constitutes 3 to 8 percent of the epidermal cells and functions as a macrophage by processing and presenting antigens to inflammatory cells such as T lymphocytes.[1]

Dermis

The epidermis and dermis interface in an undulating pattern. The projections of epidermis are known as *rete ridges*. The intervening projections of dermal connective tissue are known as *dermal papillae*. The dermis is divided into papillary dermis and reticular dermis. The papillary dermis occurs between the rete ridges and extends for a short distance beneath the tips of the rete ridges. The papillary dermis stains pale pink with the hematoxylin and eosin (H&E) stain and contains delicate collagen fibers, some of which are oriented perpendicularly or obliquely to the surface of the epidermis. Beneath the papillary dermis, the reticular dermis contains thick, deeply eosinophilic collagen fibers that are oriented parallel to the surface of the skin. Deep to the reticular dermis is the subcutaneous fat, which is divided into distinct lobules by thin septa of connective tissue. Fascia is immediately deep to the subcutaneous fat.

A superficial vascular plexus of arterioles, venules, and capillaries is present in the superficial dermis. A deep vascular plexus of arteries and veins occurs in the deep dermis and superficial subcutaneous fat and is connected to the superficial plexus by connecting vessels. The dermal vessels are often accompanied by nerves.

Adnexa

A distinctive feature of skin is the presence of a variety of adnexal structures. Eccrine sweat glands are widely distributed and function to control body temperature through the evaporation of sweat. They are composed of an intraepidermal duct, which empties directly onto the skin surface; a dermal duct; and a glandular portion, which is located in the deep dermis. The coiled glandular portion is surrounded by a narrow zone of subcutaneous fat. The apocrine sweat glands are most numerous in the axillae and the groin. The glandular portion of the apocrine sweat glands is larger and has larger lumina than the eccrine glands. The apocrine duct empties into the upper portion of a hair follicle or directly onto the skin surface. The third major adnexal structure of the skin is the pilosebaceous apparatus, which is composed of a hair follicle, a sebaceous gland, an arrector muscle, and in some parts of the body an apocrine gland. Sebaceous glands are numerous on the face but are also present on all parts of the body except the palms and soles. The multilobular glands have a single peripheral row of germinative cells that divide and produce the sebaceous cells that make up the bulk of the lobules. Sebaceous cells have a small centrally placed nucleus and foamy cytoplasm. Sebaceous glands are holocrine glands; that is, the sebaceous cells degenerate and become the secretory material that is discharged into the follicular lumen. The deepest portion of the hair follicle is the hair bulb, which surrounds a dermal hair papilla containing blood vessels and nerves. Just above the hair papilla is the matrix, a rapidly dividing area that produces the hair shaft. The hair follicle is surrounded by an inner root sheath and an outer root sheath. The arrector muscle extends from the deep portion of the hair follicle or hair bulb to the undersurface of the epidermis. Contractions of these smooth muscles produce the clinical appearance of goose bumps. Smooth muscle also occurs in the areola of the nipples and the tunica dartos of the external genitalia. Striated muscle in the skin is generally limited to the facial and platysma muscles.

CLINICOPATHOLOGIC CORRELATION

In no other area of anatomic pathology is the correlation of clinical information more important in arriving at the correct diagnosis than in the inflammatory dermatoses. Many cases that appear to be nonspecific dermatitis histologically can be accurately diagnosed when clinical information is used. For example, lichen striatus histologically shows a subacute or chronic dermatitis. However, a linear pruritic rash extending down the entire length of an arm or leg in a young individual, when combined with these histologic features, is typical of lichen striatus. The subepidermal bullae in dermatitis herpetiformis at times are nonspecific. However, a clinical history of grouped, pruritic vesicles on the elbows and interscapular area is characteristic of dermatitis herpetiformis and should stimulate a search for neutrophils within dermal papillae at the margins of the subepidermal bullae. When histologic changes do not support the clinical information, additional levels through the tissue or additional biopsies may be indicated. At times, the clinical differential diagnosis may be incorrect, and the pathologist should not hesitate to discuss impressions with the clinician before issuing the pathology report.

GENERAL RULES FOR EXAMINING THE SLIDE

The histologic diagnosis of an inflammatory dermatosis is best made by examining the pattern of inflammation and categorizing it with a specific group of diseases. In most cases, the inflammatory pattern is best evaluated by looking at the slide at low magnification. To prevent confusion, high magnification should be used only when something specific is being observed in greater detail. A few general rules are helpful in evaluating biopsy specimens of the inflammatory skin diseases: (1) look at all slides as unknowns, (2) evaluate the slide grossly against a contrasting background and note the inflammatory pattern, (3) look at all sections on each slide, and (4) look at each slide in a systematic manner, starting with the stratum corneum and progressing to the subcutaneous fat.

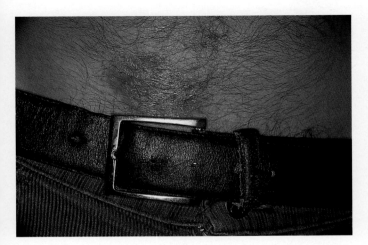

Fig. 16-1. Allergic contact dermatitis. This localized dermatitis was caused by an allergy to nickel in the belt buckle.

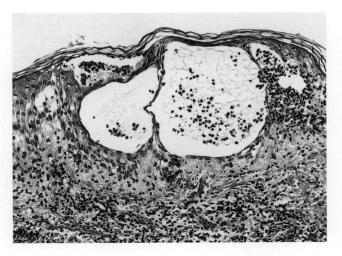

Fig. 16-2. Spongiotic dermatitis (acute dermatitis). Intraepidermal spongiotic vesicles contain acute and chronic inflammatory cells. A patchy infiltrate of mononuclear cells surrounds small vessels in the upper dermis.

INFLAMMATORY REACTION PATTERNS

Epidermal Reaction Patterns

Spongiotic Dermatitis

Spongiotic dermatitis is characterized by intercellular edema that produces separation of the cells of the malpighian layer, often resulting in the formation of microabscesses or bullae. The prickles or desmosomes between epidermal cells appear prominent and stretched in the presence of spongiosis. The epidermis is often mildly acanthotic, whereas the dermis shows vascular dilatation and a patchy perivascular infiltrate of mononuclear cells. Skin diseases that commonly produce spongiotic dermatitis include allergic contact dermatitis, nummular dermatitis, pityriasis rosea, autoeczematous dermatitis, dyshidrotic dermatitis, incontinentia pigmenti, and a variety of other eczematous processes.

Allergic Contact Dermatitis

The prototype of spongiotic dermatitis is allergic contact dermatitis caused by skin contact with allergens such as poison ivy, nickel in jewelry, or topical medications. Typically, the skin is erythematous and edematous with small vesicles and crusting. The distribution of the rash in contact dermatitis is often characteristic with nickel dermatitis occurring on the earlobes, neck, fingers, and wrists in areas of contact with jewelry (Fig. 16-1). Poison ivy occurs on exposed portions of the body and often shows linear vesicles where the broken leaf or stem of the plant has brushed against the skin. Allergic contact dermatitis of the hands and feet typically involves the dorsal aspects with sparing of the keratotic palms and soles. It should be kept in mind that any allergen can be transferred to the eyes or geni-

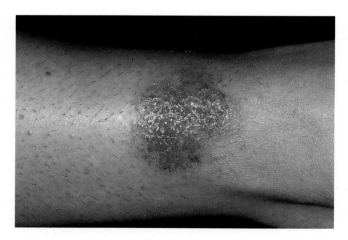

Fig. 16-3. Nummular eczema. This corn-shaped patch on the leg shows erythema and vesicles.

talia after contact with the hands. Of equal importance is that the allergen may be something to which the patient has been exposed for years. Once contact allergy to a chemical develops, the potential to react to that chemical persists for many years.

The epidermis shows hyperkeratosis and parakeratosis with mild to moderate acanthosis and spongiosis. The prickles between epidermal cells are easily visible and intraepidermal spongiotic microabscesses occur (Fig. 16-2). The surface of the epidermis may be covered with crust and cellular debris. The small vessels of the papillary dermis are dilated, and a perivascular infiltrate of lymphocytes and histiocytes is present. Occasionally, eosinophils may be present but often they are absent. Spongiosis and exocytosis of lymphocytes into the epidermis are present within 6 hours after exposure to an allergen in experimental contact dermatitis.[2]

Nummular Dermatitis

Nummular dermatitis shows coin-shaped patches of dermatitis (Fig. 16-3) involving predominantly the extremities in a symmetric pattern. The legs and the dorsal aspects of the hands are commonly affected. The coin-shaped areas, which appear swollen and elevated above the surface of the surrounding skin, are often studded with tiny vesicles, which can be seen clinically. Crusting and secondary infection are common. Often the surrounding skin appears dry and scaly.

The epidermis shows hyperkeratosis and crusting. A characteristic change is the presence of spotty parakeratosis manifested by small mounds of parakeratotic scale occurring in an interrupted pattern across the surface of the epidermis. Moderate acanthosis and spongiosis occur, often with the formation of spongiotic microabscesses (Fig. 16-4). The dermis contains a patchy perivascular infiltrate of lymphocytes, histiocytes, and eosinophils. Diseases associated with spotty parakeratosis include nummular dermatitis, pityriasis rosea, pityriasis lichenoides chronica, seborrheic dermatitis, autoeczematous dermatitis, guttate psoriasis, and pityriasis rubra pilaris.

Pityriasis Rosea

Pityriasis rosea typically involves the trunk and proximal extremities of young healthy adults in the second or third decade of life. An initial lesion known as a herald patch often precedes the main rash by 1 to several days (Fig. 16-5). Multiple scaly papules and plaques with an oval appearance tend to show a symmetric dermatome pattern. When the patient's back is observed from a distance the rash may have a characteristic "Christmas tree" distribution. Individual oval patches have a peripheral collarette of fine scale. The rash of pityriasis rosea generally lasts 4 to 6 weeks and rarely recurs. Although a viral etiology has been suggested, the exact cause remains unknown.

The stratum corneum shows mild hyperkeratosis and spotty parakeratosis (Fig. 16-6). The epidermis is mildly acanthotic with elongation of rete ridges. Spongiosis is usually focal and may occur beneath a mound of parakeratosis. Small spongiotic vesicles occur in half of the cases.[3] A patchy infiltrate of lymphocytes surrounds dilated dermal vessels, which often show extravasation of red blood cells.

Autosensitization Dermatitis

Autoeczematous dermatitis, also known as an id reaction, is thought to represent an allergic eczematous reaction to an acute dermatitis on another part of the body, although the specific antigens have not been identified.[4] Often the primary process is stasis dermatitis[5] or acute vesicular tinea pedis. When the primary eruption is treated, the id reaction clears spontaneously. Common manifestations of an id reaction are facial eczema and a vesicular eruption of the hands and forearms. When the primary dermatitis involves the hands and feet, the id reaction may extend proximally up the extremities. Erythema, edema, vesicles, and crusting are common.

The epidermis is often crusted and shows spotty parakeratosis. There is variable acanthosis associated with spongiotic vesi-

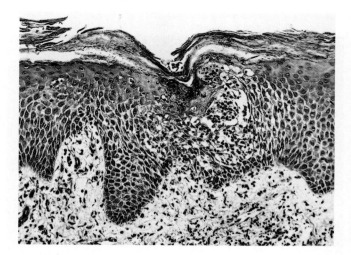

Fig. 16-4. Nummular dermatitis. Both acanthosis and spongiosis with exocytosis of lymphocytes into the epidermis are present. Spongiosis causes the prickles between epidermal cells to appear prominent and small spongiotic microabscesses are present.

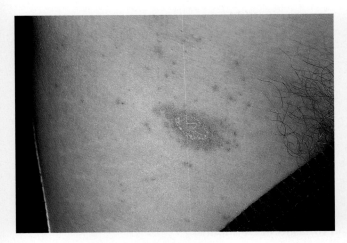

Fig. 16-5. Pityriasis rosea. This elliptical herald patch on the trunk often precedes the more extensive rash.

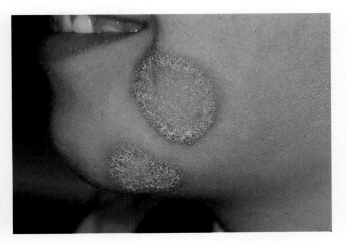

Fig. 16-7. Dermatophyte infection. This ringworm of the face was caused by contact with a cat.

cles and exocytosis of lymphocytes. Edema of the papillary dermis is prominent and may resemble early subepidermal bulla formation. A perivascular infiltrate within the superficial dermis consists of lymphocytes and histiocytes with occasional eosinophils.

Dyshidrotic Dermatitis

Dyshidrotic dermatitis or dyshidrosis is a common form of eczema that is characterized by tiny deep-seated vesicles along the margins of the fingers and toes and on the palms and soles.[6] The rash is characterized by a waxing and waning course that often shows exacerbations during times of emotional stress. The vesicular lesions progress through pustular, erosive, and scaly stages and finally resolve within a period of 1 to 3 weeks, only to recur at a later time.

There is focal hyperkeratosis with parakeratosis. Spongiosis

is often prominent with the formation of small and large intraepidermal vesicles. Erosions and crusting may be present. A perivascular infiltrate within the superficial dermis consists of lymphocytes, eosinophils, and occasional neutrophils.

Dermatophyte Infection

Dermatophyte infections, particularly of the feet and intertriginous areas, may show vesicles and pustules with or without accompanying scale. Small pustules are also occasionally seen with monilia infections. Involvement of the trunk, extremities, or face may produce annular, scaly lesions; hence the name ringworm (Fig. 16-7).

Hyperkeratosis and parakeratosis are often associated with intraepidermal spongiotic vesicles.[7] Neutrophils are present within the vesicles and often produce small pustules within the stratum corneum (Fig. 16-8). The perivascular infiltrate in the

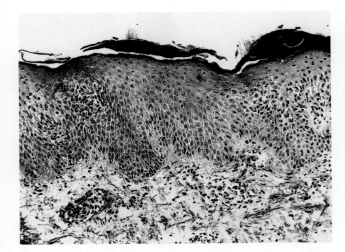

Fig. 16-6. Pityriasis rosea. Small mounds of parakeratosis (spotty parakeratosis) are associated with mild acanthosis, spongiosis, and exocytosis of inflammatory cells. A superficial perivascular infiltrate of lymphocytes is often associated with extravasation of red blood cells.

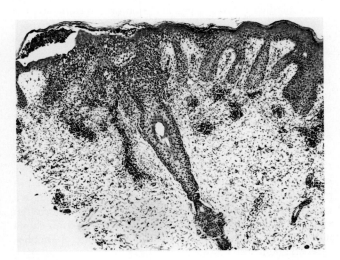

Fig. 16-8. Pustular tinea infection. A subcorneal pustule contains neutrophils. The adjacent epidermis shows acanthosis, spongiosis, and exocytosis of inflammatory cells. PAS stain demonstrated hyphae within the pustule and the stratum corneum.

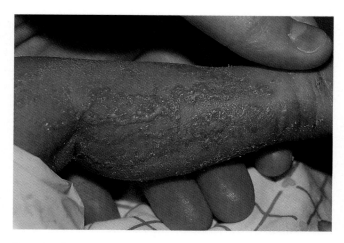

Fig. 16-9. Incontinentia pigmenti. The first stage shows linear vesicles on the extremities from birth to 2 weeks of age.

superficial dermis includes lymphocytes, histiocytes, and some neutrophils. Periodic acid-Schiff (PAS) stain with diastase predigestion demonstrates fungal hyphae within the stratum corneum and pustules.

Incontinentia Pigmenti

Incontinentia pigmenti is a sex-linked dominant disorder that affects predominantly females.[8] Males are involved so severely that they are usually aborted. The skin eruption, which has three stages, begins between birth and 2 weeks of age with erythema and linear vesiculation that involves mainly the extremities (Fig. 16-9). The second stage, from 2 to 6 weeks of age, is characterized by verrucous nodules predominantly on the extremities that may heal with atrophy and hypopigmentation. Atypical cases may present with verrucous lesions at birth. The third stage, which begins between 12 and 26 weeks of age, shows splashes of macular pigmentation on the trunk and less often the extremities. The brown pigmentation is often arranged in a whorled pattern resembling marble cake. By early adulthood, most of the pigmentary changes have resolved. Although most infants with incontinentia pigmenti show only cutaneous involvement, some may have severe mental retardation and other congenital abnormalities of the skeletal system, central nervous system (CNS), eyes, and teeth.[9]

Hyperkeratosis and parakeratosis are absent or mild. There is mild acanthosis associated with prominent spongiosis of the epidermis and exocytosis of large numbers of eosinophils into the spongiotic vesicles (Fig. 16-10). This inflammatory pattern, known as eosinophilic spongiosis, was originally described in pemphigus vulgaris.[10] Eosinophilic spongiosis may be seen in a number of other disorders. Dyskeratotic keratinocytes are often scattered within the epidermis. The superficial dermis shows mild papillary edema and a perivascular infiltrate of lymphocytes and numerous eosinophils.

Differential Diagnosis of Spongiotic Dermatitis

It is often not possible to distinguish between allergic contact dermatitis, dyshidrotic dermatitis, autoeczematous dermatitis,

and nummular dermatitis on the basis of the histologic changes. With clinical correlation, however, the distinction can usually be made. Small mounds of parakeratosis (spotty parakeratosis) are seen predominantly in pityriasis rosea, nummular dermatitis, pityriasis lichenoides chronica, seborrheic dermatitis, and pityriasis rubra pilaris. Eosinophilic spongiosis is a reaction pattern characterized by eosinophils within a spongiotic epidermis.[11] Although this reaction is characteristic of incontinentia pigmenti, it may also be seen in a number of other disorders. Dermal eosinophils are almost uniformly present in nummular dermatitis, autoeczematous dermatitis, and allergic drug eruptions but are uncommon in allergic contact dermatitis, pityriasis rosea, seborrheic dermatitis, and pityriasis lichenoides chronica.

Psoriasiform Dermatitis

Psoriasiform dermatitis is characterized by prominent parakeratosis and by acanthosis with uniform elongation and clubbing of rete ridges. Neutrophils can often be seen extravasating from dilated vessels of the papillary dermis.[12] Exocytosis of neutrophils into the epidermis is associated with parakeratosis and Munro's microabscesses. Although a large number of inflammatory dermatoses may show a psoriasiform reaction pattern, psoriasiform changes are most characteristic of psoriasis, Reiter's syndrome, seborrheic dermatitis, pityriasis rubra pilaris, and chronic neurodermatitis.[13]

Psoriasis

Psoriasis is a chronic papulosquamous disease that typically involves the scalp, groin, and extensor aspects of the extremities. Occasionally patients with psoriasis develop generalized erythroderma. Psoriasis and Reiter's syndrome are exacerbated by infection with the human immunodeficiency virus (HIV).[14,15] The typical lesion is a beefy-red plaque of the elbows or knees that is covered by a thick silvery scale (Fig. 16-11). Kinetic studies of skin in patients with psoriasis show a rapid turnover

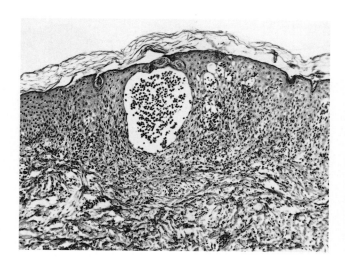

Fig. 16-10. Incontinentia pigmenti. An intraepidermal spongiotic vesicle contains numerous eosinophils. Spongiosis and exocytosis of eosinophils are present in the adjacent epidermis.

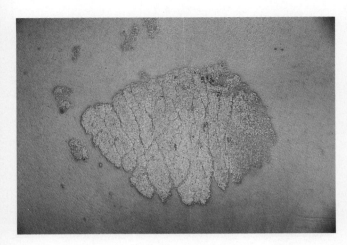

Fig. 16-11. Psoriasis. A geographic red plaque is covered by a thick silvery scale.

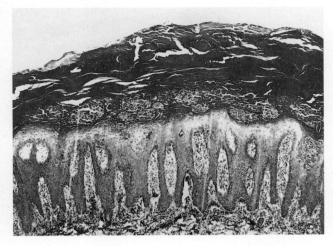

Fig. 16-13. Pustular psoriasis. There is marked hyperkeratosis, parakeratosis, and regular acanthosis of the epidermis with clubbing and fusion of rete ridges. Immediately superficial to the stratum malpighii are numerous spongiform pustules of Kogoj.

rate of psoriatic epidermis.[16,17] Psoriasis may occur in areas of trauma such as scratches (Koebner phenomenon). Discrete pitting of the fingernails and toenails is common. Psoriatic arthritis characteristically affects the distal interphalangeal joints, but larger joints may also be involved. The rheumatoid factor test is negative. Guttate psoriasis is characterized by the sudden onset of numerous 4 to 5 mm papular scaly lesions following an infection with beta-hemolytic streptococcal infection.[18] Other variants of psoriasis include a pustular eruption localized to the palms and soles (pustular psoriasis of Barber) and an acute widespread pustular eruption associated with marked constitutional symptoms (pustular psoriasis of von Zumbusch)[19] (Fig. 16-12).

A biopsy specimen of a plaque of psoriasis shows marked hyperkeratosis, parakeratosis, and a thin or absent granular cell layer. There is uniform acanthosis with elongation, clubbing, and fusion of rete ridges. Dermal papillae appear edematous and contain dilated vessels. The malpighian layer is thinned over the dermal papillae, and exocytosis of neutrophils frequently

occurs in this area. In about 75 percent of the biopsy specimens, Munro's microabscesses containing pyknotic neutrophils are present in the stratum corneum.[20] A patchy perivascular infiltrate of lymphocytes, histiocytes, and a variable number of neutrophils is localized to the superficial dermis. The classic changes just described are only present in a relatively small percentage of biopsy specimens.[21] In pustular psoriasis, numerous neutrophils are present in the superficial malpighian layers and the stratum corneum. There are subcorneal pustules containing neutrophils and Munro's microabscesses may be numerous. Neutrophils within the superficial malpighian layer often produce a sponge-like appearance due to intracellular edema and the presence of residual plasma membranes of keratinocytes. These multilocular pustules seen in pustular psoriasis have been

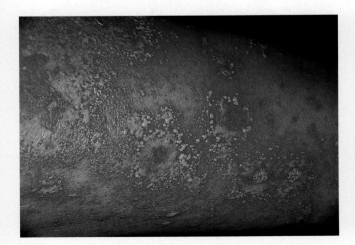

Fig. 16-12. Pustular psoriasis of von Zumbusch. Tiny pustules stud a fiery red rash in a patient with fever and leukocytosis.

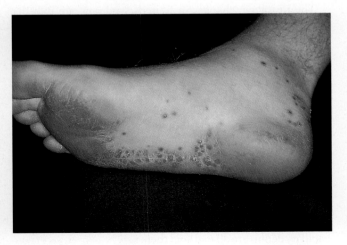

Fig. 16-14. Reiter's syndrome. Keratoderma blenorrhagica of the sole causes hyperkeratosis and pustules.

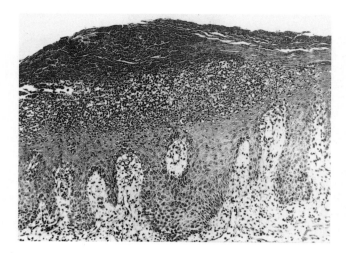

Fig. 16-15. Reiter's syndrome. The hyperkeratosis, parakeratosis, and spongiform pustules within the superficial epidermis are indistinguishable from pustular psoriasis.

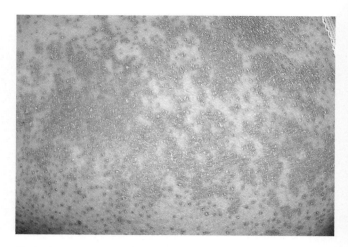

Fig. 16-16. Pityriasis rubra pilaris. Follicular papules coalesce into plaques with islands of spared skin.

referred to as spongiform pustules of Kogoj (Fig. 16-13). In guttate psoriasis the parakeratosis often occurs in discrete mounds and the rete ridge elongation is pronounced.

Reiter's Syndrome

Reiter's syndrome is characterized by the triad of arthritis, urethritis, and conjunctivitis. Some cases may be associated with diarrhea rather than with urethritis. Approximately 80 percent of affected patients have mucocutaneous lesions, including an acral eruption that resembles pustular psoriasis of the palms and soles.[22] The eruption of the palms and soles has been called keratoderma blenorrhagica (Fig. 16-14). Additional characteristic features include nail dystrophy, geographic tongue, and an erythematous, pustular eruption of the corona of the glans penis known as balanitis circinata. Arthritis is frequently the most prominent component of the syndrome. Reiter's syndrome, pustular psoriasis, and psoriatic arthritis are associated with an increased incidence of HLA-B27 antigen.[14]

The histologic changes in Reiter's syndrome are indistinguishable from pustular psoriasis (Fig. 16-15). Spongiform pustules are common. Biopsy specimens of geographic tongue and balanitis circinata also show spongiotic pustules.[23–25]

Seborrheic Dermatitis

Seborrheic dermatitis produces an erythematous scaly eruption of the scalp and less often of the eyebrows, nasolabial folds, presternal area, and groin. Dandruff and itching are the main symptoms. Severe seborrheic dermatitis is occasionally associated with Parkinson's disease.

The histologic changes resemble psoriasis but are less well developed.[26] The epidermis shows hyperkeratosis and parakeratosis, which may be spotty in nature. Mild to moderate acanthosis is produced by rete ridge elongation; however, clubbing and fusion are less marked than in psoriasis. Small vessels in the papillary dermis are dilated, and there may be exocytosis of neutrophils and lymphocytes into the epidermis. Lymphocytes surround small vessels in the superficial dermis.

Pityriasis Rubra Pilaris

Pityriasis rubra pilaris often begins as a scaly eruption of the face and scalp resembling seborrheic dermatitis.[27] Patients develop pink, finely scaly plaques of the trunk and extremities that coalesce leaving intervening islands of normal skin (Fig. 16-16). Other characteristic features include a yellowish keratoderma of the palms and soles and the presence of spiny papules at the openings of hair follicles, which are most prominent on the dorsal aspects of the fingers and in the scalp. Like psoriasis, the epidermal turnover rate is increased. A familial form of pityriasis rubra pilaris has its onset in childhood, whereas the more common acquired type usually begins in middle age.[28] The familial form persists for years, whereas the acquired form improves or clears in 75 percent of patients.[29]

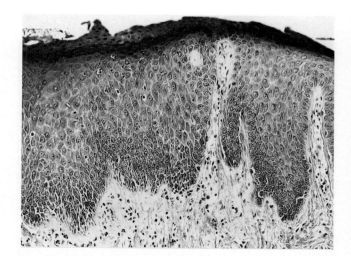

Fig. 16-17. Neurodermatitis. There is hyperkeratosis, parakeratosis and irregular acanthosis without significant spongiosis. There is focal exocytosis of lymphocytes into the epidermis.

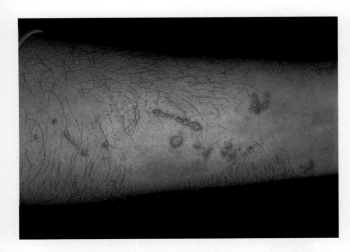

Fig. 16-18. Lichen planus. Koebner's phenomenon is demonstrated by linear scaly papules in response to a minor scratch.

There is hyperkeratosis; however, parakeratosis may be mild or absent. Keratin plugs within hair follicles may project above the surface of the adjacent stratum corneum. The epidermis at the shoulders of involved hair follicles shows spotty parakeratosis, which is referred to as shoulder parakeratosis. The acanthosis and rete ridge elongation are less marked than in psoriasis, and the granular layer is present. The neutrophils and microabscesses of psoriasis are usually absent. There is a mild perivascular infiltrate of lymphocytes in the superficial dermis.

Chronic Neurodermatitis

Chronic neurodermatitis or lichen simplex chronicus shows sharply demarcated plaques of scaly, lichenified, hyperpigmented skin with excoriations. A common site of involvement in men is the lateral leg above the ankle, where as in women the posterior neck and lateral aspects of the arms are more commonly affected.

There is hyperkeratosis and variable parakeratosis. Moderate to marked acanthosis is present, but spongiosis is usually absent or minimal (Fig. 16-17). The acanthosis is often of a psoriasiform type with elongation and clubbing of rete ridges. Neutrophilic microabscesses generally do not occur,[30] and the perivascular infiltrate in the superficial dermis is predominantly mononuclear. There is focal exocytosis of lymphocytes into the epidermis. A characteristic feature is thickening of collagen fibers in the papillary dermis. These reactive fibers are oriented perpendicular to the skin surface. Therefore, chronic neurodermatitis shows hyperplasia of three layers of skin: the stratum corneum, the malpighian layer, and the collagen of the papillary dermis.

Differential Diagnosis of Psoriasiform Dermatitis

Although the histologic changes in psoriasis and Reiter's syndrome are indistinguishable, the clinical features usually allow the proper diagnosis to be made. Spotty parakeratosis in the presence of psoriasiform epidermal changes suggests the diagnosis of seborrheic dermatitis or guttate psoriasis. The histologic diagnosis of pityriasis rubra pilaris can be made 40 to 50

percent of the time based predominantly on follicular plugging and spotty parakeratosis at the shoulders of hair follicles. Thickened collagen fibers in the papillary dermis favor the diagnosis of neurodermatitis. Other disorders such as nummular dermatitis, dyshidrotic dermatitis, and atopic dermatitis may also produce psoriasiform changes.

Lichenoid Dermatitis

Disorders classified as lichenoid dermatitis have epidermal basal cell damage as a primary event and may be associated with other features of lichen planus such as a band-like infiltrate of inflammatory cells that interacts with the epidermis.[31,32] Because of damage to basal zone melanocytes, pigmentary incontinence is common.

Lichen Planus

Lichen planus is characterized by pruritic flat-topped papules that may coalesce to form small plaques. The margins of the papules are often angulated, giving them a polygonal shape. The papules of lichen planus are violaceous and often have a surface with a lacy white pattern known as Wickham's striae.[33] Koebner's phenomenon, the reproduction of the rash by minor trauma such as scratching, occurs in lichen planus as it does in psoriasis (Fig. 16-18). Lichen planus most often involves the volar aspects of the wrists, the trunk, and the mucous membranes of the mouth and genitalia. Approximately two-thirds of the patients with clinically typical lichen planus experience spontaneous involution with a duration of approximately 8 to 15 months.[34–36] Atypical forms of lichen planus may be chronic.

A number of variants of lichen planus have been described: (1) annular lichen planus, which appears to be somewhat more common in blacks; (2) hypertrophic lichen planus,[37] which occurs as persistent, lichenified plaques of the pretibial areas; (3) atrophic lichen planus; (4) bullous lichen planus, which is most

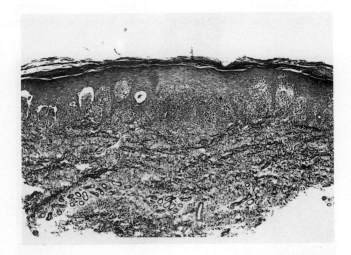

Fig. 16-19. Lichen planus. There is hyperkeratosis, plate-like acanthosis, and a band-like infiltrate of mononuclear cells. Liquefaction degeneration of the basal zone has produced small clefts (Max Joseph spaces) at the dermal-epidermal junction.

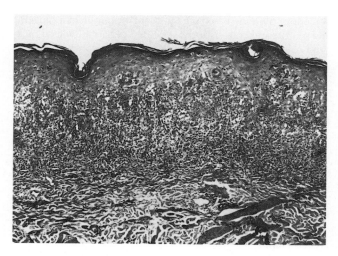

Fig. 16-20. Lichenoid drug eruption (gold). Plate-like acanthosis, liquefaction degeneration of the basal zone, and a band-like infiltrate of chronic inflammatory cells may be indistinguishable from lichen planus. The presence of parakeratosis and eosinophils are helpful distinguishing features.

often seen in individuals with acute eruptive lichen planus; (5) follicular lichen planus (lichen planopilaris), which produces scarring alopecia of the scalp and a spiny follicular eruption of the trunk and extremities due to keratin plugging of hair follicles; (6) mucosal lichen planus,[38] which produces a lacy white pattern or a white speckled pattern on the buccal mucosa with or without painful oral erosions; (7) ulcerative lichen planus,[39] which involves the soles of the feet and/or the mouth and which may be associated with typical lichen planus elsewhere; and (8) ungual lichen planus, which affects approximately 10 percent of patients and produces longitudinal ridging, pterygium formation, or even complete nail destruction.

The histologic changes of lichen planus are often diagnostic. There is hyperkeratosis; however, parakeratosis is uncommon, occurring in less than 15 percent of cases. When parakeratosis

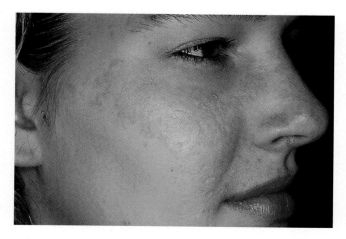

Fig. 16-21. Systemic lupus erythematosus (SLE). SLE shows an erythematous rash on sun-exposed skin of the face.

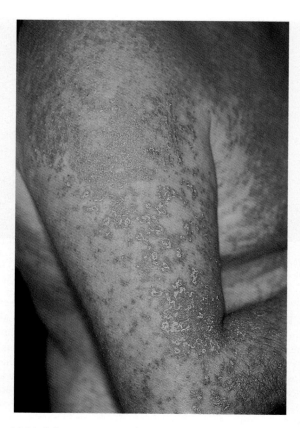

Fig. 16-22. Subacute cutaneous lupus erythematosus. This psoriasiform eruption was precipitated by sunlight exposure.

is present, it is usually mild. Hypergranulosis is present, and occasionally the granular layer may be up to one-half the thickness of the malpighian layer. The acanthosis is plate-like, and the lower margin of the epidermis shows an irregular sawtooth pattern. A key feature, liquefaction degeneration of the basal zone, is present in almost every case.[40] The dermal infiltrate is composed of lymphocytes and histiocytes and has a band-like distribution immediately beneath the basal zone (Fig. 16-19). Plasma cells, neutrophils, and eosinophils are usually absent. Extensive liquefaction degeneration may produce small clefts beneath the basal cell layer known as Max Joseph spaces. Colloid bodies, which measure 5 to 20 mm in diameter, are present in approximately 40 percent of cases of lichen planus as round eosinophilic bodies in the lower epidermis or papillary dermis. Melanin pigment is present within macrophages in the superficial dermis or free in the papillary dermis. Dilated dermal blood vessels, pigmentary incontinence, and the thickened granular layer account for the violaceous color of lichen planus papules. Immunofluorescence studies of skin show globular deposits of immunoglobulin below the dermal-epidermal junction in 95 percent of cases of lichen planus.[33]

Lichenoid Drug Eruption

Lichenoid drug eruptions are associated with gold therapy for rheumatoid arthritis.[33,41] Thiazide diuretics, chloroquine, quinidine, penicillamine, streptomycin, and arsenicals may also

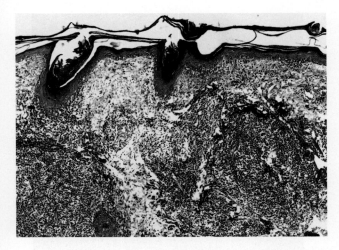

Fig. 16-23. Lupus erythematosus. There is hyperkeratosis with keratin plugging of hair follicles. Liquefaction degeneration is present at the basement membrane zone.

produce a lichenoid dermatitis. The lichenoid dermatitis caused by drugs produces a widespread violaceous papulosquamous eruption that may closely mimic lichen planus. The latent period between the beginning of administration of a drug and the appearance of the eruption is a mean of 12 months for lichenoid drug eruptions.[42]

There is hyperkeratosis with variable parakeratosis. The parakeratosis is often extensive and is a key feature in distinguishing lichenoid drug eruptions from lichen planus. There may be hypergranulosis; however, in the presence of extensive parakeratosis, the granular layer is usually thinned. Plate-like acanthosis of the epidermis is associated with liquefaction degeneration of the basal zone (Fig. 16-20), melanin pigment incontinence, the presence of colloid bodies, and a band-like dermal infiltrate. In addition to lymphocytes and histiocytes, the dermal infiltrate in lichenoid drug eruptions may contain a variable number of eosinophils and occasional plasma cells. The mixture of cell types is helpful in distinguishing lichenoid drug eruptions from lichen planus.

Lupus Erythematosus

Discoid lupus erythematosus (DLE) is a chronic scarring cutaneous eruption of sun-exposed areas.[43] Plaques of DLE typically show central hypopigmentation with a peripheral margin of hyperpigmentation. There is erythema, atrophy, telangiectasia, and keratin plugging of hair follicles. DLE often produces scarring alopecia. Most patients with DLE do not have evidence of systemic disease, although approximately 10 to 15 percent of patients with systemic lupus erythematosus (SLE) may have discoid skin lesions. The skin lesions in SLE are characterized by erythematous papules and plaques on sun-exposed skin (Fig. 16-21). Scarring is usually not a feature of the cutaneous lesions of SLE, which often appear more urticarial. A third form of lupus, subacute cutaneous lupus erythematosus (SCLE) accounts for about 10 percent of lupus cases. It is characterized by a later age of onset, prominent photosensitivity, and nonscarring skin lesions (Fig. 16-22). The skin eruption is either annular, poly-

cyclic and scaly, or psoriasiform in nature. Patients with SCLE may have negative antinuclear antibody (ANA) titers but usually have positive tests for anti-Ro/SSA autoantibody or anti-La/SSB autoantibody. Patients with SCLE usually have a good prognosis with little renal or CNS disease.

A typical skin biopsy specimen of DLE shows hyperkeratosis with absent or minimal parakeratosis. Keratin plugging is often present within dilated hair follicles, which show atrophy of follicular epithelium (Fig. 16-23). The epidermis is usually atrophic but acanthosis occasionally occurs. There is prominent liquefaction degeneration of the basal zone with melanin pigment incontinence. Colloid bodies are usually present within the epidermis or the papillary dermis. A dermal infiltrate of lymphocytes interacts with the basement membrane zone of the epidermis. The dermal infiltrate shows a patchy perivascular pattern in the superficial dermis and surrounds hair follicles in the deep and superficial dermis (Fig.16-24). The basement membrane zone often appears pink and thickened, a feature that is demonstrated even better with the PAS stain. The cutaneous lesions of SLE may show little or no hyperkeratosis and follicular plugging, but epidermal atrophy is typically present. There is liquefaction degeneration of the basal zone associated with pigmentary incontinence and colloid body formation; however, the perivascular and perifollicular dermal infiltrate is usually less marked than in DLE. Prominent vascular dilation and edema of the papillary dermis are often features of SLE. The histologic features of SCLE most closely resemble those of SLE. Two histologic features that help distinguish DLE from SLE and SCLE are the presence of hyperkeratosis and a deep dermal inflammatory infiltrate in DLE.[44] Bullous SLE has a subepidermal bulla with neutrophils that resembles the changes in dermatitis herpetiformis and linear IgA dermatosis.[45]

Lichen Nitidus

Lichen nitidus is an uncommon cutaneous disorder that affects children and young adults.[46] It is characterized by pinhead-sized, white, shiny papules that tend to be grouped on the extremities, genitals, abdomen, and breasts. Oral lesions do not occur.

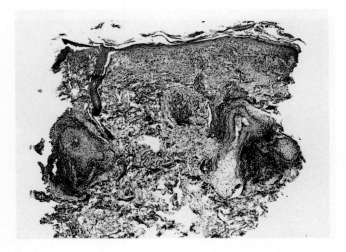

Fig. 16-24. Lupus erythematosus. The distribution of the dermal infiltrate is perivascular and periadnexal.

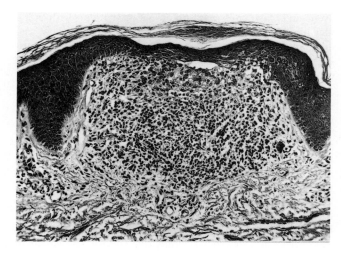

Fig. 16-25. Lichen nitidus. A focal collection of lymphocytes, histiocytes, and multinucleate cells is present between elongated rete ridges. The epidermis shows hyperkeratosis, parakeratosis, atrophy, and liquefaction degeneration.

Individual papules of lichen nitidus are often slightly elevated and show hyperkeratosis and parakeratosis. The epidermis over the center of the papule is atrophic and shows liquefaction degeneration of the basal zone (Fig. 16-25). At the margins of the papules, elongated rete ridges extend downward around the dermal infiltrate, producing a claw-like pattern. The dermal infiltrate is composed predominantly of lymphocytes and histiocytes with occasional multinucleate giant cells and epithelioid cells. The papules are usually small, occupying a space approximately the size of two to four contiguous dermal papillae. Dermal-epidermal separation over the center of the papule may occur. Immunofluorescence microscopy of skin lesions reveals deposits of subepidermal immunoglobulins similar to those of lichen planus in 80 percent of cases of lichen nitidus.[33]

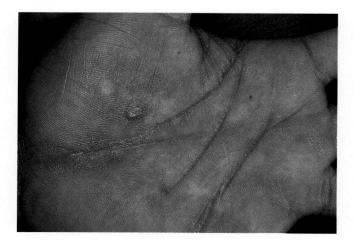

Fig. 16-26. Secondary syphilis. Brown, scaly, hyperkeratotic papules of the palm are characteristic.

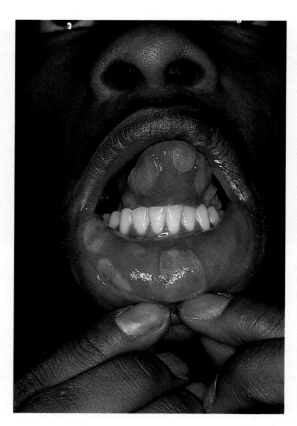

Fig. 16-27. Secondary syphilis. The same patient in Fig. 16-26 shows mucous patches of the tongue and lip

Secondary Syphilis

Although secondary syphilis may mimic a great number of cutaneous disorders, it is most often papulosquamous in character with a predilection for the palms and soles (Fig. 16-26). Widespread cutaneous lesions of secondary syphilis resemble pityriasis rosea, although pruritus is usually minimal or absent. Mucous membrane lesions are common (Fig. 16-27). The primary chancre is still present in approximately one-third of persons at the time the cutaneous rash occurs.

There is variable hyperkeratosis with parakeratosis and irregular acanthosis of the epidermis. An infiltrate of inflammatory cells often obscures the dermal-epidermal junction[47] (Fig. 16-28). Liquefaction degeneration of the basal zone is common. Deep to the band-like infiltrate, the inflammatory cells surround blood vessels that show swollen endothelial cells. Plasma cells are usually present, but in early cases of secondary syphilis they may be absent. The Warthin-Starry stain may demonstrate *Treponema pallidum* within the epidermis or in perivascular areas of the dermis. Although other patterns of inflammation occur with secondary syphilis,[47] the lichenoid pattern is most common.

Lichenoid Keratosis

Clinically, a lichenoid keratosis (lichenoid actinic keratosis, solitary lichen planus-like keratosis) may resemble an actinic

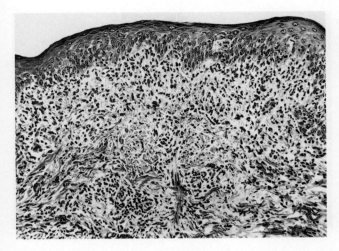

Fig. 16-28. Secondary syphilis. Mild acanthosis and a band-like infiltrate of mononuclear cells interact with the epidermis. A variable number of plasma cells are present.

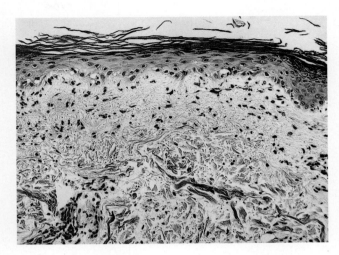

Fig. 16-29. Dermatomyositis. There is liquefaction degeneration of the basal zone associated with melanin pigment incontinence and moderate edema of the papillary dermis.

keratosis or seborrheic keratosis.[48] The characteristic lesion is a flat-topped, slightly scaly, tan to pink keratosis, which is most often located on the chest. The clinical history of a solitary keratotic lesion is very helpful in distinguishing a lichenoid keratosis from true lichen planus. Lichenoid keratoses appear to be caused by inflammation of pre-existing actinic keratoses or other forms of keratoses.

Originally described as solitary lichen planus,[49] lichenoid keratoses may exactly mimic the changes in lichen planus. In many cases, however, there is focal parakeratosis and proliferation of rete ridges with atypical keratinocytes. The atypical keratinocytes involve predominantly the deeper layers of the epidermis and are associated with loss of normal polarity of epidermal cells and individual cell dyskeratosis. Solar elastosis of dermal connective tissue is present in 70 percent of cases.[48] The liquefaction degeneration of the basal zone and the band-like infiltrate of chronic inflammatory cells closely resemble lichen planus; however, eosinophils or plasma cells are more likely to be present in a lichenoid keratosis.

Differential Diagnosis of Lichenoid Dermatitis

The pigmented purpuric dermatoses (progressive pigmentary purpura, Schamberg's disease, lichen aureus) may have a prominent lichenoid inflammatory infiltrate associated with extravasation of red blood cells (RBCs).[50] Cases of graft-versus-host disease often show epidermal atrophy with liquefaction degeneration, colloid bodies, and a lichenoid inflammatory infiltrate.[51] The helpful differential feature is the sparse nature of the infiltrate in graft-versus-host disease due to severe immunosuppression. Poikiloderma atrophicans vasculare and dermatomyositis[53] (Fig. 16-29) may cause diagnostic confusion with SLE. They generally show a sparse lichenoid infiltrate with prominent liquefaction degeneration, pigment incontinence, and vascular dilation. Parapsoriasis en plaques shows focal parakeratosis, mild spongiosis, and liquefaction degeneration of the basal layer. The early stage of cutaneous T cell

lymphoma (mycosis fungoides) cannot be differentiated from parapsoriasis en plaques.[52] Therefore, periodic skin biopsies are useful in individuals suspected clinically of having parapsoriasis en plaques. Halo nevus[54] should be included in the differential diagnosis of lichenoid dermatitis because the dense band-like infiltrate may destroy or obscure the nevus cells.

The differential diagnosis of lupus erythematosus includes lichen sclerosis et atrophicus (LS and A).[55] More than 80 percent of cases of LS and A occur in women. The disorder is characterized by pruritic, white atrophic papules that coalesce into plaques. Individual papules are polygonal and flat topped and may show keratin plugging of hair follicles (Fig. 16-30). The genitalia, neck, and trunk are sites of predilection. When LS and A involves the female genitalia, it is called kraurosis vulvae. Involvement of the glans penis is known as balanitis xe-

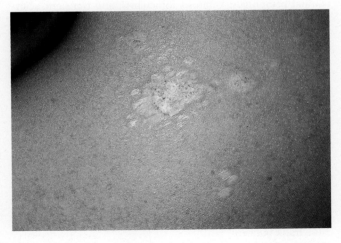

Fig. 16-30. Lichen sclerosus et atrophicus. Flat-topped white papules show keratotic follicular plugs.

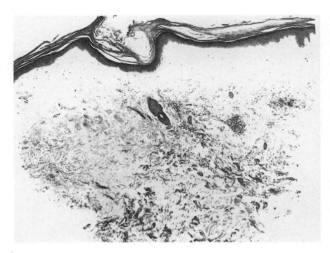

Fig. 16-31. Lichen sclerosus et atrophicus. Hyperkeratosis, follicular plugging, and epidermal atrophy are present. A band of pale-staining edematous connective tissue is present within the superficial dermis.

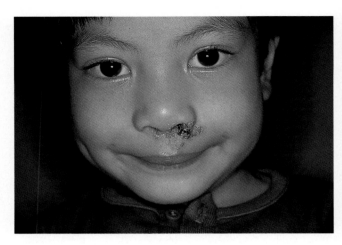

Fig. 16-32. Impetigo. Superficial vesicles around the nares break open to produce erosions and crust.

rotica obliterans. Histologically, LS and A shows prominent hyperkeratosis, resulting in a stratum corneum that may be thicker than the atrophic malpighian layer (Fig. 16-31). Follicular plugging is a common finding. Liquefaction degeneration of the basal zone is associated with incontinence of melanin pigment and in some cases with subepidermal bulla formation. The superficial third of the dermis shows a pale pink amorphous zone in which elastic fibers are absent with the Verhoeff-van Gieson Stain. Dilated blood vessels and a few inflammatory cells may be present in the edematous area. Deep to the area of edema is a band-like infiltrate of mononuclear cells.

Intraepidermal Bullous Dermatoses

Intraepidermal blisters may be produced by a variety of mechanisms: (1) epidermal necrolysis in the staphylococcal scalded skin syndrome; (2) acantholysis in pemphigus, benign chronic familial pemphigus, keratosis follicularis, and transient acantholytic dermatosis; and (3) spongiosis in allergic contact dermatitis (discussed earlier). Viral blisters may show necrolysis, acantholysis, and spongiosis. When biopsying a bullous disease, a newly formed blister should always be selected.

Impetigo

Although most cases of impetigo were previously believed to be produced by beta-hemolytic streptococci,[56] *Staphylococcus aureus* is now recognized as the most common causative agent. The superficial pustules (which occur most often on the face and hands) rapidly break, leaving erosions with honey-colored crusts (Fig. 16-32). The disorder affects predominantly children and young adults. Streptococcal impetigo may be associated with glomerulonephritis if caused by a group A streptococcus with an M antigen.[57] Staphylococcal impetigo is more likely to cause frank bullae.

In impetigo caused by beta-hemolytic streptococci the roof of the blister is formed by delicate stratum corneum. The bulla

contains numerous neutrophils and within the first few hours after onset is more properly termed a pustule (Fig. 16-33). In impetigo caused by S. *aureus* the blister is formed by the same toxin that produces staphylococcal scalded skin syndrome. The blister occurs through or beneath the granular cell layer. A few acantholytic epidermal cells may be seen in the blister cavity in either form of impetigo. The malpighian layer shows moderate spongiosis and exocytosis of lymphocytes and neutrophils. A patchy perivascular infiltrate of lymphocytes, histiocytes, and neutrophils is present in the superficial dermis. Older lesions may show only erosions covered by crust and cellular debris.

Staphylococcal Scalded Skin Syndrome

Staphylococcal scalded skin syndrome is an acute febrile disease seen predominantly in infants and children.[58] It is produced by

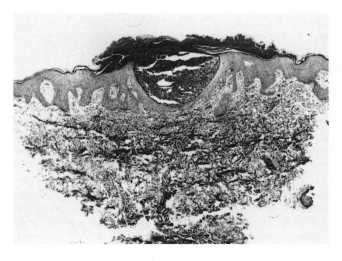

Fig. 16-33. Impetigo. A subcorneal pustule contains numerous neutrophils. The epidermis is covered by a layer of crust.

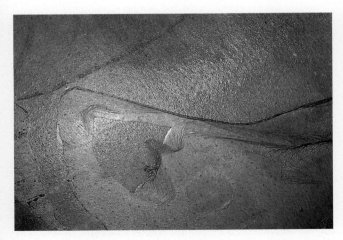

Fig. 16-34. Staphylococcal scalded skin syndrome. The toxin produces peeling of a thin layer of epidermis resembling a scald.

coagulase-positive *S. aureus*, which is often of phage group 2, type 71. The organisms are present in the nasopharynx or throat and produce a toxin that produces painful erythema, followed by desquamation of large sheets of epidermis[59] (Fig. 16-34). When treated with appropriate antibiotics, the prognosis in infants and children is good. An expanded staphylococcal scalded skin syndrome is now recognized that includes localized bullous impetigo, a scarlatiniform eruption, and the scalded skin syndrome, all of which are produced by the same staphylococcal toxin. Staphylococcal scalded skin syndrome occurs rarely in adults[60,61] in which case the prognosis for survival is guarded because the patients may be immunosuppressed or have a serious underlying disease.

The initial change is an intraepidermal blister that forms through or beneath the granular cell layer. Later the entire superficial portion of the epidermis shows extensive necrosis (Fig.

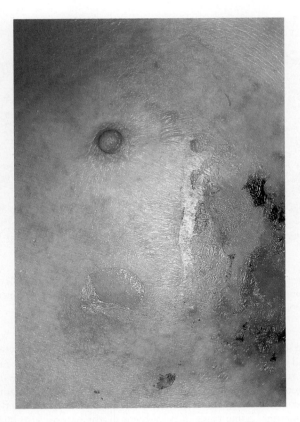

Fig. 16-36. Pemphigus vulgaris. Because the blister roof is thin, most patients present with erosions and flaccid blisters.

16-35). The malpighian layer at the floor of the blister is relatively uninvolved, and the dermis shows only a scant inflammatory infiltrate. The use of exfoliative cytology or frozen sections makes possible rapid distinction from Stevens-Johnson syndrome, which shows full-thickness epidermal necrosis.[62]

Pemphigus Erythematosus and Pemphigus Foliaceus

Pemphigus erythematosus produces a crusted erythematous rash predominantly on the face and scalp.[63] The eruption is often confused clinically with seborrheic dermatitis or lupus erythematosus. In pemphigus foliaceus, the individual lesions are similar[64]; however, more extensive areas of the scalp, face, and trunk may be involved, at times producing a resemblance to exfoliative dermatitis. It is likely that pemphigus erythematosus represents a limited form or initial stage of pemphigus foliaceus. Oral lesions are uncommon in both pemphigus erythematosus and pemphigus foliaceus, and the prognosis is much better than in pemphigus vulgaris.

The histologic changes in pemphigus erythematosus and pemphigus foliaceus are identical. Acantholysis of epidermal cells produces a superficial blister, which usually occurs just beneath the granular cell layer.[65] The roof of the blister may be lost in processing. Acantholytic cells are few in number. Often, small collections of pyknotic, dyskeratotic cells are seen in the granular layer, particularly at the openings of hair follicles or sweat ducts. The small vessels of the superficial dermal plexus

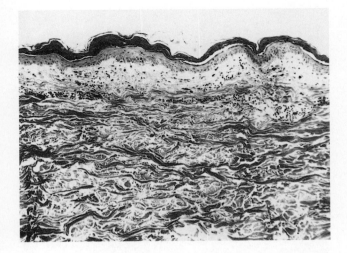

Fig. 16-35. Staphylococcal scalded skin syndrome. The superficial portion of the epidermis is necrotic and amorphous. A sparse perivascular infiltrate of lymphocytes is present in the superficial dermis.

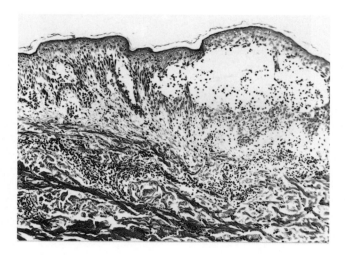

Fig. 16-37. Pemphigus vulgaris with eosinophilic spongiosis. An intraepidermal blister containing numerous eosinophils shows both spongiosis and acantholysis. The adjacent epidermis shows prominent spongiosis and exocytosis of eosinophils.

are surrounded by variable numbers of lymphocytes, histiocytes, and eosinophils. The pattern seen on immunofluorescence microscopy is similar to that seen in pemphigus vulgaris. The intercellular fluorescence in pemphigus erythematosus and foliaceus, however, may be limited to the superficial portion of the epidermis. Some cases of pemphigus erythematosus also have shown a granular pattern of immunofluorescence at the basement membrane zone, suggesting a relationship between this disorder and lupus erythematosus.[66]

Pemphigus Vulgaris

In approximately one-third of cases, pemphigus vulgaris begins as painful oral blisters that rapidly ulcerate. The oral lesions show little tendency to heal and are associated with difficulty eating and drinking, resulting in weight loss and dehydration. The cutaneous rash may be limited to a few lesions or may involve large areas of skin (Fig. 16-36). Because the blister roofs are thin, the blisters appear flaccid and break easily, leaving areas of erosions and crusts. Rubbing the skin gently at the margin of a blister often causes it to extend (Nikolsky sign). Before the advent of systemic corticosteroids and other immunosuppressive agents, pemphigus vulgaris was considered to be uniformly fatal. Patients with pemphigus have an increased incidence of thymoma and myasthenia gravis.[67]

Early changes in a nonbullous area may show spongiosis and exocytosis of eosinophils[11] known as eosinophilic spongiosis (Fig. 16-37). Intact blisters demonstrate acantholysis of epidermal cells producing a blister cavity that forms immediately above the basal cell layer. The roof of the blister usually appears viable; however, older lesions may show necrosis and crusting. The blister cavity contains individual acantholytic cells and clumps of acantholytic cells. Inflammatory cells within the blister cavity include lymphocytes and a variable number of eosinophils and neutrophils. Dermal papillae lined by a single row of basal cells, known as villi, project into the base of the blister cavity (Fig. 16-38). The single row of basal cells often

becomes separated from each other laterally producing the appearance of a "row of tombstones." The dermal inflammatory infiltrate is usually mild and consists of lymphocytes, and a few eosinophils. Direct immunofluorescence microscopy shows an intercellular immunofluorescence pattern. The autoantibodies are usually of the IgG class and complement is often present. Circulating autoantibodies can also be identified by the indirect immunofluorescence technique; however, their serum levels do not necessarily parallel the course of the disease. The pemphigus vulgaris antigen is a newly defined cadherin (calcium-dependent adhesion molecule) that is similar to desmoglein I, the pemphigus foliaceus antigen.[68]

Paraneoplastic Pemphigus

Paraneoplastic pemphigus is a recently described autoimmune disease characterized by painful mucosal ulcerations and skin lesions that include blisters and erosions. The clinical features are more suggestive of erythema multiforme than pemphigus vulgaris. The condition has been associated with a variety of underlying neoplasms such as non-Hodgkin's lymphoma, chronic lymphocytic leukemia, giant cell lymphoma, Castleman's tumor, and benign thymoma.[69] When associated with a malignant neoplasm, the prognosis is poor.[70]

Major histologic features include epidermal acantholysis with suprabasilar cleft or blister formation.[69] Basal layer vacuolization and dyskeratotic keratinocytes resemble that seen in erythema multiforme. Exocytosis of inflammatory cells into the epidermis is common. The acantholysis and dyskeratosis also involve the epithelium of hair follicles and sweat ducts. Melanin pigment is present in dermal macrophages. The dermal infiltrate tends to be polymorphous. Direct immunofluorescence testing shows IgG and complement deposition along the basement membrane zone and/or in an intercellular pattern similar to pemphigus. Indirect immunofluorescence using the patient's serum shows a pattern of antibody deposition typical of pemphigus vulgaris. Immunoprecipitation studies reveal autoantibodies that bind antigens with molecular weights distinc-

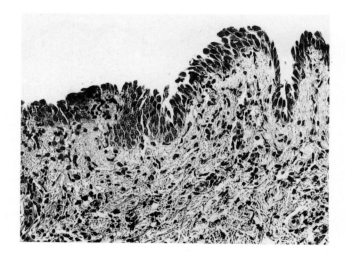

Fig. 16-38. Pemphigus vulgaris. The floor of an intraepidermal blister shows villi lined by one or two layers of epithelial cells.

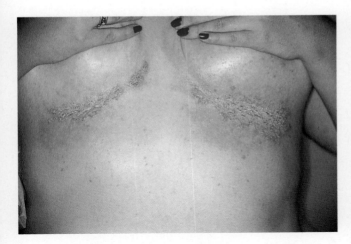

Fig. 16-39. Benign familial chronic pemphigus. These erosions under the breasts were induced by friction.

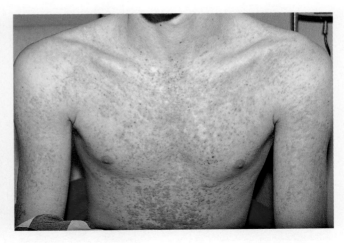

Fig. 16-41. Keratosis follicularis. Widespread keratotic papules often coalesce into scaly plaques.

tive from those of pemphigus. The antigens include desmoplakin I, desmoplakin II, and bullous pemphigoid antigen.

Benign Familial Chronic Pemphigus

Benign familial chronic pemphigus or Hailey-Hailey disease is a chronic bullous eruption that involves predominantly flexural areas such as the neck, axillae, and groin.[70] The disorder is inherited as an autosomal dominant trait and usually begins during the second decade of life. The blisters rapidly break, forming superficial crusted erosions, which become secondarily infected. The disease, which is chronic and recurrent, is aggravated by friction from tight clothing and is often worse in the summer due to heat and maceration (Fig. 16-39).

The acantholysis in Hailey-Hailey disease is marked and may involve almost the entire thickness of the epidermis. The acantholysis of large sheets of epidermal cells often produces a "dilapidated brick wall" appearance. The acantholysis typically occurs above the basal cell layer, and, as in pemphigus vulgaris,

there may be dermal papillae lined by a single layer of basal cells (villi), which extend into the base of the blister cavity. The outer root sheath of hair follicles may be involved with the acantholytic process (Fig. 16-40). Dyskeratosis of individual keratinocytes similar to that seen in Darier's disease may be present but is usually mild. The roof of the blister is viable, and few inflammatory cells are present in the blister cavity unless secondary infection is present. A mild perivascular infiltrate of lymphocytes and histiocytes is present in the superficial dermis. The results of immunofluorescence microscopy in benign familial chronic pemphigus are negative.

Keratosis Follicularis

Keratosis follicularis or Darier's disease is an autosomal dominant disorder that usually has its onset about the time of puberty. It is characterized by keratotic greasy papules and papulovesicles of the face, neck, chest, upper back, axillae, and inguinal areas[71] (Fig. 16-41). In severe cases, the entire body

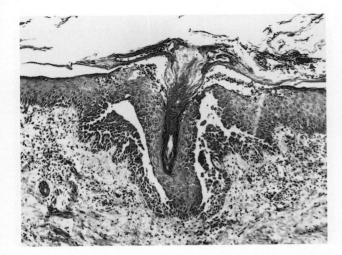

Fig. 16-40. Benign familial chronic pemphigus. Prominent acantholysis extends along the outer root sheath of a hair follicle.

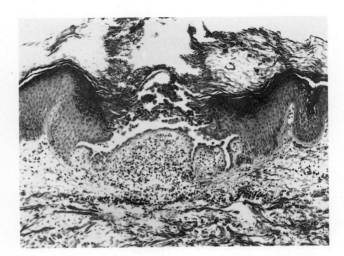

Fig. 16-42. Keratosis follicularis. A suprabasal acantholytic cleft is associated with hyperkeratosis, parakeratosis, and dyskeratotic cells.

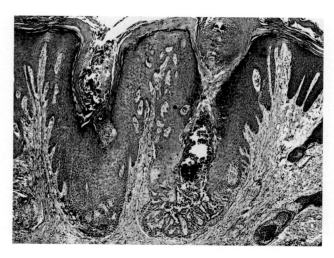

Fig. 16-43. Warty dyskeratoma. Suprabasalar acantholysis and dyskeratotic cells are present within the epithelium of a hair follicle.

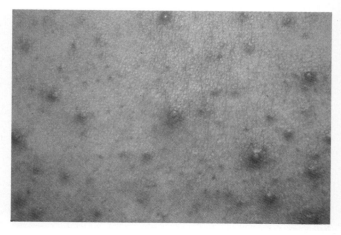

Fig. 16-45. Varicella. Numerous vesicles are in different stages of development.

surface may be affected. Involvement of the oral mucosa[72] and nails also occurs. The disease is chronic and progressive.

There is hyperkeratosis associated with parakeratosis and variable acanthosis of the epidermis. Small clefts containing acantholytic cells occur above the basal cell layer (Fig. 16-42). Two types of dyskeratotic cells are characteristic of Darier's disease. Corps ronds are large dyskeratotic cells with a central basophilic nucleus surrounded by a clear halo, and a cytoplasm that appears densely pink and homogeneous. Grains are densely basophilic with an elongated rectangular or fusiform shape, and resemble a parakeratotic cell of the stratum corneum. Upward projections of dermal papillae lined by a single layer of basaloid cells are prominent in keratosis follicularis. In hypertrophic areas of Darier's disease, the epidermis may proliferate producing pseudoepitheliomatous hyperplasia. The vesicles in Darier's disease usually remain small. Histologic changes essentially identical to Darier's disease may occur in a solitary lesion

known as a warty dyskeratoma.[73] A warty dyskeratoma resembles an enlarged hair follicle with acanthotic epithelium in which acantholytic and dyskeratotic changes of keratosis follicularis occur[74] (Fig. 16-43). The results of immunofluorescence microscopy are negative in Darier's disease and warty dyskeratoma.

Transient Acantholytic Dermatosis

Transient acantholytic dermatosis or Grover's disease typically occurs on the trunk of middle-aged or elderly men as discrete papulovesicular lesions that may itch intensely.[75,76] The patient's general health is good, and no evidence of pemphigus, Hailey-Hailey disease, or Darier's disease is present. Although original reports suggested that all cases resolved within weeks to months, it is now apparent that some cases may persist for several years.[77]

The characteristic change in transient acantholytic der-

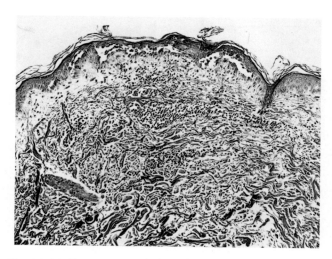

Fig. 16-44. Transient acantholytic dermatosis. Tiny suprabasalar acantholytic clefts occur in an interrupted pattern within the epidermis.

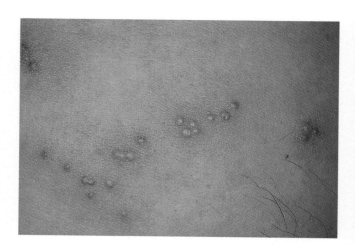

Fig. 16-46. Herpes zoster. There is a linear arrangement of vesicles with an erythematous base. Patients complain of localized pain.

matosis is a tiny suprabasal cleft containing acantholytic cells and occasionally dyskeratotic cells (Fig. 16-44). Three histologic patterns have been described, with the histologic changes resembling either pemphigus vulgaris, benign familial chronic pemphigus, or keratosis follicularis.[77] The changes in Grover's disease differ from these three disorders by showing multiple tiny discrete foci of epidermal involvement. More than one pattern may be present in an individual patient, and focal areas of spongiosis are occasionally noted. The results of immunofluorescence microscopy are negative.

Varicella, Herpes Zoster, and Herpes Simplex

Varicella or chickenpox is characterized by a widespread vesicular eruption that usually occurs in children or young adults. The vesicles and bullae are located predominantly on the trunk and face, although there may be spread to the extremities. Lesions are in all stages of development and resolution (Fig. 16-45). Re-exposure to the varicella virus or reactivation of latent varicella virus in individuals previously infected results in herpes zoster. In most cases, the virus appears to extend from cranial nerve ganglia or spinal nerve ganglia to the peripheral nerves of the skin. Usually, only one or two peripheral nerves are involved, producing a linear rash extending from the spinal cord in a dermatome distribution or involving one or more of the three branches of the trigeminal nerve. The characteristic lesions are grouped vesicles on an erythematous base, which rapidly become pustular (Fig. 16-46). The pustules heal over a 1 to 2 week period, often leaving varioliform scars. Recurrent herpes simplex infection most often involves the lips or genitalia. After the initial infection, which may be extensive or completely asymptomatic, recurrent lesions are typically localized to small groups of vesicles and pustules on an edematous swollen base (Fig. 16-47). Periodic recurrence of the lesions often is associated with fatigue, sunburn, windburn, or upper respiratory infection. Sexual contact may stimulate recurrence of genital lesions. Like herpes zoster, the virus is believed to reside in cranial nerve ganglia or dorsal root ganglia of the spinal cord with subsequent extension to the cutaneous nerves and skin.

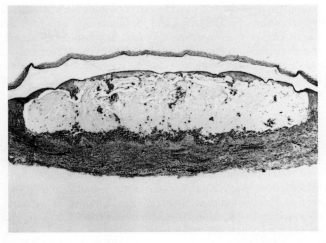

Fig. 16-48. Herpes zoster. An intraepidermal blister shows severe necrosis of epidermal cells associated with acantholysis. Multinucleate viral giant cells are often present within the vesicle.

The histologic changes in varicella, herpes zoster, and herpes simplex are essentially identical with the exception that the associated dermal inflammatory infiltrate tends to be less marked in varicella and most severe in recurrent herpes simplex.[78] An intraepidermal blister shows severe necrosis of epidermal cells with areas of spongiosis and acantholysis (Fig. 16-48). The necrosis of epidermal cells may be secondary to ballooning degeneration, which produces a marked increase in homogeneous eosinophilic cytoplasm. The ballooned epidermal cells lose their intercellular bridges and become acantholytic. Reticular degeneration results from marked intracellular edema with rupture of cell walls producing a reticulated multilocular blister. Large multinucleate viral giant cells are common in all three disorders. Eosinophilic intranuclear viral inclusions are often seen in the ballooned cells and in the multinucleate cells. The inclusions are approximately 5 mm in diameter. An intense infiltrate of lymphocytes, histiocytes, and neutrophils associated with prominent vascular dilation is most marked in herpes simplex but is also seen in herpes zoster and varicella. The intense infiltrate at the base of the blister may resemble vasculitis.

Differential Diagnosis of Intraepidermal Bullous Dermatoses

Suprabasilar acantholysis often occurs in actinic keratoses and should not be confused with acantholytic diseases such as pemphigus or Darier's disease. An important distinguishing feature is the presence of atypia of the cells of the deeper epidermis in actinic keratosis and the presence of associated actinic changes in the underlying connective tissue. It should be kept in mind that any cutaneous eruption with numerous neutrophils can produce acantholysis possibly due to the effects of lysosomal enzymes on the cohesion of epidermal cells. Pemphigus vulgaris, benign familial chronic pemphigus, and keratosis follicularis may be difficult to distinguish histologically. Of the three disorders, benign familial chronic pemphigus shows the most striking acantholysis with involvement of the full thickness of epithelium, whereas keratosis follicularis shows the most

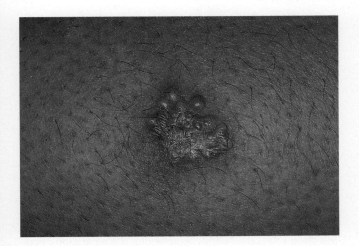

Fig. 16-47. Herpes simplex. Grouped vesicles or pustules on an erythematous base typically recur in the same area.

prominent dyskeratosis. In addition, keratosis follicularis shows hyperkeratosis, parakeratosis, and papillomatosis, which are often lacking in the other two disorders. In pemphigus vulgaris, the acantholysis is often limited to the suprabasal layer and areas of eosinophilic spongiosis may be seen. Spongiotic bullae, discussed earlier in this chapter (Fig. 16-2), are among the most common causes of intraepidermal blisters.

Subepidermal Bullous Dermatoses

When selecting a biopsy site in a patient with a bullous disease, a small relatively new lesion should be selected, and skin adjacent to the blister should be included in the biopsy specimen. Older lesions that have become necrotic, pustular, and crusted tend to show less characteristic changes. A biopsy for immunofluorescence microscopy should be from perilesional skin and should not include the blister.

Bullous Pemphigoid

Bullous pemphigoid has also been referred to as bullous disease of the aged because of its propensity to affect older individuals. Pemphigoid is a chronic, relatively benign disease that produces large tense blisters on normal-appearing or erythematous skin (Fig. 16-49). Large urticarial plaques are common. A clinical variant of pemphigoid has small grouped vesicles resembling dermatitis herpetiformis.[79] The blisters tend to involve the axillae and groin and may become quite large. Blister fluid may be clear or hemorrhagic and, unlike pemphigus vulgaris, ruptured blisters show a tendency to heal. Oral lesions are present in one-third of cases,[69] but the mouth is rarely the initial site of involvement. The duration of bullous pemphigoid is from a few months to several years, and it is uncommon for patients to die of the disease unless it is extensive. The previously reported association of bullous pemphigoid with internal malignant tumor was apparently related to the elderly population affected by both pemphigoid and cancer.[67]

A subepidermal blister shows a roof that is formed by the entire epidermis. Unlike erythema multiforme, the roof of the

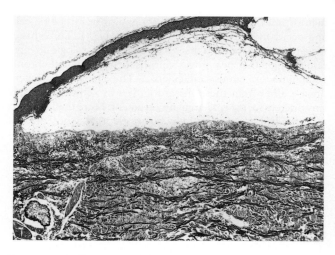

Fig. 16-50. Bullous pemphigoid. A subepidermal bulla has a roof of viable epidermis. A variable number of eosinophils are present within the blister cavity.

blister in bullous pemphigoid remains viable with minimal necrosis of epidermal cells (Fig. 16-50). The blister cavity contains serum and inflammatory cells, including many eosinophils. The extent of dermal inflammation depends on whether the blister occurred clinically on erythematous or normal-appearing skin.[80] A marked infiltrate of lymphocytes, eosinophils, and neutrophils is often present in blisters that occur on erythematous skin. Eosinophilic spongiosis is a common finding in perilesional skin, particularly if an urticarial plaque is biopsied. Blisters located on normal-appearing skin typically show a sparse perivascular infiltrate of lymphocytes and eosinophils. Immunofluorescence microscopy of skin from patients with bullous pemphigoid shows deposition of predominantly IgG, IgM, and complement in a linear pattern at the basement membrane zone. Autoantibodies can also be demonstrated in the patients' serum by the indirect immunofluorescence technique.

Herpes Gestationis

Herpes gestationis is a pruritic bullous eruption that occurs most often during the second or third trimester of pregnancy. Areas of erythema are associated with vesicles and bullae that typically begin around the umbilicus and spread to the lower abdomen and thighs[81] (Fig. 16-51). The palms, soles, and mucous membranes may be involved. Postpartum flares are common. Infant mortality does not appear to be significantly increased.

There is often marked papillary dermal edema associated with a dermal infiltrate of eosinophils and eosinophilic spongiosis. The subepidermal bulla closely resembles bullous pemphigoid. The roof of the bulla is viable and the bulla contains eosinophils. Direct immunofluorescence microscopy shows a linear deposition of C3 along the basement membrane zone and less often IgG. Like bullous pemphigoid, the separation of epidermis from dermis occurs through the lamina lucida of the basement membrane.

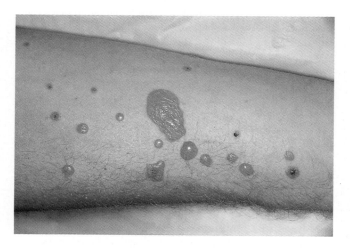

Fig. 16-49. Bullous pemphigoid. Tense blisters may occur on normal appearing skin or in areas of intense erythema.

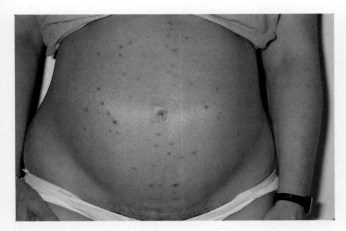

Fig. 16-51. Herpes gestationis. Erythematous papules and vesicles often begin around the umbilicus.

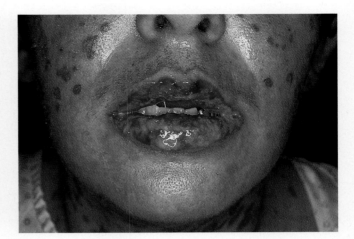

Fig. 16-53. Stevens-Johnson syndrome. In addition to the skin, the eruption may involve the mucosae of the mouth, eyes, and genitalia.

Erythema Multiforme

As the name implies, erythema multiforme may show a variety of clinical lesions, including persistent erythematous plaques, migratory erythemas, polycyclic lesions, vesicles and bullae, target lesions, and extensive mucous membrane involvement. Erythema multiforme is most common between 10 and 30 years of age and frequently follows prodromal symptoms of an upper respiratory infection. The classic cutaneous lesion of erythema multiforme is the target lesion, which has a dusky bluish center and an erythematous margin (Fig. 16-52). The hands and feet are sites of predilection. Severe erythema multiforme with mucous membrane involvement has been called erythema multiforme major or Stevens-Johnson syndrome (Fig. 16-53). Occasionally, severe Stevens-Johnson syndrome may show sloughing of large areas of the skin resembling staphylococcal scalded skin syndrome. It is controversial whether toxic epidermal necrolysis and severe erythema multiforme are part of a spectrum of disease or represent separate entities.[82] Erythema multiforme has multiple causes including infections with mycoplasma, *Histoplasma capsulatum*, and herpes simplex or reactions to drugs such as penicillin and sulfonamides. Approximately 90 percent of erythema multiforme minor is caused by recurrent herpes simplex, which usually precedes the erythema multiforme by 1 to 4 days. The erythema multiforme may recur with each episode of herpes simplex.[83]

So-called epidermal and dermal types of erythema multiforme[84] probably do not occur but represent different stages in the development of lesions. Target lesions may show different zones of involvement with predominantly epidermal centrally and dermal changes at the periphery.[85] Early or nonbullous lesions may show a relatively normal-appearing epidermis; however, dyskeratotic epidermal cells are usually present. Spongiosis with exocytosis of lymphocytes and liquefaction degeneration of the basal zone are often early changes. The

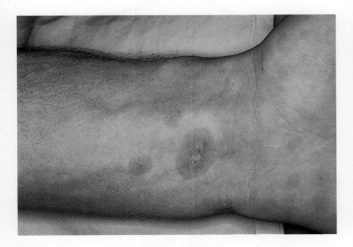

Fig. 16-52. Erythema multiforme. Target lesions have a dusky center and centrifugally spreading erythematous halo.

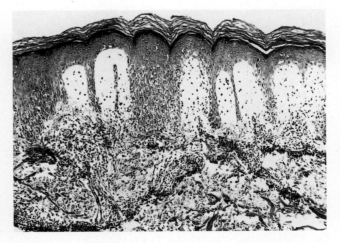

Fig. 16-54. Erythema multiforme. Biopsy of a nonbullous lesion shows marked edema of the papillary dermis associated with exocytosis of lymphocytes and individual dyskeratotic epidermal cells.

spongiosis may cause epidermal cells to appear stretched perpendicular to the skin surface.[86] In early lesions or in the erythematous margin of a target lesion, there is prominent edema of the papillary dermis (Fig. 16-54). A perivascular infiltrate of lymphocytes and histiocytes is present in the superficial dermis. Bullous lesions or the dusky centers of target lesions show subepidermal bullae with prominent necrosis of the blister roof (Fig. 16-55). Individual necrotic keratinocytes may be seen in the blister roof or sheets of necrotic keratinocytes may occur. The blister cavity contains predominantly lymphocytes, although a mixture of inflammatory cells may be present. Although extravasation of RBCs is common, true vasculitis is not seen. A variable infiltrate of lymphocytes and histiocytes surrounds small vessels in the superficial dermis. Lateral to the blister cavity, the changes may resemble those described for early or nonbullous lesions. Immunofluorescence microscopy of skin biopsy specimens shows granular deposits of immunoglobulins and complement within small vessels of the papillary dermis.[87]

Dermatitis Herpetiformis

Dermatitis herpetiformis is characterized clinically by grouped papulovesicles that are extremely pruritic[88] (Fig. 16-56). Vesicles are located symmetrically on the elbows, buttocks, and interscapular areas. Excoriations are common, and intact vesicles may be difficult to find. The eruption clinically resembles scabies. The mean age of onset is about 40 years and men are affected slightly more often than women.[88] The course is chronic with exacerbations and remissions. Although the oral mucosa is not involved, over half the patients have a syndrome characterized by gluten sensitivity, malabsorption, and villous atrophy of the jejunal mucosa. The gluten sensitivity is often asymptomatic. The villous atrophy and steatorrhea are corrected by a gluten-free diet, and if the diet can be maintained for a prolonged period of time, the cutaneous rash may also improve.[89] Sulfapyridine or sulfone drugs are effective in controlling the

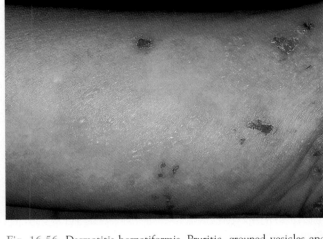

Fig. 16-56. Dermatitis herpetiformis. Pruritic, grouped vesicles and excoriations are present on the extensor aspect of the arm.

rash of dermatitis herpetiformis. Improvement is so dramatic that treatment with these drugs has been used as a diagnostic test. The drugs have no effect on the small bowel involvement.

The subepidermal blisters of older lesions may be difficult to distinguish from bullous pemphigoid. Characteristic changes, however, are seen in new lesions. A subepidermal vesicle shows a viable roof of epidermis. Early vesicles may appear multilocular. The diagnostic changes occur just lateral to the blister where there are accumulations of neutrophils within dermal papillae (Fig. 16-57). The connective tissue of the dermal papillae may show basophilic necrosis and early separation of the epidermis from the dermis producing a crescent moonshaped space. Fragmented nuclei are often seen in the dermal papillae. Although eosinophils may be present, it is the neutrophil that is the most characteristic cell in the dermal papil-

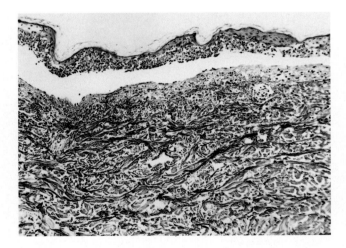

Fig. 16-55. Erythema multiforme. Biopsy of a target lesion from a patient with drug-induced Stevens-Johnson syndrome shows a subepidermal bulla with marked necrosis of the roof. Individual dyskeratotic keratinocytes can be seen in the bulla roof.

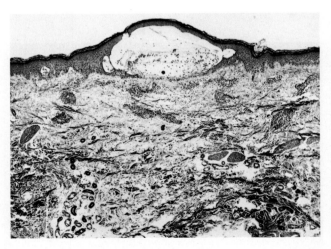

Fig. 16-57. Dermatitis herpetiformis. Adjacent to a subepidermal blister, small collections of neutrophils are present within an edematous dermal papilla. Necrosis of the connective tissue of the dermal papilla has resulted in separation from the epidermis.

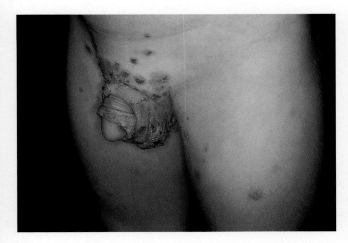

Fig. 16-58. Linear IgA dermatosis. Clusters of bullae are present in the groin of a child.

lae and the blister cavity. Within the superficial dermis, a patchy infiltrate of neutrophils, lymphocytes, and eosinophils is often noted. Immunofluorescence microscopy of a skin specimen shows deposition of IgA in a granular pattern at the basement membrane zone and/or in the papillary dermis.[90] Circulating IgA autoantibodies have been demonstrated. The diagnosis of dermatitis herpetiformis on formalin-fixed tissue

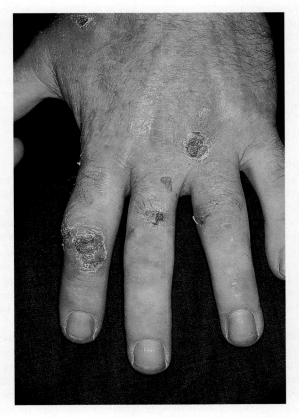

Fig. 16-59. Porphyria cutanea tarda. The dorsal hand shows ulcers and scars associated with skin fragility.

with the use of an avidin-biotin-peroxidase method has been described.[91] It has been suggested that the autoantibodies in dermatitis herpetiformis are antigluten antibodies, which may precipitate in the skin as immune complexes.[90]

Linear IgA Dermatosis

Linear IgA dermatosis was previously called chronic bullous disease of childhood[92] (Fig. 16-58). Linear IgA dermatosis occurs mainly in preschool children but may also affect adults. It clinically resembles dermatitis herpetiformis but more often has annular erythematous patches and grouped bullae that may be sausage-shaped. Gluten sensitivity is absent and the therapeutic response to sulfones is not as good as in dermatitis herpetiformis.

Neutrophils are present along the dermal-epidermal junction, with the formation of microabscesses at the tips of dermal papillae. The resulting blisters are subepidermal and contain neutrophils. Linear IgA dermatosis, dermatitis herpetiformis, and bullous systemic lupus erythematosus all show neutrophils beneath the basement membrane zone. However, in linear IgA dermatosis immunofluorescence microscopy shows a linear pattern of IgA along the basement membrane zone in contrast to the granular IgA pattern seen with dermatitis herpetiformis and the granular pattern of IgG and complement seen in bullous systemic lupus erythematosus.[45]

Porphyria Cutanea Tarda

Porphyria cutanea tarda is characterized by blisters and erosions of sun-exposed skin with secondary scarring, hyperpigmentation milia[93] (Fig. 16-59). Facial hypertrichosis is common. The skin of the chest may develop a sclerotic appearance resembling scleroderma. The photosensitivity appears to be secondary to activation of porphyrin compounds by 4,000 Å ultraviolet light (Soret band). Patients with porphyria cutanea tarda have decreased activity of hepatic uroporphyrinogen decarboxylase.[94] The condition may be precipitated by oral contraceptives or by alcohol ingestion.

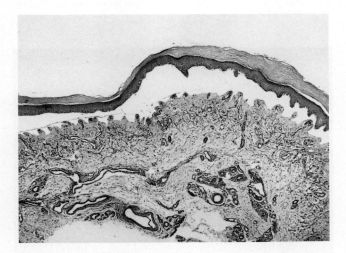

Fig. 16-60. Porphyria cutanea tarda. A biopsy of acral skin shows a subepidermal blister with festooning of dermal papillae into the floor of the blister. This PAS stain demonstrates a hyaline material around the small vessels of the dermal papillae.

Because the eruption is most common on the dorsa of the hands, the stratum corneum is often thickened in a pattern characteristic of acral skin. Linear, pink bodies in the blister roof are composed of basement membrane material and have been referred to as "caterpillar bodies." They are PAS positive and contain type IV collagen similar to the Kamino bodies of Spitz nevi.[94] The subepidermal blister is typically devoid of inflammatory cells. Inflammation is also sparse or absent in the superficial dermis. Dermal papillae protrude into the base of the blister cavity producing finger-like projections (Fig. 16-60). This finding, called "festooning," may also be seen in bullous pemphigoid, cicatricial pemphigoid, and epidermolysis bullosa. A characteristic finding in porphyria cutanea tarda is the presence of pink, hyalinized material around the small vessels of the dermal papillae. The material is PAS positive and diastase resistant and is formed by reduplications of the basement membrane of small vessels and the episodic extravasation of immunoglobulins, complement, fibrin, and other serum proteins. Immunofluorescence microscopy shows immunoglobulins and complement surrounding the small vessels of the papillary dermis[93]; however, these changes appear to be secondary to the vessel wall damage rather than the cause.

Epidermolysis Bullosa Dystrophica

Epidermolysis bullosa represents a group of genetically determined diseases that have been referred to as the mechanobullous diseases because of the production of cutaneous blisters and erosions by minor mechanical trauma.[95] The two severe dystrophic forms of the disease are inherited as either autosomal dominant or autosomal recessive traits. The onset of both diseases is at or shortly after birth, with erosions occurring on the hands, feet, knees, and diaper area after minor trauma (Fig. 16-61). Similar blisters occur in the mouth and pharynx. Many infants die within the first year of life of secondary infection or inability to sustain nutrition. In those who survive, there may be severe scarring with fusion of fingers producing club-like hands (Fig. 16-62). Scarring of the esophagus may produce esophageal stenosis.[96] Growth retardation, iron deficiency anemia, and re-

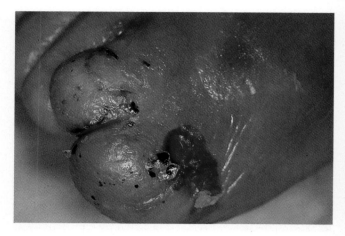

Fig. 16-62. Epidermolysis bullosa dystrophica. This adolescent's hand shows fusion and shortening of fingers with the loss of nails.

current infections are common. Squamous cell carcinomas may develop in cutaneous scars.[97]

The light microscopic changes in the dominant and recessive forms of epidermolysis bullosa dystrophica are essentially identical. The subepidermal blister shows a roof of intact and viable epidermis. There is minimal inflammation, either in the blister cavity or in the underlying dermis. Festooning may be prominent with elongated rete ridges projecting into the base of the blister cavity. Electron microscopy of the recessive form of epidermolysis bullosa shows the separation to occur just beneath the basal lamina associated with an absence of anchoring fibrils.[98] Another form of the disease, epidermolysis bullosa letalis, which occurs at birth and has similar light microscopic changes, shows separation between the plasma membrane of the basal cells and the basal lamina by electron microscopy. The results of immunofluorescence microscopy are negative in all forms of the disease.

Epidermolysis Bullosa Simplex

This form of epidermolysis bullosa is inherited as an autosomal dominant trait and often does not appear until early childhood. However, blisters may be present at birth. The mechanically induced blistering is milder than with the dystrophic forms and is typically limited to the feet and hands. The blisters heal without scarring. Biopsies of fresh lesions or of experimentally induced lesions show cytolysis and vacuolization of the basal cells with the subsequent bulla located above the basement membrane. It is now clear that epidermolysis bullosa simplex results from specific point mutations in the genes for keratin 5 or 14.[99]

Differential Diagnosis of Subepidermal Bullous Dermatoses

Cicatricial pemphigoid or benign mucous membrane pemphigoid may represent a variant of bullous pemphigoid with predominant involvement of the mucous membranes and secondary scarring.[100] The histologic changes are essentially identical to bullous pemphigoid, although dermal fibrosis may be more prominent. Herpes gestationis is a severely pruritic bullous eruption that occurs during the second or third trimester or in the im-

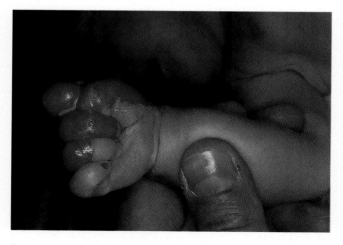

Fig. 16-61. Epidermolysis bullosa dystrophica. A newborn shows loss of the epidermis of the hand caused by minor friction.

mediate postpartum period.[101] In 50 percent of patients the rash begins on the abdomen in a periumbilical distribution. Herpes gestationis produces a subepidermal blister with eosinophils that is usually indistinguishable from bullous pemphigoid. Immunoflourescence microscopy of skin biopsies in herpes gestations shows deposition of the third component of complement and, less often, IgG at the dermal-epidermal junction. The important distinguishing features of the subepidermal bullous diseases are the prominence of eosinophils in the blister cavity in bullous pemphigoid and herpes gestationis; the necrosis of the blister roof with individual necrotic keratinocytes in erythema multiforme; the presence of neutrophils in the blister cavity in dermatitis herpetiformis, linear IgA dermatosis, and bullous systemic lupus erythematosus; and the presence of PAS-positive diastase-resistant material around small vessels in the papillary dermis in porphyria cutanea tarda. In addition, the characteristic immunofluorescence microscopy changes are of great value in distinguishing the various subepidermal bullous diseases.

Dermal Reaction Patterns

Perivascular Dermatitis

Artificial perivascular dermatitis or superficial and deep perivascular dematitis.[102] Clinically, they are often manifested as red annular lesions or red plaques, which have been referred to in general terms as reactive erythemas or gyrate erythemas. Most of these disorders appear to have an allergic basis. Clinically and histologically they have many overlapping features.

Urticaria is characterized by annular to polycyclic erythematous lesions that typically come and go over periods of hours.[103] Arthropod bite reactions are often referred to as papular urticaria because they show a papular area of erythema and edema with a central puncta at the site of the bite. Drug eruptions and viral exanthems typically produce widespread erythematous macular eruptions that may have an annular configuration.

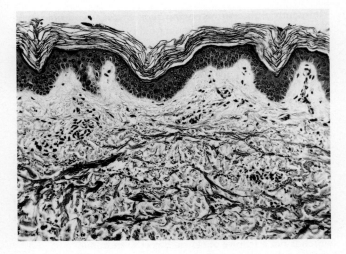

Fig. 16-63. Urticaria. The epidermis is unremarkable. Edema of the papillary dermis is associated with a sparse perivascular infiltrate of lymphocytes, histiocytes, and eosinophils.

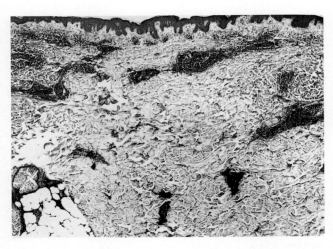

Fig. 16-64. Erythema annulare centrifugum. The epidermis is unremarkable. Dense perivascular cuffing of lymphocytes is present within both the superficial and deep dermis.

When gyrate erythemas appear to be rather fixed and change slowly over days to weeks, they have been referred to as erythema annulare centrifugum[104] or erythema perstans. These disorders have a distinct annular eyrthematous border, which may be palpable. Erythema chronicum migrans is a specific form of reactive erythema that is usually solitary and spreads cetrifugally from a central tick bite.[105] The lesions of erythema chronicum migrans, which enlarge up to 30 cm in diameter, are more common in Europe but do occur in the United States.[106] A skin biopsy of the advancing border shows a normal epidermis and a superficial and deep perivascular infiltrate of lymphocytes and plasma cells. A biopsy from the central papule may show acanthosis and spongiosis. The perivascular dermal inflitrate contains predominantly lymphocytes and eosinophils. Cases of erythema chronicum migrans in the United States are often associated with Lyme disease (described in Lyme, Connecticut), which includes arthritic, neurologic, and cardiac manifestations. The tick *Ixodes dammini* has been shown to transmit a spirochete, *Borrelia burgdorferi*, which causes the cutaneous and systemic symptoms.[107] Erythema gyratum repens consists of multiple waves of gyrate erythema that produce a clinical pattern resembling the grain of wood. The eruption is almost always associated with an internal malignat tumor. Histologically variable hyperkeratosis, parakeratosis, and spongiosis are associated with a nonspecific perivascular infiltrate of lymphocytes and occasional eosinophils.[108] Polymorphous light eruption occurs as erythematous plaques, particularly on the face and arms after sunlight exposure.[109] The eruption, which is more common in the summer, usually occurs within hours after sunlight exposure.[110] A familial form of polymorphous light eruption is common in American Indians.

Superficial perivascular dermatitis is characertized histologically by a perivascular infiltrate of inflammtory cells localized to the superficial dermal plexus. Urticaria, arthropod bite reactions, drug eruptions, and viral exanthems are examples of this type of reaction. In urticaria, the infiltrate is sparse with a mixture of cell types including lymphocytes, histiocytes, eosinophils, and occasionally neutrophils (Fig. 16-63). The pattern of superficial perivascular dermatitis with eosinophils should always suggest the possibility of an arthropod bite reaction or drug eruption. The infiltrate is predominantly lymphocytic in viral exanthems. Viral exanthems, drug eruptions, and arthropod bite reactions may also show spongiosis.

The other clinical disorders described above are more often associated with both superficial and deep perivascular dermtitis with an almost pure infiltrate of lymphocytes (Fig. 16-64). The infiltrate may be very dense and obscure the vascular lumina and endothelial cells. The presence of a dense perivascular infiltrate in the superficial and deep dermis in a biopsy specimen of facial skin with numerous pilosebaceous structures and solar elastosis should suggest the possibility of polymorphous light eruption. Cases of erythema annulare centrifugum that clinically show a peripheral collarette of scale may histologically demonstrate spotty parakeratosis and spongiosis, similar to pityriasis rosea.

Differential Diagnosis of Perivascular Dermatitis

Before a diagnosis of perivascular dermatitis is made, an attempt should be made to rule out other more specific causes of this reaction pattern. Tinea versicolor is a common superficial fungus infection in which the short hyphae and spores are refractile and can often be seen on routinely stained sections (Fig. 16-65). Dermatophyte infections such as tinea corporis also produce a superficial perivascular dermatitis but often show small foci of parakeratosis and neutrophils in the stratum corneum. The hyphae of dermatophytes usually cannot be seen with H&E-stained sections but require the use of PAS or silver methenamine stains. Progressive pigmetned purpura of Schamberg shows a superficial perivascular dermatitis with focal hemorrhage and small amounts of hemosiderin pigment. Macular forms of urticaria pigmentosa show a superficial perivascular infiltrate of mononuclear cells, which on closer examination have a centrally placed nucleus and granular gray to purple cytoplasm. A Giemsa stain is helpful in demonstrating the char-

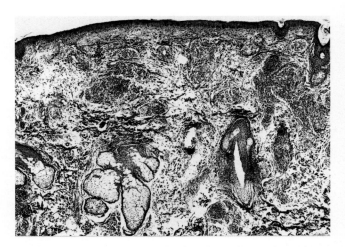

Fig. 16-66. Polymorphous light eruption. The epidermis is unremarkable. Dense patchy infiltrate of lymphocytes is oriented around blood vessels of the superficial and deep dermis.

acteristic mast cell granules. Lymphoma cutis and leukemia cutis often produce a superficial and deep perivascular infiltrate. In chronic lymphocytic leukemia or in well differentiated lymphocytic lymphoma, the lymphocytes do not appear atypical, and it may be extremely difficult to make the correct diagnosis without additional clinical information. Jessner's lymphocytic infiltrate is often listed in the differential diagnosis of superficial and deep perivascular dermatitis. It is possible that Jessner's lymphocytic infiltrate, which produces erythematous plaques or annular infiltrated lesions of the upper trunk or face, represents a variant of polymorphous light eruption (Fig. 16-66) or discoid lupus erythematosus. Occasionally, biopsy specimens of the lesions of lupus erythematosus show little or no epidermal change.

Neutrophilic Dermatoses

The neutrophilic dermatoses include Sweet's syndrome, pyoderma gangrenosum, and rheumatoid neutrophilic dermatosis. Sweet's syndrome (acute febrile neutrophilic dermatosis) is characterized by the abrupt onset of tender or painful erythematous plaques or nodules with frequent bulla formation[111] (Fig. 16-67). The patients are typically middle-aged women who have fever and malaise. There is a peripheral blood neutrophilia and the sedimentation rate is elevated. There is no response to systemic antibiotics but a dramatic improvement follows treatment with systemic corticosteroids.

The epidermis in Sweet's syndrome is often spongiotic and papillary dermal edema may be marked. The dermis contains sheets of neutrophilis with variable leukocytoclasis but no vascuiltis. Some cases of Sweet's syndrome have been associated with leukemia, particularly acute myelogenous leukemia. In most cases associated with leukemia the patient is anemic, which is not a feature of classic Sweet's syndrome.

The early lesions of pyoderma gangrenosa may closely mimic Sweet's syndrome but the clinical course is distinctive and in later lesions the infiltrate is more polymorphous and may be

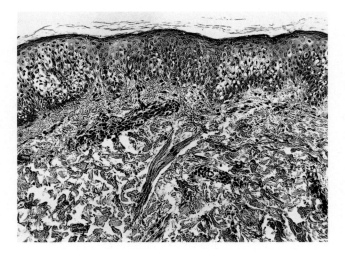

Fig. 16-65. Tinea versicolor. There is mild hyperkeratosis, acanthosis, and spongiosis of the epidermis. PAS stain revealed spores and short plump hyphae.

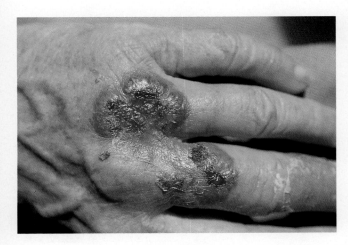

Fig. 16-67. Sweet's syndrome. The dorsal hand shows tender, edematous, hemorrhagic lesions with ulceration.

granulomatous. Rheumatoid neutrophilic dermatosis occurs in association with severe rheumatoid arthritis as symmetric erythematous papules, plaques, and/or vesicles over joints and the dorsal aspects of the hands.[112] The areas of dermal neutrophilic infiltrate tend to be smaller, superficial, and more circumscribed than in Sweet's syndrome. Other conditions such as cellulitis, bowel bypass syndrome, and disseminated gonococcemia may present with dermal neutrophilic infiltrates.

Vasculitis

Vasculitis, which is characterized by the inflammation of small or large blood vessels, may have a broad spectrum of clinical manifestations involving the skin and/or internal organs. In addition to primary destruction of vessel walls, secondary changes such as hemorrhage, thrombosis, and necrosis of tissue supplied by the vessels occur. Vasculitis may be subclassified based on the type of inflammation: (1) neutrophilic, (2) lymphocytic, or (3) granulomatous. Types of vasculitis that involve predomi-

nantly neutrophilic inflammation of vessels include leukocytocalstic vasculitis, erythema elevatum diutinum, infections vasculitis, and periarteritis nodosa. Lymphocytic vasculitis appears to be a feature of some cases of pityriasis lichenoides et varioliformis acute (Mucha-Habermann disease). Granulomatous vasculitis is seen in allergic granulomatosis, Wegener's granulomatosis, and giant cell arteritis.

Leukocytoclastic Vasculitis

Leukocytoclastic vasculitis or allergic vasculitis is characterized by two major clinical syndromes. Henoch-Schönlein purpura is a disorder of children in which prodormal symptoms are followed by abdominal pain, joint pain, and palpable purpura of the skin, mainly of the lower extremities. Leukocytoclastic vasculitis of adults has a more varied clinical picture. It may involve only the skin, only visceral organs, or both. The numerous causes include bacterial, viral, and mycoplasma infections; drug eruptions; and collagen vascular diseases.[113] The characteristic skin lesion in both children and adults in palpable purpura, which has a predilection for the legs (Fig. 16-68). Urticarial vasculitis shows relatively fixed urticarial lesions with fine purpura. Serum complement levels are typically depressed.

The epidermis in leukocytoclastic vasculitis varies from normal to necrotic depending on the severity of the vascular changes. The characteristic vascular changes involve the small postcapillary venules of the superficial vascular plexus. Vessel walls are necrotic, neutrophils are present within and around vessel walls, and the walls appear to be thickened by deposits of eosinophilic fibrin (Fig. 16-69). Leukocytoclasis or nuclear dust results from the frgementation of the nuclei of neutrophilis. Often, there is hemorrhage and thrombosis of the small vessels. At times, there may be evidence of perivascular fibrosis. In severe cases, the adjacent connective tissue and epidermis may be completely necrotic. Leukocytoclastic vasculitis is an immune complex disease that results when antigen and immunoglobu-

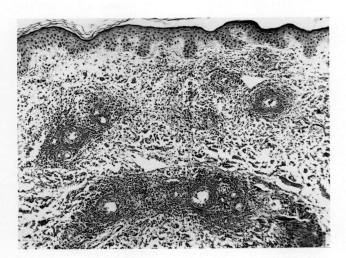

Fig. 16-69. Leukocytoclastic vasculitis. Small blood vessels of the superficial dermis show necrosis of their walls, which are infiltrated by neutrophils. The vessel walls contain fibrin and the surrounding dermis shows leukocytoclasis (nuclear dust).

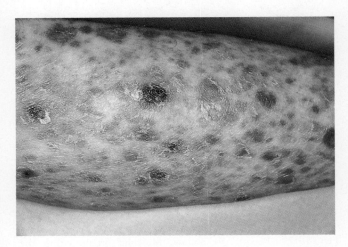

Fig. 16-68. Leukocytoclastic vasculitis. Palpable purpura are present on the leg in this patient with an allergy to sulfa.

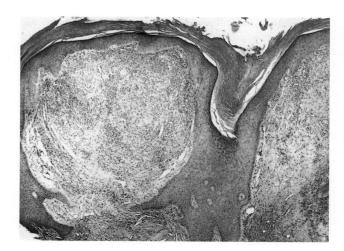

Fig. 16-70. Erythema elevatum diutinum. There is hyperkeratosis, acanthosis, and papillomatosis of the epidermis associated with a dense perivascular dermal infiltrate of neutrophils. The dermal connective tissue appears fibrotic.

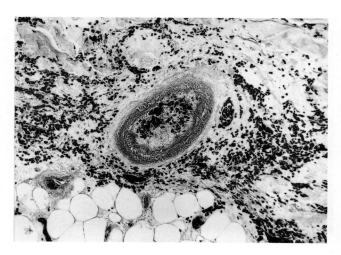

Fig. 16-72. Pseudomonas vasculitis. Blood vessel in the deep dermis shows a hazy thickening of its wall due to infiltration by organisms. The surrounding dermis shows marked hemorrhage but only a sparse inflammatory infiltrate.

lin combine with complement producing complexes within vascular lumina. Direct immunofluorescence of skin samples in leukocytoclastic vasculitis shows granular deposits of IgM or IgG and complement within small vessels of the superficial dermis. In Henoch-Schönlein purpura, the immunoglobulin deposited in the vessel walls is predominantly IgA.

Erythema Elevatum Diutinum

Erythema elevatum diutinum is a rare disease that appears to represent a chronic form of leukocytoclastic vasculitis.[114] Red to brown plaques and nodules involve the dorsa of the hands and feet, as well as the elbows and knees. The disease tends to persist for a number of years.

The epidermis shows variable acanthosis (Fig. 16-70). Neutrophils and nuclear dust are present around and within the

walls of small dermal vessels. A few lymphocytes, eosinophils, and plasma cells may also be present. Endothelial cells appear swollen, and there are deposits of fibrin within vessel walls.[115] Focal extravasation of RBCs may be noted. Fibrosis of dermal connective tissue is more marked than in classic leukocytoclastic vasculitis, and in the late stages of erythema elevatum diutinum the fibrosis may replace the inflammatory infiltrate.

Infectious Vasculitis

Gonococcal and meningococcal infections may produce an acute febrile illness with cutaneous lesions characterized by acral pustules on an erythematous base. Tiny purpura may be present around the edges of the pustules.

The epidermis is often necrotic and infiltrated by neutrophils. Small vessels of the superficial dermis and mid-dermis

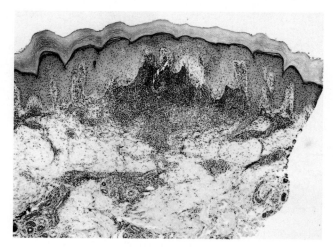

Fig. 16-71. Gonococcemia. Biopsy of acral skin shows intense neutrophilic infiltration and hemorrhage in the superficial dermis.

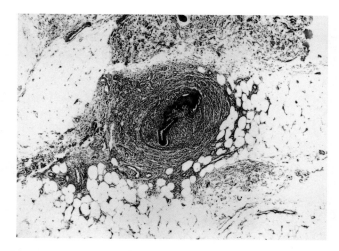

Fig. 16-73. Periarteritis nodosa. Muscular artery within the subcutaneous fat is infiltrated by neutrophils and lymphocytes with partial occlusion of its lumen. There is prominent perivascular fibrosis.

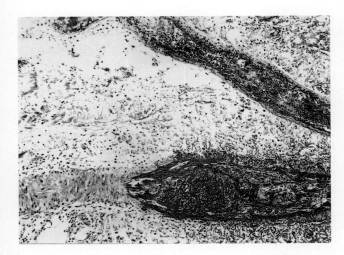

Fig. 16-74. Periarteritis nodosa. Blood vessels in the deep dermis are sectioned longitudinally and show the segmental nature of the involvement.

are surrounded and infiltrated by massive collections of neutrophils associated with nuclear dust, hemorrhage, and vessel wall necrosis (Fig. 16-71). Hemorrhage subepidermal bullae may occur.[116] Organisms are usually not demonstrable by special stains but can be demonstrated by immunofluorescence microscopy.

Pseudomonas or staphylococcal septicemia occurs most often in terminally ill or immunosuppressed individuals. Necrotic ulcers known as ecthyma gangrenosum are characteristic of pseudomonas sepsis.

The epidermis and superficial dermis may be necrotic and pale staining. Inflammatory cells are characteristically sparse or absent. Vessel walls appear thickened and necrotic and have a hazy blue appearance with H&E stain[117] (Fig. 16-72). There may be extensive hemorrhage. Closer examination of the vessel walls with a tissue Gram stain (Brown and Brenn) shows that the blue color noted on H&E stain is caused by the presence of massive numbers of organisms.

Periarteritis Nodosa

Periartertitis nodosa is a form of leukocytoclastic vasculitis that involves small- and medium-sized muscular arteries. The disorder, which is more common in men, affects the kidneys, heart, gastrointestinal tract, liver, lungs, and CNS. Approximately 10 percent of cases of systemic periarteritis nodosa involve the skin, although a purely cutaneous form of the disease also occurs.[118] Immune complexes of hepatitis B surface antigen may play a role in the pathogenesis of some cases of periarteritis nodosa.[119]

The epidermis varies from normal to ulcerated. At the junction of the deep dermis and subcutaneous fat, small and medium-sized arteries show increased thickness of their walls, which are infiltrated with neutrophils (Fig. 16-73). The vessel walls are partially necrotic, and there is thrombosis, hemorrhage, and nuclear dust. The media of the vessels may be replaced by granulation tissue or fibrosis, and the lumina may be partly or completely obliterated. The vascular inflammation is

often segmental, with intervening segments of normal-appearing vessel wall (Fig. 16-74). The surrounding connective tissue shows a mixed inflammatory infiltrate, which often includes many eosinophils.

Pityriasis Lichenoides et Varioliformis Acuta

Pityriasis lichenoides et varioliformis acuta (PLEVA) or Mucha-Habermann disease often begins in children and young adults. Papulovesicular lesions become hemorrhagic and necrotic (Fig. 16-75) and heal over a period of approximately 2 weeks, leaving small scars that resemble the scars of varicella. New lesions continue to develop for years.

The epidermis varies from normal to necrotic (Fig. 16-76). When inflammation is intense, a wedge-shaped area of necrosis of epidermis and superficial dermal connective tissue is present. A dense infiltrate of lymphocytes often completely obscures blood vessels of the superficial dermis and mid-dermis.[120] Lymphocytes and extravasated RBCs extend into the overlying epidermis. The basement membrane zone of the epidermis may be involved in a pattern suggestive of lichen planus.

Allergic Granulomatosis and Angiitis

Allergic granulomatosis of Churg and Strauss is characterized by asthma, pulmonary infiltrates, blood and tissue eosinophilia, mononeuropathy or polyneuropathy, paranasal sinus abnormalities, and a cutaneous rash composed of papules, nodules, purpuric lesions, and ulcers.[121] Cardiac involvement, renal failure, and CNS disease are common causes of death. Most patients with Churg Strauss syndrome have positive tests for P-ANCA, a type of autoantibody with specificity for myeloperoxidase.[122]

The walls of small and medium-sized muscular arteries are infiltrated by neutrophils and show fibrinoid necrosis. Granulomas containing a central area of necrotic collagen and cellular debris are present in the dermis and subcutaneous fat. The necrotic areas are surrounded by epithelioid cells, multinucleate giant cells, and mononuclear inflammatory cells. Eosinophils are often numerous.[123] A small necrotic vessel may be seen in the center of the granulomatous inflammation.

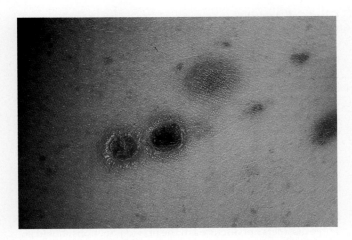

Fig. 16-75. Pityriasis lichenoides et varioliformis acuta. Lesions in different stages of development include hemorrhagic papules and ulcers.

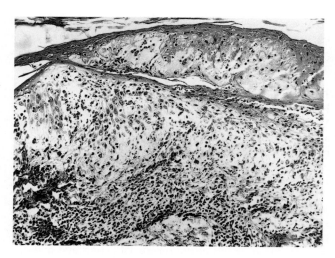

Fig. 16-76. Pityriasis lichenoides et varioliformis acuta. Focally necrotic epidermis is covered with crust and cellular debris. Dense infiltrates of lymphocytes obscure dermal blood vessels and are associated with exocytosis of lymphocytes and red blood cells.

Wegener's Granulomatosis

Necrotizing lesions of the upper and lower respiratory tract, widespread necrotizing vasculitis, and necrotizing glomerulitis with death from renal failure are the main features of Wegener's granulomatosis. The disease may begin as ulcerative lesions of the nose and oral cavity.[124] Cutaneous papulonecrotic lesions and ulcers are present in 25 to 50 percent of cases. About 90 percent of patients with active, untreated Wegener's granulomatosis have positive tests for C-ANCA, autoantibodies that are specific for protease 3.[122]

Depending on the degree of dermal inflammation, the epidermis may be normal or necrotic. Leukocytoclastic vasculitis is present in 31 percent of skin biopsies.[125] The connective tissue contains granulomas with extensive basophilic degeneration of collagen and a mixed infiltrate of eosinophils, plasma cells, and lymphocytes. Multinucleate giant cells are common. A variable amount of hemorrhage is present.

Giant Cell Arteritis

Pain and erythema over the temporal arteries of elderly individuals are the classic symptoms of giant cell arteritis.[126] Inflammation of the vessels may result in extensive areas of scalp necrosis.[127] Involvement of the retinal arteries can produce blindness. Vessels of the heart and brain may also be involved.

The arteries show destruction of internal elastic lamina with partial or complete occlusion of the lumina. Macrophages and multinucleate giant cells are present within the vessel walls and appear to surround altered elastic tissue. Different segments of the vessel walls appear to be involved unevenly in the inflammatory process. The Verhoeff-van Gieson elastic stain is helpful in defining the presence of altered elastic tissue.

Differential Diagnosis of Vasculitis

Three disorders not discussed in the previous sections should be considered in the differential diagnosis of neutrophilic vasculitis. Granuloma faciale consists clinically of solitary or multiple infiltrated facial nodules with a red-brown color and prominent follicular openings.[128] Ectatic vessels in the superficial dermis are surrounded by a "sea of neutrophils" with a lesser number of eosinophils and mononuclear cells. The infiltrate is separated from the epidermis and appendages by grenz zones of uninvolved collagen. Although nuclear dust is common, true vessel wall inflammation and necrosis are generally absent. Acute febrile neutrophilic dermatosis (Sweet's syndrome), which affects mainly women, is characterized by multiple tender red plaques of the face and/or extremities associated with fever and leukocytosis.[129,130] A dense dermal infiltrate of neutrophils may be angiocentric but is often diffuse. A few eosinophils and mononuclear cells are present. Although there may be considerable nuclear dust, true vasculitis is absent. Livedo vasculitis (atrophie blanche, segmental hyalinizing vasculitis) produces recurrent painful ulcerations of the ankles and lower legs that heal with white atrophic scars and patchy hyperpigmentation.[131] The course is chronic, with exacerbations during the winter or summer. Small vessels of the superficial dermis show marked thickening of their walls by a dense pink hyalin material that is PAS positive and diastase resistant. There is often endothelial proliferation and thrombosis, but the inflammatory infiltrate is sparse and predominantly mononuclear.

Granulomatous Dermatitis

Granulomatous dermatitis can be subclassified into necrobiotic, sarcoidal, and infectious types. The three major forms of necrobiotic granulomas are granuloma annulare, necrobiosis lipoidica, and rheumatoid nodules. Sarcoidal granulomas may be produced by sarcoidosis, tuberculoid leprosy, and reactions to silica, beryllium, and zirconium. Certain foreign body granulomas may be confused with sarcoidosis or granuloma annulare. Infectious granulomas produce pseudoepitheliomatous hyperplasia and granulomatous inflammation. This pattern is seen mainly in deep fungal infections, in atypical acid-fast bacterial infections, and in noninfectious disorders such as iododerma and bromoderma.

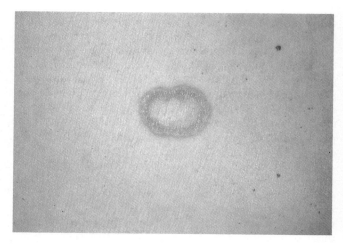

Fig. 16-77. Granuloma annulare. Atypical lesions produced by a ring of coalescing pink papules. Unlike ringworm, there is no scale.

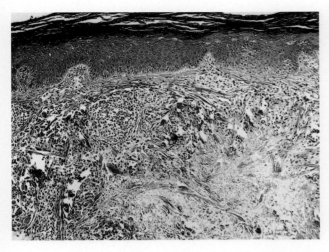

Fig. 16-78. Granuloma annulare. Stellate area of necrobiotic collagen within the upper dermis is surrounded by histiocytes and lymphocytes.

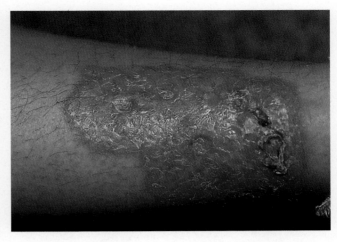

Fig. 16-80. Necrobiosis lipoidica. A red-yellow plaque with focal ulceration is present on the pretibial area of a diabetic.

Granuloma Annulare

Granuloma annulare is characterized by flesh-colored asymptomatic papules that often occur in a ring-like or circinate pattern (Fig. 16-77) on the dorsal aspects of the hands or feet. Generalized,[132] perforating,[133] and subcutaneous forms[134] of granuloma annulare also occur. The disorder affects mainly children and young adults. Most cases clear spontaneously within approximately 2 years, however, the generalized form is often persistent.

The epidermis in granuloma annulare is usually normal. Discrete stellate areas of necrobiosis within the superficial dermis are surrounded by lymphocytes, histiocytes, and epithelioid cells in a palisaded pattern (Fig. 16-78). The necrobiotic collagen varies from granular to wispy and stains somewhat basophilic with the H&E stain. Remnants of collagen fibers can be recognized in the necrobiotic areas. Multinucleate giant

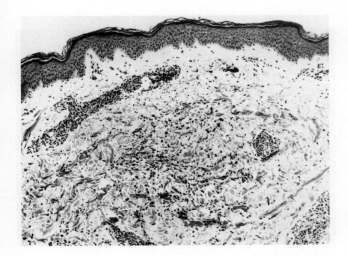

Fig. 16-79. Granuloma annulare. Single file arrangement of mononuclear cells between collagen bundles is associated with indistinct areas of necrobiosis.

cells are often present but are usually few in number. A dense lymphocytic cuffing of small vessels in the superficial dermis is a common feature. The interstitial variant of granuloma annulare may show only a single file arrangement of histiocytes between collagen bundles in a pattern that has been referred to as the "busy dermis" collagen (Fig. 16-79). Necrobiosis my be subtle in this type of granuloma annulare. IgM and complement have been found in small dermal vessels in about one-third of the cases,[135] however, the pathogenesis remains uncertain.

Necrobiosis Lipoidica

Necrobiosis lipoidica may begin as erythematous nodules on the lower extremities resembling erythema nodosum. With time the skin becomes atrophic and yellow, producing confluent plaques with hyperpigmented margins (Fig. 16-80). Telangiectatic vessels can be seen beneath the skin surface. In approximately 15 percent of cases, areas other than the legs are involved such as the arms, trunk, and face.[136] Diabetes mellitus is present or will eventually develop in 60 to 80 percent of patients with necrobiosis lipoidica.[136]

The necrobiosis in necrobiosis lipoidica is located in the deep dermis and subcutaneous fat (Fig. 16-81). Large elliptical areas of necrobiosis are oriented parallel to the surface of the skin. The necrobiotic connective tissue varies from a wispy bluish appearance to necrotic to eosinophilic and hyalinized in various cases. Granulomatous inflammation with multinucleate giant cells and vascular changes characterized by dense perivascular infiltrates of mononuclear cells are more prominent than in granuloma annulare (Fig. 16-82). Plasma cells are often present.

Rheumatoid Nodule

Rheumatoid nodules occur in adults with seropositive rheumatoid arthritis and active joint disease. They are rare in children with Still's disease. Rheumatoid nodules are nontender and occur over extensor aspects of joints. Similar nodules have been found in the lung, meninges, and heart valves. Rheumatoid nodules may occur in lupus erythematosus.[137] The lesions of

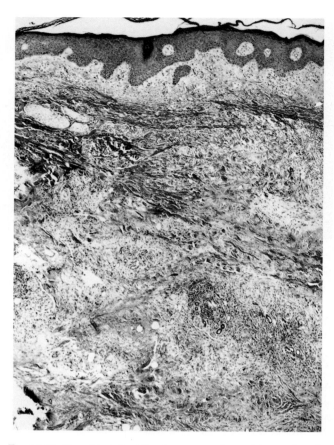

Fig. 16-81. Necrobiosis lipoidica. Large areas of necrobiosis within the deep dermis and subcutaneous fat are oriented parallel to the surface epithelium.

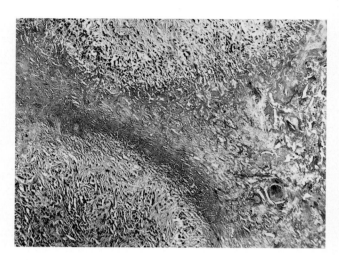

Fig. 16-83. Rheumatoid nodule. Zone of relatively complete necrobiosis is surrounded by histiocytes and epithelioid cells in a palisaded pattern. Multinucleate giant cell is present.

subcutaneous granuloma annulare (pseudorheumatoid nodules) in children[138] show histologic features that may be confused with rheumatoid nodules.

The necrobiotic connective tissue in rheumatoid nodules is deeper than in granuloma annulare or necrobiosis lipoidica. The epidermis is often not present in the biopsy specimen because the deep nodules are usually removed by general surgeons. The areas of necrobiosis are large and sharply circumscribed (Fig. 16-83). Palisading of epithelioid cells around the necrobiotic area is usually well developed. The necrobiosis tends to be complete, with few collagen fibers remaining. Occasionally, small amounts of calcium may be present within the necrobiotic tissue.

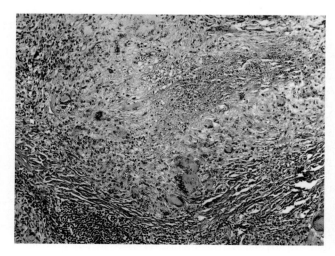

Fig. 16-82. Necrobiosis lipoidica. Area of necrobiotic connective tissue is surrounded by a palisaded infiltrate of epithelioid cells and multinucleate giant cells.

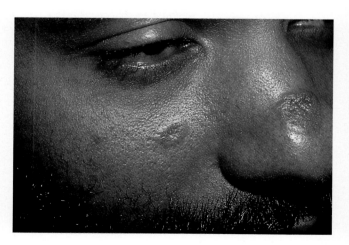

Fig. 16-84. Sarcoidosis. The facial papules may have an annular appearance.

Sarcoidosis

Sarcoidosis is a systemic granulomatous disease of unknown etiology that affects predominantly lymph nodes, lungs, eyes, and skin. Cutaneous lesions, which are present in about 25 percent of patients, most often occur as papules and nodules on the face and head (Fig. 16-84). Translucent raised brown papules occur around the eyes or on the nose. Scarring alopecia is an unusual complication.[139] About 15 to 20 percent of patients with sarcoidosis develop erythema nodosum on the legs.

The epidermis is normal or is effaced by the underlying granulomas. Distinct granulomas composed predominantly of epithelioid cells are surrounded by a narrow rim of lymphocytes (Fig. 16-85). Caseation necrosis is usually absent, but small foci of caseation necrosis occasionally occur. Multinucleate giant cells are common and may contain asteroid bodies.[140] Round, laminated, calcified Schaumann bodies occasionally are present within the giant cells. The granulomatous infiltrate may fill the dermis and extend into the subcutaneous fat.

Tuberculoid Leprosy

Tuberculoid leprosy is a variant of leprosy in which host cell-mediated immunity is generally intact and the number of organisms are few.[141] Clinical lesions are characterized by annular plaques with central clearing and variable hypopigmentation. The margins of the plaques are scaly, and there is cutaneous anesthesia in the center of the plaque. Peripheral nerves that run through the plaque may be palpably enlarged. Patients with pure tuberculoid leprosy often have only one or a few lesions. The prognosis for cure with appropriate drug therapy is excellent.

The epidermis is normal or shows mild hyperkeratosis and parakeratosis. Well circumscribed sarcoidal granulomas are present throughout the dermis (Fig. 16-86). The granulomas are surrounded by a sparse infiltrate of lymphocytes. A small num-

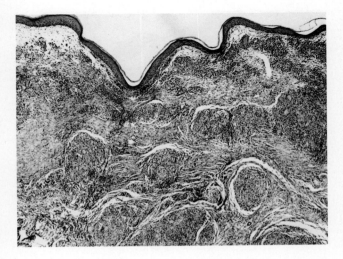

Fig. 16-85. Sarcoidosis. Numerous distinct granulomas are present throughout the dermis. Lymphocytes are sparse, and caseation necrosis is absent.

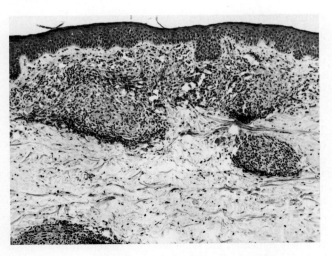

Fig. 16-86. Tuberculoid leprosy. Granulomas surrounded by a narrow rim of lymphocytes are present in the superficial dermis. Exocytosis of lymphocytes into the epidermis is present.

ber of lymphocytes may extend from the dermis into the epidermis. Cutaneous nerves in the deep dermis are almost completely obliterated by the granulomatous process. Fite's acid-fast stain may demonstrate a rare organism, but often it is negative. Lepromatous leprosy differs from the tuberculoid form by having large numbers of foamy histiocytes (Virchow cells) in the dermis, less severe nerve destruction, and numerous acid-fast bacteria when stained with the Fite stain.

Silica, Beryllium, and Zirconium Granulomas

Silica granulomas result from the contamination of wounds with particles of glass or soil that contain silicon dioxide or from the contamination of surgical wounds with talcum powder, which contains magnesium silicate. Typically, the inflammatory response does not occur until months or years after the exposure.[142] Zirconium contained in deodorant preparations[143] or poison ivy medications[144] is a rare cause of a papular eruption. Systemic berylliosis resulting from the inhalation of beryllium particles may produce a papular skin rash. Localized beryllium granulomas due to contamination of lacerations with beryllium from fluorescent light tubes are now quite rare.

Silica granulomas may be indistinguishable from sarcoidosis, although typically the granulomatous inflammation is more diffuse, with histiocytes, epithelioid cells, and multinucleate giant cells. Often, crystalline particles of silica can be observed in the dermis. Polarized light examination enhances the identification of the particles, which are doubly refractile. The granulomas produced by zirconium are indistinguishable from those of sarcoidosis, but the small zirconium particles are not detectable by polarized light examination. The cutaneous granulomas of systemic berylliosis are also indistinguishable from sarcoidosis.[145] Beryllium granuloma secondary to inoculation of beryllium into the skin often shows extensive areas of caseation necrosis surrounded by a tuberculoid granulomatous infiltrate. The epidermis may be acanthotic or ulcerated.

Foreign Body Granulomas

The most common cause of granulomatous inflammation on the face is a foreign body reaction to keratin secondary to a ruptured epidermoid cyst or acne lesion. The diagnosis of sarcoidosis should not be made when a single biopsy specimen from the face shows granulomatous inflammation.

Within the dermis are collections of epithelioid cells, histiocytes, lymphocytes, and foreign body giant cells (Fig. 16-87). The multiple nuclei of foreign body giant cells tend to be clustered in one portion of the cytoplasm. Foreign material may be present within the cytoplasm of multinucleate giant cells or within the granulomatous infiltrate. The delicate keratin fibers are often fibrillar in appearance and resemble "corn flakes on edge." Epithelium from the wall of the ruptured cyst and occasionally microabscesses containing acute inflammatory cells may be present. Although the keratin of the stratum corneum is doubly refractile, the small amounts of keratin in a foreign body reaction may be difficult to demonstrate with polarized light.

Infectious Granulomas

Infectious granulomas of the skin produced by deep fungal infections or atypical acid-fast bacterial infection typically pro-

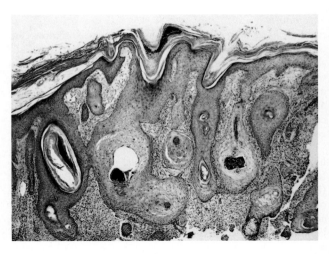

Fig. 16-88. Iododerma. Hyperkeratosis, papillomatosis, and irregular acanthosis are associated with intraepidermal neutrophilic microabscesses and a granulomatous dermal infiltrate.

duce verrucous nodules or plaques that may have small pustules studding their surfaces. An excellent review of this subject has been published by Conant et al.[146] Systemic ingestion of halogens such as iodide[147] and bromide produces cutaneous lesions that are clinically and histologically similar to deep fungal granulomas (Fig. 16-88).

The epidermis shows hyperkeratosis, parakeratosis, and papillomatosis. Marked irregular acanthosis produces pseudoepitheliomatous hyperplasia (Fig. 16-89). Microabscesses containing neutrophils and mononuclear inflammatory cells are present within the acanthotic epithelium and within the dermis. The dermis contains scattered epithelioid cells, multinucleate giant cells, histiocytes, and lymphocytes. Distinct granu-

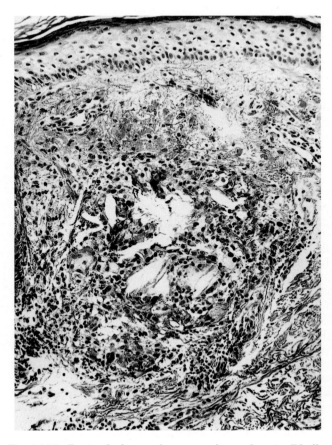

Fig. 16-87. Foreign body granuloma secondary to keratin. Fibrillar collections of keratin are surrounded by lymphocytes, histiocytes, and foreign body giant cells.

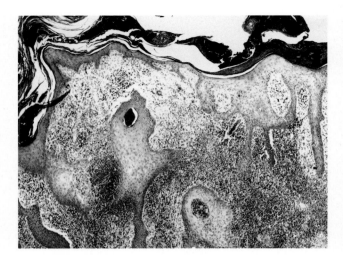

Fig. 16-89. Sporotrichosis. There is hyperkeratosis, acanthosis, and pseudoepitheliomatous hyperplasia of the epidermis. Intraepithelial microabscesses contain neutrophils. Organisms are difficult to identify in the granulomatous infiltrate without special stains.

lomas are occasionally seen; however, caseation necrosis is uncommon in deep fungal infections. The organisms that produce deep fungal infections are often visible on H&E-stained sections but are easier to identify with the silver methenamine stain and with the PAS reaction following predigestion with diastase to remove glycogen particles. Deep fungal infections and acid-fast bacterial infections may also produce palisading granulomas that may resemble granuloma annulare.[148]

Differential Diagnosis of Granulomatous Dermatitis

Tuberculosis verrucosa cutis may show epitheliomatous and granulomatous changes similar to the deep fungal infections. In cutaneous tuberculosis, however, the granulomatous inflammation tends to be less polymorphous than in the deep fungal infections. In tuberculosis verrucosa cutis, caseation necrosis may be slight to moderate, and organisms usually cannot be identified with acid-fast stains. Foreign body granulomas may show a mixed inflammatory infiltrate similar to that of deep fungal infections and halogen eruptions. However, the presence of foreign material and/or the presence of distinctive foreign body giant cells should help to distinguish foreign body reactions from deep fungal infections. Swimming pool granuloma due to infection with Mycobacterium marinum[149] also produces chronic verrucous cutaneous plaques that show epithelial hyperplasia, neutrophilic microabscesses within the epidermis, and a mixed inflammatory infiltrate in the dermis (Fig. 16-90). Epithelioid cells and giant cells are often present; however, distinct tubercle formation is uncommon and caseation necrosis is slight or absent. M. marinum is difficult to identify in tissue with the Ziehl-Neelsen stain but is easily cultured on Löwenstein-Jensen media at 32°C. The budding yeast of sporotrichosis are difficult to identify in skin with special stains but are easily cultured on Sabouraud's agar.

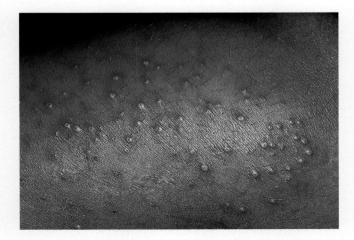

Fig. 16-91. Folliculitis. Each pustule is pierced by a hair shaft.

Folliculitis

Bacterial Folliculitis

Most cases of folliculitis are the result of infection with S. aureus. Folliculitis can be divided into superficial and deep forms. Superficial folliculitis is characterized by small pustules situated at the openings of hair follicles and frequently pierced by a hair shaft (Fig. 16-91). This form of folliculitis is known as impetigo Bockhart. More often, staphylococcal folliculitis also involves a deeper portion of the follicle and adjacent dermis. A red tender nodule centered around a hair follicle is referred to as a furuncle. Recurrent furunculosis tends to involve the buttocks and thighs and may be associated with diabetes mellitus. A larger

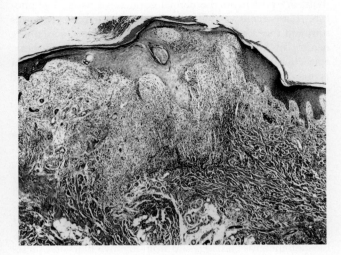

Fig. 16-90. Swimming pool granuloma. Irregular acanthosis of the epidermis is associated with a dermal infiltrate of lymphocytes, histiocytes, epithelioid cells, and multinucleate giant cells.

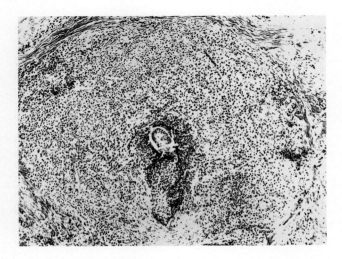

Fig. 16-92. Deep folliculitis. Intradermal hair shaft surrounded by a neutrophilic microabscess and a lymphohistiocytic infiltrate.

furuncle, which involves several hair follicles producing a boggy purulent mass, is known as a carbuncle.

Superficial folliculitis produces a subcorneal pustule located at the mouth of the hair follicle. This pustule is often pierced by a hair shaft, but this is difficult to demonstrate histologically. An inflammatory infiltrate of neutrophils, lymphocytes, and histiocytes surrounds the upper portion of the follicle and may infiltrate follicular epithelium. In deep folliculitis, a dense perifollicular infiltrate of neutrophils, lymphocytes, and histiocytes extends into the follicular epithelium. The follicular epithelium may rupture with extrusion of the hair shaft and keratin into the surrounding dermis and the formation of neutrophilic microabscesses and a foreign body granulomatous reaction (Fig. 16-92). In carbuncles, a massive dermal infiltrate of acute and chronic inflammatory cells, including plasma cells and foreign body giant cells, is centered around several hair follicles, which show destruction of follicular epithelium.

Fungal Folliculitis

Dermatophyte infections may involve the hair follicles of the scalp or head. The manifestations vary from a dry scaly eruption with breakage of hair shafts to a severe inflammatory process with boggy infiltrated plaques (kerion) and subsequent scarring alopecia. Distinct erythematous perifollicular papules and nodules occurring on the extremities or scalp secondary to a dermatophyte infection of hair follicles are known as Majocchi's granulomas.

The epidermis shows hyperkeratosis, parakeratosis, and variable acanthosis. Fungal hyphae and/or arthrospores are seen on or within the hair shaft (Fig. 16-93). Occasionally, hyphae are also seen in the adjacent stratum corneum with special stains. The location of arthrospores on the surface of the hair shaft (ectothrix) or within the hair shaft (endothrix) and the size of the arthrospores (small or large) are important clues for species identification. Follicular epithelium is often acanthotic and is infiltrated by inflammatory cells. Focal rupture of follicular ep-

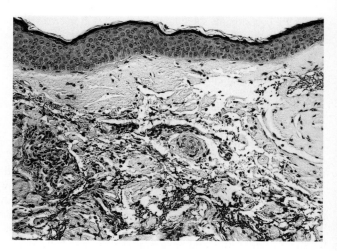

Fig. 16-94. Primary systemic amyloidosis. Amorphous masses of amyloid are present within the superficial dermis.

ithelium is associated with neutrophilic abscesses and foreign body granulomatous inflammation in the adjacent dermis.[150] Special stains such as silver methenamine or the PAS reaction are helpful in further delineating the extent of the fungal infection.

Folliculitis Decalvans

Folliculitis decalvans occurs predominantly on the scalp of black men and is characterized by perifollicular papules, pustules, and abscesses that produce boggy masses and destruction of hair follicles. Draining sinuses, inflammatory nodules, and cutaneous atrophy are common features.

Numerous hair follicles within the dermis show inflammation of follicular epithelium with lymphocytes, histiocytes, and neutrophils. There is rupture of follicular epithelium, and hair shafts are present in the dermal connective tissue. Lymphocytes, plasma cells, epithelioid cells, and foreign body giant cells surround the displaced hair shafts. Microabscesses containing neutrophils and sinus tracts with walls composed of acanthotic epithelium are often present. There is considerable fibrosis of dermal connective tissue with the formation of hypertrophic scars or keloids.

Differential Diagnosis of Folliculitis

Pityrosporum ovale is a common yeast that occupies hair follicles of the head and upper trunk. Pityrosporum folliculitis shows follicular hyperkeratosis, inflammation of follicular epithelium, dermal abscesses, and PAS-positive budding yeast in the follicular lumen and in the dermis.[151] It is important to recognize *P. ovale* and not to confuse it with dermatophyte infections. Folliculitis keloidalis (acne keloidalis) characteristically produces inflammatory papules at the nape of the neck in black men. Pseudofolliculitis barbae results from ingrown hairs and subsequent inflammation in the beard areas of black males. The histologic changes in folliculitis keloidalis and pseudofolliculitis barbae may be identical to folliculitis decalvans.

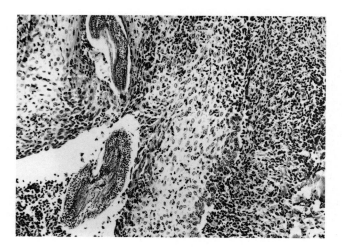

Fig. 16-93. Fungal folliculitis. Small spores can be seen within the hair shaft of an inflamed follicle.

Cutaneous Deposits

Systemic Amyloidosis

Primary Systemic Amyloidosis. The cutaneous lesions of primary systemic amyloidosis are characterized by coalescing papules and nodules with a smooth surface and a translucent appearance.[152] Lesions are commonly located around the eyes and in the perianal area. Petechiae and purpura may follow minor cutaneous trauma. The distribution of amyloid in primary systemic amyloidosis and in myeloma-associated amyloidosis is identical and includes the skin, tongue, heart, gastrointestinal tract, nerves, and carpal ligaments. The skin is involved in approximately 25 percent of cases, whereas the tongue is infiltrated and enlarged in 40 percent.[153]

Eosinophilic masses of amorphous material are deposited within the dermis and subcutaneous fat (Fig. 16-94). The dermal papillae appear enlarged and rounded due to fissured masses of amyloid that may press against the epidermis. A few fibroblasts may be present within the amyloid. Melanin pigment is often present in macrophages in the papillary dermis. Deposits of amyloid surround dermal vessels and encase eccrine sweat glands. There is often extravasation of RBCs from the affected vessels. In the subcutaneous fat, amyloid infiltrates the walls of blood vessels (Fig. 16-95) and surrounds individual fat cells producing characteristic amyloid rings. A number of recent articles have described the structure and origin of the amyloid fibrils.[154,155]

Secondary Systemic Amyloidosis. Skin lesions are rare in secondary systemic amyloidosis. Amyloid deposits are typically found in the kidneys, liver, spleen, and adrenals.[156,157] Patients may develop hepatomegaly, proteinuria, and uremia. Secondary systemic amyloidosis is associated with a chronic inflammatory process such as tuberculosis, leprosy, rheumatoid arthritis, osteomyelitis, stasis ulcers, hidradenitis suppurativa, or epidermolysis bullosa.

Skin biopsy specimens usually do not show deposits of amyloid in secondary systemic amyloidosis.

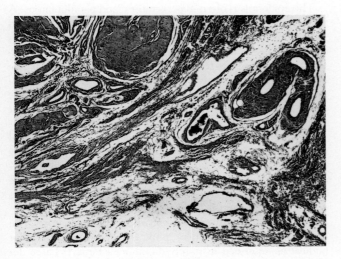

Fig. 16-95. Primary systemic amyloidosis. Blood vessels in the deep dermis are encased by dense deposits of amyloid.

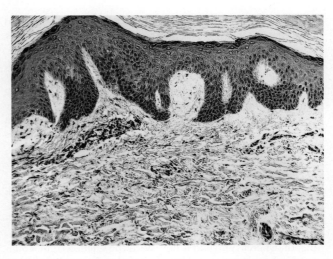

Fig. 16-96. Lichen amyloidosus. There is mild hyperkeratosis and acanthosis of the epidermis. Dermal papilla is enlarged and club-shaped due to small deposits of amyloid.

Localized Amyloidosis

Lichen amyloidosus usually involves the pretibial areas, where it produces a scaly, papular, confluent rash that may be intensely pruritic.[158] The eruption persists for many years and is refractory to treatment.

The epidermis shows a variable amount of hyperkeratosis and acanthosis. Small globules of amyloid are limited to the papillary dermis (Fig. 16-96). The amyloid may be separated from the epidermis by a narrow grenz zone of collagen or appear to be in direct contact with the epidermal basement membrane. Small amounts of melanin are present in dermal macrophages. Occasionally, the amyloid deposits in several adjacent dermal papillae coalesce to form larger aggregates. The amyloid is often fissured and contains a few fibroblasts and capillaries.

In macular amyloidosis, the interscapular or pretibial areas are involved with pruritic, symmetric, brownish, reticulated macules. This type of localized amyloidosis appears to represent an early stage of lichen amyloidosus.[159] Rubbing or scratching the lesions of macular amyloidosis may produce the hyperkeratotic papules of lichen amyloidosus. In contrast to systemic forms of amyloidosis, the amyloid in the lichenoid and macular forms of cutaneous amyloidosis results from filamentous degeneration of epidermal cells that are discharged into the papillary dermis.[160]

The epidermis is normal. The small amounts of amyloid that are deposited at the tips of dermal papillae resemble colloid bodies. The histologic changes are subtle and easily overlooked. The presence of melanin pigment in dermal macrophages is a helpful sign and should stimulate a careful search for amyloid deposits.

In nodular (tumefactive) amyloidosis one or several nodules occur mainly on the legs, but they have also been reported on the trunk and genitalia. Collections of plasma cells are present and the amyloid is produced locally by these cells. The type of amyloid is identical to that seen in primary systemic amyloid. Myeloma is usually absent.

Large masses of amyloid are present within the dermis and subcutaneous fat.[158,161] Nodular aggregates of plasma cells are present.

A variety of cutaneous tumors such as basal cell carcinoma, Bowen's disease, and seborrheic keratosis may contain deposits of amyloid.[158] Clinically, the lesions are not distinguishable from tumors that do not contain amyloid.

Small amounts of amyloid are typically present in the stroma of the tumors. Amyloid deposits are not present in blood vessels or in the surrounding dermis.

Special Stains and Procedures for Amyloidosis

In addition to the characteristic distribution and the pale pink fissured appearance of amyloid, several special stains and procedures may be helpful in distinguishing amyloid from other material. With polarized light examination, collagen is birefringent, whereas amyloid is not. With the Giemsa stain, collagen is pink and amyloid is blue. The Verhoeff-van Gieson stain stains collagen red and amyloid yellow. With the PAS reaction, collagen is pale pink, whereas amyloid is red. Amyloid stains metachromatically (red) with crystal violet or methyl violet stains. With the alkaline Congo red stain, amyloid is orange. A very helpful diagnostic feature is the apple green color (dichromatic) of amyloid with the alkaline Congo red stain and polarized light. Amyloid is brightly fluorescent with the thioflavin T stain utilizing fluorescence microscopy. Waldenström's macroglobulinemia may produce cutaneous deposits that mimic amyloid. However, by immunofluorescence microscopy the material can be shown to be predominantly IgM.

Colloid Milium

Colloid milium is a sunlight-induced disease that produces translucent papules on the dorsa of the hands and face of adults. A rare juvenile form is not related to sunlight exposure.[162]

The epidermis is often elevated and effaced by large masses of homogeneous fissured material in the dermal papillae. The colloid is separated from the epidermis by a thin grenz zone of

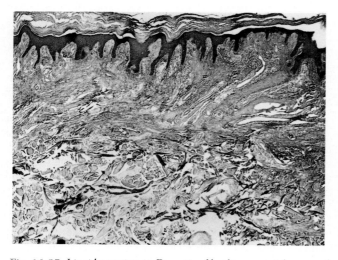

Fig. 16-97. Lipoid proteinosis. Deposits of hyaline material surround dermal vessels and are oriented perpendicular to the epidermis.

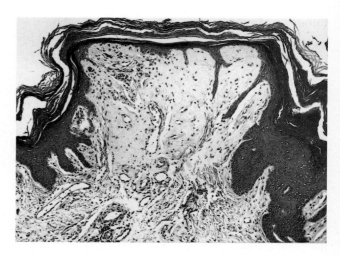

Fig. 16-98. Erythropoietic protoporphyria. Collections of hyaline material encase small vessels of the papillary dermis. Epidermis appears hyperkeratotic and papillomatous.

connective tissue. The eosinophilic fissured aggregates may contain small vessels and a variable number of fibroblasts. Amyloid and colloid can be differentiated by electron microscopy. The straight, nonbranching fibrils of amyloidosis are 70 to 100 Å in diameter. Colloid fibers are of a similar width but show branching and anastomosing. Colloid is most likely produced by fibroblasts.[163] The staining properties of colloid are similar to amyloid.[164]

Hyalinoses

Lipoid proteinosis (hyalinosis cutis et mucosae) is an autosomal recessive disorder that usually begins in infancy. Translucent waxy papules are present along the eyelid margins and around the mouth. The tongue, mucous membranes, and vocal cords are infiltrated, and the infants have a characteristic hoarse cry. Similar deposits affect the gastrointestinal tract, vagina, testis, eye, brain, and kidney.[165]

The epidermis is often hyperkeratotic and papillomatous. A pink hyalin material surrounds blood vessels, sweat glands, and hair follicles (Fig. 16-97). Rarely, diffuse dermal involvement is noted. Because of the periadnexal distribution of the hyalin material, it is often oriented perpendicular to the epidermis. The deposits produce a positive PAS reaction and are diastase resistant. The material is metachromatic with the toluidine blue stain. Fat stains on frozen sections show small droplets of fat within the hyalin material.

Erythropoietic protoporphyria is inherited as an autosomal dominant trait. It manifests in childhood as burning and itching of the skin after ultraviolet light exposure. Sun-exposed skin becomes papular, lichenified, and indurated. The dorsa of the hands and face are typical sites of involvement. Massive deposits of protoporphyrin in the liver may result in fatal cirrhosis.[166]

The epidermis shows hyperkeratosis and papillomatosis. The epidermis may contain linear, pink, PAS-positive "caterpillar bodies" as described in porphyria cutanea tarda.[94] Large deposits of a pink hyalin material are present around blood vessels in the superficial dermis (Fig. 16-98). There is little tendency

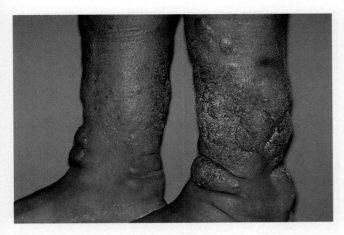

Fig. 16-99. Pretibial myxedema. Indurated plaques and nodules of the lower legs occurred in a patient with a history of Graves' disease.

for the hyalin to surround adnexal structures as in lipoid proteinosis.[167] Unlike porphyria cutanea tarda, subepidermal bullae are rare in erythropoietic protoporphyria. The hyalin material stains red with the PAS reaction and is diastase resistant. Porphyria cutanea tarda, variegate porphyria, and coproporphyria show much smaller amounts of hyalin material around small vessels in the papillary dermis. Immunofluorescence of the hyalin material in the porphyrias is positive for immunoglobulin and complement but is believed to be a secondary phenomenon related to damage and reduplication of the basement membrane of small dermal vessels associated with the leakage of serum proteins.[168]

Mucinoses

Pretibial Myxedema. Pretibial myxedema occurs in patients with hyperthyroidism (Graves' disease), especially in those individuals with exophthalmos and increased serum levels of long-acting thyroid stimulator (LATS).[169] Yellow, waxy, indurated nodules and plaques of the pretibial area (Fig. 16-99) often occur after successful treatment of the hyperthyroidism. The surface of the skin lesion may appear dimpled or scaly. The presence of a thick, stringy, dermal mucin may be obvious at the time of the biopsy.

The epidermis may show hyperkeratosis and acanthosis but is often normal. The rete ridge pattern tends to be effaced by large amounts of dermal mucin. A narrow, subepidermal grenz zone of relatively normal connective tissue separates the epidermis from massive amounts of mucin within the dermis. Collagen fibers and fibroblasts are few in number, and the dermis appears to be replaced by a pale blue wispy material or by empty spaces where mucin has been removed during processing (Fig. 16-100). The fibroblasts have a delicate fusiform or stellate shape. The mucin, which is predominantly hyaluronic acid, stains blue with the alcian blue stain at pH 2.5 but does not stain at pH 0.4. The mucin is metachromatic with the toluidine blue stain at pH 3.0 and stains positively for mucin with the colloidal iron and mucicarmine stains.

Generalized Myxedema. Patients with hypothyroidism or generalized myxedema have a dull appearance with puffy facies and pale, dry, often scaly skin. They have dry brittle hair and loss of lateral eyebrows. Their palms are yellow due to deposition of carotene in the stratum corneum.

Routinely stained sections appear relatively normal except for mild hyperkeratosis. Careful examination shows slightly increased spaces between dermal collagen fibers. Occasionally, a bluish wispy material is seen in these spaces, but the mucin is often removed during processing. The presence of dermal hyaluronic acid can usually be demonstrated with the special stains described for pretibial myxedema.[170]

Papular Mucinosis. Clinical variants of papular mucinosis are known as scleromyxedema and lichen myxedematosus. Scleromyxedema shows leonine facies and diffuse thickening of the skin.[171] In contrast to scleroderma, the skin is freely movable. In papular mucinosis, discrete papules are present (Fig. 16-101), whereas in lichen myxedematosus the papular eruption may have a lichenified appearance. In all forms of papular mucinosis, an abnormal IgG with a slow electrophoretic migration is present in the serum.[172] The abnormal immunoglobulin, which is thought to be produced in the bone marrow by plasma cells, almost always has delta-1-type light chains.[173]

The epidermis may be normal or show hyperkeratosis and acanthosis. Focal collections of mucin are present within the superficial dermis and are often separated by intervening areas of relatively normal connective tissues. In contrast to the other mucinoses, the number of fibroblasts is significantly increased in the areas of mucin deposition. The mucin is hyaluronic acid and stains similarly to that described for pretibial myxedema. At autopsy, the mucin content of the internal organs is not found to be increased.

Scleredema of Buschke. Scleredema of Buschke, also known as scleredema adultorum, is characterized by diffuse nonpitting

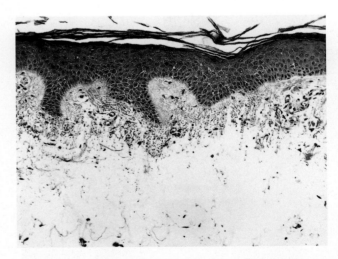

Fig. 16-100. Pretibial myxedema. The epidermis is unremarkable. Except for a narrow zone immediately deep to the epidermis, the entire dermis appears pale staining and contains fusiform and stellate fibroblasts.

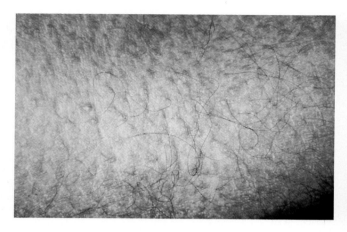

Fig. 16-101. Papular mucinosis. Sheets of brown papules are present in a patient with a monoclonal gammopathy.

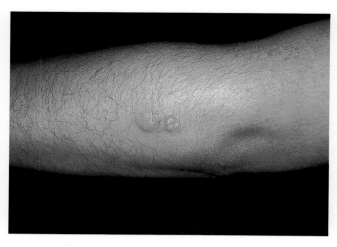

Fig. 16-103. Cutaneous focal mucinosis. The skin-colored papules are asymptomatic.

induration of the skin of the face, neck, and upper trunk and often follows an infectious episode such as influenza. In most patients, the eruption resolves over a period of months. Diabetes mellitus is a commonly associated disease.[174,175]

The dermis appears normal on superficial examination. The overall thickness of the dermis is often greatly increased, and spaces are present between collagen fibers similar to those seen in generalized myxedema. The spaces contain hyaluronic acid, which is demonstrated with special stains as described for pretibial myxedema. Often the amount of mucin is so small that the special stains fail to demonstrate any abnormality. The secretory portions of eccrine sweat glands are located in the mid-dermis, and it appears that new collagen is laid down beneath the glands, replacing a portion of the subcutaneous fat.

Digital Mucous Cyst. A solitary translucent, slightly fluctuant cyst on the distal finger proximal to the fingernail or directly over the distal interphalangeal joint is characteristic of a digital mucous cyst (Fig. 16-102). The cysts may be slightly tender and, if punctured, drain a thick mucinous material. Injection of the interphalangeal joint with methylene blue dye demonstrates a communication between the cysts and the joint space.[176]

The epidermis is effaced by a large area of pale-staining mucin within the superficial dermis and mid-dermis. Fusiform and stellate fibroblasts are present within the mucin, which may appear bluish and stringy. Older lesions tend to develop cleft-like spaces between the mucin and the surrounding connective tissue, producing a large, sharply circumscribed cyst.[177]

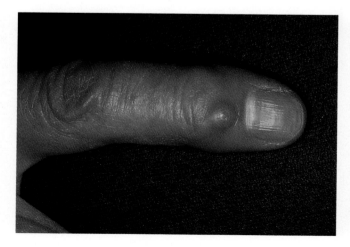

Fig. 16-102. Digital mucous cyst. This skin-colored to translucent papule occurred suddenly over the distal interphalangeal joint.

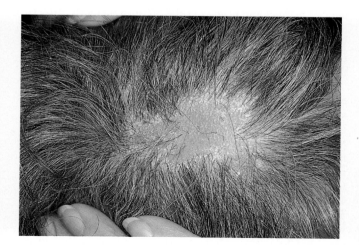

Fig. 16-104. Follicular mucinosis. This boggy plaque of the scalp is associated with alopecia.

Occasionally, the cystic space is lined by macrophages or granulation tissue. In lesions that have drained to the surface periodically, the cyst may have the appearance of being partly intraepidermal. Occasionally, synovium can be identified in the base of the cyst.

Mucocele. A solitary translucent cyst of the lower lip is characteristic of a mucous cyst (mucocele).[178] Minor trauma, such as biting the lip, causes rupture of a salivary duct, resulting in the extravasation of sialomucin into the surrounding connective tissue. The translucent papules often resolve spontaneously.

Ill-defined areas of mucin are present within the connective tissue. The mucin has a bluish amorphous to stringy appearance. In older lesions, a cystic space is lined by a wall of granulation tissue and inflammatory cells. Much mucin may be removed during processing. Mucin is phagocytized by macrophages, giving them a foamy appearance. Often a dilated salivary duct can be seen entering the cyst. The sialomucin stains positively with the PAS reaction and is diastase resistant. The alcian blue stain is positive at pH 2.5 but negative at pH 4.0. The material is not metachromatic with the toluidine blue stain. It is resistant to digestion with hyaluronidase but is removed with sialidase.

Cutaneous Focal Mucinosis. Cutaneous focal mucinosis or cutaneous myxoma occurs as a solitary asymptomatic nodule (Fig. 16-103) on the head, trunk, or extremities.[179] There is no association with systemic disease and surgical excision is curative.

The epidermis is effaced by a nonencapsulated collection of mucin within the upper dermis and mid-dermis. The mucinous area is pale staining and contains fusiform and stellate fibroblasts. Mucin that has not been removed during processing has a pale blue, wispy or stringy appearance. The histologic appearance is similar to that of a digital mucous cyst except that there

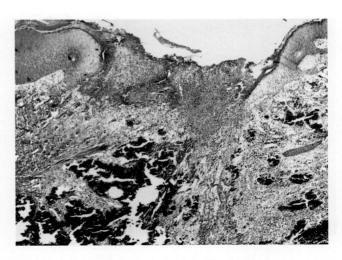

Fig. 16-106. Dystrophic calcification. Dark-staining deposits of calcium are being eliminated from the skin through an ulcerated epidermis.

is less tendency to form a sharply circumscribed cystic space with retraction of the mucin from the surrounding connective tissue. The mucin is hyaluronic acid and stains with special stains as described for pretibial myxedema.

Follicular Mucinosis. Follicular mucinosis or alopecia mucinosa occurs mainly on the face, neck, and upper trunk and is characterized by grouped follicular papules or red, raised, boggy plaques[180] (Fig. 16-104). Alopecia is not obvious if the eruption occurs on glabrous skin. About 20 percent of cases of follicular mucinosis are associated with an underlying lymphoma, most often mycosis fungoides. Follicular mucinosis that is not associated with mycosis fungoides usually resolves in 2 months to 2 years.[181]

The epithelium of hair follicles appears greatly thickened and infiltrated by a pale-staining, bluish, wispy material (Fig. 16-105). Large cystic spaces often develop within the follicular epithelium. Some follicular epithelial cells are fusiform in shape. The mucin is hyaluronic acid and stains in a manner similar to that described for pretibial myxedema. In cases of follicular mucinosis associated with lymphoma, atypical cells are present within the surrounding dermis. In mycosis fungoides, Pautrier's microabscesses are often present within the epidermis associated with a band-like dermal infiltrate of atypical mononuclear cells and a variable number of eosinophils.

Calcinosis Cutis

Dystrophic Calcification. In dystrophic calcification, the serum calcium and phosphorus levels are normal, and the calcification occurs secondary to previous tissue damage. Scleroderma, dermatomyositis,[182] granulomatous inflammation, and subcutaneous fat necrosis are often associated with dystrophic calcification.

Irregular deposits of a granular basophilic material are present in the dermis or subcutaneous fat (Fig. 16-106). Granulomatous inflammation may be present around the calcium particles.

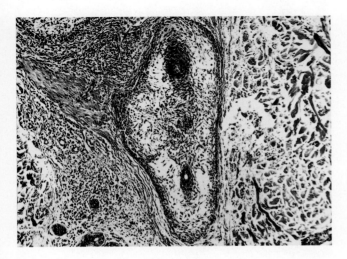

Fig. 16-105. Follicular mucinosis. The epithelium of a hair follicle shows pale-staining areas of mucin deposition associated with fusiform cells.

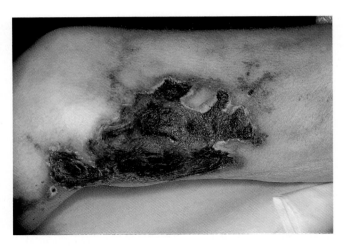

Fig. 16-107. Metastatic calcification. Livedo reticularis and ulceration are associated with extensive medial calcification of blood vessels.

Metastatic Calcification. The serum calcium and/or phosphorus levels are elevated and their product is usually over 80. Metastatic calcification may be associated with primary hyperparathyroidism, hypervitaminosis D, the milk alkali syndrome, osteomyelitis, metastatic carcinoma to bone, and renal failure with secondary hyperparathyroidism.[183] Massive calcium deposits within blood vessels of the extremities may be visible on radiographs. In renal failure with secondary hyperparathyroidism, the deposits of calcium within the media of vessels may be associated with extensive areas of skin necrosis[184] (Fig. 16-107). In patients with metastatic calcification, the vessels of the kidneys, lungs, and spleen are involved more often than the skin.

Calcium deposits are present within the media of dermal and subcutaneous blood vessels (Fig. 16-108). Focal collections of calcium may be present in the surrounding connective tissue. In cases associated with skin necrosis, the connective tissue is necrotic and amorphous.

Subepidermal Calcified Nodule. A solitary, hard, painless nodule on the face or extremities of a child is characteristic of a subepidermal calcified nodule. It has been suggested that this lesion represents dystrophic calcification in a pre-existing nevus or adnexal tumor. An elevated concentration of calcium in sweat has been reported.[185]

Focal collections of calcification within the upper dermis occur in nests resembling the pattern of a nevus. Occasionally, residual nuclei are visible within the calcified material. A foreign body granulomatous reaction may occur.

Scrotal Calcinosis. Solitary or multiple firm nodules of the scrotum (Fig. 16-109) are usually noted during the first or second decade of life. Clinically, the lesions resemble epidermoid cysts, which also occur on the scrotum.

Although originally considered idiopathic,[186] scrotal calcinosis appears to represent dystrophic calcification occurring in

ruptured or in inflamed epidermoid cysts.[187] Several patients have now been observed showing both epidermoid cysts and scrotal calcification with transitions occurring between the two disorders.

Special Stains for Calcium. The von Kossa stain is often used to identify calcium; however, it is nonspecific because it stains carbonate and phosphate salts of calcium and other minerals. Uric acid may therefore stain with the von Kossa stain. Carbonate and phosphate salts stain black with the von Kossa stain. A more specific stain for calcium is the alizarin red stain, which stains calcium red or orange-red.

Gout

Gouty tophi occur on the fingers, toes, elbows, and ears. Large tophi may discharge a chalky white material. Tophi are radiolucent but may show secondary calcification.[188]

The epidermis may be normal or may show hyperkeratosis and acanthosis. Occasionally, the epidermis is ulcerated, and uric acid is discharged to the surface. Formalin fixation removes uric acid from the tissues and produces an amorphous pale-staining appearance in the areas of uric acid deposition (Fig. 16-110). Often, however, residual uric acid is present as gray-black, needle-shaped crystals that are present in circumscribed masses.

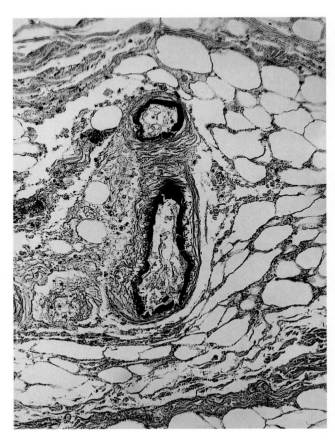

Fig. 16-108. Metastatic calcification. Blood vessels within the subcutaneous fat show large amounts of calcium within their media.

The masses of uric acid are usually surrounded by a foreign body granulomatous reaction. Uric acid crystals are brightly birefringent with polarized light. The von Kossa stain for carbonate and phosphate salts may be positive.

Xanthomas

Cutaneous xanthomas associated with hyperlipidemia may be due to an inherited defect of lipid metabolism[189] (Fig. 16-111). More often, the lipid abnormality is secondary to another systemic disease such as diabetes mellitus, pancreatitis, nephrotic syndrome, hypothyroidism, or liver disease. Only about one-third of the patients with xanthelasma have elevated serum lipids. Eruptive xanthomas, characterized by erythematous yellow papules that appear suddenly over the trunk and extremities, are consistently associated with hypertriglyceridemia.[190] Plane xanthomas are often seen with biliary cirrhosis. Diffuse normolipemic plane xanthomas may be a cutaneous sign of multiple myeloma.[191]

It is usually not possible to distinguish histologically between the various types of xanthomas except for eruptive xanthomas and xanthelasma as noted below. The epidermis shows effacement of the rete ridge pattern by the dermal infiltrate, which contains many histiocytes with foamy cytoplasm (foam cells, xanthoma cells). The cytoplasm of the histiocytes is pale stain-

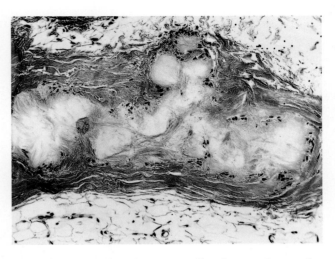

Fig. 16-110. Gout. Amorphous to crystalline deposits of uric acid are surrounded by epithelioid cells.

ing, increased in amount, and vacuolated due to the presence of numerous lipid droplets. Sudan black B, oil red O, and scarlet red stains of frozen sections demonstrate that the cytoplasmic droplets are lipid. Xanthomas may contain a variable number of fibroblasts, lymphocytes, and multinucleate giant cells. An objective diagnosis of xanthelasma can often be made if the epidermis shows the delicate features of eyelid skin and striated muscle is present deep to the infiltrate of foamy histiocytes. The foamy histiocytes typically surround a dilated blood vessel. Two features that should suggest the possibility of the eruptive form of xanthomas are the presence of a significant lymphocytic infiltrate and extracellular lipid (Fig. 16-112). The differential diagnosis of xanthomas includes lepromatous leprosy, solitary or eruptive histiocytomas,[192,193] juvenile xanthogranuloma, and histiocytosis X.

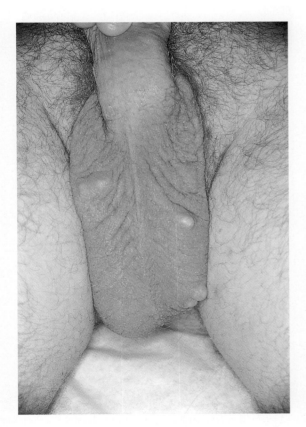

Fig. 16-109. Scrotal calcinosis. Firm scrotal nodules appear during the second or third decade of life.

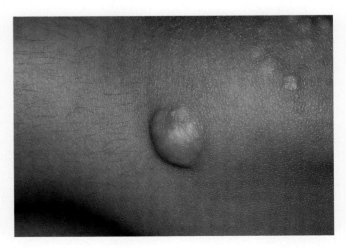

Fig. 16-111. Xanthomas. This 6-year-old boy with yellow nodules had familial hypercholesterolemia.

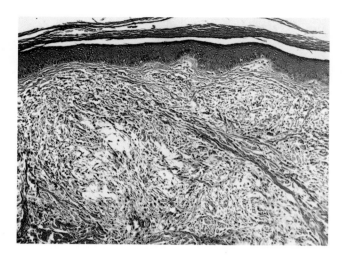

Fig. 16-112. Eruptive xanthoma. Small collections of extracellular lipid are associated with an infiltrate of lymphocytes and foamy histiocytes.

Subcutaneous Reaction Patterns

Panniculitis

Erythema Nodosum

Erythema nodosum is characterized by painful, tender nodules (Fig. 16-113) mainly on the anterior aspects of the lower legs.[194] Females are involved three times as often as males, and the 15- to 25-year-old age group is most commonly affected. The tender cutaneous nodules are often associated with prodromal symptoms of fever, arthralgia, or leg pain. The nodules rarely ulcerate and heal without scarring. Beta-hemolytic streptococcal infection and sarcoidosis are the most common causes of erythema nodosum in the United States, although in approximately 50 percent of cases there is no demonstrable cause. Deep fungal infections such as coccidioidomycosis and histoplasmosis are also causes of erythema nodosum. Drugs appear to be much less common causative agents than infection.

The epidermis and upper portions of the dermis are usually normal. Biopsy specimens of early lesions show lymphocytes and neutrophils in the interlobular septa of the subcutaneous fat. The walls of small veins may be thickened and surrounded by inflammatory cells, but true vasculitis is usually absent. In more mature lesions of erythema nodosum, the septa between fat lobules become greatly thickened with fibrous connective tissue. Focal collections of histiocytes and multinucleate giant cells arranged around minute slits in the septae are referred to as Miescher's granulomas. Lymphocytes and histiocytes predominate, and neutrophils are usually absent. The inflammatory process typically extends only for a short distance into the fat lobules. In late lesions, fibrosis of fat septa may occur with trapping of giant cells; however, there is no significant atrophy of fat lobules.

Subacute Nodular Migratory Panniculitis

Subacute nodular migratory panniculitis occurs mainly in women as nodules and plaques on the lower legs. Lesions persist for several years, and nodules may enlarge to form plaques.[195] The condition may represent a chronic form of erythema nodosum.[196]

The histologic changes in subacute nodular migratory panniculitis are essentially indistinguishable from erythema nodosum.

Weber-Christian Disease

Weber-Christian disease or relapsing febrile nodular nonsuppurative panniculitis produces recurrent crops of nodules and plaques that may involve the trunk as well as the extremities. The nodules are tender and resemble abscesses. Individual lesions heal, leaving depressed scars.[197] Patients are ill with fever, malaise, and arthralgias. Inflammation of visceral fat may produce symptoms of an acute abdomen. The existence of Weber-Christian disease is controversial as some cases turn out to have factitial panniculitis or other forms of panniculitis.

Early lesions show infiltration of entire fat lobules predominantly with neutrophils, producing changes that resemble an

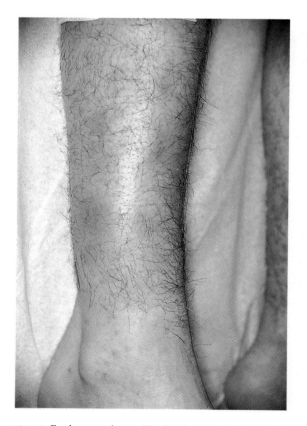

Fig. 16-113. Erythema nodosum. Tender, deep red nodules of the lower legs had a sudden onset.

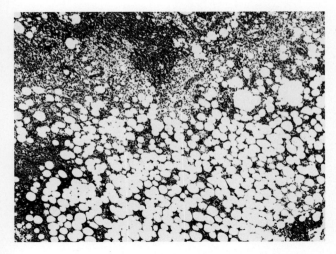

Fig. 16-114. Weber-Christian disease. Panlobular infiltrate of inflammatory cells surrounds individual lipocytes.

acute infection (Fig. 16-114). Later, macrophages predominate and ingest fat from damaged lipocytes, producing abundant foamy cytoplasm.[198] Interlobular septa are generally intact. In late stages, the fat lobules may be replaced by fibrous tissue. Blood vessels within the subcutaneous fat show thickening of their walls and are surrounded by patchy infiltrates of lymphocytes. A few multinucleate giant cells may be present.

Erythema Induratum

Erythema induratum is a rare form of panniculitis that produces inflammatory nodules on the calves. The nodules tend to break down and drain purulent material. Erythema induratum is considered a form of cutaneous tuberculosis in which *Mycobacterium tuberculosis* or its products disseminate during transient bacteremia to areas of vascular stasis.[199] Evidence of previous pulmonary or renal tuberculosis may be present, but most patients do not have clinically active disease. Delayed skin test reactions to mycobacterial antigens are positive. The term *nodular vasculitis* has been suggested for those cases in which there is no evidence of tuberculosis.[200]

The epidermis and upper dermis are often normal. A granulomatous infiltrate containing lymphocytes, histiocytes, epithelioid cells, and giant cells extends into fat lobules and replaces subcutaneous fat. Distinct tubercles may be present. There are focal areas of caseation necrosis and vascular changes characterized by vessel wall thickening, fibrinoid necrosis, and vascular inflammation. Some veins and venules may be surrounded by granulomatous inflammation.

Subcutaneous Fat Necrosis of the Newborn

Otherwise healthy infants of either sex may be affected during the neonatal period by subcutaneous fat necrosis.[201] Deep-seated nodules and plaques involve the back, cheeks, arms, thighs, and buttocks.[202] Some lesions are movable and have sharply defined margins. Several cases of subcutaneous fat necrosis have been associated with hypercalcemia.[203]

The epidermis and upper dermis are normal. Basophilic areas of fat necrosis are associated with the presence of needle-like crystals within fat cells. When clusters of fat cells are involved, the crystals have a radial arrangement. The fat is infiltrated by lymphocytes, histiocytes, epithelioid cells, and multinucleate giant cells. Interlobular septa are often thickened, and deposits of calcium occur within the fat lobules. In frozen sections, the crystals within fat cells are seen to be doubly refractile by polarized light examination. The von Kossa stain may be helpful in demonstrating the presence of calcium deposits.

Sclerema Neonatorum

Sclerma neonatorum is an uncommon disorder that affects premature or debilitated infants within the first few days of life. The skin is smooth, cool, tense, hard, and purplish. Firm induration of the skin begins on the thighs and legs but may involve the entire body except for the palms, soles, and scrotum.[204] Body movement and respiration may be hindered, and infants frequently develop pneumonia. In the past, up to 75 percent of infants with this disorder died; however, preventing a reduction in body temperature by using heated incubators for premature infants may prevent sclerema neonatorum.

The histologic changes in the fat in sclerema neonatorum are similar to subcutaneous fat necrosis of the newborn except that fat necrosis is minimal or absent. Clusters of fat cells are filled with needle-like clefts, which on frozen section are shown to be occupied by doubly refractile crystals. The crystals do not stain with fat stains. Interconnecting bands of fibrous tissue and focal collections of mononuclear inflammatory cells are seen in the fat. Calcium deposits are usually absent in sclerema neonatorum.

Pancreatic Fat Necrosis

Pancreatitis or pancreatic carcinoma may result in elevated levels of serum lipase with the resulting breakdown of fat in the skin, joints, and viscera. Tender nodules and plaques on the lower extremities tend to break down and drain an oily material. Polyarthritis, pleural effusions, and abdominal pain may result from widespread inflammation of fat.[205]

The subcutaneous fat shows focal areas of fat necrosis associated with the presence of ghost-like fat cells with thickened walls and no nuclei.[206] The basophilic areas of fat necrosis often contain calcium granules. The areas of fat necrosis may contain extravasated RBCs, as well as a polymorphic infiltrate of neutrophils, lymphocytes, histiocytes, and foreign body giant cells.

Lupus Panniculitis

Unlike the other forms of panniculitis, lupus panniculitis (lupus profundus) shows a predilection for the face, upper arms, and buttocks.[207] Lupus panniculitis may occur with either discoid or systemic lupus erythematosus. Cutaneous lesions may be preceded by trauma. The skin overlying the inflammatory nodules and plaques may be normal or show scaly atrophic lesions characteristic of discoid lupus erythematosus. Nodules that resolve leave clinically depressed areas in the skin secondary to atrophy of subcutaneous fat.

The epidermis may be normal or may show changes of discoid lupus erythematosus, which include hyperkeratosis, follic-

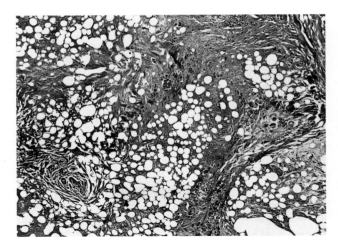

Fig. 16-115. Lupus erythematosus panniculitis. Panlobular infiltrate of inflammatory cells is associated with hyalinization of connective tissue and replacement of fat lobules.

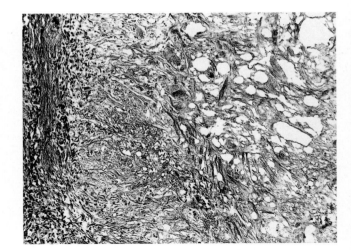

Fig. 16-117. Sclerosing lipogranuloma. Empty vacuoles from which an oily material has been dissolved during processing are associated with hyalinization of connective tissue and a granulomatous infiltrate.

ular plugging, and atrophy of the epidermis. Liquefaction degeneration of the basal zone is associated with melanin pigment incontinence and the presence of colloid bodies within the epidermis or superficial dermis. A patchy infiltrate of lymphocytes surrounds small dermal blood vessels and pilosebaceous structures. Two patterns of inflammation are seen in the subcutaneous fat. Early lesions may show only a dense patchy infiltrate of lymphocytes surrounding blood vessels in the deep dermis and upper subcutaneous fat. More advanced lesions show necrosis of fat lobules with replacement by eosinophilic hyalinized connective tissue (Fig. 16-115). The hyalinized connective tissue may run in thick bands that tend to be oriented parallel to the surface of the skin. Inflamed vessels are seen within the subcutaneous fat, and a variable number of plasma cells are present. Immunofluorescence microscopy often shows the deposition of immunoglobulins and complement in a granular pattern along the basement membrane zone.

Scleroderma

Localized scleroderma or morphea characteristically produces indurated erythematous to hyperpigmented plaques on the trunk.[208] Plaques are often surrounded by an erythematous, purple border. In systemic scleroderma, the indurated skin is not well circumscribed as in morphea and more often involves the face and acral portions of the extremities.[209] The skin over the fingers appears shiny and smooth (Fig. 16-116), and there may be ulcerations of the fingertips. Cutaneous telangiectasia and calcium deposits occur. Sclerosis of the esophagus causes difficulty in swallowing, and there may be involvement of the gas-

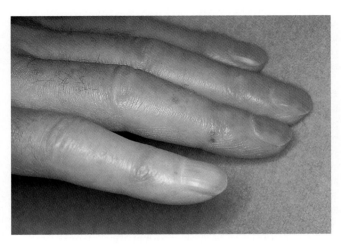

Fig. 16-116. Scleroderma. The fingers show shiny skin and mat-like telangiectasias.

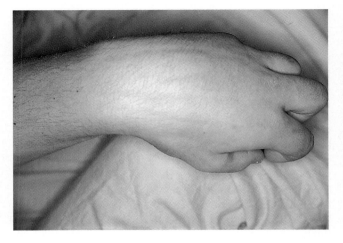

Fig. 16-118. Fasciitis with eosinophilia. Flexion of the wrist has produced the groove sign over a tendon. Skin induration occurred after strenuous weight lifting.

trointestinal tract, lungs, and kidneys with malabsorption, dyspnea, and uremia.

Inflammation is more prominent in morphea than in systemic scleroderma. Dense patches of lymphocytes occur around small vessels and eccrine sweat glands at the dermal-subcutaneous junction. In later lesions of morphea and in systemic scleroderma, the inflammatory infiltrate is mild, and the subcutaneous fat is replaced by dense fibrous connective tissue, which surrounds and entraps eccrine sweat glands.[210] The normal layer of fat around sweat glands is absent and the glands appear to be located in the mid-dermis. The connective tissue deep to the sweat glands stains pale pink with the H&E stain, consistent with new collagen. Hair follicles are often destroyed, and the overall thickness of the dermis appears increased. The dermal collagen appears compact and homogeneous with few spaces between collagen fibers. Electron microscopic examination of the deep dermis reveals active fibroblasts and an increased percentage of young collagen fibrils.[211] The young collagen fibrils show less of a tendency to be oriented parallel to the surface of the skin than the more mature collagen of the reticular dermis.

Factitial Panniculitis

Factitial panniculitis may result from mechanical trauma, thermal injuries, or injection of foreign material into the subcutaneous fat.[212] Although any part of the body may be involved, bizarre cases of inflammation of the fat of breasts and genitalia should raise suspicion of factitial panniculitis. Foreign material such as milk, paraffin oil, drugs, and paint have been injected.

Inflammation within fat lobules may show a mixture of abscesses containing neutrophils associated with areas of granulomatous inflammation. The presence of foreign material in the subcutaneous fat is diagnostic but may be difficult to document. Polarized light examination should be used in all cases of undiagnosed panniculitis.[212] Collections of calcium may be seen in the subcutaneous fat with the von Kossa stain. Paraffin oil injected into the skin shows numerous clear vacuoles with the appearance of Swiss cheese. A mixed inflammatory infiltrate may surround individual vacuoles. The oil is dissolved from the vacuoles during processing. Sclerosis of connective tissue associated with the oil vacuoles produces a reaction pattern referred to as sclerosing lipogranuloma[213] (Fig. 16-117). Drugs such as pentazocine are particularly likely to produce sclerosis of subcutaneous fat.

Differential Diagnosis of Panniculitis

There is considerable overlap in the histologic changes seen in panniculitis, and often a specific diagnosis cannot be made. It is helpful to subclassify panniculitis into septal panniculitis and lobular panniculitis. Septal panniculitis is exemplified by erythema nodosum, by far the most common cause of panniculitis, and subacute nodular migratory panniculitis, which may be a variant of erythema nodosum. The other forms of panniculitis discussed in the previous sections are lobular. Lobular panniculitis often results in replacement of fat cells with clinical atrophy. Many cases initially diagnosed as Weber-Christian disease have been found to be factitial panniculitis,[214] so a careful search for foreign material and polarized light examination should be a part of the evaluation of every case of panniculitis.

In some cases, a descriptive diagnosis such as lobular panniculitis with granulomatous inflammation may be the most specific diagnosis that can be made. Superficial migratory thrombophlebitis may mimic panniculitis but shows an inflammatory infiltrate within the wall of a large vein at the junction of the dermis and subcutaneous fat.[200] The vessel is often thrombosed.

Fasciitis

Fasciitis with eosinophilia (Shulman's syndrome) is characterized by the sudden onset of edema and induration of the skin (Fig. 16-118) of the hands, arms, and legs with sparing of the face and fingers.[215] The skin changes are often preceded by some form of strenuous physical exercise. The involved skin often has a cobblestoned or dimpled appearance and cannot be mobilized. The skin may show pigmentary changes and loss of hair. Laboratory findings include an increased number of circulating eosinophils, an elevated erythrocyte sedimentation rate, and hypergammaglobulinemia.

Skin biopsies in fasciitis with eosinophilia should be deep enough to include the full thickness of the subcutaneous fat and deep fascia. A patchy infiltrate of lymphocytes, histiocytes, and plasma cells may be present at the junction of the deep dermis and subcutaneous fat. In 15 to 20 percent of cases, there is fi-

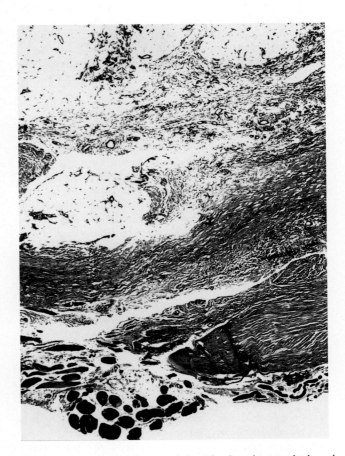

Fig. 16-119. Fasciitis with eosinophilia. The deep fascia is thickened and contains a sparse infiltrate of mononuclear cells.

brosis of the deep dermis beneath the level of eccrine sweat glands similar to that seen in morphea and scleroderma. The most typical histologic changes are a marked thickening of the deep fascia and infiltration of the fascia with lymphocytes, histiocytes, and a variable number of plasma cells[215] (Fig. 16-119). In about half of the cases, eosinophils are present in the fascia. The thickened fascia tends to replace the overlying subcutaneous fat.

Differential Diagnosis of Fasciitis

Fasciitis with eosinophilia is generally considered a variant of scleroderma. At least 50 percent of deep biopsy specimens of scleroderma also show thickening of the subcutaneous fascia.[216]

GLOSSARY OF TERMS

Only the most commonly used pathologic terms in dermatopathology are defined.

Acantholysis: loss of cohesion of cells of the malpighian layer. The rupture of desmosomes connecting epidermal cells results in intraepidermal vesicles.

Acanthosis: increased thickness of the malpighian layer.

Adnexal structures: the pilosebaceous units, eccrine sweat glands, and apocrine sweat glands. Also known collectively as adnexae or appendages.

Apoptosis: a distinctive mode of programmed cell death that typically affects individual epithelial cells and does not evoke an inflammatory response. The colloid bodies of lichen planus and lupus erythematosus are apoptotic bodies.[217]

Basement membrane zone: a narrow zone present immediately deep to the epidermal basal cells, which is visible by light microscopy using the periodic acid-Schiff reaction. The basement membrane zone is not identical to the basal lamina, which is visible by electron microscopy.

Bulla: a cavity or blister within or beneath the epidermis. A bulla smaller than 5 mm in diameter is called a vesicle.

Colloid bodies: deeply eosinophilic, round to oval bodies within the epidermis or the superficial dermis. Most, if not all, colloid bodies appear to result from the degeneration of epidermal cells. Synonyms include hyaline bodies, eosinophilic bodies, and Civatte bodies.

Crust: tissue fluid that has coagulated on the skin surface. Most often seen in acute inflammatory diseases.

Dyskeratosis: abnormal keratinization of squamous cells. It may occur as individual cell dyskeratosis or dyskeratosis of groups of cells. Dyskeratosis may be seen in inflammatory diseases and in benign or malignant tumors.

Exocytosis: the migration of inflammatory cells into the epidermis.

Festooning: the projection of prominent dermal papillae into the base of a subepidermal bulla cavity.

Follicular plugging: the occlusion and dilation of the openings of hair follicles by increased amounts of keratin.

Grenz zone: a marginal zone of uninvolved connective tissue that often separates the epidermis or the adnexa from an inflammatory or infiltrative process.

Hyperkeratosis: thickening of the stratum corneum.

Liquefaction degeneration: degeneration of the basal cells and the basement membrane zone with the formation of clear vacuoles. Also called hydropic degeneration.

Microabscesses: small abscesses within the epidermis that are not visible grossly. Munro's microabscesses of psoriasis contain pyknotic neutrophils and most often occur in the keratin layer. Spongiotic microabscess characteristic of acute dermatitis occurs within the malpighian layer due to intercellular edema. Pautrier's microabscesses of mycosis fungoides are sharply circumscribed spaces within the malpighian layer containing atypical mononuclear cells.

Necrobiosis: an alteration of dermal collagen characterized by basophilia and incomplete necrosis so the fibrillar nature of the connective tissue may still be appreciated. Necrobiosis differs from caseation necrosis, which produces more complete tissue death and in which the necrotic tissue appears amorphous. A third form of cell death, apoptosis, usually affects individual epithelial cells and results in the formation of colloid bodies.

Papillomatosis: irregular undulation of the outer surface of the epidermis produced by outward projection of epidermis and associated connective tissue.

Parakeratosis: retention of nuclei within the stratum corneum.

Pigmentary incontinence: a displacement of melanin pigment from the basal cell layer into dermal macrophages or into the connective tissue of the superficial dermis. It follows liquefaction degeneration or other alteration of the basement membrane zone.

Pseudoepitheliomatous hyperplasia: marked reactive proliferation of epidermis mimicking carcinoma.

Pustule: an intraepidermal or subepidermal cavity containing neutrophils. It may result from secondary changes in a preexisting bulla.

Pyknosis: shrinkage of nuclei.

Spongiosis: edema occurring between epidermal cells that may progress to spongiotic microabscesses and bullae.

Villi: elongated dermal papillae that project into the floor of a bulla cavity and are covered by a single layer of basal cells.

REFERENCES

1. Katz SI: The role of Langerhans' cells in immunity. Arch Dermatol 116:1361–1362, 1980
2. Fisher JP, Cooke RA: Experimental toxic and allergic contact dermatitis. II. A histopathologic study. J Allergy 29:411–428, 1958
3. Bunch LW, Tilley JC: Pityriasis rosea. Arch Dermatol 84:79–86, 1961
4. Walzer RA: Autoimmunity and cutaneous disease. Med Clin North Am 49:769–782, 1965
5. Whitfield A: Lumelian lectures on some points in the aetiology of skin diseases. Lancet 2:122–127, 1921
6. Young E: Dyshidrotic (endogenous) eczema. Dermatologica 129:306–310, 1964
7. Graham JH: Superficial fungal infections. pp. 137–268. In Graham JH, Johnson WC, Helwig EB (eds): Dermal Pathology. Harper & Row, Hagerstown, MD, 1972
8. Machado-Pinto J, Golitz LE: Incontinentia pigmenti. pp. 1725–1728. In Arndt KA, LeBoit PE, Robinson JK, Wintroub BU (eds): Cutaneous

Medicine and Surgery, An Integrated Program in Dermatology. WB Saunders, Philadelphia, 1996

9. Carney RG Jr: Incontinentia pigmenti: a world statistical analysis. Arch Dermatol 112:535–542, 1976

10. Emmerson RW, Wilson-Jones E: Eosinophilic spongiosis in pemphigus. Arch Dermatol 97:252–257, 1968

11. Ruiz E, Dng JS, Abell EA: Eosinophilic spongiosis: a clinical, histologic and immunopathologic study. J Am Acad Dermatol 30:973–976, 1994

12. Pinkus H: Psoriasiform tissue reactions. Aust J Dermatol 8:31–35, 1965

13. Pinkus H, Mehregan AH: Psoriasiform tissue reactions. pp. 125–139. In: A Guide to Dermatohistopathology. Appleton & Lange, E. Norwalk, CT, 1976

14. Obuch ML, Maurer TA, Becker B, et al: Psoriasis and human immunodeficiency virus infection. J Am Acad Dermatol 27:667–673, 1992

15. Duvie M, Johnson T, Rapini R, et al: Acquired immunodeficiency syndrome-associated psoriasis and Reiter's syndrome. Arch Dermatol 123:1622–1632, 1987

16. Weinstein GD, Van Scott EJ: Autoradiographic analysis of turnover times of normal and psoriatic epidermis. J Invest Dermatol 45:257–262, 1965

17. Weinstein GD, Frost P: Abnormal cell proliferation in psoriasis. J Invest Dermatol 50:254–259, 1968

18. Telfer NR, Chalmers RJG, Whale K, et al: The role of streptococcal infection in the initiation of guttate psoriasis. Arch Dermatol 128:39–42, 1992

19. Baker H, Ryan TJ: Generalized pustular psoriasis: a clinical and epidemiological study of 104 cases. Br J Dermatol 80:771–793, 1968

20. Gordon M, Johnson WC: Histopathology and histochemistry of psoriasis. I. The active lesion and clinically normal skin. Arch Dermatol 95:402–407, 1967

21. Cox AJ, Watson W: Histologic variations in lesions of psoriasis. Arch Dermatol 106:503–506, 1972

22. Engleman EP, Weber HM: Reiter's syndrome. Clin Orthop 57:19–29, 1968

23. Weinberger HJ, Ropes MW, Kulka JP, et al: Reiter's syndrome—clinical and pathological observations: a long-term study of 16 cases. Medicine (Baltimore) 41:35–91, 1962

24. Kulka JP: The lesions of Reiter's syndrome. Arthritis Rheum 5:195–201, 1962

25. Pindborg JJ, Gorlin RJ, Asboe-Hansen G: Reiter's syndrome. Oral Surg 16:551–560, 1963

26. Pinkus H, Mehregan AH: The primary histologic lesion of seborrheic dermatitis and psoriasis. J Invest Dermatol 46:109–116, 1966

27. Gross DA, Landau JW, Newcomer VD: Pityriasis rubra pilaris: report of a case and analysis of the literature. Arch Dermatol 99:710–716, 1969

28. Vanderhooft SL, Francis JS, Holbrook KA, et al: Familial pityriasis rubra pilaris. Arch Dermatol 131:448–453, 1995

29. Davidson CL Jr, Winkelmann RK, Kierland RR: Pityriasis rubra pilaris: a follow up study of 57 patients. Arch Dermatol 100:175–178, 1969

30. Shaffer B, Beerman H: Lichen simplex chronicus and its variants. Arch Dermatol Syph 64:340–351, 1951

31. Pinkus H: Lichenoid tissue reactions: a speculative review of the clinical spectrum of epidermal basal cell damage with special reference to erythema dyschromicum perstans. Arch Dermatol 107:840–846, 1973

32. Weedon D: The lichenoid tissue reaction. J Cutan Pathol 12:279–281, 1985

33. Fellner MJ: Lichen planus. Int J Dermatol 19:71–75, 1980

34. Altman J, Perry HO: The variations and course of lichen planus. Arch Dermatol 84:179–191, 1961

35. Samman PD: Lichen planus: an analysis of 200 cases. Trans St Johns Hosp Dermatol Soc 46:36–38, 1961

36. Tompkins JK: Lichen planus: a statistical study of 41 cases. Arch Dermatol 71:515–519, 1955

37. Haber H, Sarkany I: Hypertrophic lichen planus and lichen simplex. Trans St Johns Hosp Dermatol Soc 41:61, 1958

38. Shklar G: Erosive and bullous oral lesions of lichen planus. Arch Dermatol 97:411–416, 1968

39. Cram DL, Kierland RR, Winkelmann RK: Ulcerative lichen planus of the feet. Arch Dermatol 93:692–701, 1966

40. Black MM: What is going on in lichen planus? Clin Exp Dermatol 2:303–310, 1977

41. Pennys NS, Ackerman AB, Gottlieb NL: Gold dermatitis: a clinical and histopathological study. Arch Dermatol 109:372–376, 1974

42. Halevy S, Shai A: Lichenoid drug eruptions. J Am Acad Dermatol 29:249–255, 1993

43. Prystowsky SD, Herndon JH Jr, Gillian JN: Chronic cutaneous lupus erythematosus (DLE): a clinical and laboratory investigation of 80 patients. Medicine (Baltimore) 55:183–191, 1976

44. David KM, Bennion SD, DeSpain JD, et al: Clinical, histologic and immunofluorescent distinctions between subacute cutaneous lupus erythematosus and discoid lupus erythematosus. J Invest Dermatol 99:251–257, 1992

45. Tsuchida T, Furue M, Kashiwado T, et al: Bullous systemic lupus erythematosus with cutaneous mucinosis and leukocytoclastic vasculitis. J Am Acad Dermatol 31:387–390, 1994

46. Weiss RM, Cohen AD: Lichen nitidus of the palms and soles. Arch Dermatol 104:538–540, 1971

47. Jeerapaet P, Ackerman AB: Histologic patterns of secondary syphilis. Arch Dermatol 107:373–377, 1973

48. Goette DK: Benign lichenoid keratosis. Arch Dermatol 116:780–782, 1980

49. Lumpkin LR, Helwig EB: Solitary lichen planus. Arch Dermatol 93:54–55, 1966

50. Abramovits W, Landau JW, Lowe NJ: A report of two patients with lichen aureus. Arch Dermatol 116:1183–1184, 1980

51. Kruger GRF, Berard CW, DeLellis RA, et al: Graft-versus-host disease: morphologic variation and differential diagnosis in 8 cases of HL-A matched bone marrow transplantation. Am J Pathol 63:179–292, 1971

52. Kikuchi A, Naka W, Harada T, et al: Parapsoriasis en plaques: its potential for progression to malignant lymphoma. J Am Acad Dermatol 29:419–422, 1993

53. Janis JF, Winkelmann RK: Histopathology of the skin in dermatomyositis. Arch Dermatol 97:640–650, 1968

54. Wayte DM, Helwig EB: Halo nevi. Cancer 22:69–90, 1968

55. Bergfeld WF, Lesowitz SA: Lichen sclerosus et atrophicus. Arch Dermatol 101:247–248, 1970

56. Dajani AS, Ferrieri P, Wanamaker L: Endemic superficial pyoderma in children. Arch Dermatol 108:517–522, 1973

57. Kaplan EL, Anthony BF, Chapman SS, et al: Epidemic acute glomerulonephritis associated with type 49 streptococcal pyoderma: I. clinical and laboratory findings. Am J Med 48:9–27, 1970

58. Lowney ED, Baublis JV, Kreye GM, et al: The scalded skin syndrome in small children. Arch Dermatol 95:359–369, 1967

59. Melish ME, Glasgow LA: The staphylococcal scalded-skin syndrome. N Engl J Med 282:1114–1119, 1970

60. Levine G, Norden CW: Staphylococcal scalded-skin syndrome in an adult. N Engl J Med 287:1339–1340, 1972

61. Rothenberg R, Renna FS, Drew TM, et al: Staphylococcal scalded skin syndrome in an adult. Arch Dermatol 108:408–410, 1973

62. Elias PM, Fritsch P, Epstein EH Jr: Staphylococcal scalded skin syndrome. Clinical features, pathogenesis, and recent microbiological and biochemical developments. Arch Dermatol 113:207–219, 1977

63. Bean SF, Lynch FW: Senear-Usher syndrome (pemphigus erythematosus). Arch Dermatol 101:642–645, 1970

64. Perry HO: Pemphigus foliaceus. Arch Dermatol 83:52–72, 1961

65. Furtado TA: Histopathology of pemphigus foliaceus. Arch Dermatol 80:66–71, 1959

66. Chorzelski T, Jablonska S, Blaszczyk M: Immunopathological

investigation in Senear-Usher syndrome (coexistence of pemphigus and lupus erythematosus). Br J Dermatol 80:211–217, 1968

67. Callen JP: Internal disorders associated with bullous disease of the skin. J Am Acad Dermatol 3:107–119, 1980

68. Amagai M, Klaus-Kortum V, Stanley JR: Autoantibodies against a novel epithelial cadherin in pemphigus vulgaris, a disease of cell adhesion. Cell 67:869–877, 1991

69. Horn TD, Anhalt GJ: Histologic features of paraneoplastic pemphigus. Arch Dermatol 128:1091–1095, 1992

70. Camisa C, Helm TN, Lin YC: Paraneoplastic pemphigus: a report of three cases including one long-term survivor. J Am Acad Dermatol 27:547–553, 1992

71. Gottlieb SK, Lutzner MA: Darier's disease. Arch Dermatol 107:225–230, 1973

72. Weathers DR, Olansky S, Sharpe LO: Darier's disease with mucous membrane involvement. Arch Dermatol 100:50–53, 1969

73. Szymanski FJ: Warty dyskeratoma. Arch Dermatol 75:567–572, 1957

74. Tanay A, Mehregan AH: Warty dyskeratoma. Dermatologica 138:155–164, 1969

75. Grover RW: Transient acantholytic dermatosis. Arch Dermatol 101:426–434, 1970

76. Grover RW: Transient acantholytic dermatosis: electron microscope study. Arch Dermatol 104:26–37, 1971

77. Chalet M, Grover R, Ackerman AB: Transient acantholytic dermatosis. Arch Dermatol 113:431, 1977

78. McSorley J, Shapiro L, Brownstein MH, et al: Herpes simplex and varicella-zoster: comparative histopathology of 77 cases. Int J Dermatol 13:69–75, 1974

79. Gruber GG, Owen LG, Callen JP: Vesicular pemphigoid. J Am Acad Dermatol 3:619–622, 1980

80. Eng AM, Moncada B: Bullous pemphigoid and dermatitis herpetiformis: histopathologic differentiation of bullous pemphigoid and dermatitis herpetiformis. Arch Dermatol 110:51–57, 1978

81. Holms RC, Black MM: Herpes gestationes. Dermatol Clin 1:195–203, 1983

82. Bastuji-Gorin S, Rzany B, Stern RS, et al: Clinical classification of cases of toxic epidermal necrolysis, Stevens-Johnson syndrome, and erythema multiforme. Arch Dermatol 129:92–96, 1993

83. Howland WW, Golitz LE, Huff JC, Weston WL: Erythema multiforme: clinical, histopathologic and immunologic study. J Am Acad Dermatol 10:438, 1984

84. Orfanos CE, Schaumburg-Lever G, Lever WF: Dermal and epidermal types of erythema multiforme: a histopathological study of 24 cases. Arch Dermatol 109:682–688, 1974

85. Ackerman AB, Pennys NS, Clark WH: Erythema multiforme exudativum: distinctive pathological process. Br J Dermatol 84:554–566, 1971

86. Pinkus H, Mehregan AH: Erythema exudativum multiforme. pp. 160–161. In: A Guide to Dermatohistopathology. Appleton & Lange, East Norwalk, CT, 1976

87. Kazmierowski JA, Wuepper KD: Erythema multiforme: immune complex vasculitis of the superficial cutaneous microvasculature. J Invest Dermatol 71:366–369, 1978

88. Smith JB, Tulloch JE, Meyer LJ, et al: The incidence and prevalence of dermatitis herpetiformis in Utah. Arch Dermatol 128:1608–1610, 1992

89. Fry L, Seah PP, Riches DJ, et al: Clearance of skin lesions in dermatitis herpetiformis after gluten withdrawal. Lancet 1:288–291, 1973

90. Katz SI, Strober W: The pathogenesis of dermatitis herpetiformis. J Invest Dermatol 70:63–75, 1978

91. Zaenglein AL, Hafer L, Helm KF: Diagnosis of dermatitis herpetiformis by an avidin-biotin-peroxidase method. Arch Dermatol 131:571–573, 1995

92. Chorzelski TP, Jablonska S: IgA linear dermatosis of childhood (chronic bullous disease of childhood). Br J Dermatol 101:535–542, 1979

93. Epstein JH, Tuffanelli DL, Epstein WL: Cutaneous changes in the porphyrias. Arch Dermatol 107:689–698, 1973

94. Egbert BM, LeBoit PE, McCalmont T, et al: Caterpillar bodies: distinctive basement membrane-containing structures in blisters of porphyria. Am J Dermatopathol 15:199–202, 1993

95. Bauer EA, Briggaman RA: The mechanobullous diseases (epidermolysis bullosa). pp. 334–347. In Fitzpatrick TB, Eisen AZ, Freedberg IM, et al (eds): Dermatology in General Medicine. McGraw-Hill, New York, 1979

96. Schuman BM, Arciniegas E: The management of esophageal complications of epidermolysis bullosa. Am J Dig Dis 17:875–880, 1972

97. Chorney JA, Shroyer KR, Golitz LE: Malignant melanoma and a squamous cell carcinoma in recessive dystrophic epidermolysis bullosa. Arch Dermatol 129:1212, 1993

98. Briggaman RA, Wheeler CE Jr: Epidermolysis bullosa dystrophica–recessive: a possible role of anchoring fibrils in the pathogenesis. J Invest Dermatol 65:203–211, 1975

99. Coulombe P, Hutton ME, Letai A, et al: Point mutations in human 14 genes of epidermolysis bullosa simplex patients. Genetic and functional analyses. Cell 66:1301–1311, 1991

100. Bean SF: Cicatricial pemphigoid. Immunofluorescent studies. Arch Dermatol 110:552–555, 1974

101. Shornick JK: Pemphigoid (Herpes) gestationes. pp. 29–36. In Black MM, McKay M, Brande P (eds): Color Atlas and Text of Obstetric and Gynecologic Dermatology. Mosby-Wolfe, London, 1995

102. Ackerman AB: Histologic Diagnosis of Inflammatory Skin Diseases. Lea & Febiger, Philadelphia, 1978

103. Monroe EW, Jones HE: Urticaria. Arch Dermatol 113:80–90, 1977

104. Shelley WB: Erythema annulare centrifugum due to Candida albicans. Br J Dermatol 77:383–384, 1965

105. Scrimenti RJ: Erythema chronicum migrans. Arch Dermatol 102:104–105, 1970

106. Melski JW, Reed KD, Mitchell PD, et al: Primary and secondary erythema migrans in central Wisconsin. Arch Dermatol 129:709–716, 1993

107. Hardin JA, Steere AC, Malawista SE: Immune complexes and the evolution of Lyme arthritis: dissemination and localization of abnormal C1q binding activity. N Engl J Med 301:1358–1363, 1979

108. Boyd AS, Neldner KH, Mentor A: Erythema gyratum repens: a paraneoplastic syndrome. J Acad Dermatol 26:757–762, 1992

109. Epstein JH: Polymorphous light eruption. J Am Acad Dermatol 3:329–343, 1980

110. Jansen CT: The natural history of polymorphous light eruptions. Arch Dermatol 115:165–169, 1979

111. von den Driesch P: Sweet's syndrome (acute febrile neutrophilic dermatosis). J Am Acad Dermatol 31:535–556, 1994

112. Lowe L, Kornfeld B, Clayman J, et al: Rheumatoid neutrophilic dermatosis. J Cutan Pathol 19:48–53, 1992

113. Jennette CJ, Milling DM, Falk RJ: Vasculitis affecting the skin: a review. Arch Dermatol 130:899–906, 1994

114. Yiannias JA, El-Azhary RA, Gibson LE: Erythema elevatum diutinum: a clinical and histopathologic study of 13 patients. J Am Acad Dermatol 26:38–44, 1992

115. LeBoit PE, Yen TS, Wintraub B: The evaluation of lesions in erythema elevatum diutinum. Am J Dermatopathol 8:392–402, 1986

116. Ackerman AB: Hemorrhagic bullae in gonococcemia. N Engl J Med 282:793–794, 1970

117. Morgaretten W, Nakai H, Landing BH: Significance of selective vasculitis and the "bone marrow" syndrome in pseudomonas septicemia. N Engl J Med 265:773–776, 1961

118. Diaz-Perez JL, Winkelmann RK: Cutaneous periarteritis nodosa. Arch Dermatol 110:407–417, 1974

119. Michalak T: Immune complexes of hepatitis B surface antigen in the pathogenesis of periarteritis nodosa: a study of seven necropsy cases. Am J Pathol 90:619–632, 1978

120. Szymanski FJ: Pityriasis lichenoides et varioliformis acuta: histopathological evidence that it is an entity distinct from parapsoriasis. Arch Dermatol 79:7–15, 1959

121. Churg J, Strauss L: Allergic granulomatosis, allergic angiitis, and periarteritis nodosa. Am J Pathol 27:277–301, 1951

122. Jennette JC, Falk RJ: Anti-neutrophil cytoplasmic autoantibodies and associated diseases: a review. Am J Kidney Dis 15:517–529, 1990

123. Strauss L, Churg J, Zak FG: Cutaneous lesions of allergic granulomatosis. J Invest Dermatol 17:349–359, 1951

124. Patten SF, Tomecki KJ: Wegener's granulomatosis: cutaneous and oral mucosal disease. J Am Acad Dermatol 28:710–718, 1993

125. Barksdale SK, Hallahan CW, Kerr GS, et al: Cutaneous pathology in Wegener's granulomatosis: a clinicopathologic study of 75 biopsies in 46 patients. Am J Surg Pathol 19:161–172, 1995

126. Hamilton CR Jr, Shelley WM, Tumulty PA: Giant cell arteritis: including temporal arteritis and polymyalgia rheumatica. Medicine 50:1–27, 1971

127. Barefoot SW, Lund HZ: Temporal (giant-cell) arteritis associated with ulcerations of the scalp. Arch Dermatol 93:79–83, 1966

128. Pedace FJ, Perry HO: Granuloma faciale: a clinical and histopathologic review. Arch Dermatol 94:387–395, 1966

129. Sweet RD: An acute febrile dermatosis. Br J Dermatol 76:349–356, 1964

130. Goldman GC, Moschella SL: Acute febrile neutrophilic dermatosis (Sweet's syndrome). Arch Dermatol 103:654–660, 1971

131. Bard JW, Winkelmann RK: Livedo vasculitis: segmental hyalinizing vasculitis of the dermis. Arch Dermatol 96:489–499, 1967

132. Dicken CH, Carrington SG, Winkelmann RK: Generalized granuloma annulare. Arch Dermatol 99:556–563, 1969

133. Owens DW, Freeman RG: Perforating granuloma annulare. Arch Dermatol 103:64–67, 1971

134. Rubin M, Lynch FW: Subcutaneous granuloma annulare: comment on familial granuloma annulare. Arch Dermatol 93:416–420, 1965

135. Dahl MV, Ullman S, Goltz RW: Vasculitis in granuloma annulare: histopathology and direct immunofluorescence. Arch Dermatol 113:463–467, 1977

136. Muller SA, Winkelmann RK: Necrobiosis lipoidica diabeticorum: a clinical and pathological investigation of 171 cases. Arch Dermatol 93:272–281, 1966

137. Duboid EL, Friou GJ, Chandor S: Rheumatoid nodules and rheumatoid granulomas in systemic lupus erythematosus. JAMA 220:515–518, 1972

138. Draheim JH, Johnson LC, Helwig EB: A clinicopathologic analysis of "rheumatoid" nodules occurring in 54 children. Am J Pathol 35:678, 1959

139. Golitz LE, Shapiro L, Hurwitz E, et al: Cicatricial alopecia of sarcoidosis. Arch Dermatol 107:758–760, 1973

140. Azar HA, Lunardelli C: Collagen nature of asteroid bodies of giant cells in sarcoidosis. Am J Pathol 57:81–92, 1969

141. Ridley DS, Jopling WH: Classification of leprosy according to immunity: a five-group system. Int J Leprosy 34:255–273, 1966

142. Shelley WB, Hurley HJ: The pathogenesis of silica granulomas in man: a non-allergic colloidal phenomenon. J Invest Dermatol 34:107–123, 1960

143. Shelley WB, Hurley HJ: The allergic origin of zirconium deodorant granulomas. Br J Dermatol 70:75–101, 1958

144. Baler GR: Granulomas from topical zirconium in poison ivy dermatitis. Arch Dermatol 91:145–148, 1965

145. Stoeckle JD, Hardy HL, Weber AL: Chronic beryllium disease: long-term follow-up of sixty cases and selective review of the literature. Am J Med 46:545–561, 1967

146. Conant NF, Smith DT, Baker RD, et al: Manual of Clinical Mycology. 3rd Ed. WB Saunders, Philadelphia, 1971

147. Rosenberg FR, Einbinder J, Walzer RA, et al: Vegetating iododerma: an immunologic mechanism. Arch Dermatol 105:900–905, 1972

148. Su WPD, Kuechle MK, Peters MS, et al: Palisading granulomas caused by infectious diseases. Am J Dermatopathol 14:211–215, 1992

149. Jolly HW Jr, Seabury JH: Infections with Mycobacterium marinum. Arch Dermatol 106:32–36, 1972

150. Graham JH, Johnson WC, Burgoon CF Jr, et al: Tinea capitis: a histopathological and histochemical study. Arch Dermatol 89:528–543, 1964

151. Potter BS, Burgoon CF Jr, Johnson WC: Pityrosporum folliculitis. Arch Dermatol 107:388–391, 1973

152. Brownstein MH, Helwig EB: The cutaneous amyloidoses. II. Systemic forms. Arch Dermatol 102:20–28, 1970

153. Rukavina JG, Block WD, Jackson CE, et al: Primary systemic amyloidosis: review and experimental, genetic and clinical study of 29 cases with particular emphasis on familial form. Medicine 35:239–334, 1956

154. Glenner GG: Amyloid deposits and amyloidosis: the beta-fibrilloses. N Engl J Med 302:1283–1292; 1333–1343, 1980

155. Hashimoto K, Kobayashi H: Histogenesis of amyloid in the skin. Am J Dermatopathol 2:165–171, 1980

156. Brownstein MH, Helwig EB: Systemic amyloidosis complicating dermatoses. Arch Dermatol 102:1–7, 1970

157. Brownstein MH, Helwig EB: Secondary systemic amyloidosis: analysis of underlying disorders. South Med J 64:491–496, 1971

158. Brownstein MH, Helwig EB: The cutaneous amyloidoses. I. Localized forms. Arch Dermatol 102:8–19, 1970

159. Brownstein MH, Hashimoto K: Macular amyloidosis. Arch Dermatol 106:50–57, 1972

160. Kumakiri M, Hashimoto K: Histogenesis of primary localized cutaneous amyloidosis: sequential change of epidermal keratinocytes to amyloid via filamentous degeneration. J Invest Dermatol 73:150–162, 1979

161. Ratz JL, Bailin PL: Cutaneous amyloidosis: a case report of the tumefactive variant and a review of the spectrum of clinical presentations. J Am Acad Dermatol 4:21–24, 1981

162. Ebner H, Gebhart W: Colloid milium: light and electron microscopic investigations. Clin Exp Dermatol 2:217–226, 1977

163. Hashimoto K, Katzman RL, Kang AH, et al: Electron microscopical and biochemical analysis of colloid milium. Arch Dermatol 111:49–59, 1975

164. Graham JH, Marques AS: Colloid milium: a histochemical study. J Invest Dermatol 49:497–507, 1967

165. Caplan RM: Visceral involvement in lipoid proteinosis. Arch Dermatol 95:149–155, 1967

166. Wells MM, Golitz LE, Bender BJ: Erythropoietic protoporphyria with hepatic cirrhosis. Arch Dermatol 116:429–432, 1980

167. van der Walt JJ, Heyl T: Lipoid proteinosis and erythropoietic protoporphyria: a histological and histochemical study. Arch Dermatol 104:501–507, 1971

168. Haber LC, Bickers DR: The porphyrias: basic science aspects, clinical diagnoses and management. pp. 9–47. In Malkinson FD, Pearson RW (eds): Year Book of Dermatology. Year Book Medical, Chicago, 1975

169. Lynch PJ, Maize JC, Sisson JC: Pretibial myxedema and nonthyrotoxic thyroid disease. Arch Dermatol 107:107–111, 1973

170. Gabrilove JL, Ludwig AW: The histogenesis of myxedema. J Clin Endocrinol 17:925–932, 1957

171. Feldman P, Shapiro L, Pick AI, et al: Scleromyxedema: a dramatic response to melphalan. Arch Dermatol 99:51–56, 1969

172. McCarthy JT, Osserman E, Lombardo PC, et al: An abnormal serum globulin in lichen myxedematosus. Arch Dermatol 89:446–450, 1964

173. Harris RB, Perry HO, Kyle RA, et al: Treatment of scleromyxedema with melphalan. Arch Dermatol 115:295–299, 1979

174. Cohn BA, Wheeler CE Jr, Briggaman RA: Scleredema adultorum of Buschke and diabetes mellitus. Arch Dermatol 101:27–35, 1970

175. Fleischmajer R, Faludi G, Krol S: Scleredema and diabetes mellitus. Arch Dermatol 101:21, 1970

176. Newmeyer WL, Kilgore ES Jr, Graham WP 3d: Mucous cysts: the dorsal distal interphalangeal joint ganglion. Plast Reconstr Surg 53:313–315, 1974

177. Johnson WC, Graham JH, Helwig EB: Cutaneous myxoid cyst. JAMA 191:15–20, 1965

178. Lattanand A, Johnson WC, Graham JH: Mucous cyst (mucocele): a clinicopathologic and histochemical study. Arch Dermatol 101:673–678, 1970

179. Johnson WC, Helwig EB: Cutaneous focal mucinosis: a clinicopathologic and histochemical study. Arch Dermatol 93:13–20, 1966

180. Pinkus H: Alopecia mucinosa. Arch Dermatol 76:419–426, 1957

181. Emmerson RW: Follicular mucinosis: a study of 47 patients. Br J Dermatol 81:395–413, 1969

182. Muller SA, Winkelmann RK, Brunsting LA: Calcinosis in dermatomyositis. Arch Dermatol 79:669–673, 1959

183. Golitz LE, Fields JP: Metastatic calcification with skin necrosis. Arch Dermatol 106:398–402, 1972

184. Dahl PR, Winkelmann RK, Connolly SM: The vascular calcification-cutaneous necrosis syndrome. J Am Acad Dermatol 33:53–58, 1995

185. Shmunes E, Wood MG: Subepidermal calcified nodules. Arch Dermatol 105:593–597, 1972

186. Shapiro L, Platt N, Torres-Rodriguez VM: Idiopathic calcinosis of the scrotum. Arch Dermatol 102:199–204, 1970

187. Swinehart JM, Golitz LE: Scrotal calcinosis: dystrophic calcification in epidermoid cysts. Arch Dermatol 118:985–988, 1982

188. Lichtenstein L, Wayne Scott H, Levin MH: Pathologic changes in gout: survey of eleven necropsied cases. Am J Pathol 32:871–895, 1956

189. Fleischmajer R, Dowlati Y, Reeves JRT: Familial hyperlipidemias: diagnosis and treatment. Arch Dermatol 110:43–50, 1974

190. Schreiber MM, Shapiro SI: Secondary eruptive xanthoma. Type V hyperlipoproteinemia. Arch Dermatol 100:601–603, 1969

191. Moschella SL: Plane xanthomatosis associated with myelomatosis. Arch Dermatol 101:683–687, 1970

192. Winkelmann RK, Muller SA: Generalized eruptive histiocytoma. Arch Dermatol 88:586–596, 1963

193. Taunton OD, Yeshurun D, Jarratt M: Progressive nodular histiocytoma. Arch Dermatol 114:1505–1508, 1978

194. Sanchez YE, Vico S, de Diego V: Miescher's radial granuloma. A characteristic marker of erythema nodosum. Am J Dermatopathol 11:434–442, 1989

195. Perry HO, Winkelmann RK: Subacute nodular migratory panniculitis. Arch Dermatol 89:170–179, 1964

196. Fine RM, Meltzer HD: Chronic erythema nodosum. Arch Dermatol 100:33–38, 1969

197. Christian HA: Relapsing febrile nodular nonsuppurative panniculitis. Arch Intern Med 41:338–351, 1928

198. Milner RDG, Mitchinson MJ: Systemic Weber-Christian disease. J Clin Pathol 18:150–156, 1965

199. LaCour-Andersen S: Erythema induratum (Bazin) treated with isoniazid. Acta Derm Venereol (Stockh) 50:65–68, 1970

200. Montgomery H, O'Leary PA, Barker NW: Nodular vascular diseases of the legs: erythema induratum and allied conditions. JAMA 128:335–341, 1945

201. Weary PE, Graham GF, Selden RF Jr: Subcutaneous fat necrosis of the newborn. South Med J 59:960–965, 1966

202. Chen TH, Shewmake SW, Hansen DD, et al: Subcutaneous fat necrosis of the newborn: a case report. Arch Dermatol 117:36–37, 1981

203. Thomsen RJ: Subcutaneous fat necrosis of the newborn and idiopathic hypercalcemia. Arch Dermatol 116:1155–1158, 1980

204. Kellum RE, Ray TL, Brown GR: Sclerema neonatorum: report of case and analysis of subcutaneous and epidermal-dermal lipids by chromatographic methods. Arch Dermatol 97:372–380, 1968

205. Potts DE, Mass MF, Iseman MD: Syndrome of pancreatic disease, subcutaneous fat necrosis and polyserositis: case report and review of literature. Am J Med 58:417–423, 1975

206. Szymanski F, Bluefarb SM: Nodular fat necrosis and pancreatic disease. Arch Dermatol 83:224–229, 1961

207. Tuffanelli DL: Lupus erythematosus panniculitis (profundus): clinical and immunological studies. Arch Dermatol 103:231–242, 1971

208. Christianson HB, Dorsey CS, O'Leary PA, et al: Localized scleroderma: a clinical study of two hundred and thirty-five cases. Arch Dermatol 74:629–639, 1956

209. Tuffanelli DL, Winkelmann RK: Sustemic scleroderma: a clinical study of 727 cases. Arch Dermatol 84:359–371, 1961

210. Fleischmajer R, Damiano V, Nedwich A: Alteration of subcutaneous tissue in scleroderma. Arch Dermatol 105:59–66, 1972

211. Fleischmajer R, Nedwich A: Generalized morphea. I. Histology of the dermis and subcutaneous tissue. Arch Dermatol 106:509–514, 1972

212. Forstrom L, Winkelmann RK: Factitial panniculitis. Arch Dermatol 110:747–750, 1974

213. Urbach F, Wine SS, Johnson WC, et al: Generalized paraffinoma (sclerosing lipogranuloma). Arch Dermatol 103:277–285, 1971

214. Ackerman AB, Mosher DT, Schwamm HA: Factitial Weber-Christian syndrome. JAMA 198:731–736, 1966

215. Golitz LE: Fasciitis with eosinophilia: the Shulman syndrome. Int J Dermatol 19:552–555, 1980

216. Botet MV, Sanchez JL: The fascia in systemic scleroderma. J Am Acad Dermatol 3:36–42, 1980

217. Weedon D, Searle J, Kerr JF: Apoptosis: its nature and implications for dermatopathology. Am J Dermatopathol 1:133–144, 1979

17

Tumors of the Skin

Bruce D. Ragsdale
George F. Murphy

EPIDERMAL TUMORS

Epidermal tumors are generally composed of either squamoid or basaloid cells. They numerically predominate over the skin appendage tumors and other neoplasms to be discussed. Seemingly endless variations in architecture and disconcerting atypia pose diagnostic problems in routine material. For example, chronically inflamed keratoses acquire reactive changes that may superficially mimic carcinoma.

Criteria for differentiation of reactive alterations from true dysplasia and anaplasia within keratinocytes must be prefaced by definitions of terms. *Dysplasia* refers to cytologic and architectural characteristics with some, but not all, of the characteristics of malignant tumors. Enlarged and hyperchromatic nuclei and disordered maturation are implicit in the term dysplasia. *Anaplasia* refers to the prototypical malignant cell, which is devoid of histologic signs of differentiation. There are nuclear features of malignant tumors, but the term has no specific connotation in regard to cell size. *Atypia* simply means not typical or not normal. The term atypia is often applied to cellular changes other than dysplasia; for example, the reactive changes such as nuclear enlargement and nucleolar prominence of an inflamed epithelial neoplasm or a re-epithelializing ulcer base and the cytotoxic alterations of virally infected or metabolically poisoned cells.

The gross pathology of epithelial neoplasms is diverse and an essential element of accurate diagnosis. Abundant scale may predominate over squamous cell carcinomas due to accelerated cell cycling or impaired desquamation. A wide variety of epidermal neoplasms may mimic melanocytic tumors because of pigment incorporated into, although not produced by, their epithelial elements (e.g., pigmented basal cell carcinomas and seborrheic keratoses). Neoplasms within or directly beneath the epidermis, especially those with associated inflammation and scale, may resemble a form of dermatitis, as in superficial forms of basal cell carcinoma and squamous cell carcinoma in situ, and lichenoid keratoses.

The evolution of epidermal tumors over time depends on the individual lesion. Some seborrheic keratoses remain stable for long periods. Others undergo inflammatory regression into nondescript residual zones of verrucous epidermal hyperplasia. True warts attracting host immune responses, or simple loss of viral activity over time, can eventuate in a verrucous keratosis without specific findings of active human papillomavirus

(HPV) effect. Focal hyperkeratotic verrucous epidermal lesions are thus a final common product of a variety of senescent benign keratoses (Fig. 17-1A). Epithelial malignant tumors,[1] such as most basal cell carcinomas, may have an indolent course, with extremely slow locally invasive progression over time. The more aggressive invasive squamous cell carcinomas will grow inexorably if left untreated, and if tumor size and invasive depth increase significantly, metastases may occur. An excellent overview of pitfalls in tumor margin analysis emphasizes the importance of thinking "in three dimensions, even though the microscope slides are viewed in only two."[2]

Developmental Overgrowths

Epidermal Nevi and Hamartomas

Epidermal nevi and *hamartomas* are local or regional aberrations that arise during growth and development. Some are congenital (i.e., present at birth).[3–5]

Epidermal nevi occur in localized and generalized forms. Localized epidermal nevi can appear as linear streaks anywhere on the body. They are formed by coalescent, often hyperkeratotic papules. Most are asymptomatic, but the persistently inflamed variant (i.e., *inflammatory linear verrucous epidermal nevi* [ILVEN]) may be pruritic. ILVEN is a rather uncommon dermatosis that typically has an early average age of onset, and is unilateral, localized, pruritic, and relatively refractory to treatment. Atypical presentations of ILVEN have also been described and include late onset in life, widespread involvement, and response to treatment.[6] ILVEN represents a clonal dysregulation in growth, probably secondary to an inflammatory stimulus.[7] *Generalized ("systematized") epidermal nevi* exist as patterns of multiple streaks, often in parallel, which are either unilateral or bilateral. In some instances, large segments of the skin surface are involved. Such "systematized" epidermal nevi may be associated with mental retardation, seizures, and neural deafness, and/or other anomalies.[8]

The papillary epidermal hyperplasia characterizing epidermal nevi is both exophytic and endophytic. The constituent benign keratinocytes are arranged in normal stratified pattern with all layers represented. Various reaction patterns (epidermolytic hyperkeratosis, focal acantholytic dyskeratosis, and cornoid lamella formation) all may be present in epidermal nevi at times to an extent that obscures the basic lesion. Misdi-

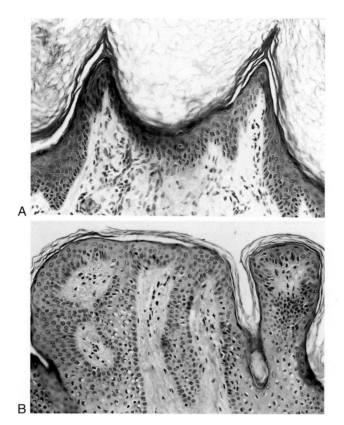

Fig. 17-1. **(A)** Verrucous epidermal hyperplasia and **(B)** epidermal nevus. The former is a final common pathway for verrucae and a variety of benign keratoses; the latter may resemble seborrheic keratosis.

agnosis as seborrheic keratosis is likely if the young age of the patient is not known. However, the base of the epidermal thickening tends to be more undulant than the relatively flat or convex deep border of the common seborrheic keratosis. Also, epidermal nevi may contain adnexal or mesenchymal components not usual in seborrheic keratosis (Fig. 17-1B). These subtle alterations of the associated superficial dermal connective tissue or anomalous follicular differentiation suggest that the lesions represent cutaneous hamartomas with epidermal predominance. Epidermal nevi composed exclusively of papillary epidermal hyperplasia are easily confused with old verrucae, acanthosis nigricans, and a number of other less common conditions. Carcinomatous change is rare.[9]

Acanthosis Nigricans

Acanthosis nigricans is a verrucous epidermal hyperplasia that is a non-neoplastic, plaque-like, intertriginous skin change sometimes acquired as a sign of visceral malignant tumor and some other clinical states.[10–12] It is mentioned here to enter the differential with epidermal nevi and papillomatous variants of seborrheic keratosis. Clinical information is essential to accurate diagnosis.

Acanthomatous Tumors

Benign acanthoma has been used as a generic term for lesions featuring epidermoid keratinization (seborrheic keratosis), granular degeneration (epidermolytic acanthoma), coronoid lamellation (porokeratosis), absence of keratinization (clear cell acanthoma), and prominent acantholytic suprabasal clefts (acantholytic acanthoma).[13]

Seborrheic Keratosis

Seborrheic keratosis is a lesion of the middle-aged and elderly and most often will appear as multiple benign, localized, neoplastic proliferations of basaloid keratinocytes with hyperkeratosis and possibly hyperpigmentation.[14–18] They arise spontaneously and are most numerous on the trunk; extremities, head, and neck are commonly involved. Upon direct examination, seborrheic keratoses are clinically flat, coin-like plaques from several millimeters to centimeters, with a uniform tan to dark brown color, and a velvety to granular surface. Small, pore-like ostia impacted with keratin are helpful in differentiating these pigmented lesions from melanomas. *Dermatosis papulosa nigra*[19] is a small, polypoidal multicentric form typically on the face of black patients. *Stucco keratosis* is a lower leg variant with chevron folded keratin above church spire projections of nonatypical hyperplastic epidermis.[20] Explosive onset of hundreds of seborrheic keratoses in association with internal malignant tumor constitutes the sign of Leser-Trélat and may be stimulated by growth factors related to the visceral tumor.

Microscopically, seborrheic keratoses are exophytic and sharply demarcated from the adjacent epidermis (Fig. 17-2). Redundant small uniform basaloid cells, probably due to a maturation defect, account for the thickening. Supportive dermal stroma typically forms a hyalinized mantle along the basal cell layer and its recognition is a helpful diagnostic feature in minute curettings (Fig. 17-2, inset). Excessive surface keratin accumulation descends into the lesion as small keratin-filled pseudohorn cysts and becomes loculated within the abnormal epithelium as horn cysts. Pseudohorn cysts represent the keratin-filled ostia that are conspicuous grossly on the surface of the lesion.

Additional variant forms include irritated (inflamed) seborrheic keratosis, seborrheic keratosis with intraepidermal epithelioma or "clonal" patterns, and adenoid seborrheic keratosis (Fig. 17-3). When inflamed, the basaloid cells accumulate more cytoplasm and undergo squamous differentiation, forming whirling squamous clusters termed *squamous eddies* because they resemble eddy currents in water. These irritated seborrheic keratoses may be confused with squamous cell carcinoma due to reactive nuclear changes and eddy pattern. Some papillations may be infarcted.

Inverted follicular keratosis[21] is a seborrheic keratosis that involves hair follicles, mainly on the face of the elderly, especially the eyelid, tending to proliferate in an endophytic manner and exhibiting squamous differentiation and "squamous eddies"[22] in association with inflammation. Alternatively, this lesion is regarded as a unique keratotic lesion of the infundibular portion

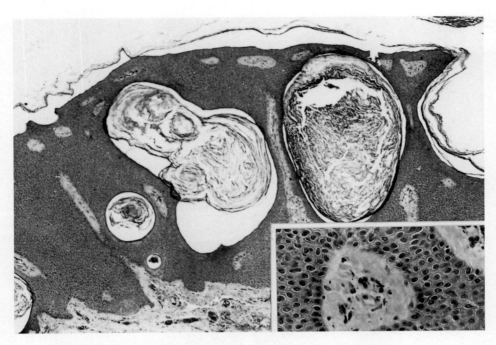

Fig. 17-2. Seborrheic keratosis. Note prominent horn cysts and pseudohorn cysts; inset shows typical hyalinized stromal mantle directly beneath the basal cell layer of this tumor.

of the hair follicle[23] or a form of wart.[24] *Pigmented seborrheic keratoses* are common; their basaloid keratinocytes carry the excess pigment without conspicuous intervening melanocytes. *Melanoacanthoma*[25] is a relatively uncommon seborrheic keratosis with many pigmented, dendritic, benign melanocytes among relatively amelanotic, neoplastic, basaloid epithelial cells.

Seborrheic keratoses are indolent neoplasms easily treated by curettage or local destruction. Their major significance is their propensity to mimic other lesions. The frequent excision of clinically odd and inflamed seborrheic keratoses to rule out more aggressive lesions is justified based on this consideration. Malignant change is almost anecdotal, but any practitioner can soon assemble examples complicated by[26] or adjacent to basal and squamous cell carcinomas. This may be a further rationale for supporting the excision of suspicious seborrheic keratoses.

Large Cell Acanthoma

Large cell acanthoma is a macular light tan to dark brown lesion of sun-exposed skin most often found on the forehead.[27] The keratinocytes of the atrophic, acanthotic, or even verrucous epidermis have enlarged nuclei and overall size, often appreciated only after comparison to adjacent normal skin or adnexa (Fig. 17-4A). Although hyperdiploid by photocytometry,[28] there is no cellular atypia, pointing away from the proposal that large cell acanthoma is really a variant of actinic keratosis.[29] It may be best regarded an intraepidermal neopla-

sia[30–32] with little or no tendency for progression to invasive carcinoma, or perhaps part of the spectrum of solar lentigo.[33]

Clear Cell Acanthoma

Acanthoma is a generic term used for "benign tumors of epidermal keratinocytes".[34–37] This relatively uncommon, usually solitary epidermal proliferation most often arises on the legs of middle-aged and older patients. It characteristically has an eroded, oozing, erythematous surface. The clinician may be concerned about basal cell carcinoma, pyogenic granuloma, or eccrine poroma. They grow slowly and are usually smaller than 2 cm in diameter.

Histologically, the abnormal epidermis constituted by clear cell acanthomas is very sharply demarcated from adjacent normal epidermis (Fig. 17-4B). Periodic acid-Schiff (PAS) stain confirms abundant cytoplasmic glycogen as the cause of the clear cytoplasm. Melanin pigment is diminished or absent in most,[38] an apparent defect in melanocyte-keratinocyte melanin transfer. Downward proliferations of glycogenated squamoid cells extend as elongated rete ridges. This and percolation of neutrophils within intercellular spaces of the tumor and within overlying parakeratotic scale may mimic psoriasis. Dilated vessels in thinned dermal papillae may reach the eroded surface. However, psoriasis does not exhibit prominent cytoplasmic glycogenation or abrupt demarcation. Eccrine poromas will show ductular differentiation. Seborrheic keratoses lack the prominent and vascularized dermal papillae and usually retain focal basaloid differentiation. Clear cell acanthomas do not form horn or pseudohorn cysts.

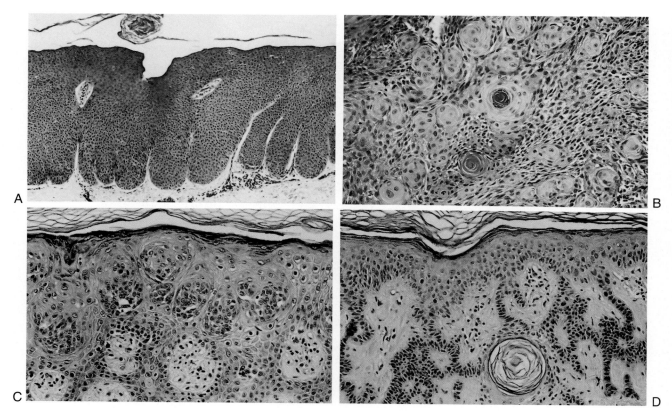

Fig. 17-3. Variant forms of seborrheic keratosis. Variants include **(A)** acanthotic form; **(B)** irritated seborrheic keratosis with numerous "squamous eddies"; **(C)** clonal pattern with nests of neoplastic cells aggregated within the epidermis; and **(D)** adenoid pattern.

Fibroepithelial Polyps

Fibroepithelial polyps is a generic term for skin tags, acrochordon, pedunculated fibroma, and squamous papilloma and connotes neoplasms that commonly occur with advancing age on the trunk, axilla, head, and neck skin. They may be sessile or pedunculated, and are soft, skin-colored, and slow growing. Eruptive fibroepithelial polyps may accompany the abrupt onset of other benign epidermal neoplasms (e.g., seborrheic keratoses), and then consideration should be given to the possibility of production of epidermal growth factors by remote primary neoplasia.

Fibroepithelial polyps have a mantle of variably reactive epidermis covering a protuberant fibrovascular core. Within the core is fibrous and adipose tissue with occasional nerve fibers. They are confused clinically with polypoidal types of melanoma, neurofibromas, polypoid dermal nevi, and pedunculated hemangiomas. They are common cosmetic problems, and are also excised for ulceration or spontaneous infarction, which may lead to pain and abrupt change in color. These details should be noted in a report when they substantiate clinical reasons for removal.

The *acquired (digital) fibrokeratoma* is a hyperkeratotic projection with collagenous core occurring mainly around interphalangeal joints.

Keratoacanthoma

Keratoacanthomas generally involve the skin of the face or dorsal aspects of the upper extremities in general, sun-exposed surfaces.[39–43] Males are afflicted with three or four times the frequency of females. These initially small keratotic papules enlarge rapidly over a few weeks or months. Mature tumors are from 1 to 2.5 cm and crater-like with a central keratotic plug. Keratoacanthomas on the nose, the ear, or the vermilion border of the lip and those that arise in subungual skin[44] also may be locally destructive. Extension into underlying skeletal muscle, perineural invasion, or even blood vessel invasion are possible.[45–47] Their natural history in a normal host is spontaneous regression[48] to a slightly depressed, annular scar.[48,49] Giant keratoacanthomas are quite rare, may exceed 5 cm in diameter, and are locally destructive. Numerous eruptive lesions characterize the Gtyzbowski type, and multiple ulcerating tumors with atypical distribution are seen in the Ferguson-Smith type.[50]

At low magnification, this exophytic and endophytic neoplasm typically has a cup shape (Fig. 17-5A). The central crater is filled with eosinophilic laminated keratin that may be inconspicuous in early lesions or suboptimal sections. The well defined overhanging rim of the crater consists of stretched hyperplastic or effaced nonatypical epidermis. Proliferating lobules and prongs of epithelium may extend from the base into the

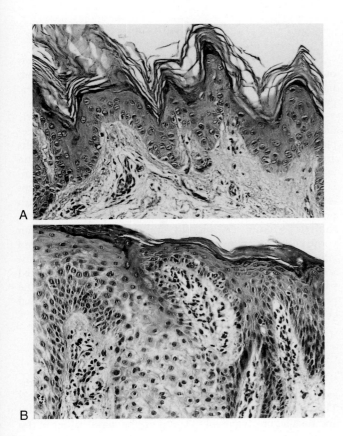

Fig. 17-4. (A) Large cell acanthoma and (B) clear cell acanthoma. Note relative size of cells forming large cell acanthoma (Fig. A) when compared to normal keratinocytes (represented on right side of Fig. B). Also observe abrupt transition separating glycogenated clear cell acanthoma (left, Fig. B) from normal epidermis (right, Fig. B). Both panels are photographed at identical magnification.

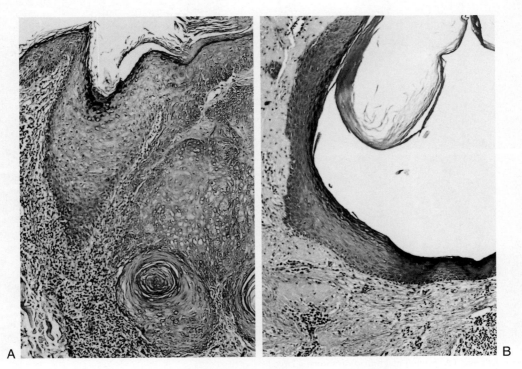

Fig. 17-5. Keratoacanthoma. (A) Early proliferative epithelial stage and (B) regressing stage characterized by surrounding scar-like fibrovascular proliferation.

reticular dermis between collagen bundles, but bilateral symmetry is generally maintained. With regression, the proliferative epithelial component becomes less prominent, eventually flattening out above a layer of scar-like fibrovascular proliferation (Fig. 17-5B).

The higher power histopathology is also distinctive. The large squamous epithelial cells have abundant cytoplasmic glycogen conferring a glassy quality (Fig. 17-6A). Cells at the periphery of proliferating lobules are more basaloid, with some degree of nuclear atypia invariably present. A rare atypical mitotic figure does not preclude the diagnosis. These cells have uniformly large, ovoid nuclei with smooth, regular contours and peripherally marginated chromatin that forms a thin, uniform band along the nuclear membrane. The delicately dispersed heterochromatin surrounds prominent, eosinophilic nucleoli. Keratin formation is "abrupt," without an intervening granular layer. Neutrophils typically infiltrate the intercellular spaces and accumulate in some of the deeper keratin pearl formations (Fig. 17-6B). Transepithelial elimination of elastic fibers may correlate with early lesional regression and is proposed to favor keratoacanthoma over a well differentiated squamous cell carcinoma. It is frequently impossible, however, to diagnose keratoacanthoma based on histology alone[42,51] and even atypical mitoses do not distinguish it from cancer.[52] Recently the movement to regard keratoacanthoma as a variant of squamous cell carcinoma[53,54] has gained popularity (i.e., "squamous cell carcinoma, keratoacanthomatous type").

Dyskeratoma

Dyskeratoma also called isolated follicular keratosis, occurs on sun-exposed, hair-bearing surfaces of adults.[55] Oral lesions have been described.[56] These solitary, elevated, keratotic papules or nodules occasionally have an umbilicated center.

On low power examination, a well demarcated, endophytic proliferation of squamous epithelium may appear to have replaced pre-existing hair follicles (Fig. 17-7A). Suprabasal clefts are formed by acantholysis and the resultant rounded and dyskeratotic acantholytic cells take two forms. Many are enlarged and strongly eosinophilic with perinuclear halos (corps ronds). Others are small, densely eosinophilic, and ovoid with pyknotic, flattened nuclei in association with a partially acantholytic stratum granulosum and parakeratotic stratum corneum (corps grains) (Fig. 17-7B). Similar acantholysis and altered cells are found in Darier's disease, best excluded by clinical history. Underlying superficial dermis has an exaggerated papillomatous pattern presumably due to downgrowth of the persisting single layer of adherent intact nonacantholytic basal cells.

Verrucae

Among four major clinical types of verrucae or warts, verrucae vulgaris and filiform warts are the most common.[57–59] These circumscribed, papillomatous, hyperkeratotic papules and nodules are commonly located on the dorsal aspect of the

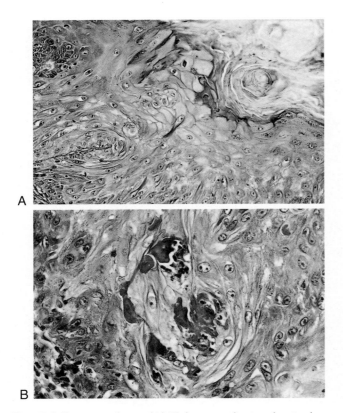

Fig. 17-6. Keratoacanthoma. **(A)** Higher magnification showing large "glassy" cells with "abrupt" keratinization, and **(B)** foci of forming neutrophil microabscesses associated with dyskeratotic cells.

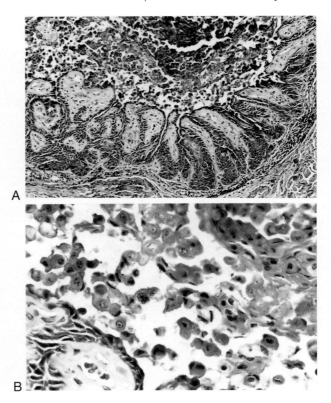

Fig. 17-7. Warty dyskeratoma. **(A)** Low magnification and **(B)** higher magnification showing characteristic corps ronds and corps grains.

hands and fingers. Any part of the body surface may be affected. Plantar warts are generally solitary or multiple, poorly defined, hyperkeratotic, painful lesions on the sole of the foot, often involving a pressure point. Flat warts (i.e., verruca plana) usually occur as multiple, skin-colored papules in linear distribution on the dorsa of the hands and feet. *Epidermodysplasia verruciformis* is a rare autosomal recessive inherited defect in helper T cell function that confers a particular susceptibility to papillomavirus. These patients develop flat warts that may evolve into dysplasias and indolent carcinomas, especially in sun-exposed or irradiated sites (e.g., on the forehead).[60] *Condyloma acuminatum* appears as a verrucous, cauliflower-like excrescence on anogenital or surrounding skin. *Bowenoid papulosis* is a form of spontaneously resolving genital wart with full-thickness epidermal anaplasia. It is distinguished clinically from squamous cell carcinoma in situ by anogenital occurrence in younger individuals, smaller expanse, multiplicity, and specific site (e.g., shaft of penis for bowenoid papulosis versus glans for carcinoma).[61,62] Molecular hybridization studies show HPV type 16 in these lesions.[63] Clinical types of HPV infection are determined by regional differences in their sites of occurrence, and also by the type of virus that elicits each lesion.

Microscopically, *verruca vulgaris* has crown-like, radiating, fibrovascular spires covered by hyperkeratotic scale, typically with parakeratosis at the tips of each spire (Fig. 17-8A). Dilated vessels within the exaggerated dermal papillae that are the cores of the epithelial projections extend close to the lesional surface. Cells in superficial epidermis have a type of koilocytotic change caused by ballooning cytoplasmic degeneration, manifest as cytoplasmic pallor and clearing. However, a more specific finding is the pallor and dispersion of chromatin imparting a steel gray tinctorial property to the nuclei of the upper epidermal layers. This appearance represents replacement of chromatin with aggregates of HPV particles. Above this zone is a widened stratum granulosum with enlarged coarse keratohyalin granules, many of which have rounded contours rather than normal stellate outlines.

The excessive keratin over verrucae commonly contains agglutinated red cell groups. Careful study often finds these are in dilated stromal core vessels of infarcted, pinched-off papillomatous spire tips.

Plantar warts have an endophytic architecture, perhaps dictated by pressure of ambulation. Numerous epithelial downgrowths tapering inward are covered by dense hyperkeratotic and parakeratotic scale. Abundant irregular, densely eosinophilic cytoplasmic keratin inclusions affecting the uppermost viable epidermal layers create a picture known as *mermecia*. Flat warts also show the viral cytopathic changes of verruca vulgaris, but have much less papillomatosis and hyperkeratosis.

Condylomata show alternating exophytic and endophytic growth of squamous epithelium about branching fibrovascular cores (Fig. 17-8B). Their early stages can resemble seborrheic keratoses or fibroepithelial polyps, but even then, careful study finds perinuclear cytoplasmic clearing, some hyperchromatic nuclear enlargement and irregularity, and multinucleation of the upper epidermal layers (i.e., koilocytosis). Mitotic activity may be brisk and frozen in metaphase in lesions that have been recently treated with podophyllin.

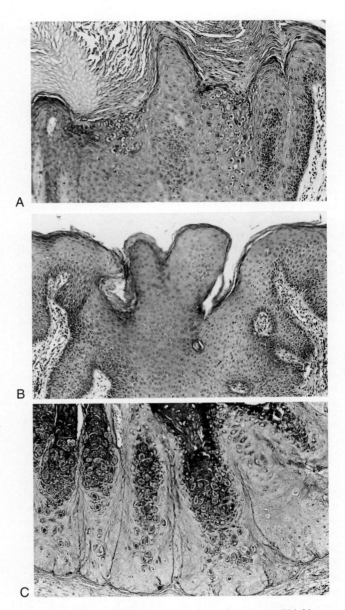

Fig. 17-8. Forms of commonly encountered verrucae. **(A)** Verruca vulgaris, **(B)** condyloma acuminatum, and **(C)** molluscum contagiosum.

Immunohistochemistry for HPV antigens and in situ hybridization for viral message may be used for documentation of HPV in tissue. HPV types 16 and 18 in anogenital warts are associated with potential subsequent development of neoplasia of the uterine cervix.

Verrucae commonly spontaneously regress via inflammatory changes akin to a delayed hypersensitivity reaction. Others will lose viral cytopathic changes and persist as localized residua that are very commonly biopsied and diagnosed as *verrucous epidermal hyperplasia consistent with remote HPV effect*. This is a reasonable approach when lesions clinically still resemble verrucae and when dilated dermal vessels still remain within dermal cores that define residual epithelial spires. Some verrucae age by developing squamous eddies similar to those in irritated seborrheic keratoses[64] and inverted follicular keratosis. Some develop glycogenation, thus resembling the picture of trichilemmoma.

Molluscum Contagiosum

Molluscum contagiosum is a common pox virus-induced cutaneous proliferation presenting as multiple, small grouped papules anywhere on the body surface but often affecting facial skin.[65] These dome-shaped papules have central umbilication around a cornified plug. Microscopy shows them to be endophytic epithelial downgrowths involving coalescent follicular infundibula (Fig. 17-8C). Diagnostic molluscum bodies are within the cornified material that fills the central crater as well as within the cytoplasm of the contiguous viable keratinocytes. These round to ovoid, bubbly aggregates of variably eosinophilic material tend to become less eosinophilic and increasingly basophilic as they ascend. Molluscum bodies should not be confused with irregular, densely eosinophilic aggregates of cytoplasmic keratin typical of plantar verrucae, corps grains and ronds, or colloid bodies. The simulation of these other structures by molluscum bodies may be greater as these viral lesions involute. Giant lesions of or extensive skin involvement by molluscum contagiosum suggest the possibility of acquired immunodeficiency syndrome (AIDS).

Actinic Keratosis

Multiple lesions of *actinic keratosis* are typically less than 1 cm and found on sun-exposed skin of middle-aged or older individuals.[66–71] Clinically and histologically similar dysplasias may result from nonactinic factors such as chronic ingestion of arsenicals. An increased incidence in renal transplant patients favors their lip region.[72] Systemic or topical chemotherapy (e.g., with 5-fluorouracil [FU]) may make them clinically more apparent and seemingly numerous due to accentuated erythema. Scales impart a roughened sandpaper-like texture. Some are pigmented, erythematous, or surmounted by horn-like scale and mimic melanocytic neoplasms, dermatoses, or invasive carcinomas. *Actinic cheilitis* is actinic keratosis involving the vermilion border of the lip.

Dysplasia of the lower epidermal layers is a histologic hallmark of actinic keratosis, first in the basal cell layer and then in more advanced lesions in overlying layers of the stratum spinosum (Fig. 17-9A). This dysplasia is characterized by enlarged, irregularly shaped nuclei with diffuse hyperchromasia or coarsely clumped nuclear chromatin. Maturation and orderly cellular positions are perturbed. The granular layer is generally absent except at and around follicular ostea. Atypical parakeratotic scale contains tightly aggregated, plump nuclear remnants with diffuse hyperchromasia. This may alternate across the specimen with orthokeratin columns emerging from sun-sheltered adnexa. Massive keratin build-up may be observed and correlate clinically as a cutaneous horn.[73] Atypical parakeratotic scale may be the only diagnostic clue when superficial

currettings consist only of stratum corneum and fail to provide the entire thickness of the epidermis. Of course, underlying squamous cell carcinoma cannot be excluded without viable epidermis in the sample.

Morphologic variants of actinic keratosis (AK) can be designated. Microscopically, the epidermal layer may be only three or four cells thick (atrophic AK) (Fig. 17-9A) or thickened (hyperplastic or hypertrophic AK) (Fig. 17-9B). Acantholytic AK lacks intercellular cohesion, and clefts or spaces within the abnormal epidermis contain rounded acantholytic cells[74] remi-

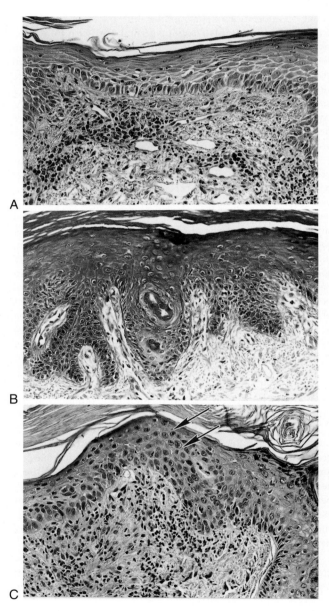

Fig. 17-9. Variant forms of actinic keratosis showing **(A)** a characteristic lesion with atypia of the lower epidermal layers; **(B)** a proliferative variant with endophytic tongues of atypical epithelium; and **(C)** actinic keratosis with focal transition to squamous cell carcinoma in situ (arrows).

niscent of pemphigus vulgaris. Pigmented AKs appear clinically as heavily pigmented macular lesions, and microscopically have a component of pigmented dendritic melanocytes.[75] Absence of downward projections composed of pigmented keratinocytes and cellular atypia distinguish pigmented AK from solar lentigo. The discohesion, coarse keratohyalin granulation, and compact hyperkeratosis of the change known as epidermolytic hyperkeratosis distinguishes epidermolytic AK.[76] The underlying dermis typically shows a variable elastosis and inflammation. In some lesions, the degree of inflammation is intense, and overt cytotoxic alterations are along the basal cell layer (lichenoid actinic keratoses).[77] Whether these variants have different biologic potential is unclear.

Some actinic keratoses progress to squamous cell carcinoma or basal cell carcinoma but with unknown frequency.[66,78] Most are clinically indolent and many may not become locally aggressive tumors within the lifetime of the host. Almost 75 percent of actinic keratoses accumulate p53 protein, presumably as a result of mutation, and this correlates with the degree of atypia.[79] Zones of full-thickness dysplasia warrant designation as actinic keratosis with focal squamous cell carcinoma (Fig. 17-9C). More pronounced and longitudinally extensive full-thickness cellular atypia with marked dyskeratosis and abnormal mitoses has been termed "bowenoid AK," but any pathologic behavioral difference from squamous cell carcinoma in situ (see below) is insignificant. Invasive squamous cell carcinoma arising in actinic cheilitis is prone to produce fatal metastases, unlike the indolent local cancers arising in actinic keratosis of other sites.

Actinic keratoses in youth lacking underlying elastosis should arouse suspicion of xeroderma pigmentosa or forms of albinism. Actinic keratoses also may be prominently developed in renal transplant patients and in other immunocompromised states.

Squamous Cell Carcinoma

Squamous cell carcinoma in situ (SCCIS) favors sun-exposed skin, although non-sun-exposed sites may also be affected (Bowen's disease).[80–83] Squamous cell carcinomas of the skin can also complicate xeroderma pigmentosa, epidermodysplasia verruciformis, and cutaneous scars and sinus tracts. It can be induced by certain chemical exposures (e.g., arsenic, coal tars, soot, and oils). The risk is dose dependent in psoralens and longwave ultraviolet light (PUVA)-treated psoriatic patients[84] and is elevated in human immunodeficiency virus (HIV) infection.[85] The in situ form may give rise to invasive lesions but is not a requirement for the development of invasive squamous cell carcinoma. SCCIS appears clinically as one or several well demarcated, erythematous, and sometimes hyperkeratotic plaques. Mucosal involvement creates zones of white, thickened epithelium, a nonspecific appearance also caused by various unrelated hyperkeratotic disorders also referred to clinically as leukoplakia. SCCIS involving the glans penis is sometimes called "erythroplasia of Querat."

SCCIS is a morphologic spectrum[86] ranging from atrophy, through acanthotic to verrucous variants. The hallmark is epidermal replacement by atypical keratinocytes proliferating at all levels[82] (Fig. 17-10). Maturation from the basal cell layer to the stratified squamous epithelial layer is lacking or defective. The "intraepidermal epithelioma" pattern consists of malignant keratinocytes nested within the epidermis and sharply juxtaposed to adjacent, normal-appearing epidermal cells. The "pagetoid type" must be distinguished from intraepidermal epithelioma (clonal seborrheic keratosis), melanoma in situ, Paget's disease, and hidroacanthoma simplex (intraepidermal eccrine poroma). The stratum corneum is thickened and densely parakeratotic, and stratum granulosum is generally absent. Superficial dermis contains dilated and more numerous vessels, fibrosis, and a chronic inflammatory infiltrate, possibly representing a localized immune response. Bowenoid papulosis would be in the differential diagnosis in anogenital location.[87–89]

Invasive squamous cell carcinoma (SCC) is usually an indurated, sometimes ulcerated plaque or nodule surmounted by hyperkeratotic scale. Well differentiated, cup-shaped SCC may be clinically indistinguishable from keratoacanthoma. In the early phases of invasive SCC, elongate rete composed of cytologically malignant cells protrude into a variably fibrotic and vascularized papillary dermis (Fig. 17-11A). Increasing complexity and irregularity of these extensions and individually invasive cells produce sheets, strands, fascicles, and nests of tumor that infiltrate the dermis more deeply and evoke an exuberant fibroblastic response. This tumor stroma is important in differentiating invasive components of SCC from reactive processes

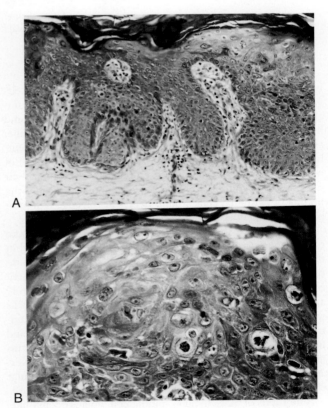

Fig. 17-10. Squamous cell carcinoma in situ. **(A)** Complete replacement of the epidermal layer by malignant cells. **(B)** Cytologic anaplasia and numerous mitoses, some atypical.

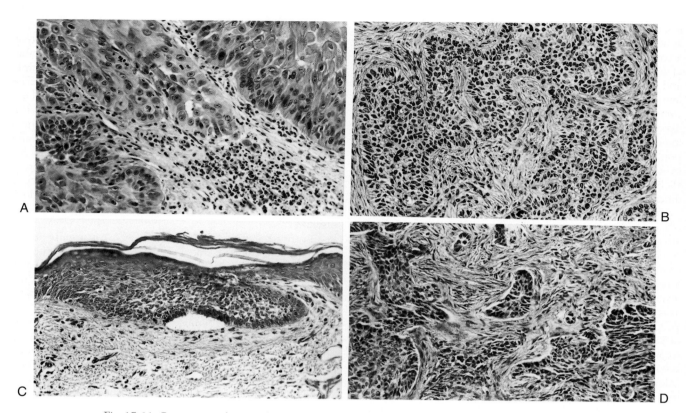

Fig. 17-11. Comparison of various forms of cutaneous carcinoma. (A) Invasive squamous cell carcinoma; (B) nodular basal cell carcinoma; (C) superficial multicentric type basal cell carcinoma; and (D) sclerosing type basal cell carcinoma.

(e.g., *pseudoepitheliomatous hyperplasia*).[90,91] The invasive cells vary from well to poorly differentiated, but some degree of nuclear atypia is always observed. Atypical nuclei are enlarged and hyperchromatic; nucleoli may be prominent and acidophilic, chromatin is delicate and evenly distributed, and nuclear membranes are uniformly thin and smoothly contoured. Nuclei of reactive keratinocytes may approach this appearance but their nucleoli are basophilic. Re-excision perineural extension is the finding of epithelial cells around nerves at the edge of a prior biopsy site and does not connote persistent neoplasm.[92]

Keratinization, the hallmark of differentiation of squamous tumors, takes two forms. Small, laminated keratin cysts within the tumor lobules (i.e., pearl formation) recapitulate maturation to corneocytes in normal epidermis and do not represent tumor necrosis. Single-cell keratinization (i.e., dyskeratosis) appears as sporadic, brightly hypereosinophilic shrunken cells with condensed pyknotic or karyolytic nuclei. Poorly differentiated tumors may show little or no ability to form keratin, and immunohistochemistry for low molecular weight cytokeratins may be required for definitive histogenetic classification. Keratin subclasses expressed are not so much related to cellular changes as they are to levels of differentiation.[93,94]

Rare forms of SCC include spindle cell, angiosarcoma-like, acantholytic, verrucous, and lymphoepithelioma-like carcinoma. *Spindle cell* variants often infiltrate a highly reactive stroma insidiously, such that differentiation of malignant epithelial and reactive stromal elements is not always possible.[95] Demonstration of cytokeratin and epithelial membrane-associated antigen (EMA) is helpful because true cutaneous mesenchymal malignant tumors including atypical fibroxanthoma will be negative.[96] *Angiosarcoma-like* or "*pseudovascular*" SCC appears as a nonhealing ulcer or crusted nodule similar to ordinary SCC and can be distinguished from true angiosarcoma by keratin and EMA positivity, as well as absence of reactivity for CD34 and CD31.[97–99]

Acantholysis also may produce a *pseudoglandular* pattern mimicking adenocarcinoma, but is distinguished by eosinophilic rounded (acantholytic) cells in the false lumens and carcinoembryonic antigen (CEA) negativity.[100] Perhaps 60 percent of sweat gland malignant tumors are S-100 positive, but SCC is not. *Adenosquamous carcinomas* of the skin are aggressive mucin-producing and gland-forming lesions.[101] Adenosquamous carcinomas with demonstrable mucin production tend to arise multifocally from epidermis, have a relatively flat surface, and are highly infiltrative. Their perineural invasion and sclerosis makes complete resection difficult.[101,102] Adenosquamous carcinomas arising on the glans penis have been interpreted as tumors of bimodal origin from surface squamous epithelium and from embryologically misplaced mucous glands of the perimeatal region of glans mucosa.[103] *Verrucous squamous cell carcinoma*[104] is deeply invasive, extending blunt, club-like lobules of minimally atypical yet malignant squamous epithelial cells into underlying connective tissue. Depth of penetration, the expansive nature of the endophytic epithelial tongues, and foci of clear-cut dysplasia, most evident along the deep pushing border, are important clues to avoid misdiagnosis as hyperplasia,[105] wart, or condyloma. *Lymphoepithelioma-like squamous cell carcinoma* is a neoplasm of sheets and scattered single polygonal to rounded neoplastic epithelial cells with no histologically discernible keratinization within a lymphocyte-rich stroma.[106,107] It may be a primitive adenexal malignant tumor, because features of incipient sweat gland and/or follicular differentiation can be seen.[106,108] Immunohistochemical reactions for keratin bring the carcinoma cells out sharply in the characteristic, often volumetrically predominant reactive background of small lymphocytes. This histology is similar to lymphoepithelial carcinomas arising in nasopharyngeal epithelium but increasingly reported in other sites (e.g., urinary bladder). Therefore, metastatic origin of this skin pattern should be excluded. Other squamous cell carcinomas have been described as *papillary*,[109] *signet ring*,[110] and *clear cell*[111] types.

Superficially invasive squamous cell carcinomas only occasionally metastasize.[112] Regional node metastases occur in less than 5 percent in tumors larger than 2 cm with invasion into reticular dermis. Tumors that recur are generally thicker, involving the lower half of dermis or deeper. Neglected tumors can be fatal.[113,114]

Basal Cell Carcinoma

The common *basal cell carcinoma* (BCC) is a well-circumscribed, tan-red plaque or a pearly, tan-gray papule relatively devoid of scale.[115–123] It occurs predominantly on the sun-exposed skin and in proportion to the number of pilosebaceous units, a fact in line with its apparent attempt to differentiate toward adnexal structures, particularly pilosebaceous units.[121,124,125] Numerous telangiectatic blood vessels course over the tumor papule or nodule. The superficial multicentric variety is a relatively large, erythematous, scaling plaque that may be confused with SCCIS, radial growth phase melanoma, or even an inflammatory dermatosis. Most BCCs are small at the time of clinical attention, but chronic neglect of this indolent neoplasm results in large, locally destructive tumors ("rodent ulcers") with invasion of underlying soft tissue and even bone.[126] Tumors that reach the central nervous system (CNS) can cause lethal meningitis. Metastases are exceptional[127,128] and about 65 percent are to regional lymph nodes. Basosquamous tumors (see below) with perineural spread in sunlight-protected skin are more likely to account for metastases.[129–131]

Individual lesions in the autosomal dominant basal cell nevus syndrome (multiple nevoid basal cell carcinoma syndrome, Gorlin's syndrome)[132–134] may appear as early as the second year of life involving face, neck, and back more than other sites. The tumors are indistinguishable on histopathologic examination from ordinary basal cell carcinomas induced by sunlight. BCC is rare in blacks.[135]

Microscopy discloses well defined foci of atypical basaloid cells arising from the undersurface of the epidermis or sides of follicular epithelium. In given samples, nests and nodules of basaloid tumor cells within the superficial and/or deep dermis may

have no apparent connection to benign epithelial structures. The low power impression of deep basophilia is due to sparsity and pallor of cytoplasm and crowded elongate cells at the periphery are arranged in a dense palisade (Fig. 17-11B). The central uniform population of nested basal cells has round to ovoid nuclei, coarsely clumped nuclear chromatin patterns, and occasional mitotic figures. Nucleoli are not prominent, an important feature in keratotic tumors showing a deceptive degree of squamous differentiation. Mitoses and individual cell necrosis are typical, the latter recognized as grouped rounded nuclear fragments. These details help in the distinction from basaloid variants of trichoepithelioma. The characteristic reactive stroma of BCC has abundant acid mucopolysaccharides; this and a paucity of hemidesmosomes contribute to the tendency for tumor cell groups to pull away from stroma at their periphery as a consequence of tissue preparation. This "separation artifact" is an important diagnostic trait. Discontinuous labeling of the basement membrane around tumor cell nests with antibodies against laminin, collagen types IV and V, and bullous pemphigoid antigen indicate disruption of this structure and is more prominent in aggressive neoplasms.[136] The stroma has a variable infiltration by mononuclear inflammatory cells and possibly amyloid.[137,138] BCCs are positive for keratin (particularly low molecular weight type) and usually negative for involucrin.[139,140] Most overexpress p53 protein.[141]

Adnexal differentiation is common. The neoplasm is an imperfect simulation of the relation between germinative hair matrix epithelium and the supportive mucinous follicular mesenchyme of the papilla. Sebaceous differentiation, abortive eccrine duct formation associated with epithelial mucinosis,[142] and inner and outer root sheath development all may be focally observed. Mucinous stroma, separation artifact, mitotic activity, and individual cell necrosis all assist in differentiating BCC with prominent adnexal differentiation from benign appendage tumors. Also, EMA positivity will be restricted to areas of divergent differentiation, in contrast to diffuse reaction in glandular or sebaceous neoplasms.

Specific histologic variants of BCC are frequently encountered. *Infundibulocystic BCCs* show upper follicular differentiation. They have sharp circumscription with smooth margins, superficial location, small cysts containing cornified cells lined by infundibular epithelium, no follicular bulbs and papillae, and no highly fibrotic stroma.[143] The *superficial-multicentric type* and *sclerosing (morpheaform) type* both are frequently ill-defined clinically, and histologically discontinuous in single profiles (Fig. 17-11C & D). These characteristics engender a risk of unanticipated inadequate excision and consequent local regrowth,[144–146] and consequently it is advised to designate these variant forms in a surgical pathology report. Multiple plates of neoplastic basaloid cells originate from the basal cell layer of the epidermis in the superficial multicentric type. A characteristic mucinous stroma underlies each bud, from which there often is separation artifact. The sclerosing or morpheaform type of BCC consists of ill-defined cords and streams of cuboidal to fusiform basal cells in a desmoplastic cellular stroma. Many of the epithelial cell groups have a pinched or compressed appearance as if the stroma exerts vice-like pressure. Associated proliferating fibroblasts may create a pseudosarcomatous appearance (*sarcomatoid BCC*). The evaluation of margins of such

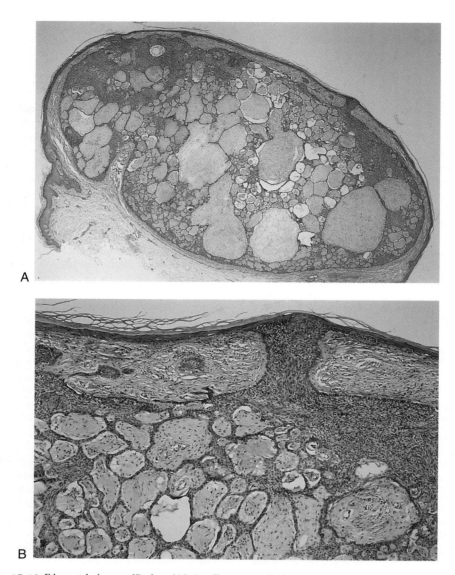

Fig. 17-12. Fibroepithelioma of Pinkus. **(A)** A well circumscribed proliferation of basaloid cells **(B)** extends into fibrous stroma as thin strands in a lace-like pattern.

lesions may be facilitated by immunohistochemistry. *Cystic BCCs* form as a result of necrosis or overabundant central production of epithelial mucin. Some BCCs contain abundant melanin pigment (*pigmented BCC*).[147] Additional variants[148] with descriptive titles are *infiltrative-adamantinoid, signet ring cell,*[149] *clear cell,*[150] *adenoid, pilar-keratotic/organoid, granular cell,*[151] tumors with hyalin inclusions,[152] and participation in "collision tumors."[153] As defined by the World Health Organization in 1980,[154] metatypical carcinoma (MTC) is similar to BCC but lacks peripheral nuclear palisading in cellular lobules and is composed of cells with larger nuclei and abundant cytoplasm as well as, occasionally, a spindle cell appearance and focally prominent intercellular bridges. MTC has a more aggressive behavior than BCC.[155] Basosquamous differentiation imparts a histologic appearance intermediate between BCC and SCC.[155] These more aggressive *metatypical-squamoid* and

basosquamous subtypes contain atypical squamous cells and tend to label with bcl-2 protein (functioning in controlling apoptosis)[156] and BER-EP4 (monoclonal antibody directed against a cell surface glycoprotein on some epithelial cells), whereas most SCCs are negative.[157] Although antibodies to keratin 17 stain BCC, especially the palisaded cells, MTC cases always express a very low level of keratin 8 and 17. MTC and recurrent BCC have higher labeling for proliferating cell nuclear antigen (PCNA) compared to primary BCC.[154]

Most SSCs express Ulex europaeus agglutinin I lectin-binding sites whereas BCCs will not.[158] CEA, a cell surface glycoprotein, is found on normal sweat gland epithelium and related neoplasms, but not on most BCC variants except rare ones with eccrine differentiation (*"eccrine epithelioma"*).[159] An extremely well differentiated BCC, the *fibroepithelioma of Pinkus* (Fig. 17-12), presents as a static polypoid thigh or low back lesion

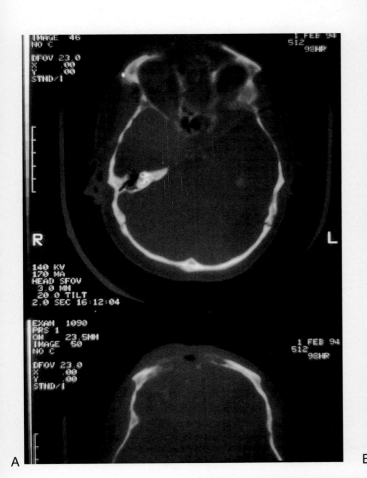

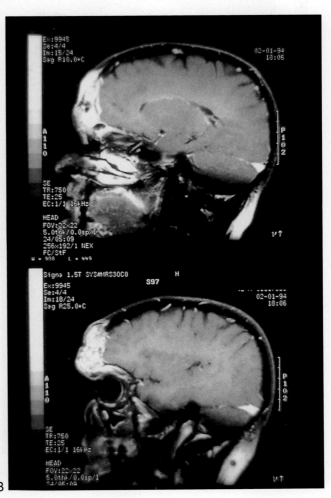

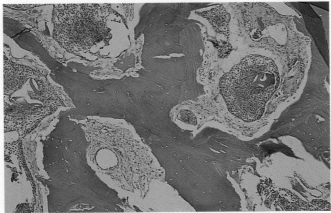

Fig. 17-13. Basal cell carcinoma invading bone. (A) CT scan and (B) MRI study show osteolysis and a high signal mass, respectively, affecting frontal calvarium. (C) Histopathologically, basal cell carcinoma nests have incited fibrovascular marrow transformation and osteoclastic erosion of frontal bone. The invaded bone beneath a 4 cm ulcerated tumor developing for 5 years was resected with the overlying skin. (*Figure continues.*)

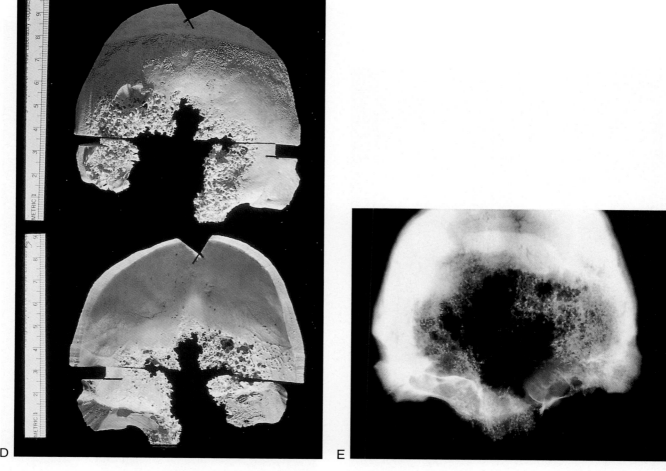

Fig. 17-13 *(Continued)*. **(D)** The resected portion of calvarium is positioned to show outer (top) and inner (bottom) aspects. **(E)** Its specimen radiograph shows osteolysis.

consisting of numerous anastomosing cords of well differenti-ated basaloid cells that arise from the epidermis and extend in lacy fashion into a delicate fibrovascular stroma.[160] The fi-broadenoma-like pattern may be due to eccrine duct spread.[160]

BCCs are found at excision margins in perhaps 5 percent, yet only about one-third of these will recur in the following 2 to 5 years.[161] Therefore, re-excision for positive margins is not nec-essarily mandatory. Widely dispersed vs. tightly clustered nests may be a better predictor of local recurrence than simply tumor at a margin.[144] Neglected BCC invading bone can lead to slow but extensive osteolysis (Fig. 17-13).

Mohs micrographic surgery[162–164] is a popular technique for treatment of larger and recurrent BCCs. As originally de-scribed, it employed "chemical cauterization" with zinc chlo-ride paste, but this step has been replaced by sharp excision op-eratively and en face frozen section technique. Additional slabs are cut from the defect walls in areas where tumor is seen in the sections; many Mohs surgeons employ their own technician and interpret the sections themselves.

ADNEXAL TUMORS

Mastery of adnexal tumor[165–167] diagnosis is challenging by virtue of the enormous number of individual tumors and their variant forms, the complicated nomenclature,[168] and the fre-quency of differentiation along two or more adnexal lines in the same tumor.[169–171] Histogenesis is the antiquated assumption that the appearance of a tumor is indicative of the cell or tissue type from which it arose ("cell of origin"). The phenotype(s) that a proliferating neoplastic population is differentiating to-ward is now the basis for assigning names according to how closely the growth patterns resemble some recognizable normal cell type(s) or structure(s). In general, adnexal tumors of the skin do not derive directly from mature appendageal epithe-lium; rather, they originate from multipotential stem cells and differentiate along adnexal pathways. This explains why many adnexal tumors imprecisely resemble their mature counterparts and how multiple differentiation pathways may be expressed simultaneously in the same lesion. Benign adnexal tumors showing an admixture of follicular, eccrine, sebaceous, and/or apocrine adnexal differentiation, such as pilosebaceous units in combination with either eccrine and/or apocrine elements, are rare but a source of diagnostic confusion. It is speculated that this represents multidirectional differentiation involving pluripotential cells of the epidermis or of adnexal structures.[172] Differentiation is likely governed not only by genetic potential, but also field influences such as regional vascularity and microenvironmental influences of the epidermis, dermis, or subcutis.

To expedite differential diagnosis, cutaneous adnexal neoplasms can be classified according to architectural patterns: (1) partially and fully cystic tumors; (2) tumors forming small nests, cords, and ducts; (3) tumors forming sheets and large nodules; and (4) infiltrative, malignant tumors (Fig. 17-14). This approach partitions a limited number of diagnostic possibilities in each pattern group. An adnexal neoplasm that does not conform completely to diagnostic criteria need not represent a new or rare entity. It is more likely to be a variant of a known tumor or one with hybrid features (e.g., the blending of spiradenoma and cylindroma in one tumor). Such lesions should be described as exhibiting mixed features.

A decision as to the benign or malignant nature of a specific tumor relies on the usual parameters of conspicuous and/or abnormal mitotic activity, necrosis, asymmetry, irregularly permeative invasive growth, and perineural or endovascular extension. These favor malignant tumor, although exceptions exist.

Certain adnexal tumors occur as part of well recognized syndromes associated with internal disease, for example, trichilemmomas and sebaceous epitheliomas as harbingers of breast (Cowden's syndrome) and gastrointestinal (Muir-Torre syndrome) carcinoma. Certain adnexal tumors may be inherited, occurring as multiple lesions (e.g., cylindroma) that require clinical monitoring, follow-up, and often, repeated surgical intervention. The Brooke-Speigler syndrome is an autosomal dominantly inherited disease characterized by the development of multiple trichoepitheliomas and cylindromas. These patients may also develop BCCs and spiradenomas.[171] Some adnexal tumors arise in lesions potentially programmed for accelerated neoplastic change, for example, a syringocystadenoma arising in a nevus sebaceus, a hamartoma that also frequently gives rise to BCC.

The gross pathology of adnexal tumors is often unimpressive. Similar skin-colored papules and nodules, solitary or multiple, may be created by dissimilar neoplastic tissue patterns. Cystic and solid tumors are generally firm. Mineralized tumors may be rock hard. The diagnosis may be forecast by extruded tumor products. For example, a trichofolliculoma has a central pore from which a wooly tuft of white hair shafts protrudes. Pain may be a clue to diagnosis because only a subset of tumors is painful (e.g., eccrine spiradenoma). Poor demarcation, asymmetry, and ulceration should arouse suspicion of a malignant tumor and the desirability of inking margins of excision.

Histopathology often can be interpreted in terms of normal appendageal differentiation. Pale cell (clear cell) change due to cytoplasmic glycogen generally recapitulates the normally glycogenated follicular outer root sheath or the embryonic acrosyringium. An accumulation of cytoplasmic fat vacuoles that indent the nucleus is a typical feature of sebaceous differentiation. The stroma of some adnexal tumors consists of a distinctive, fibrotic, eosinophilic mantle that envelops the epithelial elements. Recognition of this typical stroma assists in differentiating many basaloid adnexal neoplasms from basal cell carcinoma. Eccrine tumors commonly feature a nearly acellular hyalinized eosinophilic stroma with dilated thin-walled vessels (e.g., eccrine poroma).

Histology may change with the passage of time and altered local influences. The trichilemmal cyst, with age and possibly under inflammatory stimuli, may transform into a proliferating trichilemmal cyst and eventually into the solid pilar tumor of the scalp.

Partially and Fully Cystic Adnexal Tumors

Epidermal Inclusion Cyst

Most *epidermal inclusion cysts* form as a result of progressive cystic ectasia of the infundibulum of the hair follicle (follicular infundibular cysts).[173-175] This follows mechanical occlusion of the follicular orifice or inflammation or scarring of the follicle, as in cystic acne. Therefore, they represent retention cysts rather than true inclusion cysts. A minority, especially on extremities, result from epithelium implanted at sites of trauma. A very few arise as congenital inclusions along lines of embryonic closure. Follicular infundibular cysts clinically are dermal or subcutaneous, skin-colored, firm nodules of variable size, most often of the head, neck, and trunk, although any hair-bearing site may be involved. Post-traumatic inclusion cysts are most often acral. Exquisitely painful upon rupture, these cysts often are shelled out, and unless the entire lining is removed, may recur. Milia cysts are minute, spontaneously arising, follicular infundibular cysts involving vellus hairs of the face. Secondary milia may result from superficial dermal scarring or following blistering with dermal involvement.

Histologically, large, round to elongate tubular, keratin-filled cavities within the dermis may abut or extend into the subcutaneous fat. Communication with a pore-like epidermal ostium may be retained in early follicular infundibular cysts, but is lacking in post-traumatic epidermal inclusion cysts. The central accumulation of loosely packed keratin lamellae tends to fall out during processing. This is in contrast to the trichilemmal cyst, discussed below, which is filled with homogeneous, eosinophilic material. The epidermal cyst wall resembles surface epidermis and follicular infundibular epithelium; the epidermis-like epithelial lining has a well developed granular cell layer (Fig. 17-15A). Extrusion of keratin into the adjacent dermis provokes a foreign body type granulomatous response, frank abscess formation or edematous granulation tissue, and later, cicatrix. Scattered crinkled anucleate squames within inflammatory granulation tissue and histiocytes may be the only clue a dermal "abscess" is the site of recent cyst rupture.

Pilar Sheath Acanthoma

Pilar sheath acanthomas are usually dome-shaped, smaller than 1 cm in diameter tumors, with a central keratin-filled plug.[176,177]

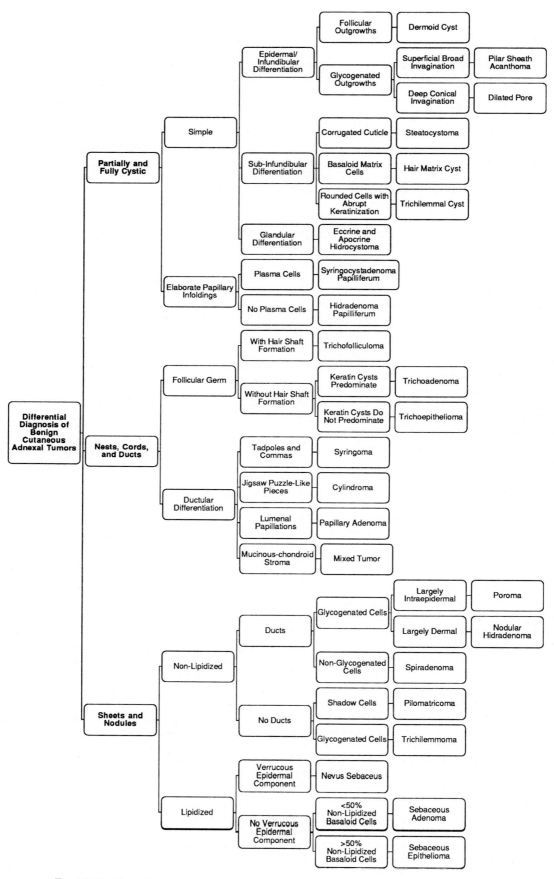

Fig. 17-14. Algorithmic approach to differential diagnosis of benign cutaneous adnexal tumors.

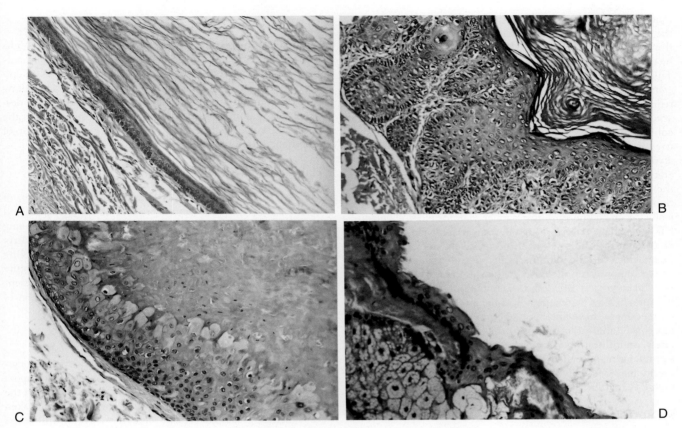

Fig. 17-15. Common cystic adnexal tumors of skin. (A) Epidermal inclusion (follicular infundibular) cyst;
(B) pilar sheath acanthoma; (C) trichilemmal cyst; and (D) steatocystoma. See text for details.

They tend to affect the facial skin of the middle-aged to elderly. This follicular infundibular cystic tumor characteristically occurs on the upper lip. The dilated pore of Winer, also likely to be facial, has a less elaborate epithelial component and extends deeper in conical form into the dermis.

The pilar sheath acanthoma is a relatively broad, shallow keratin-filled invagination that in tangential sections appears as a mid-dermal cyst. Its flattened mural keratinocytes produce keratin through a granular cell layer. Outer portions of the wall are pale, glycogenated, squamous cells resembling epithelium of the follicular outer root sheath (Fig. 17-15B). This is arranged in numerous elaborate, finger-like, serpiginous, and plate-like extensions into the surrounding dermis and occasionally even into the subcutis. The outermost layer of basal cells that surrounds these proliferations focally may appear to palisade. Small horn cysts containing laminated keratin may be observed within the proliferating epithelial elements and abortive secondary follicle formation is rarely seen. The surrounding stroma is a delicate fibrous matrix without conspicuous mucinous ground substance.

Dilated Pore

The *dilated pore of Winer*[178] is a conical infundibular acanthoma that appears as a small follicular keratotic plug (i.e., comedone) centrally within a skin-colored papule or small nodule on the head or neck. It has no age predisposition, and occasionally will be multiple. Its characteristic funnel or cone shape originates superficially as a dilated follicular infundibulum and extends inferiorly in a tapering fashion into the deep dermis and occasionally into the subcutis. Plate- and finger-like projections of squamous follicular epithelium similar to that of pilar sheath acanthoma extend from the external aspect.

Trichilemmal Cyst

The vast majority of *trichilemmal cysts*, also called pilar cysts, sebaceous cysts, or wens, are from the scalp.[122] Their lining can often can be shelled out and will be submitted without surrounding dermis. If ruptured, they extrude a cheesy, foul-smelling grumous material.

These differ from the infundibular cyst by having cohesive, homogeneously eosinophilic contents composed of keratin and lipid, frequently with cholesterol cleft formation and granular dystrophic mineralization. The content is low in sulfur-containing amino acids and thus is distinct from hair cortex. The outer layer of basaloid cells and multiple inner layers of large, pale pink, glycogenated squamous cells evolve into the central keratinaceous material without an intervening granular cell layer (Fig. 17-15C). This is described as "abrupt," or trichilemmal, keratinization. The cells lining the cyst tend to protrude into the central keratin product with rounded apical cell contours like cobblestones in contrast to the flattened interface of the granulated squamous cells that line infundibular cysts. That this is a neoplastic rather than hyperplastic lesion is supported by the finding of a nondiploid DNA content in some cases.[179] Thickening within the cyst wall permits the designation *proliferating trichilemmal cyst*.[180] Over many years this keratinocyte redundancy plus granulation tissue ingrowth deleting the keratin may result in large, bulky, solid tumors that ulcerate and contain zones of pressure necrosis (*pilar tumor of the scalp*). The irregularly lobulated interior and variable reactive nuclear atypia may arouse concern over malignant tumor. The proliferating trichilemmal cyst (PTC) is thought to be derived from the outer root sheath of anagen hair follicles with differentiation toward the infundibular and matrical segments. They typically occur on the posterior part of scalp of elderly women. PTCs may have relatively high mitotic activity and focal areas of dyskeratosis leading to confusion with squamous cell carcinoma. However, the smooth, regular, noninvasive perimeter of a pilar tumor, when included in the specimen, is unlike invasive squamous cell carcinoma. A nondiploid DNA content can be found by flow cytometry.[179] Malignant PTCs, with capacity for metastases, have areas of higher mitotic rate, marked pleomorphism, and infiltration into the surrounding stroma. Yet, rarely, an infiltrating carcinoma extends from the periphery of a proliferating pilar tumor[181–183] and rarely this is a spindle cell carcinoma.[184] Usually there is a gradual transition between benign PTC pattern and a clearly malignant histology.

Steatocystoma

Steatocystomas are rubbery, 1 to 3 cm dermal nodules that may be solitary or multiple (steatocystoma multiplex),[185,186] with an autosomal dominant pattern of inheritance. Their sites are predominantly presternal, upper arms, axillae, and scrotum. Steatocystomas may become gradually more numerous over time, and total body involvement has been described. They contain an odorless fluid that is mostly lost during removal and processing. Therefore, they appear histologically as a collapsed cystic space within the mid-dermis with corrugated infoldings of the cyst wall. The wall is composed of a single external layer of basaloid cells and several internal layers of squamoid cells that mature into a thin eosinophilic keratin layer (i.e., cuticle) resembling the duct of the normal sebaceous gland (Fig. 17-15D). Mature sebaceous lobules are within the epithelial layer or compressed just outside the cyst wall. Small or abortive hair follicles may protrude into surrounding dermis. If small hair shafts project into the lumen, *vellus hair cyst* is the diagnosis.

Eruptive Vellus Hair Cysts

Eruptive vellus hair cysts are usually a pediatric problem between the ages of 4 and 18 years, characterized by 1 to 2 mm skin-colored to variably pigmented follicular papules.[137] These round or dome-shaped lesions may have central puncta, umbilication, or hyperkeratotic crusts. Infundibular occlusion may be responsible for these mid- to upper dermal keratinizing cysts filled with lamellar keratin and small-diameter hair shafts. Cyst breakdown may produce a foreign body reaction. Spontaneous resolution within a few months to years is the rule.

Dermoid Cyst

A differential diagnostic consideration for squamous-lined cysts is the *dermoid cyst*.[188] This shows sebaceous and follicular outgrowths from what otherwise would be characterized as an epidermal inclusion cyst. They arise from skin remnants left along embryonic fusion lines. The characteristic location of the dermoid cyst is along the lines of embryonic closure such as the outer eyebrow, midline along nasal bridge, scalp, floor of mouth, or anterior neck.

Hair Matrix Cyst

The wall of a *hair matrix cyst* is composed of multiple layers of basaloid cells around a central product of closely aggregated keratin lamellae. Most are in the skin of children and young adults. The basaloid elements of the wall resemble hair matrix epithelium of pilomatricoma. Small microcysts resembling abortive follicular canals may be within the cyst wall. Rupture provokes granulomatous inflammation. Some may represent early stages of pilomatricomas analogous to the evolution of trichilemmal cysts into pilar tumors.

Hidrocystomas, Apocrine and Eccrine Types

Apocrine cystadenoma is a synonym for the apocrine hidrocystoma, a cystic, nonpapillary, nontubular adenoma with apocrine features.[189–191] These appear as blue-black nodules on the face, head, neck, and upper trunk. Their color may be mistaken for malignant melanoma.[192] Size varies from several millimeters to several centimeters. Men and women are equally affected, and patients average 55 years in age. A single cystic cavity within the superficial to mid-dermis is lined by one to several layers of cuboidal to columnar secretory cells resembling epithelium of the apocrine secretory coil (Fig. 17-16). Finely granular, eosinophilic cytoplasm pinches off at the cell apex into the chamber (decapitation secretion). Small epithelial tufts lacking the fibrovascular cores of true papillae may protrude into the cystic chamber. Duct-like spaces may be formed within epithelial bridges around the chamber. The cyst is

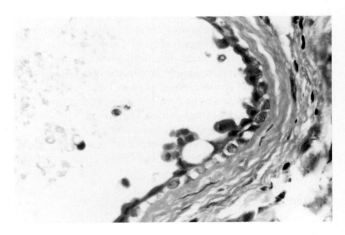

Fig. 17-16. Apocrine hidrocystoma showing characteristic papillary epithelial projections.

bound by an outermost single layer of flattened myoepithelial cells. Eosinophilic proteinaceous material, sometimes containing cholesterol clefts, may be present within the cyst cavity. Small apocrine cystadenomas that involve the inner and outer canthus of the palpebral border of the lower eyelid are often referred to as Moll gland cysts.

Apocrine cytologic features, multiple cell layers to the lining, and frond formation differentiate apocrine cystadenoma from *eccrine hidrocystoma*, a passive ectasia of the eccrine duct with chronic obstruction. These are most common over the face as small dome-shaped translucent papules, sometimes multiple over cheeks and eyelids. They may enlarge with heat stress and immediately disappear upon incision as clear fluid escapes. One or two layers of small cuboidal cells line the chamber and a connection to eccrine ducts from below may be evident.

Ciliated Cysts

Ciliated columnar cells comprising part of the wall of a cyst[193] bring up a differential diagnosis, including *cutaneous ciliated cyst* (in deep dermis or subcutaneous fat of lower extremities in young women),[194] *median raphe cyst* (a cystic anomaly near glans penis), *omphaloenteric polyp* (with intestinal crypt epithelium beneath epidermis of umbilicus), *bronchogenic cyst* (on chest or back with pseudostratified, ciliated epithelium containing goblet cells),[195] and *cutaneous endosalpingiosis* (multiple brown papules averaging 5 mm in diameter develop after a salpingectomy around the umbilicus, but not necessarily within the laparotomy incision scar; each papule contains beneath an intact epidermis a unilocular cyst with papillary projections into the lumen; oviduct type epithelium of columnar cells, some of them ciliated and others secretory thus resembling that in cutaneous ciliated cysts).[196] *Branchial cleft cysts* occur near the ear and on the neck (see Chs. 32 and 60).

Syringocystadenoma Papilliferum

Syringocystadenoma papilliferum, a benign, partially cystic, adnexal neoplasm (also known as papillary syringadenoma) has apocrine and eccrine differentiation.[197–200] Most occur on the face and scalp as skin-colored, often verrucous and scaling nodules or as verrucous, crusted plaques. One-third arise in a pre-existing nevus sebaceus. If this complication arises in early life, the appearance is that of moist keratotic nodules within the verrucous plaques, which may show a linear or zosteriform distribution. Syringocystadenoma papilliferum not associated with nevus sebaceus usually occurs at or following puberty, a milestone when nevus sebaceus on its own tends to enlarge and become more apparent.

As is implicit in its name, syringocystadenoma papilliferum is a cystic neoplasm with numerous papillary infoldings within the mid-dermis. The overlying epidermis exhibits a slightly verrucous surface with hyperkeratosis. The superficial portion of the cyst lining may be composed of keratinizing squamous cells continuous with adjacent epidermal hyperplasia such that the cyst cavity and the epidermal surface communicate. The cyst lining and the lining of the luminal papillary projections are at least two cell layers thick (Fig. 17-17A). The innermost layer of columnar epithelial cells exhibits the apocrine characteristic of

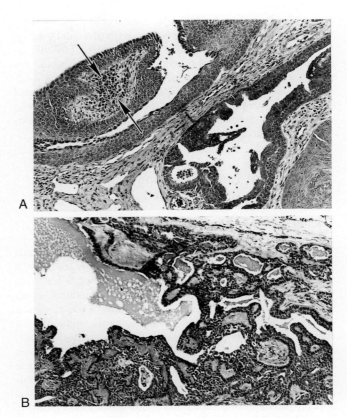

Fig. 17-17. **(A)** Syringocystadenoma papilliferum and **(B)** hidradenoma papilliferum. Note similarity between the two tumors, although the former characteristically has aggregates of plasma cells within its stroma (Fig. A, arrows).

focal decapitation secretion. Outermost are basaloid to cuboidal cells, and where these form three or more cell layers, small duct-like lumina are frequent. In the fibrovascular stroma are prominent plasma cells, an important differential diagnostic feature. These are predominantly of the IgG and IgA classes.[200,201] Dilated and hyperplastic apocrine glands may be in the stroma subjacent to this cystic tumor and serve as a reminder to seek a precursor nevus sebaceus.

Hidradenoma Papilliferum

Hidradenoma papilliferum[202] is characteristically a tumor of white women over 30 years of age, on labia majora, perineal and perianal skin, or more rarely, the skin of the nipple, eyelid,[203] or external ear canal. Clinically it will appear as a solitary, freely movable, skin-colored nodule, millimeters to several centimeters in diameter. Microscopically, the tumor consists of a large epithelium-lined cyst within the mid-dermis surrounded by a fibrovascular mantle. Absence of an inflammatory, plasma cell-rich stroma allows the distinction from syringocystadenoma, even at low power magnification (Fig. 17-17B). The superficial portion may be lined by a single layer of flattened squamous epithelial cells, occasionally in continuity with the epidermis. Most of the lining consists of two layers of cuboidal to columnar epithelium with apocrine type decapitation secretion and underlying cuboidal myoepithelial cells. Cyst wall protrudes into the lumen at numerous foci as fibrovascular papillae that are an extension of the fibrovascular mantle. Epithelial infoldings within individual papilla may impart a glandular appearance. *Tubulopapillary hidradenoma* conceptualizes a spectrum of lesions, including tubular apocrine adenoma and papillary eccrine adenoma[204] and these are also closely related to syringocystadenoma papilliferum.[205] Tubular apocrine adenoma occurs most often on the scalp.[206]

Adnexal Tumors Forming Nests, Cords, and Ducts

Trichoepithelioma and Trichoadenoma

Trichoepithelioma incompletely recapitulates the pilosebaceous apparatus.[207–209] This benign neoplasm has solitary (nonhereditary) and multiple (autosomal dominant) forms. Solitary tumors appear as pale, skin-colored papules and nodules, sometimes reaching 2 cm in diameter. Facial skin of adults is most commonly involved. Clinically it is frequently confused with basal cell carcinoma. In the multiple form, numerous skin-colored papules and nodules smaller than 1 cm develop on the face, scalp, neck, and upper trunk with a particular predilection for nasolabial folds and preauricular regions. The onset of multiple lesions often occurs during childhood and then persists and progresses during adulthood. Both solitary and multiple forms show radiating buds, nests, and anastomosing cords of basaloid cells within the mid-dermis invested within a fibrotic stroma (Fig. 17-18A). Basaloid buds resemble hair matrix and papillary mesenchymal bodies represent the attempt to form the papillary mesenchyme responsible for hair follicle induction.[210] Multiple, small, keratin-filled cysts tend to appear within the epithelial nests, particularly within the more superficial dermal nests. When these horn cysts predominate and are of nearly equal diameter, and when the basaloid component is minimal, the diagnosis is appropriately *trichoadenoma*.[211] This variant occurs as small, solitary nodules on the face and occasionally on the trunk.

Desmoplastic trichoepithelioma[212,213] is a nodular usually solitary variant of trichoepithelioma smaller than 1 cm and often affecting the face of young women. A typical central depression can clinically resemble the morpheaform variant of basal cell carcinoma. Histologically, desmoplastic trichoepithelioma consists of small cords and nests of basaloid cells compressed and distorted by a dense, sclerotic stroma.[212] Of value in ruling out BCC, especially the morphea-like form,[214] are the absence of mitoses, individual cell necrosis, and mucinous stroma without foci of separation artifact from lesional epithelium; also there is EMA positivity (75 percent), in contrast to BCC variants, which are negative. Occasional lesions of solitary trichoepithelioma cannot reliably be distinguished from keratotic BCC, and complete excision is wise.

Trichofolliculoma

Trichofolliculoma, a highly differentiated neoplastic proliferation of actively trichogenic epithelium, recapitulates all por-

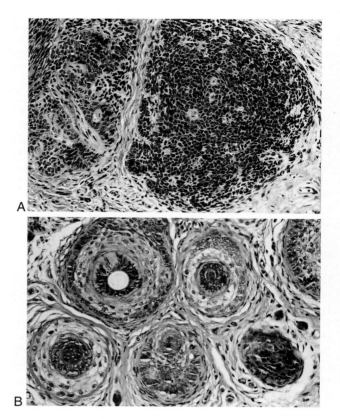

Fig. 17-18. **(A)** Trichoepithelioma and **(B)** trichofolliculoma. Observe that while the former consists of nests of basaloid cells within a fibrotic stroma, the latter more closely recapitulates various components of hair follicle formation.

tions of the pilosebaceous complex.[215] It clinically appears as a solitary, skin-colored, 3 to 5 mm nodule that frequently has a central pore or crater from which a wooly tuft of small white hairs may emerge. Histologically, this dilated follicular infundibulum-like pore (i.e., primary follicle) communicates with the epidermal surface and contains laminated keratin and often multiple small hair shafts (Fig. 17-18B). Numerous secondary follicles consisting of either rudimentary bulbs of basaloid cells or outer and inner root sheath epithelium bud at the base of this plug within the mid-dermis, producing a radiating pattern. Focal lipidization within the follicular wall, hair matrix and papilla formation, and trichogenesis are variably present. The stroma is fibrotic, and well demarcated from the adjacent dermis. Trichofolliculoma may be considered a well differentiated counterpart of trichoepithelioma.

Tumor of the Follicular Infundibulum

Tumor of the follicular infundibulum is a small lesion that resembles a superficial basal epithelioma but is comparatively innocuous.[216] Anastomosing columns of rather light-staining outer root sheath type cells form a shelf or fenestrated plate, remaining attached to overlying epidermis at multiple points (Fig. 17-19). Mitoses and apoptosis are inconspicuous.

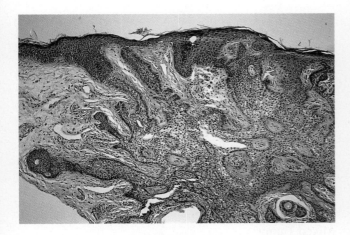

Fig. 17-19. Tumor of the follicular infundibulum. A benign basaloid cell proliferation has multiple points of connection with epidermis. There is a tendency for peripheral palisading.

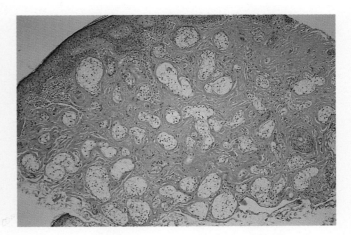

Fig. 17-20. Clear cell syringoma. The tumor consists of variably sized rounded groups of clear cells.

Syringoma

Syringoma is a benign adnexal tumor of well differentiated eccrine ductular elements.[217] These are small (1 to 3 mm in diameter), asymptomatic, skin-colored papules that may be solitary but often are multiple, especially on the face of genetically predisposed individuals. Women are preferentially affected by multiple lesions that begin at puberty and continue to form during adult life. Syringoma commonly involves lower eyelids, cheeks, axillae, lower abdomen, and vulva, but rarely acral areas. Eruptive syringomas are primarily in children as successive crops on the anterior aspect of the body surface. Linear syringomas are grouped in discrete linear or unilateral zones, a distribution paralleling some epidermal nevi. Histologically, numerous small cords and nests form discrete, symmetric aggregates within the mid-dermis. These often appear to originate from overlying keratin-filled cystic epidermal invaginations. The cytokeratin content of tumor cells suggests syringoma differentiates toward the portion of the sweat duct located in the upper dermis and lower epidermis (the "sweat duct ridge").[218] The stroma is well developed, collagenous, and eosinophilic. Characteristically, some epithelial nests have contours reminiscent of tadpoles or commas. Ductular lumina within many of the nests may contain homogeneous, eosinophilic, PAS-positive, diastase-resistant secretions. Clear cell syringomas designate a histologic variant with the same basic architecture but composed of highly glycogenated ductular epithelial cells[219] (Fig. 17-20).

Eccrine Syringofibroadenoma

Eccrine syringofibroadenoma is a sponge-like tumor that on section has thin strands and septae of small cuboidal cells separated by much fibrovascular stroma. By electron microscopy, the ducts have a keratinization pattern similar to luminal acrosyringial cells. This suggests origin of the tumor in deranged acrosyringial development in which the luminal cells predominate over the peripheral cells.[220]

Cylindroma

Cylindroma, a benign, histologically primitive adenoma, is regarded as showing apocrine differentiation.[221–223] It may occur either as a solitary lesion or as multiple, dominantly inherited[224] scalp nodules. Solitary cylindromas tend to involve the face and scalp of older adults with only 10 percent occurring on other sites.[225] Multiple lesions frequently begin as nondescript, firm, skin-colored scalp nodules. Over time, new cylindromas form, and older lesions grow and coalesce to produce a bizarre turban-like mass ("turban tumor").

Sections will show numerous ovoid to polygonal nests of basaloid cells within the superficial and deep dermis. Its epithelial nests are arranged in close approximation to form a well circumscribed but nonencapsulated tumor mass and have a tendency to mold against one another like pieces of a jigsaw puzzle (Fig. 17-21). The nests are composed of two cell types, small basaloid cells and larger pale cells, both of which contain

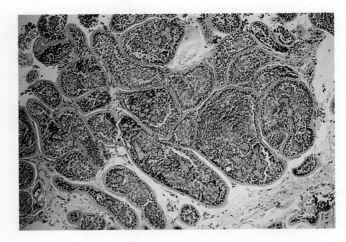

Fig. 17-21. Cylindroma. Closely approximated tumor cell groups resemble puzzle pieces. Eosinopilic material in the nests is continuous with the delimiting basement membrane material.

rounded nuclei without atypia. A distinctive thickened layer of hyalinized eosinophilic collagen and a continuous basement membrane of uniform thickness surrounds each nest. Small, round, hyalinized, eosinophilic bodies interspersed among tumor cells are focally continuous with the PAS-positive basement membrane that surrounds individual nests of tumor cells. Small, duct-like lumina are usually present within tumor nests.[223] These cellular and matrix components are nearly identical to those of eccrine spiradenoma, although the architectures of these two are quite different. The ultrastructural and immunohistochemical features fit differentiation toward the intradermal coiled portion of the eccrine sweat duct of eccrine sweat glands[223,226,227] with myoepithelial cell participation.[222] Malignant change is rare and limited for all practical purposes to the multiple lesion cases.[228,229]

Papillary Eccrine Adenoma

Papillary eccrine adenoma is a rare, solitary nodular sweat gland tumor, and is also known as tubulopapillary hidradenoma; it has a predilection for hands and feet but does occur elsewhere. Individuals with darkly pigmented skin are preferentially affected.[230] It is typically 0.5 to 2 cm in diameter. Lesions may be present for many months or years prior to excision, and recurrence after treatment is rare. This well circumscribed, symmetric proliferation of variably dilated ducts exhibits focally prominent, intraluminal, papillary, epithelial projections.[206,231,232] (Fig. 17-22). The low power appearance may suggest a benign breast lesion, especially intraductal hyperplasia, within the su-

perficial and deep dermis, not continuous with the overlying epidermis. Amorphous and granular eosinophilic secretions are in many of the duct lumens, occasionally coexistent with small, keratin-filled cysts. Adenomatous regions consist of variably spaced ducts and glands lined by one to several layers of cuboidal epithelium. Both ductular and glandular structures are formed. Immunoreactivity for S-100 protein, CEA, and EMA is consistent with differentiation toward the secretory epithelium of sweat glands.[206,231] Eosinophilic fibrovascular stromal tissue distinguishes it from dermal endometriosis, which has a more cellular stroma. The tumor may recur locally but does not metastasize. The more aggressive variant that occurs primarily on the digits of the hand, *aggressive digital papillary adenocarcinoma*, is discussed below as a variant of eccrine carcinoma.

Mixed Tumor

Mixed tumor of skin (chondroid syringoma) is a benign appendage tumor with the diagnostic feature of a myxochondroid stroma supporting eccrine and apocrine epithelial structures.[233,234] These firm, skin-colored, intradermal or subcutaneous nodules are most often on the head and neck and between 0.5 and 3 cm in diameter. The overlying skin may be fixed to the nodule.

Histologic sections present relatively well circumscribed, symmetric, ovoid to lobulated tumors within the superficial to deep dermis. The epithelium may consist of branching small to dilated ducts or be entirely composed of small solid cords and small ducts formed by cells resembling those of a syringoma. The cuboidal epithelial cells form small tubular ducts, more

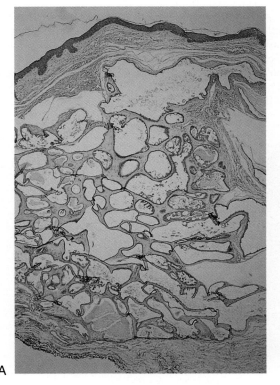

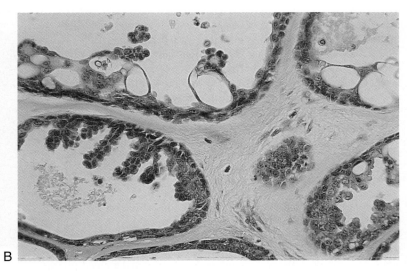

A   B

Fig. 17-22. Papillary eccrine adenoma. **(A)** Multiple small cystic spaces are crowded in dermis. **(B)** Constituent poroid cells form small papillations.

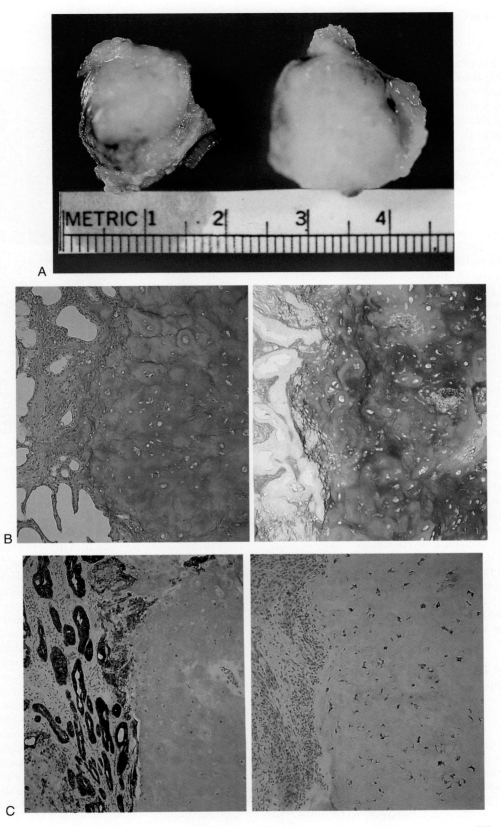

Fig. 17-23. Mixed tumor of skin. **(A)** Myxoid and chondroid matrix causes some translucency. **(B)** Basophilic cartilage matrix (left) stains for sulfated mucopolysacharide with aldehyde fuchsin at low pH (right). **(C)** Duct elements label darkly for keratin (left). Cells in the chondroid matrix react for S-100 protein, as expected for chondrocytes (right).

elaborate branching tubular lumina, and dilated cystic ducts and have a variable outer layer of flattened myoepithelial cells. The inner layer cells express cytokeratin, CEA, and EMA. The outer cell layer is positive for vimentin, S-100 protein, NSE, and, occasionally, glial fibrillary acidic protein.[235-237] The cystic spaces are frequently filled with PAS-positive, diastase-resistant material. Apocrine-like secretions have occasionally been observed, although the ducts show mostly eccrine differentiation by routine light microscopic criteria. The stroma varies from vaguely eosinophilic to basophilic and may appear to represent loose reactive fibrous tissue, pale hyalinized fibrous tissue, myxoid tissue, or solid hyaline cartilage (Fig. 17-23). Study of many cases suggests sequential evolution within the stroma over time. Initially delicate stellate fibroblast-like cells possibly related to ductal myoepithelial cells[238] are suspended in alcian blue-positive, hyaluronidase-resistant acid mucopolysaccharide (myxoid stroma). Acquisition of cytoplasmic lipid by these stromal cells may scatter mature signet ring fat cells within the myxoid background. In some lesions, the synthesis and secretion of stromal matrix components are more complete, creating solid hyaline cartilage populated by cells in lacunae showing ultrastructural features of true chondrocytes and S-100 positivity.

Although the vast majority of mixed tumors do not recur after surgical excision, seeding and regrowth of stromal and epithelial elements may occur, especially as a consequence of incomplete curettage. Symmetry and noninfiltrative pattern of growth are important features in differentiating benign mixed tumors from the rarely encountered malignant variant.[239] Malignant chondroid syringoma (also known as malignant mixed tumor of the skin) tends to appear as a rapidly growing nodule on an extremity. It may arise de novo or, rarely, from a benign chondroid syringoma.[240] Histologically, malignant chondroid syringoma is composed of epithelial structures with glandular differentiation and carcinomatous features, embedded in a mucinous stroma with spindled mesenchymal cells and areas of chondroid differentiation. Unlike biphasic synovial sarcoma, in which both components express cytokeratins, only its epithelial structures are cytokeratin positive. When this malignant variant metastasizes, it generally does so as an adenocarcinoma, leaving behind any tendency to form chondroid stroma.

Adnexal Tumors Forming Sheets and Nodules, Nonlipidized

Poroma

Poroma, a benign, usually solitary appendage tumor, is characterized by cellular differentiation toward the intraepidermal portion of the eccrine coil (acrosyringium).[241-243] The majority of these lesions occur on or near the palms and soles, where eccrine gland density is highest. Other areas where it may arise are head, neck, and trunk. Patients are generally middle-aged. The lesions are firm to rubbery, dome-shaped, verrucous or pedunculated nodules that rarely exceed 2 to 3 cm. They are intrinsically painless, but arouse concern because of their tendency to erode, with oozing, crusting, and occasionally frank ulceration.

Poromas are endophytic growths composed of lobular plates

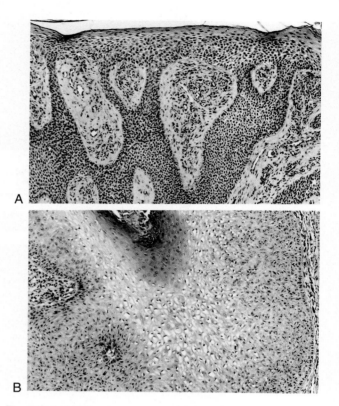

Fig. 17-24. **(A)** Eccrine poroma and **(B)** trichilemmoma. Although both tumors show endophytic growth of glycogenated cells, only the former show duct formation.

of cells that expand initially from the epidermis into the papillary dermis, and sometimes into the reticular dermis (Fig. 17-24). Their richly vascular stroma with foci of dilated and tortuous vessels should suggest the diagnosis when combined with uniform "poral" epithelial cell sheets. The intraepidermal edges of a poral tumor are sharply delineated from the more darkly eosinophilic keratinocytes of adjacent normal epidermis. They are polygonal squamoid cells, generally smaller than midepidermal keratinocytes, with inconspicuous intercellular bridges. Mitotic figures and individual cell necrosis are rare. The pallor of their cytoplasm is due to their glycogen content. The predominant cell has ultrastructural, enzymatic, histochemical, and immunohistochemical findings similar to cells of the acrosyringium.[241,244] Small eccrine duct lumens lined by a PAS-positive cuticle and sometimes a spiraling architecture should be sought and are diagnostically helpful in most poromas. EMA positivity is expected.[245] The term *dermal duct tumor* is used for tumors of similar structure situated entirely in the dermis. Their differentiation is toward the dermal portion of the sweat gland duct and like poroma, they may bear much melanin pigment.

Hidroacanthoma simplex[246,247] distinguishes poromas that display superficial intraepidermal epithelioma pattern of growth. It does not represent an entity that is biologically different from classic poroma, and thus represents one of several epithelial tumors that may show this architecture.

Trichilemmoma

Trichilemmomas are clinically verrucous, hyperkeratotic, or smooth papules ranging from a few millimeters to occasionally more than 1 cm. Facial skin is the common site, most often the nose, cheek, and upper lip. Multiple trichilemmomas occur in an autosomal dominant condition referred to as Cowden's syndrome,[248] strongly associated with carcinoma of the breast in females. Other manifestations of this syndrome are benign verrucous and lichenoid keratotic tumors of the hands and feet (acral keratoses), punctate keratoses of the palms and soles, papillomatosis of the lips and oral mucosa, and scrotal tongue.

This well defined lobular proliferation of glycogenated epithelium may originate at the shoulder of a follicular orifice and can include a portion of a pilosebaceous unit at its base (Fig. 17-24). More advanced tumors are devoid of identifiable pre-existing pilar structure. The verrucous surface may show increased scale production and therefore parakeratosis. A plate-like lobular downgrowth extends into a fibrovascular stroma. The most peripheral layer is basaloid and may show palisading. A thickened, hyalinized, stromal mantle surrounds this basaloid layer. The constituent large squamous cells have pale pink cytoplasm filled with PAS-positive glycogen. Old verrucae, generally devoid of HPV-related cytopathology, may acquire cytoplasmic glycogen and mimic the features of trichilemoma. Trichilemomas may be differentiated from ordinary verrucae by their localization about follicular infundibula, basaloid palisading at the periphery of tumor lobules, and development of a thickened, hyalinized basement membrane. The idea that all trichilemmomas are the result of HPV infection is not sustained by molecular hybridization to detect the viral genome.[249]

Desmoplastic trichilemmoma has irregular extensions of cells derived from the outer root sheath epithelium projecting into sclerotic collagen bundles, mimicking invasive carcinoma.[250]

Nodular Hidradenoma

Nodular hidradenomas, also called solid cystic hidradenoma, clear cell hidradenomas, and eccrine acrospiromas, are benign adnexal neoplasms showing eccrine acrosyringeal differentiation.[251–254] These usually solitary, asymptomatic, intradermal nodules commonly measure between 0.5 and 2 cm in diameter. They have no strong site predilection, although many are described on the face, scalp, chest, and abdomen. Smooth, normal skin covers the mass, which has variable coloration from red to blue. Superficial ulceration is an occasional cause for presentation, although this feature should also raise the possibility of malignant tumor.

The mass is composed of multiple coalescent nodules surrounded by a collagenous pseudocapsule within the superficial and deep dermis (Fig. 17-25A). Occasional lesions extend to involve the subcutaneous fat. Continuity with the overlying epidermis may or may not be seen, and when it is present, tends not to show the extensive intraepidermal origin that persists in deep poromas. Clear cell change as a result of cytoplasmic glycogenation may be inconspicuous or prominent as zonal pallor. When prominent, clear cell changes may be distinguished from metastatic hypernephroma by ductal differentiation, which is conspicuous in some and must be sought in others, as

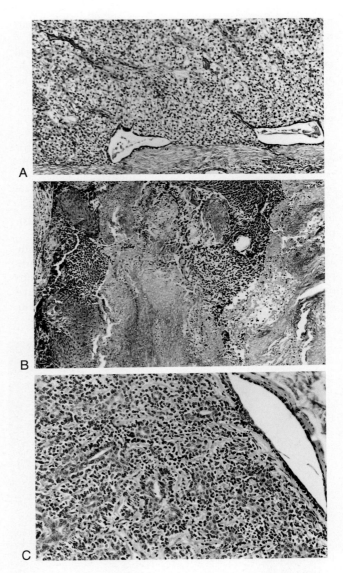

Fig. 17-25. (A) Nodular hidradenoma with clear cell change, (B) pilomatricoma showing juxtaposition of basaloid and shadow cells, and (C) edge of eccrine spiradenoma showing prominent duct formation directly beneath the enveloping capsule. Note similar duct formation in inferior portion of nodular hidradenoma.

well as relative sparsity of highly vascularized stroma. Small branching, tubular ducts and large, cyst-like ducts are lined by cuboidal epithelial cells or columnar secretory cells, respectively. Immunohistochemical reactivity for keratin, EMA, CEA, S-100 protein, and vimentin is expected.[254] Condensed, eosinophilic, hyalinized stroma forms a mantle at the periphery and often extends into the tumor as trabeculae. Solid portions of the tumor are composed of a variable admixture of small basaloid to squamoid polyhedral and fusiform cells often exhibiting distinct plasma membranes. Although tumor nuclei may be hyperchromatic and exhibit coarsely clumped chromatin, marked pleomorphism and frequent or atypical mitoses are not observed. If present, the tumor should be considered to have a potential for aggressive behavior. A zonal or diffuse pattern or necrosis also suggests a malignant variant.

Nodular hidradenomas may occasionally reform after local excision. Associated distortion and fibrosis may impede the diagnostic interpretation when the histology of the primary lesion is unknown or unavailable.

Pilomatricoma

Also known as the *calcifying epithelioma of Malherbe*, pilomatricomas are solitary, 0.5 to 3 cm firm, deep-seated dermal or subcutaneous nodules that often occur in children and adolescents and have a predilection for face and upper extremities.[255–258] Multiple lesions and familial patterns of occurrence are possible. The hereditary type has been linked to myotonic dystrophy.[259]

The proliferative elements of pilomatricomas are mitotically active. Basaloid cells resembling hair matrix are particularly prominent in early tumors (Fig. 17-25B). These grade into sheets of so-called shadow cells. Nuclear atypia or infiltrative growth patterns are restricted to the rare malignant variants (pilomatrix carcinoma). Shadow cells are eosinophilic squamous cells resembling hair cortex that have lost their nuclei, leaving ovoid, clear zones centrally within the cytoplasm, hence their name. As lesions age, shadow cells predominate or are present exclusively. Dystrophic calcification within sheets of shadow cells eventually attracts osteoclast-like giant cells that erode Howship's lacunae-like spaces in this anachronistic nonviable epithelium. Application of lamellar bone by osteoblasts emerging from the fibrovascular stroma may occur, completing a sequence paralleling enchondral ossification. Transepidermal elimination or perforation[256] can lead to "dermal osteomyelitis." Diagnosis by needle biopsy is possible.[260] Unusual clinical variants are large, extruding or perforating, multiple eruptive, familial, and malignant (pilomatic carcinoma).[261–264]

Spiradenoma

Spiradenomas are 1 to 2 cm, solitary or rarely multiple intradermal nodules that are usually found in children and young adults.[265] Any site is possible, but many are on the trunk and

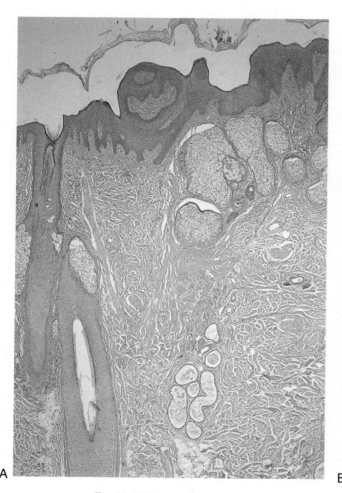

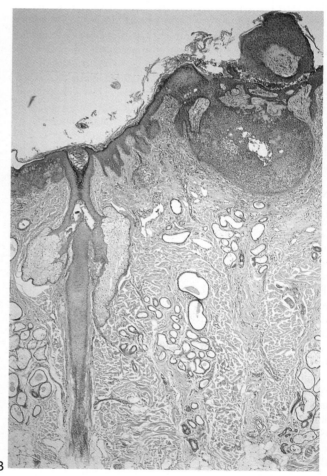

Fig. 17-26. Nevus sebaceus. **(A)** Beneath a slightly papillomatous surface are prominent sebaceous glands; deeper are apocrine units (center, bottom). **(B)** Early basal cell carcinoma has complicated another example of this lesion.

extremities. The dome-shaped, skin-colored nodules are classically painful,[266] perhaps explained by an often elaborate network of unmyelinated axons and Schwann cells within the stroma.

On a slide, an *eccrine spiradenoma* is a well circumscribed, round to ovoid, basophilic nodule or group of nodules with variable vascularity, located within a loose fibrovascular dermal stroma (Fig. 17-25C). Adjacent nodules may coalesce. Small nests resembling cylindroma are rarely nearby. The epithelial cells are characteristically closely packed and consist of three cell types. Most numerous is a large cell with a round to ovoid nucleus with evenly dispersed pale chromatin and a scant rim of cytoplasm. A second cell type, admixed with the first to form poorly defined cords, is smaller and has a round, hyperchromatic, lymphocyte-like nucleus and inconspicuous cytoplasm. The third cell type and the least apparent is only focally present in some spiradenomas; this cuboidal to flattened epithelial cell forms eccrine type ducts.[267] Origin is thought to be from the lower portion of the eccrine duct.[265,268,269]

The thin, encapsulating stromal mantle is composed of hyalinized connective tissue variably permeated by small, unmyelinated axons. Small branching stromal septa may extend from this mantle into the tumor parenchyma. Minute rounded fragments of hyalinized basement membrane material or stromal matrix appear to be progressively incorporated into the tumor nodule. These hyalinized bodies tend to become evenly distributed throughout the neoplasm, an appearance simulated only by one other adnexal tumor, the cylindroma. A heavy diffuse lymphocytic infiltration, mainly of T cells, may occur.[270] Malignant transformation is rare.

Adnexal Tumors Forming Sheets and Nodules, Lipidized

Nevus Sebaceus

Nevus sebaceus represents hamartomatous sebaceous overgrowth beneath a seborrheic keratosis-like zone of epidermal hyperplasia.[271–273] Anomalous pilar and/or apocrine differentiation and hamartomatous stromal overgrowths are frequently associated (Fig. 17-26). These congenital plaques most often affect scalp or facial skin. Prepubertal lesions with minimal sebaceous activity present as zones of localized alopecia. Peripubertal and postpubertal lesions acquire plaque-like elevation and a yellow hue in addition to the alopecia as a result of sebaceous growth. Nevus sebaceus may show sebaceous lobules that empty directly onto a verrucous epidermal surface. Anomalous hair germ-like pilar structures, apocrine metaplasia, and hamartomatous fibrovascular stromal redundancies in some lesions indicate they are developmental aberrations.

Sebaceous Hyperplasia

Sebaceous hyperplasia forms small, non-neoplastic, pale to yellow papules generally on the face of an older individual.[274] Chronically sun-exposed skin of whites is most vulnerable. Central umbilication is characteristic. Biopsy is often performed to exclude basal cell carcinoma. Multiple lobules of normal-appearing but abnormally superficial sebaceous glands are arranged in a redundant grape-like distribution around the central sebaceous duct (Fig. 17-27A). The central wide duct explains the umbilication. Even shave biopsies show benign glands too superficially located due to budding of lobules above a horizontal plane that approximate the origin of the sebaceous duct. The outer nonlipidized basaloid cell layer in lobules is not increased in hyperplasia as it is in the neoplasms.

Benign Sebaceous Neoplasms

Sebaceous adenomas and epitheliomas are relatively uncommon, usually solitary, tan-yellow papules that occur on the facial skin of middle-aged and older individuals.[275] They are often con-

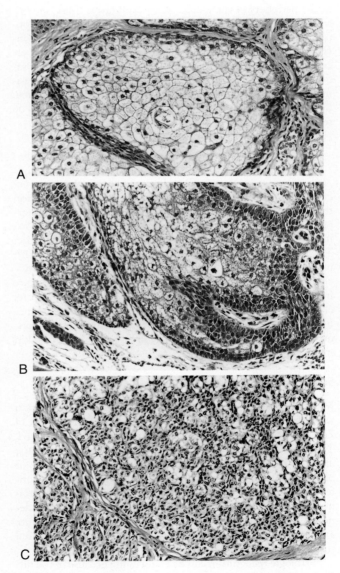

Fig. 17-27. (A) Sebaceous hyperplasia, (B) sebaceous adenoma, and (C) sebaceous epithelioma. The sebaceous epithelioma is depicted at a lower magnification to enhance assessment of relative distribution of lipidized and nonlipidized cellular elements.

fused with BCC clinically. Sebaceous epitheliomas can bleed and ulcerate, increasing the suspicion that they represent more aggressive tumors. Sebaceous adenomas and epitheliomas when multiple are associated with an internal malignant tumor in a small percentage of patients in the Muir-Torre syndrome.[276–278] Low grade colonic adenocarcinoma is the best known intercurrent malignant tumor.

Sebaceous adenomas and epitheliomas are well circumscribed lobular epithelial proliferations that originate from the overlying epidermis. They are characteristically surrounded by a fibrotic, eosinophilic stroma. Sebaceous adenomas consist of multiple, coalescent, sebaceous glands, some of which may show rudimentary or abortive formation of individual lobules and dilated ducts. The predominant central cells are well lipidized with fine vacuoles filling the cytoplasm. Basaloid cells at the periphery of the lobules are several layers thick, in contrast to the single basaloid layer in normal or hyperplastic lobules, and they may displace foamy cells in the central regions (Fig. 17-27B). Sebaceous epitheliomas have more than 50 percent basaloid cells (Fig. 17-27C). Lipidized cells may be only individually scattered throughout the tumor lobules. Neither tumor has nuclear atypia, the hallmark of sebaceous carcinoma, but considerable mitotic activity in the basaloid regions may be seen in either.

Adnexal Carcinoma

Carcinomas primary in the skin may show sebaceous, eccrine, or apocrine differentiation, at times with a perfection that allows them to be recognized as the malignant counterparts of previously discussed benign adnexal tumors.[279,280] Unlike most SCCs and BCCs, they have a tendency to metastasize. Their rarity and patterns lead to confusion histologically with metastatic carcinoma. Electron microscopy and immunohistochemistry are not particularly useful in distinguishing primary from secondary carcinomatous tumors of the skin. Therefore, clinical information becomes central. A solitary epithelial malignant tumor present for more than 6 months is usually primary. A rapidly evolving neoplastic disease involving the skin in crops is probably metastatic.

Sebaceous Carcinoma

Most *sebaceous carcinomas* occur on the eyelid, in association with the meibomian glands of the tarsus and the glands of Zeis.[281–284] The upper eyelid in women is commonly involved. These nodular, often ill-defined, firm lesions are asymptomatic and may be mistaken for chalazion, partially ruptured cysts, or blepharoconjunctivitis. Size exceeding 1 cm in diameter confers a poorer prognosis than smaller lesions. Sebaceous carcinoma may also be associated with multiple facial sebaceous adenomas, basal and squamous cell carcinomas, keratoacanthomas, and visceral carcinomas, particularly of the gastrointestinal tract (i.e., Muir-Torre syndrome).

Histologic recognition can be challenging because of the difficulty of becoming familiar with the normal histology of the periocular and ocular tissues,[285] and also subtle sebaceous malignant tumors can be seen. Sebaceous carcinomas have a vaguely lobular configuration. Many infiltrate as irregular

tongues and small clusters of malignant cells into the dermis, subcutis, and skeletal muscle. Tumor cells are frequently large and squamoid in appearance, or show basaloid differentiation with only inconspicuous lipidization (Fig. 17-28A). The latter must be distinguished from BCCs with sebaceous differentiation[286] and the former from SCCs with hydropic changes.[287] When carcinoma in a periorbital site is suspected or found at frozen section, additional cuts should be saved on glass slides for fat stains. Zones of necrosis, marked nuclear atypia, and abnormal mitotic figures are common. Pagetoid growth of tumor cells in the epidermis or conjunctiva also extends widely and confers

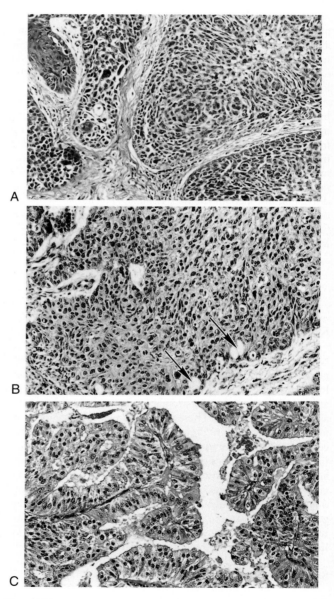

Fig. 17-28. Variants of adnexal carcinoma. **(A)** Sebaceous carcinoma with primarily squamous features and abortive lipidization, **(B)** eccrine carcinoma growing as sheets of squamoid cells with only focal duct formation (arrows), and **(C)** well differentiated apocrine carcinoma showing characteristic papillary architecture.

a poorer prognosis, as does multicentric involvement, lack of differentiation (i.e., sparse lipidization), necrosis, lack of lymphocytic reaction,[288] wide local infiltration, and vascular or orbital bone invasion. Metastases first affect regional lymph nodes of the periauricular, submaxillary, and cervical chains. Visceral spread may follow.

Eccrine Carcinoma

Eccrine carcinoma is a very rare tumor, but relatively frequent with respect to most other variants of adnexal carcinoma, and has a high rate of metastatic spread.[289,290] Clinicopathologic correlation has delineated several subtypes and presentations[291] that are important to recognize as primary skin tumors.

Ductal eccrine carcinoma[292] may initially appear as an infiltrative poroma (porocarcinoma) or present the histology of a moderately differentiated adenocarcinoma. Eccrine porocarcinoma favors extremities, particularly legs and feet, at any age (usually adults) without gender predilection. Cords and lobules of polygonal tumor cells permeate dermis at the asymmetric sides. Contiguity with benign eccrine structures or with the overlying epidermis is variable. A cribriform growth of atypical cells, some squamoid, with frequent mitoses and necrosis is classic. Nuclear atypia is always evident. At least focal spiraling ductular structures, duct formation lined by cuticular material, and/or zones of cytoplasmic glycogenation and also intraepidermal cells in discrete aggregates, often centered on acrosyringial pores, are useful clues to eccrine differentiation (Fig. 17-28B). Foci of squamous differentiation are unusual findings in eccrine adnexal neoplasms but may have the histologic features of well differentiated squamous cell carcinoma.[293] The stroma may be fibrotic, hyalinized, highly myxoid, or even frankly mucinous. Distinction from metastatic adenocarcinoma, especially of breast and lung origin, can be difficult, especially for less differentiated tumors. Ductular differentiation with PAS-positive cuticle formation is strong evidence against metastatic tumor. Nonetheless, exclusion of an extracutaneous primary adenocarcinoma by history and radiologic means should be pursued. One-third of ductal eccrine carcinomas will metastasize[294] and a similar number are fatal.

Microcystic adnexal carcinoma (MAC), or sclerosing sweat duct carcinoma,[295,296] is increasingly considered a sclerosing variant of ductal eccrine carcinoma. The facial (e.g., upper lip) skin of middle-aged and elderly women is particularly at risk from this rare tumor. Simply arriving at a malignant interpretation requires sensitivity to subtle nuclear hyperchromaticity and rare mitoses. Cords and small nests of rather uniform cuboidal to polygonal squamoid cells are extremely infiltrative and prone to perineural and perivascular extension. Characteristically, cell and nest size decreases with dermal descent. MAC type I has pilar-type microcysts. MAC type II has narrow ("syringoid") tubular profiles. The differential includes morpheaform basal cell carcinoma, desmoplastic trichoepithelioma, and adenosquamous carcinoma of skin. The marked tendency for recurrence accrues from the difficulty in clinical assessment of margins during excision. Therefore, Mohs surgery is contraindicated. Neglected or multiply recurrent tumors may mutilate and require massive resections including bone to eradicate them.

Mucinous eccrine carcinoma[297] resembles colloid carcinoma of breast and gut, favoring skin of face and proximal trunk, elderly adults, and males 2:1. Cords and clumps of cohesive polygonal tumor cells are surrounded by pools of PAS- and mucicarmine-positive mucus. The myxoid stroma of mixed tumor of the skin is sulfated and therefore stains with aldehyde fuchsin. Immunohistochemical results suggest differentiation toward eccrine secretory coil.[298] Exclusion of primary visceral carcinomas is often impossible by histology alone because of the extreme variety with which such tumors spread to skin. This gelatinous tumor recurs in about 30 percent of cases but only very rarely spreads.

Clear cell hidradenocarcinoma (malignant nodular hidradenoma)[299] also favors head, neck, and extremities of adults. This low grade malignant tumor resembles metastatic clear cell carcinoma of kidney, lung, and genital tract. It recurs in perhaps one-third of cases, but rarely metastasizes.

Trichilemmal carcinoma[294,300–303] is a slow-growing epidermal papule, indurated plaque, or nodule predilecting sun-exposed, hair-bearing skin. Solid, lobular, or trabecular growth patterns are formed by malignant epithelial cells with features of outer root sheath differentiation, including abundant glycogen-rich, clear cytoplasm, foci of pilar type keratinization, and peripheral palisading of cells with subnuclear vacuolization. Cytologic atypia is overt. Pagetoid intraepidermal spread may be seen. Despite brisk mitotic activity, recurrence and metastases are uncommon and conservative surgical excision with clear margins is adequate.[300,302]

Adenoid cystic carcinoma in the skin[304–306] can be considered primary, because embolic spread from visceral tumors with this pattern is virtually unknown. Skin of face and scalp of elderly patients of either sex feature skin-colored nodules or plaques. Perfectly round spaces formed by malignant epithelial cells and containing basophilic basement membrane-like material occur in the cribriform type and tubular variants. Confusion with adenoid basal cell carcinoma is the most frequent pitfall. Cutaneous extension from a parotid tumor or scar recurrence might be ruled out in specific body sites. This indolent, nonaggressive tumor extends avidly in perineural spaces and therefore recurs in 20 percent of cases. Metastases are very rare.

The *papillary digital adenocarcinoma*[307] forms a spectrum with papillary eccrine adenoma. The tumor arises on distal extremities, especially digits, of adult males. The painless enlarging masses are likely to have been present for several months or years. Macropapillae project into microcysts lined by atypical epithelial cells, and such areas may merge with more cellular regions of moderately differentiated adenocarcinoma. Metastatic papillary carcinoma from breast, lung, thyroid, and gonad may come to mind. Low ("aggressive digital papillary") and high grade variants are distinguished by degree of pleomorphism, mitotic rate, and necrosis, and fulfill expected differences in local recurrence and metastases.

Malignant eccrine spiradenoma (sweat gland carcinoma ex eccrine spiradenoma)[308,309] is an extremely rare exception to the rule that sweat gland carcinomas arise de novo, unassociated with a benign precursor neoplasm. Diagnosis hinges on a clinical history of rapid growth in relation to a long-standing cutaneous nodule, corroborated by finding remnants of the antecedent spiradenoma beside a typically sharply demarcated adjacent carcinoma. The malignant tumor may resemble breast cancer, carcinosarcoma, and spindle cell or anaplastic polygonal cell tumors. The high grade histology has a low potential for metastases but local recurrence may follow.

Mucoepidermoid (low grade adenosquamous) carcinoma[310,311] histologically identical to that of salivary glands may occur as a primary dermal malignant tumor (see Ch. 33).

Apocrine Carcinoma

Apocrine adenocarcinomas are solitary or multiple, solid to cystic masses from 1 cm to greater than 5 cm.[312,313] Males, usually over 40 years, exceed women with this rare malignant tumor by 5:3. Axillae and the anogential areas are most often the tumor site. Ear canal and eyelid involvement result from malignant change involving ceruminous and Moll apocrine-type glands, respectively. Rarely this cancer arises in a nevus sebaceus. Clinically the tumors have a red to purple coloration, possibly with ulceration. Most have been present for less than 1 year. Histologically, apocrine carcinomas have complex glandular patterns composed of one to several layers of epithelial cells that may form intraluminal fronds or exhibit cribriform patterns with lumenal bridging or coalescent nested areas (Fig. 17-28C). Apocrine differentiation is signified by abundant granular eosinophilic cytoplasm and at least focal decapitation secretion. Poorly differentiated areas show solid sheets or nests of malignant cells that may be suspected as apocrine only by virtue of abundant granular eosinophilic cytoplasm. The cytoplasm contains PAS-positive, diastase-resistant granules and, often, iron-positive granules. Nuclear atypia, frequent and often atypical mitoses, and single cell or zonal necrosis are all unlike granular cell tumor, which some apocrine carcinomas may superficially resemble. A spectrum of histologic patterns from normal apocrine glands through glands with atypia and in situ apocrine carcinoma may border the invasive and frankly malignant apocrine epithelium. Stromal fibrosis and hyalinization are frequent. In general, this is a slow-growing neoplasm, but the prognosis is guarded because more than one-third of patients with apocrine carcinoma die from the tumor, which spreads to regional nodes and distant sites.

MELANOCYTIC TUMORS

Melanocytic hyperplasias and neoplasms are commonly removed for cosmetic and diagnostic reasons. Most are benign. Many may be confused clinically and histologically with malignant melanoma (hereafter referred to simply as melanoma), the most common potentially fatal neoplasm of the skin. It is now increasingly appreciated that numerous melanoma variants may impersonate either benign nevi or other nonmelanocytic tumors. Clinical detection of early lesions has shown recent advances. Perhaps due to lifestyles or the changing environment, especially as they pertain to sun exposure, the incidence and mortality of melanoma have risen sharply during recent years. All of these realities have resulted in increased clinical screening and biopsy of early precursor lesions and, in consequence,

identification of lesions with significant premalignant or malignant potential.

Melanocytes are migratory, neural crest-derived cells whose precursor melanoblasts migrate to the periderm, develop dendritic shape, and normally are evenly and sparsely dispersed in the basal cell layer of the epidermis. The same cells also give rise to peripheral neurons and Schwann cells,[314] explaining the spectrum of features bridging benign melanocytic and neural lesions.[315,316] This is exemplified by neurotization (schwannian differentiation) in acquired melanocytic nevi, pigmented neurofibromas, and melanocytic schwannomas, and the association of leptomeningeal melanocytes with giant congenital melanocytic nevi.[317] One melanocyte per 10 contiguous basal keratinocytes in truncal skin, not chronically actinically damaged, is taken as normal melanocytic density. Their normal function is to synthesize photoprotective melanin pigment. Delicate melanosome-laden dendrites extend between keratinocytes toward the epidermal surface and transfer melanosomes to keratinocytes through the process of cytocrinia.

Clinically diffuse hyperpigmentation (e.g., tanning) and macular foci of cutaneous darkening (e.g., lentigines) involve benign hyperplasia of melanocytes and are associated histologically with an increase in the ratio of melanocytes to basal keratinocytes (>1:10). Often melanization of the basal cell layer is increased with thinning and elongation of the rete ridges. Planar hyperplasia of melanocytes within the basal cell layer is referred to as *lentiginous hyperplasia* ("lenticula," Latin for a lentil-shaped spot). Nested proliferation represents growth of discrete clusters of melanocytes. A symmetric pattern of growth and tendency for eventual involution are characteristics of benign melanocytic proliferations. Proliferation and migration are normal abilities of melanocytes, as seen in regenerating epidermis and repigmenting areas in vitiligo.[318,319] Similarly, upward or lateral migration of melanocytes within the epidermis (pagetoid spread) does not necessarily connote malignant tumors.[320]

Melanocytic atypia encompasses both abnormal or unusual architectural and individual cell appearances, but neither necessarily connotes a premalignant alteration. This is because nevi recurring in scars, nevi with aging (i.e., "ancient") changes, and nevi with deep, penetrating patterns are, under this view, atypical. It is those nevi that share some degree of architectural and cellular similarity with melanoma that are categorized as dysplastic and should be regarded as potentially premalignant.

Melanocytic lesions are distinguished by their ability to synthesize melanin pigment and color the clinical picture. Freckles and simple lentigines are tan-brown macules with rounded, relatively uniform borders. Early melanomas may be macular or very slightly raised, but they show more variegation in pigmentation (from brown to blue-gray to tan) and are irregular, often featuring notched borders. These alarming details contrast with the appearance of ordinary acquired nevi, which are papules or small nodules of uniform color from flesh tones to brown to black. Melanin pigment below epidermis determines the hue of blue nevi, imparting a blue-black color that may be confused with heavily pigmented vertical growth phase melanoma. Entirely amelanotic tumors are skin-colored. Those with host responses against normal and neoplastic melanocytes may show uniform or asymmetric vitiligo-like regions that enlarge beyond the limits of the original lesion (e.g., halo nevi and regressing melanoma, respectively). Congenital nevi often are accompanied by associated hamartomatous anomalies in the surface epidermis, adnexae, or underlying connective tissue, and therefore present as verrucous, hypertrichotic plaques. Dermoscopy (epiluminescent microscopy) is a clinical tool involving magnification of the clinical lesion after mineral oil coating of its surface. This may bring out additional details for which the clinician will request an explanation.[321]

Sample size in relation to the whole lesion as well as clinical context must be kept in mind and fully understood in the evaluation of pigmented lesions.[322] Small biopsy specimens from the periphery of an acral melanoma that contain proliferations resembling lentiginous nevi may not uncommonly show on complete excision radial growth phase melanoma. Nevi from acral and genital skin, as well as the superficial components of many congenital nevi, show architectural features reminiscent of dysplastic nevi or even melanoma, and may result in overdiagnosis of malignant tumors unless clinical site is considered.

Melanocytic Hyperplasia

An *ephelid* or freckle merely represents hyperactivity of melanocyte pigment donation to adjacent keratinocytes. Simple freckles are light tan, uniform, 2 to 4 mm, pigmented macules with slightly irregular borders on sun-exposed body surfaces. True hyperplasia is represented by the common *lentigo* or lentigo simplex. Lentigines are poorly circumscribed, tan or brown, slightly variegated 4 to 10 mm macules preferentially on sun-exposed skin. These occur indolently with advancing age, or suddenly after actinic damage (solar lentigo). Multiple lentigines may rapidly appear with psoralens and UV therapy (i.e., PUVA freckles). Multiple lentigines occur in the Peutz-Jeghers syndrome, centrofacial lentiginosis, Moynahan's syndrome, LEOPARD syndrome, Charley's syndrome, and xeroderma pigmentosa.[323] Lentigines are larger and more variegated than true freckles, and thus more often biopsied to exclude melanocytic dysplasia or radial growth phase melanoma, such as lentigo maligna. Certain lentigines are deeply pigmented, for example, the lower lip *labial macule* and *genital lentiginosis*.[324] Lentigo-like hyperpigmentation with increased density of terminal hairs constitutes the acquired hamartoma, *Becker's nevus*.

A freckle appears microscopically as basal cell hyperpigmentation, often with accentuation in rete ridges. Melanocytes are normal in number, and most of the melanin pigment is in basal keratinocytes. In addition to basal cell layer hyperpigmentation, a lentigo has noncontiguous melanocytic hyperplasia. Rete ridges may be slightly thinned and elongated, and the underlying dermis may show mild fibrosis and melanin pigment incontinence. Solar lentigo has dermal elastosis and lentiginous melanocytic hyperplasia with secondary epidermal rete hyperplasia, the latter occasionally simulating a reticulated seborrheic keratosis, possibly with admixed zones of epidermal atrophy.[325]

Melanocytic Nevi

Common Acquired Nevi

Nevus cells or nevocytes are round, uniform cells that contain centrally located nuclei with delicate chromatin patterns, inconspicuous nucleoli, and occasional nuclear pseudoinclusions. Pseudoinclusions are invaginations of cytoplasm producing a rounded, pale, eosinophilic body within a nucleus when viewed in a thin cross-section. Common acquired melanocytic nevi are by convention divided into junctional, compound, and dermal. These distinctions are biologically insignificant. The traditional view of a common acquired nevus begins with a noncontiguous lentiginous melanocytic hyperplasia, most often on sun-exposed skin, appearing as a regular tan macule (i.e., lentigo). In the process of nevus cell transformation, nests or theques of rounded nevus cells form along the dermal-epidermal interface. Three or more nevus cells constitute a nest. Over time, nevus cell nests bud from the intraepidermal lentiginous source into the superficial dermis, forming a compound nevus. The nested junctional component tends to be lost as dermal nevus cells extend into the deeper layers, a process often accompanied by various degrees of maturation proportional to dermal depth (Fig. 17-29). Maturing cords of relatively nonpigmented nevus cells develop into fascicles and organoid aggregates, the deepest of these assuming cytologic and histochemical characteristics of neural tissue. Maturation also entails decrease in size of nevus cells proportional to depth of descent into the dermis. Most nevi undergo gradual involution.[327,328] Very old nevi may become entirely neural in appearance, with or without admixed mature fat or amyloid.[329] Some are alleged to explain certain skin tags and some angiofibromas (e.g., fibrous papules), neither with residual nevus cells.

Junctional nevi are relatively flat, radially symmetric zones of hyperpigmentation. Nests of uniform, small, round nevus cells tend to be equally spaced at the tips of rete ridges. It is proposed that some junctional nevi arise from regions of lentiginous melanocytic hyperplasia and there may be residual hyperplasia

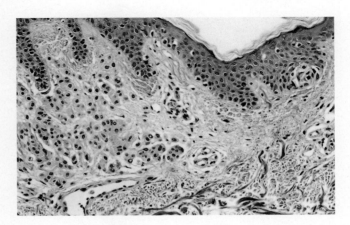

Fig. 17-29. Compound acquired melanocytic nevus showing characteristic intraepidermal nest (right) and early dermal component (left).

of benign melanocytes along the dermal-epidermal junction (i.e., lentiginous junctional nevus). *Compound and dermal nevi* are sharply circumscribed, pigmented papules. Dome-shaped elevation is attributable to the nevus cells forming dermal nests and cords. The percentage of nevi with junctional components decreases as patient age increases.[328,330] Superficial aggregates of nevus cells with rounded nuclei slightly smaller than a keratinocyte and prominent cytoplasm capable of melanin pigment synthesis are termed *epithelioid* or *type A nevus cells*. Cords of tyrosinase-negative nevus cells incapable of pigment synthesis in deeper dermis are smaller in cell diameter and are termed *type B nevus cells*. The deepest fusiform cells with histochemical profiles akin to neural tissue are *neural* or *type C nevus cells*. Very old dermal nevi devoid of residual epidermal (i.e., junctional) components may be composed exclusively of type C cells ("neuronevi")[331] and may be confused with neurofibromas, but neurofibromas have small interspersed nerve twigs, and nevi do not.

A change in size, border configuration, and/or color is a common cause for clinical concern about a pigmented lesion, leading to its excision. The most frequent microscopic explanation is a "shoulder" area of lentiginous junctional melanocytic proliferation without cellular atypia beyond the edge of the underlying dermal component, precluding a diagnosis of dysplastic nevus. This may represent reactivation of radial junctional proliferation typical of the earlier active growth phase of a benign nevus.

Nevi with very active melanin synthesis and pigment transfer to keratinocytes can arouse clinical concern because of a dark color correlating microscopically with conspicuous transepidermal elimination of melanin into stratum corneum. Historic suspicion of pigmented nevi on palms and soles leads to biopsies showing mainly junctional nevocyte nests.[332] Nevi on palms and soles tend to remain junctional throughout life.

The more recently described *deep penetrating nevus*[333] most often occurs on the head, neck and shoulder, and is commonly confused with blue nevus. They are wedge- or tack-shaped (Fig. 17-30A), and, unlike blue nevi, usually have nests of nevus cells at the dermal-epidermal junction. The dermal component varies from variably pigmented spindle and epithelioid cell morphology to smaller, acquired nevic cell differentiation; dendritic pigmented cells are not present. The most pigmented cells are generally melanophages recognized by lack of dendritic extensions and nuclear features of histiocytes (Fig. 17-30B). Gradual diminution in nevus cell size in deeper dermis (maturation) is subtle or incomplete, and thus easily leads to confusion with malignant melanoma. Table 17-1 summarizes the points of distinction between cellular blue nevus, deep penetrating nevus, and nodular malignant melanoma. When more heavily pigmented cells are more conspicuous within the deeper confines of a compound or dermal nevus, this constitutes the inverted type A pattern. Mitotic activity is absent or rare. Individual cell necrosis is not present. Nuclear chromatin is delicate and uniform nuclear membranes are thin.

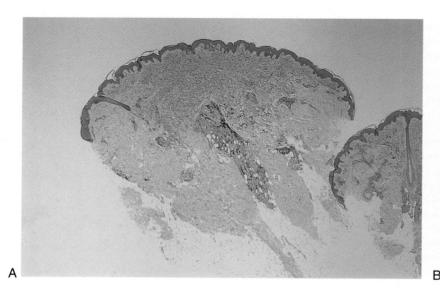

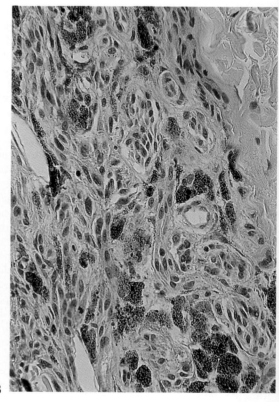

A   B

Fig. 17-30. Deep penetrating nevus. **(A)** An extension of nevus cells passes downward in fat related to a follicle. **(B)** The most heavily pigmented cells in the extension are melanophages; nevocytes are plump.

Table 17-1. Differential Diagnosis of Cellular Blue Nevus, Deep Penetrating Nevus, and Nodular Malignant Melanoma

Disorder	Clinical Appearance	Architecture	Cytology
Cellular blue nevus	Blue-black papule or nodule on lumbosacral skin	Asymmetric, with endophytic extension into subcutis	Dendritic, pigmented nevus cells and epithelioid, nonpigmented nevus cells
Deep penetrating nevus	Blue-black papule or nodule on head, neck, or upper extremity	Asymmetric, with endophytic extension into subcutis	Nondendritic, pigmented melanophages and epithelioid, variably pigmented nevic cells
Nodular melanoma	Blue-black nodule anywhere on body surface	Asymmetric	Atypia, mitoses, cellular necrosis

Nevi in genital skin may show larger junctional nests composed of somewhat atypical and dyscohesive melanocytes. Acral nevi may show pagetoid extension of benign-appearing nevus cells, but this is limited to the zone directly over prominent junctional nests. Transepidermal elimination of junctional melanocytic nevus cell nests is said to be more common in juvenile nevi than in adult nevi and may simulate intraepidermal pagetoid growth of melanoma[334] (Fig. 17-31). Tempering the significance of these findings by consideration of the site of occurrence and patient age is analogous to the considered evaluation of cartilaginous tumors of the skeleton.

Nevi are commonly excised when irritated or ulcerated by trauma or inflamed, either diffusely with mononuclear cells[335] or focally as by rupture of an internal follicle or included cyst. Cysts spatially concurrent with nevi are mainly of epidermoid (follicular infundibular) type, but dermoid cyst, trichilemmal cyst, hidrocystoma, or steatocystoma may be found.[336] The head and neck are most often the location of these composite lesions, which can undergo rapid enlargement, hemorrhage, or ulceration, arousing concern over melanoma. Nevi may have focal epidermal necrosis or impetiginization. Healing may produce superficial scar that modifies color. Such changes justify excision and should be noted in the report.

Congenital Nevi

So-called congenital melanocytic nevi may be found on as many as 1 percent of all newborns and are generally less than 1.5 cm.[337] However, because they are hamartomas, they may become grossly apparent or prominent months or years after birth. Malformations of other cutaneous structures frequently coexist. Congenital nevi of intermediate size are larger than 1.5 cm but do not cover large skin areas. Large (giant) congenital nevi exceed 144 cm² and may involve the cutaneous surface like an article of clothing ("garment" or "bathing trunk" nevi). They tend to distribute along a dermatome. Association with meningeal or cerebral melanosis is seen in the neurocutaneous melanosis syndrome[338] or may occur as a component of melanophacomatosis. Giant congenital nevi can rapidly extend[339] but also have a documented tendency for malignant degeneration; therefore, removal is generally indicated if feasible.[340] Alternatively, close clinical follow-up and biopsy of regions of pigmentation or induration is sometimes instituted.

Microscopically, confidence in designating a nevus as congenital rather than a common acquired nevus rises in proportion to the number of the following details that are observed[341]: (1) clinical lesion broader than 1 cm; (2) associated verrucous

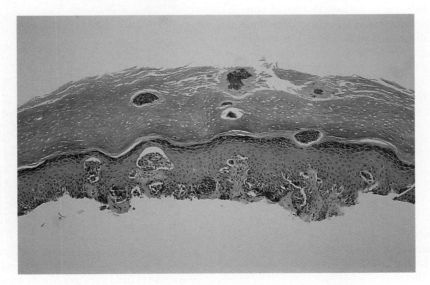

Fig. 17-31. Junctional nevus with transepidermal elimination of benign nevus cell nests.

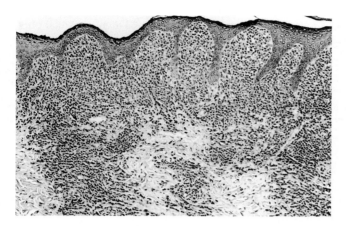

Fig. 17-32. Congenital melanocytic nevus showing typical permeative growth of nevus cells within the reticular dermal matrix.

or seborrheic keratosis-like epidermal hyperplasia; (3) some degree of anomalous architecture (e.g., bridging of adjacent rete ridges) of the intraepidermal nevus cells; (4) extensive infiltration of the mid to lower dermis and even into subcutaneous fat (Fig. 17-32); (5) dermal nevus cells forming nests within adnexal structures (e.g., eccrine ducts, hair follicles, sebaceous glands, or pilar muscles) or infiltrating perineurium; and (6) dermal nevus cells herniating into lymphatic spaces, a pseudoinvasive pattern. The specificity, sensitivity, and significance of these features for congenital origin are disputed because similar findings occur in some acquired nevi.[342]

The risk for melanoma in small congenital nevi is minimal in childhood, but increases to about 4.6 percent in adulthood.[343] Small congenital nevi may be a more frequent substrate for development of melanoma than previously recognized.[344] Melanoma in giant congenital nevi is on the order of 6 percent lifetime risk,[345] with a bimodal age of incidence in the first 5 years of life and again in early adult life.[343,346]

Regions of nodularity and color variation within large congenital nevi should be biopsied to exclude malignant change. This can arise from either the intraepidermal or dermal nevus component. Histologically there may be nuclear pleomorphism with occasional mitoses, cellular atypia, and necrosis. These features are significant if found in a sharply demarcated expansile nodule that has notable mitotic activity or an intraepidermal component with architectural features of melanoma. They must be distinguished from expansile aggregates of uniform nevocytes in the midst of the dermal component of congenital nevi; these benign "proliferative nodules" show few mitoses, no necrosis, and mature at the edges so as to blend with the adjacent nevic cells.

Blue Nevi

Common *blue nevi* are 2 to 10 mm, symmetric, blue-black, dome-shaped papules with smooth peripheral borders.[347–349] The hue of blue nevi results from filtration of the brown color of melanin pigment in the dermis through overlying dermis and epidermis (the Tyndall effect).

At low magnification, blue nevi generally appear as symmet-

ric admixtures of pigmented dendritic melanocytes and nonpigmented spindle cells (i.e., fibroblasts) within the superficial or superficial and deep dermis. A key finding is particulate melanin granules within thin dendrites and distinguishes blue nevus cells from pigment-laden melanophages (Fig. 17-33A). The term *combined nevus* is applied to the histologic admixture of blue nevus with conventional acquired melanocytic dermal nevus.[350–352]

A *cellular blue nevus* is a relatively large, 1 cm to several centimeters, blue-black, nodular tumor often located in the lumbosacral skin of young adults.[353,354] The histologic profile typically involves the full thickness of the reticular dermis, often in dumbbell configuration due to an expansile nodule in deep dermis, occasionally bulging against fat. Dendritic cells at the periphery indistinguishable from a common blue nevus are an important clue to diagnosis. Plump crowded spindle and epithelioid cells predominate toward the center (Fig. 17-33B). These areas may contain heavily pigmented spindle cells, although epithelioid cells contain less melanin pigment. They also have enlarged nuclei occasionally with prominent nucleoli but with consistently thin, uniform nuclear membranes and delicate chromatin. Collagen sclerosis may warrant the designation *desmoplastic blue nevus*.[355] One or more mitosis per square millimeter, which is about 10 high power fields, warrants the designation of *atypical cellular blue nevus* if melanoma is ex-

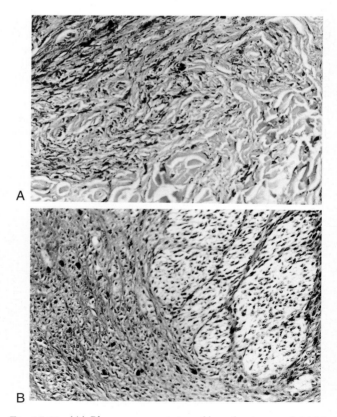

Fig. 17-33. **(A)** Blue nevus consisting of heavily pigmented, highly dendritic melanocytes, and **(B)** cellular blue nevus in which the blue nevus pattern (left) is juxtaposed with relatively nonpigmented cellular micronodules of large, pale nevic cells (right).

cluded. Complete excision and close follow-up may be indicated for any tumor not fulfilling all of the characteristic clinical and histologic criteria for cellular blue nevus.

The concept of a malignant blue nevus,[356–358] whether a melanoma arising in a blue nevus or a malignant tumor with most of the morphologic features of cellular blue nevus ("blue melanoma"),[359] is a problematic area in need of clarification.

Halo Nevus

A *halo nevus* (leukoderma aquisitum centrifugum) is distinguished by a centripetally enlarging hypopigmented peripheral zone around a 2 to 10 mm well circumscribed tan-brown papule.[360,361] The location is generally the trunk. An apparent higher frequency during summer probably relates to tanning accentuating the surrounding zone of depigmentation, so the lesion is more conspicuous. Multiple halo nevi are not uncommon. Most disappear over several months, leaving a zone of hypopigmentation that eventually repigments.

The pathobiology is a cytotoxic host response to a pre-existing acquired melanocytic nevus. This is manifest as a heavy symmetric lymphocytic infiltrate within the dermal component of a compound melanocytic nevus surrounding individual nevus cells. This cytotoxic attack may result in nevus cell injury and death. Cellular alterations secondary to injury and necrosis should not be interpreted as dysplasia or evidence of malignant tumor. Heavy infiltration by lymphocytes may completely obscure nevus cells such that they are apparent only after careful scrutiny or when they are decorated by an S-100 protein reaction. Melanophages in the upper dermis follow nevus cell destruction.

Spindle and Epithelioid Cell Nevus (Spitz Nevus)

The *spindle and epithelioid cell (Spitz) nevus* is mainly found on children and young adults.[362–365] Common locations are head, neck, and upper extremities. Because they are minimally pigmented, the associated stromal vascularity dominates the clinical appearance and lesions may mimic hemangioma or pyogenic granuloma. Multiple grouped Spitz nevi or single central tumors with peripheral satellites constitute clinical variants.

An original term for these tumors composed of plump melanocytes was "benign juvenile melanoma" because of an alarming histology but innocuous follow-up.[366,367] A prominent dermal component is usual, but some are purely junctional and others are exclusively dermal. It is their symmetry under low power magnification that is most unlike melanoma. A helmet shape with flat base, or a tapering of the dermal component resembling an inverted triangle are common configurations, symmetric about a central axis. The commonly associated epidermal hyperplasia creates angular extensions of keratinocytes between the commonly coalescent fascicles of plump lesional melanocytes (Fig. 17-34A). These fascicles seem suspended like bunches of bananas, or appear to "rain down" into dermis. Crescentic clefts commonly open between these nests of fusiform to epithelioid nevus cells and adjacent keratinocytes.[368,369] Pagetoid spread of single or grouped cells in the overlying hyperplastic epidermal layer may be seen, although significant involvement of the level of the stratum granulosum is generally

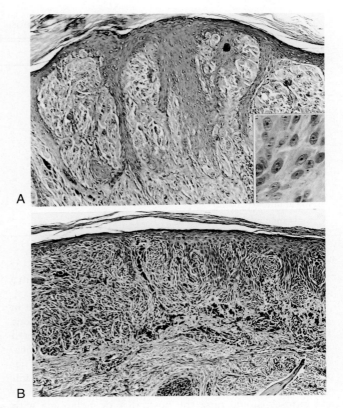

Fig. 17-34. **(A)** Spindle and epithelioid cell nevus and **(B)** pigmented spindle cell nevus. Note the characteristic epidermal hyperplasia and enlarged epithelioid nevic cells with delicate chromatin patterns (Fig. A, inset) in the spindle and epithelioid cell nevus, and the characteristic melanophage response at the base of the pigmented spindle cell nevus.

absent. Predominantly intraepidermal growth characterizes the rare pagetoid Spitz nevus.[364]

The diagnostically misleading large nuclei in Spitz nevus are euploid, in contrast to malignant melanoma, an appearance that probably relates to nuclear mRNA or nucleolar proteins.[370] Unlike the nuclear heterogeneity in melanomas, Spitz nevus nuclei tend to be roughly the same size in the same horizontal plane. Most cells have single prominent nucleoli often rendered even more conspicuous by an encircling or bordering clear zone. Nuclear membranes are uniformly thin and smoothly contoured, surrounding delicate, evenly dispersed chromatin. Cytoplasm, unlike that of melanoma, is not granular but consists of a fine net-like array of amphophilic material superimposed on a pale pink background. Ultrastructurally, this correlates with abundant ribosomes between mitochondria and other larger organelles. Eosinophilic anucleate bodies along the dermal-epidermal junction (so-called Kamino bodies) are believed to represent the necrotic residua of effete nevus cells of the intraepidermal component. They are therefore analogous to the colloid bodies seen in conditions in which basal keratinocytes undergo necrosis. Supportive connective tissue is often vascularized and hyalinized, particularly superficially. Exclusively dermal Spitz nevi represent older lesions in which predominantly epithelioid nevus cells with the previously de-

Table 17-2. Differential Diagnosis of Spitz Nevus and Nodular Melanoma

Spitz Nevus	Nodular Melanoma
Smaller (often <6 mm in diameter)	Larger (often >6 mm in diameter)
Symmetric	Often asymmetric
Epidermal layer hyperplastic	Epidermal layer normal or thinned
Fascicular, raining-down cellular orientation	Random cellular axes
Variable pagetoid spread with upper epidermal layers unaffected	Often marked pagetoid spread with involvement of stratum granulosum
Maturation present	Maturation absent
Tendency to form Kamino bodies	Kamino bodies rare or absent
Mitoses rare, especially in deep layers	Mitoses common, involving deep layers
Atypical mitoses absent	Atypical mitoses may be present
Cytoplasm amphophilic, net-like	Cytoplasm eosinophilic, granular

scribed cellular appearances tend to be scattered singly within a dense fibrotic stroma.[371]

A tendency for maturation results in a gradual decrease in cell size as nevus cells grow more deeply into the dermis. Along the deep border, individual Spitz cells typically are scattered singly rather than in the invasive nests likely with melanoma. Mitotic activity may be found among the more superficial nevus cells, is not frequent, and should be distinguished from mitoses in keratinocytes with intercellular bridges. Deep or atypical mitoses should raise the possibility of melanoma with spindle and epithelioid cell features. The term *atypical Spitz nevus* has been popularized for lesions with excessive pagetoid spread, an unusually high mitotic rate, or expansile architecture within the dermal component. Conservative complete excision is generally recommended for Spitz nevi, because local recurrence[372] complicated by scar tissue may further increase chances of misdiagnosis. Table 17-2 presents differences between Spitz nevi and nodular melanoma.

Pigmented Spindle Cell Nevus

The *pigmented spindle cell nevus of Reed* is a variant of Spitz nevus, but its distinctive clinical and histopathologic features justify its separate discussion.[373,374] This relatively small, well circumscribed, uniformly pigmented, dark brown-black nevus is characteristically but not exclusively found on the lower extremities of young adult women. Unlike the Spitz nevus, involvement of the head and neck is very rare. Most are between 3 and 10 mm and have smooth, well defined borders. Deep color and occasionally rapid growth are the source of clinical concern about melanoma. Under low magnification these usually symmetric, dome-shaped lesions expand only to the superficial dermal layers.[375] The lesional cells are fusiform, often with fascicular, coalescent growth as in an ordinary Spitz, but lacking prominent crescent clefts[376] (Fig. 17-34B). Intraepidermal mitoses may be present but dermal mitoses should raise the possibility of melanoma. Single cell pagetoid spread is seldom prominent although entire junctional nests may undergo transepidermal elimination. Variable numbers of markedly pigmented melanophages admixed with the papillary and superficial reticular dermal component are a constant accompaniment

contributing to the clinically disturbing pigmentation. As with conventional Spitz, there is some maturation with depth. The stroma may be fibrotic and focally may resemble the lamellar fibroplasia of dysplastic nevi.

Recurrent Melanocytic Nevi

Incomplete excision of a nevus, even a pure intradermal nevus, may be followed by local regrowth of typically pigmented intraepidermal nevus nests.[377,378] *Recurrent nevi* often show irregularities in pigmentation and contour that, along with the rapid clinical reappearance and growth, cause alarm and prompt additional sampling. However, the clinically rapid return of pigmentation at a site of previous nevus excision is unlike the longer delay when melanoma regrows at the site of excision.[379,380]

Recurrent nevi tend to be greater than 6 mm in diameter with confluence and variability in size and shape of intraepidermal nests, occasional foci of pagetoid growth, and foci of heavy melanin pigmentation. Nests generally predominate over single cells. Mitoses are seldom observed. There is little or no cellular atypia. There is nested and occasional single cell proliferation of nevus cells along a dermal-epidermal interface of a thinned epidermal layer devoid of rete ridges above a dermal scar. An important feature is absence of extension of the intraepidermal proliferation beyond the limits of the underlying scar, even if junctional activity was not present in the original excision.[381] This suggests a stimulatory influence of scar on nevus cells paralleling epidermal hyperplasia over dermatofibroma. Dermal nevic cells may be entrapped and distorted in the laminated superficial scar ("nevus entrapment"). The potentially alarming architectural disarray of the intraepidermal component is balanced by banal nuclear characteristics to avoid a malignant interpretation of these "pseudomelanomas".[382]

Melanocytic Dysplasia and Dysplastic Nevi

Morphologic, antigenic, functional, and genomic data comprise a growing body of evidence supporting the view that at least some benign melanocytic proliferations undergo stepwise alterations that progress from minimally dysplastic lesions to malignant tumors.[383–385] *Dysplastic melanocytic nevi* (DMN) have been shown to be indicators of an increased risk of developing malignant melanoma[386] especially when multiple and/or when in persons with immediate relatives who have had melanoma.[387,388] The hereditary melanoma trait has been localized to a single gene on the short arm of chromosome 1.[389] Patients with the multiple dysplastic nevus syndrome show chromosome instability and abnormal DNA repair after exposure to ultraviolet light.[390] In this hereditary autosomal dominant condition, an individual may have hundreds of DMN and is likely to develop one or more primary melanomas.[391] A patient with multiple DMN and at least two first-degree family members with malignant melanoma qualifies as having the syndrome. Although DMN occur in up to 5 percent of white adults in the United States,[392,393] at least 17 percent of adults with melanoma outside the familial melanoma setting have one or more DMN.[302,394–401] Furthermore, melanomas have a demonstrable contiguous DMN in 20 to 30 percent of cases.[392,402–409]

DMN usually develop in adolescence or early adulthood and, unlike common nevi, new lesions may occur throughout life.[410] The trunk is the characteristic location, but the scalp and extremities are also involved.[387,411] DMN can be diagnosed with confidence only by clinicopathologic correlation. Clinical criteria are (1) diameter usually between 5 and 12 mm, (2) macular component with indistinct, fading edges mandatory, (3) papular component often present and central within the macule, (4) variegated tan-brown color on pink background, and (5) impalpable, irregular, ill-defined border.

Only a minority of excised clinically atypical nevi fulfill the microscopic criteria for dysplastic nevus.[412,413]

Histologically, enlarged, coalescent nests of nevus cells show random cytologic atypia, defined as occasional enlarged melanocytes with prominent, hyperchromatic, irregular nuclei (Fig. 17-35). Accompanying reactive stromal changes include superficial mononuclear infiltrates and superficial dermal fibroplasia.

Previously variable histologic criteria for dysplastic nevus[414] finalized by the World Health Organization Melanoma Program[415,416] are based on those of Elder et al.[417] Both of the major and two of the minor criteria are required.[418,419]

Major criteria include the following:

1. Basilar proliferation of at least focally cytologically atypical nevomelanocytes, extending three or more rete ridges beyond a dermal melanocytic component (so-called shoulder)
2. A pattern of intraepidermal melanocytic proliferation as one of two types, lentiginous or epithelioid cell (architectural atypia)

Minor criteria include

1. Concentric eosinophilic fibrosis (condensed papillary dermal collagen outlining epidermal rete ridges) or lamellar fibroplasia (delicate layers of collagen fibers and elongate fibroblasts parallel to the epidermal surface, situated beneath tips of epidermal rete)
2. Dermal neovascularization

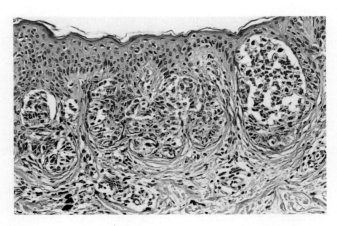

Fig. 17-35. Dysplastic nevus. Observe the enlarged, dyshesive nests with focal cytologic atypia, coalescence of nests across adjacent rete ridges, and prominent lamellar fibrosis within the underlying papillary dermis.

3. Dermal inflammatory response: lymphohistiocytic infiltrates with or without melanophages
4. Fusion of rete ridges

The melanocytic atypia is most often "random," that is, only occasional cells show enlarged nuclei with angular contours and dense hyperchromasia.[420] Dysplastic nevi with random cytologic atypia included in the criteria for inclusion are diploid by flow cytometry and image analysis techniques.[421] Cytoplasm of these cells tends to have a muddy, gray-brown or coarsely granular melanization. Cytologic atypia can be graded by judging the degree of overall increase in melanocyte size and nuclear size compared to normal, the degree of nuclear hyperchromasia and irregularity of shape, and display of prominent nucleoli. Distinction of severe from only mild or moderate atypia may be useful. Cytologic atypia is not among the defining criteria of what has been called "Clark's nevus"[422,423] and so this term is not synonymous with dysplastic nevus or the earlier term for this lesion, the B-K mole.[387] Clinical studies omitting cytologic atypia as part of the definition of the dysplastic nevus are likely to find less or no correlation with melanoma risk and may account for the erroneous assertion that dysplastic nevi are the most common form of acquired nevi.[422,424]

"Architectural atypia" includes extension ("bridging") of nevus cells between adjacent rete, nevus cell nests along sides of rete or in inter-rete spaces rather than only at rete tips as is usual for ordinary acquired nevi, and expansive nests and a very few single benign-appearing cells rising into the epidermal layer. The January 1992 NIH Consensus Development Conference on early melanoma[425] suggested discontinuance of the term "dysplastic nevus" in preference for "nevus with architectural disorder and melanocytic atypia" along with a statement describing the degree of melanocytic atypia. Discohesive infiltration of the epidermis by atypical melanocytes is not a feature of DMN.

A biopsy showing a portion of a dysplastic nevus that extends to the margin leaves significant uncertainty as to whether more significant changes are nearby. Therefore, in this situation, conservative but complete excision of the entire lesion should be considered. It is important to recognize that any melanocytic proliferation may have architectural atypia or cytologic atypia, or both, without fully meeting the criteria for a dysplastic nevus. Such lesions should be diagnosed descriptively (e.g., lentigo with cytologic atypia, compound nevus with architectural abnormality).

Fully evolved dysplastic nevi in patients with clinical signs that are compatible with multiple large atypical nevi are diagnosed as *lentiginous compound dysplastic nevi*. The lentiginous pattern describes a type of melanocytic hyperplasia with striking proliferation of nevomelanocytes along the dermal-epidermal junction usually associated with elongate tapered rete ridges. When the clinical history is not available or supportive, it should be mentioned in the report that nevi with this histology may occur as isolated lesions without established potential for further dysplastic or malignant change. DMN in individuals with clinical signs consistent with the dysplastic nevus (i.e., heritable melanoma) syndrome[426] but with no family or personal history of melanoma probably have a low prospective lifetime risk (<10 percent) for the development of melanoma. However, DMN in patients with clinical signs consistent with the dysplastic nevus syndrome and a family or personal history of melanoma have a significant lifetime risk for malignant transformation, and such patients must be monitored closely for detection of early changes in curative stages of tumor progression.[427]

Melanoma

Melanoma, a malignant tumor of melanocytes, is currently increasing in incidence more rapidly than any other cancer in the United States.[428–433] At current rates, 1 person in 128 in the United States will develop a malignant melanoma in his or her lifetime. Most melanomas arise after puberty in sun-exposed skin of whites, particularly those with fair complexion. Most reports currently agree that 20 to 30 percent of all melanomas arise in association with pre-existing nevi.[434] Yet large-scale removal of nevi is unlikely to have a major impact on the rising incidence of malignant melanoma.[344]

The minimum width of normal tissue margin in the primary excision sufficient to reduce local regrowth remains the subject of research and opinion.[435–439] Survival in melanoma is unrelated to the width of the margins.[440–443] Removal of underlying fascia is no longer deemed mandatory.[444] Radical lymph node dissection is recommended if regional lymph nodes are clinically considered to be involved. Although this cancer is diagnosable at a stage when surgical care is possible in nearly every instance, the death rate has doubled in the last 30 years.[445]

Radial Growth Phase Melanoma (Nontumorigenic)

Early melanoma tends to grow centrifugally within the epidermis and occasionally as single and clustered cells directly beneath the basement membrane (radial growth), and does not form expansile nests or nodules, even at the microscopic level (nontumorigenic growth). At this stage, malignant cells found in the papillary dermis constitute microinvasive or level II melanoma. Individual dermal nest size at this stage does not exceed those in the epidermis. Radial growth phase melanoma is generally a clinically benign, nonmetastasizing tumor, and complete removal is curative.

With progression, tumor cells more vigorously enter and grow in the dermis (vertical growth phase); expansive and coalescent nests and nodules are formed (tumorigenic growth).[446]

The presence or absence of a radial growth phase is the basis for the traditional subclassification of melanoma. Lesions that show little or no evidence of radial growth (<3 rete ridges) at the periphery of a vertical growth phase nodule are termed *nodular melanomas*. Of course, in some of these, a pre-existent radial component has been obliterated by more rapid vertical growth. Radial growth either at the shoulder of a vertical growth phase nodule or as pure radial growth phase disease is divided into three categories: superficial spreading melanoma (SSM), lentigo maligna melanoma (LMM), and acral lentiginous mucosal melanoma (ALMM). Table 17-3 contrasts these entities.

SSM in its radial growth phase forms an enlarging plaque that may or may not take origin in a pre-existing nevus.[447] Typical lesions are larger than 1 cm, have an irregular notched border, and have a variegated pink-tan-brown color. Common complaints precipitating presentation are rapid increase in size or deepening of color in a pre-existing lesion,[447,448] development of pink-white zones within already pigmented lesions, lo-

Table 17-3. Types of Radial Growth Phase Melanoma

Differential Feature	Superficial Spreading	Lentigo Maligna	Acral-Lentiginous/Mucosal
Site	Trunk, legs, arms	Face, head	Hands, feet, mucosae
Age	Young to middle-aged	Elderly	Variable
Gross appearance	Irregular, variegated plaque	Deeply pigmented macule	Deeply pigmented macule
Time-course	Months to several years	One to several decades	Months to several years
Vertical growth sign	Nodule within plaque	Nodule within macule	Often macule remains unchanged
Architecture	Nested and pagetoid intraepidermal spread	Lentiginous intraepidermal spread; epidermal atrophy	Lentiginous intraepidermal spread; epidermal hyperplasia
Cytology	Epithelioid; nuclei vesicular	Variable (often fusiform); nuclei hyperchromatic	Variable (often fusiform); nuclei hyperchromatic

calized pruritis or pain likely related to an altered host response, or ulceration and bleeding. Biopsies are often submitted with a differential including seborrheic keratosis, pigmented actinic keratosis, lentigo, or dysplastic nevus.

SSM in its radial growth phase consists of nested and single cell (pagetoid) spread[449] of universally atypical epithelioid melanocytes within a normal or slightly hyperplastic epidermal layer (Fig. 17-36). Atypical pagetoid cells usually involve all layers of the epidermis, including stratum granulosum, a very important distinction from similar spread in Spitz nevi and dysplastic nevi. Entire nests may rise through epidermis and their desiccated remnants appear in stratum corneum. SSM cells are round to oval with variably pigmented, granular cytoplasm. Nuclei are large, irregular in size and shape, with prominent, often eosinophilic nucleoli and coarsely aggregated heterochromatin and irregularly thickened nuclear membranes. By contrast, Spitz nevus cells have delicate heterochromatin, often displaced around a clear perinucleolar vacuole, with thin, uniform nuclear membranes and finely reticulated amphophilic cytoplasm. The dusty or muddy melanization of melanoma, particularly within the intraepidermal component, is shared by some dysplastic nevi. The diagnostic threshold from melanocytic dysplasia (e.g., dysplastic nevus) to radial growth phase melanoma of the superficial spreading type varies between consultants. Some consultants avoid the phrase malignant melanoma in situ altogether, preferring terms like melanocytic intraepithelial neoplasia (MIN), premalignant melanosis, atypical (intraepidermal, premalignant) melanocytic hyperplasia, and melanocytic dysplasia.[450] Useful criteria are summarized in Table 17-4. Radial growth phase melanoma may be exceedingly focal within a nevus, perhaps appearing in only one profile of a serially blocked biopsy. Most SSM in the radial phase of growth show some host response, consisting of infiltrative lymphocytic inflammatory regression or melanin pigment incontinence. Papillary dermal fibrosis with vascular prominence and ectasia are the mesenchymal sequelae of regression and may signify previously more extensive dermal involvement. Therefore, this is among the features that should be reported in a note.

Radial growth phase melanoma of the *lentigo maligna* (LM)

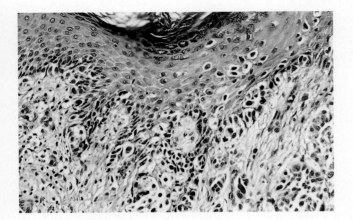

Fig. 17-36. Melanoma in situ with nested and pagetoid spread of malignant melanocytes within a thickened epidermal layer.

Table 17-4. Differential Diagnosis of Superficial Spreading Melanoma in Radial Growth Phase and Dysplastic Nevus

Dysplastic Nevus	Superficial Spreading Melanoma
Often <1 cm	Often >1 cm
Rete ridges thin and elongated	Rete ridges attenuated
Nests predominate over single cells	Single cells predominate over nests
Pagetoid spread minimal	Pagetoid spread prominent
Intraepidermal mitoses rare	Intraepidermal mitoses in one-third of lesions
Most cells not atypical	Most cells atypical
Dermal cells smaller than epidermal cells	Dermal cells similar to epidermal cells

type mainly occurs on chronically sun-damaged skin, especially facial of elderly individuals. The clinical lesions are deeply pigmented, irregular macules resembling an ink stain ("Hutchinson's melanotic freckle"). They characteristically persist with little or no change for many years before clinically nodular vertical growth supervenes, quite unlike radial growth phase of SSM. Histologically, proliferating cells in LM grow in lentiginous fashion radially above the basement membrane in the atrophic epidermal layer.[451] Contiguous growth replaces the basal cell layer of epidermis and extends down the infundibulum of hair follicles and occasionally eccrine ducts. Cytologically the cells of LM are fusiform to stellate, with marked retraction around malignant cells. Their cytoplasm is inconspicuous, as are nucleoli in the variably sized hyperchromatic nuclei. Single cell infiltration of the papillary dermis in radial growth phase lesions alter the diagnostic designation to lentigo maligna melanoma.

Acral lentiginous mucosal melanoma (ALMM) comprises approximately 10 percent of melanomas in whites.[452] It is the most prevalent melanoma in people of Asian or African descent, although the incidence of plantar involvement in North America is equal in blacks and whites,[453] arguing for the importance of a complete cutaneous and mucosal examination in general medical or dermatologic screening evaluation. ALMM has a peak incidence in the sixth decade, occurring most often on plantar, palmar, subungual, and periungual skin, and mucocutaneous junction of the oral and nasal cavities, genitalia, and anus.[454,455] The radial growth phase of ALMM appears as a deeply pigmented macule with an irregular border.[456] Vertical growth often proceeds without producing a nodule or other obvious change in the pre-existing macule.

ALMM in the radial phase of growth shares histologic features with LM except that ALMM generally has more bizarre intraepidermal melanocytes and associated epithelial hyperplasia rather than atrophy. Both LM and ALMM may form nest-like aggregates on a lentiginous pattern prior to dermal microinvasion, and this can resemble a DMN. However, DMN are generally smaller (<1 cm) than melanomas in radial growth phase and DMN cells show random rather than universal atypia in the intraepidermal compartment.

Vertical Growth Phase Melanoma (Tumorigenic)

When melanoma cells invade the dermis and grow to form mitotically active expansile (tumorigenic) nodules, the vertical growth phase has begun. Tumorigenic dermal nodules exceed the diameter of the largest intraepidermal nest. Tumorigenic nodules arising within SSM and LM types of radial growth appear clinically as papules and nodules within a macular or plaque-like field of pre-existing hyperpigmentation. The dermal nodules often form eccentrically beneath the superficial radial growth region (Fig. 17-37). For accuracy in assessing depth, the entire vertical growth phase nodule must be carefully sectioned and submitted in toto.

The *Clark system* divides melanoma into levels I and II, which connote radial growth, and levels III through V, which describe vertical growth.[457] Level I indicates in situ (pure intraepidermal) spread, and level II indicates in situ plus penetration into the papillary dermis. Level III indicates filling and expansion of papillary dermis; level IV represents extension into the reticular dermis; level V is reserved for extension into subcutaneous fat or deeper. In one series,[458,459] the

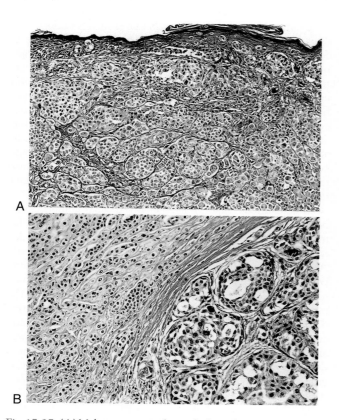

Fig. 17-37. **(A)** Melanoma, vertical growth phase showing replacement of superficial and deep dermis by coalescent nests of malignant melanocytes beneath a zone of in situ epidermal spread. **(B)** Cytologically, the melanoma cells (right) are distinct from residual dermal nevic cells (left).

5 year disease-free survival after surgery was as follows: level II invasion, 100 percent; III, 88 percent; IV, 66 percent IV, 15 percent.

The *Breslow thickness* records the depth of invasion expressed in millimeters from the overlying stratum granulosum or base of an ulcerated tumor to the deepest tumor cell. This measurement underestimates thickness to an unknown degree when a tumor is ulcerated or when the specimen is a shave biopsy with tumor extending to the base of the shave. The measurement will be overestimated if sections are oriented and sectioned tangentially. In all such situations, the measurement should be qualified by an explanatory note. Serial sectioning is likely to find a greater maximal tumor thickness than random or step sections.[460] The risk of recrudescent disease is low for lesions less than 0.76 mm, intermediate for 0.76 to 1.5 mm thickness and high for thickness over 1.5 mm[461] The corresponding 5 year disease-free survival is 98 percent for the low risk group, 44 to 63 percent for the high risk, and in between for intermediate risk.[459,462–464] "Thin" melanomas (<0.76 mm) can produce metastases and death.[465,466] The standard parameter of thickness measurement has its detractors,[467] especially against the concept of natural prognostic groupings, categories, or "breakpoints"[468] based on this measurement. Recently, methods for calculating tumor volume have been devised[469] and tested, some finding better correlation with survival.[470]

Vertical growth phase melanoma usually features epithelioid malignant melanocytes. Rare variants show spindle cell and nevus cell (small cell) morphology. Failure to mature with dermal penetration, the deepest cells being roughly the same size and shape as the more superficial cells, is a regular feature. Cytoplasm is usually granular with variable to absent pigment. Adjacent cells commonly show very different degrees of melaninization. Nuclei are enlarged, irregular, and often angulated. Nuclear membranes are irregularly thickened with coarsely clumped, "vesicular" chromatin. Nucleoli are large and often eosinophilic. Mitotic activity, usually evident deep within the vertical growth phase nodule, is unusual in even the largest and more cellular benign nevi. A lymphoid response at the base of the nodule occasionally infiltrates into the tumor and surrounds individual tumor cells. If this immunoreaction forms a continuous band under the tumor, the lymphoid infiltrate is "brisk"; if it is discontinuous, it is described as "nonbrisk." Tumor nodules that are separated from the main tumor by normal reticular dermis (microscopic "satellites"), as well as vascular invasion, should be sought in biopsy and re-excision specimens because they are a poor prognostic feature. Satellite nodules are likely lodged lymphatic emboli near the primary tumor. Cutaneous and subcutaneous metastases located between the primary melanoma and regional lymph nodes are termed *in-transit metastases* and usually indicate systematic disease.[471]

The pathology report of a melanoma is most useful if it includes the essential information in a brief diagnostic statement. Additional information of proven or potential use in formulating prognosis or treatment protocols can be added as a brief note. For example:

Diagnosis: Malignant melanoma, superficial spreading type, vertical growth phase present, invasive to Clark's level IV, measured depth 1.40 mm; biopsy margins free of tumor by at least 0.5 cm.

Note: The vertical growth phase nodule is arising in association with a partially regressed radial growth phase of the superficial spreading type. It is composed of epithelioid cells with numerous (>5/mm²) mitoses and has a brisk lymphoid infiltrate at its base. The tumor is contiguous with a compound melanocytic nevus with features of the dysplastic type. Blood vascular or lymphatic invasion and satellite spread distant from the main nodule are not observed.

As mentioned, metastases may follow excision of vertical growth phase lesions in proportion to thickness.[457,472,473] Tables are available to calculate the prospect of survival based on tumor thickness and several other variables.[474-478] Low mitotic rate, presence of brisk lymphocytic infiltration of the vertical growth phase nodule, relative thinness of the vertical growth phase nodule (<1.70 mm), location on the extremities, and female gender are all favorable prognostic indicators. Recurring thin melanomas more frequently involved head and neck sites, occurred in male patients, and showed Clark's level III and IV. This may relate to the specific problems of surgical management and the greater sun exposure in the head and neck.[479] For practical purposes, a disease-free interval of 10 years is considered a cure of melanoma; late recurrence, although reported even beyond 25 years, is extremely rare.[480,481]

Special Stains and Immunohistochemical Markers for Melanoma

Argentaffin silver stains for melanin (e.g., Fontana-Masson) are based on the reducing properties of melanin granules.[482] They can reveal finely dispersed granules not conspicuous in routine sections and also confirm that a brown pigment is melanin rather than hemosiderin. Polyclonal heteroantisera to the fetal neural protein S-100 are expected to show nuclear and cytoplasmic reactivity in well over 90 percent of melanocytic proliferations, regardless of whether they are benign or malignant.[483] Most S-100-positive but nonmelanocytic malignant neoplasms are carcinomas; their masquerade is belied by simultaneous reactivity for keratin and epithelial membrane antigen.

Keratin positivity is shown by perhaps 1 in 100 melanomas, partly explained by use of high concentrations of antikeratin antibodies.[484] HMB 45 was originally raised to a metastatic melanoma from an axillary lymph node.[485] The HMB-45 antigen is suggested to have a 10 kd molecular weight and has been localized to a glycoprotein in premelanosomal vesicles that is related to the tyrosinase system.[486] This is why the amelanotic neoplasms may be negative. In melanomas, about 89 percent of cases will contain this marker. Current commercial preparations of HMB 45 label only 40 to 50 percent of all melanomas but are valuable because immunoreactivity can be confidently equated with melanocytic differentiation. NK1/C3 cross reacts with nonmelanocytic proliferations, but positive labeling in the context of vimentin positivity but keratin- and EMA-negativity constitutes strong support for the diagnosis of a melanocytic lesion regardless of the results of concurrent HMB-45 immunostains.

Less Common Melanoma Variants

Regressing melanoma[487-489] is a diagnostic challenge only when regression is complete or nearly so. Regression is most familiar as skin-colored, pink, or gray-blue regions developing within the radial growth phase of a pre-existing melanoma. Completely regressed primary melanomas may be indistinguishable from normal skin, and may be detected only with aid of a Wood's light. The histologic hallmark of regression is papillary dermal deposition of loose, edematous collagen containing increased numbers of ectatic vessels. Numerous melanophages and residual clusters of lymphocytes are typically entrapped within this abnormal connective tissue. Lymphocytes may sometimes align along the dermal-epidermal interface, facilitating basal cell layer destruction similar to that of lichenoid keratoses. When this is the only picture in a biopsy or excision specimen of a focal skin lesion suspected to be melanoma, multiple levels should be obtained in search of small clusters of residual malignant melanocytes. Occasionally detection of residual malignant cells is facilitated by immunohistochemistry for S-100 protein and HMB-45 melanoma-associated antigen.

Small cell melanoma, also referred to as melanoma with nevus cell change and nevoid melanoma,[490] often occurs focally within vertical growth phase melanomas and therefore may be difficult to distinguish from precursor nevus. Small cell change near or at the base of a vertical growth phase nodule may mimic maturation. Small melanoma cells are differentiated from nevus cells by the diffuse hyperchromasia of their nuclei and the invariable mitotic activity. Also, at least focal gradual transition to larger malignant cells is also a helpful detail.

Spindle cell melanoma with its desmoplastic[491-495] and neurotropic[496] melanoma subtypes is a vertical growth phase pattern that often arises within the LM and ALMM types of radial growth. Histologically, recognition may be tricky because spindle cell melanoma tends to diffusely and insidiously infiltrate the collagenous reticular dermal stroma rather than enlarging as tumorigenic nodules. An important low power magnification clue is the frequent presence of lymphoplasmacytic aggregates at the most peripheral extent of the vertical growth phase nodule. Spindle cell melanoma cells generally do not display vesicular chromatin patterns or prominent nucleoli. Rather, they have enlarged, elongated, somewhat angulated nuclei with diffuse hyperchromasia. Many nuclei are extremely bland and may be overlooked as fibrocytic. Desmoplastic spindle cell melanoma (Fig. 17-38A) has associated proliferating plump fibroblasts and collagen deposition (Fig. 17-38B), further camouflaging individual tumor cells that may be accentuated with S-100 (Fig. 17-38C) but only rarely with HMB 45. Detection of an atypical lentiginous intraepidermal melanocytic growth over the spindle cell population is important because amelanotic spindle cell melanoma may mimic nonmelanocytic spindle cell tumors. Neurotropic spindle cell melanoma may show fascicles of atypical spindle cells at various angles to the epidermis, mimicking true neural differentiation (Fig. 17-39). Extensive infiltration of nerves is a hallmark feature. Perineural and in-

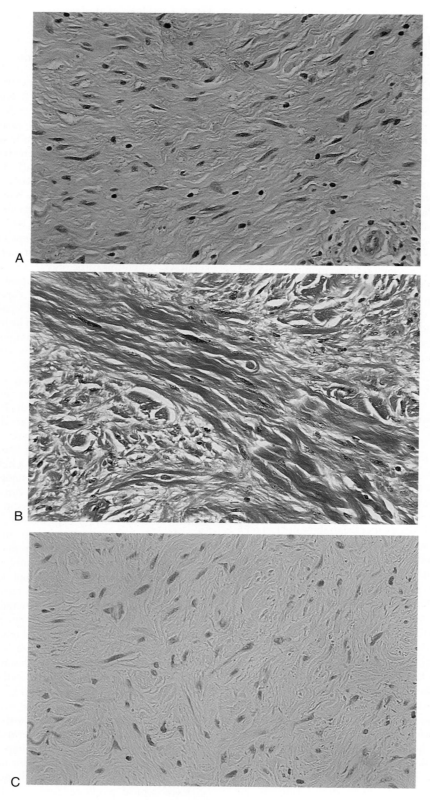

Fig. 17-38. Desmoplastic melanoma. **(A)** Rather bland, small spindle cells constitute this example. **(B)** Much collagen has been added to dermis around tumor cells (trichrome). **(C)** The S-100 reaction weakly labels tumor cells, distinguishing them from fibroblasts.

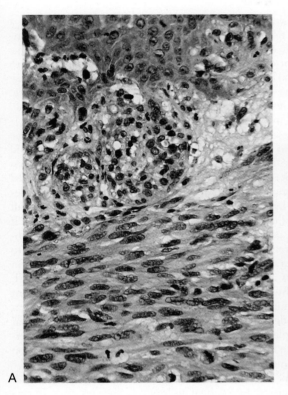

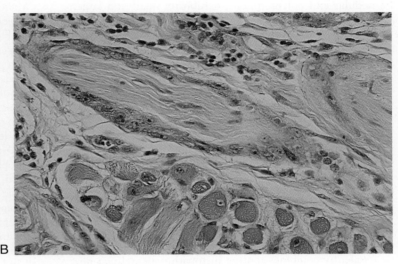

Fig. 17-39. Neurotropic melanoma. (A) A nested junctional component is a clue this is not a neural tumor. (B) Perineural growth can carry tumor well beyond grossly apparent borders.

traneural extension partly explain the need for wide excision to achieve local control.

Poorly differentiated, high grade sarcomatoid melanomas, including amelanotic sarcomatoid acral lentiginous melanomas, may have areas of osteoblastic and/or chondroblastic differentiation with strong S-100 protein reactivity in cells that appear responsible for the matrix products.[497] Some melanomas may be nearly obscured by myxoid stroma.[498,499] Others have osteoclast-like giant cells.[500] S-100 is negative in MFH and this is of help in excluding MFH because only a fraction of 1 percent of melanomas will be negative for S-100 protein. That HMB 45 reacts with only 22 percent of spindle cell melanoma[501,502] has important implications for the evaluation of cutaneous spindle cell tumors that may mimic sarcomas.

Borderline and minimal deviation melanomas represent a biologically valid concept so misunderstood, it is not presently of practical utility. By early definitions these were conceived to be biologically low grade neoplasms that seldom metastasized but had a tendency for local recurrence.[503] Their architecture was generally that of level III ("borderline") or level IV to V ("minimal deviation") tumorigenic melanomas without fully evolved cytologic anaplasia or high mitotic rates. This subset likely represents well differentiated melanoma variants.

"Splitters" will file some melanomas under additional descriptive labels: subungual,[504] balloon cell,[505] signet ring,[506] adenoid/pseudopapillary, hemangiopericytoid, pleomorphic, and rhabdoid.[507,508] As in some nevi, suggestive differentiation

toward Schwann cells, tactile corpuscles, ganglion cells, and other neuroid structures may be seen.[509,510]

TUMORS OF LYMPHOID AND MARROW-DERIVED CELLS

Lymphoproliferative Disorders

Appreciation of the skin as a lymphoid organ is the necessary basis for understanding cutaneous immunity and lymphoproliferative neoplasms.[511–513] The skin is the residence of specialized lymphocytes, histiocytes, and mast cells that comprise skin-associated lymphoid tissue (SALT).[514,515] This forms an integrated reactive system with draining lymph nodes. Benign dysplastic proliferations and frank malignant tumors of indigenous lymphohistiocytic constituents of skin commonly present diagnostic difficulties, particularly when there is no associated lymph node involvement.

There are parallels between the general histology of reactive and neoplastic lymphoid infiltrates of skin and lymphoid trafficking patterns in lymph nodes. Normal lymphocyte traffic into and out of nodal tissues occurs across subcapsular microvessels known as high endothelial venules. This central specialization of certain vascular segments is recapitulated in normal and reactive T cell trafficking in skin, where inflammatory cells tend to cluster about dermal venules. Their margination and transvascular migration are now explainable in the terms and concepts of molecular pathology. Migration away from venules to produce an interstitial pattern, on the other hand, is regarded as often abnormal and is typically observed in both T and B cell lymphomas. In normal and reactive lymph nodes, B cells are clustered within follicles and show a spectrum of maturation. Accordingly, reactive B cells infiltrates in the skin may be nodular and polymorphous, exhibiting small and large, cleaved and noncleaved stages of differentiation. Lymphomas of B cells may also attempt to recapitulate the nodular architecture of normal follicles, although the proliferating cells are monomorphic, representing a clone arrested at a single stage of B cell ontogeny.

Skin infiltration by lymphoma is relatively common. The incidence of skin lesions related to Hodgkin's disease is less than 5 percent[516,517] and for non-Hodgkin's lymphoma, up to about 20 percent.[518] Of 465 patients with Hodgkin's disease, 3.4 percent had "specific" cutaneous involvement as single or multiple dermal or subcutaneous nodules.[519] One study found cutaneous lesions as the first sign of lymphoma in 5 percent of 1,269 patients.[518] The distinction of metastatic versus primary involvement is difficult, particularly because in either situation there is likely to be infiltration of the epidermis and dermis by atypical and malignant lymphohistiocytic cells with cytologic and architectural patterns not seen in lymph nodes. Accurate diagnosis frequently combines routine histopathology, refined microscopy (1-μm-section analysis), immunohistochemistry, and molecular analytical techniques. Markers used for hematopoietic differentiation are divided into those that identify most hematopoietic cells and those that react only with B or T cell populations.[520]

Relatively new sophisticated molecular biologic techniques for the analysis of clonal lymphoid proliferations are of considerable help in reducing the uncertainty of diagnosis in selected cases (see Ch. 20).

Except for cutaneous T cell lymphoma (CTCL), most non-Hodgkin's lymphomas involving the skin cannot be accurately subclassified based on skin biopsy specimens alone. Often such specimens serve to alert the clinician of the probability of a lymphoproliferative disorder, whereas definitive classification may have to be delayed until lymphadenopathy is sampled or marrow examination is performed.

The clinical appearance of cutaneous lymphoma varies with the presence or absence of epidermal involvement. In early CTCL, the malignant T cell infiltration of the epidermis results in alterations in keratinization. The resulting erythematous, scaling plaques may be confused with psoriasis, chronic eczematous dermatitis, and other forms of dermatitis. Nonepidermotropic T cell lymphomas and B cell lymphomas tend to form deep, typically plum-colored nodules covered by an unremarkable or smooth, glistening epidermal surface. Benign lymphoid hyperplasia within the dermis frequently results in clinically indistinguishable nodules.

Cutaneous Lymphoid Hyperplasia (Pseudolymphoma, Lymphocytoma Cutis)

Typical lesions in cutaneous lymphoid hyperplasia are single or multiple coalescent erythematous nodules, often located on the face or scalp.[521-528] These tend to be firm and covered by a smooth, nonscaling epidermal surface. These nonpainful, spontaneously emerging lesions persist for many weeks or months. Linear or clustered configurations suggest florid reactions to arthropod bites that are often unrecalled. Others are a response to trauma and other uncertain stimuli.[529] Because hyperplastic clinical lesions are indistinguishable from B cell lymphoma, biopsy is frequently performed for further differentiation.

Microscopic examination finds symmetric infiltration of the superficial and deep dermis by cellular aggregates of lymphoid cells (Fig. 17-40). The infiltrate may extend into subcutaneous fat. Epidermis and papillary dermis are generally uninvolved (i.e., a grenz zone is present). Adnexal structures are not destroyed. Lymphoid follicles may have peripheral rims of small lymphoid cells (i.e., T cells) with inconspicuous cytoplasm. If there are germinal centers, they contain a spectrum of differentiation from cells with small cleaved and noncleaved nuclei to large cleaved and noncleaved nucleated cells. Confidence in diagnosis rises with additional heterogeneity, such as with eosinophils, plasma cells,[530] immunoblasts with prominent central nucleoli, and tingible body macrophages with basophilic debris in their cytoplasm. Additional features in, but not completely specific for, benign lesions are vascular proliferation, predominantly perivascular or periadnexal distribution of the infiltrate, and prominent epidermal hyperplasia.[531]

Immunohistochemical findings favoring benignancy of small cell and mixed deep dermal infiltrates include less than 75 percent B cells with a relatively even admixture of T lymphocytes, absence of light chain monotypism, low (<30 percent) proliferative index, and lack of coexpression of CD5/CD19 or CD20/CD43.[532] Larger lymphoid cells may be reactive for the Ki-1 antibody.[533] Some cases have had a monotypic plasma cell population.[534] Molecular genetic analysis may help exclude lymphoma.[535]

Granulomatous foci should be searched under polarized light for associated birefringent material consistent with residua of insect (e.g., bee) stingers or arthropod (e.g., tick) mouth parts responsible for local antigen injection. Numerous eosinophils and zones of fibrosis in a background of persistent lymphoid hyperplasia should bring to mind insect bite reactions. Zones of follicular rupture suggest pilar obstruction with dermal extrusion of noxious follicular contents (i.e., pseudolymphomatous folliculitis).

In most cases, the course is benign, spontaneously clearing or resolving after antibiotic or radiotherapy. There are reports of some cases that progressed to malignant lymphoma.[536]

Lymphocytic Dysplasia, "Parapsoriasis," and Cutaneous T Cell Lymphoma

Change in pattern over time is an important feature in the progression of CTCL, which passes through stages not unlike the dysplastic nevus-melanoma sequence.[537-543] Early lesions clinically and histologically indistinguishable from chronic dermatitis may have only subtle abnormalities in architecture (i.e., interstitial papillary dermal trafficking pattern). Some of these lesions eventually become epidermotropic CTCL with clonal T cell populations proliferating horizontally within the epidermal layer in an analogy to radial growth phase melanoma. In time, T cells begin to grow deeply into the dermis, where destructive

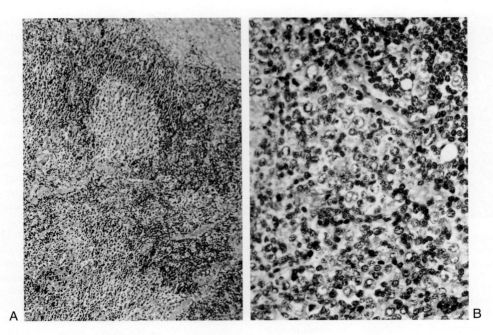

Fig. 17-40. Cutaneous lymphoid hyperplasia. (A) Note germinal center formation at scanning magnification and (B) polymorphous admixture of large and small lymphoid follicular center cell elements.

nodules may form, an event that brings to mind the emergence of vertical growth within a superficial melanoma. As with melanoma, deep dermal growth correlates with a tendency for lymphomatous dissemination.

Classic CTCL (*mycosis fungoides*) generally evolves through defined clinical stages: premalignant dysplasia ("parapsoriasis"), then the patch, plaque, and tumor stages. The dysplastic and patch stages are barely raised erythematous areas, often with adherent scale. Location on the trunk and extremities is frequent. Unlike benign dermatitis, early CTCL is often refractory to topical anti-inflammatory medications, and the resultant clinical concern often leads to biopsy. Plaque-stage CTCL lesions are raised, indurated, and variable in color, ranging from pink to red to brown-purple. The typical well defined plaques, frequently with figurate borders, have more prominent scaling and pruritis than the patch stage. Plaques of CTCL may arise de novo or may derive from pre-existing patches. Patches and plaques of CTCL are relatively indolent. They may progress slowly over many years without systemic spread or the formation of tumoral nodules. Tumor-stage nodules eventually develop if lesions remain untreated. The dome-shaped nodules are firm, often affecting the face, scalp, and body folds. They may be indistinguishable from the nodules of B cell lymphoma. The nodular stage portends the potential for visceral dissemination and a poor prognosis. Tumor nodules arise de novo in the "d'emblee" form[544] of CTCL and in human T cell leukemia/lymphoma virus-1 (HTLV-1) associated disease (see below). Generalized skin erythema and scaling (i.e., erythroderma) may occur during any of the three stages of CTCL or may be the first presenting manifestation. Erythroderma associated with high numbers of circulating tumor cells in the peripheral blood constitute the Sézary's syndrome,[545] which may be simulated by erythrodermic forms of psoriasis, contact or atopic dermatitis,

seborrheic dermatitis, and pityriasis rubra pilaris.[546,547] Sézary cells have PAS-positive cytoplasmic granules.

CTCL in its earliest stages (i.e., dysplastic and plaque stages), when it is most easily and effectively treated, is often difficult to diagnose,[548] and multiple samples of various skin sites at one time or of representative lesions sequentially over time may be required. Dysplastic-stage and patch-stage CTCL may initially resemble a low grade inflammatory dermatitis with lymphocytes in perivascular array within the papillary dermis. The minimally hyperplastic epidermal layer exhibits focal hyperkeratosis or parakeratosis. Closer inspection reveals variable numbers of atypical lymphocytes diffusely throughout the papillary dermis and within the epidermis individually and rarely as small aggregates. Three important clues should be sought in early stages of evolving T cell malignant tumor: lymphocytes in the basal zone of epidermis not associated with intercellular edema (i.e., spongiosis); intraepidermal lymphocytes with nuclear atypia consisting of hyperchromasia and contour irregularities (in patch-stage, but not often in dysplastic stages); and papillary dermal fibrosis of randomly arranged, coarse, collagen fibers replacing the normally delicate fibrils of the papillary dermis.

The plaque stage may be diagnosed from routine histopathology alone. A band-like infiltrate of lymphocytes in the lower papillary and upper reticular dermis tends to be polymorphous. Participating enlarged lymphoid cells contain markedly hyperchromatic nuclei with irregular, convoluted nuclear membranes (Fig. 17-41). Occasional immunoblast-like cells and even simulants of Reed-Sternberg variants occur with plasma cells, and variable numbers of eosinophils. Clustered cells within the nonspongiotic epidermis consist of atypical lymphocytes forming Pautrier microabscesses within lacunae resulting from mucinous epidermal change. Similar infiltration may involve appendages, particularly hair follicles. Accompanying ex-

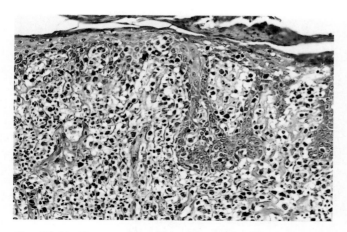

Fig. 17-41. Cutaneous T cell lymphoma, plaque stage, showing prominent epidermotropic spread of malignant lymphocytes in small aggregates (Pautrier microabscesses).

tensive mucinous inflation may produce localized hair loss (i.e., alopecia mucinosa). CTCL on face or scalp may predominantly or exclusively involve hair follicles and spare the interfollicular epidermis.[549] Granulomatous,[550,551] bullous,[552] and subcutaneous[553] forms are described.

The papillary dermis and epidermis are generally spared in the nodular or nonepidermotrophic stage. Sheets and confluent aggregates of tightly compacted lymphoid cells infiltrate dermis, displacing or destroying vessels and appendages. Their nuclear contours may be jagged, cleaved, or convoluted. Large, immunoblast-like cells are frequent.[554] Transformed variants[555] may be indistinguishable from B cell tumors, which also typically do not involve epidermis. This histopathology is to be distinguished from subcutaneous T cell lymphoma presenting as deep-seated nodules, most frequently on the extremities.[553]

Diagnostic aids include 1 μm sections to assess nuclear convolutions in epidermotropic T cells. These show to best advantage the intricate "cerebriform" nuclear convolutions that constitute the requisite cytologic atypia in early epidermotropic T cell lymphoma. Cell marker analysis using immunoperoxidase reagents coupled to monoclonal antibody probes highlight phenotypically abnormal T cells, selectively concentrated in the epidermal layer. Whereas the early dermal component is often a mix of a minority of malignant T cells, the neoplastic intraepidermal clones tend to be exclusively of the CD4 helper subtype, often lacking one or more of the pan-T cell maturation antigens of mature T cells (e.g., CD2, CD3, or CD5).[556] Molecular detection for T cell receptor gene rearrangements also may be useful, particularly when coupled with polymerase chain reaction (PCR) amplification techniques to enhance sensitivity when only small numbers of suspect cells are present.[557]

In disease limited to the skin, treatment choices include total skin electron beam irradiation, topical chemotherapy, and PUVA.[558–561] Nodal and visceral involvement occurs eventually in perhaps 50 to 75 percent of mycosis fungoides cases. The polymorphism of the infiltrate and continuing presence of cells with cerebroid nuclei is generally retained.[562,563] Alternatively, their may be a changed pattern such as large cell lymphoma[564–566] or Hodgkin's disease.[567] Table 17-5 contrasts T cell lymphoma, B cell lymphoma, and benign lymphoid hyperplasia.

Granulomatous Slack Skin

Granulomatous slack skin is a peculiar form of CTCL with an indolent course and is closely related to MF.[568,569] Asymptomatic red or violet plaques with atrophic surfaces usually develop in the axillary and groin regions. The plaques often enlarge to form pendulous folds resembling cutis laxa. Histologically, lymphomatous and granulomatous changes are intermingled. Clonal infiltrates of helper T cells similar to those in MF attract a granulomatous component that mediates massive dermal elastolysis. Hodgkin's disease evolves in some cases.

Table 17-5. Features of T and B Cell Lymphomas and Benign Lymphoid Hyperplasia

Feature	T Cell Lymphoma[a]	B Cell Lymphoma	Benign Lymphoid Hyperplasia
Epidermal involvement	+/−	−	−
Polymorphic infiltrate	+/−	−	+
True germinal centers	−	−	+/−
Pseudogerminal centers[b]	−	+/−	−
Cerebriform nuclei	+	−	+/−
T cell infiltrate	+	−	+/−
Abnormal T cell antigen expression	+	−	−
B cell infiltrate	−	+	+/−
Monotypic immunoglobulin expression	−	+	−

+, present; −, absent; +/−, present or absent.
[a] Nonepidermotropic variants may be indistinguishable from B cell lymphoma by routine morphologic criteria.
[b] May be seen as "growth centers" in well differentiated small B cell lymphocytic lymphoma.

Woringer-Kolopp Disease

Also known as *pagetoid reticulosis*, Woringer-Kolopp disease is a T cell cutaneous proliferation that consists of a monomorphic intraepidermal infiltrate of cells with cerebroid nuclei resembling the cells in mycosis fungoides and the Sézary's syndrome. However, it forms a solitary erythematosquamous patch and evolves very slowly.[570–572]

Adult T Cell Leukemia/Lymphoma

Adult T cell leukemia/lymphoma (ATLL) is a clinical variant of CTCL that results from HTLV-1 retrovirus infection occurring in scattered outbreaks worldwide.[573–575] It is clinically characterized by explosive onset of variably sized, firm, confluent nodules on the trunk and extremities. Plaques, papules, and nonexfoliative erythroderma may also be seen. A few scattered nodules may progress to hundreds of deforming tumors within several weeks. In contrast to classic CTCL, visceral involvement is to be anticipated from the outset, with dissemination through the bloodstream to lymph nodes, bone marrow, gastrointestinal tract, lungs, leptomeninges, and liver. Lytic bone lesions, hypercalcemia, and elevated serum alkaline phosphatase are often observed at presentation. Histologically, most ATLL resembles nonepidermotropic CTCL, some being indistinguishable from plaque-stage disease. In the peripheral blood, ATLL cells have hyperlobated rather than cerebriform nuclear contours.

Lymphomatoid Vasculitis

Lymphocytes, like melanocytes and many other cell types, demonstrate early stages of tumor progression that may be recognized by routine light microscopy. *Lymphomatoid vasculitis*[576] connotes a group of disorders characterized by cutaneous infiltration by dysplastic lymphocytes, variable injury to involved dermal vessels, and a tendency for some lesions to demonstrate evolution into frank lymphoma. It may be divided clinically and pathologically into at least three disorders: lymphomatoid papulosis, lymphomatoid granulomatosis, and angioimmunoblastic lymphadenopathy involving the skin.

Lymphomatoid papulosis,[577–584] the most commonly encountered of the three, is a primary cutaneous disorder characterized by a chronic clinical course of recurrent erythematous to hemorrhagic papules and nodules that may ulcerate and generally regress with scarring. The trunk and extremities are most frequently involved, and males out number females by 2:1. This chronic condition consists of successive erythematous to hemorrhagic papules and nodules that may ulcerate and generally regress with scarring. Systemic examination should find no extracutaneous disease, although a significant minority of patients will evolve to lymphoma, and close follow-up is recommended. Low power examination discloses a wedge-shaped coalescence of angiocentric mononuclear cell infiltrates (Fig. 17-42A). The overlying epidermis is hyperplastic or ulcerated. Focal epidermotropism resembling CTCL may be observed. The polymorphous infiltrate is an admixture of variably activated lymphocytes, histiocytes, eosinophils, and Reed-Sternberg-like cells in type A but not in B (Fig. 17-42B). Similar Reed-Sternberg-like cells may also be observed in regressing atypical histiocytosis, but lymphomatoid papulosis contains only occasional clusters of these cells and fails to exhibit tumoral dermal infiltration or florid epidermal hyperplasia. Associated and distinctive "dysplastic lymphocytic vasculitis" consists of endothelial swelling, vacuolization, and focal necrosis in association with intense angiocentric infiltration.

Cell marker studies in lymphomatoid papulosis indicate the atypical cells often have elevated helper/suppressor T cell ratios and defects in mature pan-T cell antigen expression not unlike CTCL. The Reed-Sternberg-like cells react positively for Ki-1, and show strong expression of interleukin-2 receptors or T cell activation complex (TAC). Arthropod bite reactions should not have a Ki-1-positive population.[581] T cell receptor gene rearrangements also can be demonstrated, supporting the view that lymphomatoid papulosis is really an indolent, regressing form of skin lymphoma.[585,586]

Lymphomatoid granulomatosis affects individuals within a wide age range, although most cases occur between the third and fifth decades, and there is a male preponderance of 1.7:1. Cutaneous lesions are usually erythematous, asymptomatic, and vary from maculopapules to annular plaques to nodules. Ulcers are commonly present. Although lymphomatoid granulomatosis characteristically affects the lungs, up to 60 percent of the cases show cutaneous involvement, and cutaneous lesions occasionally may occur before pulmonary manifestations of the disease. "Bottom heavy," predominantly T cell infiltrates composed of large lymphoid cells with prominently cleaved nuclei form angiocentric nodules (Fig. 17-43).

Angioimmunoblastic lymphadenopathy with dysproteinemia is a systemic disorder characterized by generalized lymphadenopathy, hepato- and splenomegaly, fever, anemia, and polyclonal gammopathy. Individuals in the sixth or seventh decades are generally affected, and there is no sex predilection. Cutaneous manifestations are present in over one-third of the cases and may precede the development of lymph node enlargement. The lesions tend to be polymorphous, consisting of pruritic maculopapular rashes to papular and nodular eruptions. Perivascular, superficial, and deep polymorphous infiltrates include many plasmacytoid cells and immunoblasts, hence numerous B cells are present.

Regressing Atypical Histiocytosis

Regressing atypical histiocytosis is a rare condition first thought to represent a proliferation of histiocytes that formed recurrent noduloulcerative lesions in the skin, often of extremities.[587,588] Most patients are young to middle-aged adults without gender predilection. The single or multiple 2 to 10 cm lesions frequently ulcerate. Formation is rapid, often in weeks, followed by spontaneous regression and then recurrence over a period of many months to years. Aggressive disease eventually supervenes in most cases, favoring the view that regressing atypical histiocytosis is really a regressing prodromal evolutionary phase of a fixed T cell lymphoproliferative disorder.

Exuberant epidermal hyperplasia over dense expansile dermal aggregates of anaplastic tumor cells is the expected picture. Even low power evaluation raises the possibility of hematopoietic malignant tumor. The preponderant large, atypical

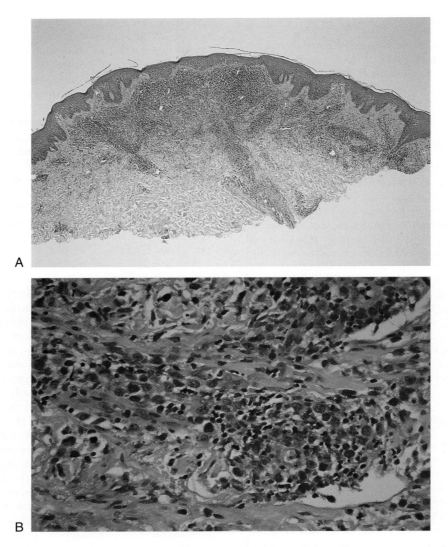

Fig. 17-42. Lymphomatoid papulosis. **(A)** A wedge-shaped angiocentric infiltrate is composed of a **(B)** polymorphous infiltrate including activated lymphocytes. (Courtesy of Dermatopathology Services, Birmingham, AL.)

mononuclear cells often have amphophilic cytoplasm, highly pleomorphic nuclei, irregular contours, vesicular nuclear chromatin, and prominent, centrally located nucleoli. A reactive inflammatory component and exuberant granulation tissue may infiltrate the lesion, perhaps followed by perilesional fibrosis, focal tumor cell necrosis, and focal infiltration by eosinophils. The majority of proliferating cells have aberrant T cell antigenic profiles and rearrangements of T cell receptor beta and gamma chain genes, indicating T cell lineage. High numbers of atypical cells also may express the Ki-1 activation antigen, a marker also expressed by true Reed-Sternberg cells.

Cutaneous B Cell Lymphoma

Primary cutaneous B cell lymphoma is a relatively rare disorder characterized by progressive, often multifocal infiltration of the dermis and subcutis by malignant lymphocytes with B cell phenotype.[589–593] Single or grouped, red, violaceous, or plum-colored, nonpruritic plaques or nodules result. Epidermal scaling is unusual in cutaneous B cell lymphoma in contrast to CTCL. The head, neck, and trunk are most often involved. This may be an expression of generalized disease or may be the only tumor manifestation.[594,595] Some cases occur in human immunodeficiency virus (HIV)-infected patients or or those with organ transplants.[596,597] Accurate recognition is important because B cell lymphoma of skin does not have a favorable prognosis[598–600]; it has a complete remission rate of 29.5 percent and a mortality rate of 71.4 percent.[599]

Histology typically presents diffuse or nodular infiltration of the entire dermis except the papillary portion (Fig. 17-44). A malignant dermal B cell infiltrate may be monomorphous or dimorphous. Either is unlike reactive B cell processes, which are composed of a spectrum of lymphocyte maturational stages and associated nonlymphoid inflammatory cells. Although primary

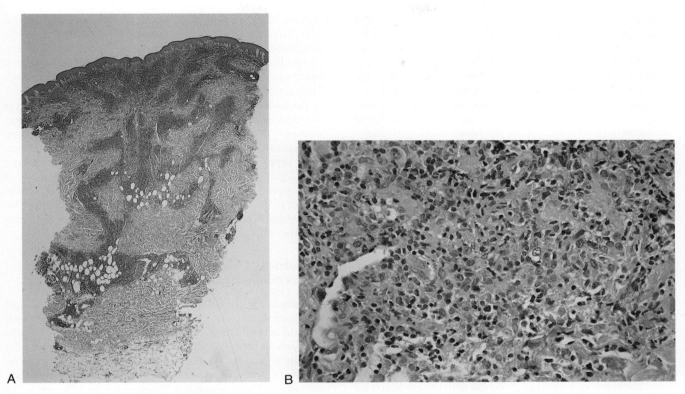

Fig. 17-43. Lymphomatoid granulomatosis. (A) Angiocentric nodules span the entire dermis. (B) Large lymphocytes participate in a vaguely granulomatous infiltrate. (Courtesy of Dermatopathology Services, Birmingham, AL.)

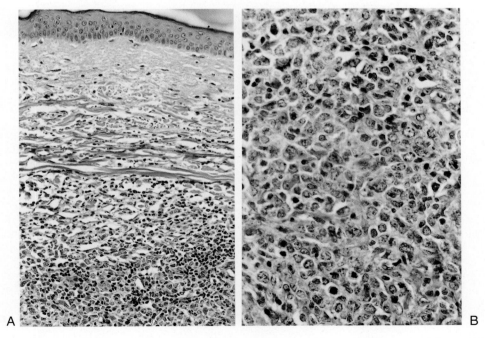

Fig. 17-44. Cutaneous B cell lymphoma. (A) Note the sparing of the epidermis and superficial dermis and (B) the monomorphous cytology of the large, atypical lymphoid cells forming the infiltrate.

nodal patterns and cellularity may be recapitulated in the skin of the same patient, there are so many exceptions that classification based on skin biopsy alone is inappropriate. Any of the well known types of cutaneous B cell lymphoma can produce skin lesions (see Ch. 20 for classification). Features that should alert the examiner to the possibility of lymphoma include surrounding and destruction of adnexal structures by the infiltrate, blood vessel involvement with wall destruction, and linear arrangement of atypical lymphocytes between collagen fibers.

Small lymphocytic lymphoma in skin is composed of nearly normal-sized lymphocytes in a nodular or diffuse interstitial pattern. The monomorphous infiltrating cells have dense chromatin, inconspicuous nucleoli, and scant cytoplasm. In some of these cases, diagnosis as "cutaneous lymphocytic infiltrate" or "small lymphocytic proliferation" is as far as one can go and the clinician should be alerted to pursue the possibility of lymphoma.[601,602] With plasmacytoid lymphocytic lymphoma, many tumor cells have features intermediate between small lymphocytes and plasma cells. Small PAS-positive intranuclear inclusions (i.e., Dutcher bodies) are typically found. *Follicular center cell (FCC) lymphomas* comprise up to one-third of cutaneous non-Hodgkin's lymphomas. Diffuse and nodular patterns in the skin can be formed by cells with small cleaved, large cleaved, and admixed FCC lymphomas, cytologically quite like their nodal counterparts. Monomorphous aggregates of small and/or large cleaved lymphocytes may be blended with reactive T cell components, leading to confusion with benign lymphoid hyperplasias, and sometimes necessitating multiple biopsies if a malignant tumor is strongly suspected. *Small noncleaved cell* (including Burkitt's lymphoma) and *large noncleaved cell lymphomas* are almost always diffuse, superficial and deep, monomorphic lymphoid infiltrates with sparing of the epidermis. In *B cell immunoblastic lymphoma*, the proliferation features immunoblast-like cells often showing plasmacytoid differentiation. These large cells contain rounded nuclei with peripherally marginated chromatin, prominent nucleoli, and abundant amphophilic, pyroninophilic cytoplasm. Intermixed neoplastic plasma cells and large immunoblasts are typical and exclude large noncleaved FCC lymphoma.

Because B cell lymphomas may be indistinguishable from nonepidermotropic cutaneous T cell lymphoma, immunohistochemical distinction is often necessary and may be accomplished on formalin-fixed, paraffin-embedded tissue. Monotypic kappa or lambda light chain expression by cells favors a clonal process that is likely malignant, although sensitivity of this approach usually requires frozen tissue sections. Molecular studies to determine the presence of immunoglobulin gene rearrangements may be performed from paraffin and are highly sensitive when PCR is employed for amplification.

Angiotropic Lymphoma (Malignant Angioendotheliomatosis)

As reflected in the earlier name, *angiotropic lymphoma* is a rare condition that was originally believed to be a diffuse neoplastic endothelial proliferation.[603–606] Most patients are over 40 years old, without gender predilection. The initial skin involvement appears as erythematous or violaceous nodules and plaques resembling erythema nodosum or other forms of panniculitis. Numerous small hyperchromatic lymphocytes are adherent to the endothelium of dilated dermal vascular channels with or without fibrin thrombi (Fig. 17-45).

This rare subset of lymphoma is characterized by an unusual expression of adhesive ligands that bond circulating tumor cells to the endothelial surface. Cell marker studies and gene rearrangements confirm the lymphoid nature of the adherent cell

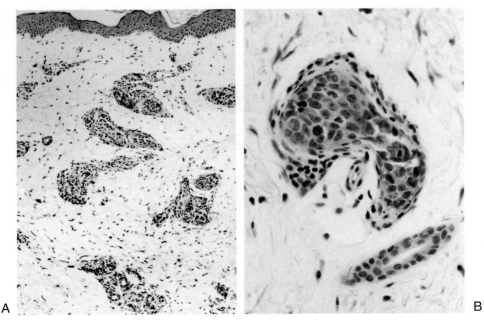

Fig. 17-45. Angiotropic lymphoma (malignant angioendotheliomatosis), showing (A) an inflammatory pattern at low magnification characterized by (B) intralumenal plugging by large, malignant lymphoid cells at higher magnification. (Courtesy of Dermatopathology Services, Birmingham, AL.)

population. Either a T or B cell phenotype may be found. Central nervous system symptoms and a fatal outcome are associated. This diagnostic term is not to be confused with "angiocentric lymphoma," which is a malignant T cell neoglasm of different microscopic appearance and with a different organ distribution (see Ch. 20).

Anaplastic Large Cell Lymphoma

Cutaneous anaplastic large cell (Ki-1) lymphoma (ALCL) is generally a neoplasm of the elderly, remaining localized to the skin in approximately 75 percent.[607–614] This is in contrast to anaplastic large cell lymphomas arising in noncutaneous sites tending to affect children and adolescents and that characteristically rapidly disseminate. Even in the 25 percent of cutaneous cases that spread to extracutaneous sites, the overall 4 years survival exceeds 90 percent. A biopsy presents a dense deep dermal infiltrate consisting of sheets of predominantly large angioplastic lymphocytes extending into subcutaneous fat, usually accompanied by admixture of reactive white cells including eosinophils (Fig. 17-46). Pseudoepitheliomatous hyperplasia commonly accompanies the infiltrate. Mitoses are numerous. Reed-Sternberg-like cells are likely. The Ki-1 antibody detects CD30 on cryostat sections. The Ber H2 antibody detects a formalin-resistant epitope of CD30 in the form of diffuse membrane staining as well as paranuclear dot-like reaction.

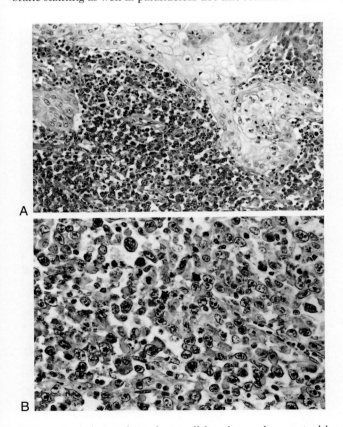

Fig. 17-46. (A) Anaplastic large cell lymphoma characterized by dermal infiltration without significant epidermotropism of large anaplastic lymphoid cells, **(B)** some of which show multinucleation. An identical picture may be seen in lesions with clinical characteristics of so-called regressing atypical histiocytosis.

Ki-1 lymphoma may present clinical diagnostic difficulties because of its resemblance to benign dermatoses, heightened by the tendency for some lesions (formerly classified as regressing atypical histiocytosis) to remit temporarily. The differential diagnosis of CD30+ cells in the dermis includes (1) primary or secondary cutaneous CD30+ ALCL, (2) cutaneous CD30+ large cell lymphoma that has progressed from another type of cutaneous lymphoma (e.g., mycosis fungoides), and (3) lymphomatoid papulosis. Cohesive sheets of CD30+ cells are not expected in the latter. Beyond these considerations, the differential diagnosis of ALCL and other anaplastic tumors may be long. Myxoid stroma and spindle cell change mimic sarcoma, sarcomatoid carcinoma, and melanoma. The separation from "syncytial" nodular sclerosing Hodgkin's disease is particularly difficult, especially because approximately 15 percent of ALCL lack CD45 immunoreactivity in paraffin sections. EMA is positive in a significant number of cases leading to possible confusion with anaplastic metastatic carcinoma, especially because LCA is occasionally negative in paraffin-embedded tissues. Seventy percent are T cell tumors, 20 percent B cell, and 10 percent "null cell" lymphomas. Approximately 15 percent lack CD45 immunoreactivity in paraffin sections. ALCL may represent the end of a spectrum of T cell proliferations with lymphomatoid papulosis and mycosis fungoides showing a continuum of changes leading to ALCL. Loss of cytokine receptors, in particular transforming growth factor (TGF)-beta may relate to this progression.[615] The observations that Epstein-Barr virus and HTLV-1 are potent inducers of CD30 expression in lymphoid cells in vitro has led to the association of these two viruses with Ki-1 lymphoma.

Tumors of Marrow-Derived Cells

Leukemia Cutis

Cutaneous infiltration by leukemia is relatively common and is associated with a poor prognosis.[616–623] The approximate incidence of skin involvement is 8 percent of patients with chronic lymphocytic leukemia, 11 percent of patients with acute myelocytic leukemia, 6 percent of patients with acute lymphocytic leukemia, 5 percent of patients with chronic myelocytic leukemia, and 10 percent of patients with monocytic leukemia. Leukemia cutis may precede or occur concomitantly with the diagnosis of systemic leukemia. Therefore a skin biopsy specimen may be useful in detecting the leukemia and facilitating its evaluation. Leukemia cutis can present as macules, papules, plaques, nodules, ecchymoses, palpable purpura, or ulcerative lesions. The various types of leukemia have stronger associations with certain skin changes. Erythroderma and bullae are a feature of chronic lymphocytic leukemia. Granulocytic leukemia tends to produce multiple large cutaneous tumors, often on the trunk, and is usually a manifestation of recurrence in treated patients or a late development as part of a wider dissemination.[623] Acute myelocytic leukemia may produce myeloblastomas or granulocytic sarcomas, which, when green from the elevated myeloperoxidase levels in the leukemic cells, are termed *chloromas*. Misdiagnosis as large cell lymphoma or metastatic anaplastic carcinoma is common. Pernio-like plaques of leukemia cutis on the distal nose and fingers may be the first evidence of myelomonocytic leukemia, which only rarely seems to produce leukemia cutis. Mucocutaneous involvement is particularly common in patients with monocytic leukemia,[622] varying from papules to plum-colored nodules that may ulcerate or become bullous, and in the oral cavity as gingival infiltrations. Adult T cell leukemia often infiltrates the dermis and subcutis. Its cutaneous manifestations occur in up to 75 percent of patients, varying from subtle maculopapules and plaques to large and ulcerative tumors, and are not dependent on the subtype of adult T cell leukemia, its pathologic features, or its survival time. Specific cutaneous infiltrates are seen in 25 to 30 percent of infants with congenital leukemia, usually evident as widespread, firm, blue, red, or violaceous nodules ("blueberry muffin baby," a description also employed for congenital neuroblastoma) and often preceding other manifestations of the leukemia by up to 4 months.

Perivascular and interstitial leukemic infiltrates are best subclassified by the special methods of hematopathology reviewed in Chapter 21. The infiltrate may mimic benign dermatoses when in a perivascular pattern, or lymphoma, generally of B cell type, when nodular or diffuse.

Noticing circulating malignant lymphocytes within blood vessels is a helpful detail in the otherwise uncertain distinction of chronic lymphocytic leukemia from small cell lymphocytic lymphoma. Chronic granulocytic leukemia enters skin as a spectrum of cells between mature and immature myeloid forms as well as occasional eosinophilic myeloblasts. The myeloblasts of acute granulocytic leukemias may be mistaken for large cell lymphoma cells or even histiocytic infiltrates.

Langerhans Cell Histiocytosis

Langerhans cell histiocytosis[624–627] is considered a disorder of altered immunity, analogous to sarcoidosis, wherein a collection of a cell population causes local damage.[627] Normally there are no Langerhans cells in the dermis in the absence of inflammation. The stimulus for pathologic Langerhans collections may be some toxic or infectious agent(s). Skin involvement is uncommon. Patients do well unless overtreated. The diffuse form of cutaneous involvement, more common in young children involving scalp, face, trunk, and intertriginous areas, may be dismissed as seborrheic dermatitis. Rarely, large localized masses may occur.

The three main clinical variants are collectively called *histiocytosis X*. *Eosinophilic granuloma*, the initial member and localized form of this group of disorders, was originally described as solitary lytic bone lesions. Infants and children are the usual victims with more than 40 percent of the localized form occurring between ages 5 and 15 years,[628] but the condition may persist into adulthood. Males are affected twice as often as females. Cutaneous lesions and mucosal lesions are uncommon, appearing as multiple, crusted papules or as solitary or multiple nodules. The face and scalp are more common cutaneous locations. Ulcerated granulomatous lesions may afflict the buccal mucous membranes or inguinal, perineal, or vulvar regions. Multiple synchronous or metachronous lesions appear in a minority of cases. The patients are usually young adults or children over 6 years of age. In adults skin involvement is a rare, benign, although chronic illness, primarily with genital ulcerations and widespread granulomatous and ulcerating lesions in the intertriginous regions.

Hand-Schüller-Christian disease is a rare chronic and disseminated variant that affects young children typically 2 to 10 years of age and only occasionally adults. Classically it produces the triad of exophthalmos, diabetes insipidus, and cranial deposits, but so can some other diseases such as tuberculosis. Multiple skeletal and extraosseous lesions may coexist with palpable defects involving the calvarium. Perhaps 40 percent of patients have skin lesions. The chest, axillae, and groin are most frequently involved, showing maculopapular and red to brown nodules and ulcers with a predisposition for the axillae and perineum.

Letterer-Siwe disease, the acute disseminated form, is described in adults but is almost exclusively limited to young children, often younger than age 3. Skin lesions are the first sign of the disorder in virtually all patients. Maculopapular and erythematous lesions frequently show a seborrheic distribution. Multiple organ system involvement is common. The skeletal defects are similar to Hand-Schüller-Christian disease, or there may be none. Prognosis is exceedingly poor, and most succumb within 2 years.

The above Langerhans cell histiocytosis lesions show considerable histologic overlap. The proliferation may be band-like within the superficial dermis, nodular and deep, or diffuse throughout the upper and mid-dermis (Fig. 17-47). Epider-

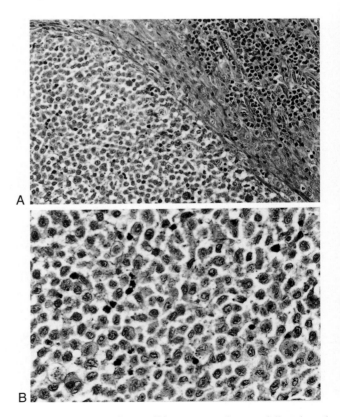

Fig. 17-47. **(A)** Langerhans cell histiocytosis showing diffuse dermal infiltration by large pale Langerhans cells with zones of fibrosis and eosinophil infiltration. **(B)** Note the characteristic cytology with ample cytoplasm and nuclear cleft formation.

motropism is frequent, paralleling perhaps the preferred residence of normal Langerhans cells. Follicles may also be heavily infiltrated, particularly in the axilla and groin. Individual tumorous Langerhans cells have noticeable cytoplasm and characteristic reinform, centrally notched or longitudinally furrowed nuclei resembling a coffee bean. Cytologic atypia and mitotic activity may be seen, but do not reliably correlate with biologic behavior or the clinical syndromes. An admixture of eosinophils is generally but not invariably observed. Some lesions are devoid of eosinophils, and the diffuse infiltrate is not particularly granulomatous. Multinucleated cells with foreign body giant cell type oval nuclei or Langhans type nuclei may occur, some accumulating cytoplasmic vacuoles conferring a xanthomatous appearance.

Normal and pathologic Langerhans cells are positive for S-100 protein, but so are melanocytes and activated histiocytes as well as some carcinoma cells (e.g., some ductal carcinomas of breast). Detection of the more specific indicator of Langerhans cell histiocytosis cells, the CD1a antigen on the cell surface, requires fresh frozen or Michel-fixed and frozen tissue sections and monoclonal antibody reagents to this antigenic determinant (e.g., Leu 6 antibody). Setting aside tissue properly for this test and possible electron microscopy should occur at the time of biopsy acquisition or frozen section evaluation. Monoclonal antibody O10 for paraffin-embedded samples is promising.[629] Characteristic tennis racquet-shaped Birbeck granules within the cytoplasm are a specific ultrastructural finding in Langerhans cells, but of unknown function. Normal DNA content and occurrence of spontaneous remissions favor histiocytosis X being an aberrant reactive process (i.e., hyperplasia) rather than a neoplasm.

"Non-X" Infantile Histiocytoses

There are several rare histiocytoses that may be confused with histiocytosis X.[628,630,631] *Hashimoto-Prizker disease* or congenital self-healing reticulohistiocytosis[632] afflicts infants at birth or soon after with crops of a dozen or more inflammatory nodules that spontaneously regress. The infants generally have no systemic manifestations. Some may have transient pancytopenia and elevated liver function tests. Dermal and subcutaneous lesions show a mononuclear cell infiltrate, occasionally with epidermotropism and ulceration. The invading cells are more phagocytic than those of histiocytosis X and have rounded reinform nuclei rather than infolded nuclear contours. These aggregated histiocytes have abundant ground-glass cytoplasm and converge to form giant cells. Birbeck granules may be detected ultrastructurally. The infiltrating cells have surface CD1a antigen and are S-100 positive. Ten to 25 percent of cells have Birbeck granules, another feature shared with Langerhans cells, and also large concentrically laminated electron-dense bodies representing mitochondrial involution during "self-healing." It has been suggested that Hashimoto-Pritzker disease is an unusual congenital variant of histiocytosis X with a variable clinical outcome.

Cephalic histiocytosis[633,634] produces numerous flat macules and small papules limited to the head and neck in young children. Facial involvement is nearly a constant finding. Over years these flatten, become pigmented, and resolve. The upper dermal histiocytic infiltrate has cells with irregular nuclei and sparse cytoplasm without foam cell change or multinucleated giant cells. The cells are CD1a and S-100 negative. Although lacking Birbeck granules, 5 to 30 percent of histiocytes have comma- or worm-shaped bodies formed of two parallel membranes. This may actually be a localized form of generalized eruptive histiocytosis[635] or an aborted phase of juvenile xanthogranuloma.[636]

"Non-X" Adult or Adolescent Histiocytoses

Indeterminate cell proliferative disorder,[637,638] also known as nodular non-X histiocytosis and generalized eruptive histiocytoma, features numerous papules or small nodules that may coalesce. This is an extremely rare condition. The face and extremities of adults are most often involved, without visceral infiltration. A dense monomorphous histiocytic infiltrate in the papillary and mid-dermis is intermingled with a few lymphocytes with some tendency for perivascular nesting. The S-100 reaction is positive. There are no Birbeck granules at the ultrastructural level, but large numbers of dense and irregularly laminated bodies are sometimes clustered together in cytoplasm.

Hereditary progressive mucinous histiocytosis[639] is an autosomal dominant condition of early adolescence showing only skin involvement by nodules less than 1 cm in diameter. These increase in number without spontaneously regressing. Spindled and stellate histiocytes are accompanied by occasional giant cells. Stromal collagen bundles are separated by abundant mucin showing acid mucopolysaccharide with increased metachromasia.

Eosinophilic histiocytosis (EH)[640] as originally described[641] creates recurrent ulcerative papules and nodules with disease duration from a few to many years. Marked pruritis is usual. A superficial and deep mixed perivascular inflammatory infiltrate shows numerous eosinophils, histiocytoid cells, lymphocytes, and large mononuclear cells with atypical hyperchromatic nuclei. Most of the lymphocytes and large mononuclear cells with atypical nuclei label with UCHL-1 (T cell marker). The histiocytoid cells react for S-100 and are dendritic, both in the epidermis and the dermis, and are likely Langerhans cells without reinform nuclei or multinucleated variants. Spongiosis, lymphocytic exocytosis, epidermal hyperplasia, and papillary dermal edema are accompanying features. The Reed-Sternberg-like cells found in lymphomatoid papulosis type A are absent and there is no labeling for Ki-1. Controversy continues as to whether EH is an unusual Ki-1-negative variant of lymphomatoid papulosis or a unique entity. Large numbers of eosinophils may lead to the misdiagnosis of arthropod bite reaction.

Xanthoma disseminatum[642] is a rare, benign mucocutaneous xanthomatosis of unknown cause affecting the skin, oropharynx, and sometimes larynx. It predominantly afflicts young adult males. Bone lesions are infrequent. Lesions may number in the hundreds and consist of closely set, round to oval, yellow-orange to mahogany brown or purple papules, nodules, and plaques. These are mainly on the face, flexor surfaces of the neck, antecubital fossae, periumbilical area, perineum, and genitalia. Other sites and upper respiratory tract involvement may be as high as 40 percent and can eventuate in respiratory difficulty. Microscopically, the infiltrate looks inflammatory, being composed of xanthoma (foam) cells, eosinophilic histiocytes, numerous Touton giant cells, and various white cells. Over time there is a decrease in large histiocytes and an increase in foam cells. The course is chronic but benign with a tendency for spontaneous regression.

True Histiocytomas

The most common purely histiocytic infiltrates of skin are the xanthogranuloma and reticulohistiocytoma. Xanthomas associated with hyperlipoproteinemia are discussed in Chapter 61.

Xanthogranuloma[643–646] most frequently involves infants and young children, hence the modifier *juvenile xanthogranuloma*; however, adults are also affected. Systemic lipid abnormalities are absent. One to several red to yellow papules or nodules on the head and upper trunk arise in infancy, or occasionally are present at birth or affect a child or adult. Sex incidence is equal. Visceral (e.g., pulmonary) and ocular (iris) lesions are reported, the latter possibly being complicated by hemorrhage. Histologically, symmetric aggregates of infiltrating cells form a dome-shaped papule within the superficial and mid-dermis. Extension into the subcutaneous fat may occur in some lesions. In early lesions, histiocytes without lipid are accompanied by few lymphocytes and eosinophils. Later, lipid-laden cells and multinucleated cells, including foreign body and Touton type giant cells, increase and dominate (Fig. 17-48A). Touton giant cells with wreath-like nuclear arrangement are lacking in tumoral xanthomas, which are composed predominantly of mononuclear foam cells. Most cases show positivity for alpha-1-antichymotrypsin, lysozyme, and other putative histiocytic markers.[647] One variant is composed predominantly of spindle cells. Xanthogranulomas usually involute within 1 year, but can persist for several years.

Reticulohistiocytoma[648] is a benign dermal proliferation of histiocytes with distinctive copious pink, ground-glass cytoplasm generally affecting middle-aged women. One or a few nodules are usually located on the head and neck, from 0.5 to 2.0 cm.

These well defined, symmetric dermal nodules often attenuate overlying epidermis. Neither xanthogranuloma nor reticulohistiocytoma is associated with inductive epidermal hyperplasia as with dermatofibroma, which can have vacuolated plump cells. The concomitant and distinctive histiocytes have tumor cells containing one or more nuclei and bright pink, PAS-positive, finely granulated cytoplasm due to large lysosomes, conferring a ground-glass appearance (Fig. 17-48B). Early lesions may have a background of acute and chronic inflammatory cells similar to xanthogranulomas. As the lesion ages, giant cells other than Touton type lie in lacunae outlined by fibrous tissue. There is no cholesterol storage or Birbeck granules.

Multicentric reticulohistiocytosis[649,650] features numerous firm yellow-tan papules and nodules on face, arms, and hands plus intermittent fevers and destructive arthritis (also known as lipoid dermatoarthritis). The same histiocyte with ground-glass cytoplasm occupies synovium and subchondral bone, admixed with inflammatory cells. The main proliferating cells have "histiocytes" markers. There is no other significant involvement other than skin and joints. This multicentric disease tends to lose its activity after several years.

Most disorders termed malignant histiocytosis or pure histio-

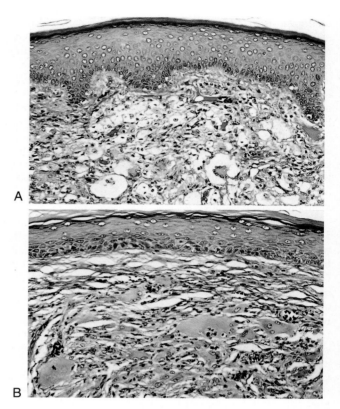

Fig. 17-48. (A) Xanthogranuloma showing characteristic Touton type giant cells and **(B)** reticulohistiocytoma characterized by multinucleated cells with typical ground-glass cytoplasm.

cytic lymphoma are in reality transformed T lymphocytic processes.

Mastocytosis

Mast cell proliferations create a spectrum of cutaneous and sometimes extracutaneous clinical disorders that can be divided conceptually into localized cutaneous and systemic forms.[651–653] *Urticaria pigmentosa* is the localized form, predominantly occurring in children and accounting for more than 50 percent of all cases. Usually multiple, solitary mastocytomas are noted shortly after birth. *Telangiectasia macularis eruptiva* (TMEP) is an adult form of cutaneous disease accounting for less than 1 percent of mastocytosis cases (Fig. 17-49). Even with so-called localized disease, most patients have subclinical mast cell aggregates in their bone marrow (mast cell microgranulomas). *Systemic mastocytosis*, with infiltration of many extracutaneous organs, including the gastrointestinal tract, constitutes 10 percent of cases and favors adults. Unlike localized cutaneous disease, the prognosis is often poor. Aggressive mastocytosis tends to lack skin involvement. The syndrome called lymphadenopathic mastocytosis with eosinophilia featuring pronounced eosinophilia, hepatosplenomegaly, and lymphadenopathy is in this subset of systemic mastocytosis. *Mast cell leukemia* is the fourth and rarest category, recognized by

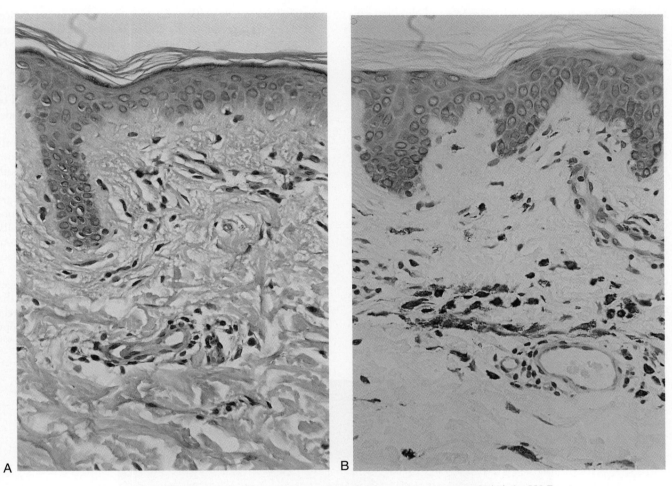

Fig. 17-49. Telangiectasia macularis eruptiva perstans (adult urticaria pigmentosa). **(A)** An H&E stain and **(B)** Giemsa show numerous variably degranulated mast cells within the papillary dermis.

numerous immature mast cells in peripheral blood and fulminant course.

Solitary mastocytomas appear as one or several tan-brown nodules that may be pruritic or blister. In urticaria pigmentosa, multiple and widely distributed lesions consist of round to oval, red-brown, nonscaling urticarial papules and small plaques. In systemic mastocytosis, similar skin lesions are associated with florid mast cell infiltration of bone marrow, gastrointestinal tract, liver, spleen, and lymph nodes, possibly predicted by bone or abdominal pain, nausea, vomiting, diarrhea, lymphadenopathy, vascular instability, headache, and/or psychiatric manifestations.

Urticaria pigmentosa in children features tumorous accumulations of mast cells within the superficial and mid-dermis and may be concentrated around papillary dermal vessels, band-like in superficial dermis or nodular, even reaching subcutaneous fat. With TMEP, the mast cell hyperplasia is about vessels of the superficial dermal capillary venules. The tightly packed oval cells have pale-staining, faintly granular pink cytoplasm. Under low power magnification there is a resemblance to nevus cells because of the consistent central localization of the uni-

form round nuclei. The cytoplasmic granules are conspicuous when stained with Bismarck green or metachromatic reagents such as toluidine blue or Giemsa and exclude other lymphoproliferative processes. Degranulation as a result of the biopsy technique may leave few granules to stain. The Leder reaction will be positive.

Adult forms may be extraordinarily subtle with only slight increases in the numbers of mast cells about superficial vessels. This might be mimicked by chronic urticaria, prolonged antigen contact, recurrent flushing, or anaphylaxis, or in scleroderma. However, these other conditions are unlikely to show dendritic and fusiform mast cells within intervenular connective tissue in an interstitial pattern as in mastocytosis. Also, in adult forms of mastocytosis, the individual mast cells are rounded rather than dendritic with Giemsa stain. In all types, eosinophils may be attracted, perhaps as a result of chemotactic factors, by degranulating mast cells. Acutely, mast cell degranulation evokes dermal edema and lymphatic ectasia similar to ordinary urticaria. When chronically sustained, there will be variable degrees of dermal fibrosis. Solitary lesions with much dermal fibrosis are called *sclerosing mastocytomas*. Elevated plasma or urinary histamine or histamine metabolites raise the suspicion of mastocytosis, but are not diagnostic.[654]

PRIMARY MESENCHYMAL TUMORS

General Considerations

Mesenchymal tumors arising in the skin and subcutaneous tissue include benign and malignant proliferations of vascular elements (endothelial cells, pericytes, and glomus cells), smooth muscle cells, dermal matrix cells (fibroblasts, dendrocytes, and mucoblasts),[655] cells popularly regarded as fibrohistiocytic and also adipose, and neural and related supporting cells.[656] Many mesenchymal proliferations in the skin have counterparts in extracutaneous tissues (e.g., leiomyomas, neuromas), but with distinctive clinical and histologic features warranting separate discussion.[657]

Hamartoma is a useful term for a malformation of mesenchymal elements normally expected in the dermis but disordered or anomalous in differentiation, structural organization, or quantity (i.e., too much or too little) of cellular elements.

The clinical appearance of some lesions can be misleading, such as a dermatofibroma with stimulated hyperpigmentation excised to exclude melanoma. Awareness of common clinical mimicries is important if the origins of the clinician's differential diagnosis involving biologically different processes is to be understood and explained in the report.

Because mesenchymal tumors can be quite heterogeneous, it is desirable to submit multiple sections, particularly of morphologically diverse areas. Margins of primary excisions should be inked to obtain sections that reflect the adequacy or inadequacy of surgical removal.

Experience soon teaches that certain features are particularly helpful in determining phenotypic expression, a phrase conceptually preferable to "cell of origin." For example, smooth muscle cells tend to have nuclei with rounded or flattened ends, whereas the ends of nuclei of neural and fibroblastic tumors are more pointed. Neural tumors have nuclear pseudoinclusions and a wavy, undulant profile in contrast to fibroblastic cells, which generally show neither. Endothelial cells tend to form blood-filled spaces and occasional intracellular lumenal vacuoles (Fig. 17-50).

Most studies show only 50 to 90 percent of given tumor types contain reactivity for the specific marker tested. Therefore, the significant lesson to be relearned is that one may make a correct diagnosis in the face of a negative marker. Light microscopy alone remains the most important test for diagnosis.[482,658]

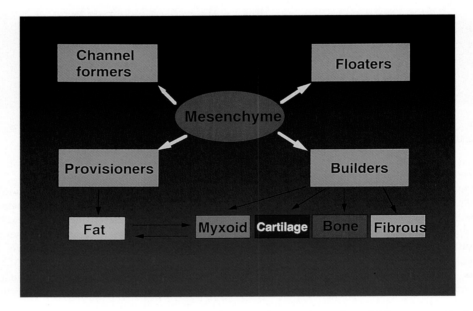

Fig. 17-50. Modulation diagram. Uncommitted mesesenchyme is the product of differentiation. Further adoption of specific function might best be termed *modulation*. Consequent extracellular matrix can be collagen dominant (fibrous or osseous) or mucopolysaccharide dominant (chondroid or myxoid). A signet ring fat cell represents the end product of storage of cytoplasmic fat that begins as multiple small vacuoles in cells. Fully modulated cells can, under altered influences (metabolic, mechanical [e.g., trauma, friction] and/or vascular [increased arterial flow vs. venous congestion]), regress to undifferentiated-appearing spindle or round cells easily mistaken for fibroblasts or lymphocytes, respectively, then adopt other functions reflected in a new cytomorphology. Through this process, mesenchyme forms channels (blood vessels) through which cellular elements float (lymphohematopoietic elements). Cells specializing in building the body structure produce a spectrum of matrices ranging from collagen dominant (fibrous and osseous) to mucopolysaccharide predominant (cartilage and myxoid). Accumulation of cytoplasmic fat stores ("provisions") creates adipose tissue. Cells with mixed features of "builders" and "provisioners" are not uncommon in reactive-reparative processes, just as mesenchymal tumors commonly illustrate more than one modulational potential.

There still are definitively diagnostic features in a fair percentage of sarcomas and immunohistochemistry results taken out of context can be very misleading.

Generalizations about the natural history of mesenchymal tumors cannot be made. Certain entities grow symmetrically larger over time, stabilize, and even eventually involute. Others show well defined stages of tumor progression.

Vascular Tumors

Table 17-6 presents a classification of vascular lesions.[659]

Vascular Hyperplasias

Vascular hyperplasia entails proliferation of endothelial cells that line dermal vessels and also neovascularization involving growth of entire vascular channels. Both frequently accompany inflammatory and reparative processes, and when exuberant,

Table 17-6. A Classification of Vascular Hyperplasias and Neoplasms That May Be Encountered in the Skin

Vascular hyperplasias
    Acroangiodermatitis
    Intravascular papillary endothelial hyperplasia
    Angiokeratomas of corporis diffusum (Fabry), digital (Mibelli), Fordyce, and solitary papular types
Endothelial tumors of blood and lymph vessels
    Benign
        Hemangioma
            Angiokeratoma circumscripta
            Capillary hemangioma
            Pyogenic granuloma (lobular capillary hemangioma)
            Cavernous hemangioma
            Sinusoidal hemangioma
            Arteriovenous hemangioma
            Microvenular hemangioma
            Glomeruloid hemangioma
            Acquired tufted hemangioma (angioblastoma)
            Targetoid hemangioma
            Epithelioid hemangioma (angiolymphoid hyperplasia with eosinophilia, histiocytoid hemangioma)
        Lymphangiomas (circumscriptum, cavernosum, progressive)
        Lymphangioendothelioma
        Angiomatosis and lymphangiomatosis
    Intermediate
        Epithelioid hemangioendothelioma
        Kaposiform hemangioendothelioma
        Retiform hemangioendothelioma
        Endovascular papillary angioendothelioma
        Spindle cell hemangioendothelioma
    Malignant
        Kaposi's sarcoma
        Angiosarcoma
        Lymphangiosarcoma
Perivascular tumors
    Benign
        Benign hemangiopericytoma
        Glomus tumor
    Malignant
        Malignant hemangiopericytoma
        Malignant glomus tumor

may be confused with neoplasia. Examples discussed are acroangiodermatitis and intravascular papillary endothelial hyperplasia (IPEH; also known as vegetant intravascular hemangioendothelioma or Masson tumor). Accurate histologic recognition of these disorders is important because they may be confused with angiosarcoma and certain histologic variants of Kaposi's sarcoma.

Acroangiodermatitis[660] is an exaggerated form of stasis dermatitis most often seen in the lower extremities of elderly individuals. It is hyperpigmented, purpuric, and indurated and so is clinically confused with Kaposi's sarcoma, chronic dermatitis, or epidermal and dermal neoplasia. An ill-defined plaque within the superficial dermis (Fig. 17-51A) is formed by numerous small, rounded proliferating vessels lined by plump endothelial cells. Proliferating vessels arranged in small clusters and aggregates extend from the level of the normal superficial vascular plexus as glomeruloid structures into dermal papillae (Fig. 17-51B) exhibiting hemosiderin, edema, and fibrosis.

Intravascular papillary endothelial hyperplasia (IPEH)[661–664] is most often a lesion of the dermis of the head, neck, and distal extremity (i.e., hand) of middle-aged and older women. It is usually slow growing as nondescript nodules less than 2 cm, often enclosed within an apparently traumatically distorted or ectatic vascular lumen within the mid- to deep dermis. It can also be seen as a limited pattern in large organizing hematomas and in organizing thrombi in veins and cavernous hemangiomas. Microscopically, numerous minute sheets and papillary projections composed of nearly acellular collagen and residual unorganized fibrin are covered by a single layer of flattened endothelium. Mitotic figures are rare, and nuclear atypia is not observed. Advance of this cellular dissecting variant of recanalization and organization into the provoking thrombus follows lines of Zahn and this explains the papillary structure. Over time, the pattern tends to solidify into a rounded hyalinized hypocellular collagenous nodule with persistent interstitial capillary channels and some hemosiderin staining.

Angiokeratomas[665] are blue-black superficial lesions composed of dilated, thin-walled, dermal vessels that invaginate upward into a hyperplastic, verrucous epidermal layer. The dark color may invite biopsy to exclude melanoma. Attenuation of superficial dermis makes the channel or channels appear to lie within basal epidermis. Angiokeratomas occur in five clinical settings: (1) angiokeratoma corporis diffusum signifies diffuse cutaneous involvement associated with Fabry's disease; (2) Mibelli type, probably autosomal dominant, occurs on the dorsa of the fingers and toes; (3) scrotal lesions are typical of Fordyce type, also arising on penis, vulva, or upper thighs; (4) solitary papular angiokeratoma (Fig. 17-52) favors lower extremity, often with focal trauma history; (5) angiokeratoma circumscriptum, the only variant seen at birth, favors females, appearing as cystic nodules coalescing as plaques or in linear configuration, enlarging with the patient. Only the latter is a true hemangioma. The others are vascular telangiectasias.

Hemangiomas

Hemangiomas are acquired or congenital.[666] *Congenital hemangiomas* show a predilection for the head and neck of female infants, although any site may be affected. Strawberry hemangiomas are small, bosselated, and intensely red. Most are

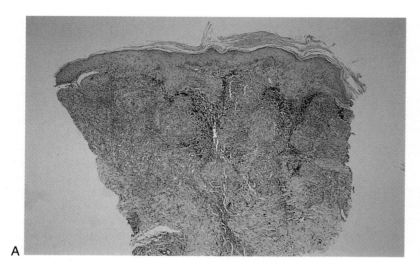
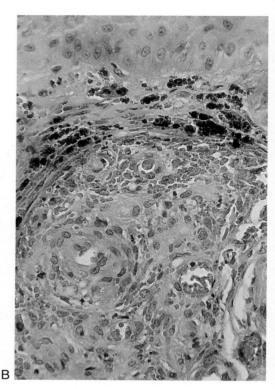

Fig. 17-51. Acroangiodermatitis. **(A)** A dermal plaque is composed of clustered vascular aggregates **(B)** protruding as glomeruloid structures into dermal papillae.

capillary hemangiomas that completely regress spontaneously by fibrosis within the first decade of life. Larger congenital lesions may produce significant deformity. They typically do not involute, and tend to infiltrate deeply. Larger vascular chambers of cavernous hemangiomas may be associated with multiple enchondromas (Maffucci's syndrome), involvement of the gastrointestinal tract as well as the skin (blue rubber bleb nevus syndrome), or consumption coagulopathy as a result of intralesional thrombosis (Kasabach-Merritt syndrome). Angiomatous lesions can be components of multisystem anomaly syndromes.[667] Small capillary hemangiomas are commonly acquired in middle-aged and older individuals, especially on the face, neck, and trunk. These bright red, symmetric, dome-shaped papules have been called "senile hemangiomas."

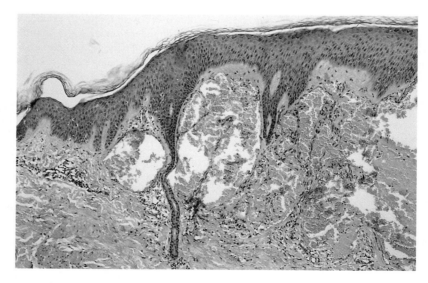

Fig. 17-52. Solitary angiokeratoma. This vascular telangiectasia consists of several dilated channels separated from hyperplastic epidermis by little or no compressed dermal remnant.

Microscopically, *capillary hemangiomas* are dermal groups of rounded vessels, lined by flattened endothelial cells devoid of mitotic activity. Congenital lesions are more lobulated with numerous small vessels and an associated proliferation of plump pericytes that can be alarming until their lack of cellular variation and atypia registers. Progressive luminal ectasia may appear in acquired lesions with age, while walls remain thin. Hemangiomas with capillary, arterial, and venous components can be subclassified according to the predominant or various vessel types of which they are comprised (e.g., venous or arteriovenous hemangiomas).

Lobular capillary hemangioma[668,669] has been long known as "pyogenic granuloma" because of clinical resemblance to polypoid granulation tissue when ulcerated. This lesion is most frequently situated on mucosal membranes or on distal extremities, particularly around nails, but has deep dermal, entirely subcutaneous or intravascular variants.[670] It can occur in port wine stains.[671] Common features are rapid growth, size less than 2 cm, and pedunculation. An early lobular capillary hemangioma is often an ulcerated proliferation of rounded, anastomosing vessels and pericytes with lobular architecture, embedded within a markedly edematous stroma that may contain both neutrophils and mononuclear cells. Mitotic figures may be prominent, but atypical (e.g., tripolar) mitoses are not observed. Older lesions show less inflammatory change and edema. Rare clustered and disseminated[672,673] variants are reported. Simple excision is curative, though a few reform locally. Trunk lesions may recur as multiple satellites.[674] Bacillary angiomatosis,[675] the infection by *Rochalimaea* species, showing fragmented neutrophils and clumps of silver-positive organisms should be excluded.

Cavernous hemangiomas are more extensive, deeply expansile, and less well circumscribed within the dermis. Their ectatic channels have somewhat thicker walls than capillary hemangiomas. Intraluminal thrombi in various states of organization and/or phleboliths are often found.

The sinusoidal variant of cavernous hemangioma (*sinusoidal hemangioma*)[676] more frequently affects adult females, is usually on limbs and trunk, with a special predilection for the subcutaneous tissue of the breast. The low power pattern shows a lobular tumor with large thin-walled vessels similar to a cavernous hemangioma. Its special feature is the interconnecting markedly dilated, congested, thin-walled channels in a sinusoidal pattern, with minimal or no intervening stroma. This creates a prominent pseudopapillary pattern reminiscent of Masson's tumor. The lining luminal cells are in a single layer, perhaps with slight pleomorphism. The multicellular layering and organizing thrombi seen in angiosarcoma are absent, nor is there dissection along collagen planes or prominent mitoses. Ossification may be found. Complete excision is curative.

The *arteriovenous hemangioma*[677,678] (acral arteriovenous tumor) is usually solitary, averaging 5 mm, with a male predilection (2.5:1) and peak incidence in the sixth decade. Location in decreasing likelihood is face (especially perioral), proximal extremities, and trunk. Duration for a few years is typical as they do not spontaneously involute. This well circumscribed dermal and/or subcutaneous neoplasm pushes dermal adnexae aside and consists of large, interconnected channels with fused fibromuscular walls characteristically lacking organized elastic lamellae. Typically, many of the veins may show excessive elaboration of basophilic sulfated mucopolysaccharide similar to the mural change in traumatized vein walls.

Microvenular hemangioma[679] presents as asymptomatic red or purple papules, plaques, or nodules up to 1 cm in children and young adults, most commonly on an extremity. Histopathology features irregular branching blood vessels of fairly uniform small caliber distributed throughout the dermis.[680] Diameters are so small that lumens may be inconspicuous and Kaposi's sarcoma is simulated. However, there is no significant atypia and a sparse inflammatory infiltrate at most.

Glomeruloid hemangioma[681,682] occurs mainly on the trunk of middle-aged adults and in association with POEMS syndrome (polyneuropathy, organomegaly, endocrinopathy, M-protein, skin lesions). At low magnification, these multiple small papules will appear as a vascular proliferation in the superficial dermis or in clusters throughout the dermis resembling either a capillary or tufted hemangioma. At higher power, ectatic vessels contain one or more small capillaries, thus creating the appearance of a glomerulus. Eosinophilic globules surrounding the vessels may be immunoglobulin from the serum within pericytes.

Acquired *tufted hemangiomas* (angioblastomas)[683-688] appear as red-blue patches, usually on the shoulders and upper back near the base of the neck of children or young adults. This very slowly growing progressive lesion appears clinically as ill-defined red or brown macules, papules, and nodules. Regression is not reported and tenderness is common. Microscopically multiple ovoid lobules of pericyte proliferation occur within the mid- and lower dermis or superficial subcutis. This constitutes the classically described "cannonball" distribution of vascular lobules. The name derives from semilunar channels into which more cellular regions ("tufts") protrude.[685,686] Cellular atypia is absent and mitoses are rare. The spindle cell component of nodular Kaposi's sarcoma is absent. Complete excision is often impossible.

The *targetoid hemangioma*[689-692] is mainly encountered in children to young adults without strong site predilection. At some point in its very slow evolution, it comes to resemble a concentrically ringed target. Although its endothelial cells are only modestly atypical and minimally mitotic, two features may bring to mind Kaposi's sarcoma or other more aggressive vascular neoplasms: dissecting type growth through dermal collagen and/or adipose tissue and papillary intravascular endothelial cell profiles in racemose vascular lumina. Marked hemosiderin deposition at the advancing edge constituting one of the rings may not be a helpful feature in making the distinction if only a central punch biopsy is submitted. Chronic inflammatory cells are scattered between the channels. Simple excision is curative.

Epithelioid hemangioma[693-695] is also known as *angiolymphoid hyperplasia with eosinophilia*,[696] and is one of several lesions grouped into a dissimilar group of lesions collectively referred to as *histiocytoid hemangiomas*.[697-699] Most often it will appear as an asymptomatic, pale red, sessile nodule or a plaque on the head, especially around the ear or on the neck or limbs of middle-aged women. This poorly circumscribed proliferation of lumen-forming epithelioid endothelial cells is accompanied by variable inflammation in superficial and deep dermis. Enlarged nuclei of the channel-forming cells have vesicular chromatin and conspicuous nucleoli. Mitoses are infrequent. Cytoplasm is eosinophilic to amphophilic, imparting an epithelioid or, to some, a histiocytoid appearance. Lumens may not be formed in ill-defined cords and aggregates of these plump endothelial cells. Admixed eosinophils are numerous and lymphoid aggregates, even follicles, are not unusual at the periphery. More than 60 percent are intimately associated with a large vessel that shows mural damage or rupture, or both. This implies at least some are reactive processes. About one-third recur, but virtually none has metastasized. Regression is rare, so surgical excision is reasonable.

Kimura's disease is an inflammatory condition formerly thought identical with epithelioid hemangioma[700,701] and primarily seen in young men of Asian descent.[702] Multiple dense lymphoid aggregates with prominent germinal centers, eosinophils, and thin-walled vessels lined by attenuated endothelial cells involve the head and neck and less often the trunk and limbs. Pruritis and pain are typical. Lymphadenopathy and peripheral blood eosinophilia are frequent.[703]

Lymphangioma

Lymphangiomas[704] consist of thin-walled dermal vessels, often within the most superficial dermis, filled with proteinaceous fluid and occasional lymphocytes (Fig. 17-53). Red cells may become admixed during biopsy. Hemangiomas may mimic lymphangioma if they seem to have empty channels due to gravitational separation of red cells from plasma, or because blood drains out at biopsy. Cutaneous lymphangiomas usually present in infancy, most before age 5.[705] In *lymphangioma circumscriptum*[706] an asymptomatic tumor present at birth or in early childhood, lymphatic channels in superficial dermis herniate into a hyperplastic epidermal layer evoking variable hyperkeratosis analogous to angiokeratoma. Clinically, one or several patches of small translucent vesicles resemble multiple small blisters. Chamber distention fluctuates with the efficiency of local lymphatic drainage. *Lymphangioma cavernosum* is a small or large lesion constituted by fluid-filled endothelial-lined spaces in skin or subcutaneous tissue, sometimes with lymphoid infiltrates. The commonest location is the neck (cystic hygroma). *Progres-*

sive lymphangioma[707] affects children or young adults as well defined pink to brown macules or plaques resembling a bruise on extremities or trunk. They tend to slowly enlarge, predominantly in the superficial dermis but may extend deeper, even into subcutaneous tissue. Its vessels are oriented horizontally in the superficial dermis and become smaller in the deeper dermis. As with the other lymphangiomas, the channels have a single endothelial lining layer without tuft formation or atypia,[708] but the anastomosing channels simulate angiosarcoma. The lymphangioma-like form of Kaposi's sarcoma should also be excluded.[709] The benign lymphangioendothelioma[710] is characterized by a greater cellularity.

Glomus Tumor and Variants

Glomus tumors[711–714] and the ectatic channel variant known as *glomangioma* (Fig. 17-54) may occur as solitary or multiple, often painful nodules with predilection for skin of the extremities. The neoplastic glomus cell resembles its normal counterpart, being rounded with moderate quantities of eosinophilic cytoplasm, and a small, rounded, centrally disposed nucleus. The uniform tumor cell proliferation, often with equidistant nuclear position, is an extravascular accumulation, with smooth muscle features demonstrable by electron microscopy or immunohistochemistry. *Glomangioleiomyoma* is an uncommon variant of glomus tumor in which elongate mature smooth muscle cells are admixed with glomus cells. The few cases of *malignant glomus tumor* have been only locally invasive, and metastases exceedingly rare.[715–717]

Borderline Vascular Tumors

In parallel with the terminology popular for tumors of other organs (e.g., ovary), a borderline category of low grade endothelial tumors reluctant to metastasize can be set aside. This would contain at least four members.

Epithelioid hemangioendothelioma (EH)[718–720] is a rare, nodular, tan to pink, deep dermal or subcuticular lesion rarely found

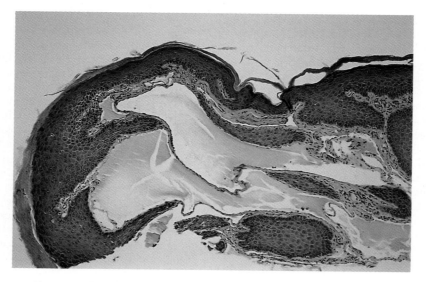

Fig. 17-53. Lymphangioma. Proteinaceous fluid fills dilated dermal channels.

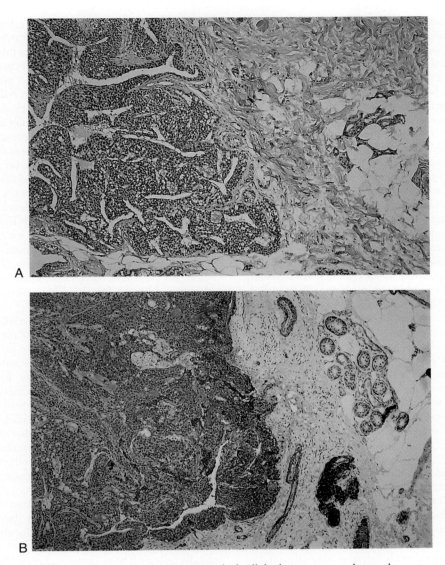

Fig. 17-54. Glomangioma. **(A)** A well circumscribed cellular lesion is grouped around tortuous vascular channels. **(B)** The glomus cells are reactive for smooth muscle actin, unlike adjacent epithelium of sweat gland coils.

in virtually any site. EH with cutaneous presentation is anecdotal. Concomitant involvement of underlying bone suggests bone origin with superficial extraosseous extension. Solitary cutaneous involvement has little precedent.[720] The tumor arises in young or middle-aged adults and slowly but progressively enlarges, ranging from less than 1 cm to more than 20 cm at diagnosis. Its polygonal or rounded cells arranged in sheets, cords, or nests is easily mistaken for metastatic adenocarcinoma or a fatty tumor because of intracellular lumens creating a signet ring appearance. Red cells should be sought in these spaces. Also, the tumor may be contiguous to or in a large vessel. Bland round to oval nuclei are of fairly uniform size and mitoses are infrequent. A myxoid stroma stains positively for sulfated mucopolysaccharide with the aldehyde fuchsin stain at low pH. This matrix simulates chondroid but has its parallel in basophilic thickening within injured walls of traumatized large

vessels. Weibel-Palade bodies and intercellular junctions bordered by membrane flaps and pinocytotic vesicles are ultrastructural features shared with benign endothelial cells. Immunohistochemistry finds positivity for factor VIII antigen, Ulex europeus I binding (UEA), CD31 and CD34, and vimentin. This tumor is now known to occur in liver, lung (formerly "hyalinizing intravascular bronchoalveolar tumor"), and bone (formerly "angioglomoid sarcoma"). When tumor is in skin and also in these organs, the question of metastasis vs. multifocality may be insoluble.[721] Local recurrence follows excision in about 25 percent. Metastases occur in perhaps 20 percent, with a fatal outcome in less than 10 percent.

Kaposiform hemangioendothelioma[722] is exclusively found in children and adolescents, located in superficial skin or deep soft tissue. The Kasabach-Merritt or lymphangiomatosis syndromes may be associated. The distinctive histology consists of tubular and capillary caliber vessels in jumbled array, admixed with fascicles of spindle cells and glomeruloid nests of polygonal cells. Features resembling Kaposi's sarcoma are hyaline intracytoplasmic globules, extravasated, fragmented red blood cells, and only modest atypia and mitotic activity. Cytoplasmic vacuoles are common. CD34 should be positive and UEA negative. Feasibility of surgical excision depends on lesion depth. The tumor can regrow locally, metastasize regionally, and kill if deep and massive.

The *retiform hemangioendothelioma*[723] has a wide range of age incidence but favors young adults with extremity location. The lesions present as 2 to 9 cm dermal and subcutaneous masses. Microscopically, arborizing elongated blood vessels (retiform pattern) have endovascular papillae with collagenous cores. Hobnail monomorphic endothelial cells have scant cytoplasm, no mitoses, and mild or no cellular atypia. A prominent lymphocytic infiltrate is characteristic.

The *endovascular papillary angioendothelioma*,[724,725] known under the convenient eponym Dabska tumor, is an extremely rare endothelial tumor with equal sex incidence afflicting children and adolescents. This plaque-like red-brown lesion of trunk and extremities is centered in mid-dermis and subcutis. Distinctive intravascular papillations are formed by polygonal, moderately variable, plump endothelial cells covering eosinophilic globules of PASD-positive basement membrane material. Mature lymphocytes are attracted and held, implying surface receptors similar to so-called high endothelial cells. Much of the lesion may resemble a deep lymphangioma. Similar histology may be found in regional lymph nodes, possibly representing metastatic spread. The local regrowth rate is 50 percent but no fatalities are recorded following surgical removal.

Spindle cell hemangioendothelioma is a more recently described low grade endothelial tumor[726] resembling both a cavernous hemangioma and the tumor stage of Kaposi's sarcoma. This tumor, typically of extremities, is more common in males (2:1). It has arisen within the chronic lymphedema of Milroy's disease (essential lymphedema due to lymphatic hypoplasia) and with Maffucci's syndrome (skeletal enchondromatosis with soft tissue hemangiomas). The process has a long clinical evolution with local regrowth in as many as 70 percent of cases. Careful assessment of margins may not prevent this, because it is a multifocal tumor in perhaps one-half the cases. Metastases are not reported prior to irradiation and some argue it is a non-neoplastic lesion.[727–730]

Kaposi's Sarcoma

Kaposi's sarcoma, a multifocal angioproliferative process, occurs in two very different forms: one indolent and the other aggressive.[731–740] The indolent form[741] affects elderly individuals, particularly of Southern European descent, and Ashkenazi Jews. The aggressive form arises in a background of immunosuppression, especially AIDS[739,742–744] and tends to have a more erratic distribution and wider variety of clinical appearance. African cases have additional clinical forms.[745]

Whether Kaposi's sarcoma is a hyperplastic or a neoplastic process is debated.[746] Most are found diploid by flow cytometry, favoring hyperplasia.[747] Transfection experiments and DNA sequence data showing herpesvirus 6 episomes in tumor cells[748–750] support a neoplastic nature despite the rarity of finding embolic neoplastic cells in transit in peripheral blood.

An early lesion may appear as an intensely erythematous, nonblanching plaque mimicking subcutaneous bleeding or a petechial papule. Patches progress to purpuric plaques sometimes appearing at sites of trauma. In AIDS,[751] facial involvement is a common initial site with predilection for the nose. Late in the course, hemorrhagic nodules appear and may ulcerate. Both forms of Kaposi's sarcoma present a clinical diagnostic challenge at any stage, but particularly in association with AIDS where the differential diagnosis includes a number of uncommonly encountered infectious and neoplastic disorders. Because of the implications of the diagnosis, it must be made cautiously, particularly in the early, less developed stages. Disorders that commonly may be confused with Kaposi's can be summarized by stage: (1) patch stage: bruise or ecchymoses; progressive pigmentary purpura (Schamberg disease); postinflammatory hyperpigmentation; localized vasculitis; (2) plaque and nodular stage: angiosarcoma; sarcoidosis; cutaneous amyloidosis; lymphoma and benign lymphoid hyperplasia; atypical dermatofibroma; vascularized scar.

Early *patch-stage* Kaposi's presents a subtle increase in cellularity around the superficial vascular plexus and periadnexal adventitia (Fig. 17-55A). This is due to ill-defined proliferations of bland-appearing spindle cells, some of which appear to form vascular slits or angulated spaces. The papillary dermis is spared in early lesions. A distinctive feature of this angiocentric spindle cell proliferative process is to form a mantle about hair follicles and sweat glands.[752] In these locations, new vascular channels may surround pre-existent ones ("promontory sign"). Hemosiderin may be scattered through the lesion. Dilated lymphatics and inflammatory cells consisting of lymphocytes and plasma cells in small aggregates may be at the periphery.

Plaque and nodular lesions have denser cellular aggregates of spindle cells within the dermis. In part, these often retain regions of bland spindle cells with nuclear pallor and delicate chromatin distribution. Nearby and signifying more advanced disease are spindle cells with more coarsely clumped heterochromatin than typically found in patch or plaque disease, and mitotic figures are usually identified. In fully developed nodular lesions, proliferating cells form expansile sheets and nodules that contain characteristic slit-like spaces containing erythrocytes tightly crowded single file within these spaces (boxcar arrangement). This stage might be confused with a primary spindle cell mesenchymal neoplasm in which recent hemorrhage has occurred, especially leiomyosarcoma. Diagnostically useful hyaline globules within cytoplasm of proliferating Kaposi's spindle cells are PAS positive, and are believed to represent membrane residues from phagocytized erythrocytes[753] (Fig. 17-55B). Unlike dermatofibrosarcoma protuberans, there is no reaction for factor XIIIa. There is inconsistent expression of factor VIII antigen and UEA labeling, with more frequent staining for CD31[754,755] and CD34. Only a minority (about 15 percent) of Kaposi's sarcomas composed predominantly of spindle cells show reactivity for any vascular determinants, supporting the view that they begin as endothelial proliferations[756] and evolve toward an indeterminant cell lineage.[658,659]

Unlike stasis dermatitis and acroangiodermatitis, the initial channels in Kaposi's sarcoma are irregular and angulated. Their

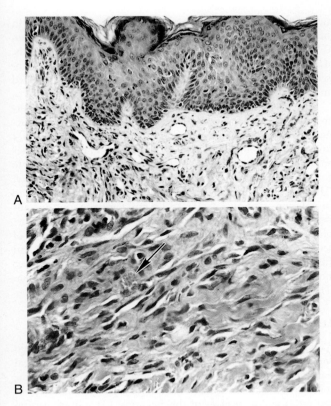

Fig. 17-55. Kaposi's sarcoma, showing (A) typical proliferation of bland spindle cells about pre-existing superficial dermal vessels, and (B) formation by these cells of slit-like spaces within dermal connective tissue. Also note characteristic hyaline globules (arrow) within the cytoplasm of a spindle cell.

course is predetermined by growth along reticular dermal collagen bundles enveloping them. The involvement of the periadnexal adventitia is also unlike stasis change. When inflammatory reaction predominates, the vascular components are easy to overlook. Superficial inflammatory dermatoses and secondary syphilis may be considered. Plasma cells are rare in the former; atypical vascular spaces lined by flat, nonobliterative endothelial cells are unusual in the latter. Kaposi's sarcoma can be simulated in small samples of targetoid hemangioma, some hemangioendotheliomas, "sclerosing hemangioma" (vascular variant of dermatofibroma), proliferating scars, bacillary angiomatosis, and verruga peruana.

Prognosis relates to type: localized "Mediterranean"—0 percent mortality from tumor; regionally aggressive disease—35 percent mortality at 5 years; generalized—100 percent fatal. Visceral involvement can predate skin lesions or occur without them.[757]

Angiosarcoma

Most cutaneous *angiosarcomas* arise de novo on skin of the head and neck of elderly individuals,[758–762] particularly men (2:1). Single or multiple dusky, erythematous plaques enlarge and eventually develop nodules that may ulcerate.

Cutaneous angiosarcomas dissect between collagen fibers to produce poorly circumscribed and asymmetric zones of dermal hypercellularity. Dilated lymphatic spaces and infiltrates of

lymphocytes may be at the periphery. Early and lower grade ("hemangioma-like") angiosarcomas form angulated and irregular vascular spaces, not all of which are filled with blood. Sarcomatous endothelial cells form one or more layers and often redundantly bulge into the lumen, perhaps as small papillations (Fig. 17-56). Cribriform aggregations or solid sheets of anaplastic epithelioid cells may mimic metastatic carcinoma and fusiform cells of other sarcomas. The atypical nuclei are markedly hyperchromatic and irregular in contour. They have prominent nucleoli, enhancing the mimicry of carcinoma. Occasional atypical mitotic figures can be found. Cytoplasm is scant in flattened cells and single cells lining some channels, but copious in "hob nail" luminal cells, spindle, epithelioid,[763,764] pleomorphic, and granular cell[765] variations. Reticulin stain is helpful by outlining complex amalgamated vascular boundaries by staining basement membrane within the solid aggregates of tumor cells. Ultrastructural characteristics of endothelial cells can be sought, such as cytoplasmic Weibel-Palade bodies, pericellular basement membrane, and pinocytotic vesicles.[766]

Factor VIII-associated antigen can be demonstrated by immunohistochemistry in most cases of angiosarcoma but it may be limited to the better differentiated areas. "Aberrant" cytokeratin positivity is not unexpected.[764,767,768] CD31, a 130 kd membrane-bound glycoprotein (gp IIa) belonging to the immunoglobulin supergene family, also known as platelet-endothelial cell adhesion molecule (PECAM-1)[754,755,769] is a sensitive marker for endothelial neoplasms.[770–773]

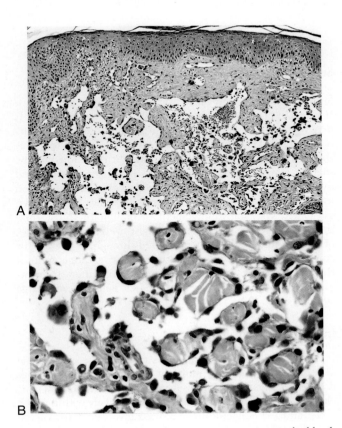

Fig. 17-56. (A) Angiosarcoma showing anastomosing irregular blood-filled spaces within the superficial and deep dermis. (B) These spaces are lined by plump, hyperchromatic endothelial cells.

CD34 is a 110 kd transmembrane glycoprotein present on human hematopoietic progenitor cells and vascular endothelial cells. The function of CD34 is still unclear but there is evidence that it plays a role in cell adhesion and possibly in signal transduction. Frequently used antibodies reactive in paraffin tissue are QBEND10 and MY10. This marker has been found to be very sensitive for neoplasms with endothelial differentiation.[774] In one study, CD34 decorated 70 percent of angiosarcomas, 90 percent of Kaposi's sarcomas, and 100 percent of epithelioid hemangioendotheliomas.[775] Indeed, CD34 often stains neoplastic endothelial cells more strongly than normal endothelium.[776]

Tumors likely to be confused with angiosarcoma include metastatic poorly differentiated carcinoma, primary adenoid and acantholytic squamous cell carcinoma,[777] malignant melanoma, and epithelioid sarcoma.[778] Angioproliferative states that mimic angiosarcoma include epithelioid and targetoid hemangioma, intravascular papillary endothelial hyperplasia, and Kaposi's sarcoma.

Only perhaps 15 percent of patients will survive 5 years or more after diagnosis of angiosarcoma. Mortality at 15 months is 50 percent. The most common cause of death is local tumor effect and hemorrhage, although distant metastases are likely with survival for more than 15 months.

The *endothelial sarcomas arising in chronic lymphedema,*[761] such as upper extremities following radical mastectomy (i.e., the Stewart-Treves syndrome) may have mixed features of angiosarcoma and lymphangiosarcoma. Showers of red-purple nodules may develop in the edematous skin.

Muscle Tumors

Smooth Muscle Hamartoma

Smooth muscle hamartoma is usually one patch several centimeters in diameter, most commonly in the lumbar region. It may be present at birth or arise in childhood or early adulthood (L5). Usually there are small, follicular papules throughout the patch, although the entire lesion may be slightly elevated. The patch shows hyperpigmentation and hypertrichosis in some patients, indicating that this lesion forms a spectrum with Becker's nevus.[779] There is no known associated systemic involvement or malignant transformation.[780] Numerous thick, long, straight, well defined bundles of smooth muscle fibers are scattered throughout the dermis and extend in various directions. The arrangement of the smooth muscle bundles in the dermis differs from piloleiomyoma, in which the smooth muscle bundles form a large aggregate.

Infantile Myofibromatosis

Infantile myofibromatosis[781] includes two variants of the same disorder: (1) congenital multiple myofibromatosis—fibrous nodules confined to the skin, subcutaneous tissue, skeletal muscle, and bone with spontaneous regression likely within 1 to 2 years; and (2) congenital generalized myofibromatosis—visceral lesions also present, conferring a high mortality rate within the first few months of life, usually as a result of obstruc-

tion of a vital organ, failure to thrive, debility, or infection. In both, firm, skin-colored to red-purple nodules, averaging from 0.5 to 1.5 cm in greater diameter, are in dermis and subcutis, usually at birth, mainly on the trunk, head, and neck. Microscopically, fibroblasts and plumper myofibroblasts are arranged in interlacing bundles or in a whorled pattern.

A *myofibroma* can occur in children and adults as a small dermal or subcutaneous lesion without site predilection, with circumscribed, lobulated, or plexiform configuration and cellular composition similar to the infantile lesions. These solitary lesions are several times more common than the above multiple forms but similarly favor the upper body including oral cavity. They are firm, scar-like dermal and subcutaneous white-gray to pink lesions that average 0.5 to 1.5 cm. Larger lesions may ulcerate. Microscopically, plump spindle cells form sharply marginated short bundles and nodules, a pattern reminiscent of leiomyoma. Special stains show features of both myoblastic and fibroblastic cell types. Vimentin and actin will be found, but not desmin or S-100 protein. The latter excludes neurofibroma. The prominent myxoid matrix of nodular fasciitis is lacking.

Leiomyoma and Angioleiomyoma

Common dermal and subcutaneous tumors composed of benign smooth muscle cells are classified into five important clinical variants: (1) multiple piloleiomyomas and (2) solitary piloleiomyoma, both arising from arrectores pilorum muscles, often on extensor surfaces of the forearms; (3) solitary genital leiomyoma, arising from the dartoic, vulvar, or mamillary muscle; (4) solitary angioleiomyoma, arising from the muscle of veins; and (5) leiomyomas with additional mesenchymal elements.[780,782–785]

Multiple *piloleiomyomas*[786] are by far the most common type of leiomyoma. They appear as small, firm, red or brown intradermal nodules arranged in a group or linear array. Often two or more areas are affected. Usually, but not always, the lesions are tender and give rise spontaneously to occasional attacks of pain[787] attributed to muscular contractions. Solitary piloleiomyomas are intradermal nodules up to 2 cm in diameter. Most of them are tender or painful. *Solitary genital leiomyomas* are intradermal, on the scrotum, the labia majora, or rarely, the nipple. Most genital leiomyomas are asymptomatic.

Piloleiomyomas, whether multiple or solitary, and genital leiomyomas have a similar histologic appearance. They are poorly demarcated and are composed of interlacing bundles of smooth muscle fibers with varying amounts of admixed collagen (Fig. 17-57A). The neoplastic muscle fibers are generally straight, with little or no waviness; they contain centrally located, thin, very long, blunt-edged nuclei without notable mitoses (Fig. 17-57B). The muscle bundles are only slightly more eosinophilic than collagen, and thus are often difficult to distinguish from collagen bundles, despite cytologic differences. The nuclei of smooth muscle cells are blunted and one end is often flattened, unlike the tapering nuclei of fibrocytes. Smooth muscle cells often have a clear perinuclear zone, especially in cross-section, whereas fibrocytes do not. The differentiation between muscle and collagen bundles is facilitated with one of the collagen stains. With the aniline blue stain, muscle stains red and collagen blue. With a trichrome stain (Fig. 17-57C),

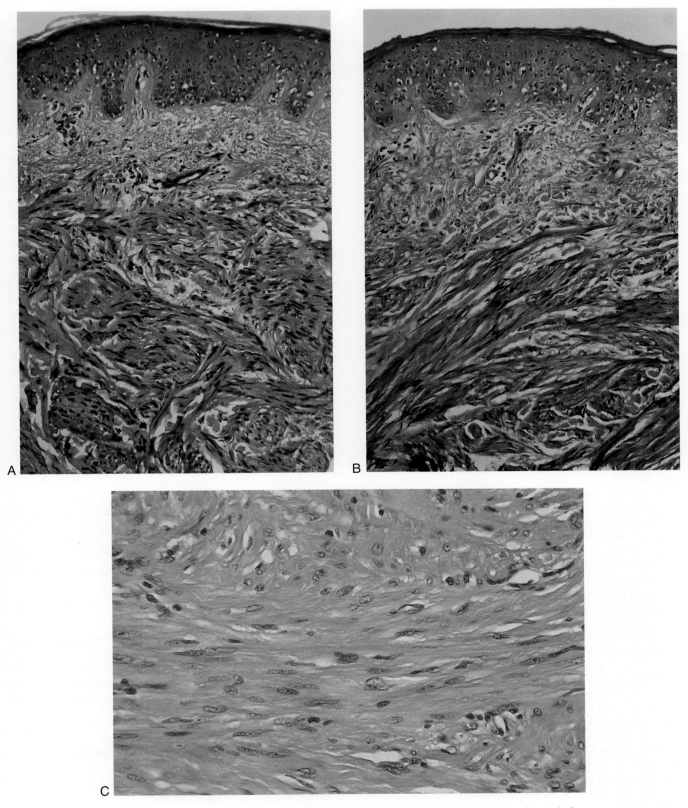

Fig. 17-57. (A) Piloleiomyoma consisting of poorly demarcated interlacing bundles of smooth muscle that, unlike fibroblasts, (B) have copious red-staining cytoplasm with trichrome stain. (C) Typically on cross-sectioning, the muscle bundles show clear perinuclear zones.

muscle is dark red, and collagen is green or blue. Intracytoplasmic myofibrils often can be visualized as longitudinal striations in H&E sections and more easily if stained with phosphotungstic acid-hematoxylin.

Solitary *angioleiomyomas* are usually subcutaneous. They uncommonly exceed 4 cm. The lower extremities are the most common site. Pain and tenderness are present in most, but not all.[787,788]

Angioleiomyomas differ from the other types of leiomyoma by being encapsulated, having only a small amount of intralesional collagen, and by having conspicuous vascular channels. Angioleiomyomas have been subdivided into a capillary or solid type, a cavernous type, and a venous type depending on the predominant channel configuration.[789] Tumor cells spiral off from the walls of the variably sized vascular channels, such that the nodule may appear fenestrated or sieve-like. The *angiolipoleiomyoma*[790] is a rare acquired asymptomatic acral lesion of adults, usually male, in which mature lipomatous fat is added to the histology of angioleiomyoma. *Lipoleiomyomas* have admixed fat.[791]

Superficial Leiomyosarcoma

Superficial leiomyosarcomas include those arising in dermis and subcutaneous tissues, but not those in deeper soft tissue or body spaces.[792–796] *Vulvar* and *scrotal leiomyosarcomas* tend to be larger and better circumscribed than those in skin or subcutaneous location. Their traditional inclusion under the general heading of cutaneous leiomyosarcoma has been challenged.[796] Strong prognostic correlations follow location in dermis (cutaneous leiomyosarcoma) as compared to subcutaneous leiomyosarcoma. The former is traditionally thought of as arising from pilar muscles, correlating with higher occurrence on extensor surfaces where hair is abundant. Subcutaneous leiomyosarcomas tend to have a prominent vascularity and are assumed to arise from vascular walls,[797] analogous to angioleiomyomas. Cutaneous leiomyosarcomas present as firm dermal nodules that usually span less than 2 cm in diameter, most commonly in the 50 to 70 age range. Males are predilected 2 to 3:1. The skin is depressed or discolored in cutaneous leiomyosarcoma, as opposed to the subcutaneous variant, in which the skin is uninvolved and freely movable over the nodule.

In both locations, superficial leiomyosarcomas are asymmetric, consisting of infiltrative tumor fascicles with zones of hypercellularity standing out as increased nuclear density with variably eosinophilic myoplasm and collagenous stroma. Full-thickness colonization of the dermis and infiltration of the subcutis by destructive, pushing fascicles may occur (Fig. 17-58A). Less differentiated regions exhibit multinucleation and bizarre nuclear forms. Better differentiated zones retain elongated nuclei with blunt ends typical of smooth muscle cells (Fig. 17-58B). Nuclei have coarsely clumped heterochromatin. Mitoses should be easily found. The number of mitoses may be high in anaplastic areas even when there will be no metastases.[798]

The *epithelioid variant of leiomyosarcoma*, composed of round to oval cells with abundant eosinophilic cytoplasm, may be confused with a variety of primary and metastatic neoplasms. Some tumors have clear cell (leiomyoblastomatous) features.[799]

The presence of bizarre giant cells in leiomyosarcoma may cause a resemblance to malignant fibrous histiocytoma.[798]

However, at least in some areas, there are greatly elongated, thin, blunt-ended nuclei characteristic of smooth muscle cells. Also, demonstration of the enhancement of longitudinal striation due to myofibrils by staining with trichrome or phosphotungstic acid-hematoxylin will aid in the distinction. The same holds true of subcutaneous leiomyosarcomas, in which the presence of endothelial-lined vessels may suggest a hemangiopericytoma. Immunohistochemical staining of deparaffinized sections shows expression of desmin in all cutaneous leiomyosarcomas and of muscle-specific actin in the great majority.[800] Only about half of the subcutaneous leiomyosarcomas show a significant number of tumor cells that are positive for desmin and actin.[801] Smooth muscle actin is a monoclonal antibody against alpha smooth muscle actin.[802] These smooth muscle markers may be demonstrated in "myofibroblastic" lesions such as nodular fasciitis and therefore are not absolute diagnostic criteria. Some hold that ultrastructural study is a more reliable means for definite identification. Electron microscopic examination has shown that the tumor cells have the characteristics of smooth muscle cells even when there is marked nuclear atypicality.[798] Thus, the tumor cells show skeins of intermediate filaments punctuated by dense bodies, subplasmalemmal plaques, pinocytotic vesicles, and external pericellular lamina.[798,803–805]

Tumors confined to the dermis are amenable to surgical eradication, but because up to 50 percent recur, adequate excision should be confirmed by careful pathologic evaluation of all margins. Dermal tumors rarely metastasize to regional lymph nodes. Death from the purely cutaneous form is an anecdotal occurrence.[806] By contrast, subcutaneous leiomyosarcomas may cause hematogenous metastases, especially to the lungs, and lead to death in about one-third of the patients.[793,807] No correlation seems to exist between the degree of histologic malignancy of the tumor and metastases, which occur in up to 40 percent of cases.[792] DNA content, as determined by flow cytometry, was a strong predictor of metastatic potential in one study.[808] Purely subcutaneous leiomyosarcomas must be differentiated from leiomyosarcomas involving skeletal muscle or fascia, which are nearly always fatal.[801] Involvement of underlying fascia or skeletal muscle is a harbinger of likely metastases.[801]

Rhabdomyosarcoma

Rhabdomyosarcoma, the most common soft tissue sarcoma in children, adolescents, and young adults, may occur as a skin or submucosal nodule in the orbital/eyelid area, nasal/oropharyngeal region, or ear/mastoid location.[809–812] Presentation in the skin is unusual, accounting for less than 1 percent of reported cases.

Fibrous and So-Called Fibrohistiocytic Tumors

Hyperplasias and Hamartomas

Keloids are abnormal hyperplasias of collagen-forming fibroblasts generally representing excessive and sustained post-traumatic scar formation. Some occur spontaneously. Individuals of

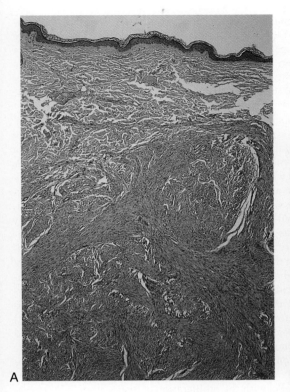

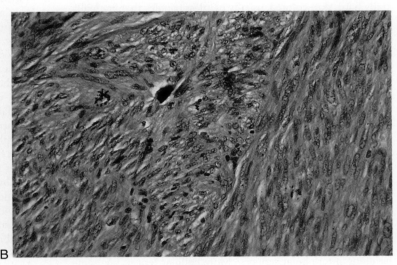

Fig. 17-58. **(A)** Superficial leiomyosarcoma showing interlacing bundles of smooth muscle cells in dermis beneath the epidermal layer and **(B)** variable cytologic atypia with mitotic activity.

African ancestry are especially prone. The early stages of these nodules can be erythematous, then may acquire progressive pigmentation over time. A keloid shows irregular proliferation of fibroblasts and deposition of collagen bundles within dermis with the characteristic feature of broad, eosinophilic, hyalinized collagen bundles. It will be negative for both CD34 and factor XIIIa. A hypertrophic scar[813] resembles a keloid in that the proliferating fascicles of fibroblasts are randomly oriented. In ordinary scars, hyalinized collagen bundles typical of keloid are entirely lacking. Recrudescence is much higher for keloids than for hypertrophic scars. Fibroblasts and collagen strands in hypertropic scars are aligned parallel to the epidermal surface. With cutaneous scars and keloids, there should be passing consideration to exclude an initial or recurrent manifestation of dermatofibrosarcoma protuberans (CD34+) and also aggressive fibromatosis (extra-abdominal desmoid tumor), the latter featuring increased interstitial mast cells.

A connective tissue hamartoma or *collagen nevus*[814] is a palpable abnormal aggregate of fibroblasts and collagen bundles in the dermis. Participation of abnormal vessels and even nerve bundles indicates that the proliferation is in reality a developmental anomaly rather than a response to injury or a neoplasm. Exophytic *elastic nevi* are also described.[815] *Pleomorphic fibroma* with bizarre cells scattered in a dense collagenous background, and *sclerosing (sclerotic) fibroma*, a well circumscribed, markedly hypocellular heavy collagenous deposit,[816] can occur in dermis. Multiple sclerotic fibromas are a marker for Cowden's disease.[817]

Angiofibromas are common, subtle, solitary skin-colored papules on the face, especially the nose (fibrous papules).[818] In tuberous sclerosis, multiple angiofibromas, erroneously termed adenoma sebaceum, may develop. They consist of superficial and mid-dermal proliferations of fibroblasts and small vessels, sometimes associated with concentric fibrosis about hair follicles (Fig. 17-59). Plump stellate cells within the superficial dermis are typical.

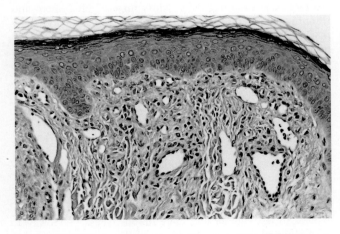

Fig. 17-59. Fibrous papule (angiofibroma). Note telangiectatic superficial vessels and plump connective tissue cells.

Dermal Fibroxanthomas (Dermatofibromas and So-Called Cutaneous Fibrous Histiocytomas)

Dermal fibroxanthomas are common neoplasms most often removed from young and middle-aged adults, and have slight female predominance.[819–821] Many are on the lower extremity, although any skin surface with the possible exception of scalp may be involved. These small and slow-growing lesions are initially hard, skin colored, usually painless papules that gradually and symmetrically enlarge to become tan to brown nodules. The induction of excessive pigmentation in the overlying hyperplastic epidermis causes confusion with nodular malignant melanoma. The Fitzpatrick sign is evoked by pinching the lesion: nodular melanomas will bulge outward, whereas dermatofibromas commonly dimple inward because they are bound to deep dermis and subcutaneous fat.

Dermatofibromas are symmetric, unencapsulated proliferations of small stellate fibroblasts admixed with vacuolated cells within the mid-dermis (Fig. 17-60). Benign-appearing, factor XIIIa-positive fibroblasts typically infiltrate among and surround individual reticular dermal collagen bundles that appear compact and round in cross-section and highlighted by shrinkage artifact. The edges of the focal lesion are indistinct because of the spiky interdigitation of its fibrocellular substance with surrounding dermis. Larger lesions or those situated near or at the dermal-subcutaneous boundary extend rays a short way into fat along interlobular septa.[822] More cellular lesions are composed of plump fibroblasts with occasional mitotic figures. Atypical mitoses are not seen. When cellularity wanes centrally, it is replaced by coarse compact and hyalinized collagen bundles. Multinucleated giant cells with copious eosinophilic or clear vacuolated cytoplasm, perhaps of Touton type, when present, tend to be located across the superficial region of the lesion. Some lesions have many small vessels and conspicuous hemosiderin throughout the tumor nodule, a variant sometimes going by the antiquated term sclerosing hemangioma[823] (Fig. 17-60H). The overlying epidermis characteristically undergoes hyperplastic thickening with elongate slender rete possibly terminating in basaloid hyperplasia resembling primary follicular germ or basal cell carcinoma. This may be interpreted as induction of pilar epithelium by the tumor.[824] Sebaceous induction may also be seen. When hyperpigmented, these epidermal extensions have been likened to "dirty fingers." Effacement and thinning of epidermis is only occasionally seen, and under low power examination, suggests an alternate diagnosis such as neurofibroma. Very rarely, the overlaying epidermis shows squamous cell carcinoma in situ.[825] Deep dermatofibromas may be distinguished from small dermatofibrosarcoma protuberans lesions by lack of "honeycomb" infiltration of fat and by factor XIIIa positivity and no reaction with CD34.[822,826–831]

Extensive variation in proportions of fibroblastic and vacuolated, plump "histiocytic" cells and giant cells in the same or different tumors suggests a microscopic morphologic spectrum. It seems a reasonable assumption that this apparant "histological spectrum of benign histiocytomas of the skin is made up of morphological variants of a neoplasm initially cellular with scant fibrous stroma and conspicuous storiform pattern which evolves to less cellular and more fibrous types."[832] However, neither morphologic nor statistical evidence has verified this evolutional hypothesis. Some steadfastly maintain that dermatofibromas are sclerosing inflammations.[833] The significant percentage of dermal dendrocytes in dermatofibromas[830] can be used as an argument favoring the inflammatory "reactive" nature of this process in the skin with an initial proliferative response of the same cells and, later, a secondary residual sclerotic process.[834]

Although used in several dermatopathology texts and articles as a synonym for dermatofibroma, a case can be made for reserving the term *cutaneous fibrous histiocytoma* (Fig. 17-61) for lesions with more conspicuous vacuolated and rounded cells admixed with plump fibroblasts featuring more variation in nuclear size and staining. Rather than histiocytic in differentiation, the vacuolated cells may be filled with fat and/or constipated with mucopolysaccharides normally produced by fibroblasts for the dermal ground substance. Distinct multinodularity and/or obvious subcutaneous involvement in a tumor with the more cellular, monotonously storiform features of benign fibrous histiocytoma described in soft tissue sites distinguishes *cutaneous fibrous histiocytoma* from the common dermatofibroma.[835] These larger dermal lesions, unlike conventional dermatofibromas, have a significant (perhaps 15 percent) rate of local regrowth if subtotally excised. They may be looked on as completing a spectrum between fibrocollagenous dermatofibroma and (with increasing atypia) atypical fibroxanthoma.

In parallel with the proliferation of histiocytoma/fibrous histiocytoma variants in soft tissue, an outpouring of papers has presented various subtypes, generally comprising less than 2 percent of large series of these lesions. Their sufficiently distinctive clinical appearances and/or recurrence rates are delineated in arguments to set them aside under special designations[836,837]

1. *Cellular fibrous histiocytoma* was applied by Calonje et al[838] to tumor variants with larger overall size, higher cellularity, more fascicular architecture, focal smooth muscle-like appearance, moderate mitotic rate, focal areas of necrosis or infarction, common extension into subcutis, and limited cellular polymorphism. These are said to recur in 26 percent of cases.

2. *Aneurysmal ("angiomatoid") fibrous histiocytoma,*[839,840] usually encountered on extremities, has large, blood-filled tissue spaces that may account for half the tumor volume. It is proposed that it is most likely to develop from "hemosiderin histiocytoma" (sclerosing hemangioma). Misdiagnosis as a vascular neoplasm is a common pitfall.

3. *Epithelioid cell histiocytoma* (epithelioid benign fibrous histiocytoma) clinically simulates pyogenic granuloma or Spitz nevus. This lesion has a uniform cell type and density with 50 to 80 percent of the constituent cells being large and epithelioid with prominent cytoplasm conferring angular outlines. Multinucleation without nuclear atypia or frequent mitoses is expected. Spitz nevus (because of plump polygonal cell composition and an epithelial collarette) and reticulohistiocytoma (but without eosinophils) are the main differentials. Two of 40 in two series recurred.[841,842]

4. *Storiform variant of fibrous histiocytoma*[843] is to be distinguished from DFSP.

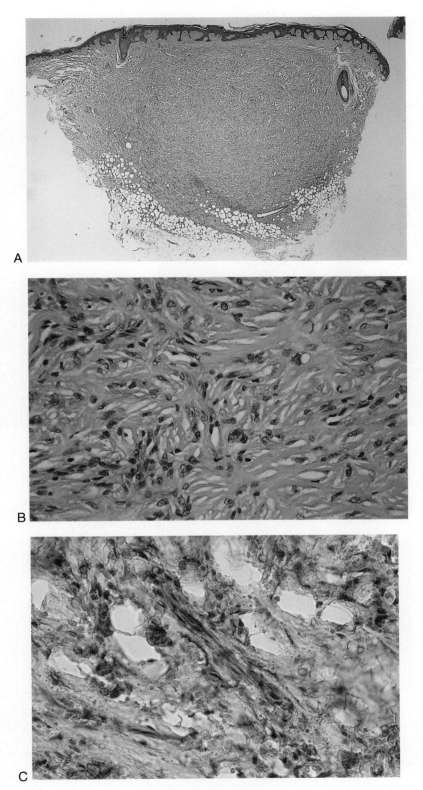

Fig. 17-60. Dermatofibroma. (A) Marked epidermal hyperplasia overlies a zone of dermal spindle cell proliferation with (B) storiform pattern and containing (C) neutral lipid (oil red O stain). (*Figure continues.*)

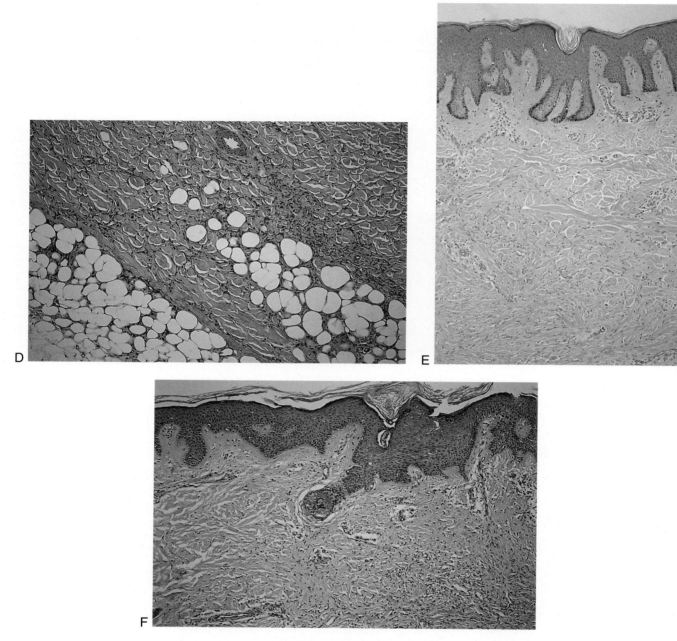

Fig. 17-60 (*Continued*). (**D**) An infiltrative pattern of bland fibroblasts surrounds individual thickened collagen bundles at the base of the tumor as it extends into fat with wedge-shaped extensions, tending to follow interlobular septa. (**E**) Elongate rete over the tumor tend to be hyperpigmented and (**F**) induction of hair germ or (**G**) sebaceous glands may be seen. (**H**) The sclerosing hemangioma variant has prominent small vessels, foamy cells, and hemosiderin. (*Figure continues.*)

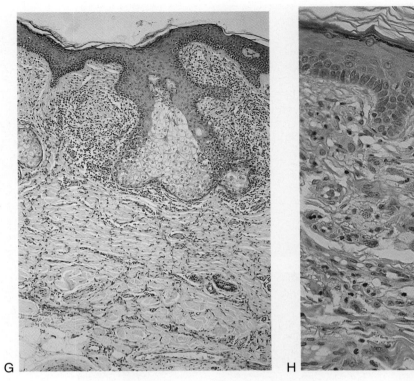

Fig. 17-60 (*Continued*).

5. *Palisading cutaneous histiocytoma*[844] has nuclear palisading and Verocay-like bodies that resemble schwannoma, in addition to the more typical features of the "fibrous variant of cutaneous fibrous histiocytoma." It is typically a dome-shaped nodule on digits. Positive results for factor XIIIa and vimentin suggest connective tissue differentiation for this tumor.[845]

6. *Atypical cutaneous fibrous histiocytoma*[846] resembles atypical fibroxanthoma.

7. The *atypical "pseudosarcomatous" variant*[847] (sometimes called dermatofibroma with "monster" cells[833]) contains scattered, bizarre, pleomorphic cells of multinucleate or histiocyte-like type in a conventional dermatofibroma backdrop. The pleomorphism is attributed to "degenerative change." The authors propose that many of the so-called atypical fibroxanthomas reported to arise on the limbs or trunk of young adults are probably examples of this lesion.

8. *Ossifying dermatofibroma* has osteoclast-like giant cells.[848]

9. *Clear cell dermatofibroma* features 80 percent or more markedly vacuolated cells. Perhaps 1 percent of dermatofibromas will have similar clear cell change in a minor part (<10 percent) of the infiltrate.[849]

10. *"Giant" dermatofibromas* are 5 cm or larger and occur most frequently on the legs.[850]

The proliferating spindle cells in "benign fibrous histiocytoma" react for vimentin, but are generally negative for lysozyme and other histiocyte markers. "The term "histiocyte" is often used as a crutch by physicians and pathologists in diagnosing unusual problems."[627] Headington[851] has vigorously argued that the term "histiocyte" is obsolete as it has been applied uncritically to cells of different types and different lineage. Wick et al[482] sum up the argument that the nosologic premise of the "fibrohistiocytic" category is "badly flawed," nay, a house of cards, and that there are no reliable and exclusive markers of "fibrohistiocytic" or "dendrocytic" cells. Even those studies finding reactivity with monoclonal antimacrophage antibodies in cutaneous "benign fibrous histiocytomas" admit that the positive cells may be a reactive infiltrate and not the neoplastic component.[852] Factor XIIIa positivity, in parallel with dermal dendrocytes, and lack of reactivity with MAC 387 have suggested the alternate designation *dermal dendrocytoma* despite their divergence in regard to CD34 (dendrocytes frequently positive; dermatofibromas negative).[853,854] This assertion is contested by those who find only a minority of cells at the periphery reacting for factor XIIIa and who deem these reactive.[842]

Dermatomyofibroma

The *dermatomyofibroma* is a benign, plaque-like proliferation of fibroblasts and myofibroblasts in dermis, predilecting the shoulder region including axillae and upper arm of young adults, especially women.[855,856] Keloid is likely to be the clinical diagnosis. Well defined elongate fascicles of slender spindle cells are arranged predominantly parallel to the skin surface in reticular

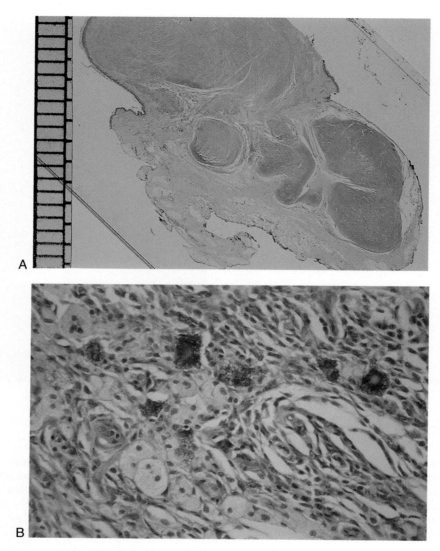

Fig. 17-61. Cutaneous fibrous histiocytoma. **(A)** A polypoid and multinodular dermal tumor with satellite-like foci is composed of **(B)** fibroblasts, foamy cells, and hemosiderin-laden multinucleate giant cells.

dermis (Fig. 17-62). In contrast to dermatofibroma, the spindle cells are factor XIIIa negative. Plaque-stage dermatofibrosarcoma protuberans is more basophilic under low power due to cellular crowding, and generally actin negative. Diffuse neurofibroma lacks parallel orientation of cells and is S-100 positive. By electron microscopy, myofibroblasts and undifferentiated mesenchymal cells accompany fibroblasts in dermatomyofibroma. Conservative excision is curative.

Dermatofibrosarcoma Protuberans

Dermatofibrosarcoma protuberans is a low grade, highly infiltrative dermal sarcoma that arises in the third and fourth decades and has a slight male predilection.[857–861] It is more likely to occur on the chest, back, and thighs. Initially firm, skin colored plaques eventually become lobulated, exophytic nodules associated with red-blue coloration of the overlying epidermis. The

tumor tends to be much larger than a dermatofibroma or cutaneous fibrous histiocytoma, but size alone is not an absolute criterion. Ulceration may occur.

Microscopically this asymmetric, expansile, infiltrating cellular tumor tends to fill dermis, usually with extension into the underlying subcutaneous fat. The proliferating cells have very little variation in nuclear size and contour, but this is obscured by the nuclei being discoid rather than spindle shaped (Fig. 17-63). Therefore, they appear pale and round or, alternatively, dark and ellipsoidal, depending on orientation relative to section plane. A tight, repetitive pinwheel-like storiform growth pattern is better appreciated with a reticulin stain. Unlike dermatofibroma, there is no conspicuous interspersed mature collagen. Cells with foamy cytoplasm, hemosiderin-laden macrophages, and multinucleated giant cells should be absent or inconspicuous. Unlike normal dermal dendrocytes and the cells of dermatofibroma, factor XIIIa is negative. The mode of

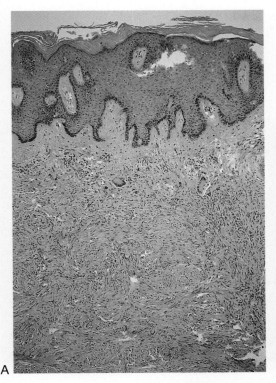
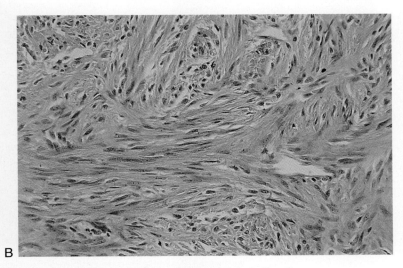

Fig. 17-62. Dermatomyofibroma. **(A)** Epidermal hyperplasia **(B)** overlies fascicles of slender spindle cells with more eosinophilic cytoplasm than the cells of dermatofibroma.

infiltration of subcutaneous fat is distinctive. Diffuse infiltration around single adipocytes creates a pattern variously called the "honeycomb" or "sandwich sign" (Fig. 17-63C). Mitotic figures are infrequent and atypical mitoses may be seen. Multinucleated tumor cells or necrosis are rare. Diagnosis by fine needle aspiration is possible.[862]

Immunostaining of conventional DFSP finds vimentin and CD34[830] positive, whereas S-100, desmin, and muscle-specific actin are negative.[827,863,864] As previously mentioned, CD34 is a useful discriminant between DFSP (88 percent positive)[829] and dermatofibroma (negative in most studies). Thirty percent recur locally after simple excision. Metastases are uncommon but more likely with a high mitotic rate (>8/hpf) and significant fibrosarcomatous areas.

Variants of DFSP include the myxoid (alcian blue-positive),[865] fibrosarcomatous,[866,867] or "dedifferentiated" (CD34–),[868,869] plaque-like (CD34+), DFSP with giant cell fibroblastoma-like differentiation, granular cell,[870] atrophic,[871] and pigmented (Bednar) types. Plaque-like DFSP has dermal and subcutaneous tumor cell bands oriented parallel to the epidermis. DFSP and giant cell fibroblastoma (GCF) predominate in different age groups, but there are cases of DFSP that contain areas that closely resemble GCF.[872] Some cases of GCF have recurred as[873] or transformed into[874,875] DFSP. It has been proposed that GCF is a juvenile form of DFSP.[876] Occasionally, DFSP will evolve toward the pattern of malignant fibrous histiocytoma.[869] The Bednar tumor[877] has small deposits of melanin

pigment in occasional tumor cells that accept Fontana-Masson stain, causing confusion with primary spindle cell melanocytic tumors; however, most cells are negative for S-100 protein. Only about 60 cases of Bednar tumor have been reported.[878] Some have developed fibrosarcomatous areas and metastasized.[879]

Atypical Fibroxanthoma

Atypical fibroxanthoma (AFX)[657,880–887] should be used to denote a pleomorphic mesenchymal predominantly dermal tumor no more than 2 cm in diameter (Fig. 17-64A), usually occurring on the actinic-damaged skin of elderly persons or occasionally on the trunk or extremities of younger individuals. Similar tumors have been reported at sites of irradiation.[888] Epidermis will be elevated, effaced, and possibly attenuated to the point of ulceration by an extremely pleomorphic and plump spindle cell proliferation. The bizarre, haphazardly arranged tumor cells have copious eosinophilic cytoplasm that may be vacuolated by neutral fat and ground substance-like mucopolysaccharide. Large irregular, extremely hyperchromatic nuclei feature multipolar (Fig. 17-64B) and asymmetric mitoses. The spindle cell variant of AFX lacks pleomorphism, has a brisk mitotic rate, traps adnexal structures, and frequently has a prominent collarette of compressed adnexal epithelium.[889] An inflammatory infiltrate and focal osteoid and osteoclast-like giant cells[890] may be found. The atypical cells of AFX form a nodule

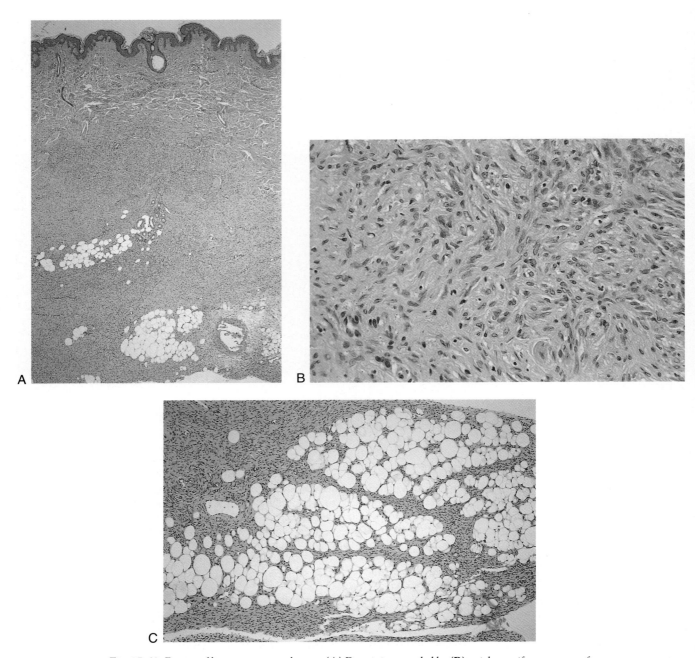

Fig. 17-63. Dermatofibrosarcoma protuberans. **(A)** Dermis is expanded by **(B)** a tight storiform pattern of stubby plump spindle cells **(C)** demonstrating characteristic "honeycomb-like" infiltration of subcutaneous fat. (Compare to Fig. 17-60D). (Courtesy of Jeffery Warner.)

that will appear independent from epidermal keratinocytes and melanocytes and this alone should point away from considerations of squamous cell carcinoma and melanoma. Despite bizarre nuclear pleomorphism, most of these neoplasms are diploid on flow cytometry.[885] Immunohistochemistry is helpful in the further distinction of AFX from anaplastic spindle cell squamous cell carcinoma and spindle cell melanoma. AFX is variably positive for alpha-1-antichymotrypsin and negative for S-100 protein (melanomas are positive) and negative for

cytokeratin (carcinomas are variably positive), EMA, and desmin. CD68 cannot be used as a diagnostic criterion for tumors with malignant fibrous histiocytoma pattern, nor does it lend any weight to the putative histiocytic origin of these tumors because it is expected in any cells exhibiting phagolysosomes or lysosome-like granules indicating phagocytosis or autophagy.[891] Alpha-1-antitrypsin, alpha-1-antichymotrypsin, cathepsin-B, and factor XIIIa (focal) may be positive.

Clear cell AFX exists as a variant and, even more than con-

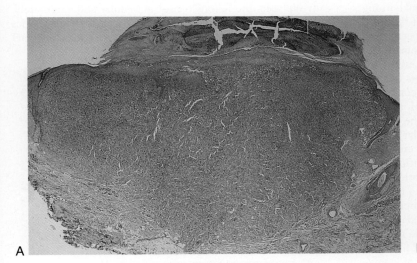

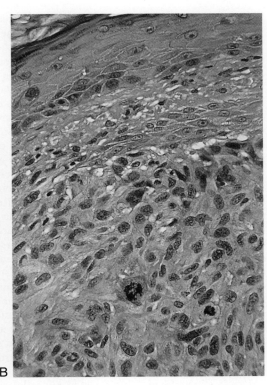

Fig. 17-64. Atypical fibroxanthoma. **(A)** An ulcerated dermal nodule consists of **(B)** large, plump, fusiform cells with bizarre mitotic figures.

ventional AFX, might be mistaken for renal cell carcinoma, a keratin-negative tumor that not uncommonly metastasizes to the skin especially of the scalp and that can be pleomorphic with spindle cells. Renal carcinoma tends to have a very vascular stroma, unlike AFX.

Small size and superficial location are likely the factors confirming an excellent prognosis. Metastases from AFX are exceptional,[892,893] but complete excision is desirable to avoid local recurrences.[894] Currently, the term "superficial MFH" is often used synonymously for the skin lesion christened AFX by Helwig[895] in 1961. This is because AFX and pleomorphic MFH share an identical histologic picture. However, this practice ignores the guidelines of Headington et al[896] that the latter should be "large" (greater than 1 cm), the requirement of Silvis et al[897] that it be "centered in the deep dermis and invade the superficial subcutis," and of Enzinger and Weiss[898] that it display deep invasion, necrosis, or vascular invasion. These are the features that confer the risk of metastases. Therefore they seem valid criteria on which to assign a clinically relevant name to individual lesions. Use of the term *superficial MFH* without explanation for small dermal lesions can result in unnecessarily extensive surgery and radiation or chemotherapy often employed for MFH arising in deep soft tissues. Larger tumors with aggressive behavior manifest by extensive subcuticular involvement, penetration of fascia and muscle, necrosis, or vascular invasion have a definite risk of recurrence and metastases and warrant diagnosis as MFH.

Interestingly, objective evidence for the central role of ultra-

violet (UV) radiation in the development of AFX has recently been presented, involving mutations of cytosine bases in the p53 gene.[899] This is the first in vivo demonstration of solar UV-induced mutations in a human mesenchymal neoplasm and likely further distinguishes AFX from true MFH. The concept of the histiocytic nature of this group of tumors has as its cornerstone a dated tissue culture report that would not pass peer review today[900] and the biologic veracity of the term "malignant fibrous histiocytoma" has been increasingly challenged of late.

Neural Tumors

Neural Hyperplasias

Traumatic neuromas[901,902] are tangles of nerve twigs in accentuated fibrous tissue creating firm nodules at sites of previous trauma to peripheral nerves. These disorganized wayward redundant regenerative attempts may be associated with localized pain and anesthesia. *Morton's neuroma*[903–906] is a misnomer used to describe this painful pedal neuralgia that most commonly appears as a benign enlargement of the third common digital branch of the medial plantar nerve located between, and often distal to, the third and fourth metatarsal heads. Ironically this entity was named after T.G. Morton of Philadelphia, who thought that it occurred about the fourth metatarsophalangeal articulation because of irritation from its fibular osseous neighbor.[907] The distal third intermetatarsal space is the most common location of Morton's neuroma. An intermetatarsal neuroma can also occur in other spaces, usually the second and rarely the first or fourth. It is found more frequently in women than in men, with ages ranging from 18 to 60 years of age. However, it is most commonly diagnosed between the fourth and fifth decades. The patient is likely to be overweight. Transient stretching and crushing are probably etiologic. The pain classically presents as a paroxysmal burning sensation. It is most often localized to the region of the third and fourth plantar metatarsal heads. A resected specimen is fusiform. Morton's neuroma is neither a true neuroma nor a neoplasm. The term "neuroma" refers only to tumorous nodules that are formed by hyperplasia of both neurities (axons) and of sheath (Schwann) cells. Morton's neuroma consists of endoneural and neural edema; perineural, epineural, and endoneural fibrosis and hypertrophy; hyalinization of the walls of endoneural blood vessels; subintimal and perivascular fibrosis that may lead to occlusion of local blood vessels; mucinous changes endoneurally and perineurally; demyelination with axonal loss; and Renaut body (hyalin granule) formation, usually in a subperineural location. Renaut bodies are a nonspecific response to nerve trauma, particularly to compression. More specific to Morton's neuroma are endoneural edema and demyelination. An intermetatarsal bursa with sterile reactive changes such as mural vascular prominence and/or fibrinous surface exudate is frequently associated, but cellular inflammation is not expected.

Neurofibroma and Schwannoma

Neurofibromas and schwannomas (neurilemomas) are benign proliferations of perineural supporting cells (i.e., Schwann cells). Neurofibromas develop from nerves and can affect any cutaneous surface.[908,909] The age range is wide. They appear as skin-colored, soft papules, nodules, or pedunculated tumors commonly mistaken for melanocytic nevi or acrochordons. They are most often solitary and unassociated with systemic disease. A multitude of lesions over much of the body surface can develop in neurofibromatosis, type I (von Recklinghausen's disease). Schwannomas (neurilemomas) affect middle-aged adults, generally on the skin of the head, neck, and extremities. They are generally solitary and painless, creating flesh-colored papules and nodules. (See Ch. 59 for more discussion.)

Neurofibromas appear microscopically as well defined, nonencapsulated, often exophytic dermal neoplasms formed of small, variably cellular aggregates of benign-appearing spindle cells randomly oriented or in parallel, embedded within a loose fibrillary, eosinophilic matrix (Fig. 17-65A). Acid mucopolysaccharide in the background accounts for loose structure and, if excessive, confers a myxoid quality and translucency to the gross specimen. Tumor cells have bland nuclear chromatin patterns, often wavy nuclear contour, and are devoid of mitotic activity. Unlike neurotized nevi, axons forming nerve twigs pass through the spindle cell component composed mostly of Schwann cells. Neurofibromas contain numerous mast cells also seen in heavily neurotized nevi but serving as a useful distinction from dermatofibromas. Plexiform neurofibromas that connote von Recklinghausen neurofibromatosis are

recognized as cellular and hypertrophied nerve trunks that ramify like tentacles within the reticular dermis. The *cellular (atypical) neurofibroma* features pleomorphic cellularity but without mitoses.

Schwannomas (also known as neurilemomas, neurinomas, and neurolemomas) are encapsulated tumors of the dermis that often extend into or primarily arise in the subcutis. They may be plexiform and simulate plexiform neurofibroma.[910] Classically biphasic, the lesions consist of cellular and, alternately, loose myxoid zones of spindle cells with nuclear characteristics similar to those of neurofibromas. In Antoni type A (cellular)

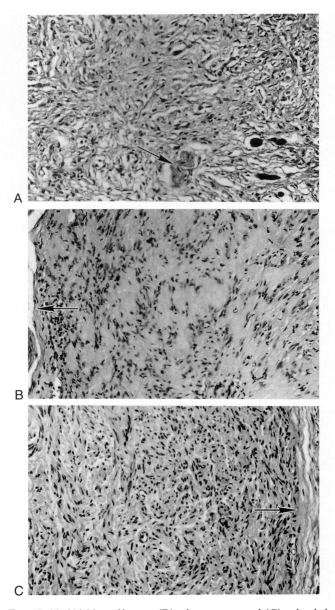

Fig. 17-65. (A) Neurofibroma, (B) schwannoma, and (C) palisaded encapsulated neuroma. Note nerve fiber within the spindle cell matrix of neurofibroma (Fig. A, arrow), and the well defined peripheral borders of schwannoma and palisaded encapsulated neuroma (Fig. B & C, arrows).

areas, spindle cell nuclei may align in parallel. Two parallel rows of these palisaded nuclei constitute a Verocay body (Fig. 17-65B). Zones of more randomly oriented spindle cells within an abundant mucinous background constitute Antoni B areas. In older persistent lesions, isolated nuclei may become large and dark staining but no mitoses are found, unlike those with malignant change.[911] This has become popularized as "ancient change." More densely cellular lesions with pleomorphism but few if any mitoses are termed cellular schwannomas.[912] Origin from a nerve may be demonstrated in any of these variants.

Palisaded Encapsulated Neuroma

Palisaded encapsulated neuroma is a distinctive clinicopathologic entity that favors the mucocutaneous junctions of facial skin of middle-aged patients without gender predilection.[913–915] They form solitary, painless skin-colored papulonodules often mistaken for cysts. Low magnification of the section shows an encapsulated, nodular tumor composed of spindle cells within the dermis. Constituent uniform benign-appearing spindle cells are usually arranged in coalescent fascicles[916] and typically show evidence of poorly formed palisaded aggregates (Fig. 17-65C). Mitoses and necrosis are absent. Unmyelinated axons, unlike neurofibromas and neurilemomas, comprise at least half the volume, balancing the Schwann cell and fibroblastic elements.

An S-100 reaction separates this from other well demarcated benign spindle cell tumors such as leiomyomas. A Bodian stain will bring out the high concentration of axons, which argues against other well circumscribed benign neural lesions of the dermis (e.g., neurilemoma).

Multiple Mucosal Neuromas

Pink pedunculated nodules developing in early childhood or present at birth on all accessible mucosal surfaces (oral mucosa, lips, tongue, conjunctivae) have a strong association with medullary carcinoma of the thyroid and pheochromocytoma.[917,918] The fully expressed syndrome is variously designated multiple endocrine neoplasia (MEN) IIb or III and features a marfanoid somatotype with muscle wasting. Hypertrophied mucosal nerves may resemble palisaded encapsulated neuromas. Focal macular pigmentations may be present. Deletions on chromosome 20p are described.[919]

Granular Cell Tumor

Granular cell tumor is most common in middle-aged women and favors location on the extremities and tongue.[920] Ten percent of patients have multiple neoplasms. These painless, skin-colored, nondescript nodules grow slowly and are often present for some time before histologic diagnosis. Overlying verrucous mucosal thickening or epidermal pseudoepitheliomatous hyperplasia may be confused with invasive squamous cell carcinoma, particularly in superficial samples.

These are poorly demarcated, lobulated collections of infiltrating plump, rounded cells with small, eccentrically located round nuclei. The characteristic granular pink cytoplasm has coarse and fine granules that ultrastructurally are lysosomes and laminated membranous aggregates similar to myelin bodies (Fig. 17-66). The larger PAS-positive granules are termed *an-*

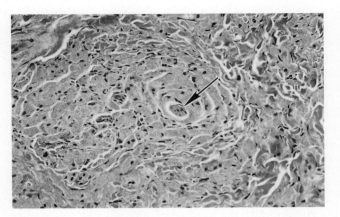

Fig. 17-66. Granular cell tumor showing plump cells with finely granular cytoplasm seemingly arising within the perineural region that surrounds a small dermal nerve twig (arrow).

gulate bodies. Continuity with nerves, especially at the periphery, combines with S-100 immunoreactivity to indicate these are Schwann cells,[921] perhaps with an enzymatic deficiency leading to lipid constipation. Granular cells should not be mistaken for xanthoma cells, which have finely vacuolated rather than granular cytoplasm. Mitoses are not expected. Malignant variants are controversial.[922]

The *plexiform granular cell tumor*[923] presents as a plaque on extremities, more often in children than adults. Fascicles of plump cells are prominently aggregated around nerve bundles in the dermis and subcutis. Sarcoidosis and leprosy are ruled out by S-100 positivity. Pseudoepitheliomatous hyperplasia is not present with this variant. Such a skin tumor with plexiform pattern raises the differential of neurofibroma,[924] neurilemoma,[925,926] palisaded encapsulated neuroma, ossifying plexiform tumor,[927] plexiform xanthoma,[928] plexiform xanthomatous tumor,[929] plexiform spindle cell nevus (deep penetrating nevus), and plexiform fibrohistiocytic tumor (see below).

Malignant Peripheral Nerve Sheath Tumor

Malignant peripheral nerve sheath tumor (MPNST) is a term now popularized for sarcomas previously called malignant schwannoma and neurofibrosarcoma.[930] In addition to their propensity to arise in type I neurofibromatosis patients,[931] they also occur sporadically. MPNST is discussed in more detail in Chapter 59. EMA positivity in as many as 42 percent[932] reflects a perineural cell element.[933] S-100 protein can be identified in 50 to 70 percent of MPNST. Glial fibrillary acidic protein (GFAP) is an intermediate filament that has been shown to be aberrantly expressed by peripheral Schwann cells, nerve sheath tumors, and chondroid tissue. HMB 45 stains rare spindle and epithelioid MPNSTs.[934,935]

Neuroendocrine Carcinoma

Neuroendocrine carcinoma is also known as *trabecular carcinoma* because of growth pattern and as *Merkel cell carcinoma*.[936–941]

This is primarily a tumor of the elderly, affecting men and women equally. The tumor cells duplicate many features of Merkel cells, which normally inhabit the epidermal basal cell layer in low numbers. However, tumor location, with more than half in the head and neck and the remainder on the extremities, buttocks, and other sites, is unlike the predominant palm, digit, and dorsal foot location of normal Merkel cells. Patients generally describe a lesion enlarging within several months but occasional tumors have been present a couple of years at initial presentation. They are pink to red and between 0.5 and 9.0 cm, appearing as a raised, tender, nodular tumor. Ulceration and superficial hemorrhage are frequent. If not mistaken for a boil or blood blister, the clinical differential may include hemangioma, lymphoma, or angiosarcoma.

Histologically, the small neoplastic cells may appear to be lymphocytes because of round, dark-staining nuclei and extremely scant cytoplasm. Bouin's fixation enhances argyrophilia with the Grimelius reaction. These asymmetric tumors have an infiltrative border at the periphery. Most have a nodular or diffuse cellular arrangement enhancing the mimicry of lymphoma. A minority have a partial or total nested, cordforming, or trabecular pattern. Most tumors are large enough to extend into subcutaneous fat (Fig. 17-67A). The round to slightly ovoid nuclei often have a central clearing similar to unbuffered formalin artifact (Fig. 17-67B). Nucleoli are absent or inconspicuous. Frequent mitotic activity and frequent individual cell and zonal necrosis are conspicuous malignant features. A few show epidermotrophic pagetoid invasion of epidermis.[942] There may be an associated in situ or invasive squamous cell carcinoma with or without eccrine or basal cell features; this suggests multidirectional ectodermal differentiation.[943–945]

Distinctive ultrastructural characteristics are dense-core neurosecretory granules between 80 and 200 nm, as in normal Merkel cells, and intercellular junctions, unlike lymphoma. Aggregated bundles of intermediate microfilaments in juxtanuclear location correlate with "button-like" or "dot-like" paranuclear positivity for cytokeratin (Fig. 17-67C), not found in nonendocrine small cell carcinomas[482] and only rarely in superficial primitive neuroectodermal tumors (neuroblastoma).[946] The keratin is predominantly type 20.[947] Other immunohistochemical parameters are positivity for neuron-specific enolase and quite likely also with epithelial membrane antigen, chromogranin A,[948] and also synaptophysin and neuropeptides such as bombesin. No reactivity is usually found for S-100, glial fibrillary acidic protein, actin, or vimentin. Focal reactivity may be found for chromogranin, vasoactive intestinal peptide, pancreatic polypeptide, calcitonin, substance P, somatostatin, adrenocorticotropic hormone, and other peptide hormones. A negative CEA reaction is expected, whereas 50 percent of secondary small cell carcinomas are positive for CEA.[482]

The combination of clinical setting (isolated lesion in a nonsmoker) and the histologic, immunohistochemical,[949] and ultrastructural details[950] mentioned above will separate neuroendocrine carcinomas from lymphoma, small cell melanoma variants, and metastatic neuroblastoma or small cell carcinoma from extracutaneous sites.

Merkel cell carcinomas have a marked tendency for recurrence after primary excision, which therefore should be exten-

sive. More than half have lymph node metastases at diagnosis or within several years after, with 30 to 40 percent showing distant metastases. Associated ectopic endocrinopathy such as elevated serum adrenocorticotropic hormone or calcitonin is very rare, in contrast to small cell undifferentiated carcinoma of the lung.

Neurothekeoma (Nerve Sheath Myxoma, Lobular Neuromyxoma, Perineural Myxoma, Pacinian Neurofibroma)

Neurothekeoma is a somewhat controversial tumor that has phenotypic features of supportive perineural cells.[951–955] It can arise at any age, but most patients are young and female. Most are solitary and on the skin of the face, shoulders, or upper extremities. They are skin-colored to erythematous soft nodules from 0.5 to 2 cm that grow slowly as well demarcated, lobulated tumors with fibrous septations that expand mid-dermis, sparing a grenz zone. Some are subcutaneous but only very rarely are they in deep soft tissue. At one end of this spectrum, neuroid spindle cells with vesicular nuclei and single small nucleoli are separated by acid mucopolysaccharide, with lobulation defined by fibrous septa (*nerve sheath myxoma*).[956–958] At the other end is *cellular neurothekeoma*, composed of bundles of epithelioid cells in scant myxoid stroma, and with less plexiform compartmentalization.[959] Epithelioid tumor cells with prominent eosinophilic cytoplasm may be few or predominate and feature nuclear irregularity, moderate size variation, hyperchromasia, and mitotic activity. Necrosis and invasive destruction of dermis or appendages are not found. It is suspected that over time, lesions acquire more mucopolysaccharide and lose their epithelioid component. Focal pleomorphism, a few giant cells, and normal mitotic figures are frequently seen. Calcification[960] as well as metaplastic osteoid and chondroid are possible. Unlike melanocytes, the epithelioid cells of cellular neurothekeoma do not show S-100 protein[959] and contain no melanin. Unlike melanocytic nevi, there is no maturation or junctional component. HMB 45 is negative. NK 1-C3, a melanocyte marker, was diffusely positive in a series in which three cases also had SMA (but not desmin) positivity, leading to the suggestion that cellular neurothekeomas are actually epithelioid pilar smooth muscle lesions.[961] In spite of atypia, this benign lesion only rarely recurs.

Tumors of Adipose Tissue

Lipomatous Hamartomas

Nevus lipomatosus superficialis[962–964] consists of multiple, brown-yellow, coalescent nodules that form a cerebriform skin surface along the skin folds of the flank, buttocks, and upper portion of the posterior thigh. Other sites such as thorax or abdomen are rarely affected. These are congenital hamartomas, although they may not become apparent until early adulthood. Rather than being collagenous, the lower and mid-dermis are filled with mature fat. The epidermis may be thrown into a verrucous or bosselated pattern.

The term *pedunculated lipofibroma* was proposed by Mehregan

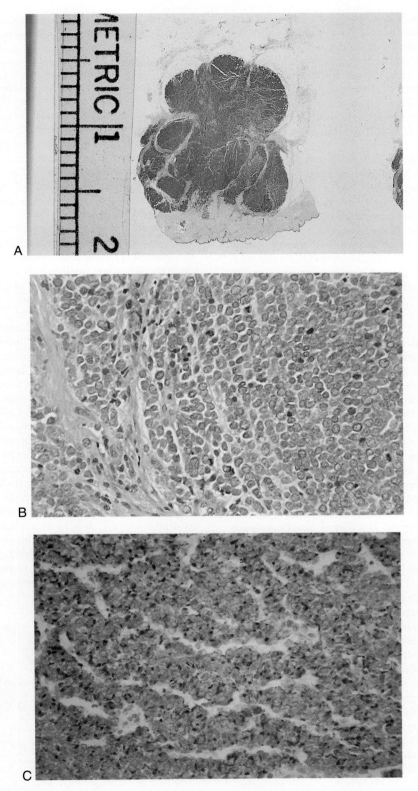

Fig. 17-67. Neuroendocrine (Merkel cell) carcinoma of the skin. (A) A lobulated tumor expands from dermis into subcutaneous fat. (B) Malignant cells with characteristic pale nuclei, single cell necrosis, and mitotic activity have a vague trabecular pattern. (C) Dot-like positivity for keratin is characteristic.

et al[965] for lesions previously described as solitary nevus lipomatosus cutaneous superficialis, or solitary lipofibroma.[966] Age of onset is predominantly after the third decade. The lesions are most common on buttock and upper thigh, but also occur on the back, shoulder, knee, neck, and ear. In the multiple lesion clinical form, lesions are present at birth or develop in the first three decades of life. Distribution is usually linear or along the lines of skin folds. The site of predilection is the pelvic girdle, most commonly the buttock, sacral, and coccygeal regions, and upper thigh.

Acrochordons tend to be smaller, predilect intertriginous areas, and do not entrap adnexal structures. The mature adipocytes in nevus lipomatosus have been variously attributed to the mature degenerative changes in the dermal collagen and elastic tissue, displacement of subcutaneous adipose tissue into the dermis, and differentiating lipoblasts originating from the dermal blood vessels. Ultrastructural studies[967] note the close proximity of the fat cells to the vasculature and the differentiation of immature lipoblasts through a multivesicular stage into mature fat cells as in fetal adipogenesis.

Lipoma

Lipomas are common neoplasms of subcutaneous fat, frequently encountered by dermatopathologists.[963] Rare and exotic subtypes are numerous. In the space allowed, only the more commonly encountered variants can be mentioned. For additional information, Chapter 18 can be consulted.

Ordinary lipomas are soft, nodular tumors that occur in adults. They are often confused with cysts or other subcutaneous tumors. *Myolipomas* of soft tissue are rarely subcutaneous.[969] *Cutaneous angiomyolipoma* is rare, occurring mainly in men in their 50s, and presenting as a single painless subcutaneous nodule on an extremity.[970] Unlike the better known HMB 45-positive[971,972] renal tumor with the same name, they are independent of tuberous sclerosis and pulmonary lymphangiomyomatosis. The *adenolipoma* is a dermal or subcutaneous variant of the common lipoma containing incorporated sweat glands.[973]

In two rare conditions, multiple lipomas composed of mature fat cells arise in adult life. They are adiposis dolorosa or Dercum's disease, in which there are tender circumscribed or diffuse fatty deposits,[974] and benign symmetric lipomatosis, which is characterized by the gradual development of many large, coalescent, asymptomatic lipomas, mainly on the trunk and arms and beginning in early adulthood.[975] In some instances, referred to as Madelung's disease, the lipomas are present especially in the region of the neck in a "horse-collar" distribution.[976] Occasionally, benign symmetric lipomatosis is inherited as an autosomal dominant trait.

By definition, lipomas contain mature adipocytes as a principal component. They tend to be surrounded by a thin connective tissue capsule and are composed often entirely of normal fat cells that are indistinguishable from the fat cells in the subcutaneous tissue. Occasional "hibernoma-like" cells or multivesicular cells around foci of necrosis should not be misinterpreted as malignant lipoblasts. Substantial basophilic mucopolysaccharide may fill regions of the tumor and recommends the term *myxolipoma*. Focal chondroid and/or osteoid

production have no significance other than underscoring the common ancestry of functional mesenchymal cells.

Angiolipoma

Angiolipomas usually occur as encapsulated subcutaneous lesions and may be mistaken for cysts.[977,978] As a rule, they arise in young adults. The forearm is the single most common location for this tumor, which is more often multifocal than solitary. Clinically, they resemble ordinary lipomas except for their greater tendency to be multiple and to be tender or painful.

Inapparent at the gross level, angiolipomas show sharp encapsulation, numerous small caliber vascular channels containing characteristic microthrombi, and variable amounts of mature adipose tissue (Fig. 17-68). These thrombi are well demonstrated by phosphotungstic acid-hematoxylin staining,[978] and are likely artifacts of removal because they show no organization. The degree of vascularity is quite variable, ranging from only a few small angiomatous foci to lesions with a predominance of dense vascular and stromal tissue. The angiomatous foci are composed in part of well formed, dilated capillaries engorged with erythrocytes. Other capillaries appear tortuous and have poorly formed lumina and prominent proliferation of pericytes. Perivascular fibrosis may be prominent.

By way of differential diagnosis, angiolipomas with prominent perithelial fibrocytes may bring to mind spindle cell lipoma, which, however, lacks the conspicuous capillary channels with fibrin thrombi. Hybrid lesions with mixed features of both entities may be encountered. Cellular angiolipomas composed almost entirely of vascular channels and prominent spindle cells and pericytes are sometimes confused with Kaposi's sarcoma, angiosarcoma, or solid tumors such as those of smooth muscle. Subcutaneous position, encapsulation, septation, small size, diminutive nonatypical endothelial cells, microthrombi, some admixed mature fat, and clinical presentation in healthy individuals help to exclude a malignant diagnosis.[979] *Nodular-cystic fat necrosis*[980] is a non-neoplastic condition in which necrotic fat lobules become palpably firm with fibrous encapsulation and detach, becoming movable, perhaps over substantial distances, beneath the skin. Due to regional reactive vascular prominence, it is thought that some prior examples have been included in series of angiolipoma.[981]

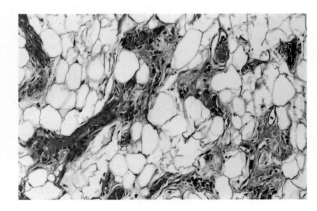

Fig. 17-68. Angiolipoma consisting of mature adipose tissue through which course anastomosing vessels containing microthrombi.

The term infiltrating angiolipoma as formerly used by Dionne and Seemayer[982] and Puig et al[983] is synonymous with intramuscular angioma,[984] which usually has abundant mature fat between the vascular channels; by convention, this volumetrically predominant fat is not acknowledged in the name *intramuscular hemangioma*. Within the stromal fat supporting arterial, capillary, and venous channels are splayed skeletal muscle fibers. This fatty vascular tumor may be encountered in superficial muscles of the face and neck, and has an approximate 20 percent local regrowth rate.

Hibernoma

Hibernoma is a benign, moderately firm, solitary, subcutaneous tan or red-brown tumor generally measuring between 3 and 12 cm in diameter, but occasionally larger.[985,986] Although usually asymptomatic, it is occasionally tender. Hibernomas may appear in childhood and slowly increase in size,[987] but more commonly they arise in adulthood. This rare tumor arises most frequently in the subcutis of the shoulder girdle, posterior neck, and axilla, but not all hibernomas occur at sites where brown fat is normally located, such as the abdomen. Clinically hibernomas are indistinguishable from lipomas and similarly have no tendency to recur locally.

Histologic examination reveals that the tumor is divided into numerous lobules by well vascularized connective tissue. In contrast to ordinary lipoma of white fat, the highly vascular nature of the tumor is readily apparent in most sections. The tumor cells are round to polygonal and are closely apposed to one another within the lobules.[987] Small rounded cells with finely granular eosinophilic cytoplasm are filled with mitochondria. Larger multivacuolated (xanthomatous) fat cells are called "mulberry cells"; these predominate but, as vacuoles merge, larger univacuolated fat cells appear. The incomplete modulation of the mulberry cells may be due to underdeveloped enzyme systems.[988]

Hibernomas are to be distinguished from granular cell tumors, which have no lipid vacuoles, and also certain forms of round cell liposarcoma, which usually contain diagnostic multivacuolar eosinophilic lipoblasts.

Spindle Cell Lipoma

Spindle cell lipoma occurs on the posterior neck and shoulders of middle-aged men.[989,990] This well circumscribed admixture of mature adipocytes and uniform, collagen-forming spindle cells has a slightly mucinous matrix in which mast cells are scattered. CD34 strongly labels most cells in spindle cell lipoma and accentuates their highly dendritic morphology. It should not be confused with liposarcomas, especially the mitotically active spindle cell liposarcoma, because it is easily cured by local excision.

Other variants of lipoma are uncommonly encoutered in the skin (see Ch. 18).

Lipoblastoma and Lipoblastomatosis

Lipoblastoma is an uncommon solitary circumscribed variant of lipoma arising in the subcutaneous fat between the time of birth and 7 years of age.[991–993] The slowly growing tumor may reach considerable size. About 70 percent occur in limbs, mostly in the lower extremities.[994]

Of two basic forms, *lipoblastoma* is relatively superficial and encapsulated.[993] *Lipoblastomatosis* is deeply situated, poorly circumscribed, and tends to grow into the surrounding tissue spaces and musculature.[988] Both commonly present as a painless nodule or mass, affecting boys twice as frequently as girls. Peripheral immature lipoblasts with fat vacuoles of various size and central mature fat cells containing a single, large fat vacuole are characteristic whether the tumor is deeply or superficially situated. The size of the lipoblasts varies. Most of them contain a single vacuole that is variable in size but smaller than that found in mature fat cells. This vacuole displaces the nucleus against the cytoplasmic membrane.[988] Nonvacuolated cells that are spindle shaped or stellate are seen in the mucinous stroma. Fibrous septa partition lobules in the circumscribed form.

Only the age of the patient, abundance of lipoblasts, absence of atypical mitoses,[995] and a sometimes subtle lobularity afford distinction from liposarcoma, especially the myxoid type.[996] Despite the cellular immaturity, prognosis is excellent after simple excision for lipoblastoma and wide local excision for diffuse lipoblastomatosis. Cellular maturation has been described in serial biopsies over time.

Liposarcoma

Although *liposarcomas* constitute 15 to 20 percent of all soft tissue sarcomas, they only rarely arise in the subcutaneous fat.[997,998] Most commonly, they originate in the intermuscular fascial planes, with a special predilection for the thighs. From a fascial plane, they extend to the subcutaneous tissue. Liposarcomas arise de novo and for practical purposes do not develop from lipomas. The average age of onset is 50 years. Apparent gross circumscription of the lesion may offer false hope of eradication by simply shelling out the tumor. In reality, liposarcomas extend microscopic pseudopod-like extensions that commonly insinuate between fascial planes. Occasionally, small satellite nodules become separated from the lobulated sarcomatous mass, leading to an erroneous impression of multicentricity.

The cells of liposarcoma bear a close resemblance to different stages in the development of fat and are found in variable proportions as a function of histologic subtype, but show a much greater individual variability. Four types of liposarcoma are generally recognized, with differing prognosis[999]: (1) well differentiated lipoma-like, (2) well differentiated and poorly differentiated myxoid, (3) round cell, and (4) pleomorphic liposarcoma.

There are three closely related *subtypes of well differentiated liposarcoma*: (1) well differentiated "lipoma-like," (2) well differentiated inflammatory, and (3) well differentiated sclerosing liposarcoma. Well differentiated liposarcomas are low grade and may regrow locally but do not metastasize. Therefore, the term *atypical lipoma* has been introduced for the subcutaneous form of well differentiated liposarcoma. This is the form of liposarcoma most likely to be biopsied by dermatologists.

Atypical lipomas in subcutis rarely recur and are usually cured by local excision. Because of this benign course Evans[1000] has suggested an even less committal designation for this neoplasm, *atypical lipomatous tumor.* It has been recommended that this term be restricted to subcutaneous tumors, especially when of small size with minimal atypical changes.[1001] Atypical lipoma histologically features distended fat cells with slight variation in size and shape, with interspersed occasional lipoblasts. Broad fibrous septa containing cells with enlarged, hyperchromatic atypical nuclei are a characteristic feature. Complete excision with small margins of surrounding tissues may be adequate treatment. "Dedifferentiation" (outgrowth of a high grade sarcoma pattern in the initial specimen or recurrence) is extremely rare, in contrast to this event in retroperitoneal well differentiated liposarcoma.

The hallmark of all liposarcoma variants is the *lipoblast*. To designate a cell as a lipoblast, it must show the ability to synthesize and accumulate non-membrane-bound lipid in the cytoplasmic matrix. Acceptable malignant lipoblasts are quite variable in appearance, but their common morphologic denominator is well demarcated cytoplasmic lipid that displaces or indents one or more irregular hyperchromatic nuclei. The nucleus conforms to the contour of the lipid droplet, creating an apparent delicate scalloping of the nuclear membrane. Hyperchromaticity and variability from lipoblast to lipoblast support a malignant diagnosis. Benign fat necrosis, myxoid change in structural fat, lipogranuloma, lymphoma with signet ring changes, and carcinoma can contain vacuolated cells that mimic lipoblasts. Lesions such as pleomorphic lipoma and lipoblastoma illustrate that even unequivocal lipoblasts do not always signal malignant tumors. A lipid stain often aids in the diagnosis. The demonstration of neutral lipid in cells with special stains (e.g., Sudan black, oil red O) on frozen sections of tumor tissue is insufficient for a diagnosis of liposarcoma unless lipoblasts are also found. Many other mesenchymal tumors, especially after irradiation, and some carcinomas (e.g., of kidney and adrenal) routinely contain fat.

The main utility of immunohistochemistry in the diagnosis of liposarcoma is one of exclusion because no specific or useful immunohistochemical marker has been found for malignant fatty tumors.

Tumors of Bone

Osteoma Cutis

Most patients with extensive foci of ossification in the skin usually have *Albright's hereditary osteodystrophy* (pseudohypoparathyroidism type Ia and pseudopseudohypoparathyroidism). These patients have deficient end organ response to parathyroid hormone (PTH), with hypocalcemia, hyperphosphatemia, and elevated serum PTH. Cutaneous bone formation in 24 to 47 percent occurs as numerous widespread osteomas with a predilection for periarticular regions.[1002] This is in addition to phenotypic features including short stature and skeletal anomalies.

There are four groups of patients with osteoma cutis, with the osteomas focal or regional in all but the first group: (1) widespread osteomas since birth or early life, but without evidence of Albright's hereditary dystrophy[1003]; (2) a single, large, plaque-like osteoma present since birth either in the skin of the scalp or in the skin or subcutaneous tissue of an extremity[1004,1005]; (3) a single small osteoma arising in later life in various locations[1004] and in some instances showing transepidermal elimination of bony fragments; and (4) multiple miliary osteomas of the face of women.[1006]

Single small *dermal osteomas* are not uncommon incidental findings in the vicinity of basal cell carcinomas and older nevi. Primary osteoma cutis can be a syndrome component.[1007] The multiple miliary facial cases have been interpreted as metaplastic ossification within acne scars.[1008] However, the absence of acne vulgaris among the patients in the older age group and the presence in one case of miliary osteomas also in the scalp, where acne does not occur,[1009] raises the possibility that the acne vulgaris is coincidental.

In osteoma cutis, mature lamellar bone appears as an island (or continent) in dermal collagen. They tend to be round or oval and with time undergo central remodeling involving osteoclastic removal of bone substance and establishment of a minute marrow cavity. Plump flattened spindle or stellate cells around the surface may resemble periosteum and are functional osteoblasts slowly creating new osteoid. A minority of these persist to be included as resident osteocytes in the mineralized matrix. In situ hybridization techniques indicate that given appropriate stimulation, indigenous fibroblasts have the ability to modulate into osteoblastic cells, which have the same properties as osteoblasts, such as high alkaline phosphatase activity and a high expression of osteonectin.[1010]

Subungual Exostosis

Subungual exostoses are projections from terminal phalanges (Fig. 17-69) and are probably stimulated by local trauma or inflammation and may painfully elevate nail and periungual skin, perhaps ulcerating, to be mistaken for primary infection.[1011] Toe location is much more common than finger and first or second digits are favored. An adequate biopsy will show chondrometaplasia of parosteal soft tissue and even dermal fibroblasts, followed by enchondral ossification along the deeper aspect facing bone; by this process, the bony stalk is built out. Radiographic correlation provides confirmation of the histopathologic impression.[1012] By contrast, a phalangeal osteochondroma will take origin from the metaphyseal region rather than terminal phalangeal tuft.

Osteosarcoma Primary in Skin

Occasional reports establish the ability of a matrix-producing sarcoma to arise in dermis that resembles the primary osteosarcoma of bone.[1013] In suspected instances, careful exclusion of an occult bone sarcoma as by bone scan is imperative.

Rare Cutaneous Tumors with Mesenchymal Differentiation

Carcinosarcoma refers to the coexistence of a clear-cut carcinoma and sarcomatous elements intermingled in the same tumor[1014–1016] and also spindle cell squamous cell carcinomas with a sharp segregation between the epithelial and the vimentin-positive sarcoma-like components.[1014]

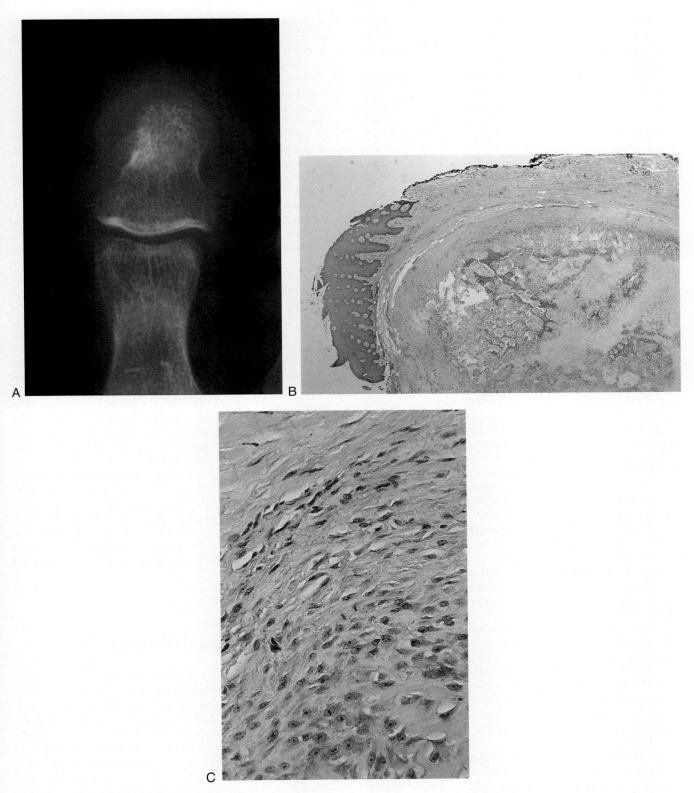

Fig. 17-69. Subungual exostosis. (A) A vague radiodensity extends from the left border of the terminal phalanx of the great toe. (B) A chondro-osseous proliferation elevating epidermis (C) extending from the phalanx appears to accrete at its growing surface through modulation of dermal fibroblasts into matrix-producing cells.

Regarding cutaneous cartilage tumor, although rare *dermal chondroid nodules* are reported,[1017] most cartilage tumors encountered by dermatologists will be *chondromas of soft tissue* and are likely to be in digits (see Ch. 18).

Ectopic meningothelial hamartoma[1018] is a predominantly occipital scalp or midline back lesion usually presenting in childhood or shortly after birth, with equal sex incidence. This is a more or less well circumscribed solitary nodule in skin and subcutaneous tissue commonly deemed clinically a cyst or hemangioma. There is no connection to underlying bone. There is no intracranial mass as is usually found with meningioma extending through calvarium.[1019] This deeply situated tumor consists of a disorganized mixture of medium-sized blood vessels, nerves, and variably prominent strands and nests of cuboidal, epithelioid eosinophilic cells in a pseudoinfiltrative pattern between collagen bundles. Artifactual clefts lined by epithelioid cells may bring to mind angiosarcoma but the cells are more uniform. Laminated mineralizations and reactive giant cells may be found. The cells are reactive for EMA and vimentin and have meningothelial features by electron microscopy. By contrast, *cutaneous heterotopic meningothelial nodules*,[1020] also known as type I cutaneous meningiomas,[1021,1022] are discrete small subcutaneous nodules only of meningothelial elements, commonly with psammoma bodies, collagen, and small nerves but without the other mesenchymal hamartomatous elements; an abnormality of spinal closure or cranial fusion may coexist.

Epithelioid sarcoma[1023–1025] is generally an acral malignant tumor of young adults. It may mimic granulomatous inflammation because of its festooned arrangement of cells superficially resembling plump histiocytes around necrobiotic centers. The fibroma-like variant lacks this necrosis and is instead composed of deceptively bland fibrohistiocytic and myoid cells arranged in a fibroma-like or dermatofibroma-like pattern with an affinity for bone involvement. The conventional and fibroma-like variants share clinical presentation as an indolent acral lesion, ultrastructural features,[1026,1027] and positivity for vimentin and low molecular weight keratin.[1028] Multiple recurrences and late metastases, possibly epidermotrophic, are typical, leading to fatality in 30 to 50 percent of all cases.

Giant cell fibroblastoma[1029] is a superficial rare fibroblastic tumor occurring mainly in very young male patients in various locations. Highly atypical cells are scattered in a hypocellular sclerotic background. Some regions may be quite cellular and have thick-walled vessels. Distinctive very wide spaces are incompletely lined by factor VIII-negative lesional fibroblasts. Frequently mistaken for sarcoma, this lesion should also be distinguished from a neurofibroma with ancient change, diffuse neurofibroma (paraneurofibroma), liposarcoma lacking a capillary network, and a peculiar angiosarcoma. Half of the patients experience local regrowth of this nonmetastasizing tumor that some[1030] regard as a childhood variant of dermatofibrosarcoma protuberans.

Perineurioma[1031–1033] is a rare, benign, soft tissue tumor mainly of women and is usually situated deeply in soft tissue. It resembles neurofibroma except for spindle cell arrangement in short fascicles, often in a storiform pattern. Its cells resemble those of the normal perineurium, in both conventional stains and by immunohistochemistry. The latter or ultrastructural

study are necessary for confident diagnosis. EMA but not S-100 protein can be demonstrated. By electron microscopy, the cells have elongate processes invested by basal laminal and have pinocytotic vesicles.

Plexiform fibrohistiocytic tumor[1034] is a lesion of children and young adults. Nondescript dermal nodules, frequently on an upper extremity, have two patterns that may be mixed: fibrohistiocytic, with osteoclast-like cells; and fibroblastic, resembling fibromatosis. Tumor nodules are circumscribed by short fascicles of fibroblastic cells that intersect slightly or extend randomly out into soft tissue creating a plexiform growth pattern; over one-third recur and local lymph node metastases are reported.[1035]

Regarding *solitary fibrous tumor of the skin*,[1036] dermis and subcutaneous tissues are among the extrapleural locations this distinctive spindle cell neoplasm can be located. Spindle cells with large, oval to spindled vesicular nuclei and moderate amounts of eosinophilic cytoplasm are between abundant bands of collagen. Mitoses are rare. There may be pattern overlap with synovial sarcoma, fibrosarcoma, schwannoma, and leiomyosarcoma, but keratin, EMA, S-100, and smooth muscle markers are not found. Collagen IV is demonstrable.

Superficial angiomyxoma[1037,1038] appears as an exophytic dermal lesion with variable subcutaneous involvement. It is a poorly circumscribed tumor with lobular outline. Similar to its better known counterpart in the pelvic retroperitoneum, it is extensively myxomatous with a network of numerous small blood vessels. Stellate or bipolar cells and muciphages populate the matrix with or without epithelial elements. Its tendency for local recurrence is substantial, especially with epithelium. Consideration should be given to the presence of a systemic syndrome (Charney's, NAME, LAMB).

Superficial malignant fibrous histiocytoma as mentioned above is a term applied to cutaneous and subcutaneous sarcomas larger than AFX and with a tendency to involve deeper structures. A trend toward revised nomenclature for tumors previously regarded as variants of MFH (itself formerly called "malignant fibroxanthoma" or "fibroxanthosarcoma") has begun with a preference for "myxofibrosarcoma" rather than myxoid MFH.[1039]

METASTATIC TUMORS TO SKIN

Cutaneous metastases occur in up to 9 percent of all cancer patients.[1040–1045] The frequencies of various tumor types in metastatic skin disease parallels the specific solid tumor incidence in each sex.[1045] A skin lesion as the harbinger of an occult malignant neoplasm is an opportunity to detect a potentially treatable cancer before other evidence of it is present, to modify therapy as appropriate to the tumor stage, or possibly to use the cutaneous lesion as a source of easily accessible tumor cells for specific therapy.[1040] This situation is more likely in males because of their higher frequency of lung and renal cancers, which invade blood vessels early on. Overall, breast carcinoma is the most frequent in women, accounting for approximately two-thirds of all metastases, followed by colon, melanoma, lung, ovaries, and sarcoma and others. In men, lung cancer is the most common primary, accounting for about one-fourth of all cases of cutaneous metastasis, followed by colon cancer; melanoma; oropharyngeal, renal, and gastric carcinomas; sarcoma; and others. It is reported that skin metastases tend to be close to the site of the primary tumor, for example, chest with lung cancer, abdominal wall with gastrointestinal primaries, and lower back with renal carcinomas.[1046] Skin involvement by lymphoma/leukemia appears in about 7 percent of cases and was discussed previously in this chapter.

Cutaneous involvement by cancer can occur by direct extension from the primary tumor or by local or distant metastasis. Metastatic cancer clearly does not localize in random fashion, because in 75 percent of men the sites are head, neck, anterior chest, and abdomen, together accounting for only 25 percent of the body surface.[1046] In women, 75 percent are on the anterior chest and abdomen, together comprising less than 20 percent of the skin surface. The abdominal wall is the single most common site for appearance of a metastasis from an unknown primary, with lung cancer being the most frequent type. Physical factors determining the localization of cutaneous metastases include peculiarities of vascular supply[1047,1048] and perhaps segmental temperature. Batson's valveless vertebral venous plexus parallels and is interconnected with the portal, caval, and pulmonary venous systems, and is a caudal route for tumor emboli.[1049]

The clinical configuration of metastatic cutaneous malignant tumors is quite variable in terms of size and shape, color (skin tone to hemorrhagic), and epidermal coverage (flat, elevated, invaded, or ulcerated). There may be mimicry of simple edema, inflammation, fibrosis, vasculitis, or nearly the full spectrum of primary cutaneous tumors.[1050] The main clinical forms include diffuse dermal lymphatic spread, nodular aggregates within the dermis, and predominant desmoplastic response. Diffuse lymphatic dissemination produces edema and inflammation that, in the extreme, appear as brawny induration with a peau d'orange epidermal surface change. The latter results when superficial dermal edema occurs about follicular ostia, rendering them prominent and patulous. Tumor emboli within blood vessels can produce telangiectasias or overt zones of infarctive tissue necrosis. Desmoplasia stimulated by tumor is a firm induration, even a woody hard depression. Sometimes cutaneous metastases disappear spontaneously, probably because the skin provides a poor site for their growth.

There is no single common histology. Without resorting to special laboratory work, most can be classified no further than adenocarcinoma, squamous cell carcinoma, or undifferentiated carcinoma. Carcinomas that infiltrate the dermis unassociated with any epithelial or adnexal structures can be considered typical but several types have special proclivities. For example, both metastatic carcinomas and cutaneous metastases from melanomas can infiltrate the epidermal layer, closely mimicking primary skin tumors. A marked desmoplastic reaction can obscure tumor cells. Rather than evolving through defined and progressive stages, as do many primary malignant counterparts, metastatic tumors simply enlarge in size or undergo partial necrosis over time.

REFERENCES

1. Marks R: An overview of skin cancers. Incidence and causation. Cancer 75:607–612, 1995
2. Rapini RP: False-negative surgical margins. Adv Dermatol 10:137–148, 1995
3. Su WPD: Histopathologic varieties of epidermal nevus. A study of 160 cases. Am J Dermatopathol 4:161–170, 1982
4. Basler RSW, Jacobs SI, Taylor WB: Ichthyosis hystrix. Arch Dermatol 114:1059–1060, 1978
5. Ackerman AB: Histopathlogic concept of epidermolytic hyperkeratosis. Arch Dermatol 102:253–259, 1970
6. Goldman K, Don PC: Adult onset of inflammatory linear verrucous epidermal nevus in a mother and her daughter. Dermatology 189:170–172, 1994
7. Welch M, Smith KJ, Skelton HG, Turiansky G: Inflammatory linear verrucous epidermal nevus in patients with positive results of tests for human immunodeficiency virus 1. Cutis 55:365–368, 1995
8. Stosiek N, Hornstein OP, Hiller D, Peters KP: Extensive linear epidermal nevus associated with hemangiomas of bones and vitamin-D-resistant rickets. Dermatology 189:278–282, 1994
9. Levin A, Amazon K, Rywlin AM: A squamous cell carcinoma that developed in an epidermal nevus. Report of a case and a review of the literature. Am J Dermatopathol 6:51–55, 1984
10. Matsuoka LY, Wortsman J, Goldman J: Acanthosis nigricans. Clin Dermatol 11:21–25, 1993
11. Schwartz RA: Continuing medical education: acanthosis nigricans. J Am Acad Dermatol 1–19, quiz 20–22, 1994
12. Hud J Jr, Cohen JB, Wagner JM, Cruz PD Jr: Prevalance and significance of acanthosis nigricans in an adult obese population. Arch Dermatol 128:941–944, 1992
13. Megahed M, Scharffetter-Kochanek K: Acantholytic acanthoma. Am J Dermatopathol 15:283–285, 1993
14. Nindl A, Nakagawa H, Furue M, Ishibashi Y: Simple epithelial cytokeratin expression in seborrheic keratosis. J Cutan Pathol 19:415–422, 1992
15. Holdiness MR: The sign of Leser-Trelat. Int J Dermatol 25:564–572, 1986
16. Ellis DL, Kafka SP, Chow JC, et al: Melanoma, growth factors acanthosis nigricans, the sign of Leser-Trelat, and multiple acrochordons. A possible role for alpha-transforming growth factor in cutaneous paraneoplastic syndromes. N Engl J Med 317:1582–1587, 1987
17. Mevorah B, Michima Y: Cellular response of seborrheic keratosis following croton boil irritation and surgical trauma. Dermatologica 131:452–464, 1965
18. Zhu WY, Leonardi C, Kinsey W, Penneys NS: Irritated seborrheic keratoses and benign verrucous acanthomas do not contain papillomavirus DNA. J Cutan Pathol 18:449–452, 1991
19. Hairston MA Jr, Reed RJ, Derbes VJ: Dermatosis papulosa nigra. Arch Dermatol 89:655–658, 1964
20. Shall L, Marks R: The pathology and pathogenesis of stucco keratosis. Br J Dermatol, suppl. 117:32–33, 1987
21. Mehregan AH: Inverted follicular keratosis is a distinct follicular tumor. Am J Dermatopathol 5:467–470, 1983
22. Sim-Davis D, Marks R, Wilson Jones E: The inverted follicular keratosis. A surprising variant of seborrheic wart. Acta Derm Venereol (Stockh) 56:337–344, 1976
23. Mehregan AH: Inverted follicular keratosis. Arch Dermatol 89:229–235, 1964
24. Spielvogel RL, Austin C, Ackerman AB: Inverted follkeratosis is not a specific keratosis but a verruca vulgaris (or seborrheic keratosis) with squamous eddies. Am J Dermatopathol 5:427–442, 1983

25. Prince C, Mehregan AH, Hashimoto K, Plotnick H: Large melanoacanthomas: a report of five cases. J Cutan Pathol 11:309–317, 1984

26. Monteagudo JC, Jorda E, Ferencio C, Llombart-Bosch A: Squamous cell carcinoma in situ (Bowen's disease) arising in seborrheic keratosis; three lesions in two patients. J Cutan Pathol 16:348–352, 1989

27. Argenyi ZB, Huston BM, Argenyi EE, et al: Large-cell acanthoma of the skin. A study by image analysis cytometry and immunohistochemistry. Am J Dermatopathol 16:140–144, 1994

28. Fand SB, Pinkus H: Polypoidy in benign epidermal neoplasia. J Cell Biol 47:59a–60a, 1970

29. Rahbari H, Pinkus H: Large cell acanthoma. One of the actinic keratoses. Arch Dermatol 114:49–52, 1978

30. Sanchez Yus E, del Rio E, Requena L: Large-cell acanthoma is a distinctive condition. Am J Dermatopathol 14:140–147, 1992

31. Rabinowitz AD, Inghirami G: Large-cell acanthoma. A distinctive keratosis. Am J Dermatopathol 14:136–138, 1992

32. Weinstock MA: Large-cell acanthoma. Am J Dermatopathol 14:133–134, 1992

33. Roewert HJ, Ackerman AB: Large-cell acanthoma is a solar lentigo. Am J Dermatopathol 14:122–132, 1992

34. Cotton DWK, Mills PM, Stephenson TJ, Underwood JCE: On the nature of clear cell acanthomas. Br J Dermatol 117:569–574, 1987

35. Baden TJ, Woodley DT, Wheeler CE Jr: Multiple clear cell acanthoma. Case report and delineation of basement membrane zone antigens. J Am Acad Dermatol 16:1075–1078, 1987

36. Hashimoto T, Inamoto N, Nakamura K: Two cases of clear cell acanthoma: an immunohistochemical study. J Cutan Pathol 15:27–30, 1988

37. Brownstein MH: The benign acanthomas. J Cutan Pathol 12:172–188, 1985

38. Langer K, Wuketich S, Konrad K: Pigmented clear cell acanthoma. Am J Dermatopathol 16:134–139, 1994

39. Schwartz RA: Keratoacanthoma. J Am Acad Dermatol 30:1–19, 1994

40. Kern WH, McGray MK: The histopathologic differentiation of keratoacanthoma and squamous cell carcinoma of the skin. J Cutan Pathol 7:318–325, 1980

41. Chalet MD, Connors RC, Ackerman AB: Squamous cell carcinoma and keratoacanthoma: criteria for histologic differentiation. J Dermatol Surg 1:16–17, 1975

42. Pilch H, Weiss J, Heubner C, Heine M: Differential diagnosis of keratoacanthomas and squamous cell carcinomas: diagnostic value of DNA image cytometry and p53 expression. J Cutan Pathol 21:507–513, 1994

43. Royds JA, Stephenson TJ, Silcocks PB, Bleehen SS: Proliferating nuclear antigen immunostaining in keratoacanthoma and squamous cell carcinoma of the skin. Pathologica 86:612–616, 1994

44. Allen CA, Stephens M, Steel WM: Subungual keratoacanthoma. Histopathology 25:181–183, 1994

45. Calonje E, Wilson Jones E: Intravascular spread of keratoacanthoma. An alarming but benign phenomenon. Am J Dermatopathol 14:414–417, 1992

46. Janecka IP, Wolff M, Crikelair F, Cosman B: Aggressive histological features of keratoacanthoma. J Cutan Pathol 4:342–348, 1978

47. Lapius NA, Helwig EB: Perineural invasion by keratoacanthoma. Arch Dermatol 116:791–793, 1980

48. Blessing K, al Nafussi A, Gordon PM: The regressing keratoacanthoma. Histopathology 24:381–384, 1994

49. Rossman RE, Freeman RG, Knox JM: Multiple keratocanthoma. Arch Dermatol 89:374–381, 1964

50. Kingman J, Callen JP: Keratoacanthoma. A clinical study. Arch Dermatol 120:736–740, 1984

51. Cain CT, Niemann TH, Argenyi ZB: Keratoacanthoma versus squamous cell carcinoma. An immunohistochemical reappraisal of p53 protein and proliferating cell nuclear antigen expression in keratoacanthoma-like tumors. Am J Dermatopathol 17:324–331, 1995

52. Giltman LI: Tripolar mitosis in a keratoacanthoma. Acta Derm Venereol (Stockh) 61:362–363, 1981

53. Hodak E, Jones RE, Ackerman AB: Solitary keratoacanthoma is a squamous cell carcinoma. Three examples with metastases. Am J Dermatopathol 15:332–342, 1993

54. Sleater JP, Beers BB, Stephens CA, Hendricks JB: Keratoacanthoma. A deficient squamous cell carcinoma? Study of bcl-2 expression. J Cutan Pathol 21:514–519, 1994

55. Tanay A, Mehregan AH: Warty dyskeratoma. Dermatologica 138:155–174, 1969

56. Harrist TJ, Murphy GF, Mihm MC Jr: Oral warty dyskeratoma. Arch Dermatol 116:929–931, 1980

57. Lutzner MA: The human papillomaviruses. Arch Dermatol 119:631–635, 1983

58. McCance DJ: Human papillomaviruses and cancer. Biochem Biophys Acta 823:195–205, 1986

59. Jaworsky C, Murphy GF: Special techniques in dermatology. Arch Dermatol 125:963–974, 1989

60. Kaspar TA, Wagner RF Jr, Jablonska S, et al: Prognosis and treatment of advanced squamous cell carcinoma secondary to epidermodysplasia verruciformis: a worldwide analysis of 11 patients. J Dermatol Surg Oncol 17:237–240, 1991

61. Howell JB: Nevoid basal cell carcinoma syndrome. Profile of genetic and environmental factors in oncogenesis. J Am Acad Dermatol 11:98–104, 1984

62. Lutzer MA: Epidermodysplasia verruciformis. An autosomal recessive disease characterized by viral warts and skin cancer. A model for viral oncogenesis. Bull Cancer 65:169–182, 1978

63. Yabe Y, Yasui M, Yoshino N, et al: Epidermodysplasia verruciformis: viral particles in early malignant lesions. J Invest Dermatol 71:225–228, 1978

64. Zhu WY, Leonardi C, Kinsey W, Penneys NS: Irritated seborrheic keratoses and benign verrucous acanthomas do not contain papillomavirus DNA. J Cutan Pathol 18:449–452, 1991

65. Reed RJ, Parkinson RP: The histogenesis of molluscum contagiosum. Am J Surg Pathol 1:161–166, 1977

66. Sober AJ, Burstein JM: Precursors to skin cancer. Cancer, 75 suppl. 2:645–650, 1995

67. Sim CS, Slater S, McKee PH: Mutant p53 expression in solar keratosis. An immunohistochemical study. J Cutan Pathol 19:302–308, 1992

68. Brownstein MH, Rabinowitz AD: The precursors of cutaneous squamous cell carcinoma. Int J Dermatol 18:1–16, 1979

69. James MP, Wells GC, Whimster IW: Spreading pigmented actinic keratosis. Br J Dermatol 98:373–379, 1978

70. Cataldo E, Doku HC: Solar chelitis. J Dermatol Surg Oncol 7:989–995, 1981

71. Hirsch T, Marmelzat WL: Lichenoid actinic keratosis. Dermatol Int 6:101–103, 1967

72. King GN, Healy CM, Glover MT, et al: Increased prevalence of dysplastic and malignant lip lesions in renal-transparent recipients. N Engl J Med 332:1052–1057, 1995

73. Yu RC, Pryce DW, MacFarlane AW, Stewart TW: A histopathological study of 643 cutaneous horns. Br J Dermatol 124:449–452, 1991

74. Carapeto FJ, Garcia Perez A: Acantholytic keratosis. Dermatologica 148:233–239, 1974

75. Subrt P, Jorizzo JL, Apisarnthanarax P, et al: Spreading pigmented actinic keratosis. J Am Acad Dermatol 8:63–67, 1983

76. Ackerman AB, Reed RJ: Epidermolytic variant of solar keratosis. Arch Dermatol 107:104–106, 1973

77. Tan CY, Marks R: Lichenoid solar keratosis prevalence and immunologic findings. J Invest Dermatol 79:365–367, 1982

78. Marks R, Rennie G, Selwood T: The relationship of basal cell carcinomas and squamous cell carcinomas to solar keratoses. Arch Dermatol 124:1039–1042, 1988

79. Sim CS, Slater S, McKee PH: Mutant p53 expression in solar keratosis. An immunohistochemical study. J Cutan Pathol 19:302–308, 1992

80. McGibbon DH: Malignant epidermal tumours. J Cutan Pathol 12:224–238, 1985

81. Fleming ID, Amonette R, Monagham T, Fleming MD: Principles of management of basal and squamous cell carcinoma of the skin. Cancer 75:699–704, 1995

82. Kossard S, Rosen R: Cutaneous Bowen's disease. An analysis of 1001 cases according to age, sex and site. J Am Acad Dermatol 27:406–410, 1992

83. Penneys NS, Bogaert M, Serfling U, Sisto M: The proliferative population in cutaneous Bowen's disease includes all epidermal layers abstracted. J Cutan Pathol 18:383, 1991

84. Stern RS, Laird N, Melski J, et al: Cutaneous squamous-cell carcinoma in patients treated with PUVA. N Engl J Med 310:1156–1161, 1984

85. Wang C-Y, Brodland DG, Su WPD: Skin cancers associated with acquired immunodeficiency syndrome. Mayo Clin Proc 70:766–772, 1995

86. Strayer DS, Santa Cruz DJ: Carcinoma in situ of the skin: a review of histopathology. J Cutan Pathol 7:244–259, 1980

87. Wade TR, Kopf AW, Ackerman AB: Bowenoid papulosis of the penis. Cancer 42:1890–1903, 1978

88. Ulbright TM, Stehman FB, Roth LM, et al: Bowenoid dysplasia of the vulva. Cancer 59:2910–2919, 1982

89. Hahn A, Loning T, Hoos A, Henke P: Immunohistochemistry (S-100, KL1) and human papillomavirus DNA hybridization on morbus Bowen and bowenoid papulosis. Virchows Arch [A] 413:113–122, 1988

90. Civatte J: Pseudo-carcinomatous hyperplasia. J Cutan Pathol 12:214–223, 1985

91. Gattuso P, Candel AC, Castelli MJ, et al: Pseudoepitheliomatous hyperplasia in chronic cutaneous wounds. A flow cytometric study. J Cutan Pathol 21:312–315, 1994

92. Stern JB, Haupt HM: Reexcision perineural invasion. Am J Surg Pathol 14:183–185, 1990

93. Perkins W, Campbell I, Leigh IM, Mackie RM: Keratin expressions in normal skin and epidermal neoplasms demonstrated by a panel of monoclonal antibodies. J Cutan Pathol 19:476–482, 1992

94. Watanabe S, Ichikawa E, Takahashi H, Otsuka F: Changes of cytokeratin and involucrin expression in squamous cell carcinomas of the skin during progression to malignancy. Br J Dermatol 132:730–739, 1995

95. Smith KJ, Skelton HG III, Morgan AM, et al: Spindle cell neoplasms coexpressing cytokeratin and vimentin (metaplastic squamous cell carcinoma). J Cutan Pathol 19:286–293, 1992

96. Silvis NG, Swanson PE, Manivel JC, et al: Spindle-cell and pleomorphic neoplasms of the skin. Am J Dermatopathol 10:9–19, 1988

97. Banerjee S, Eyden B, Wells S, et al: Pseudoangiosarcomatous carcinoma. A clinicopathologic study of seven cases. Histopathology 21:13–24, 1992

98. Nappi O, Wick MR, Pettinato G, et al: Pseudovascular adenoid squamous cell carcinoma of the skin: a neoplasm that may be mistaken for angiosarcoma. Am J Surg Pathol 16:429–438, 1992

99. Cox NH, Long ED: Pseudoangiosarcomatous squamous cell carcinoma of skin. Histopathology 22:295–296, 1993

100. Wick MR, Pettinato G, Nappi O: Adenoid (acantholytic) squamous carcinoma of the skin, abstracted. J Cutan Pathol 15:351, 1988

101. Weidner N, Foucar E: Adenosquamous carcinoma of the skin. An aggressive mucin- and gland-forming carcinoma. Arch Dermatol 12:775–779, 1985

102. Banks ER, Cooper PH: Adenosquamous carcinoma of the skin: a report of 10 cases. J Cutan Pathol 18:227–234, 1991

103. Cubilla AL, Ayala MT, Barreto JE, et al: Surface adenosquamous carcinoma of the penis. A report of three cases. Am J Surg Pathol 20:156–160, 1996

104. Schwartz RA: Verrucous carcinoma of the skin and mucosa. J Am Acad Dermatol 32:1–21, 1995

105. Kim J, Su W, Kurtin P, Ziesmer S: Marjolin's ulcer. Immunohistochemical study of 17 cases and comparison with common squamous cell carcinoma and basal cell carcinoma. J Cutan Pathol 19:278–285, 1992

106. Carr KA, Bulengo-Ransby SM, Weiss LM, Nickoloff BJ: Lymphoepithelioma-like carcinoma of the skin. A case report with immunophenotypic analysis and in situ hybridization for Epstein-Barr viral genoma. Am J Surg Pathol 16:909–913, 1992

107. Requena L, Sanchez Yus E, Jimenez E, Roo E: Lymphoepithelioma-like carcinoma of the skin: a light-microscopic and immunohistochemical study. J Cutan Pathol 21:541–548, 1994

108. Wick MR, Swanson PE, LeBoit PE, et al: Lymphoepithelial-like carcinoma of the skin with adnexal differentiation. J Cutan Pathol 18:93–102, 1991

109. Landman G, Taylor RM, Friedman KJ: Cutaneous papillary squamous cell carcinoma. A report of two cases. J Cutan Pathol 17:105–110, 1990

110. Cramer SF, Heggeness LM: Signet-ring squamous cell carcinoma. Am J Clin Pathol 91:488–491, 1989

111. Requena L, Sanchez M, Requena I, et al: Clear cell squamous cell carcinoma. A histologic, immunohistologic, and ultrastructural study. J Dermatol Surg Oncol 17:656–660, 1991

112. Lund HZ: How often does squamous cell carcinoma metastasize? Arch Dermatol 92:635–637, 1965

113. Perez GL, Randle HW: Natural history of squamous cell carcinoma of the skin: case report. Cutis 55:34–36, 1995

114. Panayiotou BN, Aravindan N, Sinka SK, Ryatt K: Cutaneous SCC: metastases with a predilection for lungs 6 years after excision of the primary tumour. Br J Clin Pract 49:107–108, 1995

115. Southwick GJ, Schwartz RA: The basal cell nevus syndrome. Disasters occurring among a series of thirty-six patients. Cancer 44:2294–2305, 1979

116. Murphy GF, Krizinski PA, Myzak LA, Ershier WB: Local immune response in basal cell carcinoma: characterization by transmission electron microscopy and T6 monoclonal antibody. J Am Acad Dermatol 8:477–485, 1983

117. Guillen FJ, Day CL Jr, Murphy GF: Expression of activation antigens on T cells infiltrating basal cell carcinomas. J Invest Dermatol 85:203–206, 1985

118. Metcalf JS, Maize JC: Histopathologic considerations in the management of basal cell carcinoma. Semin Dermatol 8:259–265, 1989

119. Sexton M, Jones DB, Maloney ME: Histologic pattern analysis of basal cell carcinoma. J Am Acad Dermatol 23:1118–1126, 1990

120. Ryan JF: Basal cell carcinoma and chronic venous stasis. Histopathology 14:657–659, 1989

121. Miller SJ: Biology of basal cell carcinoma. Parts I and II. J Am Acad Dermatol 24:1–13, 161–175, 1991

122. Shimizu N, Ito M, Tazawa T, Sato Y: Immunohistochemical study on keratin expression in certain cutaneous epithelial neoplasms. Basal cell carcinoma, pilomatricoma, and seborrheic keratosis. Am J Dermatopathol 11:534–540, 1989

123. Kirihara Y, Haratake J, Horie A: Clinicopathological and immunohistochemical study of basal cell carcinoma with reference to the features of basement membrane. J Dermatol 19:161–169, 1992

124. Rosai J: Basal cell carcinoma with follicular differentiation, letters to the editor I and II. Am J Dermatopathol 10:457–458, 1988; 11:479–480, 1989

125. Graham PG, McGavran MH: Basal-cell carcinomas and sebaceous glands. Cancer 17:803–806, 1964

126. Sahl WJ: Basal cell carcinoma: influence of tumor size on mortality and morbidity. Int J Dermatol 34:319–321, 1995

127. von Domarus H, Stevens PJ: Metastatic basal cell carcinoma. J Am Acad Dermatol 10:1043–1060, 1984

128. Snow SN, Sahl W, Lo JS, et al: Metastatic basal cell carcinoma. Report of five cases. Cancer 73:328–335, 1994

129. Mehregan AH: Aggressive basal cell epithelioma on sunlight-protected skin. Report of eight cases, one with pulmonary and bone metastases. Am J Dermatopathol 5:221–229, 1983

130. Farmer ER, Helwig EB: Metastatic basal cell carcinoma. A clinicopathologic study of seventeen cases. Cancer 46:748–757, 1980

131. Lopez De Faria J, Navarrete MA: The histopathology of the skin basal cell carcinoma with areas of intermediate differentiation. A metatypical carcinoma. Pathol Res Pract 187:978–985, 1991

132. Pratt MD, Jackson R: Nevoid basal cell carcinoma syndrome: a 15-year follow-up of cases in Ottawa and the Ottawa Valley. J Am Acad Dermatol 16:964–970, 1987

133. Howell JB: Nevoid basal cell carcinoma syndrome. Profile of genetic and environmental factors in oncogenesis. J Am Acad Dermatol 11:98–104, 1984

134. Howell JB, Anderson DE: The nevoid basal cell carcinoma syndrome. Arch Dermatol 118:824–826, 1982

135. Chorun L, Norris JE, Gupta M: Basal cell carcinoma in blacks: a report of 15 cases. Ann Plast Surg 33:90–95, 1994

136. De Rosa G, Barra E, Guarino M, et al: Fibronectin, laminin, type IV collagen distribution, and myofibroblastic stromal reaction in aggressive and nonaggressive basal cell carcinoma. Am J Dermatopathol 16:258–267, 1994

137. Looi LNM: Localized amyloidosis in basal cell carcinoma. A pathologic study. Cancer 52:1833–1836, 1983

138. Satti MB, Azzopardi JG: Amyloid deposits in basal cell carcinoma of the skin. J Am Acad Dermatol 22:1082–1087, 1990

139. Heyderman E, Grahm RM, Chapman DV, et al: Epithelial markers in primary skin cancer. An immunoperoxidase study of the distribution of epithelial membrane antigen (EMA) and carcinoembryonic antigen (CEA) in 65 primary skin carcinomas. Histopathology 8:423–434, 1984

140. Said JW, Sassoon AF, Shintaku IP, Banks-Schlegel S: Involucrin in squamous and basal cell carcinomas of the skin. An immunohistochemical study. J Invest Dermatol 82:449–452, 1984

141. Shea CR, McNutt NS, Volkenandt M, et al: Overexpression of p53 protein in basal cell carcinomas of human skin. Am J Pathol 141:25–29, 1992

142. Heenan PJ, Bogle MS: Eccrine differentiation in basal cell carcinoma. Invest Dermatol 100:295S–299S, 1993

143. Walsh N, Ackerman AB: Infundibulocystic basal cell carcinoma: a new described variant. Mod Pathol 3:599–608, 1990

144. Seidman JD, Berman JJ, Moore GW: Basal cell carcinoma. Importance of histologic discontinuities in the evaluation of resection margins. Mod Pathol 4:325–330, 1991

145. Dixon AY, Lee SH, McGregor DH: Histologic evolution of basal cell carcinoma recurrence. Am J Dermatopathol 13:241–247, 1991

146. Dixon AY, Lee SH, McGregor DH: Histologic features predictive of basal cell carcinoma recurrence. Results of a multivariate analysis. J Cutan Pathol 20:137–142, 1993

147. Maloney ME, Jones DB, Sexton FM: Pigmented basal cell carcinoma. Investigation of 70 cases. J Am Acad Dermatol 27:74–78, 1992

148. Johnson TM, Tschen J, Ho C, et al: Unusual basal cell carcinomas. Cutis 54:85–92, 1994

149. White GM, Barr RJ, Liao SY: Signet ring cell basal cell carcinoma. Am J Dermatopathol 13:288–292, 1991

150. Barr RJ, Alpern KS, Santa Cruz DJ, Fretzin DF: Clear cell basal cell carcinoma: an unusual degenerative variant. J Cutan Pathol 20:308–316, 1993

151. Garcia P, Lopez Carreira M, Martinez-Gonzalez MA, et al: Granular cell basal cell carcinoma. Light microscopy, immunohistochemical and ultrastructural study. Virchows Arch [A] 422:173–177, 1993

152. James CL: Basal cell carcinoma with hyaline inclusions. Pathology 27:97–100, 1995

153. Boyd AS, Rapini RP: Cutaneous collision tumors. An analysis of 69 cases and review of the literature. Am J Dermatopathol 16:253–257, 1994

154. Kazantseva IA, Khlebnikova AN, Babaev VR: Immunohistochemical study of primary and recurrent basal cell and metatypical carcinomas of the skin. Am J Dermatopathol 18:35–42, 1996

155. Lopes De Faria J, Navurrete MA: The histopathology of the skin: basal cell carcinoma with areas of intermediate differentiation. Pathol Res Pract 187:978–985, 1991

156. Morales-Ducret CR, van de Rijn M, Smoller BR: bcl-2 expression in primary malignancies of the skin. Arch Dermatol 131:909–912, 1995

157. Tellechea O, Reis JP, Domingues JC, Baptista AP: Monoclonal antibody Ber EP4 distinguishes basal-cell carcinoma from squamous-cell carcinoma of the skin. Am J Dermatopathol 15:452–455, 1993

158. Heng MC, Fallon-Friedlander S, Bennett R: Expression of Ulex europaeus agglutin I lectin-binding sites in squamous cell carcinomas and their absence in basal cell carcinomas. Indicator of tumor type and differentiation. Am J Dermatopathol 14:216–219, 1992

159. Nogita T, Ohta A, Hidano A, et al: Basal cell carcinoma with eccrine differentiation. J Dermatol 22:111–115, 1995

160. Stern JB, Haupt HM, Smith RRL: Fibroepithelioma of Pinkus. Eccrine duct spread of basal cell carcinoma. Am J Dermatopathol 16:585–587, 1994

161. Gooding CA, White G, Yatsuhashi M: Significance of marginal extension in excised basal cell carcinoma. N Engl J Med 273:923–924, 1965

162. Headington JT: A dermatopathologist looks at Mohs micrographic surgery, editorial. Arch Dermatol 126:950–951, 1990

163. Mikhail GR (ed): Mohs Micrographic Surgery. WB Saunders, Philadelphia, 1991

164. Miller PK, Roenigk RK, Brodland DG, Randle HW: Cutaneous micrographic surgery. Mohs procedure. Mayo Clin Proc 67:971–980, 1992

165. Murphy GF, Elder DE: Non-Melanocytic Tumors of the Skin. Armed Forces Institute of Pathology, Washington, DC, 1991

166. Smith KJ, Skelton HG, Holland TT: Recent advances and controversies concerning adnexal neoplasms. Dermatol Clin 10:117–160, 1992

167. Mehregan AH: Hair follicle tumors of the skin. J Cutan Pathol 12:189–195, 1985

168. Massa MC, Medenica M: Cutaneous adnexal tumors and cysts: a review. Pathol Annu 22:225–276, 1987

169. Buchi ER, Peng Y, Eng AM, Tso MO: Eccrine acrospiroma of the eyelid with onocytic, apocrine and sebaceous differentiation. Further evidence of pluripotentiality of the adnexal epithelia. Eur J Ophthalmol 1:187–193, 1991

170. Sanchez Yus E, Requena L, Simon P, Sanchez M: Complex adnexal tumor of the primary epithelial germ with distinct patterns of superficial epithelioma with sebaceous differentiation, immature trichoepithelioma, and apocrine adenocarcinoma. Am J Dermatopathol 14:245–252, 1992

171. Weyers W, Nilles M, Eckert F, Schill W-B: Spiradenomas in Brooke-Speigler syndrome. Am J Dermatopathol 15:156–161, 1993

172. Wong T-Y, Suster S, Cheek RF, Mihm MC: Benign cutaneous adnexal tumors with combined folliculosebaceous, apocrine and eccrine differentiation. Clinicopathologic and immunohistochemical study of eight cases. Am J Dermatopathol 18:124–136, 1996

173. Massa MC, Medenica M: Cutaneous adnexal tumors and cysts: A review. Part 1. Tumors with hair follicle differentiation and cysts related to different parts of the hair follicle. Pathol Annu 20:189–233, 1985

174. Hashimoto K, Mehregan AH, Kumakiri M: Tumors of Skin Appendages. Butterworths, Boston, 1987

175. Rahbari H: Epidermoid cysts with seborrheic verruca-like cyst walls. Arch Dermatol 118:326–328, 1982

176. Bhawan J: Pilar sheath acanthoma: a new benign follicular tumor. J Cutan Pathol 6:438–440, 1979

177. Mehregan AH, Brownstein MH: Pilar sheath acanthoma. Arch Dermatol 114:1495–1497, 1978

178. Winer IH: The dilated pore, a trichoepithelioma. J Invest Dermatol 23:181–188, 1954

179. Sleater J, Beers B, Stefan M, et al: Proliferating trichilemal cyst. Report of four cases, two with nondiploid DNA content and increased proliferation index. Am J Dermatopathol 15:423–428, 1993

180. Sakamoto F, Ito M, Nakamura A, Sato Y: Proliferating trichilemmal cyst with apocrine-acrosyringeal and sebaceous differentiation. J Cutan Pathol 18:137–141, 1991

181. Reed RJ, Lamar LM: Invasive hair matrix tumors of the scalp. Arch Dermatol 94:310–316, 1966

182. Rutty GN, Richman PI, Laing JH: Malignant change in trichilemmal cysts. A study of cell proliferation and DNA content. Histopathology 21:465–468, 1992

183. Amaral AL, Nascimento AG, Goellner JR: Proliferating pilar (trichilemmal) cyst. Report of two cases, one with carcinomatous transformation and one with distant metastases. Arch Pathol Lab Med 108:808–810, 1984

184. Mori O, Hachisuka H, Sasai Y: Proliferating trichilemmal cyst with spindle cell carcinoma. Am J Dermatopathol 12:479–484, 1990

185. Brownstein MH: Steatocystoma simplex. A solitary steatocystoma. Arch Dermatol 118:409–411, 1982

186. Klingman AM, Kirchbaum JKD: Steatocystoma multiplex. A dermoid tumor. J Invest Dermatol 42:383–387, 1964

187. Mayron R, Grimwood RE: Familial occurrence of eruptive vellus hair cysts. Pediatr Dermatol 5:94–96, 1988

188. Brownstein MH, Helwig EB: Subcutaneous dermoid cysts. Arch Dermatol 107:237–239, 1973

189. Fukuda M, Kato H, Hamada T: Apocrine hidrocystoma. A report of five cases and review of the Japanese literature. J Dermatol 16:315–320, 1989

190. Murayama N, Tsuboi R, Unno K, Ogawa H: Multiple eccrine hidrocystomas. Br J Dermatol 131:585–586, 1994

191. Yasaka N, Iozumi K, Nashiro K, et al: Bilateral periorbital eccrine hidrocystoma. J Dermatol 21:490–493, 1994

192. Milum EA: A solitary pigmented tumor of the face. Arch Dermatol 127:572–575, 1991

193. Kurban RS, Bhawan J: Cutaneous cysts lined by nonsquamous epithelium. Am J Dermatopathol 13:509–517, 1991

194. Trotter SE, Rassi DM, Saad M, et al: Cutaneous ciliated cyst occurring in a male. Histopathology 25:492–493, 1994

195. Muramatsu T, Shirai T, Sakamoto K: Cutaneous bronchogenic cyst. Int J Dermatol 29:143–144, 1990

196. Dore N, Landry M, Cadotte M, Suchurch W: Cutaneous endosalpingiosis. Arch Dermatol 116:909–912, 1980

197. Mammino JJ, Bidmar DA: Syringocystadenoma papilliferum. Int J Dermatol 30:763–766, 1991

198. Marrogi AJ, Wick MR, Dehner LP: Benign cutaneous adnexal tumors in childhood and young adults, excluding pilomatrixoma: review of 28 cases and literature. J Cutan Pathol 18:20–27, 1991

199. Premalatha S, Rao NR, Yesudian P, et al: Segmental syringocystadenoma papilliferum in an unusual location. Int J Dermatol 24:520–521, 1985

200. Vanatta PR, Bangert JL, Freeman RG: Syringocystadenoma papilliferum. A plasmacytotropic tumor. Am J Surg Pathol 9:678–683, 1985

201. Mambo NC: Immunohistochemical study of the immunoglobulin classes of the plasma cells in papillary syringadenoma. Virchows Arch [A] 397:1–6, 1982

202. van der Putte SC: Mammary-like glands of the vulva and their disorders. Int J Gynecol Pathol 13:150–160, 1994

203. Santa Cruz DJ, Prioleau PG, Smith ME: Hidradenoma papilliferum of the eyelid. Arch Dermatol 117:55–56, 1981

204. Fox SB, Cotton DWK: Tubular apocrine adenoma and papillary eccrine adenoma: entities or unity? Am J Dermatopathol 14:149–154, 1992

205. Ishiko A, Shimizu H, Inamoto N, Nakmura K: Is tubular apocrine adenoma a distinct clinical entity? Am J Dermatopathol 15:482–487, 1993

206. Magahed M, Hölzle E: Papillary eccrine adenoma. A case report with immunohistochemical examination. Am J Dermatopathol 15:150–155, 1993

207. Wiley EL, Milchgrub S, Freeman RG, Kim ES: Sweat gland adenomas. Immunohistochemical study with emphasis on myoepithelial differentiation. J Cutan Pathol 20:337–343, 1993

208. Headington JT: Tumors of the hair follicle. Am J Pathol 85:479–514, 1976

209. Takei Y, Fukushiro S, Ackerman AB: Criteria for histologic differentiation of desmoplastic trichoepithelioma (sclerosing epithelial hamartoma) from morphea-like basal cell carcinoma. Am J Dermatopathol 7:207–221, 1985

210. Brooke JD, Fitzpatrick JE, Golitz LE: Papillary mesenchymal bodies. A histologic finding useful in differentiating trichoepitheliomas from basal cell carcinoma, abstracted. J Cutan Pathol 14:350, 1987

211. Rahbari H, Mehregan A, Pinkus H: Trichoadenoma of Nikolowski. J Cutan Pathol 4:90–98, 1977

212. Brownstein MH, Shapiro L: Desmoplastic trichoepithelioma. Cancer 40:2979–2986, 1977

213. Hunt SJ, Kilzer B, Santa Cruz DJ: Desmoplastic trichilemmoma. Histologic variant resembling invasive carcinoma. J Cutan Pathol 17:45–52, 1990

214. Leppard BJ, Sanderson KV: The natural history of trichilemmal cysts. Br J Dermatol 94:379–390, 1976

215. Smith SR, Brady JG: Stump the experts. Trichofolliculoma. Dermatol Surg 21:581, 652, 1995

216. Mehregan AH: Infundibular tumors of the skin. J Cutan Pathol 11:387–395, 1984

217. Hashimoto K, Gross BG, Lever WF: Syringoma: histochemical and electron microscopic studies. J Invest Dermatol 47:150–166, 1966

218. Eckert F, Nilles M, Schmid U, Altmannsberger M: Distribution of cytokeratin polypeptides in syringomas. An immunohistochemical study on paraffin-embedded material. Am J Dermatopathol 14:115–121, 1992

219. Feibelman CE, Maize JC: Clear cell syringoma. Am J Dermatopathol 6:139–150, 1984

220. Ishida-Yamamoto A, Iizuka H: Eccrine syringofibroadenoma (Mascaro). An ultrastructural and immunohistochemical study. Am J Dermatopathol 18:207–211, 1996

221. Cardenas AA, Norton SA, Fitzpatrick JE: Solitary violaceous nodule on the face. Arch Dermatol 129:498–499, 501, 1993

222. Tellechea O, Reis JP, Ilheu O, Poiares Baptista A: Dermal cylindroma. An immunohistochemical study of thirteen cases. Am J Dermatopathol 17:260–265, 1995

223. Penneys N, Kaiser M: Cylindroma expresses immunohistochemical markers linking it to eccrine coil. J Cutan Pathol 20:40–43, 1993

224. Gerretsen AL, Beemer FA, Deenstra W, et al: Familial cutaneous cylindromas: investigations in five generations of a family. J Am Acad Dermatol 33:199–206, 1995

225. Crain RC, Helwig EB: Dermal cylindroma (dermal eccrine cylindroma). Am J Clin Pathol 35:504–515, 1961

226. Cotton DWK, Braye SG: Dermal cylindromas originate from the eccrine sweat gland. Br J Dermatol 111:53–61, 1984

227. Kallioinen M: Immunoelectron microscope demonstration of the basement membrane components laminin and type IV collagen in the dermal cylindroma. J Pathol 147:97–102, 1985

228. Gerretsen AL, van der Putte SC, Deenstra W: Cutaneous cylindroma with malignant transformation. Cancer 72:1618–1623, 1993

229. Lo JS, Peschen M, Snow SN, et al: Malignant cylindroma of the scalp. J Dermatol Surg Oncol 17:897–901, 1991

230. Rulon DB, Helwig EB: Papillary eccrine adenoma. Arch Dermatol 113:596–598, 1977

231. Aloi F, Pich A: Papillary eccrine adenoma. A histopathological and immunohistochemical study. Dermatologica 182:47–51, 1991

232. Nova MP, Kress Y, Jennings TA, et al: Papillary eccrine adenoma and low-grade eccrine carcinoma. A comparative histologic, ultrastructural, and immunohistochemical study. Surg Pathol 3:179–188, 1990

233. Mills SE: Mixed tumor of the skin: a model of divergent differentiation. J Cutan Pathol 11:382–386, 1984

234. Ferreiro JA, Nascimento AG: Hyaline-cell rich chondroid syringoma. A tumor mimicking malignancy. Am J Surg Pathol 19:912–917, 1995

235. Banerjee SS, Harris M, Eyden BP, et al: Chondroid syringoma with hyaline cell change. Histopathology 22:235–245, 1993

236. Hasseb-el-Naby HM, Tam S, White WL, Ackerman AB: Mixed tumors of the skin. A histological and immunohistochemical study. Am J Dermatopathol 11:413–428, 1989

237. Iglesias FD, Forcelledo FF, Sanchez TS, et al: Chondroid syringoma. A histological and immunohistochemical study of 15 cases. Histopathology 17:311–318, 1990

238. Wiley EL, Milchgrub S, Freeman RG, Kim ES: Sweat gland adenomas. Immunohistochemical study with emphasis on myoepithelial differentiation. J Cutan Pathol 20:337–343, 1993

239. Trown K, Heenan PJ: Malignant mixed tumor of the skin (malignant chondroid syringoma). Pathology 26:237–243, 1994

240. Metzler G, Schaumburg-Lever G, Hornstin O, Rassner G: Malignant chondroid syringoma. Immunohistopathology. Am J Dermatopathol 18:83–89, 1996

241. Watanabe S, Mogi S, Ichikawa E, et al: Immunohistochemical analysis of keratin distribution in eccrine poroma. Am J Pathol 142:231–239, 1993

242. Kakinuma H, Miyamoto R, Iwasawa U, et al: Three subtypes of poroid neoplasia in a single lesion. Eccrine poroma, hidroacanthoma simplex, and dermal duct tumor. Histologic, histochemical, and ultrastructural findings. Am J Dermatopathol 16:66–72, 1994

243. Goldner R: Eccrine poromatosis. Arch Dermatol 101:606–608, 1970

244. Hashimoto K, Lever WF: Eccrine poroma. Histochemical and electron microscopic studies. J Invest Dermatol 43:237–247, 1964

245. Takanashi M, Urabe A, Nakayama J, Hori Y: Distribution of epithelial membrane antigen in eccrine poroma. Dermatologica 183:187–190, 1991

246. Mehregan AH, Lauson DN: Hidroacanthoma simplex. Arch Dermatol 100:303–305, 1969

247. Rahbari H: Hidroacanthoma simplex. A review of 15 cases. Br J Dermatol 109:219–225, 1983

248. Shapiro SD, Lambert CW, Schwartz RA: Cowden's disease. A marker for malignancy. Int J Dermatol 27:232–237, 1988

249. Leonardi CL, Zhu WY, Kinsey WH, Penneys NS: Trichilemmomas are not associated with human papillomavirus DNA. J Cutan Pathol 18:193–197, 1991

250. Crowson AN, Magro CM: Basal cell carcinoma arising in association with desmoplastic trichilemmoma. Am J Dermatopathol 18:43–48, 1996

251. Johnson BL Jr, Helwig EB: Eccrine acrospiroma. A clinicopathologic study. Cancer 23:641–657, 1969

252. Cohen PR, Tschen JA: A painlessly enlarging scalp nodule. Arch Dermatol 128:547–550, 1992

253. Hernandez-Perez E, Cestoni-Parducci R: Nodular hidradenoma and hidradenocarcinoma. A 10-year review. J Am Acad Dermatol 12:15–20, 1985.

254. Haupt HM, Stern JB, Berlin SJ: Immunohistochemistry in the differential diagnosis of nodular hidradenoma and glomus tumor. Am J Dermatopathol 14:310–314, 1992

255. Hashimoto K, Nelson RG, Lever WF: Calcifying epithelioma of Malherbe: histochemical and electron microscopic studies. J Invest Dermatol 47:391–408, 1966

256. Marogi AJ, Wick MR, Dehner LP: Pilomatrical neoplasms in children and young adults. Am J Dermatopathol 14:87–94, 1992

257. Kaddu S, Beham-Schmid C, Soyer HP, et al: Extramedullary hematopoiesis in pilomatricomas. Am J Dermatopathol 17:126–130, 1995

258. Solanki P, Ramzy I, Durr N, Henkes D: Pilomatrixoma. Cytologic features with differential diagnostic considerations. Arch Pathol Lab Med 111:294–297, 1987

259. Chiaramonti A, Gilgor RS: Pilomatricoma associated with myotonic dystrophy. Arch Dermatol 114:1363–1365, 1978

260. Ortiz J, Garcia Macias C, Abad M, et al: Pilomatrixoma: a description of two cases diagnosed by fine-needle aspiration. Diagn Cytopathol 12:155–157, 1995

261. Panico L, Manivel JC, Pettinato G, et al: Pilomatrix carcinoma. A case report with immunohistochemical findings, flow cytometric comparison with benign pilomatrixoma and review of the literature. Tumori 80:308–314, 1994

262. Sau P, Lupton GP, Graham JH: Pilomatrix carcinoma. Cancer 71:2491–2498, 1993

263. Gould E, Kurzon R, Kowalczyk AP, Saldana M: Pilomatrix carcinoma with pulmonary metastasis. Report of a case. Cancer 54:370–372, 1984

264. Hanly MG, Allsbrook WC, Pantazis CG, et al: Pilomatrical carcinosarcoma of the cheek with subsequent pulmonary metastases. A case report. Am J Dermatopathol 16:196–200, 1994

265. Mambo NC: Eccrine spiradenoma: clinical and pathologic study of 49 tumors. J Cutan Pathol 10:312–320, 1983

266. Naversen DN, Trask DM, Watson FH, Burket JM: Painful tumors of the skin: "LEND AN EGG." J Am Acad Dermatol 20:298–300, 1993

267. Watanabe S, Horose M, Sato S, Jakahashi H: Immunohisto-chemical analysis of cytokeratin expression in eccrine spira-denoma: similarities to the transitional portions between secretory segments and coiled ducts of eccrine glands. Br J Dermatol 131:799–807, 1994

268. Hashimoto K, Gross BG, Nelson RG, Lever WF: Eccrine spiradenoma. Histochemical and electron microscopic studies. J Invest Dermatol 46:347–365, 1966

269. Munger BL, Berghorn BM, Helwig EB: A light and electron microscopic study of a case of multiple eccrine spiradenoma. J Invest Dermatol 38:289–297, 1962

270. van den Oord JJ, De Wolf-Peeters C: Perivascular spaces in eccrine spiradenoma. A clue to its histological diagnosis. Am J Dermatopathol 17:266–270, 1995

271. Mehregan AH: Sebaceous tumors of the skin. J Cutan Pathol 12:196–199, 1985

272. Alessi E, Sala F: Nevus sebaceus. A clinicopathologic study of its evolution. Am J Dermatopathol 8:27–31, 1986

273. Alessi E, Wong SN, Advani HH, Ackerman AB: Nevus sebaceous is associated with unusual neoplasms. An Atlas. Am J Dermatol 10:116–127, 1988

274. Kudoh K, Hosokawa M, Miyazawa T, Tagami H: Giant solitary sebaceous gland hyperplasia clinically simulating epidermoid cyst. J Cutan Pathol 15:396–398, 1988

275. Rulon DB, Helwig EB: Cutaneous sebaceous neoplasms. Cancer 33:82–102, 1974

276. Schwartz RA, Goldberg DJ, Mahmood F, et al: The Muir-Torre syndrome: a disease of sebaceous and colonic neoplasms. Dermatologica 178:23–28, 1989

277. Paraf F, Sasseville D, Watters AK, et al: Clinicopathological relevance of the association between gastrointestinal and sebaceous neoplasms. The Muir-Torre syndrome. Hum Pathol 26:422–427, 1995

278. Burgdorf WHC, Pitha J, Fahmy A: Muir-Torre syndrome. Histologic spectrum of sebaceous proliferation. Am J Dermatopathol 8:202–208, 1986

279. Berg JW, McDivitt RW: Pathology of sweat gland carcinoma. Pathol Annu 3:123–144, 1968

280. Steffen C, Ackerman AB: Intraepidermal epithelioma of Borst-Jadassohn. Am J Dermatopathol 7:5–24, 1985

281. Rao NA, Hidayat AA, McLean IW, Zimmerman LE: Sebaceous carcinomas of the ocular adnexa. A clinicopathologic study of 104 cases, with five-year follow-up data. Human Pathol 13:113–122, 1982

282. Wick MR, Goellner JR, Wolfe JT III, Su WP: Adnexal carcinomas of the skin. II. Extraocular sebaceous carcinomas. Cancer 56:1163–1172, 1985

283. Ansai S, Hashimoto H, Aoki T, et al: A histochemical and immunohistochemical study of extra-ocular sebaceous carcinoma. Histopathology 22:127–133, 1993

284. Bailet JW, Zimmerman MC, Arnstein DP, et al: Sebaceous carcinoma of the head and neck. Case report and literature review. Arch Otolaryngol Head Neck Surg 118:1245–1249, 1992

285. Piest KL, Lloyd WC, Wulc AE: Dermatopathology of the ocular adnexa. pp. 445–466. In Murphy GF Dermatopathology. WB Saunders, Philadelphia, 1995

286. Friedman KJ, Boudreau S, Farmer ER: Superficial epithelioma with sebaceous differentiation. J Cutan Pathol 14:193–197, 1987

287. Kuo T: Clear cell carcinoma of the skin. Am J Surg Pathol 4:573–583, 1980

288. Hasebe T, Mukai K, Yamaguchi N, et al: Prognostic value of immunohistochemical staining for proliferating cell nuclear antigen, p53, and c-erbB-2 in sebaceous gland carcinoma and sweat gland carcinoma: comparison with histopathological parameter. Mod Pathol 7:37–43, 1994

289. Cooper PH: Carcinomas of sweat glands. Pathol Annu 22:83–124, 1987

290. Santa Cruz DJ: Sweat gland carcinomas: a comprehensive review. Semin Diagn Pathol 4:38–74, 1987

291. Alessi E, Caputo R: Syringomatous carcinoma of the scalp presenting as a slowly enlarging patch of alopecia. Am J Dermatopathol 15:503–505, 1993

292. Urso C, Paglierani M, Bondi R: Histologic spectrum of carcinomas with eccrine ductal differentiation (sweat-gland ductal carcinomas). Am J Dermatopathol 15:435–440, 1993

293. Peña J, Suster S: Squamous differentiation in malignant eccrine poroma. Am J Dermatopathol 15:492–496, 1993

294. Kolde G, Macher E, Grundmann E: Metastasizing eccrine porocarcinoma. Report of two cases with fatal outcome. Pathol Res Pract 187:477–481, 1991

295. Cooper PH: Sclerosing carcinomas of sweat ducts (microcystic adnexal carcinoma). Arch Dermatol 122:261–264, 1986

296. Nickoloff BJ, Fleischmann HE, Carmel J, et al: Microcystic adnexal carcinoma. Immunohistologic observations suggesting dual (pilar and eccrine) differentiation. Arch Dermatol 122:290–294, 1986

297. Snow SN, Reizner GT: Mucinous eccrine carcinoma of the eyelid. Cancer 70:2099–2104, 1992

298. Eckert F, Schmid U, Hardmeier T, Altmannsberger M: Cytokeratin expression in mucinous sweat gland carcinomas. An immunohisto-chemical analysis of four cases. Histopathology 21:161–165, 1992

299. Wong TY, Suster S, Nogita T, et al: Clear cell eccrine carcinomas of the skin. A clinicopathologic study of nine patients. Cancer 73:1631–1643, 1994

300. Wong TY, Suster S: Tricholemmal carcinoma. A clinicopathologic study of 13 cases. Am J Dermatopathol 16:463–473, 1994

301. Hunt SJ, Abell E: Malignant hair matrix tumor ("malignant trichoepithelioma") arising in the setting of multiple hereditary trichoepithelioma. Am J Dermatopathol 13:275–281, 1991

302. Boscaino A, Terracciano LM, Donofrio V, et al: Tricholemmal carcinoma. A study of seven cases. J Cutan Pathol 19:94–99, 1992

303. Reis JP, Tellechea O, Cunha MF, Baptista AP: Trichilemmal carcinoma. Review of 8 cases. J Cutan Pathol 20:44–49, 1993

304. Seab JA, Graham JH: Primary cutaneous adenoid cystic carcinoma. J Am Acad Dermatol 17:113–118, 1987

305. Fukai K, Ishii M, Kobayashi H, et al: Primary cutaneous adenoid cystic carcinoma. Ultrastructural study and immunolocalization of types I, III, IV, and V collagens and laminin. J Cutan Patol 17:374–380, 1990

306. Cooper PH, Adelson GL, Holthaus WH: Primary cutaneous adenoid cystic carcinoma. Arch Dermatol 120:774–777, 1984

307. Kao GF, Helwig EB, Graham JH: Aggressive digital papillary adenoma and adenocarcinoma. A clinicopathological study of 57 patients, with histochemical, immunopathological, and ultrastructural observations. J Cutan Pathol 14:129–146, 1987

308. Biernat W, Wozniak L: Spiradenocarcinoma. A clinicopathologic and immunohistochemical study of three cases. Am J Dermatopathol 16:377–382, 1994

309. Wick MR, Swanson PE, Kaye VN, Pittelkow MR: Sweat gland carcinoma ex eccrine spiradenoma. Am J Dermatopathol 9:90–98, 1987

310. Landman G, Farmer ER: Primary cutaneous mucoepidermoid carcinoma. Report of a case. J Cutan Pathol 18:56–59, 1991

311. Friedman KJ: Low-grade primary cutaneous adenosquamous (mucoepidermoid) carcinoma: report of a case and review of the literature. Am J Dermatol 11:43–50, 1989

312. Paties C, Taccagni GL, Papotti M, et al: Apocrine carcinoma of the skin. A clinicopathologic, immunocytochemical, and ultra-structural study. Cancer 71:375–381, 1993

313. Nishikawa Y, Tokusashi Y, Saito Y, et al: A case of apocrine adenocarcinoma associated with hamartomatous apocrine gland hyperplasia of both axillae. Am J Surg Pathol 18:832–836, 1994

314. LeDouarin NM: Cell line segregation during peripheral nervous system ontogeny. Science 231:1515–1522, 1986

315. Ito K, Takeuchi T: The differentiation in-vitro of the neural crest cells of the mouse embryo. J Embryol Exp Morph 84:49–62, 1984

316. Quevedo WC, Fleischmann RD: Developmental biology of mammalian melanocytes. J Invest Dermatol 75:116–120, 1980

317. Slaughter JC, Hardman JM, Kempe LG, Earle KM: Neurocutaneous melanosis and leptomeningeal melanomatosis in children. Arch Pathol 88:298–304, 1969

318. Breathnach AS: Melanocytes in early regenerated human epidermis. J Invest Dermatol 35:245–251, 1960

319. Staricco RG: Mechanism of migration of the melanocytes from the hair follicle into the epidermis following dermabrasion. J Invest Dermatol 36:99–104, 1961

320. Ainsworth AM, Folberg R, Reed RJ, Clark WH Jr: Melanocytic nevi, melanocytomas, melanocytic dysplasias, and uncommon forms of melanoma. pp. 167–208. In Clark WH, Godlman LI, Mastrangelo MJ (eds): Human Malignant Melanoma. Grune & Stratton, Orlando, FL, 1979

321. Yadav S, Vossaert KA, Kopf AW, et al: Histopathologic correlates of structures seen on dermoscopy (epiluminescence microscopy). Am J Dermatopathol 15:297–305, 1993

322. Bhuta S: Electron microscopy in the evaluation of melanocytic tumors. Semin Diagn Pathol 10:92–101, 1993

323. Mooi WJ, Krausz T: Biopsy pathology of melanocytic disorders. Biopsy Pathology Series 17, Chapman & Hall, London, 1992

324. Barnhill RL, Albert LS, Shama SK, et al: Genital lentiginosis: a clinical and histopathologic study. J Am Acad Dermatol 22:453–460, 1990

325. Mehregan AH: Lentigo senilis and its evolution. J Invest Dermatol 65:429–433, 1975

326. Elder D, Clark W, Elenitsas R, et al: The early and intermediate precursor lesions of tumor progression in the melanocytic system. Common acquired nevi and atypical (dysplastic) nevi. Semin Diagn Pathol 10:18–35, 1993

327. Stegmaier OC: Natural regression of the melanocytic nevus. J Invest Dermatol 32:413–419, 1959

328. Lund HZ, Stobbe GD: The natural history of the pigmented nevus. Factors of age and anatomic location. Am J Pathol 25:1117–1147, 1949

329. MacDonald DM, Black MM: Secondary localized cutaneous amyloidosis in melanocytic naevi. Br J Dermatol 103:553–556, 1980

330. Stegmaier OC, Montgomery H: Histopathologic studies of pigmented nevi in children. J Invest Dermatol 20:51–64, 1953

331. Masson P: Giant neuro-naevus of the hairy scalp. Ann Surg 93:218–222, 1931

332. Fallowfield ME, Collina G, Cook MG: Melanocytic lesions of the palm and sole. Histopathology 24:463–467, 1994

333. Cooper PH: Deep penetrating (plexiform spindle cell) nevus. A frequent participant in combined nevus. J Cutan Pathol 19:172–180, 1992

334. Kantor GR, Wheeland RG: Transepidermal elimination of nevus cells. A possible mechanism of nevus involution. Arch Dermatol 123:1371–1374, 1987

335. Benz G, Holzel D, Schmoeckel C: Inflammatory cellular infiltrates in melanocytic nevi. Am J Dermatopathol 13:538–542, 1991

336. Cohen PR, Rapini RP: Nevus with cyst. A report of 93 cases. Am J Dermatopathol 15:229–234, 1993

337. Walsh MY, MacKie RM: Histological features of value in differentiating small congenital melanocytic naevi from acquired naevi. Histopathology 12:145–154, 1988

338. Kadonaga JN, Frieden IJ: Neurocutaneous melanosis. Definition and review of the literature. J Am Acad Dermatol 24:747–755, 1991

339. Angelucci D, Natali PG, Americo PL, et al: Rapid perinatal growth mimicking malignant transformation in a giant congenital melanocytic nevus. Hum Pathol 22:297–300, 1991

340. Ruiz-Maldonado R, Tamayo L, Laterza AM, Duran C: Giant pigmented nevi. Clinical, histopathologic, and therapeutic considerations. J Pediatr 120:906–911, 1992

341. Mark GJ, Mihm MC Jr, Liteplo MG et al: Congenital melanocytic nevi of the small and garment type: clinical, histologic and ultrastructural studies. Hum Pathol 4:395–418, 1973

342. Rhodes AR, Silverman RA, Harrist TJ, Melski JW: A histologic comparison of congenital and acquired nevomelanocytic nevi. Arch Dermatol 121:1266–1273, 1985

343. Rhodes AR, Sober AJ, Day CL, et al: The malignant potential of small congenital nevocellular nevi. An estimate of association based on a histologic study of 234 primary cutaneous melanomas. J Am Acad Dermatol 6:230–241, 1982

344. Harley S, Walsh N: A new look at nevus-associated melanomas. Am J Dermatopathol 18:137–141, 1996

345. Lorentzen M, Pers M, Bretteville-Jensen G: The incidence of malignant transformation in giant pigmented nevi. Scand J Plast Reconstr Surg 71:163–167, 1977

346. Illig L, Weidner F, Hundeiker M, et al: Congenital nevi less than or equal to 10 cm as precursors to melanoma. 52 cases, a review, and a new conception. Arch Dermatol 121:1274–1281, 1985

347. Gonzalez-Campora R, Galera-Davidson H, Vazquez-Ramirez FJ, Diaz-Cano S: Blue nevus: classical types and new related entities. A differential diagnostic review. Pathol Res Pract 190:627–635, 1994

348. Cochran A, Bailly C, Paul E, Dolbeau D: Nevi, other than dysplastic and spitz nevi. Semin Diagn Pathol 10:18–35, 1993

349. Dorsey CS, Montgomery H: Blue nevus and its distinction from mongolian spot and the nevus of Ota. J Invest Dermatol 22:225–236, 1954

350. Fletcher V, Sagebiel RW: The combined nevus. pp. 273–283. In Ackerman AB (ed): Pathology of Malignant Melanoma. Masson, New York, 1981

351. Leopold JG, Richards DB: The interrelationship of blue and common nevi. J Pathol 95:37–43, 1968

352. Pulitzer DR, Martin PC, Cohen AP, Reed RJ: Histologic classification of the combined nevus. Analysis of the variable expression of melanocytic nevi. Am J Surg Pathol 15:1111–1122, 1991

353. Rodriquez HA, Ackerman LV: Cellular blue nevus—clinicopathologic study of forty-five cases. Cancer 21:393–405, 1968

354. Lambert WC, Brodkin RH: Nodal and subcutaneous cellular blue nevi—a pseudometastasizing pseudomelanoma. Arch Dermatol 120:367–370, 1984

355. Michal M, Kerekes Z, Kinkor Z, et al: Desmoplastic cellular blue nevi. Am J Dermatopathol 17:230–235, 1995

357. Nakano S, Groth W, Gartmann H, Steigleder GK: Malignant blue nevus with metastases to lung. Am J Dermatopathol 10:436–441, 1988

358. Pich A, Chiusa L, Margaria E, Aloi F: Proliferative activity in the malignant cellular blue nevus. Hum Pathol 24:1323–1329, 1993

359. Temple-Camp CRE, Saxe N, King H: Benign and malignant cellular blue nevus. A clinicopathologic study of 30 cases. Am J Dermatopathol 10:289–296, 1988

360. Wayte DM, Helwig EB: Halo nevi. Cancer 22:69–90, 1968

361. Swanson JL, Wayte DM, Helwig EB: Ultrastructure of halo nevi. J Invest Dermatol 50:434–437, 1968

362. Piepkorn M: On the nature of histologic observations: the case of the Spitz nevus. J Am Acad Dermatol 32:248–254, 1995

363. Binder S, Asnong C, Paul E, Cochran A: The histology and differential diagnosis of Spitz nevus. Semin Diagn Pathol 10:36–46, 1993

364. Busam KJ, Barnhill RL: Pagetoid Spitz nevus. Intradermal Spitz tumor with prominent pagetoid spread. Am J Surg Pathol 19:1061–1067, 1995

365. Barnhill RL, Barnhill MA, Berwick M, Mihm MC: The histologic spectrum of pigmented spindle cell nevus. A review of 120 cases with emphasis on atypical variants. Hum Pathol 22:52–58, 1991

366. Spitz S: Melanomas of childhood. Am J Pathol 24:591–609, 1948

367. Allen AC: Juvenile melanomas of children and adults and melanocarcinomas of children. Arch Dermatol 82:325–335, 1960

368. Kamino H, Misheloff E, Ackerman AB, et al: Eosinophilic gobules in Spitz's nevi—new findings and a diagnostic sign. Am J Dermatopathol 1:319–324, 1979

369. Kamino H, Jagirdar J: Fibronectin in eosinophilic globules of Spitz's nevi. Am J Dermatopathol 6:313–316, 1984

370. Vogt T, Stolz W, Glabl A, et al: Multivariate DNA cytometry discriminates between Spitz nevi and malignant melanomas because large polymorphic nuclei in Spitz nevi are not aneuploid. Am J Dermatopathol 18:142–150, 1996

371. Barr RJ, Morales RV, Graham JH: Desmoplastic nevus—a distinct histologic variant of mixed spindle cell and epithelioid cell nevus. Cancer 47:557–564, 1980

372. Gambini C, Rongioletti F: Recurrent Spitz nevus. Case report and review of the literature. Am J Dermatopathol 16:409–413, 1994

373. Ainsworth AM, Folberg R, Reed RJ, Clark WH Jr: Pigmented spindle cell tumor. In p. 179. Clark WH, Goldman LI, Mastrangelo MJ (eds): Human Malignant Melanoma. Grune Stratton, Orlando, FL, 1979

374. Sau P, Graham JH, Helwig EB: Pigmented spindle cell nevus. Arch Dermatol 120:1615, 1984

375. Sagebiel RW, Chinn EK, Egbert BM: Pigmented spindle cell nevus: clinical and histologic review of 90 cases. Am J Surg Pathol 8:645–653, 1984

376. Smith NP: The pigmented spindle cell tumor of Reed: an under-diagnosed lesion. Sem Diagn Pathol 4:75–87, 1987

377. Sexton M, Sexton CW: Recurrent pigmented melanocytic nevus. A benign lesion, not to be mistaken for malignant melanoma. Arch Pathol Lab Med 115:122–126, 1991

378. Estrada JA, Pierard-Franchimont C, Pierard GE: Histogenesis of recurrent nevus. Am J Dermatopathol 12:370–372, 1990

379. Schoenfeld RJ, Pinkus H: The recurrence of nevi after incomplete removal. Arch Dermatol 78:30–35, 1958

380. Curley RK, Fallowfield ME, Cook MG, Marsden RA: Effect of incisional biopsy on subsequent histology of melanocytic naevi. Br J Dermatol 123:504–506, 1990

381. Cox AJ, Walton RG: The induction of junctional changes in pigmented nevi. Arch Pathol 79:428–434, 1965

382. Kornberg R, Ackerman AB: Pseudomelanoma. Recurrent melanocytic nevus following partial surgical removal. Arch Dermatol 111:1588–1590, 1975

383. Roth ME, Grant-Kels JM, Ackerman AB, et al: The histopathology of dysplastic nevi. Continued controversy. Am J Dermatopathol 13:38–51, 1991

384. Clark WH Jr, Elder DE, Guerry D IV: Dysplastic Nevi and malignant melanoma. pp. 684–756. In Farmer ER, Hood AF (eds): Pathology of the Skin. Appleton & Lange, E. Norwalk, CT, 1990

385. Clark WH Jr, Elder DE, Guerry D IV et al: A study of tumor progression: the precursor lesions of superficial spreading and nodular melanoma. Hum Pathol 15:1147–1165, 1984

386. Rhodes AR, Harrist TJ, Day CL, et al: Dysplastic melanocytic nevi in histologic association with 234 primary cutaneous melanomas. J Am Acad Dermatol 9:563–574, 1983

387. Clark WH Jr, Reimer RR, Greene M, et al: Origin of familial melanomas from heritable melanocytic lesions. "The B-K mole syndrome." Arch Dermatol 114:732–738, 1978

388. Halpern AC, Guerry D IV, Elder DE, et al: Dysplastic nevi as risk markers of sporadic (nonfamilial) melanoma: a case-control study. Arch Dermatol 127:995–999, 1991

389. Bale SJ, Dracopoli NC, Tucke MA, et al: Mapping the gene for hereditary cutaneous malignant melanoma-dysplastic nevus to chromosome 1p. N Engl J Med 320:1367–1372, 1989

390. Sanford KK, Tarone RE, Parshad R, et al: Hypersensitivity to G2 chromatid radiation damage in familial dysplastic naevus syndrome. Lancet 2:1111–1116, 1987

391. Greene MH, Goldin LR, Clark WH Jr, et al: Familial cutaneous malignant melanoma: autosomal dominant trait possibly linked to the Rh locus. Proc Natl Acad Sci USA 80:6071–6075, 1983

392. Rhodes AR, Harrist TJ, Day CL, et al: Dysplastic melanocytic nevi in histologic association with 234 primary cutaneous melanomas. J Am Acad Dermatol 9:563–574, 1983

393. Crutcher WA, Sagebiel RW: Prevalence of dysplastic naevi in a community practice. Lancet 1:728–729, 1984

394. Kelly JW, Holly EA, Shpall PN, Ahn DK: The distribution of melanocytic naevi in melanoma patients and control subjects. Australas J Dermatol 30:1–8, 1989

395. Elder DE, Goldman LI, Goldman SC, et al: The dysplastic nevus syndrome: a phenotypic association of sporadic cutaneous melanoma. Cancer 46:1787–1794, 1980

396. Grob JJ, Andrac L, Ramano MH, et al: Dysplastic naevus in non-familial melanoma. A clinicopathological study of 101 cases. Br J Dermatol 118:745–752, 1988

397. English DR, Menz J, Heenan PJ, et al: The dysplastic naevus syndrome in patients with cutaneous malignant melanoma in Western Australia. Med J Aust 145:194–198, 1986

398. Rhodes AR, Sober AJ, Mihm MC Jr, Fitzpatrick TB: Possible risk factors for primary cutaneous malignant melanoma. Clin Res 28:252A, 1980

399. Nordlund JJ, Kirkwood J, Forget BM, et al: Demographic study of clinically atypical (dysplastic) nevi in patients with melanoma and comparison subjects. Cancer Res 45:1855–1861, 1985

400. Scheibner A, Milton GW, McCarthy WH, et al: Multiple primary melanoma—a review of 90 cases. Aust J Dermatol 23:1–8, 1982

401. Barnhill RL, Roush GC: Histopathologic spectrum of clinically atypical melanocytic nevi. II. Studies of nonfamilial melanoma. Arch Dermatol 126:1315–1318, 1990

402. Clark WH Jr, Elder DE, Guerry D IV, et al: A study of tumor progression: the precursor lesions of superficial spreading and nodular melanoma. Hum Pathol 15:1147–1165, 1984

403. Cook MG, Robertson I: Melanocytic dysplasia and melanoma. Histopathology 9:647–658, 1985

404. Duray PH, Ernstoff MS: Dysplastic nevus in histologic contiguity with acquired nonfamilial melanoma. Arch Dermatol 123:80–84, 1987

405. McGovern VJ, Shaw HM, Milton GW: Histogenesis of malignant melanoma with an adjacent component of the superficial spreading type. Pathology 17:251–254, 1985

406. Black WC: Residual dysplastic and other nevi in superficial spreading melanoma: clinical correlations and association with sun damage. Cancer 62:163–173, 1988

407. Gruber SB, Barnhill RL, Stenn KS, Roush GC: Nevomelanocytic proliferations in association with cutaneous malignant melanoma: a multivariate analysis. J Am Acad Dermatol 21:773–780, 1989

408. Marks R, Dorevitch AP, Mason G: Do all melanomas come from "moles?" A study of the histological association between melanocytic naevi and melanoma. Australas J Dermatol 31:77–80, 1990

409. Hastrup N, Osterlind A, Drzewiecki KT, Hou-Jensen K: The presence of dysplastic nevus remnants in malignant melanomas: a population-based study of 551 malignant melanomas. Am J Dermatopathol 13:378–385, 1991

410. Halpern AC, Guerry D IV, Elder DE, et al: Natural history of dysplastic nevi. J Am Acad Dermatol 29:51–57, 1993

411. Tong AK, Murphy GF, Mihm MC Jr: Dysplastic nevus: a formal histogenetic precursor of malignant melanoma. pp. 10–18. In Mihm MC, Murphy GF, Kaufman N (eds): Pathobiology and recognition of malignant melanoma. Williams & Wilkins, Baltimore, 1988

412. Black WC, Hunt WC: Histologic correlations with the clinical diagnosis of dysplastic nevus. Am J Surg Pathol, 14:44–52, 1990

413. Peter RU, Worret WI, Nickolay-Kiesthardt J: Prevalence of dysplastic nevi in healthy young men. Int J Dermatol 31:327–330, 1992

414. Ackerman AB, A bad-Casintahan MFA, Robinson MJ: Dysplastic nevus: message or massage? Dermatopathol Pract Concept 1:63–66, 1995

415. Clemente C, Cochran A, Elder DE, et al: Histopathologic diagnosis of dysplastic nevi: concordance among pathologists convened by the WHO Melanoma Program. Hum Pathol 22:313–319, 1991

416. Cramer SF: Histopathologic and clinical criteria for definition of dysplastic nevi, letter. Hum Pathol 22:842–843, 1991

417. Elder DE, Green MH, Guerry D IV, et al: The dysplastic nevus syndrome: our definition. Am J Dermatopathol 4:455–460, 1982

418. Smoller BR, Egbert BM: Dysplastic nevi can be diagnosed and graded reproducibly. A longitudinal study. J Am Acad Dermatol 27:399–402, 1992

419. Hastrup N, Clemmensen OJ, Spaun E, Sondergaard K: Dysplastic naevus. Histological criteria and their inter-observer reproducibility. Histopathology 24:503–509, 1994

420. Barnhill RL, Roush GC, Duray PH: Correlation of histologic architectural and cytoplasmic features with nuclear atypia in atypical (dysplastic) nevomelanocytic nevi. Hum Pathol 21:51–58, 1990

421. Sangueza OP, Hyder DM, Bakke AC, White CR Jr: DNA determination in dysplastic nevi. A comparative study between flow cytometry and image analysis. Am J Dermatopathol 15:99–105, 1993

422. Ackerman AB, Magana-Garcia M: Naming acquired melanocytic nevi. Unna's, Miescher's, Spitz's, Clark's. Am J Dermatopathol 12:193–209, 1990

423. Ackerman AB, Cerroni L, Kerl H: Pitfalls in the Histopathologic Diagnosis of Malignant Melanoma. Lea & Febiger, Philadelphia, 1994

424. Roth ME, Grant-Kels JM, Ackerman AB, et al: The histopathology of dysplastic nevi. Continued controversy. Am J Dermatopathol 13:38–51, 1991

425. NIH Consensus Conference: Statement on diagnosis and treatment of early melanoma, January 27–29, 1992. Am J Dermatopathol 15:34–43, 1993

426. Ponz de Leon M: Hereditary melanoma and dysplastic nevus syndrome. Recent Results Cancer Res 136:94–109, 1994

427. Carey W Jr, Thompson CJ, Synnestvedt M, et al: Dysplastic nevi as a melanoma risk factor in patients with familial melanoma. Cancer 74:3118–3125, 1994

428. Barnhill R, Mihm M: The histopathology of cutaneous malignant melanoma. Semin Diagn Pathol 10:47–75, 1993

429. Ceballos PI, Ruiz-Maldonado R, Mihm MC Jr: Melanoma in children. N Engl J Med 332:656–662, 1995

430. Kang S, Barnhill R, Mihm M, Sober A: Multiple primary cutaneous melanomas. Cancer 70:1911–1916, 1992

431. Clark WH, Evans HL, Everett MA, et al: Early melanoma. Histologic terms. J Cutan Pathol 18:477–479, 1991

432. Elder DE, Guerry D IV, Epstein MN, et al: Invasive malignant malanomas lacking competence for metastasis. Am J Dermatopathol, suppl. 6:55–61, 1984

433. Friedman RJ, Rigel DS, Kopf AW: Malignant melanoma in the 1990's: the continued importance of early detection and the role of the physician examination and self-examination of the skin. CA Cancer J Clin 41:201–206, 1991

434. Stolz W, Schmoekel C, Landthaler M, Braun-Falco O: Association of early malignant melanoma with nevocytic nevi. Cancer 63:550–555, 1989

435. O'Rourke MG, Bourke C: Recommended width of excision for primary malignant melanoma. World J Surg 19:343–345, 1995

436. Drzewiecki KT, Andersson AP: Local melanoma recurrences in the scar after limited surgery for primary tumor. World J Surg 19:346–349, 1995

437. Brown CD, Zitelli JA: The prognosis and treatment of true local cutaneous recurrent malignant melanoma. Dermatol Surg 21:285–290, 1995

438. Landthaler M, Braun-Falco O, Leitl A, et al: Excisional biopsy as the first therapeutic procedure versus primary wide excision of malignant melanoma. Cancer 64:1612–1616, 1989

439. Zitelli JA, Moy RL, Abell E: The reliability of frozen sections in the evaluation of surgical margins for melanoma. J Acad Dermatol 24:102–106, 1991

440. Ackerman AB, Scheiner AM: How wide and deep is wide and deep enough? A critique of surgical practice in excisions of primary cutaneous malignant melanoma. Hum Pathol 14:743–744, 1983

441. Cosimi AB, Sober AJ, Mihm MC, Fitzpatrick TB: Conservative surgical management of superficially invasive cutaneous melanoma. Cancer 53:1256–1259, 1984

442. Heenan PJ, English DR, Holman CDJ, Armstrong BK: The effects of surgical treatment on survival and local recurrence of cutaneous malignant melanoma. Cancer 69:421–426, 1992

443. Urist MM, Balch CM, Soong S-J, et al: The influence of surgical margins and prognostic factors predicting the risk of local recurrence in 3445 patients with primary cutaneous melanoma. Cancer 55:1398–1402, 1985

444. Stahlin JS Jr: Malignant melanoma: an appraisal. Surgery 64:1149–1157, 1968

445. Kopf AW, Rigel DS, Friedman RJ: The rising incidence and mortality rate of malignant melanoma. J Dermatol Surg Oncol 8:760–761, 1982

446. Herlyn M, Balaban G, Bennicelli J, et al: Primary melanoma cells of the vertical growth phase: similarities to metastatic cells. J Natl Cancer Inst 74:283–289, 1985

447. Tajima Y, Nakajrma T, Sugano I, et al: Malignant melanoma within an intradermal nevus. Am J Dermatopathol 16:301–306, 1994

448. Hastrup N, Osterlind A, Drzewiecki KT, Hou-Jensen K: The presence of dysplastic nevus remnants in malignant melanomas. A population-based study of 551 malignant melanomas. Am J Dermatopathol 13:378–385, 1991

449. Fallowfield ME, Cook MG: Pagetoid infiltration in primary cutaneous melanoma. Histopathology 20:417–420, 1992

450. Rywlin AM: Intraepithelial melanocytic neoplasia (IMN) versus intraepithelial atypical melanocytic proliferation (IAMP). Am J Dermatopathol 10:92–93, 1988

451. Clark WH, Mihm MC: Lentigo maligna and lentigo-maligna melanoma. Am J Pathol 55:39–67, 1969

452. Kerl H, Hödl S, Stettner H: Acral lentiginous melanoma. pp. 217–242. In Ackerman AB (ed): Pathology of Malignant Melanoma. Masson New York, 1981

453. Stevens NG, Liff JM, Weiss NS. Plantar melanoma: is the incidence of melanoma of the sole of the foot really higher in blacks than whites? Int J Cancer 45:691–693, 1990

454. Paladugu RR, Winberg CD, Yonemoto RH: Acral lentiginous melanoma. A clinicopathologic study of 36 patients. Cancer 52:161–168, 1983

455. Arrington JH, Reed RJ, Ichinose H, Krementz ET: Plantar lentiginous melanoma. A distinct variant of human cutaneous malignant melanoma. Am J Surg Pathol 1:131–143, 1977

456. Ridgeway CA, Hieken TJ, Ronan SG, et al: Acral lentiginous melanoma. Arch Surg 130:88–92, 1995

457. Buttner P, Garbe C, Bertz J, et al: Thickness and importance of Clark's level for prognostic classification. Cancer 75:2499–2506, 1995

458. Wanebo HJ, Fortner JG, Woodruff J, et al: Selection of the optimum surgical treatment of stage I melanoma by depth of microinvasion: use of the combined microstage technique (Clark-Breslow). Ann Surg 182:302–315, 1975

459. Wanebo HJ, Woodruff J, Fortner JG: Malignant melanoma of the extremities. A clinicopathologic study using levels of invasion (microstage). Cancer 35:666–676, 1975

460. Solomon A, Ellis C, Headington J: An evaluation of vertical growth in superficial spreading melanomas by sequential serial microscopic sections. Cancer 52:2338–2341, 1983

461. Breslow A: Tumor thickness, level of invasion and node dissection in stage I cutaneous melanoma. Ann Surg 182:572–575, 1975

462. Balch CM, Murad TM, Soong S-J, et al: A multifactorial analysis of melanoma. Prognostic histopathological features comparing Clark's and Breslow's staging methods. Ann Surg 188:732–742, 1978

463. Breslow A: Thickness, cross-sectional areas and depth of invasion in the prognosis of malignant melanoma. Ann Surg 172:902–908, 1970

464. Breslow A, Cascinelli N, van der Esch EP, Morabito A: Stage I melanoma of the limbs. Assessment of prognosis by levels of invasion and maximum thickness. Tumori 64:273–284, 1978

465. Naruns PL, Nizze JA, Cochran AJ, et al: Recurrence potential of thin primary melanomas. Cancer 57:545–548, 1986

466. Woods JE, Soule EH, Creagan ET: Metastasis and death in patients with thin melanomas (less than 0.76 mm). Ann Surg 198:63–64, 1983

467. Green M, Ackerman B: Thickness is not an accurate gauge of prognosis of primary cutaneous melanoma. Am J Dermatopathol 15:461–473, 1993

468. Day C, Lew R, Mihm M Jr, et al: The natural break points for primary

tumor thickness in clinical stage I melanoma. N Engl J Med 305:1155, 1981

469. Bahmer FA, Hantirah S, Baum H-P: Rapid and unbiased estimation of the volume of cutaneous malignant melanoma using Cavalieri's principle. Am J Dermatopathol 18:159–164, 1996

470. Friedman RJ, Rigel DS, Kopf AW, et al: Volume of malignant melanoma is superior to thickness as a prognostic indicator. Preliminary observation. Dermatol Clin 9:643–648, 1991

471. Roses DF, Harris MN, Rigel D, et al: Local and intransit metastases following definitive excision for primary cutaneous malignant melanoma. Ann Surg 198:65–69, 1983

472. Spellman JE Jr, Driscoll D, Velez A, Karakousis C: Thick cutaneous melanoma of the trunk and extremities: an institutional review. Surg Oncol 3:335–343, 1994

473. Robert M, Wen D, Cochran A: Pathological evaluation of the regional lymph nodes in malignant melanoma. Semin Diagn Pathol 10:102–115, 1993

474. Clark WH Jr, Elder DE, Guerry D IV, et al: Model predicting survival in stage I melanoma based on tumor progression. J Natl Cancer Inst 81:1893–1904, 1989

475. Garbe C, Buttner P, Burg G, et al: Primary cutaneous melanoma. Prognostic classification of anatomic location. Cancer 75:2492–2498, 1995

476. Sugihara T, Yoshida T, Kokubu I, et al: Prognostic evaluation of cutaneous malignant melanoma based on the pTNM classification. J Dermatol 21:953–959, 1994

477. Garbe C, Buttner P, Bertz J, et al: Primary cutaneous melanoma. Identification of prognostic groups and estimation of individual prognosis for 5093 patients. Cancer 75:2484–2491, 1995

478. Thorn M, Ponten F, Bergstrom R, et al: Clinical and histopathologic predictors of survival in patients with malignant melanoma. A population-based study in Sweden. J Natl Cancer Inst 86:761–769, 1994

479. Vilmer C, Bailly C, LeDoussal V, et al: Thin melanomas with unusual aggressive behavior: a report of nine cases. J Am Acad Dermatol 34:439–444, 1996

480. Kelly J, Marsden S, Sagebiel R: Frequency and duration of patient follow-up after treatment of a primary malignant melanoma. J Am Acad Dermatol 13:756–760, 1985

481. McCarthy N, Shaw H, Thompson J, et al: Time and frequency of recurrence of cutaneous stage I malignant melanoma with guidelines for follow-up study. Surg Gynecol Obstet 166:497–502, 1988

482. Wick MR, Swanson PE, Ritter JH, Fitzgibbon JF: The immunohistology of cutaneous neoplasia: a practical perspective J Cutan Pathol 20:481–497, 1993

483. Argenyi ZB, Cain C, Bromley C, et al: S-100 protein-negative malignant melanoma. Fact or fiction? A light-microscopic and immunohistochemical study. Am J Dermatopathol 16:233–240, 1994

484. Zarbo RJ, Gown AM, Nagle RB, et al: Anomalous cytokeratin expression in malignant melanoma. Mod Pathol 3:494–501, 1990

485. Gown AM, Vogel AM, Hoak D, et al: Monoclonal antibodies specific for melanocytic tumors distinguish subpopulations of melanocytes. Am J Pathol 123:195–203, 1986

486. Adema GJ, deBoer AJ, Hullenaar R, et al: Melanocyte lineage specific antigens recognized by monoclonal antibodies NKI-beteb, HMB-50, and HMB-45 are encoded by a single c DNA. Am J Pathol 143:1579–1585, 1993

487. Avril MF, Charpentier P, Margulis A, Guillaume JC: Regression of primary melanoma with metastases. Cancer 69:1377–1381, 1992

488. Smith JL Jr, Stehlin JS Jr: Spontaneous regression of primary malignant melanomas with regional metastases. Cancer 18:1399–1415, 1965

489. Chang P, Knapper WH: Metastatic melanoma of unknown primary. Cancer 49:1106–1111, 1982

490. Wong TY, Suster S, Duncan LM, Mihm MC: Nevoid melanoma: a clinicopathological study of seven cases of malignant melanoma mimicking spindle and epithelioid cell nevus and verrucous dermal nevus. Hum Pathol 26:171–179, 1995

491. Skelton HG, Smith KJ, Laskin WB, et al: Desmoplastic malignant melanoma. J Am Acad Dermatol 32:717–725, 1995

492. Weinzweig N, Tuthill RJ, Yetman RJ: Desmoplastic malignant melanoma: a clinicohistopathologic review. Plast Reconstr Surg 95:548–555, 1995

493. Bruijn JA Mihm MC, Barnhill RL: Desmoplastic melanoma. Histopathology 20:197–206, 1992

494. Anstey A, Cerio R, Ramnarain N, et al: Desmoplastic malignant melanoma. An immunocytochemical study of 25 cases. Am J Dermatopathol 16:14–22, 1994

495. Spitz JL, Silvers DN: Desmoplastic melanoma (or is it merely cicatrix?) arising at the site of biopsy within a conventional melanoma: pitfalls in the diagnosis desmoplastic melanoma. Cutis 55:40–44, 1995

496. Carlson JA, Dickersin GR, Sober AJ, Barnhill RL: Desmoplastic neurotropic melanoma. A clinicopathologic analysis of 28 cases. Cancer 75:478–494, 1995

497. Lucas DR, Tazelaar HO, Unni KK, et al: Osteogenic melanoma. A rare variant of malignant melanoma. Am J Surg Pathol 17:400–409, 1993

498. Prieto VG, Kanik A, Salob S, McNutt NS: Primary cutaneous myxoid melanoma: immunohistologic clues to a difficult diagnosis. J Am Acad Dermatol 30:335–339, 1994

499. Bhuta S, Mirra JM, Cochran AJ: Myxoid malignant melanoma. A previously undescribed histologic pattern noted in metastatic lesions and a report of four cases. Am J Surg Pathol 10:203–211, 1986

500. Denton KJ, Stretch J, Athanasou N: Osteoclast-like giant cells in malignant melanoma. Histopathology 20:179–180, 1992

501. Anstey A, Cerio R, Ramnarain N, et al: Desmoplastic malignant melanoma. An immunocytochemical study of 25 cases. Am J Dermatopathol 16:14–22, 1994

502. Cochran AJ: Melanoma markers: biological and diagnostic considerations. pp. 35–49. In Mihm MC Jr, Murphy GF, Kaufman N (eds): Pathobiology and Recognition of Malignant Melanoma. Williams & Wilkins, Baltimore, 1988

503. Muhlbauer JI, Margolis RJ, Mihm MC, Reed RJ: Minimal deviation melanoma: a histological variant of cutaneous malignant melanoma in its vertical growth phase. J Invest Dermatol 30:63–65, 1983

504. Blessing K, Kernohan NM, Park KGM: Subungual malignant melanoma. Clinicopathological features of 100 cases. Histopathology 19:425–430, 1991

505. Kao GF, Helwig EB, Graham JH: Balloon cell malignant melanoma of the skin. A clinicopathologic study of 34 cases with histochemical, immunohistochemical, and ultrastructural observations. Cancer 69:2942–2952, 1992

506. Sheibani K, Battifora H: Signet-ring cell melanoma. A rare morphologic variant of malignant melanoma. Am J Surg Pathol 12:28–34, 1988

507. Bittesini L, Dei Tos AP, Fletcher CD: Metastatic malignant melanoma showing a rhabdoid phenotype. Further evidence of a non-specific histological pattern. Histopathology 20:167–170, 1992

508. Chang ES, Wick MR, Swanson PE, Dehner LP: Metastatic malignant melanoma with "rhabdoid" features. Am J Clin Pathol 102:426–431, 1994

509. DiMaio SM, Mackay B, Smith JL Jr, Dickerson GR: Neurosarcomatous transformation in malignant melanoma. An ultrastructural study. Cancer 50:2345–2354, 1982

510. Reed RJ, Leonard DD: Neurotropic melanoma. A variant of desmoplastic melanoma. Am J Surg Pathol 3:301–311, 1979

511. Murphy GF, Mihm MC Jr: Benign, dysplastic and malignant lymphoid infiltrates of the skin: an approach based on pattern analysis. pp. 123–141. In Murphy GF, Mihm MC Jr (eds):

Lymphoproliferative Disorders of The skin. Butterworths, Boston, 1986

512. Isaacson PG, Norton AJ (eds): Cutaneous lymphomas. pp. 131–191. In Isaacson PG, Norton AJ (eds): Extranodal Lymphoma. Churchill Livingstone, Edinburgh, 1994

513. Willemze R, Beljaards RC, Meijer CJ, Rijlaarsdam JR: Classification of primary cutaneous lymphomas. Historical overview and perspectives. Dermatology, suppl. 189, 2:8–15, 1994

514. Giannotti B, Santucci M: Skin-associated lymphoid tissue (SALT)-related B-cell lymphoma (primary cutaneous B-cell lymphoma). Arch Dermatol 129:353–355, 1993

515. Bailey EM, Ferry JA, Harris NL, et al: Low-grade B-cell lymphoma of mucosa-associated lymphoid tissue type of skin and soft tissue: a study of 15 primary and secondary cases. Lab Invest 70:44A, 1994

516. Gordon RA, Lookingbill DP, Abt AB: Skin infiltration in Hodgkin's disease. Arch Dermatol 116:1038–1040, 1980

517. Sioutos N, Keri H, Murphy SB, Kadin ME: Primary cutaneous Hodgkin's disease: unique clinical, morphologic, and immunophenotypic findings. Am J Dermatopathol 16:2–8, 1994

518. Rosenberg SA, Diamond HD, Jaslowitz B, et al: Lymphosarcoma: a review of 1269 cases. Medicine 40:31–76, 1961

519. White RW, Patterson JW: Cutaneous involvement in Hodgkin's disease. Cancer 55:1136–1145, 1985

520. Wallace ML, Smoller BR: Immunohistochemistry in diagnostic dermatopathology. J Am Acad Dermatol 34:163–183, 1996

521. MacDonald DM: Histopathological differentiation of benign and malignant cutaneous lymphocytic infiltrates. Br J Dermatol 107:715–718, 1982

522. Smolle J, Torne R, Soyer HP, Kerly H: Immunohistochemical classification of cutaneous pseudolymphomas. Delineation of distinct patterns. J Cutan Pathol 17:149–159, 1990

523. Schmid U, Eckert F, Griesser H, et al: Cutaneous follicular lymphoid hyperplasia with monotypic plasma cells. Am J Surg Pathol 19:12–20, 1995

524. McNutt NS: Cutaneous lymphohistiocytic infiltrates simulating malignant lymphoma. pp. 256–285. In Murphy GF, Mihm MC Jr (eds): Lymphoproliferative Disorders of the Skin. Butterworths, Boston, 1986

525. Sangueza OP, Yadav S, White CR, Braziel RM: Evolution of B-cell lymphoma from pseudolymphoma. A multidisciplinary approach using histology, immunohistochemistry, and Southern blot analysis. Am J Dermatopathol 14:408–413, 1992

526. Smoller BR, Glusac EJ: Histologic mimics of cutaneous lymphoma. Pathol Annu 30:123–141, 1995

527. Hurt MA, Santa Cruz DJ: Cutaneous inflammatory pseudotumor: lesions resembling "inflammatory pseudotumors" or "plasma cell granulomas" of extracutaneous sites. Am J Surg Pathol 14:764–773, 1990

528. Cerio R, MacDonald DM: Benign cutaneous lymphoid infiltrates. J Cutan Pathol 12:442–452, 1985

529. Caro WA, Helwig EB: Cutaneous lymphoid hyperplasia. Cancer 24:487–502, 1969

530. Toonstra J, van der Putte SCJ: Plasmacytoid monocytes in Jessner's lymphocytic infiltration of the skin. A valuable clue for the diagnosis. Am J Dermatopathol 13:321–328, 1991

531. Rijlaarsdam JU, Meijer CJLM, Willemze R: Differentiation between lymphadenosis benign cutis and primary cutaneous follicular center cell lymphomas. A comparative clinicopathologic study of 57 patients. Cancer 65:2301–2306, 1990

532. Ritter JH, Adesokan PN, Fitzgibbon JF, Wick MR: Paraffin section immunohistochemistry as an adjunct to morphologic analysis in the diagnosis of cutaneous lymphoid infiltrates. J Cutan Pathol 21:481–493, 1994

533. Eckert F, Schmid U, Kaudewitz P, et al: Follicular lymphoid hyperplasia of the skin with high content of Ki-positive lymphocytes. Am J Dermatopathol 11:345–352, 1989

534. Schmid U, Eckert F, Griesser H, et al: Cutaneous follicular lymphoid hyperplasia with monotypic plasma cells. A clinicopathologic study of 18 patients. Am J Surg Pathol 19:12–20, 1995

535. Wechsler J, Bagot M, Henni T, et al: Gene analysis in 18 cases of cutaneous lymphoid infiltrates of uncertain significance. Arch Pathol Lab Med 119:157–162, 1995

536. Wood GS, Ngan B-Y, Tung R, et al: Clonal rearrangements of immunoglobulin genes and progression to B cell lymphoma in cutaneous lymphoid hyperplasia. Am J Pathol 135:13–19, 1989

537. Yamamura T, Aozasa K, Sano S: The cutaneous lymphomas with convoluted nucleus. Analysis of thirty-nine cases. J Am Acad Dermatol 10:796–803, 1984

538. McNutt NS, Crain WR: Quantitative electron microscopic comparison of lymphocyte nuclear contours in mycosis fungoides and in benign infiltrates in skin. Cancer 47:698–709, 1981

539. Murphy GF: Cutaneous T cell lymphoma. pp. 131–155. In Fenoglio C(ed): Advances in Pathology. Vol. 1. Year Book Medical, Chicago, 1988

540. Knobler RM, Edelson RL: Lymphoma cutis. T-cell type. pp. 184–187. In Murphy GF, Mihm MC Jr (eds): Lymphoproliferative disorders of the skin. Butterworths, Boston, 1986

541. Barcos M: Mycosis fungoides. Diagnosis and pathogenesis. Am J Clin Pathol 99:452–458, 1993

542. LeBoit PE: Variants of mycosis fungoides and related cutaneous T-cell lymphomas. Semin Diagn Pathol 8:73–81, 1991

543. Willemze R, Beljaards RC, Meijer CJ: Classification of primary cutaneous T-cell lymphomas. Histopathology 24:405–415, 1994

544. Blasik LG, Newkirk RE, Dimond RL, Clendenning WE: Mycosis fungoides d'emblee. A rare presentation of cutaneous T-cell lymphoma. Cancer 49:742–747, 1982

545. Bueschner SA, Winkelmann RK: Sézary syndrome. A clinicopathologic study of 39 cases. Arch Dermatol 119:979–986, 1983

546. Shapiro PE, Pinto FJ: The histologic spectrum of mycosis fungoides/Sézary syndrome (cutaneous T-cell lymphoma). A review of 222 biopsies, including newly described patterns and the earliest pathologic changes. Am J Surg Pathol 18:645–667, 1994

547. Kuzel TM, Roenigk HH Jr, Rosen ST: Mycosis fungoides and the Sézary syndrome. A review of pathogenesis, diagnosis, and therapy. J Clin Oncol 9:1298–1313, 1991

548. King-Ismael D, Ackerman AB: Guttate parapsoriasis/digitate dermatosis (small plaque parapsoriasis) is mycosis fungoides. Am J Dermatopathol 14:518–530, 1992

549. Lacour JP, Castanet J, Perrin C, Ortonne JP: Follicular mycosis fungoides. A clinical and histologic variant of cutaneous T-cell lymphoma. Report of two cases. J Am Acad Dermatol 29:330–334, 1993

550. Argenyi ZB, Goeken JA, Piette WW, Madison KC: Granulomatous mycosis fungoides. Clincopathologic study of two cases. Am J Dermatopathol 14:200–210, 1992

551. LeBoit PE, Zackheim HS, White CR Jr: Granulomatous variants of cutaneous T-cell lymphoma. The histopathology of granulomatous mycosis fungoides and granulomatous slack skin. Am J Surg Pathol 12:83–95, 1988

552. Kartsonis J, Brettschneider F, Weissman A, Rosen L: Mycosis fungoides ballosa. Am J Dermatopathol 12:76–80, 1990

553. Mehregan DA, Su WP, Kurtin PJ: Subcutaneous T-cell lymphoma. A clinical, histopathologic, and immunohistochemical study of six cases. J Cutan Pathol 21:110–117, 1994

554. Brooks B, Sorensen FB, Thestrup-Pedersen K: Estimates of nuclear volume in plaque and tumor-stage mycosis fungoides. A new prognostic indicator. Am J Dermatopathol 16:599–606, 1994

555. Wood GS, Bahler DW, Hoppe RT, et al: Transformation of mycosis fungoides. T-cell receptor beta gene analysis demonstrates a common clonal origin for plaque-type mycosis fungoides and CD30+ large-cell lymphoma. J Invest Dermatol 101:296–300, 1993

556. Ralfkiaer E: Immunohistologic markers for the diagnosis of cutaneous lymphomas. Sem Diagn Pathol 8:62–72, 1991

557. Lessin SR, Rook AH, Rovera G: Molecular diagnosis of cutaneous T-cell lymphoma: polymerase chain reaction amplification of T-cell antigen receptor beta-chain gene rearrangements. J Invest Dermatol 96:299–302, 1991

558. Epstein EH Jr, Levin DL, Croft JD Jr, Lutzner MA: Mycosis fungoides. Survival, prognostic features, response to therapy, and autopsy findings. Medicine 15:61–72, 1972

559. Hamminga L, Hermans J, Noordijk EM, et al: Cutaneous T-cell lymphoma. Clinicopathological relationships, therapy and survival in ninety-two patients. Br J Dermatol 107:145–156, 1982

560. Kemme DJ, Bunn PA Jr: State of the art therapy of mycosis fungoides and Sezary syndrome. Oncology 6:31–42, 1992

561. Van Scott EJ, Kalmanson JD: Complete remissions of mycosis fungoides lymphoma induced by topical nitrogen mustard (HN2). Control of delayed hypersensitivity in HN2 by desensitization and by induction of specific immunologic tolerance. Cancer 32:18–30, 1973

562. Long JC, Mihm MC: Mycosis fungoides with extra-cutaneous dissemination. A distinct clinicopathologic entity. Cancer 34:1745–1755, 1974

563. Rappaport H, Thomas LB: Mycosis fungoides. The pathology of extracutaneous involvement. Cancer 34:1198–1229, 1974

564. Cerroni L, Rieger E, Hodl S, Kerl H: Clinicopathologic and immunologic features associated with transformation of mycosis fungoides to large-cell lymphoma. Am J Surg Pathol 16:543–552, 1992

565. Chan WC, Griem ML, Grozea PN, et al: Mycosis fungoides and Hodgkin's disease occurring in the same patient. Report of three cases. Cancer 44:1408–1413, 1979

566. Scheen SR III, Banks PM, Winkelmann RK: Morphologic heterogeneity of malignant lymphomas developing in mycosis fungoides. Mayo Clin Proc 59:95–106, 1984

567. Simrell CR, Boccia RV, Longo DL, Jaffe ES: Coexisting Hodgkin's disease and mycosis fungoides. Immunohistochemical proof of its existence. Arch Pathol Lab Med 110:1029–1034, 1986

568. LeBoit PE: Granulomatous slack skin. Dermatol Clin 12:375–389, 1994

569. Balus L, Manente L, Remotti D, et al: Granulomatous slack skin. Report of a case and review of the literature. Am J Dermatopathol 18:199–206, 1996

570. Degreef H, Holvoet C, Van Vloten WA, et al: Woringer-Kolopp disease. An epidermotropic variant of mycosis fungoides. Cancer 38:2154–2165, 1976

571. Deneau DG, Wood GS, Beckstead J, et al: Woringer-Kolopp disease (pagetoid reticulosis). Four cases with histopathologic ultrastructural, and immunohistologic observations. Arch Dermatol 120:1045–1051, 1984

572. Lever WF: Localized mycosis fungoides with prominent epidermotropism. Woringer-Kolopp disease. Arch Dermatol 113:1254–1256, 1977

573. Lichtman AH, Mihm MC Jr, Murphy GF: The role of retroviruses in cutaneous T-cell lymphomas. p. 205. In Murphy GF, Mihm MC Jr (eds): Lymphoproliferative Disorders of the Skin. Butterworths, Boston, 1986

574. Arai E, Chow KC, Li Cy, et al: Differentiation between cutaneous form of adult T cell leukemia/lymphoma and cutaneous T cell lymphoma by in situ hybridization using a human T cell leukemia virus-1 DNA probe. Am J Pathol 144:15–20, 1994

575. Hall WW: Human T cell lymphotropic virus type 1 and cutaneous T cell leukemia/lymphoma. J Exp Med 180:1581–1585, 1994

576. Harrist TJ, Murphy GF, Mihm MC Jr: Lymphomatoid vasculitis: a subset of lymphocytic vasculitis. p. 115. In Moschella SL (ed): Dermatology Update: Reviews for Physicians. Elsevier, New York, 1982

577. Sanchez NP, Pittelkow MR, Muller SA, et al: The clinicopathologic spectrum of lymphomatoid papulosis: study of 31 cases. J Am Acad Dermatol 8:81–94, 1983

578. Weiss LM, Wood GS, Ellisen LW, et al: Clonal T-cell populations in pityriasis lichenoides et varioliformis acuta (Mucha-Habermann disease). Am J Pathol 126:417–421, 1987

579. Kadin ME: Lymphomatoid papulosis and associated lymphomas. how are they related? Arch Dermatol 129:351–353, 1993

580. Karp DL, Torn TD: Lymphomatoid papulosis. J Am Acad Dermatol 30:379–395, 1994

581. Smoller BR, Longacre TA, Warnke RA: Ki-1 (CD-30) expression in differentiation of lymphomatoid papulosis from arthropod bite reactions. Mod Pathol 5:492–496, 1992

582. el-Azhary RA, Gibson LE, Kurtin PJ, et al: Lymphomatoid papulosis: a clinical and histopathologic review of 53 cases with leukocyte immunophenotyping, DNA flow cytometry, and T-cell receptor gene rearrangement studies. J Am Acad Dermatol 30:210–218, 1994

583. Cockerell CJ, Stetler LD: Accuracy in diagnosis of lymphomatoid papulosis. Am J Dermatopathol 13:20–25, 1991

584. Kadin ME: Lymphomatoid papulosis. Am J Dermatopathol 17:197–208, 1995

585. Kadin ME, Vonderheid EC, Sako D, et al: Clonal composition of T cells in lymphomatoid papulosis. Am J Pathol 126:13–17, 1987

586. Weiss LM, Wood GS, Trela M, et al: Clonal T-cell populations in lymphomatoid papulosis. Evidence of a lymphoproliferative origin for a clinically benign disease. N Engl J Med 315:475–579, 1986

587. Headington JT, Roth MS, Schnitzer B: Regressing atypical histiocytosis: a review and critical appraisal. Semin Diagn Pathol 4:28–37, 1987

588. Turner ML, Gilmour HM, McLaren KM, et al: Regressing atypical histiocytosis. Report of two cases with progressions to high grade T-cell non-Hodgkin's lymphoma. Hematol Pathol 7:33–47, 1993

589. Wood GS, Burke JS, Horning S, et al: The immunologic and clinicopathologic heterogeneity of cutaneous lymphomas other than mycosis fungoides. Blood 62:464–472, 1983

590. Kurtin P, Murphy GF, Mihm MC Jr: Lymphoma cutis: B-cell type. pp. 142–159. In Murphy GF, Mihm MC Jr (eds): Lymphoproliferative Disorders of the Skin. Butterworths, Boston, 1986

591. Rijaarsdam JU, Willemze R: Primary cutaneous B-cell lymphomas. Leuk Lymphoma 14:213–218, 1994

592. Nagatani T, Miyazawa M, Matsuzaki T, et al: Cutaneous B-cell lymphoma—a clinical, pathological and immunohistochemical study. Clin Exp Dermatol 18:530–536, 1993

593. Santucci M, Pimpinelli N, Arganini L: Primary cutaneous B-cell lymphoma. A unique type of low-grade lymphoma. Clinicopathologic and immunologic study of 83 cases. Cancer 67:2311–2326, 1991

594. Charlotte F, Wechsler J, Joly P, et al: Nonepidermotropic cutaneous lymphomas. A histopathological and immunohistological study of 52 cases. Arch Pathol Lab Med 118:56–63, 1994

595. Holbert JM Jr, Chesney TMcC: Malignant lymphoma of the skin. A review of recent advances in diagnosis and classification. J Cutan Pathol 9:133–168, 1982

596. Burns MK, Kennard CD, Dubin HV: Nodular cutaneous B-cell lymphoma of the scalp in the acquired immunodeficiency syndrome. J Am Acad Dermatol 25:933–936, 1991

597. McGregor JM, Yu CC, Lu QL, et al: Post-transplant cutaneous lymphoma. J Am Acad Dermatol 29:549–554, 1993

598. Willemze R, Kaudewitz P, Berti E, et al: Primary CD30 (Ki-1) positive large cell lymphomas: definition and differential diagnostic aspects. pp. 265–273 In: Lambert WC, Giannotti B, van Vloten WA (ed): Basic Mechanisms of Physiologic and Aberrant Lymphoproliferation in the Skin. Plenum Press, New York, 1994

599. Santucci M, Pimpinelli N: Cutaneous B-cell lymphoma: a SALT-related tumor? pp. 301–315. In Lambert WC, Giannotti B, van

Vloten WA: (eds): Basic Mechanisms of Physiologic and Aberrant Lymphoproliferation in the Skin. Plenum Press, New York, 1994

600. Rijaarsdam U, Bakels V, van Oostveen JW, et al: Changing concepts on cutaneous pseudo-B-cell lymphomas and their relationship to cutaneous B-cell lymphomas. pp. 355–361. In Lambert WC, Giannotti B, van Vloten WA (eds): Basic Mechanisms of Physiologic and Aberrant Lymphoproliferation in the Skin. Plenum Press, New York, 1994

601. Evans HL, Winkelmann RK, Banks PM: Differential diagnosis of malignant and benign cutaneous lymphoid infiltrates. A study of 57 cases in which malignant lymphoma had been diagnosed or suspected in the skin. Cancer 44:699–717, 1979

602. Fisher ER, Park EJ, Wechsler HL: Histologic identification of malignant lymphoma cutis. Am J Clin Pathol 65:149–158, 1976

603. Bhawan J, Wolff SM, Ucci AA, Bhan AK: Malignant lymphoma and malignant angioendotheliomatosis: one disease. Cancer 55:570–576, 1985

604. Demier T, Dail DH, Aboulafia DM: Four varied cases of intravascular lymphomatosis and a literature review. Cancer 73:1738–1745, 1994

605. Di Giuseppe JA, Nelson WG, Seifter EJ, et al: Intravascular lymphomatosis. A clinicopathologic study of 10 cases and assessment of response to chemotherapy. J Clin Oncol 12:2573–2579, 1994

606. Perniciaro C, Winkelmann R K, Daoud MS, Su W PD: Malignant angioendotheliomatosis is an angiotropic intravascular lymphoma. Am J Dermatopathol 17:242–248, 1995

607. Kinney MC, Greer JP, Glick AD et al: Anaplastic large-cell Ki-1 malignant lymphomas. Pathol Annu 26:1–24, 1991

608. Krishnan J, Tomaszewski M, Kao G: Primary cutaneous CD30-positive anaplastic large-cell lymphoma. Report of 27 cases. J Cutan Pathol 20:193–202, 1993

609. DeBruin PC, Beljaards RC, Van Heerde P, et al: Differences in clinical behavior and immunophenotype between primary cutaneous and primary nodal anaplastic large cell lymphoma of T-cell or null cell phenotype. Histopathology 23:127–135, 1993

610. Beljaards RC, Kaudewitz P, Berti E, et al: Primary cutaneous CD30-positive large cell lymphoma: definition of a new type of cutaneous lymphoma with a favorable prognosis. Cancer 71:2097–2104, 1993

611. Willemze R, Beljaards RC: Spectrum of primary cutaneous CD30 (Ki-1)-positive lymphoproliferative disorders. A proposal for classification and guidelines for management and treatment. J Am Acad Dermatol 28:973–980, 1993

612. Ratnam KV, Su WP, Zeismer SC, Li CY: Value of immunohistochemistry in the diagnosis of leukemia cutis. Study of 54 cases using paraffin-section markers. J Cutan Pathol 19:193–200, 1992

613. Kurtin PJ, Di Caudo DJ, Habermann TM, et al: Primary cutaneous large cell lymphomas. Morphologic, immunophenotypic, and clinical features of 20 cases. Am J Surg Pathol 18:1183–1191, 1994

614. Camisa C, Helm TN, Sexton C, Tuthill R: Ki-1-positive anaplastic large-cell lymphoma can mimic benign dermatoses. J Am Acad Dermatol 29:696–700, 1993

615. Kadin ME, Cavaille-Coll MW, Gertz R, et al: Loss of receptors for transforming growth factor β in human T-cell malignancies. Proc Natl Acad Sci 91:6002–6006, 1994

616. Su WPD, Buechner SA, Li CY: Clinicopathologic correlations of leukemia cutis. J Am Acad Dermatol 11:121–128, 1984

617. Buechner SA, Li CY, Su WPD: Leukemia cutis: a histopathologic study of 42 cases. Am J Dermatopathol 7:109–119, 1985

618. Desch JK, Smoller BR: The spectrum of cutaneous disease in leukemias. J Cutan Pathol 20:407–410, 1993

619. Spencer PS, Helm TN: Skin metastases in cancer patients. Cutis 39:119–121, 1987

620. Baer MR, Barcos M, Farrell H, et al: Acute myelogenous leukemia with leukemia cutis. Eighteen cases seen between 1969 and 1986. Cancer 63:2192–2200, 1989

621. Greenwood R, Barker DJ, Tring FC, et al: Clinical and immunohistological characterization of cutaneous lesions in chronic lymphocytic leukemia. Br J Dermatol 113:447–453, 1985

622. Sepp N, Radaszkiewicz T, Meijer CJ, et al: Specific skin manifestations in acute leukemia with monocytic differentiation. A morphologic and immunohistochemical study of 11 cases. Cancer 71:124–132, 1993

623. Kaiserling E, Horny HP, Geerts ML, Schmid U: Skin involvement in myeogenous leukemia. Morphologic and immunophenotypic heterogeneity of skin infiltrates. Mod Pathol 7:771–779, 1994

624. Harrist TJ, Bhan AK, Murphy GF, et al: Histiocytosis X: in situ characterization of cutaneous infiltrates using monoclonal antibodies and heteroantibodies. Am J Clin Pathol 79:294–300, 1983

625. Murphy GF, Harrist TJ, Bhan AK, Mihm MC: Distribution of T cell antigens in histiocytosis X cells. Quantitative immunoelectron microscopy using monoclonal antibodies. Lab Invest 48:90–97, 1983

626. Ben-Ezra JM, Koo CH: Langerhans' cell histiocytosis and malignancies of the M-PIRE system. Am J Clin Pathol 99:464–471, 1993

627. Lieberman PH, Jones CR, Steinman RM, et al: Langerhans cell (eosinophilic) granulomatosis. A clinicopathologic study encompassing 50 years. Am J Surg Pathol 20:519–552, 1996

628. Broadbent V, Gadner H, Komp DM, Ladisch S: Histiocytosis syndromes in children: II. Approach to the clinical and laboratory evaluation of children with Langerhans cell histiocytosis. Med Pediatr Oncol 17:492–495, 1989

629. Emile J-F, Wechsler J, Brousse N, et al: Langerhan's cell histiocytosis: definitive diagnosis with the use of monoclonal antibody O10 on routinely paraffin-embedded samples. Am J Surg Pathol 19:636–641, 1995

630. Marrogi AJ, Dehner LP, Coffin CM, Wick MR: Benign cutaneous histiocytic tumors in childhood and adolescence, excluding Langerhans' cell proliferations. A clinicopathologic and immunohistochemical analysis. Am J Dermatopathol 14:8–18, 1992

631. Caputo R, Alessi E, Berti E: Cutaneous histiocytoses in children. Histopathologic, ultrastructural, and immunohistochemical findings. Prog Surg Pathol 10:111–126, 1989

632. Herman LE, Rothman KF, Harawi S, Gonzalez-Serva A: Congenital self-healing reticulohistiocytosis. A new entity in the differential diagnosis of neonatal papulovesicular eruptions. Arch Dermatol 126:210–212, 1990

633. Gianotti F, Caputo R, Ermacora E, Gianni E: Benign cephalic histiocytosis. Arch Dermatol 122:1038–1043, 1986

634. Roper SS, Spraker MK: Cutaneous histiocytosis syndromes. Pediatr Dermatol 3:19–30, 1986

635. Umbert I, Winkelmann RK: Eruptive histiocytoma. J Am Acad Dermatol 20:958–964, 1989

636. Gianotti R, Alessi E, Caputo R: Benign cephalic histiocytosis: a distinct entity or a part of a wide spectrum of histiocytic proliferative disorders of children? A histopathological study. Am J Dermatopathol 15:315–319, 1993

637. Winkelmann RK: Cutaneous syndrome of non-X histiocytosis: a review of the macrophage-histiocytic diseases of the skin. Arch Dermatol 117:667–672, 1981

638. Wood GS, Haber RS: Novel histiocytoses considered in the context of histiocyte subset differentiation. Arch Dermatol 129:210–214, 1993

639. Bork K, Hoede N: Hereditary progressive mucinous histiocytosis in women. Arch Dermatol 124:1225–1229, 1988

640. Helton JL, Maize JC: Eosinophilic histiocytosis. Histopathology and immunohistochemistry. Am J Dermatopathol 18:111–117, 1996

641. McLeod WA, Winkelmann RK: Eosinophilic histiocytosis: a variant form of lymphomatoid papulosis or a disease sui generis? J Am Acad Dermatol 13:952–958, 1985

642. Szekeres E, Tiba A, Korom I: Xanthoma disseminatum: a rare

condition with non-X, non-lipid cutaneous histiocytopathy. J Dermatol Surg Oncol 14:1021–1024, 1988

643. Sonoda T, Hashimoto H, Enjoji M: Juvenile xanthogranuloma. Clinicopathologic analysis and immunohistochemical study of 57 patients. Cancer 56:2280–2286, 1985

644. Janney CG, Hurt MA, Santa Cruz DJ: Deep juvenile xanthogranuloma: subcutaneous and intramuscular forms. Am J Surg Pathol 15:150–159, 1991

645. Zelger B, Cerio R, Orchard G, Wilson-Jones E: Juvenile and adult xanthogranuloma: a histological and immunohistochemical comparison. Am J Surg Pathol 18:126–135, 1994

646. Caputo R, Grimalt R, Gelmetti C, Cottoni F: Unusual aspects of juvenile xanthogranuloma. J Am Acad Dermatol suppl. 29:868–870, 1993

647. Marrogi AJ, Dehner LP, Coffin CM, Wick MR: Benign cutaneous histiocytic tumors in childhood and adolescence, excluding Langerhans' cell proliferations. A clinicopathologic and immunohistochemical analysis. Am J Dermatopathol 14:8–18, 1992

648. Zelger B, Cerio R, Soyer HP, et al: Reticulohistiocytoma and multicentric reticulohistiocytosis: histopathologic and immunophenotypic distinct entities. Am J Surg Pathol 16:577–584, 1994

649. Heathcote JG, Guenther LC, Wallace AC: Multicentric reticulohistiocytosis: a report of a case and a review of the pathology. Pathology 17:601–608, 1985

650. Mangi MH, Mufti GJ: Multicentric reticulohistiocytosis. Detailed immunophenotyping confirms macrophage origin. Am J Surg Pathol 14:687–693, 1990

651. Mihm MC, Clark WH, Reed RJ, Caruso MG: Mast cell infiltrates in the skin and the mastocytosis syndrome. Hum Pathol 4:231–239, 1973

652. DiBaco RS, DeLeo VA: Mastocytosis and the mast cell. J Am Acad Dermatol 7:709–722, 1982

653. Lannert K, Parwaresch MR: Mast cells and mast cell neoplasia: a review. Histopathology 3:349–365, 1979

654. Friedman BS, Steinberg SC, Meggs WJ, et al: Analysis of plasma histamine levels in patients with mast cell disorders. Am J Med 87:649–654, 1989

655. Cawley EP, Lupton CH Jr, Wheeler CE, McManus TFA: Examination of normal and myxedematous skin. Arch Dermatol 76:537–544, 1957

656. Enzinger FM, Weiss SW: Soft Tissue Tumors. 3rd Ed. Mosby, St. Louis, 1995

657. Fletcher CDM, McKee PH: Sarcomas—a clinicopathological guide with particular reference to cutaneous manifestation. Clin Exp Dermatol 9:451–465, 1984

658. Swanson PE, Wick MR: Immunohistochemical evaluation of vascular neoplasms. Clin Dermatol 9:243–253, 1991

659. Silverman RA: Hemangiomas and vascular malformation. Pediatr Clin North Am 38:811–834, 1991

660. Strutton G, Weedon D: Acro-angiodermatitis. A simulant of Kaposi's sarcoma. Am J Dermatopathol 9:85, 1987

661. Kuo T, Sayers P, Rosai J: Masson's "vegetant intravascular hemangioendothelioma": a lesion often mistaken for angiosarcoma. Cancer 38:1227–1236, 1976

662. Stewart M, Smoller BR: Multiple lesions of intravascular papillary endothelial hyperplasia (Masson's lesion). Arch Pathol Lab Med 118:315–316, 1994

663. Clearkin KP, Enzinger FM: Intravascular papillary endothelial hyperplasia. Arch Pathol Lab Med 100:441–444, 1976

664. Albrecht S, Kahn HJ: Immunohistochemistry of intravascular papillary endothelial hyperplasia. J Cutan Pathol 17:16–21, 1990

665. Paller AS: Metabolic disorders characterized by angiokeratomas and neurologic dysfunction. Neurol Clin 5:441–446, 1987

666. Mulliken JB: Cutaneous vascular anomalies Semin Vascu Surg 6:204–218, 1993

667. Del Rio R, Alsina M, Monteagudo J, et al: POEMS syndrome and multiple angioproliferative lesions mimicking generalized histiocytomas. Acta Derm Venereol 74:388–390, 1994

668. Nichols GE, Gaffey MJ, Mills SE, Weiss LM: Lobular capillary hemangioma: an immunohistochemical study including steroid hormone receptor status. Am J Clin Pathol 97:770–775, 1992

669. LeBoit PE: Lobular capillary proliferation. The underlying process in diverse benign cutaneous vascular neoplasms and reactive conditions. Semin Dermatol 8:298–310, 1990

670. Cooper PH, McAllister HA, Helwig EB: Intravenous pyogenic granuloma. Am J Surg Pathol 3:221–228, 1979

671. Swerlick RA, Cooper PH: Pyogenic granuloma (lobular capillary hemangioma) within port wine stains. J Am Acad Dermatol 8:627–630, 1983

672. Torres JE, Sanchez JL: Disseminated pyogenic granuloma developing after an exfoliative dermatitis. J Am Acad Dermatol 32:280–282, 1995

673. Nappi O, Wick MR: Disseminated lobular capillary hemangioma (pyogenic granuloma). A clinicopathologic study of two cases. Am J Dermatopathol 8:379–385, 1986

674. Warner J, Wilson Jones E: Pyogenic granuloma recurring with multiple satellites. A report of 11 cases. Br J Dermatol 80:218–227, 1968

675. LeBoit PE: Bacillary angiomatosis. Mod Pathol 8:218–222, 1995

676. Calonje E, Fletcher CDM: Sinusoidal hemangioma. A distinctive benign vascular neoplasm within the group of cavernous hemangiomas. Am J Surg Pathol 15:1130–1135, 1991

677. Connelly MG, Winkelmann RK: Acral arteriovenous tumor. A clinicopathologic review. Am J Surg Pathol 9:15–21, 1985

678. Koutlas JG, Jessurun J: Arteriovenous hemangioma. A clinicopathologic and immunohistochemical study. J Cutan Pathol 21:343–349, 1994

679. Hunt SJ, Santa Cruz DJ, Barr RJ: Microvenular hemangioma. J Cutan Pathol 18:235–240, 1991

680. Aloi F, Tomasini C, Pippione M: Microvenular hemangioma. Am J Dermatopathol 15:534–538, 1993

681. Chan JK, Fletcher CD, Hicklin GA, Rosai J: Glomeruloid hemangioma. A distinctive cutaneous lesion of multicentric Castleman's disease associated with POEMS syndrome. Am J Surg Pathol 14:1036–1046, 1990

682. Rongioletti F, Gambini C, Lerza R: Glomeruloid hemangioma. A cutaneous marker of POEMS syndrome. Am J Dermatopathol 16:175–178, 1994

683. Alessi E, Bertani E, Sala F: Acquired tufted angioma. Am J Dermatopathol 8:426–429, 1986

684. Calonje E, Fletcher CDM: New entities in cutaneous soft tissue tumors. Pathologica 8:1–15, 1993

685. Padilla RS, Orkin M, Rosai J: Acquired "tufted" angioma (progressive capillary hemangioma). A distinctive clinicopathologic entity related to lobular capillary hemangioma. Am J Dermatopathol 9:292–300, 1987

686. Wilson-Jones EW, Orkin M: Tufted angioma (angioblastoma). A benign progressive angioma, not to be confused with Kaposi's sarcoma or low grade angiosarcoma. J Am Acad Dermatol 20:214–225, 1989

687. Bernstein EF, Kantor G, Howe N, et al: Tufted angioma of the thigh. J Am Acad Dermatol 31:307–311, 1994

688. Hebeda CL, Scheffer E, Starink TM: Tufted angioma of late onset. Histopathology 23:191–193, 1993

689. Santa Cruz CD, Aronberg J: Targetoid hemosiderotic hemangioma. J Am Acad Dermatol 19:550–558, 1988

690. Rapini RP, Gollitz LE: Targetoid hemosiderotic hemangioma. J Cutan Pathol 17:233–235, 1990

691. Vion B, Frenk E: Targetoid hemosiderotic hemangioma. Dermatology 184:300–302, 1992

692. Morganroth GS, Tigelaar RE, Longley BJ, et al: Targetoid hemangioma associated with pregnancy and the menstrual cycle. J Am Acad Dermatol 32:282–284, 1995

693. Olsen TG, Helwig EB: Angiolymphoid hyperplasia with eosinophilia. A clinicopathological study of 116 patients. J Am Acad Dermatol 12:781–796, 1985

694. Fetsch JF, Weiss SW: Observations concerning the pathogenesis of epithelioid hemangioma (angiolymphoid hyperplasia). Mod Pathol 4:449–455, 1991

695. Allen PW: Angiolymphoid hyperplasia with eosinophilia. Histopathology 19:387, 1991

696. Rosai J: Angiolymphoid hyperplasia with eosinophilia of the skin. Its nosological position in the spectrum of histiocytoid hemangioma. Am J Dermatopathol 4:175–184, 1982

697. Rosai J, Gold J, Landy R: The histiocytoid hemangiomas. A unifying concept embracing several previously described entities of skin, soft tissues, large vessels, bone, and heart. Hum Pathol 10:707–730, 1979

698. Allen PW, Ramakrishna B, MacCormac LB: The histiocytoid hemangiomas and other controversies. Path Annu 2:51–87, 1992

699. Tsang WY, Chan JK: The family of epithelioid vascular tumors. Histopathology 8:187–212, 1993

700. Kuo TT, Shih LY, Chan HL: Kimura's disease. Involvement of regional lymph nodes and distinction from angiolymphoid hyperplasia with eosinophilia. Am J Surg Pathol 12:843–854, 1988

701. Chun SI, Ji HG: Kimura's disease and angiolymphoid hyperplasia with eosinophilia: clinical and histopathologic differences. J Am Acad Dermatol 27:954–958, 1992

702. Googe PB, Harris NL, Mihm MC Jr: Kimura's disease and angiolymphoid hyperplasia with eosinophilia: two distinct histopathologic entities. J Cutan Pathol 14:263–271, 1987

703. Urabe A, Tsuneyoshi M, Enjoji M: Epithelioid hemangioma versus Kimura's disease: a comparative clincopathologic study. Am J Surg Pathol 11:758–766, 1987

704. Flanagan BP, Helwig EB: Cutaneous lymphangioma. Arch Dermatol 113:24–30, 1977

705. Peachey R, Whimster I: Lymphangioma of skin. A review of 65 cases. Br J Dermatol 83:519–527, 1970

706. Whimster JW: The pathology of lymphangioma circumscriptum. Br J Dermatol 94:473–486, 1976

707. Zhu WY, Penneys NS, Reyes B, et al: Acquired progressive lymphangioma. J Am Acad Dermatol 813–815, 1991

708. Watanabe M, Kishiyama K, Ohkawara A: Acquired progressive lymphangioma. J Am Acad Dermatol 8:663–667, 1983

709. Gange RW, Jones EW: Lymphangioma-like Kaposi's sarcoma. A report of three cases. Br J Dermatol 100:327–334, 1979

710. Jones EW, Winkelmann RK, Zachary CB, Reda AM: Benign lymphangioendothelioma. J Am Acad Dermatol 23:229–235, 1990

711. Kaye VM, Dehner LP: Cutaneous glomus tumor. A comparative immunohistochemical study with pseudoangiomatous intradermal melanocytic nevi. Am J Dermatopathol 13:2–6, 1991

712. Dervan PA, Tobbia IN, Casey M, et al: Glomus tumours: an immunohistochemical profile of 11 cases. Histopathology 14:483–491, 1989

713. Porter PL, Bigler SA, McNutt M, Gown AM: The immunophenotype of hemangiopericytomas and glomus tumors, with special reference to muscle protein expression: an immunohistochemical study and review of the literature. Mod Pathol 4:46–52, 1991

714. Heys SD, Brittenden J, Atkinson P, Eremin O: Glomus tumour: an analysis of 43 patients and review of the literature. Br J Surg 79:345–347, 1992

715. Gould EW, Manivel JC, Albores-Saavedra J, Monforte H: Locally infiltrative glomus tumors and glomangiosarcomas: a clinical, ultrastructural, and immunohistochemical study. Cancer 65:310–318, 1990

716. Noer H, Krogdahl A: Glomangiosarcoma of the lower extremity. Histopathology 18:365–366, 1991

717. Brathwaite CD, Poppiti RJ: Malignant glomus tumor. A case report with widespread metastases in a patient with multiple glomus body hamartomas. Am J Surg Pathol 20:233–238, 1996

718. Weiss SW, Enzinger FM: Epithelioid hemangioendothelioma: a vascular tumor often mistaken for a carcinoma. Cancer 50:970–981, 1982

719. LeBoit PE: Self assessment—1993. Epithelioid hemangioendothelioma. J Cutan Pathol 21:570, 1994

720. Resnik K, Kantor G, Spielvogel R, Ryan E: Cutaneous epithelioid hemangioendothelioma without systemic involvement. Am J Dermatopathol 15:272–276, 1993

721. Bollinger BK, Laskin WB, Knight BC: Epithelioid hemangioendothelioma with multiple site involvement: literature review and observations. Cancer 73:610–615, 1994

722. Zukerberg LR, Nickoloff BJ, Weiss SW: Kaposiform hemangioendothelioma of infancy and childhood. An aggressive neoplasm associated with Kasabach-Merritt syndrome and lymphangiomatosis. Am J Surg Pathol 17:321–328, 1993

723. Calonje E, Fletcher CDM, Wilson Jones E, Rosai J: Retiform hemangioendothelioma: a distinctive form of low-grade angiosarcoma delineated in a series of 15 cases. Am J Surg Pathol 18:115–125, 1994

724. Manivel JC, Wick MR, Swanson PE, et al: Endovascular papillary angioendothelioma of childhood: a vascular lesion possibly characterized by "high" endothelial cell differentiation. Hum Pathol 17:1240–1244, 1986

725. Morgan J, Robinson MJ, Rosen LB, et al: Malignant endovascular papillary angioendothelioma (Dabska tumor). A case report and review of the literature. Am J Dermatopathol 11:64–68, 1989

726. Weiss SW, Enzinger FM: Spindle cell hemangioendothelioma. A low-grade angiosarcoma resembling a cavernous hemangioma and Kaposi's sarcoma. Am J Surg Pathol 10:521–530, 1986

727. Fletcher CD: The non-neoplastic nature of spindle cell hemangioendothelioma. Am J Clin Pathol 98:545–546, 1992

728. Imayama S, Murakamai Y, Hashimoto H, Hori Y: Spindle cell hemangioendothelioma exhibits the ultrastructural features of reactive vascular proliferation rather than of angiosarcoma. Am J Clin Pathol 97:279–287, 1992

729. Battocchio S, Facchetti F, Brisigotti M: Spindle cell haemangioendothelioma: further evidence against its proposed neoplastic nature. Histopathology 22:296–298, 1993

730. Fletcher CDM, Beham A, Schmid C: Spindle cell haemangioendothelioma: a clinicopathological and immunohistochemical study indicative of a non- neoplastic lesion. Histopathology 18:291–301, 1991

731. Beckstead JH, Wood GS, Fletcher V: Evidence for the origin of Kaposi's sarcoma from lymphatic endothelium. Am J Pathol 119:294–300, 1985

732. Dictor M: Kaposi's sarcoma. Origin and significance of lymphaticovenous connections. Virchows Arch 409:23–35, 1986

733. Nickoloff BJ, Griffiths CEM: Factor XIIIa-expressing dermal dendrocytes in AIDS-associated cutaneous Kaposi's sarcoma. Science 243:736–35, 1989

734. DeDobbeleer G, Godfrine S, Andre J, et al: Clinically uninvolved skin in AIDS. Evidence of atypical dermal vessels similar to early lesions observed in Kaposi's sarcoma. J Cutan Pathol 14:154–157, 1987

735. Safai B, Mike V, Giraldo G, et al: Association of Kaposi's sarcoma with second primary malignancies: possible etiopathogenic implications. Cancer 45:1472–1479, 1980

736. Finesmith TH, Shrum JP: Kaposi's sarcoma. Int J Dermatol 33:755–762, 1994

737. Chor PJ, Santa Cruz DJ: Kaposi's sarcoma. A clinicopathologic review and differential diagnosis. J Cutan Pathol 19:6–20, 1992

738. Auerbach H, Brooks JJ: Kaposi's sarcoma: neoplasia or hyperplasia. Surg Pathol 2:19–28, 1989

739. Ziegler JI, Templeton AC, Vogel CL: Kaposi's sarcoma. A comparison of classical, endemic, and epidemic forms. Sem Oncol 11:46–52, 1984

740. Friedman-Birnbaum R, Bergman R, Bitterman-Deutsch O, Weltfriend S: Classic and iatrogenic Kaposi's sarcoma. Histopathological patterns as related to clinical course. Am J Dermatopathol 15:523–527, 1993

741. Ron IG, Kuten A, Wigler N, et al: Classical disseminated Kaposi's sarcoma in HIV-negative patients: an unusually indolent subtype. Br J Cancer 68:775–776, 1993

742. Krigel RL, Friedman-Kien AE: Epidemic Kaposi's sarcoma. Semin Oncol 17:350–360, 1990

743. Jones RR, Spaull J, Spry C, Jones EW: Histogenesis of Kaposi's sarcoma in patients with and without acquired immune deficiency syndrome (AIDS). J Clin Pathol 39:742–749, 1986

744. Stein M, Spencer D, Kuten A, Bezwoda W: AIDS-related Kaposi's sarcoma: a review. Isr J Med Sci 30:298–305, 1994

745. Taylor JF, Templeton AC, Vogel CL, et al: Kaposi's sarcoma in Uganda. A clinicopathological study. Int J Cancer 8:122–135, 1971

746. Auerbach HE, Brooks JJ: Kaposi's sarcoma. Neoplasia or hyperplasia? Surg Pathol 2:19–28, 1989

747. Fukunaga M, Silverberg SG: Kaposi's sarcoma in patients with acquired immune deficiency syndrome. A flow cytometric DNA analysis of 26 lesions in 21 patients. Cancer 66:758–764, 1990

748. Ioachim HL, Dorsett B, Melamed J, et al: Cytomegalovirus, angiomatosis, and Kaposi's sarcoma. New observations of a debated relationship. Mod Pathol 5:169–178, 1992

749. Kaaya EE, Parravicini C, Sundelin B, et al: Spindle cell ploidy and proliferation in endemic and epidemic African Kaposi's sarcoma. Eur J Cancer 28A:1890–1894, 1992

750. Seigal B, Levinton-Kriss S, Schiffer A, et al: Kaposi's sarcoma in immunosuppression. Possibly the result of a dual viral infection. Cancer 65:492–498, 1990

751. Allen PJ, Gillespie DL, Redfield RR, Gomez ER: Lower extremity lymphedema caused by acquired immune deficiency syndrome-related Kaposi's sarcoma. Case report and review of the literature. J Vasc Surg 22:178–181, 1995

752. Ruszezak ZB, Mayer-DaSilva A, Orfanos CE: Kaposi's sarcoma in AIDS. Multicentric angioneoplasia in early skin lesions. Am J Dermatopathol 9:388–398, 1987

753. Kao GF, Johnson FB, Sulica VI: The nature of hyaline (eosinophilic) globules and vascular slits of Kaposi's sarcoma. Am J Dermatopathol 12:256–267, 1990

754. Parums DV, Cordell JL, Micklem K et al JC70: a new monoclonal antibody that detects vascular endothelium associated antigen on routinely processed tissue sections. J Clin Pathol 43:752–757, 1990

755. Kuzu I, Bicknell R, Harris AL, et al: Heterogeneity of vascular endothelial cells with relevance to diagnosis of vascular tumours. J Clin Pathol 45:143–148, 1992

756. Zhang Y-M, Bachmann S, Hemmer C, et al: Vascular origin of Kaposi's sarcoma. Expression of leukocyte adhesion molecule-1, thrombomodulin, and tissue factor. Am J Pathol 144:51–59, 1994

757. Sunter JP: Visceral Kaposi's sarcoma. Occurrence in a patient suffering from celiac disease. Arch Pathol Lab Med 102:543–545, 1978

758. Girard C, Johnson WC, Graham JH: Cutaneous angiosarcoma. Cancer 26:868–883, 1970

759. Bhutto AM, Uehara K, Takamiyagi A, et al: Cutaneous malignant hemangioendothelioma: clinical and histopathological observations of nine patients and a review of the literature. J Dermatol 22:253–261, 1995

760. Holden CA, Wilson Jones E: Angiosarcoma of the face and scalp. J R Soc Med, 78 suppl. 11:30–31, 1985

761. Capo V, Ozzello L, Fenoglio CM, et al: Angiosarcomas arising in edematous extremities, immunostaining for factor VIII-related antigen and ultrastructural features. Hum Pathol 16:144–145, 1985

762. Haustein UF: Angiosarcoma of the face and scalp. Int J Dermatol 30:851–856, 1991

763. Marrogi AJ, Hunt SJ, Santa Cruz DJ: Cutaneous epithelioid angiosarcoma. Am J Dermatopathol 12:350–356, 1990

764. Prescott RJ, Banerjee SS, Eyden BP, Haboubi NY: Cutaneous epithelioid angiosarcoma: a clinicopathological study of four cases. Histopathology 25:421–430, 1994

765. Hitchcock MG, Hurt MA, Santa Cruz DJ: Cutaneous granular cell angiosarcoma. J Cutan Pathol 21:256–262, 1994

766. Murphy GF, Dickerson GR, Harrist TJ, Mihm MC: The role of diagnostic electron microscopy in dermatology. p. 370. In Moschella S (ed): Dermatology Update. Reviews for Physicians. Elsevier, New York, 1982

767. Gray MH, Rosenberg AE, Dickersin GR, Bhan AK: Cytokeratin expression in epithelioid vascular neoplasms. Hum Pathol 21:212–217, 1990

768. Palman C, Brooks JJ, LiVolsi VA: Aberrant expression of cytokeratin in vascular tissue and tumors. Lab Invest 3:77A, 1990

769. Newman PJ, Berndt MC, Gorski J, et al: PECAM-1 (CD31) cloning and relation to adhesion molecules of the immunoglobulin gene superfamily. Science 247:1219–1222, 1990

770. DeYoung B, Swanson PE, Sirgi KE, CD31 immunoreactivity is specific for endothelial differentiation in human neoplasms. Lab Invest 6:5A, 1993

771. DeYoung BR, Wick MR, Fitzgibbon JF, et al: CD31: an immunospecific marker for endothelial differentiation in human neoplasms. Appl Immunohistochem 1:97–100, 1993

772. Miettinen M, Lindenmayer AE, Chaubal A: Endothelial cell markers CD31, CD34, and BNH9 antibody to H- and Y-antigens—evaluation of their specificity and sensitivity in the diagnosis of vascular tumors and comparison with von Willebrand factor. Mod Pathol 7:82–90, 1994

773. Longacre TA, Rouse RV: CD31: a new marker for vascular neoplasia. Adv Anat Pathol 1:16–20, 1994

774. Suster S, Wong TY: On the discriminatory value of anti-HPCA-1 (CD-34) in the differential diagnosis of benign and malignant cutaneous vascular proliferations. Am J Dermatopathol 16:355–363, 1994

775. Van De Rijn M, Rouse RV: CD34: a review. Appl Immunohistochem 2:71–80, 1994

776. Traweek ST, Kandalaft PL, Mehta P, Battifora H: The human hematopoietic progenitor cell antigen (CD34) in vascular neoplasia. Am J Clin Pathol 96:25–31, 1991

777. Nappi O, Wick MR, Pettinato G, et al: Pseudovascular adenoid squamous cell carcinoma of the skin. A neoplasm that may be mistaken for angiosarcoma. Am J Surg Pathol 16:429–438, 1992

778. von Hochstetter AR, Meyer VE, Grant JW, et al: Epithelioid sarcoma mimicking angiosarcoma. The value of immunohistochemistry in the differential diagnosis. Virchows Arch [A] 418:271–278, 1991

779. Urbanek RW, Johnson WC: Smooth muscle hamartoma associated with Becker's nevus. Arch Dermatol 114:104–106, 1978

780. Gagne EJ, Su WPD: Congenital smooth muscle hamartoma of the skin. Pediatr Dermatol 10:142–145, 1993

781. Parker RK, Mallory SB, Baker GF: Infantile myofibromatosis. Pediatr Dermatol 8:129–132, 1991

782. Fisher WC, Helwig B: Leiomyomas of the skin. Arch Dermatol 88:510–520, 1963

783. Bronson DM, Fretzin DF, Farrell LN: Congenital pilar and smooth muscle nevus. J Am Acad Dermatol 8:111–114, 1983

784. Slifman NR, Harrist TJ, Rhodes AR: Congenital arrector pili hamartoma. Arch Dermatol 121:1034–1037, 1985

785. Darling TN, Kamino H, Murray JC: Acquired cutaneous smooth muscle hamartoma. J Am Acad Dermatol 28:844–845, 1993

786. Straka BF, Wilson BB: Multiple papules on the leg: multiple piloleiomyomas. Arch Dermatol 127:1717, 1720, 1991

787. Montgomery H, Winkelmann RK: Smooth muscle tumors of the skin. Arch Dermatol 79:32–41, 1959

788. MacDonald DM, Sanderson KV: Angioleiomyoma of the skin. Br J Dermatol 91:161–168, 1974

789. Hachisuga T, Hashimoto H, Enjoji M: Angioleiomyoma. A clinicopathological reappraisal of 562 cases. Cancer 54:126–130, 1984

790. Fitzpatrick JE, Mellette JR, Hwang RJ, et al: Cutaneous angiolipoleiomyoma. J Am Acad Dermatol 23:1093–1098, 1990

791. Scurry JP, Carey MP, Targett CS, Dowling JP: Soft tissue lipoleiomyoma. Pathology 23:360–362, 1991

792. Dahl I, Angervall L: Cutaneous and subcutaneous leiomyosarcoma. A clinicopathologic study of 47 patients. Pathol Eur 9:307–315, 1974

793. Fields JP, Helwig EB: Leiomyosarcoma of the skin and subcutaneous tissue. Cancer 47:156–169, 1981

794. Yamamura T, Takada A, Higashiyama M, Yoshikawa K: Subcutaneous leiomyosarcoma. Br J Dermatol 124:252–257, 1991

795. Jegasothy BV, Gilgor RS, Hull DM: Leiomyosarcoma of the skin and subcutaneous tissue. Arch Dermatol 117:478–481, 1981

796. Newman PL, Fletcher CD: Smooth muscle tumors of the external genitalia: clinicopathologic analysis of a series. Histopathology 18:523–529, 1991

797. Varela-Duran J, Oliva H, Rosai J: Vascular leiomyosarcoma. The malignant counterpart of vascular leiomyoma. Cancer 44:1684–1691, 1979

798. Headington JT, Beals TF, Niederhuber JE: Primary leiomyosarcoma of skin: a report and critical appraisal. J Cutan Pathol 4:308–317, 1977

799. Suster S: Epithelioid leiomyosarcoma of the skin and subcutaneous tissue. Clinicopathologic immunohistochemical, and ultrastructural study of five cases. Am J Surg Pathol 18:232–240, 1994

800. Swanson PE, Stanley MW, Scheithauer BW, et al: Primary cutaneous leiomyosarcoma. J Cutan Pathol 15:129–141, 1988

801. Hashimoto H, Daimaru Y, Tsuneyoshi M, Enjoji M: Leiomyosarcoma of the external soft tissue. Cancer 57:2077–2088, 1986

802. Skalli O, Ropraz P, Trzeciak A, et al: A monoclonal antibody against alpha-smooth muscle actin: a new probe for smooth muscle differentiation. J Cell Biol 103:2787–2796, 1986

803. Manivel JC, Wick MR, Dehner LP: Non-Vascular Sarcomas of the Skin. Pathology of Unusual Malignant Cutaneous Tumors. Marcel Dekker, New York, pp. 211–279, 1985

804. Seifert HW: Ultrastructural investigation on cutaneous angioleiomyoma. Arch Dermatol Res 271:91–99, 1981

805. Lundgren L, Kindblom LG, Seidal T, Angervall L: Intermediate and fine cytofilaments in cutaneous and subcutaneous leiomyosarcomas. APMIS 99:820–828, 1991

806. Wascher RA, Lee MY: Recurrent cutaneous leiomyosarcoma. Cancer 70:490–492, 1992

807. Phelan JT, Sherer W, Mesa P: Malignant smooth-muscle tumors (leiomyosarcomas) of soft-tissue origin. N Engl J Med 266:1027–1030, 1962

808. Oliver GF, Reiman HM, Gonchoroff NJ, et al: Cutaneous and subcutaneous leiomyosarcoma. Br J Dermatol 124:252–257, 1991

809. Schmidt D, Fletcher CDM, Harms D: Rhabdomyosarcomas with primary presentation in the skin. Pathol Res Pract 189:422–427, 1993

810. Wiss K, Solomon AR, Raimer SS: Rhabdomyosarcoma presenting as a cutaneous nodule. Arch Dermatol 124:1687–1690, 1988

811. Schmitt FC, Bittencourt A, Mendonca N, Dorea M: Rhabdomyosarcoma in a congenital pigmented nevus. Pediatr Pathol 12:93–98, 1992

812. Wong T-Y, Suster S: Primary cutaneous sarcomas showing rhabdomyoblastic differentiation. Histopathology 26:25–32, 1995

813. Ehrich HP, Desmouliere A, Diegelmann RF, et al: Morphological and immunochemical differences between keloid and hypertrophic scar. Am J Pathol 145:105–113, 1994

814. Uitto J, Santa Cruz DJ, Eisen AZ: Connective tissue nevi of the skin. Clinical genetic and histopathologic classification of hamartomas of the collagen, elastin and proteoglycan type. J Am Acad Dermatol 3:441–461, 1980

815. Fork HE, Sanchez RL, Wagner RF Jr, Raimer SS: A new type of connective tissure nevus: isolated exophytic elastoma. J Cutan Pathol 18:457–463, 1991

816. Shitabata PK, Crouch ED, Fitzgibbon JF, et al: Cutaneous sclerotic fibroma. Immunohistochemical evidence of a fibroblastic neoplasm with ongoing type I collagen synthesis. Am J Dermatopathol 17:339–343, 1995

817. Requena L, Gutierrez J, Sanchez Yus ES: Multiple sclerotic fibromas of the skin. A cutaneous marker of Cowden's disease. J Cutan Pathol 19:346–351, 1992

818. Cerio R, Rao BK, Spaull J, Wilson Jones E: An immunohistochemical study of fibrous papule of the nose: 25 cases. J Cutan Pathol 16:194–198, 1989

819. Vilanova JR, Flint A: The morphological variations of fibrous histiocytoma. J Cutan Pathol 1:155–164, 1974

820. Goette DK, Helwig EB: Basal cell carcinoma and basal cell carcinoma-like changes overlying dermatofibroma. Arch Dermatol 111:589–592, 1975

821. Li D-F, Iwasaki H, Kikuchi M, et al: Dermatofibroma: superficial fibrous proliferation with reactive histiocytes: a multiple immunostaining analysis. Cancer 74:66–73, 1994

822. Zelger B, Sidoroff A, Stanzl U, et al: Deep penetrating dermatofibroma versus dermatofibrosarcoma protuberans. A clinicopathologic comparison. Am J Surg Pathol 18:677–686, 1994

823. Gross RE, Wolbach BS: Sclerosing hemangioma. Am J Pathol 19:533–552, 1943

824. Dalziel K, Marks R: Hair follicle-like change over histiocytomas. Am J Dermatopathol 8:462–466, 1986

825. Herman KL, Kantor GR, Katz SM: Squamous cell carcinoma in-situ overlying dermatofibroma. J Cutan Pathol 17:385–387, 1990

826. Aiba S, Tabata N, Ishii H, et al: Dermatofibrosarcoma protuberans is a unique fibrohistiocytic tumour expressing CD34. Br J Dermatol 127:79–84, 1992

827. Kutzner H: Expression of the human progenitor cell antigen CD34 (HPCA-1) distinguishes dermatofibrosarcoma protuberans from fibrous histiocytoma in formalin-fixed, paraffin-embedded tissue. J Am Acad Dermatol 28:613–617, 1993

828. Weiss SW, Nicholoff BJ: CD34 is expressed by a distinctive cell population in peripheral nerve, nerve sheath tumors, and related lesions. Am J Surg Pathol 17:1039–1045, 1993

829. Cohen PR, Rapini RP: Dermatofibroma and dermatofibrosarcoma protuberans: differential expression of CD34 and factor XIIIa, letter. Am J Dermatopathol 16:573–574, 1994

830. Abenoza P, Lillemoe T: CD34 and Factor XIIIa in the differential diagnosis of dermatofibroma and dermatofibrosarcoma protuberans. Am J Dermatopathol 15:429–434, 1994

831. Kamino H, Jacobson M: Dermatofibroma extending into the subcutaneous tissue. Differential diagnosis from dermatofibrosarcoma protuberans. Am J Surg Pathol 14:1156–1164, 1990

832. Gonzalez S, Duarte I: Benign fibrous histiocytoma of the skin: a morphologic study of 290 cases. Pathol Res Pract 174:379–391, 1982

833. Tamada S, Ackerman AB: Dermatofibroma with monster cells. Am J Dermatopathol 9:380–387, 1987

834. Ackerman AB, Ragaz A: Dermatofibroma. The Lives of Lesions: Chronology in Dermatopathology. Mason, New York, 37–45, 1984

835. Franquemont DW, Cooper PH, Shmookler BM, Wick MR: Benign fibrous histiocytoma of the skin with potential for local recurrence: a tumor to be distinguished from dermatofibroma. Mod Pathol 3:158–163, 1990

836. Calonje E, Fletcher CD: New entities in cutaneous soft tissue tumors. Pathologica 85:1–15, 1993

837. Calonje E, Fletcher CDM: Cutaneous fibrohistiocytic tumors: an update. Adv Anat Pathol 1:2–15, 1994

838. Calonje E, Mentzel T, Fletcher CD: Cellular benign fibrous histiocytoma. Clinicopathologic analysis of 74 cases of a distinctive variant of cutaneous fibrous histiocytoma with frequent recurrence. Am J Surg Pathol 18:668–676, 1994

839. Santa Cruz DJ, Kyriakos M: Aneurysmal ("angiomatoid") fibrous histiocytoma of the skin. Cancer 47:2053–2061, 1981

840. Calonje E, Fletcher CDM: Aneurysmal benign fibrous histiocytoma: clinicopathological analysis of 40 cases of a tumor frequently misdiagnosed as a vascular neoplasm. Histopathology 26:323–331, 1995

841. Wilson Jones E, Cerio R Smith NP: Epithelioid cell histiocytoma: a new entity. Br J Dermatol 120:185–195, 1989

842. Singh Gomez C, Calonje E, Fletcher CDM: Epithelioid benign fibrous histiocytoma of skin: clinico-pathologic analysis of 20 cases of a poorly known variant. Histopathology 24:123–129, 1994

843. Vilanova JR, Flint A: The morphological variations of fibrous histiocytomas. J Cutan Pathol 1:155–164, 1974

844. Schwob VS, Santa Cruz DJ: Palisading cutaneous fibrous histiocytomas. J Cutan Pathol 13:403–407, 1986

845. Helm KF, Helm T, Helm F: Palisading cutaneous fibrous histiocytoma. An immunohistochemical study demonstrating differentiation from dermal dendrocytes. Am J Dermatopathol 156:559–561, 1993

846. Leyva WH, Santa Cruz DJ: Atypical cutaneous fibrous histiocytoma. Am J Dermatopathol 8:467–471, 1986

847. Beham A, Fletcher CDM: Atypical "pseudosarcomatous" variant of cutaneous benign fibrous histiocytoma: report of eight cases. Histopathology 17:167–169, 1990

848. Kuo TT, Chan HL: Ossifying dermatofibroma with osteoclast-like giant cells. Am J Dermatopathol 16:193–195, 1994

849. Zelger BW, Steiner H, Kutzner H: Clear cell dermatofibroma. Case report of an unusual fibrohistiocytic lesion. Am J Surg Pathol 20:483–491, 1996

850. Requena L, Farina MC, Fuente C, et al: Giant dermatofibroma. A little known clinical variant of dermatofibroma. J Am Acad Dermatol 30:714–718, 1994

851. Headington JT: The histiocyte in memorium editorial. Arch Dermatol 122:532–533, 1986

852. Soini Y: Cell differentiation in benign cutaneous fibrous histiocytomas. An immunohistochemical study with antibodies to histiomonocytic cells and intermediate filament proteins. Am J Dermatopathol 12:134–140, 1990

853. Sueki H, Whitaker D, Buchsbaum M, Murphy GF: Novel interactions between dermal dendrocytes and mast cells in human skin. Implications for hemostasis and matrix repair (see comments). Lab Invest 69:160–172, 1993

854. Cerio R, Spaull JR, Wilson Jones E: Histiocytoma cutis: a tumour of dermal dendrocytes (dermal dendrocytoma). Br J Dermatol 120:197–206, 1989

855. Kamino H, Reddy VB, Gero M, Greco MA: Dermatomyofibroma: a benign cutaneous, plaque-like proliferation of fibroblasts and myofibroblasts in young adults. J Cutan Pathol 19:85–93, 1992

856. Colomé MI, Sanchez RL: Dermatomyofibroma: report of two cases. J Cutan Pathol 21:371–376, 1994

857. Taylor HB, Helwig EB: Dermatofibrosarcoma protuberans. Cancer 15:717–725, 1961

858. Parker TL, Zitelli JA: Surgical margins for excision of dermatofibrosarcoma protuberans. J Am Acad Dermatol 32:233–237, 1995

859. Kahn LB, Saxe N, Gordon W: Dermatofibrosarcoma protuberans with lymph node and pulmonary metastases. Arch Dermatol 114:599–601, 1978

860. Koh CK, Ko CB, Bury HP, Wyatt EH: Dermatofibrosarcoma protuberans. Int J Dermatol 34:256–260, 1995

861. Minoletti F, Miozzo M, Pedeutour F, et al: Involvement of chromosomes 17 and 22 in dermatofibrosarcoma protuberans. Genes Chromosom Cancer 13:62–65, 1995

862. Powers CN, Hurt MA, Frable WJ: Fine-needle aspiration biopsy. Dermatofibrosarcoma protuberans. Diagn Cytopathol 9:145–150, 1993

863. Leong AS, Lim MH: Immunohistochemical characteristics of dermatofibrosarcoma protuberans. Appl Immunohistochem 2:42–47, 1994

864. Dominguez-Malagon HR, Ordonez NG, Mackay B: Dermatofibrosarcoma protuberans. Ultrastructural and immunocytochemical observations. Ultrastruct Pathol 19:281–290, 1995

865. Frierson HF, Cooper PH: Myxoid variant of dermatofibrosarcoma protuberans. Am J Surg Pathol 7:445–450, 1983

866. Wrotnowski U, Cooper PH, Shmookler BM: Fibrosarcomatous change in dermatofibrosarcoma protuberans. Am J Surg Pathol 12:287–293, 1988

867. Ding J, Hashimoto H, Enjoji M: Dermatofibrosarcoma protuberans with fibrosarcomatous areas. A clinicopathologic study of nine cases and a comparison with allied tumors. Cancer 64:721–729, 1989

868. Connelly JH, Evans HL: Dermatofibrosarcoma protuberans: a clinicopathologic review with emphasis of fibrosarcomatous areas. Am J Surg Pathol 16:921–925, 1992

869. O'Dowd J, Laidler P: Progression of dermatofibrosarcoma protuberans to malignant fibrous histiocytoma. Report of a case with implications for tumor histogenesis. Hum Pathol 19:368–370, 1988

870. Banerjee SS, Harris M, Eyden BP, Hamid BNA: Granular cell variant of dermatofibrosarcoma protuberans. Histopathology 17:375–378, 1990

871. Zelger BW, Ofner D, Zelger BG: Atrophic variants of dermatofibroma and dermatofibrosarcoma protuberans. Histopathology 26:519–528, 1995

872. Beham A, Fletcher CD: Dermatofibrosarcoma protuberans with areas resembling giant cell fibroblastoma: report of two cases. Histopathology 17:165–167, 1990

873. Pitt MA, Coyne JD, Harris M, McWilliam LJ: Dermatofibrosarcoma protuberans recurring as a giant cell fibroblastoma with subsequent fibrosarcomatous change. Histopathology 24:197–198, 1994

874. Allen PW, Zwi J: Giant cell fibroblastoma transforming into dermatofibrosarcoma protuberans. Am J Surg Pathol 16:1127–1128, 1992

875. Shmookler BM: Giant cell fibroblastoma transforming into dermatofibrosarcoma protuberans, reply. Am J Surg Pathol 16:1128–1129, 1992

876. Michal M, Zamecnik M: Giant cell fibroblastoma with a dermatofibrosarcoma protuberans component. Am J Dermatopathol 14:549–552, 1992

877. Ding J, Hashimoto H, Sugimoto T, et al: Bednar tumor (pigmented dermatofibrosarcoma protuberans). An analysis of six cases. Acta Pathol Jpn 40:744–754, 1990

878. Lopez JI, Elizade JM, Fdez-Larrinoa A: Pigmented dermatofibrosarcoma protuberans (Bednar tumor). Dermatology 184:281–282, 1992

879. Onoda N, Tsutsumi Y, Kakudo K, et al: Pigmented dermatofibrosarcoma protuberans (Bednar tumor). An autopsy case with systemic metastases. Acta Pathol Jpn 40:935–940, 1990

880. Fretzin DFJ, Helwig EB: Atypical fibroxanthoma of the skin. A clinicopathologic study of 140 cases. Cancer 31:1541–1552, 1973

881. Oshiro Y, Fukuda T, Tsuneyoshi M: Atypical fibroxanthoma versus benign and malignant fibrous histiocytoma: a comparative study of their proliferative activity using MIB-1, DNA flow cytometry, and p53 immunostaining. Cancer 75:1128–1134, 1995

882. Longacre TA, Smoller BR, Rouse RV: Atypical fibroxanthoma: multiple immunohistologic profiles. Am J Surg Pathol 17:1199–1209, 1993

883. Dahl I: Atypical fibroxanthoma of the skin. A clinicopathological study of 57 cases. Acta Pathol Microbiol Scand [A] 84:183–197, 1976

884. Wick MR, Fitzgibbon J, Swanson PE: Cutaneous sarcomas and sarcomatoid neoplasms of the skin. Semin Diagn Pathol 10:148–158, 1993

885. Worrell TJ, Ansari Q, Ansari J, Cockerell C: Atypical fibroxanthoma. DNA ploidy analysis of 14 cases with possible histogenetic implications. J Cutan Pathol 20:211–215, 1993

886. Enzinger FM: Atypical fibroxanthoma and malignant fibrous histiocytoma. Am J Dermatopathol 1:185, 1979

887. Enzinger FM: In reply (questions to the Editorial Board). Am J Dermatopathol 2:185, 1979

888. Rachmaninoff N, McDonald JR, Cook JC: Sarcoma-like tumors of the skin following irradiation. Am J Clin Pathol 36:427–437, 1961

889. Calonje E, Wadden C, Wilson Jones E, Fletcher CDM: Spindle cell non-pleomorphic atypical fibroxanthoma: analysis of a series and delineation of a distinct variant. Histopathology 22:247–254, 1993

890. Val-Bernal JF, Corral J, Fernandez F, Gomez-Bellnert C: Atypical fibroxanthoma with osteoclast-like giant cells. Acta Derm Venerol 74:467–470, 1994

891. Kaiserling E, Xiao JC, Ruck P, Horny HP: Aberrant expression of macrophage-associated antigens (CD68 and Ki-M1P) by Schwann cells in reactive neoplastic neural tissue. Light- and electron-microscopic findings. Mod Pathol 6:463–468, 1993

892. Glavin FL, Cornwell ML: Atypical fibroxanthoma of the skin metastatic to a lung. Am J Dermatol 7:57–63, 1985

893. Helwig EB, May D: Atypical fibroxanthoma of the skin with metastasis. Cancer 57:368–376, 1986

894. Brown MD, Swanson NA: Treatment of malignant fibrous histiocytoma and atypical fibrous xanthomas with micrographic surgery. Dermatol Surg Oncol 15:1287–1292, 1989

895. Helwig EB: Atypical fibroxanthoma. In: Tumor Seminar Proceedings of 18th Annual Tumor Seminar of San Antonio Society of Pathologists, 1961. Tex J Med 59:664–667, 1963

896. Headington JT, Niederhuber JE, Repola DA: Primary malignant fibrous histiocytoma of the skin. J Cutan Pathol 5:329–338, 1978

897. Silvis NG, Swanson PE, Manivel JC, Spindle-cell and pleomorphic neoplasms of the skin. Am J Dermatopathol 10:9–19, 1988

898. Enzinger FM, Weiss SW: Soft Tissue Tumors. 3rd Ed. Mosby, St. Louis, p. 354, 1995

899. Dei Tos AP, Maestro R, Doglioni C, et al: Ultraviolet-induced p53 mutations in atypical fibroxanthoma. Am J Pathol 145:11–17, 1994

900. Ozzello L, Stout AP, Murray MR: Cultural characteristics of malignant histiocytomas and fibrous xanthomas. Cancer 16:311–344, 1963

901. Argenyi ZB: Recent developments in cutaneous neural neoplasms. J Cutan Pathol 20:97–108, 1993

902. Argenyi ZB, Santa Cruz D, Bromley C: Comparative light-microscopic and immunohistochemical study of traumatic and palisaded encapsulated neuromas of the skin. Am J Surg Pathol 14:504–510, 1992

903. Bartolomei FJ, Wertheimer SJ: Intermetatarsal neuromas: distribution and etiologic factors. J Foot Surg 22:279–282, 1983

904. Meachim G, Abberton JJ: Histological findings in Morton's metatarsalgia. J Pathol 103:209–217, 1971

905. Reed RJ, Bliss BO: Morton's neuroma. Regressive and productive intermetatarsal elastofibrositis. Arch Pathol 95:123–129, 1973

906. Scotti TM: The lesion of Morton's metatarsalgia (Morton's toe). Arch Pathol 63:91, 1957

907. Morton TG: A peculiar and painful affliction of the fourth metatarsophalangeal articulation. Am J Med Sci 71:37–45, 1876

908. Megahed M: Histopathological variants of neurofibroma. A study of 114 lesions. Am J Dermatopathol 16:486–495, 1994

909. Requena L, Sanqueza OP: Benign neoplasms with neural differentiation: a review. Am J Dermatopathol 17:75–96, 1995

910. Woodruff JM, Funkhouser JW, Marshall ML, et al: Plexiform (multinodular) schwannoma. A tumor simulating the plexiform neurofibroma. Am J Surg Pathol 7:691–697, 1983

911. Woodruff JM, Selig AM, Crowley K, Allen PW: Schwannoma (neurilemoma) with malignant transformation. A rare, distinctive peripheral nerve tumor. Am J Surg Pathol 18:882–895, 1994

912. Megahed M, Ruzieka T: Cellular schwannoma. Am J Dermatopathol 16:418–421, 1994

913. Reed ML, Jacoby RA: Cutaneous neuroanatomy and neuropathology. Am J Dermatopathol 5:335–362, 1983

914. Fletcher CDM: Solitary circumscribed neuroma of the skin (so-called palisaded, encapsulated neuroma). A clinico-pathological and immunohistochemical study. Am J Surg Pathol 13:574–580, 1989

915. Albrecht S, Kahn HJ, From L: Palisaded encapsulated neuroma: an immunohistochemical study. Mod Pathol 2:403–406, 1989

916. Argenyi ZB, Cooper PH, Santa Cruz DJ: Plexiform and other unusual variants of palisaded encapsulated neuroma. J Cutan Pathol 20:34–39, 1993

917. Williams ED, Pollock DJ: Multiple mucosal neuromata with endocrine tumours: a syndrome allied to von Rechlinghausen's disease. J Pathol 91:71–80, 1966

918. Khairi MRA, Dexter RN, Burzynski N, Johnston CC Jr: Mucosal neuroma, pheochromocytoma, and medullary thyroid carcinoma: MEN type III. Medicine 54:89–112, 1975

919. Fryns JP, Chrzanowska K: Mucosal neuromata syndrome [MEN type IIb (III)]. J Med Genet 25:703–706, 1988

920. Apisarnthanarax P: Granular cell tumor: an analysis of 16 cases and review of the literature. J Am Acad Dermatol 5:171–182, 1981

921. Kurtin PJ, Bonin DM: Immunohistochemical demonstration of the lysosome-associated glycoprotein CD68 (KP-1) in granular cell tumors and schwannomas. Hum Pathol 25:1172–1178, 1994

922. Al-Sarraf M, Loud A V, Vaitkevicius VK: Malignant granular cell tumor. Histochemical and electron microscopic study. Arch Pathol 91:550–558, 1971

923. Lee J, Bhjawan J, Wax F, Farber J: Plexiform granular cell tumor: a report of two cases. Am J Dermatopathol 16:537–541, 1994

924. Jurecka W: Plexiform neurofibroma of the skin. Am J Dermatopathol 10:209–217, 1988

925. Kao GF, Laskin WB, Olsen TG: Solitary cutaneous plexiform neurilemmoma (schwannoma): a clinicopathologic, immunohisto-chemical, and ultrastructural study of 11 cases. Mod Pathol 2:20–26, 1989

926. Rongioletti F, Drago F, Rebora A: Multiple cutaneous plexiform schwannomas with tumors of the central nervous system. Arch Dermatol 125:431–432, 1989

927. Rooney MT, Nacimento AG, Tung RLK: Ossifying plexiform tumor: report of a cutaneous ossifying lesion with histologic features of neurothekeoma. Am J Dermatopathol 16:189–192, 1994

928. Beham A, Fletcher CDM: Plexiform xanthoma: an unusual variant. Histopathology 19:565–567, 1991

929. Michal M: Plexiform xanthomatous tumor. A report of three cases. Am J Dermatopathol 16:532–536, 1994

930. Wick MR, Swanson PE, Scheithauer BW, et al: Malignant peripheral nerve sheath tumor: an immunohistochemical study of 62 cases. Am J Clin Pathol 87:425–433, 1987

931. Dabski C, Reiman H, Muller S: Neurofibrosarcoma of skin and subcutaneous tissues. Mayo Clin Proc 65:164–282, 1990

932. Hirose T, Hasegawa T, Kudo E, et al: Malignant peripheral nerve sheath tumors: an immunohistochemical study in relation to ultrastructural features. Hum Pathol 23:865–870, 1992

933. Theaker JM, Fletcher CD: Epithelial membrane antigen expression by the perineurial cell: further studies of peripheral nerve lesions. Histopathology 14:581–592, 1989

934. Johnson TL, Lee MW, Meis JM, et al: Immunohistochemical characterization of malignant peripheral nerve sheath tumors. Surg Pathol 4:121–135, 1991

935. Shimizu S, Teraki Y, Ishiko A, et al: Malignant epithelioid schwannoma of the skin showing partial HMB-45 positivity. Am J Dermatopathol 15:378–384, 1993

936. Visscher D, Cooper PH, Zarbo RJ, Crissman JD: Cutaneous neuroendocrine (Merkel cell) carcinoma: an immunophenotypic, clinicopathologic, and flow cytometric study. Mod Pathol 2:331–338, 1989

937. Smith DE, Anderson PJ, Bielamowicz S, et al: Cutaneous neuroendocrine (Merkel cell) carcinoma. A report of 35 cases. Am J Clin Oncol 18:199–203, 1995

938. Gould VE, Moll R, Moll I, et al: Neuroendocrine (Merkel) cells of the skin: hyperplasia, dysplasias, and neoplasms. Lab Invest 52:334–353, 1985

939. Haag ML, Glass LF, Fenske WA: Merkel cell carcinoma. Diagnosis and treatment. Dermatol Surg 21:669–683, 1995

940. Ratner D, Nelson BR, Brown MD, Johnson TM: Merkel cell carcinoma. J Am A cad Dermatol 29:143–156, 1991

941. Bayrou O, Avril MF, Charpentier P, et al: Primary neuroendocrine carcinoma of the skin. Clinicopathologic study of 18 cases. J Am Acad Dermatol 24:198–297, 1991

942. LeBoit PE, Crutcher WA, Shapiro PE: Pagetoid intraepidermal spread in Merkel cell (primary neuroendocrine) carcinoma of the skin. Am J Surg Pathol 16:584–592, 1992

943. Gomez LG, DiMaio S, Silva EG, Mackay B: Association between neuroendocrine (Merkel cell) carcinoma and squamous carcinoma of the skin. Am J Surg Pathol 7:171–177, 1983

944. Gould E, Albores-Saavedra J, Dubner N, et al: Eccrine and squamous differentiation in Merkel cell carcinoma. An immunohistochemical study. Am J Surg Pathol 12:768–772, 1988

945. Heenan PJ, Cole JM, Spagnolo DV: Primary cutaneous neuroendocrine carcinoma (Merkel cell tumor). An adnexal epithelial neoplasm. Am J Dermatopathol 12:7–16, 1990

946. Van Nguyen A, Argenyi ZB: Cutaneous neuroblastoma. Peripheral neuroblastoma. Am J Dermatopathol 15:7–14, 1993

947. Miettinen M: Keratin 20. Immunohistochemical marker for gastrointestinal, urothelial, and Merkel cell carcinomas. Mod Pathol 8:384–388, 1995

948. Brinkschmidt C, Stolze P, Faharenkamp AG, et al: Immunohistochemical demonstration of chromogranin A, chromogranin B, and secretoneurin in Merkel cell carcinoma of the skin. An immunohistochemical study on 18 cases suggesting two types of Merkel cell carcinoma. Appl Immunohistochem 3:37–44, 1995

949. Shah IA, Netto D, Schlageter MO, et al: Neurofilament immunoreactivity in Merkel-cell tumors. A differentiating feature from small-cell carcinoma. Mod Pathol 6:3–9, 1993

950. Sibley RK, Dehner LP, Rosai J: Primary neuroendocrine (Merkel cell?) carcinoma of the skin. A clinicopathologic and ultrastructural study of 43 cases. Am J Surg Pathol 9:95–108, 1985

951. Gallager RL, Helwig EB: Neurothekeoma—a benign cutaneous tumor of neural origin. Am J Clin Pathol 74:759–764, 1980

952. Husain S, Silvers DN, Halpern AJ, McNutt NS: Histologic spectrum of neurothekeoma and the value of immunoperoxidase staining for S-100 protein in distinguishing it from melanoma. Am J Dermatopathol 16:496–503, 1994

953. Henmi A, Sato H, Wataya T, et al: Neurothekeoma. Report of a case with immunohistochemical and ultrastructural studies. Acta Pathol 36:1911–1919, 1986

954. Holden CA, Wilson-Jones E, MacDonald DM: Cutaneous lobular neuromyxoma. Br J Dermatol 106:211–215, 1982

955. Ilsoda M, Katayama M: Neurothekeoma. Cutis 41:255–256, 1988

956. Pulitzer DR, Reed RJ: Nerve-sheath myxoma (perineurial myxoma). Am J Surg Pathol 7:409–421, 1985

957. Blumberg AK, Kay S, Adelaar RS: Nerve sheath myxoma of digital nerve. Cancer 63:1215–1218, 1989

958. Angervall L, Kindblom L-G, Haglid K: Dermal nerve sheath-myxoma. A light and electron microscopic, histochemical and immunohistochemical study. Cancer 53:1752–1759, 1984

959. Barnhill RL, Mihm M: Cellular neurothekeoma. A distinctive variant of neurothekeoma mimicking nevomelanocytic tumors. Am J Surg Pathol 14:113–120, 1990

960. Goette DK: Calcifying neurothekeoma. J Dermatol Surg Oncol 12:958–960, 1986

961. Calonje E, Wilson-Jones E, Smith NP, Fletcher CDM: Cellular "neurothekeoma". An epithelioid variant of pilar leiomyoma? Morphological and immunohistochemical analysis of a series. Histopathology 20:397–404, 1992

962. Ragsdale BD, Dupree WB: Fatty neoplasms. pp. 254–278. In Bogumill GP, Fleegler EJ (eds): Tumors of the Hand and Upper Limb. Churchill Livingstone, Edinburgh, 1993

963. Dotz W, Prioleau PG: Nevus lipomatosus cutaneous superficialis: a light and electron microscopic study. Arch Dermatol 120:376–379, 1984

964. Hendricks WM, Limber GK: Nevus lipomatosus superficialis. Cutis 29:183–185, 1982

965. Mehregan AH, Tavafolghi V, Ghandchi A: Nevus lipomatosus cutaneous superficialis (Hoffman-Zurhelle). J Cutan Pathol 2:307–313, 1975

966. Field LM: A giant pendulous fibrolipoma. J Dermatol Surg Oncol 8:54–55, 1982

967. Reymond JL, Stoebner P, Amblard P: Nevus lipomatosus cutaneous superficialis: an electron microscopic study of four cases. J Cutan Pathol 7:295–301, 1980

968. Osment LS: Cutaneous lipomas and lipomatosis. Surg Gynecol Obstet 127:129–132, 1968

969. Meis JM, Enzinger FM: Myolipoma of soft tissue. Am J Surg Pathol 15:121–125, 1991

970. Mehregan DA, Mehregan DR, Mehregan AH: Angiomyolipoma. J Am Acad Dermatol 27:331–333, 1992

971. Chan JKC, Tsang WYW, Pau MY, et al: Lymphangiomyomatosis and angiomyolipoma: closely related entities characterized by hamartomatous proliferation of HMB-45-positive smooth muscle. Histopathology 22:445–455, 1993

972. Kaiserling E, Krober S, Xiao J-C, Schaumburg-Lever G: Angiomyolipoma of the kidney. Immunoreactivity with HMB-45. Light-and electron-microscopic findings. Histopathology 25:41–48, 1994

973. Hitchcock MG, Hurt MA, Santa Cruz DJ: Adenolipoma of the skin: a report of nine cases. J Am Acad Dermoatol 29:82–85, 1993

974. Blomstrand R, Juhlin L, Nordenstam H, et al: Adiposis dolorsa associated with defects of lipid metabolism. Acta Derm Venereol (Stockh) 51:243–250, 1971

975. Enzi G. Multiple symmetric lipomatosis: an update clinical report. Medicine (Baltimore) 63:56–64, 1984

976. Uhlin SR: Benign symmetric lipomatosis. Arch Dermatol 115:94–95, 1979

977. Howard WR, Helwig EB: Angiolipoma. Arch Dermatol 82:924–931, 1960

978. Dixon AY, McGregor DH, Lee SH: Angiolipomas: an ultrastructural clinicopathological study. Hum Pathol 12:737–747, 1981

979. Hunt SJ, Santa Cruz DJ, Barr RJ: Cellular angiolipoma. Am J Surg Pathol 14:75–81, 1990

980. Hurt MA, Santa Cruz DJ: Nodular cystic fat necrosis. A reevaluation of the so-called mobile encapsulated lipoma. Am J Acad Dermatol 21:493–498, 1989

981. Sahl WJ Jr: Mobile encapsulated lipomas. Formerly called angiolipomas. Arch Dermatol 114:1684–1686, 1978

982. Dionne GP, Seemayer TA: Infiltrating lipomas and angiolipomas revisited. Cancer 33:732–738, 1974

983. Puig L, Moreno S, DeMoragas JM: Infiltrating angiolipoma. J Dermatol Surg Oncol 12:617–619, 1986

984. Allen PW, Enzinger FM: Hemangiomas of skeletal muscle: an analysis of 89 cases. Cancer 29:8–22, 1972

985. Muszynski CA, Robertson DP, Goodman JC, Baskin DS: Scalp hibernoma: case report and literature review. Surg Neurol 42:343–345, 1994

986. Dardick I: Hibernoma: a possible model of brown fat histogenesis. Hum Pathol 9:321–329, 1978

987. Novy FG Jr, Wilson JW: Hibernomas, brown fat tumors. Arch Dermatol 73:149–157, 1956

988. Vellios F, Baez J, Shumacker HB: Lipoblastomatosis: a tumor of fetal fat different from hibernoma. Am J Pathol 34:1149–1159, 1958

989. Enzinger FM, Harvey DJ: Spindle cell lipoma. Cancer 36:1852–1859, 1975

990. Fletcher C, Martin-Bates E: Spindle cell lipoma: a clinicopathological study with some original observation. Histopathology 11:803–817, 1987

991. Greco MA, Garcia RL, Vuletin JC: Benign lipoblastomatosis. Ultrastructure and histogenesis. Cancer 45:511–515, 1980

992. Sawyer JR, Parsons EA, Crowson ML, et al: Potential diagnostic implications of breakpoints in the long arm chromosome 8 in the lipoblastoma. Cancer Genet Cytogenet 76:39–42, 1994

993. Chung EB, Enzinger FM: Benign lipoblastomatosis. An analysis of 35 cases. Cancer 32:483–492, 1973

994. Coffin CM, Williams RA: Congenital lipoblastoma of the hand. Pediatr Pathol 12:857–864, 1992

995. Chaudhuri B, Ronan SG, Ghosh L: Benign lipoblastoma. Cancer 46:611–614, 1980

996. Mentzel T, Calonje E, Fletcher CDM: Lipoblastoma and lipoblastomatosis: A clinicopathological study of 14 cases. Histopathology 23:527–533, 1993

997. Enterline HT, Culberson JD, Rochlin DB, et al: Liposarcoma. Cancer 13:932–950, 1960

998. Enzinger FM, Winslow DJ: Liposarcoma: a study of 103 cases. Virchows Arch (Pathol Anat) 335:367–388, 1962

999. Chang HR, Hajdu SI, Collin C, Brennan MF: The prognostic value of histologic subtypes in primary extremity liposarcoma. Cancer 64:1514–1520, 1989

1000. Evans HL: Liposarcomas and atypical lipomatous tumors: a study of 66 cases followed for a minimum of 10 years. Surg Pathol 1:41–54, 1988

1001. Enzinger FM, Weiss SW: Soft Tissue Tumors. 3rd Ed. CV Mosby, St Louis, 1995

1002. Prendiville JS, Lucky AW, Mellory SB et al: Osteoma cutis as a presenting sign of pseudohypoparathyroidism. Pediatr Dermatol 9:11–18, 1992

1003. O'Donnell TF Jr, Geller SA: Primary osteoma cutis. Arch Dermatol 104:325–326, 1971

1004. Burgdorf W, Nasemann T: Cutaneous osteomas: a clinical and histopathologic review. Arch Dermatol Res 260:121–135, 1977

1005. SanMartin O, Alegre V, Martinez-Aparicio A: et al: Congenital platelike osteoma cutis: case report and review literature. Pediatr Dermatol 10:182–186, 1993

1006. Boneschi V, Alessi E, Brambilla L: Multiple miliary osteomas of the face. Am J Dermatopathol 15:268–271, 1993

1007. Ruggieri M, Pavone V, Smilari P, et al: Primary osteoma cutis—multiple café-au-lait spots and woolly hair anomaly. Pediatr Radiol 25:34–36, 1995

1008. Moritz DL, Elewski B: Pigmented post acne osteoma cutis in a patient treated with minocycline: report and review of the literature. J Am Acad Dermatol 24:851–853, 1991

1009. Helm F, De La Pava S, Klein E: Multiple miliary osteomas of the skin. Arch Dermatol 96:681–682, 1967

1010. Oikarinen A, Tuomi M-L, Kallionen M, et al: A study of bone formation in osteoma cutis employing biochemical, histochemical and in situ hybridization techniques. Acta Derm Venereol (Stockh) 2:172–174, 1992

1011. Jetmalani SN, Rich P, White CR Jr: Painful solitary subungual nodule. Subungual exostosis (SE). Arch Dermatol 128:849, 852, 1992

1012. Goettmann S, Drape JL, Idy-Peretti I, et al: Magnetic resonance imaging: a new tool in the diagnosis of tumors of the nail apparatus. Br J Dermatol 130:701–710, 1994

1013. Kuo TT: Primary osteosarcoma of the skin. J Cutan Pathol 19:151–155, 1992

1014. Izaki S, Hirai A, Yoshizawa Y, et al: Carcinosarcoma of the skin. Immunohistochemical and electron microscopic observations. J Cutan Pathol 20:272–278, 1993

1015. Leen EJ, Saunders MP, Vallum DI, Keen CE: Carcinosarcoma of skin. Histopathology 26:367–371, 1995

1016. McKee PH, Fletcher CDM, Stavrinos P, Pambakian H: Carcinosarcoma arising in eccrine spiradenoma. A clinicopathologic and histochemical study of two cases. Am J Dermatopathol 12:335–343, 1990

1017. Ando K, Goto Y, Herabayashi N, et al: Cutaneous cartilaginous tumor. Dermatol Surg 21:339–341, 1995

1018. Suster S, Rosai J: Hamartoma of the scalp with ectopic meningothelial elements. A distinctive benign soft tissue lesion that may simulate angiosarcoma. Am J Surg Pathol 14:1–11, 1990

1019. Huggins TJ, Ragsdale BD, Schnapf DJ, et al: Radiologic-pathologic correlation from the Armed Forces Institute of Pathology. Calvarial invasion by meningioma. Radiology 141:709–713, 1981

1020. Theaker JM, Fletcher CDM, Tudway AJ: Cutaneous heterotopic meningeal nodules. Histopathology 16:475–479, 1990

1021. Lopez DA, Silvers DN, Helwig EB: Cutaneous meningiomas. A clinicopathologic study. Cancer 34:728–744, 1974

1022. Serwatka LM, Mellete JR: Cutaneous meningioma. J Dermatol Surg Oncol 10:896–900, 1984

1023. Zanolloi MD, Wilmoth G, Shaw J, et al: Epithelioid sarcoma: clinical and histologic characteristics. J Am Acad Dermatol 26:302–305, 1992

1024. Pastel-Levy C, Bell DA, Rosenberg AE, et al: DNA flow cytometry of epithelioid sarcoma. Cancer 70:2823–2826, 1992

1025. Heenan PJ, Quirk CJ, Papadimitriou JM: Epithelioid sarcoma: a diagnostic problem. Am J Dermatopathol 8:95–104, 1986

1026. Fisher C: Epithelioid sarcoma: the spectrum of ultrastructural differentiation in seven immunohistochemically defined cases. Hum Pathol 19:265–275, 1988

1027. Ishida T, Oka T, Matsushita H, Machinami R: Epithelioid sarcoma: an electron-microscopic immunohistochemical and DNA flow cytometric analysis. Virchows Arch A Pathol Anat Histopathol 421:401–408, 1992

1028. Mirra JM, Kessler S, Bhuta S, Eckardt J: The fibroma-like variant of epithelioid sarcoma. A fibrohistiocytic/myoid cell lesion often confused with benign and malignant spindle cell tumors. Cancer 69:1382–1395, 1992

1029. Dymock R, Allen P, Stirling J, et al: Giant cell fibroblastoma: distinctive recurrent tumor of childhood. Am J Surg Pathol 11:263–271, 1987

1030. Smookler BM, Enzinger FM, Weiss SW: Giant cell fibroblastoma. A juvenile form of dermatofibrosarcoma protuberans. Cancer 64:2154–2161, 1989

1031. Mentzel T, DeiTos AP, Fletcher CD: Perineurioma (storiform perineurial fibromas): clinicopathological analysis of four cases. Histopathology 25:261–267, 1994

1032. Weidner N, Nasr A, Johnston J: Plexiform soft tissue tumor composed predominantly of perineurial fibroblasts (perineuroma). Ultrastruct Pathol 17:251–262, 1993

1033. Tsang WY, Chan JK, Chow LT, Tse CC: Perineuroma: an uncommon soft tissue neoplasm distinct from localized hypertrophic neuropathy and neurofibroma. Am J Surg Pathol 16:756–763, 1992

1034. Giard F, Bonneau R, Raymond GP: Plexiform fibrohistiocytic tumor. Dermatologica 183:290–293, 1991

1035. Enzinger FM, Zhang RY: Plexiform fibrohistiocytic tumor presenting in children and young adults. An analysis of 65 cases. Am J Surg Pathol 12:818–826, 1988

1036. Goodlad JR, Fletcher CDM: Solitary fibrous tumour arising at unusual sites: analysis of a series. Histopathology 19:515–522, 1991

1037. Wilk M, Schmoeckel C, Kaiser HW, et al: Cutaneous angiomyxoma: a benign neoplasm distinct from cutaneous focal mucinosis. J Am Acad Dermatol 33:352–355, 1995

1038. Allen PW, Dymock RB, MacCormac LB: Superficial angiomyxomas with and without epithelial components. Report of 30 tumors in 28 patients. Am J Surg Pathol 12:519–530, 1988

1039. Mentzel T, Calonje E, Wadden C, et al: Myxofibrosarcoma. Clinicopathologic analysis of 75 cases with emphasis on the low-grade variant. Am J Surg Pathol 20:391–405, 1996

1040. Schwartz RA: Continuing Medical Education. Cutaneous metastatic disease. J Am Acad Dermatol 33:161–182, 1995

1041. Schwartz RA: Histopathologic aspects of cutaneous metastatic disease. J Am Acad Dermatol 33:649–657, 1995

1042. McKee PH: Cutaneous metastases. J Cutan Pathol 12:239–250, 1985

1043. Aguilar A, Schoendorff C, Lopez Redondo MJ, et al: Epidermotropic metastases from internal carcinomas. Am J Dermatopathol 13:452–458, 1991

1044. Spencer SP, Helm TN: Skin metastases in cancer patients. Cutis 39:119–121, 1987

1045. Brownstein MH, Helwig EG: Metastatic tumors of skin. Cancer 29:1298–1307, 1972

1046. Brownstein MH, Helwig EG: Patterns of cutaneous metastasis. Arch Dermatol 105:862–868, 1972

1047. Balakrishnan C, Noorily MJ, Prasad JK, Wilson RF: Metastatic adenocarcinoma in a recent burn scar. Burns 20:371–372, 1994

1048. Boyd AS, Rapini RB: Cutaneous collision tumors. An analysis of 69 cases and review of the literature. Am J Dermatopathol 16:253–257, 1994

1049. Batson OV: The role of the vertebral veins in metastatic processes. Ann Intern Med 16:38–45, 1942

1050. Youngberg GA, Berro J, Young M, Leicht SS: Metastatic epidermotropic squamous carcinoma histologically simulating primary carcinoma. Am J Dermatopathol 11:457–465, 1989

18

Soft Tissue Tumors

Jorge Albores-Saavedra
Ruby Delgado
Frank Vuitch

Soft tissue tumors constitute a heterogeneous group of neoplasms in terms of clinical presentation, morphologic features, and clinical behavior. They arise from the extraskeletal mesenchymal tissues, which lie between the epidermis and the parenchymal organs. Tumors arising from the lymphoid system and from the supporting tissues of specific organs and viscera are not included in this group. Neuroectodermally derived peripheral nerve tumors, however, have been included traditionally among the soft tissue tumors because they present similar problems with regard to diagnosis and treatment (these are discussed in detail in Ch. 59).

CLINICAL ASPECTS

Symptomatology

A soft tissue tumor is usually manifested as a painless mass that interferes with the function and/or cosmetic well-being of the patient. Very few soft tissue tumors are associated with the production of biologically active substances. Among the rare systemic manifestations, the hypoglycemic and osteomalacia-rickets syndromes have been studied most extensively.[1–3]

Symptoms may not reflect the biologic behavior of the tumor. In general, however, rapidly growing soft tissue neoplasms that are fixed to surrounding tissues or that invade or destroy adjacent structures must be considered malignant neoplasms until proved otherwise.

Soft tissue tumors of the abdominal cavity and retroperitoneum frequently produce signs and symptoms by means of displacement, compression, or obstruction. Most benign soft tissue neoplasms are well demarcated and sometimes encapsulated. However, some benign tumors and pseudotumors may mimic sarcomas because of their infiltrative growth patterns. The stimulus for the growth of some benign soft tissue tumors or hamartomas may originate early in embryonic and fetal development, before definitive tissue and organ boundaries are established; therefore, these tumors may involve many structures, mimicking the insinuative growth of sarcomas. Hemangiomas and lymphangiomas of childhood are conspicuous examples of this type of growth pattern.

Benign and malignant soft tissue tumors may be components of heritable syndromes. Renal angiomyolipomas, pulmonary lymphangiomyomas, and cardiac rhabdomyomas are associated with tuberous sclerosis.[4,5] The coexistence of fibromatosis and colonic polyposis constitutes part of Gardner's syndrome, which is inherited as a dominant trait.[6] The multiple symmetric lipomatoses, including familial cervical lipodysplasia, are associated with metabolic disorders, whereas the multiple cutaneous leiomyomata of pilar origin and neurofibromatosis (von Recklinghausen's disease) may be complicated by the development of sarcomas.[7] A small percentage of lipomas and angiolipomas are multiple and genetically determined but do not become malignant.[8] Patients with Werner's syndrome, a rare autosomal recessive disorder characterized by shortness of stature and premature aging, often develop a variety of soft tissue sarcomas.[9] Patients with the Li-Fraumeni syndrome, a rare and yet important family cancer syndrome, are at risk for the development of soft tissue sarcomas.[10,11]

DIAGNOSTIC PROCEDURES

The images of soft tissue tumors on routine radiologic examination are often too vague to permit precise definition of the lesion. Magnetic resonance imaging (MRI) and computed tomography (CT) offer superior soft tissue contrast and enable staging with greater confidence. Because of the multiplanar imaging capability, MRI is superior to CT in providing accurate anatomic perspective, compartmentalization, extent and outline of the tumor, its effects on surrounding tissues, and its relationship with adjacent structures, including bone, joints, neurovascular bundles, and visceral organs in the case of deep-seated lesions. Routine x-ray and CT are superior to MRI only in the identification and evaluation of calcifications. The pattern of calcification may eliminate the confusion between myositis ossificans and soft tissue sarcomas. The presence of calcifications in a clinically malignant soft tissue tumor may reduce the diagnostic possibilities to synovial sarcomas, chondrosarcomas, and osteosarcomas. Angiography adds information concerning invasion and compression or destruction of local blood vessels, and aids the surgeon by providing a vascular map of the tumor and the limb or region in which it resides. Angiographic study is required for clinical assessment of certain vascular malformations and neoplasms. Preferably, the heavily vascularized segments of malignant soft tissue tumors delineated by this procedure should be biopsied as they likely represent the least differentiated portions of the lesion. CT remains the modality of choice when evaluating for visceral metastases. MRI is used for post-therapeutic surveillance and detection of residual or recurrent tumor once enough time, approximately 3 months, is allowed for postoperative and/or postradiation changes to resolve or stabilize.

The determination of the biologic nature of a soft tissue tumor rests on the histologic evaluation of representative sections of the entire tumor. For small tumors, 3 cm or less, an excisional biopsy is advocated as a diagnostic and therapeutic procedure. For the latter, a rim of surrounding normal tissues should be included, as marginal excisions often result in recurrences. In larger lesions, an incisional biopsy is indicated. Whether this is accomplished through a transcutaneous needle biopsy or an open biopsy, it is imperative that the biopsy is representative of the lesion, as it dictates the definitive treatment to follow. Multiple incision biopsies may be necessary to establish the diagnosis. In general, biopsy of the edges should be avoided as soft tissue tumors frequently elicit inflammatory, edematous, and/or fibrous host responses, as well as nonspecific degenerative changes. Similarly, superficial biopsies of ulcerated soft tissue tumors should be avoided. Imaging studies may prove invaluable in targeting diagnostic areas and avoiding areas of necrosis or hemorrhage.

Fine needle aspiration (FNA) has become a primary diagnostic procedure in the clinical management of soft tissue tumors.[12–16] Diagnostic accuracy is essentially the same as that of needle core biopsy.[17] Preparation of both alcohol-fixed and air-dried smears optimizes cytologic assessment, as nuclear detail is better appreciated on hematoxylin and eosin (H&E) or Papanicolaou (Pap) stains, whereas some cytoplasmic and stromal features are more apparent on metachromatic stains. Definitive diagnostic criteria exist for the precise identification of many soft tissue lesions, including granular cell tumor, alveolar soft part sarcoma, biphasic synovial sarcoma, rhabdomyosarcoma, liposarcoma, and pleomorphic lipoma. Alternatively, salient cytomorphologic features may place the lesion within a differential diagnostic category: myxoid, spindled, pleomorphic, epithelioid, or small round cell (Appendices 18-1 to 18-3). Subclassification within these categories, particularly spindle cell tumors, may be very difficult.[18] However, the most elemental information provided by FNA, the exclusion of a malignant lymphoma or carcinoma, is in itself of maximum clinical value. FNA is also a reliable and practical means for obtaining material for ancillary studies of diagnostic and/or prognostic value such as electron microscopy, cytogenetics, molecular analysis, and flow cytometry. In addition, immunohistochemistry may be performed routinely on cytologic smears and cell blocks when indicated. Diagnostic material can be obtained in about 90 percent of soft tissue tumors, and diagnostic accuracy of distinguishing benign from malignant lesions exceeds 90 percent.[12] Exfoliative cytology may be utilized when soft tissue sarcomas invade or metastasize to visceral organs or serous cavities. However, tumor cell morphology may be altered dramatically (e.g., spindle cells tend to become rounded in serous effusions).[16]

Frozen section diagnosis of soft tissue tumors is a routine procedure that may be followed by definitive surgery. To avoid serious mistakes, the pathologist should have broad experience not only with these tumors and with the technique, but with the complete clinical information regarding each case as well. Otherwise, it is preferable not to undertake definitive treatment on the basis of that diagnostic procedure. However, frozen sections should still be performed in order to determine adequacy of the tissue for definitive diagnosis and in preparation for other diagnostic techniques, such as immunohistochemistry, cytogenetics, and electron microscopy.

THE PATHOLOGIST'S APPROACH TO THE STUDY OF SOFT TISSUE TUMORS

The pathologic assessment of soft tissue tumors should yield the information required to prognosticate biologic behavior and to plan the course of treatment. Size, histologic classification, histologic grading, lymphatic or blood vessel invasion, the presence of satellite nodules, and adequacy of surgical excision margins are important features that should be included in surgical pathology reports. Soft tissue tumors are renowned for their morphologic heterogeneity, which mandates adequate sampling.

Although the majority of soft tissue tumors can be recognized with conventional stains, in some cases, ancillary diagnostic procedures such as immunohistochemistry, electron microscopy, cytogenetics, and molecular genetics are required to establish the correct diagnosis.

Traditionally pathologists have used a variety of special stains to assist in establishing tumor histogenesis. Unfortunately, the substances demonstrated by these techniques are nonspecific and with few exceptions are of little help in the diagnosis. Moreover, the advent of immunohistochemistry has led to a marked reduction in the number of special stains used by surgical pathologists.

IMMUNOHISTOCHEMISTRY

The value of immunoperoxidase stains lies in their judicious use and interpretation. The sophistication of immunoperoxidase techniques, especially improved methods of antigen retrieval, has resulted in increased sensitivity of the commonly employed antibodies, requiring a refamiliarization with their specificity. Awareness of the noted advantage of some fixatives for staining certain antigens may be of benefit in selecting the proper fixative and/or antibody, and may influence the interpretation of the immunostains. In addition to these and other general principles, some comments pertaining to the immunohistochemistry of soft tissue tumors are worthy of mention.

The intermediate filament, vimentin, has been overemphasized as a mesenchymal marker; however, it is frequently positive in lymphomas, melanomas, and some carcinomas. Its ubiquitous nature may be used to assess the immunoreactivity of the tissue section examined.

The plasticity of the mesenchyme and the participation of the ectoderm during its early stages of development, may pro-

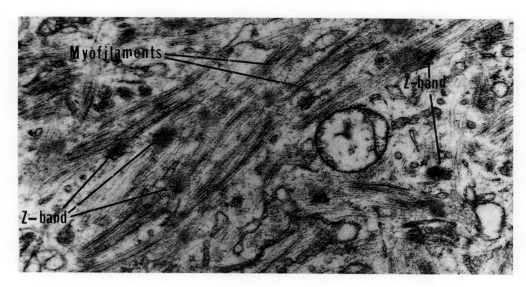

Fig. 18-1. Rhabdomyosarcoma. Portion of the cytoplasm of a malignant rhabdomyoblast showing thick and thin filaments and Z-band material.

vide an explanation for the immunoreactivity to epithelial markers (cytokeratin and epithelial membrane antigen) encountered in the following lesions: (1) biphasic and monophasic synovial sarcoma, (2) epithelioid sarcoma, (3) epithelioid phenotypes of certain sarcomas (e.g., epithelioid angiosarcoma, (4) tumors exhibiting divergent differentiation (e.g., desmoplastic round cell tumor), and (5) reactive and neoplastic myofibroblasts. Cytokeratin positivity has also been detected in leiomyosarcoma and malignant fibrohistiocytoma, malignant melanoma,[19] and malignant melanoma of soft parts (clear cell sarcoma).[20]

Reactivity for the antibody HMB 45, widely used as a melanoma-specific marker, also characterizes a peculiar smooth muscle phenotype that is an integral component of angiomyolipoma.[21]

The antibody CD34, originally recognized as a hematopoietic progenitor cell marker, also stains vascular endothelium, deep dermal dendrocytes, and dendritic cells of the endoneurium. Despite this antigenic diversity, CD34 has proven to be of value in specific diagnostic situations such as (1) confirming the diagnosis of solitary fibrous tumor,[22] (2) distinguishing between dermatofibrosarcoma protuberans and dermatofibroma,[23] (3) identifying benign and malignant endothelial lesions, (4) identifying benign nerve sheath tumors, as antigenicity tends to be lost in malignant ones,[24] and (5) differentiating epithelioid sarcoma from carcinoma.[25]

Within the soft tissue tumors, immunoreactivity for S-100 protein is shared by those having a lipomatous, neural, or cartilaginous origin. In general, such immunoreactivity varies from intense and diffuse in the benign tumors to weak or focal in the malignant ones. Perhaps its greatest value lies in ruling out a malignant melanoma, including the malignant melanoma of tendon and aponeurosis (clear cell sarcoma), when coupled with HMB-45 antibody.

Knowledge of the sequential expression of differentiation markers may be relevant in selecting the appropriate antibody. For example, alveolar and embryonal rhabdomyosarcoma are usually immunoreactive for desmin and muscle-specific actin, whereas staining for myoglobin, which is expressed later in embryonic myogenesis, would be expected in the better differentiated areas of the tumors in which rhabdomyoblasts with abundant cytoplasm are found.[26] At the other extreme of the spectrum, monoclonal antibodies to the nuclear product of MyoD1, a myogenic regulatory gene expressed at an early stage of striated muscle differentiation, help characterize both primitive childhood rhabdomyosarcoma[27] and adult pleomorphic rhabdomyosarcoma.[28]

Strong diffuse homogeneous staining for antibodies to the cell surface glycoprotein MIC2 (013, HBA71 and 12E7) seems to characterize Ewing sarcoma/peripheral neuroectodermal tumor (PNET).[29] However, heterogeneous staining for these antibodies has been reported in a subset of rhabdomyosarcomas, lymphoblastic lymphomas, and in desmoplastic small round cell tumors.[25,30] Therefore, the findings should be interpreted in the context of immunohistochemical panels appropriate for the evaluation of small round cell tumors. Immunoreactivity for MIC2 has also been noted in hemangiopericytomas, solitary fibrous tumor, synovial sarcoma, leiomyosarcoma, and malignant fibrous histiocytoma, and is therefore of limited value in the differential diagnosis of spindle cell tumors.[25,30a]

Immunohistochemistry has also provided a practical means for evaluating the expression of nuclear proliferation-associated antigens,[31] oncogene and tumor suppressor gene proteins,[32] and other markers of potential prognostic significance.

ELECTRON MICROSCOPY

Ultrastructural evaluation of soft tissue tumors permits resolution of a number of problems in differential diagnosis. It is particularly helpful in determining the neuroectodermal, mesenchymal, lymphoreticular, or melanocytic nature of undiffer-

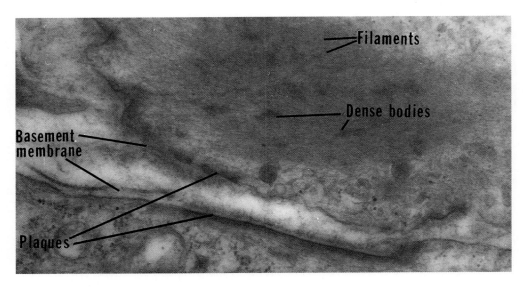

Fig. 18-2. This leiomyosarcoma is characterized by orderly arranged actin filaments with interspersed dense bodies and condensation plaques in the cytoplasmic portion of the plasma membrane.

entiated small cell tumors. Cellular junctions, primitive neurofibrils, and neurosecretory granules are found in neuroblastomas and primitive neuroectodermal tumors; abundant glycogen particles in Ewing's sarcoma; premelanosomes and melanosomes in melanomas; actin and myosin filaments and Z-band material in rhabdomyosarcomas; scant numbers of cytoplasmic organelles, absence of junctional attachments, and pseudopodial projections in malignant lymphomas.[33]

Most examples of rhabdomyosarcoma, leiomyosarcoma, myofibroblastic lesions, and neurogenic sarcoma can be recognized by electron microscopy.

Parallel arrays of actin and myosin filaments and rudimentary sarcomeres are the minimal criteria for the diagnosis of rhabdomyosarcoma.[34–36] The number and arrangement of these proteins depend on the stage of development of the rhabdomyoblasts and are in direct relationship to the degree of differentiation of the tumor (Fig. 18-1). Only in the most mature rhabdomyoblasts are they present in sufficient number and aligned in a manner so as to replicate mature skeletal muscle, forming cross-striations visible by light microscopy.

Ultrastructurally, neoplastic smooth muscle cells contain longitudinal arrays of actin filaments in association with dense bodies, condensation plaques on the cytoplasmic side of the plasma membrane, and pinocytotic vesicles (Fig. 18-2). These structures are diagnostic and their development is related to the degree of differentiation of the tumor.[37] Myofibroblasts contain

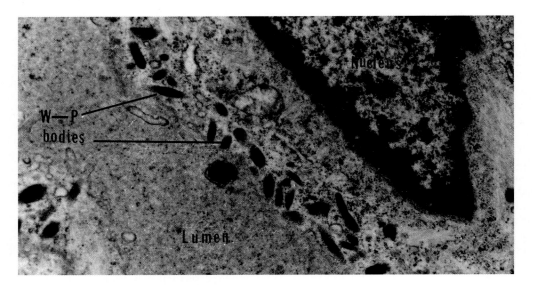

Fig. 18-3. Normal endothelial cells and capillary lumen. Distinct elongated electron-dense formations, the Weibel-Palade bodies, are specifically found in vascular endothelial cells.

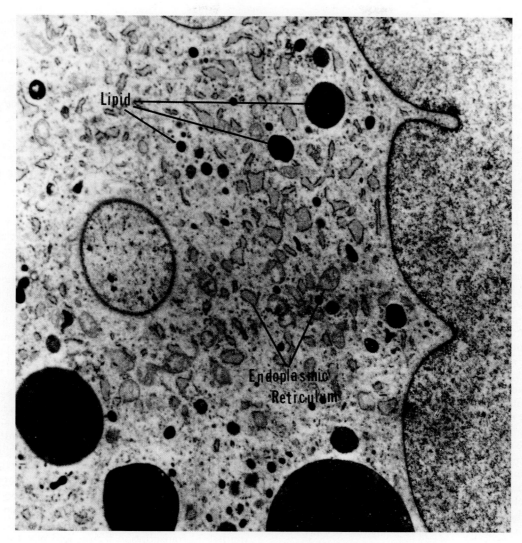

Fig. 18-4. Liposarcoma. Numerous variable-sized non-membrane-bound lipid droplets in close association with endoplasmic reticulum are indicative of the lipogenic nature of this neoplastic cell.

in addition to the ultrastructural smooth muscle markers a well developed rough endoplasmic reticulum. Because the immunohistochemical profile of myofibroblasts is indistinguishable from that of smooth muscle cells or fibroblasts, electron microscopy is the best tool for identification.[38]

The longitudinally striated rod-shaped bodies described by Weibel and Palade are intracytoplasmic components specific for endothelial cells (Fig. 18-3). Therefore, the demonstration of these bodies in neoplastic cells permits identification of that cell line. However, Weibel-Palade bodies are rarely seen in angiosarcomas.[33]

Bundles of microtubules associated with neurosecretory granules in a tumor of small round cells joined by occasional desmosomes are characteristic of neuroblastomas. By contrast, the discovery of longitudinally arranged microtubules and elongated cytoplasmic processes in a spindle cell sarcoma establishes the neurogenic nature of the tumor. Intracytoplasmic fat is al-

most always present in relatively large amounts in liposarcomas and fibrous histiocytomas, adding to the difficulties in the differential diagnosis of these two lesions, which also may mimic each other at the light microscopic level[33] (Fig. 18-4).

Electron microscopic examination of soft tissue tumors presents some disadvantages, including the requirements of proper fixation and sampling, availability of instrumentation, and technical and professional expertise, in addition to the attendant expense.

CLASSIFICATION AND GRADING OF SOFT TISSUE TUMORS

As our diagnostic tools continue to proliferate, become more sophisticated, and are more readily available, it has become possible to phenotype most soft tissue tumors. This permits classification of these lesions into homogeneous groups, although morphologic dissimilarities are often apparent within any given group of tumors. Accordingly, as recommended by the World Health Organization (WHO)[39] we currently group these neoplasms on the basis of their cellular line of differentiation (fibrous tissue, adipose tissue, muscle tissue, blood vessels, lymph vessels, and synovial tissue) and, as a separate group, soft tissue tumors with distinct clinicopathologic manifestations but uncertain phenotype. Likewise, we describe fibrous histiocytic-tumors as a single group because of their frequency, clinicopathologic relevance, and disputed histogenesis. Other histogenetically different tumors that share morphologic features with soft tissue lesions, such as tumors of peripheral nerves and mesotheliomas, are described in Chapters 30 and 49.

The basis for histopathologic diagnosis of sarcomas resides in the discovery of a gradation in maturation from primitive mesenchymal cells to those cellular elements mimicking mature mesenchymal tissue. This general principle is based on the belief that sarcomas originate not from dedifferentiation of mature cells but from primitive mesenchymal tissue, which, in its neoplastic growth and differentiation, replicates embryologic stages of development of the various normal mesenchymal tissues, as has been shown in rhabdomyosarcomas, leiomyosarcomas, and liposarcomas. This common ancestry (primitive mesenchymal cell) may explain the histologic similarities among these different types of tumors. In addition to the histologic type, patient age, grade, stage, and anatomic location of the tumor are also important parameters in determining prognosis of, and therapy for, soft tissue sarcomas. According to the degree of cellularity, cellular pleomorphism, mitotic activity, and necrosis, sarcomas can be divided into three histologic grades that correlate well with prognosis.[40–42] Although this grading system can be applied to most sarcomas (fibrosarcoma, leiomyosarcoma, synovial sarcoma, extraskeletal chondrosarcoma), it is apparent that the grade of some tumors is closely linked to the histologic type. Such is the case with alveolar rhabdomyosarcoma, Ewing's sarcoma, and epithelioid angiosarcomas, which are uniformly high grade, whereas dermatofibrosarcoma protuberans and myxoid liposarcoma are low grade tumors.

Table 18-1. Cytogenetic Heterogeneity in Adipose Tissue Lesions and Morphologic Correlates

Lipoblastoma[52]	Rearrangement of 8q
Hibernoma[53]	Abnormalities in 11q
Lipoma[a]	t(various;12)(various;q13–15)
Spindle and pleomorphic lipoma[54]	Loss of chromosome 16 material
Well differentiated liposarcoma[a]	Ring chromosomes and giant marker chromosomes, with chromosome 12-derived sequences
Myxoid/round cell liposarcoma[b]	t(12;16)(q13;p11)
Pleomorphic liposarcoma[a]	Complex karyotypes

[a] See text for references.
[b] See Table 18-2 for references.

Several staging systems for soft tissue sarcomas were designed in the recent past, but their prognostic power was considered insufficient when tested in a series of soft tissue sarcomas excised with wide surgical margins.[43] A new model with four risk factors has been developed and found useful for prognostic purposes. According to this system, the key risk factors for death due to tumor are male sex, grade III to IV malignant tumor, tumor necrosis, and tumor size over 10 cm.[40]

CYTOGENETICS AND MOLECULAR GENETICS

Cytogenetics and molecular genetics have yielded remarkable insights into the field of soft tissue neoplasia. The great majority of soft tissue tumors have clonal chromosomal abnormalities, some of which are tumor-specific translocations. The molecular characterization of such abnormalities has unveiled recurrent as well as novel genes and molecular pathways that appear to be preferentially involved in or critical to the genesis of soft tissue tumors.[44–50] Different abnormal karyotype categories with clinicopathologic correlates have emerged, and are discussed below. Several of these may be found in a single histogenetic tumor type[51] (Table 18-1) reflecting the multiple tumorigenic pathways that may be operative in soft tissues. Conversely, certain types of chromosomal aberrations may characterize groups of tumors with similar behavior, regardless of their histogenetic origin.[55]

Tumor-specific reciprocal chromosomal translocations have been identified in a diverse group of soft tissue sarcomas (Table 18-2) and are considered diagnostic. Because these translocations are frequently the only cytogenetic abnormality found, it is possible that they represent a key event in tumorigenesis. The common denominator in these translocations is the formation of chimeric genes (constructs of the rearranged genes) encoding hybrid transcription factors and novel fusion proteins. Many of these fusion proteins, containing juxtaposed functional domains usually found in separate proteins, function as potent "oncogenic" transcriptional activators[62] that by enhanced expression of target genes lead to reproducible aberrant differentiation (sarcomas). Because variant chromosomal translocations involving different translocation partners have been found for a single tumor type (i.e., alveolar rhabdomyosarcoma) (Table 18-2), it is conceivable that they give rise to similar chimeric transcription factors that alter expression of a common group of target genes.[63] On the other hand, molecular diversity of the standard chromosome translocations is constantly being identified and its morphologic and biologic consequence and clinical significance explored. Thus in the case of synovial sarcoma, subtle differences in breakpoint positions correlate with tumor phenotypes: a breakpoint in Xp11.21 correlates with a monophasic synovial sarcoma, whereas a breakpoint in Xp11.23 is found in biphasic synovial sarcomas.[66]

Variable chromosomal translocations have been encountered in about two-thirds of typical lipomas and proves that chromosomal aberrations are not solely associated with malignant tu-

Table 18-2. Tumor-Specific Chromosomal
Translocations

Ewing sarcoma[56]	t(11;22)(q24;q11.2–12)	**EWS**/*FLI-1*
	t(21;22)(q22;q12)	**EWS**/*ERG*
	t(7;22)(p22;q12)	**EWS**/*ETV-1*
Desmoplastic small round cell tumor[57,58]	t(11;22)(p13;q12)	**EWS**/*WT-1*
Clear cell sarcoma[59]	t(12;22)(q13–14;q12)	**EWS**/*ATF-1*
Extraskeletal myxoid chondrosarcoma[60,61]	t(9;22)(q21;q11–12)	**EWS**/*CHN*
Alveolar rhabdomyosarcoma[62–64]	t(2;13)(q35;q14)[a]	*PAX3/FKHR*
	t(1;13)(p36;q14)	*PAX7/FKHR*
Synovial sarcoma[65,66]	t(X;18)(p11.2;q11.2)	*SYT/SSX*
Myxoid and round cell/liposarcoma[67,68]	t(12;16)(q13;p11)	**TLS-FUS/** *CHOP*
Rhabdoid tumor[69]	t(11;22)(p15.5;q11.23)[b]	?
Hemangiopericytoma[70]	t(12;19)(q13;q13.3)	?

[a] Also found in the solid variant of alveolar rhabdomyosarcoma.
[b] Isolated case.

EWS and TLS/FUS (in bold) are genes with <u>RNA-binding domains</u> that are <u>replaced</u> by DNA-binding domains of their translocation partners. Because they are ubiquitously expressed, they are believed to mediate the *enhanced transcriptional activation potential* of the fusion protein.[48] FLI-1, ERG, ETV-1, WT-1, ATF-1, PAX3, PAX7, FKHR, and CHOP (italicized) are transcription factor encoding genes with <u>DNA-binding domains</u> that are <u>integrated</u> into the chimeric gene. Some such as FLI-1 and WT-1 are developmentally regulated, and are thought to confer *target specificity* (i.e., site, tissue, age) to the transcriptional activity generated by the fusion protein.[48]

CHN is a member of the steroid/thyroid receptor gene superfamily.

A portion of SSX exhibits homology with a transcriptional repressor domain.

SYT appears to be a *novel* gene, heretofore not sharing homology with any known gene sequence.

mors. Although significantly the chromosomal region 12q14-15 seems to be constantly involved, the rearrangements may be both intra-and interchromosomal, more or less complex, and have a variety of translation partners.[71,72] The 12q14-15 chromosomal breakpoint in lipomas demonstrates disruption of the HMGI-C gene, an architectural factor that functions in transcriptional regulation, and because it is rearranged in a benign neoplastic process it is speculated that it may be involved in adipogenesis.[44]

Ring chromosomes and giant marker chromosomes are vehicles for low level genomic amplification of selected sequences. They seem to characterize low grade sarcomas, having been identified in myxoid malignant fibrous histiocytoma, well differentiated liposarcoma,[55,73,74] and dermatofibrosarcoma protuberans.[75] The ring chromosomes in well differentiated liposarcoma contain chromosome 12-derived sequences, whereas those in dermatofibrosarcoma protuberans are composed of interspersed sequences from chromosomes 17 and 22. Of interest, a 17;22 translocation has been reported in giant cell fibroblastoma, further strengthening the histogenetic association of this tumor with dermatofibrosarcoma protuberans.[76]

Trisomies have been found in lesions with favorable prognosis such as congenital fibrosarcoma[77] and aggressive fibromatosis.[78] Trisomies involving chromosomes 11, 17, 20, and 8 have been found in the former, and 8 and 20 in the latter. In particular the presence of trisomy 8 may be a predictor of recurrence in desmoid tumors. It is presumed that the resultant extra copy of genes promotes cell proliferation. Although these findings appear to substantiate the neoplastic nature of fibromatosis, clonal chromosomal abnormalities have also been detected in conditions regarded as reactive in origin such as proliferative and nodular fasciitis.[79]

Complex karyotypes with multiple clonal chromosomal aberrations are seen in high grade sarcomas including pleomorphic malignant fibrous histiocytoma[80] and pleomorphic liposarcoma.[51,73] They reflect an advanced malignant state and mirror the phenotypic complexity. Interestingly amidst these complex karyotypes, malignant fibrous histiocytomas with a 19+ marker chromosome appear to have an increased relapse rate.[80]

Other cytogenetic findings of significance include a recurrent structural abnormality involving band q25 of chromosome 17 in alveolar soft part sarcoma, which may be implicated in the development of this enigmatic tumor.[81]

Secondary aberrations that accompany primary cytogenetic changes are probably an indication of clonal evolution and tumor progression.[82] They are more evident in recurrences or metastases.

Standard *cytogenetics* can reveal a wide variety of chromosomal alterations; however, it is limited by the requirement of fresh viable tumor cells obtained under sterile conditions and the need to establish tissue culture with the risk of overgrowth by stromal elements. *Molecular cytogenetic analyses*, generally referred to as *FISH* (fluorescent in situ hybridization) involves the detection of DNA sequences by hybridization with probes that recognize either localized chromosome regions or whole chromosomes. FISH is very effective in demonstrating chromosomal translocations, abnormal chromosome copy number, chromosomal deletions and gene amplification, and can be performed on fresh or paraffin-embedded material.[83] The most sensitive molecular assay for detecting chromosomal translocations is *RT-PCR* (reverse-transcriptase polymerase chain reaction), which detects chimeric transcripts by means of primer pairs derived from the genes involved in the chromosomal translocation.[58] RT-PCR has identified translocations not apparent at the cytogenetic level[49] as well as translocation-bearing circulating tumor cells in peripheral blood.[84] Its main drawback is the requirement for intact mRNA in snap-frozen tissue and the variability of some rearrangements. *DNA-based PCR* assays applicable to archival material are in development.[48] Monoclonal antibodies to tumor-specific translocation products may be forthcoming.

Amplification or activation of the dominant oncogenes and loss or inactivation of the recessive tumor suppressor genes have been implicated independently or in combination, in tumor genesis and progression. The best studied of the *tumor suppressor genes* in soft tissue tumors are p53 and the related MDM2, whose protein product binds to and inactivates p53, and the retinoblastoma gene. Alterations of the p53 gene are a common event in soft tissue sarcomas,[85–88] and is best illustrated in the Li-Fraumeni syndrome, characterized by a

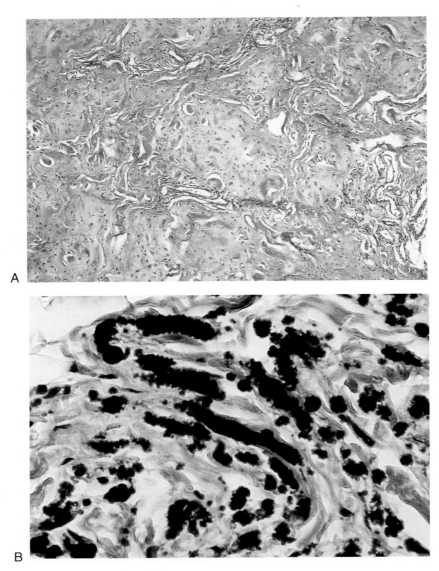

Fig. 18-5. **(A)** Elastofibroma. Hypocellular eosinophilic matrix containing thickened elastic fibers and globules. **(B)** Elastic tissue stain reveals characteristic serrated appearance of the altered elastic fibers.

germline mutation of p53 and the frequent occurrence of sarcomas. Nuclear overexpression of p53 protein, detected by immunohistochemistry, correlates closely with the histologic tumor grade.[85,88] The mutations of p53 in soft tissue sarcomas have been found to be quite heterogeneous both in their distribution throughout the gene and in the type of genetic alterations that result.[86] Furthermore, the dominance of p53 mutations with null nuclear protein expression appears to be unique to soft tissue sarcomas.[87] Focal nuclear p53 immunoreactivity has been noted in reactive and benign soft tissue lesions, and is thought to be the result of accumulation of wild type rather than mutated p53.[89] Amplification of MDM2 gene, mapped to 12q13–14, has been seen with high frequency in atypical lipomas/well differentiated liposarcomas, and correlates with the presence of ring chromosomes previously discussed.[90] There is also a suggestion that MDM2 overexpression may participate in tumor progression.[91] Not unexpectedly, tumors that simultaneously coexpress p53 and MDM2 are strongly associated with a poor outcome.[92] Alterations in retinoblastoma (Rb) gene are postulated to be common primary events in human sarcomas, which may be involved in tumorigenesis or early phases of tumor progression. In one study, Rb expression detected by immunohistochemistry did not influence outcome,[93] whereas in another, DNA alterations of Rb-1 gene correlated with a high tumor grade.[94] Regarding specific tumors, loss of a tumor suppressor gene at 11p15.5, the locus involved in the Beckwith-Wiedemann syndrome, may be the molecular basis of embryonal rhabdomyosarcoma[95] and other tumors associated with this syndrome. Loss and/or inactivation of the APC (adenomatosis polyposis coli) gene appears to be a primary event in the development of desmoid tumors and is found in both sporadic ones and in those associated with Gardner syndrome.[96] Studies of *oncogene* participation in soft tissue sarcomas are limited. Amplification of *c-myc* has been found in diverse soft tissue sarcomas, amplification of *c-fms* oncogene was detected only in liposarcomas,[97] and *H-ras-1* mutations may be relevant in embryonal rhabdomyosarcoma and malignant fibrous histiocytoma.[98]

Autonomous or neoplastic growth may result from the simultaneous coexpression of a *growth factor* and its *receptor*, through a mechanism known as autocrine/paracrine growth. Several growth factors and their corresponding receptors have been found to be coexpressed in soft tissue tumors of many histologic types, suggesting their contribution to sarcomagenesis.[45] There is also compelling evidence that an autocrine/paracrine mechanism of proliferation may play a major role in the development of the Kaposi's sarcoma lesion.[99] Briefly, the purported cytokine-driven phenotypic conversion of the endothelial cell, which constitutively expresses the scatter factor receptor (SF-R), into the Kaposi's sarcoma cell, leads to the endogenous production of the scatter factor (SF), thus establishing a self-promoting autocrine/paracrine loop. Similarly the vascular endothelial growth factor (VEGF) and its receptor have been implicated in the genesis of angiosarcoma.[100]

Advances in developmental biology have identified critical genes whose expression defines or precedes tissue or cell lineage differentiation. Identification of early stage lineage-specific genes may prove useful as *molecular differentiation markers* for the characterization of primitive or undifferentiated tumors. A case in point is the diagnostic utility of MyoD1, a myogenic regulatory gene, in identifying rhabdomyosarcomas among pediatric small round cell tumors[101] and adult pleomorphic sarcomas.[102]

FIBROUS TISSUE TUMORS

Nuchal Fibroma

Nuchal fibroma is a subcutaneous firm rubbery lesion that is poorly demarcated and occurs most commonly in the posterior neck of young adult males.[103] Microscopically nuchal fibroma is composed of dense hypocellular fibrous tissue containing small clusters of perivascular inflammatory cells. The dense hyalinized fibrous tissue often extends into adjacent fat and small nerves. In contrast to elastofibroma, there are no elastic fibers in nuchal fibromas.

Elastofibroma

The rare elastofibroma is usually found in the infrascapular region of elderly patients and consists of abundant dense fibrous tissue containing few fibroblasts and myofibroblasts as well as numerous serrated elastic fibers and globules[104,105] (Fig. 18-5). It has also been described adjacent to the greater trochanter, the ischial tuberosity, and in the foot. Although these lesions

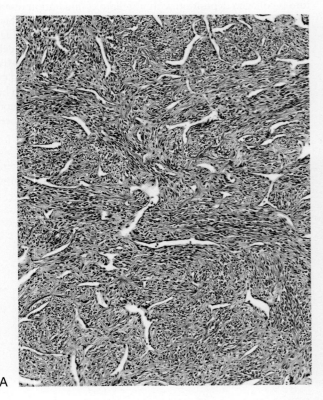

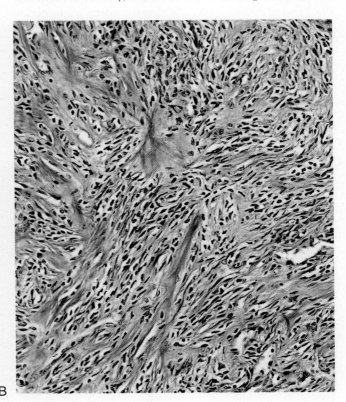

Fig. 18-6. (A) Hemangiopericytic pattern in a solitary fibrous tumor showing fascicles of spindle cells. (B) Zones of collagen deposition with a stellate configuration resembling amianthoid fibers.

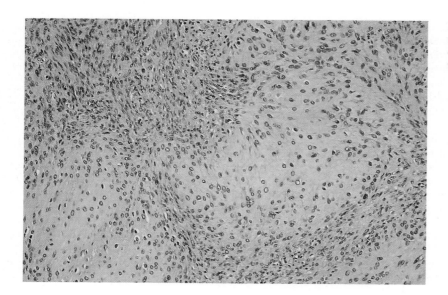

Fig. 18-7. Juvenile aponeurotic fibroma. Plump oval fibroblasts in a cord-like arrangement separated by a collagenous stroma. Foci of noncalcified chondroid differentiation are seen.

have been thought to be reactive or degenerative and the result of mechanical stress, their precise pathogenesis has not been determined. A single example of gastric elastofibroma associated with a chronic peptic ulcer has been recorded.[106] Collagens I, II, and III have been demonstrated in elastofibroma.[107]

FNA reports of elastofibroma describe scant cellularity, including few adipocytes, striated elastic fibers, and spindled fibroblasts, with admixed large aggregates of homogeneous matrix showing distinct borders. Within the matrix fragments are serrated globular crystal-like aggregates, described as "fern-like" or "braid-like," which stain strongly for elastin.[108]

Solitary Fibrous Tumor

Solitary fibrous tumors have long been recognized in the pleura, but their occurrence in many other sites including the soft tissues has been documented only recently.[109–111] These

benign mesenchymal tumors are usually small, well demarcated, and involve the superficial tissues of the head and neck, back, buttock, orbit, and groin. Microscopically, fascicles of spindle cells predominate, but focal hemangiopericytic, herringbone, and storiform patterns are often present (Fig. 18-6A). Stromal sclerosis, which is a constant feature, determines cell density. Sclerotic areas are hypocellular, whereas less fibrotic stromal foci are hypercellular. A characteristic but unusual feature is collagen deposition with a stellate configuration resembling amianthoid fibers similar to those seen in myofibroblastomas of lymph nodes (Fig. 18-6B). There is mild cytologic atypia and mitotic figures are not common. The neoplastic cells show positive reactivity for vimentin and CD34 and negative staining for factor VIII-related antigen, S-100 protein, and cytokeratins. Solitary fibrous tumors have been confused with hemangiopericytoma and less frequently with neurogenic tumors.

FNA of one intrapulmonary solitary fibrous tumor has been

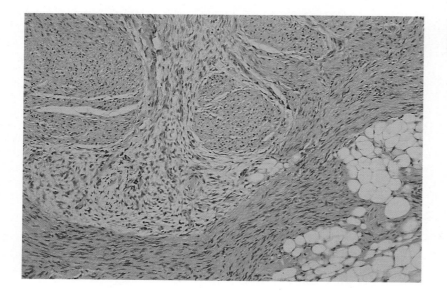

Fig. 18-8. Fibrous hamartoma of infancy. Characteristic histologic pattern showing primitive mesenchyme, fibrous trabeculae, and mature adipose tissue.

reported.[112] Smears showed moderate cellularity of spindled fibroblast-like cells singly and in loosely cohesive clusters with haphazard overlapping, lack of polarity, and bland evenly distributed chromatin.

Fibroma of Tendon Sheath

Fibromas of tendon sheath are slow-growing, well demarcated nodular lesions, usually measuring less than 2 cm in greatest dimension.[113–117] They occur predominantly in the distal portion of the upper extremities of young adult males. Attachment to tendons and tendon sheaths is seen in some cases. Histologic features include an abundant fibrous matrix containing fascicles of fibroblasts and myofibroblasts.[118,119] Significant variations in cellularity are encountered; some lesions are hypercellular whereas others are paucicellular. Although characteristic slit-like vascular spaces are found in most cases, fasciitis-like changes with a focal storiform pattern have occasionally been described. Because of these changes, some authors have suggested that this lesion is related to nodular faciitis. There is no nuclear pleomorphism and only occasional mitotic figures are present. Recurrence may occur following incomplete excision.

Juvenile Aponeurotic Fibroma

Juvenile aponeurotic fibroma (calcifying fibroma) is a rare infiltrating fibroblastic proliferation that affects preferentially the hands and feet of children and adolescents and often recurs following local excision.[120–122] The tumor is densely cellular, and consists of plump fibroblasts and dense collagen fibers as well as islands of chondroid tissue with foci of calcification, which distinguishes this lesion from palmar and plantar fibromatosis (Fig. 18-7). However, calcification may not occur in infants. Mature bone trabeculae are seen in a few cases. Aponeurotic fibromas have also been reported in adults, in sites other than the palms and soles. Multiple primary tumors have also been reported.[123]

Fibrous Hamartoma of Infancy

Fibrous hamartoma of infancy occurs predominantly during the first 2 years of life, affecting the deep dermis and subcutaneous tissue of the axilla, shoulder, back, upper arm, or scrotum.[124–128] Despite its benign nature, it may be confused with sarcomas or aggressive fibromatosis or with other benign lesions such as aponeurotic fibroma, dermatofibroma, or nodular fasciitis. Fibrous hamartoma of infancy can be distinguished, however, by its distinctive histology, consisting of an admixture of mature adipose tissue, interlacing bundles of fibroblasts and myofibroblasts, and islands of primitive mesenchyme composed of loosely arranged spindle or stellate cells (Fig. 18-8). This growth pattern is interrupted in areas of some lesions by dense, wavy bands of collagen with interspersed fibrocytes. Local recurrence has occasionally been reported and the recurrences usually appear more fibrotic than the primary tumor.

Juvenile Nasopharyngeal Angiofibroma

Juvenile nasopharyngeal angiofibroma is a highly vascular fibrous tumor that occurs almost exclusively in adolescent boys. It arises in the posterior superior nasal cavity and usually involves the nasal septum, the nasopharynx, and the pterygoid region by the time it produces symptoms of unilateral nasal obstruction and hemorrhage.[129–131] The tumor is locally expansive, growing into the soft tissues of the retropharyngeal area through the openings between the bones of the posterior face and the base of the skull and eroding the bone to break into the regional sinuses, the orbit, and in some advanced cases, the base of the cranium. This pattern of growth produces characteristic radiographic changes.[132] Histologically, it is composed of a fibrous stroma with varying amounts of collagenous fibrous tissue arranged in irregular interwoven or myxomatous patterns (Fig. 18-9). Stellate and elongate fibrocytes and myofibroblasts are the predominant stromal cells. The tumor is richly endowed with small and large endothelium-lined vascular channels whose walls contain no elastic fibers and few irregularly

Fig. 18-9. Juvenile nasopharyngeal angiofibroma. Bland spindled and stellate cells in abundant collagenous stroma surround vascular structures that lack muscular walls.

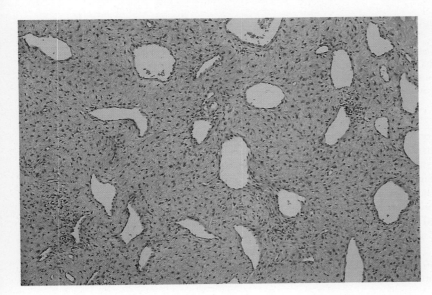

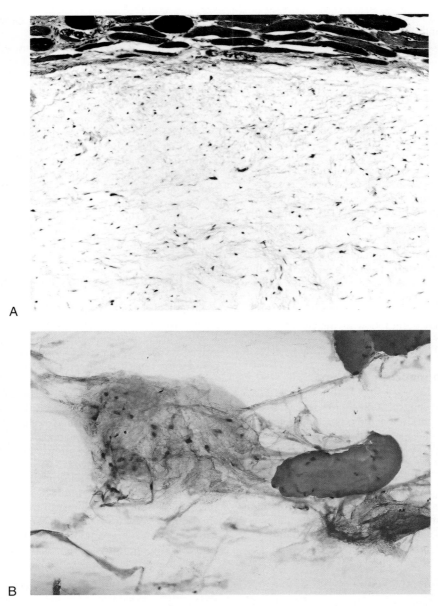

Fig. 18-10. **(A)** Intramuscular myxoma. A well circumscribed intramuscular nodule composed of fibroblast-like cells lying in a myxoid stroma. **(B)** Fine needle aspiration of intramuscular myxoma shows a paucicellular smear with abundant semitransparent fibrillar background myxoid matrix, scattered skeletal muscle cells, and bland spindled and stellate cells. (H&E.)

arranged smooth muscle cells. The relative rigidity of the fibrous stroma and the lack of vascular mural contractile elements are thought to be important factors in the pathogenesis of the sometimes massive, uncontrollable hemorrhages. Trauma to these lesions, including that of biopsies, has been associated with life-threatening hemorrhages; therefore, if necessary, biopsies of suspicious posterior polypoid nasal masses in young men are best done in the operating room with blood available for transfusion.

Recurrences after surgery are frequent because of the insinuative growth of the tumor into inaccessible places in the head.

Surgery is the most successful treatment[133,134]; irradiation is reserved for residual and recurrent tumor beyond the reach of the surgeon's knife. Because these lesions tend to occur predominantly in the hormonally turbulent environment of the adolescent boy, attempts have been made to relate either their pathogenesis or treatment, or both, to sex hormones.[135] Treatment with estrogens has succeeded in reducing tumor size in some, but not all, patients. Significant numbers of testosterone receptors, but not estradiol or progesterone receptors, have been demonstrated in juvenile nasopharyngeal angiofibromas. Abnormal sexual maturity and serum hormone levels have not

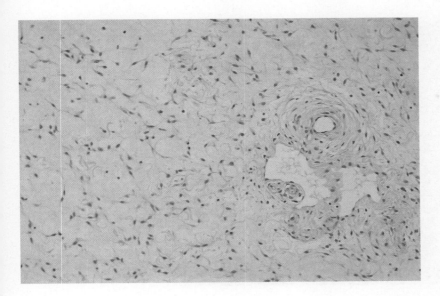

Fig. 18-11. Aggressive angiomyxoma composed of cytologically bland stellate cells in a myxoid matrix and variable-sized vessels with perivascular fibrous condensation.

been found in the few isolated cases studied specifically. The tumor may regress as the patient gets older, but treatment is necessary for the adolescent boy for whom one cannot risk the morbidity of invasive growth or the possibility of massive hemorrhage from the tumor.

Intramuscular Myxoma

Intramuscular myxoma, an uncommon benign fibroblastic tumor, must be distinguished from other myxoid neoplasms, notably myxoid liposarcoma and aggressive angiomyxoma. Most myxomas arise in the large muscles of the thigh, pelvic girdle, and shoulder and on gross examination appear as well circumscribed gelatinous nodules; few are completely encapsulated.[136-138] Fewer than 10 percent of myxomas are multiple and associated with fibrous dysplasia of adjacent bones.[139] The tumor cells are spindle-shaped or stellate, having drawn-out cytoplasmic processes and lying in an abundant mucoid matrix (Fig. 18-10A). The degree of cellularity and vascularization varies from tumor to tumor but most of them appear hypocellular and poorly vascularized. Electron microscopic studies have shown that the principal cell of intramuscular myxomas is similar to a fibroblast.[140]

FNA of intramuscular myxoma shows abundant metachromatic myxoid background material containing sparse scattered bland spindled and stellate cells.[141,142] Smears show few small blood vessels or adipocytes, but may contain skeletal muscle cells. The spindled cells have ovoid nuclei with uniform chromatin distribution, and may have long intertwined cytoplasmic processes resulting in a fibrillar appearance (Fig. 18-10B). The low cellularity, lack of nuclear atypia, and semitransparent nature of the background myxoid matrix allow distinction from malignant myxoid lesions.[143]

Aggressive Angiomyxoma

Aggressive angiomyxoma is a locally recurring nonmetastasizing fibroblastic tumor that occurs preferentially in the soft tissues of the pelvis, vulva, and perineum of adult women.[144-150] Several cases involving the scrotum, spermatic cord, inguinal region, and pelvis of men have been documented.[151] The tumor is poorly demarcated, has a gelatinous surface, and can measure more than 15 cm in diameter. It is composed of cytologically bland spindle and stellate cells with virtually no mitotic figures growing in a myxoid and sometimes fibrotic stroma that contains numerous blood vessels (Fig. 18-11). The neoplastic cells show consistent reactivity for vimentin and variable reactivity for muscle-specific actin and desmin. Occasionally the blood vessels may show a focal plexiform pattern reminiscent of myxoid liposarcoma. A perivascular inflammatory infiltrate is seen in some cases.

Angiomyofibroblastoma has been described as a vulvar lesion resembling angiomyxoma, but with higher cellularity and vascular density and better circumscription.[152]

Dermatofibrosarcoma Protuberans

No other tumor can better exhibit the formation of a storiform pattern than dermatofibrosarcoma protuberans (DFSP)[153-155] (Fig. 18-12A). This slow-growing dermal and subcutaneous tumor has a tendency to recur following conservative or incomplete excision. It is seen most often in the chest wall, extremities, and head and neck of young adults and adolescents, but it may occur at any age and in other anatomic sites. Metastases are exceptional. Microscopically, plump fibroblasts exhibit a prominent storiform pattern. The tumor cells, which usually show positive reactivity for CD34, extend into the subcutaneous adipose tissue along septa and between fat cells or in a distinct multilayered pattern. These patterns of extension are useful in distinguishing DFSP from deep dermatofibroma,[156] which is CD34 negative and factor XIIIa positive.[157] Focal myxoid changes are sometimes seen, more often in local recurrences than in the primary tumors. Fibrosarcomatous areas with the characteristic herringbone pattern have been described in 15 to 20 percent of DFSP.[158-160] These fibrosarcomatous changes can be seen in the primary lesion or in

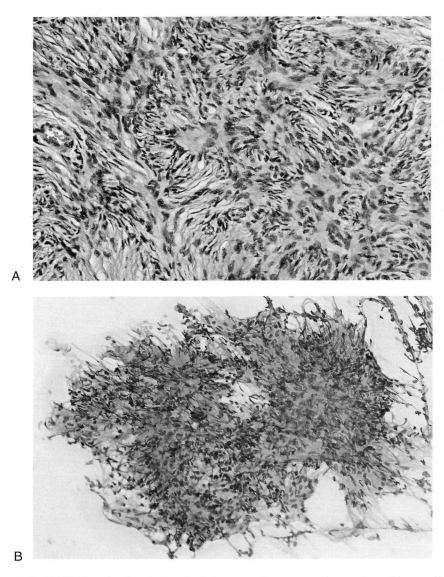

Fig. 18-12. **(A)** Uniform slender spindle cells displaying storiform pattern characteristic of dermatofibrosarcoma protuberans. **(B)** Fine needle aspiration smear from dermatofibrosarcoma protuberans demonstrates a highly cellular cohesive compact cluster of uniform spindle cells with storiform architecture. (H&E.)

recurrences. Recognition of this variant of DFSP is important because it has a greater propensity for the development of distant metastases.[160] Likewise, DFSP may show foci of giant cell fibroblastoma, suggesting a close relationship between these two tumors.[161,162] In fact, it has been proposed that giant cell fibroblastoma represents the juvenile form of DFSP.[163] Rarely these tumors contain melanin-bearing cells with dendritic processes; this is the so-called Bednar tumor, which follows a clinical course similar to that of conventional DFSP.[164]

FNA yields cellular aspirates with cohesive metachromatic fibrillar stromal fragments, usually without a myxoid background.[165] The tumor cells are both cohesive in compact storiform clusters, in which all nuclei are arranged radially from a central focus, as well as dispersed singly. Cells in clusters have ill-defined cytoplasmic borders, whereas discohesive cells show

bipolar cytoplasmic processes or have stripped cytoplasm. All cells show tapered to oval nuclei with delicate chromatin and inconspicuous nucleoli. Only one cell type is present, without inflammatory elements, although entrapped adipose tissue may be seen. Vascular structures are not prominent (Fig. 18-12B).

Giant Cell Fibroblastoma

Giant cell fibroblastoma is a rare and distinctive fibrous tumor of childhood and adolescence that usually arises in the superficial soft tissues, often recurs following local excision, but does not metastasize.[166–172] It is well circumscribed and microscopically consists of varying proportions of cellular solid areas and sinusoidal-like spaces, both containing fibroblastic cells as

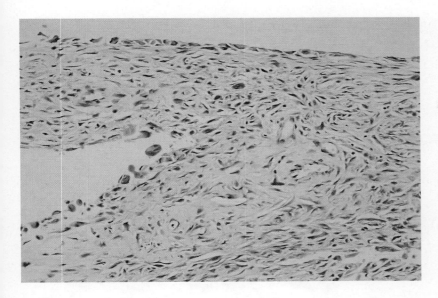

Fig. 18-13. Giant cell fibroblastoma. Vascular-like spaces lined by mononuclear and multinucleated giant cells are surrounded by fibroblastic cells.

well as multinucleated floret-like cells[170] (Fig. 18-13). Giant cross-striated fibrils probably representing short-spacing collagen have been observed ultrastructurally in both the spindle and multinucleated cells.[169] A close relationship between giant cell fibroblastoma and dermatofibrosarcoma protuberans has been stressed in recent years.[167,172]

Low Grade Fibromyxoid Sarcoma

Because of its bland cytomorphology and myxoid features this low grade sarcoma is often confused with benign lesions such as nodular fasciitis, myxoid neurofibroma, intramuscular myxoma, or fibromatosis. However, fibromyxoid sarcoma often recurs following conservative excisions and after many years a significant number of patients develop pulmonary metastases.[173–177] The tumor most often affects the extremities, neck, buttocks, and chest wall of middle-aged adults. It is deeply seated, well demarcated, pale yellow, and myxoid. Microscopically, hypocellular fibrotic foci alternate with more cellular myxoid areas (Fig. 18-14A). However, this tumor lacks the nodular growth pattern that is characteristic of myxofibrosarcoma. The neoplastic cells are spindle-shaped or stellate with oval hyperchromatic nuclei and poorly defined, pale

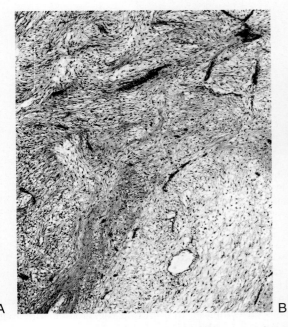

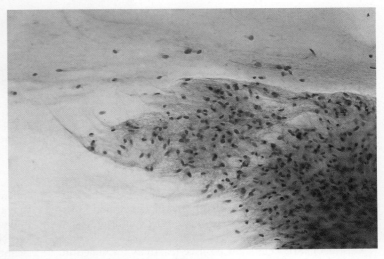

Fig. 18-14. (A) Low grade fibromyxoid sarcoma. Myxoid areas alternate with collagenized areas. A rich vascular network is noted. (B) Fine needle aspiration of low grade fibromyxoid sarcoma shows a tissue fragment of mildly pleomorphic spindle cells with bipolar cytoplasmic tags in a myxoid background. (Papanicolaou.)

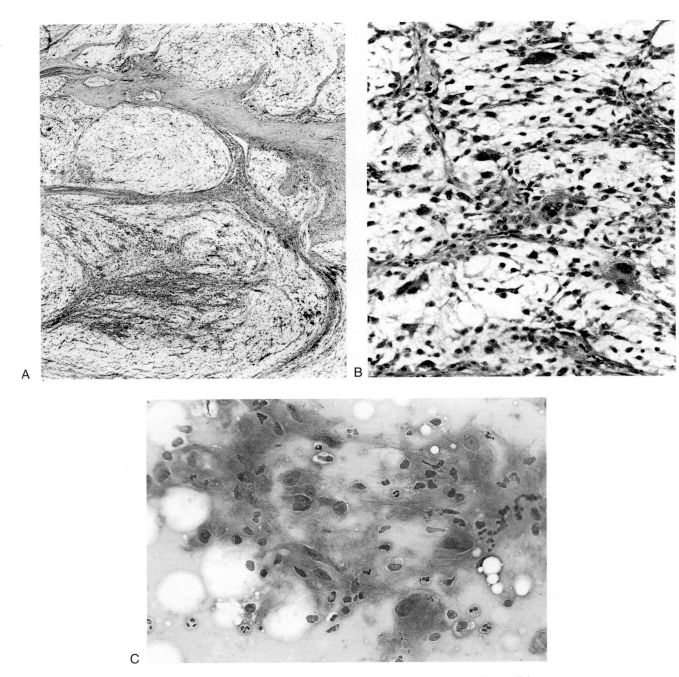

Fig. 18-15. **(A)** Characteristic nodular growth pattern of myxofibrosarcoma. **(B)** Hypocellular area containing curvilinear blood vessels and scattered pleomorphic cells in myxofibrosarcoma. **(C)** Fine needle aspiration of myxofibrosarcoma shows semitransparent metachromatic myxoid matrix containing moderately pleomorphic spindled and rounded cells. (Diff-Quik.)

eosinophilic cytoplasm. A rich vascular network and perivascular arrangement of tumor cells is seen in some tumors. Mitotic figures are uncommon. The tumor usually infiltrates adjacent fat and skeletal muscle.

Most neoplastic cells show positive reactivity for vimentin. Occasionally, some cells express reactivity for actin and desmin reflecting focal myofibroblastic differentiation.[176] By electron

microscopy the neoplastic cells have features of fibroblasts. We have karyotyped two low grade fibromyxoid sarcomas and found no chromosome abnormalities.

FNA smears reveal mildly pleomorphic spindled nuclei with scant bipolar cytoplasm in a myxoid background, with fragments of blood vessels within and separate from tumor cell clusters. Nuclear features were not readily recognized as malignant

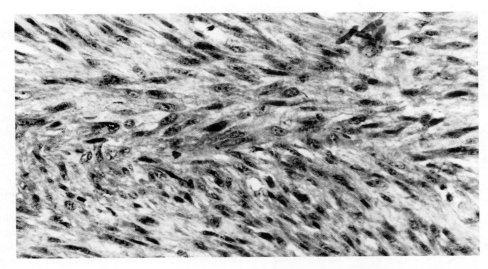

Fig. 18-16. Malignant spindle cells arranged in a herringbone pattern often seen in fibrosarcoma.

in one case we have seen, or in a report of the closely related lesion, myxofibrosarcoma[178] (Fig. 18-14B).

Myxofibrosarcoma (Malignant Fibrous Histiocytoma, Myxoid Type)

The classification of myxoid malignant fibrous histiocytoma has been questioned in recent years in view that immunohistochemical and ultrastructural studies have failed to prove a histiocytic phenotype.[179,180] We therefore believe this entity should be included among the fibroblastic tumors. This tumor is characterized by a nodular growth pattern and myxoid areas of variable extent containing prominent curvilinear blood vessels (Fig. 18-15A & B). In low grade neoplasms the myxoid foci are usually hypocellular and alternate with moderately cellular areas. The cells are fusiform or stellate and contain hyperchromatic nuclei. Few mitotic figures and lack of necrosis are additional features. High grade myxofibrosarcomas are less myxoid and consist of densely cellular fascicles of spindle cells admixed with multinucleated giant cells, both showing marked nuclear pleomorphism. A focal storiform pattern, numerous mitotic figures, and areas of necrosis are common findings. The neoplastic cells are immunoreactive for vimentin and occasionally for actin. Ultrastructurally, the cells have a fibroblastic phenotype.[180–183] Approximately 55 percent of the tumors recur and 25 percent metastasize, especially to the lungs and lymph nodes. DNA ploidy analysis does not correlate with outcome.[179,184] Myxofibrosarcoma is one of the most common malignant soft tissue tumors in the extremities of elderly subjects.[179,185–187] Tumors involving the superficial soft tissues are smaller, more common, and have a better prognosis than deepseated neoplasms.[179,186,187]

In the low grade lesions, FNA shows metachromatic background myxoid material containing vascular fragments and mildly pleomorphic spindle cells, resembling the low grade fibromyxoid sarcoma. Higher grade lesions show more obvious chromatin irregularities and nuclear pleomorphism in the spin-

dle cells, as well as admixed bizarre multinucleated tumor giant cells[188,189] (Fig. 18-15C).

Fibrosarcoma

Although once considered frequent neoplasms, increasing awareness of the existence of other fibrosarcomatoid neoplasms and pseudoneoplasms has made it apparent that fibrosarcomas are uncommon. This is particularly the case if the histologic diagnosis of this neoplasm is restricted to densely cellular tumors composed of malignant spindle cells exhibiting a herringbone pattern[190–192] (Fig. 18-16). Using this criterion, it is possible to separate fibrosarcomas from fibromatosis, fibrohistiocytic tumors, myofibromatoses, nodular faciitis, proliferative myositis, and other reactive myofibroblastic proliferations with similar histologic features. Fibrosarcomas are vimentin positive and rarely express low molecular weight cytokeratin and muscle-specific actin indicating a myofibroblastic component.[193] This immunohistochemical profile does not allow distinction between fibromatosis and fibrosarcoma or between monophasic synovial sarcoma and fibrosarcoma. Approximately 25 percent of fibrosarcomas overexpress p53 protein.[192] By electron microscopy, in addition to fibroblasts, a myofibroblastic component is seen in one-third of the cases.[194] From a review of the recent literature, the following statements can be made:

1. Fibrosarcomas arise in both the superficial and deep soft tissues of the extremities, chest wall, and head and neck.[190–192]
2. The tumor is less common and less aggressive in children and should be treated conservatively.[195–198] In fact, metastases have not been documented in infantile fibrosarcomas. Moreover, rarely these tumors may regress spontaneously.[199–200]
3. Cellular fibromatosis and fibrosarcomas in children are probably the same neoplastic entity.[193,196] This is further

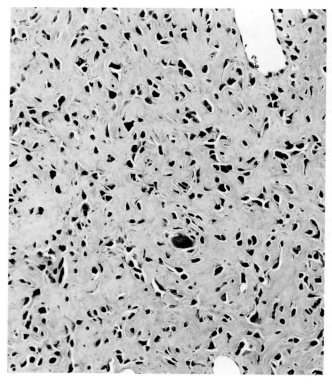

Fig. 18-17. Ovoid cells with scant to clear cytoplasm embedded in a sclerotic stroma typify sclerosing epithelioid fibrosarcoma.

substantiated by the recent demonstration that both share the same cytogenetic abnormalities.[193,201–203]

4. In adults, the tumor often recurs following limited excisions and is able to metastasize; therefore, a more aggressive surgical treatment is indicated. Approximately 60 percent of the patients die with metastases within 5 years after surgical therapy.[190]

5. Marked cellular pleomorphism is not a feature of fibrosarcoma.

6. Fibrosarcomas spread almost exclusively through vascular channels, and metastases appear most often in the lungs.

FNA smears from fibrosarcomas are cellular, with mildly pleomorphic spindled nuclei in fascicular aggregates and singly, with scattered dense stromal fragments but not myxoid background. The features are essentially indistinguishable from low grade malignant peripheral nerve sheath tumors.

Sclerosing Epithelioid Fibrosarcoma

This recently described histologically distinctive variant of fibrosarcoma has been confused with carcinomas and other malignant tumors, especially synovial sarcomas and melanomas.[204] It is composed of relatively small round or ovoid cells with clear cytoplasm arranged in cords or nests and embedded in a sclerotic stroma (Fig. 18-17). The tumors arise preferentially in the deep soft tissues of the extremities of adult patients.[204,205] Approximately 50 percent of the patients develop local recurrence and 40 percent distant metastases. The tumors show positive reactivity for vimentin. Less frequently they are positive for epithelial membrane antigen (50 percent), S-100 protein (25 percent), neuron-specific enolase (14 percent), and cytokeratin (14 percent). Ultrastructurally the cells exhibit features of fibroblasts.

FIBROMATOSES

Fibromatoses are considered a large family of fibroblastic proliferations with similar biologic behavior.

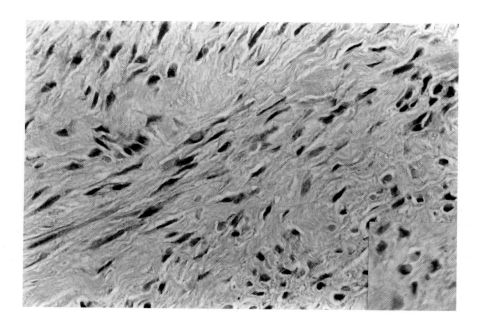

Fig. 18-18. Infantile digital fibroma. Some fibroblasts contain large eosinophilic inclusions (seen in cross-section in inset).

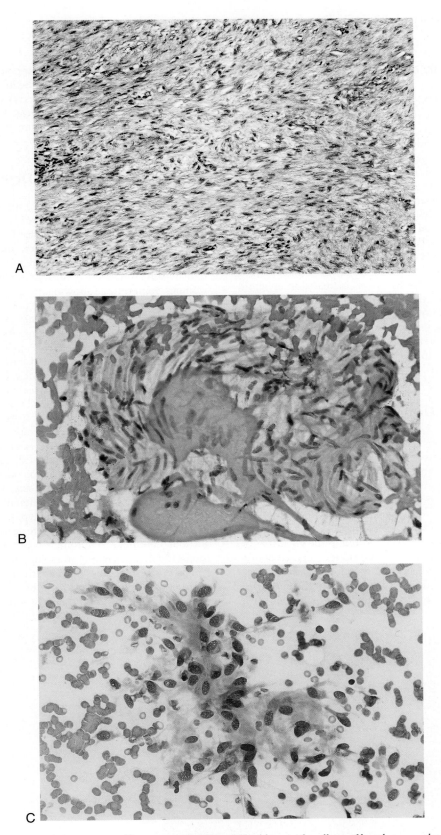

Fig. 18-19. (A) Aggressive fibromatosis. Bundles of fibroblasts with collagen fibers between them. (B) Fine needle aspiration smear of desmoid tumor demonstrates a fascicular bundle of elongated uniform spindle cells showing bipolar cytoplasmic processes and entrapped skeletal muscle. (H&E.) (C) Another desmoid tumor shows less cohesive cells with plumper ovoid nuclei and scant metachromatic matrix on Fine needle aspiration. (Diff-Quik.)

Palmar, Plantar, and Penile Fibromatosis

Palmar fibromatosis (Dupuytren's contracture),[206–208] plantar fibromatosis (Ledderhose's disease),[209] and penile fibromatosis (Peyronie's disease),[210,211] form cellular fibroblastic and myofibroblastic nodules and plaques that infiltrate the deep dermis and underlying tendons, aponeurotic (palmar and plantar) and facial (penile) structures from which they arise. Patients are usually young adults but children and elderly subjects are also affected. Severe contractures of the fibrous masses can lead to distressing dysfunction best treated surgically by partial or complete excision of the tumors and release of the engulfed tendons and fascia. Palmar fibromatosis may occur in patients who have Peyronie's disease, and both palmar and plantar fibromatoses have been found to occur in the same person. The incidence of palmar fibromatosis is increased in epileptic and diabetic patients.[212] Although trauma has often been associated with these conditions, it has not been proved an etiologic factor. By contrast, genitourinary tract infections and administration of beta-adrenergic blocking agents have been cited as etiologic factors in the development of Peyronie's disease.[213]

Infantile Digital Fibromatosis

Infantile digital fibromatosis (recurrent digital fibroma of childhood) is an infiltrative cellular fibrous tumor that almost always involves the toes and fingers of infants and young children.[214,215] The red or tan dermal tumor usually arises on the dorsa of the tips of the digits, can infiltrate into the periosteum, and may recur following incomplete excision. Although lesions outside the digits including the breast have been described,[216,217] they have not been reported in the great toes or thumbs. Histologically, digital fibromatosis is composed of myofibroblasts that contain diagnostic round eosinophilic cytoplasmic inclusions usually located at one pole of the elongated nucleus (Fig. 18-18). Ultrastructurally, these inclusions have

been found to be composed of amorphous granular material and numerous actin filaments.[218–220] The inclusions show a hollow-like pattern of peripheral reactivity for muscle-specific actin.[217,218] These observations suggest that defective regulation of cellular filament architecture plays a role in the development of the inclusions.[217,218]

Fibromatosis (Desmoid)

Fibromatoses (desmoid tumors) are locally infiltrative fibroblastic proliferations akin to sarcomas in their growth but lacking the capability to metastasize.[221] They commonly arise in the abdominal wall, extremities, and mesentery, but they have been described in many other anatomic sites.[222–225] There is a definite prevalence of abdominal desmoids in young women, sometimes following pregnancies, whereas extra-abdominal desmoids have no sex predilection. The shoulder girdles, chest wall, extremities, and mesentery are the most common extra-abdominal locations. As is the case with most soft tissue tumors, their etiology is unknown, although genetic predisposition, trauma, hormonal stimuli, and other factors have been implicated in their development.[225] Estrogen exposure has been implicated on the basis of population studies, response to antiestrogen therapy, and the occasional demonstration of estrogen receptors in tumor tissue.[225,226] Desmoids form bulky gray-white masses that infiltrate skeletal muscles and often recur following conservative surgical excision. The presence of desmoid in the abdominal wall, mesentary, or retroperitoneum in association with colonic adenomatosis (polyposis) constitutes part of *Gardner's syndrome*, which is inherited as a dominant trait.[227] According to different series, 2 to 29 percent of patients with adenomatosis (polyposis) of the colon develop mesenteric fibromatosis that is more aggressive than in patients without Gardner's syndrome.[228] Mesenteric and retroperitoneal fibromatosis may grow rapidly and form large masses that compress and sometimes infiltrate the intestinal wall leading to obstruction. Pelvic fibromatosis, on the other hand, may be confused with an ovarian tumor or infiltrate the urinary blad-

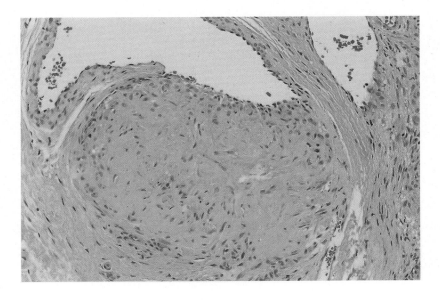

Fig. 18-20. Nodular appearance of myofibroma with peripherally placed myofibroblasts, associated with dilated vascular spaces.

der, vagina, or rectum. Desmoid tumors of children are histologically similar to those of adults, although they are more common in boys than in girls and are usually located in the extremities or head and neck.[229,230] Regardless of their location, desmoid tumors are composed of fascicles of fibroblasts and myofibroblasts in a collagenous stroma[231] (Fig. 18-19A). Extensive myxoid areas are seen more often in mesenteric fibromatosis. The lack of cytologic atypia and mitotic figures distinguishes desmoids from fibrosarcomas.

FNA of desmoid tumors shows scanty to moderate cellularity, with frequent damaged cells, including naked nuclei.[232,233] Some fibroblasts are intact with spindle-shaped nuclei and distinct bipolar cytoplasm. The nuclei are oval to elongated with finely dispersed chromatin and inapparent nucleoli. Clusters of spindled cells oriented in "school of fish" fascicles may be encountered (Fig. 18-19B & C). Fragments of fibrillar collagen and small blood vessels may be noted, along with atrophic skeletal muscle cells, which mimic multinucleated tumor giant cells. If the aspirate from a desmoid tumor is unusually cellular, it may be confused with nodular fasciitis; if many fibrous tissue fragments are present, neurofibroma enters the differential diagnosis. Unlike these lesions, desmoid tumors lack a myxoid matrix. Neurofibromas are paucicellular on FNA, and show elongated twisted nuclei in loose clusters and singly. Desmoids also lack nuclear palisades and contrasting Antoni A and B areas, which are cytologic and histologic features of neurilemoma.[234] Schwannoma cells appear in branching clusters with syncytial cytoplasm, and elongated nuclei with pointed ends, which may include enlarged atypical forms representing degenerative ("ancient") change. The background in tissue fragments of schwannoma is fibrillar in cellular areas, and more myxoid with histiocytes in Antoni B areas. Aspirates of desmoid tumors show bland uniform spindle cells with collagenous stroma, lacking mitoses, necrosis, or atypia, which may result in underdiagnosis as a scar, in contrast to the locally aggressive nature of these neoplasms. FNA appearance of variant forms of fibromatoses (e.g., fibromatosis colli) resembles that of desmoid tumors.

Congenital Myofibromatoses

Congenital myofibromatoses may appear as solitary or multiple nodules. When multiple the nodules affect the soft tissues, bones, and viscera of newborns and children.[235–239] The condition is almost always fatal in infants who have visceral involvement, especially when the lungs are affected. The viscera involved in congenital generalized fibromatosis include the gastrointestinal (GI) tract, lungs, heart, kidneys, and many other organs. The central nervous system (CNS) is affected only by invasion from osseous or dural lesions. The solitary lesion (myofibroma) is a nodule measuring 1 to 2 cm in greatest dimension that involves the skin, muscle, or bone. Microscopically the lesions are composed of fascicles of myofibroblasts that are vimentin and actin positive. Intravascular growth is a common feature (Fig. 18-20). Cellular areas with a hemangiopericytic pattern are often seen. Infants with congenital myofibromatosis without visceral involvement have a good prognosis, for their tumors will regress spontaneously over a few months. Solitary myofibromatosis can occur in adults.[240]

Juvenile Hyaline Fibromatosis

Juvenile hyaline fibromatosis is an exceedingly rare hereditary disorder characterized by fibroblastic proliferation and the production of abundant hyalinized ground substance.[241–244] Clinically the patients are usually children under 5 years of age with multiple slowly growing subcutaneous nodules, hypertrophic gingiva, and radiolucent bone lesions.[243] The basic abnormality appears to be a metabolic disturbance in the formation of collagen, probably caused by insufficient macromolecular organization of collagen molecules.[243]

Fibromatosis Colli

Fibromatosis colli is a locally infiltrative mass of the sternocleidomastoid muscle of infants that disappears within 3 to 4 months, either producing little or no deformity of the muscle or forming fibrous scar tissue, which can eventuate in torticollis (wry neck) by contracture.[245] The lesion rarely appears before 2 weeks of age, and it is in the early tumor stage that the infiltrative fibroblastic growth characteristic of fibromatosis is seen. The cytologic appearance by FNA at this stage is also identical to other fibromatoses. Intrauterine factors including trauma have been suggested as causes of fibromatosis colli. Birth trauma such as breech delivery, previously thought to be a primary cause, may be actually secondary to intrauterine development of the lesion that subsequently interferes with the proper movement and placement of the head before delivery.

Idiopathic Gingival Fibromatosis

Idiopathic gingival fibromatosis, a benign fibrous proliferation of the gingiva that appears first in childhood or adolescence, is an autosomal dominant heritable disorder that is sometimes associated with hypertrichosis and mental retardation.[246,247] The localized form can be excised without difficulty. However, when the fibromatosis involves the gingival tissues, the hard palate, the maxilla, and the mandible, complete surgical removal is difficult. If not removed, the tumor may enlarge to fill the oral cavity and oropharynx, resulting in death by starvation.

FIBROHISTIOCYTIC TUMORS

A number of fibrohistiocytic tumors such as dermatofibromas, atypical fibroxanthomas, epithelioid histiocytomas, and reticulohistiocytomas arise in the dermis and are discussed in detail under skin tumors (see Ch. 17).

Deep Juvenile Xanthogranuloma

A benign cutaneous histiocytic lesion of infancy, juvenile xanthogranuloma has also been described in the deep soft tissues.[248–250] The cutaneous lesions that can be single or multiple are often located in the head and neck and undergo spontaneous involution.[248,249] The deep-seated lesions also occur in children but involve the subcutaneous tissue and skeletal muscle. They are well demarcated, measuring up to 2 cm in greatest dimension. Microscopically, there is a proliferation of histiocytic cells with

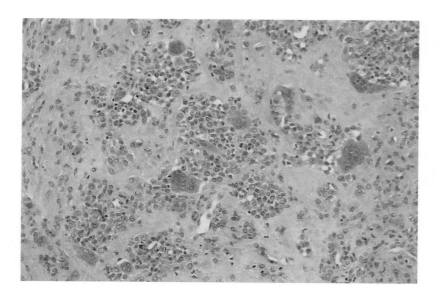

Fig. 18-21. Giant cell tumor of tendon sheath. Multinucleated and mononuclear cells in a hyalinized stroma.

abundant foamy or eosinophilic cytoplasm and bland vesicular nuclei. Scattered Touton giant cells are seen in some cases. Admixed with the mononuclear histiocytes are eosinophils, lymphocytes, and plasma cells. Infiltration of skeletal muscle fibers by the histiocytes and inflammatory cells should not be interpreted as a sign of malignant tumors. The immunohistochemical profile of the lesion supports macrophagic-myofibroblastic differentiation. In contrast to histiocytosis X, juvenile xanthogranuloma lacks Birbeck granules on electron microscopic study.

Giant Cell Tumor of Tendon Sheath (Localized Nodular Tenosynovitis)

Giant cell tumors of tendon sheath are relatively small (2 to 3 cm) nodules most commonly seen in the hands of young adults, although they do occur in other anatomic sites.[251,252] These slow-growing, well circumscribed, lobulated, yellow nodules are associated with tendons and are not attached to the skin. A rare diffuse infiltrating variant has also been described. About 10 percent of them produce cortical erosion of the underlying bone.[253] Microscopically, they contain variable numbers of histiocyte-like mononuclear cells, multinucleated osteoclastic giant cells, and lipid-laden histiocytes (Fig. 18-21). Immunohistochemical observations indicate that both the mononuclear cells and the multinucleated giant cells are of histiocytic derivation.[254] Some of these tumors are densely cellular, whereas others are predominantly fibrotic and hyalinized. Mitotic figures and blood vessel invasion are rare and do not correlate with malignant clinical behavior. Local recurrence is seen in about 15 percent of cases. We are unable to separate the

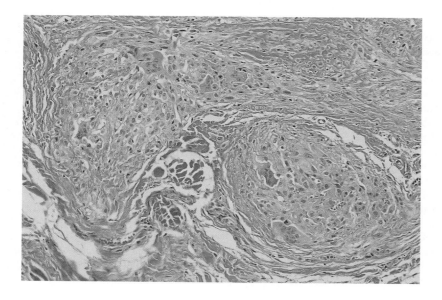

Fig. 18-22. Typical plexiform fibrohistiocytic tumor showing fascicles of fibroblastic spindle cells intermixed with nodules of epithelioid histiocyte-like cells containing osteoclast type giant cells.

malignant giant cell tumor of tendon sheath from the malignant fibrous histiocytoma, giant cell type.[255,256]

FNA smears of giant cell tumor of tendon sheath are highly cellular, with a dispersed mixture of multinucleated osteoclast-like giant cells, polygonal mononuclear cells resembling osteoblasts, and hemosiderin-laden macrophages.[257] The mononuclear cells show uniform rounded eccentric nuclei with fine chromatin and small nucleoli, as well as a perinuclear pale zone, probably Golgi apparatus, without vacuolization.

Plexiform Fibrohistiocytic Tumor

Plexiform fibrohistiocytic tumor is a lesion of low malignant potential occurring in children.[258] It recurs in one-third of the cases and on rare occasions metastasizes to regional lymph nodes. The most common location is the upper extremity, especially the shoulder and forearm. The lesion characteristically involves the deep dermis and subcutaneous tissue. The tumor is composed of nodules of epithelioid histiocyte-like cells containing scattered osteoclast type giant cells, and fascicles of fibroblastic spindle cells, both components intermixed in a plexiform arrangement (Fig. 18-22). Predominantly fibroblastic and predominantly histiocytic forms are reported. Fine needle aspiration smears show disassociated fibroblasts and histiocyte-like cells with abundant granular to vacuolated cytoplasm, and round to oval nuclei.[259] Scattered bi- or multinucleated osteoclast-like cells are also seen. The spindle and histiocyte-like cells have a similar immunophenotype and ultrastructural appearance, showing features between histiocytes and myofibroblasts.[260] That is, the tumor cells are immunoreactive for alpha-1-antitrypsin, alpha-1-antichymotrypsin, and alpha-smooth muscle-specific actin, and show an abundance of lysosomes and filopodia, in combination with peripheral thin filaments with dense bodies. The osteoclast-like giant cells stain with the macrophage antibody CD68. A complex chromosomal abnormality is reported in one case.[261] This lesion is often confused with plexiform neurofibroma, fibrous hamartoma of infancy, fibromatosis, and solitary myofibroma.

Angiomatoid Fibrous Histiocytoma

Angiomatoid fibrous histiocytoma is a low grade malignant fibrous histiocytoma that occurs predominantly in the extremities, trunk, and head and neck region of adolescents, children, and young adults.[262,263] In addition to the mass, a small number of patients developed systemic symptoms such as anemia, fever, and polyclonal gammopathy. Most tumors involve the superficial soft tissues, are well demarcated, often surrounded by a fibrous pseudocapsule, and show cystic degeneration. Histologically, they are characterized by nodules or sheets of bland spindle-shaped and rounded cells, vascular-like spaces, and a lymphoplasmacytic infiltrate (Fig. 18-23). Rarely the inflammatory infiltrate is so pronounced and diffuse as to obscure the neoplastic cells. Old and recent hemorrhage is a constant feature. In about one-half of the tumors the neoplastic cells show positive reactivity for CD68, suggesting a histiocytic phenotype.[264] Ultrastructural studies have also suggested histiocytic differentiation.[265–267] Positive reactivity for muscle-specific actin and desmin in approximately 20 percent of the cases probably reflects a myofibroblastic component.[268] In the largest series published so far, less than 20 percent of the tumors recurred and 1 percent metastasized to distant sites.[262] The recurrence rate was higher in head and neck tumors and distant metastases occurred in only one deep-seated lesion.

In one series,[267] 2 of 20 cases had FNA, which showed cellular smears with stromal fragments and mixed fibroblastic and atypical histiocyte-like cells in loose clusters and singly, with admixed mature lymphocytes, plasma cells, and occasional eosinophils. Mitotic figures and multinucleated giant cells were rare.

Storiform-Pleomorphic Malignant Fibrous Histiocytoma

Storiform-pleomorphic malignant fibrous histiocytoma is the most common soft tissue sarcoma of adults over age 50, with most cases involving the musculature of the extremities (especially the thigh), and the retroperitoneum. Following aggressive surgery, local recurrences develop in about 25 percent, and distant metastases in about one-third.[269] The characteristic histologic features of storiform-pleomorphic malignant fibrous histiocytoma are also seen, sometimes extensively, in other pleomorphic malignant tumors, such as pleomorphic liposarcoma, dedifferentiated chondrosarcoma, malignant schwannoma, and sarcomatoid carcinoma. In one study,[270] more than one-half the cases diagnosed as malignant fibrous histiocytoma by light microscopy were reclassified when analyzed by thorough tissue sampling, immunohistochemistry, and electron microscopy, because they showed some differentiation other than fibroblastic or myofibroblastic.

The storiform-pleomorphic type contains, in addition to histiocytes and fibroblasts arranged in a storiform pattern, multi-

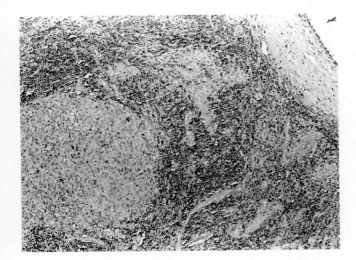

Fig. 18-23. Three components of angiomatoid fibrous histiocytoma: nodules of histiocytes, a lymphoplasmacytic infiltrate, and vascular-like spaces.

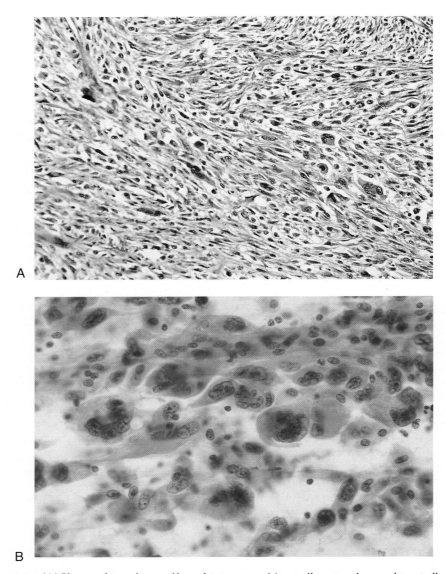

Fig. 18-24. **(A)** Pleomorphic malignant fibrous histiocytoma. Mitotically active pleomorphic spindle cells in a somewhat fascicular arrangement with numerous scattered bizarre giant cells. **(B)** Fine needle aspiration of malignant fibrous histiocytoma, storiform-pleomorphic type, shows extremely pleomorphic mononuclear and multinucleate cells in a cluster, with coarse chromatin clumping. (Papanicolaou.)

nucleated giant cells and strap cells with abundant eosinophilic cytoplasm resembling rhabdomyoblasts.[271–273] These cells have large pleomorphic and hyperchromatic nuclei and may contain cytoplasmic lipid droplets (Fig. 18-24A). Mitotic figures are common. Inflammatory cells, mainly lymphocytes and plasma cells, are always present in this tumor. Occasionally, polymorphonuclear leukocytes, eosinophils, and even lipid-laden histiocytes may also be present.

By FNA, clusters and dispersed cells are seen, sometimes with background necrotic debris. The mononuclear spindle cells have coarse chromatin, irregular nuclear contours, and relatively common atypical mitotic figures. Plump rounded mononuclear and multinucleate tumor giant cells with abundant, often vacuolated cytoplasm also show malignant nuclear features[274] (Fig. 18-24B).

Giant Cell Malignant Fibrous Histiocytoma

The giant cell type, with a histologic appearance resembling that of a giant cell tumor of bone, has been described in the superficial and deep soft tissues of the extremities, head, and neck.[275–277] The neoplastic giant and mononuclear cells are arranged in different sized nodules, which on occasion contain

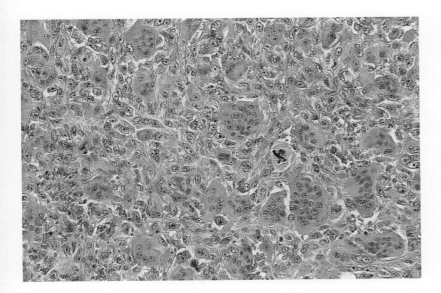

Fig. 18-25. Osteoclast type giant cells and malignant mononuclear histiocyte-like cells are characteristic of giant cell malignant fibrous histiocytoma.

osteoid and mature bone trabeculae (Fig. 18-25). FNA demonstrates the same admixture of mildly pleomorphic mononuclear cells and osteoclastic giant cells.[278] The superficial neoplasms arise in the subcutaneous tissue, fascia, or dermis and may appear as skin tumors, whereas the deep-seated tumors involve skeletal muscle, fascia, and tendons. Their size and anatomic location correlate well with prognosis. Superficial giant cell tumors are smaller than the deep ones and may recur after limited local excision, but in general they are less aggressive than the larger, deep-seated ones, which often metastasize and may lead to the death of the patient. It should be kept in mind that a variety of sarcomas including leiomyosarcomas may contain reactive osteoclast-like giant cells and focally simulate this tumor.

Inflammatory (Xanthomatous) Malignant Fibrous Histiocytoma

The inflammatory malignant fibrous histiocytoma, described originally in the retroperitoneum as xanthogranuloma, consists of mononuclear and multinucleated histiocytic cells and a mixed population of inflammatory cells, chiefly xanthomatous histiocytes, polymorphonuclear leukocytes, lymphocytes, and plasma cells.[279] For this reason, it may be confused with xanthogranulomatous inflammation. However, the cytologic atypia present in the histiocytic cells permits separation. Some of the histiocytic cells may have multilobed nuclei with prominent nucleoli, thus resembling Reed-Sternberg cells. Multinucleated giant cells often contain polymorphonuclear leukocytes in their cytoplasm. When the giant cells die the polymorphonuclear leukocytes become extracellular and form small microabscesses (Fig. 18-26A). Tumor cells produce a neutrophilic and eosinophilic factor that explains the non-neoplastic inflammatory component.[280] This tumor occurs most often in the retroperitoneum but may also be found in the extremities. A patient presented with a leukemoid reaction probably caused by myelopoietic activity by the tumor.[281] Despite its deceptively benign microscopic appearance, local recurrence has been reported in about one-half the patients and distant metastasis in one-third.

FNA specimens reveal the same mixed inflammatory cell elements, which may partially obscure the dissociated large atypical cells, whose cytoplasm may contain neutrophils and whose nuclei are large and multilobed, with open chromatin and prominent nucleoli[282] (Fig. 18-26B).

LIPOMATOUS TUMORS

Lipoma

Benign tumors composed entirely of mature adipose tissue occur at all ages and are the most common soft tissue tumors. They are slow growing, relatively small, and often located in the subcutaneous tissue. By contrast, intramuscular, mesenteric, mediastinal, and retroperitoneal lipomas are less common and are larger than those located in the subcutis.[283,284] Moreover, these deep-seated tumors often extend to adjacent tissues and may recur following local excision, raising the clinical suspicion of liposarcoma.[285–289] Although most lipomas are separated from surrounding tissues by thin fibrous capsules, some have an infiltrative growth pattern, such as intramuscular lipomas, in which skeletal muscle fibers are separated and flattened by the tumor.[286–289] The presence of a tumor mass and absence of a clinical history of muscle disease helps distinguish intramuscular lipoma from muscle replacement by fat in severe muscle atrophy. Focal myxoid changes in lipomas may lead to confusion with liposarcoma. Rarely osseous metaplasia occurs in lipomas.[289]

Familial lipomas are multiple, sometimes symmetric, and not infrequently associated with metabolic disorders, especially hypercholesterolemia.[288] Regional lipomatosis of the extremities has been associated with gigantism.

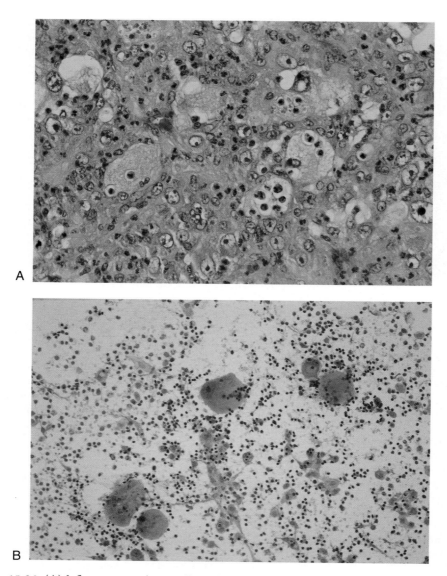

Fig. 18-26. **(A)** Inflammatory malignant fibrous histiocytoma. Malignant mononuclear and xanthoma cells with phagocytosed acute inflammatory cells. **(B)** Fine needle aspiration smear of inflammatory malignant fibrous histiocytoma demonstrates very large bizarre tumor cells with prominent nucleoli, in a mixed inflammatory cell background. (H&E.)

Excessive growth of mature adipose tissue having infiltrative properties and involving extensive portions of the trunk or extremities is known as *diffuse lipomatosis.* Although clinically this condition may simulate liposarcoma, microscopically it resembles an ordinary lipoma.

Adipose tissue tumors of the joints associated with synovia (*lipoma arborescens*) and tendon sheaths are thought to represent reactive inflammatory lesions because of their relatively frequent association with trauma, chronic tenosynovitis, or arthritis.

The FNA specimen from a lipoma is viscous, oily fluid with soft yellow tissue fragments. FNA smears from lipoma show mature adipocytes in clusters, as well as lipid droplets in the back-

ground released from ruptured cells.[290–292] FNA or other trauma may cause patchy fat necrosis in lipomas, but the resultant histiocytic infiltrate should not be mistaken for lipoblasts at subsequent excision. Entrapped atrophic skeletal muscle cells on FNA smears from intramuscular lipoma should be distinguished from multinucleated tumor giant cells.

Angiolipoma

Angiolipoma are solitary or multiple asymptomatic or painful subcutaneous nodules.[293] Some, especially the multiple ones, are genetically determined and inherited as an autosomal dominant trait.[294,295] Microscopically, the focal angiomatous

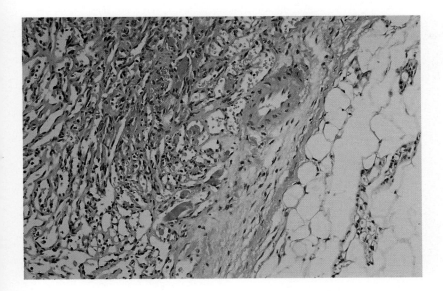

Fig. 18-27. Cellular angiolipoma. Cellular component consisting of a marked proliferation of vascular channels lined by spindled endothelial cells (left) juxtaposed to typical angiolipoma (right). Note characteristic fibrin microthrombi.

component consists of small vessels lined by prominent endothelial cells and often containing erythrocytes and fibrin thrombi. Infiltrating angiolipomas are found in skeletal muscle and may form large masses in the extremities or paravertebral region.[296] Rarely the vascular component of angiolipomas is hypercellular and obliterates the adipose tissue (Fig. 18-27). Hyperplastic endothelial cells may become spindly and the tumor can be confused with Kaposi's sarcoma or angiosarcoma.[297]

Prominent branching vascular structures may be found in aspirates from angiolipomas, as they are in myxoid liposarcomas. However, the adipocytes of angiolipomas are monomorphic and univacuolated with bland peripheral nuclei, as they are in ordinary lipomas.

Myolipoma

Tumors composed of mature adipose tissue and smooth muscle have been designated *myolipomas*.[298] These tumors are larger than ordinary lipomas and occur within the abdominal cavity or retroperitoneum. Occasionally they are found in the subcutaneous tissue. Microscopically, the smooth muscle component usually predominates and shows positive reactivity for muscle actin and desmin. Deep-seated lesions have been confused with liposarcoma.

Angiomyolipoma

Angiomyolipomas are composed of variable proportions of mature fat, blood vessels, and smooth muscle. Thought to be hamartomas, they are found more frequently in the kidney than in any other anatomic location, with the liver second.[299–302] They have been described in association with tuberous sclerosis and pulmonary lymphangiomyomatosis. Angiomyolipomas are usually single except in patients with tuberous sclerosis, in whom renal tumors may be multiple and bilateral. The classic angiomyolipoma is easy to recognize. The adipose tissue is ma-

ture, the smooth muscle cells are not atypical, and the blood vessels show thick walls, which lack elastic tissue and are prone to hemorrhage. However, some angiomyolipomas may be large, cellular, and show epithelioid smooth muscle cells, numerous multinucleated giant cells, and strap cells with cytologic atypia, features that mimic malignant fibrous histiocytoma, leiomyosarcoma, or liposarcoma[302] (Fig. 18-28). Characteristically the smooth muscle cells of angiomyolipomas are HMB-45 positive, a feature that is useful in the diagnosis of the atypical forms.[302] Renal angiomyolipomas with lymph node involvement interpreted as multicentric foci rather than metastases have been reported.[303,304] One case with distant metastases and another with renal vein invasion have also been documented.[305]

FNA of angiomyolipoma yields cellular smears, with a variable proportion of mature adipocytes and bundles of smooth muscle cells. As noted histologically, some cases will show pleomorphic or epithelioid smooth muscle cells. Vascular structures are not prominent on FNA.[306,307]

Myelolipoma

Myelolipoma, a tumor-like lesion composed of a mixture of mature fat and bone marrow, is most often seen in the adrenal glands, although it has been reported rarely in the soft tissues of the presacral region and retroperitoneum.[308–311] Most patients with myelolipomas are asymptomatic. The tumors vary in size from microscopic foci to large masses.[312] A few myelolipomas have been reported in association with endocrine abnormalities such as Cushing's syndrome or Addison's disease.[313] A few of these tumors have had features of both myelolipoma and adrenocortical adenoma.[314]

Chondroid Lipoma

A rare and unique type of lipoma showing chondroid differentiation has recently been added to the list of benign adipose tissue tumors.[315–317] Because the tumor cells bear some resem-

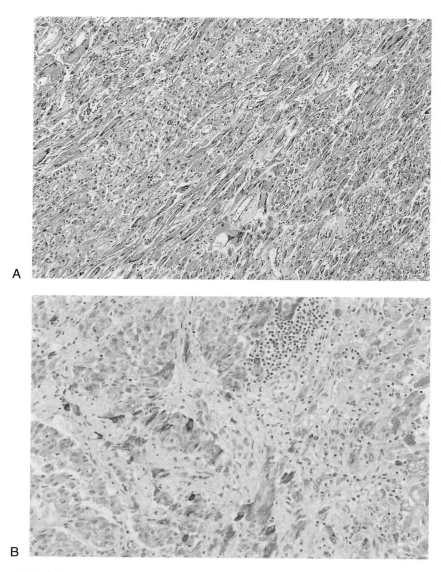

Fig. 18-28. **(A)** Atypical angiomyolipoma containing multinucleated strap cells resembling rhabdomyoblasts. This variant of angiomyolipoma is often confused with liposarcoma or malignant fibrous histiocytoma. **(B)** HMB-45-positive cells of atypical angiomyolipoma.

blance to lipoblasts and chondrocytes and show mild cytologic atypia, chondroid lipoma has been confused with liposarcoma and chondrosarcoma. The vacuolated cells contain both fat and glycogen and are reactive for vimentin, S-100 protein, and focally for cytokeratin. Ultrastructurally, cells sharing features of mature adipocytes, lipoblasts, and chondroblasts are found.[317]

Hibernoma

Hibernomas are uncommon benign adipose tissue tumors composed of cells that biochemically and histologically resemble brown fat.[318–321] A few examples of the malignant counterpart of hibernoma have been recorded.[322,323] Brown adipose tissue is present in relatively large amounts in certain animals that

hibernate, and is metabolically quite different from white adipose tissue, thought to be important in the production of nonshivering thermogenesis in some animals.[318] It is found in various locations in the adult human but is more abundant in fetuses and infants. Hibernomas occur most often in the scapular region, mediastinum, and upper thorax, and are usually 5 to 10 cm in diameter. Hibernomas have a unique, easily identifiable light microscopic appearance; they consist of round to polygonal multivacuolated cells with centrally located nuclei (Fig. 18-29). These cells are clustered in a lobular pattern around the numerous blood vessels of the tumor. Ultrastructurally, numerous mitochondria are present in the cytoplasm of brown fat and hibernoma cells, even those cells with large unilocular fat vacuoles, which at the light microscopic level re-

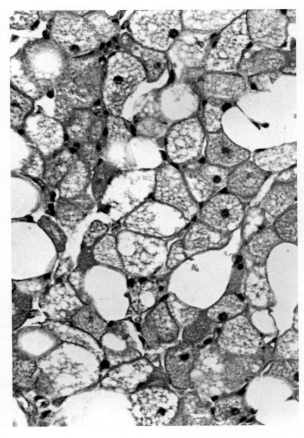

Fig. 18-29. Large multivacuolated cells of hibernoma.

semble the lipocytes of white adipose tissue. Scanty endoplasmic reticulum and small Golgi apparatus further distinguish the cells of the hibernoma and brown fat from those of fetal or adult white adipose tissue.[319] Biochemically, the same types of lipids are found in hibernomas and lipomas but are present in different proportions. This is interpreted to reflect the relatively large number of mitochondria in the hibernoma cell as compared with those of the white adipose cells constituting the lipoma.[324]

On FNA smears, hibernomas demonstrate the diagnostic brown fat cells with multiple uniform cytoplasmic vacuoles and central bland round nuclei, as well as admixed capillaries and univacuolated adipocytes.[325,326]

Lipoblastomatosis

Lipoblastomatosis, a benign adipose tissue tumor of children, is characterized by lobules containing a variable proportion of mature fat cells and lipoblasts in different stages of development (Fig. 18-30). Myxoid changes and a prominent capillary network are commonly present.[327–332] A circumscribed form (benign lipoblastoma) is confined to the subcutaneous tissue, whereas the diffuse form (diffuse lipoblastomatosis) tends to infiltrate muscle and may recur following local excision. Because

of the rarity of liposarcomas under age 15, lipoblastomatosis should always be a strong diagnostic consideration in adipose tissue tumors of children.

The few cytologic reports describe cellular fibrofatty tissue fragments containing mono- and multivacuolated lipoblasts, as well as numerous stellate and spindled cells in a myxomatous background.[333] The nuclei show bland chromatin, although they may be scalloped or displaced by cytoplasmic lipid vacuoles, or show pseudoinclusions. Cohesive clusters of lipoblasts may be traversed by ramifying capillaries.

Spindle Cell Lipoma and Pleomorphic Lipoma

Spindle cell lipoma and pleomorphic lipoma are benign lesions that share common features, including their occurrence as solitary, painless, slow-growing masses located on the shoulder, posterior neck, or upper back of adult males, commonly 40 years or older.[334–337] Both tumors involve the subcutis and are well circumscribed and encapsulated like ordinary lipoma, but are more pale and firm on cut surface.[334–337]

Microscopically, spindle cell lipoma is composed of an admixture of mature adipocytes, uniform spindle cells, and bundles of brightly eosinophilic collagen fibers[334,335,338,339] (Fig.

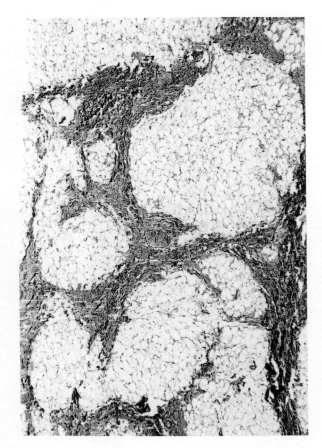

Fig. 18-30. Lipoblastomatosis showing the characteristic lobulation of the fetal type of adipose tissue.

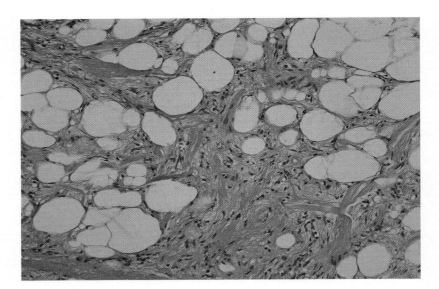

Fig. 18-31. Spindle cell lipoma composed of short fascicles of spindle cells with collagen fibers admixed with mature adipose tissue.

18-31). The fibroblast-like spindle cells are oriented in short fascicles and may occupy a portion or most of the tumor (cellular variant of spindle cell lipoma). For the most part, the vascular component is inconspicuous; however, some lesions may have a marked hemangiopericytic appearance or mimic a vascular neoplasm.[340,341] Prominent myxoid stromal change and degeneration may also be present. Pleomorphic lipoma, on the other hand, receives its name from the presence of bizarre multinucleated giant cells having peripherally arranged hyperchromatic nuclei and deeply eosinophilic central cytoplasm, the so-called floret-type giant cells[336,337] (Fig. 18-32). These cells are dispersed in a fibromyxoid matrix and alternate with hyalin collagen fibers, mature adipocytes, and occasional lipoblasts. Transitional forms between spindle cell and pleomorphic lipoma are not uncommon. By immunohistochemistry, S-100 protein stains the mature adipocytes, whereas the spindle cells are negative and the pleomorphic cells may show weak intracytoplas-mic positivity.[342] Ultrastructural studies suggest that both the spindle and pleomorphic multinucleated cells that characterize these tumors are prelipoblastic mesenchymal cells.[343] The anatomic site and superficial location distinguishes these two lesions from well differentiated liposarcoma/atypical lipoma.

Reports of FNA from spindle cell lipomas and pleomorphic lipomas describe good correlation with histologic features, namely admixed fusiform fibroblast-like cells in the former, and multinucleate floret-type giant cells associated with mature adipocytes in the latter.[292]

Liposarcoma

Liposarcoma is the second most common sarcoma surpassed only by malignant fibrous histiocytoma. It occurs almost exclusively in adults. The major sites of involvement are the ex-

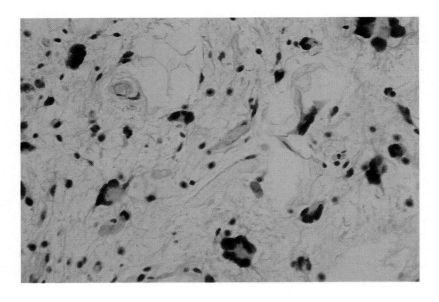

Fig. 18-32. Floret-like giant cells with peripheral placed hyperchromatic nuclei and eosinophilic cytoplasm characterize pleomorphic lipoma.

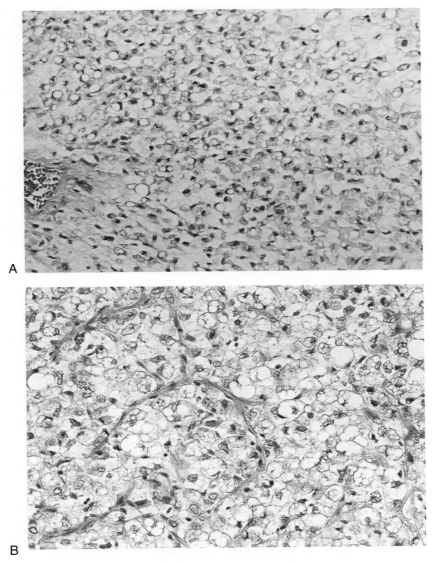

Fig. 18-33. **(A)** Lipoblasts. Univacuolated signet ring cell type. **(B)** Typical multivacuolated lipoblasts with indentation of hyperchromatic nucleus.

tremities, particularly the medial thigh and popliteal fossa, the retroperitoneum, the inguinal region, and the spermatic cord. Tumors involving the extremities usually occur between the third and fifth decades. Those arising in deep soft tissues, especially the retroperitoneum, present at a later peak age, between the fifth and seventh decades, and attain a larger size. Liposarcomas comprise a clinically and morphologically heterogeneous group of lesions[344–355] that recapitulate different stages in the development of normal adipose tissue. Based on natural history and histomorphology, and supported by recent cytogenetic findings,[356,357] three main categories are recognized[353]: (1) myxoid liposarcoma, and combined myxoid and round cell liposarcoma, (2) well differentiated liposarcoma/atypical lipoma and dedifferentiated liposarcoma, and (3) pleomorphic liposarcoma. Based solely on clinical behavior, myxoid liposarcoma

and well differentiated liposarcoma are low grade lesions that recur frequently and may undergo transformation to their high grade counterparts, round cell liposarcoma and dedifferentiated liposarcoma, respectively. The latter two and pleomorphic liposarcoma are high grade lesions with a propensity to metastasize. The low grade liposarcoma are long-standing lesions, with rapid growth indicating evolution to a higher grade. Grossly, liposarcomas are well circumscribed, often encapsulated, and have a lobulated pattern. The cut surface varies from pale yellow and gelatinous to gray-white and firm, reflecting its fat content and cellular composition. Traditionally, the distinctive feature of liposarcomas has been the lipoblast in any of its usual forms[355]: primitive cells with fine cytoplasmic vacuolation, small univacuolated or "signet ring cell" type (Fig. 18-33A), the typical multivacuolated cells with central scalloped hyperchro-

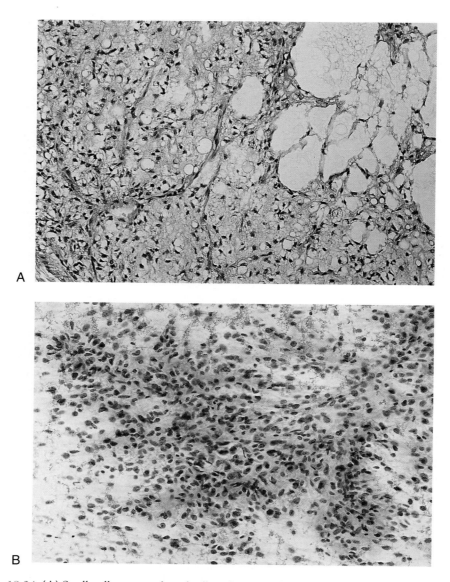

Fig. 18-34. **(A)** Small stellate mesenchymal cells and primitive lipoblasts in a myxoid stroma and a delicate plexiform capillary pattern characterize myxoid liposarcoma. Myxoid pools (upper right) are a frequent finding. **(B)** Fine needle aspiration of myxoid and round cell liposarcoma shows relatively uniform cells with small nuclei and abundant pale cytoplasm adherent to capillaries and dyshesive into the myxoid background. (H&E.)

matic nucleus (Fig. 18-33B), and large univacuolated cells resembling the mature adipocyte. However, given the existence of lipoblast-like cells (e.g., vacuolated endothelial cells, capillaries, lipid-laden macrophages, signet ring cell lymphoma[358]), the lipoblast cannot be relied upon as the single criterion, nor is it required for the diagnosis of liposarcoma if other characteristic features described below are present.

Myxoid and round cell liposarcomas commonly involve the soft tissues of the lower extremities. Myxoid liposarcoma is characterized by small, primitive, spindle-shaped, stellate or angulated mesenchymal cells, lipoblasts in varying early stages of differentiation, abundant myxoid matrix, and a delicate plexiform capillary pattern (Fig. 18-34A). The myxoid change may be prominent with the formation of mucin pools. Round cell liposarcoma consists of sheets or cords of uniform small round cells with eosinophilic cytoplasm, hyperchromatic nuclei, and frequent mitoses. Scattered lipoblasts or transitional cells having finely vacuolated or granular cytoplasm resembling brown fat are also found (Fig. 18-35). Round cell liposarcoma is almost always seen arising in a background of myxoid liposarcoma, and rarely occurs in pure form. According to a recent clinicopathologic study[359] a round cell component of greater than 5 percent in a myxoid liposarcoma predicts an adverse outcome and qualifies this lesion as a high grade combined myxoid and round cell liposarcoma.

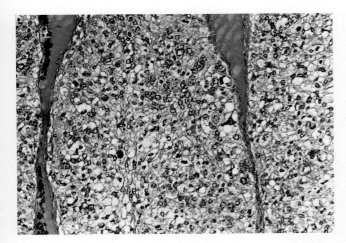

Fig. 18-35. Round cell component of a mixed type of liposarcoma is seen. The cells are cohesive and have a vacuolated cytoplasm.

Well differentiated liposarcoma and atypical lipoma are morphologically indistinguishable lesions. The term *atypical lipoma* is applied to tumors arising in the deep subcutis and superficial soft tissues because they have demonstrated an indolent behavior, recurring infrequently.[346,347,350] By contrast, well differentiated liposarcoma refers to tumors arising in the deep soft tissues of the extremities, inguinal region, or retroperitoneum that commonly recur and may dedifferentiate.[346,347,350,360,361] Two main subtypes of well differentiated liposarcoma are known: lipoma-like (adipocytic) and sclerosing. As its name implies, *lipoma-like liposarcoma* is composed largely of mature adipocytes showing variation in cell size and atypical hyperchromatic nuclei (atypical adipocytes) (Fig. 18-36), accompanied by typical lipoblasts, floret giant cells, and bizarre multinucleated stromal cells in fibrous septae. In *sclerosing liposarcoma*, the lipomatous areas alternate with fibrous bands containing scattered atypical hyperchromatic stromal cells. A third subtype, *inflammatory liposarcoma*, is confined to the retroperitoneum and is associated with a prominent lymphoplasmacytic infiltrate, mimicking an inflammatory pseudotumor. Well differentiated liposarcomas associated with a benign or malignant smooth muscle component have been reported,[362,363] and should be distinguished from the dedifferentiated liposarcoma, described below. Osseous and cartilaginous metaplasia also occur. The clinical behavior of well differentiated liposarcoma is strongly influenced by location.[361,364] Although survival rates vary, 5 year survival rates of 100 percent have been reported for the superficially located atypical lipomas, decreasing to 71 percent for the well differentiated liposarcomas located in deep soft tissues of the extremities and to 31 percent for those arising in the retroperitoneum. Parenthetically, these findings and cytogenetic studies (discussed earlier) provide support to the idea that liposarcomas are not derived from lipomas, which are largely subcutaneous and have a different karyotypic profile.

Dedifferentiated liposarcoma refers to a nonlipogenic high grade sarcoma associated with or juxtaposed to a well differentiated liposarcoma.[351,361,365–371] The dedifferentiated component usually has the appearance of a malignant fibrous histiocytoma or a fibrosarcoma; however, heterologous elements including rhabdomyosarcoma and leiomyosarcoma have been noted.[365–368] Dedifferentiation may occur in the primary tumor or in recurrences, and its incidence appears to correlate with the duration of the lesion.[361] Therefore, it is more commonly seen in tumors arising in the retroperitoneum and the inguinal region, but is not site dependent and can occur in extremities and subcutis.[361,365] Dedifferentiated liposarcoma, although high grade, bears a better prognosis than other pleomorphic sarcomas.[365] If present only focally, it may not have an impact on prognosis and may even be absent in subsequent recurrences.[351,361]

An uncommon variant of well differentiated liposarcoma has been recognized by some authors under the term *spindle cell liposarcoma*.[353,372] It is characterized by the presence of relatively bland spindle cells arranged in short fascicles or whorls, in addition to a well differentiated liposarcomatous component. Although frequently located in the subcutaneous tissues of the shoulder girdle or upper limbs, it has a behavior somewhere between atypical lipoma and well differentiated liposarcoma.

Pleomorphic liposarcoma occurs mainly in the extremities and is characterized by bizarre giant and multinucleated lipoblasts, intracytoplasmic eosinophilic globules, and foci of undifferentiated pleomorphic spindled and rounded cells (malignant fibrohistiocytoma-like).

In addition to the above, liposarcomas of *mixed* type or no specific type are encountered. Myxoid change or degeneration may occur in any histologic type of liposarcoma, and should not be misconstrued as diagnostic of a myxoid liposarcoma. For the latter, all other unequivocal distinguishing features must be present. In general, thorough sampling of liposarcomas is mandatory to identify a high grade component.

All major histologic types of liposarcoma have been found in the anterior mediastinum, although well differentiated and myxoid liposarcomas are the most common.[373]

Liposarcomas in children are rare, predominantly of myxoid type, and carry an excellent prognosis.[374,375]

Ultrastructurally, malignant lipoblasts replicate the various embryonic stages of development of adipose tissue.[376–383] The

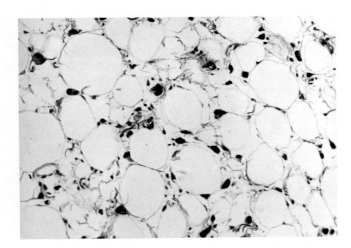

Fig. 18-36. Well differentiated liposarcoma. Many adipocytes contain large hyperchromatic nuclei.

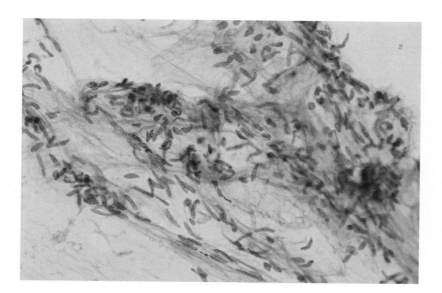

Fig. 18-37. Fine needle aspiration of leiomyoma shows bland spindled nuclei, some in tandem rows, with syncytial and bipolar cytoplasm. (Papanicolaou.)

precursor is a spindle-shaped or stellate perivascular primitive mesenchymal cell that resembles an immature fibroblast. As it migrates away from the capillary, this cell begins lipoblastic differentiation evidenced by the appearance of non-membrane-bound fine lipid droplets in the cytoplasm. These lipid droplets later coalesce into a single intracytoplasmic vacuole that displaces the nucleus to the periphery, the signet ring lipoblast, or into multiple large intracytoplasmic vacuoles that indent a centrally placed nucleus. These late lipoblasts display in addition surface pinocytotic vesicles and a discontinuous external lamina. Primitive non-fat-storing mesenchymal cells, fibroblasts, and myofibroblastic tumor cells are additional components in well differentiated, dedifferentiated, pleomorphic, and spindle cell liposarcomas.

Immunohistochemistry is usually not useful in liposarcomas. S-100 protein antibodies stain mature adipocytes and well differentiated lipoblasts, but reactivity is generally focal and weak in less differentiated liposarcomas and is nonspecific.

On FNA, liposarcomas[384-386] are characterized by the presence of atypical multivacuolated lipoblasts. Specific subtypes show characteristic features cytologically. Well differentiated (lipoma-like) liposarcoma shows predominantly mature adipocyte clusters, with variable numbers of mononuclear or multinucleate cells with nuclear anaplasia. Myxoid liposarcoma demonstrates a background of mesenchymal mucin, a branching capillary network, and clusters of monovacuolated and atypical multivacuolated lipoblasts (Fig. 18-34B). The cellularity of myxoid liposarcoma on FNA tends to be high, and the matrix is semitranslucent and sometimes fibrillar, similar to myxofibrosarcoma (low grade malignant fibrous histiocytoma), in contrast to the opaque matrix of chondrosarcomas, which contains lacunar cells. Nuclear atypia is less pronounced in myxoid liposarcomas than myxofibrosarcoma, and a branching capillary pattern is prominent in myxoid liposarcoma.[386] Round cell liposarcoma also shows a background of mesenchymal mucin, but the highly cellular lesion shows moderate pleomorphism of round to ovoid nuclei in clusters or as dyshesive individual cells. Monovacuolated lipoblasts are also frequent.

Pleomorphic liposarcoma contains spindled fibroblast-like cells, rounded histiocyte-like cells, and pleomorphic multinucleated giant cells that may be impossible to distinguish from malignant fibrous histiocytoma on cytologic grounds.

SMOOTH MUSCLE TUMORS

The most frequent sites of smooth muscle tumors are the uterus, the GI tract, and, to a lesser extent, the retroperitoneum, muscles of the skin, and the walls of small and large blood vessels.

Leiomyoma

Cutaneous leiomyomas are dermal or subcutaneous nodules, often painful, that usually measure less than 2 cm. They can be single or multiple. They arise most frequently from the arrector pili muscles of the extremities and have been reported to be familial.[387-389] The patients are usually adolescent or young adults but affected children have also been reported. Recurrence after excision may be due to incomplete removal of the lesion. Solitary lesions of the nipple, vulva, and scrotum arise from the smooth muscle around the areola and the dartos.[390-391] Other solitary leiomyomas originate from the smooth muscle of blood vessel walls; these lesions have a prominent vascular component and should be considered *angiomyomas* or *angioleiomyomas*.[392] They are more common in the extremities of adult females and have been divided into three histologic subtypes: capillary, cavernous, and venous types. Leiomyomas are well demarcated, and show spindle cells with cigar-shaped nuclei and tapering eosinophilic cytoplasm (Fig. 18-37). The cells form fascicles that intersect at right angles, with some fascicles cut on end and others cut longitudinally. The stroma may be hyalinized or show focal myxoid changes.

Leiomyomas are exceedingly rare in deep soft tissues.[393-397]

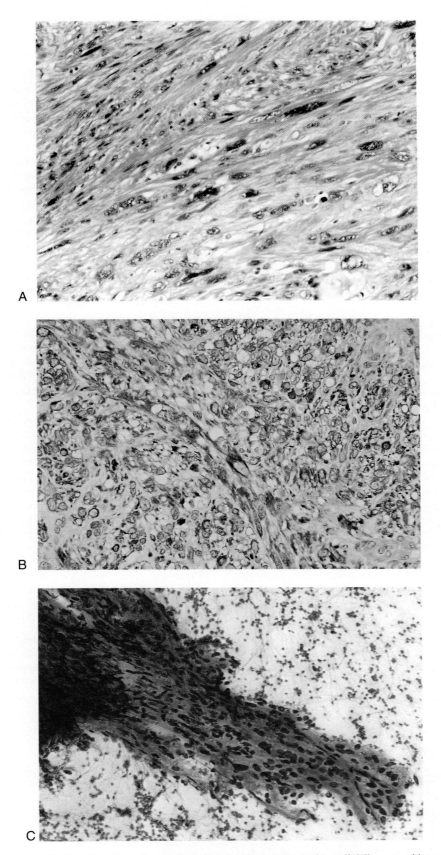

Fig. 18-38. **(A)** Bundles of neoplastic smooth muscle cells are seen in this well differentiated leiomyosarcoma. **(B)** Intense cytoplasmic positivity for desmin in a high grade leiomyosarcoma. **(C)** Fine needle aspiration of leiomyosarcoma shows slightly pleomorphic nuclei in a tissue cluster with tandem rows, as well as stripped nuclei in the background. (Diff-Quik.)

These smooth muscle tumors are larger than the superficial ones, and they may become calcified. Cellularity, cytologic atypia, and mitotic activity are the best parameters separating leiomyomas from leiomyosarcomas of soft tissues. In some cases, however, these features may be unreliable, as in other anatomic locations. Moreover, some leiomyomas may contain bizarre cells with large hyperchromatic nuclei and multinucleated giant cells; these features have been interpreted as being of degenerative nature. Most *epithelioid leiomyomas (leiomyoblastomas)* occur in the GI tract and the uterus. They are exceedingly rare in the soft tissues.

Leiomyosarcoma

According to anatomic site, leiomyosarcomas are divided into three groups: deep, superficial (cutaneous), and those arising from the walls of large blood vessels. Most deep leiomyosarcomas occur in the retroperitoneum, omentum, or mesentery. They are most common in females between 40 and 60 years of age and can be quite large. Retroperitoneal tumors may infiltrate the kidney, colon and other viscera, making surgical resection impossible.

Cutaneous leiomyosarcomas are less common and smaller than the deep ones and are low grade malignant tumors.[398] Most of these tumors are solitary, painful nodules. They may appear at any age and at any anatomic site but occur preferentially in the lower extremities, and are more common on the extensor than the flexor aspects of the extremities.

Rarely, leiomyosarcomas arise from the walls of blood vessels, especially the large veins of the extremities.[399–401] Most of these tumors exhibit intraluminal growth with invasion of the vessel wall and adjacent soft tissues. For this reason, venography, arteriography, and CT are important tools in preoperative diagnosis and planning of surgical treatment.

Despite the fact that leiomyosarcomas show several growth patterns and variable degrees of differentiation, the histologic diagnosis is not difficult because most of these tumors contain well differentiated areas in which smooth muscle cells forming fascicles can be easily identified (Fig. 18-38A). Distinction of cellular leiomyomas from well differentiated leiomyosarcomas is a much more difficult task. The mitotic index is not always a reliable diagnostic criterion and other features such as size, anatomic location, cellularity, and cytologic atypia must be taken into account.

Most of these tumors are composed of fascicles of well differentiated smooth muscle cells. However, leiomyosarcomas with extensive myxoid features, a hemangiopericytic pattern (vascular leiomyosarcoma), and pleomorphic giant cells resembling pleomorphic rhabdomyosarcoma or malignant fibrous histiocytoma have been described.[401] Epithelioid leiomyosarcomas are exceedingly rare in the soft tissues. Not infrequently, leiomyosarcomas show more than one histologic growth pattern. Ultrastructural studies are helpful in demonstrating cytoplasmic features akin to those present in normal smooth muscle. Myofilaments, however, are scanty and not universally present and are seen only in a small percentage of the neoplastic cells. The recognition of leiomyosarcoma can now be assisted by the demonstration of smooth muscle antigens such as desmin and muscle-specific actin by immunohistochemistry[402,403] (Fig. 18-38B). Like synovial sarcoma and epithelioid sarcoma, leiomyosarcoma can also express cytokeratin and epithelial membrane antigen.[403]

Prognosis correlates well with the size and anatomic location of the leiomyosarcoma. Most patients with tumors of the retroperitoneum and veins of the extremities have large tumors and die as a result of metastases.[404–406] By contrast, cutaneous leiomyosarcomas are relatively small and often recur following local excision, but rarely metastasize.

FNA of leiomyoma and leiomyosarcoma may yield scant or abundantly cellular smears.[407,408] Benign and low grade malignant lesions may be difficult to distinguish; both show oval and elongated nuclei in cohesive clusters of spindle cells. Leiomyomas tend to have more syncytial densely staining cytoplasm, whereas low grade leiomyosarcomas have more loose groupings and single cells with scant cytoplasm, including stripped nuclei. Nuclei may be arranged in parallel rows representing palisades

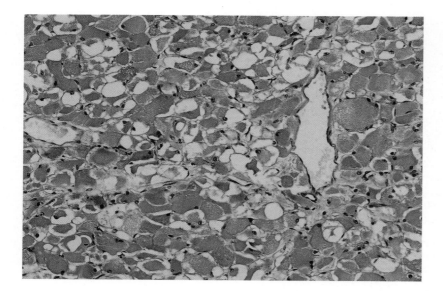

Fig. 18-39. Adult rhabdomyoma. The tumor is composed of polygonal cells with voluminous granular eosinophilic cytoplasm and small peripherally placed nuclei. Cytoplasmic vacuolation is evident.

(though Verocay bodies of fibrillar cytoplasm as seen in neurilemoma[409] are absent), and in tandem rows resembling train boxcars. The nuclei tend to have indentations, suggesting segmentation due to longitudinal contraction, blunted ends, finely granular chromatin, and inconspicuous nucleoli (Fig. 18-38C). Blood vessels may be seen within the cell clusters. Some cases show admixed stromal collagen fibrils or myxoid matrix in the background. High grade leiomyosarcomas demonstrate spindle cells and multinucleate giant cells with conspicuous nuclear atypia, coarse chromatin clumping, pleomorphism, and lack of cohesion. Necrotic debris and stripped nuclei are also common features. Epithelioid smooth muscle tumors are exceedingly rare in soft tissues but are apt to be confused with epithelial neoplasms on FNA.[407] Epithelioid leiomyomas show cohesive clusters with abundant syncytial cytoplasm, uniform rounded nuclei, and fine chromatin without nucleoli. Epithelioid leiomyosarcomas demonstrate loose groups and solitary cells with rounded nuclei of variable sizes containing coarse chromatin, some with nucleoli, and scant or stripped cytoplasm.

TUMORS OF STRIATED MUSCLE

Rhabdomyoma

Despite the large mass and ubiquity of skeletal muscles, rhabdomyomas are among the rarest benign soft tissue tumors and are found almost exclusively in the head and neck, vagina, vulva, and anus. Rhabdomyomas rarely occur as multiple lesions and occasionally recur after incomplete resection.

Two distinctive histologic types are recognized: the *adult* and the *fetal*. The adult type rhabdomyoma is more common and occurs almost exclusively about the head and neck (oral cavity, pharynx, and larynx) of adult men,[410–414] whereas fetal rhabdomyomas have a broader anatomic distribution and occur in men, women, and children.[415] The *adult rhabdomyoma* is easy to recognize because it is composed of large, round to polygonal cells similar to mature skeletal muscle fibers (Fig. 18-39). The abundant cytoplasm is eosinophilic and granular and contains peripherally arranged vacuoles. In other cells, thin strands of cytoplasm extend between the vacuoles to the distinct cell boundaries, producing the characteristic spider appearance. Intracytoplasmic glycogen, dissolved during routine tissue processing, results in the vacuolated appearance of the tumor cells. Longitudinal and cross-striations can be seen in occasional cells, and the organization of myofibrils into highly organized sarcomeres is observed readily with electron microscopy. Eosinophilic crystalline structures arranged in haphazard fashion in the cells of adult rhabdomyomas are hypertrophied, densely packed Z bands. By immunohistochemistry the cells show positive reactivity for muscle-specific actin, desmin, and myoglobin.[412] FNA smears of adult type rhabdomyoma reveal large polygonal cells with sharply defined cell borders, abundant granulated or striated cytoplasm, and uniform round peripheral nuclei. Some cells are multinucleated, resembling mature skeletal muscle.[414,416] Cytoplasmic rod-shaped inclusions may be seen. Spider cells are not a feature of FNA smears.

The *fetal rhabdomyoma* is composed of fascicles of densely packed spindle cells resembling the various developmental stages of striated skeletal muscle.[415] The cellular variant of fetal rhabdomyoma is confined to the head and neck of children and has been misdiagnosed as sarcoma because of its cellularity and mild pleomorphism, but the paucity of mitoses and the circumscribed growth of the tumor distinguish it from sarcomas. Unlike those of the adult rhabdomyoma, the nuclei of the fetal type are small and uniform. In some tumors, the cells are dispersed in a myxoid stroma. The immunohistochemical profile of the fetal variant is similar to that of the adult type of rhabdomyoma. The vaginal and vulvar rhabdomyomas are mainly myxoid fetal rhabdomyomas.

Cardiac rhabdomyomas, most likely hamartomas rather than neoplasms, are usually multiple, and affect newborns and infants. These tumors occur predominantly in males and can cause sudden death. They are frequently associated with tuberous sclerosis or coexist with other congenital cardiac malformations.[417] Cases not associated with tuberous sclerosis or congenital heart disease have also been documented. Cardiac rhabdomyomas are composed of large cells with clear glycogen-rich cytoplasm and spider cells, both of which show diffuse positivity for myoglobin, actin, desmin, and vimentin.

Rhabdomyosarcoma

In contrast to liposarcomas, rhabdomyosarcomas are more frequent in children, adolescents, and young adults. In fact, rhabdomyosarcoma is the most common soft tissue sarcoma in the pediatric age group. Regardless of their histologic appearance, rhabdomyosarcomas are high grade malignant tumors. They grow rapidly and often develop hematogenous spread to the lungs and other viscera. Lymph node metastases are also common, especially in the alveolar type, reaching an incidence at autopsy as high as 74 percent of patients dying of the disease. In spite of this aggressive biologic behavior, modern multimodality therapy has considerably improved the survival rate of patients with these tumors, especially the embryonal, botryoid, and spindle cell types. On the basis of their microscopic features, five histologic types have been described: embryonal, botryoid, spindle cell, alveolar, and pleomorphic.[418–420] The botryoid and spindle cell types may be regarded as subtypes of the embryonal category.

Embryonal Type

The embryonal rhabdomyosarcoma, the most common variant, occurs most often in the head and neck and especially in the orbit of children. Other common sites are the deep soft tissues of the extremities and the urogenital tract.[421] In hollow organs—urinary bladder, vagina, biliary tract—they form characteristic edematous, polypoid masses (*sarcoma botryoides*). Rarely, embryonal rhabdomyosarcomas occur in adults or are congenital.[422] The histologic appearance varies from one tumor to another and in different fields of the same tumor, from round cells with hyperchromatic nuclei and scanty cytoplasm to elongate or strap-shaped cells displaying centrally placed vesicular or hyperchromatic nuclei and abundant acidophilic cytoplasm with

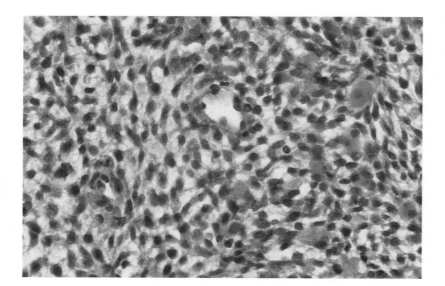

Fig. 18-40. Undifferentiated primitive cells and scattered rounded rhabdomyoblasts in an embryonal rhabdomyosarcoma.

cross-striations (Fig. 18-40). Myxoid areas containing stellate cells are common and may predominate in some tumors. Most embryonal and botryoid rhabdomyosarcomas show positive reactivity for muscle-specific actin and desmin. Only the well differentiated areas containing large rhabdomyoblasts with abundant cytoplasm show positive reactivity for myoglobin.[423–425] With multimodality therapy 67 percent of patients with embryonal and 95 percent of patients with *botryoid rhabdomyosarcoma* survived 5 years.[426] When the tumor is composed predominantly of spindle cells arranged in fascicular and storiform patterns and the stroma shows varying degrees of fibrosis the term *spindle cell rhabdomyosarcoma* is used.[420,427,428] This tumor has been confused with leiomyosarcoma, although cross-striations are often seen in the spindle cells. Spindle cell rhabdomyosarcoma also has a favorable prognosis.[418,419]

Alveolar Type

Alveolar rhabdomyosarcomas appear predominantly in adolescents and young adults, are more common in the extremities than in the head and neck, and comprise the most aggressive variant.[429,430] They are composed primarily of round cells with scanty cytoplasm, vesicular or hyperchromatic nuclei, and prominent nucleoli; occasional myoglobin-positive cells exhibit abundant cytoplasm, and multinucleated giant cells with peripheral wreath-like nuclei may be seen in some tumors. The cellular elements are characteristically separated by fibrous connective tissue septa forming an alveolar pattern. The peripheral cells are attached to the septa and the discohesive central cells appear "floating" in the center of the alveoli (Fig. 18-41). In some tumors, however, discohesiveness does not occur and the alveoli are filled with tumor cells producing a solid growth pattern. A characteristic translocation, t(2;13) (q35;q14) has been reported in most alveolar rhabdomyosarcomas.[431] Approximately 54 percent of patients survive 5 years or longer when multimodality therapy is used.[419]

Pleomorphic Type

Because pleomorphic rhabdomyosarcoma frequently cannot be distinguished from pleomorphic leiomyosarcoma, malignant fibrous histiocytoma, and pleomorphic liposarcoma on histologic grounds alone, it is essential to use immunohistochemical stains and sometimes electron microscopy for correct identification. The pleomorphic variant is the rarest form of rhabdomyosarcoma and occurs predominantly in the extremities of adult patients, usually over 60 years of age.[432–435] It is a clinically aggressive neoplasm. More than 50 percent of the patients die with distant metastases. The tumor is composed of large spindle-shaped and multinucleated giant cells, both having abundant eosinophilic cytoplasm (Fig. 18-42A). Pleomorphic rhabdomyosarcomas usually show positive reactivity for vimentin and muscle-specific actin. Less frequently they stain for desmin and myoglobin (Fig. 18-42B). Electron microscopy reveals Z-band material arranged in rudimentary sarcomeres.

FNA of embryonal and alveolar rhabdomyosarcomas[436–439] yields cellular smears with predominantly small mildly pleomorphic cells, and scattered larger cells, including bi- and multinucleate forms. Diagnostic tadpole or ribbon-shaped rhabdomyoblasts are not found in most cases, but other small round blue cell tumors of childhood generally lack bi- and multinucleate cells, so their presence is a useful diagnostic clue (Fig. 18-42C). Nuclei tend to be hyperchromatic with thickened membranes, but nucleoli are usually inconspicuous. Some cases show nuclear molding (resembling neuroblastoma), tigroid background (resembling seminoma and Ewing's sarcoma), cytoplasmic vacuoles (resembling Ewing's sarcoma and Burkitt's lymphoma), and cytoplasmic fragments that resemble lymphoglandular bodies. Bare nuclei are common, with small cells having scant cytoplasm, and only intermediate and larger cells showing more abundant well defined eosinophilic cytoplasm. Metachromatic stromal fragments and necrotic cells may be present. Cytologic distinction between alveolar and embryonal subtypes is unreliable unless intact alveolar structures or characteristic wreath-like multinucleate cells are seen.[439]

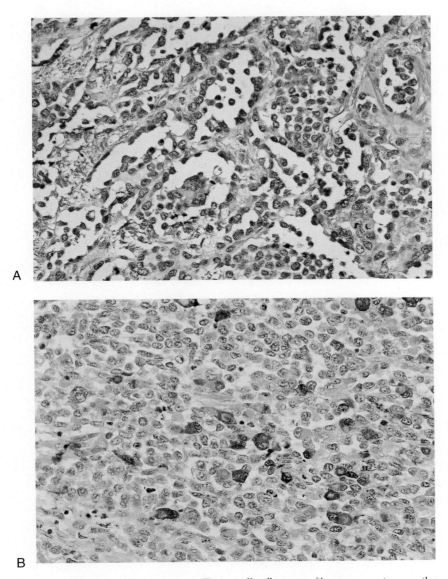

Fig. 18-41. **(A)** Alveolar rhabdomyosarcoma. Tumor cells adherent to fibrous septae circumscribe central loose aggregates of small round tumor cells resulting in distinctive alveolar pattern. **(B)** Better differentiated rhabdomyoblasts demonstrate strong immunopositivity for myoglobin.

TUMORS OF BLOOD VESSELS

Hemangioma

Most benign vascular tumors arise in the skin and subcutaneous tissues, but no organ or tissue is exempt.[440,441] Hemangiomas are primarily tumors of infancy and childhood. Some are evident at birth; relatively few become manifest after the age of 30 years. Females are afflicted slightly more frequently than males, but males can predominate in some of the clinical syndromes that include vascular tumors.[442–444] Certain types of benign vascular tumors are associated with familial disease.

Benign vascular tumors of the mucosal surfaces, including hemangiomas, hereditary hemorrhagic telangiectasia (Rendu-Osler-Weber disease), and arteriovenous malformations, frequently produce acute and chronic hemorrhage and, sometimes, resultant anemia. The association of giant cavernous hemangiomas with thrombocytopenia and extensive purpura, the Kasabach-Merritt syndrome, was first described in 1940 in an infant boy whose purpura disappeared when sclerosis of the hemangioma was accomplished by means of radiation therapy.[442] More recent studies have shown this syndrome to be a consumptive coagulopathy with reactive fibrinolysis and traumatic intravascular hemolysis.[445–447] The precise mechanism of the coagulopathy is unknown. Platelet sequestration has been demonstrated in the tumor, but other coagulation abnormalities seem to be operative.

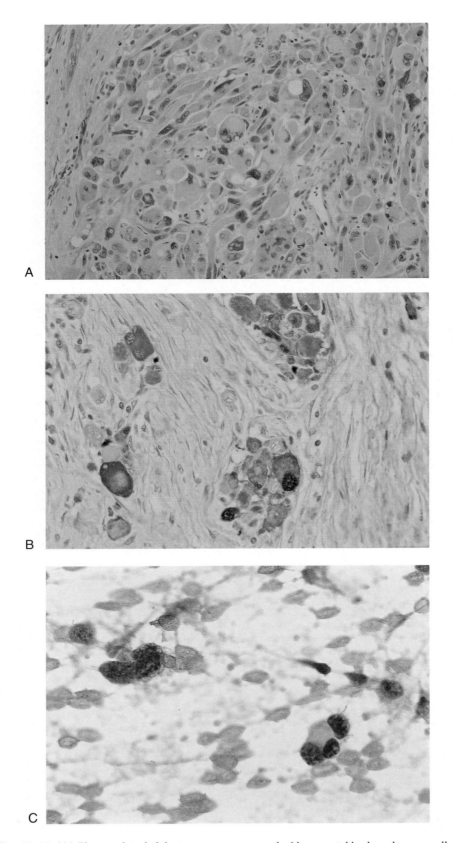

Fig. 18-42. **(A)** Pleomorphic rhabdomyosarcoma composed of large variably shaped tumor cells with deeply eosinophilic cytoplasm and hyperchromatic nuclei. **(B)** Immunoreactivity for myoglobin confirms skeletal muscle origin. **(C)** Fine needle aspiration smear of embryonal rhabdomyosarcoma demonstrates pleomorphic small cells with hyperchromatic nuclei, including multinucleate cells, one with more abundant well defined eosinophilic cytoplasm. (H&E.)

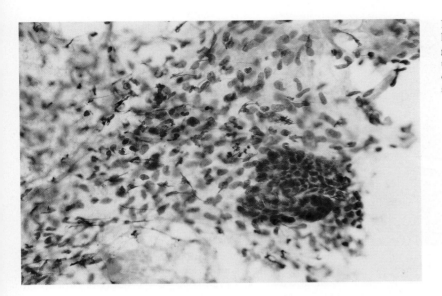

Fig. 18-43. Fine needle aspiration of intraparotid cellular hemangioma in a young child ("infantile hemangioendothelioma") shows a densely cellular cluster of uniform bland spindled nuclei focally forming small caliber vascular channels, with an entrapped ductal structure. (H&E.)

Skeletal and soft tissue gigantism associated with vascular tumors seems to depend on the presence of arteriovenous fistulas in the tumor mass.[448,449] The most extreme clinical manifestations of these problems are exemplified by the Klippel-Trenaunay and Parkes-Weber syndromes, which include extensive cutaneous capillary hemangiomas of the extremities, usually the legs, with superficial varicose veins and hypertrophy of the bones of the affected part. Angiography can sometimes demonstrate arteriovenous fistulas that can be ligated to control the gigantism. Unlike the continuing gigantism that occurs sometimes with lipomatosis or neurofibromatosis, the growth of the soft tissues, bones, and sometimes the hemangiomas arrests when the patient reaches the third decade of life.

Cellular Hemangioma of Infancy

Cellular capillary hemangiomas are the most common vascular tumors. They are found most frequently in infants and children, especially in the head and neck.[450–453] These tumors are multilobular, densely cellular, and composed of small capillary channels, each lined by a single layer of endothelial cells. Frequently, the vascular channels are obliterated by plump endothelial cells leading to the formation of solid areas. This histologic pattern has led to the designation benign "juvenile" hemangioendothelioma. The tumor may grow rapidly, infiltrate adjacent tissues, and mitoses and papillary tufts may be present, features that sometimes lead to confusion of these lesions with malignant vascular tumors. The lack of anastomosing channels is helpful in distinguishing hemangiomas from angiosarcomas, as is the patient's age, because angiosarcomas are very rare in children.[454] Most of the cellular capillary hemangiomas regress spontaneously.

On FNA, hemangiomas yield a bloody aspirate, even from a single needle thrust, and may contain scattered bland spindled nuclei of endothelial cells with indistinct cell borders or bare nuclei. Cellular hemangiomas of infancy show more densely cellular clusters of uniform spindled cells forming small lumens[455] (Fig. 18-43).

Acquired tufted angioma is histologically similar to cellular hemangioma but occurs in older patients.[456–457] Some of the vascular channels at the periphery of the lobules have a slit-like architecture, and because of this, tufted angioma has been confused with Kaposi's sarcoma. Likewise, targetoid hemosiderotic hemangiomas[458] may also be confused with the patch stage of Kaposi's sarcoma. Grossly the lesion shows an ecchymotic halo. Another exceedingly rare cutaneous vascular lesion is glomeruloid hemangioma, which is associated with multicentric Castleman's disease and POEMS syndrome (polyneuropathy, organomegaly, endocrinopathy, M protein [plasmacytosis], and skin lesions).[459–461]

Pyogenic Granuloma

Pyogenic granulomas, first thought to be reactive granulation tissue formed as a result of pyogenic infection, are now recognized as a variant of capillary hemangioma. When they occur on a cutaneous or mucosal surface, they can be distorted by secondary ulceration and granulation tissue formation. Histologically, the capillaries are arranged in lobules separated by fibrous connective tissue containing small veins and arteries.[462,463] Each lobule is fed by a large vessel, often with a muscular wall. Infiltrates of inflammatory cells are most dense adjacent to areas of ulceration and granulation tissue. A collarette of acanthotic epithelium may surround the base of the pyogenic granuloma, especially in lesions of the lip and oral mucosa. Classically, these lesions have been described as polypoid, but sessile nodules and more deep-seated lesions have also been reported. Pyogenic granulomas occur on the skin, especially that of the extremities and external genitalia, and the mucosal surfaces of the oral cavity and nose. Intravenous pyogenic granulomas involving medium-sized and small veins of the head and neck and upper extremity are small painless nodules.[464,465] They seem to arise out of the venous wall, perhaps from the vasa vasorum in the larger vessels.[465] Pyogenic granulomas are benign lesions but recurrences with satellite lesions have occurred after surgical removal and cauterization.[466]

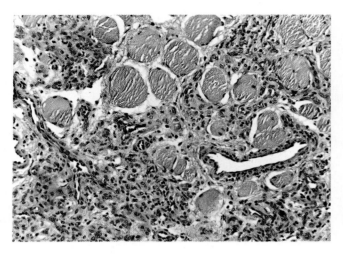

Fig. 18-44. Intramuscular hemangioma. Capillaries lined by prominent endothelial cells infiltrate skeletal muscle fibers.

Cavernous Hemangioma

Cavernous hemangiomas are composed of dilated channels lined by endothelial cells. Their walls may contain pericytes, fibroblasts, and collagen, but not in the regular arrangement seen in normal venules and arterioles. Capillary and cavernous hemangiomas of the skin are components of several clinical syndromes, as described previously. A variant of superficial cavernous hemangioma composed of interconnected dilated blood vessels has been named *sinusoidal hemangioma*.[467] Because of the anastomosing vascular channels and the occasional prominent pseudopapillary pattern, it has been confused with angiosarcoma. However, the flat endothelial cells that line the blood vessels show no atypical changes.

Arteriovenous Hemangioma

Although arteriovenous hemangiomas are most commonly found in adults, many authors consider these lesions congenital anomalies rather than true neoplasms.[468–470] Superficial and deep lesions occur. They consist of large veins and arteries with irregularly thickened walls. Arteriovenous hemangiomas may be associated with hypertrophy of the extremity. Not infrequently, these lesions are associated with dystrophic calcification and organizing thrombi.

Venous Hemangioma

Venous hemangioma is composed of thickened blood vessels that can still be recognized as veins. However, the smooth muscle of the wall is disorganized and extends into the adjacent soft tissue. Organizing thrombi occlude the lumen of some of the abnormal veins. Venous hemangiomas in the feet of children may be associated with Turner's syndrome.[471]

Intramuscular Hemangioma

Intramuscular hemangiomas can be predominantly capillary, cavernous, arteriovenous, or more commonly a mixture of these types. They are found most frequently in the lower extremities of

children and young adults and characteristically infiltrate skeletal muscle, nerves, and vascular walls.[472–475] The capillary type of intramuscular hemangioma appears to be more frequent in the muscles of the head and neck (Fig. 18-44). Because of their infiltrating nature, local recurrence due to incomplete excision is common.[474] Those tumors that invade through fascia into adjacent muscles, periosteum, and subcutaneous tissue must be distinguished from extensive regional hemangiomatosis. Careful physical examination and angiography are invaluable diagnostic tools in these situations. Anatomic location and histologic type of intramuscular hemangiomas do not correlate with local recurrence.

Hemangiomatosis

The term *hemangiomatosis* has recently been applied to vascular lesions usually affecting extensive portions of the body in a contiguous fashion.[476–478] A mixture of vascular channels including capillary and cavernous vessels as well as large veins characterize this lesion, which may infiltrate fibrofatty tissue, skeletal muscle, and even bone. The majority of patients are children or young adults. Local recurrence is common and is probably due to incomplete excision.[478]

Epithelioid Hemangioma

The epithelioid hemangioma, also known as *angiolymphoid hyperplasia with eosinophilia*, is a distinctive benign vascular tumor seen most often in the face and scalp of young per-

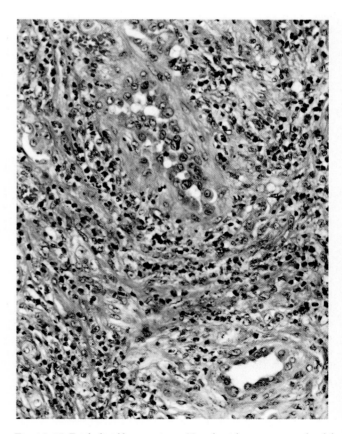

Fig. 18-45. Epithelioid hemangioma. Vessels with prominent cuboidal endothelial cells are surrounded by inflammatory elements.

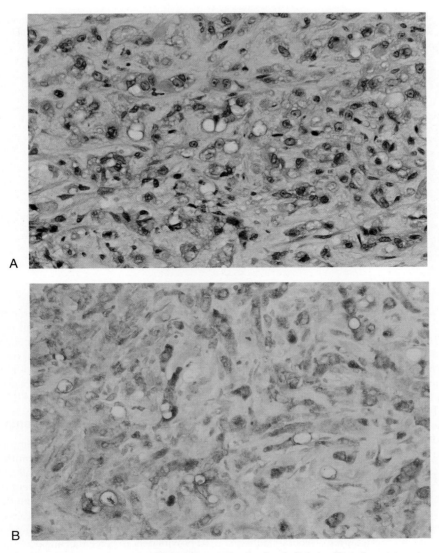

Fig. 18-46. (A) Epithelioid hemangioendothelioma. Cords of endothelial cells with incipient intracytoplasmic lumina in a hyaline matrix. (B) The tumor cells are immunoreactive for factor VIII-related antigen.

sons.[479–482] The lesion appears as small papules or dermal or subcutaneous nodules measuring less than 2 cm in diameter. Occasionally, it may arise within a blood vessel, especially a vein. Microscopically, one sees proliferation of small blood vessels, each lined by large epithelioid endothelial cells (Fig. 18-45). An inflammatory infiltrate of variable extent, containing lymphocytes and eosinophils, is usually present. This tumor can be separated from *Kimura's disease* on morphologic grounds.[483,484] A vascular proliferation termed *bacillary angiomatosis* resembling epithelioid hemangioma but containing a neutrophilic infiltrate and rickettsiae organisms easily identified with the Warthin-Starry stain has been reported in acquired immunodeficiency syndrome (AIDS) patients.[485,486]

Epithelioid Hemangioendothelioma

Epithelioid hemangioendothelioma, a distinctive low grade malignant neoplasm, first described in the lung as "intravascular bronchioloalveolar tumor," is composed of large epithelioid vacuolated endothelial cells that grow predominantly in anastomosing cords and nests; for this reason, it is often confused with metastatic carcinoma (Fig. 18-46A). However, at least in some areas, the tumor cells are vasoformative and line small vascular channels. The hyalinized stroma usually contains myxoid foci superficially resembling chondroid matrix. The endothelial nature of the tumor has been well documented both by immunohistochemical methods and by electron microscopy. Tumor cells are immunoreactive for factor VIII-related antigen, Ulex europaeus lectin, CD31, CD34, and occasionally for cytokeratin (Fig. 18-46B). By electron microscopy, Weibel-Palade granules and intracytoplasmic lumina as well as intercellular junctions and basal lamina are seen. Superficial and deep tumors have been recognized in the extremities, head and neck, and chest wall and mediastinum of adult patients.[487–490] Superficial tumors involve the subcutis and may

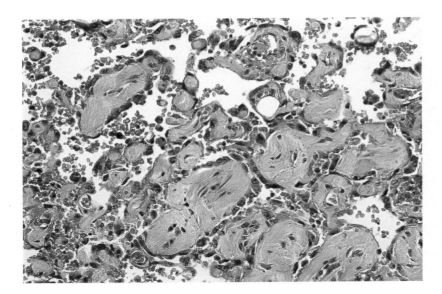

Fig. 18-47. Interanastomosing vascular channels lined by hyperchromatic atypical endothelial cells characteristic of angiosarcoma.

appear as skin tumors. The deep ones infiltrate skeletal muscle. Approximately one-half of these tumors appear to arise from the walls of blood vessels, especially veins, and exhibit angiocentric features. About 20 percent of epithelioid hemangioendotheliomas give rise to metastases in lungs, bones, and lymph nodes. Epithelioid hemangioendothelioma may also occur as a primary neoplasm of the liver, bone, and other visceral organs.

FNA of epithelioid hemangioendothelioma shows small groups and single epithelioid cells with slightly pleomorphic nuclei and generally moderate amounts of cytoplasm. The cells usually show vacuolation or intranuclear pseudoinclusions.[490]

Spindle Cell Hemangioendothelioma

Spindle cell hemangioendothelioma is a recently recognized benign vascular tumor that is occasionally seen in association with Maffucci's syndrome.[491–495] The tumor, which occurs in the superficial soft tissues of the extremities of young adults,

combines histologic features of cavernous hemangioma and Kaposi's sarcoma.[491,492] More than half of the cases arise within veins. Although local recurrence is common, and initial reports described it as a low grade malignant tumor,[491] metastases have not been documented. It is important to distinguish it from Kaposi's sarcoma because spindle cell hemangioendothelioma has not been found in association with AIDS.

Angiosarcoma

Angiosarcoma is a highly malignant tumor, most commonly located in the head and neck, extremities, and trunk of elderly patients.[496–501] Children are rarely affected.[502] In the head and neck the tumors often arise in the dermis and present as purple macular lesions whereas in the extremities they are deep-seated hemorrhagic neoplasms. Other anatomic locations include the breast, liver, adrenal gland, thyroid, spleen, and kidney.[503–505] Approximately 15 percent of angiosarcomas are multicentric.[500]

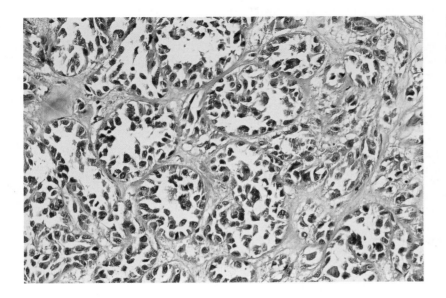

Fig. 18-48. Epithelioid angiosarcoma. Empty vascular spaces are lined by neoplastic epithelioid endothelial cells. The pattern of growth and the cytologic features closely resemble adenocarcinoma.

Microscopically, angiosarcomas are characterized by interconnecting, often deceptively benign channels lined by the neoplastic, cytologically atypical endothelial cells (Fig. 18-47). These neoplastic channels freely infiltrate surrounding structures, usually following perivascular and perineural spaces. In the skin, they infiltrate around skin adnexa and between individual collagen fibers. On occasion, tumor cells may form solid cords of cytokeratin-positive epithelioid cells closely resembling carcinoma, *epithelioid angiosarcoma*[503] (Fig. 18-48) Undifferentiated spindle-shaped cells may predominate in some areas. Intracytoplasmic lumen formation is a useful feature in the differential diagnosis. Besides the extensive local growth, metastases develop primarily in the lungs, with a relatively high incidence of lymphatic spread. When the endothelial nature of the lesion is difficult to ascertain, electron microscopy may be of some help.

Immunoperoxidase stains for endothelial markers including factor VIII-related antigen, Ulex europaeus lectin, CD31, and CD34 are valuable in clarifying the histologic nature of the tumors with a predominantly epithelioid solid pattern of growth. A number of cases of radiation-induced angiosarcomas have been reported.[500] Others have been associated with chronic lymphedema or deposition of foreign material.[506] Size, anatomic location, and tumor grade are important prognostic factors; overall, however, the prognosis is poor. Local recurrence is common (60 percent) and the 5 year survival rate for patients with angiosarcoma is 24 percent.[500]

Angiosarcomas associated with severe chronic lymphedema appear in the upper extremities several years after radical mastectomy or in the lower extremities with primary or secondary lymphedema. Some of these tumors appear to be preceded by the development of dermal lymphangiomatosis, a nodular proliferation of small lymphatic channels lined by normal-appearing endothelial cells. The tumor usually appears as single or multiple cutaneous nodules covered by purple skin.

FNA of angiosarcoma yields mostly blood, but careful examination reveals pleomorphic hyperchromatic oval-to-spindle cells lying singly and in small clusters, often with stripped cytoplasm.[507] The cells may show longitudinal nuclear grooves, cytoplasmic vacuoles and projections, and binucleation.

Kaposi's Sarcoma

Kaposi's sarcoma (KS) is considered an endemic disease in African countries.[508,509] It was relatively rare in the United States until the advent of the epidemic of AIDS.[510] Epidemiologic and molecular pathology studies have suggested that sporadic African and AIDS-associated Kaposi's sarcoma may be caused by human herpesvirus 6 or 8.[511–514] Human herpesvirus 8 DNA was identified in 92 percent of Kaposi's sarcoma tissue specimens from sporadic and AIDS-KS patients by the polymerase chain reaction.[514] Other endothelial lesions and skin lesions in immunosuppressed patients did not contain amplifiable Kaposi's sarcoma herpesvirus DNA, indicating that the above findings cannot be explained on the basis of disseminated viral infection.[514] Kaposi's sarcoma has also been reported to occur in association with other immunodeficiency states.[509] In organ transplant recipients, this tumor may account for 5 percent of all malignant tumors in the post-transplantation period. In 15 to 20 percent of AIDS patients, Kaposi's sarcoma develops; this figure is even higher in patients who die of AIDS. In addition to skin lesions, involvement of the GI tract, lymph nodes, and lungs is common in these patients. However, AIDS patients rarely die as a result of Kaposi's sarcoma.

Sporadic Kaposi's sarcoma is manifested by one or multiple purpuric plaques in the distal portions of the extremities of elderly patients. Later the lesions become darker, nodular, and eventually ulcerate. In about 15 percent of cases, the lesion is solitary and may be confused with pyogenic granuloma. Some

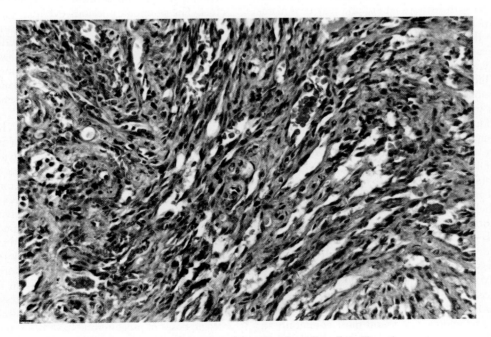

Fig. 18-49. Slit-like vascular spaces and fascicles of spindle cells in Kaposi's sarcoma.

patients with the sporadic type of Kaposi's sarcoma also develop lesions in lymph nodes, mucous membranes, and viscera.

Microscopically, the typical lesion is characterized by a proliferation of spindle-shaped cells that grow in a fascicular arrangement with intervening clefts or vascular channels (Fig. 18-49). The early patch and plaque stages, which consist of small dilated capillaries surrounded by inflammatory cells, are difficult to recognize. The late stage mimics fibrosarcoma. A number of cells have been implicated in the histogenesis of Kaposi's sarcomas. The spindle cells usually show reactivity for a variety of endothelial markers, including factor VIII-related antigen, Ulex europaeus lectin, CD34, and CD31, thus supporting the endothelial nature of this neoplasm.[515,516] Whether these cells derive from vascular or lymphatic vessels is still a matter of debate.[517,518]

The association of multicentric Castleman's disease and Kaposi's sarcoma has been documented in recent years. These two rare lesions may appear simultaneously and may even coexist in the same lymph node.[519]

On FNA, Kaposi's sarcoma shows clusters of hyperchromatic twisted spindle cells with scant cytoplasm in a bloody background.[520]

TUMORS OF LYMPHATIC VESSELS

Cystic Lymphangioma

Cystic lymphangiomas (cystic hygromas) occur most commonly in the neck and upper mediastinum but can form large masses in the axillary and inguinal areas, retroperitoneum, omentum, mesentery, liver, and spleen.[521–525] They are seen most frequently in the young pediatric age group (60 percent under the age of 5 years). Some cystic hygromas are congenital, occur in association with hydrops fetalis, and may be a manifestation of Turner's syndrome.[523,525,526] Cystic lymphangiomas located in the neck occur predominantly in newborns and infants, whereas those found elsewhere can present at any age. Abdominal lymphangiomas often become manifest in the second decade of life, arise in the mesentery, and may cause intestinal obstruction or infarction. Retroperitoneal lymphangiomas also occur in young adults and often displace adjacent organs such as kidney, pancreas, colon, or duodenum. Only rarely do cystic lymphangiomas infiltrate adjacent tissues, making their complete excision difficult or impossible. Cystic lymphangiomas are multilocular and contain clear or chylous fluid. Hemorrhage, inflammation secondary to rupture, and infection can change the character of the fluid. The cysts are lined with attenuated endothelial cells that usually show reactivity for factor VIII-related antigen, CD31, and CD34 and bind Ulex europaeus. The walls of the lymphatic cysts are composed of fibrous connective tissue containing scattered, irregularly arranged thin layers of smooth muscle. Cystic lymphangiomas can occasionally be confused with cystic mesotheliomas. However, mesothelial cells are cytokeratin positive and do not stain for endothelial markers.

Superficial lymphangiomas are found most commonly in adults and present as small cutaneous vesicles, so-called lym-phangioma circumscriptum, or as dermal nodules.[527] Because some of these lesions develop as a complication of chronic lymphedema, it is not clear whether they represent lymphangiectasis or true neoplasms of lymphatic vessels.

Lymphangiomatosis

Extensive multicentric involvement of a portion of the body by lymphangioma is known as *lymphangiomatosis*. This condition occurs preferentially in infants and children and may affect the extremities, the trunk, or the viscera.[528–532] Some patients develop bone lesions. Patients with extensive visceral lesions are associated with poor prognosis.[531] Complex anastomosing cavernous, and cystic lymphatic vessels infiltrate the affected tissues.

Lymphangiomyoma (Lymphangiomyomatosis)

Lymphangiomyomas are distinctive hamartomatous lesions characterized by a proliferation of lymphatic vessels and smooth muscle and found almost exclusively in women of childbearing age.[533–536] The localized form of the lesion has been designated *lymphangiomyoma* whereas the extensive or multicentric variant is referred to as *lymphangiomyomatosis*. Because angiomyolipomas occur in association with lymphangiomyomatosis, some have suggested that this lesion is a component of the tuberous sclerosis syndrome.[537,538] The lesions involve the thoracic duct, pulmonary lymphatics, and mediastinal and retroperitoneal lymph nodes and lymphatic vessels. Patients with pulmonary lesions usually present with pneumothorax, hemoptysis, or chylous effusion whereas those with abdominal or retroperitoneal involvement have chylous ascites. The pulmonary lesions eventually progress to honeycombing, respiratory insufficiency, and death. Grossly, the single or multiple lesions are nodular or cylindrical masses that can be spongy, cystic, or rubbery. They may measure up to 15 cm in diameter but are usually smaller, measuring up to only a few centimeters. In some patients, the entire lymphatic chain from thorax to abdomen may be involved. The end-stage pulmonary disease has a honeycomb appearance.

The lesion is histologically distinctive, characterized by the presence of narrow and broad fascicles of smooth muscle derived from the walls of anastomosing lymphatic channels, which are lined by a single layer of endothelial cells. The smooth muscle cells are immunoreactive for muscle actin and occasionally for desmin. Likewise, the smooth muscle cells of lymphangiomyomatosis have shown reactivity with the HMB-45 antibody. Foci of lymphoid tissue, sometimes containing germinal centers, can be seen in many of these lesions.

The strong tendency of these lesions to occur in young women suggests an etiologic relationship with ovarian function and, more specifically, with estrogens. In fact, estrogen and progesterone receptors have occasionally been found in some of these lesions.[539–543] With this in mind, castration and pharmacologic doses of progesterone have been used, with some success, to diminish the size of the pulmonary and abdominal le-

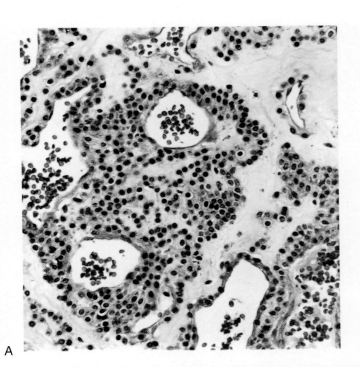

A

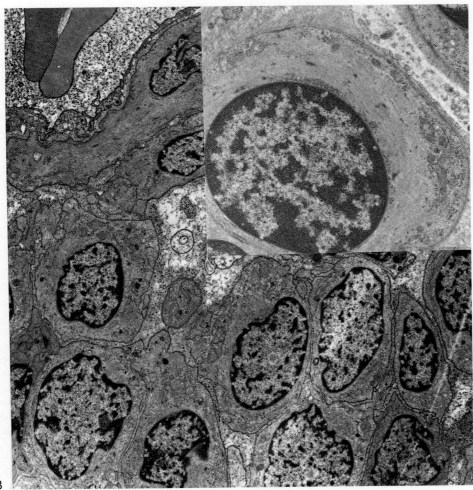

B

Fig. 18-50. **(A)** Numerous blood vessels surrounded by round epithelioid cells. The stroma is hyalinized. Glomus tumor. **(B)** Ultrastructurally, this tumor is composed of round cells with cytoplasmic features of smooth muscle. Insert clearly shows elements of smooth muscle, particularly the orderly arranged filaments with dense bodies.

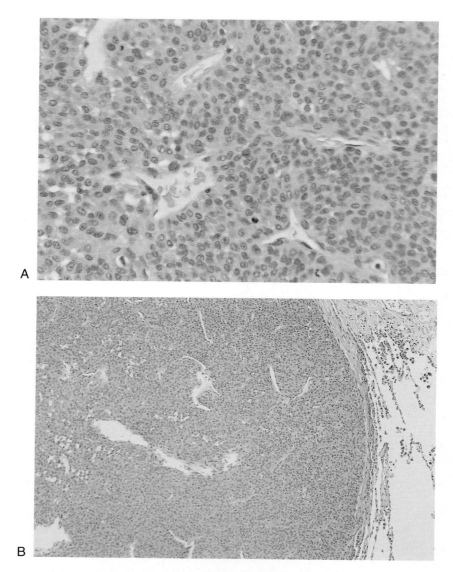

Fig. 18-51. **(A)** Malignant glomus tumor. Small vascular channels are surrounded by trabeculae of epithelioid cells some of which show nuclear atypia. **(B)** Pulmonary metastasis of tumor shown in Fig. A.

sions and to control the formation of effusions. However, tamoxifen has been reported to worsen the course of the disease.[544] Dietary fat manipulation and surgical bypass procedures have also been used to treat the ascites that so often complicates the lives of the women with this disease.

PERIVASCULAR TUMORS

Glomus Tumor

Glomus tumors are composed of epithelioid smooth muscle cells similar to those of the glomus body, a specialized arteriovenous shunt involved in thermoregulation. Benign, locally infiltrative, and malignant forms have been described.[545] Be-

nign glomus tumors are composed of sheets, nests, or trabeculae of clear, polygonal epithelioid cells surrounding open vascular channels (Fig. 18-50A). When vascular channels are dilated, the term *glomangioma* is used. Glomus cells show immunoreactivity for vimentin and muscle actin.[546] Numerous cytoplasmic filaments and pinocytotic vesicles are constant ultrastructural features[547] (Fig. 18-50B). Dilated unmyelinated axons course through the connective tissue between the groups of tumor cells, and are easily found in cutaneous lesions, but are not seen in visceral glomus tumors. Mast cells are scattered throughout the lesions and may participate in the regulation of blood flow by their production of vasoactive amines. The connective tissue stroma frequently is hyalinized or myxoid.

Benign glomus tumors are small nodules or plaque-like lesions located in the skin, especially in the subungual parts of the fingers, but they occur also in the deep soft tissues, bone, and in many organs where, unlike the cutaneous lesions, they are seldom associated with pain. They can be single or multiple.[548–550] The stomach is the most frequent site of visceral involvement,[551,552] but intestinal,[553] pulmonary, and intravascular glomus tumors have been described.[554] The vast majority of glomus tumors are solitary, well circumscribed, and benign. Sporadic multiple glomus tumors occur.[548,549] Multiple and familial glomus tumors inherited as an autosomal dominant trait have also been reported.[555,556] Infiltrative glomus tumors are usually larger than the benign ones, measuring up to 12 cm in diameter.[545,557]

A single report of FNA of an axillary glomus tumor[558] described confusion with epithelial cells and was misdiagnosed as ectopic breast lobules. The smears were cellular, with tight clusters and less cohesive sheets of medium-sized polygonal cells and stripped nuclei. Nuclei were round to oval, with fine chromatin, and cytoplasm was poorly defined, with some delicate wisps of metachromatic material. Thin-walled blood vessels criss-crossed the cell clusters, and mast cells were noted.

Glomangiosarcoma

Glomangiosarcoma, an exceedingly rare malignant variety of glomus tumor, has now been well documented.[545,559,560] It is highly cellular and shows mild to moderate cytologic atypia with numerous mitotic figures; it invades surrounding tissues but rarely metastasizes. We have now seen two malignant glomus tumors that have metastasized. One of these was located in the esophagus and the other in the dermis (Fig. 18-51). The histologic diagnosis of glomangiosarcoma can be facilitated by identification of the malignant component as well as areas of conventional glomus tumor. Glomangiosarcoma may be confused with other malignant round cell neoplasms such as Ewing's sarcoma, primitive neuroectodermal tumors, rhabdomyosarcoma, and carcinoid tumors.[545,553]

Hemangiopericytoma

Hemangiopericytomas are composed of a branching network of blood vessels surrounded by sheets of polygonal, round, or spindle cells, thought to be derived from the vascular pericyte[561,562] (Fig. 18-52). It is important to bear in mind that with one exception (endothelial tumors) all benign and malignant soft tissue tumors may display a focal hemangiopericytic pattern, which can confuse the pathologist. Solitary fibrous tumor, mesenchymal chondrosarcoma, vascular leiomyosarcoma, and synovial sarcoma are most often confused with hemangiopericytomas. We therefore believe that hemangiopericytoma is a diagnosis of exclusion. The immunohistochemical profile of the tumor lacks specificity. It stains with vimentin and CD34 but is negative with muscle-specific actin and desmin.[563,564] Ultrastructurally the tumor cells are usually surrounded by varying amounts of basal lamina, but rarely contain cytoplasmic filaments, with dense bodies and pinocytic vesicles, features that link them to smooth muscle cells.[565]

Hemangiopericytomas are primarily tumors of adults that occur anywhere in the body, including the meninges[566] and viscera, but are most common in the deep soft tissues of the lower extremities, retroperitoneum, and head and neck. Retroperitoneal hemangiopericytomas have rarely been associated with hypoglycemia.[567] Familial hemangiopericytomas have been described. In infants and very young children, "congenital or infantile hemangiopericytomas" tend to occur more frequently in subcutaneous tissues of the head and neck or within the parotid gland, where they exhibit an almost uniformly benign behavior.[561,568,569]

Benign and malignant forms of hemangiopericytomas have been described, although biologic behavior is often difficult to predict based on morphologic features. Large tumors with foci of necrosis, increased mitotic rate, cellularity, and anaplasia are more likely to exhibit malignant biologic behavior. The 5 year survival rate is approximately 70 percent for patients with hemangiopericytomas of soft tissue.[561] Metastases are primarily hematogenous, but lymph node metastases have been reported. Not uncommonly, recurrences and metastases appear initially 5 to 10 years after treatment. Long-term survival, even in the presence of metastases, is not unusual. However, some patients succumb soon after diagnosis because of extensive local and metastatic growth of the neoplasm. DNA analysis by flow cytometry does not correlate with outcome.[570,571]

Fig. 18-52. Hemangiopericytoma. Staghorn-like vessels are surrounded by a proliferation of pericytes having oval to angulated nuclei and indistinct cytoplasmic borders.

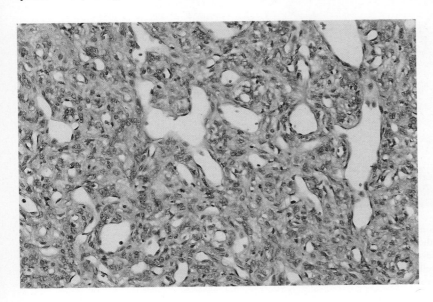

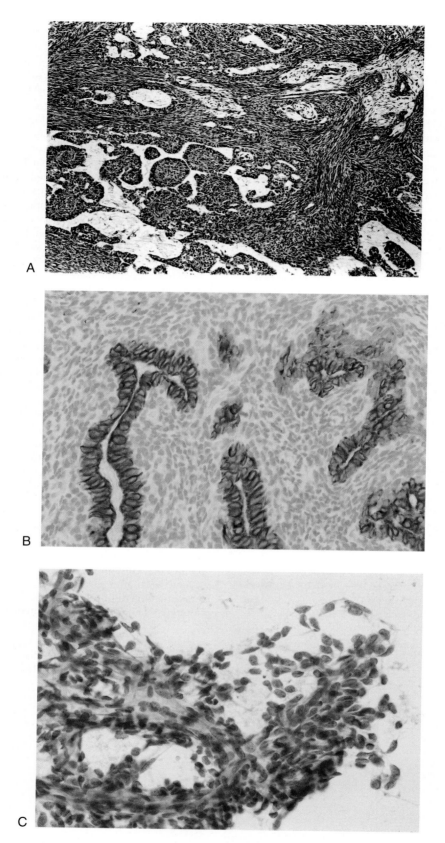

Fig. 18-53. **(A)** Both the fibrosarcomatous and the epithelial components of this synovial sarcoma are clearly seen. **(B)** Cytokeratin stains the epithelial component of a biphasic synovial sarcoma. **(C)** Fine needle aspiration of synovial sarcoma reveals abundant uniform spindle cells in a branching tissue fragment containing vascular structures, as well as individual dispersed nuclei. Chromatin is uniform and nuclear features are deceptively bland. (Papanicolaou.)

By FNA, hemangiopericytoma shows knobby clusters of ovoid to spindle cells, as well as single cells with ill-defined finely granular cytoplasm.[572,573] Chromatin tends to be evenly distributed, without prominent nucleoli, and with variable numbers of scattered mitotic figures. Vascular structures are seen within the tissue clusters.

TUMORS OF TENOSYNOVIAL TISSUES

Synovial Sarcoma

Synovial sarcomas do not arise from synovial membranes, but are formed by two types of cells that resemble normal synovial cells. These tumors are most commonly found in the lower extremities of young adults, but they have also been reported in children and elderly patients.[574–576] Likewise, they have been described in many other anatomic sites, including the head and neck, chest wall, retroperitoneum, and mediastinum.[577] Microscopically, synovial sarcomas may exhibit a biphasic morphology with a variable proportion of spindle-shaped and epithelial cells. The spindle-shaped cells usually predominate and are arranged in fascicles, whereas the epithelial cells form glands, cords, nests, or papillary structures (Fig. 18-53A). Focal squamous differentiation occurs in some cases.[578] The existence of monophasic synovial sarcomas, composed entirely of spindle cells or epithelial cells, is now widely accepted.[574,575] Extensive calcification, osteoid and bone formation is seen in some tumors.[579,580] In terms of immunohisto-

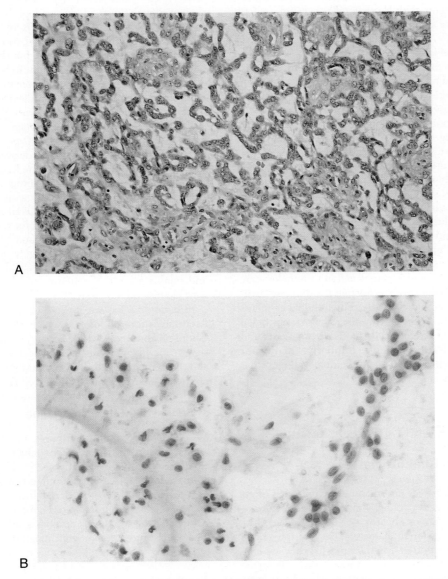

Fig. 18-54. (A) Lace-like growth pattern of extraskeletal myxoid chondrosarcoma. Anastomosing cords of chondroblasts in a myxoid matrix. (B) Fine needle aspiration of myxoid chondrosarcoma shows two clusters of relatively uniform rounded tumor cells, one group in cords resembling epithelial cells, and the other group dispersed in a dense myxoid matrix. (Papanicolaou.)

chemistry, both the epithelial and the spindle cell types are keratin- and epithelial membrane antigen positive[581–583] (Fig. 18-53B), although only a small proportion of spindle cells express these epithelial markers. Positive reactivity for carcinoembryonic antigen has also been shown in some of these tumors. Electron microscopic studies tend to give credence to the existence of monophasic, fibrosarcoma-like synovial sarcomas, because the monophasic tumors are ultrastructurally identical to the spindle cell component of biphasic synovial sarcomas.[582,583] Most synovial sarcomas show a balanced translocation t(18;X) (p11.2; q11.2).[584,585] Patients having predominantly glandular biphasic tumors with a low mitotic index have a longer disease-free interval than do those with highly mitotic or purely monophasic tumors.[586] The 5 year survival rate for the former tumors is more than 90 percent and about 40 percent for the latter group. Patients with densely calcified and ossified synovial sarcomas have a better prognosis than those with noncalcified tumors.[579,580]

FNA smears of synovial sarcoma are very cellular, with a predominance of bipolar spindle cells showing small to medium-sized ovoid to spindled nuclei. Irregular branching tumor tissue fragments are characteristic, containing vascular structures and many tightly packed overlapping cells arranged in strands or rows, as well as large numbers of single dispersed similar nuclei in the background (Fig. 18-53C). The chromatin is bland and evenly distributed, with small inconspicuous nucleoli, and usually at least a few mitotic figures. Pleomorphism is usually absent, and even in biphasic tumors, most of the tumor cells on FNA specimens appear mesenchymal, with some cases showing small acinar-like structures or cylindrical epithelial cells at the edges of spindle cell clusters.[587] Cytoplasm of the spindled and ovoid cells is scant and delicate, seen as thin uni- or bipolar processes, or stripped entirely from naked nuclei. Mast cells may be seen.

In the abdominal wall and inguinal region of females, care should be taken to consider endometriosis in the differential diagnosis of masses with biphasic spindle and epithelial elements on smear.[588] Endometriosis shows crowded columnar epithelial clusters, bland spindled stromal cells in tissue fragments and singly, and hemosiderin pigment. Similarly, malignant mesothelioma may produce a chest or abdominal wall mass that resembles synovial sarcoma cytologically.[589,590]

CARTILAGE AND BONE TUMORS

Chondroma

Chondromas of soft tissues are uncommon and most often seen in the hands and feet of young adults.[591,592] Some are associated with tendons, tendon sheaths, or joint capsules. Most are solitary and small (< 3 cm in diameter), but multiple chondromas have also been reported. Microscopically, they are lobulated and densely cellular and may show considerable cytologic atypia.[593–595] Because of these features, they have been confused with chondrosarcomas. However, these tumors follow a benign clinical course. Some may recur following local excision, but so far metastases have not been recorded.

Chondrosarcoma

Several distinct clinicopathologic types of extraskeletal chondrosarcomas are recognized in the soft tissues, with myxoid and mesenchymal chondrosarcomas being the most common.

Myxoid Chondrosarcoma

Myxoid chondrosarcomas occur mainly in the deep tissues of the extremities of adults, but may arise in other anatomic locations.[596–600] They are well circumscribed and multinodular, with a lobulated microscopic pattern; the myxoid lobules are separated by connective tissue bands of variable thickness. The round or elongated tumor cells usually have hyperchromatic or vesicular nuclei with scanty acidophilic cytoplasm, and often form interconnecting cords (Fig. 18-54A). They show positive reactivity for S-100 protein and occasionally stain for cytokeratin. Hyaline cartilage is not seen, but the stroma is rich in sulfated mucopolysaccharides resistant to hyaluronidase digestion, a feature that permits separation from other myxoid mesenchymal tumors such as liposarcoma. Electron microscopic studies have confirmed the cartilaginous nature of these tumors, as well as those referred to as *chordoid sarcomas*.[601–603] Once considered to be low grade, approximately 50 percent of myxoid chondrosarcomas metastasize and cause death of the patients, usually many years after diagnosis.[604] In one large series, larger size and older age were significant adverse prognostic factors.[598]

FNA specimens are cellular, showing loosely cohesive clusters and cords of medium-sized cells in a metachromatic myxoid matrix (Fig. 18-54B). The matrix tends to present as fragments that are dense and opaque and contain embedded cells. Tumor cells are ovoid and relatively uniform with eccentric rounded nuclei, occasionally clefted, showing fine chromatin and small nucleoli. Vascularity and hyaline cartilage matrix with lacunae are not seen.[605–607]

In paraspinal masses, myxoid chondrosarcoma must be differentiated from chordoma, which also has a myxoid matrix. Chordoma has more varied sizes and shapes of cells, including signet ring-like cells and large vacuolated physaliferous cells, and the neoplastic cells show immunoreactivity for keratin and epithelial membrane antigen, as well as S-100 protein.[606,608]

Mesenchymal Chondrosarcoma

Mesenchymal chondrosarcoma is a histologically distinctive malignant soft tissue tumor, thought to derive from primitive cartilage-forming mesenchyme.[609] The patients are often young adults with tumors commonly located in the thigh, retroperitoneum, or orbit.[610,611] Intracranial and intraspinal mesenchymal chondrosarcomas have also been reported.[612–614] Clinically, these tumors are more aggressive than the myxoid type of chondrosarcoma,[615] although their clinical course is often protracted and metastases may occur many years after diagnosis.[616] The 5 year survival rate for patients with mesenchymal chondrosarcoma is around 50 percent but the 10 year survival rate is only 27 percent.[611] Grossly, the tumors are usually calcified, lobulated, and exhibit hemorrhage, necrosis, and cystic degeneration. The calcifications are seen radiographically.[616]

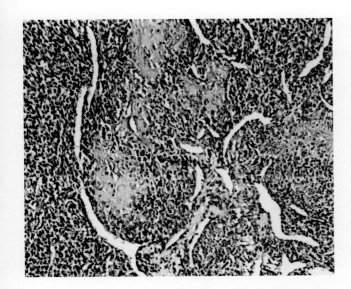

Fig. 18-55. Mesenchymal chondrosarcoma. Small undifferentiated cells, foci of hyaline cartilage, and numerous capillaries are characteristic features.

Their characteristic microscopic appearance includes closely packed undifferentiated round to oval cells, numerous vascular channels, and islands of well differentiated cartilage that are S-100 protein positive[617] (Fig. 18-55). Most tumors are diploid.[612] Occasionally the small round undifferentiated cells stain for glial fibrillary acidic protein.[612]

By FNA, the hallmark feature is the presence of dual populations of small undifferentiated cells and well differentiated hyaline cartilage. The small round cells may form compact clusters, with nuclear molding and irregular granular chromatin; the cartilage shows dense fragments of metachromatic fibrillar matrix containing polygonal cells with vacuolated cytoplasm in lacunae.[618,619]

Although usually a bone lesion, plasmacytoma may present as a soft tissue mass, most often near the vertebral column. The plasma cells may be well differentiated or more immature and pleomorphic. A surprising degree of clustering into three-dimensional balls surrounded by delicate blood vessels may be seen on FNA, which may lead to confusion with the immature cells of mesenchymal chondrosarcoma, or with metastatic carcinoma.[620]

Other Chondrosarcomas

Well differentiated and clear cell chondrosarcomas are exceedingly rare in soft tissues; therefore, little is known about their natural history. The embryonal chondrosarcoma first described in the nasoethmoidal region of children is also very rare.[621] Only seven examples of this distinctive type of chondrosarcoma have been reported in soft tissues.[622,623]

Osteogenic Sarcoma

Extraskeletal osteogenic sarcomas are extremely rare. In contrast to those that are primary in bone, the extraskeletal lesions are more common in adults and practically nonexistent during the first two decades of life.[624] These tumors are more common in the extremities and retroperitoneum.[625–627] Like osteosarcoma of bone, the soft tissue osteosarcoma exhibits a broad morphologic spectrum, with areas resembling malignant fibrous histiocytoma, fibrosarcoma, and schwannoma. However, all contain varying amounts of neoplastic osteoid, bone, and cartilage, permitting their recognition. Nearly two-thirds of patients die with lung and bone metastases.[627] The most important consideration in differential diagnosis is myositis ossificans.

PLURIPOTENTIAL MESENCHYMAL TUMORS

Mesenchymoma

The recognition that a variety of soft tissue tumors may differentiate along several cell lines and have more than one component including bone, cartilage, and skeletal muscle explains the rarity with which the diagnosis of mesenchymoma is made by surgical pathologists. Liposarcomas that show osteoid, bone, cartilage, and smooth muscle are no longer included among the mesenchymomas. Likewise, tumors that contain cartilage, bone, small undifferentiated cells, and a hemangiopericytic pattern are designated mesenchymal chondrosarcoma. We believe the term *mesenchymoma* will eventually be abandoned by surgical pathologists.

Ectomesenchymoma

An exceedingly rare malignant soft tissue tumor termed *ectomesenchymoma* has recently been described. It is characterized by the admixture of ganglion cells, neuroblasts, and mesenchymal elements, usually rhabdomyoblasts.[628–631]

MISCELLANEOUS TUMORS

Granular Cell Tumor

Granular cell tumors are yellow or yellow-tan, firm nodules found in the dermis and subcutaneous tissue of the extremities, chest wall, and head and neck. Other anatomic locations include tongue, oral cavity, GI and respiratory tracts, biliary tree, genitourinary tract, central and peripheral nervous systems, uterus, vulva, and breast.[632–634] Most patients are adults but adolescents and children may also be affected. Gingival granular cell tumors have a predilection for newborns.[635] The familial occurrence of granular cell tumors has been documented.[636] Females are more commonly affected than males and black Americans seem to be affected disproportionally. Benign, atypical, and malignant granular cell tumors have been described. Benign granular cell tumors rarely measure more than 1 to 2 cm in diameter but can recur following incomplete excision. Some are multiple and multifocal. Pseudoepitheliomatous hyperpla-

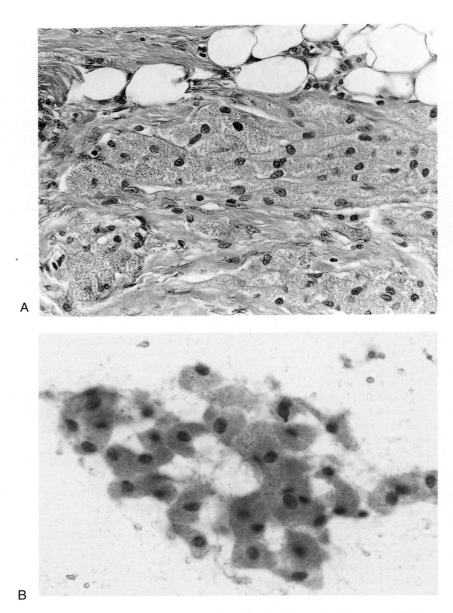

Fig. 18-56. (A) Granular cell tumor. Large granular cells are infiltrating adipose tissue. **(B)** Fine needle aspiration of granular cell tumor shows a loose cluster and single cells, which range from polygonal to elongated, with abundant coarsely granular cytoplasm. Nuclei are small, round, and uniform. (Papanicolaou.)

sia may be prominent in the epithelium overlying these tumors. The round to polygonal cells have a distinctive, coarsely granular eosinophilic cytoplasm, with indistinct borders (Fig. 18-56A). The cytoplasmic granules are associated with histochemical reactions characteristic of lysosomes; when viewed through the electron microscope, the cytoplasm is crowded with numerous secondary lysosomes packed with various kinds of material and cytoplasmic debris. The nuclei are small, round, and hyperchromatic. Nucleoli are small or not visible. Mitotic figures are not seen. Granular cell tumors show immunoreactivity for vimentin, S-100 protein, neuron-specific enolase, and myelin basic protein.[637–639]

The same features are seen in FNA smears. The aspirates are generally surprisingly cellular considering the indurated texture of the tumor. Loose clusters and single cells, which range from polygonal to spindled, show abundant cytoplasm with indistinct borders filled with coarse granules that are eosinophilic as well as periodic acid-Schiff (PAS) positive and diastase resistant.[640] The nuclei are usually small, round, eccentric, and uniform, without prominent nucleoli (Fig. 18-56B). The cells may be mistaken for histiocytes but the cytoplasm lacks vacuoles or pigment, and the nuclei are rounder and denser.

The histogenesis of the granular cell tumor is still debated. The anatomic relationship and frequent association of granular cells with peripheral nerves and the ultrastructural and immunohistochemical features of the cells are used to support the argument that most of these lesions are of Schwann cell origin. Some granular cell tumors are of smooth muscle derivation.[641]

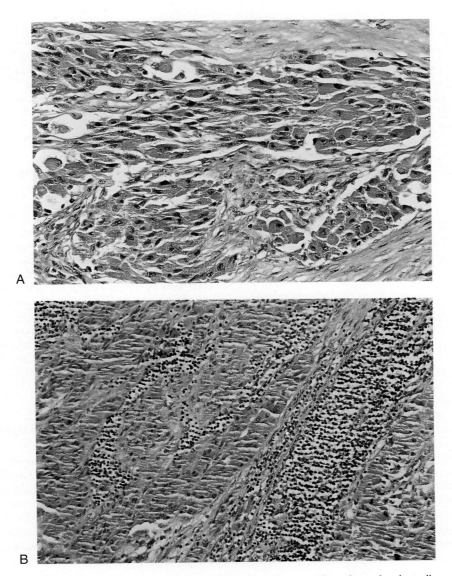

Fig. 18-57. (A) Malignant granular cell tumor of the perineal region. The polygonal and spindle granular cells show large nuclei and prominent nucleoli. (B) Metastasis of granular cell tumor shown in Fig. A. The nodal metastasis appears better differentiated than the primary tumor.

Epithelial tumors such as ameloblastomas may have a component of granular cells.[642] DESP and angiosarcoma may also contain granular cells.[643]

Malignant Granular Cell Tumor

Malignant granular cell tumors are usually larger than benign ones.[643,644,644a] Histologically, they consist of polygonal or round granular cells with large nuclei, and prominent nucleoli, as well as fascicles of atypical spindle cells (Fig. 18-57). Mitotic figures may be seen in malignant granular cell tumors, in contrast to their virtual absence in the benign form. We have seen invasion of the skin by the malignant granular cells mimicking junctional activity (epidermotropism). In the largest series published to date, 63 percent of the patients either died of disease or were living with metastases.[644a] Widespread lymphatic and hematogenous metastases have been major factors in causing the deaths of these patients, occurring usually within 2 years of the diagnosis.

Granular cell tumors with histologic features intermediate between the benign and the malignant forms have been designated atypical. They usually follow a benign clinical course.

Ossifying Fibromyxoid Tumor

The cell phenotype of ossifying fibromyxoid tumor, a recently described distinctive soft tissue tumor, has not been elucidated.[645–647] It usually occurs in the subcutaneous tissue or within skeletal muscle of the extremities of patients between 50 and 80 years of age. Ossifying fibromyxoid tumors are well demarcated, firm, and usually ossified at the periphery, often measuring less than 5 cm in diameter. Most follow a benign clinical

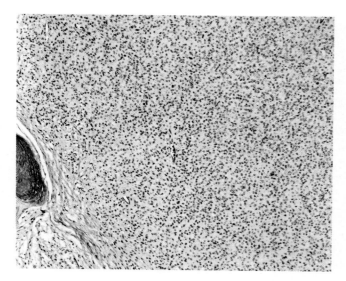

Fig. 18-58. Ossifying fibromyxoid tumor composed of monotonous sheets of uniform small cells with eosinophilic cytoplasm and round to oval nuclei. Note peripherally placed mature bone trabecula.

course, but some recur following incomplete excision. Moreover, malignant examples have rarely been reported.[648] Histologically the tumor exhibits a lobular pattern of growth and is surrounded by a fibrous capsule. Mature bony trabeculae present within the capsule form an incomplete shell in 80 percent of the tumors. The remaining tumors lack bone formation. The densely cellular lobules contain round, polygonal, and spindle cells that are uniform in size and show small round nuclei and clear or eosinophilic cytoplasm (Fig. 18-58). Prominent myxoid areas with a trabecular pattern mimic myxoid chondrosarcoma. Rarely osteoid, cartilage, and osteoclast-like giant cells are identified in the central portion of the mass. Mild cytologic atypia and few mitotic figures are seen. The malignant form of the tumor may show more nuclear atypia and a greater number of mitotic figures (Fig. 18-59). These features together with osteoid deposition between tumor cells may result in misdiagnosis of osteosarcoma. The immunohistochemical profile is nonspecific and includes positive reactivity for vimentin, S-100 protein, glial fibrillary protein, and Leu-7.[649] Actin and desmin reactivity has been reported in some cases. Although electron microscopy has failed to show a specific cell type, a Schwann cell origin has been suggested.[650]

Pleomorphic Hyalinizing Angiectatic Tumor of Soft Parts

Pleomorphic hyalinizing angiectatic tumor is an unusual but distinctive mesenchymal tumor of uncertain lineage that is characterized by fascicles of spindled and pleomorphic cells interspersed with hyalinized ectatic vessels.[651] Despite the degree of cellularity and pleomorphism that these lesions may attain, mitotic activity is negligible. Intracellular hemosiderin deposition and intranuclear cytoplasmic inclusions are common findings. Most of the tumors reported have shown infiltrative margins. Pleomorphic hyalinizing angiectatic tumor occurs in adults and usually involves the subcutaneous tissues of the lower extremity. It behaves clinically as a low grade sarcoma with a propensity for local recurrence. It also may express CD34 immunoreactivity.

Alveolar Soft Part Sarcoma

The term *alveolar soft part sarcoma*, coined by Christopherson et al,[652] emphasizes the characteristic histologic appearance of a distinctive tumor consisting of groups of neoplastic cells displaying an organoid or alveolar pattern resulting from septation of the mass by thin bands of fibrovascular tissue (Fig. 18-60A). Alveolar soft part sarcoma has been subjected to many ultrastructural and immunohistochemical studies, yet its histogenesis remains unknown.[653–655] Approximately one-half of the tumors

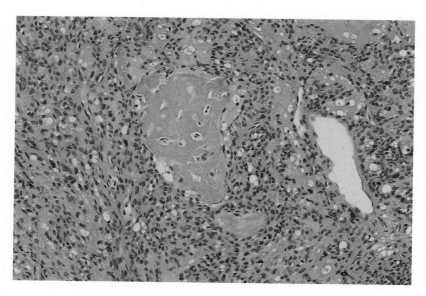

Fig. 18-59. Malignant ossifying fibromyxoid tumor showing hypercellularity, cytologic atypia, and foci of osteoid, reminiscent of a low grade osteosarcoma.

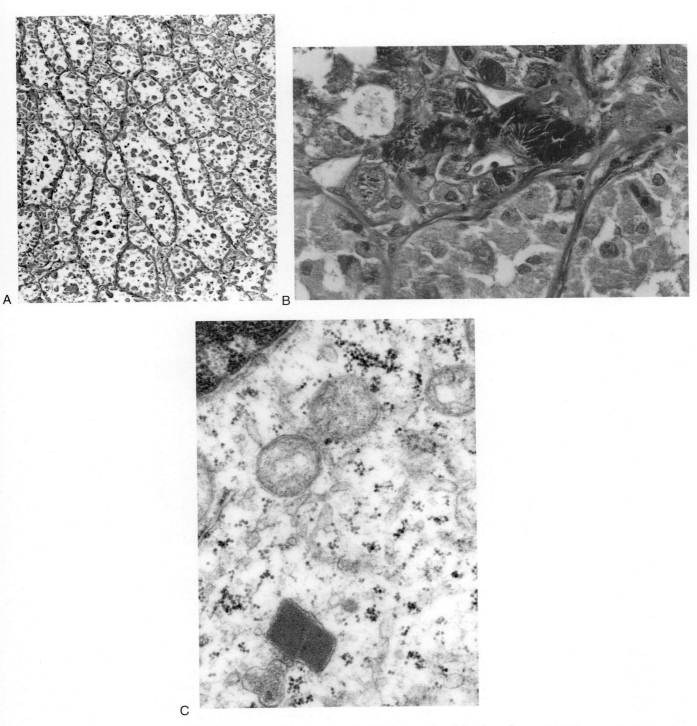

Fig. 18-60. **(A)** Characteristic alveolar pattern and cell composition of alveolar soft part sarcoma are clearly shown. **(B)** PAS-positive diastase-resistant rod-shaped crystals diagnostic of alveolar soft part sarcoma. **(C)** Alveolar soft part sarcoma. Intracytoplasmic-rhomboid crystals are a characteristic ultrastructural feature of this tumor. (*Figure continues.*)

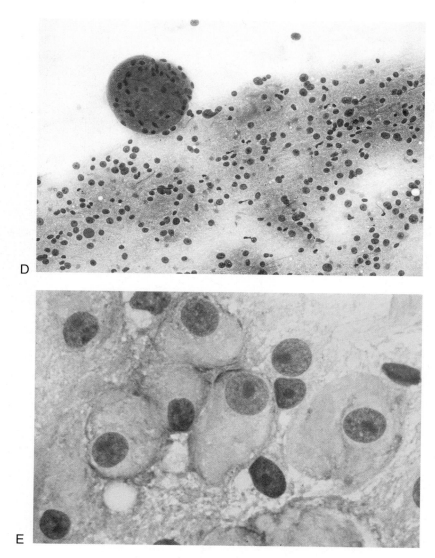

Fig. 18-60 *(Continued).* **(D)** Fine needle aspiration smear of alveolar soft part sarcoma demonstrates large cells, both singly (often bare nuclei) and in an alveolar ball-like aggregate. **(E)** High power of fine needle aspiration shows cells with finely granular cytoplasm. Nuclei are round with open chromatin and single prominent nucleoli. (Diff-Quik.)

show positive reactivity for desmin, suggesting skeletal muscle differentiation. However, myoglobin and muscle actin stains are consistently negative. Although expression of myogenic regulatory proteins such as MyoD1 has been demonstrated by some authors,[656,657] recent studies have failed to confirm this observation.[658] The tumor cells have abundant eosinophilic cytoplasm, and some contain characteristic PAS-positive intracytoplasmic crystalloids readily defined with the electron microscope (Fig. 18-60B & C). A three-dimensional model of the crystalloids prepared by digital image analysis of electron micrographs by computer has shown a filamentous structure similar to that of actin.[659] Most tumors appear in the thighs of young adults.[660] In children, they are more frequent in the head and neck.[661] In

adults, unusual sites include the stomach, pituitary gland, and the uterus.[662,663] Although these tumors exhibit a fairly uniform histologic pattern and few mitoses, they often spread via the blood stream. The survival for patients who presented without metastases was 60 percent at 5 years, 38 percent at 10 years, and 15 percent at 20 years.[660] The most frequent site of metastasis was the lung followed by bone and brain.

FNA smears of alveolar soft part sarcoma show large cells, both singly and in large alveolar aggregates associated with thin-walled vascular structures. The cytoplasm is abundant and finely granular; nuclei are central and round, with open chromatin and prominent nucleoli (Fig. 18-60D & E). Bare nuclei are also seen, due to fragility of the cytoplasm.[664,665]

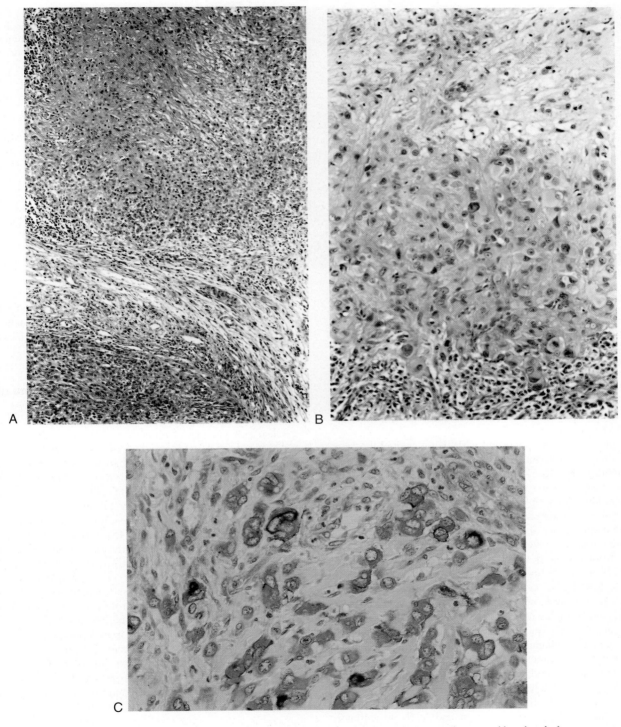

Fig. 18-61. (A) Epithelioid sarcoma. Two nodules surrounded by lymphocytes and separated by a band of connective tissue. One of the nodules shows central necrosis. (B) Higher magnification of nodule of epithelioid sarcoma showing malignant histiocytic-like cells surrounded by inflammatory cells. (C) Tumor cells in epithelioid sarcoma show immunoreactivity for epithelial membrane antigen.

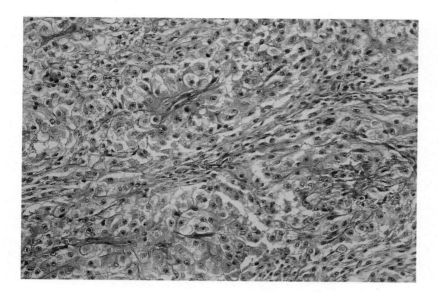

Fig. 18-62. Malignant melanoma of soft parts. Nests of uniform round to spindled cells with eosinophilic to clear cytoplasm, vesicular nucleus, and prominent basophilic nucleoli. Melanin pigment is present.

Epithelioid Sarcoma

Epithelioid sarcoma is a morphologically distinct soft tissue neoplasm that characteristically affects the distal parts of the extremities of young adults.[666] Rarely, the tumor occurs in children.[667] The neoplasm usually appears as single or multiple nodules in the dermis; these nodules enlarge rapidly and ulcerate the skin, thus mimicking abscesses or nonspecific ulcers clinically. Deeper lesions form larger nodules that infiltrate tendons and aponeuroses.

Neoplastic cells are polygonal with dense acidophilic cytoplasm and are grouped in nodules with central necrosis or hyalinization (Fig. 18-61A & B). Because of this feature the tumor is often confused with necrobiotic granulomas such as rheumatoid nodules. Spindle-shaped cells sometimes cluster at the periphery of the nodules; when they become numerous, the histologic appearance of the lesion may be confused with that of a fibrosarcoma. Moreover, tumor cells may form cords or nests in the midst of a dense desmoplastic reaction, enhancing the epithelioid appearance and mimicking squamous cell carcinoma. Multinucleated giant cells are occasionally present. The neoplastic cells usually show positive reactivity for cytokeratin, vimentin, and epithelial membrane antigen[668–671] (Fig. 18-61C). Less frequently they stain for muscle-specific actin, desmin, S-100 protein, neurofilaments, and carcinoembryonic antigen.[672]

Epithelioid sarcomas follow a protracted course. Local recurrences are common and metastases are most often blood-borne to the lungs, although lymph node metastases are relatively frequent. A more rapid clinical course is associated with proximal or axial tumor locations, increased size and depth of the tumor, hemorrhage, many mitotic figures, necrosis, or vascular invasion.[673] The 5 year survival rate is close to 70 percent, but decreases to 50 percent at 10 years. Although of unknown histogenesis, based on immunohistochemical and ultrastructural findings a synovial or fibrohistiocytic derivation has been suggested.[674,675]

FNA cytology of epithelioid sarcoma yields smears with dissociated and loosely clustered large polygonal cells showing dense eosinophilic cytoplasm, eccentric round nuclei with open chromatin (some bi- or multinucleate), and usually evident nucleoli. The tumor cells are apt to be mistaken for carcinoma cells.[676]

Clear Cell Sarcoma (Malignant Melanoma of Tendons and Aponeuroses)

Clear cell sarcoma of tendons and aponeuroses (*malignant melanoma of soft parts*) is a rare neoplasm, primarily of the foot and knee region of young adults, where it attaches firmly to tendons and aponeuroses.[677–684] It is formed by groups and fascicles of predominantly round and spindle cells with clear cytoplasm (Fig. 18-62). Scattered multinucleated giant cells are occasionally seen. About 70 percent of these tumors contain melanin. Most are S-100 protein and HMB-45 positive.[685–689] When examined electron microscopically the neoplastic cells contain premelanosomes indicating that these tumors are malignant melanomas of soft tissue. However, unlike the garden varieties of malignant melanoma, clear cell sarcomas are deep, are always associated with tendons or aponeuroses, and lack epidermal involvement. Moreover, these tumors show a specific translocation t(12;22) (q13;q12) not found in melanomas.[690–694] About 50 percent of patients die of their metastatic disease.

By FNA, clear cell sarcoma shows dispersed round to plump spindled cells with granular cytoplasm that may contain melanin pigment, and eccentric round nuclei with prominent nucleoli and intranuclear pseudoinclusions.[695,696]

Ewing's Sarcoma and Primitive Neuroectodermal Tumor

Ewing's sarcoma and primitive neuroectodermal tumor (PNET) are two highly malignant closely related neoplasms. In fact, some believe they may represent two morphologic expressions of a single nosologic entity.[697] Ewing's sarcoma patients

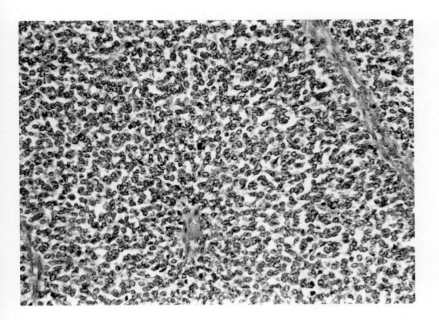

Fig. 18-63. Extraskeletal Ewing's sarcoma. Sheets of small round cells with little cytoplasm are present. The stroma is scant and contains some small blood vessels.

are usually children, adolescents or young adults; the tumor is exceedingly rare after the age of 40 years.[698,699] PNETs also occur in children but the age range of patients is broader with a mean of 18 years.[700] Some cases occur in patients over 50 years of age. Both tumors are more common among males and arise preferentially in the paraspinal region, chest wall, and extremities.[698–701] Some PNETs originate from nerve trunks of the extremities or chest wall, a feature not seen in Ewing's sarcoma. Microscopically Ewing's sarcoma is composed of small undifferentiated cells that contain glycogen, a substance that is absent in most PNETs (Fig. 18-63). Rosette or pseudorosette formation, a characteristic feature of PNET, is lacking in Ewing's sarcoma, which often show geographic necrosis (Fig. 18-64). Both

tumors stain with monoclonal antibody HBA71 and O13, which react with the cell surface glycoprotein P30/32 MIC2.[702] Moreover, these tumors share a characteristic cytogenetic abnormality t(11;22)(q24;q12) further strengthening the hypothesis that they are closely related histogenetically. The 5 year survival rates for patients with Ewing's sarcoma and PNET are 65 percent[699] and 30 percent, respectively.[700] Therefore, prognostically their separation is justified.

Ewing's sarcoma is more often primary within bone than within soft tissues, although bone tumors may show a large component of soft tissue extension at presentation. Therefore, any case of suspected soft tissue Ewing's sarcoma should have nearby bones carefully evaluated for involvement.

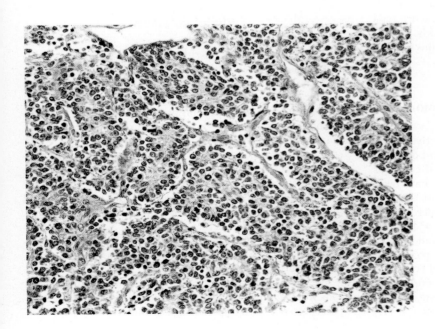

Fig. 18-64. Primitive neuroectodermal tumor (PNET) of sciatic nerve. Organoid pattern in a small round cell neoplasm showing pseudorosettes and a fibrillary background. Compare with Ewing's sarcoma (Fig. 18-63).

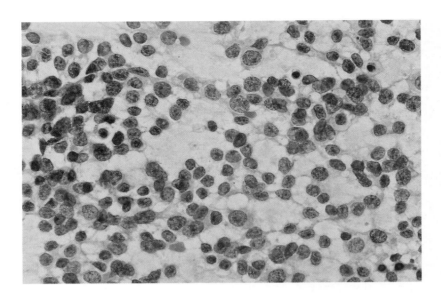

Fig. 18-65. Fine needle aspiration of Ewing's sarcoma shows large numbers of relatively uniform small round cells with even chromatin, lacking prominent nucleoli or nuclear molding. (H&E.)

FNA smears from Ewing's sarcoma and PNET are cellular, showing uniform round cells, about twice the size of mature lymphocytes, with round nuclei that have evenly distributed chromatin.[703–705] (Fig. 18-65). The cells of Ewing's sarcoma lack obvious nucleoli and nuclear molding. Cytoplasmic borders are generally well defined, and cytoplasmic vacuoles, when present, represent glycogen pools. A "tigroid" background, similar to seminoma, may also be seen due to the abundant glycogen.[703] By contrast, nuclear molding and occasional Homer-Wright rosettes are features of FNA smears of PNET.[704]

FNA features of neuroblastoma that assist in differential diagnosis from these two lesions are the presence of fibrillary neuropil, prominent nuclear molding and Homer-Wright rosettes, differentiating ganglion cells, and clinical features.[705] FNA features of non-Hodgkin's lymphomas in children (most often lymphoblastic and Burkitt's types) are cell dissociation, scant blue cytoplasm on Romanowsky type stains, lymphoglandular bodies and tingible body macrophages in the background, and positive immunostains for lymphoid markers.[705]

Desmoplastic Small Round Cell Tumor

Desmoplastic small round cell tumor is a distinctive highly malignant round cell neoplasm that shows divergent differentiation and occurs preferentially in the abdominal cavity of young adult males.[706–712] Extra-abdominal tumors have been documented with increasing frequency.[713] Most patients have a palpable abdominal mass that can involve the peritoneum diffusely. Of 23 patients in one series, 16 died of widespread metastases, 5 were alive with evidence of disease, and only 1 patient had no evidence of recurrence.[709] Microscopically the tumors consist of nests or trabeculae of small round or spindle cells embedded in a dense fibrous stroma (Fig. 18-66A). The neoplastic cells coexpress epithelial and mesenchymal markers, especially keratin and desmin (Fig. 18-66B & C). Al-though one-half of the tumors stain for neuron-specific enolase, none shows reactivity for chromogranin. Ultrastructurally the neoplastic cells contain aggregates of intermediate filaments. A characteristic t(11;22)(p13;q11.2) reciprocal translocation has been found in several examples of desmoplastic small round cell tumor.[714]

One FNA case report of desmoplastic small round cell tumor described clusters of uniform round to polygonal cells with prominent nucleoli and moderate amounts of cytoplasm often showing a perinuclear globule.[715] By contrast, other reports describe loose clusters and single cells with scant cytoplasm, slightly variable nuclear sizes and shapes, finely granular chromatin, and inconspicuous nucleoli.[716,717] Desmoplastic stroma is not a feature of FNA smears.

Rhabdoid Tumor

Rhabdoid tumor was first described as a distinctive highly malignant round cell neoplasm of the kidney.[718] However, subsequent studies established that many neoplasms of epithelial, lymphoid, endocrine, melanocytic neuroepithelial, and mesenchymal origin may have a rhabdoid phenotype.[719–724] This phenotype consists of eosinophilic or hyaline cytoplasmic inclusions that have been recognized on FNA material.[725] Ultrastructurally the inclusions are composed of whorls of intermediate filaments that show variable reactivity for vimentin, cytokeratin, epithelial membrane antigen, and desmin.[726] Leiomyosarcomas, rhabdomyosarcomas, and epithelioid and synovial sarcomas may show focal rhabdoid features.[726] Therefore, extrarenal rhabdoid tumor should be a diagnosis of exclusion. Soft tissue rhabdoid tumors occur both in adults and children and have a poor prognosis. Less than 50 percent of the patients survive 5 years or longer.

FNA cytology shows clusters of uniform round to polygonal cells with prominent nucleoli and moderate amounts of cytoplasm, often showing a perinuclear globule.[725,727]

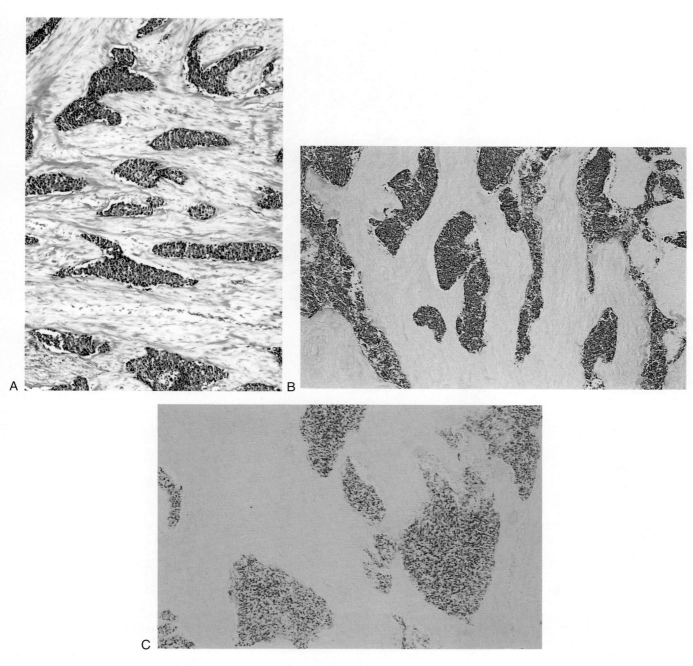

Fig. 18-66. **(A)** Irregular nests of undifferentiated tumor cells enveloped by a dense fibrous stroma, define desmoplastic small round cell tumor. **(B)** Cytokeratin reactivity in desmoplastic small round cell tumor. **(C)** Desmin reactivity in small round cell tumor shown in Fig. B. (Figs. B and C courtesy of Carlos Manivel M.D.)

TUMOR-LIKE LESIONS
Nodular Fasciitis, Proliferative Fasciitis, Proliferative Myositis, and Related Lesions

Nodular fasciitis, a common soft tissue pseudosarcoma, is a rapidly growing lesion arising in association with the deep cutaneous or muscle fascia of the proximal extremities, trunk, or head.[728–730] These lesions are usually small (about 2 cm in diameter), but they may measure up to 6 cm and have infiltrating borders. Microscopically, the cellular lesions with a prominent storiform pattern and increased mitotic activity may be confused with sarcoma, especially malignant fibrous histiocytoma.[731–733] These biologically benign proliferations can be correctly diagnosed by recognizing their characteristic combination of anatomic features: the usual anatomic locations; the

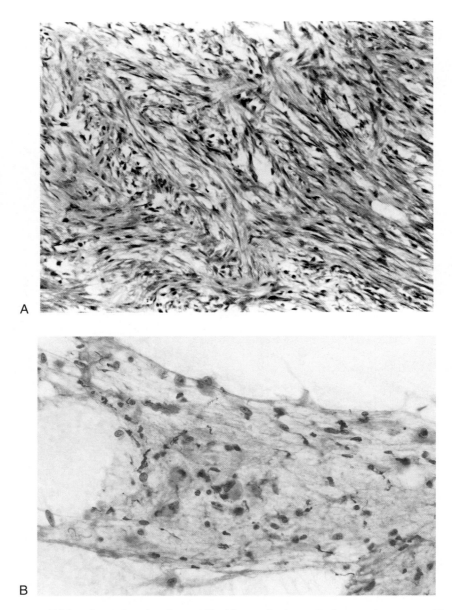

Fig. 18-67. (A) Interlacing fascicles of young fibroblasts and microcystic degeneration are noted in this nodular fasciitis. (B) Fine needle aspiration of nodular fasciitis shows a fibrillar semitransparent myxoid background containing plump spindle cells and rare rounded ganglion-like cells, with admixed lymphocytes. (Papanicolaou.)

radial arrangement of the numerous vascular channels in the mass, reflecting a reparative process; the admixture of fibroblasts and myofibroblasts with bland nuclei, occasional multinucleated giant cells, lymphocytes, and plasma cells; and the myxomatous stroma with microcyst formation (Fig. 18-67A). Focally some lesions show keloid-like strands of collagen. The spindle cells of nodular fasciitis are vimentin positive and often express muscle-specific actin and smooth muscle actin, which reflect myofibroblastic differentiation. Rarely desmin-positive cells have been reported.[732] Nodular fasciitis may also develop within blood vessels, further suggesting a malignant behavior.

However, these examples of intravascular fasciitis behave in the same manner as the conventional form.[734] Another variant, *cranial fasciitis*, occurs exclusively in the cranium of infants and children and usually produces a large defect in the outer table of the skull.[735] Subcutaneous lesions that have prominent populations of large fibroblasts that resemble ganglion cells have been called *proliferative fasciitis* because of their resemblance to proliferative myositis, another inflammatory tumor thought to be related to trauma.[736,737] In *proliferative myositis*, bands of bizarre fibroblasts and ganglion-like cells separate and atrophy but do not destroy groups of muscle fibers[737] (Fig. 18-

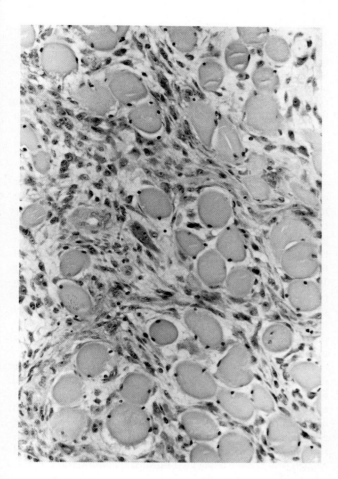

Fig. 18-68. Proliferative myositis. Young fibroblasts and ganglion-like cells dissociate skeletal muscle fibers.

68). This lesion is most often seen in muscles of the shoulder girdle and trunk, and patients have a mean age of 50 years, although it has also been reported in children.[738]

FNA of nodular fasciitis shows a prominent background of mesenchymal mucin. Smears generally are moderately to abundantly cellular, depicting large plump myofibroblasts, both dyshesive and in tissue fragments rich in cytoplasmic fibrils and mucosubstances[739–741] (Fig. 18-67B). The nuclei are oval with finely dispersed chromatin, although occasionally they are enlarged and hyperchromatic. Small nucleoli are common, and mitotic figures may be identified, as can occasional binucleate cells and rounded ganglion-like cells (as in proliferative fasciitis/myositis). An admixture of lymphocytes and occasional lipid-laden macrophages can be seen. If material obtained is less cellular than usual, distinction from desmoid tumor may be difficult. Because of the presence of atypical cells, low grade myxofibrosarcoma may be a consideration. In the appropriate clinical setting, with characteristic cytologic findings, nonsurgical management results in spontaneous resolution, usually within 4 weeks.[741]

Proliferative fasciitis and proliferative myositis resemble nodular fasciitis cytologically on FNA, although the larger rounded ganglion-like cells are more numerous in the latter le-

sion.[742–744] These ganglion-like cells have abundant lightly basophilic cytoplasm, eccentric large round nuclei with smooth membranes and even chromatin, and prominent eosinophilic nucleoli. Admixed multinucleate skeletal muscle cells, which may be atrophic, are encountered in proliferative myositis, and can be confused with tumor giant cells. All these lesions share FNA features typical of mesenchymal repair.[745]

Pseudosarcomatous Myofibroblastic Proliferations

A heterogeneous group of myofibroblastic proliferations that clinically and pathologically mimic sarcomas has been described in different anatomic locations. Numerous descriptive terms have been employed to designate these lesions. Their clinicopathologic heterogeneity is probably a reflection of the different etiologic factors and the anatomic locations. Some of these lesions appear following surgical trauma and are a manifestation of abnormal repair (*postoperative spindle cell nodule*).[746] Others, such as those involving the lymph nodes, spleen, and liver are Epstein-Barr virus-related lesions[747] (*inflammatory pseudotumors*). In the gallbladder, inflammatory pseudotumor has been associated with autoimmune disorders.[748] The etiologic factors are not known in the pseudosarcomatous proliferation of the urinary bladder in children, although a bacterial in-

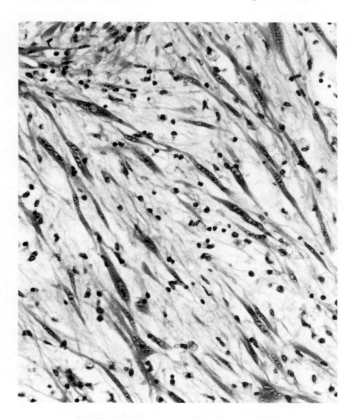

Fig. 18-69. Pseudosarcomatous myofibroblastic proliferation. Loose haphazardly arranged bipolar myofibroblasts with vesicular nuclei and prominent nucleoli in a myxoid background with scattered inflammatory cells.

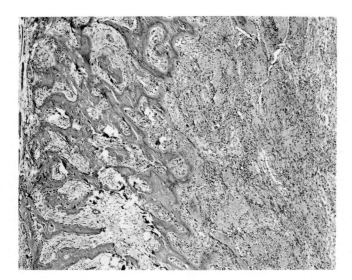

Fig. 18-70. Zonal growth pattern of myositis ossificans: central zone of fibroblastic proliferation, intermediate zone of collagen and osteoid deposition, on a peripheral zone of osteoid trabeculae rimmed by osteoblasts.

fection has been suspected.[749–751] Multifocality is not a feature of these bladder lesions. The intra-abdominal, retroperitoneal, pulmonary, and soft tissue lesions are the largest. Moreover, they may be multicentric, recur, and cause polyclonal gammopathy (*inflammatory fibrosarcoma, inflammatory myofibroblastic tumor, plasma cell granuloma*).[752–756] Their etiology is unknown. Microscopically two basic patterns are recognized. One group of lesions resembles nodular fasciitis and consists of plump myofibroblasts set in a myxoid stroma (Fig. 18-69). The myofibroblasts have abundant eosinophilic cytoplasm and vesicular nuclei with prominent nucleoli. The predominant inflammatory cells are eosinophils and polymorphonuclear leukocytes. Stromal fibrosis is rare. Another pattern seen more often in retroperitoneal, intra-abdominal, and pulmonary lesions consists of fascicles of myofibroblasts, numerous lymphocytes and plasma cells, and a fibrotic or hyalinized stroma. Some lesions show a mixture of these two patterns. Our experience suggests that these are benign locally invasive lesions. Those located in the abdomen, the retroperitoneum, or the deep soft tissues show potential for persistent local growth and local recurrence.[755]

Atypical Decubital Fibroplasia

Atypical decubital fibroplasia is another reactive pseudosarcomatous fibroblastic and myofibroblastic proliferation that occurs preferentially in physically debilitated and immobilized patients.[757] The most common anatomic locations are soft tissues of shoulder, chest wall, sacrum, buttock, and thigh, where decubitus ulcers are most common. Microscopically there is a proliferation of atypical fibroblasts and myofibroblasts embedded in a myxoid stroma containing dilated thin-walled vascular channels. Fibrinoid necrosis is common.

Calcifying Fibrous Pseudotumor

The rare and distinctive calcifying fibrous pseudotumor, also known as fibrous tumor with psammoma bodies, affects predominantly young adults and children.[758,759] The most common anatomic locations are the extremities, back, neck, and in-

guinal region. The lesion is well demarcated, measuring up to 15 cm in greatest dimension. Microscopically, it is characterized by abundant hypocellular hyalinized fibrous tissue containing lymphocytes and plasma cells as well as psammoma bodies and dystrophic calcifications. Occasional multinucleated giant cells and lymphoid follicles are noted in some cases. Calcifying fibrous pseudotumors may represent the end stage of the pseudosarcomatous myofibroblastic proliferations described above.

Myositis Ossificans

Myositis ossificans is a lesion that closely simulates osteosarcoma. About one-half of patients have a history of trauma before the appearance of the mass. The muscles of the thigh are commonly affected, but the lesion may be seen in any muscle group.[760] A periosteal reaction is seen in many cases. Ossification can be demonstrated roentgenographically 4 to 6 weeks after trauma. Microscopically, three zones can be identified (Fig. 18-70). The first, in the central portion of the mass, is composed of atypical spindle cells with mitotic figures. Osteoid and cartilage are seen in the middle zone and mature bone trabeculae form the periphery of the lesion. We have seen two examples of myositis ossificans that regressed spontaneously several months after needle core biopsy diagnosis.

By FNA, myositis ossificans shows spindle cells and myxoid matrix similar to nodular fasciitis, if the central zone is sampled. Fragments of dense metachromatic osteoid matrix, plump plasmacytoid osteoblasts sometimes showing prominent nucleoli, and multinucleate osteoclastic giant cells also may be seen. Experienced Scandinavian cytopathologists have advocated nonsurgical management, resulting in spontaneous resolution, although others have advocated histologic confirmation.[761,762]

Juxta-Articular Myxoma

Juxta-articular myxoma is a specific variant of myxoma associated with cyst formation that occurs in the vicinity of large joints, primarily the knee.[763] Trauma is thought to play a role in its development. Most cases have occurred in adult males, presenting as enlarging painful masses. The lesion is predominantly located in the subcutaneous tissue but may extend to adjacent dermis, musculature, and juxta-articular soft tissues. Microscopically, juxta-articular myxoma is composed of fibroblast-like cells with small hyperchromatic nuclei and delicate cytoplasmic processes within a myxoid matrix. The overall appearance is that of a variably collagenized myxoma with ganglion cyst-like spaces, and is readily recognized as benign. However, large infiltrating or hypercellular lesions with nodular fasciitis-like areas may be mistaken for a myxofibrosarcoma, or any other of the low grade myxoid sarcomas. Despite its benign nature, complete conservative excision is recommended as these lesions are prone to recur.

Retroperitoneal Fibrosis

Retroperitoneal fibrosis is a poorly defined entity capable of producing a large fibrous mass that may lead to ureteral obstruction, hydronephrosis, and renal failure.[764–772] The disease affects predominantly men in the fifth or sixth decades of life but has been described in children.[765] Mediastinal fibrosis, sclerosing cholangitis, Reidel's thyroiditis, and orbital pseudotumor

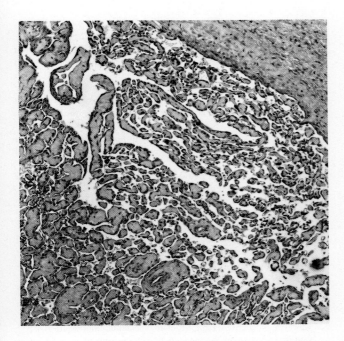

Fig. 18-71. Intravascular papillary endothelial hyperplasia. Fibrotic vein containing endothelium-covered papillary fronds. Part of the fibrotic wall of the vein is seen.

have been linked with retroperitoneal fibrosis, suggesting a systemic process.[764] The etiology of the disease is unknown but has been associated with infections, trauma, hemorrhage, atherosclerosis, and certain drugs. Serotonin, produced by carcinoid tumors, the ergot derivative methysergide, and more recently bromocriptine have been associated with retroperitoneal fibrosis.[764,767,771] Withdrawal of these substances may be followed by regression of the fibrosis. An autoimmune pathogenetic mechanism has been suggested for those cases of retroperitoneal fibrosis apparently not associated with obvious causes. Microscopically there is fibrosis with extensive hyalinization and interspersed spindle cells, most of which express the immunophenotype of a tissue macrophage.[764] Some investigators have proposed that the vasculitis and perivasculitis present in some of the lesions may be related to antigen-antibody complex-induced vascular damage. Methysergide and the few other drugs associated with this disease are thought to act as haptens to initiate the immune response. Probably the closest relationship these lesions have with neoplasia is their similarity to certain retroperitoneal, mesenteric, and mediastinal cancers, especially lymphomas, that can elicit an exuberant desmoplastic reaction in the host. The correct diagnosis of cancer may elude the surgeon and pathologist unless many deep biopsy specimens of the fibrous mass are obtained.

Organizing Thrombi and Papillary Endothelial Hyperplasia

Organizing thrombi in which the endothelial cells grow in fascicles can mimic Kaposi's sarcoma. We have seen rare capillary hemangiomas composed of fascicles of spindle-shaped endothelial cells closely simulating Kaposi's sarcoma. The lobular pattern in these hemangiomas helps one to distinguish them from Kaposi's sarcoma (Albores-Saavedra J, unpublished obser-

vations). Exuberant endothelial proliferations arranged in papillary patterns can occur in vascular thrombi and less frequently in hematomas and in hemangiomas.[773,774] This lesion, known as *Masson's hemangioma, vegetative intravascular hemangioendothelioma,* or *papillary endothelial hyperplasia,* is thought to represent organization of a thrombus or a hematoma with exuberant endothelial cell proliferation.[775,776] In its late stage, it may simulate an angiosarcoma (Fig. 18-71). Two forms of papillary endothelial hyperplasia have been described. The primary form is usually associated with a vascular thrombus and rarely with a hematoma, whereas the secondary type constitutes a component of another lesion such as hemangioma, schwannoma, pyogenic granuloma, or lymphangioma.[776,777] Primary papillary endothelial hyperplasia occurs commonly in subcutaneous tissue and, less frequently, in the dermis. The most common locations are the fingers and the head and neck, followed by the extremities. The location of the secondary type is determined by the underlying disease process.

Other Tumor-Like Lesions

In the past the injection of silica was used for the treatment of hernias and elicited an exuberant fibrohistiocytic reaction that closely resembles a malignant fibrous histiocytoma.[778]

An atypical spindle cell proliferation resembling a mesenchymal neoplasm caused by *Mycobacterium avium-intracellulare* has been described in AIDS patients.[779]

Tumoral calcinosis, an idiopathic disorder characterized by the periarticular deposition of calcium, may form large soft tissue masses in the vicinity of large joints that radiologically can be confused with chondrosarcoma. Microscopically, it consists of a central zone of amorphous or granular calcified material, bordered by a florid proliferation of mono- and multinucleated histiocytes, osteoclast-like giant cells and fibroblasts in the active phase, and by fibrous tissue in the inactive phase.[780]

SOFT TISSUE SARCOMA-LIKE MALIGNANT NEOPLASMS

A number of malignant neoplasms primarily discussed in other chapters of this book morphologically mimic soft tissue sarcomas and on rare occasion may present as soft tissue lesions clinically. Examples of these lesions, in addition to visceral sarcomas, are spindle cell (sarcomatoid) carcinomas, metaplastic carcinomas, myoepithelial carcinomas, and sarcomatous overgrowth of biphasic tumors (e.g., malignant phyllodes tumor and cystic nephroma). In midline lesions one may encounter immature mesenchymal components or sarcomatous transformation of teratomas. In the mediastinum, a spindle cell thymoma or other primary thymic neoplasms may simulate a soft tissue tumor. The intranodal origin of a vascular leiomyosarcoma, reticulum cell sarcoma, or sclerosing lymphoma may not be readily apparent. Extranodal lymphomas and other hematologic carcinomas may have a primary soft tissue location. Malignant mesotheliomas represent a distinct category of soft tissue tumors and should be appropriately recognized. Finally and more important, it behooves pathologists to remember the morphologic diversity of malignant melanoma up front.

REFERENCES

1. Cotterill AM, Holly JMP, Davies SC, et al: The insulin-like growth factors and their binding proteins in a case of non-islet cell tumor-associated hypoglycemia. J Endocrinol 131:303–311, 1991

2. Evans DJ, Azzopardi JG: Distinctive tumors of bone and soft tissue causing acquired vitamin-D-resistant osteomalacia. Lancet 1:353–354, 1972

3. Weidner N, Santa-Cruz D: Phosphaturic mesenchymal tumors. A polymorphous group causing osteomalacia or rickets. Cancer 59:1442–1454, 1987

4. Bissada M, White JH, Sun CN, et al: Tuberous sclerosis complex and renal angiomyolipoma. Urology 6:105–113, 1975

5. Taylor RS, Joseph DB, Kohaut EC, et al: Renal angiomyolipoma associated with lymph node involvement and renal cell carcinoma in patients with tuberous sclerosis. J Urol 141:930–932, 1989

6. Burke AP, Sobin LH, Shekitka KM, et al: Intra-abdominal fibromatosis. A pathologic analysis of 130 tumors with comparison of clinical subgroups. Am J Surg Pathol 14:335–341, 1990

7. Guccion JG, Enzinger FM: Malignant schwannoma with von Recklinghausen's neurofibromatosis. Virchows Arch [A] 383:43–57, 1979

8. Kurzweg FT, Spencer R: Familial multiple lipomatosis. Am J Surg 82:726–729, 1951

9. Usui M, Ishui S, Yamawaki S, Hirayama T: The occurrence of soft tissue sarcomas in three siblings with Werner's syndrome. Cancer 54:2580–2586, 1984

10. Li FP, Fraumeni JF Jr: Soft tissue sarcomas, breast cancer and other neoplasms: a familial syndrome. Ann Intern Med 71:747–752, 1969

11. Maulkin D: P53 and the Li-Fraumeni syndrome. Biochem Biophys Acta 1198:197–213, 1994

12. Willén H, Akerman M, Carlen B: Fine needle aspiration (FNA) in the diagnosis of soft tissue tumours; a review of 22 years experience. Cytopathology 6:236–247, 1995

13. Miralles TG, Gosalbez F, Menendez P, et al: Fine needle aspiration cytology of soft tissue lesions. Acta Cytol 30:671–678, 1986

14. Campora RG, Arias-Munoz G, Otal-Salaverri C, et al: Fine needle aspiration cytology of primary soft tissue tumors. Morphologic analysis of the most frequent types. Acta Cytol 36:905–917, 1992

15. Layfield LJ, Anders KH, Glasgow BJ, et al: Fine needle aspiration of primary soft tissue lesions. Arch Pathol Lab Med 110:420–424, 1986

16. Hajdu SI: Diagnosis of soft tissue sarcomas on aspiration smears, editorial. Acta Cytol 40:607–608, 1996

17. Bennert KW, Abdul-Karim FW: Fine needle aspiration cytology vs. needle core biopsy of soft tissue tumors. A comparison. Acta Cytol 38:381–384, 1994

18. Powers CN, Berardo MD, Frable WJ: Fine-needle aspiration biopsy: pitfalls in the diagnosis of spindle-cell lesions. Diagn Cytopathol 10:232–241, 1994

19. Zarbo RJ, Gown AM, Nagle RB, et al: Anomalous cytokeratin expression in malignant melanoma. Mod Pathol 3:494–501, 1990

20. Mooi WJ, Deenik W, Peterrse JL, et al: Keratin immunoreactivity in melanoma of soft parts (clear cell sarcoma). Histopathology 27:61–65, 1995

21. Pea M, Bonetti F, Zamboni G, et al: Melanocyte marker HMB-45 is regularly expressed in angiomyolipomas of the kidney. Pathology 23:185–188, 1991

22. Suster S, Nascimiento AG, Miettinen M, et al: Solitary fibrous tumors of soft tissue. A clinicopathologic and immunohistochemical study of 12 cases. Am J Surg Pathol 19:1257–1266, 1995

23. Abenoza P, Lillemoe T: CD34 and Factor XIIIa in the differential diagnosis of dermatofibroma and dermatofibrosarcoma protuberans. Am J Dermatopathol 15:429–434, 1993

24. Weiss SW, Nickoloff BJ: CD-34 is expressed by a distinctive cell population in peripheral nerve, nerve sheath tumors, and related lesions. Am J Surg Pathol 17:1039–1045, 1993

25. Weiss SW, Brooks JSJ (eds): Soft Tissue Tumors. Monographs in Pathology. No. 38. Williams & Wilkins, Baltimore, 1996

26. Parham DM, Webber B, Holt H, et al: Immunohistochemical study of childhood rhabdomyosarcomas and related neoplasms: results of an Intergroup Rhabdomyosarcoma Study Project. Cancer 67:3072–3080, 1991

27. Dias P, Parham DM, Shapiro DN, et al: Myogenic regulatory protein (MyoD1) expression in childhood solid tumors: diagnostic utility in rhabdomyosarcoma. Am J Pathol 137:1283–1291, 1990

28. Wesche WA, Fletcher CD, Dias P, et al: Immunohistochemistry of MyoD1 in adult pleomorphic soft tissue sarcomas. Am J Surg Pathol 19:261–269, 1995

29. Ambros IM, Ambron PF, Strehl S, et al: MIC2 is a specific marker for Ewing's sarcoma and peripheral primitive neuroectodermal tumors. Cancer 67:1886–1893, 1991

30. Perlman EJ, Dickman PS, Askin FB, et al: Ewing's sarcoma—routine diagnostic utilization of MIC2 analysis. A pediatric oncology group/children's cancer group intergroup study. Hum Pathol 25:304–307, 1994

30a. Renshaw AA: 013 (CD99) in spindle cell tumors. Appl Immunohistochem 3:250–256, 1995

31. Swanson SA, Brooks JJ: Proliferation markers Ki-67 and p105 in soft tissue lesions: correlation with DNA flow cytometric characteristics. Am J Pathol 137:1491–1500, 1990

32. Kawai A, Noguchi M, Beppu Y, et al: Nuclear immunoreaction of p53 protein in soft tissue sarcomas. A possible prognostic factor. Cancer 73:2499–2505, 1994

33. Erlandson RA: Diagnostic Transmission Electron Microscopy of Tumors. Lippincott-Raven, Philadelphia, 1994

34. Morales AR, Fine G, Horn RC Jr: Rhabdomyosarcoma: an ultrastructural appraisal. Pathol Annu 7:81–106, 1972

35. Mieraue GW, Favara BE: Rhabdomyosarcoma in children: ultrastructural study of 31 cases. Cancer 46:2035–2040, 1980

36. Agnamanolis DP, Dasu S, Krill CE Jr: Tumors of skeletal muscle. Hum Pathol 17:778–795, 1986

37. Erlandson RA: The ultrastructural distinction between rhabdomyosarcoma and other undifferentiated "sarcomas". Ultrastruct Pathol 11:83–101, 1987

38. Albores-Saavedra J, Manivel JC, Essenfeld H, et al: Pseudosarcomatous myofibroblastic proliferations in the urinary bladder of children. Cancer 66:1234–1241, 1990

39. Weiss S: Histologic Typing of Soft Tissue Tumors. World Health Organization, Geneva, 1994

40. Rooser B, Attewell R, Berg N, et al: Prognostication in soft tissue sarcoma. A model with four risk factors. Cancer 61:817–823, 1988

41. Costa J, Wesley RA, Glatstein E, et al: The grading of soft tissue sarcomas. Results of a clinico-pathologic correlation in a series of 163 cases. Cancer 53:530–541, 1984

42. Condre JM, Bui NB, Bonochon F, et al: Histopathologic grading in spindle cell soft tissue sarcomas. Cancer 61:2305–2309, 1988

43. Rooser B, Attewell R, Rydholm A: The staging of soft-tissue sarcomas. Int Orthop 11:339–343, 1987

44. Cooper CS: Translocations in solid tumors. Curr Opin Genet Develop 6:71–75, 1996

45. Pollock RE: Molecular determinants of soft tissue sarcoma proliferation, review. Semin Surg Oncol 10:315–322, 1994

46. Fletcher JA: Cytogenetics and experimental models of sarcomas, review. Curr Opin Oncol 6:367–371, 1994

47. Bridge JA: Cytogenetics and experimental models of sarcomas, review. Curr Opin Oncol 7:333–339, 1995

48. Ladanyi M: The emerging molecular genetics of sarcoma translocations, review. Diagn Mol Pathol 4:162–173, 1995

49. Barr FG, Chatten J, D'Cruz CM, et al: Molecular assays for chromosomal translocations in the diagnosis of pediatric soft tissue sarcomas. JAMA 273:553–557, 1995

50. Sreekantaiah C, Ladanyi M, Rodriguez E, et al: Chromosomal aberra-

tions in soft tissue tumors. Relevance to diagnosis, classification, and molecular mechanisms, review. Am J Pathol 144:1121–1134, 1994

51. Fletcher CD, Akerman M, Dal Cin P, et al: Correlation between clinicopathological features and karyotype in lipomatous tumors. A report of 178 cases from the Chromosomes and Morphology (CHAMP) Collaborative Study Group. Am J Pathol 148:623–630, 1996

52. Fletcher JA, Kozakewich HP, Schoenberg ML, et al: Cytogenetic findings in pediatric adipose tumors: consistent rearrangement of chromosome 8 in lipoblastoma. Genes Chromosom Cancer 6:24–29, 1993

53. Mrozek K, Karakousis CP, Bloomfield CD: Band 11q13 is nonrandomly rearranged in hibernomas, review. Genes Chromosom Cancer 9:145–147, 1994

54. Mandahl N, Mertens F, Willen H, et al: A new cytogenetic subgroup in lipomas: loss of chromosome 16 material in spindle cell and pleomorphic lipomas. J Cancer Res Clin Oncol 120:707–711, 1994

55. Orndal C, Mandahl N, Rydholm A, et al: Supernumerary ring chromosomes in five bone and soft tissue tumors of low or borderline malignancy. Cancer Genet Cytogenet 60:170–175, 1992

56. Denny CT: Gene rearrangements in Ewing's sarcoma, review. Cancer Invest 14:83–88, 1996

57. Gerald WL, Rosai J, Ladanyi M: Characterization of the genomic breakpoint and chimeric transcripts in the EWS-WT1 gene fusion of desmoplastic small round cell tumor. Proc Natl Acad Sci USA 92:1028–1032, 1995

58. de Alava E, Ladanyi M, Rosai J, et al: Detection of chimeric transcripts in desmoplastic small round cell tumor and related developmental tumors by reverse transcriptase polymerase chain reaction. A specific diagnostic assay. Am J Pathol 147:1584–1591, 1995

59. Zucman J, Delattre O, Desmaze C, et al: EWS and ATF-1 gene fusion induced by t(12;22) translocation in malignant melanoma of soft parts. Nat Genet 4:341–345, 1993

60. Clark J, Benjamin H, Gill S, et al: Fusion of the EWS gene to CHN, a member of the steroid/thyroid receptor gene superfamily, in a human myxoid chondrosarcoma. Oncogene 12:229–235, 1996

61. Stenman G, Andersson H, Mandahl N, et al: Translocation t(9;22)(q22;q12) is a primary cytogenetic abnormality in extraskeletal myxoid chondrosarcoma. Int J Cancer 62:398–402, 1995

62. Fredericks WJ, Galili N, Mukhopadhyay S, et al: The PAX3-FKHR fusion protein created by the t(2;13) translocation in alveolar rhabdomyosarcomas is a more potent transcriptional activator than PAX3. Mol Cell Biol 15:1522–1535, 1995

63. Davis RJ, D'Cruz CM, Lovell MA, et al: Fusion of PAX7 to FKHR by the variant t(1;13)(p36;q14) translocation in alveolar rhabdomyosarcoma. Cancer Res 54:2869–2872, 1994

64. Parham DM, Shapiro DN, Downing JR, et al: Solid alveolar rhabdomyosarcomas with the t(2;13). Report of two cases with diagnostic implications. Am J Surg Pathol 18:474–478, 1994

65. Clark J, Rocques PJ, Crew AJ, et al: Identification of novel genes, SYT and SSX, involved in the t(X;18)(p11.2;q11.2) translocation found in human synovial sarcoma. Nat Genet 7:502–508, 1994

66. Renwick PJ, Reeves BR, Dal Cin P, et al: Two categories of synovial sarcoma defined by divergent chromosome translocation breakpoints in Xp11.2, with implications for the histologic sub-classification of synovial sarcoma. Cytogenet Cell Genet 70:58–63, 1995

67. Knight JC, Renwick PJ, Cin PD, et al: Translocation t(12;16) (q13;p11) in myxoid liposarcoma and round cell liposarcoma: molecular and cytogenetic analysis. Cancer Res 55:24–27, 1995

68. Kuroda M, Ishida T, Horiuchi H, et al: Chimeric TLS/FUS-CHOP gene expression and the heterogeneity of its junction in human myxoid and round cell liposarcoma. Am J Pathol 147:1221–1227, 1995

69. Besnard-Guerin C, Cavenee W, Newsham I: The t(11;22) (p15.5;q11.23) in a retroperitoneal rhabdoid tumor also includes a regional deletion distal to CRYBB2 on 22q. Genes Chromosom Cancer 13:145–150, 1995

70. Sreekantaiah C, Bridge JA, Rao UN, et al: Clonal chromosomal ab-

normalities in hemangiopericytoma. Cancer Genet Cytogenet 54:173–181, 1991

71. Sreekantaiah C, Leong SP, Sandberg AA: Complex cytogenetic changes in benign neoplasms. Report of six lipomas. Cancer Genet Cytogenet 47:113–130, 1990

72. Sreekantaiah C, Leong SP, Karakousis CP, et al: Cytogenetic profile of 109 lipomas. Cancer Res 51:422–433, 1991

73. Sreekantaiah C, Karakousis CP, Leong SP, et al: Cytogenetic findings in liposarcoma correlate with histopathologic subtypes. Cancer 69:2484–2495, 1992

74. Suijkerbuijk RF, Olde Weghuis DE, Van den Berg M, et al: Comparative genomic hybridization as a tool to define two distinct chromosome 12-derived amplification units in well-differentiated liposarcomas. Genes Chromosom Cancer 9:292–295, 1994

75. Pedeutour F, Simon MP, Minoletti F, et al: Ring 22 chromosomes in dermatofibrosarcoma protuberans are low-level amplifiers of chromosome 17 and 22 sequences. Cancer Res 55:2400–2403, 1995

76. Craver RD, Correa H, Kao YS, et al: Aggressive giant cell fibroblastoma with a balanced 17;22 translocation. Cancer Genet Cytogenet 80:20–22, 1995

77. Schofield DE, Fletcher JA, Grier HE, et al: Fibrosarcoma in infants and children. Application of new techniques. Am J Surg Pathol 18:14–24, 1994

78. Fletcher JA, Naeem R, Xiao S, et al: Chromosome aberrations in desmoid tumors. Trisomy 8 may be a predictor of recurrence [see comments]. Cancer Genet Cytogenet 79:139–143, 1995

79. Sawyer JR, Sammartino G, Baker GF, et al: Clonal chromosome aberrations in a case of nodular fasciitis. Cancer Genet Cytogenet 76:154–156, 1994

80. Rydholm A, Mandahl N, Heim S, et al: Malignant fibrous histiocytomas with a 19p+ marker chromosome have increased relapse rate. Genes Chromosomes Cancer 2:296–299, 1990

81. van Echten J, van den Berg E, van Baarlen J, et al: An important role for chromosome 17, band q25, in the histogenesis of alveolar soft part sarcoma. Cancer Genet Cytogenet 82:57–61, 1995

82. Orndal C, Mandahl N, Rydholm A, et al: Chromosomal evolution and tumor progression in a myxoid liposarcoma, review. Acta Orthop Scand 61:99–105, 1990

83. Nagao K, Ito H, Yoshida H: Chromosomal translocation t(X;18) in human synovial sarcomas analyzed by fluorescence in situ hybridization using paraffin-embedded tissue. Am J Pathol 148:601–609, 1996

84. Peter M, Magdelenat H, Michon J, et al: Sensitive detection of occult Ewing's cells by the reverse transcriptase-polymerase chain reaction. Br J Cancer 72:96–100, 1995

85. Kawai A, Noguchi M, Beppu Y, et al: Nuclear immunoreaction of p53 protein in soft tissue sarcomas. A possible prognostic factor. Cancer 73:2499–2505, 1994

86. Toguchida J, Yamaguchi T, Ritchie B, et al: Mutation spectrum of the p53 gene in bone and soft tissue sarcomas. Cancer Res 52:6194–6199, 1992

87. Wadayama B, Toguchida J, Yamaguchi T, et al: p53 expression and its relationship to DNA alterations in bone and soft tissue sarcomas. Br J Cancer 68:1134–1139, 1993

88. Wang J, Coltrera MD, Gown AM: Abnormalities of p53 and p110RB tumor suppressor gene expression in human soft tissue tumors: correlations with cell proliferation and tumor grade. Mod Pathol 8:837–842, 1995

89. Dei Tos AP, Doglioni C, Laurino L, et al: p53 protein expression in non-neoplastic lesions and benign and malignant neoplasms of soft tissue. Histopathology 22:45–50, 1993

90. Nilbert M, Rydholm A, Willen H, et al: MDM2 gene amplification correlates with ring chromosome in soft tissue tumors. Genes Chromosomes Cancer 9:261–265, 1994

91. Nakayama T, Toguchida J, Wadayama B, et al: MDM2 gene amplification in bone and soft-tissue tumors: association with tumor pro-

gression in differentiated adipose-tissue tumors. Int J Cancer 64:342–346, 1995

92. Cordon-Cardo C, Latres E, Drobnjak M, et al: Molecular abnormalities of mdm2 and p53 genes in adult soft tissue sarcomas. Cancer Res 54:794–799, 1994

93. Karpeh MS, Brennan MF, Cance WG, et al: Altered patterns of retinoblastoma gene product expression in adult soft-tissue sarcomas. Br J Cancer 72:986–991, 1995

94. Wunder JS, Czitrom AA, Kandel R, et al: Analysis of alterations in the retinoblastoma gene and tumor grade in bone and soft-tissue sarcomas. J Natl Cancer Inst 83:194–200, 1991

95. Besnard-Guerin C, Newsham I, Winqvist R, et al: A common region of loss of heterozygosity in Wilms' tumor and embryonal rhabdomyosarcoma distal to the D11S988 locus on chromosome 11p15.5. Hum Genet 97:163–170, 1996

96. Miyaki M, Konishi M, Kikuchi-Yanoshita R, et al: Coexistence of somatic and germ-line mutations of APC gene in desmoid tumors from patients with familial adenomatous polyposis. Cancer Res 53:5079–5082, 1993

97. Castresana JS, Barrios C, Ruiz J, et al: Sporadic amplification of the c-fms proto-oncogene in human musculoskeletal sarcomas. Anticancer Res 13:807–810, 1993

98. Wilke W, Maillet M, Robinson R: H-ras-1 point mutations in soft tissue sarcomas. Mod Pathol 6:129–132, 1993

99. Polverini PJ, Nickoloff BJ: Role of scatter factor and the c-met protooncogene in the pathogenesis of AIDS-associated Kaposi's sarcoma, review. Adv Cancer Res 66:235–253, 1995

100. Hashimoto M, Ohsawa M, Ohnishi A, et al: Expression of vascular endothelial growth factor and its receptor mRNA in angiosarcoma. Lab Invest 73:859–863, 1995

101. Dias P, Parham DM, Shapiro DN, et al: Myogenic regulatory protein (MyoD1) expression in childhood solid tumors: diagnostic utility in rhabdomyosarcoma. Am J Pathol 137:1283–1291, 1990

102. Wesche WA, Fletcher CD, Dias P, et al: Immunohistochemistry of MyoD1 in adult pleomorphic soft tissue sarcomas. Am J Surg Pathol 19:261–269, 1995

103. Balachandran K, Allen PW, MacCormac LB: Nuchal fibroma. A clinicopathological study of nine cases. Am J Surg Pathol 19:313–317, 1995

104. Järvi OH, Saxen E, Hopsu-Havu VK, et al: Elastofibroma. A degenerative pseudotumor. Cancer 23:42–47, 1969

105. Peters JL, Fisher CS: Elastofibroma. J Thorac Cardiovasc Surg 75:836–838, 1978

106. Enjoji M, Sumiyoshi K, Sueyoshi K: Elastofibromatous lesion of the stomach in a patient with elastofibroma dorsi. Am J Surg Pathol 9:233–237, 1985

107. Madri JA, Dise CA, LiVolsi VA, et al: Elastofibroma dorsi: an immunochemical study of collagen content. Hum Pathol 12:186–190, 1981

108. Pisharodi LR, Cary D, Bernacki EG Jr: Elastofibroma dorsi: diagnostic problems and pitfalls. Diagn Cytopathol 10:242–244, 1994

109. Suster S, Nascimento AG, Miettinen M, et al: Solitary fibrous tumors of soft tissue. A clinicopathologic and immunohistochemical study of 12 cases. Am J Surg Pathol 19:1257–1266, 1995

110. Goodlad JR, Fletcher CDM: Solitary fibrous tumor arising at unusual sites: analysis of a series. Histopathology 19:515–522, 1991

111. Dorfman DM, Dickersin GR, Rosenberg AE, et al: Solitary fibrous tumor of the orbit. Am J Surg Pathol 18:281–287, 1994

112. Caruso RA, LaSpada F, Gaeta M, et al: Report of an intrapulmonary solitary fibrous tumor: fine-needle aspiration cytologic findings, clinicopathological, and immunohistochemical features. Diagn Cytopathol 14:64–67, 1996

113. Chung EB, Enzinger FM: Fibroma of tendon sheath. Cancer 44:1945–1954, 1979

114. Lundgren LG, Kindblom LG: Fibroma of tendon sheath. A light and electron microscopic study of 6 cases. Acta Pathol Microbiol Immunol Scand 92:401–409, 1984

115. Cooper PH: Fibroma of tendon sheath. J Am Acad Dermatol 11:625–628, 1984

116. Hashimoto H, Tsuneyoshi M, Daimaru Y, et al: Fibroma of tendon sheath: a tumor of myofibroblasts: a clinicopathologic study of 18 cases. Acta Pathol Jpn 35:1099–1107, 1985

117. Humphreys S, McKee PH, Fletcher CDM: Fibroma of tendon sheath: a clinicopathologic study. J Cutan Pathol 13:331–338, 1986

118. Sarma DP, Weilbaecher TG, Rodriguez FH Jr: Fibroma of tendon sheath. J Surg Oncol 32:230–232, 1986

119. Pulitzer DR, Martin PC, Reed RJ: Fibroma of tendon sheath. A clinicopathologic study of 32 cases. Am J Surg Pathol 13:472–479, 1989

120. Keasbey LE: Juvenile aponeurotic fibroma (calcifying fibroma). A distinctive tumor arising in the palms and soles of young children. Cancer 6:338–346, 1953

121. Allen PW, Enzinger FM: Juvenile aponeurotic fibroma. Cancer 26:857–867, 1970

122. Goldman RL: The cartilage analogue of fibromatosis (aponeurotic fibroma). Further observations based on 7 new cases. Cancer 26:1325–1331, 1970

123. Hassel B: Calcifying aponeurotic fibroma: a case of multiple primary tumours: case report. Scand J Plast Reconstruct Hand Surg 26:115–118, 1992

124. Enzinger FM: Fibrous hamartoma of infancy. Cancer 18:241–248, 1965

125. Greco MA, Schinella RA, Vuletin JC: Fibrous hamartoma of infancy. An ultrastructural study. Hum Pathol 15:717–723, 1984

126. Groisman G, Kerner H: A case of fibrous hamartoma of infancy in the scrotum, including immunohistochemical findings. J Urol 144:330–333, 1990

127. Paller AS, Gonzalez-Cruzzi F, Sherman JO: Fibrous hamartoma of infancy: eight additional cases and a review of the literature. Arch Dermatol 125:88–92, 1989

128. Fletcher CD, Powell G, Van Noorden S, et al: Fibrous hamartoma of infancy: a histochemical and immunohistochemical study. Histopathology 12:65–70, 1988

129. Fu Y-S, Perzin KH: Nonepithelial tumors of the nasal cavity, paranasal sinus, and nasopharynx: a clinicopathologic study. I. General features and vascular tumors. Cancer 33:1275–1288, 1974

130. Neel HB III, Whicker JH, Devine KD, et al: Juvenile angiofibroma: review of 120 cases. Am J Surg 126:547–556, 1973

131. Hicks JL, Nelson JF: Juvenile nasopharyngeal angiofibroma. Oral Surg Oral Med Oral Pathol 35:807–817, 1973

132. Gonsalves CG, Briant TDR: Radiologic findings in nasopharyngeal angiofibromas. J Can Assoc Radiol 29:209–215, 1978

133. Rodriguez H: a new surgical approach to nasopharyngeal angiofibroma. Cancer 19:458–460, 1966

134. Chandler JR, Goulding R, Moskowitz L, et al: Nasopharyngeal angiofibroma: staging and management. Ann Otol Rhinol Laryngol 93:322–327, 1984

135. Lee DA, Rao BR, Meyer JS, et al: Hormonal receptor determination in juvenile nasopharyngeal angiofibromas. Cancer 46:547–551, 1980

136. Enzinger FM: Intramuscular myxoma: a review and follow-up study of 34 cases. Am J Clin Pathol 43:104–113, 1965

137. Rosin RD: Intramuscular myxomas. Br J Surg 60:122–124, 1973

138. Kindblom LG, Stener B, Angervall L: Intramuscular myxoma. Cancer 34:1737–1744, 1974

139. Ireland DC, Soule EH, Irvins JC: Myxoma of somatic soft tissues: a report of 58 patients, 3 with multiple tumor and fibrous dysplasia of bone. Mayo Clin Proc 48:401–410, 1973

140. Feldman PS: A comparative study including ultrastructure of intramuscular myxoma and myxoid liposarcoma. Cancer 43:512–525, 1979

141. Akerman M, Rydholm A: Aspiration cytology of intramuscular myxoma. Acta Cytol 27:505–510, 1983

142. Caraway NP, Staerkel GA, Fanning CV, et al: Diagnosing intramus-

cular myxoma by fine-needle aspiration: a multidisciplinary approach. Diagn Cytopathol 11:255–261, 1994

143. Wakely PE, Geisinger KR, Cappellari JO, et al: Fine-needle aspiration cytopathology of soft tissue: chondromyxoid and myxoid lesions. Diagn Cytopathol 12:101–105, 1995

144. Allen PW, Dymock RB, MacCormac LB: Superficial angiomyxomas with and without epithelial components. Report of 30 tumors in 28 patients. Am J Surg Pathol 12:519–530, 1988

145. Begin LR, Clement PB, Kirk ME, et al: Aggressive angiomyxoma of pelvic soft parts: a clinicopathologic study of nine cases. Hum Pathol 16:621–628, 1985

146. Hilgers RD, Pai R, Bartow SA, et al: Aggressive angiomyxoma of the vulva. Obstet Gynaecol 68:60S–62S, 1990

147. Sementa AR, Gambini C, Borgiani L, et al: Aggressive angiomyxoma of the pelvis and perineum: report of a case with immunohistochemical and electron microscopic study. Pathologica 81:463–469, 1989

148. Steeper TA, Rosai J: Aggressive angiomyxoma of the female pelvis and perineum: report of nine cases of a distinctive type of gynecologic soft tissue neoplasm. Am J Surg Pathol 7:463–475, 1983

149. Fetsch JF, Laskin WB, Lefkowitz M, et al: Aggressive angiomyxoma. A clinicopathologic study of 29 female patients. Cancer 78:79–90, 1996

150. Woods SDS, Essex WB, Hughes ESR: Aggressive angiomyxoma of the female pelvis. Aust NZ J Surg 57:687–688, 1987

151. Tsang WYW, Chan JKC, Lee KC, et al: Aggressive angiomyxoma. A report of four cases occurring in men. Am J Surg Pathol 16:1059–1065, 1992

152. Fletcher CD, Tsang WY, Fisheer C, et al: Angiomyofibroblastoma of the vulva. A benign neoplasm distinct from aggressive angiomyxoma. Am J Surg Pathol 16:373–382, 1992

153. Taylor HB, Helwig EB: Dermatofibrosarcoma protuberans. A study of 115 cases. Cancer 15:717–725, 1962

154. McPeak CJ, Cruz T, Nicastri AD: Dermatofibrosarcoma protuberans: an analysis of 86 cases—five with metastasis. Ann Surg 166:803–813, 1967

155. Fletcher CDM, Evans BJ, Macartney JC, et al: Dermatofibrosarcoma protuberans: a clinicopathological and immunohistochemical study with a review of the literature. Histopathology 9:921–938, 1985

156. Kamino H, Jacobson M: Dermatofibroma extending into the subcutaneous tissue. Differential diagnosis from dermatofibrosarcoma protuberans. Am J Surg Pathol 14:1156–1164, 1990

157. Zelger B, Sideroff A, Stanzl U, et al: Deep penetrating dermatofibroma versus dermatofibrosarcoma protuberans. A clinicopathologic comparison. Am J Surg Pathol 18:677–686, 1994

158. Wrotnowski U, Cooper PH, Shmookler BM: Fibrosarcomatous change in dermatofibrosarcoma protuberans. Am J Surg Pathol 12:287–293, 1988

159. Ding J, Hashimoto H, Enjoji M: Dermatofibrosarcoma protuberans with fibrosarcomatous areas. A clinicopathologic study of nine cases and a comparison with allied tumors. Cancer 64:721–729, 1989

160. Connelly JH, Evans HL: Dermatofibrosarcoma protuberans. A clinicopathologic review with emphasis on fibrosarcomatous areas. Am J Surg Pathol 16:921–925, 1992

161. Beham A, Fletcher CDM: Dermatofibrosarcoma protuberans with areas resembling giant cell fibroblastoma: report of two cases. Histopathology 17:165–167, 1990

162. Alguacil-Garcia A: Giant cell fibroblastoma recurring as dermatofibrosarcoma protuberans. Am J Surg Pathol 15:798–801, 1991

163. Shmookler BM, Enzinger FM, Weiss SW: Giant cell fibroblastoma. A juvenile form of dermatofibrosarcoma protuberans. Cancer 64:2154–2161, 1989

164. Dupree WB, Langloss JN, Weiss SW: Pigmented dermatofibrosarcoma protuberans (Bednar tumor). A pathologic, ultrastructural, and immunohistochemical study. Am J Surg Pathol 9:630–639, 1985

165. Powers CN, Hurt MA, Frable WJ: Fine needle aspiration biopsy: dermatofibrosarcoma protuberans. Diagn Cytopathol 9:145–150, 1993

166. Shmookler BM, Enzinger FM: Giant cell fibroblastoma: a peculiar childhood tumor, abstracted. Lab Invest 46:76A, 1982

167. Shmookler BM, Enzinger FM, Weiss SW: Giant cell fibroblastoma: a juvenile form of dermatofibrosarcoma protuberans. Cancer 64:2154–2161, 1989

168. Abdul-Karim FW, Evans HL, Silva EG: Giant cell fibroblastoma: a report of three cases. Am J Clin Pathol 83:165–170, 1985

169. Yang AH, Chen BF: Intracytoplasmic giant cross-striated fibrils in giant cell fibroblastoma. Histopathology 27:383–385, 1995

170. Pinto A, Hwang WS, Wong AL, et al: Giant cell fibroblastoma in childhood. Immunohistochemical and ultrastructural study. Mod Pathol 5:639–642, 1992

171. Chou P, Gonzalez-Crussi F, Mangkorkanok M: Giant cell fibroblastoma. Cancer 63:756–762, 1989

172. Zámecník M, Michal M: Giant cell fibroblastoma with pigmented dermatofibrosarcoma protuberans component. Am J Surg Pathol 18:736–740, 1994

173. Evans HL: Low-grade fibromyxoid sarcoma. A report of two metastasizing neoplasms having a deceptively benign appearance. Am J Clin Pathol 88:615–619, 1987

174. Evans HL: Low grade fibromyxoid sarcoma. A report of 12 cases. Am J Surg Pathol 17:595–600, 1993

175. Devaney DM, Dervan P, O'Neill S, et al: Low grade fibromyxoid sarcoma. Histopathology 17:463–479, 1990

176. Goodlad JR, Mentzel T, Fletcher CDM: Low grade fibromyxoid sarcoma: clinicopathological analysis of eleven new cases in support of a distinct entity. Histopathology 26:229–238, 1995

177. Nichols GE, Cooper DH: Low-grade fibromyxoid sarcoma: case report and immunohistochemical study. J Cutan Pathol 21:356–362, 1994

178. Merck C, Hagmar B: Myxofibrosarcoma. Acta Cytol 24:137–144, 1980

179. Mentzel T, Calonje E, Wadden C, et al: Myxofibrosarcoma. Clinicopathologic analysis of 75 cases with emphasis on the low-grade variant. Am J Surg Pathol 20:391–405, 1996

180. Fukuda T, Tsuneyoshi M, Enjoji M: Malignant fibrous histiocytoma of soft parts: an ultrastructural quantitative study. Ultrastruct Pathol 12:117–129, 1988

181. Kindblom LG, Merck C, Angervall L: The ultrastructure of myxofibrosarcoma. A study of 11 cases. Virchows Arch A Pathol Anat Histol 381:121–139, 1979

182. Hirose T, Sano T, Hizawa K: Ultrastructural study of the myxoid area of malignant fibrous histiocytomas. Ultrastruct Pathol 12:621–630, 1988

183. Wood GS, Beckstead JH, Turner RR, et al: Malignant fibrous histiocytoma tumor cells resemble fibroblasts. Am J Surg Pathol 10:323–335, 1986

184. Becker RL, Venzon D, Lack EE, et al: Cytometry and morphometry of malignant fibrous histiocytoma of the extremities. Prediction of metastasis and mortality. Am J Surg Pathol 15:957–964, 1991

185. Angervall L, Kindblom LG, Merck C: Myxofibrosarcoma. A study of 30 cases. Acta Pathol Microbiol Scand (A) 85:127–140, 1977

186. Merck C, Angervall L, Kindblom LG, et al: Myxofibrosarcoma. A malignant soft tissue tumor of fibroblastic-histiocytic origin. A clinicopathologic and prognostic study of 110 cases using a multivariate analysis. APMIS, suppl. 282, 91:1–40, 1983

187. Weiss SW, Enzinger FM: Myxoid variant of malignant fibrous histiocytoma. Cancer 39:1672–1685, 1977

188. Merck C, Hagmar B: Myxofibrosarcoma. Acta Cytol 24:137–144, 1980

189. Walaas L, Angervall L, Hagmar B, et al: A correlative cytologic and histologic study of malignant fibrous histiocytoma: an analysis of 40 cases examined by fine needle aspiration cytology. Diagn Cytopathol 2:46–54, 1986

190. Scott SM, Reiman HM, Pritchard DJ, et al: Soft tissue fibrosarcoma: a clinicopathologic study of 132 cases. Cancer 64:925–931, 1989

191. Iwasaki H, Enjoji M: Infantile and adult fibrosarcomas of the soft tissues. Acta Pathol Jpn 29:377–388, 1979

192. Oshiro Y, Fukuda T, Tsuneyoshi M: Fibrosarcoma versus fibromatoses and cellular nodular fasciitis. A comparative study of their proliferative activity using proliferating cell nuclear antigen, DNA flow cytometry and p53. Am J Surg Pathol 18:709–712, 1994

193. Schofield DE, Fletcher JA, Grier HE, et al: Fibrosarcoma in infants and children. Application of new techniques. Am J Surg Pathol 18:14–24, 1994

194. Suh CH, Ordoñez NG, Mackay B: Fibrosarcoma: observations of the ultrastructure. Ultrastruct Pathol 17:221–229, 1993

195. Balsaver AM, Butler JJ, Martin RG: Congenital fibrosarcoma. Cancer 20:1607–1616, 1967

196. Chung EB, Enzinger FM: Infantile fibrosarcoma. Cancer 38:729–739, 1976

197. Soule EH, Pritchard DJ: Fibrosarcoma in infants and children. Cancer 40:1711–1721, 1977

198. Gonzalez-Crussi F, Wiederhold MD, Sotelo-Avila C: Congenital fibrosarcoma. Presence of a histiocytic component. Cancer 46:77–86, 1980

199. Madden NP, Spicer RD, Allibore EB, et al: Spontaneous regression of neonatal fibrosarcoma. Br J Cancer, suppl. 18:S72–75, 1992

200. Wilson MB, Stanley W, Sens D, et al: Infantile fibrosarcoma — a misnomer? Pediatr Pathol 10:901–907, 1990

201. Dal Cin P, Brock P, Casteels-van Daele M, et al: Cytogenetic characterization of congenital or infantile fibrosarcoma. Eur J Pediatr 150:579–581, 1991

202. Adam LR, Davison EV, Malcolm AJ, et al: Cytogenetic analysis of a congenital fibrosarcoma. Cancer Genet Cytogenet 52:37–41, 1991

203. Mandahl N, Heim S, Rydholm A, et al: Nonrandom numerical chromosome aberration (+8, +11, +17, +20) in infantile fibrosarcoma. Cancer Genet Cytogenet 40:137–139, 1989

204. Meis-Kindblom JM, Kindblom L-G, Enzinger FM: Sclerosing epithelioid fibrosarcoma. A variant of fibrosarcoma simulating carcinoma. Am J Surg Pathol 19:979–993, 1995

205. Reid R, Barrett A, Hamblen DL: Sclerosing epithelioid fibrosarcoma. Histopathology 28:451–455, 1996

206. Ushijima M, Tsuneyoshi M, Enjoji M: Dupuytren type fibromatoses: a clinicopathological study of 62 cases. Acta Pathol Jpn 34:991–1001, 1984

207. Iwasaki H, Muller H, Stutte JH, et al: Palmar fibromatosis (Dupuytren's contracture: ultrastructural and enzyme histochemical studies of 43 cases. Virchows Arch [A] 405:41–53, 1989

208. Murrell GA: An insight into Dupuytren's contracture. Ann R Coll Surg Engl 74:156–160, 1992

209. Aviles E, Arlen M, Miller T: Plantar fibromatosis. Surgery 69:117–120, 1971

210. Chesney J: Peyronie's disease. Br J Urol 47:209–218, 1975

211. Bodner H: Peyronie's disease revisited. Int Surg 63:69–71, 1978

212. Arafa M, Noble SG, Royle SG, et al: Dupuytren's and epilepsy revisited. N Hand Surg 17:221–226, 1992

213. Pryor JP, Khan O: Beta blockers and Peyronie's disease, letter. Lancet 1:331, 1979

214. Reye RDK: Recurring digital fibrous tumours of childhood. Arch Pathol 80:221–228, 1965

215. Rosenberg HS, Stenback WA, Spjut HJ: The fibromatoses of infancy and childhood. Perspect Pediatr Pathol 4:269–348, 1978

216. Purdy LJ, Colby TV: Infantile digital fibromatosis occurring outside the digit. Am J Surg Pathol 8:787–790, 1984

217. Pettinato G, Manivel JC, Gould EW, et al: Inclusion body fibromatosis of the breast. Two cases with immunohistochemical and ultrastructural findings. Am J Clin Pathol 101:714–718, 1994

218. Iwasaki H, Kikuchi M, Ohtsuki I, et al: Infantile digital fibromatosis. Identification of actin filaments in cytoplasmic inclusions by heavy meromyosin binding. Cancer 52:1653–1661, 1983

219. Zina AM, Rampini E, Fulcheri E, et al: Recurrent digital fibromatosis of childhood. An ultrastructural and immunohistochemical study of two cases. Am J Dermatopathol 8:22–26, 1986

220. Mukai M, Torikata C, Iri H, et al: Immunohistochemical identification of aggregated actin filaments in formalin-fixed paraffin-embedded sections: study of infantile digital fibromatosis by a new pretreatment. Am J Surg Pathol 16:110–115, 1992

221. Allen PW: The fibromatoses: a clinicopathologic classification based on 140 cases. Am J Surg Pathol 1:255–270, 1977

222. Gansar GF, Markowitz IP, Cerise EJ: Thirty years of experience with desmoid tumors at Charity Hospital. Am Surg 53:318–319, 1987

223. Reitamo JJ, Hayry P, Nykyri E, et al: The desmoid tumor. I. Am J Clin Pathol 77:665–673, 1982

224. Hayry P, Reitamo JJ, Vihko R, et al: The desmoid tumor. III. Am J Clin Pathol 77:681–685, 1982

225. Reitamo JJ, Scheinin TM, Hayry P: The desmoid syndrome. New aspects in the cause, pathogenesis and treatment of desmoid tumor. Am J Surg 151:230–237, 1986

226. Procter H, Singh L, Baum M, et al: Response of multicentric desmoid tumors to tamoxifen. Br J Surg 74:401–403, 1987

227. Burke AP, Sobin LH, Shekitka KM, et al: Intra-abdominal fibromatosis. A pathologic analysis of 130 tumors with comparison of clinical subgroups. Am J Surg Pathol 14:335–341, 1990

228. Burke AP, Sobin LH, Shekitka KM: Mesenteric fibromatosis. A follow-up study. Arch Pathol Lab Med 114:832–835, 1990

229. Ayala AG, Ro JY, Goepfert H, et al: Desmoid fibromatosis: a clinicopathologic study of 25 children. Semin Diagn Pathol 3:138–150, 1986

230. Rock MG, Pritchard DJ, Reiman HM, et al: Extraabdominal desmoid tumors. J Bone Joint Surg [Am] 66:1369–1374, 1984

231. Enzinger FM, Shiraki M: Musculo-aponeurotic fibromatosis of the shoulder girdle (extra-abdominal desmoid). Analysis of thirty cases followed up for ten or more years. Cancer 20:1131–1140, 1967

232. Zaharopoulos P, Wong J: Fine needle aspiration cytology in fibromatoses. Diagn Cytopathol 8:73–78, 1992

233. Raab SS, Silverman JF, McLeod DL, et al: Fine needle aspiration biopsy of fibromatoses. Acta Cytol 37:323–328, 1993

234. Dahl I, Hagmar B, Idvall I: Benign solitary neurilemoma (schwannoma): a correlative cytological and histological study of 28 cases. Acta Pathol Microbiol Immunol Scand 92:91–101, 1984

235. Rosenberg HS, Stenback WA, Spjut HG: The fibromatoses of infancy and childhood. Perspect Pediatric Pathol 4:269–348, 1978

236. Briselli MF, Soule EH, Gilchrist GS: Congenital fibromatosis. Report of 18 cases of solitary and 4 cases of multiple tumors. Mayo Clin Proc 55:554–562, 1980

237. Roggli VL, Kim H-S, Hawkins, E: Congenital generalized fibromatosis with visceral involvement. Cancer 45:954–960, 1980

238. Fletcher CD, Achu P, Van Noorden S, et al: Infantile myofibromatosis: a light microscopic, histochemical and immunohistochemical study suggesting true smooth muscle differentiation. Histopathology 11:245–258, 1987

239. Chung EB, Enzinger FM: Infantile myofibromatosis: a review of 59 cases with localized and generalized involvement. Cancer 48:1807–1818, 1981

240. Daimaru Y, Hashimoto H, Enjoji M: Myofibromatosis in adults (adult counterpart of infantile myofibromatosis). Am J Surg Pathol 13:859–865, 1989

241. Kitano Y: Juvenile hyalin fibromatosis. Arch Dermatol 112:86–88, 1976

242. Woyke S, Domagala W, Markiewicz D: A 19 year follow-up of multiple juvenile fibromatosis. J Pediatr Surg 19:302–306, 1984

243. Remberger K, Krieg T, Kunze D, et al: Fibromatosis hyalinica multiplex (juvenile hyaline fibromatosis): light microscopic, electron microscopic, immunohistochemical and biochemical findings. Cancer 56:614–624, 1985

244. Woyke A, Domagala W, Olszuvski WW: Ultrastructure of a fibromatosis hyalinica multiplex juvenilis. Cancer 26:1157–1168, 1970

245. Rosenberg HS, Stenback WA, Spjut HG: The fibromatoses of infancy and childhood. Perspect Pediatric Pathol 4:269–348, 1978

246. Cuestas-Carnero R, Barnancini CA: Hereditary gingival fibromatosis associated with hypertrichosis: report of five cases in one family. J Oral Maxillofac Surg 46:415–420, 1988

247. Bakaren G, Scully C: Hereditary gingival fibromatosis in a family with Zimmerman-Laband syndrome. J Oral Pathol Med 20:457–463, 1991

248. Sonoda T, Hashimoto H, Enjoji M: Juvenile xanthogranuloma. Clinicopathologic analysis and immunohistochemical study of 57 patients. Cancer 56:2280–2286, 1985

249. Winkelmann RK, Oliver GF: Subcutaneous xanthogranulomatosis: an inflammatory non-X histiocytic syndrome (subcutaneous xanthomatosis). J Am Acad Dermatol 21:924–929, 1989

250. Janney CG, Hurt MA, Santa-Cruz DJ: Deep juvenile xanthogranuloma. Subcutaneous and intramuscular forms. Am J Surg Pathol 15:150–159, 1991

251. Jones FE, Soule EH, Coventry MB: Fibrous xanthoma of synovium (giant-cell tumor of tendon sheath, pigmented nodular synovitis). A study of one hundred and eighteen cases. J Bone Joint Surg [Am] 51:76–86, 1969

252. Ushijima M, Hashimoto H, Tsuneyoshi M, et al: Giant cell tumor of the tendon sheath (nodular tenosynovitis). A study of 207 cases to compare the large joint group with the common digit group. Cancer 57:875–884, 1986

253. Kindblom LG, Gunterberg B: Pigmented villonodular synovitis involving bone. J Bone Joint Surg [Am] 60:830–832, 1978

254. Wood GS, Beckstead JH, Medeiros JL, et al: The cells of giant cell tumor of tendon sheath resemble osteoclasts. Am J Surg Pathol 12:444–452, 1988

255. Kahn LB: Malignant giant cell tumor of the tendon sheath. Ultrastructural study and review of the literature. Arch Pathol Lab Med 95:203–208, 1973

256. Castens HP, Howell RS: Malignant giant cell tumor of tendon sheath. Virchows Arch [A] 382:237–243, 1979

257. Wakely PE Jr, Frable WJ: Fine-needle aspiration biopsy cytology of giant-cell tumor of tendon sheath. Am J Clin Pathol 102:87–90, 1994

258. Enzinger FM, Zhang R: Plexiform fibrohistiocytic tumor presenting in children and young adults. An analysis of 65 cases. Am J Surg Pathol 12:818–826, 1988

259. Angervall L, Kindblom LG, Lindholm S, et al: Plexiform fibrohistiocytic tumor. Report of a case involving preoperative aspiration cytology and immunohistochemical and ultrastructural analysis of surgical specimens. Pathol Res Pract 188:350–356, 1992

260. Hollywood K, Holley MP, Fletcher CDM: Plexiform fibrohistiocytic tumor: clinicopathological, immunohistochemical and ultrastructural analysis in favor of a myofibroblastic lesion. Histopathology 19:503–513, 1991

261. Smith S, Fletcher CDM, Smith MA, et al: Cytogenetic analysis of a plexiform fibrohistiocytic tumor. Cancer Genet Cytogenet 48:31–34, 1990

262. Costa MJ, Weiss SW: Angiomatoid malignant fibrous histiocytoma. A long-term follow up study of 108 cases with evaluation of histologic predictors of outcome. Am J Surg Pathol 14:1126–1132, 1990

263. Enzinger FM: Angiomatoid malignant fibrous histiocytoma. A distinctive fibrohistiocytic tumor of children and young adults simulating a vascular neoplasm. Cancer 44:2147–2157, 1979

264. Smith MEF, Costa MJ, Weiss SW: Evaluation of CD68 and other histiocytic antigens in angiomatoid malignant fibrous histiocytoma. Am J Surg Pathol 15:757–763, 1991

265. Sun C-CJ, Toker C, Breitenecker R: An ultrastructural study of angiomatoid fibrous histiocytoma. Cancer 49:2103–2111, 1982

266. Wegmann W, Heitz PU: Angiomatoid malignant fibrous histiocytoma. Evidence for the histiocyte origin of tumor cells. Virchows Arch [A] 406:59–66, 1985

267. Pettinato G, Manivel JC, De Rosa G, et al: Angiomatoid malignant fibrous histiocytoma: cytologic, immunohistochemical, and flow cytometric study of 20 cases. Mod Pathol 3:479–487, 1990

268. Fletcher CDM: Angiomatoid "malignant fibrous histiocytoma." An immunohistochemical study indicative of myoid differentiation. Hum Pathol 22:563–568, 1991

269. Pezzi CM, Rawlings MS Jr, Esgro JJ, et al: Prognostic factors in 227 patients with malignant fibrous histiocytoma. Cancer 69:2098–2103, 1992

270. Fletcher CD: Pleomorphic malignant fibrous histiocytoma: fact or fiction? A critical reappraisal based on 159 tumors diagnosed as pleomorphic sarcoma. Am J Surg Pathol 16:213–228, 1992

271. Kempson RL, Kyriakos M: Fibroxanthosarcoma of the soft tissues: a type of malignant fibrous histiocytoma. Cancer 29:961–976, 1972

272. Kearney MM, Soule EH, Ivins JC: Malignant fibrous histiocytoma. A retrospective study of 167 cases. Cancer 45:167–178, 1980

273. Taxy JB, Battifora H: Malignant fibrous histiocytoma. An electron microscopic study. Cancer 40:254–267, 1977

274. Walaas L, Angervall L, Hagmar B, et al: A correlative cytologic and histologic study of malignant fibrous histiocytoma: an analysis of 40 cases examined by fine needle aspiration cytology. Diagn Cytopathol 2:46–54, 1986

275. Guccian JG, Enzinger FM: Malignant giant cell tumor of soft parts: an analysis of 32 cases. Cancer 29:1518–1529, 1972

276. Alguacil-Garcia A, Unni KK, Goelner JR: Malignant giant cell tumor of soft parts; ultrastructural study of four cases. Cancer 40:244–253, 1977

277. Gould E, Albores-Saavedra J, Roth M, et al; Malignant giant cell tumor of soft parts presenting as a skin tumor. Am J Dermatopathol 11:197–201, 1989

278. Angervall L, Hagmar B, Kindblom L, et al: Malignant giant cell tumor of soft tissues. A clinicopathologic, cytologic, ultrastructural, angiographic, and microangiographic study. Cancer 47:736–747, 1981

279. Kyriakos M, Kempson RL: Inflammatory fibrous histiocytoma: an aggressive and lethal lesion. Cancer 37:1584–1606, 1976

280. Isoda M, Yasumoto S: Eosinophil chemotactic factor derived from a malignant fibrous histiocytoma. Clin Exp Dermatol 11:253–258, 1986

281. Takahashi K, Kimura Y, Naito M, et al: Inflammatory fibrous histiocytoma presenting leukemoid reaction. Pathol Res Pract 184:498–502, 1989

282. Walaas L, Angervall L, Hagmar B, et al: A correlative cytologic and histologic study of malignant fibrous histiocytoma: an analysis of 40 cases examined by fine needle aspiration cytology. Diagn Cytopathol 2:46–54, 1986

283. Signen RD, Bregman D, Klausner S: Giant lipoma of the mesentery: report of an unusual case and review of the literature. Am Surg 42:595–597, 1976

284. Weitzner S, Blumenthal BI, Moynihan PC: Retroperitoneal lipoma in children. J Pediatr Surg 14:88–91, 1979

285. Bennhoff DF, Wood JW: Infiltrating lipomata of the head and neck. Laryngoscope 88:839–840, 1978

286. Bjerregaard P, Hagen K, Daugaard S, et al: Intramuscular lipoma of the lower limb: long term follow-up after local resection. J Bone Joint Surg [Br] 71:812–816, 1989

287. Banny JM, Bilbao MK, Hodges CV: Pelvic lipomatosis: a rare cause of suprapubic mass. J Urol 109:592–595, 1973

288. Kindblom LG, Angervall L, Stener B, et al: Intermuscular and intramuscular lipomas and hibernomas; clinical, roentgenologic, histologic, and prognostic study of 46 cases. Cancer 33:754–762, 1974

289. Fletcher CD, Martin-Bates E: Intramuscular and intermuscular lipoma: neglected diagnoses. Histopathology 12:275–287, 1988

290. Walaas L, Kindblom LG: Lipomatous tumors: a correlative cytologic and histologic study of 27 tumors examined by fine needle aspiration cytology. Hum Pathol 16:6–18, 1985

291. Akerman M, Rydholm A: Aspiration cytology of lipomatous tumors: a 10-year experience at an Orthopedic Oncology Center. Diagn Cytopathol 3:295–302, 1987

292. Willén H, Akerman M, Carlen B: Fine needle aspiration (FNA) in the diagnosis of soft tissue tumours; a review of 22 years experience. Cytopathology 6:236–247, 1995

293. Howard WR, Helwig ER: Angiolipoma. Arch Dermatol 82:924–931, 1960

294. Belcher RW, Czarnetzki BM, Carney JF: Multiple (subcutaneous) angiolipomas. Clinical, pathologic and pharmacologic studies. Arch Dermatol 110:583–587, 1974

295. Gorlin RJ: Some soft tissue heritable tumors. Birth Defects 12:72–79, 1976

296. Lin JJ, Lin F: Two entities in angiolipoma: a study of 459 cases of lipoma with review of the literature on infiltrating angiolipoma. Cancer 34:720–727, 1974

297. Hunt SJ, Santa Cruz DJ, Barr RJ: Cellular angiolipoma. Am J Surg Pathol 14:75–79, 1990

298. Meis JM, Enzinger FM: Myolipoma of soft tissue. Am J Surg Pathol 15:121–125, 1991

299. Tong YC, Chieng PU, Tsa TC, et al: Renal angiomyolipoma: report of 24 cases. Br J Urol 66:585–589, 1990

300. Farrow GM, Harrison EG, Utz DC: Renal angiomyolipoma: a clinicopathologic study of 32 cases. Cancer 22:564–570, 1968

301. Heckle W, Osterhage HR, Frohmuller HG: Diagnosis and treatment of renal angiomyolipoma. Urol Int 42:201–206, 1987

302. Ashfaq R, Weinberg AG, Albores-Saavedra J: Renal angiomyolipomas and HMB-45 reactivity. Cancer 71:3091–3097, 1993

303. Sant GR, Ucci AA Jr, Meares EM Jr: Multicentric angiomyolipoma: renal and lymph node involvement. Urology 28:111–113, 1986

304. Manabe T, Moriya T, Kimoto M: Benign renal angiomyolipoma with regional lymph node involvement in renal angiomyolipoma. J Urol 128:1292–1296, 1982

305. Ferry JA, Malt RA, Young RH: Renal angiomyolipomas with sarcomatous transformation and pulmonary metastases. Am J Surg Pathol 15:1083–1088, 1991

306. Wadih GE, Raab SS, Silverman JF: Fine needle aspiration cytology of renal and retroperitoneal angiomyolipoma. Report of two cases with cytologic findings and clinicopathologic pitfalls in diagnosis. Acta Cytol 39:945–950, 1995

307. Tallada N, Martinez S, Raventos A: Cytologic study of renal angiomyolipoma by fine-needle aspiration biopsy: report of four cases. Diagn Cytopathol 10:37–40, 1994

308. Fowler MR, Alba JM, William RB, et al: Extraadrenal myelolipomas compared with extramedullary hematopoietic tumors: a case of presacral myelolipoma. Am J Surg Pathol 6:363–374, 1982

309. Massey GS, Green JB, Marsh WL: Presacral myelolipoma. Cancer 60:403–406, 1987

310. Burrows S, Drake WM Jr, Singley TL: Large retroperitoneal myelolipoma associated with acute myelogenous leukemia. Am J Clin Pathol 52:733–737, 1969

311. Hunter SB, Schemakewitz EH, Patterson C, et al: Extraadrenal myelolipoma; a report of two cases. Am J Clin Pathol 97:402–404, 1992

312. Wilhelmus JL, Schrodt GR, Alberhasky MT, et al: Giant adrenal myelolipoma. Arch Pathol Lab Med 105:532–535, 1981

313. Bennett BD, McKenna TJ, Hough AJ, et al: Adrenal myelolipoma associated with Cushing's disease. Am J Clin Pathol 73:443–447, 1980

314. Vyberg M, Sestoft L: Combined adrenal myelolipoma and adenoma associated with Cushing's syndrome. Am J Clin Pathol 86:541–545, 1986

315. Meis JM, Enzinger FM: Chondroid lipoma. A unique tumor simulating liposarcoma and myxoid chondrosarcoma. Am J Surg Pathol 17:1103–1112, 1993

316. Nielsen GP, O'Connell JX, Dickersin GR, et al: Chondroid lipoma, a tumor of white fat cells. A brief report of two cases with ultrastructural analysis. Am J Surg Pathol 19:1272–1276, 1995

317. Kindblom L-G, Meis-Kindblom JM: Chondroid lipoma. An ultrastructural and immunohistochemical analysis with further observations regarding its differentiation. Hum Pathol 26:706–715, 1995

318. Dardrik IU: Hibernoma: a possible model of brown fat histogenesis. Hum Pathol 9:321–329, 1978

319. Levine GD: Hibernoma: an electron microscopic study. Hum Pathol 3:351, 1972

320. Rigor VU, Goldstone SE, Jones J, et al: Hibernoma: a case report and discussion of a rare tumor. Cancer 57:2207–2211, 1986

321. Ahn C, Harvey JC: Mediastinal hibernoma a rare tumor. Ann Thorac Surg 50:828–831, 1990

322. Albores-Saavedra J, Larraza O, Alonso-Ruiz P: Hibernoma maligno con metastasis pulmonares. Patologia 18:193–203, 1980

323. Enterline HT, Lowry LD, Richman AV: Does malignant hibernoma exist? Am J Surg Pathol 3:265–271, 1979

324. Jeanrenaud B: Lipid components of adipose tissue. p. 169. In: Handbook of Physiology. American Physiological Society, Washington DC, 1965

325. Hashimoto CH, Cobb CJ: Cytodiagnosis of hibernoma. A case report. Diagn Cytopathol 3:326–329, 1987

326. Walaas L, Kindblom LG: Lipomatous tumors: A correlative cytologic and histologic study of 27 tumors examined by fine needle aspiration cytology. Hum Pathol 16:6–18, 1985

327. Vellios F, Baez J, Shumacker HB: Lipoblastomatosis: a tumor of fetal fat different from hibernoma. Am J Pathol 34:1149–1159, 1958

328. Chung EB, Enzinger FM: Benign lipoblastomatosis: an analysis of 35 cases. Cancer 32:482–492, 1973

329. Alba Greco M, Garcia RL, Vuletin JC: Benign lipoblastomatosis: ultrastructure and histogenesis. Cancer 45:511–515, 1980

330. Hanada M, Tokuda R, Ohnishi Y, et al: Benign lipoblastoma and liposarcoma in children. Acta Pathol Jpn 36:605–612, 1986

331. Gaffney EF, Vellios F, Hargreaves HK: Lipoblastomatosis: ultrastructure of two cases and relationship to human fetal white adipose tissue. Pediatr Pathol 5:207–216, 1986

332. Jimenez JF: Lipoblastoma in infancy and childhood. J Surg Oncol 32:238–244, 1986

333. Dharan M, Siplovich L: Intraoperative cytology of lipoblastoma. A case report. Acta Cytol 37:563–565, 1992

334. Enzinger FM, Harvey DA: Spindle cell lipoma. Cancer 36:1852–1859, 1975

335. Angervall L, Dahl I, Kindblom LG, et al: Spindle cell lipoma. Acta Pathol Microbiol Scand 84:477–487, 1976

336. Shmookler BM, Enzinger FM: Pleomorphic lipoma: a benign tumor simulating liposarcoma. A clinicopathologic analysis of 48 cases. Cancer 47:126–133, 1981

337. Azzopardi JG, Iocco J, Salm R: Pleomorphic lipoma: a tumour simulating liposarcoma. Histopathology 7:511–523, 1983

338. Bolen JW, Thorning D: Spindle-cell lipoma: a clinical, light- and electron-microscopical study. Am J Surg Pathol 5:435–441, 1981

339. Fletcher CDM, Martin-Bates E: Spindle cell lipoma: a clinicopathological study with some original observations. Histopathology 11:803–817, 1987

340. Warkel RL, Rehme CG, Thompson WH: Vascular spindle cell lipoma. J Cutan Pathol 9:113–118, 1982

341. Hawley IC, Krausz T, Evans DJ, et al: Spindle cell lipoma—a pseudoangiomatous variant. Histopathology 24:565–569, 1994

342. Beham A, Schmid C, Hodi S, et al: Spindle cell and pleomorphic lipoma: an immunohistochemical study and histogenetic analysis. J Pathol 158:219–222, 1989

343. Pitt MA, Roberts IS, Curry A: Spindle cell and pleomorphic lipoma: an ultrastructural study. Ultrastruct Pathol 19:475–480, 1995

344. Enzinger FM, Winslow DJ: Liposarcoma. A study of 103 cases. Virchows Arch [A] 335:367–388, 1962

345. Kindblom L-G, Angervall L, Svendsen P: Liposarcoma. A clinicopathologic, radiographic and prognostic study. Acta Pathol Microbiol Scand Sect A Suppl 253:1–71, 1975

346. Evans HL, Soule EH, Winklemann RK: Atypical lipoma, atypical intra-

muscular lipoma and well differentiated retroperitoneal liposarcoma. A reappraisal of 30 cases formerly classified as well differentiated liposarcoma. Cancer 43:574–584, 1979

347. Evans HL: Liposarcoma. A study of 55 cases with reassessment of its classification. Am J Surg Pathol 3:507–523, 1979

348. Hashimoto H, Enjoji M: Liposarcoma: a clinicopathologic subtyping of 52 cases. Acta Pathol Jpn 32:933–948, 1982

349. Bolen JW, Thorning D: Liposarcomas: a histogenetic approach to the classification of adipose tissue neoplasms. Am J Surg Pathol 8:3–17, 1984

350. Azumi N, Curtis J, Kempson RL, et al: Atypical and malignant neoplasms showing lipomatous differentiation. A study of 11 cases. Am J Surg Pathol 11:161–183, 1987

351. Evans HL: Liposarcomas and atypical lipomatous tumors: a study of 66 cases followed for a minimum of 10 years. Surg Pathol 1:41–54, 1988

352. Chang HR, Hajdu SI, Collin C, et al: The prognostic value of histologic subtypes in primary extremity liposarcoma. Cancer 64:1514–1520, 1989

353. Mentzel T, Fletcher CDM: Lipomatous tumours of soft tissues: an update. Virchows Arch 427:353–363, 1995

354. Weiss SW: WHO Histologic Typing of Soft Tissue Tumors. 2nd Ed. Springer-Verlag, New York, 1994

355. Enzinger FM, Weiss SW: Liposarcoma. pp. 431–466. In Enzinger FM, Weiss SW (eds): Soft Tissue Tumors. CV Mosby, St. Louis, 1995

356. Sreekantaiah C, Karakousis CP, Leong SP, et al: Cytogenetic findings in liposarcoma correlate with histopathologic subtypes. Cancer 69:2484–2495, 1992

357. Fletcher CD, Akerman M, Dal Clin P, et al: Correlation between clinicopathological features and karyotype in lipomatous tumors. A report of 178 cases from the Chromosome and Morphology (CHAMP) Collaborative Study Group. Am J Pathol 148:623–630, 1996

358. Mathur DR, Ramdeo IN, Sharma SP, et al: Signet ring cell lymphoma simulating liposarcoma—a case report with brief review of literature, review. Indian J Cancer 25:52–55, 1988

359. Smith TA, Easley KA, Goldblum JR: Myxoid/round cell liposarcoma of the extremities. A clinicopathologic study of 29 cases with particular attention to extent of round cell liposarcoma. Am J Surg Pathol 20:171–180, 1996

360. Kindblom L-G, Angervall L, Fassina AS: Atypical lipoma. Acta Pathol Microbiol Scand Sect A 90:27–36, 1982

361. Weiss SW, Rao VK: Well-differentiated liposarcoma (atypical lipoma) of deep soft tissue of the extremities, retroperitoneum and miscellaneous sites. A follow-up study of 92 cases with analysis of the incidence of "dedifferentiation." Am J Surg Pathol 16:1051–1058, 1992

362. Evans HL: Smooth muscle in atypical lipomatous tumors. A report of three cases. Am J Surg Pathol 14:714–771, 1990

363. Suster S, Wong TY, Moran CA: Sarcomas with combined features of liposarcoma and leiomyosarcoma: study of two cases of an unusual soft-tissue tumor showing dual lineage differentiation. Am J Surg Pathol 17:905–911, 1993

364. Lucas DR, Nascimento AG, Sanjay BK, et al: Well-differentiated liposarcoma. The Mayo Clinic experience with 58 cases. Am J Clin Pathol 102:677–683, 1994

365. McCormick D, Mentzel T, Beham A, et al: Dedifferentiated liposarcoma: a clinicopathologic analysis of 32 cases suggesting a better prognostic subgroup among the pleomorphic sarcomas. Am J Surg Pathol 18:1213–1223, 1994

366. Snover DC, Sumner HW, Dehner LP: Variability of histologic pattern in recurrent soft tissue sarcomas originally diagnosed as liposarcoma. Cancer 49:1005–1015, 1982

367. Tallini G, Erlandson RA, Brennan MF, et al: Divergent myosarcomatous differentiation in retroperitoneal liposarcoma. Am J Surg Pathol 17:546–556, 1993

368. Evans HL, Khurana KK, Kemp BL, et al: Heterologous elements in the dedifferentiated component of dedifferentiated liposarcoma. Am J Surg Pathol 18:1150–1157, 1994

369. Hashimoto H, Daimaru Y, Tsuneyoshi M, et al: Soft tissue sarcoma with additional anaplastic components. A clinicopathologic and immunohistochemical study of 27 cases. Cancer 66:1578–1589, 1990

370. Meis JM: Dedifferentiation in bone and soft tissue tumors: a histological indicator of tumor progression. Part 1. Pathol Annu 1:37–62, 1991

371. Coindre JM, de Loynes B, Bui NB, et al: Dedifferentiated liposarcoma: a clinicopathologic study of 6 cases. Ann Pathol 12:20–28, 1992

372. Dei Tos AP, Mentzel T, Newman PL, et al: Spindle cell liposarcoma: a hitherto unrecognized variant of liposarcoma: analysis of six cases. Am J Surg Pathol 18:913–921, 1994

373. Klimstra DS, Moran CA, Perino G, et al: Liposarcoma of the anterior mediastinum and thymus. A clinicopathologic study of 28 cases. Am J Surg Pathol 19:782–791, 1995

374. Shmookler BM, Enzinger FM: Liposarcoma occurring in children. An analysis of 17 cases and review of the literature. Cancer 52:567–574, 1983

375. Castleberry RP, Kelly DR, Wilson ER, et al: Childhood liposarcoma. Report of a case and review of the literature. Cancer 54:579–584, 1984

376. Gould VE, Jao W, Gould NS, et al: Electron microscopy of adipose tissue tumors: comparative features of hibernomas, myxoid and pleomorphic liposarcomas. Pathobiol Annu 9:339–357, 1979

377. Lagace R, Jacob S, Seemayer TA: Myxoid liposarcoma: an electron-microscopic study: biological and histogenic considerations. Virchows Arch (Pathol Anat) 384:159–172, 1979

378. Kindblom L-G, Säve-Södebergh J: The ultrastructure of liposarcoma: a study of 10 cases. Acta Pathol Microbiol Scand 87:109–121, 1979

379. Battifora H, Nunez-Alonso C: Myxoid liposarcoma: study of ten cases. Ultrastruct Pathol 1:157–169, 1980

380. Fu YS, Parker FG, Kaye GI, et al: Ultrastructure of benign and malignant adipose tissue tumors. Part 1, Pathol Annu 15:67–89, 1980

381. Rossouw DJ, Cinti S, Dickersin GR: Liposarcoma: an ultrastructural study of 15 cases. Am J Clin Pathol 85:649–667, 1985

382. Erlandson RA: Ultrastructural features of specific human neoplasms. pp. 475–481. In: Diagnostic Transmission Electron Microscopy of Tumors. Lippincott-Raven, Philadelphia 1994

383. Suzuki T: Ultrastructural characteristics of a pleomorphic liposarcoma: a possible involvement of myofibroblasts. Acta Pathol Jpn 37:843–852, 1987

384. Walaas L, Kindblom LG: Lipomatous tumors: a correlative cytologic and histologic study of 27 tumors examined by fine needle aspiration cytology. Hum Pathol 16:6–18, 1985

385. Akerman M, Rydholm A: Aspiration cytology of lipomatous tumors: a 10-year experience at an Orthopedic Oncology Center. Diagn Cytopathol 3:295–302, 1987

386. Wakely PE, Geisinger KR, Cappellari JO, et al: Fine-needle aspiration cytopathology of soft tissue: chondromyxoid and myxoid lesions. Diagn Cytopathol 12:101–105, 1995

387. Klopfer HW, Krafchuk J, Dubes V, et al: Hereditary multiple leiomyoma of the skin. Am J Hum Genet 10:48–52, 1958

388. Fisher WC, Helwig EB: Leiomyomas of the skin. Arch Dermatol 88:510–520, 1963

389. Smith LJ Jr: Tumors of the corium. p. 533. In Helwig EB, Mostofi FK (eds): The Skin. International Academy of Pathology Monograph. Williams & Wilkins, Baltimore, 1971

390. Nascimento AG, Karas M, Rosen PP, et al: Leiomyoma of the nipple. Am J Surg Pathol 3:151–154, 1979

391. Newman PL, Fletcher CDM: Smooth muscle tumours of the external genitalia: clinicopathologic analysis of a series. Histopathology 18:523–529, 1991

392. Hachisuga T, Hashimoto H, Enjoji M: Angioleiomyoma. A clinico-pathologic reappraisal of 562 cases. Cancer 54:126–130, 1984

393. Goodman AH, Briggs RC: Deep leiomyoma in an extremity. J Bone Joint Surg [Am] 47:529–532, 1965

394. Ledesma-Medina J, Oh KS, Girdany BR: Calcification in childhood leiomyoma. Radiology 135:339–341, 1980

395. Drew EJ: Large leiomyoma of the upper extremity. Am J Surg 112:938–940, 1966

396. Goodman AH, Briggs RC: Deep leiomyoma of an extremity. J Bone Joint Surg 47A:529–532, 1965

397. Kilpatric SE, Mentzel T, Fletcher CDM: Leiomyoma of deep soft tissue. Clinicopathologic analysis of a series. Am J Surg Pathol 18:576–582, 1994

398. Fields JP, Helwig EB: Leiomyosarcomas of the skin and subcutaneous tissue. Cancer 47:156–169, 1981

399. Berlin O, Stener B, Lars-Gunner K, Angervall L: Leiomyosarcoma of venous origin in the extremities. Cancer 54:2147–2159, 1984

400. Leu HJ, Makek M: Intramural venous leiomyosarcomas. Cancer 57:1395–1400, 1986

401. Varela-Duran J, Oliva H, Rosai J: Vascular leiomyosarcoma. The malignant counterpart of vascular leiomyoma. Cancer 44:1684–1691, 1979

402. Tsukada T, Tippens D, Gordon D, et al: HHF 35, a muscle actin-specific monoclonal antibody: I. Immunocytochemical and biochemical characterization. Am J Pathol 126:51–60, 1987

403. Miettinen M: Immunoreactivity for cytokeratin and epithelial membrane antigen in leiomyosarcoma. Arch Pathol Lab Med 112:637–640, 1988

404. Wile AG, Evans HL, Romsdahl MM: Leiomyosarcoma of soft tissue. A clinicopathologic study. Cancer 48:1022–1032, 1981

405. Shmookler BM, Lauer DH: Retroperitoneal leiomyosarcoma. A clinico-pathologic analysis of 36 cases. Am J Surg Pathol 7:269–280, 1983

406. Hashimoto H, Daimaru Y, Tsuneyoshi M, et al: Leiomyosarcoma of the external soft tissues: a clinicopathologic, immunohistochemical, and electron microscopic study. Cancer 57:2077–2088, 1986

407. Tao LC, Davidson DD: Aspiration biopsy cytology of smooth muscle tumors. Acta Cytol 37:300–308, 1993

408. Dahl I, Hagmar B, Angervall L: Leiomyosarcoma of the soft tissue. A correlative cytological and histological study of 11 cases. Acta Pathol Microbiol Scand [A] 89:285–291, 1981

409. Dahl I, Hagmar B, Idvall I: Benign solitary neurilemoma (schwannoma): a correlative cytological and histological study of 28 cases. Acta Pathol Microbiol Immunol Scand 92:91–101, 1984

410. DiSant' Agnese PA, Knowles DM: Extracardiac rhabdomyoma: a clinicopathologic study and review of the literature. Cancer 46:780–789, 1980

411. Fu YS, Perzin KH: Non-epithelial tumors of the nasal cavity, paranasal sinuses, and nasopharynx: a clinicopathological study. V. Skeletal muscle tumors (rhabdomyoma and rhabdomyosarcoma). Cancer 37:367–372, 1976

412. Gibas Z, Miettinen M: Recurrent parapharyngeal rhabdomyoma: evidence of neoplastic nature of the tumor from cytogenetic study. Am J Surg Pathol 16:721–728, 1992

413. Hamper K, Renninghoff J, Schafer H: Rhabdomyoma of the larynx recurring after 12 years: immunohistochemistry and differential diagnosis. Arch Otorhinolaryngol 246:222–226, 1989

414. Vuong PN, Neveux Y, Balaton A, et al: Adult type rhabdomyoma of the palate. Cytologic presentation of two cases with histologic and immunologic study. Acta Cytol 34:413–419, 1990

415. Dehner LP, Enzinger FM, Font RL: Fetal rhabdomyoma: an analysis of nine cases. Cancer 30:160–166, 1972

416. Tani E, Ersöz C, Silversward C, et al: Rhabdomyoma: primary diagnosis by fine needle aspiration (FNA) cytology and immunocytochemistry. Cytopathology 6:204–208, 1995

417. Burke AP, Virmani R: Cardiac rhabdomyoma: a clinicopathologic study. Mod Pathol 4:70–74, 1991

418. Newton WA, Gehan EA, Webber BL: Classification of rhabdomyosarcomas and related sarcomas. Pathologic aspects and proposal for a new classification. An Intergroup Rhabdomyosarcoma Study. Cancer 76:1073–1085, 1995

419. Wijnaendts LCD, Linden VD, Van Unnik AJM, et al: Histopathological classification of childhood rhabdomyosarcomas: relationship with clinical parameters and prognosis. Hum Pathol 25:900–907, 1994

420. Tsokos M, Webber B, Parham D, et al: Rhabdomyosarcoma: a new classification scheme related to prognosis. Arch Pathol Lab Med 116:847–855, 1992

421. Raney RB, Tefft M, Lawrence W, et al: Paratesticular sarcoma in childhood and adolescence: a report from the Intergroup Rhabdomyosarcoma Studies I and II, 1973–1983. Cancer 60:2337–2343, 1987

422. Lloyd RV, Hajdu SI, Knapper WH: Embryonal rhabdomyosarcoma in adults. Cancer 51:557–565, 1983

423. de Jong AS, van Kessel-van Vark M, Albus-Lutter CE, et al: Skeletal muscle actin as tumor marker in the diagnosis of rhabdomyosarcoma in childhood. Am J Surg Pathol 9:467–474, 1985

424. Parham DM, Webber B, Hold H, et al: Immunohistochemical study of childhood rhabdomyosarcomas and related neoplasms: results of an Intergroup Rhabdomyosarcoma Study project. Cancer 67:3072–3080, 1991

425. Dias P, Parham DM, Shapiro DN, et al: Myogenic regulatory protein (MyoD1) expression in childhood solid tumors: diagnostic utility in rhabdomyosarcoma. Am J Pathol 137:1283–1291, 1990

426. Lack EE, Parez-Atayde AR, Schuster SR: Botryoid rhabdomyosarcoma of the biliary tree. Am J Surg Pathol 5:643–652, 1981

427. Cavazzana AO, Schmidt D, Ninfo V, et al: Spindle cell rhabdomyosarcoma: a prognostically favorable variant of rhabdomyosarcoma. Am J Surg Pathol 16:229–235, 1992

428. Leuschner I, Newton WA, Schmidt D, et al: Spindle cell variants of embryonal rhabdomyosarcoma in the paratesticular region: a report of the Intergroup Rhabdomyosarcoma Study. Am J Surg Pathol 17:221–230, 1993

429. Horn RC, Enterline HT: Rhabdomyosarcoma: a clinicopathologic study of 39 cases. Cancer 11:181–199, 1958

430. Enzinger FM, Shiraki M: Alveolar rhabdomyosarcoma: an analysis of 110 cases. Cancer 24:18–31, 1969

431. Douglass EC, Rowe ST, Valentine M, et al: Variant translocations of chromosome 13 in alveolar rhabdomyosarcoma. Genes Chromosom Cancer 3:480–482, 1991

432. Albores-Saavedra J, Martin RG, Smith JL: Rhabdomyosarcoma. A study of 35 cases. Ann Surg 157:186–197, 1963

433. Schürch W, Bégin LR, Seemayer TA, et al: Pleomorphic soft tissue myogenic sarcomas of adulthood. Am J Surg Pathol 20:131–147, 1996

434. Gaffney EF, Dervan PA, Fletcher CD: Pleomorphic rhabdomyosarcoma in adulthood. Analysis of 11 cases with definition of diagnostic criteria. Am J Surg Pathol 17:601–609, 1993

435. Hollowood K, Fletcher CD: Rhabdomyosarcoma in adults. Semin Diagn Pathol 11:47–57, 1994

436. Seidal T, Walaas L, Kindblom LG, Angervall L: Cytology of embryonal rhabdomyosarcoma: a cytologic, light microscopic, electron microscopic, and immunohistochemical study of seven cases. Diagn Cytopathol 4:292–299, 1988

437. Seidal T, Mark J, Hagmar B, Angervall L: Alveolar rhabdomyosarcoma: a cytogenetic and correlated cytological and histological study. Acta Pathol Microbiol Immunol Scand 90:345–354, 1982

438. Akhtar M, Ali MA, Bakry M, et al: Fine needle aspiration biopsy diagnosis of rhabdomyosarcoma: cytologic, histologic, and ultrastructural correlations. Diagn Cytopathol 8:465–474, 1992

439. Almeida M, Stastny JF, Wakely PE, et al: Fine-needle aspiration biopsy of childhood rhabdomyosarcoma: reevaluation of the cytologic criteria for diagnosis. Diagn Cytopathol 11:231–236, 1994

440. Hoehn JG, Farrow GM, Devine KD, et al: Invasive hemangioma of the head and neck. Am J Surg 120:495–500, 1970

441. Johnson WC: Pathology of cutaneous vascular tumors. Int J Dermatol 15:239–270, 1976

442. Rodriguez-Erdmann F, Button L, Murray JE, et al: Kasabach-Merritt syndrome: coagulo-analytical observations. Am J Med Sci 261:9–15, 1971

443. Kasabach HH, Merritt KK: Capillary hemangioma with extensive purpura. Am J Dis Child 59:1063–1067, 1940

444. Henley JD, Danielson CFM, Rothenberger SS, et al: Kasabach-Merritt syndrome with profound platelet support. Am J Clin Pathol 99:628–630, 1993

445. de Prost Y, Teillac D, Bodemer C, et al: Successful treatment of Kasabach-Merritt syndrome with pentoxifylline. J Am Acad Dermatol 25:854–855, 1991

446. Wind MS, Pillari G: Deep soft tissue hemangioma of infancy: Kasabach-Merritt syndrome. NY State J Med 79:373–374, 1979

447. Esterly NB: Kasabach-Merritt syndrome in infants. J Am Acad Dermatol 8:504–513, 1983

448. Goidanick IF, Campanancci M: Vascular hamartomata and infantile angioectatic osteohyperplasia of the extremities. J Bone Joint Surg [Am] 44:815–820, 1962

449. Lofland GK, Filston HC: Giant cutaneous hemangioma associated with axillary arteriovenous fistula causing congestive heart failure in the newborn infant. J Pediatr Surg 22:458–460, 1987

450. Nagao K, Matsuzaki O, Shigematsu H, et al: Histopathologic studies of benign infantile hemangioendothelioma of the parotid gland. Cancer 46:2250–2256, 1980

451. Gonzalez-Crussi F, Reyes-Mugica M: Cellular hemangiomas (hemangioendotheliomas) in infants: light microscopic, immunohistochemical, and ultrastructural observations. Am J Surg Pathol 15:769–778, 1991

452. Pasyk KA, Grabb WC, Cherry GW: Cellular haemangioma: light and electron microscopic studies of two cases. Virchows Arch (Pathol Anat) 396:103–126, 1982

453. Coffin CM, Dehner LP: Vascular tumors in children and adolescents: a clinicopathologic study of 228 tumors in 222 patients. Part 1, Pathol Annu, 28:97–120, 1993

454. Kauffman SL, Stout AP: Malignant hemangioendothelioma in infants and children. Cancer 14:1186–1196, 1961

455. Hilborne LH, Glasgow BJ, Layfield LJ: Fine needle aspiration cytology of juvenile hemangioma of the parotid gland: a case report. Diagn Cytopathol 3:152–155, 1987

456. Padilla RS, Orkin M, Rosai J: Acquired "tufted" angioma (progressive capillary hemangioma). A distinctive clinicopathologic entity related to lobular capillary hemangioma. Am J Dermatopathol 9:292–300, 1987

457. Jones EW, Orkin M: Tufted angioma (angioblastoma). A benign progressive angioma, not to be confused with Kaposi's sarcoma or low-grade angiosarcoma. J Am Acad Dermatol 20:214–225, 1989

458. Rapini RP, Golitz LE: Targetoid hemosiderotic hemangioma. J Cutan Pathol 17:233–235, 1990

459. Chan JK, Fletcher CD, Hicklin GA, et al: Glomeruloid haemangioma. A distinctive cutaneous lesion of multicentric Castleman's disease associated with POEMS syndrome. Am J Surg Pathol 14:1036–1046, 1990

460. Ishikawa O, Nihei Y, Ishikawa H: The skin changes of POEMS syndromes. Br J Dermatol 117:523–526, 1987

461. Kanitakis J, Roger H, Soubrier M, et al: Cutaneous angiomas in POEMS syndrome. An ultrastructural and immunohistochemical study. Arch Dermatol 124:695–698, 1988

462. De Kaminsky AR, Otero AC, Kaminsky CA, et al: Multiple disseminated pyogenic granuloma. Br J Dermatol 98:461–464, 1978

463. Mills SE, Cooper PH, Fechner RE: Lobular capillary hemangioma: the underlying lesion of pyogenic granuloma: a study of 73 cases from the oral and nasal mucous membranes. Am J Surg Pathol 4:471–479, 1980

464. Cooper PH, McAllister HA, Helwig EB: Intravenous pyogenic granuloma: a study of 18 cases. Am J Surg Pathol 3:221–228, 1979

465. Ulbright TM, Santa Cruz DJ: Intravenous pyogenic granuloma. Case report with ultrastructural findings. Cancer 45:1646–1652, 1980

466. Warner J, Jones EW: Pyogenic granuloma recurring with multiple satellites: a report of 11 cases. Br J Dermatol 80:218–227, 1968

467. Calonje E, Christopher DM, Fletcher DM: Sinusoidal hemangioma. A distinctive benign vascular neoplasm within the group of cavernous hemangiomas. Am J Surg Pathol 15:1130–1135, 1991

468. Connelly MG, Winkelmann RK: Acral arteriovenous tumor: a clinicopathologic review. Am J Surg Pathol 9:15–21, 1985

469. Girard C, Graham JH, Johnson WC: Arteriovenous hemangioma (arteriovenous shunt): a clinicopathological and histochemical study. J Cutan Pathol 1:73–87, 1974

470. Rusin LJ, Harrell ER: Arteriovenous fistula. Cutaneous manifestations. Arch Dermatol 112:1135–1138, 1976

471. Weiss SW: Pedal hemangioma occurring in Turner's syndrome: an additional manifestation of the syndrome. Hum Pathol 19:1015–1018, 1988

472. Allen PW, Enzinger FM: Hemangiomas of skeletal muscle: an analysis of 89 cases. Cancer 29:8–22, 1972

473. Angervall L, Nilsson L, Stener B, et al: Angiographic, microangiographic, and histologic study of vascular malformation in striated muscle. Acta Radiol 7:65–70, 1968

474. Beham A, Fletcher CDM: Intramuscular angioma: a clinicopathologic analysis of 74 cases. Histopathology 18:53–59, 1991

475. Cohen AJ, Youkey JR, Clagett GP: Intramuscular hemangioma. JAMA 249:2680–2684, 1983

476. Holden KR, Alexander F: Diffuse neonatal hemangiomatosis. Pediatrics 46:411–421, 1970

477. Howat AJ, Campbell PE: Angiomatosis: a vascular malformation of infancy and childhood. Pathology 19:377–382, 1987

478. Rao VK, Weiss SW: Angiomatosis of soft tissue: an analysis of the histologic features and clinical outcome in 51 cases. Am J Surg Pathol 16:764–771, 1992

479. Wells GC, Whimster IW: Subcutaneous angiolymphoid hyperplasia with eosinophilia. Br J Dermatol 81:1–15, 1969

480. Wilson-Jones E, Blehen SS: Inflammatory angiomatous nodules with abnormal blood vessels occurring about the ears and scalp (pseudo or atypical pyogenic granuloma). Br J Dermatol 81:804–816, 1969

481. Olsen TG, Helwig EB: Angiolymphoid hyperplasia with eosinophilia: a clinicopathologic study of 116 patients. J Am Acad Dermatol 12:781–796, 1985

482. Fetsch JF, Weiss SW: Observations concerning the pathogenesis of epithelioid hemangioma (angiolymphoid hyperplasia). Mod Pathol 4:449–455, 1991

483. Urabe A, Tsuneyoshi M, Enjoji M: Epithelioid hemangioma versus Kimura's disease. A comparative clinicopathologic study. Am J Surg Pathol 11:758–766, 1987

484. Chan JKC, Hui PK, Ng CS, et al: Epithelioid haemangioma (angiolymphoid hyperplasia with eosinophilia) and Kimura's disease in Chinese. Histopathology 15:557–574, 1989

485. Leboit P, Berger TG, Egbert BM, et al: Bacillary angiomatosis: the histopathology and differential diagnosis of a pseudoneoplastic infection in patients with human immunodeficiency virus disease. Am J Surg Pathol 13:909–913, 1989

486. Relman DA, Loutit JS, Schmidt TM, et al: The agent of bacillary angiomatosis: an approach to the identification of uncultured pathogens. N Engl J Med 323:1573–1578, 1990

487. Weiss SW, Enzinger FM: Epithelioid hemangioendothelioma. A vascular tumor often mistaken for a carcinoma. Cancer 50:971–981, 1982

488. Weiss SW, Ishak KG, Dail DH, et al: Epithelioid hemangioendothelioma and related lesions. Semin Diagn Pathol 3:259–287, 1986

489. Suster S, Moran CS, Koss MN: Epithelioid hemangioendothelioma of the anterior mediastinum. Clinicopathologic, immunohistochemical and ultrastructural analysis of 12 cases. Am J Surg Pathol 18:871–881, 1994

490. Pettinato G, Insabato L, De Chiara A, et al: Epithelioid hemangioendothelioma of soft tissue, fine needle aspiration cytology, electron microscopy and immunohistochemistry of a case. Acta Cytol 30:194–200, 1986

491. Weiss SW, Enzinger FM: Spindle cell hemangioendothelioma, a low-grade angiosarcoma resembling a cavernous hemangioma and Kaposi's sarcoma. Am J Surg Pathol 10:521–530, 1986

492. Perkins PL, Weiss SW: Spindle cell hemangioendothelioma: an analysis of 78 cases with reassessment of its pathogenesis and biologic behavior. Am J Surg Pathol 20:1196–1204, 1996

493. Scott GA, Rosai J: Spindle cell hemangioendothelioma. Report of seven additional cases of a recently described vascular neoplasm. Am J Dermatopathol 10:281–288, 1988

494. Fay JT, Schow SR: A possible case of Maffuci's syndrome. J Oral Surg 26:739–744, 1968

495. Fanburg JC, Meis-Kindblom JM, Rosenberg AE: Multiple enchondromas associated with spindle-cell hemangioendotheliomas. An overlooked variant of Maffuci's Syndrome. Am J Surg Pathol 19:1029–1038, 1995

496. Hodgkinson DJ, Soule EH, Woods JE: Cutaneous angiosarcoma of the head and neck. Cancer 44:1106–1113, 1979

497. Maddox JC, Evans HL: Angiosarcoma of skin and soft tissue: a study of 44 cases. Cancer 1907–1921, 1981

498. Holden CA, Spittle MF, Jones EW: Angiosarcoma of the face and scalp, prognosis and treatment. Cancer 59:1046–1057, 1987

499. Lydiatt WM, Shaha AR, Shah JP: Angiosarcoma of the head and neck. Am J Surg 168:451–454, 1994

500. Mark RJ, Poen JC, Tran LM, et al: Angiosarcoma. A report of 67 patients and a review of the literature. Cancer 77:2400–2406, 1996

501. Karpeh MS, Caldwell C, Gaynor JJ, et al: Vascular soft-tissue sarcomas: an analysis of tumor-related mortality. Arch Surg 126:1474–1481, 1991

502. Selby DM, Stocker JT, Ishak KG: Angiosarcoma of the liver in childhood: a clinicopathologic and follow-up study of 10 cases. Pediatr Pathol 12:485–498, 1992

503. Fletcher CDM, Beham A, Bekir S, et al: Epithelioid angiosarcoma of deep soft tissue: a distinctive tumor readily mistaken for an epithelial neoplasm. Am J Surg Pathol 15:915–924, 1991

504. Wenig BM, Abbondanzo SL, Heffess CS: Epithelioid angiosarcoma of the adrenal glands. A clinicopathologic study of nine cases with a discussion of the implications of finding "epithelial-specific" markers. Am J Surg Pathol 18:62–73, 1994

505. Eusebi V, Carcangiu ML, Dina R, et al: Keratin-positive epithelioid angiosarcoma of thyroid: a report of four cases. Am J Surg Pathol 14:737–747, 1990

506. Jennings TA, Petterson L, Axiotis CA, et al: Angiosarcoma associated with foreign body material. A report of three cases. Cancer 62:2436–2444, 1988

507. Abele JS, Miller T: Cytology of well-differentiated and poorly differentiated hemangiosarcoma in fine needle aspirates. Acta Cytol 26:341–348, 1982

508. Friedman-Kien AE, Saltzman BR: Clinical manifestations of classical, endemic African, and epidemic AIDS-associated Kaposi's sarcoma. J Am Acad Dermatol 22:1237–1250, 1990

509. Wahman A, Melnick SL, Rhame FC, et al: The epidemiology of classic, African, and immunosuppressed Kaposi's sarcoma. Epidemiol Rev 13:178–199, 1991

510. Des Jarlais DC, Marmor M, Thomas P, et al: Kaposi's sarcoma among four different AIDS risk groups. N Engl J Med 310:1119, 1984

511. Kempf W, Adams V, Pfaltz M, et al: Human herpesvirus type 6 and cytomegalovirus in AIDS-associated Kaposi's sarcoma: no evidence for an etiological association. Hum Pathol 26:914–919, 1995

512. Chang Y, Cesarman E, Pessin MS, et al: Identification of herpesvirus-like DNA sequences in AIDS-associated Kaposi's sarcoma. Science 266:1865–1869, 1994

513. Jin Y, Tsai ST, Yan JJ: Detection of Kaposi's sarcoma-associated herpesvirus-like DNA sequence in vascular lesions. A reliable diagnostic marker for Kaposi's sarcoma. Am J Clin Pathol 105:360–363, 1996

514. Dictor M, Rambech E, Way D, et al: Human herpesvirus 8 (Kaposi's sarcoma associated herpesvirus) DNA in Kaposi's sarcoma lesions, AIDS Kaposi's sarcoma cell lines, endothelial Kaposi's sarcoma simulators, and the skin of immunosuppressed patients. Am J Pathol 148:2009–2016, 1996

515. Ordoñez NG, Batsakis JG: Comparison of Ulex europaeus lectin and factor VIII-related antigen in vascular lesions. Arch Pathol Lab Med 108:129–132, 1984

516. Miettinen M, Lindenmayer EA, Chaubal A: Endothelial cell markers CD31, CD34, and BNH9 antibody to H and Y antigens. Evaluation of their specificity and sensitivity in the diagnosis of vascular tumors and comparison with von Willebrand factor. Mod Pathol 78:82–90, 1994

517. Beckstead JH, Wood GS, Fletcher V: Evidence for the origin of Kaposi's sarcoma from lymphatic endothelium. Am J Pathol 119:294–300, 1985

518. Dorfman RF: Kaposi's sarcoma: evidence supporting its origin from the lymphatic system. Lymphology 21:45–52, 1988

519. Rywlin AA, Rosin L, Cabello B: Coexistence of Castleman's disease and Kaposi's sarcoma. Report of a case and a speculation. Am J Dermatopathol 5:277–281, 1983

520. Hales M, Bottles K, Miller T, et al: Diagnosis of Kaposi's sarcoma by fine-needle aspiration. Cancer 88:20–25, 1987

521. Bratu M, Brown M, Carter M, et al: Cystic hygroma of the mediastinum in children. Am J Dis Child 119:348–351, 1970

522. Barrana KG, Freeman NV: Massive infiltrating cystic hygroma of the neck in infancy. Arch Dis Child 38:523–531, 1973

523. Chervenak FA, Isaacson G, Blakemore KJ: Fetal cystic hygroma. Cause and natural history. N Engl J Med 309:822–825, 1983

524. Emery PJ, Bailey CM, Evans JNG: Cystic hygroma of the head and neck: a review of 37 cases. J Laryngol Otol 98:613–619, 1984

525. Byrne J, Blanc WA, Warburton D, et al: The significance of cystic hygroma in fetuses. Hum Pathol 15:61–67, 1984

526. Carr RF, Ochs RH, Ritter DA, et al: Fetal cystic hygroma and Turner's syndrome. Am J Dis Child 140:580–593, 1986

527. Prioleau PG, Santa Cruz DJ: Lymphangioma circumscripta following radical mastectomy and radiation therapy. Cancer 42:1989–1991, 1978

528. Asch MJ, Cohen AH, Moore TC: Hepatic and splenic lymphangiomatosis with skeletal involvement. Surgery 76:334–338, 1974

529. Bell A, Simon BK: Chylothorax and lymphangiomas of bone: unusual manifestation of lymphatic disease. South Med J 71:459–463, 1978

530. Ramani P, Shah A: Lymphangiomatosis: histologic and immunohistochemical analysis of four cases. Am J Surg Pathol 17:329–335, 1993

531. Tazelaar HD, Kerr D, Yousem SA, et al: Diffuse pulmonary lymphangiomatosis. Hum Pathol 24:1313–1322, 1993

532. Hilliard RI, McKendry JBJ, Phillips MJ: Congenital abnormalities of the lymphatic system. A new clinical classification. Pediatrics 86:988–994, 1990

533. Cornog JL, Enterline HT: Lymphangiomyoma: a benign lesion of chyliferous lymphatics synonymous with lymphangiopericytoma. Cancer 19:1909–1930, 1966

534. Bhattacharyya AK, Balogh K: Retroperitoneal lymphangioleiomyomatosis: a 36-year benign course in a postmenopausal woman. Cancer 56:1144–1146, 1985

535. Carrington C, Cugell D, Gaensler E, et al: Lymphangioleiomyomatosis: physiologic-pathologic-radiologic correlations. Am Rev Respir Dis 116:977–995, 1977

536. Cagnano M, Benharroch D, Geffen DB: Pulmonary lymphangi-oleiomyomatosis: report of a case with associated multiple soft tissue tumors. Arch Pathol Lab Med 115:1257–1259, 1991

537. Kaku T, Toyoshima S, Enjoji M: Tuberous sclerosis with pulmonary and lymph node involvement: relationship to lymphangiomyomatosis. Acta Pathol Jpn 33:395–402, 1983

538. Lack EE, Dolan MF, Finisio J, et al: Pulmonary and extrapulmonary lymphangioleiomyomatosis; report of a case with bilateral renal an-giomyolipomas, multifocal lymphangioleiomyomatosis, and a glial polyp of the endocervix. Am J Surg Pathol 10:650–657, 1986

539. Bretnani MM, Carvalho RR, Saldiva PH, et al: Steroid receptors in pulmonary lymphangiomyomatosis. Chest 85:96–100, 1984

540. Berger U, Khaghani A, Pomerance A, et al: Pulmonary lymphangi-oleiomyomatosis and steroid receptors: an immunohistochemical study. Am J Clin Pathol 93:609–614, 1990

541. Colley MH, Geppert E, Franklin WA: Immunohistochemical detec-tion of steroid receptors in a case of pulmonary lymphangioleiomy-omatosis. Am J Surg Pathol 13:803–807, 1989

542. Luna CM, Gene R, Jolly EC, et al: Pulmonary lymphangiomyomato-sis associated with tuberous sclerosis: treatment with tamoxifen and tetracycline-pleurodesis. Chest 88:473–476, 1985

543. Ohori NP, Yousem SA, Sonmez-Alpan E, et al: Estrogen and proges-terone receptors in lymphangioleiomyomatosis, epithelioid heman-gioendothelioma, and sclerosing hemangioma of the lung. Am J Clin Pathol 96:529–534, 1991

544. Tomasian A, Greenberg MS, Rumerman H: Tamoxifen for lymphan-gioleiomyomatosis. N Engl J Med 306:745–746, 1982

545. Gould EW, Manivel JC, Albores-Saavedra J, et al: Locally infiltrative glomus tumors and glomangiosarcomas: a clinical, ultrastructural, and immunohistochemical study. Cancer 65:310–318, 1990

546. Schurch W, Skalli O, Lagace R, et al: Intermediate filament proteins and actin isoforms as markers for soft-tissue tumor differentiation and origin. III. Hemangiopericytomas and glomus tumors. Am J Pathol 136:771–786, 1990

547. Tsuneyoshi M, Enjoji M: Glomus tumor. A clinicopathologic and electron microscopic study. Cancer 50:1601–1607, 1982

548. Conant MA, Winsenfeld SL: Multiple glomus of the skin. Arch Der-matol 103:481–485, 1971

549. Goodman TF, Abele DC: Multiple glomus tumors: a clinical and elec-tron microscopic study. Arch Dermatol 103:11–23, 1971

550. Heys SD, Brittenden J, Atkinson P, et al: Glomus tumor: an analysis of 43 patients and review of the literature. Br J Surg 79:345–347, 1992

551. Warner KE, Haidak GL: Massive glomus tumor of the stomach: 20-year follow-up and autopsy findings. Am J Gastroenterol 79:253–255, 1984

552. Salima H, Modlin IM, West AB: Multiple glomus tumors of the stom-ach with intravascular spread. Am J Surg Pathol 16:291–299, 1992

553. Hamilton CW, Shelburne JD, Bossen EH, et al: A glomus tumor of the jejunum masquerading as a carcinoid tumor. Hum Pathol 13:859–861, 1982

554. Googe PB, Griffin WC: Intravenous glomus tumor of the forearm. J Cutan Pathol 20:359–363, 1993

555. Landerthaler M, Braun-Falco O: Congenital multiple plaque-like glo-mus tumors. Arch Dermatol 126:1203–1207, 1990

556. Tran LP, Velanovich V, Kaufmann CR: Familial multiple glomus tu-mors: report of a pedigree and literature review. Ann Plast Surg 32:89–92, 1994

557. Wood WS, Dimmick JE: Multiple infiltrating glomus tumors in chil-dren. Cancer 1680–1685, 1977

558. Holck S, Bredesen JL: Solid glomus tumor presenting as an axillary mass. Report of a case with morphologic study, including cytologic characteristics. Acta Cytol 40:555–562, 1996

559. Noer H, Krogdahl A: Glomangiosarcoma of the lower extremity. Histopathology 18:365–366, 1991

560. Brathwaite CD, Poppiti RJ Jr: Malignant glomus tumor. A case report of widespread metastases in a patient with multiple glomus body hamartomas. Am J Surg Pathol 20:233–238, 1996

561. Enzinger FM, Smith BH: Hemangiopericytoma: an analysis of 106 cases. Hum Pathol 7:61–82, 1976

562. McMaster M, Soule E, Irving J: Hemangiopericytoma: a clinico-pathologic study and long term follow-up of 60 patients. Cancer 36:2232–2244, 1975

563. Nappi O, Ritter JH, Pettinato G, et al: Hemangiopericytoma: histopathological pattern or clinicopathologic entity? Semin Diagn Pathol 12:221–232, 1995

564. Porter PL, Bigler SA, McNutt M, et al: The immunophenotype of he-mangiopericytomas and glomus tumors, with special reference to mus-cle protein expression: an immunohistochemical study and review of the literature. Mod Pathol 4:46–52, 1991

565. Dardick I, Hammar SP, Scheithauer BW: Ultrastructural spectrum of hemangiopericytoma: a comparative study of fetal, adult and neoplas-tic pericytes. Ultrastruct Pathol 13:111–134, 1989

566. Mena H, Ribas JL, Pezeshkpour GH, et al: Hemangiopericytoma of the central nervous system: a review of 94 cases. Hum Pathol 22:84–91, 1991

567. Cotterill AM, Holly JMP, Davies SC, et al: The insulin-like growth factors and their binding proteins in a case of non-islet-cell tumor-as-sociated hypoglycemia. J Endocrinol 131:303–311, 1991

568. Bayley PV, Weber TR, Tracy TF Jr: Congenital hemangiopericytoma: an unusual vascular neoplasm. Surgery 114:936–941, 1993

569. Virden CP, Lynch FP: Infantile hemangiopericytoma: a rare cause of a soft tissue mass. J Pediatr Surg 28:741–743, 1993

570. Fukunaga M, Shimoda T, Nikaido T, et al: Soft tissue vascular tumors: a flow cytometric DNA analysis. Cancer 71:2233–2241, 1993

571. Finn WG, Goolsby CL, Rao MS: DNA flow cytometric analysis of he-mangiopericytoma. Am J Clin Pathol 101:181–185, 1994

572. Nickels J, Koivuniemi A: Cytology of malignant hemangiopericy-toma. Acta Cytol 23:119–125, 1979

573. Nguyen G-K, Neifer R: The cells of benign and malignant heman-giopericytomas in aspiration biopsy. Diagn Cytopathol 1:327–331, 1985

574. Soule EH: Synovial sarcoma. Am J Surg Pathol 10:78–82, 1986

575. Evans HL: Synovial sarcoma: a study of 23 biphasic and 17 probable monophasic examples. Pathol Annu 15:309–313, 1980

576. Schmidt D, Thum P, Harms D, et al: Synovial sarcoma in children and adolescents. A report from the Kiel Pediatric Tumor Registry. Cancer 67:1667–1672, 1991

577. Witkin GB, Miettinen M, Rosai J: A biphasic tumor of the medi-astinum with features of synovial sarcoma. Am J Surg Pathol 13:490–499, 1989

578. Mirra JM, Wang S, Bhuta S: Synovial sarcoma with squamous differ-entiation of its mesenchymal glandular elements. Am J Surg Pathol 8:791–796, 1984

579. Varela-Duran J, Enzinger FM: Calcifying synovial sarcoma. Cancer 50:345–352, 1982

580. Milchgrub S, Ghandur-Mnaymneh L, Dorfman HD, et al: Synovial sarcoma with extensive osteoid and bone formation. Am J Surg Pathol 17:357–363, 1993

581. Corson JM, Weiss LM, Banks-Schlegel SP, et al: Keratin proteins in and carcinoembryonic antigen in synovial sarcomas: an immunohis-tochemical study of 24 cases. Hum Pathol 15:615–621, 1984

582. Ordoñez NG, Mahfouz SM, Mackay B: Synovial sarcoma: an im-munohistochemical and ultrastructural study. Hum Pathol 21:733–749, 1990

583. Tsuneyoshi M, Yokoyama K, Enjoji M: Synovial sarcoma: a clinico-pathologic and ultrastructural study of 42 cases. Acta Pathol Jpn 33:23–28, 1983

584. Gilgenkrantz S, Chery M, Teboul M, et al: Sublocalization of the X break point in the translocation (x;18)(p11.2; q11.2) primary change in synovial sarcoma. Oncogene 5:1063–1066, 1990

585. Clark J, Rocques PJ, Crew AJ, et al: Identification of novel genes SYT and SSX involved in the t(x;18)(p11.2; q11.2) translocation found in synovial sarcoma. Nat Genet 7:502–505, 1994

586. Cagle LA, Mirra JM, Storm FK, et al: Histologic features relating to prognosis in synovial sarcoma. Cancer 59:1810–1814, 1987

587. Akerman M, Willen H, Carlen B, et al: Fine needle aspiration (FNA) of synovial sarcoma—a comparative histological-cytological study of 15 cases, including immunohistochemical, electron microscopic and cytogenetic examination and DNA-ploidy analysis. Cytopathology 7:187–200, 1996

588. Ashfaq R, Molberg KH, Vuitch F: Cutaneous endometriosis as a diagnostic pitfall of fine needle aspiration biopsy. A report of three cases. Acta Cytol 38:577–581, 1994

589. Sterrett G, Whitaker D, Shilkin KB, et al: Fine needle aspiration cytology of malignant mesothelioma. Acta Cytol 31:185–193, 1987

590. Tao LC: Aspiration biopsy cytology of mesothelioma. Diagn Cytopathol 5:14–21, 1989

591. Lichtestein L, Goldman RL: Cartilage tumors in soft tissues, particularly in the hand and foot. Cancer 17:1203–1208, 1964

592. Dahlin DC, Salvador AH: Cartilaginous tumors of the soft tissues of the hands and feet. Mayo Clin Proc 49:721–726, 1974

593. Chung EB, Enzinger FM: Chondroma of soft parts. Cancer 41:1414–1424, 1978

594. Humphreys S, Pambakian H, McKee PH, et al: Soft tissue chondroma—a study of 15 tumors. Histopathology 10:147–159, 1986

595. Reiman HM, Dahlin DC: Cartilage- and bone-forming tumors of the soft tissues. Semin Diagn Pathol 3:288–305, 1986

596. Enzinger FM, Shiraki M: Extraskeletal myxoid chondrosarcoma: an analysis of 39 cases. Hum Pathol 3:421–435, 1972

597. Ueda Y, Okada Y, Nakanishi I: Cellular variant of extraskeletal myxoid chondrosarcoma of abdominal wall: a case report with comparative immunohistochemical study on cartilaginous collagenous proteins in various myxoid mesenchymal tumors. J Cancer Res Oncol 118:147–151, 1992

598. Meis YM, Martz KL: Extraskeletal myxoid chondrosarcoma: a clinicopathologic study of 120 cases, abstracted. Mod Pathol 5:9A, 1992

599. Abramovici LG, Steiner GC, Bonar F: Myxoid chondrosarcoma of soft tissue and bone: a retrospective study of 11 cases. Hum Pathol 26:1215–1220, 1995

600. Dedick K: Embryonal form of extraskeletal myxoid chondrosarcoma with intermediate filament positive hyaline-like globules. Zentralbl J Pathol 138:312–315, 1992

601. Wolford J, Bedetti C: Skeletal myxoid chondrosarcoma with microtubular aggregates within rough endoplasmic reticulum. Arch Pathol Lab Med 112:77–81, 1988

602. DeBlois G, Wang S, Kay S: Microtubular aggregates within rough endoplasmic reticulum: an unusual ultrastructural feature of extraskeletal myxoid chondrosarcoma. Hum Pathol 17:469–475, 1986

603. Payne C, Dardick I, MacKay B: Extraskeletal myxoid chondrosarcoma with intracisternal microtubules. Ultrastruct Pathol 18:257–261, 1994

604. Saleh G, Evans HL, Ro JY, et al: Extraskeletal myxoid chondrosarcoma: a clinicopathologic study of ten patients with long term follow-up. Cancer 70:2827–2830, 1992

605. Niemann TH, Bottles K, Cohen MB: Extraskeletal myxoid chondrosarcoma: fine-needle aspiration biopsy findings. Diagn Cytopathol 11:363–366, 1994

606. Wakely PE, Geisinger KR, Cappellari JO, et al: Fine-needle aspiration cytopathology of soft tissue: chondromyxoid and myxoid lesions. Diagn Cytopathol 12:101–105, 1995

607. Jones H, Ozua PO, Lee DM: The diagnosis of extraskeletal myxoid chondrosarcoma by fine needle aspiration. Cytopathology 6:273–276, 1995

608. Kontozoglou T, Qizilbash AH, Sianos J, et al: Chordoma: cytologic and immunocytochemical study of four cases. Diagn Cytopathol 2:55–61, 1986

609. Lichtenstein L, Bernstein D: Unusual benign and malignant chondroid tumors of bone. Cancer 12:1142–1157, 1959

610. Dabska M, Huvos AG: Mesenchymal chondrosarcoma in the young: a clinicopathologic study of 19 patients with explanation of histogenesis. Virch Arch A Pathol Anat Histopathol 399:88–104, 1983

611. Nakashima Y, Unni KK, Shives TC, et al: Mesenchymal chondrosarcoma of bone and soft tissue. A review of 111 cases. Cancer 57:2444–2454, 1986

612. Rushing EJ, Armonda RA, Ansari Q, et al: Mesenchymal chondrosarcoma. A clinicopathologic and flow cytometric study of 13 cases presenting in the central nervous system. Cancer 77:1884–1890, 1996

613. Rushing EJ, Mena H, Smirniotopoulos JG: Mesenchymal chondrosarcoma of the cauda equina. J Clin Neuropathol 14:150–153, 1995

614. Scheithauer BW, Rubinstein LJ: Meningeal mesenchymal chondrosarcoma; report of 8 cases and review of the literature. Cancer 42:2744–2752, 1978

615. Fu YS, Kay S: A comparative ultrastructural study of mesenchymal chondrosarcoma and myxoid chondrosarcoma. Cancer 33:1531–1542, 1974

616. Shapeero LG, Vanel D, Couanet D, et al: Extraskeletal mesenchymal chondrosarcoma. Radiology 186:819–823, 1993

617. Swanson PE, Lillemoe TJ, Manivel JC, et al: Mesenchymal chondrosarcoma. An immunohistochemical study. Arch Pathol Lab Med 114:943–948, 1990

618. Doria MI, Wang HH, Chinoy MJ: Retroperitoneal mesenchymal chondrosarcoma. Report of a case diagnosed by fine needle aspiration cytology. Acta Cytol 34:529–532, 1990

619. González-Cámpora R, Otal-Salaverri C, Pascual AG, et al: Mesenchymal chondrosarcoma of the retroperitoneum. Report of a case diagnosed by fine needle aspiration biopsy with immunohistochemical, electron microscopic demonstration of S-100 protein in undifferentiated cells. Acta Cytol 39:1237–1243, 1995

620. Das DK, Gupta SK, Sehgal S: Extramedullary plasma cell tumors: diagnosis by fine needle aspiration cytology. Diagn Cytopathol 2:248–251, 1986

621. Albores-Saavedra J, Angeles-Angeles A, Ridaura C, et al: Embryonal chondrosarcoma in children. Patologia 15:153–162, 1977

622. Jessurun J, Rojas ME, Albores-Saavedra J: Congenital extraskeletal embryonal chondrosarcoma. Case report. J Bone Joint Surg [Am] 64:293–296, 1982

623. Hachitanda Y, Tsuneyoshi M, Daimaru Y, et al: Extraskeletal myxoid chondrosarcoma in young children. Cancer 61:2521–2526, 1988

624. Allan CS, Soule EH: Osteogenic sarcoma of the somatic soft tissues. Clinicopathologic study of 26 cases and review of literature. Cancer 27:1121–1133, 1971

625. Huvos AG: Osteogenic sarcoma of bones and soft tissues in older persons: a clinicopathologic analysis of 117 patients older than 60 years. Cancer 57:1442–1449, 1986

626. Sordillo PP, Hajdu SI, Magill GB, et al: Extraosseous osteogenic sarcoma: a review of 48 patients. Cancer 51:727–734, 1983

627. Chung EB, Enzinger FM: Extraskeletal osteosarcoma. Cancer 60:1132–1142, 1987

628. Kawamoto EH, Weidner N, Agostini RM, et al: Malignant ectomesenchymoma of soft tissue. Report of two cases and review of the literature. Cancer 59:1791–1802, 1987

629. Karcioglu Z, Someren A, Mathes SJ: Ectomesenchymoma: a malignant tumor of migratory neural crest (ectomesenchyme) remnants showing ganglionic, Schwannian, melanocytic and rhabdomyoblastic differentiation. Cancer 39:2486–2496, 1977

630. Cozzutto C, Cornelli A, Bandelloni R: Ectomesenchymoma: report of two cases. Virchows Arch 398:185–195, 1982

631. Kodet R, Kashuri N, Marsden HB, et al: Gangliorhabdomyosarcoma: a histopathological and immunohistochemical study of three cases. Histopathology 10:181–193, 1986

632. Lack EE, Worsham GF, Callihan MD, et al: Granular cell tumor: a clinicopathologic study of 110 patients. J Surg Oncol 13:301–316, 1980

633. Paskin DL, Hull JD: Granular cell myoblastoma: a comprehensive review of 15 years' experience. Ann Surg 175:501–503, 1972

634. Lindberg G, Saboorian H, Housini I, et al: The clinico-pathologic spectrum of granular cell tumors. Lab Invest 74:9A, 1996

635. Lack EE, Worsham GF, Callihan MD, et al: Gingival granular cell tumor of the newborn (congenital "epulis"): a clinical and pathologic study of 21 patients. Am J Surg Pathol 5:37–46, 1981

636. Murray DE, Seman E, Utzinger W: Granular cell myoblastomas in successive generations. J Surg Oncol 1:193–197, 1969

637. Mukai M: Immunohistochemical localization of S-100 protein and peripheral nerve myelin proteins (P2 protein and PO protein) in granular cell tumors. Am J Pathol 112:139–146, 1983

638. Nakazato Y, Ishizeki J, Takahashi K, et al: Immunohistochemical localization of S-100 protein in granular cell myoblastoma. Cancer 49:1624–1628, 1982

639. Slavin RE, Christie JD, Swedo J, et al: Locally aggressive granular cell tumor causing priapism of the crus of the clitoris. A light and ultrastructural study, with observations concerning the pathogenesis of fibrosis of the corpus cavernosum in priapism. Am J Surg Pathol 10:497–507, 1986

640. Franzen S, Stenkvist B: Diagnosis of granular cell myoblastoma by fine needle aspiration biopsy. Acta Pathol Microbiol Scand 72:391–395, 1968

641. Christ ML, Ozzello L: Myogenous origin of a granular cell tumor of the urinary bladder. Am J Clin Pathol 56:736–749, 1971

642. Tandler B, Rosai EP: Granular cell ameloblastoma: Electron microscopic observation. J Oral Pathol 6:410–412, 1977

643. Sinsir A, Osborne BM, Grunbaum E: Malignant granular cell tumors: a case report and review of the recent literature. Hum Pathol 27:853–858, 1996

644. Robertson AJ, Mcintosh W, Lamont P, et al: Malignant granular cell tumour (myoblastoma) of the vulva: report of a case and review of the literature. Histopathology 5:69–79, 1981

644a.Fanburg JC, Meis-Kindblom JM, Kindblom LG: Malignant atypical and multicentric granular cell tumors: Diagnostic criteria and clinicopathologic correlation. Lab Invest 74:6A, 1996

645. Enzinger FM, Weiss SW, Liang CY: Ossifying fibromyxoid tumor of soft parts. A clinicopathological analysis of 59 cases. Am J Surg Pathol 13:817–827, 1989

646. Miettinen M: Ossifying fibromyxoid tumor of soft parts. Additional observations of a distinctive soft tissue tumor. Am J Clin Pathol 95:142–149, 1991

647. Yoshida H, Minamizaki T, Yumoto T, et al: Ossifying fibromyxoid tumor of soft parts. Acta Pathol Jpn 41:480–486, 1991

648. Kilpatrick SE, Ward WG, Mozes M, et al: Atypical and malignant variants of ossifying fibromyxoid tumor: clinicopathologic analysis of 6 cases. Am J Surg Pathol 19:1039–1046, 1995

649. Schofield JB, Krausz T, Stamp GWH, et al: Ossifying fibromyxoid tumor of soft parts: immunohistochemical and ultrastructural analysis. Histopathology 22:101–112, 1993

650. Fisher C, Hedges M, Weiss SW: Ossifying fibromyxoid tumor of soft parts with stromal cyst formation and ribosome-lamella complexes. Ultrastruct Pathol 18:593–600, 1994

651. Smith MEF, Fisher C, Weiss SW: Pleomorphic hyalinizing angiectatic tumor of soft parts. A low-grade neoplasm resembling neurilemoma. Am J Surg Pathol 20:21–29, 1996

652. Christopherson MW, Foote FWJ, Stewart FW: Alveolar soft-part sarcomas: structurally characteristic tumors of uncertain histogenesis. Cancer 5:100–111, 1952

653. Mukai M, Torikata C, Shimoda T, et al: Alveolar soft-part sarcoma. Assessment of immunohistochemical demonstration of desmin using paraffin sections and frozen sections. Virchows Arch A Pathol Anat Histopathol 414:503–509, 1989

654. Ordoñez NG, Ro JY, Mackay B: Alveolar soft-part sarcoma. An ultrastructural and immunocytochemical investigation of its histogenesis. Cancer 63:1721–1736, 1989

655. Miettinen M, Ekfors T: Alveolar soft-part sarcoma. Immunohistochemical evidence of muscle cell differentiation. Am J Clin Pathol 93:32–38, 1990

656. Rosai J, Dias P, Parham DM, et al: MyoD1 protein expression in alveolar soft-part sarcoma as confirmatory evidence of its skeletal muscle nature. Am J Surg Pathol 15:974–981, 1991

657. Sciot R, Dal-Cin P, De-Vos R, et al: Alveolar soft-part sarcoma: evidence for its myogenic origin and for the involvement of 17q25. Histopathology 23:439–444, 1993

658. Wang NP, Bacchi CE, Jiang JJ, et al: Does alveolar soft-part sarcoma exhibit skeletal muscle differentiation? An immunocytochemical and biochemical study of myogenic regulatory protein expression. Mod Pathol 9:496–506, 1996

659. Mukai M, Tarikata C, Iri H, et al: Alveolar soft part sarcoma. An elaboration of a three dimensional configuration of the crystalloids by digital image processing. Am J Pathol 116:398–406, 1984

660. Lieberman PH, Brennan MF, Kimmel M, et al: Alveolar soft-part sarcoma. A clinico-pathologic study of half of a century. Cancer 63:1–13, 1989

661. Simmons WB, Haggerty HS, Ngan B, et al: Alveolar soft-part sarcoma of the head and neck: a disease of children and young adult. Int J Pediatr Otorhinolaryngol 17:139–153, 1989

662. Yagihashi S, Yagihashi N, Hase Y, et al: Primary alveolar soft-part sarcoma of stomach. Am J Surg Pathol 15:399–406, 1991

663. Bots GT, Tijssen CC, Wijnalda D, et al: Alveolar soft-part sarcoma of the pituitary gland with secondary involvement of the right cerebral ventricle. Br J Neurosurg 2:101–107, 1988

664. Shabb N, Sneige N, Fanning CV, et al: Fine needle aspiration cytology of alveolar soft part sarcoma. Diagn Cytopathol 7:293–298, 1991

665. Persson S, Willems JS, Kindblom LG, et al: Alveolar soft part sarcoma. An immunohistochemical, cytologic and electron-microscopic study and a quantitative DNA analysis. Virchows Arch Pathol Anat Histopathol 412:499–513, 1988

666. Enzinger FM: Epithelioid sarcoma. A sarcoma simulating a granuloma or a carcinoma. Cancer 26:1029–1041, 1970

667. Schmidt D, Harms D: Epithelioid sarcoma in children and adolescents. An immunohistochemical study. Virch Arch A 410:423–431, 1987

668. Chase DR, Enzinger FM, Weiss SW, et al: Keratin in epithelioid sarcoma. An immunohistochemical study. Am J Surg Pathol 8:435–441, 1984

669. Gerharz CD, Moll R, Meister P, et al: Cytoskeletal heterogeneity of an epithelioid sarcoma with expression of vimentin, cytokeratins, and neurofilaments. Am J Surg Pathol 14:274–283, 1990

670. Daimaru Y, Hashimoto H, Tsuneyoshi M, et al: Epithelial profile of epithelioid sarcoma. An immunohistochemical analysis of eight cases. Cancer 59:134–141, 1987

671. Manivel JC, Wick MR, Dehner LP, et al: Epithelioid sarcoma. An immunohistochemical study. Am J Clin Pathol 87:319–326, 1987

672. Blewitt RW, Aparicio SGR, Bird CC: Epithelioid sarcoma: a tumor of myofibroblasts. Histopathology 7:573–584, 1983

673. Chase DR, Enzinger FM: Epithelioid sarcoma. Diagnosis, prognostic indicators, and treatment. Am J Surg Pathol 9:241–263, 1985

674. Tsuneyoshi M, Enjoji M, Shinohara N: Epithelioid sarcoma: a clinicopathologic and electron microscopic study. Acta Pathol Jpn 30:411–420, 1980

675. Fisher ER, Horvat B: The fibrocytic derivation of the so-called epithelioid sarcoma. Cancer 30:1074–1081, 1972

676. Pohar-Marinsek Z, Zidar A: Epithelioid sarcoma in FNAB smears. Diagn Cytopathol 11:367–372, 1994

677. Enzinger FM: Clear cell sarcoma of tendons and aponeurosis. An analysis of 21 cases. Cancer 18:1163–1174, 1965

678. Kindblom LG, Lodding P, Angervall L: Clear cell sarcoma of tendons and aponeuroses; an immunohistochemical and electron microscopic analysis indicating neural crest origin. Virchows Arch [A] 401:109–128, 1983

679. Chung EB, Enzinger FM: Malignant melanoma of soft parts. A re-assessment of clear cell sarcoma. Am J Surg Pathol 7:405–413, 1983

680. Eckardt JJ, Pritchard DJ, Soule EH: Clear cell sarcoma: a clinico-pathologic study of 27 cases. Cancer 52:1482–1488, 1983

681. Lucas DR, Nascimento AG, Sim FH: Clear cell sarcoma of soft tissues: Mayo Clinic experience with 35 cases. Am J Surg Pathol 16:1197–1204, 1992

682. Montgomery EA, Meis JM, Ramos AG, et al: Clear cell sarcoma of tendons and aponeuroses: a clinicopathologic study of 58 cases with analysis of prognostic factors. Int J Surg Pathol 1:89–99, 1993

683. Pavlidis NA, Fisher C, Wiltshaw E: Clear-cell sarcoma of tendons and aponeuroses: a clinicopathologic study. Presentation of six additional cases with review of the literature. Cancer 54:1412–1417, 1984

684. Sara AS, Evans HL, Benjamin RS: Malignant melanoma of soft parts (clear cell sarcoma): a study of 17 cases, with emphasis on prognostic factors. Cancer 65:367–374, 1990

685. Hasegawa T, Hirose T, Kudo E, et al: Clear cell sarcoma: an im-munohistochemical and ultrastructural study. Acta Pathol Jpn 39:321–327, 1989

686. Swanson PE, Wick MR: Clear cell sarcoma: an immunohistochemi-cal analysis of six cases and comparison with other epithelioid neo-plasms of soft tissue. Arch Pathol Lab Med 113:55–60, 1989

687. Epstein AL, Martin AO, Kempson R: Use of a newly established hu-man cell line (SU-CCS-I) to demonstrate the relationship of clear cell sarcoma to malignant melanoma. Cancer Res 44:1265–1274, 1984

688. Benson JD, Kraemer BB, Mackay B: Malignant melanoma of soft parts: an ultrastructural study of four cases. Ultrastruct Pathol 8:57–70, 1985

689. Mukai M, Torikata C, Iri H, et al: Histogenesis of clear cell sarcoma of tendons and aponeuroses: an electron microscopic, biochemical, enzyme histochemical, and immunohistochemical study. Am J Pathol 114:264–272, 1984

690. Mrozek K, Karakousis CP, Perez-Mesa C, et al: Translocation t(12;22)(q13;q12.2-12.3) in clear cell sarcoma of tendons and aponeuroses. Genes Chromosom Cancer 6:249–252, 1993

691. Bridge JA, Sreekantaiah C, Neff JR, et al: Cytogenetic findings in clear cell sarcoma of tendons and aponeuroses: malignant melanoma of soft parts. Cancer Genet Cytogenet 52:101–106, 1991

692. Rodriguez E, Sreekantaiah C, Reuter VE, et al: t(12;22)(q13;q13) and trisomy 8 are nonrandom aberrations in clear cell sarcoma. Cancer Genet Cytogenet 64:107–110, 1992

693. Stenman G, Kindblom LG, Angervall L: Reciprocal translocation t(12;22)(q13;q13) in clear cell sarcoma of tendons and aponeuroses. Genes Chromosom Cancer 4:122–127, 1992

694. Travis JA, Bridge JA: Significance of both numerical and structural chromosomal abnormalities in clear cell sarcoma. Cancer Genet Cy-togenet 64:104–106, 1992

695. Caraway NP, Fanning CV, Wojcik EM, et al: Cytology of malignant melanoma of soft parts: fine needle aspirates and exfoliative speci-mens. Diagn Cytopathol 9:632–638, 1993

696. Almeida MM, Nunes AM, Frable WJ: Malignant melanoma of soft tissue. A report of three cases with diagnosis by fine needle aspiration cytology. Acta Cytol 38:241–246, 1994

697. Dehner LP: Primitive neuroectodermal tumor and Ewing's sarcoma. Am J Surg Pathol 17:1–13, 1993

698. Angervall L, Enzinger FM: Extraskeletal neoplasm resembling Ew-ing's sarcoma. Cancer 36:240–251, 1975

699. Shimada H, Newton WA Jr, Soule EH, et al: Pathologic features of extraosseous Ewing's sarcoma: a report from the Intergroup Rhab-domyosarcoma Study. Hum Pathol 19:442–453, 1988

700. Marina NM, Etcubanas E, Parham DM, et al: Peripheral primitive neuroectodermal tumor (peripheral neuroepithelioma) in children. A review of the St. Jude experience and controversies in diagnosis and management. Cancer 64:1952–1960, 1989

701. Askin FB, Rosai J, Sibley RK, et al: Malignant small cell tumor of the thoracopulmonary region in childhood. A distinctive clinicopatho-logic entity of uncertain histogenesis. Cancer 43:2438–2451, 1979

702. Weidner N, Tjoe J: Immunohistochemical profile of monoclonal an-tibody O13: antibody that recognizes glycoprotein p30/32^{MIC2} and is useful in diagnosing Ewing's sarcoma and peripheral neuroepithe-lioma. Am J Surg Pathol 18:486–494, 1994

703. Akhtar M, Ali MA, Sabbah R: Aspiration cytology of Ewing's sar-coma. Light and electron microscopic correlations. Cancer 56:2051–2060, 1985

704. Kumar PV: Fine needle aspiration cytologic findings in malignant small cell tumor of the thoracopulmonary region (Askin tumor). Acta Cytol 38:702–706, 1994

705. Silverman JF, Joshi VV: FNA biopsy of small round cell tumors of childhood: cytomorphologic features and the role of ancillary studies. Diagn Cytopathol 10:245–255, 1994

706. Ordóñez NG, Zirkin R, Bloom RE: Malignant small-cell epithelial tu-mor of the peritoneum coexpressing mesenchymal-type intermediate filaments. Am J Surg Pathol 13:413–421, 1989

707. Gonzalez-Crussi F, Crawford SE, Sun C-CJ: Intraabdominal desmo-plastic small-cell tumors with divergent differentiation. Am J Surg Pathol 14:633–642, 1990

708. Gerald WL, Miller HK, Battifora H, et al: Intra-abdominal desmo-plastic small round-cell tumor. Report of 19 cases of a distinctive type of high-grade polyphenotypic malignancy affecting young individu-als. Am J Surg Pathol 15:499–513, 1991

709. Ordonez NG, El-Naggar AK, Ro JY, et al: Intra-abdominal desmo-plastic small cell tumor: a light microscopic, immunocytochemical, ultrastructural, and flow cytometric study. Hum Pathol 24:850–855, 1993

710. Layfield LJ, Lenarsky C: Desmoplastic small cell tumors of the peri-toneum coexpressing mesenchymal and epithelial markers. Am J Clin Pathol 96:536–543, 1991

711. Norton J, Monaghan P, Carter RL: Intra-abdominal desmoplastic small cell tumour with divergent differentiation. Histopathology 19:560–562, 1991

712. Variend S, Gerrard M, Norris PD, et al: Intra-abdominal neuroecto-dermal tumour of childhood with divergent differentiation. Histopathology 18:45–51, 1991

713. Prat J, Matias-Guiu X, Algaba F: Desmoplastic small round cell tu-mor. Am J Surg Pathol 16:306–307, 1992

714. Rodriguez E, Sreekantaiah C, Gerald W, et al: A recurring transloca-tion, t(11;22) (p13;q11.2), characterizes intra-abdominal desmoplas-tic small round-cell tumors. Cancer Genet Cytogenet 69:17–21, 1993

715. Setrakian S, Gupta PK, Heald K, et al: Intraabdominal desmoplastic small round cell tumor. Report of a case diagnosed by fine needle as-piration cytology. Acta Cytol 36:373–376, 1992

716. Caraway NP, Fanning CV, Amato RJ, et al: Fine-needle aspiration of intra-abdominal desmoplastic small cell tumor. Diagn Cytopathol 9:465–470, 1993

717. El-Kattan I, Redline RW, El-Naggar AK, et al: Cytologic features of intraabdominal desmoplastic small round cell tumor. A case report. Acta Cytol 39:514–520, 1995

718. Beckwith JB, Palmer NF: Histopathology and prognosis of Wilms' tumor: results from the first National Wilms' Tumor Study. Cancer 41:1937–1948, 1978

719. Sotelo-Avila C, Gonzalez-Crussi F, DeMello D, et al: Renal and ex-trarenal rhabdoid tumors in children: a clinicopathologic study of 14 patients. Semin Diagn Pathol 3:151–163, 1986

720. Parham DM, Weeks DA, Beckwith JB: The clinicopathologic spec-trum of putative extrarenal rhabdoid tumors. Am J Surg Pathol 18:1010–1029, 1994

721. Sola-Perez J, Perez-Guillermo M, Bas-Bernal A, et al: Malignant rhabdoid tumor of soft tissues: a cytopathological and immunohisto-chemical study. Diagn Cytopathol 8:369–373, 1992

722. Ushigome S, Shimoda T, Nikaido T, et al: Histopathologic diagnostic and histogenetic problems in malignant soft tissue tumors: reassessment of malignant fibrous histiocytoma, epithelioid sarcoma, malignant rhabdoid tumor, and neuroectodermal tumor. Acta Pathol Jpn 42:691–706, 1992

723. Weeks DA, Beckwith JB, Mierau GW, et al: Renal neoplasms mimicking rhabdoid tumor of kidney. Am J Surg Pathol 15:1042–1054, 1991

724. Weeks DA Jr, Beckwith JB, Mierau GW: Rhabdoid tumor: an entity or a phenotype? Arch Pathol Lab Med 113:113–114, 1989

725. Drut R: Malignant rhabdoid tumor of the kidney diagnosed by fine-needle aspiration cytology. Diagn Cytopathol 6:124–126, 1990

726. Wick MR, Ritter JH, Dehner LP: Malignant rhabdoid tumor. A clinicopathologic review and conceptual discussion. Semin Diagn Pathol 12:233–248, 1995

727. Akhtar M, Kfoury H, Haider A, et al: Fine-needle aspiration biopsy diagnosis of extrarenal malignant rhabdoid tumor. Diagn Cytopathol 11:271–276, 1994

728. Konwaler BE, Keasbey L, Kaplan L: Subcutaneous pseudosarcomatous fibromatosis (fasciitis). Am J Clin Pathol 25:241–252, 1955

729. Dahl I, Angervall L, Magnusson S, et al: Nodular fasciitis. Acta Pathol Microbiol Scand [A] 79:681–682, 1971

730. Bernstein KE, Lattes R: Nodular (pseudosarcomatous) fasciitis, a nonrecurrent lesion. Cancer 49:1668–1678, 1982

731. Price EB, Silliphant WM, Shuman R: Nodular fasciitis: a clinicopathological analysis of 65 cases. Am J Clin Pathol 35:122–136, 1961

732. Montgomery EA, Meis JM: Nodular fasciitis. Its morphologic spectrum and immunohistochemical profile. Am J Surg Pathol 15:942–948, 1991

733. Shimizu S, Hashimoto H, Enjoji M: Nodular fasciitis: an analysis of 250 patients. Pathology 16:161–166, 1984

734. Patchefsky AS, Enzinger FM: Intravascular fasciitis: a report of 17 cases. Am J Surg Pathol 5:29–36, 1981

735. Lauer DH, Enzinger FM: Cranial fasciitis of childhood. Cancer 45:401–406, 1980

736. Chung EB, Enzinger FM: Proliferative fasciitis. Cancer 36:1450–1458, 1975

737. Meister P, Konrad EA, Buckmann FW: Nodular fasciitis and proliferative myositis as variants of one disease entity. Invest Cell Pathol 2:277–281, 1979

738. Montgomery EA, Meis JM, Frizzera G: Proliferative fasciitis and myositis of childhood. Am J Surg Pathol 16:364–372, 1992

739. Dahl I, Akerman M: Nodular fasciitis. A correlative cytologic and histologic study of 13 cases. Acta Cytol 25:215–222, 1981

740. Gonzalez-Campora R, Otal-Salaverri C, Hevia-Vazquez A, et al: Fine needle aspiration in myxoid tumors of the soft tissues. Acta Cytol 34:179–191, 1990

741. Stanley MW, Skoog L, Tani EM, et al: Nodular fasciitis: spontaneous resolution following diagnosis by fine-needle aspiration. Diagn Cytopathol 9:322–324, 1993

742. Lundgren L, Kindblom LG, Willems J, et al: Proliferative myositis and fasciitis. A light and electron microscopic, cytologic, DNA-cytometric and immunohistochemical study. APMIS 100:437–448, 1992

743. Chow LTC, Chow WH, Lee JCK: Fine needle aspiration (FNA) cytology of proliferative fasciitis: report of a case with immunohistochemical study. Cytopathology 6:349–357, 1995

744. Jacobs JC: Aspiration cytology of proliferative myositis. A case report. Acta Cytol 39:535–538, 1995

745. James LP: Cytopathology of mesenchymal repair. Diagn Cytopathol 1:91–104, 1985

746. Proppe KH, Scully RE, Rosai J: Postoperative spindle cell nodules of genitourinary tract resembling sarcomas. A report of eight cases. Am J Surg Pathol 8:101–108, 1984

747. Arber DA, Kamel OW, Van de Riju M, et al: Frequent presence of the Epstein-Barr virus in inflammatory pseudotumor. Hum Pathol 26:1093–1098, 1995

748. Albores-Saavedra J, Henson DE, Klimstra D: Tumors of the gallbladder, extrahepatic bile ducts and ampulla of Vater. Fascicle 23, 3rd Ed. Armed Forces Institute of Pathology, Washington, DC (in press)

749. Albores-Saavedra J, Manivel JC, Essenfield H, et al: Pseudosarcomatous myofibroblastic proliferations in the urinary bladder of children. Cancer 66:1234–1241, 1990

750. Lundgren L, Aldenborg F, Angervall L, et al: Pseudomalignant spindle cell proliferations of the urinary bladder. Hum Pathol 25:181–191, 1994

751. Hojo H, Newton WA, Hamoudi AB, et al: Pseudosarcomatous myofibroblastic tumor of the urinary bladder in children: a study of 11 cases with review of the literature. Am J Surg Pathol 19:1224–1236, 1995

752. Anthony PP: Inflammatory pseudotumour (plasma cell granuloma) of lung, liver and other organs. Histopathology 23:501–503, 1993

753. Hollowood K, Fletcher CDM: Pseudosarcomatous myofibroblastic proliferations of the spermatic cord ("proliferative funiculitis")—histologic and immunohistochemical analysis of a distinctive entity. Am J Surg Pathol 16:448–454, 1992

754. Pettinato G, Manivel KC, De Rosa N, et al: Inflammatory myofibroblastic tumor (plasma cell granuloma). Clinicopathologic study of 20 cases with immunohistochemical and ultrastructural observations. Am J Clin Pathol 94:538–546, 1990

755. Coffin CM, Watterson J, Priest J, et al: Extrapulmonary inflammatory myofibroblastic tumor: a clinicopathologic and immunohistochemical study of 84 cases. Am J Surg Pathol 19:859–872, 1995

756. Meis JM, Enzinger FM: Inflammatory fibrosarcoma of the mesentery and retroperitoneum. A tumor closely simulating inflammatory pseudotumor. Am J Surg Pathol 15:1146–1156, 1991

757. Montgomery EA, Meis JM, Mitchell MS, et al: Atypical decubital fibroplasia. A distinctive fibroblastic pseudotumor occurring in debilitated patients. Am J Surg Pathol 16:708–715, 1992

758. Fetsch JF, Montgomery EA, Meis JM: Calcifying fibrous pseudotumor. Am J Surg Pathol 17:502–508, 1993

759. Rosenthal NS, Abdul-Karim FW: Childhood fibrous tumor with psammoma bodies. Arch Pathol Lab Med 112:798–800, 1988

760. Ackerman LW: Extra-osseous localized non-neoplastic bone and cartilage formation (so-called myositis ossificans). J Bone Joint Surg [Am] 40:279–298, 1958

761. Rööser B, Herrlin K, Rydholm A, Akerman M: Pseudomalignant myositis ossificans. Clinical, radiologic, and cytologic diagnosis in five cases. Acta Orthop Scand 60:457–460, 1989

762. Wakely PE Jr, Almeida M, Frable WJ: Fine-needle aspiration biopsy cytology of myositis ossificans. Mod Pathol 7:23–25, 1994

763. Meis JM, Enzinger FM: Juxta-articular myxoma: a clinical and pathological study of 65 cases. Hum Pathol 23:639–646, 1992

764. Hughes D, Buckley PJ: Idiopathic retroperitoneal fibrosis is a macrophage-rich process. Implications for its pathogenesis and treatment. Am J Surg Pathol 17:482–490, 1993

765. Chan SL, Johnson HW, McLaughlin MG: Idiopathic retroperitoneal fibrosis in children. J Urol 122:103–104, 1977

766. Comings DE, Shub KB, Van Eyes J, et al: Familial multifocal fibrosclerosis. Ann Intern Med 66:884–892, 1967

767. Kains JPD, Hardy JC, Chevalier C, et al: Retroperitoneal fibrosis in two patients with Parkinson's disease treated with bromocriptine. Acta Clin Belg 45:306–310, 1990

768. Lee I: Human fibroblasts in idiopathic retroperitoneal fibrosis express HLA-DR antigens. J Korean Med Sci 6:279–283, 1991

769. Mitchinson MJ: Aortic disease in retroperitoneal and mediastinal fibrosis. J Clin Pathol 25:287–293, 1972

770. Mitchinson MJ: The pathology of idiopathic retroperitoneal fibrosis. J Clin Pathol 25:681–689, 1970

771. Murphy F, Pichard R: Bromocriptine-associated retroperitoneal fibrosis presenting with testicular retraction. Br J Urol 64:318–319, 1989

772. Osborne BM, Butler JJ, Bloustein P, et al: Idiopathic retroperitoneal fibrosis (sclerosing retroperitonitis). Hum Pathol 18:735–739, 1987

773. Salyer WR, Salyer DC: Intravascular angiomatosis. Development and distinction from angiosarcoma. Cancer 36:995–1001, 1975

774. Kuo T-T, Sayers P, Rosai J: "Masson's vegetant intravascular hemangioendothelioma:" A lesion often mistaken for angiosarcoma. Study of seventeen cases located in the skin and soft tissues. Cancer 38:1227–1236, 1976

775. Clearkin KP, Enzinger FM: Intravascular papillary endothelial hyperplasia. Arch Pathol Lab Med 100:441–444, 1976

776. Hashimoto H, Daimaru Y, Enjoji M: Intravascular papillary endothelial hyperplasia: a clinicopathologic study of 91 cases. Am J Dermatopathol 5:539–546, 1983

777. Kuo T, Gomez LG: Papillary endothelial proliferation in cystic lymphangiomas. A lymphatic vessel counterpart of Masson's vegetant intravascular hemangioendothelioma. Arch Pathol Lab Med 103:306–308, 1979

778. Weiss SW, Enzinger FM, Johnson FB: Silica reaction simulating fibrous histiocytoma. Cancer 42:2738–2743, 1978

779. Umlas J, Federman M, Crawford C, et al: Spindle cell pseudotumor due to *Mycobacterium avium-intracellulare* in patients with acquired immunodeficiency syndrome (AIDS). Positive staining of mycobacteria for cytoskeleton filaments. Am J Surg Pathol 15:1181–1187, 1991

780. Slavin RE, Wen J, Kumar D, et al: Familial tumoral calcinosis: a clinical, histopathologic, and ultrastructural study with an analysis of its calcifying process and pathogenesis. Am J Surg Pathol 17:788–802, 1993

Appendix 18-1. Fine Needle Aspiration of Spindle Cell Soft Tissue Lesions

	Cellular Hemangioma	Schwannoma	Leiomyoma	Fibromatosis Desmoid	DFSP	Synovial Sarcoma	Leiomyosarcoma	MFH
Peak age	Child	20–50 yr	Adolescent, young adult	Child or young adult	25–40 yr	15–35 yr	Adult	50–70 yr
Common locations	Head and neck	Nerve	Dermis, extremity	Abdominal wall, sternocleidomastoid, musculoaponeurosis	Dermal	Extremity, near joint	Retroperitoneum, dermal, large veins of extremity	Extremity, retroperitoneum
Cellularity	Moderate	Moderate	Moderate	Moderate	High	Very high	High	High
Background	Bloody	Clean	Clean	Clean, collagen	Metachromatic fibrous stromal fragments	Clean	± necrosis, sometimes myxoid	± necrosis
Cell pattern	Clusters, lumens	Dense and loose areas, palisades	Palisades, tandem rows	Loose clusters and single cells	Storiform clusters, single cells	Fascicles, single cells	Fascicles, rows, palisades, single cells	Storiform
Cell types	Spindled	Spindled, elongated	Spindled, vessels in clusters	Spindled, plump, elongated, skeletal muscle	Spindled, monomorphic	Spindled, vessels in clusters, ± epithelial clusters	Spindled, rarely epithelioid, vessels in clusters	Spindled, rounded, multinucleate
Cytoplasm	Scant, bipolar	Syncytial, Verocay bodies	Syncytial, abundant	Tags, bipolar processes	Fibrillary, syncytial in clusters	Scant tags	Discrete, eosinophilic, stripped	Vacuolated, bipolar
Nuclei	Even chromatin	Twisted shapes, dense chromatin, pseudoinclusions	Blunted, cigar-shaped, finely granular chromatin	Bland, fine chromatin	Uniform, finely granular chromatin	Uniform, granular chromatin, mitotic figures	Blunt spindled, coarsely granular chromatin, sometimes pleomorphic	Pleomorphic, bizarre chromatin
Nucleoli	Inconspicuous	Inconspicuous	Inconspicuous	Inconspicuous	Inconspicuous	Inconspicuous	Small	Yes
Special	Factor VIII-related protein	Degenerative pleomorphism, S-100 protein	Actin, desmin	Actin	CD34	Keratin, EMA	Actin, desmin	Osteoclasts, mixed inflammatory cells

Abbreviations: DFSP, dermatofibrosarcoma protuberans; MFH, malignant fibrous histiocytoma; EMA, epithelial membrane antigen.

Appendix 18-2. FNA of Myxoid Soft Tissue Lesions

	Nodular Fasciitis	Intramuscular Myxoma	Myxoid Liposarcoma	Myxofibrosarcoma (Myxoid MFH)	Myxoid Chondrosarcoma	Chordoma
Peak age	20–35 yr	Adult	40–60 yr	Over 40 yr	Adult	40–60 yr
Common locations	Superficial extremity	Thigh, shoulder, buttock muscles	Deep extremity or retroperitoneum	Deep extremity or retroperitoneum	Deep extremity	Base of skull, sacrococcygeal
Cellularity	Moderate	Low	Moderate-high	Moderate-high	Moderate-high	High
Background	Myxoid, fibrillar, semitransparent	Myxoid, fibrillar, semitransparent	Myxoid, fibrillar, semitransparent	Myxoid, fragments, semiopaque	Myxoid, fragments, semiopaque	Myxoid, fragments, semiopaque
Cell pattern	Storiform	Scattered randomly	Plexiform vasculature	Curvilinear vasculature	Cords, clusters	Single and clusters in matrix
Cell types	Spindled, ovoid, ganglion-like, lymphs, histiocytes	Spindled, stellate, skeletal muscle	Lipoblasts, single and clustered on vasculature	Spindled, multinucleate	Round, medium-sized	Moderately pleomorphic
Cytoplasm	Bipolar processes and tags	Bipolar processes and tags	Multivacuolated, rounded	Bipolar processes	Scant, embedded in matrix	Abundant, vacuolated (signet ring-like, physaliferous)
Nuclei	Dark to finely granular chromatin	Uniform, bland chromatin	Scalloped contours, hyperchromatic	Pleomorphic, coarse chromatin	Uniform, fine chromatin	Central, ovoid, fine chromatin
Nucleoli	Small	Inconspicuous	Small	Larger	Small	Small
Special	Rapid onset post-trauma		S-100 protein		S-100 protein, hyaluronidase-resistant sulfated mucopolysaccharide	S-100 protein, keratin, EMA

Abbreviations: MFH, malignant fibrous histiocytoma; EMA, epithelial membrane antigen.

Appendix 18-3. FNA of Epithelioid Soft Tissue Lesions

	Granular Cell Tumor	Clear Cell Sarcoma	Epithelioid Sarcoma	Alveolar Soft Part Sarcoma	Plasmacytoma
Peak age	30–60 yr	20–40 yr	10–35 yr	15–35 yr	Over 40 yr
Common locations	Tongue, dermis, breast	Deep, distal leg	Dermal or tendon nodules, distal extremity	Leg or head and neck	Near bone, paravertebral
Cellularity	Moderate	Moderate	Moderate	High	High
Background	Clean	Clean	± necrotic debris	Clean	Clean
Cell patterns	Loose clusters and single	Dispersed	Dissociated	Dispersed and alveolar balls	Dispersed and clusters
Cell types	Polygonal to spindled	Round to plump spindled	Polygonal, large	Polygonal, very large, thin-walled vessels	Variably uniform to pleomorphic, vascular septa with clusters
Cytoplasm	Marked coarse eosinophilic granularity, indistinct borders	Finely granular	Densely eosinophilic	Abundant, granular, fragile	Basophilic, perinuclear hof
Nuclei	Round, uniform dense chromatin	Eccentric, round, finely granular chromatin, pseudoinclusions	Eccentric, round, open chromatin, some binucleate	Central, round, open chromatin, bare nuclei	Eccentric, round, clockface clumpy chromatin, ± binucleate
Nucleoli	Inconspicuous	Prominent	Evident	Prominent	Variable
Special	PAS, S-100 protein	Melanin, S-100 protein, HMB 45	Keratin	PAS+ crystals	Kappa/lambda

Abbreviation: PAS, periodic acid-Schiff.

19

The Breast

Steven G. Silverberg
Shahla Masood

Lesions of the mammary gland, by virtue of their incidence, constitute one of the most important chapters in a text on human pathology, and the major topic of mammary pathology is the diagnosis of malignant tumors. In several regions of the world, malignant breast tumors constitute the most common group of cancers among women, and men are by no means exempt from them. In the United States, for example, approximately 18 percent of all malignant tumors are breast cancers, representing the most important cause of death by cancer in women; in absolute figures, this means approximately 46,000 deaths per year.[1]

It is nonetheless important to understand the benign lesions, whether they are tumoral or not. These lesions manifest their own specific characteristics and require equally specific treatments. Furthermore, an intimate knowledge of benign breast lesions facilitates the differential diagnosis between them and malignant lesions. Consequently, the discussion in this chapter covers both the benign and the malignant morphologic alterations of the human breast.

In recent years, the role of the diagnostic surgical pathologist has become not only to diagnose a breast lesion as benign or malignant, but equally to assay the prognosis of both. Among benign lesions, the pathologist must distinguish those with widely varying risks of subsequent development of breast cancer. Among breast carcinomas, some will almost always be cured by conservative treatment, whereas others will require extensive multimodality therapy for even a reasonable chance of extended survival. A major role of the pathologist is to establish, by both traditional histopathologic observation and the use of an array of new and sophisticated tests—among which the pathologist must choose the most appropriate—the prognosis and, by extension, the appropriate treatment for each individual case.

The cytopathologist is also playing an increasingly more important role in the management of breast disease. As radiologic technical improvements result in the identification of smaller and more subtle mammary lesions, fine needle aspiration (FNA)—often performed and always interpreted by the cytopathologist—becomes a more important tool in deciding which patients need to undergo formal biopsy and, in the case of those lesions diagnosed definitively as carcinoma by FNA, enables definitive treatment to be undertaken in many cases without the additional expense and time consumed by a tissue biopsy.

The signs, symptoms, and sometimes even the morphologic manifestations of an intraparenchymal mass are often discrete, requiring a multidisciplinary approach for their proper interpretation. The information provided by pathologists, based on the study of histologic and cytologic specimens, is of maximum value only when integrated with both radiologic and clinical findings. Recent texts have emphasized the importance of this multidisciplinary approach.[2,3] Only in this manner can we ensure efficient and precise diagnosis and diminish possible recurrences or metastases. As an example, let us remind both the clinician and the pathologist that it is the responsibility of the latter to determine whether a specimen sent to him by the clinician is an adequate and representative one, or whether it is necessary to obtain another, as well as to decide for what studies the tissue will be submitted. The requirement for well preserved, high quality specimens is one about which the pathologist must be intransigent, because such a requirement will prove considerably less blameworthy than an erroneous diagnosis.

EMBRYOLOGY AND HISTOLOGY

The understanding and correct interpretation of the morphologic lesions of mammary tissue require a knowledge of the normal histologic structures and their embryologic origins.

The early embryo produces a ventral, linear, ectodermal thickening extending from the axillary region to the inguinal region, along both sides of the midsagittal plane. These thickenings are the milk ridges. By the ninth week of embryonic development, these ridges persist only in the pectoral region, where the ectoderm undergoes further thickening and produces solid cords of cells that burrow into the underlying mesenchyme[4,5] (Fig. 19-1).

Near the end of the embryonic period, these cords become hollow and thus constitute the future mammary gland parenchyma: the lactiferous sinus, the lactiferous ducts, and the secretory alveoli.[5,6] The stroma of the future mammary gland includes tissue situated around the lobar glandular formations; this is the intralobar connective tissue. Beyond the limits of the intralobar connective tissue, the stroma is denser and constitutes the interlobar connective tissue. The resting gland consists of approximately 15 to 25 lobes separated by the dense interlobar fibrous septa. Each lobe is subdivided into lobules that

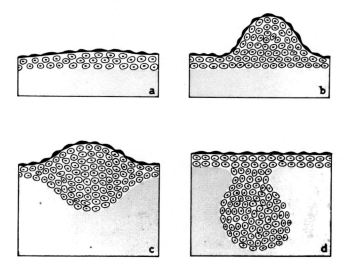

Fig. 19-1. Embryonic development of the mammary gland. (a) Ectoderm. (b & c) Thickening of ectoderm. (d) Solid ectodermal cord invading the underlying mesenchyme.

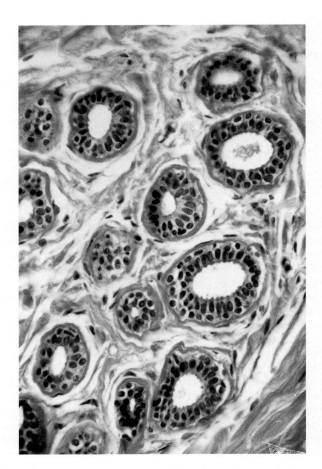

Fig. 19-2. Normal mammary gland. Lactiferous ducts and the surrounding connective tissue are shown.

represent the functional units of the mammary parenchyma. A surface ectodermal thickening, pushed anteriorly by the mesenchyme, constitutes the nipple, which is surrounded by a pigmented ectodermal zone called the areola. Ultrastructurally, the walls of the glandular system consist of a basal lamina, a discontinuous layer of myoepithelial cells, and two layers of columnar cells. The columnar cells possess numerous microvilli on the luminal surface as well as between the cells, and the myoepithelial cells are characterized by an abundant contractile fibrillar cytoplasmic apparatus.[7,8] These myoepithelial cells are well demonstrated immunohistochemically by their staining with antibodies to muscle-specific actin or S-100 protein.

During gestation, the fetal mammary gland undergoes hormonal stimulation of maternal origin, producing signs of secretory activity that regress at birth.[9] At puberty, under the influence of sexual hormones, the female mammary gland acquires its ultimate maturation: the development of the lactiferous duct system and the process of lobulation occur simultaneously with a proliferation of the surrounding connective and adipose tissues (Fig. 19-2).

During the period of sexual activity, the mammary gland reacts to the influences of the hormonal cycle, and the glandular system thus undergoes a cellular proliferation during the estrogenic phase, followed by discrete secretory activity at the end of the cycle.[9,10] Concomitant with these changes, the intralobular connective tissue increases its capacity to bind water, particularly near the end of the cycle. This phenomenon explains the impression of heaviness and fullness experienced by many women in the premenstrual period.

During periods of lactation, under the action of different hormones (estrogens, progesterone, prolactin, and others such as cortisol and insulin), the acinar cells undergo a marked secretory differentiation and the lobules become hyperplastic and

crowded (Fig. 19-3). The interlobular septa are markedly thinned. Colostrum production and subsequently milk production occur at the distal part of the glandular system, the cellular activities of which thus comprise protein and lipid synthesis. Once secreted, ejection of the milk requires sucking, oxytocin secretion, and myoepithelial cell contraction. After menopause, the lobules become atrophic and the excretory ducts undergo cystic degenerative dilation. The surrounding stroma manifests a loss of cellularity accompanied by fibrosis.[11]

MACROSCOPIC ANATOMY

The mammary gland is a glandular system surrounded by fibroadipose tissue that rests on a musculoconnective tissue bed. The gland is covered by the epidermis. Centrally located is the nipple, a cylindrical excrescence, which is surrounded by a circular, pigmented area called the areola; the tubercles of Montgomery[12] are specialized sebaceous glands of the areola that enlarge during pregnancy and lactation. The arteries of the mammary gland are branches of the internal mammary, exter-

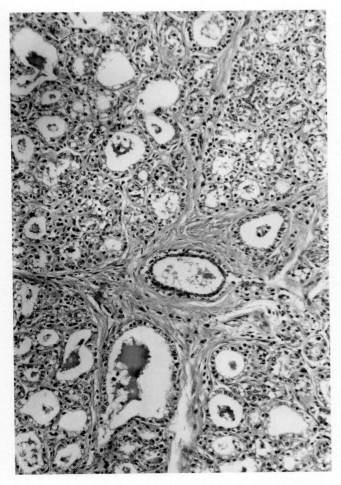

Fig. 19-3. Lactating mammary gland, secretory differentiation of acinar cells. Note the structural difference between the secretory acini and the lactiferous ducts.

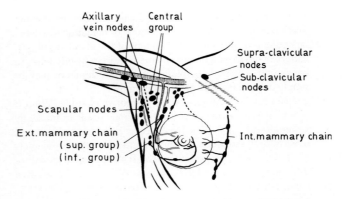

Fig. 19-4. Structure of the lymphatic system of the mammary gland.

nal mammary, and intercostal arteries. The veins are the axillary, internal mammary, and intercostal veins.

The structure of the lymphatic system has a direct influence on the mode of dissemination of tumors (Fig. 19-4). The cutaneous lymphatics and some of the perilobular, perialveolar, and ductal lymphatic pathways drain into the areolar plexus.[13,14] Three main lymphatic groups arise from the plexus: the external, internal, and inferior groups. Most of the deep lymphatics bypass the areolar plexus and drain into these groups. The external mammary lymphatics terminate in the external mammary nodes. These nodes are in continuity with the different axillary groups: the scapular nodes, the central nodes, the axillary vein nodes, and the subclavicular nodes. From there, large lymphatic trunks drain into the jugular-subclavian venous system. The interpectoral nodes described by Rotter are of little significance and are usually not dissected unless the pectoralis major muscle is removed. The internal mammary lymphatics drain into the internal mammary nodes between the costal car-

tilages. These nodes surround the internal mammary vessels and are usually small. They receive some drainage from the lateral half of the breast. Connecting lymphatics between the left and right lymphatic chains exist at the level of the first costal interspace. The inferior mammary lymphatics empty into the anterior pectoral, axillary, and subclavicular nodes. When the lymphatic drainage is blocked by metastases, retrograde lymphatic spread develops, explaining various metastatic locations such as the opposite axilla and the liver. Intramammary lymph nodes are frequently aspirated or removed as mammographically detected masses.[15]

CONGENITAL ABNORMALITIES

Like other organs, the mammary glands can present congenital anomalies resulting from improper embryonic development:

Athelia: lack of nipple; generally occurs with amastia, both rare
Amastia: absence of the mammary gland; can be uni- or bilateral
Polythelia: the presence of supernumerary nipples
Polymastia: presence of supernumerary mammary glands (polymastia and polythelia result from the persistence of portions of the milk ridge that normally undergo involution)

NEUROENDOCRINE ANOMALIES

The normal development of the mammary gland is under the influence of the neuroendocrine system. When this stimulation is absent or disturbed, abnormalities occur:

Precocious development of the breast occurs as part of the clinical presentation of premature—although normal—

adolescence. Rarely, it is associated with estrogen-producing ovarian tumors, lutein cysts, or tumors of the adrenal cortex.

Micromastia is insufficient development of the gland at puberty. Failure of development can be due to ovarian insufficiency or congenital adrenal hyperplasia, or the development may be simply delayed because of late menarche.

Macromastia is hypertrophy of the mammary gland.[16] When it occurs, it is generally at puberty and may result in markedly voluminous breasts. This hypertrophy is due to an abnormal sensitivity to estrogenic hormones and is sometimes symmetric. The microscopic structure reveals a remarkable growth of the connective and adipose tissues. A few cases of massive breast hypertrophy have been reported during pregnancy.

Gynecomastia is the unilateral or bilateral development of the mammary gland in the male. When it occurs, it is usually at puberty or in old age. This anomaly is discussed in detail later in the section on pathologic conditions of the male breast.

BASIC TECHNIQUES OF HANDLING BREAST SPECIMENS

The main types of specimens submitted to the pathologist in various breast disorders are from needle aspirations, from incisional and excisional biopsies, from the different techniques of mastectomy, and from therapeutic local excisions or re-excisions.

An accurate description of the gross appearance of the specimen is an essential step in the evaluation of breast disease, because it can be made only once, while the specimen is fresh. A good description must be sufficiently detailed so anyone familiar with pathology can visualize the specimen on the basis of the report alone. Careful palpation of the specimen is of great importance for detection of any malignant lesion.

The examination includes the gathering of the following information: the weight, the dimensions, the number of fragments, and the description of each fragment. More specifically, this description gives the following details: color, consistency, infiltration of the surrounding tissues, and appearance of the different slices obtained through the specimen. Any pathologic condition, such as cysts, fibrosis, inflammation or hemorrhagic foci, necrosis, firm areas, and granular degeneration with chalky streaks, should be noted. The presence of microcalcifications detected by mammography should be confirmed by specimen radiography. If the presence of an intraductal papilloma is suspected, the main lactiferous ducts should be opened lengthwise and a careful excision of the papilloma with surrounding tissues performed. If the search for papilloma is negative, transverse sections should be made and totally embedded.

Imprints or smears of the lesion are made to obtain fine details of the cytologic structures. Needle aspiration biopsies are studied similarly. Two methods can be used: the air-dried smear stained with a Giemsa or similar technique or the wet-smear technique with fixation in 95 percent alcohol. Both methods are satisfactory, but the second technique gives better nuclear detail and allows comparison with tissue biopsy specimens.

These imprints provide information that is complementary to histologic slides.[17,18]

When an immediate frozen section examination is requested, if the pathologist concurs, the most suspicious area of the specimen is carefully selected. The fragments must be thin (<0.5 cm in thickness) in order to obtain readable frozen sections. After freezing and sectioning, the fragment is placed in fixative. The number of blocks of tissue taken from a given specimen for frozen section examination depends on the circumstances, with diffuse or ill-defined lesions requiring more sections for accuracy.

The detection of asymptomatic anomalies such as lobular carcinoma in situ depends on the number of blocks examined, but the chance of correctly diagnosing lobular carcinoma in situ is low, about 18 percent.[19] If the lesion has been detected by mammography, and no grossly detectable lesion is present, or if the only lesion is less than 1.0 cm in greatest diameter, a frozen section should not be performed except in unusual circumstances.[20,21] In any event, difficulties will be encountered with certain lesions, such as lobular carcinoma in situ, intraductal papilloma, and well differentiated papillary carcinoma. In many of these cases, intraoperative smears or imprints may be easier to interpret than frozen sections[17,18]; in other instances, it is wiser to wait for paraffin-embedded permanent sections in order to avoid a false positive or a false negative result.

How extensively should an excisional biopsy specimen be sampled for microscopic examination? The answer to this question depends both the size of the specimen and the reason for which it was obtained. Small biopsies (those that can be cut in their entirety into 6 to 8 tissue blocks or fewer) should be submitted in toto for microscopy. In the case of larger specimens, sampling that is both cost effective and diagnostically sufficient consists of (1) 10 blocks of fibrous (as opposed to fatty) parenchyma in grossly lesion-free specimens removed for the indication of a palpable mass[22]; or (2) all regions of radiographic calcification (confirmed by specimen radiographs) and fibrous parenchyma in mammographically directed biopsies without a palpable or visible mass.[23] If a clinically palpable or nonpalpable mass is detected at gross examination of the specimen, the mass should be submitted in its entirety unless it has been demonstrated intraoperatively to be a fibroadenoma, in which case less extensive sampling may suffice. All specimens should be inked to demonstrate margins before they are sectioned.

Mastectomy Specimens

When dealing with a simple mastectomy specimen, the description must include the appearance of the nipple and skin and the localization and description of pathologic foci. The biopsy incision, when present, should be opened, and any residual tumor should be sought. The following fragments are typically sampled: the nipple, the region beneath the nipple, the tumor and any abnormal macroscopic lesions, as well as the presumably normal parenchyma. A recent study has suggested that routine sampling of normal parenchyma in quadrants distal to the main lesion or biopsy cavity may be eliminated.[24]

The frequency of nipple involvement by breast cancer varies according to the number of sections taken from the area. Taking a cylindrical block 1 cm deep containing the nipple and the areola, and performing 14 horizontal sections has demonstrated that the percentage of nipple involvement increases significantly and may attain 50 percent. Therefore, the risk of leaving a malignant focus in the nipple area can be important when subcutaneous mastectomy techniques are used. If the nipple has been removed, however, its extensive examination by the pathologist adds little except time and expense.

The dissection of the axillary tail is important because lymph nodes may be found even if there had been no formal dissection of the axilla. The remaining fragments of the specimen can then be fixed and retained for possible further examination.

Sectioning of fresh breast tissue is not easy, particularly when there is marked fatty infiltration. Different methods have been proposed to overcome this difficulty, among which are partial freezing or fixation until the tissues are firm enough to be sliced. These techniques are particularly used when large sections of breast parenchyma are needed (e.g., for comparison with mammography results).

In radical mastectomy (a less frequently performed procedure in recent years), the examination of the mammary gland is followed by a careful dissection of the axillary fat. The nodes are usually divided into three groups: those lateral to and below the pectoralis minor, those behind and within the borders of the muscle, and those above or medial to the muscle. The most medial nodes are near the apex of the axilla. Sometimes nodes are found between the pectoralis minor and the excised fragment of the pectoralis major (Fig. 19-5). Lymph nodes that are dissected out without their respective muscles should be identified with respect to their position and should be so labeled by the surgeon. In the much more frequently performed modified radical mastectomy, the pectoralis muscles are not removed, and only level I and some level II lymph nodes are obtained. The nodes identified by the pathologist at the apex of the axillary dissec-

tion specimen may be submitted for microscopic examination separately and the results reported independently.

The most widely used method for detection of metastases is based on careful palpation and removal of lymph nodes present in the axillary fat tissue. This is preferred to the more time consuming and perhaps more sophisticated method that uses alcohol to clear the adipose tissue. Although this method finds many more small lymph nodes, these rarely add significantly to the number of positive nodes. All the nodes should be dissected, labeled, and embedded.

The number of nodes recovered from the axillary region of a modified radical mastectomy varies from 0 to 70 or more. These variations are at least in part due to anatomic differences. It is important to remember that approximately 30 to 40 percent of clinically normal nodes exhibit metastases histologically. Also, enlarged, suspicious lymph nodes may reveal merely a massive fatty infiltration or lymphoid hyperplasia.

Clinical staging is based partially on the presence of palpable lymph nodes. The currently widely accepted clinical TNM staging system is presented in Table 19-1. Pathologic expression of the nodes is expressed in the pN portion of the classification.

Mastectomy scars often become the site of tumor recurrence; any suspicious modification of a scar should be removed and examined microscopically, because granulomatous reaction to suture material may simulate carcinoma.

Local Excision (Lumpectomy, Tylectomy, Quadrantectomy) Specimens

In many centers in North America and Europe, many if not most patients with primary operable breast cancer are now treated by a breast-conserving local excision with or without radiotherapy. The choice of such therapy over mastectomy depends in part on the evaluation by the pathologist of the initial excision specimen. It is crucial in these cases to (1) record the gross dimensions of the tumor before removing any of it for special studies, such as hormone receptor assays or flow cytometry; (2) carefully note the gross relationship of the tumor to the resection margins; and (3) mark the surface of the specimen with some type of ink, which must be dried before the specimen is incised. We have found the resection margins in these cases to be often extremely difficult to evaluate microscopically, despite the employment of one of the suggested techniques of cutting and embedding[25,26]; nevertheless, surgeons usually request that a statement appear in the final pathology report describing the adequacy of resection. The tumor differentiation (grade), extent of intraductal carcinoma within and/or adjacent to an infiltrating carcinoma, and presence or absence of lymphatic invasion adjacent to or distant from the primary tumor are also important determinations that will influence subsequent management. Even if the initial excision is not intended as the final operative treatment, many patients will obtain a second opinion after this excision, and some will decide not to have further surgery. Therefore, the information specified above and summarized in more detail in references 25 and 26 should be supplied in every case.

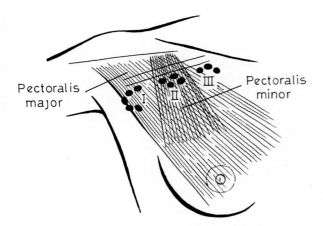

Fig. 19-5. Dissection of axillary nodes. The nodes are divided into three groups according to anatomic location with respect to the pectoralis muscles.

Pectoralis major

Pectoralis minor

Table 19-1. American Joint Committee on Cancer (AJCC) Staging System for Breast Cancer, 1992 Revision

Primary tumor (T)
    Tx—Primary tumor cannot be assessed
    T0—No evidence of primary tumor
    Tis—Carcinoma in situ: intraductal carcinoma, lobular carcinoma in situ, or Paget's disease of the nipple with no tumor
    T1—Tumor 2 cm or less in greatest dimension
        T1a—0.5 cm or smaller
        T1b—More than 0.5 cm but not more than 1 cm in greatest dimension
        T1c—More than 1 cm but not more than 2 cm in greatest dimension
    T2—Tumor more than 2 cm but not more than 5 cm in greatest dimension
    T3—Tumor more than 5 cm in greatest dimension
    T4—Tumor of any size with direct extension to chest wall or skin
        T4a—Extension to chest wall
        T4b—Edema (including peau d'orange), ulceration of the skin of the breast, or satellite skin nodules confined to the same breast
        T4c—Both (T4a and T4b)
        T4d—Inflammatory carcinoma
Regional lymph nodes (N)
    Clinical classification
        Nx—Regional lymph nodes cannot be assessed (e.g., previously removed)
        N0—No regional lymph node metastasis
        N1—Metastasis to one or more movable ipsilateral axillary node
        N2—Metastasis to one or more ipsilateral axillary lymph node fixed to one another or to other structures
        N3—Metastases to ipsilateral internal mammary lymph node(s)
    Pathologic (pN) classification
        pNx—Regional lymph node metastasis cannot be assessed
        pN0—No regional lymph node metastasis
        pN1—Metastasis to one or more movable ipsilateral axillary node
            pN1a—Only micrometastasis (none larger than 0.2 cm)
            pN1b—Metastasis to one or more lymph node, any of which is larger than 0.2 cm
                pN1bi—Metastases in one to three lymph nodes, any of which is larger than 0.2 cm in greatest dimension
                pN1bii—Metastases to four or more lymph nodes, any of which is larger than 0.2 cm and all of which are less than 2 cm in greatest dimension
                pN1biii—Extension of tumor beyond the capsule of a lymph node metastasis less than 2 cm in greatest dimension
                pN1biv—Metastasis to a lymph node 2 cm or more in greatest dimension
        pN2—Metastasis to ipsilateral axillary lymph nodes that are fixed to one another or to other structures
        pN3—Metastasis to one or more ipsilateral internal mammary lymph node
Distant metastases (M)
    Mx—Presence of distant metastases cannot be assessed
    M0—No distant metastasis
    M1—Distant metastasis (including metastases to one or more ipsilateral supraclavicular node)

Stage Grouping

Stage	TNM grouping
0	Tis, N0, M0
I	T1, N0, M0
IIA	T0, N1, M0
	T1, N1, M0
	T2, N0, M0
IIB	T2, N1, M0
	T3, N0, M0
IIIA	T0, N2, M0
	T1, N2, M0
	T2, N2, M0
	T3, N1, M0
	T3, N2, M0
IIIB	T4, any N, M0
	Any T, N3, M0
IV	Any T, any N, M1

(From American Joint Committee on Cancer,[565] with permission.)

METHODS OF DIAGNOSIS

Clinical Method

The medical history and physical examination of the breast are essential steps in diagnosis. The clinical signs of primary breast neoplasms are few. In the overwhelming majority of cases, there is a painless breast mass and, less frequently, nipple discharge or erosion, skin retraction, or an axillary mass. The differential diagnosis between benign and malignant lesions relies on more elaborate diagnostic methods such as mammography and sonography, but most of all on tissue examination. Education of the public about the fundamental facts of cancer and self-examination of the breast also represents an important factor in the early detection of breast disease.

Mammography

Mammography is basically a soft tissue radiologic examination of the breast that is now an indispensable part of the workup of breast lesions. Perhaps its main asset is its ability to detect clinically impalpable malignant lesions. This new technology has modified the way in which surgical specimens should be handled. Stereotactic localization of the radiographic abnormalities is followed by pathologic examination of the identified areas. This procedure correlates the radiographic abnormalities with the histologic images: microcalcifications and epithelial and stromal alterations. When the lesion is grossly imperceptible or measures less than 1.0 cm in greatest diameter, frozen section examination should not be performed, in order to obtain good quality permanent sections.[20,21] A radiogram of the surgical specimen enables the pathologist to identify with certainty that the lesion present in the preoperative mammogram was localized and properly processed for microscopic examination.[23,25,26]

The recognition of microcalcifications is important. Table 19-2 summarizes the sources of interpretative error in the evaluation of biopsies directed by microcalcifications.[27] In the absence of microcalcifications, soft tissue densities may be more difficult to localize and interpret pathologically. Careful comparison of pre- and postoperative radiograms will contribute to solve the problem.

The efficiency of mammography to detect in situ carcinomas, both intralobular and intraductal, is well demonstrated and is responsible for the higher percentage of these lesions in biopsies performed for suspicious mammograms than in those performed for palpable masses.[28]

Ultrasonography

Ultrasonography does not replace mammography for the detection of subclinical malignant tumors. It is useful in the characterization of lesions in dense mammary parenchyma and in the differential diagnosis between cystic and solid masses.[29]

Table 19-2. Problems and Solutions in Evaluation of Mammographically Directed Biopsies

No confirmation of microcalcifications in the specimen radiograph
    Mammographic abnormalities inadequately localized or surgical sample misdirected
    Definite absence of microcalcifications in the preoperative mammograms
    Microcalcifications located in the dermis; ellipse of skin should be embedded
    Inadequate x-ray equipment does not reveal microcalcifications in the specimen radiograph
Presence of noncorresponding microcalcifications in the specimen radiograph
    Microcalcifications do not correspond to those detected preoperatively: mammogram review or rebiopsy if calcifications are still present
    Microcalcifications have not been excised entirely: additional biopsy
    Microcalcifications seen in specimen represent talc or other radiopaque contaminant
Specimen radiograph demonstrates the presence of a lesion, but microcalcifications not identified in microscopic sections
    Microcalcifications are composed of oxalate crystals: use polarization lenses
    Microcalcifications have not been removed by the biopsy: x-ray paraffin blocks and remaining fixed tissue (if any)
    Microcalcifications lie deeper in block: cut deeper, x-ray block
    Microcalcifications have been leached by acidic fixative or shattered out of section: check pH of fixative and with the histotechnologist for knife chatter

(Data from Lagios.[27])

Galactography

Galactography is another diagnostic radiologic procedure. A radiopaque medium is injected into the main lactiferous ducts, and mammograms are taken. It is a useful technique for detection of any tumor lesion in the main ducts.[30]

Other Techniques

New methods of breast lesion imaging include magnetic resonance imaging (MRI), positron emission tomography (PET), and single photon emission imaging computed tomography (SPECT).[31] All of these and others may become clinically more important in the future.

Fine Needle Aspiration (Aspiration Cytology)

The history of the use of breast fine needle aspiration biopsy (FNAB) dates back to the 19th century. Martin and Ellis,[32] at the Memorial Hospital for Cancer and Allied Diseases in New York, were the first to report their experience with this procedure in 1930. Since then, many other reports have appeared in the literature emphasizing the importance of FNAB in the evaluation of patients with breast lesions. The changes in the medical economy in the United States, and the emphasis on cost containment, have been a major factor in stimulating interest in the use of FNAB in this country.[33,34]

Other advantages of FNAB include minimal physical and psychological discomfort to the patient. FNAB is a procedure that is easily accepted by a woman, which may lead to an earlier detection of breast cancer. FNAB relieves the anxiety of a woman with benign breast disease by providing a rapid diagnosis. In malignant circumstances, FNAB allows a woman to actively participate in treatment planning. In addition, FNAB may serve as a therapeutic procedure when a cyst is encountered. Furthermore, FNAB is an attractive alternative to surgical biopsy in evaluation of local chest wall recurrences, lymph node metastases, and in inoperable conditions. FNAB is also often the only diagnostic procedure for presurgical chemotherapy and/or radiotherapy regimens.

The fear of an erroneous diagnosis leading to an unnecessary mastectomy is considered the major factor for the existing differences in the practice of FNAB. To overcome this problem, the diagnostic accuracy of FNAB must approach that of frozen sections. Furthermore, due to the multidisciplinary nature of FNAB procedure and the existing differences among different institutions in regard to the approach to FNAB, there are difficulties in the interpretation of the reported results in the literature. This is best reflected by the wide range of reported diagnostic accuracy (50 to 95 percent) in the literature. In our review of the reported results on the diagnostic accuracy of FNAB of nonpalpable breast lesions in 3,000 cases with histologic follow-up, the diagnostic accuracy ranged from 68 to 100 percent.[35]

Based on the reports in the literature and our own experience, the diagnostic accuracy of breast FNAB significantly improves when a pathologist examines the patient and performs the procedure.[36,37] Proficiency in the biopsy technique, smear preparation, and interpretation of the cytomorphology are the key factors for a successful FNAB. The result of a breast FNAB is influenced by the number of needle biopsies in an individual lesion. There is strong evidence that the number of aspirations positively influences the cell yield as well as the diagnostic accuracy of FNAB of the breast.[38,39] In one study, the sensitivity of FNAB increased from 61 percent with one aspirate to 91 percent with three aspirates.[39] Availability of an immediate microscopic evaluation of FNAB smears also reduces the number of insufficient cases and enhances the diagnostic accuracy of this procedure.[40] With the clinical information correlated, this assessment may result in repeat aspiration in the same setting in the case of inadequate specimens or in cases where there is incompatibility of the results with the clinical findings. In addition, recognition of the presence of a malignant tumor via an immediate assessment of the direct smears guides specimen triage for tumor marker studies and prognostic tests.

Attempts to render a diagnosis on breast aspirates that are markedly limited in cellularity or are obscured by blood, necrosis, inflammatory exudate, or drying artifact often lead to an incorrect diagnosis. Both the nature of the lesion (including small size, marked fibrosis, and extensive necrosis) and the experi-

ence of the aspirator may limit the value of the specimen obtained.

The standard criteria for a "diagnostic aspirate" are not yet well defined. Providing that the cells are well preserved and they are not obscured by blood and/or inflammatory cells, Kline[41] considers a breast aspirate to be satisfactory when there are more than three to six epithelial cell groups per slide. Sneige[42] recognizes the cellularity to be adequate when there are more than four to six well visualized cell groups. The criteria for adequacy of cytologic specimens for nonpalpable breast lesions are also variable. Dowlatshahi et al[43] recommended the presence of more than six epithelial clusters of more than 10 cells each to be considered a sufficient sample. Layfield et al[44] consider aspirates as insufficient when less than 25 epithelial cells are present per slide. A consensus of these and other criteria has recently been published.[567]

General Considerations in Interpretation of Breast Fine Needle Aspirations

Because the breast consists of major lactiferous ducts, branched ducts, lobules, and connective tissue stroma, it is not unusual to find coexisting adipose tissue, epithelial cells, and stromal components in breast fine needle aspirates. In benign conditions, the cellularity is generally low or moderate and the epithelial cells are arranged in clusters and small groups with myoepithelial cells present. Typically, cytologic atypia and nuclear changes are minimal. By contrast, fine needle aspirates of malignant breast disease are usually characterized by cellular aspirates in an isolated dispersed cell pattern. Anisonucleosis, chromatin clumping, nuclear membrane abnormalities, and necrosis are common cellular features in fine needle aspirates of malignant breast tumors. These cellular characteristics are, in general, reliable indicators of most benign and malignant breast disease. However, there are exceptions, such as high cellularity in lactating adenoma and insignificant atypia in well differentiated breast carcinoma.

Thus, interpretation of breast fine needle aspirates should be based on multiple parameters and not on single criteria. In addition, the new technologies such as cytometry, ploidy study, and molecular testing should not be used as a sole diagnostic measure in differentiation between benign and malignant breast disease.

False Negative Results

Generally tumors with extensive necrosis and fibrosis and those with size of less than 1 cm give rise to false negative diagnosis. Fibrosis is the most important reason for the false negative diagnosis in breast cytology. This may be due to desmoplasia, scar tissue, or radiation. A desmoplastic reaction to tumor is commonly seen in lobular carcinoma as well as ductal carcinoma. However, because the cells in lobular carcinoma are small, they may be missed or misinterpreted as lymphocytes. Another reason for a false negative diagnosis is the presence of well differentiated breast tumors such as tubular, mucinous, and papillary carcinoma and those with insignificant atypia such as lobular carcinoma and the monomorphic type of ductal carcinoma seen in some elderly patients.[39] Malignant tumors associated with a cystic lesion also have a high potential for false negative diagnosis. These tumors often present a hemorrhagic fluid, but rarely they may appear with a clear fluid and no residual mass.

Poor technique resulting in a missed target is an increasingly frequent problem and another important cause of false negative diagnosis. In a review of the literature, the range of false negative breast FNAB in palpable breast lesions varied from 1 to 31 percent with an average rate of 10 percent.[45] This rate definitely can be reduced by gaining experience in the technique as well as interpretation of breast cytology.

False Positive Results

False positive diagnosis should not occur because of its dramatic clinical implications, particularly in institutions where no frozen section confirmation is required for positive breast aspirates. A conclusive diagnosis of malignant tumor in breast FNAB should be reported only in those cases where there are sufficient cytologic criteria for a malignant tumor and no other reason or explanation for the atypia exists. It is absolutely essential for the pathologist interpreting breast aspirates to be familiar with benign and reactive conditions that give rise to significant atypia. These include ruptured cyst, fibrocystic change, fat necrosis, organizing hematoma, atypical fibroadenoma, gynecomastia, granulation tissue, pregnancy-related and lactational change, papilloma, tubular adenoma, atypical hyperplasia, mucocele-like lesions, changes induced by radiotherapy and chemotherapy, and epithelial hyperplasia in phyllodes tumors.[42,46,47] False positive findings have ranged from 0 to 11 percent, but in experienced hands, the range has been reduced to 0.1 to 0.2 percent, which is similar to that reported for frozen section examination.[48]

Reporting and Management System

The results of FNABs are reported as insufficient, negative (benign), inconclusive (suspicious), or positive for malignant tumor. An "insufficient" diagnosis refers to those cases in which there is no or minimal cellular material or the cells are obscured by blood, inflammatory cells, or necrotic debris or are distorted by drying artifact. In these situations, repeat aspiration or excisional biopsy is recommended. Carnoy's solution may be used to lyse the obscuring red blood cells prior to staining.

Smears containing adequate numbers of well preserved benign cells are reported as negative or benign. Benign diagnoses are further specified as to the type of lesion (e.g., fibrocystic change, fibroadenoma, inflammatory conditions). The cytologic findings in these cases are correlated with clinical and mammographic findings. Some investigators still believe that a negative breast FNAB does not exclude the presence of a malignant tumor and should be followed by an open biopsy. However, evaluations based on the combined findings of physical examination, mammography, and FNAB (the so-called triple test) have shown a diagnostic accuracy of 99 percent for breast cancer when all three tests were in agreement.[49,50] Thus, this combination may assist in avoiding unnecessary surgery, especially in young women. By contrast, despite a negative FNAB, when there are any suspicious clinical or mammographic findings, an open biopsy is indicated.

Breast fine needle aspirates that show cells with significant cytologic atypia and/or architectural changes, but quantitatively insufficient for malignant tumor, are reported as inconclusive or suspicious. These cases need an excisional biopsy or a confirmatory frozen section to establish the final diagnosis. Aspirations that show conclusive cytologic evidence for malignant tumor are reported as positive (malignant) with further specification of the type of the lesion and nuclear grading. This diagnosis justifies definitive therapy unless the clinical and mammographic findings are not in agreement with the positive FNAB results. In such cases, confirmation of cancer by a frozen section is recommended prior to definitive treatment.

Because the distinction between in situ and invasive lesions cannot be made on breast cytology alone, if the status of tumor invasion is therapeutically important, this can be achieved by core biopsy or surgical excision of the lesion. It cannot be overemphasized that the success of breast FNAB depends on the experience of the cytopathologist. In pathology practices where the number of breast fine needle aspirates are low and/or the pathologist is not experienced in the interpretation of breast FNAB, frozen section confirmation is recommended before any definitive treatment.

Core Needle Biopsy

Needle biopsy techniques such as the Tru-Cut needle and the speed drill biopsy procedures produce a core of tissue and are preferred by some pathologists to the aspiration cytology method, which, according to them, gives greater numbers of false negative and false positive diagnoses. However, this opinion is not shared by all investigators.

One situation in which core biopsy appears to be superior to FNAB is in the management of some mammographically detected nonpalpable lesions. Sneige[51] has recently reviewed the results of published series of ultrasound and mammographically guided FNAB and stereotactic core biopsies in this clinical situation. She concluded that core biopsy (or directed excisional biopsy) was necessary in cases with microcalcifications but no mass, but FNA could be utilized initially for cases with a nonpalpable mass. She emphasized that, with core biopsies as with our discussion of FNAB above, a surgical biopsy should be performed if needle biopsy results do not correlate with mammographic findings or if an insufficient sample is obtained. In her review of a total of over 700 stereotactic core biopsies in seven reported series, sensitivity ranged from 71 to 100 percent, and insufficient samples from 0 to 17 percent; in all but one report, however, the latter figure was 6 percent or less.

Excisional Biopsy

Excisional biopsy is the most definitive diagnostic method for most breast lesions. The reliability of the frozen section examination is indeed excellent in the hands of well trained and experienced pathologists, the accuracy being above 95 percent in published series.[52–54] However, because breast biopsies today are generally not followed immediately by definitive therapy, and because a higher proportion of cancers are impalpable and often noninvasive, many pathologists are performing progressively fewer-frozen section examinations on these specimens. In most of these cases, it is more appropriate to wait for the results of the examination of good paraffin-embedded sections of the biopsy specimen than to depend on the results of frozen section examination.

The danger of tumor dissemination initiated by a biopsy procedure or enhanced by a delay between diagnosis and treatment has been extensively discussed.[55] To avoid any risk, an excisional biopsy of all suspicious lesions should be performed, and adequate treatment should be started without delay after the pathologic report has been obtained. If these recommendations are followed, the prognosis is comparable in series of patients who have immediate major surgery and patients who undergo major surgery after a few days delay.

Processing of the excisional biopsy specimen and preparation of the surgical pathology report have been discussed above.

INFLAMMATORY LESIONS

Acute Mastitis

Acute mastitis generally occurs during periods of lactation. Predisposing factors include fissures of the nipple and hypertrophy of either the functional components or the lymphatics of the mammary gland. *Staphylococcus aureus* and *Streptococcus* are the most common etiologic agents, and thus the prognosis of this disease has considerably improved with the development of antibiotic therapy.

Clinically, acute mastitis manifests as usual inflammation: the breast is edematous, painfully swollen, and red. There may be a discharge from the nipple. Microscopically, we observe neutrophilic and histiocytic inflammatory infiltration, as well as vascular congestion and edema of the lactiferous ducts and surrounding stroma. There also may be zones of necrosis, which lead to abscess formation.[56]

Cytologically, acute mastitis presents with abundant neutrophils, a few histiocytes, and a necrotic background. A few reactive epithelial cells are also present. Occasionally, the degree of cytologic atypia due to inflammation may approximate the change seen in carcinoma and present a potential diagnostic dilemma. An inflammatory background and a limited number of epithelial cells are the features that militate against a diagnosis of carcinoma.[46]

Chronic Mastitis

Chronic mastitis is a complication of the acute form. We observe lymphocytes, plasma cells, and histiocytes with variable amounts of fibrous tissue. Foreign body giant cells and epithelioid cells may be present in granulomatous lesions. Mammary duct fistula is a lesion associated with a duct lined with metaplastic squamous epithelium.[57] The presence of lymphocytes, plasma cells, and foamy cells is a constant finding around ductal cysts, ruptured or not. It is a manifestation of structural modifications and it is not related to any infection.

When lymphocytes are prominent throughout the breast

around ducts, lobules, and blood vessels, and are accompanied by lobular atrophy and sclerosis and dense keloid-like fibrosis, the condition is referred to as *lymphocytic mastopathy*[58] (Fig. 19-6). Because of the frequent association of this probably autoimmune lesion with diabetes mellitus, it is also sometimes called diabetic mastopathy.[59] Lymphoma of the breast is usually distinguishable from lymphocytic mastopathy by its more focal nature and greater cytologic atypia, as well as by immunologic and molecular studies (see below), but it has been postulated that mammary lymphomas may originate from lymphocytic mastopathy.[60]

Cytologically, the aspirates from chronic mastitis are cellular and show a mixed population of lymphocytes, plasma cells, fibroblasts, and histiocytes. Scattered clusters of epithelial cells with mild cytologic atypia induced by inflammation are also present.

Galactocele

Galactocele, which occurs during lactation, is a slowly evolving cystic degeneration of a duct with secondary inflammation and necrosis.[61] Lymphocytes are abundant in the surrounding

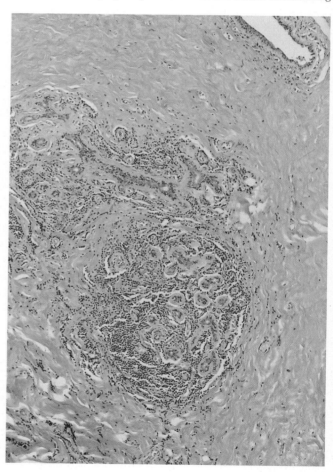

Fig. 19-6. Lymphocytic mastopathy. Note lymphocytic infiltrate cuffing atrophic ducts and lobules, and surrounding keloid-like dense fibrosis. Compare with Fig. 19-118 (malignant lymphoma).

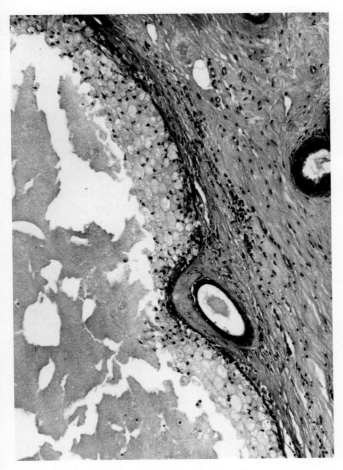

Fig. 19-7. Galactocele. Note the cystic degeneration of a duct with the presence of desquamated foamy cells.

stroma (Fig. 19-7). It has been observed in women taking oral contraceptives.

Cytologically, the aspirates consist of cyst fluid containing abundant numbers of foamy histiocytes, isolated and clusters of epithelial cells, and a few inflammatory cells admixed with lipid micelles. The background is granular and contains proteinaceous material. Occasional dispersed cells are seen. FNAB of galactocele is associated with immediate regression of the mass.[61]

Specific Chronic Mastitides

In certain cases, the lesions of chronic mastitis can be specific to the agent involved. *Tuberculous mastitis* is rare and is a complication of a primary pulmonary or lymph node tuberculosis spreading by vascular dissemination.[62] Macroscopically, soft, yellow nodules scattered in the breast tissue are observed. Abscedation of converging nodules and external fistula formation may occur. If these lesions undergo secondary fibrosis, they may macroscopically resemble tumoral lesions. Microscopically, tuberculoid granulomas with Langhans cells and central

caseation indicate the nature of the lesions; the histologic diagnosis is of course confirmed by the presence of acid-fast bacilli and a positive culture. Regional lymph nodes may reveal the presence of solitary tubercles without caseation.

Syphilitic involvement of the mammary gland is extremely rare. Those cases reported in the older literature resulted from contamination during lactation by newborns suffering from congenital syphilis. Rare cases of secondary and tertiary syphilis have been reported.[63]

Mammary gland *actinomycosis* is an infrequent disease resulting from a primary pulmonary infection. Diagnosis is made by observation of the organism within the inflammatory granulomas.

Rare cases of mammary sarcoidosis have been reported.[64] One should remember that sarcoid-like pictures can be observed in lymph nodes draining breast carcinoma. Other rare diseases include filariasis, scleroderma, blastomycosis, cryptococcosis, and histoplasmosis.

Noninfective granulomatous mastitis has also been reported. It is a diagnosis of exclusion, but is probably of autoimmune etiology and often responds to steroids.[65]

Cytologically, granulomatous mastitis is characterized by a cellular aspirate demonstrating conspicuous numbers of lymphocytes, plasma cells, and granulomas with epithelioid and multinucleated giant cells. Isolated and clusters of fibroblasts and reactive ductal epithelial cells are also present. Occasionally, necrosis may be seen. The cellular material from such aspirates should be carefully examined for the presence of acid-fast bacilli, fungi, and parasites.[62] Sarcoidosis shows no evidence of necrosis and cat-scratch disease typically demonstrates microabscess formation. Occasionally, the distinction between atypical mononuclear epithelioid histiocytes in granulomatous mastitis and neoplastic mammary epithelial cells may be difficult. Close attention to the inflammatory background and to the characteristic cytologic (and immunocytochemical, if necessary) features of the histiocytes should help to avoid false positive diagnosis by FNAB.

Fat Necrosis

Fat necrosis can occur in large breasts secondary to trauma or may be associated with carcinoma or any lesion provoking suppurative or necrotic degeneration. It is also seen following the trauma of biopsy and may be difficult to distinguish grossly from residual tumor at the biopsy site. The clinical manifestations of fat necrosis may mimic a malignant tumor and, in the past, these nodular, solid lesions were in fact, frequently misinterpreted as carcinoma.[66,67]

A history of pain and tenderness, ecchymosis, and retraction of the skin are the most common clinical features. Even the macroscopic granulomatous, nodular, yellow appearance of the lesion is suggestive of a malignant tumor. Histologically, however, the diagnosis of this benign lesion presents no problem. It is a typical inflammatory infiltrate of the fat tissue with areas of fibrosis and necrosis. Large fat vacuoles are surrounded by histiocytes. Multinucleated giant cells are present, as well as blood pigment and lipid crystals (Fig. 19-8). At a later stage, more and more fibrous tissue gradually replaces the active granulomatous

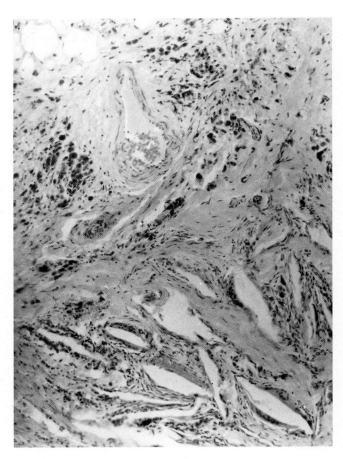

Fig. 19-8. Fat necrosis. Inflammatory granuloma with areas of fibrosis and lipid crystals surrounded by multinucleated giant cells.

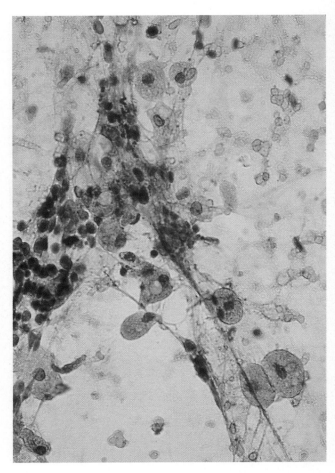

Fig. 19-9. Cellular debris, inflammatory cells, small vessels, and lipid-laden macrophages in an aspirate of fat necrosis. (Papanicolaou stain, × 400.)

process. Typical calcified formations, which represent the walls of cysts, are often observed on mammograms.

The description of fat necrosis illustrates rather well the necessity of performing a biopsy of every suspicious lesion before major surgery. The skin retraction, the suspicious macroscopic appearance, and the calcifications are all misleadingly suggestive of malignant tumor, and, without histologic proof, such lesions could be misinterpreted and an unnecessary mastectomy could be performed.

Cytologically, fat necrosis presents predominantly with fat, amorphous debris, foamy macrophages, neutrophils, lymphocytes, plasma cells, fibroblasts, and fragments of fibrous tissue and small vessels. Macrophages have abundant vacuolated cytoplasm. Multinucleated giant cells may also be present (Fig. 19-9). Scattered ductal epithelial cells may show conspicuous cytologic atypia and potentially lead to a false positive diagnosis of cancer. The cells in fat necrosis, however, are usually present in cohesive sheets and rarely represent the majority of cellular elements as they do in carcinoma. Fat necrosis may coexist with cancer. Thus, lesions displaying fat necrosis should be carefully sampled. Also considered in the differential diagnosis

is hibernoma of the breast, which is rare and does not have abundant inflammatory cells.

Plasma Cell Mastitis (Mammary Duct Ectasia)

Plasma cell mastitis was described in 1923 by Bloodgood, who called it varicocele tumor, and subsequently by Adair,[68] who called it plasma cell mastitis. Haagensen suggested the term *mammary duct ectasia*. Although plasma cell mastitis is not a frequent lesion, its correct interpretation by the pathologist is extremely important, as its clinical and macroscopic manifestations can closely resemble those of carcinomas. The formation of a firm lump and possibly a retraction of the nipple may erroneously suggest the diagnosis of tumor. A serous, purulent, or bloody discharge from the nipple can be observed. Plasma cell mastitis occurs at menopause in multiparous women. Its etiology is not known, but this seems to be a lesion of the aging breast. Its high incidence has been confirmed by studies of autopsy material in which 25 percent of supposedly normal breasts in fact showed plasma cell mastitis. The treatment is local surgical excision.

Grossly, there is a firm, poorly defined mass measuring up to 5 cm in diameter. The cut surface reveals a yellow or white granular tissue with dilated ducts that contain brown granular or creamy necrotic material. Compression of the dilated ducts expels this material.

Histologically, this lesion represents a progressive dilation of the main lactiferous ducts with chronic inflammatory lesions and foreign body granuloma formation. The granulomas occur around the necrotic cellular debris and lipids released by the damaged and ruptured ducts (Fig. 19-10). The dilated ducts are lined by flattened cells and contain foamy macrophages, neutrophils, lymphocytes, and sometimes numerous plasma cells. Neutral fat and crystalline lipid bodies are found in this material. There is marked periductal fibrosis often accompanied by a surrounding lymphocytic or plasma cell infiltration. A sarcoidlike reaction has been described in a few cases. Microscopically, there is no difficulty diagnosing this lesion and thus ruling out the clinical suspicion of a malignant tumor.

Cytologically, plasma cell mastitis is characterized by a predominant population of plasma cells and granulomas and the absence of acid-fast bacilli, fungi, and other causative agents. Lymphocytes, fibroblasts, and other mononuclear inflammatory cells are also present.

Recurrent Subareolar Granuloma

Recurrent subareolar granuloma or abscess is a particular form of chronic mastitis associated with lactation. It consists of an inflammatory alteration of the subareolar ducts with recurrent abscess formation and possibly secondary skin fistula. The cystic lesion is lined by stratified squamous epithelium. Careful removal of the involved area is adequate treatment.

Cytologically, subareolar granuloma shows a cellular aspirate with an inflammatory background, foreign body type giant cells, macrophages, and clusters of reactive ductal epithelial

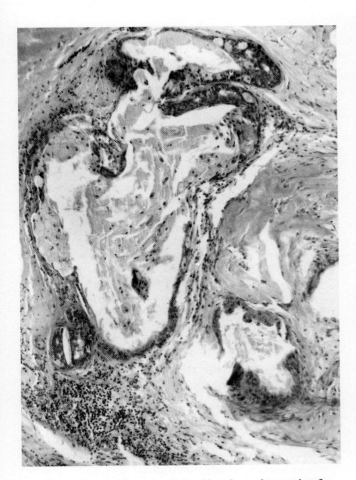

Fig. 19-10. Plasma cell mastitis. Dilated lactiferous ducts with inflammatory infiltrate and giant cell granulomas around cellular debris and lipids.

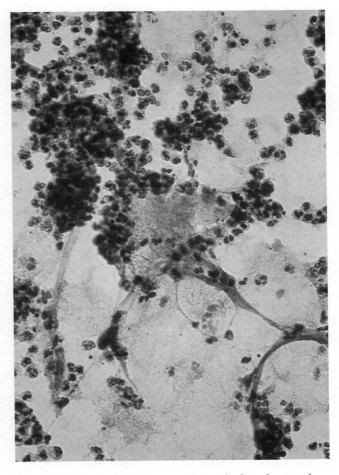

Fig. 19-11. Direct smear from an aspirate of subareolar granuloma demonstrating numerous neutrophils and a few anucleate squamous cells. (Papanicolaou stain, × 200.)

cells.[69] The defining cytologic feature of this entity is the presence of nucleated squamous cells, keratinous material, and metaplastic and parakeratotic squamous cells (Fig. 19-11). Similar to other inflammatory processes, subareolar granuloma demonstrates some of the potential diagnostic pitfalls for a positive diagnosis of a malignant tumor, which include the presence of atypical ductal epithelial cells and atypical squamous cells and evidence of exuberant granulation tissue formation. In such cases, the presence of an inflammatory background and keratinous material should alert one to refrain from making a diagnosis of carcinoma. Included in the differential diagnosis is ruptured epidermal inclusion cyst arising in the skin. The peripheral location of the epidermal inclusion cyst easily separates this lesion from subareolar granuloma, which is centrally located. Precise diagnosis of subareolar abscess has major clinical implications because this lesion requires surgical excision of the abscess and the associated sinus tract and ducts.

Mammary Subcutaneous Phlebitis

Mammary subcutaneous phlebitis (Mondor's disease) is characterized by superficial thoracic vein thrombophlebitis.[70] The cause is unknown and it occurs more frequently in women. Clinically, it occurs as a painful superficial cord beneath the skin of the mammary region. Microscopically, there is thrombosis of the subcutaneous veins with secondary fibrosis of the vein wall. Strictly speaking, Mondor's disease is not a mastitis but is included in this chapter because it may represent a problem in differential diagnosis.

Cosmetic Mammary Injections and Implants

For cosmetic reasons, various materials (oils, paraffin wax, epoxy resin, silicone compounds) have been injected or otherwise introduced into human breasts.[71] These substances are in general well tolerated, but they may also provoke the formation of an inflammatory reaction with chronic abscesses, giant cell foreign body granulomas, necrosis, and cutaneous fistulas.

The existence of a tender, firm nodule combined with the clinical history will suggest the diagnosis. The histologic examination shows a foreign body granuloma surrounded by more or less pronounced inflammatory reaction. Involvement of the thoracic wall and even the pleural cavity by the inflammatory process has been reported.

More important than injections in current practice are mammary implants, which have been introduced either for mammary augmentation or reconstruction after partial or total mastectomy. It is estimated that approximately 2 million women have received these implants since the early 1960s.[72] The most common of these implants consist of liquid silicone surrounded by an elastomere shell (Fig. 19-12). The implants are removed, often after many years, either because of rupture or leakage of their contents or of fear of the patient concerning the frequently reported but generally poorly documented relationship of these implants to various systemic diseases.[73] The implants are often removed with a surrounding fibrous capsule, formed as

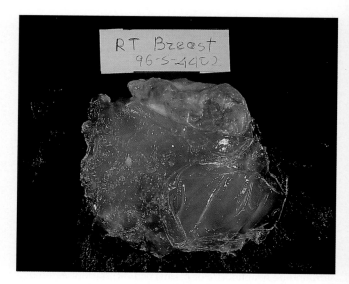

Fig. 19-12. Silicone implant removed from breast. Note gel leakage and adjacent capsule.

a reactive process, which may include foamy macrophages and foreign body giant cells containing refractile but not birefringent material consistent with silicone gel, as well as other inflammatory cells and often a reaction with features of synovial metaplasia[74–76] (Fig. 19-13).

The College of American Pathologists has recommended that each institution receiving implants removed for any reason develop a written policy for their storage or return to patients, with each implant being photographed, weighed, and carefully described grossly (including any identifying inscriptions and a statement on the integrity of its envelope). Any attached capsule or other tissue should also be measured and described grossly and submitted for microscopic examination. The implant should be sterilized if it is to be returned to the patient and should be delivered in a sealed container with a biohazard label.[77]

Infarction

Infarction can be related to different clinical conditions. It may appear during pregnancy and lactation. The lesion is usually small with well defined borders and arises in the parenchyma or in benign tumors (fibroadenomas) or intraductal papillomas. The pathogenesis is not clear; because there is no evidence of vascular anomaly or history of trauma, an abnormally elevated metabolic activity of the mammary parenchyma has been suggested. In older women, it can be associated with thromboembolic diseases, with cases of Wegener's granulomatosis, and with anticoagulant therapy.[78,79] Massive necrosis of the parenchyma has been described, particularly with use of dicumarol derivatives.

The histologic appearance is characterized by ischemic necrosis with or without hemorrhage. The lesion is of practical importance because it can grossly mimic carcinoma, and the

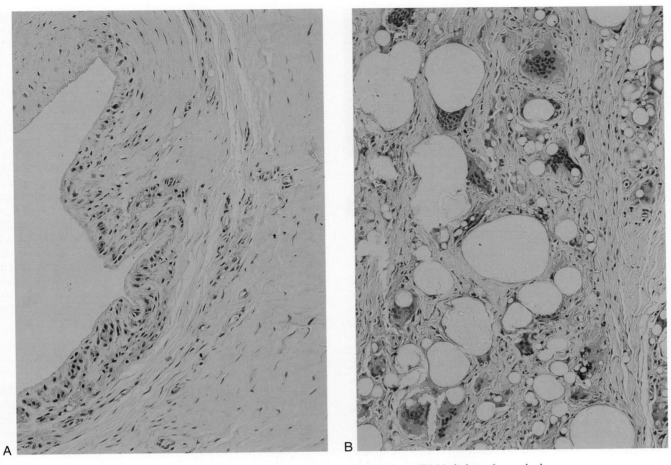

Fig. 19-13. **(A)** Capsule of silicone implant, with synovial metaplasia. **(B)** Underlying foreign body reaction with large spaces, some containing silicon particles.

pathologist must therefore be aware of this differential diagnosis.

FIBROCYSTIC MASTOPATHY

The wide variety of terms (cystic hyperplasia, Reclus' disease, Schimmelbusch's disease, mammary dysplasia, mastodynia, fibroadenosis, Brodie's cystic disease, fibrous dysplasia, chronic cystic mastitis, fibrous mastopathia) found in the literature describing fibrocystic change reflects its extreme polymorphism and the difficulty of integrating so many varied lesions under one simple heading. This is why various attempts at precise pathologic classification have been made.[80]

The etiology of fibrocystic mastopathy—the most common lesion of the breast—remains only partially understood. All we can say at present is that the histologic structures of the mammary tissue are submitted to different influences and factors that may permanently modify them. Genetic background, hormonal balance, age, parity, lactation history, and possibly viruses and psychosomatic illnesses can all influence the mor-

phology of the mammary glands.[81] The existence of hormonal factors is suggested by various clinical and experimental findings: for example, the lesion develops at an age when the mammary gland has already been exposed to long estrogenic stimulation, and experimental estrogen injections induce the development of cysts in the mammary gland of the rhesus monkey.

Fibrocystic mastopathy is a common condition among young women and the incidence rate increases with age, reaching a peak at about 40 to 45 years of age. Clinically, the patient reports the presence of a poorly defined mass often accompanied by discomfort and tenderness and aggravated during the premenstrual period. The lesion may appear in a localized or a diffuse form, and frequently, both mammary glands are involved. Clinical examination reveals the beads on a string sign, that is, one or several fine nodules of different sizes. Mammography reveals microcalcifications and other pathologic radiologic findings.

Macroscopically, the lesion is characterized by the dense, often glistening appearance of the involved tissue, with the presence of a variable number of blue or yellow cysts of different sizes (Fig. 19-14). Sclerosing adenosis appears as a moderately

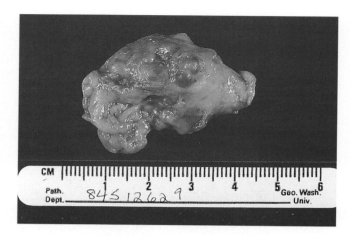

Fig. 19-14. Gross appearance of fibrocystic mastopathy.

firm, lobular, circumscribed mass; the section reveals lobulated gray-white granular tissue. A careful search for any area suggestive of cancer must be performed; more specifically, the presence of fine, granular, dense tissue with chalky yellow streaks is highly suspicious.

It is time to reconsider histologically the old concept of fibrocystic "disease," described by Reclus and Schimmelbusch almost a century ago, and to separate definite benign lesions from a spectrum of proliferative epithelial lesions, some of which are related to neoplasia.[82–91] The benign lesions, which could be named *functional mastopathies*, are very common. They represent physiologic alterations due to cyclic or unbalanced hormonal stimulations or mammary tissue hypersensitive to normal hormonal activity. Therefore, the term *disease* should be abandoned to qualify these alterations, which include cysts of various sizes, duct ectasia, stromal fibrosis, sclerosing adenosis, and apocrine change.

When proliferative epithelial changes are present, we are dealing with the *proliferative form of fibrocystic mastopathy*. The proliferative changes are seen in the ductal system or the lobules, or both, and current classifications rely on a system of grading of the different degrees of proliferative changes or hyperplasias[82–91] (Table 19-3). The grading goes from mild to severe in terms of epithelial proliferation, loss of cell polarity, number of cell layers, and cellular atypias, and is further subdivided by the unit(s) (ducts, lobules) involved. It is important to evaluate the presence and the severity of the hyperplasia because they enable the assignment of the patient to a specific risk category for the development of carcinoma. From the abundant literature available on benign mastopathy and its relationship to breast cancer risk, it is now imperative that the pathologist grade the severity of the hyperplasia and discuss the findings with the surgeon to arrive at the optimal treatment.

A few rules should be followed to adopt a coherent attitude toward the management of this frequent breast pathology. The breast biopsy material should be totally examined and the precise location of mammographic anomalies identified, usually by specimen radiography. The pathologist and the clinician should carefully discuss the therapeutic program and agree on the significance of the terms adopted to describe the lesions.

The specific components of the fibrocystic complex are discussed individually, but it should be remembered that various combinations of these components are almost always present in every specimen.

Lactiferous Cysts

Lactiferous cysts represent the most minimal changes observed in fibrocystic mastopathy. They are small and disseminated in the parenchyma, and their number and size vary greatly. These cysts develop as the result of the dilation of ducts or as the multiplication and expansion of terminal ductules (blunt duct adenosis, columnar alteration of lobules, unfolded lobules) (Fig. 19-15). They are lined by a flattened, cuboidal, or columnar epithelium, which may reveal degenerative cellular alterations. The desquamated cells in the cystic fluid exhibit a characteristic, finely vacuolar, abundant pale cytoplasm and small, round, regular nuclei. Abundant lipids can be detected in the cytoplasm. Necrosis with accumulation of cellular debris may result in cholesterol crystal formation with secondary fibrosis. Necrosis and secondary calcification may be observed in the cyst epithelium.

Stromal Fibrosis

Fibrosis is a constant feature of fibrocystic mastopathy. The modified epithelial structures are surrounded by variable amounts of dense and poorly cellular stroma; collagen fibers are abundant (Fig. 19-15). Epithelial proliferation seems to stimulate this stromal growth.

Adenosis

Adenosis is a proliferation of ductules and acini with the persistence of structures suggesting the lobular disposition observed in the normal gland. This proliferation may be accom-

Table 19-3. Classifications of Proliferative Mastopathy

Black et al[84]	Wellings et al[85]	Page et al[86]
1: Normal	Grade I	Normal
2: Hyperplasia	Grade II	Hyperplasia without atypia
3: Distinct but minimal atypia	Grade III	Atypical hyperplasia (mild, moderate, or severe)
4: Atypia suggestive of in situ carcinoma	Grade IV	DCIS or LCIS
5: Atypia consistent with in situ carcinoma	Grade V (DCIS or LCIS)	

Abbreviations: DCIS, ductal carcinoma in situ; LCIS, lobular carcinoma in situ.

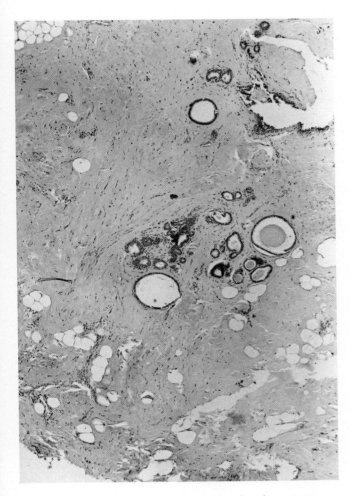

Fig. 19-15. Fibrocystic disease. Rare cystic ductal structures surrounded by stromal fibrosis are shown.

panied by variable degrees of myoepithelial hyperplasia and fibrosis. There may be an increased number of cellular layers above the basal lamina; cellular atypias are very mild, a characteristic that helps differentiate this from more severe lesions such as atypical hyperplasia and in situ or infiltrating carcinoma. The presentation of a lobular pattern and the presence of numerous myoepithelial cells (demonstrable by actin or S-100 protein immunoreactivity) are also useful for the distinction from carcinoma. Apocrine metaplasia may be present (*apocrine adenosis*).[92]

Some subclassifications have been proposed to qualify particular images. Sclerosing adenosis, the most common type, is discussed in detail below. In *florid adenosis* the ductal proliferation is particularly evident and is associated with myoepithelial proliferation and fibrosis. Multiple foci of the lesions are commonly observed and they are rather well circumscribed. Blunt duct adenosis is characterized by lobular dilation with varying degrees of cellular proliferation, and is now more commonly referred to as *unfolding lobules*. The term *nodular adenosis* has been proposed to describe a lesion consisting of a nodular proliferation of tubules of relatively uniform size and the absence of the

whorled arrangement usually provoked by marked fibrosis. Nodular adenosis should not be confused with tubular carcinoma. The absence of a double-layered epithelium with myoepithelial cells and the presence of cellular atypia and intraductal epithelial bridging are morphologic criteria in favor of carcinoma.[92] By contrast, in *microglandular adenosis* (MGA), the lesion usually presents as a mass, a lobular disposition is not observed, and other markers of the fibrocystic complex are often absent.[92,93] Histologically, one sees small round glands haphazardly extending through fibrous and adipose tissue (Fig. 19-16). The glands are lined by a single layer of uniform cells, often with clear cytoplasm, and usually contain dense, eosinophilic, periodic acid-Schiff (PAS)-positive material in their lumina. The main differential diagnosis is with tubular carcinoma, in which the glands also lack myoepithelial cells but are less uniformly round, do not contain dense intraluminal material, and provoke a sclerosing response (see below).[92,93] Atypical variants of MGA and carcinomas arising within them have been reported.[94,95]

Sclerosing Adenosis

Sclerosing adenosis is proliferation of the ductules accompanied by a marked interstitial fibrosis that breaks up the epithelial structures into distorted glandular formations. A false appearance of invasion of the stroma by epithelial cells is thus created.[96] Occasionally, the lesion can be recognized as a clinically palpable mass measuring 0.4 to 2.5 cm in diameter. Grossly, this lesion is firm, nodular, poorly demarcated, and shows a gray-white cut surface. Light brown areas are often present. These gross features of *adenosis tumor*[97] are suggestive of carcinoma; two criteria, however, will differentiate the two. The typical yellow-white steaks of carcinoma are absent and sclerosing adenosis is never as hard as carcinoma.

More often, foci of sclerosing adenosis are discovered microscopically in the context of fibrocystic changes. At low magnification, they constitute dense cellular foci disseminated in the parenchyma (Fig. 19-17). The individual cells have a normal

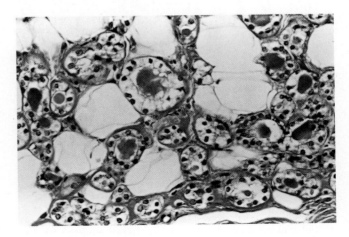

Fig. 19-16. Microglandular adenosis. Uniform small, round glands extend through mammary fat without a stromal response. Glands are lined by a single layer of clear cells and contain intraluminal dense eosinophilic material.

size and regular form except for the alterations provoked by compression and distortion (Fig. 19-18). Mitoses are rare. Participation of myoepithelial cells in this lesion can always be demonstrated. A florid epithelial cell phase is followed by a sclerotic phase (Fig. 19-19) where the epithelial structures are buried in an abundant, dense, hyalinized connective tissue (the number of elastic fibers is not significantly modified).[98] Calcifications and necrosis may be seen. Foci of sclerosing adenosis may be present in perineural spaces; they should not be misinterpreted as a malignant infiltration.[99]

Sclerosing adenosis may constitute a difficult diagnostic problem on frozen section, and a wrong diagnosis of carcinoma may be made if the pathologist is not aware of the particular microscopic appearance of this lesion. Intraoperative smears or imprints, however, are easily interpretable as benign. Disorders of ovarian function have been suggested as causally related, although clinical data do not always confirm the existence of hormonal anomalies. Numerous pregnancies, suppression of lactation, and irregularities of menstruation have been reported to

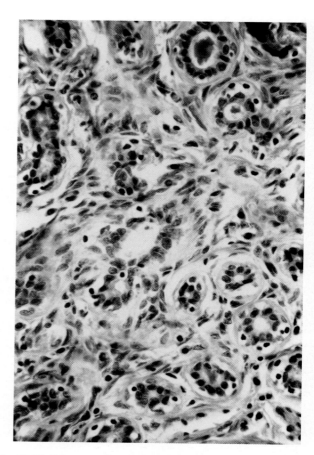

Fig. 19-18. Sclerosing adenosis. Detail showing bimorphic appearance and lack of atypia.

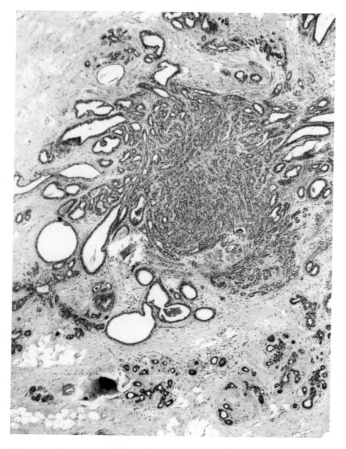

Fig. 19-17. Sclerosing adenosis. Note the dense cellular area composed of epithelial structures modified by the stromal proliferation. This should not be misinterpreted as a malignant proliferation. Retained lobular configuration and peripheral dilation are characteristic and useful findings, as are lack of cytologic atypia and mitotic activity.

support this hypothesis. Sclerosing adenosis may indicate a slightly elevated risk for the development of carcinoma.[100,101]

Apocrine Metaplasia

Apocrine metaplasia[102] is characterized by the presence of large ductal cells with round, small nuclei and an abundant, pale eosinophilic cytoplasm. A typical feature is the presence of some cells bearing a bulging apical pole, called gasoline pump cells or apocrine blebs. These cells either line dilated ducts or can be seen in papillary proliferations (Fig. 19-20). Electron microscopy has shown that they are proliferative and secretory cells with numerous mitochondria, which account for the eosinophilia.[103] A good immunohistochemical marker of apocrine metaplasia is gross cystic disease fluid protein (GCDFP-15).[92] This type of metaplasia is more frequent in benign lesions, and focal apocrine metaplasia is seen virtually exclusively in benign conditions. Intraductal and infiltrating apocrine carcinomas do, however, exist (see below). The etiology of this metaplasia remains controversial.

Radial Sclerosing Lesion

Radial sclerosing lesion is also known as indurative mastopathy, radial scar, benign sclerosing ductal proliferation, nonencapsulated sclerosing lesion, sclerosing papillary proliferation, and sclerosing adenosis with pseudoinfiltration. The various synonyms proposed to qualify this rather common lesion justify our perplexity concerning the genesis of the alterations.[96,104,105]

The lesion consists of a central area of sclerosis with engulfed haphazardly arranged ducts around this central core. The central area has a radial disposition and may be surrounded by adenosis, intraductal papillary proliferations, and epithelial hyperplasia (Fig. 19-21). The central scar contains collagen and elastic fibers. The ductal structures maintain their two cell layers, except when epithelial cells are altered by sclerosis and elastosis. Multiple and bilateral locations have been observed.

The distorted and irregular disposition of the glandular structures explains our concern when a diagnostic decision has to be

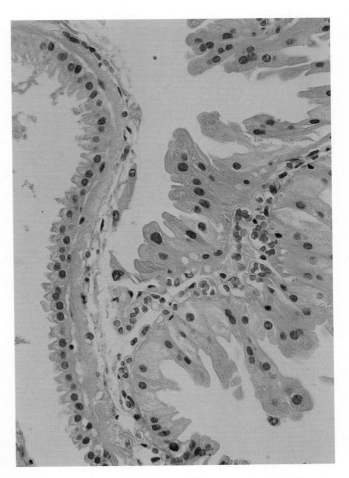

Fig. 19-20. Apocrine metaplasia. Papillary intraductal proliferation lined by cells with voluminous brightly eosinophilic cytoplasm and enlarged atypical nuclei.

made. The main difficulty lies in the confusion with tubular carcinoma. The absence of cellular atypia and mitoses, the persistence of a double-layered epithelium, and the characteristic circumscription of the lesion are in favor of benignity. The histogenesis of this lesion is a matter of controversy; some investigators have suggested that it represents a proliferation of terminal ducts and lobules accompanied by occlusive fibrosis of ductal laminae. Radial scar is usually associated with fibrocystic changes. Divergent views on the significance of scar lesions have been expressed in the literature, but opinions are generally in favor of their benign evolution.

Epithelial Proliferation or Hyperplasia

Under the heading epithelial proliferation or hyperplasia we gather all degrees of ductal epithelial proliferation that can be observed in fibrocystic mastopathy. It includes the lesions mentioned as duct, lobular, and papillomatoid hyperplasia, adenomatosis, and epitheliosis (the term used by British patholo-

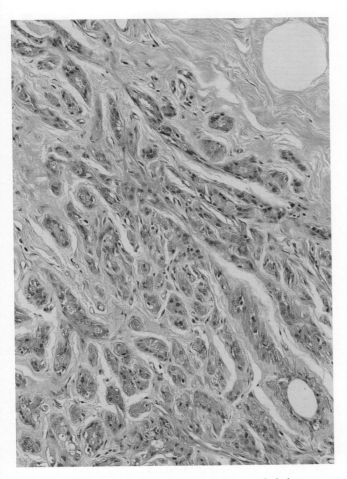

Fig. 19-19. Sclerosing adenosis. Distortion of the epithelial structures by interstitial fibrosis is seen.

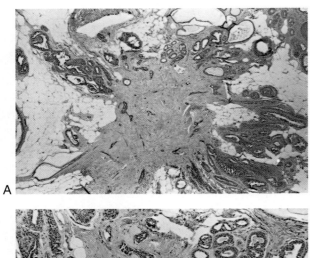

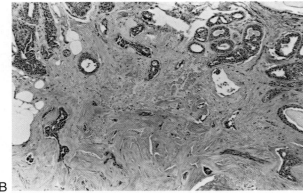

Fig. 19-21. Radial sclerosing lesion. **(A)** Central sclerosis surrounded by radially arranged ducts, many of which are hyperplastic. **(B)** Sclerotic center of lesion at higher magnification contains entrapped pseudoinfiltrative ducts.

gists).[106] When the proliferation is moderate and not accompanied by cellular atypia, the benign character of the lesion is evident. The recognition of an atypical hyperplasia is important, as we now have pertinent data showing that these patients are subject to a greater risk of developing cancer, in the range of about 4 to 5 times that of women with breast biopsies showing no proliferative changes.[86–91] The variety of terms proposed to characterize these proliferations is a source of confusion among pathologists; therefore it is to be desired that a clear definition of every term used should be expressed.

The best definition of ductal hyperplasia is one that demands a proliferation of cells within the duct lumen, defined by more than the usual single layer of ductal epithelial cells and underlying layer of myoepithelial cells. Although proliferations of the myoepithelial cell layer do occur, the usual intraductal hyperplasia involves primarily the inner ductal epithelial layer. The continued presence of myoepithelial cells—usually obvious by routine light microscopy, but demonstrable if necessary by either immunohistochemistry or electron microscopy—is one of the features used to distinguish benign hyperplastic processes from intraductal carcinoma (ductal carcinoma in situ [DCIS]).

Architecturally, in typical intraductal hyperplasia there are solid cell nests as well as complicated ridges, tufts, arcades, fen-

estrated sheets, and papillary proliferations (Figs. 19-22 to 19-25). An important feature is that the lumina formed are irregular in both size and shape, with numerous compressed slit-like spaces. This differs from the lumina of the cribriform pattern of DCIS, in which the spaces are round, regular, and appear uniformly punched out. If papillae are formed, they generally are supported by central fibrovascular connective tissue cores, unlike the papillae composed solely of tumor cells in micropapillary DCIS.

At higher magnification, the cells are generally small and irregularly shaped, with a tendency for the nuclei to be ovoid or somewhat spindled (Figs. 19-26 and 19-27). These cells are usually admixed with more rounded ones, so that the general impression is one of a lack of cellular uniformity. The cells tend to form swirls or to stream through septa between lumina. The cytologic features of malignant tumors (nuclear hyperchromasia, chromatin clumping, prominent nucleoli, mitotic figures) are absent or present only focally. When enlarged and atypical nuclei are present, they are often located in cells showing the cytoplasmic features of apocrine metaplasia, as described above,

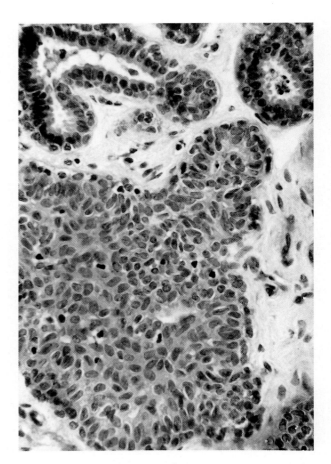

Fig. 19-22. Ductal hyperplasia. Note the solid cellular growth without marked cellular atypia; partial obliteration of the ductular lumen by cellular proliferation; and absence of cellular atypia and mitoses (high magnification).

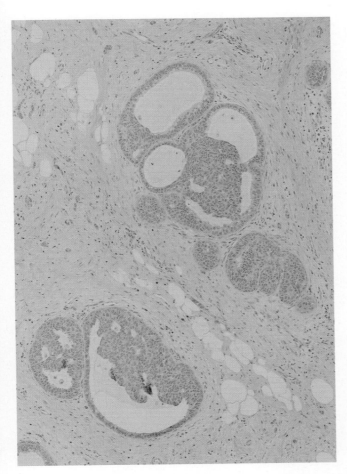

Fig. 19-23. Ductal hyperplasia without atypia. Solid cellular proliferations with some irregular slit-like spaces partially fill small ducts.

and this focal apocrine change within a ductal proliferation is a good indicator of benignity (Fig. 19-20).

The ducts containing proliferative lesions may undergo focal or extensive sclerosis, sometimes obscuring the well demarcated peripheral boundaries of individual ducts[107,108] (Figs. 19-28 and 19-29). In these cases, an appearance difficult to distinguish from epithelial invasion into the surrounding stroma may be created. Two useful hints for distinguishing this appearance from DCIS with focal true stromal invasion are that the cellular proliferation itself lacks the characteristic architectural and cytologic features of DCIS and the surrounding sclerosis is generally of a dense hyaline type rather than the looser, somewhat myxoid, often inflamed, myofibroblastic stroma initiated by an infiltrating carcinoma.

Although it is deceptively easy to think of *atypical ductal hyperplasia* (ADH) as any intraductal hyperplasia with a degree of architectural or cytologic atypia, in fact such a definition would lead to overdiagnosis of this condition and blunting of its clinical implication—a four- to fivefold increased risk of subsequent development of carcinoma.[86–91] Therefore, it is manda-

tory to define ADH as a lesion that almost but not quite satisfies the qualitative and quantitative criteria for DCIS. Thus, unless we have to seriously consider the diagnosis of DCIS in a ductal proliferative lesion, we do not make the diagnosis of ADH. Because several different patterns of DCIS exist, these are considered in more detail later in this chapter, and lesions of ADH that differ qualitatively from them are also discussed there. The most common pattern of ADH is one that architecturally, at low magnification, evokes the suspicion of DCIS, but cytologically shows at least some of the irregularity, spindling, streaming, and/or swirling mentioned above as characteristic of ductal hyperplasia without atypia. Because the best validated criteria for DCIS demand that the lesion involve at least two complete duct profiles, another pattern of ADH is one in which classic criteria for low grade DCIS are met, but only in a single duct or portions of one or more ducts.

The discussion of ductal hyperplasia and its atypical form leads into the question of whether similar lesions can be defined in the lobules of the breast. Atypical lobular hyperplasia (ALH) is a well characterized lesion that—like ADH—is best diag-

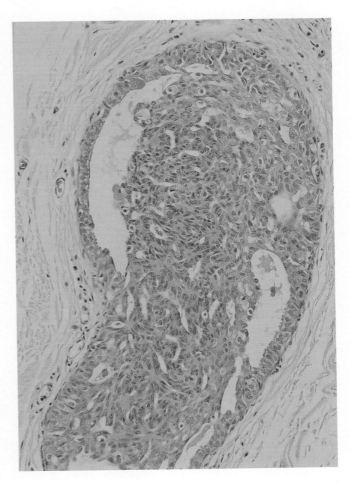

Fig. 19-24. Ductal hyperplasia without atypia. Irregularity in size and shape of lumina within the intraductal proliferation is emphasized here, as are cell streaming and lack of nuclear atypia.

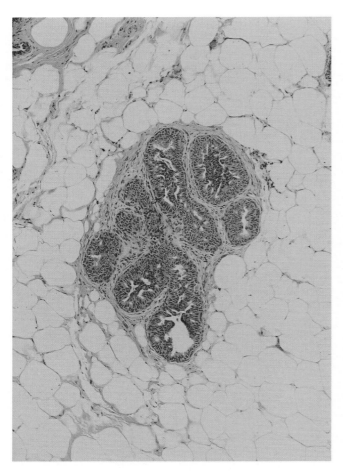

Fig. 19-25. Ductal hyperplasia without atypia. Low power view emphasizes irregularity of newly formed spaces within original duct lumina.

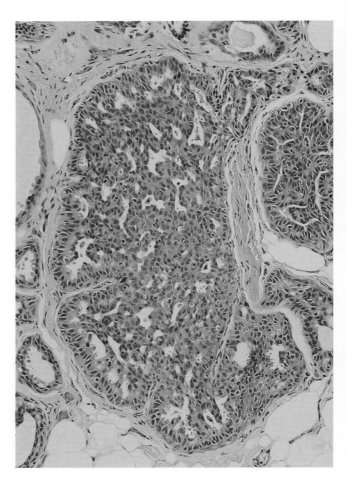

Fig. 19-26. Ductal hyperplasia without atypia. Note bimorphic cell population, lack of nuclear atypia, and irregularly sized and shaped intraluminal spaces.

nosed by its close resemblance to, without quite meeting the criteria of, lobular carcinoma in situ (LCIS). These two lesions are discussed in more detail later in this chapter. Whether a *lobular hyperplasia* without atypia exists is the subject of some controversy, with some authors accepting this diagnosis and others denying it. Carter[109] both accepts and illustrates the lesion, and also defines it as intralobular proliferation of cells that are not appreciably enlarged or atypical, do not distend the lobules, and are accompanied by at least some myoepithelial cells. This lesion, so defined, appears to be uncommon, to be unassociated with fibrocystic changes, and to be of unknown clinical significance.

All these ductal and lobular hyperplastic lesions, as well as DCIS and LCIS, are usually diagnosed in the absence of a palpable mass, unless the mass is related to other fibrocystic changes. In current practice, they are usually seen in biopsies performed for mammographically suspicious microcalcifications. The calcifications may be located pathologically either within the hyperplastic or malignant lesion or adjacent to it in foci of sclerosing adenosis or some other totally benign condition. The pathologist should comment not only on the fact that

microcalcifications are present in the surgically excised specimen, but also on their location in lesional or serendipitously associated tissue, because the exact location may be useful in subsequent mammographic follow-up of the patient.

Premalignant Significance

As mentioned above and shown in Table 19-4, the subsequent risk of developing carcinoma after a benign breast biopsy varies with the lesion or lesions diagnosed in the biopsy specimen. It has generally been accepted that, in the absence of proliferative disease, there is no increased risk, although some recent studies suggest that even this statement may not be true.[100,101] In any event, significant risk is generally considered to reside only in those breasts harboring proliferative changes, and particularly those with either atypical hyperplasia—whether ductal or lobular—or DCIS or LCIS.[86-91] A few caveats concerning these statistics should be raised, however. First, it must be remembered that these data have been validated only for diagnoses made using the standardized

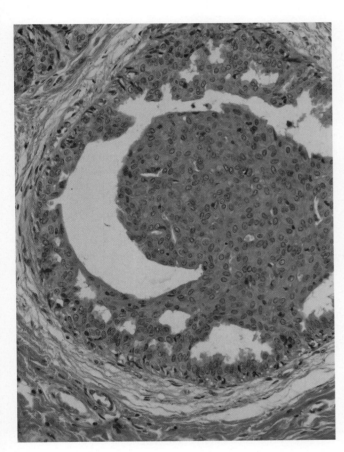

Fig. 19-27. Ductal hyperplasia without atypia. Solid proliferation extending into lumen shows prominent swirling of uniform cells with somewhat ovoid nuclei.

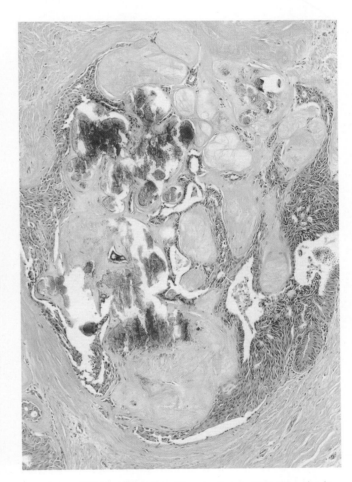

Fig. 19-28. Sclerosing ductal proliferative lesion. Note dense hyaline sclerosis within and around the duct, creating a pseudoinfiltrative appearance.

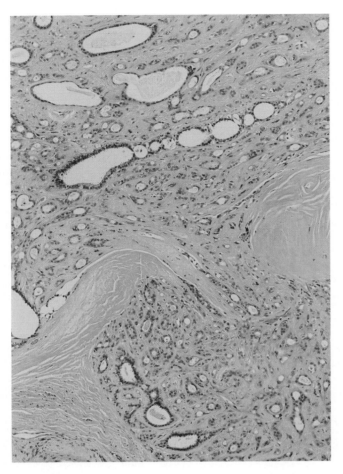

Fig. 19-29. Sclerosing ductal proliferative lesion. The proliferation it-self is architecturally and cytologically benign.

Table 19-4. Relative Risk of Breast Cancer Development After Benign Breast Biopsy[a]

No proliferative changes	1.0
Proliferative changes without atypia	1.5–2
Atypical hyperplasia	4–5
Carcinoma in situ	8–10

[a] Consensus of studies in references 86 to 91; assumes no further treatment or prophylaxis after biopsy, and average of 10 to 15 years of follow-up.

histopathologic criteria that are discussed in this chapter. Thus, for example, a more loosely applied diagnosis of atypical ductal or lobular hyperplasia will be associated with considerably less risk than that quoted here. Second, these data have been generated in a statistically significant manner only for women in the age range of 35 to 55 years, and only for a follow-up period of 10 to 15 years. Thus, we do not know whether the same risks can be quoted for, for example, 30 year follow-up of ADH in a 25-year-old woman. Finally, it is extremely important to remember that the relative risk figures quoted are relative to an absolute risk of 2 percent cancer development in 10 to 15 years of follow-up. Thus, the four to five times relative risk that sounds horrendous when quoted this way is only an 8 to 10 percent absolute risk, and the long-term survival rate for cancers developing in closely monitored patients is probably in the range of 75 to 80 percent. Thus, the absolute risk of dying of breast cancer for a 50-year-old woman with a diagnosis of ADH, if nothing more is done other than close follow-up, is probably in the range of 1 to 2 percent. If statistics are presented in this manner to patients, they will probably provoke consid-

erably less panic than if they are presented simply as relative risk factors.

It should also be remembered that the risks quoted above can be magnified by other factors, such as a positive family history of breast cancer, specifically in the presence of abnormalities of the BRCA-1 gene. These and other epidemiologic risk factors for breast cancer are discussed in more detail below.

Finally, two additional points should be raised. The first is that, although we present the diagnostic criteria for the spectrum of intraductal lesions as if they were easily reproducible, in fact even experts can have difficulty in the differential diagnosis of these lesions.[110] It is clear, however, that far greater consensus can be reached if the criteria for each diagnosis are universally understood and applied,[111] and also if histologic sections of high quality are available. The need for the latter again underlines the injunction mentioned above against performing frozen sections in the absence of a gross lesion in a breast biopsy (or in the presence of a grossly intraductal lesion), because freezing artifact will make the permanent sections even more problematic.

Second, the difficulty in separating the intraductal lesions microscopically is mirrored in recent molecular biologic studies, which have emphasized that some alterations thought to represent part of the malignant phenotype can be present not only in DCIS and LCIS, but in some atypical hyperplasias—and rarely even lesions diagnosed as hyperplasia without atypia—as well.[112–115] Thus, perhaps premalignant or even malignant changes develop in some lesions before they are detectable by our usual microscopic criteria.

Cytomorphology of Fibrocystic Change, High Risk Proliferative Lesions, and Premalignant Breast Disease

Although it is now possible to separate breast lesions histopathologically into benign, premalignant, and malignant categories, and despite the reliability of breast FNAB in separating benign from malignant lesions, the cytologic features of premalignant lesions have not yet been well defined.

With increase in utilization of FNAB for the diagnosis of palpable and nonpalpable breast lesions, it is almost essential to differentiate low risk benign changes from those known to be

Table 19-5. Cytologic Grading System for Interpretation of Mammographically Guided Fine Needle Aspiration Biopsies

Cellular Arrangement	Cellular Pleomorphism	Myoepithelial Cells	Anisonucleosis	Nucleoli	Chromatin Clumping	Score
Monolayer	Absent	Many	Absent	Absent	Absent	1
Nuclear overlapping	Mild	Moderate	Mild	Micronucleoli	Rare	2
Clustering	Moderate	Few	Moderate	Micro and/or rare macronucleoli	Occasional	3
Loss of cohesion	Conspicuous	Absent	Conspicuous	Predominantly macronucleoli	Frequent	4

(From Masood et al,[119] with permission.)

associated with a high risk of a subsequent malignant tumor. Recognition of the spectrum of changes seen in high risk lesions by FNAB can also assist in identification of clinically occult proliferative breast disease in women with a family history of breast cancer. This provides an effective means of selecting suitable patients for chemopreventive trials. Subsequently, the aspirates from these patients can be used for monitoring of surrogate endpoint biomarkers in these trials.[116–118] In addition, using the same diagnostic terminology for breast FNAB as is commonly used in diagnostic histopathology would also offer a significant advantage if it could be accurately applied.

In a prospective study utilizing mammographically guided fine needle aspirates in 100 nonpalpable breast lesions, one of us (SM) assessed the reliability of a cytologic grading system to define the cytologic features of proliferative and nonproliferative breast disease and to differentiate between benign, premalignant, and malignant breast lesions.[119] We developed a cytologic grading system evaluating the aspirates for their cellular arrangement, the degrees of cellular pleomorphism and anisonucleosis, presence of myoepithelial cells and nucleoli, and the chromatin pattern. Values ranging from 1 to 4 were assigned to each criterion, and a score based on the sum of the individual values was calculated for each case. With scores ranging from 6 to 24, the cases were divided into nonproliferative breast disease without atypia (score 6 to 10), proliferative breast disease without atypia (score 11 to 14), proliferative breast disease with atypia (score 15 to 18), and cancer (score 19 to 24) (Table 19-5). Comparing the cytologic interpretation to the reported histologic diagnosis obtained from needle localization biopsies, we found a high degree of concordance between the results.[119]

We believe that, by using strict cytologic criteria, it may be possible to define the continuous spectrum of changes in breast lesions and separate hyperplasia from neoplasia.[119,120]

Nonproliferative Breast Disease

The cell yield in these aspirates is variable and depends on the nature of the lesion. In noncystic lesions, the aspirate is scanty or moderate. Frequently, the aspirate consists of clusters of monotonous small uniform-appearing epithelial cells arranged in monolayered sheets with a honeycomb pattern. Foam cells, apocrine cells, single naked cells, and fragments of stromal cells are frequently observed. The cells have regular nuclei with a fine chromatin pattern. Nucleoli are not commonly seen. Myoepithelial cells are easily identified (Figs. 19-30 and 19-31).

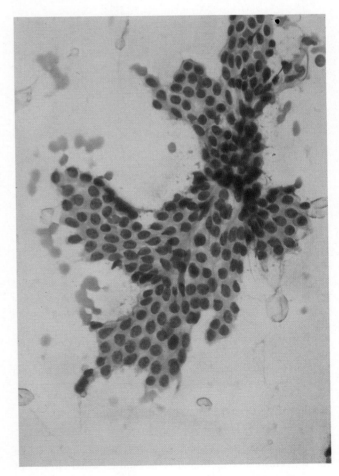

Fig. 19-30. Cytomorphology of nonproliferative breast disease characterized by a monolayered clustering of uniform population of epithelial and myoepithelial cells. (Papanicolaou stain, × 200.)

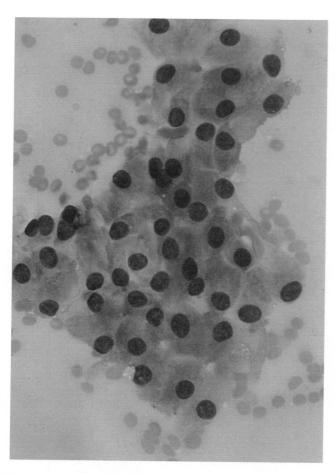

Fig. 19-31. Another view of the same case demonstrating metaplastic apocrine cells. (Diff-Quik, × 400.)

Proliferative Breast Disease Without Atypia

Proliferative breast disease differs from nonproliferative breast disease by its higher cell yield and unique cellular arrangement. The cellularity is moderate to high depending on the degree of proliferative epithelial changes. There are increased numbers of tightly cohesive groups of ductal epithelial and myoepithelial cells with some overriding of the nuclei, occasional loss of polarity, and some variability in the nuclear size. Micronucleoli may be seen. Cytologic atypia is inconspicuous. Apocrine cells, histiocytes, and occasional naked nuclei are the accompanying cells in these aspirate (Figs. 19-32 and 19-33).

Proliferative Breast Disease With Atypia (Atypical Hyperplasia)

The cellular aspirates are frequently rich and are composed of multiple clusters of epithelial cells. The crowded clusters of cells show conspicuous loss of polarity and overriding of the nuclei. Nucleoli are present and display irregular and coarse chromatin patterns. Variation in nuclear size and cellular pleomor-

phism are also present. Within the crowded atypical epithelial cells, there is morphologic evidence of myoepithelial cell differentiation (Figs. 19-34 and 19-35).

Other investigators have reported more difficulty in making these distinctions. Dziura and Bonfiglio in 1979[121] described cell changes in ductal neoplasia. Similarly, they found anisonucleosis, the presence of macronucleoli, chromatin clumping, marked nuclear overlap, and cellular disarray as cellular indicators of malignant tumor. However, only limited predictability of the degree of hyperplasia was possible with their morphologic criteria, but their samples were obtained from already excised lesions rather than FNAB of intact breasts. Bibbo et al[122] also attempted to define cytologic features of atypical hyperplasia in stereotactic FNA cytology of clinically occult malignant and high risk benign lesions. They also found some limitation in the grading of ductal hyperplasia.

In a follow-up study, we used this cytologic grading system in evaluation of palpable breast lesions in 156 consecutive FNABs.[123] Follow-up histology was available in 146 cases. The interpretation of FNAB was performed by four pathologists who

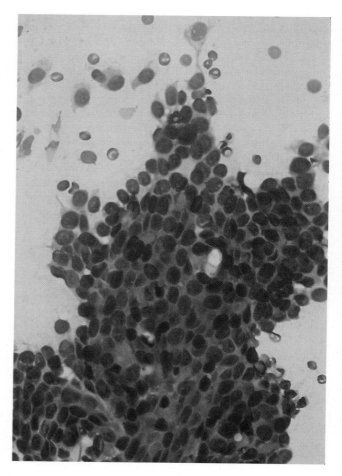

Fig. 19-32. Direct smear from an aspirate of proliferative breast disease without atypia showing crowded clusters of epithelial and myoepithelial cells with overriding of the nuclei. (Diff-Quik, × 200.)

stages of proliferative breast disease is still problematic and they refrain from making a definitive diagnosis of atypical hyperplasia or carcinoma in situ on fine needle aspirates. However, they believe that in selected cases, separation between DCIS and atypical hyperplasia is possible. They recognize atypical hyperplasia when cells are arranged in flat cohesive sheets with distinct cell borders and myoepithelial cells. By contrast, DCIS presents with single cells constituting more than 10 percent of the atypical cells, cellular dyshesion, an inflammatory background, coarsely granular chromatin, and nuclear pleomorphism. Shiels et al[127] studied the cytomorphology of 15 cases of DCIS. The absence of myoepithelial cells, and a cellular smear with conspicuous nuclear overriding and atypia, are considered by these authors to be the most important cytologic features differentiating DCIS from atypical hyperplasia.

Presently, most investigators advocate an intraoperative consultation or an excisional biopsy for any case diagnosed as atypical hyperplasia, suspicious or inconclusive for carcinoma.[120,125,128] Some of the limitations of FNAB may not necessarily be the result of our inability to recognize different enti-

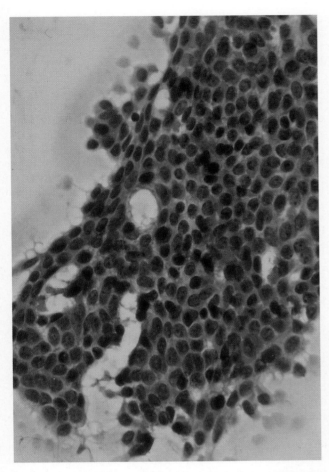

Fig. 19-33. Papanicolaou-stained smear of the same case as in Fig. 19.32 with similar features. (Original magnification × 200.)

have become familiar with the grading system by a personalized training experience. Despite the heterogeneity of sampling in palpable FNAB, particularly in larger tumors, there was a diagnostic accuracy of 95 percent. Differentiation between fibroadenoma and papillary lesions versus proliferative breast disease was not always possible. There were two cases of low grade carcinoma in situ, one case of infiltrating lobular carcinoma, and three cases of infiltrating duct carcinoma that were misinterpreted as atypical hyperplasia. Review of these cases demonstrated absence of the cellular dyshesion commonly seen in the usual mammary neoplasia. Furthermore, these tumors were low grade.

Similar limitations have been observed in a study conducted by Sneige and Staerkel.[124] The authors evaluated our grading system in a retrospective study of low grade in situ lesions of the breast. They believe that our cytologic grading system should be complemented by incorporating architectural features such as cribriform and/or micropapillary patterns in differentiation between atypical hyperplasia or noncomedocarcinoma in situ. Others[125,126] also believe that separation between various

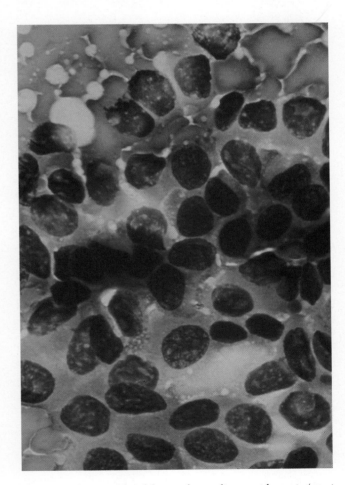

Fig. 19-34. Aspirate of proliferative breast disease with atypia (atypical ductal hyperplasia) demonstrating loosely arranged cellular pattern with nuclear atypia. Myoepithelial cells are seen as spindled cells. (Diff-Quik, × 1,000.)

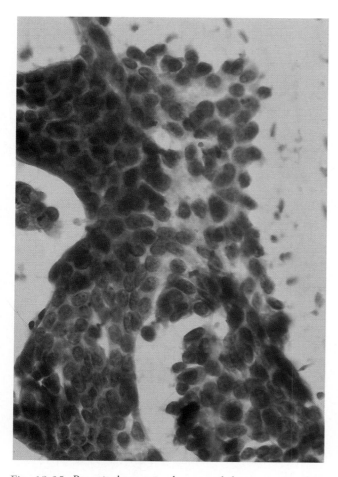

Fig. 19-35. Papanicolaou-stained smear of the same case shows marked overriding of the nuclei, anisonucleosis, and hyperchromasia. (Papanicolaou stain, × 400.)

ties. The presence of heterogeneity of individual lesions is an important factor to be considered. As an example, in a study conducted by Lennington et al in 1994,[129] the authors reviewed 100 sequentially collected DCIS cases from a consultation practice. ADHs were intermixed in 17 cases of DCIS, and mixed patterns of comedo and noncomedo type DCIS were seen in another 33 cases. In all the cases of combined ADH and DCIS, the more advanced patterns of DCIS were seen in the central portion of the lesion, whereas the ADH components were arranged peripherally.

BENIGN NEOPLASMS

Fibroadenoma

The fibroadenoma is the most frequent benign tumor of the breast. Rare before puberty, it usually appears in the 15 to 35 year age group, the greatest frequency being in the 20s. It is a slowly growing, estrogen-dependent, fibroepithelial neoplasm. Dysmenorrhea, premenstrual tension, and irregular menses are often mentioned in the clinical history of the patient, suggesting a hormonal disturbance. Clinical and pathologic studies of fibroadenomas in patients receiving oral contraceptives have been published.[130]

The fibroadenoma usually manifests as a single mass, but it may be multifocal and may occur in both breasts simultaneously. Clinically it is a circumscribed, movable mass with a firm, elastic consistency. The tumor does not adhere to adjacent tissues or the overlying skin.

There is still some debate over whether the fibroadenoma is a true neoplasm or represents hyperplastic change of both the stromal and epithelial components. Fibroadenoma and certain foci of fibrocystic mastopathy sometimes exhibit identical structures, which suggests etiologic and morphologic relationships between the two lesions. Some studies have also found fibroadenomas to be polyclonal, suggesting that they are not neoplastic.[131]

Macroscopically, the lesion is a well encapsulated, firm rubbery mass, measuring 0.5 to 5 cm in diameter. The cut section reveals a gray or pink lobulated, bulging tissue; the lobules are bordered by fibrous septa. When the epithelial elements are abundant, the color tends to be more pink or light tan. The mass is encapsulated by a thin fibrous surface (Fig. 19-36).

Microscopically, the fibroadenoma is a benign, localized proliferation of epithelial cells and fibroblasts, occurring in a voluminous and misshapen lobule. Classically, we distinguish two histologic types, which may occur alone or in combination. The *pericanalicular* form exhibits well preserved glandular structures with normal bistratified epithelium, embedded in loose connective tissue stroma whose cells tend to adopt a concentric arrangement about the glands (Fig. 19-37). Although collagen and reticulin are abundant, the number of elastic fibers is not significantly increased. Capillary vascularization is discrete. Glandular proliferation with moderate cytologic atypia can be observed, but these lesions raise no suspicion of a malignant tumor. Hyalinization, edema, and myxoid degeneration can be observed. Extensive myxoid change may cause confusion with mucinous carcinoma on FNAB, and may be associated in a familial condition with cardiac and cutaneous myxomas.[132] Neutral mucopolysaccharides have been identified in the ground

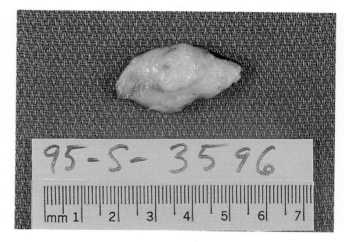

Fig. 19-36. Fibroadenoma, gross appearance.

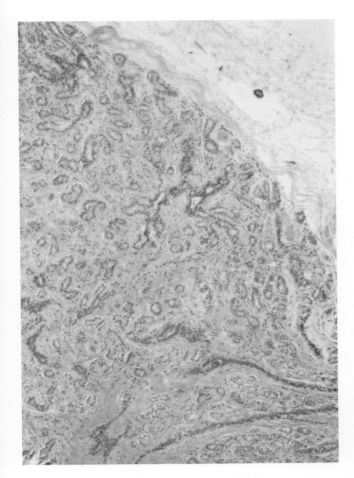

Fig. 19-37. Fibroadenoma, pericanalicular type.

Evolution and Prognosis

The growth of fibroadenoma is slow; it may take years before these lesions reach a palpable size. At menopause, fibroadenomas stabilize or regress; growth may be rapid during pregnancy, and signs of secretion have been observed during lactation.[135]

Infarction of fibroadenoma is an uncommon complication that may occur during pregnancy or lactation. The possible etiologic mechanisms are thrombosis of the feeding vessel or a relative vascular insufficiency with respect to increased metabolic activity. This complication should be borne in mind since the infarcted benign lesion may grossly simulate carcinoma.[136]

The possibility of malignant transformation of fibroadenoma has given rise to much controversy.[137,138] A few cases have been reported in the literature, the most frequent type of associated carcinoma described being lobular in situ carcinoma. The exact incidence of malignant transformation is difficult to evaluate because some carcinomas may totally replace a preexisting fibroadenoma. Because fibroadenoma is a common lesion, one can expect to observe the coincidental and simultaneous presence of fibroadenoma and carcinoma in the same breast, especially in older patients. The development of sarcoma is discussed with cystosarcoma phyllodes.

The risk of subsequent carcinoma in patients with fibroadenoma has also been investigated. Dupont and colleagues[139]

substance of the connective tissue proliferation. Squamous metaplasia with keratinized cyst formation is possible, but rare. In the *intracanalicular* form, the glandular structures are elongated and tightly compressed by a hyperplastic fibrous stroma arranged in irregular nodules (Fig. 19-38). The epithelial structures thus appear stretched out, distorted, or atrophic. The stroma may be densely or poorly cellular and rich in collagen, or it may be calcified. Acid mucopolysaccharides are present in the ground substance. Squamous, bony, and cartilaginous metaplasia as well as the presence of smooth muscle fibers have been reported.

Ultrastructural studies demonstrate that the stromal proliferation is responsible for the tumor growth.[133,134] Secretory cells generally constitute a single cell layer; the presence of occasional cilia has been reported. Myoepithelial cells whose long axis runs parallel to the basement membrane lie beneath the epithelial cells. Multilayered basal lamina may be present. These multiple layers of basal lamina may result from successive episodes of cell death and new proliferation, each new generation of cells laying down a new membrane parallel to the last. Surrounding the cellular structures are bundles of collagen fibers and aggregates of microfibrils. Myoepithelial cells retain their usual relationship to the basement membrane.[134]

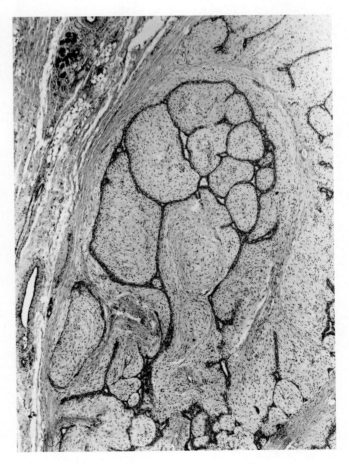

Fig. 19-38. Fibroadenoma, intracanalicular type.

concluded that patients with *complex* fibroadenomas (containing cysts, sclerosing adenosis, epithelial calcifications, and/or papillary apocrine change) or benign proliferative disease in excised parenchyma adjacent to the fibroadenoma had a three to fourfold risk of subsequent cancer, whereas patients with fibroadenomas and neither of these factors, with a negative cancer family history, showed essentially no elevated risk.

Cytology

Cytologically, the aspirates from fibroadenomas are typically cellular and demonstrate a biphasic pattern consisting of epithelial and stromal elements. The cell population consists of two different cell types. Large cells form sheets of monolayered epithelial clusters with finger-like projections in an antler-horn pattern. The second cell type, small cells with naked nuclei, may be bipolar or spindle shaped, and are admixed with epithelial cells or lie freely in the background (Figs. 19-39 and 19-40). Apocrine cells, histiocytes, and occasionally multinucleated giant cells may also be seen in smears obtained from aspirates of fibroadenoma.[140,141]

Fibroadenomas may be associated with significant cytologic atypia, resulting in a false positive diagnosis.[46,47,142] Response

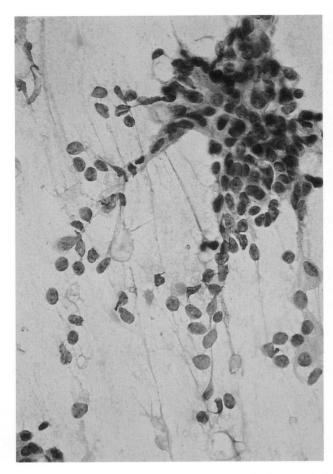

Fig. 19-40. Higher magnification of the same case displaying naked nuclei in the background and spindled myoepithelial cells within the cluster of epithelial cells. (Papanicolaou stain, × 200.)

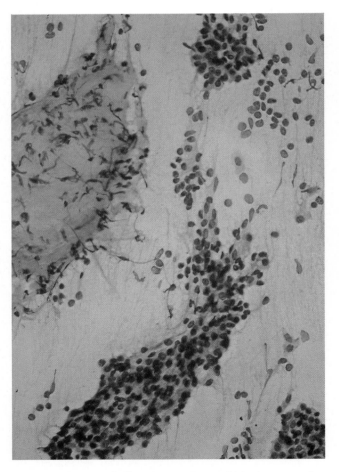

Fig. 19-39. Aspirate of a fibroadenoma showing biphasic pattern of epithelial and stromal components. (Papanicolaou stain, × 100.)

to inflammation and hormonal stimulation, presence of squamous and apocrine metaplasia, and coexistence of atypical hyperplasia are the potential causes of atypia in fibroadenomas. Pregnancy and lactational changes increase the cellularity of the smears in fibroadenomas and induce nuclear atypia and conspicuous nucleoli. In these circumstances, the cytologic features may simulate carcinoma. The absence of necrotic background and of isolated single pleomorphic epithelial cells differentiates fibroadenoma from carcinoma. Fibroadenoma may be associated with a myxoid background and this may be misdiagnosed as mucinous carcinoma. However, the presence of numerous naked nuclei, stromal fragments, and lack of cells with eccentric nuclei are the features against mucinous carcinoma.

Another diagnostic difficulty may arise in differentiation between low grade carcinoma of the breast, especially tubular carcinoma, and fibroadenoma.[143] Immunostaining for muscle-specific actin to detect myoepithelial cells in most aspirates is an important diagnostic adjunct.[144,145] Tubular carcinoma is also marked by conspicuous monomorphism due to a lack of myoepithelial cells. In addition, tubular carcinoma has complex and rigid tubular structures, fragments of elastic material, and isolated cells that retain their cytoplasm.[146]

As discussed above, carcinoma may arise adjacent to or within a breast fibroadenoma. The cytologic features in these cases vary according to the site of sampling. If only the benign component is sampled, the smears may show no evidence of a malignant tumor. This necessitates multiple sampling of breast lesions by FNA.[147]

Also included in the differential diagnosis are the spectrum of fibrocystic change, atypical hyperplasia, and papillary lesions. There are overlapping cytologic features between these entities that occasionally make the distinction difficult. According to Bottles et al,[141] the presence in fibroadenoma of well demarcated stroma containing fibrillary clusters of spindle cells is the most important differentiating feature. Linsk et al[140] advocate the use of quantitative analysis of defined cytologic criteria to differentiate between fibrocystic change and fibroadenoma. In our experience, the clinical presentation of a well defined movable mass is an important contrasting feature to the ill-defined indurated appearance of fibroproliferative lesions.

Cystosarcoma phyllodes, another biphasic tumor of the breast, should also be distinguished from fibroadenoma. The features of this tumor are discussed in detail below.

Juvenile Fibroadenoma

The juvenile fibroadenoma is a rapidly growing, often bilateral tumor of young patients. Histologically, this lesion manifests an active proliferation of the epithelial and connective tissue elements. Essentially, it is the age of the patient and the rapid growth of the lesion that characterize this type of fibroadenoma.[148,149]

Typically, the aspirates are cellular and display an almost monomorphic cellular pattern consisting of a conspicuous number of monolayered sheets and papillae that are composed of uniform, bland, columnar cells, surrounded by a few foam cells and histiocytes.

Adenoma

Mammary adenomas are well demarcated pure adenomatous proliferations of the breast tissue with a very sparse stroma. They are divided in the Atlas of Tumor Pathology[150] into tubular, lactating, apocrine and ductal adenomas, adenolipoma, and so-called pleomorphic adenoma (benign mixed tumor). These lesions are all uncommon with the exception of lactating adenoma. They appear almost exclusively in young women and are all benign. The *lactating adenoma* appear during pregnancy or lactation.[135] The closely packed cells show mitoses and cytoplasmic vacuoles (Fig. 19-41). The *tubular adenoma* shows tubular structures that are very regular in size and shape and are lined by a single layer of epithelial cells.[151] The *pleomorphic adenoma* resembles the benign mixed tumor of salivary gland.[152–154] *Adenolipomas* are best considered a type of hamartoma (see below).

The *ductal adenoma* is an uncommon and poorly understood lesion that was initially described in 1984 as a solid, usually sclerosing lesion of breast ducts.[155] The cases subsequently re-

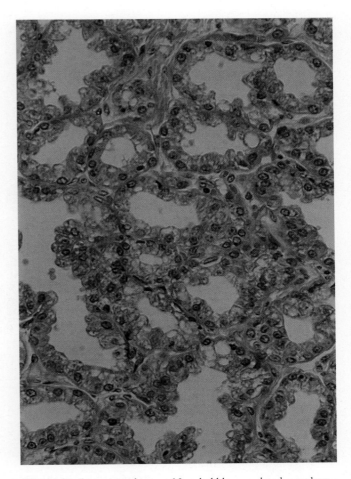

Fig. 19-41. Lactating adenoma. Note bubbly vacuolated cytoplasm.

ported by Lammie and Willis[156] often arose in major subareolar ducts, suggesting to us that these lesions are essentially sclerosing intraductal papillomas.

Cytologic Features

The most commonly encountered and best described adenoma is the lactating adenoma. These lesions yield highly cellular aspirates. The most striking features in this pregnancy-induced lesion is the presence of proteinaceous bubbly vacuoles in the background of the smear. Cytoplasmic vacuolization with fraying of the cytoplasmic borders is the representation of pregnancy-associated cytoplasmic secretion. Foamy macrophages and loose epithelial cells with uniform nuclei and prominent nucleoli are also present[157,158] (Fig. 19-42). Occasionally, aspirates contain predominantly dissociated cells. The cells have large nuclei with prominent nucleoli. These features simulate carcinoma and may lead to false positive diagnoses. Clinical history remains one of the most important factors in avoiding misdiagnosis of cancer in pregnant women. Most infiltrating carcinomas show more cellular discohesion, loss of polarity, necrosis, hyperchromasia, nuclear atypia, and anisonucleosis than lactating adenoma.[159] The diagnosis of carcinoma in pregnancy should be made only when the cell pattern and nuclear

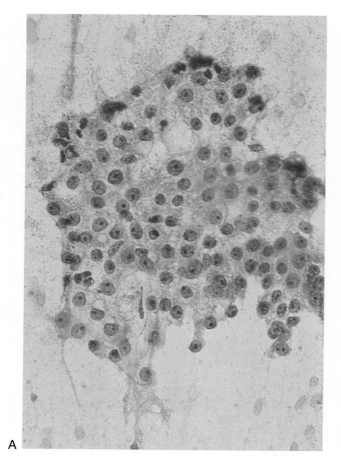 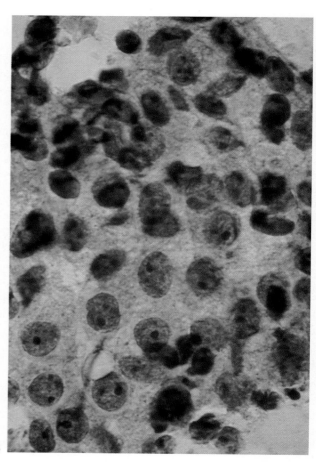

Fig. 19-42. **(A)** Direct smear from a lactating adenoma showing loosely cohesive clusters of epithelial cells in a proteinaceous background. (Papanicolaou stain, × 200.) **(B)** Higher magnification of the same case featuring reactive epithelial changes with prominent nucleoli and abundant cytoplasm with ill-defined borders. (Papanicolaou stain, × 400.)

changes are classic and clinical findings are appropriate. Suspicious lesions and those that persist after pregnancy should be further biopsied. Overall, FNAB reduces the number of unnecessary open biopsies in pregnant women.

Lactating adenoma can also mimic fibroadenoma in pregnancy. Clinically, however, lactating adenomas initially present during pregnancy, whereas fibroadenomas with lactational changes are often discovered prior to pregnancy. In contrast to fibroadenomas, naked nuclei and epithelial clusters in an antler-horn pattern are not seen in lactating adenoma.[160]

Nipple Adenoma

The nipple adenoma (subareolar papillomatosis, florid papillomatosis, papillary adenoma) is an uncommon entity observed in a wide range of age groups.[161–163] It consists of a nodule localized immediately beneath the nipple, which is often clinically misdiagnosed as carcinoma or Paget's disease. The nipple can be crusted or ulcerated. A serous or bloody discharge is fre-

quently observed. The macroscopic appearance is that of a circumscribed, solitary, solid mass.

The cut section reveals a gray or tan, soft to firm tissue. Microscopically, we observe a proliferation of ducts of variable sizes with characteristic papillary structures (Fig. 19-43). The intensity of the papillary proliferation varies from one case to another; sometimes this proliferation is very abundant and plugs the ducts, and sometimes it is absent. The ductal structures are lined by a double-layered epithelium with prominent myoepithelial cells. The nuclei may be moderately enlarged but are uniform and normochromatic. Mitotic figures are rare. Apocrine metaplasia and squamous cysts are common. Dense fibrosis may occur between the ducts, resembling the pseudoinvasive pattern encountered in sclerosing adenosis.

Despite the occasional clinical and even pathologic mimicking of a malignant tumor, and that nipple adenomas are sometimes incidental findings in breasts removed for carcinoma,[162,163] the risk of progression to cancer is minimal. This is a benign lesion that may be treated by local excision in uncomplicated cases.

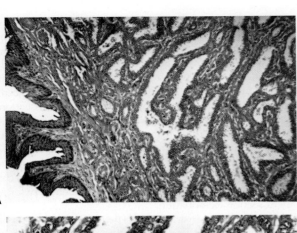

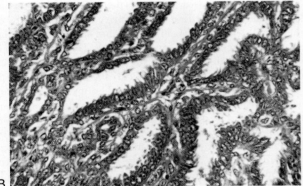

Fig. 19-43. Nipple adenoma. **(A)** Low magnification. Ductal proliferation is localized beneath the mammary skin (seen at left). **(B)** High magnification. The glandular structures are lined by columnar epithelium underlain by myoepithelium. The nuclei are regular and mitoses are absent.

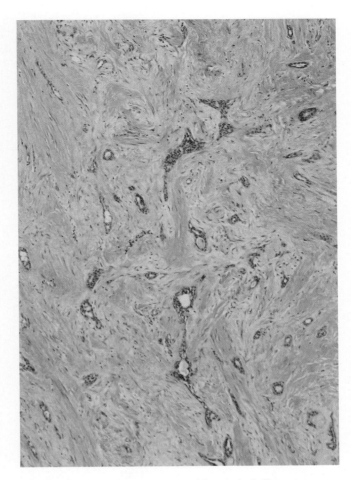

Fig. 19-44. Syringomatous adenoma of the nipple. Infiltrative comma-shaped small ducts without a stromal response. (Courtesy of Mirka W. Jones, MD, Magee-Women's Hospital, Pittsburgh, PA.)

The nipple adenoma is histologically identical to hidradenoma papilliferum of the vulva and may arise in the modified sweat glands of the areolar region. *Syringomatous adenoma* also occurs beneath the areolar region.[164] This lesion is more infiltrative and more likely to recur locally but also is benign (Fig. 19-44).

Cytologically, nipple adenomas present with a cellular aspirate with an inflammatory background. Clusters of epithelial cells forming papillae, naked nuclei, and hemosiderin-containing macrophages are the main cytologic component of nipple adenoma. Epithelial cells also may appear singly. The nuclei are uniform and contain finely distributed chromatin and inconspicuous nucleoli (Fig. 19-45). The cytologic features of this lesion, although not particularly distinctive, are sufficiently characteristic to render a correct diagnosis in the proper clinical setting.[165]

Adenomyoepithelioma

In this uncommon tumor, there is a biphasic proliferation of ducts lined by epithelial cells and surrounding polygonal to spindled myoepithelial cells, which make up the most conspicuous element (Fig. 19-46). Local recurrences have been re-

ported, but distant metastases have been seen in only one case, which had an infiltrative growth pattern, cytologically malignant cells, and a high mitotic rate.[166,167] Rare pure myoepithelial cell tumors, both benign and malignant, have also been observed.[168]

Cytologically, adenomyoepitheliomas yield a rich cellular aspirate consisting of sheets of crowded, cohesive clusters of smooth, uniform cells. The cells are round to oval with a fine chromatin pattern and are surrounded by many naked nuclei. Stromal material is scanty. Positive immunostaining of tumor cells for keratin, muscle-specific actin, and S-100 protein substantiates the diagnosis. Tumor cells also show evidence of myoepithelial cell differentiation by electron microscopy.[169]

Hamartoma

Mammary hamartomas present clinically as well demarcated, discrete, palpable or nonpalpable masses, and are usually initially thought to be fibroadenomas. However, they lack the typical microscopic growth pattern of fibroadenoma, because they contain both lobules and ducts, in addition to dense connective

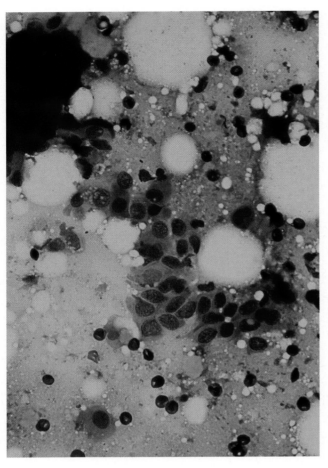

Fig. 19-45. Aspirate from a nipple adenoma showing a papilla surrounded by mononuclear inflammatory cells and macrophages. (Diff-Quik stain, × 20.)

tissue and, not infrequently, adipose tissue[170–172] (Fig. 19-47). The cytologic features are not well characterized, but should be heterogeneous and benign. Treatment is local excision.

Intraductal Papilloma

The intraductal papilloma is a benign papilliform proliferation of the ductal epithelium.[173–175] It is not a common lesion, and care must be taken to avoid misinterpreting it as carcinoma. Papillomas may be solitary or multiple; in the latter case, we speak of papillomatosis. Solitary papillomas are more frequent, and they develop in the terminal portion of a main duct. Subareolar papillomatosis, or nipple adenoma, has been discussed previously.

Intraductal papilloma may appear at any age but is more common between 30 and 50 years. The main clinical features include spontaneous or induced serous or bloody nipple discharge, the presence of a small subareolar tumor, and, more rarely, nipple retraction.

Mammography following intraductal injection of contrast

medium (galactography) helps to identify and localize intraductal papillomas. Gross examination of the surgical specimen, including a careful dissection of the ducts, reveals a soft, friable, yellow or red papilliform structure attached to the inner wall of a duct. The size varies from a few millimeters to a few centimeters in diameter. Cystic changes are occasionally produced by obstruction of the duct harboring the papilloma. Dissection of the lesion should be carefully performed by gently opening the duct with scissors; proper fixation and embedding of the specimen are essential to obtain an easily readable slide. Frozen section should be avoided if at all possible; the distinction of these lesions from intraductal carcinomas may be difficult, and tissue should be fixed properly and submitted in its entirety for permanent section examination.

Microscopic examination reveals delicate branching of papillary structures, consisting of connective tissue covered by epithelial cells (Fig. 19-48). These cells are arranged in two layers, which include myoepithelial cells (Fig. 19-49). The presence of a double row of cells is one of the morphologic criteria proposed by Kraus and Neubecker[175] to distinguish a papilloma from a papillary carcinoma. The myoepithelial cells may require immunohistochemical techniques for their demonstration.[176,177] The epithelial cells may also proliferate to form solid masses. These masses may surround empty spaces, but these are usually variable in size and shape and compressed into flattened slits by the cells, unlike the uniform round spaces in a cribriform type of intraductal carcinoma. The papillae are located in enlarged ducts, which are sometimes filled by these florid structures. When the tension within the cystic duct is high, the superficial cellular layers are flattened or exhibit small foci of erosion.

The epithelial cells resemble those of a normal duct; mitoses are rare and the nuclei are regularly oriented parallel to the long axis of the cells. Sometimes, these cells exhibit hyperplastic changes. They may be larger than normal duct cells, and the nuclei are discretely irregular and hyperchromatic. Apocrine cells may be present. In some cases, the proliferating myoepithelial cells invade and distend the connective tissue of the

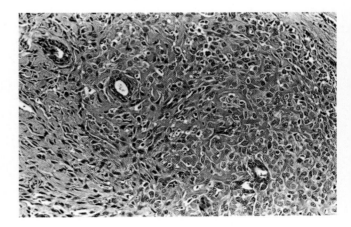

Fig. 19-46. Adenomyoepithelioma. Locally recurrent tumor contains small ductal structures engulfed by polygonal myoepithelial cells becoming spindled at periphery of nodule.

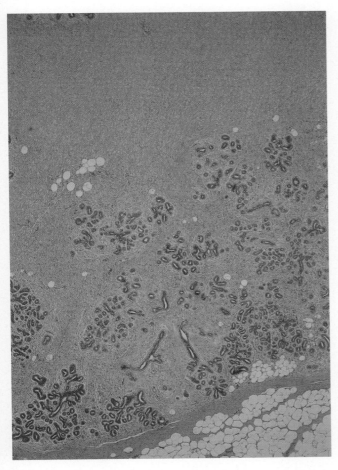

Fig. 19-47. Mammary hamartoma. Circumscribed mass of irregularly distributed mammary ducts, lobules, and stroma including adipose tissue.

papillary processes. These pictures are quite similar to those of sclerosing adenosis and can be confused with a carcinomatous infiltration.[175]

The differential diagnosis between a florid atypical papilloma and an intraductal papillary carcinoma is sometimes extremely difficult. Generally, when a diagnostic error is made, it is a false positive one rather than a false negative one, benign lesions being taken for malignant ones. Intraductal or intracystic papillary carcinomas exhibit the presence of multilayered epithelial papillae without central connective tissue cores, often with loss of nuclear polarity and cytologic atypia. The presence of a true cribriform pattern, that is, cell strands bridging the duct lumen and forming uniform round spaces, is also characteristic of a malignant tumor. Very thin stromal formations may sometimes separate the epithelial components. If fibrovascular connective tissue cores are present in a carcinoma, the cellular proliferation lacks myoepithelial cells and the atypical epithelial cells are all arranged with their long axes perpendicular to the basement membrane. Large solid proliferations favor benignity, because solid intraductal carcinomas tend to develop central necrosis,

as in comedocarcinoma. Foci of apocrine metaplasia also favor benignity.

Cytology

The cytologic diagnosis of intraductal papilloma can be made either by examining the serous or bloody nipple secretion or by FNAB of a palpable lesion. Characteristically, the smears are cellular. In a proteinaceous or bloody background, large numbers of foamy macrophages, apocrine cells, and naked nuclei are present. The epithelial cells are arranged in three-dimensional papillary clusters and are often tall columnar in appearance. Cell balls are common and some degree of cytologic atypia is frequently seen (Figs. 19-50 and 19-51). Differentiation between intraductal papilloma and well differentiated papillary carcinoma is difficult cytologically. Immunostaining for muscle specific actin to detect myoepithelial cells in intraductal papilloma is an important diagnostic adjunct.[178] Generally, however, it is best to perform surgical biopsy of breast lesions with papillary features.

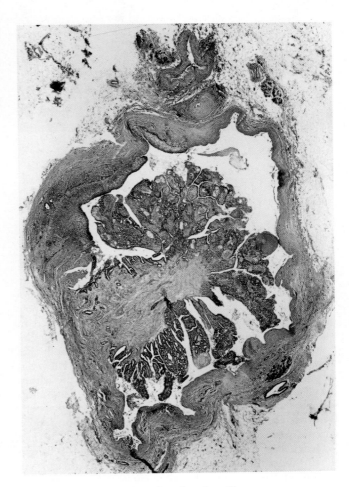

Fig. 19-48. Intraductal papilloma.

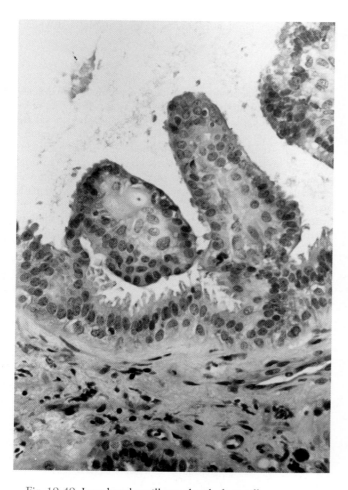

Fig. 19-49. Intraductal papilloma, detail of a papillary structure.

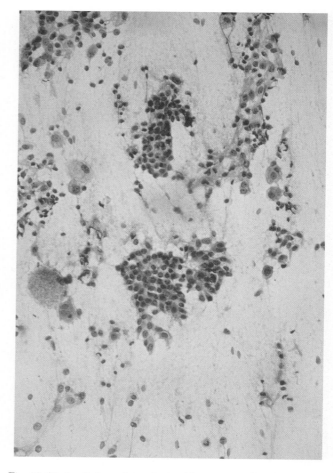

Fig. 19-50. A cellular aspirate obtained from an intraductal papilloma, showing crowded clusters of epithelial cells, macrophages, and columnar cells in a proteinaceous background. (Papanicolaou stain, × 200.)

Evolution

There is much diversity of opinion about the malignant potential of intraductal papillomas. Although the older literature maintained that patients with intraductal papilloma have a greater chance of developing cancer later, most authors now question this malignant potential. Ashikari et al[179] showed, in a retrospective study of a series of papillary carcinomas, that the prior biopsies of these patients reported as benign papillomas were in reality already malignant papillary lesions. However, foci of typical carcinoma certainly may occur focally within ductal lesions with the appearance of papillomas, and ultrastructural and histochemical studies show similarities that confirm the relationship between benign and malignant lesions and the existence of borderline cases.

Generally speaking, the evolution of these lesions is benign in most cases; thus, the pathologist must avoid overdiagnosing benign papillary lesions in fear of missing differentiated carcinoma. In any case, excision of these lesions must be complete to avoid any risk of local recurrence. Multiple papillomas probably have a greater cancer risk than solitary ones.[173,176,179–181]

Variants

Some of the variations on the theme of intraductal papilloma have already been discussed above, namely sclerosing papillomas (discussed with intraductal hyperplasia and radial scar), subareolar papillomatosis (nipple adenoma), and ductal adenoma. Another variant that should be mentioned here is *collagenous spherulosis*,[182,183] which is usually an incidental microscopic finding but may rarely present as a breast mass. This benign lesion consists of multiple intraductal acellular spherules, apparently representing basement membrane material, surrounded by small uniform myoepithelial cells (Fig. 19-52). Its differential diagnosis includes intraductal carcinoma and adenoid cystic carcinoma.

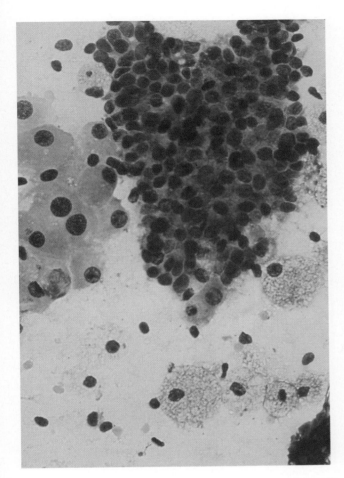

Fig. 19-51. Higher magnification of the same case as in Fig. 19-50 showing apocrine cells, epithelial cells, and foamy macrophages (Diff-Quik, × 400.)

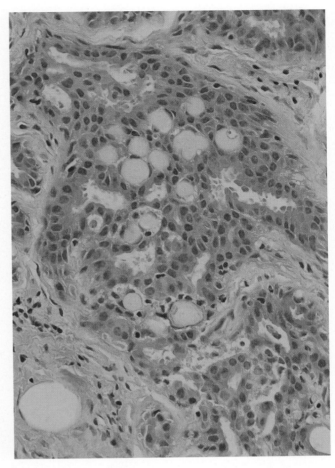

Fig. 19-52. Collagenous spherulosis. A duct contains focally calcified acellular hyaline spherules surrounded by uniform small myoepithelial cells.

Juvenile Papillomatosis

In 1980, Rosen et al[184] recognized juvenile papillomatosis as a clinicopathologic entity. The lesion is more frequent in adolescents and young women but occasionally occurs in women up to the age of menopause. There is frequently a family history of breast cancer. Clinically, it is characterized by a painless, movable, circumscribed mass that is often interpreted as a fibroadenoma. Macroscopically, juvenile papillomatosis is composed of nonencapsulated multinodular masses. Microscopically, there is cystic duct dilation with intraductal solid or papillary epithelial proliferation, often associated with fibrosis, sclerosing adenosis, apocrine metaplasia, and intraductal foamy histocytes. When the epithelial proliferation is quite marked, it should not be confused with an intraductal carcinoma. The cytologic appearance is also benign.[185] The premalignant potential of juvenile papillomatosis is not yet determined; therefore, wide excision followed by a careful follow-up is suggested.[186]

Benign Tumors of Connective Tissue

Benign tumors of the connective tissue may arise in the mammary gland. *Leiomyomas* may develop deep in the breast from the vessels or in the areola from the smooth muscle fibers present in this region. They occur in women in their fifth and sixth decades and have a slow rate of growth.[187] *Lipomas* are common, well encapsulated, palpable, soft masses that are seen in women aged 40 to 60 years. Fibromas and osteomas are exceptionally rare. Fibromatosis can occur as an infiltrative process that may recur locally.[188] Myofibroblastoma has been described as more common in the male than in the female breast.[189]

Granular cell tumor has been described in the mammary gland.[190,191] Grossly, it is a firm, round mass that adheres to adjacent tissue and may simulate a carcinoma. Microscopically, characteristic large clear cells with a granular, PAS-positive, eosinophilic cytoplasm and small round nuclei are arranged in

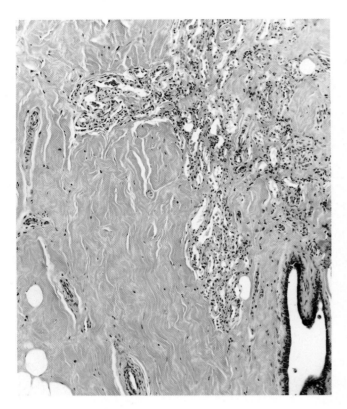

Fig. 19-53. Perilobular hemangioma.

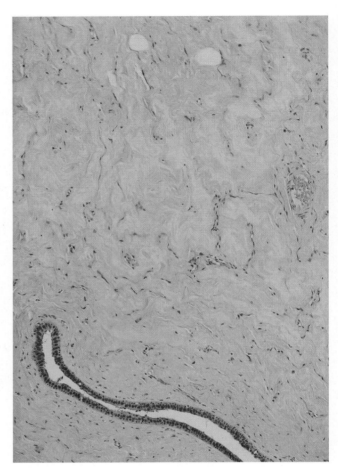

Fig. 19-54. Pseudoangiomatous hyperplasia of mammary stroma. The slit-like spaces are not lined by endothelial cells.

clumps or nests surrounded by large collagenous and reticular bundles. Ultrastructural studies reveal that these granules correspond to lysosomes. Electron microscopic and immunohistochemical investigations tend to support a nerve sheath differentiation for these tumors. Cytologically they must be distinguished from apocrine lesions. *Adenolipoma* is a hamartoma containing typical mammary lobules included in the fatty tissue. Hamartomas are discussed above.

Hemangiomas, previously thought to be rare, have been described recently as relatively common incidental microscopic findings. The most frequently encountered is the *perilobular hemangioma*, which generally measures less than 1.5 mm and is sharply circumscribed[192,193] (Fig. 19-53). Other less common benign vascular lesions include *angiomatosis*,[194] *venous hemangioma*,[195] and *hemangioma with atypical cytologic features*.[196] A related lesion that initially appeared to be of vascular origin is *pseudoangiomatous hyperplasia of mammary stroma* (PASH). This lesion was an incidental finding in 23 percent of breast biopsies in one series.[197] The slit-like spaces interspersed within keloid-like fibrosis, which are characteristic of this entity (Fig. 19-54), have been shown not to be of vascular origin by virtue of negative immunostaining for endothelial markers. As with the other benign vascular lesions mentioned above, the main clinical significance of PASH is its tendency to be confused with mammary angiosarcoma. This should usually not be a problem, because angiosarcomas almost always present as bulky infiltrative masses that are obviously malignant clinically and grossly, and contain (focally or diffusely) large, atypical, mitotically active endothelial cells (see discussion below). *Hemangiopericytoma* of the breast has also been reported.[198]

CYSTOSARCOMA PHYLLODES

A giant type of fibroadenoma was described in 1838 by Muller,[199] who used the name *cystosarcoma phyllodes* to qualify the leaf-like and fleshy gross appearance of this tumor. This term has since been consecrated by use, although it is confusing. It is essentially a fibroepithelial tumor in which the stroma or mesenchymal component shows a marked proliferation. Cystosarcoma phyllodes is also known as phyllodes tumor as well as by numerous other names.[200–205] It is a rare mammary neoplasm that appears most frequently in middle-aged women, an older age group than those with fibroadenoma, and represents approximately 1 percent of all fibroepithelial tumors of the breast.

It has been reported more rarely in younger women and in the elderly. In young women and adolescents, reports of this tumor frequently represent misdiagnoses of large juvenile fibroadenomas (see above).

Clinically, it is usually a rapidly growing, bulky tumor that may attain a diameter of 15 cm or more (Fig. 19-55). In spite of its large size and rapid growth, it does not infiltrate adjacent tissues or the overlying skin. Skin ulceration may produce a clinical condition that mimics carcinoma. The macroscopic appearance is that of a firm, nodular, usually well circumscribed tumor. Sections of the tumor reveal numerous gray-white to yellow nodules surrounded by fibrous septa that evoke a leaflike appearance. In large tumors, hemorrhagic and cystic areas and necrosis may be present. Smaller tumors may also be encountered.

Microscopic examination reveals an intracanalicular pattern of fibroadenoma-like growth with intense proliferation of the stromal cells, often displaying periductal hypercellular cuffing (Figs. 19-56 and 19-57). The stromal cells are large and elongated and reveal different degrees of cellular atypia. Foci of hyalinized or densely collagenous tissue and deposits of intercellular mucoid material may be observed.

Some tumors are classified as histologically benign (cellular fibroadenoma, periductal fibroma), whereas others are considered histologically malignant (periductal sarcoma). In the first group, the general pattern of the tumors resembles the fibroadenoma except for increased stromal cellularity. Mitoses are rare and cellular atypia is mild. In the second group, the stroma is markedly cellular, and there is a haphazard arrangement of the cells, with regions of pure stromal proliferation (stromal overgrowth).[205] All degrees of nuclear atypia and nuclear hypertrophy are present. The sarcoma-like foci reproduce the appearance of a differentiated fibrosarcoma or liposarcoma or, in the most undifferentiated cases, the structure of an anaplastic and pleomorphic sarcoma. There is increased mitotic activity. The ductal formations are distorted by the marked stromal overgrowth but exhibit no signs of a malignant tumor. Some cases may show an intense proliferative activity of the epithelial structures and even squamous metaplasia. The atypical stromal overgrowth is evident at the periphery of the tumor, where secondary infiltration of the adjacent tissues is observed. Some tumors have a mucinous matrix, which makes them resemble myxoid liposarcomas. Chondroid and osteoid metaplasia are also occasionally observed. Finally, there is a borderline group that shows intermediate alterations that are difficult to classify.

Some investigators advocate this subdivision into histologically benign and malignant categories based on criteria such as cellular atypia, mitotic activity, the type of margin (pushing or infiltrating), and the ratio of mesenchymal over epithelial tissue. Others have challenged the validity of this practice, and recommend a borderline or intermediate category, while yet others have suggested the use of proliferative indices obtained by such techniques as flow cytometry[206,207] or immunostaining for proliferating cell nuclear antigen.[208] Because the histologic grading of cystosarcomas has not proved to be a totally reliable

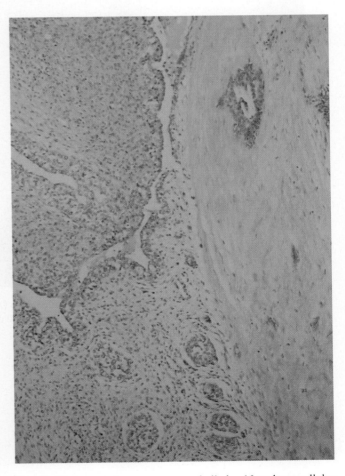

Fig. 19-56. Low grade cystosarcoma phyllodes. Note hypercellular periductal stroma with minimal atypia, and well demarcated tumor border.

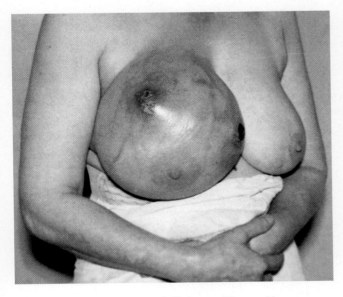

Fig. 19-55. Cystosarcoma phyllodes in a 52-year-old woman.

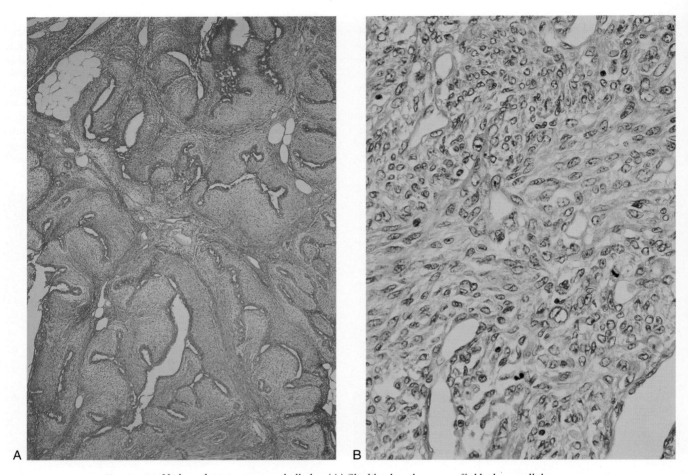

Fig. 19-57. High grade cystosarcoma phyllodes. **(A)** Slit-like ductal spaces cuffed by hypercellular stoma. **(B)** Focus of stromal overgrowth with atypia and mitotic activity.

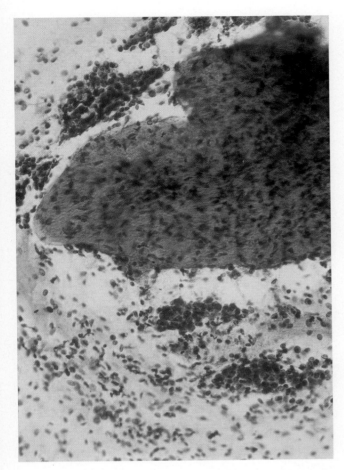

Fig. 19-58. Biphasic pattern seen in an aspirate of low grade cystosarcoma phyllodes, similar to features seen in fibroadenoma. (Papanicolaou stain, × 200.)

prediction of the clinical behavior, all these lesions should be considered potentially aggressive tumors. Those with marked cellularity, cytologic anaplasia, and high mitotic activity pose no diagnostic problem.

Cytologically, aspirates of cystosarcomas are rich in cellularity and demonstrate a distinct biphasic pattern. The epithelial component consists of a uniform population of epithelial cells forming large folded sheets with numerous naked nuclei in the background. The stromal component consists of spindle cells enmeshed in pink-staining acid mucopolysaccharide that is best demonstrated by metachromatic stains. Foam cells, macrophages, and multinucleated giant cells may also be seen[202,209-212] (Fig. 19-58). Cytologic distinction between benign cystosarcoma and fibroadenoma is not practical. Cytologic features such as the pattern of cell distribution, cellularity of stromal tissue fragments, and uniformity of stromal cells are not reliable diagnostic features.[212] Cytologic diagnosis of borderline and malignant phyllodes tumor by FNAB is possible when both clinical and cytologic features are taken into account. Borderline and malignant phyllodes tumors characteristically present with abundant cellular stromal fragments, isolated stromal cells with nuclear pleomorphism, and large folded epithelial sheets

(Fig. 19-59). Varying degrees of ductal epithelial proliferation can be seen in phyllodes tumors. Occasionally, this may lead to a false positive diagnosis of breast carcinoma.[209-211] Thus, it is advisable to perform frozen sections in cases in which phyllodes tumor is the suspected diagnosis.

Local recurrences are seen in approximately 20 percent of benign cystosarcomas,[202] but metastases are infrequent (approximately 10 percent), even in the histologically malignant group, and should not occur in the benign group. In some cases, recurrences of initially benign lesions present obviously malignant features. Metastases consist of poorly differentiated mesenchymal elements. The most common site is the lung. A few cases of metastases to axillary lymph nodes have been reported. Wide local excision is adequate treatment for the histologically benign lesions, and mastectomy is required for voluminous or histologically malignant tumors.

Electron microscopic observations of malignant cystosarcoma phyllodes are suggestive of the mesenchymal origin of this tumor.[213,214] Estrogen and progesterone receptors are present or absent according to different authors; these findings may reflect the relative amounts of epithelial and stromal components. Progesterone receptor appears to be localized predominantly in the stromal component.[215]

Malignant cystosarcoma should not be confused with fibrosarcoma. Ductal elements, which represent an integral portion of cystosarcoma phyllodes, are absent in fibrosarcoma, or may be seen as entrapped elements at the periphery of the lesion. Carcinosarcoma is a very rare lesion exhibiting both epithelial and mesenchymal malignant elements, and is discussed with metaplastic carcinomas below.

MALIGNANT TUMORS

In spite of the apparent progress made in surgery, radiotherapy, and chemotherapy, the percentage of deaths caused by breast cancer has varied little over the past 30 years. What little improvement we have made in diagnosis and treatment seems counterbalanced by an increased incidence of the disease. In the United States, it is estimated that one woman in about nine will develop breast cancer at some time in her life, and that approximately 46,000 women will die of it each year.[1-3] Thus, we can understand the importance of improving our knowledge of the etiologic risk factors, as well as of the biologic behavior of breast cancers.

The combination of modern and often sophisticated diagnostic procedures, including mammography, ultrasonography, and FNA, allows earlier diagnosis of small lesions. About one of four biopsies performed for mammographically detected nonpalpable lesions is malignant, and close to one-half of those are noninvasive, with many of the others being small invasive carcinomas—both of these types of cancers having been encountered only rarely two to three decades ago.[28] By contrast, many tumors have nevertheless advanced beyond the local stage at the time of diagnosis, and these form a majority in developing countries without sophisticated screening programs. Despite earlier diagnosis, even in the United States, the death rate for

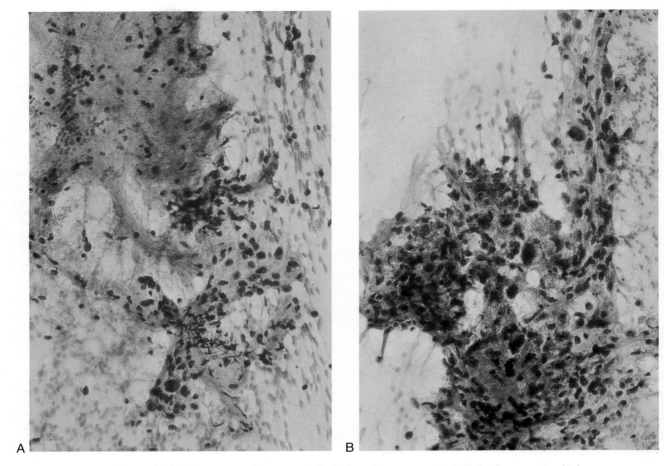

Fig. 19-59. **(A)** Direct smear from aspirate of a high grade cystosarcoma phyllodes demonstrating biphasic pattern and atypical spindle cells. (Papanicolaou stain, × 200.) **(B)** Higher magnification of the same case showing bizarre spindled tumor cells. (Papanicolaou stain, × 400.)

breast cancer has fallen only about 10 percent in the past two decades.[216]

Etiology and Risk Factors

The etiology of breast cancer remains unknown, but the large volume of information gathered in recent years, including experimental, epidemiologic, and clinical data, is progressively bringing us to a more sophisticated approach to the problem. However, the factors that are discussed should be interpreted with caution because they are not particularly strong determinants of risk, they do not have the same importance in different populations, and their effects are not additive and can seemingly be canceled out by favorable factors.

Study of the epidemiology of breast cancer is still evolving, and the reader is referred to recent texts for complete discussion of current thinking in this field.[2,3,217,218] A general summary statement might be that many of the tenets that were strongly advanced at the time of our previous edition are once again being challenged. For example, dietary fat is now thought to play a less important role than in earlier years,[219,220] the role of alcohol has yet to be determined,[221] and the exact mechanisms by which steroid hormones—both endogenous and exogenous—play their undoubted role are still not clear.[222] Although the mouse mammary tumor virus was discovered almost 60 years ago, and has played a major role in fundamental studies on the biology of breast cancer, the role of viruses in human breast cancer is still thought to be minimal.[223] Genetic factors are under increasing current scrutiny,[224,225] especially since the discovery of the two breast cancer susceptibility genes, rather unimaginatively named BRCA-1 and BRCA-2.[226,227] Mutations of these genes have thus far, however, been associated with only a small fraction of breast cancers. Although familial breast cancers occur at a younger age and are more frequently bilateral, only minor variations in tumor histopathology are seen between familial and nonfamilial cases.[228] Similarly, differences in breast cancer pathology between high risk and low risk populations (such as American white women and Japanese women) are generally minimal, although it can be demonstrated that benign proliferative breast lesions have increased in Japanese women as breast cancer has also become more prevalent.[229]

Screening and Prevention

As mammography has undergone technical, economic, and interpretative improvements over the past two decades, it has served as the basis for screening programs in the United States and other countries, with demonstrable benefits of diagnosis of "earlier" (i.e., preinvasive and small invasive) cancers and more precancerous proliferative lesions.[28,216] This has been associated with definite improvement in breast cancer mortality rates in the screened populations for women over 50 years of age,[230,231] but the results in younger women have been more controversial.[232–234] Although it is generally agreed that women between 40 and 50 years old should have annual clinical breast examinations, and that all women should be taught breast self-examination, the role of mammographic screening in the younger population is still under investigation. Preliminary data suggest that breast cancers in younger women may grow more rapidly, which impacts further on the cost/benefit ratio of screening in this population by implying that, if mammographic screening is to be performed in these women, it may need to be done more frequently.[235] The screening interval, baseline age, and possible utilization of prophylactic mastectomy in women with a strong breast cancer family history, with or without cancer susceptibility gene mutations or biopsy-proven premalignant lesions, also remain to be established.

Prevention of breast cancer in these and possibly other women at high risk is also currently under investigation.[236,237] Some of the trials either underway or contemplated involve the use of tamoxifen (an antiestrogen), vitamin A analogues and similar retinoids, dehydroepiandrosterone, monoterpenes, and isoflavonoids.[237] Follow-up studies will include both the development of breast cancer and surrogate endpoint biomarkers such as mammographic breast density, markers of breast cell proliferation or death, hormonal changes, and the like.[238–240] The results of these trials will probably not be available for at least several years.

Classification of Malignant Neoplasms

The continual development of more and more sophisticated methods of breast tissue retrieval and evaluation has significantly increased the possibility of the recognition and interpretation of very early, morphologically discrete cancerous lesions. Thus, whatever system is used to describe and classify breast cancers must be adapted to the requirements of the small and difficult borderline lesions. Various classifications of breast cancers have been devised, and each of them is subject to criticism in one way or another. A perfect classification system would ideally correlate both clinical manifestations and histologic features with prognosis. Unfortunately, no perfect classification system has yet been elaborated—either by the "lumpers" or "splitters." Therefore, we propose the use of the World Health Organization (WHO) system,[241] which has the definite advantages of worldwide distribution and which, with minor modifications, represents a decent compromise among different opinions (Table 19-6). Table 19-7 divides breast carcinomas into three groups according to prognosis. It is worth remembering that most breast cancers (65 to 75 percent) are infiltrating duct carcinomas of no specific subtype.

Lobular Carcinoma In Situ

Lobular carcinoma is an uncommon variant of mammary cancer, representing approximately 10 percent of all malignant tumors of the breast. It arises in the distal portion of the ductules of the lobular system, usually in the upper outer quadrant of the breast (the most common location of breast cancer in general). Two stages of the disease, seen with about equal frequency, can be observed: the in situ type and the infiltrating type. The infiltrating type is described later.

Lobular carcinoma in situ (LCIS) was first thoroughly described by Foote and Stewart,[242] who recognized the lesion as a special type of breast carcinoma in 1941. They pointed out the multicentricity of the lesion and its association with invasive carcinoma. Since this first description, a large number of cases have been reported.[243–249]

LCIS is associated with 0.8 to 3.6 percent of all benign epithelial lesions of the breast.[245–247] It is classically observed more or less fortuitously in biopsy specimens of mammary parenchyma removed for various other reasons, such as fibrocystic mastopathy. In recent years, more cases have been detected by mammography, but the microcalcifications leading to biopsy are frequently located in adjacent benign lesions. As the chance of discovering a focus of LCIS by blind biopsy is very

Table 19-6. World Health Organization Classification of Carcinomas of the Breast

Noninvasive
Intraductal carcinoma
With Paget's disease
Lobular carcinoma in situ
Invasive
Invasive ductal carcinoma
With Paget's disease
Invasive ductal carcinoma with a predominant intraductal component
Invasive lobular carcinoma
Medullary carcinoma
Mucinous carcinoma
Invasive papillary carcinoma
Tubular carcinoma
Adenoid cystic carcinoma
Secretory (juvenile) carcinoma
Apocrine carcinoma
Carcinoma with metaplasia
Inflammatory carcinoma (unusual clinical presentation)

(From World Health Organization,[241] with permission.)

Table 19-7. Prognosis of Breast Carcinoma Related to Histologic Type

Favorable	Intermediate	Unfavorable
Noninvasive carcinoma (DCIS, LCIS)	Infiltrating duct carcinoma	Inflammatory carcinoma
Cribriform carcinoma	Infiltrating lobular carcinoma	Lipid-rich carcinoma
Mucinous carcinoma		Metaplastic carcinoma
Medullary carcinoma	Apocrine carcinoma	
Papillary carcinoma		
Tubular carcinoma		
Adenoid cystic carcinoma		
Secretory carcinoma		

Abbreviations: DCIS, ductal carcinoma in situ; LCIS, lobular carcinoma in situ.

low, it would not be advisable to advocate routine large excision of apparently normal breast tissue merely to look for such foci. The disease is usually seen in premenopausal women.

Since the first description of this lesion, ideas about its malignant potential have varied. More recent and comprehensive data indicate that LCIS does, in fact, represent a precursor of invasive carcinoma: subsequent ipsilateral invasive carcinoma arises in approximately 10 to 15 percent of cases, with contralateral breast carcinoma in an approximately equal percent.[243–250] The relatively high percentage (36 percent) of subsequent invasive carcinoma of lobular type[248] is a good indication of the relationship that exists between in situ and invasive forms. A recent molecular study has noted loss of heterozygosity on the 11q13 chromosome in about one-half of the lesions of LCIS accompanying infiltrating lobular carcinoma, but only rarely in LCIS without invasive cancer, suggesting that some cases of LCIS may actually be preinvasive cancers whereas others may merely be markers of elevated cancer risk.[251] A clear distinction should be made between LCIS and intraductal carcinoma, since we know that the risk of subsequent invasive carcinoma at the same site is greater in the intraductal lesion, and the contralateral risk is less.[252,253] The interval between the diagnosis of LCIS and the development of ipsilateral or contralateral carcinoma varies in published series from less than 5 years to more than 30 years.

Microscopically, the lesion is characterized by intralobular proliferation of the cells lining the acini; the lumen becomes packed with cells and progressively disappears as the lobule becomes more and more distended (Fig. 19-60). Two types of cells are observed: the typical cells with small oval or round hyperchromatic nuclei, no apparent nucleoli, and pale cytoplasm (Fig. 19-60), and a rarer population of cells with large, hyperchromatic nuclei and prominent nucleoli.[254] Both cell types may be found in the same acini. Pleomorphism is usually minimal, necrosis is absent, and mitoses are extremely rare. The cells characteristically lack cohesion. Intracytoplasmic lumina containing mucinous material are observed frequently.[255] The lesion is usually limited to the acini, but terminal ducts are sometimes involved by the cellular proliferation. This is known

as pagetoid extension. The ductal cells are replaced by larger cells having a prominent round nucleus and pale cytoplasm (Fig. 19-61).

The number of lobules involved is variable. In some cases, the proliferation may be limited to a single lobule, but multicentric foci often occur, and it is necessary to evaluate multiple tissue blocks. According to Rosen,[253] at least 75 percent of a lobule should be involved in order to recognize the lesion as LCIS. Page et al[256] demand distention and filling of at least 50 percent of the acini in at least one lobular unit, and we follow this definition, with lesser extents of similar proliferation being diagnosed as atypical lobular hyperplasia (see below).

The characteristics of the disease make it difficult to recommend a definite type of treatment for LCIS. The potential risk of the coexistence or subsequent development of invasive carcinoma has suggested to some investigators in the past the most cautious attitude: total mastectomy with low axillary dissection. Subcutaneous mastectomy cannot eliminate the risk of leaving some breast tissue, especially if the nipple is not removed. Because contralateral carcinoma represents a definite risk, as stated above, some authors have suggested that a substantial contralateral biopsy or even a mastectomy be performed. However, today the usual choice is a careful, lifetime follow-up program with regular clinical and radiologic examination. The patient must be fully informed of the risks of this choice, however, because we know it cannot be totally safe until effective methods of early detection of invasive transforma-

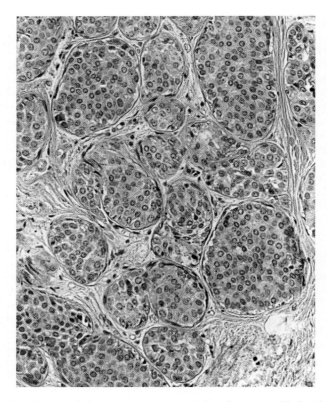

Fig. 19-60. Lobular carcinoma in situ. Enlarged acini are filled with uniform cells lacking pleomorphism or mitotic activity.

tion of LCIS become available. It is important that the patient participate in the therapeutic decision, as it is still a controversial problem.

Cytologic Findings

Because LCIS is rarely a palpable mass, FNA diagnoses of this lesion are uncommon and are usually made with mammographic localization. Aspirates of LCIS and atypical lobular hyperplasia (ALH) may show loosely cohesive groups of small uniform cells with eccentric regular nuclei and occasional intracytoplasmic lumina. The nuclei are hyperchromatic with fine chromatin clumping and occasional inconspicuous nucleoli. Occasionally, small cell groups forming "cell balls," conforming to acini of lobular neoplasia, may be seen (Fig. 19-62). The distinction between ALH, LCIS, and infiltrating lobular carcinoma (ILC) may be difficult if not impossible.[257–259] Aspirates of ILC show overlapping features but are more cellular and contain more atypical single cells. Characteristic cytomorphologic findings in ILC include low to moderate cell yield. The

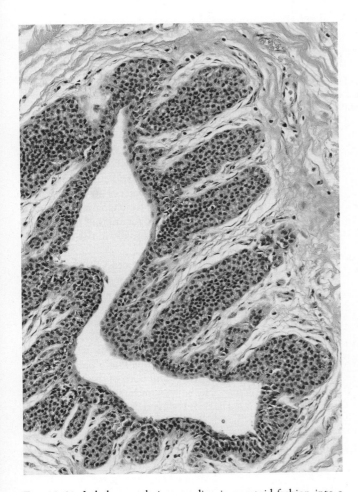

Fig. 19-61. Lobular neoplasia extending in pagetoid fashion into a duct. Intralobular growth must be evaluated to distinguish lobular carcinoma in situ from atypical lobular hyperplasia.

smears show a relatively uniform population of small to medium-sized cells. The cells have scanty ill-defined cytoplasm with an increased nuclear/cytoplasmic ratio and tend to occur in small groups, cords, or singly. The cytoplasm may contain sharply punched out vacuoles. Occasionally, signet ring forms may be seen. We believe that the cellular aspirates that contain significant numbers of small uniform cells characteristic of ILC in the presence of a suspicious mass should be diagnosed accordingly and definitive therapy undertaken. However, patients with paucicellular aspirates should undergo an excisional biopsy to establish the diagnosis.

Differential Diagnosis

LCIS should not be confused with ALH, papillomatosis or ductal hyperplasia of small ducts, or intraductal carcinoma with extension into the acini.[260] ALH is discussed below. Papillomatosis shows typical ramifying papillary structures with fibrous cores. Intraductal carcinoma in lobules shows marked cellular atypia and frequent foci of necrosis, both of which are generally lacking in LCIS, but may be present in its rare pleomorphic variant; in the latter lesion the lack of cohesiveness of the tumor cells is a helpful features.[261]

Atypical Lobular Hyperplasia

ALH is defined as a lesion that does not quite meet the diagnostic criteria for LCIS. Because we define LCIS as a proliferation of uniform abnormal cells that distends and fills at least one-half of the acini in at least one lobular unit, the definition of ALH is thus a qualitatively similar cellular proliferation that differs from LCIS by virtue of either not distending or not filling the acini, or distending and filling fewer than one-half of the acini in a single lobular unit[256] (Fig. 19-63). If residual luminal spaces are present, the acini are not filled, and if the acini are not appreciably larger than the normal acini adjacent to a suspect lesion, they are not distended. The cells, however, are essentially identical to those of LCIS.

The term *lobular neoplasia* is used in the literature both as a synonym for ALH and to cover the spectrum of ALH and LCIS.[245,256] For that reason, we prefer to avoid the use of this term, with one major exception: if we cannot clearly distinguish on a biopsy between ALH and LCIS, we use the generic term *lobular neoplasia*.

The most frequent use of this term in our experience occurs when atypical lobular proliferation is seen exclusively in a terminal duct, without involvement of the lobular unit on multiple levels of the block. Because the degree of distention and filling of the acini is thus not determinable, the distinction between ALH and LCIS cannot be made. A similar problem occurs when the process involves pre-existing lesions such as fibroadenoma or sclerosing adenosis.[262] In the case of sclerosing adenosis or other sclerosing lesions, the distinction from invasive carcinoma may be difficult.

Clinically, ALH shares with LCIS the predilection to present as an incidental finding in breast tissue removed for other reasons. It also shares with LCIS the significance as a marker of subsequent noninvasive or invasive cancer in the ipsilateral or

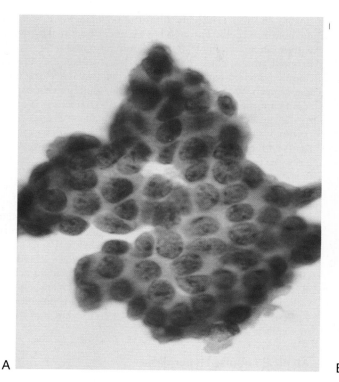 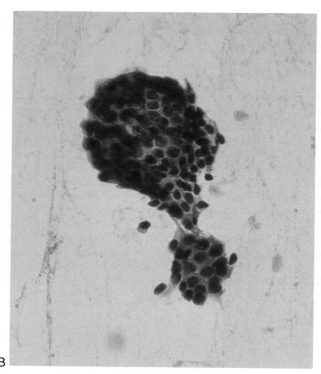

Fig. 19-62. **(A)** Cytomorphology of lobular neoplasia featuring clustering of small uniform cells with insignificant nuclear atypia. (Papanicolaou stain, × 400.) **(B)** Another view of the same case showing "cell balls" conforming to distended acini. (Papanicolaou stain, × 400.)

contralateral breast. The magnitude of this risk is generally quoted as about one-half that of LCIS (a relative risk of 4 to 5 times, or an absolute risk of 8 to 10 percent), but this risk is increased by approximately 50 percent if the lesion extends from the lobular unit into the ductal compartment of the breast (atypical lobular hyperplasia with duct extension, or ALH-DE).[263]

The *cytologic appearance* of ALH is essentially the same as that of LCIS. The lesion is even less likely to be appreciated on FNAB, however, because it is generally more limited in distribution. The main *differential diagnosis* is with LCIS, but lobular hyperplasia without atypia, unfolding lobules, and atypical ductal proliferations extending into lobules may also pose diagnostic problems.

Intraductal Carcinoma

Only a few decades ago, intraductal carcinoma (ductal carcinoma in situ [DCIS]) was a relatively infrequently seen and poorly characterized mammary lesion. In recent years, as mammographic detection has resulted in the diagnosis of more and more preinvasive carcinoma, an extensive literature on DCIS has developed, as have controversies related to its diagnosis, prognostic significance, and clinical management.[264–281] DCIS is now known to be an extremely heterogeneous lesion, with

variable clinical, pathologic, molecular biologic, and probably prognostic characteristics. For example, we now know that one form of the disease is clinically evident and characterized by a palpable tumor, a bloody nipple discharge, or an erosive nipple lesion (Paget's disease), while another form is a microscopic disease observed in breast tissue removed for another reason or detected by an abnormal mammogram, usually in the form of microcalcifications.

Similarly, the histopathologic picture of DCIS is quite variable, with some lesions—often those presenting in the clinically palpable form—composed of many closely applied ducts filled with pleomorphic large cells and exhibiting central necrosis, whereas other cases consist of no more than a few widely scattered duct profiles containing a cribriform or micropapillary arrangement of small uniform cells with minimal atypia and no necrosis.[265,266,269,271–276] These patterns, however, are not mutually exclusive, and both of them—as well as intermediate variants—may be seen in the same case, as may lesions better diagnosed as ADH or even ductal hyperplasia without atypia.

When the lesion is visible grossly, it may measure from a few millimeters to several centimeters in diameter, and is often multicentric. The ill-defined mass reveals cystic cavities filled with a creamy exudate. This gross picture suggests a lesion with comedonecrosis. The noncomedo types of DCIS, if they are grossly visible at all, generally present the appearance of a poorly defined gritty granularity that is better felt than seen,

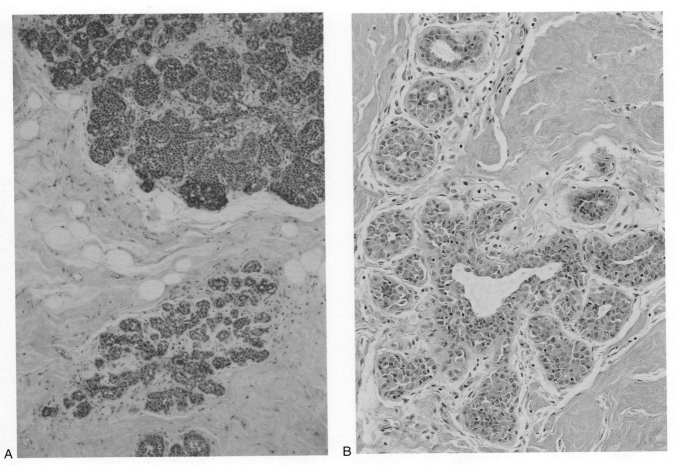

Fig. 19-63. Atypical lobular hyperplasia (ALH). **(A)** ALH on bottom contains same cells as lobular carcinoma in situ on top, but acinar distention and filling by these cells is seen only on top. **(B)** ALH involving terminal duct/lobular unit in another case: residual lumina are present in most acini.

and marks the site of mammographically detected microcalcifications.

Microscopically, intraductal carcinoma is characterized by a neoplastic growth within the mammary ducts. The major histologic variants are, in order of increasing cytologic atypia, the cribriform, micropapillary, solid, and comedo types, but other less common variants exist as well and, as previously mentioned, two or more types may coexist side by side.[267–269,271–273,275,276] In the *cribriform* type (Figs. 19-64 and 19-65), the tumor cells form bridges over uniform spaces filling the lumen, producing a uniformly punched-out pattern referred to as "Roman bridges" or "cartwheels." Unlike the spaces in an intraductal hyperplasia, the spaces in cribriform DCIS are uniform in both size and shape, and appear rounded rather than angular and slit-like. The cells between these spaces are generally small and uniform, with minimal cytologic atypia or mitotic activity. Unlike intraductal hyperplasia there is only a single cell type within the lumen (no myoepithelial cells), and the cells do not swirl or stream within the septa and are not compressed to an ovoid or spindled shape. As with all other forms of intra-

ductal carcinoma, central necrosis may be present, but it is relatively uncommon in the cribriform type.

In the *micropapillary* pattern of DCIS, small papillae that lack connective tissue axes project into the lumen (Figs. 19-66 and 19-67). The cells in this variant are usually slightly more atypical than in the cribriform type, but still display relative uniformity and few mitotic figures. As with the cribriform type, the presence of only one type of cell within the involved lumens is an important differential diagnostic feature for the distinction from intraductal papilloma and other benign papillary lesions. The absence of fibrovascular connective tissue cores is also useful, as is the slight but definite atypia present in micropapillary DCIS.

In the *solid* type, the ductal lumens are filled by solid plugs of tumor cells showing a slight to moderate degree of nuclear pleomorphism and atypia (Fig. 19-68). Benign solid intraductal proliferations generally involve only very small duct profiles, and often display some irregular lumen formation, as well as spindling, swirling, and streaming, whereas solid DCIS is a more monotonous proliferation and exhibits greater cytologic atypia.

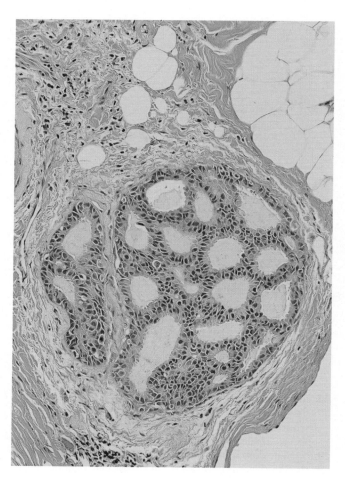

Fig. 19-64. Ductal carcinoma in situ, cribriform type. Note uniform "punched-out" spaces (compare with Figs. 19-23 to 19-27).

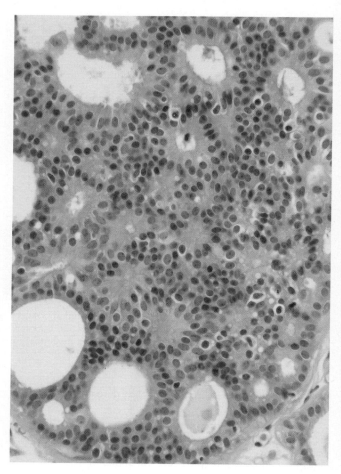

Fig. 19-65. Ductal carcinoma in situ, cribriform type. Cells are of one type, uniform, and lack more than minimal atypia. No streaming is seen between luminal spaces (compare with Figs. 19-23 to 19-27).

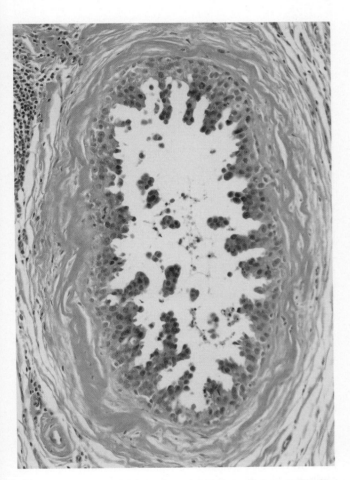

Fig. 19-66. Ductal carcinoma in situ, micropapillary type. Papillae have no connective tissue cores and are lined by cells with modest atypia.

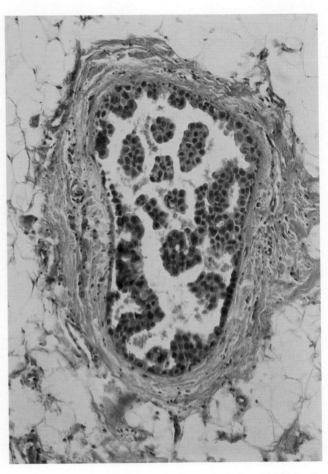

Fig. 19-67. Ductal carcinoma in situ, micropapillary type. Another case with somewhat more atypia than seen in Fig. 19-66.

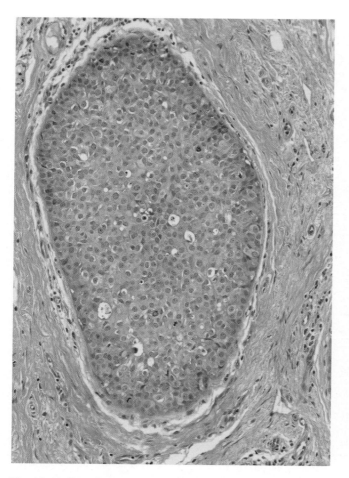

Fig. 19-68. Ductal carcinoma in situ, solid type. The marked atypia noted in comedocarcinoma (see Figs. 19-69 and 19-70) is not present.

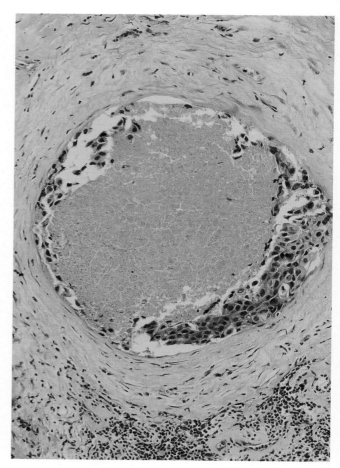

Fig. 19-69. Ductal carcinoma in situ (DCIS), comedo type. Solid growth pattern, central necrosis, and marked nuclear atypia are characteristic. The surrounding sclerosing and lymphoid reaction is typical in this type of DCIS, but may be absent and is often present in other

As with the other forms of DCIS, the solid variant may develop central necrosis, in which case it is to be distinguished from *comedocarcinoma*, the most atypical form, in which solid sheets of large, highly anaplastic cells with numerous mitotic figures (many of which may be atypical) are punctuated by foci of central tumor necrosis (Figs. 19-69 and 19-70). This is the form most likely to present as a palpable mass, tends to involve the largest number of ducts and to have the greatest tumor diameter, and is, according to most experts, the most likely to be associated with or develop into infiltrating carcinoma.

Several other histopathologic variants of intraductal carcinoma have been described. In the *papillary stratified spindle cell* type, large papillae with central connective tissue axes are lined by tall columnar cells with their nuclei perpendicular to the basement membrane (Fig. 19-71). In the pattern known as *clinging carcinoma*, a few layers of dyspolaric atypical cells line ducts with minimal architectural abnormalities[282] (Fig. 19-72). We believe that evidence for the neoplastic nature of this lesion is more poorly documented than in other forms of DCIS, and prefer to think of it as a form of atypical hyperplasia. In *cystic hypersecretory duct carcinoma*, the malignant ducts are greatly

dilated and filled with luminal dense colloid-like material[283] (Fig. 19-73). A *mucinous* variant is occasionally seen accompanying infiltrating mucinous carcinoma, and rarely in pure intraductal form; this lesion is characterized by proliferated atypical cells containing large mucin globules. Finally, intraductal carcinoma of *apocrine* type can manifest any of the growth patterns referred to above, but is also characterized by voluminous apocrine cytoplasmic differentiation within the tumor cells[284–286] (Fig. 19-74). The distinction of this lesion from benign atypical apocrine proliferations may be extremely difficult, because apocrine metaplastic cells characteristically display moderate degrees of nuclear atypia. As mentioned previously, focal apocrine differentiation within a ductal proliferative lesion is virtually always benign but a duct that is totally replaced by apocrine epithelium with nuclear atypia may be either benign or malignant. The general consensus is that the size and number of ducts involved and the degree of nuclear atypia are useful in the differential diagnosis, but reproducible diagnostic criteria are still difficult to obtain.[284–287]

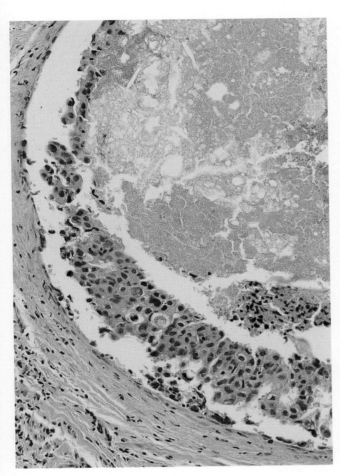

Fig. 19-70. Ductal carcinoma in situ, comedo type. High magnificationof another case to show marked (grade 3) nuclear atypia.

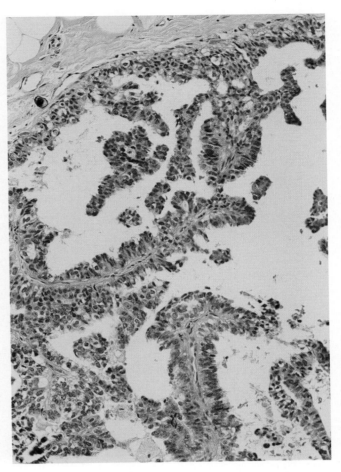

Fig. 19-71. Ductal carcinoma in situ, papillary stratified spindle cell type. The papillae are larger than in the micropapillary type and have connective tissue cores (compare with Figs. 19-66 and 19-67). Stratification, lack of myoepithelial cells, and nuclear atypia distinguish this from intraductal papilloma.

Secondary calcification of necrotic foci within DCIS is common; it is a diagnostic criterion of considerable significance in mammography, yet in itself is certainly not diagnostic histopathologically.[288] Also commonly seen are stromal fibrosis, myxoid change, and lymphoid infiltration around the involved ducts; these changes are most commonly seen in comedocarcinoma, where they may indicate stromal infiltration that is demonstrable ultrastructurally but not at the routine light microscopic level.[276,289,290]

Not only can intraductal carcinoma express stromal invasion that is not demonstrable by routine studies, but routine microscopy can suggest the presence of stromal invasion that is not really present. This *pseudoinvasion*[291–293] has been noted after previous FNAB, where it represents artifactual displacement of tumor cells by the biopsy needle (Fig. 19-75). It is also a problem, however, when DCIS develops within sclerosing lesions such as sclerosing adenosis or radial scars.[262] In these instances, it is important for the pathologist to envision the benign lesion and to be assured that the malignant cells entrapped in the sclerosing process are still consistent with an absence of true stromal invasion (Fig. 19-76).

The *cytopathologic features* of intraductal carcinoma reflect the morphologic diversity of this lesion. There are distinct differences between high grade comedocarcinomas and better differentiated DCIS of noncomedo type.

FNAB of intraductal comedocarcinoma is usually cellular and displays loosely cohesive clusters of malignant cells with individual cell necrosis and mitotic figures. Nuclear membrane abnormalities, chromatin clumping, and conspicuous nucleoli are usually present. Nuclear pleomorphism and irregularly shaped nuclei are characteristic features, and particles of calcified material may or may not be present[294–296] (Figs. 19-77 and 19-78). Aspirates from noncomedo DCIS vary in cellularity and are characterized by a monomorphic cell population of small to medium-sized epithelial cells arranged singly or as loosely cohesive clusters (Figs. 19-79 and 19-80). The cell clusters may have solid, cribriform, or papillary patterns, depending on the architecture of the lesion; there are no accompanying myoepithelial cells. This is in contrast to atypical hyperplasia,

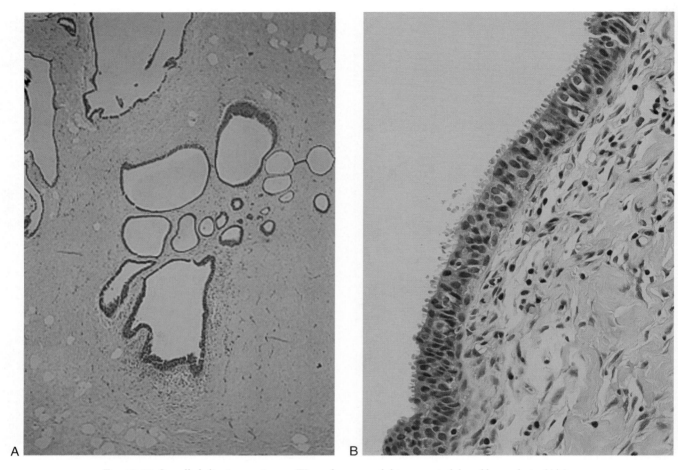

Fig. 19-72. So-called clinging carcinoma. We prefer to regard this as atypical ductal hyperplasia. (A) Low power view. (B) Detail.

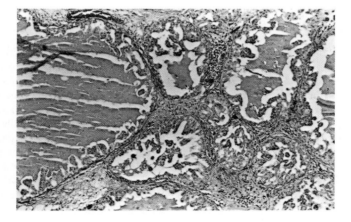

Fig. 19-73. Cystic hypersecretory duct carcinoma. Dilated ducts contain colloid-like secretory material and are lined by malignant papillae.

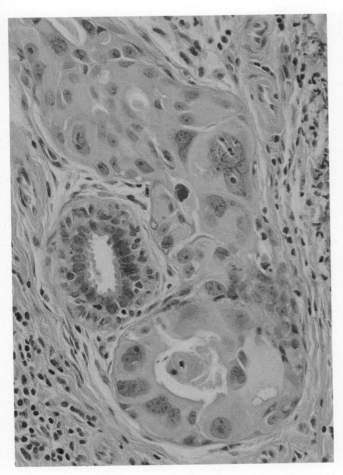

Fig. 19-74. Ductal carcinoma in situ, apocrine type. Compare bizarre cells with apocrine cytoplasm with single residual uninvolved small duct at left center. Also compare with Fig. 19-20 (benign apocrine metaplasia).

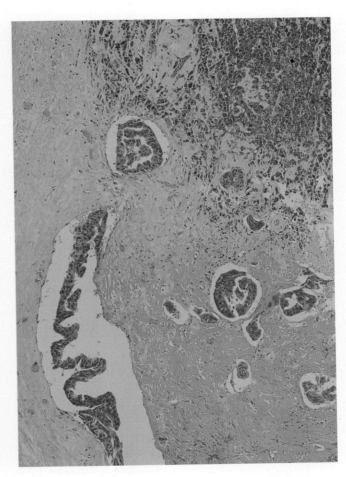

Fig. 19-75. Ductal carcinoma in situ, with pseudoinvasion after fine needle aspiration biopsy. Note relation of fragmented malignant glands to organizing hemorrhage in needle track at upper right.

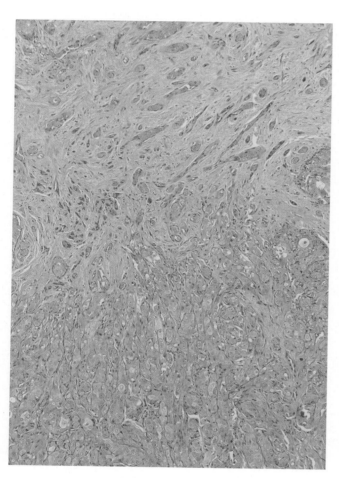

Fig. 19-76. Ductal carcinoma in situ in sclerosing adenosis. Residual benign adenosis is seen at the top.

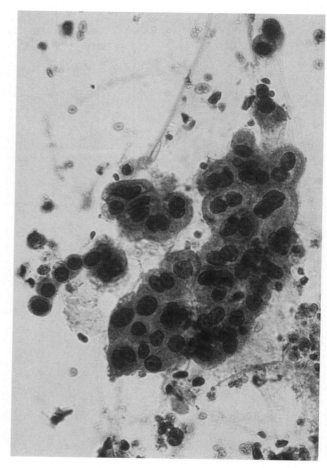

Fig. 19-77. Aspirate of a comedocarcinoma in situ featuring pleomorphic population of neoplastic epithelial cells in a necrotic background. (Diff-Quik, × 400.)

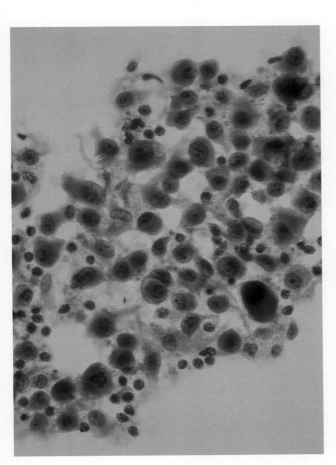

Fig. 19-78. Papanicolaou-stained smear of the same case as in Fig. 19-77 displaying individual cell necrosis characteristic of comedocarcinoma. (Papanicolaou stain, × 400.)

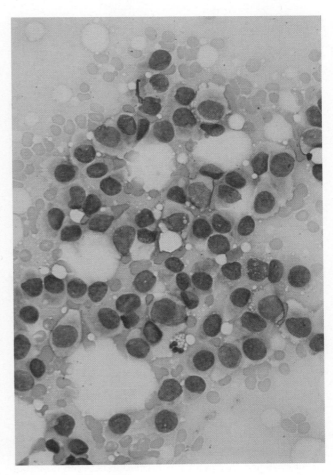

Fig. 19-79. Cytomorphology of noncomedocarcinoma in situ showing a monotonous population of epithelial cells. (Diff-Quik stain, × 200.)

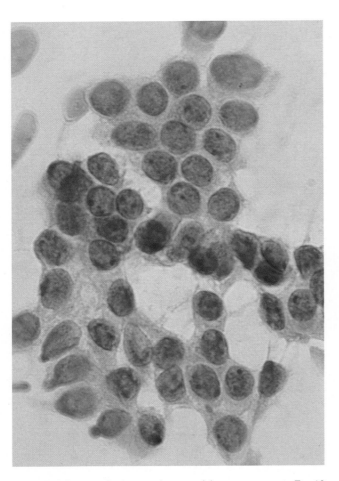

Fig. 19-80. Papanicolaou-stained smear of the same case as in Fig. 19-79, demonstrating small cells with uniform nuclei, inconspicuous nucleoli, and cribriform pattern. (Papanicolaou stain, × 400.)

in which the myoepithelial cells are seen intermingled within the groups of atypical cells and appear as part of the cellular aggregate (Figs. 19-34 and 19-35 and Table 19-5). In noncomedo DCIS microcalcific particles, foamy histiocytes, and a few isolated myoepithelial cells may be seen in the background.

Our cytologic criteria for the distinction between nonproliferative breast disease without atypia, proliferative breast disease without atypia, proliferative breast disease with atypia (atypical hyperplasia), and preinvasive carcinoma are presented in detail in the section above on fibrocystic mastopathy, and are summarized in Table 19-5.[119] The most useful features for the diagnoses of malignant lesions are increased cellularity, loss of cellular cohesion, significant pleomorphism, anisonucleosis, and a coarse chromatin pattern. Macronucleoli, when present, were associated with carcinoma, but their absence did not necessarily indicate benignity. Myoepithelial cells were absent in all cases of carcinoma, and were usually easily found in the lesser proliferative diseases, including atypical hyperplasia. Micronucleoli were commonly seen in both benign and malignant lesions and could not be used as a reliable indicator of carcinoma.

It should be noted, however, that the application of these and similar criteria has not always met with uniform success in the hands of others, and proliferative lesions—especially those with atypia—should probably be biopsied before therapeutic decisions are made.[124–126,128,297]

The cytologic features of DCIS are also often seen in invasive carcinomas. In comparing the cytomorphology of these two entities, we have not yet been able to define any specific criteria to distinguish in situ from invasive lesions. The latter, however, are generally more cellular and more frequently display conspicuous loss of cell cohesion. Assessment of tumor invasion by confirmatory surgical biopsy is our recommended procedure unless the patient has obvious locally advanced or metastatic disease.

Special Studies in Intraductal Carcinoma

Aside from morphology, attempts have been made to utilize ancillary studies to distinguish between atypical hyperplasia and carcinoma in situ, and also to predict the behavior of the latter lesion. For the most part, however, these studies have not provided information beyond that obtained from careful microscopic examination. In general terms, aneuploidy assessed by flow or image cytometry is about twice as frequent in DCIS as in ADH, but considerable overlap exists between the two conditions.[298–300] As expected, aneuploid cases of DCIS tend to be those with high grade nuclei, particularly comedocarcinomas. Morphometric studies were also not particularly useful in distinguishing atypical hyperplasia from low grade intraductal carcinoma.[300] Among oncogenes, HER-2/neu (c-erbB-2) has been the most widely studied. Immunohistochemical positivity for this oncogene is found most frequently in the comedo type of DCIS, but it is also encountered in a smaller proportion of cases of noncomedo DCIS and ADH.[301–303] Interestingly, in most studies this oncogene has been expressed in a smaller proportion of cases of infiltrating carcinoma than of DCIS.

p53 protein expression has also been investigated in the spectrum of intraductal lesions.[302,303] As with other markers, immunohistochemical expression of p53 protein is considerably more frequent in high grade or comedo DCIS. Thus, this marker also tells us that there is some difference biologically between the high grade and low grade lesions, but does not aid greatly in differential diagnosis. The monoclonal antibody B72.3 has also been mentioned as potentially diagnostically useful, particularly in fine needle aspirates.[304] However, the use of this antibody is more likely to complement the usual cytopathologic criteria than to replace or refute them. The same may be said of immunostaining for muscle-specific actin, which can be useful to identify myoepithelial cells in benign proliferative lesions at both the histopathologic and cytopathologic levels.[305–307] Immunostaining for estrogen and progesterone receptors is not particularly diagnostically useful, but, like many of the other studies, it confirms a fundamental biologic difference between low grade DCIS, which is generally positive, and the high grade comedo type lesions, which tend to be receptor negative.[301,302] Finally, newer chromosomal and molecular studies will no doubt continue to confirm the biologic differences between the different lesions, but will probably prove to be of less help in practical differential diagnosis.[308]

Evolution and Treatment

The natural history and treatment of intraductal carcinoma continue to evolve at the time of the writing of this text, but a few generally accepted conclusions may be emphasized. First, the preinvasive nature of DCIS is universally accepted, although the exact risk of progression to invasive carcinoma in untreated or inadequately treated cases remains debatable. The number of well studied cases that were treated by excisional biopsy only is small in number, and follow-up of these patients is often short. The recent data of Page et al[309] have shown that the natural history of small noncomedo lesions can last over at least two decades. Invasive carcinoma appears to develop in such lesions at a rate about 10 times that of women with no proliferative breast lesions, and to develop invariably in the same breast and at essentially the same site as that in which DCIS was discovered. In contrast to low grade DCIS, high grade lesions of comedo type are apparently more likely to progress to invasive carcinoma, and tend to do so more quickly.[267,268,271, 274–276] The diagnostic criteria for the comedo type have varied widely in different studies, however, with some authors emphasizing the presence of necrosis and others the cytologic features. We personally believe that necrosis may be the least significant differentiating factor, with the solid growth pattern and high grade nuclear morphology being better predictors of behavior.[275,276] Some of the biologic markers mentioned above are probably also important in predicting the behavior of DCIS, but it is unclear at this moment whether any of them will be more important than routine microscopic observation.

Regardless of the histologic pattern, complete surgical excision of DCIS is the recommended initial treatment.[271,277–281] However, it is still debated whether postextirpative radiotherapy is necessary for all cases or only for high grade or comedo lesions, as well as whether pathologically reported positive or negative margins should influence the decision for or against the use of radiation therapy. In general terms, postoperative radiation halves the incidence of subsequent local recurrence, and approximately 80 percent of patients whose tumors recur locally are still salvageable by appropriate treatment at that time.

The exact diagnostic criteria for and the clinical significance of *microinvasion* occurring in DCIS are also still controversial. We have defined microinvasive carcinoma as less than 10 percent invasive cancer in an otherwise intraductal lesion,[310] whereas others have either defined it by the total size of the lesion or have not used the term at all. Regardless of the definition, it is well established that metastases to the axillary lymph nodes and beyond can occur whenever stromal invasion is present in the primary tumor. The infrequent lymph node metastases reported in pure DCIS have probably developed in cases in which a small focus of invasion was missed by inadequate sectioning.[311,312] Thus, it is still controversial whether axillary node dissection is indicated in some, none, or all cases of DCIS, and how the decision is to be made in the individual patient.

Atypical Ductal Hyperplasia

Just as we have defined ALH by distinguishing it from LCIS, atypical ductal hyperplasia (ADH) should be defined as a lesion that approaches but does not quite satisfy the diagnostic criteria for DCIS. As with LCIS, low grade DCIS is defined in qualitative as well as quantitative terms. Page et al[256] demand the involvement of two complete duct profiles for the diagnosis of DCIS, whereas Tavassoli and Man[272] require that the lesion measure at least 2 mm in diameter. Because the former criterion is better validated by the studies of others, and it is easier to count than to measure, we use this definition; thus, ADH may consist of a lesion that qualitatively satisfies the criteria for DCIS but involves less than two complete duct profiles. Alternatively, ADH is diagnosed in a lesion that almost but not quite fulfills the qualitative criteria discussed above for the diagnosis of DCIS. In these cases as well, the lesion is generally well differentiated and involves only a few ducts; therefore, it is appropriate to choose the less malignant diagnosis and avoid overtreatment.

As discussed above, ADH, diagnosed in this manner, carries a risk of development of subsequent carcinoma that is intermediate between that of DCIS and that of intraductal hyperplasia without atypia. A generally quoted relative risk is four to fivefold (absolute risk 8 to 10 percent at 10 to 15 years).[313–315] Whether this risk can be lowered is currently being tested in the prevention studies referred to above.

Infiltrating Duct Carcinoma

Infiltrating duct carcinoma not otherwise specified (IDC-NOS) is the most frequent type of breast carcinoma and is thus a very common tumor. The histologic characteristics of infiltrating duct carcinoma within a given lesion can be so diversified that careful examination may reveal almost all the different types—present in different proportions—described in the morphologic classifications of the lesion. The existence of a preinvasive phase is confirmed by numerous cases in which intraductal malignant proliferations coexist with the infiltrating malignant structures.

Grossly, infiltrating duct carcinoma is characterized by a very firm, poorly defined nodule measuring from a few millimeters to several centimeters in diameter. Cut sections reveal a gray-white, slightly retracted granular tissue with small white or yellow streaks disposed in a radial fashion around the center of the nodule. (These yellow streaks are due to elastosis rather than to tumor necrosis.) The firmness, the granularity of the nodule, and its gritty consistency are constant and typical features of this tumor (Fig. 19-81). The dense and retracted appearance of the tumor is related to the abundance of the fibrous and elastic tissue. The nodule margins are irregular and adhere to the peripheral fibroadipose tissue. Mammographic studies have shown two types of tumoral outgrowth into the surrounding tissues: pushing and infiltrating.

Multiple tumor nodules can sometimes be observed grossly and are very frequent in whole-organ sections. Bilateral development also occurs and represents either two independent tu-

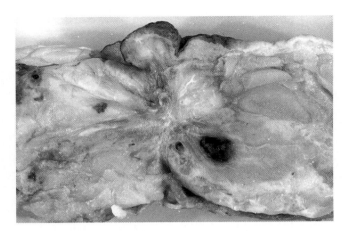

Fig. 19-81. Infiltrating duct carcinoma. Typical gross appearance of a firm, stellate, scar-like process.

mors or metastatic involvement of the contralateral breast. This distinction may be aided by immunohistochemical and molecular studies.[316–318] Skin involvement is characterized by thickening and induration.

Microscopically, the diagnosis is best made architecturally at low power magnification (Fig. 19-82). The neoplastic cells are arranged in single files, small solid clusters, tubes, long cords, large sheets, syncytia, glandular or anastomosing structures, and mixtures of all these types. The masses are irregular in size and shape and infiltrate and deform the intervening stroma, in which collagen and reticulin fibers are present. The number of elastic fibers is increased and represents an intense stromal reaction (elastosis).

The malignant cells exhibit different degrees of polymorphism. Any type of cellular structure can be found, from small regular elements with round, slightly hyperchromatic nuclei and a relatively normal nuclear/cytoplasmic ratio to anaplastic, large irregular cells with voluminous, hyperchromatic nuclei, hypertrophied nucleoli, and markedly reduced cytoplasm. Mitoses are present in variable numbers. Stromal fibrosis varies greatly in intensity. Some carcinomas reveal few neoplastic cells dispersed in abundant fibrous tissue, while others exhibit only fine fibrous strands around numerous epithelial structures (Fig. 19-83). The scirrhous type is defined by the abundance of the dense fibrous stroma in which the epithelial cells are engulfed and compressed (Fig. 19-82).

Electron microscopy shows that the neoplastic cords are always surrounded by a basal lamina. The presence of myoepithelial cells can be identified in some cases. Cartilaginous and bony metaplastic changes may occur. Foci of necrosis, myxoid degeneration, and calcification are common findings (Fig. 19-84). Benign stromal multinucleated giant cells that are phenotypically related to osteoclastic cells are also seen in some tumors.[319] When necrosis is marked, granulomatous inflammatory changes may be present, with foreign body giant cells around the necrotic tissular material. Lipid degeneration with large foamy cells may occur. Infiltration of blood vessels and lymphatics should be carefully searched for, because this finding worsens the clinical prognosis.

The multicentric cancers that are undetected clinically or grossly are by no means rare and may represent more than 10 percent of carcinomas.[316,318,320] However, the occurrence of two dominant primary lesions in the same breast is a rarity. The multicentric lesions are usually of the noninvasive type (LCIS or DCIS). This eventuality occurs more frequently in the presence of large (>5 cm in diameter) uncircumscribed primary lesions with nipple and skin involvement. The multicentricity of carcinoma is well established and explains why the treatment of this disease is still a matter of discussion. There is a discrepancy between the relatively low rate of local recurrence in the remaining breast tissue following segmental resection and the high percentage of tumor multifocality in mastectomy specimens. Absence of correlation between pathologic and clinical studies, the relatively benign evolution of occult lesions considered to be histologically malignant, and the eradication of tumor foci left in the remaining tissue by postoperative radiotherapy are some of the proposed explanations found in the literature.[320]

Although the ultrastructure of all types of malignant cells is characterized by prominent organelles, none of the modifications is absolutely specific.[289,290] For example, intracytoplasmic

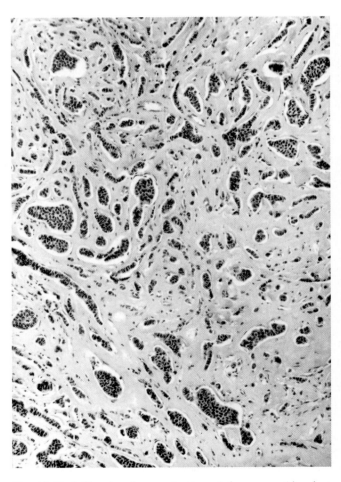

Fig. 19-82. Infiltrating duct carcinoma, scirrhous type. Abundant dense stroma compresses the epithelial structures.

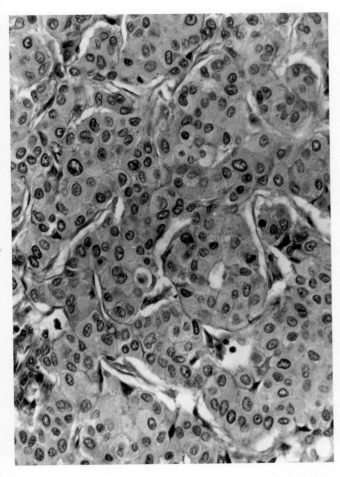

Fig. 19-83. Infiltrating duct carcinoma. Numerous glandular formations lined by large cells with hyperchromatic but relatively uniform nuclei are seen. Minimal stroma is present.

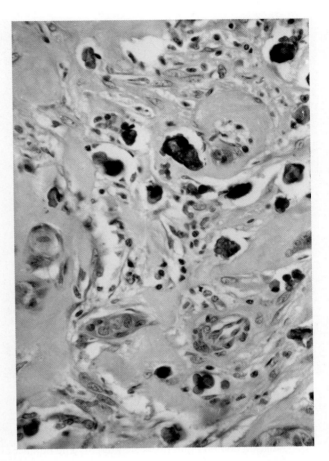

Fig. 19-84. Infiltrating duct carcinoma. Note the presence of diffuse fibrosis and numerous microcalcifications.

lumina (Fig. 19-85) have been described in all types of carcinomas but are more abundant in the infiltrating lobular type. They appear as spherical cavities of variable size and are lined by microvilli. The lumina contain electron-dense material, some of which corresponds to mucin. The presence of cilia is not frequent (Fig. 19-86). More specific alterations are mentioned in the discussion of each histologic type of tumor. Finally, it should be remembered that qualitative ultrastructural features distinguishing ducts from lobules in normal resting breasts have not been identified. This indicates that an ultrastructural differentiation between lobular and ductal carcinomas is not realistic.

Differential Diagnosis

More significant difficulties of differential diagnosis occur in the distinction between benign hyperplastic epithelial lesions and carcinoma than in the recognition of the different types of malignant tumors. This problem becomes even more complicated in frozen section examinations. A highly cellular adenosis, for example, can mimic an infiltrating duct carcinoma.

Needless to say, if doubt exists, the pathologist should resist the surgeon's impatience and defer diagnosis until adequate permanent sections can be prepared and studied. As discussed above, lesions smaller than 1.0 cm should not be frozen at all.

It should also be remembered that IDC-NOS is in some ways a diagnosis of exclusion, that is, it is a carcinoma that does not satisfy the classic criteria for any other specific type, such as lobular, tubular, medullary, and so on. In some circumstances the differential diagnosis between IDC-NOS and a specific subtype may be problematic. Our general rule is to favor IDC-NOS in these situations, because (1) it is always statistically the more common tumor and (2) grading of the tumor will still aid in establishing the prognosis, even if an especially favorable or unfavorable type is eliminated.[321–323] Indeed, a recent study has presented credible evidence that grading may be more important than typing in the great majority (if not all) of cases.[323]

Cytologic Features

The cellularity of IDC-NOS is variable and, depending on the degree of fibrous response, aspirates may be quite hypocellular. However, in most cases, infiltrating duct carcinomas are rich in cellularity and the aspirated smears show tumor cells in a dis-

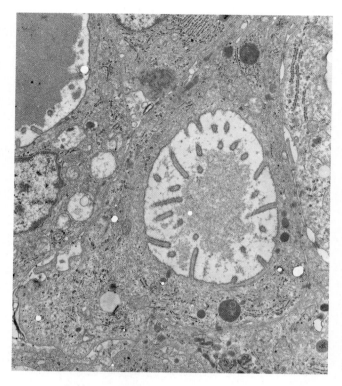

Fig. 19-85. Infiltrating duct carcinoma. Electron micrograph shows intracellular lumina with microvilli.

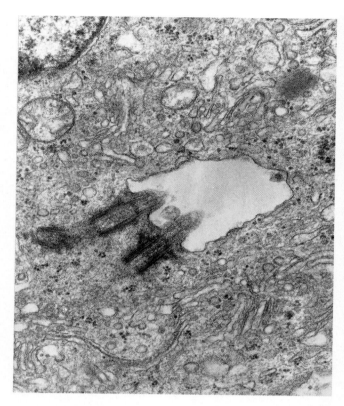

Fig. 19-86. Infiltrating duct carcinoma. Electron micrograph shows presence of cilia in an intracellular lumen.

persed cell pattern displaying various degrees of polymorphism.[324,325] Scattered individual cells and aggregates of tumor cells as three-dimensional clusters, syncytial groupings, or occasionally gland-like arrangements characterize the neoplasm (Figs. 19-87 and 19-88). The background contains cellular debris, microcalcific particles, and red blood cells. Cell size varies and ranges from relatively uniform small cells to large and markedly bizarre forms. However, the tumor cells are often pleomorphic with hyperchromatic nuclei and prominent nucleoli. Anisonucleosis is conspicuous and mitoses may also occasionally be seen. Nuclear molding and overriding and crowding of the nuclei are also common. Poorly differentiated infiltrating duct cell carcinoma can form multinucleated giant cells, often seen intermingled with mononuclear neoplastic epithelial cells.

Overall, the frequency of false negative diagnosis of infiltrating duct carcinoma is relatively low. False negative diagnosis may be due either to poor aspiration biopsy technique or the presence of prominent sclerosis in the tumor. This is best exemplified in scirrhous type infiltrating duct carcinoma, which yields hypocellular aspirates and may contain few neoplastic cells. Thus, attempts should be made to perform multiple aspirations of the lesion and remain sensitive to the adequacy of the specimen. The presence of benign epithelial cells and stromal components does not exclude the possibility of an infiltrating duct carcinoma. These elements may be introduced during aspiration via accidental sampling of surrounding breast tissue.

Prognostic Factors

Prognosis is determined by the interval to recurrence and the length of survival; therefore, treatments that delay but do not reduce the frequency of recurrence may increase the length of survival without reducing the mortality of the disease. Any information gathered by the pathologist about the prognosis of a breast cancer will help the clinician treat and follow the patient. Accurate collection, interpretation, and reporting of such information are clearly essential. Several factors are considered to have some prognostic value. The two most consistent factors that reflect the extent of the disease at the time of diagnosis and treatment are the size of the tumor and lymph node involvement.

Tumor Size

The size of the tumor is a good, although rudimentary, criterion for evaluating the duration of the disease and the survival time. However, size is not always related to the age of the lesion; growth rates may vary considerably, and doubling times from less than 30 to more than 300 days have been reported.[235] Nonetheless, the larger tumors are associated with more positive nodes, blood vessel and lymphatic dissemination, multicentricity, and short-term treatment failures. In general, this information can be safely translated in terms of poorer prognosis, but it does not provide any specific indication of rates of re-

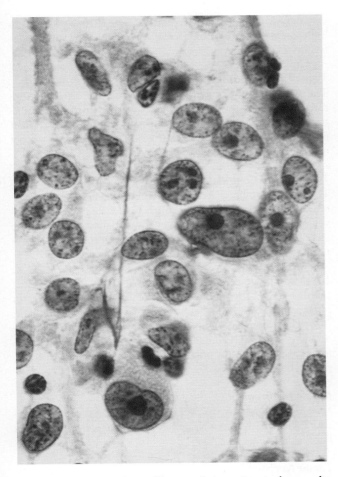

Fig. 19-87. Aspirate of an infiltrating duct carcinoma shows a dispersed cell pattern with conspicuous anisonucleosis and nuclear atypia. (Papanicolaou stain, × 1,000.)

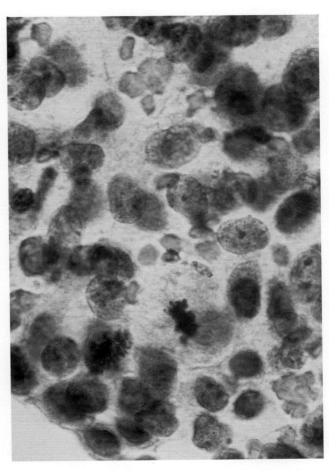

Fig. 19-88. Another view of the same case featuring a mitotic figure. (Papanicolaou stain, × 1,000.)

currence and mortality differences. Current data show that the percentage of small tumors (<1 cm in diameter) has increased in recent years, consistent with the generally earlier diagnosis of breast cancer. Even these small carcinomas, however, may be associated with nodal and distant metastases, especially if they show unfavorable prognostic features such as high tumor grade, estrogen receptor negativity, and/or lymphatic invasion.[326–329]

Lymph Node Involvement
Lymph node involvement is an important prognostic factor in mammary cancer.[330–335] Approximately 25 percent of clinically negative axillary nodes are in fact microscopically invaded by metastases. Furthermore, the number of lymph nodes detected depends on how meticulous a dissection is done on surgical specimens. More specifically, the following procedures will increase the percentage of nodal metastases found: dissection after treatment of the axillary fat with a clearing agent, histologic examination of all the nodes dissected, and sectioning of all nodes at different levels. It has been shown that, with respect to prognosis, it is more important to evaluate the absolute number of invaded nodes than the percentage of positive nodes. Pa-

tients with fewer than four involved nodes have almost as good a prognosis as those with a negative axillary dissection, whereas four or more involved nodes indicates a poor prognosis.[330]

These data suggest that careful dissection of macroscopically detectable nodes and a reasonable number of tissue sections of all suspicious nodes will procure sufficient information for evaluation of tumor evolution and, possibly, prospective epidemiologic studies. Clearing of the axillary fat[336] and keratin immunostaining[335,337] will identify more micrometastases, but the clinical significance of these is probably minimal.

Histologic Grading
Histologic grading methods have been discussed extensively, and their relative values have been confirmed by various studies.[321–323,338–340] The system recommended here has been applied to all breast carcinomas by Elston and Ellis and colleagues[323,340] and is presented in detail in Table 19-8; it involves assessments of tubule formation, nuclear pleomorphism, and mitotic activity, and is easy to perform and quite reproducible. The grade derived by this system correlates well with axillary and distant metastases and with eventual patient

Table 19-8. Combined Architectural and Cytologic Grading System for Infiltrating Duct Carcinoma

Feature	Assessment	Numeric Score[a]
Tubule formation	In >75% of tumor	1
	10%–75%	2
	<10%	3
Nuclear pleomorphism	Small, regular uniform cells	1
	Moderate increase in size and variability	2
	Marked variation	3
Mitotic counts at tumor periphery	0–9/10 HPF[b]	1
	10–19	2
	20 or more	3

[a] The three scores are added together. A final tally of 3 to 5 = grade I (well differentiated); 6 or 7 = grade II (moderately differentiated); and 8 or 9 = grade III (poorly differentiated).

[b] HPF = high power fields, defined by use of a Leitz Ortholux microscope with wide-angle eyepieces and $25\times$ objective (field area 0.274 mm^2). This must be recalculated for other microscopes.

(From Gompel and Silverberg,[566] as adapted from Elston and Ellis,[340] with permission.)

survival. Many other prognostic features such as ploidy, proliferation markers, hormone receptors, oncogenes, and others are strongly correlated with tumor grade.

Tumor Immunity

The interrelationship between tumoral tissue and normal breast tissue varies with the quality of the individual's immunologic response, which may in some manner determine clinical prognosis. Different morphologic appearances of the axillary nodes have been considered to be histologic expressions of these immunologic characteristics. The histologic patterns that have been evaluated include sinus histiocytosis, lymphocyte predominance or depletion, germinal center predominance, and absence of nodal stimulation.

Sinus histiocytosis is characterized by the presence, in the distended nodal sinusoids, of large histiocytes that resemble macrophages but do not contain phagocytosed material. Some authors have tried to correlate the prognosis with sinus histiocytosis of the lymph nodes draining the tumor.[341–343] These findings are at least partially open to question because the value of this prognostic factor seems to be counterbalanced by other tumor characteristics. Yet, in series of carcinomas showing identical characteristics, sinus histiocytosis may prove to be of some prognostic value. For example, sinus histiocytosis is related to better survival in cases of moderately or poorly differentiated carcinomas or in cases with a moderate number of nodal metastases; on the other hand, in well differentiated tumors or when nodal metastases are absent, the prognosis is good regardless of the presence or absence of sinus histiocytosis.[342] The absence of any difference in the prevalence of the other patterns mentioned previously (lymphocytic predominance or depletion, germinal center predominance, and absence of nodal

stimulation) in patients with positive or negative nodes fails to indicate any value of these factors as individual prognostic determinants.

Type of Tumor Border

The type of tumor border (the microscopic malignant structures either push the surrounding tissues aside or frankly infiltrate them) has been considered as a prognostic factor, but it provides inconclusive results that again are explained by other interfering factors, such as the histologic type.[344]

Tumor in the Contralateral Breast

The risk of developing a tumor in the contralateral breast in patients with carcinoma is significantly higher than the risk of developing a first primary in the general population.[317,345] If the second tumor is a new primary rather than a metastasis, its prognostic factors are the same as for any other breast cancer.

Local Skin Involvement

Involvement of the skin overlying the primary tumor is a factor of poor prognosis. It has been shown that a significant proportion of carcinomatous cells that invade the epidermis are colonized by melanocytes migrating downward. Melanin pigment is found dispersed in fine granules in the cytoplasm of the malignant cells.[346]

Nipple Involvement

Nipple involvement is another factor that worsens prognosis.[347] The involvement should be by invasive carcinoma, not Paget's disease.

Tumor Necrosis

There is some correlation between tumor necrosis and other factors that influence treatment failure or survival such as tumor size, histologic grade, clinical stage, histologic tumor type, and nipple involvement.[348]

Blood and Lymphatic Vessel Invasion

Blood vessel invasion occurs in approximately 5 percent of all breast carcinomas and is a bad prognostic sign.[349] Special immunohistochemical techniques for endothelial cells improve the detection of vascular spaces. Lymphatic invasion is seen more frequently, and serves predominantly as a predictor of axillary lymph nodal metastases.[350,351] It must be distinguished from retraction artifact.

Perineural Space Invasion

Invasion of perineural spaces by neoplastic cells is not uncommon and is associated with tumors showing lymphatic invasion and nodal metastases. It has also been described in sclerosing adenosis and in intraductal carcinoma.[292]

Presence of Estrogen and Progesterone Receptors

The demonstration of the presence of specific estrogen receptors (ERs) and progesterone receptors (PRs) in breast cancer tissue indicates an important association between breast cancer and the endocrine system. The practical use of receptor assay techniques can thus provide an approach to the prognostic significance of the hormonal sensitivity of breast cancer and also may help predict the response to endocrine treatments.[352–358]

Immunohistochemical techniques based on the direct recognition of the specific receptor protein by monoclonal antibodies have modified our concept of receptor pathophysiology. For example, it has been possible to demonstrate that receptors are localized in the nucleus and not in the cytoplasm, as first thought. Results of ER measurements evaluated by biochemical and immunoenzymatic methods can be compared with immunohistochemical results, with a good approximation. These techniques have also permitted the use of analyses using fine needle aspirations and will contribute to the selection of patients with potentially hormone-responsive tumors.[355,356]

Heterogeneity of the tumor cell population in terms of ERs is a frequent finding that is not fully understood. ERs have been localized in benign conditions such as fibrocystic mastopathy, fibroadenoma, and even normal breast tissue. Therefore, identification of ERs is not a specific indicator of a malignant tumor.

Quantitative evaluation of PRs, like that of ERs, can be used for prediction of clinical prognosis and choice of the proper treatment of breast cancers. It has been shown that a positive statistical correlation exists between PRs and the disease-free interval.

The group of patients whose lesions contain both ERs and PRs have a higher probability of remission following hormonal therapy than the group of patients whose lesions contain only ERs or only very low levels of the receptors. Therefore, it is important that both types of receptors should be investigated. ER and PR positivity are strongly correlated with nuclear grade, better differentiated tumors being more frequently receptor rich. However, this correlation is far from automatic, so fresh tumor tissue should be submitted for receptor analysis in every case in which this is feasible. In other cases, immunostaining can still be performed on paraffin blocks.[357]

Tumor Markers

Different tumor markers have been evaluated and correlated with clinical prognosis. Some studies tend to relate the presence of carcinoembryonic antigen (CEA) with the capability to metastasize in some tumors, but other investigations do not confirm these findings.[358] Moreover, other markers such as human chorionic gonadotrophin (hCG), placental lactogen, lactalbumin, pregnancy-specific beta-1-glycoprotein, cathepsins, growth factors, and ABH isoantigens are also described, but no definite prognostic conclusions can be drawn.[359–362]

Oncogenes

Oncogenes and receptors of growth factors are currently being investigated with the purpose of demonstrating their value as prognostic factors.[361–366] Although some oncogenes such as protein p21 or *ras* oncogene are not found exclusively in malignant mammary tissues, and thus have a moderate value in terms of clinical prediction, others such as c-erbB2 (HER2-neu) and epithelial growth factors seem to provide valuable data. Recent studies have suggested that the overexpression of certain oncogenes may be associated with a higher likelihood of metastatic disease.[365,366]

Flow and Image Cytometry

In recent years, the prognostic value of DNA analysis of cancers of the breast by flow and image cytometry has been the subject of many reports.[367] Most studies have found that a diploid histogram and a low S-phase fraction are associated with a lower rate of axillary lymph nodal metastases and a higher survival rate, compared with aneuploid high S-phase tumors.[367–369] However, the ploidy values are also correlated with such better established indices of prognosis as tumor grade and steroid hormone receptor status, so the independent significance of flow cytometry remains to be established.

Other Proliferation Markers

In addition to flow and image cytometry, estimates of proliferation rate may be obtained on fresh or fixed tumor tissues by the use of immunostaining for antibodies such as MIB-1, Ki-67, and proliferating cell nuclear antigen (PCNA), by counting of argyrophilic nucleolar organizer regions (AgNORs), and by counting mitotic figures in a variety of manners.[367–373] All of these techniques have been found to be related to prognosis in breast cancer and to one another. Because mitotic counts are part of the grading system discussed above, it is not clear whether these specialized techniques add significant prognostic information to carefully performed histologic grading.

Angiogenesis

There is evidence that tumor angiogenesis, as detected by immunohistochemical staining of endothelium followed by counting of microvessels within a tumor, is of prognostic significance in breast cancer.[374] Some recent studies, however, have suggested that it may not be an independent prognostic factor.[375,376]

Summary

As breast cancers get smaller and smaller, and as less and less money is available for medical care, there are more and more tests that can be performed on breast cancer tissues to provide prognostic information. There is no doubt that tumor stage (including primary tumor size and axillary lymph node status), tumor grade (including mitotic activity), and tumor receptor status (necessary for treatment as well as prognosis) provide a great deal of prognostic information in most cases. Which (if any) additional studies will be required to practice cost-effective medicine in the future remains to be determined.

Evolution

Local Tumor Extension

Local extension of the tumor, which can be multifocal, takes place both within and along the lactiferous ducts, in the stroma, and in the surrounding adipose tissue. The rate of local extension of the primary lesion varies from one case to another and has little influence on the probability of metastatic dissemination. Ductal carcinomas progress from in situ to invasive more rapidly than do lobular ones. The frequency of nipple involvement varies from 8 to 50 percent, depending on the study. This discrepancy is due to differences in the nipple specimen examined.

Lymphatic Dissemination

Neoplastic cells enter the lymphatic system around the tumor nodules and adjacent ducts and from there spread to the sub-areolar plexus; the external, central, and apical axillary nodes; and the internal mammary lymphatics of the inner portion of the breast (see earlier discussion of anatomy). Later, supraclavicular nodes are infiltrated, indicating disseminated disease. More distant lymphatic dissemination includes the cervical, mediastinal, and inguinal nodes. Invasion of the internal mammary chain occurs in approximately one-third of all breast cancers and is more probable in large tumors and in those with a central or medial location and axillary metastases.[377]

Hematogenous Metastases

Blood-borne metastases are common in bones, lungs, liver, ovaries, adrenals, pleura, peritoneum, pituitary, and other sites.[378–381] The most frequently involved bones are the vertebrae, pelvis, femur, humerus, skull, ribs, and clavicle.[380] Bone metastases are usually of the osteolytic type, but in about 10 percent of cases the osteoblastic type is encountered. Hypercalcemia is a frequent clinical finding in cases of bony metastases. Pulmonary metastases are usually nodular, but lymphatic dissemination can occur with carcinomatous lymphangitis. Pleural involvement with recurrent pleural effusion frequently accompanies the pulmonary infiltration.

Recurrences

Local recurrences may appear near the mastectomy scar within a few years after treatment and may involve large areas of the thoracic wall. Late recurrences are typical of breast cancer. It is not rare to diagnose recurrences or metastases 10 or even 20 years after the initial treatment. They may appear anywhere but are common in the contralateral breast,[317] possibly representing new primary foci. The explanation of this histologic behavior is not known; immunologic defense mechanisms can be suggested although there are as yet no substantial data to prove this idea. The existence of periods of survival exceeding 10 years without any treatment is another argument suggesting immunologic defense mechanisms.[382]

Other Types of Infiltrating Carcinoma

Apocrine Carcinoma

Apocrine carcinoma is an uncommon type of carcinoma.[284,383] The tumor consists of glandular structures lined by large cells with an abundant, bright, eosinophilic cytoplasm, resembling the apocrine cells of sweat glands (Fig. 19-89). The cytoplasm may be homogeneous or granular. Electron microscopic studies have not confirmed that these cells are truly apocrine in nature.[384]

Because the clinical history and the prognosis are similar to those of other infiltrating duct carcinomas, it has been proposed that we include these cases among the latter.[284,383] This tumor should not be confused with true sweat gland carcinoma, which may arise from sweat glands of the skin overlying the mammary gland. The exact frequency of this type of carcinoma is uncertain, but it certainly represents fewer than 1 percent of all breast cancers, even including some histiocytoid and lobular carcino-

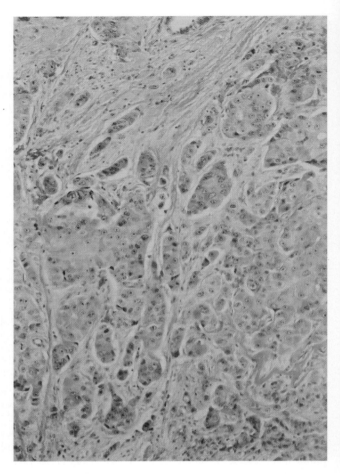

Fig. 19-89. Apocrine carcinoma. This ductal carcinoma is composed of cells with brightly eosinophilic cytoplasm. Architectural and cytologic features of a malignant tumor distinguish this lesion from apocrine metaplasia. The cells were immunoreactive for GCDFP-15 and androgen receptor and negative for estrogen and progesterone receptors, typical for both benign and malignant apocrine ductal epithelium.

mas as described below. Gross cystic disease fluid protein-15 (GCDFP-15) is an excellent immunohistochemical marker of aprocine tumor cell differentiation.[385]

Cytologically, aspirates of apocrine carcinoma yields numerous pleomorphic tumor cells. The cells have abundant basophilic to eosinophilic, granular cytoplasm. The nuclei are enlarged and vesicular and are centrally or eccentrically located. The nucleoli are prominent and may be multiple (Fig. 19-90). Apocrine carcinoma must be distinguished from hyperplastic apocrine cells seen in proliferative breast disease. Aside from the accompanying polymorphous cell population in proliferative lesions, lack of significant anisonucleosis and hyperchromasia favor a diagnosis of benign apocrine change. Included in the cytologic differential diagnosis are lipid-rich and secretory carcinomas.[386] The cytologic features of a variant of apocrine carcinoma with lipid-rich giant cells have been described.[387] Cytologically, secretory carcinoma is characterized by the presence of irregular large sheets of malignant polygonal cells with granular and vacuolated cytoplasm.[388]

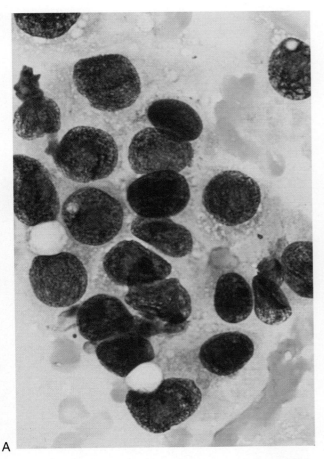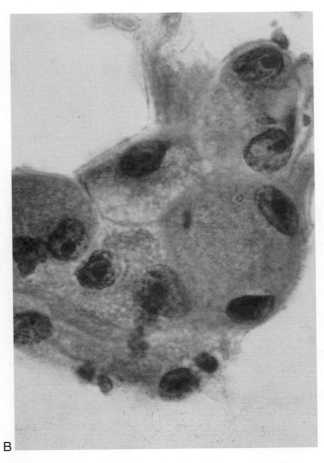

Fig. 19-90. Aspirate of an apocrine carcinoma. **(A)** The cells are pleomorphic and have abundant granular cytoplasm. (Diff-Quik, × 1,000.) **(B)** Papanicolaou-stained smear of the same case showing binucleation and presence of macronucleoli. (Papanicolaou stain, × 1,000.)

Infiltrating Lobular Carcinoma

Infiltrating lobular carcinoma (ILC), or small cell carcinoma, is a relatively uncommon form of breast cancer, accounting for approximately 5 to 10 percent of all breast carcinomas.[389–392] The peak incidence rate occurs around 50 years of age. In about 50 percent of the cases, it appears in association with LCIS.[393] It is frequently multifocal and bilateral.

Macroscopically, infiltrating lobular carcinoma is a firm, rubbery, poorly circumscribed, gray-white mass, which is indistinguishable from the much more common infiltrating duct carcinoma. Microscopically, the classic pattern is characterized by thread-like strands of small to medium-sized epithelial cells that diffusely infiltrate a dense, fibrous matrix. The tumor cells secrete mucosubstances into intracellular lumens, which are PAS positive after diastase digestion.[394] The single file cellular arrangement, also called Indian file, is characteristic of this tumor (Fig. 19-91). Sometimes the cells form concentric rings around an apparently normal dilated duct; this is called the bullseye pattern. Care must be taken not to misinterpret this arrangement as chronic mastitis, especially on a frozen section.

Another histologic pattern that has been recognized more recently is the confluent variant, in which infiltrating tumor cells (still typically small and uniform) maintain somewhat of a lobular pattern. This is currently separated into the *solid* and *alveolar* variants,[390,391,393,395–397] which are said by most but not all authors to have a less favorable prognosis than the classic type (Figs. 19-92 and 19-93). The *tubulolobular* variant (Fig. 19-94) consists of small cells forming both classic lobular structures and small tubules; it is rare but has a favorable prognosis.[398] An unfavorable prognosis, on the other hand, has been a feature of the recently described *pleomorphic lobular carcinoma*.[399] This tumor is characterized by typical lobular carcinoma architecture combined with a high nuclear grade and brightly eosinophilic cytoplasm that can be demonstrated to be of apocrine type by GCDFP-15 immunoreactivity (Fig. 19-95). A pleomorphic type of LCIS has also been described, which is difficult to distinguish from DCIS.[261]

Ultrastructural study of ILC shows the cells to be rich in organelles. The Golgi apparatus and rough endoplasmic reticulum are well developed. Ribosomes and mitochondria are abundant. The nuclei are lobulated and contain large nucleoli. Intracytoplasmic lumina are numerous and are seen at the light microscopic level as signet ring cells.

Cytologically, infiltrating lobular carcinomas present with low to moderate cell yield and a relatively uniform population

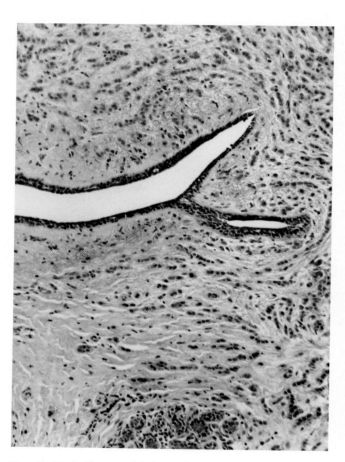

Fig. 19-91. Infiltrating lobular carcinoma. Note the single-file arrangement and swirling around normal duct.

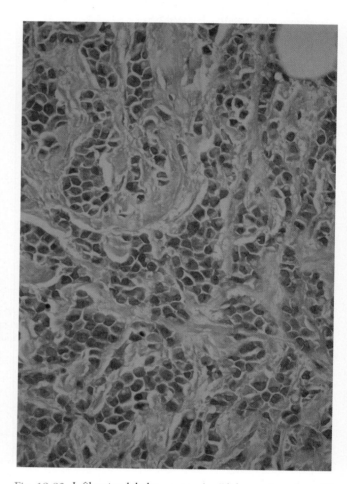

Fig. 19-92. Infiltrating lobular carcinoma, solid type. Irregular solid nests of uniform small tumor cells. (Courtesy of AR Frost, M.D., George Washington University, Washington, DC.)

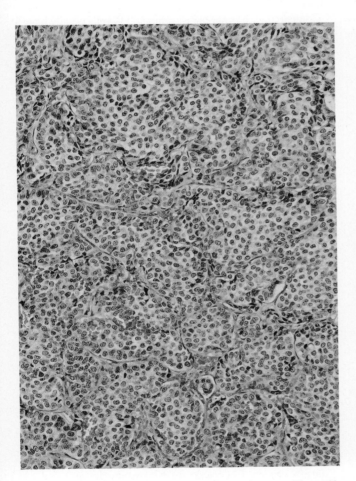

Fig. 19-93. Infiltrating lobular carcinoma, alveolar type. This infiltrating tumor forms round aggregates of uniform small cells, reminiscent of lobular carcinoma in situ.

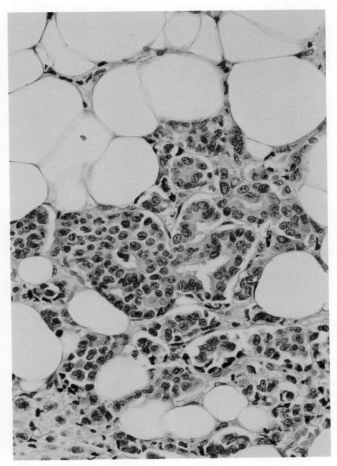

Fig. 19-94. Infiltrating tubulolobular carcinoma. Uniform small cells form lobular and tubular structures.

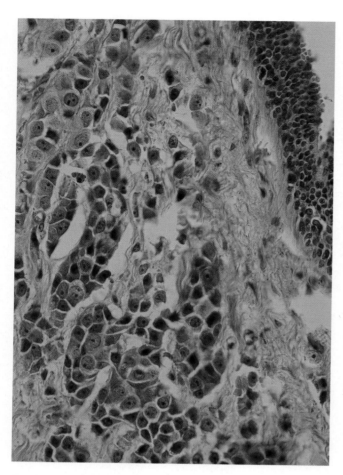

Fig. 19-95. Infiltrating pleomorphic lobular carcinoma. Large tumor cells (compare with benign duct at upper right) with high grade nuclei and eosinophilic cytoplasm grow in solid and classic lobular pattern.

of small to medium-sized cells. The cells appear singly, in small groups, single file, or in cords, and are characterized by scant ill-defined cytoplasm and a high nuclear/cytoplasmic ratio. The cytoplasm may contain sharply punched-out vacuoles and occasional signet ring forms may be seen. The nuclei have a fine chromatin pattern and small nucleoli and often are eccentric. Anisonucleosis is minimal (Fig. 19-96). In contrast to the darkly stained uniform small cells typical of classic ILC, pleomorphic lobular carcinomas show conspicuous nuclear enlargement, hyperchromasia, marked variation in cell size, and occasional nucleoli. A careful search for single files of tumor cells or the typical small cells of ILC may lead to the correct diagnosis.[400–403]

Cytomorphologic distinction between atypical lobular hyperplasia, LCIS, and an ILC may also be difficult. This is because of overlapping cytologic features seen in these entities. Thus, unless the aspirate is cellular and contains significant numbers of tumor cells with characteristic cytomorphology of ILC, one must refrain from making a definitive diagnosis and the patient must undergo an excisional biopsy. Included in the cytologic differential diagnosis are also a variety of lesions such as metastatic small cell undifferentiated tumor, carcinoid tumor

of the breast (if this exists), and low grade malignant lymphoma. Even more frequent is the problem of differential diagnosis from infiltrating duct carcinoma; one study found that the only reliable distinguishing features for the latter were coarsely granular chromatin and larger cell and nuclear size.[403]

ILCs are also considered as the major cause of false negative diagnosis of malignant tumor in breast aspirates. This is because of paucicellular aspirates, widely dispersed cells, and lack of major nuclear atypia. Thus, if the mammogram and physical examination strongly suggest carcinoma and FNAB is negative, lobular carcinoma must be ruled out.

Compared with other breast tumors, ILC cells usually have a higher percentage of positive ERs, probably related to their usual low nuclear grade.[393] Nodal metastases of this tumor usually exhibit a loose arrangement of small cells with a dense infiltration of the peripheral sinus (Fig. 19-97). This sinus catarrh pattern can thus simulate malignant lymphoma or even benign sinus histiocytosis. Study of the primary tumor will eliminate this error. Distant metastases are found with a predilection in the ovaries and uterus and the gastrointestinal tract, and particularly in the stomach, where the similarity with a primary carcinoma may lead to diagnostic difficulty. These tumors also tend to metastasize to peritoneal surfaces.[404] In some metastases, the tumor cells resemble histiocytes. Mucin stains and immunohistochemical techniques (epithelial membrane antigen and cytokeratin) may help to solve the difficulty.

Generally speaking, ILC is as lethal as the average infiltrating breast carcinoma. However, as mentioned above, the tubulolobular type is generally more favorable, and the alveolar and solid types may be—while the pleomorphic type certainly is—more aggressive. Tumors with greater than 10 percent signet ring cells and with a high S-phase fraction also appear to be prognostically unfavorable.[393,394]

Metaplastic Carcinoma

Different types of metaplasia can be seen in mammary carcinoma. All are very rare. Wargotz and colleagues[405–409] divided these cases into five categories:

1. Spindle cell carcinoma (the most common, in which the spindle cells may be deceptively lacking in atypia (Fig. 19-98A), and cytokeratin immunostaining or electron microscopy may be necessary to demonstrate the epithelial nature of the tumor cells)
2. Carcinosarcoma (the most aggressive), in which both the epithelial and stromal component appear histologically malignant (Fig. 19-98B)
3. Matrix-producing carcinoma, in which there is direct transition from carcinoma to a cartilaginous or osseous matrix without intervening spindle cells
4. Pure squamous cell carcinoma (intraductal or infiltrating) of ductal origin
5. Metaplastic carcinoma with osteoclastic giant cells

Not all authorities have accepted this classification, and many consider types 2, 3, and 5 as separate categories outside the spectrum of metaplastic carcinomas.[410–414] The main differential diagnosis of these tumors is with one another, but var-

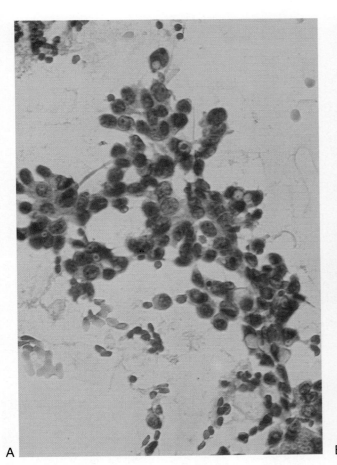
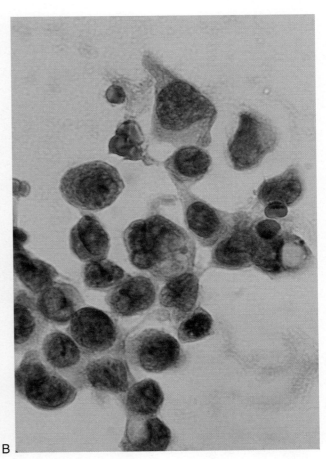

Fig. 19-96. **(A)** Aspirate of an infiltrating lobular carcinoma with small uniform cells and a few signet ring cells. (Papanicolaou stain, × 200.) **(B)** High magnification of the same case displaying a few signet rings. (Papanicolaou stain, × 400.)

ious sarcomas, benign mixed tumor of salivary gland type, squamous metaplasia in an infarcted papilloma, and benign spindle cell proliferations such as nodular fasciitis or fibromatosis must be considered depending on the type of metaplasia encountered.

Cytologically, aspirates from metaplastic carcinomas are rich in cellularity with the tumor cells seen in a myxoid background.[415-418] The mesenchymal cells are elongated, atypical, and pleomorphic. Multinucleation and mitoses are frequently seen. Also present, singly or in small groups, are round to oval atypical cells with sharply demarcated cytoplasm characteristic of carcinoma. Positive immunostaining for vimentin, cytokeratin and S-100 protein may be seen in both the epithelial and the sarcomatoid component (Figs. 19-99 and 19-100). Electron microscopic evaluation of aspirated material can also show the characteristic ultrastructural features of metaplastic carcinoma. Metaplastic carcinoma should be distinguished from pseudosarcomatous fasciitis, fibromatosis, and pure sarcomas.[419-421] Cytologically, pseudosarcomatous fasciitis and fibromatosis present with variable cellularity and contain microtissue fragments and individually arranged spindle-shaped cells that have a bland appearance. Unfortunately, most spindle cell carcinomas

are also bland, so immunohistochemical or ultrastructural studies may be essential. Pure sarcomas should also be distinguished from metaplastic carcinoma by the use of immunocytochemistry and ultrastructural studies.

Medullary Carcinoma

Medullary carcinoma represents less than 5 percent of mammary malignant tumors and shows a significantly higher survival rate at 10 years than infiltrating duct carcinoma in most studies.[422-426] Some investigators have questioned the favorable prognosis generally assigned to this particular type of carcinoma[427,428] but, if the lesion closely fits the strictly defined morphologic criteria, we agree that the prognosis is significantly more favorable. Table 19-8 summarizes the distinct morphologic criteria of typical medullary carcinoma. The atypical type exhibits some but not all features of the typical form and can probably be eliminated as a specific diagnosis if strict criteria are applied.[423,426,428] Bilaterality has been reported.

Grossly, medullary carcinoma is characterized by a soft, sometimes bulky, circumscribed mass deeply situated in the mammary gland. The cut sections reveal diffuse, gray-tan, ho-

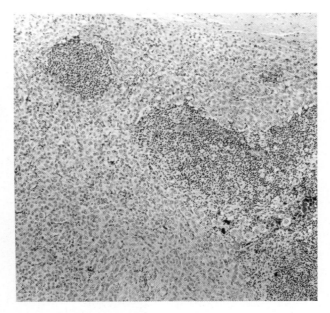

Fig. 19-97. Sinus catarrh-like pattern of lymph node metastasis in infiltrating lobular carcinoma.

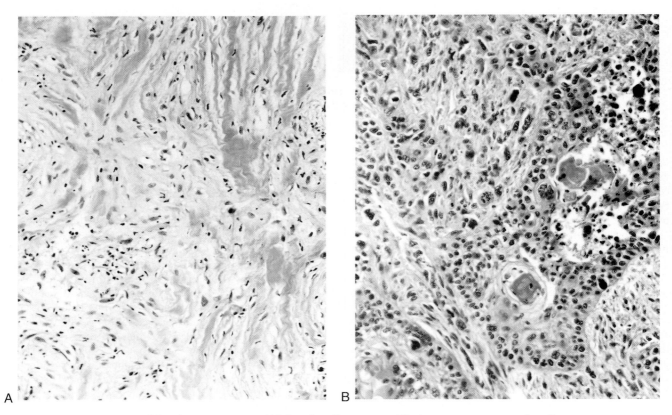

Fig. 19-98. Metaplastic carcinomas. (A) Spindle cell carcinoma. The benign-appearing spindle cells in this infiltrative lesion were immunoreactive for cytokeratins. (B) Carcinosarcoma. Both the epithelial and the stromal component appear malignant; the former contains squamous pearls.

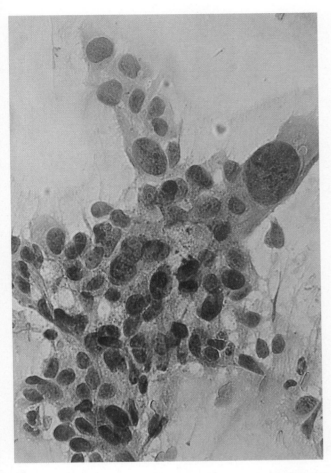

Fig. 19-99. Smear from an aspirate of metaplastic carcinoma featuring neoplastic oval, round, and spindle cells with conspicuous pleomorphism. (Papanicolaou stain, × 400.)

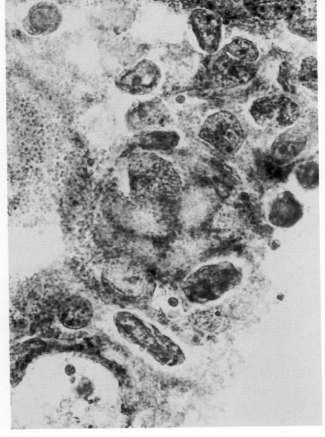

Fig. 19-100. Positive immunostaining for cytokeratin seen in cell block preparation of the same case as in Fig. 19-99. (Original magnification × 400.)

mogeneous tissue with hemorrhagic and sometimes necrotic foci. There is no skin attachment and no superficial ulceration even if the tumor is voluminous.

Microscopically, the tumor is characterized by a predominantly sheet-like growth pattern of large, polymorphic cells with round or cleaved, vesicular nuclei and prominent nucleoli (Fig. 19-101). Squamous metaplasia is seen in approximately 15 percent of cases. Cytoplasm is abundant and basophilic. Mitoses are quite frequent. Marked or moderate cellular pleomorphism is present; multinucleated cells and bizarre giant cell reactions can be observed. Calcifications are practically never encountered. No intraductal, microglandular, or papillary neoplastic component should be present in the typical case. The stroma characteristically reveals a marked lymphocytic infiltrate that may contain plasma cells. The significance of the lymphocytic infiltrate has aroused much controversy; it has been suggested that it represents a host reaction to tumor cell antigens.[429,430] As expected from the microscopic appearance, most medullary carcinomas are aneuploid with high S-phase fractions and receptor negative.[427]

The electron microscope reveals that myoepithelial cells and deposition of basal lamina are not frequent characteristics of medullary carcinoma.[431] These findings also apply to the tubular type of carcinoma, which has similarly a favorable clinical prognosis. Cytoplasmic fibrillar bundles and mitochondrial alterations have been described.[432] The frequency of axillary lymph node metastases is similar to that calculated for infiltrating duct carcinomas, but the prognosis remains more favorable even if lymph node metastases are present.[423] The 10 year survival rate for this tumor exceeds 80 percent in typical cases.

Cytologically, aspirates of medullary carcinoma are generally cellular and contain many isolated and clusters of highly anaplastic epithelial cells admixed with numerous lymphocytes and plasma cells. The background is necrotic. Tumor cells show conspicuous pleomorphism, and have enlarged nuclei, anisonucleosis, and high nuclear/cytoplasmic ratios. Multiple irregularly shaped macronucleoli are present. The cytoplasm is scant to abundant and may be finely granular (Fig. 19-102). Depending on the predominance of tumor cells or lymphoid cells, the cytologic differential diagnosis includes poorly differentiated

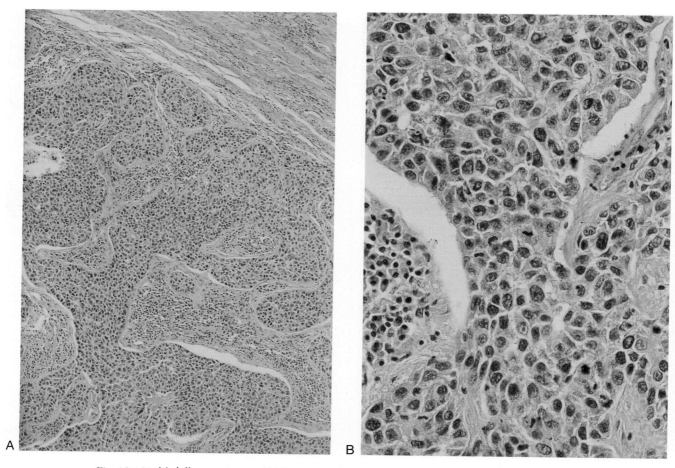

Fig. 19-101. Medullary carcinoma. **(A)** Low power photomicrograph shows pushing tumor border, "syncytial" growth pattern, and prominent lymphoid infiltration. **(B)** Detail of large pleomorphic tumor cells and lymphoplasmacytic infiltrate.

duct carcinoma with lymphocytic infiltration or malignant lymphoma. The diagnosis of medullary carcinoma should only be entertained when a well defined soft mass is aspirated and a mixed component of high grade malignant cells and lymphocytes and plasma cells is present.[433]

Papillary Carcinoma

Infiltrating papillary adenocarcinoma constitutes less than 1 percent of all mammary tumors. It is more frequent in older patients, and the mean age of diagnosis varies from 63 to 67 years. It is characterized by the proliferation of papillary structures originating within the large lactiferous ducts and invading into the mammary stroma. A bloody or serous nipple discharge is a common finding.

Grossly, papillary carcinomas are usually large, rather well demarcated masses situated in the subareolar region with hemorrhagic and cystic foci. The softness of the specimen is due to the scarcity of stroma. Microscopically, the papillary structures are seen within a variable number of ducts (noninfiltrating type) and infiltrate the adjacent stroma. The infiltration of the stroma is usually associated with a loss of papillary differentiation.

More common than infiltrating papillary carcinoma is *intracystic papillary carcinoma*.[434,435] This lesion, which is essentially an intraductal carcinoma in a cystically expanded duct, should not be considered as a form of infiltrating carcinoma.[436] At the other end of the prognostic spectrum is *micropapillary carcinoma*,[437] a highly aggressive infiltrating tumor that histologically resembles serous papillary carcinoma of the ovary (Fig. 19-103). Fortunately, this latter tumor is rare.

Characteristically, the majority of aspirates of papillary carcinoma (generally the intracystic variant) are highly cellular, with tissue fragments, small clusters of cells, a significant number of single cells, and a hemorrhagic diathesis[435,438,439] (Fig. 19-104). Necrotic debris may be seen in the background. The tumor cell population invariably has a monotonous appearance and consists of low to tall columnar cells, single papillae, and three-dimensional aggregates. The papillae are vascularized and contain a thin stromal network. Atypical bare nuclei are also present.

The cytologic distinction between papillary carcinoma and benign papillary lesions of the breast is difficult, justifying excisional biopsy unless a conclusive diagnosis of cancer can be made by demonstrating cytologically malignant single cells with a monotonous pattern. Immunocytochemistry for detection of CEA and muscle-specific actin may be helpful.

Mucinous Carcinoma

Mucin production is a frequently observed phenomenon in mammary carcinoma. Massive production of mucin, described more than a century ago by Larrey,[440] is rare and characterizes mucinous carcinoma (colloid carcinoma, gelatinous carcinoma).[441–443] The pure type appears at a later age, is associated with a longer duration of symptoms, and reveals a larger size compared with other types of carcinoma, including the mixed mucinous or colloid type. Together they represent 2 to 3 percent of all breast carcinomas.

Grossly, mucinous carcinoma is represented by a firm, irregular, well circumscribed, gelatinous or glairy mass, sometimes measuring 10 cm or more in diameter. The mucinous material is contained in numerous cystic formations, which have a translucent blue-green or gray color. When the mucinous foci are discrete, the mixed type may look like an infiltrating duct carcinoma.

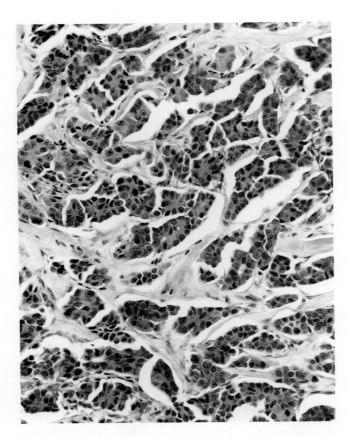

Fig. 19-103. Infiltrating micropapillary carcinoma. Note resemblance to ovarian serous carcinoma.

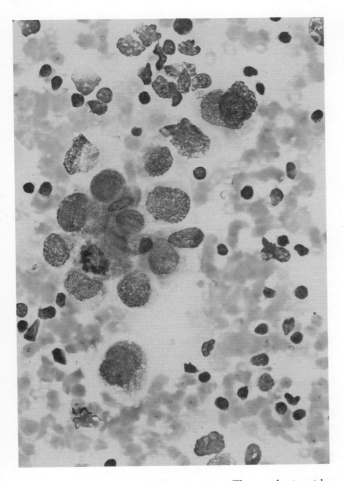

Fig. 19-102. Aspirate of medullary carcinoma. The neoplastic epithelial cells are large and pleomorphic and are surrounded by lymphocytes. (Diff-Quick × 400.)

Microscopically, the epithelial cells are arranged as clusters, cords, or individual cells separated from the stroma by abundant extracellular mucin (Fig. 19-105). The malignant cells exhibit the usual criteria of malignant tumors and reveal variable tubular differentiation; sometimes the epithelial elements are so rare that a careful search is necessary to find them. Mucicarmine, Alcian blue, and PAS reactions are positive. The pure type is characterized by well differentiated cells occurring singly or in small groups and dispersed within pools of mucin that comprise at least 50 percent of the whole tumor. The mixed type shows the concomitant presence of mucinous and other (usually infiltrating duct) elements. Even if the nonmucinous elements are rare, the tumor should be classified as mixed. The nuclear grade is low in the pure type and in the mucinous foci of the mixed type. Argyrophilic granules that ultrastructurally resemble endocrine granules have been observed in the cytoplasm.[444]

The origin of the mucinous substances has been debated. Ultrastructural studies and the presence of mucin in nodal metastases demonstrate the epithelial origin of the mucinous material.[445] Mucin production is accompanied by dilated rough endoplasmic reticulum (RER), large Golgi apparatus, and mucin granules contained within smooth membranes.

The prognosis, which is good, is better for the pure mucinous type. The incidence of regional nodal metastases is low, particularly in cases of pure mucinous carcinoma. Mixed mucinous

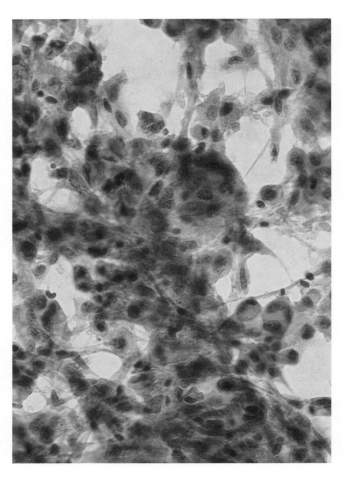

Fig. 19-104. Smear from an aspirate of intracystic papillary carcinoma featuring crowded clustering of epithelial cells forming papillae with vascular cores, lined by single-layered columnar cells. (Papanicolaou stain, × 400.)

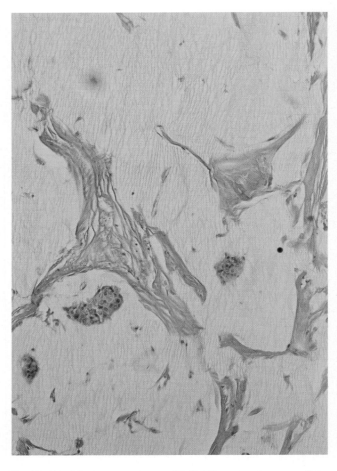

Fig. 19-105. Mucinous carcinoma. Well differentiated tumor cells in pools of extracellular mucin.

carcinomas generally metastasize as the nonmucinous component.

Differential diagnosis includes other mammary tumors with prominent mucin formation, such as infiltrating lobular carcinoma with numerous signet ring cells. The only common feature of the two tumors, however, is mucin, which is entirely intracellular rather than extracellular in the signet ring cell variant. Potentially more confusing is the so-called *mucocele-like lesion* of the breast, a mass composed of multiple cysts containing mucin, with rupture and discharge of acellular mucin into surrounding parenchyma.[443,446] Although this lesion was initially thought to be benign, more recent studies suggest that it probably represents an intraductal variant of mucinous carcinoma.

Cytologically, the aspirated material in pure mucinous carcinoma has a glistening appearance. The smear shows abundant mucin and clusters of relatively small, uniform epithelial cells with bland cytologic features. The mucin appears metachromatic in Diff-Quik and pale green to yellow in the Papanicolaou stain. Against a background of extracellular mucin, the tu-

mor cells appear in three-dimensional clusters, or as dissociated groups of cells and isolated cells. The tumor cells are relatively uniform and have wispy cytoplasm with ill-defined borders. A few signet ring forms may also be seen. The nuclei may have a vesicular pattern with mild anisonucleosis or nuclear irregularity. Macronucleoli are rare (Figs. 19-106 and 19-107).

In mixed mucinous carcinoma, the smear shows cytologic features of both mucinous and infiltrating duct or other carcinoma.[447] Mucinous carcinoma should be distinguished from mucocele-like tumors of the breast and also from myxoid fibroadenomas. Fibroadenomas characteristically have cell clusters with finger-like branching and naked nuclei in the background. Mucocele-like tumors of the breast are said to show no nuclear atypia in aspirated cells.[448]

Tubular Carcinoma

Tubular carcinoma was first described by Cornil and Ranvier in 1869.[449] Macroscopically, it is a rather hard tumor with stellate or ill-defined margins; cut sections show a gray-white color. Tu-

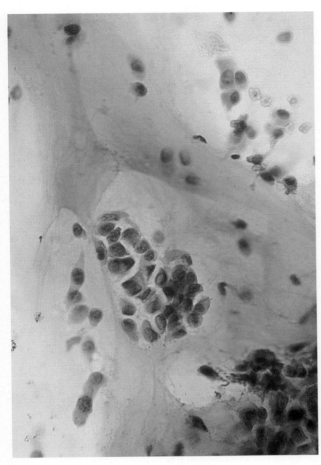

Fig. 19-106. Direct smear from an aspirate of mucinous carcinoma. The epithelial cells are seen singly and in clusters in mucoid background. (Papanicolaou stain, × 400.)

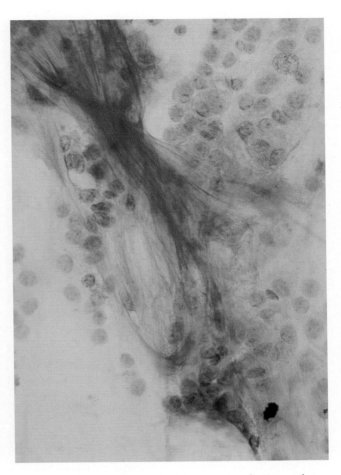

Fig. 19-107. Extracellular and cytoplasmic staining for mucin, characteristic of mucinous carcinoma. (Mucin stain × 400.)

mor size ranges from 0.2 to 4 cm,[450] but most tumors are quite small. Tubular carcinoma is an infrequent form (1 to 10 percent) of breast carcinoma, characterized by the presence of well formed regular tubules lined by a single layer of cuboidal cells and separated by a hyalinized stroma[450–456] (Fig. 19-108). The tubules are often teardrop shaped rather than uniformly round. Elastosis occurs chiefly around the tubules and the vessels. Myoepithelial cells are absent. Calcifications are frequent: more than 50 percent of cases show intraductal carcinoma, often with calcified foci.

Different histologic types have been recognized. The pure type has been described above; the sclerosing type is a small lesion characterized by haphazardly arranged tubules infiltrating into fat and connective tissue.[457] This type could represent an earlier form of the classic tubular type. In the mixed type, at least 75 percent of the infiltrating tumor is of the tubular type, although some authors permit only 50 percent.[455]

The frequency of tubular carcinoma is considerably higher (about 10 percent) in recent series that include larger proportions of smaller tumors detected by mammographic screening. The tumor is much rarer (1 percent) in series in which larger tumors detected by palpation predominate. The high incidence of

associated LCIS or ILC suggests that lobular and tubular carcinomas are two divergent types of a specialized form of secretory casein-producing carcinoma.[398] Ultrastructural studies show that the tumor cells resemble those of normal lactiferous ducts. They contain numerous bundles of filaments and reveal alterations of the basal membrane.[431,458] Cytoplasmic protrusions are present in both apical and basal poles of the cells. Myoepithelial cells are very rare, and the basal lamina is often broken or incomplete. Numerous elastic fibers are present around the tubular structures. The prognosis for this slowly growing tumor is very good when tubular elements comprise 75 percent or more of the tumor. Axillary lymph node metastases occur in up to 30 percent of cases, but are less common in small pure tubular tumors,[459] and distant metastases are rare.

Differential Diagnosis

Tubular carcinoma is a well differentiated tumor that should not be mistaken for benign lesions such as sclerosing or microglandular adenosis or radial sclerosing lesion.[92,96,104] The disorganized arrangement of the epithelial structures and the infiltration of the parenchyma surrounding the tumor are features indicative of carcinoma. The tubules are generally more widely spaced, and their lumina more dilated, than in scleros-

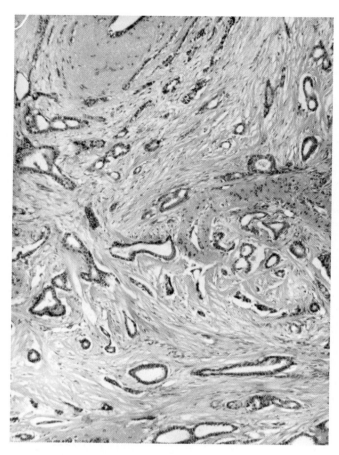

Fig. 19-108. Tubular carcinoma. Widely separated tubules lined by a single layer of small uniform cells.

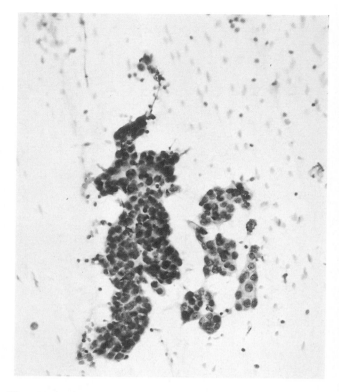

Fig. 19-109. Smear of an aspirate from a tubular carcinoma. Uniform small tumor cells are forming tubules. (Papanicolaou stain, × 200.)

ing adenosis. Prominent myoepithelial cells are not observed ultrastructurally or immunohistochemically in tubular carcinoma but are found in sclerosing adenosis. They are also absent in microglandular adenosis, but this condition lacks the reactive stroma of tubular carcinoma, and generally contain prominent intraluminal colloid-like secretory material. The basal membranes surrounding the glands are preserved in sclerosing adenosis; histochemical and electron microscopic observations show that this is not the case in tubular carcinoma.[460]

Cytologic Features

Cytologically, aspirates of tubular carcinoma are moderately cellular. The most striking feature of this entity is the structural pattern of highly cohesive, angular tubules that reflects the histologic appearance of the tumor. Tumor cells are uniform and have regularly shaped nuclei with finely dispersed chromatin and small nucleoli. Occasionally, there may be cellular atypia such as irregular, grooved nuclei, uneven deposition of chromatin on the nuclear membrane, and an occasional intracytoplasmic vacuole. Myoepithelial cells are only seen in the background (Fig. 19-109). The high rate of unsatisfactory cytologic specimens in tubular carcinoma and lack of significant cyto-

logic atypia are contributing factors to the difficulty of this diagnosis by fine needle aspirates.[461] In addition, cytomorphology resembling tubular carcinoma may also be seen in aspirates of benign lesions such as radial scars, which mammographically are very similar to small tubular carcinoma.[462] Aspirates of radial scar, however, are less cellular and show more myoepithelial cells in the background and within the clusters of epithelial cells.

Infiltrating Cribriform Carcinoma

Infiltrating cribriform carcinoma has been characterized recently.[463,464] It comprises 3 to 5 percent of all invasive breast cancers and tends to be intermediate in size between the smaller tubular carcinoma and the larger infiltrating duct carcinoma. Its gross appearance does not differ from that of these other two tumor types.

Histologically, this neoplasm displays islands of cells with punched-out spaces, identical to the picture of the cribriform pattern of intraductal carcinoma, but the irregular sizes and shapes of the islands, as well as a reactive stroma, indicate that this is an invasive tumor (Fig. 19-110). Some of the islands may be more solid, but all are characterized by a low or occasionally intermediate nuclear grade. Foci of intraductal carcinoma (often but not necessarily of cribriform type) and of tubular carcinoma are often intermixed. Cytologically there is a close resemblance to tubular carcinoma and well differentiated IDC-NOS. The tumor is virtually always diploid and ER rich.

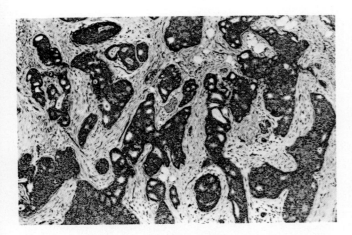

Fig. 19-110. Infiltrating cribriform carcinoma. Irregular nests of infiltrating carcinoma are punctuated by uniform punched-out spaces lined by well differentiated tumor cells.

Differential Diagnosis

The major differential diagnoses are with cribriform intraductal carcinoma and tubular or adenoid cystic carcinoma. Tubular carcinoma is distinguished by its lack of coalescence of tubules to form large islands with many lumina. The presence of basement membrane material within cystic spaces and of myoepithelial cells is necessary for the diagnosis of adenoid cystic carcinoma; this tumor is considerably rarer than infiltrating cribriform carcinoma, and electron microscopy or immunohistochemistry may be required for its diagnosis.

Prognosis

The prognosis of infiltrating cribriform carcinoma is excellent as long as this pattern comprises more than 50 percent of the invasive component of a breast cancer.[463–465] Axillary lymph node metastases (almost always to fewer than four nodes) are not uncommon, but distant metastases and death resulting from this tumor type are exceedingly rare.

Adenoid Cystic Carcinoma

The pure type of adenoid cystic carcinoma (cylindroma, ACC) is a very rare, slow-growing mammary carcinoma accounting for less than 1 percent of all breast tumors.[466–470] It is histologically identical to similar tumors of the salivary glands, bronchi, cervix, and Bartholin's gland (Fig. 19-111).

Most of these tumors appear in middle-aged women. Grossly, it is usually a firm, small tumor that does not exhibit any specific characteristic. Microscopically, the tumor shows typical glandular, round, and regular honeycombed structures lined by small cuboidal cells with round and hyperchromatic nuclei. The intraluminal material is mucicarmine positive. Electron microscopy characteristically displays the presence of true glandular structures and pseudocysts, which are extracellular compartments enclosed by tumor cells and lined by a basement membrane.[436] Basaloid cells, thought by most authors to be myoepithelial cells, are prominent in the tumor, and can be

demonstrated by immunoreactivity for muscle-specific actin. ACC should not be confused with the cribriform type of ductal carcinoma. Immunohistochemistry and electron microscopy are helpful in making this distinction, as is the fact that cribriform carcinoma is always ER rich and ACC ER negative.

The prognosis is excellent compared with the survival rate of the same type of tumor in other anatomic locations and with that of other breast cancers. Regional lymph nodal metastases have been described, as well as recurrences in the mastectomy scar, but both are rare.[470]

Cytologically, aspirates of ACC are cellular and display clusters of small cells with scant cytoplasm, hyperchromatic nuclei, and occasional micronucleoli. The tumor cells surround cores of acellular, homogeneous material that are translucent with the Papanicolaou stain and pink with the May-Grunwald-Giemsa stain (Fig. 19-112). The cytologic differential diagnosis includes infiltrating cribriform, lobular and mucinous carcinomas, carcinoid tumor, small cell undifferentiated carcinoma, lymphoma, and cribriform intraductal carcinoma.[469,471] Cellular monomorphism, the presence of extracellular metachromatic spherules, and the absence of the traditional cytologic features of malignant tumors are the distinguishing features of

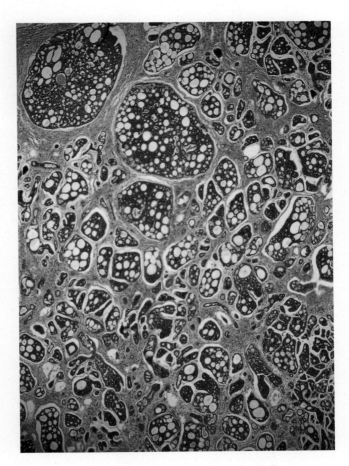

Fig. 19-111. Adenoid cystic carcinoma. Typical cylindromatous pattern.

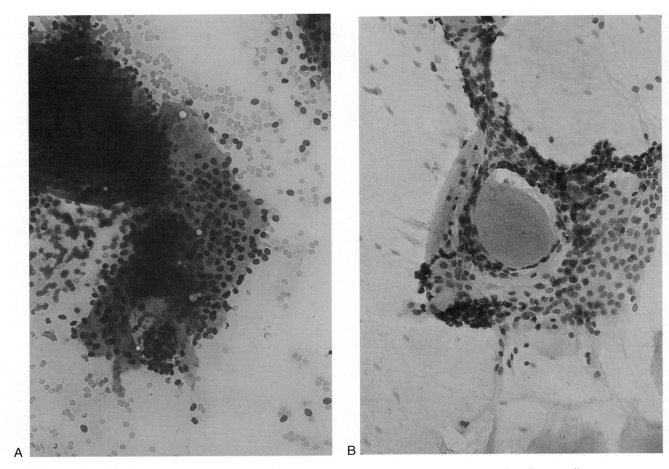

Fig. 19-112. **(A)** Diff-Quik-stained smear from an aspirate of adenoid cystic carcinoma. The cells are small and uniform and surround acellular homogeneous material. **(B)** Papanicolaou-stained smear of the same case displaying similar features. (× 400.)

ACC. ACC should also be distinguished from collagenous spherulosis. Adenoid cystic carcinoma forms a mass and presents as a palpable breast lesion, whereas collagenous spherulosis is usually an incidental finding of microscopic dimensions, associated with the spectrum of fibrocystic change. Collagenous spherulosis shows more obvious myoepithelial cells on FNAB.[472]

Lipid-Rich Carcinoma

Lipid-rich carcinoma has rarely been mentioned in the literature.[473–475] Grossly, these tumors are often less firm than the usual infiltrating duct carcinoma, and there is no retraction of the surrounding tissues. Microscopically, they are characterized by poorly differentiated masses of large cells with irregular nuclei and sometimes clear cytoplasm containing neutral lipids. Two other features characterize lipid-rich carcinoma: lymph node metastases may mimic a reticuloendotheliosis, and ocular metastases involve the eyelid and orbital soft tissues and not the retina, the usual site of ocular metastasis in breast carcinoma.

The prognosis is poor. Some authorities deny that this particular morphologic condition is a distinctive entity; they mention the presence of vacuolated cells in various conditions such as benign lesions and different types of carcinoma.[476]

Cytologically, aspirates from lipid-rich carcinoma are cellular and show loosely cohesive tumor cells.[477] The cytoplasm is abundant and has a foamy appearance. Characteristically, the cytoplasm contain single or multiple vacuoles. The nuclei have distinct nuclear membranes, a course chromatin pattern, and small nucleoli. Mild anisonucleosis is also present. Nuclear vacuoles and indentation are occasionally seen (Fig. 19-113).

The differential diagnosis includes secretory carcinoma (see next section) and infiltrating lobular carcinoma with numerous signet ring cells; in both of these tumors the intracytoplasmic material stains for mucin rather than lipid. *Histiocytoid carcinoma* is classified by Van Bogaert and Maldague[474] as a type of lipid-rich carcinoma, but newer evidence suggests that it is actually a type of apocrine carcinoma, as evidenced by immunoreactivity for GCDFP-15.[478] Both lipid-rich and histiocytoid carcinomas also must be distinguished from nonepithelial fibrohistiocytic and granular cell tumors.[478]

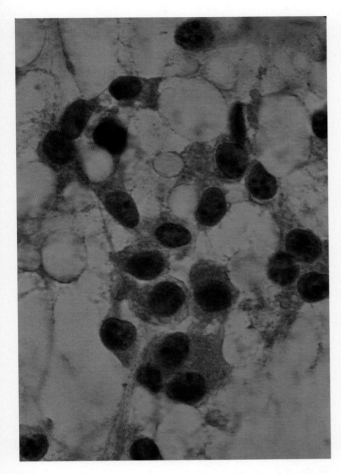

Fig. 19-113. Direct smear from an aspirate of lipid-rich carcinoma showing dispersed cell pattern. Tumor cells have abundant foamy cytoplasm. (Diff-Quik × 400.)

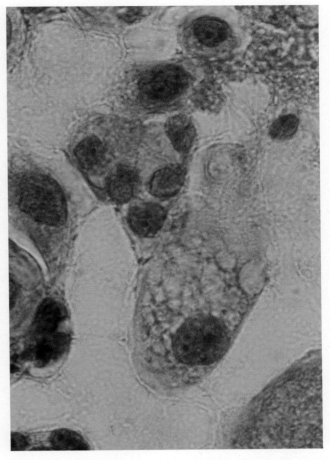

Fig. 19-114. Aspirate of a secretory carcinoma showing pleomorphic tumor cells with multiple cytoplasmic vacuoles. (Papanicolaou stain, × 1,000.)

Secretory Carcinoma

Secretory carcinoma is a rare tumor that has also been known as juvenile carcinoma, but almost one-third of reported cases have occurred in adults.[479–483] As the name suggests, the main histologic feature is the presence of voluminous intracellular and extracellular secretory material (predominantly sulfated acid mucopolysaccharide). The tumor, which is frequently grossly circumscribed, has a gray or yellow cut surface. Microscopically, the cells exhibit abundant clear or amphophilic cytoplasm and are arranged in papillary, lobular, or solid structures. Axillary nodal metastases, when they occur, contain the same secretory material. Distant metastases are rare, and the prognosis is excellent in young patients; in adults, the clinical behavior is not markedly different from that of other infiltrating carcinomas.

Cytologically, secretory carcinoma has numerous large branching sheets of neoplastic cells with cytoplasmic vacuoles and extracellular lumens.[484] The background is necrotic and there are multivacuolated lacy elements in the cytoplasm (Fig. 19-114).

Glycogen-Rich Clear Cell Carcinoma

Glycogen-rich clear cell carcinoma is also a rare variant of mammary carcinoma, with slightly over 40 cases reported to date.[485,486] It is defined as a carcinoma in which over 90 percent of the cells have abundant clear cytoplasm containing glycogen. The differential diagnosis includes primary secretory, lipid-rich, and histiocytoid carcinoma, as well as metastatic clear cell adenocarcinoma and primary or metastatic squamous cell carcinoma with clear cell features. Many glycogen-rich clear cell carcinomas have apocrine features.[486] They tend to exhibit a high nuclear grade and to be nondiploid with a high S-phase fraction,[485] and behave accordingly.

Carcinoma with Neuroendocrine Features

In 1977, Cubilla and Woodruff[487] reported eight cases of a small cell tumor of the breast that was argyrophilic by light microscopy and contained neurosecretory type granules ultrastructurally, and named this tumor primary *carcinoid tumor* of the breast. Subsequent studies have indicated that argyrophilia and neurosecretory granules, as well as immunohistochemical markers of neuroendocrine activity (neuron-specific enolase, chromogranin, synaptophysin, and others), may be seen in up to 50 percent of all breast carcinomas,[488,489] and are particularly common in mucinous carcinoma.[444] These tumors have clinical and gross features as expected for the corresponding histologic types without these neuroendocrine features, and do not appear to vary significantly in their natural history or prognosis. A small proportion of them resemble the tumors described by Cubilla and Woodruff, but identical tumors lacking neuroendocrine features are also encountered, and probably represent the alveolar type of infiltrating lobular carcinoma[390,391] (Fig. 19-93). Thus, although a true primary carcinoid of the breast may exist, it is certainly extremely rare at best.

The differential diagnosis of this problematic tumor also includes carcinoid tumor metastatic to the breast from elsewhere,[490] as well as both primary and metastatic *small cell neuroendocrine carcinomas*.[489,491] The primary type is extremely rare, resembles its bronchial counterpart, and is equally aggressive in its behavior.

Cytologically, these tumors must be distinguished from one another and from mammary lymphoma.[490,492] Immunohistochemical studies on FNA material may be necessary.

Paget's Disease

The first clinical description of Paget's disease was published by Velpeau,[493] but it was Paget who first observed the association of the skin lesion with breast cancer.[494] Paget did not recognize the cancerous nature of the skin involvement, and this finding should be credited to Jacobeus.[495] Paget's disease is a particular form of ductal carcinoma in situ accompanied by involvement of the nipple epidermis (Fig. 19-115). The major ar-

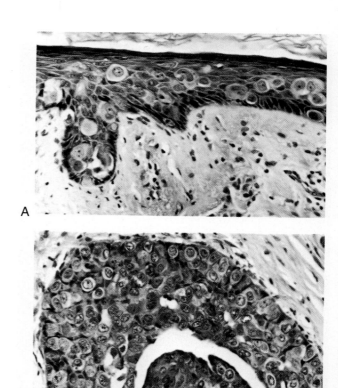

Fig. 19-116. Paget's disease. **(A)** The nipple epidermis is infiltrated by large round cells with a round nucleus and abundant clear cytoplasm. **(B)** An underlying lactiferous duct is infiltrated by the same type of neoplastic cells.

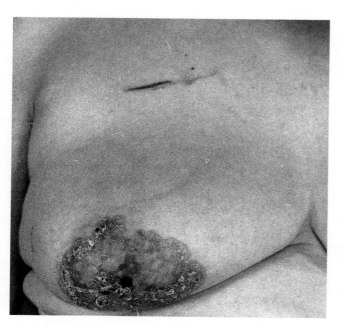

Fig. 19-115. Paget's disease, clinical appearance.

gument for considering this disease as a special form of intraductal carcinoma is the rather constant presence of a carcinoma in the depths of the mammary gland. The clinical manifestation includes crusting and erosion of the nipple, pruritus, and bloody discharge. These characteristics explain why the lesion was initially considered to be a primary skin tumor. Paget's disease accompanies less than 5 percent of all breast cancers; the peak incidence rate occurs around 50 years of age. It rarely occurs in men.[496] Microscopically, the nipple epidermis is infiltrated by large ovoid or round cells with a round nucleus and abundant clear cytoplasm (Fig. 19-116). These cells (Paget cells) may exhibit hyperchromatic irregular nuclei and mitoses. They are isolated or constitute small masses or clumps, usually located in the deeper layers of the epithelium. When the cells occur in nests, this arrangement may recall the junctional component of an amelanotic melanoma; compounding the difficulty is the fact that Paget cells may occasionally contain melanin granules.[497] However, melanoma of the nipple virtually never occurs. A form of Paget's disease in which the cells largely replace the normal squamous cells of the nipple epidermis (so-called anaplastic Paget's disease[498] occasionally occurs;

in this situation the differential diagnosis is with in situ squamous carcinoma (Bowen's disease). Again, as with melanoma, Bowen's disease of the nipple is exceedingly rare. If the diagnosis is in doubt, mucin staining (PAS with diastase digestion) and immunoreactivity for cytokeratin CAM5.2 and c-erbB-2 are characteristic of Paget cells. All of these findings should be negative in melanoma and Bowen's disease. Immunostaining for human milk fat globulin and CEA, although generally positive, has not been as consistent.[499]

Cytologically, Paget's disease is characterized by a pleomorphic population of neoplastic epithelial cells. The cells are large with centrally located nuclei and abundant clear cytoplasm. Tumor cells are seen in a background of keratinous debris, inflammatory cells, and squamous cells. The differential diagnosis (because of the location of the lesion) includes subareolar abscess and periareolar duct hyperplasias. In these cases, although some degree of atypia may be seen in epithelial cells, the clustering of cohesive aggregates of epithelial cells favors the benign nature of these lesions. Malignant melanoma, although extremely rare, may cytologically present with features similar to Paget's disease. Distinction from malignant melanoma is possible by immunocytochemistry, as discussed above.

The histogenesis of the disease is controversial. Neither histochemical techniques nor electron microscopy has definitively settled the matter. In almost all cases, if numerous serial sections of the underlying mammary parenchyma are made, the primary breast carcinoma will appear (always with an intraductal component). Also, ultrastructural studies generally confirm the great similarity between Paget cells and elements of the inner layer of the mammary ducts.[500] Thus, there is thought to be an extension of the malignant cells upward in the duct system with final infiltration of the overlying cutaneous epithelium. This theory is not unanimously accepted, and different arguments favor other sources of Paget's cells, such as malignant cells originating de novo within the epithelium of the nipple.[501] Even in the absence of microscopic evidence of the parenchymal tumor, there is a possibility that a very small focus of malignant ductal transformation is present but has escaped even a careful search. A field effect, with simultaneous primary tumors in epidermis and lactiferous ducts, is difficult to rule out, however.

The prognosis depends on the underlying mammary tumor and on the presence of metastatic regional nodes. Treatment is directed at the intraductal and/or infiltrating duct carcinoma. Primary carcinoma of the nipple is a rarity and should not be misinterpreted as Paget's disease; both basal cell and squamous carcinoma of the nipple epithelium have been described.[502]

Inflammatory Carcinoma

Inflammatory carcinoma represents the gravest and most rapidly fatal type of all mammary cancers. Luckily, it is rare.[503–507] The average duration of symptoms does not exceed a few months before the lesion becomes clinically evident. The diagnosis of inflammatory carcinoma is suggested by the clinical appearance: a large portion of the breast presents fullness, enlargement, and edema. Except for the findings encountered in Tunisia,[508] this type of carcinoma is not statistically related to pregnancy or lactation.[503] Mammography reveals an overall increased density of the breast and generalized skin thickening.

Microscopically, all the histologic varieties of carcinoma are represented in inflammatory carcinoma; the specific morphologic feature is dermal lymphatic neoplastic infiltrates accompanied by edema of the dermis and vascular dilation. The clinical features of inflammatory carcinoma are not always correlated with the presence of lymphatic tumor emboli[505] and lymphatic emboli have been reported in the absence of the clinical findings of inflammatory carcinoma.[507] Because any surgical procedure is contraindicated due to the diffuse tumoral infiltration, the diagnosis is better obtained by the less traumatic needle biopsy. The prognosis is very poor; the 5 year survival rate with surgery alone does not exceed 5 percent. However, with combined radiotherapy and chemotherapy, the current disease-free 5 year survival is in the range of 25 to 50 percent.[504]

Locally recurrent inflammatory carcinoma may present dermal lymphatic tumor emboli with or without inflammatory clinical features. Distant metastases are common.[504] Inflammatory carcinoma should not be confused with inflamed cysts, chronic subareolar disease, any true inflammatory disease of the breast, or diffuse edema and skin thickening resulting from congestive heart failure.

The Surgical Pathology Report in Cases of Breast Carcinoma

As discussed above, there are so many pathologic observations that have been reported to be of prognostic and, in many instances, therapeutic significance in breast cancer that it may become difficult for the pathologist to know which factors to mention in the final surgical pathology report. The Association of Directors of Anatomic and Surgical Pathology (ADASP), for this reason, has recommended the use of a standardized surgical pathology report and a "checklist" approach for reporting many types of cancer,[509] and they[510] and others[511] have published sample checklists for carcinoma of the breast. Table 19-9 presents the breast cancer checklist recently published by the ADASP. It should be noted that the article in which this checklist originally appeared contains an extensive discussion of the rationale behind and the specific details of various items in the checklist, and should be consulted before applying the checklist in a pathology practice.[510] Also notable is the observation that the factors reported will vary depending on the diagnosis (particularly in situ vs. invasive carcinoma) and, to a lesser extent, the type of specimen (e.g., incisional or excisional biopsy, re-excision, mastectomy) and the indication (microcalcifications, nonpalpable mass, palpable mass) for which it was obtained. It is also true that specific institutional requirements, based on consultation among the various specialists (surgeons, radiologists, radiation oncologists, medical oncologists, pathologists) participating in the care of breast cancer patients, may supplement or override the recommendations in this or any other standardized format. Nevertheless, we believe that this can at least serve as a framework on which to base a rational and complete reporting system.

Table 19-9. Breast Cancer Checklist

Name: _____			SP# _____	
Breast specimen	1. Left	2. Right		_____
	1. Excisional (for palpable mass)			
	2. Mammographic location			
	3. Incisional (includes core needle and FNA)			
	4. Re-excisional	5. Mastectomy	6. Chest wall	_____
Specimen size				_____
Tumor size(s)				_____
Tumor type				
	1. DCIS	5. Mixed NOS/ILC	9. Papillary	
	2. LCIS	6. Tubular	10. Cribriform	
	3. Infiltrating ductal (NOS)	7. Mucinous	11. Other (specify)	
	4. Infiltrating lobular	8. Medullary		_____
Grade of invasive component	1. I	2. II	3. III	_____
Gross margin	1. Free (specify distance)	2. Involved		_____
Margins invasive (specify type of margin evaluation)	1. Free (specify distance)	2. Focal	3. >Focal	4. Unevaluable _____
Margins DCIS (specify type of margin evaluation)	1. Free (specify distance)	2. Focal	3. >Focal	4. Unevaluable _____
DCIS nuclear morphology	1. High grade	2. Intermediate grade	3. Low grade	_____
DCIS patterns	1. Large area of central necrosis (comedo)			
	2. Small areas of central necrosis			
	3. Cribriform 4. Solid	5. Micropapillary 6. Papillary		
	(specify all that apply)			_____
Calcification in in situ	1. Absent	2. Prominent in DCIS	3. Focal in DCIS	
	4. In LCIS	5. Prominent in benign breast tissue		
	6. Focal in benign breast tissue			_____
Peritumoral lymphatic invasion	1. Absent	2. Present	3. Dermal	_____
Peritumoral vascular invasion	1. Absent	2. Present		_____
Extent DCIS within invasive tumor	1. Absent	2. Slight	3. Moderate-marked	
	4. Tumor primarily DCIS with focal invasion			_____
Extent DCIS adjacent to invasive tumor	1. Absent	2. Slight	3. Moderate-marked	_____
EIC status	1. EIC negative	2. EIC positive	3. EIC indeterminate	_____

Note: If a tumor is primarily DCIS with focal invasion or has a moderate or marked amount of DCIS within the infiltrating tumor and any in the adjacent tissue, it is EIC positive

Skin	1. Not sampled	2. Free	3. Invasive	4. Dermal lymphatic _____
Nipple	1. Not sampled	2. Free	3. Invasive	4. Dermal lymphatic
	5. DCIS	6. Paget's		_____
Muscle	1. Not sampled	2. Free	3. Involved	_____
Mastectomy				
Tumor location	1. Central 2. UOQ	3. UIQ	4. LOQ	5. LIQ
Multiple areas involved:	1. Central 2. UOQ	3. UIQ	4. LOQ	5. LIQ
	6. Only 1 area involved			_____
Lymph nodes (number of involved nodes in relation to total number examined)				
Total				_____
Level I				_____
Level II				_____
Level III				_____
Other (specify)				_____
Extranodal extension	1. Absent	2. Present		_____
Metastatic cancer in				_____
Nature of nontumorous breast tissue (describe)				

Comments:

Ancillary studies (results and methodology used)

Abbreviations: FNA, fine needle aspiration; DCIS, ductal carcinoma in situ; LCIS, lobular carcinoma in situ; NOS, not otherwise specified; ILC, infiltrating lobular carcinoma; EIC, extensive intraductal component; UOQ, upper outer quadrant; UIQ, upper inner quadrant; LOQ, lower outer quadrant; LIQ, lower inner quadrant. (From ADASP,[510] with permission.)

Resection Margins

The subject of resection margins in excisional biopsy or re-excision specimens is a particularly problematic one at this time. The ADASP recommends that the report should state "(1) whether sections of the margins have been taken parallel (shaved) or perpendicular to the surgical margin and (2) whether tumor is at margin (grossly or microscopically)." If tumor is not present at a margin, the distance from the closest margin should be specified.[510] The decision about how to process the specimen to examine the margins is thus left to the individual pathologist, although both the technical aspects and the significance of various distances from tumor to margin are still argued. For example, "close" margins are variably defined as less than one high power field,[512] less than or equal to 2 mm,[513] or within 1 mm,[514] and others have three groupings of less than 1, 1 to 9, and equal to or greater than 10 mm.[515] Considering additional variations in type of disease (DCIS, invasive carcinoma with an extensive intraductal component [EIC],[514] invasive carcinoma lacking EIC), treatment (with or without radiotherapy), and length of follow-up, it is no wonder that the conclusions reached on the value of examination of margins are also variable. Some authors even recommend frozen section analysis of resection margins,[516] a practice that we consider a waste of time and money. At present, we agree with the ADASP on the reporting of margins, but we realize that different clinicians may use the same results to justify different therapeutic options, and suspect that it is premature to decide which of them is correct.

Sarcomas

Sarcomas are very uncommon cancers of the breast, representing about 0.5 percent of mammary tumors.[517–520] They include all tumors originating in the mesenchymal stroma of the mammary gland. They occur in relatively elderly women and tend to undergo various types of metaplasia, which include bony and cartilaginous metaplasia and their malignant counterparts.

Fibrosarcomas and malignant fibrous histiocytomas are rapidly growing, poorly demarcated firm tumors.[521] They represent the most common mammary sarcoma unassociated with cystosarcoma phyllodes and must be distinguished from benign fibromatosis,[522] myofibroblastoma (a lesion seen primarily in male breasts),[523] metaplastic carcinoma of spindle cell type (see above), and various lesions of the subcutaneous tissue overlying the breast proper.

Microscopically, they are characterized by large bundles of fusiform cells with elongated or anaplastic hyperchromatic nuclei. The cells may be arranged in a herringbone or storiform pattern. The former was found by Jones et al[521] to be associated with a more favorable prognosis, as were low grade atypia and fewer mitoses. Isolated cases of various other sarcomas have been mentioned in the literature.[520,524,525] Osteosarcoma and chondrosarcoma must be distinguished from matrix-producing metaplastic carcinoma (see above). All of these sarcomas are characterized by hematogenous rather than lymphatic dissemination; all of them may occur postradiation,[526] and all of them must also be distinguished from malignant cystosarcoma phyllodes, in which the epithelial component may be largely replaced by sarcomatous overgrowth (see above). Thus, extensive sectioning is generally required to rule out cystosarcoma, which tends to have a more favorable prognosis.

Liposarcoma

Liposarcoma is a very unusual tumor of the breast.[527] The reported cases are large, lobulated, soft yellow tumors usually characterized by large, bizarre adipocytes and myxoid degeneration. Lymphatic and hematogenous metastases are frequent. Multiple local recurrences are observed in some cases.

Angiosarcoma

Angiosarcoma (malignant hemangioendothelioma, hemangiosarcoma) is an infrequent tumor that manifests as a rapidly growing breast mass with a blue-red discoloration of the overlying skin. It may appear in women of all ages. Microscopically, it consists of numerous irregular blood vessels in which the endothelial cells show nuclear and cytoplasmic anomalies, often separated by spindle cells. Reticulin and immunohistochemical staining confirm the endothelial location and nature of the neoplastic elements. Thrombi as well as necrotic and hemorrhagic zones are common. Hematogenous metastases are the rule. The prognosis is very poor in the high grade sarcomas but may be more favorable in the better differentiated ones[528,529] (Fig. 19-117). Mammary angiosarcoma should not be mistaken for highly vascular or acantholytic carcinoma, or for benign or malignant vascular tumors of the skin of the breast. Angiosarcomas of both the breast and the overlying skin are being reported with greater frequency in recent years after radiotherapy for breast carcinoma.[530] Although deceptively benign appearing angiosarcomas do occur, so do truly benign hemangiomas and hemangiopericytomas, which also enter into the differential diagnosis (see above). The presence of a palpable mass and of communicating vascular channels favor low grade angiosarcoma over these benign lesions.

Cytopathology of Mammary Sarcomas

As with other breast lesions, sarcomas of the breast can be diagnosed by FNAB.[531,532] Although they are rare, there are sufficient numbers of reports in the literature that define the cytomorphology of various types. Cytologically, aspirates from sarcomas are rich in cellularity and demonstrate a population of pleomorphic spindle cells with conspicuous numbers of mitoses and evidence of necrosis. Multinucleation, cytoplasmic vacuolation, and phagocytosis are common. To differentiate sarcomas of the breast from metaplastic carcinoma and carcinoma with giant cells, it is essential to use immunocytochemistry and electron microscopy. The cytopathology of sarcomas of the breast is essentially identical to that of their more common soft tissue counterparts, and is discussed in more detail in Chapter 18 of this text.

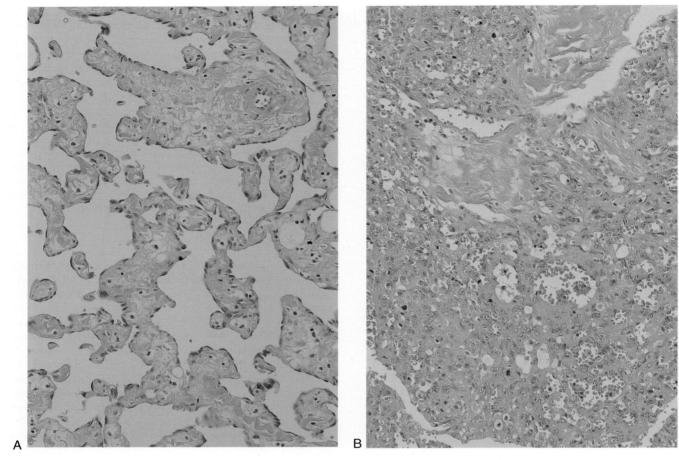

Fig. 19-117. Angiosarcoma. **(A)** Low grade focus with complex papillary architecture as the major clue to a malignant tumor; endothelial cells are increased in number but small and flat. **(B)** High grade focus in same tumor, with solid nests of anaplastic tumor cells with numerous mitotic figures.

Lymphomas and Leukemias

Different types of lymphomas and leukemic infiltrates may be observed as primary tumors of the breast. Most cases, however, represent part of the spectrum of a disseminated disease. Primary localizations manifest as a single nodule or as a diffuse infiltrative process. Microscopically, Hodgkin's disease, multiple myeloma, and various non-Hodgkin's lymphomas have been described.[533–540] The infiltrating cells extend around the ducts and lobules and infiltrate the adjacent stroma and fatty tissue (Fig. 19-118).

Lymphoid pseudotumor, or pseudolymphoma, is sometimes encountered in the breast. It is characterized microscopically by the presence of follicular germinal centers showing phagocytosis and surrounded by a lymphoid infiltrate. The follicular cells do not exhibit any cytologic alterations suspicious of a malignant tumor. Marker studies show a polyclonal population of lymphoid cells. Follow-up has been benign.[541] Lymphocytic mastopathy (see above) is also in the differential diagnosis.

Lymphoid and hematopoietic tumors must also be distinguished from infiltrating lobular carcinomas, which can also infiltrate as noncohesive small round cells. Signet ring cells with

intracellular lumina are a useful marker of lobular carcinoma. If there is any doubt, immunohistochemical staining for epithelial and leukocytic/lymphoid markers will provide the answer.

Cytologically, fine needle aspirates from malignant lymphoma of the breast, whether primary or secondary, present with a cellular sample. The tumor cells appear in a dispersed pattern and lymphoglandular bodies are seen in the background (Fig. 19-119). The cytomorphology of breast lymphoma varies according to the histologic subtype of the lesion (see Ch. 20). It ranges from a uniform monotonous cell population to a pleomorphic population of atypical lymphoid cells.

An incorrect diagnosis of carcinoma may result in unnecessary surgery, since the treatment of lymphoma is chemotherapy and/or radiotherapy. By contrast, a false negative diagnosis of chronic mastitis or fat necrosis may delay appropriate treatment. In the absence of a clinical history of a generalized lymphoma, the presence of lymphoid cells in breast aspirates may be misinterpreted as chronic mastitis, fat necrosis, medullary carcinoma, duct cell carcinoma with lymphocytic infiltration, carcinoid tumor, or primary or metastatic small cell carcinoma. Reactive processes such as Rosai-Dorfman disease, as well as unremarkable intramammary lymph nodes, can also yield a cel-

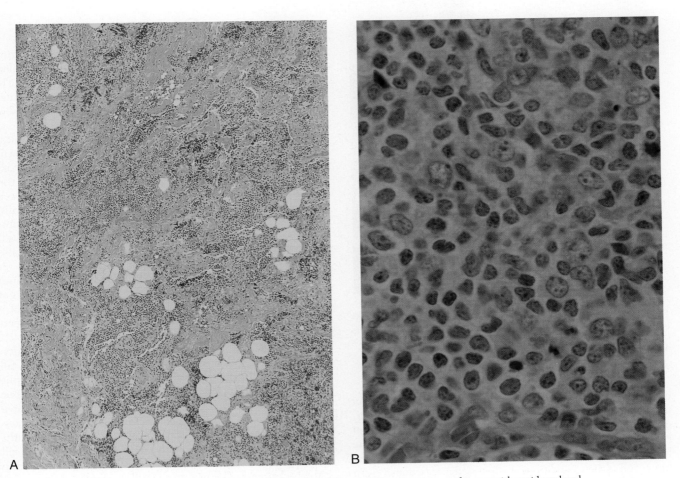

Fig. 19-118. Lymphoma of breast. **(A)** Compare diffusely infiltrative pattern of tumor with periductal and perilobular distribution of lymphocytic mastopathy (Fig. 19-6). **(B)** Detail showing lymphoid features of malignant cells.

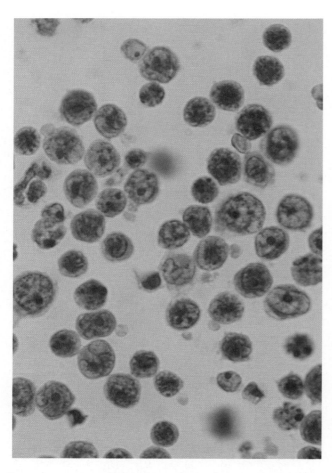

Fig. 19-119. Smear of high grade lymphoma of the breast. Sheet-like pattern of atypical lymphoid cells with high nucleocytoplasmic ratio, chromatin clumping, and conspicuous nucleoli. (Papanicolaou stain, × 400.)

lular aspirate consisting of lymphoid cells.[542] The diagnosis of malignant lymphoma is therefore usually established by immunocytochemistry and/or flow cytometry. Rare cases of Hodgkin's disease[538] and leukemic cell infiltrates[539] of the breast have also been diagnosed by FNAB; the cytologic features of all of these conditions are discussed more extensively in Chapter 20.

Metastatic Tumors

Metastatic tumors to the breast are rare.[540,543–545] Clinically, the lesion is indistinguishable from a primary tumor. The most frequent neoplasms reported (after carcinoma of the opposite breast) are melanomas, lymphomas (discussed above), carcinoma of the stomach, carcinoma of the ovary, and tumors of the nasopharyngeal region. The recognition of the metastatic nature of such lesions is important to avoid unnecessary radical surgical procedures. Usually metastatic nodules exhibit a sharp transition at the periphery with the normal breast tissue and do not reveal any in situ component. They often occur in subcuta-

neous tissue rather than in mammary parenchyma. Cytologically, metastases vary according to the primary tumor; adenocarcinomas may be difficult to distinguish from primary breast cancers.[540]

PATHOLOGIC CONDITIONS OF THE MALE BREAST

Gynecomastia

Enlargement of the male breast can occur at any time during life. During adolescence, such enlargements are generally bilateral and temporary. This temporary hypertrophy may be due to some hormonal stimulation, which usually regresses spontaneously after a few months. An increase in the plasma estradiol level has been reported in these cases.

In adults, gynecomastia is associated with various clinical conditions that will be mentioned only briefly: Cushing's syndrome; Klinefelter's syndrome; chronic liver disease; thyrotoxicosis; hypogonadism; feminizing adrenal tumors; various testicular tumors with or without steroid production; estrogen therapy; and other iatrogenic causes, such as digitalis, chemotherapeutic agents (busulfan, vincristine), and phenothiazine or other tranquilizers. It has been reported in heroin addicts and in cannabis smokers. An idiopathic origin has also been reported.[546–548] Cystosarcoma phyllodes has been reported in a case of gynecomastia,[549] as have sclerosing adenosis[550] and other fibrocystic changes[551] as well as many cases of carcinoma. Microscopically, the hypertrophy consists of a dense stromal proliferation accompanied by a variable hyperplasia of the lactiferous ducts.

Cytologically, gynecomastia shows variable cellularity. Monolayered, well organized sheets of small uniform cells, tall columnar cells, and bare nuclei are commonly seen. Apocrine metaplasia, macrophages, tissue fragments, and adipose tissue may also be present.[552,553] Gynecomastia may be associated with atypical proliferative changes and closely resemble noncomedo type DCIS and create diagnostic difficulty. Similarly, gynecomastia may occasionally show a loosely cohesive cell arrangement with atypical single epithelial cells scattered in the background. The presence of tall columnar cells may contribute to misinterpretation of the lesion as papillary carcinoma. Extreme care should be exercised to limit the diagnosis of carcinoma in a male breast to cases in which the aspirate is highly cellular and shows the obvious cytologic features of a malignant tumor.

Differential Diagnosis

Gynecomastia should not be mistaken for pseudogynecomastia, which is observed in obese patients and which consists of an adipose infiltration of the gland without epithelial or stromal proliferation.

Senescent gynecomastia appears in men over age 60; it may be unilateral or bilateral. Spontaneous regression usually occurs within a few months. A unilateral lesion should not be con-

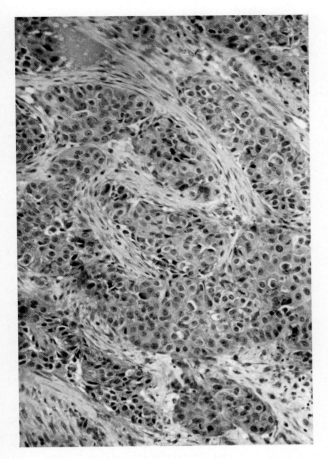

Fig. 19-120. Infiltrating duct carcinoma in a male breast.

fused with carcinoma. Microscopically, the lesion is characterized by dense fibrous proliferation with a few scattered remaining ducts.

Carcinoma of the Male Breast

Rare in those under 30 years of age, carcinoma of the breast in men arises at a later age than in women and is approximately 100 times less frequent than carcinoma of the female breast. It is more frequent in certain parts of the world such as Egypt, where it is related to chronic liver disease secondary to schistosomiasis. Hormonal factors play a probable causal role in fewer cases than in women, and radiation exposure and genetic factors may therefore be more important.[554-556] An association with Klinefelter's syndrome has been noted,[557] as well as with gynecomastia[558] and with prostatic carcinoma. The last of these associations is difficult to evaluate because of both the use of estrogens to treat prostate cancer[559] and the likelihood of prostate cancer to metastasize to the breast, where it may be confused with primary breast cancer.[560] All the histologic types of carcinoma encountered in the female breast may be seen in the male breast, but they often exhibit poorer differentiation. Familial cases have been reported.[561]

Infiltrating duct carcinoma is the most common type, but all types of carcinoma have been reported (Fig. 19-120). Their cytologic appearance is as expected.[552,553] Grossly, the tumor infiltrates the small mammary gland, as well as the skin and the pectoral fascia. Ulceration of the overlying skin is common. The prognosis is poor, probably because the small volume of the breast increases the likelihood of skin and nipple involvement, with invasion of dermal lymphatics and early metastatic spread.[562] c-erbB-2 positivity has been reported as related to prognosis,[562] but ploidy and receptor status may not be.[562,563] ERs and PRs are present in an even higher percentage than in female patients.[562,564] Treatment in most reported series has been radical mastectomy with adjuvant radiotherapy and chemotherapy.

REFERENCES

1. Wingo PA, Tong T, Bolden S: Cancer statistics, 1995. CA Cancer J Clin 45:8–30, 1995
2. Harris JR, Lippman ME, Morrow M, Hellman S (eds): Diseases of the Breast. Lippincott-Raven, Philadelphia, 1996
3. Bland KI, Copeland EM III (eds): The Breast: Comprehensive Management of Benign and Malignant Diseases. WB Saunders, Philadelphia, 1991
4. Propper A: Etude experimentale des premiers stades de la morphogenese mammaire. Ann Biol 9:267, 1970
5. Page AL, Anderson TJ: Stages of breast development. pp. 11–29. In: Diagnostic Histopathology of the Breast. Churchill Livingstone, Edinburgh, 1987
6. McCarty KS Jr, Tucker JA: Breast. pp. 893–902. In Sternberg SS (ed): Histology for Pathologists, Lippincott-Raven, Philadelphia, 1992
7. Ozzello L: Ultrastructure of the human mammary gland. Pathol Ann 6:1–60, 1971
8. Ahmed A: Atlas of the Ultrastructure of Human Breast Diseases. Churchill Livingstone, Edinburgh, 1978
9. Forsyth IA: The mammary gland. Baillieres Clin Endocrinol Metab 5:809–832, 1991
10. Vogel PM, Georgiade NG, Fetter BF, et al: The correlation of histologic changes in the human breast with the menstrual cycle. Am J Pathol 104:23–34, 1981
11. Kramer WM, Rush BF Jr: Mammary duct proliferation in the elderly. A histopathologic study. Cancer 31:130, 1973
12. Smith DM Jr, Peters TG, Donegan WL: Montgomery's areolar tubercle: a light microscopic study. Arch Pathol Lab Med 106:60–63, 1982
13. Halsell JT, Smith JR, Bentlage CR, et al: Lymphatic drainage of the breast demonstrated by vital dye staining and radiography. Ann Surg 162:221–226, 1965
14. Turner-Warwick RT: The lymphatics of the breast. Br J Surg 46:574–582, 1979
15. Egan RL, McSweeney MB: Intramammary lymph nodes. Cancer 51:1838–1842, 1983
16. Strombeck JO: Macromastia in women and its surgical treatment. A clinical study based on 1042 cases. Acta Chir Scand, suppl. 341:1–129, 1964
17. Esteban JM, Zaloudek C, Silverberg SG: Intraoperative diagnosis of breast lesions: comparison of cytologic with frozen section technics. Am J Clin Pathol 88:681–688, 1987
18. Mair S, Lash RH, Suskin D, Mendelsohn G: Intraoperative surgical specimen evaluation: frozen section analysis, cytologic examination, or both? A comparative study of 206 cases. Am J Clin Pathol 96:8–14, 1991

19. Ashikari R, Huvos AG, Snyder RE: Prospective study of noninfiltrating carcinoma of the breast. Cancer 39:435, 1977

20. Oberman HA: A modest proposal. Am J Surg Pathol 16:69–70, 1992

21. Association of Directors of Anatomic and Surgical Pathology: Immediate management of mammographically detected breast lesions. Am J Surg Pathol 17:850–851, 1993

22. Schnitt SJ, Wang HH: Histologic sampling of grossly benign breast biopsies: how much is enough? Am J Surg Pathol 13:505–512, 1989

23. Owings DV, Hann L, Schnitt SJ: How thoroughly should needle localization breast biopsies be sampled for microscopic examination? A prospective mammographic/pathologic correlative study. Am J Surg Pathol 14:578–583, 1990

24. Lester SC, Richardson A: Routine methods for examining mastectomy specimens: optimizing diagnostic/prognostic information and minimizing cost. Mod Pathol 9:19A, 1996

25. Lagios MD, Bennington JL: Protocol for the pathologic examination and tissue processing of the mammographically directed breast biopsy. pp. 23–46. In Bennington JL, Lagios MD (eds): The Mammographically Directed Biopsy. Hanley & Belfus, Philadelphia, 1992

26. Schnitt SJ, Connolly JL: Processing and evaluation of breast excision specimens: a clinically oriented approach. Am J Clin Pathol 98:125–137, 1992

27. Lagios MD: Pathologic examination and tissue processing for the mammographically directed biopsy. California Society of Pathologist, San Francisco, December 3, 1987

28. Stock RJ, Kunschner A, Mazer J, Murphy A: Mammographic localization and biopsy: the experience of a gynecologic oncology group. Gynecol Oncol 33:172–176, 1989

29. Bassett LW, Kimme-Smith C: Breast sonography. AJR 156:449–455, 1991

30. Baker KS, Davey DD, Stelling CB: Ductal abnormalities detected with galactography: frequency of adequate excisional biopsy. AJR of 162:821, 1994

31. Adler DD, Wahl RL: New methods for imaging the breast: techniques, findings, and potential. AJR 164:19, 1995

32. Martin HE, Ellis EB: Biopsy of needle puncture and aspiration. Ann Surg 92:169–181, 1930

33. Lannin DR, Silverman JF, Walker C, Pories WJ: Cost-effectiveness of fine needle aspiration of the breast. Ann Surg 203:474–480, 1986

34. Donegan WL: Evaluation of a palpable mass. N Engl J Med 327:937–942, 1992

35. Masood S: Fine needle aspiration biopsy of nonpalpable breast lesions. pp. 33–63. In Schmidt W (ed): Cytopathology Annual 1994. American Society of Clinical Pathologists Press, Chicago, 1994

36. Frable WJ: Needle aspiration biopsy: past, present and future. Hum Pathol 20:504–517, 1989

37. Hammond S, Keyhani-Rofagha S, O'Toole RV: Statistical analysis of fine needle aspiration cytology of the breast. A review of 678 cases plus 4265 cases from the literature. Acta Cytol 31:276–280, 1989

38. Pennes DR, Naylor B, Rebner M: Fine needle aspiration biopsy of the breast: influence of the number of passes and the sample size of the diagnostic yield. Acta Cytol 34:673–676, 1990

39. Patel TJ, Gartell PC, Smallwood JA, et al: Fine needle aspiration cytology of breast masses. An evaluation of its accuracy and reasons for diagnostic failure. Ann R Coll Surg Eng 69:156–159, 1987

40. Giard RWM, Hermans J: Fine needle aspiration cytology of the breast with immediate reporting of the results. Acta Cytol 37:358–360, 1993

41. Kline TS: Survey of aspiration biopsy cytology of the breast. Diagn Cytopathol 7:98–105, 1991

42. Sneige N: Fine needle aspiration of the breast: a review of 1995 cases with emphasis on diagnostic pitfalls. Diagn Cytopathol 9:106–112, 1993

43. Dowlatshahi K, Gent HJ, Schmidt R, et al: Nonpalpable breast tumors: diagnosis with stereotaxic localization and fine needle aspiration. Radiology 170:427–433, 1989

44. Layfield L, Parkinson B, Wong J, et al: Mammographically guided fine needle aspiration biopsy of nonpalpable breast lesions. Can it replace open biopsy? Cancer 68:2007–2011, 1991

45. Ulanow R, Galblum L, Carter JW: Fine needle aspiration in the diagnosis and management of solid breast lesions. Am J Surg 148:653–657, 1984

46. Kline TS: Masquerades of malignancy. A review of 4241 aspirates from the breast. Acta Cytol 25:263–266, 1981

47. Stanley MW, Tani EM, Skoog L: Fine needle aspiration of fibroadenomas of the breast with atypia. Spectrum including cases that cytologically mimic carcinoma. Diagn Cytopathol 6:375–382, 1990

48. Feldman PS, Corell JL: Fine Needle Cytology and Its Clinical Applications: Breast and Lung. American Society of Clinical Pathologists Press, Chicago, 1985

49. Hermansen C, Paulsen HS, Jensen J, et al: Diagnostic reliability of combined physical examinations, mammography, and fine needle puncture ("Triple-test") in breast tumors. Cancer 60:1866–1871, 1987

50. Silverman JF, Lannin DR, O'Brain K, Norris HT: The triage role of fine needle aspiration biopsy of palpable breast masses. Diagnostic accuracy and cost-effectiveness. Acta Cytol 31:731–736, 1987

51. Sneige N: A comparison of fine-needle aspiration, core biopsy, and needle localization biopsy techniques in mammographically detectable nonpalpable breast lesions. Pathol Case Rev 1:6–11, 1996

52. Agnantis NJ, Apostolikas N, Christodoulou I, et al: The reliability of frozen-section diagnosis in various breast lesions: a study based on 3451 biopsies. Recent results. Cancer Res 90:205, 1984

53. Fessia L, Ghiringhello R, Arisio R, et al: Accuracy of frozen section diagnosis in breast cancer detection. A review of 4436 biopsies and comparison with cytodiagnosis. Pathol Res Pract 179:61, 1984

54. Oneson RH, Minke JA, Silverberg SG: Intraoperative pathologic consultation: an audit of 1,000 recent consecutive cases. Am J Surg Pathol 13:237–243, 1989

55. Robbins GF, Bros ST: The significance of delay in relation to prognosis of patients with primary operable breast cancer. Cancer 10:338, 1957

56. Thomsen AC, Espersen T, Maigaard S: Course and treatment of milk stasis, noninfectious inflammation of the breast and infectious mastitis in nursing women. Am J Obstet Gynecol 149:492–495, 1984

57. Patey DH, Thackray AC: Pathology and treatment of mammary duct fistula. Lancet 2:871, 1958

58. Schwartz IS, Strauchen JA: Lymphocytic mastopathy: an autoimmune disease of the breast? Am J Clin Pathol 93:725–730, 1990

59. Tomaszewski JE, Brooks JSJ, Hicks D, LiVolsi VA: Diabetic mastopathy: a distinctive clinicopathologic entity. Hum Pathol 23:780–786, 1992

60. Aozasa K, Ohsawa M, Saeki K, et al: Malignant lymphoma of the breast: immunologic type and association with lymphocytic mastopathy. Am J Clin Pathol 97:699–704, 1992

61. Gupta RK, McHutchinson AGR, Dowle CS, Simpson JS: Fine needle aspiration cytodiagnosis of breast masses in pregnant and lactating women and its impact on management. Diagn Cytopathol 9:156–159, 1993

62. Gita J: Cytomorphology of tuberculosis mastitis. A report of nine cases with fine needle aspiration cytology. Acta Cytol 29:974–978, 1985

63. Whitaker HT, Moore RM: Gumma of the breast. Surg Gynecol Obstet 98:473–477, 1954

64. Banik S, Bishop PW, Ormerod LP, O'Brien TE: Sarcoidosis of the breast. J Clin Pathol 39:446–448, 1986

65. Donn W, Rebbeck P, Wilson C, Gilks B: Idiopathic granulomatous mastitis. A report of three cases and review of the literature. Arch Pathol Lab Med 118:822–825, 1994

66. Meyer JE, Silverman P, Gandbhir L: Fat necrosis of breast. Arch Surg 113:801–805, 1978

67. Clarke D, Curtis JL, Martinez A, et al: Fat necrosis of the breast simulating recurrent carcinoma after primary radiotherapy in the management of early stage breast carcinoma. Cancer 52:442–445, 1983

68. Adair FE: Plasma cell mastitis; a lesion simulating mammary carcinoma; a clinical and pathologic study with a report of ten cases. Arch Surg 26:735, 1933

69. Macansh S, Greenberg M, Barraclough B, Pacey F: Fine needle aspiration cytology of granulomatous mastitis. Report of a case and review of the literature. Acta Cytol 34:38–42, 1990

70. Catania S, Zurrida S, Veronesi P, et al: Mondor's disease and breast cancer. Cancer 69:2267–2270, 1992

71. Raven RW: Paraffinoma of the breast. Clin Oncol 7:157–161, 1981

72. Cook RR, Delongchamp RR, Woodbury M, et al: The prevalence of women with breast implants in the United States—1989. J Clin Epidemiol 48:519–525, 1995

73. Mann RD: Breast implants: the tyranny of the anecdote. J Clin Epidemiol 48:504–506, 1995

74. Kasper CS: Histologic features of breast capsules reflect surface configuration and composition of silicone bag implants. J Clin Pathol 102:655–659, 1994

75. Raso DS, Crymes LW, Metcalf JS: Histological assessment of fifty breast capsules from smooth and textured augmentation and reconstruction mammoplasty prostheses with emphasis on the role of synovial metaplasia. Mod Pathol 7:310–316, 1994

76. Chase DR, Oberg KC, Chase RL, et al: Pseudoepithelialization of breast implant capsules. Int J Surg Pathol 1:151–154, 1994

77. CAP Surgical Pathology Committee: Recommendation for the handling of prosthetic breast implants. CAP Today 8:28, 1994

78. Robitaille Y, Seemayer TA, Thelmo WL, et al: Infarction of the mammary region mimicking carcinoma of the breast. Cancer 33:1183–1189, 1974

79. Flint A, Oberman HA: Infarction and squamous metaplasia of intraductal papilloma: a benign breast lesion that may simulate carcinoma. Hum Pathol 15:764–767, 1984

80. Page DL, Vander Zwaag R, Rogers LW, et al: Relation between component parts of fibrocystic disease complex and breast cancer. J Natl Cancer Inst 61:1055, 1978

81. Vorheer H: Fibrocystic breast disease: pathophysiology, pathomorphology, clinical picture and management. Am J Obstet Gynecol 154:161–179, 1986

82. Hutter RVP: Goodbye to "fibrocystic disease." N Engl J Med 312:179–181, 1985

83. Love SM, Gelman RS, Sclen W: "Fibrocystic disease" of the breast: a non-disease? N Engl J Med 307:1010–1014, 1982

84. Black MM, Barclay TH, Cutler SJ, et al: Association of atypical characteristics of benign breast lesions with subsequent risk of breast cancer. Cancer 29:383, 1977

85. Wellings SR, Jensen HM, Marcum RG: An atlas of subgross pathology of the human breast with special reference to possible precancerous lesions. J Natl Cancer Inst 55:231, 1975

86. Page DL, Dupont WD, Rogers LW, et al: Atypical hyperplastic lesions of the female breast: a long-term follow-up study. Cancer 55:2698–2708, 1985

87. Page DL, Dupont WD: Anatomic markers of human premalignancy and risk of breast cancer. Cancer 66:1326–1335, 1990

88. Dupont WD, Parl FF, Hartmann WH, et al: Breast cancer risk associated with proliferative breast disease and atypical hyperplasia. Cancer 71:1258–1265, 1993

89. Lagios MD: Human breast precancer: current status. Cancer Surv 2:383, 1977

90. van Bogaert LJ: The proliferative behavior of the human adult mammary epithelium. Acta Cytol 23:252–257, 1979

91. Fechner RE, Mills SE: Breast Pathology: Benign Proliferations, Atypias, and In Situ Carcinomas. pp. 89–106. ASCP Press, Chicago, 1990

92. Eusebi V, Foschini MP, Betts CM, et al: Microglandular adenosis, apocrine adenosis, and tubular carcinoma of the breast. An immunohistochemical comparison. Am J Surg Pathol 17:99–109, 1993

93. Tavassoli FA, Norris HJ: Microglandular adenosis of the breast: a clinicopathologic study of 11 cases with ultrastructural observations. Am J Surg Pathol 7:731–737, 1983

94. Rosenblum MK, Purrazella R, Rosen PP: Is microglandular adenosis a precancerous disease? A study of carcinoma arising therein. Am J Surg Pathol 10:237–245, 1986

95. Popper HH, Gallagher JV, Ralph G, et al: Breast carcinoma arising in microglandular adenosis: a tumor expressing S-100 immunoreactivity. Report of five cases. Breast J 2:154–159, 1996

96. Oberman HA: Benign breast lesions confused with carcinoma. p. 1. In McDivitt RW, Oberman HA, Ozzello L, Kaufman N (eds): The Breast. Williams & Wilkins, Baltimore, 1984

97. Nielsen BD: Adenosis tumor of the breast: a clinicopathological investigation of 27 cases. Histopathology 11:1259–1275, 1987

98. Martinez-Hernandez A, Francis DJ, Silverberg SG: Elastosis and other stromal reactions in benign and malignant breast tissue. An ultrastructural study. Cancer 40:700, 1977

99. Taylor HB, Norris HJ: Epithelial invasion of nerves in benign diseases of the breast. Cancer 20:2245, 1967

100. Jensen RA, Page DL, Dupont WD, Rogers LW: Invasive breast cancer risk in women with sclerosing adenosis. Cancer 64:1977–1983, 1989

101. McDivitt RW, Stevens JA, Lee NC, et al: Histologic types of benign breast disease and the risk for breast cancer. Cancer 69:1408–1414, 1992

102. Wellings SR, Alpers CE: Apocrine cystic metaplasia: subgross pathology and prevalence in cancer-associated versus random autopsy breasts. Hum Pathol 18:381, 1987

103. Murad TM, von Haam E: The ultrastructure of fibrocystic disease of the breast. Cancer 22:587, 1968

104. Andersen JA, Carter D, Linell F: A symposium on sclerosing duct lesions of the breast. Pathol Annu 21:145–179, 1986

105. Nielsen M, Christensen L, Andersen JA: Radial scars in women with breast cancer. Cancer 59:1019–1025, 1987

106. Raju U, Crissman JD, Zarbo RJ, Gottlieb C: Epitheliosis of the breast. An immunohistochemical characterization and comparison to malignant intraductal proliferations of the breast. Am J Surg Pathol 14:939–947, 1990

107. Rickert RR, Kalisher L, Hutter RVP: Indurative mastopathy: a benign sclerosing lesion of breast with elastosis which may simulate carcinoma. Cancer 47:561, 1981

108. Fenoglio C, Lattes R: Sclerosing papillary proliferations in the female breast. Cancer 33:691, 1974

109. Carter D: Interpretation of Breast Biopsies. 3rd Ed. pp. 133–139. Lippincott-Raven, Philadelphia, 1996

110. Rosai J: Borderline epithelial lesions of the breast. Am J Surg Pathol 15:209–221, 1991

111. Schnitt SJ, Connolly JL, Tavassoli FA, et al: Interobserver reproducibility in the diagnosis of ductal proliferative breast lesions using standardized criteria. Am J Surg Pathol 16:1133–1143, 1992

112. Micale MA, Visscher DW, Gulino SE, Wolman SR: Chromosomal aneuploidy in proliferative breast disease. Hum Pathol 25:29–35, 1994

113. Visscher DW: Biomarkers of proliferative breast disease. Breast J 1:222–227, 1995

114. Walker RA: The pathology of "precancerous" breast disease. Pathol Annu 29:75–98, 1994

115. Zhuang Z, Nayar R, Merino MJ, Silverberg SG: Loss of heterozygosity (LOH) on chromosome 11q13 in lobular lesions (ALH, LCIS, ILC) of the breast using tissue microdissection and polymerase chain reaction (PCR). Mod Pathol 9:27A, 1996

116. Marshall CJ, Schumann GB, Ward JH, et al: Cytologic identification

of clinically occult proliferative breast disease in women with a family history of breast cancer. Am J Clin Pathol 95:157–165, 1991

117. Fabian CJ, Zalles C, Kamel S, et al: Biomarker and cytologic abnormalities in women at high and low risk for breat cancer. J Cell Biochem 176:152–160, 1993

118. Masood S: Standardization of immunoassays as surrogate endpoints. J Cell Biochem 19:28–35, 1994

119. Masood S, Frykberg ER, McLellan GL, et al: Prospective evaluation of radiologically detected fine needle aspiration biopsy of nonpalpable breast lesions. Cancer 66:1480–1487, 1990

120. Masood S, Frykberg ER, McLellan GL, et al: Cytologic differentiation between proliferative and nonproliferative breast disease in mammographically guided fine-needle aspirates. Diagn Cytopathol 7:581–590, 1991

121. Dziura BR, Bonfiglio TA: Needle cytology of the breast. Acta Cytol 23:332–340, 1979

122. Bibbo M, Scheiber M, Cajulis R, et al: Stereotaxic fine needle aspiration cytology of occult malignant and premalignant breast lesions. Acta Cytol 32:193–201, 1988

123. Masood S, Hardy NM, Assaf N, Lu L: Cytologic grading system in diagnosis of high risk and malignant breast lesions: merits and pitfalls. Acta Cytol 38:797–798, 1994

124. Sneige N, Staerkel GA: Fine needle aspiration cytology of ductal hyperplasia with and without atypia and ductal carcinoma in situ. Hum Pathol 25:485–492, 1994

125. Silverman J, Masood S, Ductaman BS, et al: Can FNA biopsy separate atypical hyperplasia, carcinoma in situ, and invasive carcinoma of the breast? Cytomorphologic criteria and limitations in diagnosis. Diagn Cytopathol 9:713–728, 1993

126. Abendroth CS, Wang HH, Ducatman BS: Comparative features of carcinoma in situ and atypical ductal hyperplasia of the breast on fine needle aspiration biopsy: Am J Clin Pathol 96:654–659, 1991

127. Shiels LA, Mulford D, Dawson AG: Cytomorphology of proliferative breast disease, abstracted. Acta Cytol 37:768, 1993

128. Stanley MW, Henry-Stanley MJ, Zera R: Prospective study of high risk proliferative lesions of breast duct epithelium by fine needle aspiration, abstracted. Acta Cytol 35:611, 1991

129. Lennington WJ, Jensen RA, Dalton LW, Page DL: Ductal carcinoma in situ of the breast: heterogeneity of individual lesions. Cancer 73:118–124, 1994

130. Fechner RE: Fibroadenomas in patients receiving oral contraceptives. A clinical and pathologic study. Am J Clin Pathol 53:857–864, 1970

131. Noguchi S, Aihara T, Koyama H, et al: Clonal analysis of benign and malignant human breast tumors by means of polymerase chain reaction. Cancer Lett 90:57–63, 1995

132. Carney JA, Toorkey BC: Myxoid fibroadenoma and allied conditions (myxomatosis) of the breast: a heritable disorder with special associations including cardiac and cutaneous myxomas. Am J Surg Pathol 15:713–721, 1991

133. Yeh IT, Francis DI, Orenstein JM, Silverberg SG: Ultrastructure of cystosarcoma phyllodes and fibroadenoma. A comparative study. Am J Clin Pathol 84:131–136, 1985

134. Jao W, Vasquez LT, Keh PC, et al: Myoepithelial differentiation and basal lamina deposition in fibroadenoma and adenosis of the breast. J Pathol 126:107, 1978

135. O'Hara MF, Page DL: Adenomas of the breast and ectopic breast under lactational influences. Hum Pathol 16:707–712, 1985

136. Rickert RR, Rajan S: Localized breast infarcts associated with pregnancy. Arch Pathol 97:159, 1975

137. Eusebi V, Azzopardi JG: Lobular endocrine neoplasia in fibroadenoma of the breast. Histopathology 4:413, 1986

138. Diaz NM, Palmer JO, McDivitt RW: Carcinoma arising within fibroadenomas of the breast. Am J Clin Pathol 95:614–622, 1991

139. Dupont WD, Page DL, Parl FF, et al: Long-term risk of breast cancer in women with fibroadenoma. N Engl J Med 331:10–15, 1994

140. Linsk JA, Kreuzer G, Zajicek J: Cytologic diagnosis of mammary tumors from aspiration biopsy smears—II. Studies on 210 fibroadenomas and 210 cases of benign dysplasia. Acta Cytol 16:130–138, 1972

141. Bottles K, Chan JS, Holly EA, et al: Cytologic criteria for fibroadenoma: a stepwise logistic regression analysis. Am J Clin Pathol 89:707–713, 1988

142. Chen KTK: Aspiration cytology of breast fibroadenoma with atypia. Diagn Cytopathol 82:283–288, 1992

143. Rogers LA, Lee KR: Breast carcinoma simulating fibroadenoma or fibrocystic change by fine needle aspiration. A study of 16 cases. Am J Clin Pathol 98:155–160, 1992

144. Masood S, Lu L, Assaf-Munasif N, McCaulley K: Application of immunostaining for muscle specific actin detection of myoepithelial cells in breast fine needle aspirates. Diagn Cytopathol 13:71–74, 1995

145. Fischler D, Sneige N, Ordonez N, Fornage B: Tubular cancer of the breast (TBC): cytological features in fine needle aspiration and application of monoclonal anti-α smooth muscle actin in diagnosis. Diagn Cytopathol 10:120–125, 1994

146. Deitos AP, Grustina DD, Martin DV, et al: Aspiration biopsy cytology of tubular carcinoma of the breast. Diagn Cytopathol 11:146–150, 1994

147. Gupta RK, Simpson J: Carcinoma of the breast in a fibroadenoma: diagnosis by fine needle aspiration cytology. Diagn Cytopathol 7:60–62, 1991

148. Pike AM, Oberman HA: Juvenile cellular adenofibromas. a clinicopathologic study. Am J Surg Pathol 9:730–736, 1985

149. Mies C, Rosen PP: Juvenile fibroadenoma with atypical epithelial hyperplasia. Am J Surg Pathol 11:184–190, 1987

150. Rosen PP, Oberman HA: Tumors of the mammary gland. pp. 67–72. In: Atlas of Tumor Pathology, Third Series, Fascicle 7. Armed Forces Institute of Pathology, Washington DC, 1993

151. Hertel BF, Zaloudek C, Kempson RL: Breast adenomas. Cancer 37:2891–2905, 1976

152. Willen R, Uvelius B, Camaron R: Pleomorphic adenoma in the breast of a human female. Aspiration biopsy findings and receptor determination. Case report. Acta Clin Scand 152:709–713, 1986

153. Diaz NM, McDivitt RW, Wick MR: Pleomorphic adenoma of the breast: a clinicopathologic and immunohistochemical study of 10 cases. Hum Pathol 22:1206–1214, 1991

154. Narita T, Matsuda K: Pleomorphic adenoma of the breast: case report and review of the literature. Pathol Int 45:441–447, 1995

155. Azzopardi JG, Salm R: Ductal adenoma of the breast: a lesion which can mimic carcinoma. J Pathol 144:15–23, 1984

156. Lammie GA, Willis RR: Ductal adenoma of the breast. A review of fifteen cases. Human Pathol 20:903–908, 1989

157. Gupta RK, McHutchinson AGR, Dowle CS, Simpson JS: Fine needle aspiration cytodiagnosis of breast masses in pregnant and lactating women and its impact on management. Diagn Cytopathol 9:156–159, 1993

158. Grenko RT, Lee KP, Lee KR: Fine needle aspiration cytology of lactating adenoma of the breast: a comparative light and morphometric study. Acta Cytol 34:21–26, 1990

159. Novotny DB, Maygarden SJ, Shermar RW, Frable WJ: Fine needle aspiration of benign and malignant breast masses associated with pregnancy. Acta Cytol 35:678–686, 1991

160. Finley JL, Silverman JF, Lannin DR: Fine needle aspiration cytology of breast masses in pregnant and lactating women. Diagn Cytopathol 5:255–259, 1989

161. Diaz NM, Palmer JO, Wick MR: Erosive adenomatosis of the nipple: histology, immunohistology, and differential diagnosis. Mod Pathol 5:179–184, 1992

162. Rosen PP, Caicco JA: Florid papillomatosis of the nipple: a study of 51 patients including nine with mammary carcinoma. Am J Surg Pathol 10:87–101, 1986

163. Jones MW, Tavassoli FA: Coexistence of nipple duct adenoma and

breast carcinoma: a clinicopathologic study of five cases and review of the literature. Mod Pathol 8:633–636, 1995

164. Jones MW, Norris HJ, Snyder RC: Infiltrating syringomatous adenoma of the nipple: a clinical and pathological study of 11 cases. Am J Surg Pathol 13:197–201, 1989

165. Mazzara PF, Flint A, Naylor B: Adenoma of the nipple: cytopathologic features. Acta Cytol 33:188–190, 1989

166. Rosen PP: Adenomyoepithelioma of the breast. Hum Pathol 18:1232–1237, 1987

167. Loose JH, Patchefsky AS, Hollander IJ, et al: Adenomyoepithelioma of the breast. A spectrum of biologic behavior. Am J Surg Pathol 16:868–876, 1992

168. Tavassoli FA: Myoepithelial lesions of the breast: myoepitheliosis, adenomyoepithelioma, and myoepithelial carcinoma. Am J Surg Pathol 15:554–568, 1991

169. Vielh P, Thiery JP, Validire P, et al: Adenomyoepithelioma of the breast: fine needle sampling with histologic, immunologic and electron microscopic analysis. Diagn Cytopathol 9:188–193, 1993

170. Oberman HA: Hamartomas and hamartoma variants of the breast. Semin Diagn Pathol 6:135–145, 1989

171. Davies JD, Kulka J, Mumford AD, et al: Hamartomas of the breast: six novel diagnostic features in three-dimensional thick sections. Histopathology 24:161–168, 1994

172. Daya D, Trus T, D'Souza TJ, et al: Hamartoma of the breast, an underrecognized breast lesion. A clinicopathologic and radiographic study of 25 cases. Am J Clin Pathol 103:685–689, 1995

173. Carter D: Intraductal papillary tumors of the breast. A study of 78 cases. Cancer 39:1689–1692, 1977

174. Murad TM, Contesso G, Mouriesse H: Papillary tumors of the large lactiferous ducts. Cancer 48:122–133, 1981

175. Kraus FT, Neubecker RD: The differential diagnosis of papillary tumors of the breast. Cancer 15:444–455, 1962

176. Papotti M, Gugliotta P, Ghiringello B, Bussolati G: Association of breast carcinoma and multiple intraductal papillomas: an histological and immunohistochemical investigation. Histopathology 8:963, 1984

177. Raju UB, Lee MW, Zarbo RJ, Crissman JD: Papillary neoplasia of the breast: immunohistochemically defined myoepithelial cells in the diagnosis of benign and malignant papillary breast neoplasms. Mod Pathol 2:569–576, 1989

178. Masood S, Lu L, Assaf-Munasifi N, et al: Application of immunostaining for muscle specific actin in detection of myoepithelial cells in breast fine needle aspirates. Diagn Cytopathol 13:71–74, 1995

179. Ashikari P, Huvos AG, Snyder RE, et al: A clinicopathologic study of atypical lesions of the breast. Cancer 33:310, 1974

180. Ohuchi N, Abe R, Kasai M: Possible cancerous change of intraductal papillomas of the breast: a 3-D reconstruction study of 25 cases. Cancer 54:605–611, 1984

181. Page DL, Dupont WD: Anatomic markers of human premalignancy and risk of breast carcinoma. Cancer 66:1326–1335, 1990

182. Grignon DJ, Ro JY, Mackay BN, et al: Collagenous spherulosis of the breast: immunohistochemical and ultrastructural studies. Am J Clin Pathol 91:386–392, 1989

183. Wells CA, Wells CW, Yeomans P, et al: Spherical connective tissue inclusions in epithelial hyperplasia of the breast (collagenous spherulosis). J Clin Pathol 43:905–908, 1990

184. Rosen PP, Cantrell B, Mullen DL, et al: Juvenile papillomatosis (swiss cheese disease) of the breast. Am J Surg Pathol 4:3–12, 1980

185. Ostrzega N: Nine needle aspiration cytology of juvenile papillomatosis of breast. A case report. Diagn Cytopathol 9:457–460, 1993

186. Rosen PP, Kimmel M: Juvenile papillomatosis of the breast: a follow-up study of 41 patients having biopsies before 1979. Am J Clin Pathol 93:599–603, 1990

187. Jones MW, Norris HJ, Wargotz ER: Smooth muscle and nerve sheath tumors of the breast. A clinicopathologic study of 45 cases. Int J Surg Pathol 2:85–92, 1994

188. Rosen PP, Ernsberger D: Mammary fibromatosis: a benign spindle-cell tumor with significant risk for local recurrence. Cancer 63:1363–1369, 1989

189. Wargotz ES, Weiss SW, Norris HJ: Myofibroblastoma of the breast. Sixteen cases of a distinctive benign mesenchymal tumor. Am J Surg Pathol 11:493–502, 1987

190. Demay RM, Kay S: Granular cell tumors of the breast. Pathol Annu 19:121–148, 1984

191. Ingram DL, Mossler JA, Snowhite J, et al: Granular cell tumors of the breast. Steroid receptor analysis and localization of carcinoembryonic antigen, myoglobin and S-100 protein. Arch Pathol Lab Med 108:897–901, 1984

192. Jozefczyk MA, Rosen PP: Vascular tumors of the breast. II. Perilobular hemangiomas and hemangiomas. Am J Surg Pathol 9:491–503, 1985

193. Lesueur GC, Brown R, Bhathal PS: Incidence of perilobular hemangioma in the female breast. Arch Pathol Lab Med 107:308–310, 1983

194. Rosen PP: Vascular tumors of the breast. III. Angiomatosis. Am J Surg Pathol 9:652–658, 1985

195. Rosen PP: Vascular tumors of the breast. IV. The venous hemangioma. Am J Surg Pathol 9:659–665, 1985

196. Hoda SA, Cranor ML, Rosen PP: Hemangiomas of the breast with atypical histological features: further analysis of histological subtypes confirming their benign character. Am J Surg Pathol 16:553–560, 1992

197. Ibrahim RE, Sciotto CG, Weidner N: Pseudoangiomatous hyperplasia of mammary stroma: some observations regarding its clinicopathologic spectrum. Cancer 63:1154–1160, 1989

198. Mittal KR, Gerald W, True LD: Hemangiopericytoma of breast: report of a case with ultrastructural and immunohistochemical findings. Hum Pathol 17:1181–1183, 1986

199. Muller J: Uber den feinern Bau und die Formen der Krankhaften Geschwujlste. G. Reimer, Berlin, 1838

200. Norris HJ, Taylor HB: Relationship of histologic features to behavior of cystosarcoma phyllodes. Analysis of ninety-four cases. Cancer 20:2090, 1967

201. Ward RM, Evans HL: Cystosarcoma phyllodes: a clinicopathologic study of 26 cases. Cancer 58:2282, 1986

202. Grigoni WF, Santini D, Grassigli A, et al: A clinicopathologic study of cystosarcoma phyllodes. Twenty case reports. Arch Anat Cytol Pathol 30:303–306, 1982

203. Lindqvist KD, Van Heerden JA, Weiland LH, Martin JK Jr: Recurrent and metastatic cystosarcoma phyllodes. Am J Surg 144:341–343, 1982

204. Cohn-Cedermark G, Rutqvist LE, Rosendahl I, Silfversward C: Prognostic factors in cystosarcoma phyllodes: a clinicopathologic study of 77 patients. Cancer 68:2017–2022, 1991

205. Hawkins RE, Schofield JB, Fisher C, et al: The clinical and histologic criteria that predict metastases from cystosarcoma phyllodes. Cancer 69:141–147, 1992

206. Grimes MM: Cystosarcoma phyllodes of the breast: histologic features, flow cytometric analysis, and clinical correlations. Mod Pathol 5:232–239, 1992

207. El-Naggar AK, Ro JY, McLemore D, Garnsy L: DNA content and proliferative activity of cystosarcoma phyllodes of the breast: potential prognostic significance. Am J Clin Pathol 93:480–485, 1990

208. Ng WF, Poon CSP, Alagaratnam TT, et al: Prognostic value of proliferating cell nuclear antigen in phyllodes tumor of the breast. Int J Surg Pathol 2:125–132, 1994

209. Simi U, Morrelti D, Iacconi P, et al: Fine needle aspiration cytopathology of phyllodes tumor: differential diagnosis with fibroadenomas. Acta Cytol 32:63–66, 1988

210. Silverman JF, Geisinger KR, Frable WJ: Fine needle aspiration cytology of mesenchymal tumors of the breast. Diagn Cytopathol 4:50–58, 1988

211. Dusenberry D, Frable WJ: Fine needle aspiration cytology of phyllodes tumor: potential diagnosis pitfalls. Acta Cytol 36:215–221, 1992

212. Shimizu K, Masana N, Yamada T, et al: Cytologic evaluation of phyllodes tumors as compared to fibroadenomas of the breast. Acta Cytol 38:891–897, 1994

213. Auger M, Hanna W, Kahn HJ: Cystosarcoma phyllodes of the breast and its mimics: an immunohistochemical and ultrastructural study. Arch Pathol Lab Med 113:1231–1235, 1989

214. Yeh IT, Francis DJ, Orenstein JM, Silverberg SG: Ultrastructure of cystosarcoma phyllodes and fibroadenoma: a comparative study. Am J Clin Pathol 84:131–136, 1985

215. Rao BR, Meyer JS, Fry CG: Most cystosarcoma phyllodes and fibroadenomas have progesterone receptor but lack estrogen receptor. Stromal localization of progesterone receptor. Cancer 47:2016–2021, 1981

216. Karp JE, Pinn VW: Breast cancer: a template for progress through multidisciplinary cancer research. Breast J 1:128–154, 1995

217. Spratt JS, Donegan WL, Sigdestad CP: Epidemiology and etiology. pp. 116–141. In Donegan WL, Spratt JS (eds): Cancer of the Breast. 4th Ed. WB Saunders, Philadelphia, 1995

218. Brinton LA, Devesa SS, Weber BL, et al: Etiology and pathogenesis of breast cancer. pp. 159–306. In Harris JR, Lippman ME, Morrow M, Hellman S (eds): Diseases of the Breast. Lippincott-Raven, Philadelphia, 1996

219. Howe GR: Dietary fat and breast cancer risks. An epidemiologic perspective. Cancer 74:1078–1084, 1994

220. Willett WC, Hunter DJ: Prospective studies of diet and breast cancer. Cancer 74:1085–1089, 1994

221. Schatzkin A, Longnecker MP: Alcohol and breast cancer. Cancer 74:1101–1110, 1994

222. Hulka BS, Liu ET, Lininger RA: Steroid hormones and risk of breast cancer. Cancer 74:1111–1124, 1994

223. Asch BB: Tumor viruses and endogenous retrotransposons in mammary tumorigenesis. J Mammary Gland Biol Neoplasia 1:49–60, 1996

224. Anderson DE: Familial versus sporadic breast cancer. Cancer 70:1740–1746, 1992

225. Skolnick MH, Cannon-Albright LA: Genetic predisposition to breast cancer. Cancer 70:1747–1754, 1992

226. Slovak ML, Wolman SR: Breast cancer cytogenetics: clues to genetic complexity of the disease. Breast J 2:124–140, 1996

227. Easton DF, Bishop DT, Ford D, et al: Genetic linkage analysis in familial breast and ovarian cancer: results from 214 families. Am J Hum Genet 52:678–701, 1993

228. Claus EB, Risch N, Thompson D, Carter D: Relationship between breast histopathology and family history of breast cancer. Cancer 71:147–153, 1993

229. Schnitt SJ, Jimi A, Kojiro M: The increasing prevalence of benign proliferative breast lesions in Japanese women. Cancer 71:2528–2531, 1993

230. Shapiro S: Periodic breast cancer screening in seven foreign countries. Cancer 69:1919–1924, 1992

231. Pelikan S, Moskowitz M: Effects of lead time, length bias, and false-negative assurance on screening for breast cancer. Cancer 71:1998–2005, 1993

232. Woolf SH: United States Preventive Services Task Force recommendations on breast cancer screening. Cancer 69:1913–1918, 1992

233. Baines CJ: The Canadian National Breast Screening Study. Why? What next? and So what? Cancer 76:2107–2112, 1995

234. Feig SA: Mammographic screening of women aged 40–49 years. Benefit, risk, and cost considerations. Cancer 76:2097–2106, 1995

235. Peer PGM, van Dijck JAAM, Hendriks JHCL, et al: Age-dependent growth rate of primary breast cancer. Cancer 71:3547–3571, 1993

236. Ford LG, Brawley OW, Perlman JA, et al: The potential for hormonal prevention trials. Cancer 74:2726–2733, 1994

237. O'Shaughnessy JA: Chemoprevention of breast cancer. JAMA 275:1349–1353, 1996

238. Pike MC, Spicer DV: The chemoprevention of breast cancer by reducing sex steroid exposure. J Cell Biochem, suppl. 17G:26–36, 1993

239. Christove K, Chew KL, Ljung BM, et al: Cell proliferation in hyperplastic and in situ carcinoma lesions of the breast estimated by in vivo labelling with bromodeoxyuridine. J Cell Biochem, suppl. 19:165–172, 1994

240. McKittrick R, Fabian C, Kamel S, et al: Dysplasia and other biomarker abnormalities as potential surrogate endpoint biomarkers in breast chemoprevention trials, abstracted. Proc Am Soc Clin Oncol 14:A348, 1995

241. World Health Organization: Histological Typing of Breast Tumours. 2nd Ed. International Histological Classification of Tumours. p. 19. World Health Organization, Geneva, 1981

242. Foote FW Jr, Stewart FW: Lobular carcinoma in situ. A rare form of mammary cancer. Am J Pathol 17:491–496, 1941

243. Andersen JA: Lobular carcinoma in situ. A long-term follow-up in 52 cases. Acta Pathol Microbiol Scand [A] 82:519–533, 1974

244. Newman W: Lobular carcinoma of the female breast. Report of 73 cases. Ann Surg 164:305–314, 1966

245. Haagensen CD, Lane N, Lattes R, et al: Lobular neoplasia (so-called lobular carcinoma in situ) of the breast. Cancer 42:737–769, 1978

246. Frykberg ER, Santiago F, Betsill WL Jr, O'Brien PH: Lobular carcinoma in situ of the breast. Surg Gynecol Obstet 164:285–301, 1987

247. Wheeler JF, Enterline HT, Roseman JM, et al: Lobular carcinoma in situ of the breast. Long-term follow up. Cancer 34:554–563, 1974

248. Rosen PP, Leiberman DH, Braun DW, et al: Lobular carcinoma in situ of the breast: detailed analysis of 99 patients with average follow up of 24 years. Am J Surg Pathol 2:225–251, 1978

249. Ottesen GL, Graversen HP, Blichert-Toft M, Zedeler K, et al: Lobular carcinoma in situ of the female breast. Short-term results of a prospective nationwide study. Am J Surg Pathol 17:14–21, 1993

250. Webber BL, Heise H, Neifeld JP, et al: Risk of subsequent contralateral breast carcinoma in a population of patients with in situ breast carcinoma. Cancer 47:2928–2932, 1981

251. Zhuang Z, Nayar R, Merino MJ, Silverberg SG: Loss of heterozygosity (LOH) on chromosome 11q13 in lobular lesions (ALH, LCIS, ILC) of the breast using tissue microdissection and polymerase chain reaction (PCR). Mod Pathol 9:27A, 1996

252. Betsill W, Rosen PP, Lieberman P, et al: Intraductal carcinoma. Long-term follow-up after treatment by biopsy alone. JAMA 239:1863–1867, 1978

253. Rosen PP: Lobular carcinoma in situ and intraductal carcinoma of the breast. pp. 59–105. In McDivitt RW, Oberman HA, Ozzello L, et al (eds): The Breast. Williams & Wilkins, Baltimore, 1984

254. Ludwig AS, Okagaki T, Richart RM, et al: Nuclear DNA content of lobular carcinoma in situ of the breast. Cancer 31:1553, 1973

255. Andersen JA, Vendelboe ML: Cytoplasmic mucous globules in lobular carcinoma in situ. Diagnosis and prognosis. Am J Surg Pathol 5:251, 1981

256. Page DL, Anderson TJ, Rogers LW: Epithelial hyperplasia. pp. 120–156. In Page DL, Anderson TJ (eds): Diagnostic Histopathology of the Breast, Churchill Livingstone, Edinburgh, 1987

257. Silverman J, Masood S, Ducatman BS, et al: Can FNA biopsy separate atypical hyperplasia, carcinoma in situ, and invasive carcinoma of the breast? Cytomorphologic criteria and limitations in diagnosis. Diagn Cytopathol 9:713–728, 1993

258. Kline TS, Kline IK: High risk lesions pp. 235–248. In: Guide to Clinical Aspiration Biopsy. Igaku-Shoin, New York, 1989

259. Salhany K, Page DL: Fine needle aspiration of mammary lobular carcinoma in situ and atypical lobular hyperplasia. Am J Clin Pathol 92:22–26, 1989

260. Fechner RE: Ductal carcinoma involving the lobule of the breast: a

source of confusion with lobular carcinoma in situ. Cancer 28:274–281, 1971

261. Frost AR, Tsangaris TN, Silverberg SG: Pleomorphic lobular carcinoma in situ. Pathol Case Rev 1:27–31, 1996

262. Oberman HA, Markey BA: Noninvasive carcinoma of the breast presenting in adenosis. Mod Pathol 4:31–35, 1991

263. Page DL, Dupont WD, Rogers LW: Ductal involvement by cells of atypical lobular hyperplasia of the breast: a long-term follow-up study of cancer risk. Hum Pathol 19:201–207, 1988

264. Simon MS, Schwartz AG, Martino S, Swanson GM: Trends in the diagnosis of in situ breast cancer in the Detroit metropolitan area. 1973 to 1987. Cancer 69:466–469, 1992

265. Gump FE, Jicha DL, Ozzello L: Ductal carcinoma in situ (DCIS): a revised concept. Surgery 102:790–795, 1987

266. Holland R, Hendriks JHCL, Verbeek ALM, et al: Extent, distribution, and mammographic/histological correlations of breast ductal carcinoma in situ. Lancet 335:519–522, 1990

267. Lagios MD: Duct carcinoma in situ: pathology and treatment. Surg Clin North Am 70:853–871, 1990

268. Lagios MD, Margolin FR, Westdahl PR, et al: Mammographically detected duct carcinoma in situ: frequency of local recurrence following tylectomy and prognostic effect of nuclear grade on local recurrence. Cancer 63:618–624, 1989

269. Patchefsky AS, Schwartz GF, Finkelstein SD, et al: Heterogeneity of intraductal carcinoma of the breast. Cancer 63:731–741, 1989

270. Silverstein MJ, Waisman JR, Gamagami P, et al: Intraductal carcinoma of the breast (208 cases): clinical factors influencing treatment choice. Cancer 66:102–108, 1990

271. Lagios MD: Ductal carcinoma in situ: controversies in diagnosis, biology, and treatment. Breast J 1:68–78, 1995

272. Tavassoli FA, Man Y: Morphofunctional features of intraductal hyperplasia, atypical intraductal hyperplasia, and various grades of intraductal carcinoma. Breast J 1:155–162, 1995

273. Lennington WJ, Jensen RA, Dalton LW, Page DL: Ductal carcinoma in situ of the breast. Heterogeneity of individual lesions. Cancer 73:118–124, 1994

274. Poller DN, Silverstein MJ, Galea M, et al: Ductal carcinoma in situ of the breast: a proposal for a new simplified histological classification. Association between cellular proliferation and c-erbB-2 protein expression. Mod Pathol 7:257–262, 1994

275. Moriya T, Silverberg SG: Intraductal carcinoma (ductal carcinoma in situ) of the breast. Cancer 74:2972–2978, 1994

276. Moriya T, Silverberg SG: Intraductal carcinoma (ductal carcinoma in situ) of the breast: analysis of pathologic findings of 85 pure intraductal carcinomas. Int J Surg Pathol 3:83–91, 1995

277. Fisher B, Costantino J, Redmond C, et al: Lumpectomy compared with lumpectomy and radiation therapy for the treatment of intaductal breast cancer. N Engl J Med 328:1581–1586, 1993

278. Fisher ER, Costantino J, Fisher B, et al: Pathologic findings from the National Surgical Adjuvant Breast Project (NSABP) Protocol B-17. Intraductal carcinoma (ductal carcinoma in situ). Cancer 75:310–319, 1995

279. Page DL, Lagios MD: Pathologic analysis of the National Surgical Adjuvant Breast Project (NSABP) B-17 trial. Unanswered questions remaining unanswered considering current concept of ductal carcinoma in situ. Cancer 75:1219–1222, 1995

280. Silverstein MJ, Gierson ED, Colburn WJ, et al: Can intraductal breast carcinoma be excised completely by local excision? Clinical and pathologic predictors. Cancer 73:2985–2989, 1994

281. Solin LJ, Yeh I, Kurtz J, et al: Ductal carcinoma in situ (intraductal carcinoma) of the breast treated with breast-conserving surgery and definitive irradiation. Correlation of pathologic parameters with outcome of treatment. Cancer 71:2532–2542, 1993

282. Eusebi V, Foschini MP, Cook MG, et al: Long-term follow-up of in situ carcinoma of the breast with special emphasis on clinging carcinoma. Semin Diagn Pathol 6:165–173, 1989

283. Guerry P, Erlandson RA, Rosen PP: Cystic hypersecretory hyperplasia and cystic hypersecretory duct carcinoma of the breast. Pathology, therapy, and follow-up of 39 patients. Cancer 61:1611, 1988

284. Abati AD, Kimmel M, Rosen PP: Apocrine mammary carcinoma: clinicopathologic study of 72 cases. Am J Clin Pathol 94:371–377, 1990

285. O'Malley FP, Page DL, Nelson EH, Dupont WD: Ductal carcinoma in situ of the breast with apocrine cytology: definition of a borderline category. Hum Pathol 25:164–168, 1994

286. Tavassoli FA, Norris HJ: Intraductal apocrine carcinoma: a clinicopathologic study of 37 cases. Mod Pathol 7:813–818, 1994

287. Carter DJ, Rosen PP: Atypical apocrine metaplasia in sclerosing lesions of the breast: a study of 51 patients. Mod Pathol 4:1–5, 1991

288. Foschini MP, Fornelli A, Peterse JL, et al: Microcalcifications in ductal carcinoma in situ of the breast: histochemical and immunohistochemical study. Hum Pathol 27:178–183, 1996

289. Gould VE, Miller J, Jao W: Ultrastructure of medullary, intraductal, tubular and adenocystic breast carcinomas. Comparative patterns of myoepithelial differentiation and basal lamina deposition. Am J Pathol 78:401, 1975

290. Ozzello L: Ultrastructure of human mammary carcinoma cells in vivo and in vitro. J Natl Cancer Inst 48:1043, 1972

291. Tavassoli FA, Pestaner JP: Pseudoinvasion in intraductal carcinoma. Mod Pathol 8:380–383, 1995

292. Tsang WYW, Chan JKC: Neural invasion in intraductal carcinoma of the breast. Hum Pathol 23:202–204, 1992

293. Tabbara SO: Pseudoinfiltration of ductal carcinoma in situ after fine-needle aspiration. Pathol Case Rev 1:17–21, 1996

294. Moriya T, Sidawy MK, Silverberg SG: Detection of ductal carcinoma in situ of the breast in cytologic samples. Acta Cytol 37:767, 1993

295. Malamud YR, Ducatman BS, Wang HH: Comparative features of comedo and noncomedo ductal carcinoma in situ of the breast on fine needle aspiration biopsy. Diagn Cytopathol 8:571–576, 1992

296. Sneige N, Staerkel GA: Fine needle aspiration cytology of ductal hyperplasia with and without atypia and ductal carcinoma in situ. Hum Pathol 25:485–492, 1994

297. Thomas PA, Raab SS: Fine-needle aspiration biopsy cytology of atypical ductal hyperplasia. Pathol Case Rev 1:12–16, 1996

298. Crissman JD, Visscher DW, Kubus J: Image cytophotometric DNA analysis of atypical hyperplasia and intraductal carcinomas of the breast. Arch Pathol Lab Med 114:1249–1253, 1990

299. Teplitz RL, Butler BB, Tesluk H, et al: Quantitative DNA patterns in human preneoplastic breast lesions. Anal Quant Cytol Histol 12:98–102, 1990

300. Norris HJ, Bahr GF, Mikel UV: Quantitative DNA patterns in human preneoplastic breast lesions. Anal Quant Cytol Histol 12:98–102, 1990

301. Wilbur DC, Barrows GH: Estrogen and progesterone receptor and c-erbB-2 oncoprotein analysis in pure in situ breast carcinoma: an immunohistochemical study. Mod Pathol 6:114–120, 1993

302. Poller DN, Roberts EC, Bell JA, et al: p53 protein expression in mammary ductal carcinoma in situ: relationship to immunohistochemical expression of estrogen receptor and c-erbB-2 protein. Hum Pathol 24:463–468, 1993

303. Bose S, Lesser ML, Norton L, Rosen PP: Immunophenotype of intraductal carcinoma. Arch Pathol Lab Med 120:81–85, 1996

304. Masood S: Use of monoclonal antibody B72.3 in breast fine needle aspirates. Breast Cancer Treat 14:154, 1989

305. Papotti M, Eusebi V, Gagliotta P, Bussolati G: Immunohistochemical analysis of benign and malignant papillary lesions of the breast. Am J Surg Pathol 7:451–461, 1983

306. Raju VB, Lee MW, Zarbo RJ, Crissman JD: Papillary neoplasia of the breast: immunohistochemically defined myoepithelial cells in the di-

agnosis of benign and malignant papillary breast neoplasms. Mod Pathol 20:569–576, 1989

307. Masood S, Lu L, Assaf-Munasifi N, McCaulley K: Application of immunostaining for muscle specific actin for detection of myoepithelial cells in breast fine needle aspirates. Diagn Cytopathol 13:71–74, 1995

308. Micale MA, Visscher DW, Gulino SE, Wolman SR: Chromosomal aneuploidy in proliferative breast disease. Hum Pathol 25:29–35, 1994

309. Page DL, Dupont WD, Rogers LW, et al: Continued local recurrence of carcinoma 15–25 years after a diagnosis of low grade ductal carcinoma in situ of the breast treated only by biopsy. Cancer 76:1197–1200, 1995

310. Silverberg SG, Chitale AR: Assessment of significance of proportions of intraductal and infiltrating tumor growth in ductal carcinoma of the breast. Cancer 32:830, 1973

311. Silverstein MI, Rosser RJ, Gierson ED, et al: Axillary lymph node dissection for intraductal carcinoma—is it indicated? Cancer 59:1819, 1987

312. Rosen PP: Axillary lymph node metastases in patients with occult noninvasive breast carcinoma. Cancer 46:1298, 1980

313. Tavassoli FA, Norris HJ: A comparison of the results of long-term follow-up for atypical intraductal hyperplasia and intraductal hyperplasia of the breast. Cancer 65:518–529, 1990

314. Carter CL, Corle DK, Micozzi MS, et al: A prospective study of the development of breast cancer in 16,692 women with benign breast disease. Am J Epidemiol 128:467–477, 1988

315. Page DL, Dupont WD: Anatomic markers of human premalignancy and risk of breast carcinoma. Cancer 66:1326–1335, 1990

316. Dawson PJ, Baekey PA, Clark RA: Mechanisms of multifocal breast cancer: an immunocytochemical study. Hum Pathol 26:965–969, 1995

317. Pandis N, Teixeira MR, Gerdes AM, et al: Chromosome abnormalities in bilateral breast carcinomas. Cytogenetic evaluation of the clonal origin of multiple primary tumors. Cancer 76:250–258, 1995

318. Noguchi S, Aihara T, Koyama H, et al: Discrimination between multicentric and multifocal carcinomas of the breast through clonal analysis. Cancer 74:872–877, 1994

319. Chiloso M, Bonetti F, Menestrina F, et al: Breast carcinoma with stromal multinucleated giant cells. J Pathol 152:55, 1987

320. Holland R, Veling SHJ, Mravunac M, et al: Histologic multifocality of Tis, T1–2 breast carcinomas. Implications for clinical trials of breast-conserving surgery. Cancer 56:979, 1985

321. Dalton LW, Page DL, Dupont WD: Histologic grading of breast carcinoma. A reproducibility study. Cancer 73:2765–2770, 1994

322. Robbins P, Pinder S, de Klerk N, et al: Histological grading of breast carcinomas: a study of interobserver agreement. Hum Pathol 26:873–879, 1995

323. Pereira H, Pinder SE, Sibbering DM, et al: Pathological prognostic factors in breast cancer. IV. Should you be a typer or a grader? A comparative study of two histological prognostic features in operable breast carcinoma. Histopathology 27:219–226, 1995

324. Wilkinson EJ, Franzini DA, Masood S: Cytological needle sampling of the breast: techniques and end results. pp. 475–498. In Bland KI, Copeland EM (eds): The Breast. WB Saunders, Philadelphia, 1991

325. Silverman FJ: Breast. pp. 703–770. In Bibbo M (ed): Comprehensive Cytopathology. WB Saunders, Philadelphia, 1991

326. McKinney CD, Frierson HF Jr, Fechner RE, et al: Pathologic findings in nonpalpable invasive breast cancer. Am J Surg Pathol 16:33–36, 1992

327. Leitner SP, Swern AS, Weinberger D, et al: Predictors of recurrence for patients with small (one centimeter or less) localized breast cancer (T1a,b N0 M0). Cancer 76:2266–2274, 1995

328. Russo SA, Fowble B, Fox K, et al: The identification of a subset of patients with axillary node-negative minimally invasive breast cancer

who may benefit from adjuvant systemic therapy. Breast J 1:163–172, 1995

329. Halverson KJ, Taylor ME, Perez CA, et al: Management of the axilla in patients with breast cancers one centimeter or smaller. Am J Clin Oncol 17:461–466, 1994

330. Fisher B, Bauer M, Wickerham DL, et al: Relation of number of positive axillary nodes to the prognosis of patients with primary breast cancer. Cancer 52:1551, 1983

331. Veronesi U, Rilke F, Luini A, et al: Distribution of axillary node metastases by level of invasion. Cancer 59:682, 1987

332. Weigand RA, Isenberg WM, Russo J, et al: Blood vessel invasion and axillary lymph node involvement as prognostic indicators for human breast cancer. Cancer 50:962, 1982

333. Donegan WL: Prognostic factors. Stage and receptor status in breast cancer. Cancer 70:1755–1764, 1992

334. McGuire WL, Tandon AK, Allred DC, et al: Prognosis and treatment decisions in patients with breast cancer without axillary node involvement. Cancer 70:1775–1781, 1992

335. Nasser IA, Lee AKC, Bosari S, et al: Occult axillary lymph node metastases in "node-negative" breast carcinoma. Hum Pathol 24:950–957, 1993

336. Morrow M, Evans J, Rosen PP, Kinne DW: Does clearing of axillary lymph nodes contribute to accurate staging of breast carcinoma? Cancer 53:1329, 1984

337. Trojani M, De Mascarel I, Bonichou F, et al: Micrometastases to axillary lymph nodes from carcinoma of breast: detection by immunohistochemistry and prognostic significance. Br J Cancer 55:303, 1987

338. Bloom HJG, Richardson WW: Histological grading and prognosis in breast cancer. A study of 1409 cases of which 359 have been followed for 15 years. Br J Cancer 11:359, 1957

339. Fisher ER, Gregorio RM, Fisher B: The pathology of invasive breast cancer. A syllabus derived from findings of the National Surgical Adjuvant Breast Project (protocol no. 4). Cancer 36:1, 1975

340. Elston CW, Ellis IO: Pathological prognostic factors in breast cancer. I. The value of histological grade in breast cancer: Experience from a large study with long-term follow-up. Histopathology 19:403–410, 1991

341. Fisher ER, Kotwal N, Hermann C, et al: Types of tumor lymphoid response and sinus histiocytosis. Arch Pathol Lab Med 107:222, 1983

342. Silverberg SG, Chitale AR, Hind AD, et al: Sinus histiocytosis and mammary carcinoma. Cancer 26:1177, 1970

343. Horst H-A, Horny H-P: Characterization and frequency distribution of lymphoreticular infiltrates in axillary lymph node metastases of invasive ductal carcinoma of the breast. Cancer 60:3001, 1987

344. Silverberg SG, Chitale AR, Levitt SH: Prognostic significance of tumor margins in mammary carcinoma. Arch Surg 102:450, 1971

345. Prior P, Waterhouse JAH: Incidence of bilateral tumours in a population based series of breast cancer patients. I. Two approaches to an epidemiological analysis. Br J Cancer 37:620, 1978

346. Azzopardi JG, Eusebi V: Melanocyte colonization and pigmentation of breast carcinoma. Histopathology 1:21, 1977

347. Andersen JA, Pallesen RM: Spread to the nipple and areola in carcinoma of the breast. Ann Surg 189:367, 1979

348. Fisher ER, Palekar AS, Gregorio RM, et al: Pathological findings from the national Surgical Adjuvant Breast Project (protocol no 4). IV. Significance of tumor necrosis. Hum Pathol 9:523, 1978

349. Lauria R, Perrone F, Carlomagno C, et al: The prognostic value of lymphatic and blood vessel invasion in operable breast cancer. Cancer 76:1772–1778, 1995

350. Orbo A, Stalsberg H, Kunde D: Topographic criteria in the diagnosis of tumor emboli in intramammary lymphatics. Cancer 66:972–977, 1990

351. Clement CG, Boracchi P, Andreola S, et al: Peritumoral lymphatic invasion in patients with node-negative mammary duct carcinoma. Cancer 69:1396–1403, 1992

352. Nomura Y, Miura S, Koyama H, et al: Relative effect of steroid hormone receptors on the prognosis of patients with operable breast cancer. Cancer 69:153–164, 1992

353. Baddoura FK, Cohen C, Unger ER, et al: Image analysis for quantitation of estrogen receptor in formalin-fixed paraffin-embedded sections of breast carcinoma. Mod Pathol 4:91–95, 1991

354. Traish AM, Newton AW, Styperek K, et al: Estrogen receptor functional status in human breast cancer. Diagn Mol Pathol 4:220–228, 1995

355. Masood S: Prognostic and diagnostic implications of estrogen and progesterone receptor assays in cytology. Diagn Cytopathol 10:263–267, 1994

356. Masood S: Estrogen and progesterone receptors in cytology. Diagn Cytopathol 8:475–491, 1992

357. Wilbur DC, Willis J, Mooney RA, et al: Estrogen and progesterone receptor detection in archival formalin-fixed, paraffin-embedded tissue from breast carcinoma: a comparison of immunohistochemistry with the dextran-coated charcoal assay. Mod Pathol 5:79–84, 1992

358. Esteban JM, Felder B, Ahn C, et al: Prognostic relevance of carcinoembryonic antigen and estrogen receptor status in breast cancer patients. Cancer 74:1575–1583, 1994

359. Cohen C, Sharkey FE, Shulman G, et al: Tumor-associated antigens in breast carcinomas. Prognostic significance. Cancer 60:1294, 1987

360. Castiglioni T, Merino MJ, Elsner B, et al: Immunohistochemical analysis of cathepsins D, B, and L in human breast cancer. Hum Pathol 25:857–862, 1994

361. Dabbs DJ: Correlations of morphology, proliferation indices, and oncogene activation in ductal breast carcinoma: nuclear grade, S-phase, proliferating cell nuclear antigen, p53, epidermal growth factor receptor, and c-erbB-2. Mod Pathol 8:637–642, 1995

362. Visscher DW, DeMattia F, Ottosen S, et al: Biologic and clinical significance of basic fibroblast growth factor immunostaining in breast carcinoma. Mod Pathol 8:665–670, 1995

363. Wolman SR, Pauley RJ, Mohamed AN, et al: Genetic markers as prognostic indicators in breast cancer. Cancer 70:1765–1774, 1992

364. Barnes DM, Dublin EA, Fisher CJ, et al: Immunohistochemical detection of p53 protein in mammary carcinoma: an important new independent indicator of prognosis? Hum Pathol 24:469–476, 1993

365. De Potter CR: The neu-oncogene: more than a prognostic indicator? Hum Pathol 25:1264–1268, 1994

366. Champème MH, Bièche I, Hacène K, Lidereau R: Int-2/FGF3 amplification is a better independent predictor of relapse than c-myc and c-erbB-2/neu amplifications in primary human breast cancer. Mod Pathol 7:900–905, 1994

367. Gamel JW, Meyer JS, Province MA: Proliferative rate by S-phase measurement may affect cure of breast carcinoma. Cancer 76:1009–1018, 1995

368. Sapi Z, Hendricks JB, Pharis PG, Wilkinson EJ: Tissue section image analysis of breast neoplasms. Evidence of false aneuploidy. Am J Clin Pathol 99:714–720, 1993

369. Keshgegian AA, Cnaan A: Proliferation markers in breast carcinoma. Mitotic figure count, S-phase fraction, proliferating cell nuclear antigen, Ki-67 and MIB-1. Am J Clin Pathol 104:42–49, 1995

370. Biesterfeld S, Noll I, Noll E, et al: Mitotic frequency as a prognostic factor in breast cancer. Hum Pathol 26:47–52, 1995

371. Simpson JF, Page DL: Cellular proliferation and prognosis in breast cancer: statistical purity versus clinical utility. Hum Pathol 25:331–332, 1994

372. Layfield LJ, Kerns BJM, Conlon DH, et al: Determination of proliferation index by MIB-1 immunostaining in early stage breast cancer using quantitative image analysis. Breast J 1:362–371, 1995

373. Mourad WA, Setrakian S, Hales ML, et al: The argyrophilic nucleolar organizer regions in ductal carcinoma in situ of the breast. Cancer 74:1739–1745, 1994

374. Barbareschi M, Weidner N, Gasparini G, et al: Microvessel density quantification in breast carcinomas. Assessment by light microscopy vs. a computer-aided image analysis system. Appl Immunohistochem 3:75–84, 1995

375. Costello P, McCann A, Carney D, Dervan PA: Prognostic significance of microvessel density in lymph node negative breast carcinoma. Hum Pathol 26:1181–1184, 1995

376. Goulding H, Abdul Rashid NFN, Robertson JF, et al: Assessment of angiogenesis in breast carcinoma. An important factor in prognosis? Hum Pathol 26:1196–1200, 1995

377. Wyatt JP, Sugarbaker ED, Stanton MF: Involvement of internal mammary lymph nodes in carcinoma of breast. Am J Pathol 31:143, 1955

378. de la Monte SM, Hutchins GM, Moore GW: Influence of age on the metastatic behavior of breast carcinoma. Hum Pathol 19:529, 1988

379. Ceci G, Franciosi V, Nizzoli R, et al: The value of bone marrow biopsy in breast cancer at time of diagnosis. A prospective study. Cancer 61:96, 1988

380. Viadana E, Bross IDJ, Pickren JW: An autopsy study of some routes of dissemination of cancer of the breast. Br J Cancer 27:336, 1973

381. Rubens RD: Metastatic breast cancer and its complications. Curr Opin Oncol 4:1050–1054, 1992

382. Everson TC: Spontaneous regression of cancer. Ann NY Acad Sci 114:721, 1964

383. Frable WJ, Kay S: Carcinoma of the breast. Histologic and clinical features of apocrine tumors. Cancer 21:756–763, 1968

384. Roddy HJ, Silverberg SG: Ultrastructural analysis of apocrine carcinoma of the human breast. Ultrastruct Pathol 1:385–393, 1980

385. Losi L, Lorenzini R, Eusebi V, Bussolati G: Apocrine differentiation in invasive carcinoma of the breast. Comparison of monoclonal and polyclonal gross cystic disease fluid protein-15 antibodies with prolactin-inducible protein mRNA gene expression. Appl Immunohistochem 3:91–98, 1995

386. Gupta RK, Wakefield SJ, Naran S, Dowle CC: Immunocytochemical and ultrastructural diagnosis of a rare mixed apocrine-medullary carcinoma of the breast in a fine needle aspirate. Acta Cytol 33:104–108, 1989

387. Duggan MA, Young GK, Hwang WS: Fine needle aspiration biopsy of an apocine carcinoma with multivacuolated lipid rich giant cells. Diagn Cytopathol 4:62–66, 1988

388. Nguyen G-K, Neifer R: Aspiration biopsy cytology of secretory carcinoma of the breast. Diagn Cytopathol 3:234–237, 1987

389. Dixon JM, Anderson TJ, Page DL, et al: Infiltrating lobular carcinoma of the breast. Histopathology 6:149–161, 1982

390. Martinez V, Azzopardi JG: Invasive lobular carcinoma of the breast: incidence and variants. Histopathology 3:467–488, 1979

391. Shousha S, Backhous CM, Alaghband-Zadeh J, Burn I: Alveolar variant of invasive lobular carcinoma of the breast. Am J Clin Pathol 85:1–5, 1986

392. Silverstein MJ, Lewinsky BS, Waisman JR, et al: Infiltrating lobular carcinoma. Is it different from infiltrating duct carcinoma? Cancer 73:1673–1677, 1994

393. Frost AR, Terahata S, Yeh I-T, et al: An analysis of prognostic features in infiltrating lobular carcinoma of the breast. Mod Pathol 8:830–836, 1995

394. Frost AR, Terahata S, Yeh I-T, et al: The significance of signet ring cells in infiltrating lobular carcinoma of the breast. Arch Pathol Lab Med 119:64–68, 1995

395. Du Toit RS, Locker AP, Ellis IO, et al: Invasive lobular carcinoma of the breast: the prognosis of histopathological types. Br J Cancer 60:605–609, 1989

396. DiConstanzo D, Rosen PP, Gareen I, et al: Prognosis in infiltrating lobular carcinoma: an analysis of "classical" and variant tumors. Am J Surg Pathol 14:12–23, 1990

397. Nesland JM, Grude TH, Ottestad L, Johannessen JV: Invasive lobu-

lar carcinoma of the breast: the importance of an alveolar growth pattern. Pathol Annu 27:233–247, 1992

398. Fisher ER, Gregorio RM, Redmond G, Fisher B: Tubulolobular invasive breast cancer: a variant of lobular invasive cancer. Hum Pathol 8:679–683, 1977

399. Eusebi V, Magalhaes F, Azzopardi JG: Pleomorphic lobular carcinoma of the breast: an aggressive tumor showing apocrine differentiation. Hum Pathol 23:655–662, 1992

400. Antoniades K, Spector HB: Similarities and variations among lobular carcinoma cells. Diagn Cytopathol 3:55–59, 1987

401. Leach C, Howell LP: Cytodiagnosis of classic lobular carcinoma and its variants. Acta Cytol 36:199–202, 1992

402. Dabbs DJ, Grenko RT, Silverman JF: Fine needle aspiration cytology of pleomorphic lobular carcinoma of the breast. Duct carcinoma as a diagnostic pitfall. Acta Cytol 38:923–926, 1994

403. de las Morenas A, Crespo P, Moroz K, Donnelly MM: Cytologic diagnosis of ductal versus lobular carcinoma of the breast. Acta Cytol 39:865–869, 1995

404. Lamovec J, Bracko M: Metastatic pattern of infiltrating lobular carcinoma of the breast: an autopsy study. J Surg Oncol 48:28–33, 1991

405. Wargotz ES, Norris HJ: Metaplastic carcinomas of the breast. I. Matrix-producing carcinoma. Hum Pathol 20:628–635, 1989

406. Wargotz ES, Deos PH, Norris HJ: Metaplastic carcinomas of the breast. II. Spindle cell carcinoma. Hum Pathol 20:732–740, 1989

407. Wargotz ES, Norris HJ: Metaplastic carcinomas of the breast. III. Carcinosarcoma. Cancer 64:1490–1499, 1989

408. Wargotz ES, Norris HJ: Metaplastic carcinomas of the breast. IV. Squamous cell carcinoma of ductal origin. Cancer 65:272–276, 1990

409. Wargotz ES, Norris HJ: Metaplastic carcinomas of the breast. V. Metaplastic carcinoma with osteoclastic giant cells. Hum Pathol 21:1142–1150, 1990

410. Oberman HA: Metaplastic carcinoma of the breast. A clinicopathologic study of 29 patients. Am J Surg Pathol 11:918–929, 1987

411. Kaufman MW, Marti JR, Gallager HS, et al: Carcinoma of the breast with pseudosarcomatous metaplasia. Cancer 53:1908, 1984

412. Hasleton PS, Misch KA, Vasudev KS, et al: Squamous carcinoma of the breast. J Clin Pathol 34:116–124, 1978

413. Nielsen BB, Kiaer HW: Carcinoma of the breast with stromal multinucleated giant cells. Histopathology 9:183–193, 1985

414. Tavassoli FA: Classification of metaplastic carcinomas of the breast. Part 2. Pathol Annu 27:89–120, 1992

415. Jebsen PW, Hagmar BM, Nesland JM: Metaplastic breast carcinoma: a diagnostic problem in fine needle aspiration biopsy. Acta Cytol 35:396–402, 1991

416. Kline TS, Kline IK: Metaplastic carcinoma of the breast diagnosed by aspiration biopsy cytology: report of two cases and literature review. Diagn Cytopathol 6:63–67, 1990

417. Stanley MW, Tani EM, Skoog L: Metaplastic carcinoma of the breast: fine needle aspiration cytology of seven cases. Diagn Cytopathol 5:22–28, 1989

418. Boccato P, Briani G, d'Atri C, et al: Spindle cell and cartilaginous metaplasia in a breast carcinoma with osteoclast-like stromal cells. Acta Cytol 32:75–78, 1988

419. Silverman JF, Geisinger KR, Frable WJ: Fine needle aspiration cytology of mesenchymal tumors of the breast. Diagn Cytopathol 4:50–58, 1988

420. Tani EM, Stanley MW, Skoog L: Fine needle aspiration cytology of bilateral mammary fibromatosis: report of a case. Acta Cytol 32:555–558, 1988

421. Fritsches HG, Muller EA: Pseudosarcomatous fasciitis of the breast: cytologic and histologic features. Acta Cytol 27:73–75, 1983

422. Bloom HJG, Richardson WW, Field JR: Host resistance and survival in carcinoma of the breast. A study of 104 cases of medullary carcinoma in a series of 1411 cases of breast cancer followed for 20 years. BMJ 3:181–188, 1970

423. Wargotz ES, Silverberg SG: Medullary carcinoma of the breast: a clinicopathologic study with appraisal of current diagnostic criteria. Hum Pathol 19:1340–1346, 1988

424. Ridolfi RL, Rosen PP, Port A, et al: Medullary carcinoma of the breast. A clinicopathologic study with 10 years follow-up. Cancer 40:1365, 1977

425. Rapin V, Contesso G, Mouriesse H, et al: Medullary breast carcinoma: a reevaluation of 95 cases of breast cancer with inflammatory stroma. Cancer 61:2503–2510, 1988

426. Pedersen L, Zedeler K, Holck S, et al: Medullary carcinoma of the breast: proposal for a new simplified histopathological definition. Br J Cancer 63:591–595, 1991

427. Cook DL, Weaver DL: Comparison of DNA content, S-phase fraction, and survival between medullary and ductal carcinoma of the breast. Am J Clin Pathol 104:17–22, 1995

428. Gaffey MJ, Mills SE, Frierson HF Jr, et al: Medullary carcinoma of the breast: interobserver variability in histopathologic diagnosis. Mod Pathol 8:31–38, 1995

429. Ben-Ezra J, Sheibani K: Antigenic phenotype of the lymphocytic component of medullary carcinoma of the breast. Cancer 59:2037–2041, 1987

430. Tanaka H, Hori M, Ohki T: High endothelial venule and immunocompetent cells in typical medullary carcinoma of the breast. Virchows Arch A Pathol Anat Histopathol 420:253–261, 1992

431. Gould VE, Miller J, Jao W: Ultrastructure of medullary, intraductal, tubular and adenocystic breast carcinomas. Am J Pathol 78:401–407, 1975

432. Ahmed A: The ultrastructure of medullary carcinoma of the breast. Virchows Arch [A] 388:175–186, 1980

433. Kline TS, Kannan V, Kline IK: Appraisal and cytomorphologic analysis of common carcinoma of the breast. Diagn Cytopathol 1:188–193, 1985

434. Lefkowitz M, Lefkowitz W, Wargotz ES: Intraductal (intracystic) papillary carcinoma of the breast and its variants. A clinicopathologic study of 77 cases. Hum Pathol 25:802–809, 1994

435. Corkill ME, Sneige N, Fanning T, El-Naggar A: Fine-needle aspiration cytology and flow cytometry of intracystic papillary carcinoma of breast. Am J Clin Pathol 94:673–680, 1990

436. Fisher ER, Palekar AS, Redmond C, et al: Pathologic findings from the National Surgical Adjuvant Breast Project (Protocol No. 4) VI. Invasive papillary cancer. Am J Clin Pathol 73:313–322, 1980

437. Siriaunkgul S, Tavassoli FA: Invasive micropapillary carcinoma of the breast. Mod Pathol 6:660–662, 1993

438. Baroales RH, Suhrland MJ, Stanley MW: Papillary neoplasms of the breast: fine needle aspiration findings in cystic and solid cases. Diagn Cytopathol 10:336–341, 1994

439. Nguyen CK, Redburn J: Aspiration cytology of papillary carcinoma of the breast. Diagn Cytopathol 8:511–516, 1992

440. Larrey M: Tumeur gelatiniforme ou colloide de la mamelle. Bull Soc Chir Paris 3:545, 1853

441. Rasmussen BB, Rose C, Christensen I: Prognostic factors in primary mucinous breast carcinoma. Am J Clin Pathol 87:155–160, 1987

442. Komaki K, Sakamoto G, Sugano H, et al: Mucinous carcinoma of the breast in Japan. A prognostic analysis based on morphologic features. Cancer 61:989–996, 1988

443. Fisher ER, Palekar AS, Stoner F, Costantino J: Mucocele-like lesions and mucinous carcinoma of the breast. Int J Surg Pathol 1:213–220, 1994

444. Rasmussen BB, Rose C, Thorpe SM, et al: Argyrophilic cells in 202 human mucinous breast carcinomas. Relation to histopathologic and clinical factors. Am J Clin Pathol 84:737, 1985

445. Harris M, Vasudev KS, Anfield C, et al: Mucin-producing carcinomas of the breast: ultrastructural observations. Histopathology 2:177–188, 1978

446. Ro JY, Sneige N, Sahin AA, et al: Mucocelelike tumor of the breast

associated with atypical ductal hyperplasia or mucinous carcinoma. Arch Pathol Lab Med 115:137–140, 1991

447. Stanley MW, Tani EM, Skoog L: Mucinous breast carcinoma and mixed mucinous infiltrating ductal carcinoma. A comparative cytologic study. Diagn Cytopathol 52:34–38, 1989

448. Bharagava V, Miller TR, Cohen MB: Mucocele-like tumors of the breast. Cytologic findings in two cases. Am J Clin Pathol 95:875–877, 1991

449. Cornil V, Ranvier L: Manuel d'histologie pathologique. G Bailliere, Paris, 1869

450. Carstens PHB, Greenberg RA, Francis D, et al: Tubular carcinoma of the breast. A long-term follow-up. Histopathology 9:271–280, 1985

451. Cooper HS, Patchefsky AS, Krall RA: Tubular carcinoma of the breast. Cancer 42:2334–2442, 1978

452. Oberman HA, Fidler WJ: Tubular carcinoma of the breast. Am J Surg Pathol 3:387–395, 1979

453. Tobon H, Salazar H: Tubular carcinoma of the breast. Arch Pathol Lab Med 101:310–316, 1977

454. McDivitt RW, Boyce W, Gersell D: Tubular carcinoma of the breast. Clinical and pathological observations concerning 135 cases. Am J Surg Pathol 6:401–411, 1982

455. Deos PH, Norris HJ: Well-differentiated (tubular) carcinoma of the breast. Am J Clin Pathol 78:1–7, 1982

456. Parl FF, Richardson LD: The histologic and biologic spectrum of tubular carcinoma of the breast. Hum Pathol 14:694–698, 1983

457. Andersson I: Radiographic screening for breast carcinoma. II. Prognostic considerations on the basis of a short-term follow-up. Acta Radiol [Diagn] (Stockh) 22:227–233, 1981

458. Harris M, Ahmed A: The ultrastructure of tubular carcinoma of the breast. J Pathol 123:79–83, 1979

459. Berger AC, Miller SM, Harris MN, Roses DF: Axillary dissection for tubular carcinoma of the breast. Breast J 2:204–208, 1996

460. Flotte TJ, Bell DA, Greco MA: Tubular carcinoma and sclerosing adenosis. The use of basal lamina as a differential feature. Am J Surg Pathol 4:75–77, 1980

461. Bondeson L, Lindholm K: Aspiration cytology of tubular breast carcinoma. Acta Cytol 34:15–20, 1990

462. de la Torre M, Lindholm K, Lindgren A: Fine needle aspiration cytology of tubular breast carcinoma and radial scar. Acta Cytol 38:884–890, 1994

463. Page DL, Dixon JM, Anderson TJ, et al: Invasive cribriform carcinoma of the breast. Histopathology 7:525–536, 1983

464. Venable JG, Schwartz AM, Silverberg SG: Infiltrating cribriform carcinoma of the breast: a distinctive clinicopathologic entity. Hum Pathol 21:333–338, 1990

465. Dawson PJ, Karrison T, Ferguson DJ: Histologic features associated with long-term survival in breast cancer. Hum Pathol 17:1015, 1986

466. Ro JY, Silva EG, Gallager HS: Adenoid cystic carcinoma of the breast. Hum Pathol 18:1276–1281, 1987

467. Sumpio B, Jennings T, Sullivan P, et al: Adenoid cystic carcinoma of the breast. Am Surg 205:295–301, 1987

468. Leeming R, Jenkins M, Mendelsohn G: Adenoid cystic carcinoma of the breast. Arch Surg 127:233–235, 1992

469. Zaloudek C, Oertel YC, Orenstein JM: Adenoid cystic carcinoma of the breast. Am J Clin Pathol 81:297–307, 1984

470. Peters GN, Wolff M: Adenoid cystic carcinoma of the breast: report of 11 new cases. Cancer 52:680–686, 1982

471. Stanley MW, Tani EM, Rutquist LE, Skoog L: Adenoid cystic carcinoma of the breast: diagnosis by fine needle aspiration. Diagn Cytopathol 9:184–187, 1993

472. Johnson TL, Kini SH: Cytologic features of collagenous spherulosis of the breast. Diagn Cytopathol 7:417–419, 1991

473. Ramos CV, Taylor HB: Lipid-rich carcinoma of the breast. A clinicopathologic analysis of 13 examples. Cancer 33:812–819, 1974

474. Van Bogaert LJ, Maldague P: Histologic variants of lipid-secreting carcinoma of the breast. Virchows Arch [A] 375:345–353, 1977

475. Wrba F, Ellinger A, Reiner G, et al: Ultrastructural and immunohistochemical characteristics of lipid-rich carcinoma of the breast. Virchows Arch [A] 413:381–385, 1988

476. Barwick KW, Kashgarian M, Rosen PP: Clear-cell change within duct and lobular epithelium of the human breast. Pathol Annu 17:319–328, 1982

477. Insabato L, Russo R, Cascone AM, Angrisani P: Fine needle aspiration cytology of lipid-secreting breast carcinoma. A case report. Acta Cytol 37:752–755, 1993

478. Eusebi V, Foschini MP, Bussolati G, Rosen PP: Myoblastomatoid (histiocytoid) carcinoma of the breast. A type of apocrine carcinoma. Am J Surg Pathol 19:553–562, 1995

479. Oberman HJ: Secretory carcinoma of the breast in adults. Am J Surg Pathol 4:465–470, 1980

480. Tavassoli FA, Norris HJ: Secretory carcinoma of the breast. Cancer 45:2404–2413, 1980

481. Akhtar M, Robinson C, Ali MA, et al: Secretory carcinoma of the breast in adults. Light and electron microscopic study of three cases with review of the literature. Cancer 51:2245–2254, 1983

482. Rosen PP, Cranor ML: Secretory carcinoma of the breast. Arch Pathol Lab Med 115:141–144, 1991

483. Dominguez F, Riera JR, Junco P, Sampedro A: Secretory carcinoma of the breast: report of a case with diagnosis by fine needle aspiration. Acta Cytol 36:507–510, 1992

484. d'Amore ESG, Maisto L, Gatteschi MB, et al: Secretory carcinoma of the breast. Report of a case with fine needle aspiration biopsy. Acta Cytol 30:309–312, 1986

485. Toikkanen S, Joensuu H: Glycogen-rich clear-cell carcinoma of the breast: a clinicopathologic and flow cytometric study. Hum Pathol 22:81–83, 1991

486. Hayes MMM, Seidman JD, Ashton MA: Glycogen-rich clear cell carcinoma of the breast. A clinicopathologic study of 21 cases. Am J Surg Pathol 19:904–911, 1995

487. Cubilla AL, Woodruff JM: Primary carcinoid tumor of the breast: a report of eight patients. Am J Surg Pathol 1:283–292, 1977

488. Taxy JB, Tischler AS, Insalaco SJ, Battfora H: "Carcinoid" tumor of the breast: a variant of conventional breast cancer? Hum Pathol 12:170–179, 1981

489. Papotti M, Macri L, Finzi G, et al: Neuroendocrine differentiation in carcinomas of the breast: a study of 51 cases. Semin Diagn Pathol 6:174–188, 1989

490. Lozowski MJ, Faegenburg D, Mishriki Y, Lundy J: Carcinoid tumor metastatic to breast diagnosed by fine needle aspiration: case report and literature review. Acta Cytol 33:191–194, 1989

491. Francois A, Chatikhine VA, Chevallier B, et al: Neuroendocrine primary small cell carcinoma of the breast. Report of a case and review of the literature. Am J Clin Oncol 18:133–138, 1995

492. Ku N, Ribbo M: Fine needle aspiration of mammary carcinoma with features of a carcinoid tumor. A case report with immunohistochemical and ultra-structural studies. Acta Cytol 38:73–78, 1994

493. Velpeau A: Traite des maladies du sein et de la region mammaire. Masson, Paris, 1858

494. Paget J: Disease of the mammary areola preceding cancer of the mammary gland. St Barth Hosp Rep 10:87–89, 1874

495. Jacobeus HC: Paget's disease und sein Verhaltnis zum Milchdrusen Karzinom. Virchows Arch 178:124, 1904

496. Lancer HA, Moschell SL: Paget's disease of the male breast. J Ann Acad Dermatol 7:393, 1982

497. Neubecker RD, Bradshaw RP: Mucin, melanin and glycogen in Paget's disease of the breast. Am J Clin Pathol 36:40, 1961

498. Rayne SC, Santa Cruz DJ: Anaplastic Paget's disease. Am J Surg Pathol 16:1085–1091, 1992

499. Hitchcock A, Topham S, Bell J, et al: Routine diagnosis of mammary Paget's disease: a modern approach. Am J Surg Pathol 16:58–61, 1992

500. Nadji M, Morales AR, Girtanner RE, et al: Paget's disease of the skin. Cancer 50:2203–2206, 1982

501. Lagios MD, Westdahl PR, Rose MR, et al: Paget's disease of the nipple. Cancer 54:545–551, 1984

502. Shertz WT, Balogh K: Metastasizing basal cell carcinoma of the nipple. Arch Pathol Lab Med 110:761–762, 1986

503. Levine PH, Steinhorn SC, Ries LGV, et al: Inflammatory breast cancer. The experience of the Surveillance, Epidemiology and End Results (SEER) Program. J Natl Cancer Inst 74:291–297, 1985

504. Thomas F, Arriagada R, Spielmann M, et al: Pattern of failure in patients with inflammatory breast cancer treated by alternating radiotherapy and chemotherapy. Cancer 76:2286–2290, 1995

505. Ellis DL, Teitelbaum SL: Inflammatory carcinoma of the breast: a pathologic definition. Cancer 33:1045–1047, 1974

506. Lucas FV, Perez-Mesa C: Inflammatory carcinoma of the breast. Cancer 41:1595–1605, 1978

507. Saltzstein SL: Clinically occult inflammatory carcinoma of the breast. Cancer 34:382, 1974

508. Mourali N, Muenz LR, Tabbane F, et al: Epidemiologic features of rapidly progressing breast cancer in Tunisia. Cancer 46:2741, 1980

509. Association of Directors of Anatomic and Surgical Pathology: Standardization of the surgical pathology report. Am J Surg Pathol 16:84–86, 1992

510. Association of Directors of Anatomic and Surgical Pathology: Recommendations for the reporting of breast carcinoma. Hum Pathol 27:220–224, 1996

511. Rosai J, Members of the Department of Pathology, Memorial Sloan-Kettering Cancer Center: Standardized reporting of surgical pathology diagnoses for the major tumor types. A proposal. Am J Clin Pathol 100:240–255, 1993

512. Frazier TG, Wong RWY, Rose D: Implications of accurate pathologic margins in the treatment of primary breast cancer. Arch Surg 124:37–38, 1989

513. Smitt MC, Nowels KW, Zdeblick MJ, et al: The importance of the lumpectomy surgical margin status in long term results of breast conservation. Cancer 76:259–267, 1995

514. Schnitt SJ, Abner A, Gelman R, et al: The relationship between microscopic margins of resection and the risk of local recurrence in patients with breast cancer treated with breast-conserving surgery and radiation therapy. Cancer 74:1746–1751, 1994

515. Silverstein MJ, Lagios MD, Craig PH, et al: A prognostic index for ductal carcinoma in situ of the breast. Cancer 77:2267–2274, 1996

516. Sauter ER, Hoffman JP, Ottery FD, et al: Is frozen section analysis of reexcision lumpectomy margins worthwhile? Cancer 73:2607–2612, 1994

517. Oberman HA: Sarcomas of the breast. Cancer 18:1233–1243, 1965

518. Norris HJ, Taylor HB: Sarcomas and related mesenchymal tumors of the breast. Cancer 22:22–28, 1968

519. Callery CD, Rosen PP, Kinne DW: Sarcoma of the breast—a study of 32 patients with reappraisal of classification and therapy. Ann Surg 201:527–532, 1985

520. Pollard SG, Marks PV, Temple LN, Thompson HH: Breast sarcoma: a clinicopathologic review of 25 cases. Cancer 66:941–944, 1990

521. Jones MW, Norris HJ, Wargotz ES, Weiss SW: Fibrosarcoma-malignant fibrous histiocytoma of the breast: a clinicopathological study of 32 cases. Am J Surg Pathol 16:667–674, 1992

522. Wargotz ES, Norris HJ, Austin RM, Enzinger FM: Fibromatosis of the breast. A clinical and pathological study of 28 cases. Am J Surg Pathol 11:38–45, 1987

523. Wargotz ES, Weiss S, Norris HJ: Myofibroblastoma of the breast. Sixteen cases of a distinctive mesenchymal tumor. Am J Surg Pathol 11:493–502, 1987

524. Chen KTK, Kuo T, Hoffman KD: Leiomyosarcoma of the breast. Cancer 47:1883–1886, 1981

525. Going JJ, Lumsden AB, Anderson TJ: A classical osteogenic sarcoma of the breast: histology, immunohistochemistry and ultrastructure. Histopathology 10:631–641, 1986

526. Kuten A, Sapir D, Cohen Y, et al: Postirradiation soft tissue sarcoma occurring in breast cancer patients: report of seven cases and results of combination chemotherapy. J Surg Oncol 28:168–171, 1985

527. Austin RM, Dupree WB: Liposarcoma of the breast: a clinicopathologic study of 20 cases. Hum Pathol 17:906–913, 1986

528. Merino MJ, Carter D, Berman M: Angiosarcoma of the breast. Am J Surg Pathol 7:53–60, 1983

529. Rosen PP, Kimmel M, Ernsberger D: Mammary angiosarcoma: the prognostic significance of tumor differentiation. Cancer 62:2145–2151, 1988

530. Buatti JM, Harari PM, Leigh BR, Cassady JR: Radiation-induced angiosarcoma of the breast. Case report and review of the literature. Am J Clin Oncol 17:444–447, 1994

531. Silverman JF, Geisinger KR, Frable WJ: Fine needle aspiration cytology of mesenchymal tumors of the breast. Diagn Cytopathol 4:50–58, 1988

532. Stanley MW, Tani GM, Horwitz CA, et al: Primary spindle cell sarcomas of the breast. Diagnosis of fine needle aspiration. Diagn Cytopathol 4:244–249, 1988

533. Tulesinghe PU, Anthony PP: Primary lymphoma of the breast. Histopathology 9:297–307, 1985

534. Cohen PL, Brooks JJ: Lymphomas of the breast: a clinicopathologic and immunohistochemical study of primary and secondary cases. Cancer 67:1359–1369, 1991

535. Giardini R, Piccolo C, Rilke F: Primary non-Hodgkin's lymphomas of the female breast. Cancer 69:725–735, 1992

536. Aozasa K, Ohsawa M, Saeki K, et al: Malignant lymphoma of the breast: immunologic type and association with lymphocytic mastopathy. Am J Clin Pathol 97:699–704, 1992

537. Ben Yehuda A, Steiner-Saltz D, Libson E, et al: Plasmacytoma of the breast. Unusual initial presentation of myeloma: report of two cases and review of the literature. Blut 58:169–170, 1989

538. Corrigan C, Sewell C, Martin A: Recurrent Hodgkin's disease in the breast: diagnosis of a case by fine needle aspiration and immunocytochemistry. Acta Cytol 34:669–672, 1990

539. Pettinato G, DeChiara A, Insabato L, DeRenza A: Fine needle aspiration biopsy of a granulocytic sarcoma (chloroma) of the breast. Acta Cytol 32:67–71, 1988

540. Gupta RK: Fine-needle aspiration cytology of metastatic malignancies and lymphomas involving the breast. Breast J 1:322–325, 1995

541. Lin JJ, Farha GJ, Taylor RJ: Pseudolymphoma of the breast. I. In a study of 8654 consecutive tylectomies and mastectomies. Cancer 45:973–978, 1980

542. Perez-Guillerma M, Sola-Perez J, Rodriguez-Bermejo M: Malakoplakia and Rosai-Dorfman disease: two entities of histiocytic origin infrequently localized in the female breast. The cytologic aspect in aspirates via fine needle aspiration cytology. Diagn Cytopathol 9:698–704, 1993

543. Nielsen M, Andersen JA, Henriksen FW, et al: Metastases to the breast from extramammary carcinomas. Acta Pathol Microbiol Scand [A] 89:251–256, 1981

544. McCrea ES, Johnston C, Haney DJ: Metastases to the breast. AJR 141:685–690, 1983

545. Yamasaki H, Saw D, Zdanowitz J, Faltz LL: Ovarian carcinoma metastasis to the breast: case report and review of the literature. Am J Surg Pathol 17:193–197, 1993

546. Bannayan GA, Hajdu SI: Gynecomastia: clinicopathologic study of 351 cases. Am J Clin Pathol 57:431–437, 1972

547. Carlson HE: Gynecomastia. N Engl J Med 303:795–799, 1980

548. Williams MJ: Gynecomastia. Its incidence, recognition and host characterization in 447 autopsy cases. Am J Med 34:103–112, 1963

549. Bartoli C, Zurrida SM, Clemente C: Phyllodes tumor in a male patient with bilateral gynaecomastia induced by oestrogen therapy for prostatic carcinoma. Eur J Surg Oncol 17:215–217, 1991

550. Bigotti G, Kasznica J: Sclerosing adenosis in the breast of a man with pulmonary oat cell carcinoma: report of a case. Hum Pathol 17:861–863, 1986

551. Banik S, Hale R: Fibrocystic disease in the male breast. Histopathology 12:214–216, 1988

552. Sneige N, Holder PD, Katz R, et al: Fine needle aspiration cytology of the male breast in a cancer center. Diagn Cytopathol 9:691–697, 1993

553. Das DK, Junaid TA, Mathews SB, et al: Fine needle aspiration cytology diagnosis of male breast lesions. A study of 185 cases. Acta Cytol 39:870–876, 1995

554. Mabuchi K, Bross DS, Kessler II: Risk factors for male breast cancer. J Natl Cancer Inst 74:371–375, 1985

555. Wolman SR, Sanford J, Ratner S, Dawson PJ: Breast cancer in males: DNA content and sex chromosome constitution. Mod Pathol 8:239–243, 1995

556. Casagrande JT, Hanisch R, Pike MC, et al: A case-control study of male breast cancer. Cancer Res 48:1326–1330, 1988

557. Evans DB, Crichlow RW: Carcinoma of the male breast and Klinefelter's syndrome. Is there an association? CA Cancer J Clin 37:246–251, 1987

558. Heller KS, Rosen PP, Schottenfeld D, et al: Male breast cancer: a clinicopathologic study of 97 cases. Ann Surg 118:60–65, 1978

559. Schlappack OK, Braun O, Maier U: Report of two cases of male breast cancer after prolonged estrogen treatment for prostatic carcinoma. Cancer Detect Prev 9:319–322, 1986

560. Sobin LH, Sherif M: Relation between male breast cancer and prostate cancer. Br J Cancer 42:787, 1980

561. Kozak FK, Hall JG, Baird PA: Familial breast cancer in males: a case report and review of the literature. Cancer 58:2736, 1986

562. Joshi MG, Lee AKC, Loda M, et al: Male breast carcinoma: an evaluation of prognostic factors contributing to a poorer outcome. Cancer 77:490–498, 1996

563. Gattuso P, Reddy VB, Green L, et al: Prognostic significance of DNA ploidy in male breast carcinoma. A retrospective analysis of 32 cases. Cancer 70:777–780, 1992

564. Pegoraro RJ, Nirmul D, Joubert SM: Cytoplasmic and nuclear estrogen and progesterone receptors in male breast cancer. Cancer Res 42:4812, 1982

565. American Joint Committee on Cancer: Breast. p. 149. In Beahrs OH, Henson DE, Hutter RVP, et al (eds): Manual for Staging of Cancer. 4th Ed. Lippincott-Raven, Philadelphia, 1992

566. Gompel C, Silverberg SG: Pathology in Gynecology and Obstetrics. 4th Ed. Lippincott-Raven, Philadelphia, 1994

567. National Cancer Institute: The uniform approach to breast fine needle aspiration biopsy. A synopsis. Acta Cytol 40:1120–1126, 1996

20

Lymph Nodes and Spleen

Lawrence M. Weiss
Daniel A. Arber
Karen L. Chang

PATHOLOGIC EVALUATION OF THE LYMPH NODE

Fine Needle Aspiration Biopsy

Fine needle aspiration biopsy is being increasingly used for the evaluation of lymphadenopathy.[1] It can be used to determine whether a suspected enlarged lymph node is indeed lymphoid tissue, to obtain material for special studies (including culture, immunophenotyping studies, and molecular studies), to diagnose metastatic tumors, to diagnose reactive hyperplasia or infectious lymphadenitis, to diagnose and stage Hodgkin's disease and non-Hodgkin's lymphomas, to identify residual recurrent lymphoma, and to diagnose transformation of lymphoma. The efficacy varies with the clinical situation. It is probably best applied in cases in which reactive hyperplasia is suspected, and least effective in cases in which the initial diagnosis of a non-Hodgkin's lymphoma is the primary clinical consideration.

Excisional Lymph Node Biopsy

An excised lymph node biopsy should be received fresh (and not in fixative), intact, preferably sterile, and always with complete clinical information. Placing the specimen on a dry towel or sponge will introduce artifacts. If a long period must elapse before receipt by the pathologist, the node may be placed in sterile saline, although this may introduce undesirable artifacts into subsequent frozen section studies. One should first harvest tissue for sterile studies, which may include microbiologic cultures and cytogenetic studies, if indicated. Fresh tissue for possible frozen section immunohistochemical, flow cytometric studies, and molecular studies should also be taken at this time. If a metastatic tumor is a possibility, a small piece should also be appropriately fixed for electron microscopy. Rapid frozen section evaluation may be quite helpful for determining adequacy of the tissue, establishing a tentative diagnosis, and determining which special studies may be particularly useful to obtain at once. Only a small piece of tissue should be frozen, and if nec-

essary, this piece may be kept frozen for possible future frozen section immunohistochemical studies or molecular studies. Contrary to historic belief, we find frozen section diagnosis of hematolymphoid disorders to be reliable, as long as the limitations of the technique are recognized. Cytologic characteristics are often not well appreciated in frozen sections, but touch or (as we prefer) rapidly fixed scrape preparations may demonstrate cytologic features as well as or even better than in paraffin sections. Distinctions that can usually be made in frozen sections include benign vs. malignant, hematolymphoid vs. nonhematolymphoid, Hodgkin's vs. non-Hodgkin's lymphoma, and low grade vs. high grade non-Hodgkin's lymphoma. We try to provide as much of a diagnosis as necessary for immediate clinical decisions and avoid making distinctions that are not needed rapidly. Of course, the diagnosis should always be deferred in cases in which significant doubt exists.

Prompt and proper tissue fixation is more important than choice of fixative in the preparation of good histologic sections. The sections should be thinly cut and not underfixed, as this will hinder morphologic interpretation, or overfixed, as this may hinder immunohistochemical studies. If formalin is used as the primary fixative, it should be freshly prepared and at the proper pH. Some pathologists use a second fixative, usually a metal-based fixative such as B5, for fixation of lymph nodes. Sections should be cut thinly, to better evaluate nuclear features. Hematoxylin and eosin (H&E)-stained sections are usually adequate for morphologic interpretation, but some pathologists supplement this with reticulin-van Gieson (to evaluate the architecture), Giemsa (to better visualize the nuclear features), and methyl green pyronine stains (to get a rough estimate of the RNA content of the cytoplasm).

Special Studies

In diagnostically difficult cases, H&E stained sections are usually supplemented with a panel of *paraffin section immunohistochemical studies*, with the particular selected panel components dependent on the differential diagnosis suggested by the morphologic features. A listing of many of the important leukocyte antigens easily detectable in paraffin sections is presented in

Table 20-1. Selected Useful Major Leukocyte Antigens Detectable in Paraffin Sections

Antibody	Predominant Hematolymphoid Cell Expression
Ki-67 (mib-1)	Proliferating cells
TdT	Thymic lymphoid cells and lymphoblastic neoplasms
Myeloperoxidase	Myeloid cells and myeloid leukemia
Lysozyme	Histiocytes, myeloid cells, histiocytic neoplasms, and myeloid leukemia
Immunoglobulin light and heavy chains	Plasma cells, plasma cell and plasmacytoid neoplasms, some follicular lymphomas
bcl-2	Nongerminal center B cells, most T cells, most follicular lymphomas, many low grade and some higher grade B cell lymphomas
Epithelial membrane antigen	Plasma cells and plasma cell neoplasms, many nodular L&H lymphocyte predominance, anaplastic large cell lymphoma, and T cell rich B cell lymphoma
EBV latent membrane protein	Some EBV-infected cells (most notably EBV-positive Hodgkin's cells, post-transplant lymphoproliferations, and EBV-associated infectious mononucleosis)
CD1	Thymocytes and some T lymphoblastic lymphomas, Langerhans cells, and Langerhans cell histiocytosis
CD3	T cells and many T cell lymphomas
CD8	T cytotoxic/suppressor cells, some T cell lymphoma
CD15	Myeloid cells, Hodgkin's disease, some non-Hodgkin's lymphomas
CD20	B cells and B cell lymphomas, nodular L&H lymphocyte predominance
CD21	Follicular dendritic cells, mantle and marginal zone B cells and neoplasms
CD30	Activated lymphoid cells, Hodgkin's disease, anaplastic large cell lymphoma
CD34	Progenitor cells, some myeloid leukemias, some lymphoblastic neoplasms
CD43	T cells, myeloid cells, mast cells, T cell lymphomas, some B cell lymphomas, myeloid leukemia, mast cell neoplasms
CD45/CD45RB	Hematolymphoid cells
CD45RA	B cells and subset of T cells, B cell lymphomas, nodular L&H lymphocyte predominance
CD45R0	Most T cells, histiocytes, myeloid cells, T cell lymphomas
CD57	Subset of T cells and natural killer cells, subset of T cell lymphomas
CD68	Histiocytes, myeloid cells, mast cells and neoplasms, some non-Hodgkin's lymphomas
CD79a	Immature and mature B cells and lymphomas, plasma cells and plasma cell neoplasms

Abbreviations: TdT, terminal deoxynucleotidyl transferase; L&H, lymphocytic and histiocytic; EBV, Epstein-Barr virus.
(Modified from Weiss et al,[511] with permission.)

Table 20-1. Some suggested panels are given in Table 20-2. Immunostains are helpful by providing an indication as to the immunoarchitecture and cell lineage, and by providing an assessment of cancer in some cases. Immunostains can demonstrate the B and T cell areas or show that architecture has been altered or effaced. Stains for follicular dendritic cells can indicate the presence of follicles and other structures, while antibodies such as Ki-67 can provide a measure of cell proliferation of various compartments or cell populations. Cell lineage studies that can be performed in paraffin sections help one decide between hematolymphoid vs. nonhematolymphoid, and B vs. T vs. other. Examples of immunostudies that strongly favor a diagnosis of hematolymphoid malignant tumor in paraffin sections include the demonstration of immunoglobulin light chain restriction in B cell lymphomas (usually in plasmacytoid neoplasms, but occasionally in follicular lymphomas), reactivity of follicular B cells with bcl-2 protein (in follicular lymphoma), and the aberrant coexpression of CD43, or less commonly CD45RO, with B lineage markers (in diffuse B cell lymphomas). The aberrant coexpression of CD43 may also be used to help in subclassification due to its differential expression in different subtypes of B cell lymphoma.[2]

An even wider range of antibodies can be used in *cell suspension studies* or acetone-fixed *frozen sections*[3,4] (Table 20-3). *Flow cytometry* studies are of particular use in quantitating immunoglobulin light chain ratios and in the performance of double-labeling studies. Flow cytometry studies are also used by some to determine cell proliferation and DNA content.[5-7] Studies of both have shown correlation with the grade of the

Table 20-2. Suggested Panels for Paraffin Section Immunohistochemistry

Undifferentiated neoplasm	CD45/45RB, keratin, S-100, CD30, (CD20, CD43)
Hodgkin's vs. non-Hodgkin's	CD45/45RB, CD30, CD15, CD20, CD43
Non-Hodgkin's, general	CD45/45RB, CD30, CD20, CD43
Nodular lymphocyte predominance	CD45/45RB, CD20, CD57, CD15, (epithelial membrane antigen)[a]
Follicular lymphoma	CD20, CD43, BCL-2
T cell lymphoma	CD45/45RB, CD30, CD20, CD3, CD43, (CD45RO)
Acute leukemia	CD45/45RB, CD43, CD15, CD68, CD34, myeloperoxidase, TdT
Lymphoblastic	CD43, CD3, CD79a, TdT
Diffuse B cell lymphoma	CD20, CD43, (CD79a)
Large cell lymphoma	CD20, CD3, CD43, CD30 (epithelial membrane antigen, CD45RO)
Plasmacytoid proliferations	Immunoglobulin light chains, CD20, CD43, (CD79a, immunoglobulin heavy chains)

[a] Parentheses indicate optional antibody or antibodies to be ordered with initial screening panel.
(Modified from Weiss et al,[511] with permission.)

Table 20-3. Selected Useful Major Leukocyte Antigens Detectable Only in Suspensions or Frozen Sections

Antibody	Predominant Hematolymphoid Expression
CD2	T cells and T cell lymphomas
CD4	Histiocytes and histiocytic neoplasms, T helper cells and many T cell lymphomas
CD5	T cells and many T cell lymphomas, many B small lymphocytic lymphoma/chronic lymphocytic leukemia, mantle cell lymphoma
CD7	Most T cells and T cell lymphomas, some myeloid leukemias
CD10 (CALLA)	Precursor B cells and B lymphoblastic neoplasms, many follicular lymphomas
CD11c	Histiocytes and histiocytic neoplasms, M4 and M5 myeloid leukemia, hairy cell leukemia, marginal cell lymphoma
CD16	Natural killer cells and neoplasms
CD19	B cells and B cell lymphomas
CD22	B cells and B cell lymphomas
CD23	Mantle zone B cells and most B small lymphocytic lymphoma/chronic lymphocytic leukemia
CD25 (TAC)	Activated lymphoid cells, adult T cell lymphoma/leukemia, hairy cell leukemia, most anaplastic large cell lymphomas, most Hodgkin's disease, subset of other B and T cell lymphomas
CD38	Plasma cells and plasma cell neoplasms, B and T precursor cells and lymphoblastic neoplasms
CD56	Natural killer cells and subset of T cell/natural killer lymphomas

(Modified from Weiss et al,[511] with permission.)

lymphomas as well as specific prognosis. Another advantage of flow cytometry is its applicability to fluid specimens such as aspiration biopsies, although immunocytochemical studies can be performed on cell smears. Disadvantages of flow cytometry include the difficulty in obtaining adequate numbers of cells in fibrotic tissues (particularly in extranodal sites), the inability to visualize the individual staining cells (although one can "gate" on certain populations by differential cell size and granularity), and the inability to relate the flow cytometric results to specific architectural compartments. Frozen section immunohistochemical studies have the advantage of allowing correlation of staining with architecture. However, morphology is less than optimal, and therefore it is difficult to assign accurate staining profiles to rare cell populations such as Reed-Sternberg cells, particularly when there is staining of adjacent cells. With the increased number of monoclonal antibodies reacting in cell suspension and frozen sections, one can apply additional criteria for malignant tumors.[3] These include aberrant absence of immunoglobulin (common in diffuse large cell B cell lymphoma) or other B lineage antigens (uncommon in B cell lymphoma), and the aberrant absence of T lineage antigens in peripheral T cell lymphoma. In addition, these studies may be useful in the subclassification of lymphomas. For example, the low grade B

cell lymphomas may be more easily subclassified by their differential expression of CD5, CD10, and CD23.[8,9]

Molecular studies may be helpful in selected cases. The detection of clonal immunoglobulin light and heavy chain gene and T cell receptor gene rearrangements is a very useful tool in hematopathology.[10–14] Although the identification of a monoclonal population is not completely synonymous with cancer, these studies can be very helpful in difficult cases. Antigen receptor gene rearrangements may be detected by Southern blot hybridization with a sensitivity of approximately 1 to 5 percent, but it generally requires frozen tissue and takes about 2 weeks to complete. Sufficient DNA may be obtained by fine needle aspiration biopsy.[15] Alternatively, one may also use the polymerase chain reaction (PCR), a technique that may not detect all gene rearrangements, but has a shorter turnaround time of less than 1 week and can usually be performed in tissue taken from paraffin blocks. In cases with detectable gene rearrangements, the sensitivity of PCR for the detection of lymphoma cells may be very high, but there is also a potential for false positive results as a result of contamination during the analysis. Both Southern blot hybridization and PCR can be used to accurately stage patients with known lymphoma and to identify recurrent or residual disease, with PCR having a higher potential sensitivity.[10]

Cytogenetics may be useful in diagnosis and classification of lymphoproliferations in some instances. Certain lymphomas are associated with characteristic cytogenetic abnormalities, usually translocations (see section on non-Hodgkin's lymphomas). Cytogenetic abnormalities may be detected by classic metaphase analysis after brief cell culture, by fluorescence in situ hybridization (FISH) on cells in interphase, by Southern blotting, or by PCR. Classic cytogenetics requires fresh, sterile tissue but does not require foreknowledge of the translocation being sought. FISH can be performed on paraffin sections, but one can only examine the section for one translocation at a time.[16] Both Southern blot hybridization and PCR require knowledge of the specific translocation. In the case of Southern blot hybridization, a specific probe that hybridizes to the area of the genome just adjacent to the translocation must be available, and in the case of PCR, the sequence of DNA flanking both sides of the translocation must be known. Although classic cytogenetics may reveal a characteristic translocation, the actual breakpoint may occur in widely varying locations in the genome at the molecular level. Therefore, there is a potential for false negative results by Southern blot hybridization and PCR methodologies, depending on the specific translocation. Although chromosomal translocations are specific for neoplasia when they are detected by classic cytogenetics, FISH, and Southern blotting, this may not be the case when the translocation is detected by the highly sensitive PCR. For example, the t(14;18) has been detected by PCR in tissues with reactive follicular hyperplasia from patients without a history of lymphoma.[17]

NONHEMATOPOIETIC LESIONS IN LYMPH NODES

The following is a list of the various nonhematopoietic lesions that may be encountered in lymph nodes:

Metastatic tumors
    Carcinoma
    Germ cell tumor
    Malignant melanoma
    Sarcoma
    Childhood tumors
Congenital rests and inclusions
    Epithelial
        Salivary gland
        Breast
        Thyroid
        Müllerian
    Stromal
        Müllerian
    Nevomelanocytic
        Ordinary nevus
        Blue nevus
Primary mesenchymal lesions
    Lipomatosis
    Vascular
        Vascular transformation of sinuses
        Bacillary angiomatosis
        Kaposi's sarcoma
        Intranodal hemangioma and variants
        Lymphangioma
        Hemangioendothelioma and variants
        Angiosarcoma
    Smooth muscle
        Smooth muscle proliferation of the nodal hilum
        Intranodal leiomyoma
        Angiomyomatous hamartoma
        Leiomyomatosis
        Lymphangiomyomatosis
        Angiomyolipoma
    Myofibroblast
        Inflammatory pseudotumor
        Palisaded myofibroblastoma
Protein Deposition
    Proteinaceous lymphadenopathy
    Amyloid

Metastatic Tumors

Metastatic tumors are the most frequent and most important nonhematopoietic lesions encountered in lymph nodes. In any lymph node dissection, all lymph nodes should be grossly identified and submitted for microscopic examination. The number of involved nodes, as well as the total number of lymph nodes examined should be specified. In many cases, this information should be given by the specific node group. If only one lymph node is involved, it is often useful to comment on whether the metastasis is macroscopic or microscopic (<3 mm). If the anatomic area may be treated with irradiation, one should comment on the presence of any significant extranodal soft tissue extension.[18] Whether immunohistochemical stains should be performed to facilitate detection of histologically inapparent metastases is a subject of debate.[19] It is our opinion that these studies are not usually necessary, because many studies have not demonstrated that the detection of these micrometastases has a significant impact on prognosis.

A lymph node biopsy may show an undifferentiated malignant tumor that cannot be classified by histologic examination. Application of a limited panel of immunohistochemical markers will resolve most cases (Table 20-2); a panel is necessary because tumors frequently have somewhat overlapping reactivities. Most undifferentiated tumors presenting in lymph nodes are found to represent non-Hodgkin's lymphoma. Because CD45/45RB stains about 90 percent of cases of non-Hodgkin's lymphoma, this antibody is an excellent initial screening tool for these neoplasms. The category of non-Hodgkin's lymphoma most likely to be CD45/45RB negative is anaplastic large cell lymphoma; these cases may be identified by use of CD30 antibodies.[20,21] Embryonal carcinoma may be CD30+, but that tumor should also be strongly positive for keratin. Malignant lymphomas may rarely express keratin, but the staining is usually focal, globular, and paranuclear. After malignant lymphoma, carcinoma represents the next most common neoplasm to present as an undifferentiated tumor in the lymph node. In particular, undifferentiated nasopharyngeal carcinoma may closely mimic immunoblastic lymphoma. In addition to keratin stains, in situ hybridization for Epstein-Barr virus is usually positive in this tumor.[22] Malignant melanoma may present in lymph nodes, particularly in the axillary and inguinal groups. Occasionally, small round blue cell tumors of childhood may present in lymph nodes; immunohistochemical studies, electron microscopy, and possibly specialized molecular studies may all be helpful in arriving at the correct diagnosis.

Fine needle aspiration biopsy is a highly effective method for diagnosing metastatic neoplasms in lymph nodes. Key features in the identification of carcinoma include cohesive cell groupings, common cell borders, cytoplasmic differentiation (such as mucin vacuoles or squamous features), and nuclear molding. Key features in the identification of melanoma by fine needle aspiration biopsy include abundant cytoplasm, the presence of melanin pigment, rounded or oblong nuclei, intranuclear cytoplasmic invaginations, and prominent nucleoli. Material obtained by fine needle aspiration may be subjected to immunocytochemical studies, including keratin and S-100 stains for confirmation.

Carcinoma presents in lymph nodes without a known primary in about 3 percent of cases, so-called called carcinoma of unknown origin.[23] Breast, lung, and renal carcinomas are the most common carcinomas to present in this fashion. The site of the lymph node may suggest the primary site. A neck presentation should suggest carcinoma of the upper aerodigestive tract or thyroid.[24] Even extensive head and neck examination may not reveal the primary site. An axillary presentation should suggest ipsilateral breast carcinoma; mammography may sometimes be necessary to reveal the primary lesion. However, carcinomas from the lung, skin, stomach, or pharynx may all present in an axillary node.[25] A supraclavicular presentation should suggest a lung, gastrointestinal tract, or genitourinary tract primary (particularly the ovary, in a woman).[26] An inguinal presentation should suggest carcinoma of the skin, genitourinary tract, and lower gastrointestinal tract. Immunohistochemical studies may help to identify the primary site. For example, thyroglobulin is specific for thyroid carcinoma, prostatic specific antigen and prostatic acid phosphatase are specific for prostate carcinoma, whereas estrogen receptor is positive in a restricted set of neoplasms, including breast carcinoma, carcinomas of the female genital tract, and some thyroid neoplasms. The differential diagnosis of metastatic malignant tumors is discussed in more detail in Chapter 15.

Congenital Rests and Inclusions

Not all epithelial elements found in lymph nodes represent metastatic carcinoma. Inclusions of salivary gland, breast, thyroid, and müllerian epithelium have all been described. *Inclusions of salivary gland tissue* are commonly found in adjacent lymph nodes, usually within the lymph node parenchyma. Most often, ducts alone are encountered but acini may also be seen. These inclusions may become clinically evident when they are cystically dilated, as frequently occurs in human immunodeficiency virus (HIV)-infected patients, forming so-called benign lymphoepithelial cysts.[27] These cysts may be confused with cystic variants of metastatic squamous cell carcinoma; the key feature is the cytologic atypia present in the lining cells in the latter. The salivary gland inclusions may give rise to neoplasms, the most common example being Warthin's tumor.

Inclusions of breast epithelium have been rarely reported in axillary lymph nodes, most often in the intracapsular or subcapsular regions.[28] These inclusions may undergo the same changes as normal breast epithelium, including atypical hyperplasia, carcinoma in situ, and rarely, primary carcinoma. Thyroid inclusions have also been reported in lateral cervical lymph nodes, usually in subcapsular regions. To accept a thyroid inclusion as ectopic and not metastatic, one should see completely follicular architecture with no papillary structures, psammoma bodies, or atypical nuclear features, with no suggestion of the cytology of papillary carcinoma.[29]

Inclusions of müllerian epithelium are seen within the capsule and parenchyma in 5 to 40 percent of intra-abdominal lymph nodes of females (and rarely in males), according to a large autopsy and surgical study[30] (Fig. 20-1). Occasionally, inclusions may be found within germinal centers or the sinuses. Müllerian epithelial inclusions seem to be more common in patients with epithelial tumors of the ovary, particularly borderline serous tumors. They usually consist of tubuloglandular structures lined by a single layer of epithelial cells with a distinct basement membrane. Occasionally, papillary structures can be found. Müllerian inclusions have bland nuclear features with basal orientation, differentiated cytoplasm—with the frequent presence of cilia, the lack of a stromal response, and the presence of a basement membrane, which are not features of metastases. When unaccompanied by endometrial stroma, the inclusions are sometimes termed *endosalpingiosis;* when endometrial stroma is present, the term *endometriosis* should be applied.[31] Occasionally, only stroma is present; this is most commonly seen when deciduosis is identified in pregnant women.[32]

Nevus cell inclusions are also relatively common, seen in about 3 percent of axillary node dissections by light microscopic examination, and about 5 percent of cases when S-100 staining is used[33] (Fig. 20-2). They have also been reported in inguinal and cervical lymph nodes. The inclusions are composed of cells

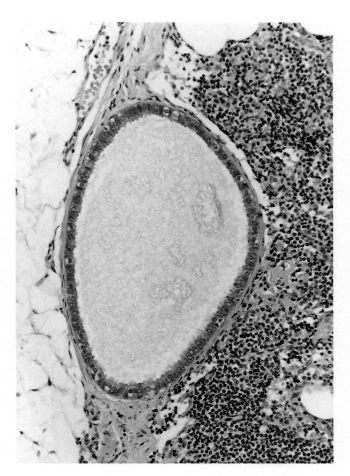

Fig. 20-1. Müllerian inclusion in a lymph node. Note the bland nuclear features and the presence of cilia.

resembling the cells of benign intradermal nevi, but inclusions resembling blue nevus have also been reported.[34] The keys to the distinction from metastatic tumor are the nevus cell inclusion's bland cytologic features, nesting architecture, and presence in the lymph node capsule in contrast to the subcapsular sinus, as more typically seen in carcinoma. Occasionally, the subcapsular sinus is involved by nevus cell inclusions, but there is virtually always more extensive involvement of the adjacent capsule.

Mesenchymal Lesions

Lipomatosis, or fatty replacement of the lymph node, is a relatively common occurrence.[35] The fatty replacement begins in the lymph node hilum, leaving a rim of normal lymphoid tissue at the outer cortex. It is usually clinically insignificant, but may be a cause of lymphadenopathy, particularly in obese individuals.

Vascular transformation of lymph node sinuses is a reactive proliferation of blood vessels in the lymph node sinuses, probably as a result of venous obstruction.[36] The vessels range from en-

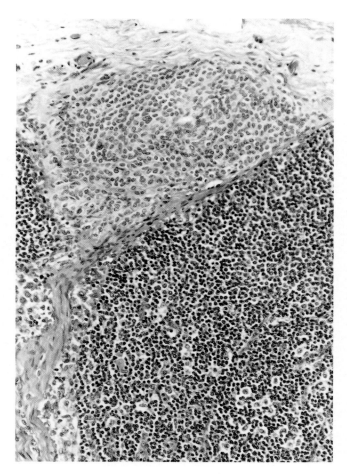

Fig. 20-2. Nevus cell inclusion. There is a nest of nevus cells in the lymph node capsule.

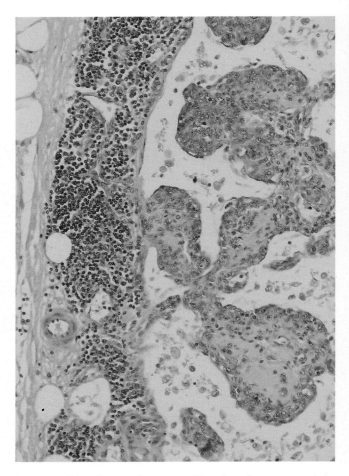

Fig. 20-3. Vascular transformation of lymph node sinuses, nodular spindle cell variant. The cells lining the spaces do not stain with epithelial markers.

dothelial-lined small dilated vascular channels through well formed blood vessels, and is generally associated with fibrosis. There is also a nodular spindle cell variant, characterized by a proliferation of spindle cells forming irregular interlacing bundles and cuffs around endothelium-lined vascular channels, most often seen in retroperitoneal lymph nodes draining carcinomas[37] (Fig. 20-3). Vascular transformation of lymph node sinuses is usually an incidental finding but occasionally may present as lymphadenopathy. Its significance lies in not confusing it with other more clinically important vascular lesions of lymph nodes. The nodular spindle cell variant must not be mistaken for lymph node involvement by metastatic carcinoma.

Bacillary angiomatosis is another reactive proliferation of blood vessels that may involve lymph nodes.[38] It is a pseudoneoplastic vascular proliferation caused by a bacterium identical or related to the cat-scratch disease bacillus. Although more common in skin, involved lymph nodes show patchy involvement by coalescent nodules of proliferating blood vessels lined by reactive endothelial cells. Admixed are scattered neutrophils and an eosinophilic material, which can be shown to represent bacilli on Warthin-Starry stain.

Kaposi's sarcoma is the most common primary vascular tumor of lymph nodes. It is usually seen in this country as a complica-

tion of HIV infection, particularly in homosexual men,[39] but is also seen as a lymphadenopathic form in children and young adults in Africa. There is strong evidence that both forms of Kaposi's sarcoma are associated with human herpesvirus (HHV)-8.[40] Lymph nodes involved by Kaposi's sarcoma may show complete effacement of architecture, one or several nodules, or subtle subcapsular involvement (Fig. 20-4). Uninvolved lymph node parenchyma may show nonspecific reactive hyperplasia or Castleman like features. Histologically, Kaposi's sarcoma involving lymph nodes is identical to that involving other organs.

Other primary vascular neoplasms of lymph node are rare and include nodal hemangioma, epithelioid hemangioma, lymphangioma, epithelioid hemangioendothelioma, spindle and epithelioid (histiocytoid) hemangioendothelioma, polymorphous hemangioendothelioma, and angiosarcoma. These neoplasms have been recently reviewed.[41,42]

There are many rare *smooth muscle proliferations* that may involve the lymph node.[35] Lymphangiomyomatosis (vascular leiomyomatosis), a proliferation of smooth muscle and lymphatics, and angiomyolipoma, a proliferation of smooth muscle, adipose tissue, and thick-walled blood vessels, are associated

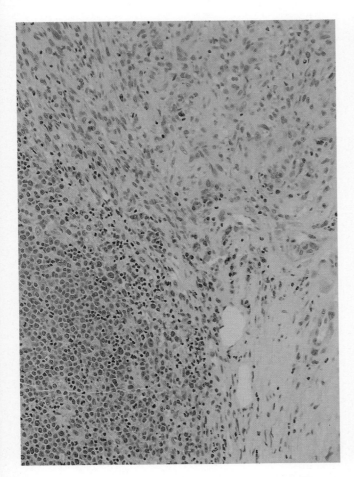

Fig. 20-4. Kaposi's sarcoma. Capsular involvement is seen in this case.

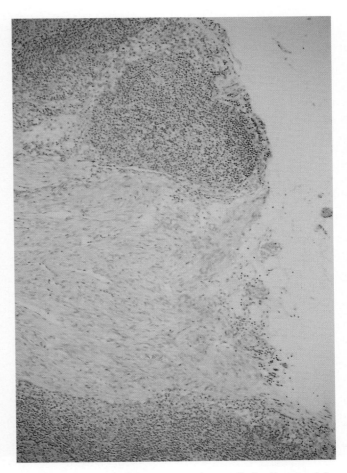

Fig. 20-5. Lymphangiomyomatosis. The spindled cells stained for smooth muscle actin and HMB-45.

with tuberous sclerosis, and share HMB-45 positivity[43] (Fig. 20-5). Smooth muscle proliferation of the nodal hilum is an irregular proliferation of smooth muscle cells, accompanied by fibrosis, limited to the hilum, and is usually found in inguinal lymph nodes.[44] Angiomyomatous hamartoma is an irregular proliferation of smooth muscle cells associated with blood vessels that also has a predilection for inguinal lymph nodes; however, it can involve all parts of the lymph node.[42] Leiomyomatosis of the lymph node consists of a proliferation of bland smooth muscle cells in the intra-abdominal lymph nodes of women.[45] Patients usually have coexisting uterine leiomyomas, although this is not always the case.

Inflammatory pseudotumor is a reactive proliferation of myofibroblasts and inflammatory cells.[46,47] Despite the similarity in the names, this disease is probably distinct from its extranodal namesakes. It usually occurs in young adults with an equal male/female ratio. Patients present with one or several moderately enlarged lymph nodes that may be matted together into larger masses up to 10 cm. There are often systemic symptoms such as fever and night sweats. The lesion is benign, but may recur. Histologically, there is infiltration of the lymph node capsule and hilum by spindled and inflammatory cells with an edematous to fibrous background (Fig. 20-6). The spin-

dled cells consist of myofibroblasts and fibroblasts, whereas the inflammatory cells are small lymphocytes, plasma cells, immunoblasts, eosinophils, neutrophils, and histiocytes. There is also a proliferation of small blood vessels. The remaining lymph node parenchyma is unremarkable and generally nonreactive. The differential diagnosis includes Kaposi's sarcoma and the spindle cell variant of atypical mycobacterial infection. Kaposi's sarcoma generally has a greater degree of cellularity, with slit-like spaces and hemorrhage. Atypical myco-bacterial infection can closely simulate inflammatory pseudotumor.[48] The clinical setting may suggest atypical mycobacterial infection; acid-fast stains will resolve any dubious cases.

Palisaded myofibroblastoma (hemorrhagic spindle cell tumor with amianthoid fibers) is a distinctive benign neoplasm showing myofibroblastic differentiation that is almost always found in inguinal lymph nodes.[49–51] It consists of a proliferation of spindle cells with bland, spindled nuclei. The cytoplasm occasionally shows intracytoplasmic globules of actin filaments. The most characteristic feature of this neoplasm is the presence of stellate areas of extracellular collagen deposition, termed *amianthoid fibers*. The spindle cells stain for vimentin, muscle-specific actin, and myosin, whereas the amianthoid fibers may stain for type I and type II collagen and actin.

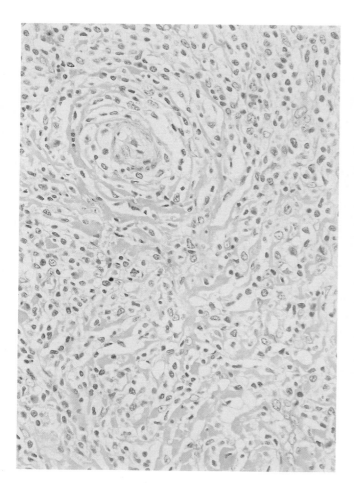

Fig. 20-6. Inflammatory pseudotumor. The capsule is fibrotic and contains a reactive lymphoid infiltrate.

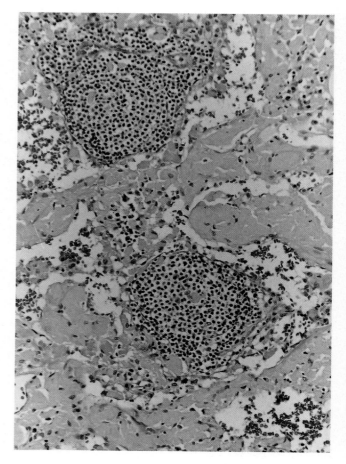

Fig. 20-7. Amyloidosis. Preferential paracortical involvement is seen in this case. The amorphous material showed apple green birefringence on Congo Red stain.

Protein Deposition

Proteinaceous lymphadenopathy, also known as angiocentric sclerosing lymphadenopathy, is a rare disease of unknown etiology.[52] It is thought to be an unusual variant of plasma cell dyscrasia. Patients have been reported to present with generalized lymphadenopathy and polyclonal hypergammaglobulinemia. Involved lymph nodes show obliteration of the normal architecture by deposition of a nonamyloid material, which appears to be composed of bundles of fine reticulin fibers. Typically, this material lines vessel walls. Lymphocytes and plasma cells are very rarely seen. The lack of light chain predominance, the paucicellularity, and the global angiosclerotic changes of proteinaceous lymphadenopathy are morphologic features not found in light chain deposition disease or multiple myeloma.

Amyloid deposits are frequently seen in the lymph nodes of patients with systemic amyloidosis.[53] Less commonly, amyloid may be identified in the lymph nodes of patients with plasmacytoma, lymphoplasmacytic lymphoma, or Castleman's disease.[54] Amyloid lymphadenopathy in the absence of systemic amyloidosis or lymphoproliferative disease is extremely rare. The morphologic features of amyloid in lymph nodes is consistent, despite the clinical presentation. The deposits may involve the walls of the lymph node vessels, may partially or completely replace the lymph node follicles, or may be diffusely present throughout the lymph node parenchyma (Fig 20-7). Congo red cytochemical staining shows the amorphous eosinophilic amyloid material to have a unique characteristic apple green birefringence. Proteinaceous lymphadenopathy can easily be distinguished from amyloid lymphadenopathy, because of the typical onion skinning on reticulin stain and lack of Congo red birefringent staining in the globular deposits of the former entity. Para-amyloid refers to a periodic acid schiff (PAS)-positive, Congo red nonbirefringent inflammatory or abnormal immunoreaction product seen in lymph nodes with angioimmunoblastic lymphadenopathy or Hodgkin's disease, or due to iatrogenic causes. The sclerosis commonly seen in inguinal and pelvic lymph nodes stains for collagen and does not show Congo red birefringence, distinguishing it from amyloid lymphadenopathy.

REACTIVE LYMPHADENOPATHY

The lymph node can undergo a variety of changes in response to reactive conditions. Broadly, these changes can be divided into two groups: lymphadenitis and lymphoid hyperplasia. The term *lymphadenitis* is used when an infectious agent is highly probable, whereas the term *lymphoid hyperplasia* is applied when it is presumed that the lymph node changes have occurred in response to antigenic stimulation without actual infectious involvement of the node. Several different patterns can be seen in lymphoid hyperplasia, including reactive follicular hyperplasia, caused by preferential stimulation of the B cell compartment of the node; reactive paracortical hyperplasia, caused by preferential stimulation of the T cell compartment; and reactive histiocytic hyperplasia, caused by preferential stimulation of the histiocytic compartment. Often, combinations of these patterns are observed, as it is unusual for one compartment to be stimulated without some involvement of the others. Nonetheless, it is useful to classify the various lymphadenopathies according to their predominant pattern of involvement. In some diseases, necrosis is the predominant histologic pattern. Granulomatous disorders are considered separately.

The following is a list of reactive lymphadenopathies:

Follicular
  Nonspecific reactive follicular hyperplasia
  Rheumatoid arthritis
  Sjögren's syndrome
  Kimura's disease
  Toxoplasmosis
  Syphilis
  Castleman's disease
  HIV-associated lymphadenopathy
  Progressive transformation of germinal centers

Paracortical
  Nonspecific reactive paracortical hyperplasia
  Viral
      Epstein-Barr
      Cytomegalovirus
      Herpes
  Drug-induced/postvaccinial
  Dermatopathic lymphadenitis

Sinus
  Sinus histiocytosis
  Monocytoid B cell hyperplasia
  Hemophagocytic syndrome
  Sinus histiocytosis with massive lymphadenopathy
  Whipple's disease
  Exogenous lipids

Extensive necrosis
  Complete necrosis/infarction
  Kikuchi's histiocytic necrotizing lymphadenitis
  Systemic lupus erythematosus
  Kawasaki disease

Granulomatous
  Noninfectious

Infectious
  Nonsuppurative
  Suppurative
      Cat-scratch disease
      Lymphogranuloma venereum
      Yersinia

Fine needle aspiration biopsy is an effective method for the evaluation of reactive lymphadenopathy, both by ruling out carcinoma and by suggesting a specific etiology to a reactive condition. Material may also be obtained for appropriate microbiologic studies. The diagnosis of reactive lymphoid hyperplasia should only be made in a setting in which adequate clinical follow-up is available. If adenopathy persists or further enlargement occurs after a reactive diagnosis has been rendered based on a fine needle aspiration biopsy, one must either repeat the aspiration biopsy or perform an open biopsy.

Reactive Follicular Hyperplasia

The follicles represent the B cell compartment of the lymph node. Unstimulated follicles are termed *primary follicles*. They consist of small B lineage lymphocytes (CD20+) that are easily seen, embedded in a network of dendritic reticulum cells that are not easily appreciated morphologically, but can always be demonstrated by appropriate immunohistochemical studies for these cells (CD21 or CD35). With the appropriate stimulation secondary follicles are formed. The most prominent feature of the secondary follicle is the germinal center. Germinal centers are composed of a mixture of small and large cleaved and noncleaved follicular center cells—a polytypic mixture of kappa- and lambda-bearing cells—with admixed CD4+, CD57+, small T lymphocytes, tingible body macrophages (CD68+), and occasionally polyclonal plasma cells, all embedded in a network of dendritic reticulum cells. In highly reactive follicles, polarization is seen, with one axis of the germinal center composed primarily of large noncleaved cells and tingible body macrophages (the dark zone), and the other axis composed primarily of small cleaved cells (the pale zone) Fig. 20-8. Surrounding the germinal center is a mantle of small B lymphocytes, which share morphologic and immunologic features with the cells that are found in the centers of primary follicles. In spleen and occasionally in abdominal lymph nodes, there is an outer layer of marginal B cells, cells with slightly irregular nuclei, a moderate rim of pale to clear cytoplasm, and occasional plasmacytoid features. The follicles are surrounded by a paracortical region that is often expanded.

Reactive follicular hyperplasia may be recognized in fine needle aspiration specimens by the presence of small cellular aggregates at low magnification, and the presence of a polymorphous population of lymphoid cells at high magnification (Fig. 20-9). Tingible body macrophages are also present.

The major differential diagnosis of reactive follicular hyperplasia is follicular lymphoma. Numerous histologic criteria have been proposed for the distinction[55,56] (Table 20-4), but one must keep in mind that no one criterion is diagnostic. In practice, one must assess many features in combination, also considering clinical factors such as the relative rarity of follicu-

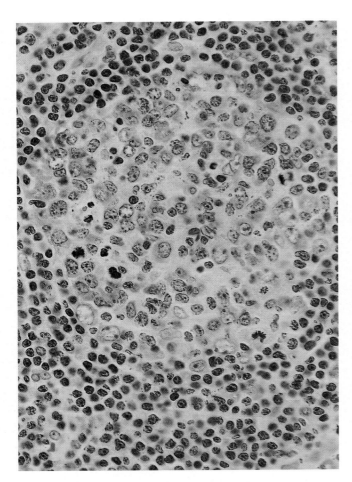

Fig. 20-8. Reactive germinal center. Note the differences in cell types at the left vs. the right; this phenomenon has been called polarization.

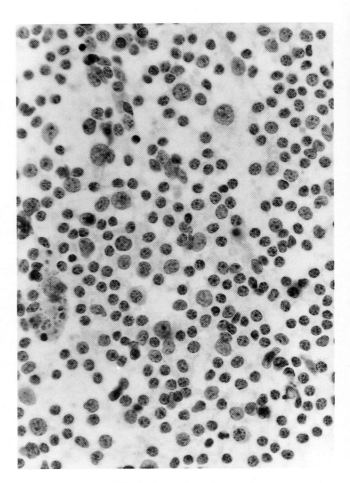

Fig. 20-9. Reactive follicular hyperplasia, fine needle aspiration. Note the mixture of lymphoid cells, with a tingible body macrophage present at the edge of the field.

lar lymphoma in patients under the age of 40. Particularly helpful histologic features include the greater density of follicles, the uniformity of size, and uniformity of cellular composition in follicular lymphoma as opposed to reactive follicular hyperplasia. In difficult cases, immunohistochemical and molecular studies may be helpful in determining the correct diagnosis (Table 20-5). The expression of bcl-2 protein in neoplastic as opposed to reactive follicles is usually very useful, with the caveat that bcl-2 protein may be negative in some follicular lymphomas, particularly follicular large cell lymphomas.[57–59] In addition, bcl-2 protein may be expressed by the T helper cells in reactive follicles; comparison of bcl-2 stains with B and T lineage stains will prevent mistaking bcl-2 reactivity of T cells for bcl-2 reactivity in follicular lymphoma. Under some conditions, the t(14;18) may be detected by PCR in reactive tissues,[17] but this is generally not a problem in protocols generally used for routine diagnosis.[60]

Other neoplasms that should be considered in the differential diagnosis include the nodular variant of mantle cell lymphoma and interfollicular Hodgkin's disease. In the nodular variant of mantle cell lymphoma, the lymphoid follicles become entirely replaced by neoplastic mantle cells, mimicking primary follicles. However, in contrast to reactive primary fol-

licles, the follicles of mantle cell lymphoma are larger and the cells comprising the neoplastic nodules usually have a greater degree of nuclear atypicality than those of primary follicles. Paraffin section immunohistochemical studies often demonstrate aberrant coexpression of CD20 and CD43 in the cells of mantle cell lymphoma[2,61] The interfollicular variant of Hodgkin's disease can closely mimic reactive follicular hyperplasia, in that both may show highly reactive germinal centers. Examination of the interfollicular areas in the former will demonstrate Reed-Sternberg cells and variants in the appropriate milieu.[62] Immunohistochemical studies will usually demonstrate positivity for CD15 and negativity for CD45 in the Hodgkin's cells of most cases of Hodgkin's disease; however, stains for CD30 may not be of use, as scattered CD30+ cells may be found in both disorders: CD30+ Reed-Sternberg cells and variants in Hodgkin's disease and CD30+ immunoblasts in reactive follicular hyperplasia.

Once a diagnosis of reactive follicular hyperplasia is established, one should attempt to identify a specific etiology. This may be possible in only a minority of cases. Nonetheless, many diseases showing reactive follicular hyperplasia have distinctive features that either allow their identification or suggest their diagnosis, prompting the appropriate confirmatory studies.

Table 20-4. Histologic Features Useful in the Distinction of Reactive Follicular Hyperplasia vs. Follicular Lymphoma

Reactive Follicular Hyperplasia	Follicular Lymphoma
Follicles limited to cortical region	Follicles present throughout the node
Follicles do not extend beyond capsule	Follicles extend beyond capsule
Low density of follicles	High density of follicles
Abundant interfollicular areas	Compressed interfollicular areas
No areas of diffuse effacement	Areas of diffuse effacement or architecture
Follicles of uneven size and shape	Follicles of similar size and shape
Mantle zone distinct	Mantle zone indistinct or absent
Mixture of cell types in germinal center	Monomorphic or polymorphic population
Tingible body macrophages present	Tingible body macrophages usually absent
Low to high mitotic rate	Low to moderate mitotic rate
Cell polarization often evident	Cell polarization absent

Nonspecific reactive follicular hyperplasia is common in the younger age groups, and generally resolves spontaneously without further consequences for the patient. By contrast, nonspecific reactive follicular hyperplasia occurring in the elderly often involves multiple lymph nodes and has been associated with concurrent or subsequent malignant lymphoma in a significant subset of cases.[63]

Rheumatoid Lymphadenopathy

Patients with rheumatoid arthritis commonly have lymphadenopathy, but biopsies are usually performed only if the lymph node reaches an unusually large size or grows at an unusually fast rate. The characteristic features of rheumatoid lymphadenopathy include a marked reactive follicular hyperplasia with a paracortical polyclonal plasmacytosis.[64,65] The reactive changes are often present throughout the lymph node and may occur outside the capsule as well. Occasionally, there is a sinusoidal hyperplasia containing numerous neutrophils. The differential diagnosis includes syphilis, the plasma cell variant of Castleman's disease, and other collagen vascular diseases, particularly Sjögren's disease. In some cases, a paracortical proliferation may predominate, mimicking a peripheral T cell lymphoma.

Sjögren's Lymphadenopathy

The lymph node findings in Sjögren's disease may be indistinguishable from rheumatoid lymphadenopathy.[66] However, the former often contains a proliferation of monocytoid B cells in the sinusoidal or paracortical regions. When extensive, these proliferations may be indistinguishable from or actually represent early low grade B cell lymphoma of mucosa-associated lymphoid tissue (MALToma). Because these proliferations often show lymphoplasmacytoid features, staining for immunoglobulin light chains may be helpful in the differential diagnosis. Evidence of aberrant coexpression of CD20 and CD43 or the identification of significant monoclonal populations on molecular analysis of the immunoglobulin genes would favor the diagnosis of lymphoma. The significance of small clonal B cell populations is not yet clear.[67]

Kimura's Lymphadenopathy

Kimura's disease is a benign chronic inflammatory disease of probable allergic etiology. It predominantly affects Asians of young to middle age, but may occasionally affect other ethnic groups and other ages. Patients usually present with subcutaneous or soft tissue masses of the head and neck, often with infiltration of the salivary gland and involvement of regional lymph nodes. However, patients may occasionally present with isolated lymphadenopathy. Laboratory studies characteristically reveal eosinophilia with increased levels of IgE.

Table 20-5. Immunohistochemical and Molecular Features Useful in the Distinction of Reactive Follicular Hyperplasia vs. Follicular Lymphoma

Reactive Follicular Hyperplasia	Follicular Lymphoma
bcl-2 protein negative in follicles	bcl-2 protein often positive in follicles
MT2 positive in follicles	MT2 sometimes negative in follicles
Polytypic immunoglobulins in follicles, often detectable in paraffin sections	Monotypic or absent immunoglobulins in follicles, usually detectable only in frozen sections
Polytypic immunoglobulin mRNA in follicles, often detectable in paraffin sections	Monotypic or absent immunoglobulin mRNA in follicles
Germline immunoglobulin genes	Monoclonal rearrangements of immunoglobulin genes
Germline bcl-2 genes by Southern blot	Rearranged bcl-2 gene in most cases
t(14;18) not detectable by classic cytogenetics	t(14;18) usually detectable by classic cytogenetics
t(14;18) usually not detectable by PCR	t(14;18) usually detectable by PCR

Involved lymph nodes usually show a characteristic triad of florid reactive follicular hyperplasia, increased vascularity, and marked eosinophilia of the paracortical regions[68–70] (Fig. 20-10). The reactive follicles frequently contain a proteinaceous material and many show prominent vascularization. Those that are highly vascularized usually show eosinophilia, which can be intense enough to form eosinophilic microabscesses. Occasionally, focal necrosis of the germinal centers can be seen. Immunohistochemical studies show large amounts of IgE on the processes of the follicular dendritic cells. The paracortical regions are also highly vascularized with numerous postcapillary venules. The most characteristic finding is marked eosinophilic infiltration, sometimes with the formation of eosinophilic abscesses. Scattered plasma cells and mast cells are also present. The sinuses also show marked eosinophilia. Other lymph node findings include the presence of polykaryocytes and focal sclerosis.

The differential diagnosis of Kimura's lymphadenopathy includes many diseases with eosinophilia, such as drug-induced lymphadenopathy, parasitic infestation, Langerhans cell histiocytosis, Hodgkin's disease, and non-Hodgkin's lymphoma with eosinophilia. In drug-induced lymphadenopathy, the primary changes are in the paracortex, which contains a mixed population including immunoblasts and plasma cells, as well as eosinophils. Parasitic infestation can usually be suggested from the history; the lymph node may show direct evidence of the organism. Langerhans cell histiocytosis preferentially involves the sinuses. Hodgkin's disease and non-Hodgkin's lymphoma with eosinophilia, particularly interfollicular variants, may be confused with Kimura's disease, but attention to the identification of atypical cytology should allow easy distinction. Kimura's disease should not be confused with *angiolymphoid hyperplasia with eosinophilia* in any way except the name.[68,70] The latter is a primary vascular proliferation characterized by an epithelioid appearance of the lining endothelial cells. Although there is often eosinophilia, the clinical picture and, most important, the histologic appearance, are otherwise markedly different.

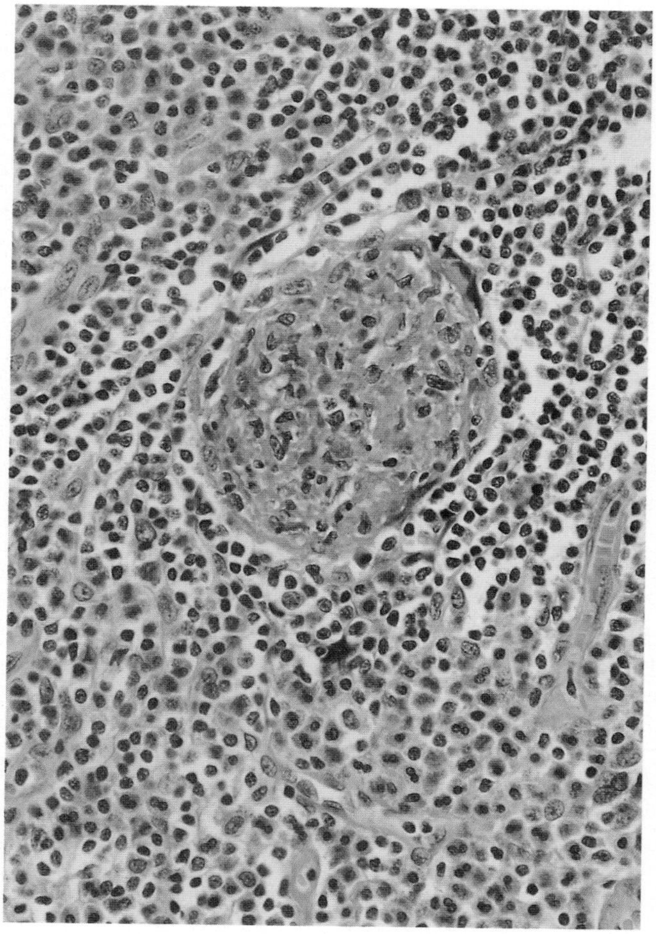

Toxoplasmic Lymphadenitis

The symptoms of toxoplasmic lymphadenitis, caused by infection with the protozoon *Toxoplasma gondii*, may range from enlargement of a solitary node, usually posterior cervical, to a generalized lymphadenopathy with fever, resembling acute infectious mononucleosis. A characteristic triad of findings is seen, including (1) florid reactive follicular hyperplasia, (2) clusters of epithelioid histiocytes, and (3) reactive monocytoid B cell proliferation in sinuses[71,72] (Fig. 20-11). This triad of findings is often found in close spatial relationship to one another. The epithelioid histiocytes are not organized into well formed granulomas, giant cells are rare if at all present, and eosinophils and necrosis are not seen. Rather, ill defined aggregates of epithelioid histiocytes are seen in paracortical areas, in the mantle zones (impinging on the germinal centers), and occasionally present within germinal centers. In addition to the characteristic triad, there is often a plasmacytosis. Only rarely can the organism be identified morphologically as intracellular trophozoites or cysts. The lymph node findings most likely represent a reaction to antigens associated with the organism rather than the organism itself, since PCR studies for *T. gondii* are usually negative in toxoplasmic lymphadenitis.[73]

The characteristic histologic triad is both a sensitive and relatively specific marker of toxoplasmic lymphadenitis, and the diagnosis should be suggested if these findings are encountered. Rarely, HIV-associated lymphadenopathy has been reported to show the triad in the absence of toxoplasmic infection, but these lymph nodes usually show other features characteristic of that disorder. In addition, leishmaniasis can cause very similar histologic findings, although the characteristic intracellular organisms can usually be identified if the histiocytes are carefully examined. The appropriate serologic studies for toxoplasmosis should be performed to confirm a diagnosis of toxoplasmic lymphadenitis.

Fig. 20-10. Kimura's disease. The germinal center shows deposition of a proteinaceous material, while the paracortical area shows intense eosinophilia.

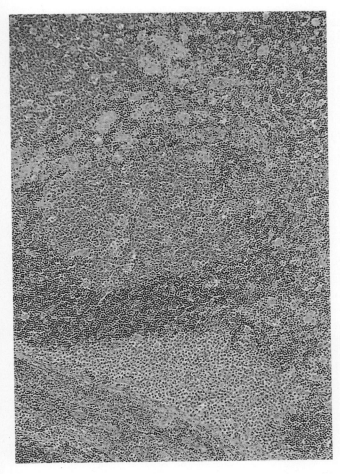

Fig. 20-11. Toxoplasmic lymphadenitis. This field shows the characteristic triad of reactive follicular hyperplasia, clusters of epithelioid histiocytes, and a reactive monocytoid B cell proliferation.

Syphilitic Lymphadenitis

Enlargement of lymph nodes occurs in primary and secondary syphilis. Follicular hyperplasia and extensive paracortical plasmacytosis are common histologic features.[74] Frequently, the capsule is fibrotic, and contains an obliterative endarteritis with a perivascular lymphoplasmacytosis. In addition, aggregates of epithelioid histiocytes or small noncaseating granulomata may be present. Spirochetes are usually identified by Warthin-Starry silver stain or by immunohistochemical studies in the walls of postcapillary venules, in areas of necrosis, or occasionally within germinal centers.

Progressive Transformation of Germinal Centers

Progressive transformation of germinal centers is a variant of nonspecific reactive follicular hyperplasia in which some follicles undergo a marked enlargement up to four times normal size[75,76] (Fig. 20-12). The enlarged follicles consist of numerous

small lymphocytes, often admixed with residual germinal center cells, the latter sometimes forming clusters. The progressively transformed germinal centers are found in a background of smaller, typical-appearing secondary lymphoid follicles, with transitional follicles usually present. Immunohistochemical studies of the small lymphocytes show the typical phenotype of polyclonal mantle zone B cells, with an expanded network of follicular dendritic cells forming the framework of the nodule.

Progressive transformation of germinal centers is more common in males and occurs in all age groups, although there is a predilection for the young. The most frequent presentation is that of an asymptomatic, solitary, enlarged lymph node, usually in the neck or inguinal region. The disease may recur in a significant subset of patients, but is otherwise not generally clinically significant. Progressive transformation of germinal centers has been reported to coexist with lymphocytic and histiocytic (L&H) lymphocyte predominance Hodgkin's disease.[77] In addition, patients with progressive transformation of germinal centers may develop L&H lymphocyte predominance, but only in a very low percentage of cases.[78]

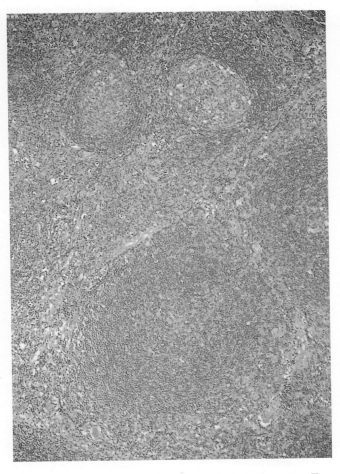

Fig. 20-12. Progressive transformation of germinal centers. Two reactive follicles are seen at top, while a progressively transformed germinal center is seen at bottom.

L&H lymphocyte predominance Hodgkin's disease represents the most important entity to be distinguished from progressive transformation of germinal centers; this differential diagnosis is discussed in the section on L&H lymphocyte predominance. Progressive transformation of germinal centers must also be distinguished from follicular lymphoma, particularly the floral variant. The progressively transformed germinal centers are generally larger than the follicles of follicular lymphoma. In addition, the background of reactive follicular hyperplasia in progressive transformation of germinal centers is different than that of follicular lymphoma, in which all the follicles are generally neoplastic. In difficult cases, immunohistochemical or molecular studies may be necessary. Occasional cases of mantle cell lymphoma may be difficult to distinguish from progressive transformation of germinal centers. The cells of mantle cell lymphoma usually have more irregular nuclear contours than the round lymphocytes in progressive transformation of germinal centers.

Castleman's Disease

Castleman's disease, also known as angiofollicular lymph node hyperplasia or giant lymph node hyperplasia, may be localized or multicentric.[79] Localized Castleman's disease can be divided into hyaline-vascular, plasma cell, transitional, and stromal rich types.[80–82] In the hyaline-vascular type of localized Castleman's disease, there is no age or sex predilection. Patients generally present with a mass that is usually asymptomatic, except from possible impingement on adjacent structures. The mediastinum is the most common site of involvement, followed by the abdomen, lung, skeletal muscle, and axillary and cervical soft tissue. The lesion is cured by surgical excision. Some cases are associated with a vascular or follicular dendritic cell neoplasm or an angiolipomatous hamartoma.[83–85]

Histologically, the hyaline vascular type of *localized Castleman's disease* shows numerous regressively transformed germinal centers (Fig. 20-13). The mantle zones are expanded and usually have an "onion-skin" appearance. The germinal centers are typically small, hypervascular, and occasionally multiple. They usually show lymphocyte depletion, with a hyalinized appearance. Penetrating vessels can sometimes be seen entering the follicle from the interfollicular region. The interfollicular region is hypervascular and is composed of a mixture of small lymphocytes, plasmacytoid monocytes, and plasma cells.[86] Occasionally, cells with large, hyperchromatic nuclei are present. In rare cases, the interfollicular areas may be markedly expanded, with increased numbers of spindled cells; these cases are more frequently present in the abdomen. The sinuses are usually obliterated and there is often a thickened capsule, with extension of the fibrosis around blood vessels. Immunohistochemical studies demonstrate that the follicles are composed predominantly of follicular dendritic cells with scattered polyclonal B cells. The interfollicular areas are composed mostly of T cells, with polyclonal plasma cells. Molecular studies show a germline configuration of lymphocyte antigen receptor genes, and no viruses have been identified.[87]

Hyaline-vascular follicles have been reported in other types of reactive follicular hyperplasia, including HIV-associated

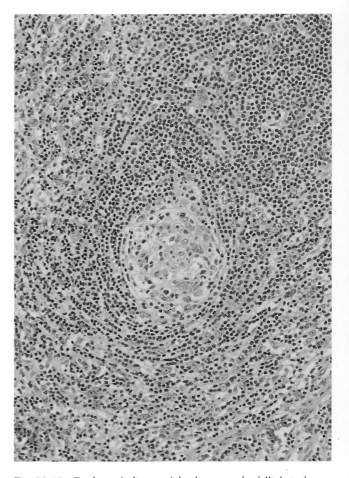

Fig. 20-13. Castleman's disease. A hyaline-vascular follicle is shown.

lymphadenopathy.[79] However, the intefollicular regions in HIV-associated lymphadenopathy tend to be more polymorphous, with greater numbers of plasma cells and immunoblasts and generally lack the intense vascularity of Castleman's disease. In hyaline-vascular Castleman's disease, capsular fibrosis is more prominent and the lymph node is usually much larger in overall size. The expanded mantle zones in hyaline-vascular Castleman's disease may also mimic mantle cell lymphoma, but the cells in the reactive mantle zones lack the cytologic atypia commonly seen in the lymphoma; immunologic studies may also be helpful in making this distinction.

The plasma cell type of localized Castleman's disease is about one-tenth as common as the hyaline-vascular type; it also does not have an age or sex predilection.[80] However, patients frequently have systemic symptoms that resolve after surgical removal of the lesion. They include fever with a raised erythrocyte sedimentation rate (ESR), sweating, and fatigue; hematologic abnormalities, including thrombocytopenia and anemia[88]; and immunologic disorders, including hyperglobulinemia and rarely myasthenia gravis. Almost all patients have increased levels of serum interleukin-6, and the symptomatology may be relieved by therapy with monoclonal interleukin-6 antibody.[89] In contrast to the hyaline-vascular type, the abdomen (particularly the small intestinal mesentery) is the most common site involved by the plasma cell type.

In the plasma cell type, the clinical mass is usually a collection of discrete, enlarged lymph nodes. The most striking histologic finding is the presence of sheets of mature plasma cells in the interfollicular regions. Other cells are few, except for occasional immunoblasts. There is no increase in vascularity. The follicles usually contain large germinal centers with mitotic figures, nuclear debris, and histiocytes. No central blood vessel is seen, and there is no hyalinization, although some follicles may be of the hyaline-vascular type. The nodal architecture is usually at least partially preserved, with patent sinuses. Immunohistochemical studies reveal the interfollicular plasma cells to be monotypic in about one-half of cases.[90] Interleukin-6 is found in the germinal center cells and immunoblasts.[91]

The differential diagnosis of the plasma cell type of Castleman's disease includes rheumatoid disease, syphilis, HIV-associated lymphadenopathy, and lymph nodes involved by or adjacent to other neoplasms (particularly Kaposi's sarcoma and Hodgkin's disease). Studies to rule out these other diseases should be performed before making a diagnosis of the plasma cell type of Castleman's disease.

Rare cases transitional between the hyaline-vascular and plasma cell types of localized Castleman's disease have been reported. The clinical features more closely resemble the hyaline-vascular type. Histologically, the follicles are mostly of the hyaline-vascular type, although hyperplastic follicles may also be present. The interfollicular regions show both marked vascularity and extensive polyclonal plasmacytosis.

Recently, a stromal-rich variant of Castleman's disease has been described.[82] The lesions tend to be large and are usually found in the abdomen or retroperitoneal soft tissue. Histologically, the interfollicular zones are enlarged in size, so that they comprise greater than 75 percent of the size of the mass. These areas are rich in spindled cells, mostly endothelial cells, histiocytes, follicular dendritic cells, and fibroblastic reticulum cells.

Multicentric Castleman's disease usually occurs in older patients and is associated with systemic manifestations.[92,93] There is multicentric lymph node enlargement, and splenomegaly is common. Patients are usually anemic and have polyclonal hypergammaglobulinemia. As a rule, there is evidence of multisystem disease, such as involvement of the liver, kidney, skin, and central nervous system. The bone marrow often shows plasmacytosis. Some patients may present with POEMS syndrome (polyneuropathy, organomegaly, endocrinopathy, M-protein, and skin symptoms).[94] In many of these patients, the disease has an aggressive course with a fatal outcome.

Histologically, the nodes resemble the plasma cell type of Castleman's disease, although some hyaline-vascular follicles may be present.[93,95] Immunohistochemical studies reveal the interfollicular plasma cells to be monotypic or polytypic. Molecular studies may show a germline configuration of the lymphocyte antigen receptor genes or may demonstrate small clonal populations of T or B cells.[96] Evidence of Epstein-Barr virus or, more recently, the Kaposi's sarcoma-associated herpesvirus (HHV-8) has been found in many cases.[96,97]

Histologic changes indistinguishable from multicentric Castleman's disease may be found in Kaposi's sarcoma and acquired immunodeficiency syndrome (AIDS). In addition, mul-

ticentric Castleman's disease may be complicated by malignant lymphoma. Therefore, studies should be done to exclude these possibilities in any patient for whom a diagnosis of multicentric Castleman's disease is being considered.

HIV-Associated Lymphadenopathy

HIV-associated lymphadenopathy is included in the section on reactive follicular hyperplasia because patients usually show some type of follicular hyperplasia at the time of lymph node biopsy. Nonetheless, it must be acknowledged that follicular involution and lymphoid depletion may sometimes be the dominant findings, although usually at a late stage in the disease course and more commonly at autopsy than in surgical specimens. Lymphadenopathy is common in HIV-infected patients. Biopsies are generally performed in this population to rule out infection or a neoplasm such as malignant lymphoma or Kaposi's sarcoma. However, persistent generalized lymphadenopathy is a part of the spectrum of HIV-associated disease, defined by the Centers for Disease Control and Prevention as lymph node enlargement of at least 3 months' duration, absence of any illness or drug use known to cause lymph node enlargement, and histologic evidence of reactive follicular hyperplasia.[98]

Three to four main stages of lymph node changes have been described.[99–102] "Explosive" reactive follicular hyperplasia represents the earliest and most common histologic finding (Fig. 20-14). In explosive reactive follicular hyperplasia, there are numerous secondary follicles distributed throughout the lymph node, with highly irregular sizes and shapes. The germinal centers frequently show polarization and contain a mixture of germinal center B cells and numerous tingible body macrophages. Typically, the mantle zones are thinned and may be entirely absent, simulating malignant lymphoma. In some follicles, the phenomenon of follicle lysis may be seen (Fig. 20-15). In follicle lysis, there is invagination of small lymphocytes into the germinal center, with separation of the clusters of germinal center cells into irregular clusters. In contrast to progressive transformation of germinal centers, the affected follicles are of normal size. This is often accompanied by follicular hemorrhage. The paracortical lymphoid tissue is often reduced in size, but is usually hypervascular and contains a mixed infiltrate including plasma cells and sometimes immunoblasts, eosinophils, and epithelioid histiocytes. Other characteristic features include a proliferation of monocytoid B cells in paracortical regions, focal dermatopathic changes, and Warthin-Finkeldey type giant cells (in follicles or the paracortical regions).[103]

Over time, floridly reactive follicles are found admixed with hyaline-vascular follicles (follicular involution) that closely resemble the characteristic follicles of the hyaline-vascular Castleman's disease. Early on, the paracortical region is diminished in size but, over time, the paracortical areas become expanded with hypervascularity and numerous plasma cells, forming a picture that closely mimics the plasma cell variant of Castleman's disease. Finally, in lymphocyte depletion, there is a generalized loss of lymphoid cells in both the follicles and paracortical regions (Fig. 20-16). The germinal centers are en-

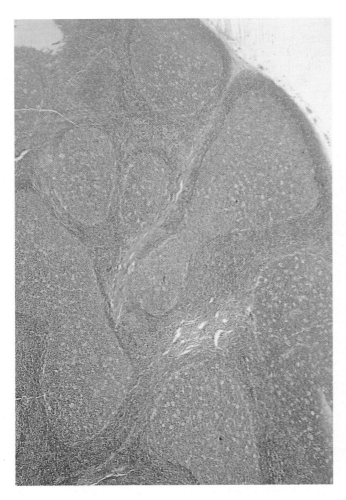

Fig. 20-14. HIV-associated lymphadenopathy. "Explosive" reactive follicular hyperplasia is seen.

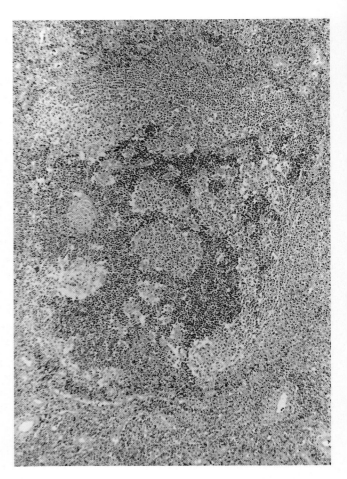

Fig. 20-15. HIV-associated lymphadenopathy. This follicle is undergoing follicle lysis.

tirely absent or reduced to skeletons of follicular dendritic cells, endothelial cells, and histiocytes. The paracortical region is also greatly diminished in size and consists of histiocytes and plasma cells, but only scattered lymphoid cells. There may be a granulomatous appearance imparted by the numerous histiocytes, a finding that should prompt appropriate special stains for *Mycobacteria avium-intracellulare* or other organisms. Due to diminution of the follicular and paracortical areas, the sinusoidal areas often appear prominent. Lymph nodes with lymphocyte depletion are generally smaller, not larger, than usual, and therefore usually not seen in surgical specimens.

In explosive reactive follicular hyperplasia, HIV can be demonstrated in the follicular dendritic cells by electron microscopy, immunohistochemical studies, or in situ hybridization; these cells represent a major reservoir of HIV in the latent phase prior to the development of AIDS.[104] In follicle lysis, a disrupted network of follicular dendritic cells can be demonstrated by immunohistochemical studies.[105] The paracortical areas have a decreased CD4/CD8 ratio, similar to that seen in the peripheral blood in these patients.

Patients with explosive reactive follicular hyperplasia or mixed reactive follicular hyperplasia with hyaline-vascular follicles are generally in the pre-AIDS state with a relatively good prognosis. Patients without follicular hyperplasia—those with follicular involution or lymphocyte depletion—have a poor prognosis and usually have clinical AIDS.

None of the above described changes is diagnostic of HIV-associated lymphadenopathy. Nonetheless, the identification of this constellation of findings should at least prompt the suggestion of this diagnosis, particularly in the appropriate clinical settings. Several phases of this disorder can show a close resemblance to the several types of Castleman's disease. If a diagnosis of HIV-associated lymphadenopathy is suspected, one should also carefully scrutinize the lymph node for concurrent infection as well as malignant neoplasms. In particular, Kaposi's sarcoma can be present as a very focal finding in the capsule of the lymph node, particularly in cases showing hyaline-vascular follicles with Castleman-like features or lymphocyte depletion. In addition, areas of concomitant non-Hodgkin's lymphoma should not be overlooked.

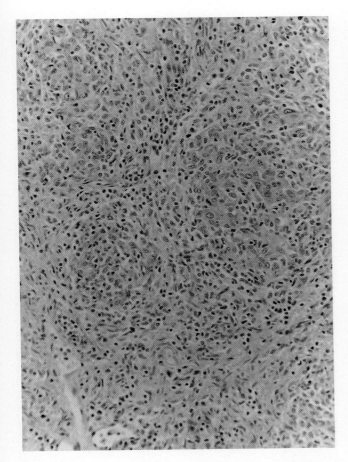

Fig. 20-16. HIV-associated lymphadenopathy. Marked lymphocyte depletion is present.

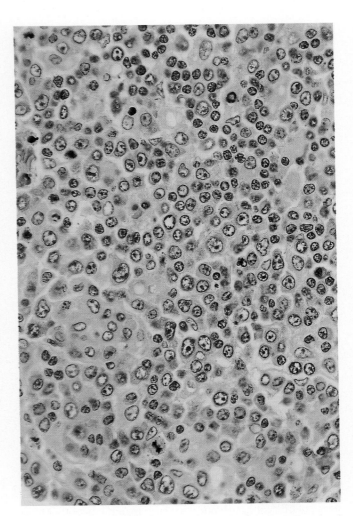

Fig. 20-17. Reactive paracortical hyperplasia. A spectrum of lymphoid differentiation, including numerous immunoblasts, is seen. This case was Epstein-Barr virus-associated acute infectious mononucleosis.

Reactive Paracortical Hyperplasia

The paracortex represents the T cell zone of the lymph node. It contains numerous T cells, with CD4+ cells generally outnumbering CD8+ cells; scattered B cells and plasma cells; histiocytes; occasional interdigitating dendritic cells (S-100 positive; no Birbeck granules) and Langerhans cells (S-100 positive; Birbeck granules); and fibroblastic reticulum cells (Fig. 20-17). In addition, there are high endothelial venules. In the unstimulated state, almost all of the lymphoid cells are small with a condensed chromatin pattern. On immune stimulation, the paracortex becomes expanded, with greater numbers of small and large B and T cells and plasma cells, giving rise to an overall mottled appearance. Many of the large cells have features of classic immunoblasts—cells with large nuclei with vesicular chromatin and prominent nucleoli. There is also a proliferation of high endothelial venules. Benign paracortical hyperplasia is virtually always accompanied by some degree of reactive follicular hyperplasia and often reactive sinus hyperplasia. Most of the time, a specific etiology cannot be determined, but some disorders are associated with characteristic or occasionally diagnostic features. Fine needle aspiration biopsy

of reactive paracortical hyperplasia reveals a polymorphous population of lymphoid cells, including small, medium, and large lymphoid cells with scattered plasma cells.

Viral Lymphadenitis

Viral lymphadenitis represents a common cause of reactive paracortical hyperplasia. Although florid reactive follicular hyperplasia may be a prominent histologic finding in early lesions, reactive paracortical hyperplasia soon becomes the dominant feature, and in some cases, overruns the follicles and leads to diffuse effacement of nodal architecture. In florid cases, focal necrosis may be present in either the follicles or the paracortical region. The sinuses may show histiocytic hyperplasia, occasionally with hemophagocytosis; a range of plasmacytoid cells, including immunoblasts; or a proliferation of monocytoid B cells. The monocytoid B cells may extend into the paracortical areas.

The differential diagnosis includes several types of malignant lymphoma. Sheets of immunoblasts may be focally present, leading to potential confusion with large cell non-Hodgkin's lymphoma. In some cases, Reed-Sternberg-like cells may be found, leading to potential confusion with Hodgkin's disease. In both situations, attention should be given to identifying overall retention of architecture (when present) and a spectrum of identifiable cell types in reactive paracortical hyperplasia. Typically, one can identify small lymphocytes, plasma cells, and plasmacytoid immunoblasts in varying numbers. In difficult cases, immunohistochemical studies may be of value, with a mixture of B and T cells with polyclonal plasmacytoid lymphocytes and plasma cells in reactive paracortical hyperplasia. By contrast, non-Hodgkin's lymphoma generally shows sheets of B cells or T cells in B and T cell lymphoma, respectively, with monotypic plasmacytoid cells or plasma cells in lymphoplasmacytic lymphomas. The immunoblasts in reactive paracortical hyperplasia usually have basophilic cytoplasm, sometimes with a paranuclear hof, basophilic nucleoli, and are CD45+ and CD15−, whereas Hodgkin's cells have amphophilic to eosinophilic cytoplasm lacking a hof, eosinophilic nucleoli, and are CD45− and CD15+. In addition, Hodgkin's cells are found in their characteristic milieu, which usually includes eosinophils and lacks a spectrum of plasmacytoid cells.

Epstein-Barr virus (EBV)-associated acute infectious mononucleosis represents a prototype of reactive paracortical hyperplasia[106–108] (Fig. 20-17). The specific diagnosis may be suggested by clinical studies, including a lymphocytosis with atypical lymphocytes and a positive mono-spot test or other EBV serologic studies. Immunohistochemical studies for EBV latent membrane protein (LMP) or in situ hybridization for Epstein-Barr early RNA (EBER) may be useful in identifying specific evidence of EBV, although one must keep in mind that other lymphoproliferations such as Hodgkin's disease and some non-Hodgkin's lymphoma may be EBV-associated and that EBV-seropositive individuals may have rare EBV-positive cells (EBER+, but LMP−) in benign lymphoid tissues.

Cytomegalovirus (CMV) in both immunocompetent and immunocompromised hosts may show features of reactive paracortical hyperplasia similar to EBV-associated infectious mononucleosis.[109,110] Although the characteristic CMV inclusions are generally easy to find in immunocompromised patients, they are usually very rare and require careful search. The infected cells are mostly T cells of both helper and suppressor phenotype. In addition to reactive paracortical hyperplasia, CMV lymphadenitis usually shows a florid reactive follicular hyperplasia with a proliferation of monocytoid B cells in sinuses that extends into the paracortex. The differential diagnosis of CMV lymphadenitis includes other causes of reactive immunoblastic hyperplasia as well as Hodgkin's disease, due to the superficial resemblance of CMV-infected cells to Reed-Sternberg cells. In addition, CMV-infected cells may be CD15+, similar to Reed-Sternberg cells.[111] Immunohistochemical studies for CMV antigens or in situ hybridization studies for CMV DNA should resolve any problematic cases.

Herpes simplex lymphadenitis is common in patients with clinically evident skin lesions, and also rarely occurs as isolated

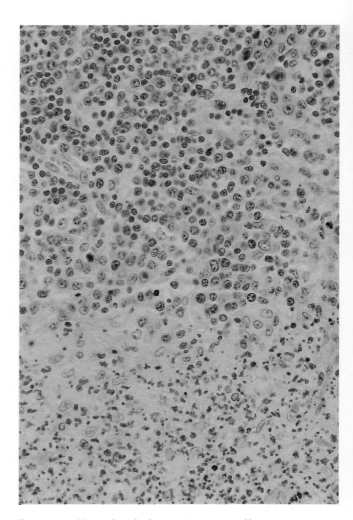

Fig. 20-18. Herpes lymphadenitis. A reactive infiltrate is seen at top, while necrosis with herpetic inclusions is seen at bottom.

lymph node enlargement.[112,113] The histologic appearance can be indistinguishable from nonspecific reactive paracortical hyperplasia. However, there is often necrosis, which may be extensive and accompanied by neutrophils and granulation tissue (Fig. 20-18). The characteristic inclusions of herpes simplex are typically found within the areas of necrosis or in the viable lymphoid tissue at the edge of the necrosis. In situ hybridization for herpes simplex DNA can provide confirmation of the diagnosis.

Drug-Induced Lymphadenopathy

A wide variety of drugs, most notably diphenylhydantoin (Dilantin), can cause lymph node enlargement.[114–116] The lymphadenopathy usually occurs within several weeks after therapy is begun, and resolves within several weeks after the medication is stopped. Typically, reactive paracortical hyperplasia is seen, usually accompanied by eosinophils. Even in the absence of the appropriate history, the presence of these two

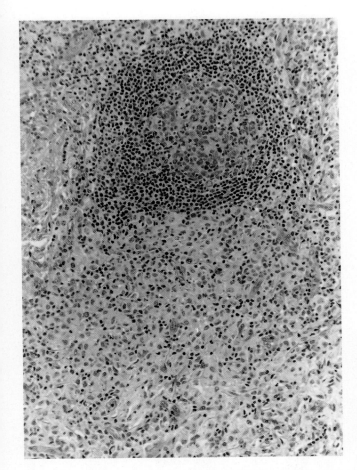

Fig. 20-19. Dermatopathic lymphadenopathy. The paracortical region is pale, due to a proliferation of cytoplasm-rich dendritic cells and macrophages.

Dermatopathic Lymphadenopathy

Dermatopathic lymphadenopathy is a special form of paracortical hyperplasia in which the predominant hyperplastic elements are the dendritic cells[117–120] (Fig. 20-19). This disorder is associated with a variety of skin disorders, particularly those that lead to disruption of the skin barrier, but interestingly has been reported in patients without clinically evident skin lesions. In dermatopathic lymphadenopathy, there is a proliferation of interdigitating dendritic cells, Langerhans cells, histiocytes, eosinophils, as well as a range of lymphoid cells, imparting a mottled appearance at low magnification. The interdigitating dendritic cells and Langerhans cells, usually not morphologically identifiable in normal lymph nodes, are easy to recognize in dermatopathic lymphadenopathy, because of their characteristic grooved nuclei. The histiocytes often (but not always) contain visible melanin pigment. The dendritic cells and melanin-laden macrophages may be easily recognized in fine needle aspiration biopsy specimens (Fig. 20-20). The lymphoid cells vary from small, round lymphocytes to small lymphocytes

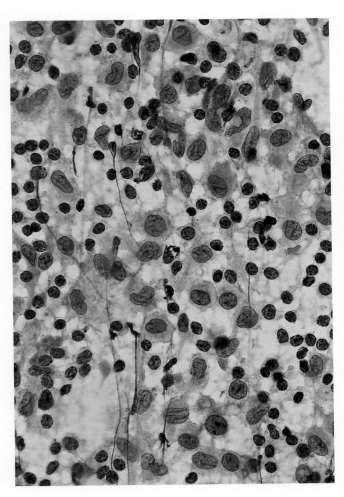

Fig. 20-20. Dermatopathic lymphadenopathy, fine needle aspiration. The characteristic grooved nuclei of interdigitating cells and Langerhans cells are easy to recognize in smear preparations.

features in combination should prompt a suggestion of drug-induced lymphadenopathy. However, the histologic findings may not be completely specific, and the findings may be indistinguishable from viral lymphadenitis or even angioimmunoblastic lymphadenopathy. Similar to viral lymphadenitis, a reactive follicular hyperplasia is often found in the early stages of drug-induced lymphadenopathy.

The differential diagnosis of drug-induced lymphadenopathy includes angioimmunoblastic lymphadenopathy, peripheral T cell lymphoma, and Hodgkin's disease, diseases that commonly have a reactive component that includes eosinophils. In contrast to these other diseases, the overall lymph node architecture is usually retained in drug-induced lymphadenopathy. In addition, the spectrum of lymphoid atypia seen in peripheral T cell lymphoma is absent in drug-induced lymphadenopathy, and the presence of numerous immunoblasts and plasma cells is unusual for Hodgkin's disease. The lymph node findings in *postvaccinial lymphadenopathy* may be indistinguishable from drug-induced lymphadenopathy. This disorder is rare now that smallpox vaccinations have been discontinued, but can be encountered following tetanus inoculations.

with irregular nuclear contours to immunoblasts. Confirmation of the diagnosis can be achieved with an S-100 stain, which should label both the interdigitating dendritic cells and Langerhans cells.

The diagnosis of dermatopathic lymphadenopathy is usually very straightforward. Although proliferating Langerhans cells are also seen in Langerhans cell histiocytosis, that disorder primarily affects the sinuses with secondary extension into the paracortical areas. The most difficult point in the differential diagnosis is the evaluation of dermatopathic nodes in patients with known or suspected mycosis fungoides, a topic covered in the section on mycosis fungoides later in this chapter.

Sinus Hyperplasia

Nonspecific Sinus Histiocytosis

Sinus histiocytosis is often seen in lymph nodes that drain the extremities and the mesentery, and in lymph nodes that drain sites of malignant tumors or of prosthesis placement.[121,122] It is often idiopathic. Morphologically, one sees uniformly sized histiocytes with cytologically bland nuclei and abundant cytoplasm that fill and distend subcapsular and trabecular lymph node sinuses. Rarely, there may be histiocytes with prominent erythrophagocytosis, particularly in the axillary lymph nodes of patients with breast cancer.[123] A rare signet ring variant of sinus histiocytosis may occur, also in the axillary lymph nodes of patients with breast cancer.[124]

Monocytoid B Cell Hyperplasia

Monocytoid B cell hyperplasia is seen in the sinuses or parasinusoidal areas in about 10 percent of reactive lymph nodes[125] (Fig. 20-21). It is almost invariably seen in toxoplasmosis,[71] and is also commonly found in HIV-associated benign lymphadenopathy, suppurative granulomatous lymphadenitis, and viral lymphadenitis.[126,127] Monocytoid B cells are medium-sized cells with small nuclei, irregular nuclear outlines, and a bland chromatin pattern. There is a moderate rim of pale to clear cytoplasm that forms distinct cell borders with adjacent cells. Usually, there are admixed neutrophils and plasma cells, and occasionally, immunoblasts can be seen. Monocytoid B cells stain for CD20 but not for bcl-2 protein, and polytypic cytoplasmic immunoglobulins can occasionally be demonstrated.

Monocytoid B cell hyperplasia may be easily confused with marginal zone B cell lymphoma (monocytoid B cell lymphoma).[128] Features favoring lymphoma include the proliferation comprising more than 50 percent of the lymph node with confluent extension into the paracortical areas, a greater degree of nuclear atypia and a higher mitotic rate, and the presence of a component of another lymphoma, such as follicular lymphoma or a malignant lymphoplasmacytic proliferation. Staining for immunoglobulin light chains and bcl-2 protein may be of value in this situation. Marginal zone B cell lymphoma has monotypic light chains and is usually bcl-2 protein positive, whereas monocytoid B cell hyperplasia has polytypic light chains and is bcl-2 protein negative.

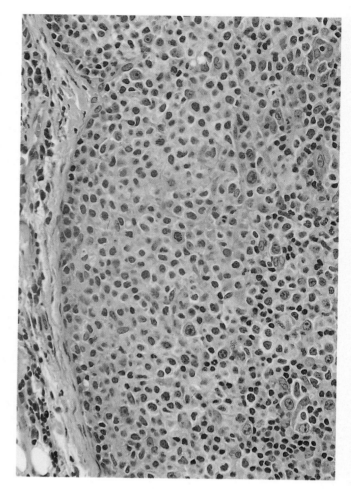

Fig. 20-21. Monocytoid B cell hyperplasia. The sinuses and parasinusoidal regions are expanded by medium-sized cells with small bland nuclei and abundant clear cytoplasm.

Infection-Associated Hemophagocytic Syndrome

Infection-associated hemophagocytic syndrome is a non-neoplastic, systemic proliferation of benign-appearing histiocytes.[129–131] It may be caused by almost any infectious agent. Most patients have a documented primary or iatrogenic (e.g., organ transplant-related) immunodeficiency. Patients usually have fever and other constitutional symptoms, hepatosplenomegaly, and generalized lymphadenopathy, and less often, a skin rash and bilateral pulmonary infiltrates. Laboratory evaluation usually reveals pancytopenia and liver function abnormalities. Infection-associated hemophagocytic syndrome is a benign, self-limiting condition. However, affected patients may die during the acute disease episode due to multisystem failure or later due to infectious complications exacerbated by their underlying immunodeficiency.[131] In addition, Epstein-Barr-associated hemophagocytic syndrome appears to be a particularly virulent form of this syndrome, affecting young children and leading rapidly to death.[132,133]

The pathologic features vary with the time that biopsies are performed. Early in the disease, lymph nodes are only partially involved by a small number of histiocytes and a marked immunoblastic proliferation. Later in the disease, one sees massive sinusoidal infiltration by benign-appearing histiocytes (Fig. 20-22). The histiocytes may show prominent hemophagocytosis and platelet phagocytosis. Germinal centers, if present, are inconspicuous.

The differential diagnosis of infection-associated hemophagocytic syndrome includes malignant lymphomas associated with benign hemophagocytosis and familial hemophagocytic lymphohistiocytosis, both of which are discussed below.

Familial Hemophagocytic Lymphohistiocytosis

Familial hemophagocytic lymphohistiocytosis is a rare and usually fatal disease that is characterized by marked lymphohistiocytic infiltration in multiple organs.[131,134] Most patients are less than 1 year old. Approximately three-fourths of cases are familial, with an autosomal recessive mode of inheritance. The infants usually present with fevers, hepatosplenomegaly, pulmonary effusions, and a skin rash. Laboratory findings include pancytopenia and a severe hypofibrinogenemia without abnor-

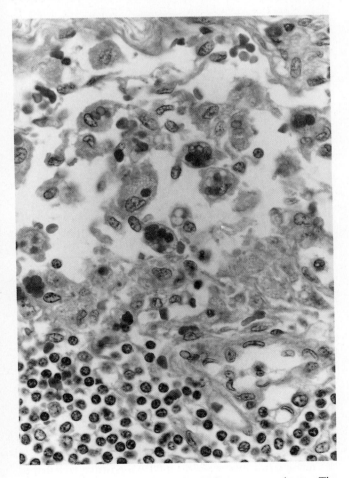

Fig. 20-22. Infection-associated hemophagocytic syndrome. The sinuses contain numerous histiocytes exhibiting erythrophagocytosis.

malities of other clotting factors. Impaired cellular and humoral immunity are features of this disorder.[135] The disease is usually rapidly fatal (within weeks), with death due to sepsis or bleeding. Rare patients have survived several months to years.

The lymph nodes and bone marrow are the most frequently involved organs, followed by the spleen, liver, and the central nervous system. Lymph nodes in patients with familial hemophagocytic lymphohistiocytosis are partially to completely effaced by a sinusoidal infiltrate of benign-appearing histiocytes, lymphocytes, and plasma cells. The histiocytosis is quite pronounced and is accompanied by prominent erythrophagocytosis as well as phagocytosis of lymphocytes and other cellular debris. Other organs of the reticuloendothelial system may also contain large numbers of hemophagocytic histiocytes.

Familial hemophagocytic lymphohistiocytosis and infection-associated hemophagocytic syndrome may be clinically and morphologically similar. In fact, they may represent the same disease, with familial hemophagocytic lymphohistiocytosis presenting as infection-associated hemophagocytic syndrome in individuals with familial immunodeficiencies.

Malignant Lymphoma with Benign Erythrophagocytosis

Malignant lymphoma with benign erythrophagocytosis refers to a condition in which lymphoma is associated with a reactive hemophagocytic disorder.[136,137] T cell lymphomas, and less often other lymphomas, may induce a marked hyperplasia of cytologically benign hemophagocytosing histiocytes.[136,138] Malignant lymphoma with benign erythrophagocytosis may present in two different ways. In the first presentation, patients with known (usually disseminated) lymphoma develop a syndrome mimicking infection-associated hemophagocytic syndrome.[136,138] Most patients do not also have a systemic infection, although in one study approximately 20 percent of such patients had active infections, predominantly of viral origin.[139] Morphologically, the lymph node sinuses are filled with abundant cytologically benign histiocytes that show erythrophagocytosis as well as phagocytosis of leukocytes and platelets.[136,138] Malignant lymphoma cells are found at anatomic sites without the histiocytic proliferation. The occurrence of erythrophagocytosis is usually a terminal event in a patient with advanced stage lymphoma.[139] In the second clinical presentation, the hemophagocytic syndrome occurs in the absence of any previously diagnosed cancer and usually prompts a search for a malignant tumour.[137] In this setting, benign hemophagocytizing histiocytes are intimately interspersed with lymphoma cells. Paraffin and frozen section immunophenotyping studies usually demonstrate a T cell lineage. The prognosis is extremely poor in most patients.

Malignant lymphoma with benign erythrophagocytosis may be confused with infection-associated hemophagocytic syndrome.[136,139] Identification of the lymphoma cells distinguishes the malignant tumor from infection-associated hemophagocytic syndrome. Also, the lymphomas are usually not associated with a systemic infection, as is infection-associated hemophagocytic syndrome. Biopsies of other organs may be needed for cases in which this distinction may be difficult.

Sinus Histiocytosis with Massive Lymphadenopathy

Sinus histiocytosis with massive lymphadenopathy (Rosai-Dorfman disease) is a rare idiopathic disease of proliferating histiocytes.[140,141] The disorder is most commonly seen in children, but the disease affects all age groups.[142] Approximately 90 percent of patients present with massive bilateral and painless cervical lymphadenopathy. Axillary, inguinal, para-aortic, and mediastinal lymph nodes may also be involved, with or without concomitant cervical disease. Solitary lymph node involvement is unusual. Extranodal sites are involved in approximately 40 percent of cases.[142–144] Constitutional symptoms are common, but hepatosplenomegaly is rare. Most afflicted patients undergo spontaneous remission, with disease manifestations gradually subsiding over several months to years.[142,145] Sinus histiocytosis with massive lymphadenopathy may cause or significantly contribute to death in a small number of patients.[142,145]

The lymph nodes are markedly enlarged and often matted together; the cut surface is a dull yellow-white. Microscopically, one sees extensive fibrosis limited to the capsule. The normal lymph node architecture is partially or completely effaced due to massively dilated sinuses, which are filled with numerous characteristic histiocytes (Fig. 20-23). The nuclei of these unique histiocytes are intermediately sized, have a vesicular chromatin pattern, and contain one to several nucleoli (Fig. 20-24). The nuclear membranes are well delineated and delicate. Cytologic atypia is unusual. The cytoplasm is abundant, amphophilic in H&E stains, and contains intact lymphocytes (termed *lymphophagocytosis* or *emperipolesis*). Less often, the histiocytes may phagocytose plasma cells, neutrophils, or red blood cells. Plasma cells are easily found in the sinuses and intrasinusal tissues. Eosinophils are not seen.

Ultrastructurally, the proliferating histiocytes contain lipid vacuoles, numerous complex filopodia, and varying numbers of lysosomes, and lack Birbeck granules. Immunohistochemical studies show that the cells express S-100 protein and other markers associated with macrophages.[146] The cells do not express the CD1 antigen found on Langerhans cells, and also lack expression of R4/23, a monoclonal antibody with high specificity for follicular dendritic cells.[147–149] Molecular studies show a germline configuration for both the immunoglobulin heavy chain gene and the beta-T cell receptor gene.[149]

The differential diagnosis includes reactive sinus histiocytosis and Langerhans cell histiocytosis (histiocytosis X), both of which may have low power appearances similar to sinus histiocytosis with massive lymphadenopathy. However, the sinuses are far more distended than in the former two disorders. Also, the histiocytes of reactive sinus histiocytosis differ cytologically from the characteristic cells of sinus histiocytosis with massive lymphadenopathy and do not uniformly express S-100 protein. Likewise, the cytologic characteristics of Langerhans cells and the presence of eosinophils help to separate Langerhans cell histiocytosis from sinus histiocytosis with massive lymphadenopathy. CD1 expression, the presence of Birbeck granules, and lack of emperipolesis in Langerhans cell histiocytosis also help differentiate Langerhans cell histiocytosis from sinus histiocytosis with massive lymphadenopathy. The differential

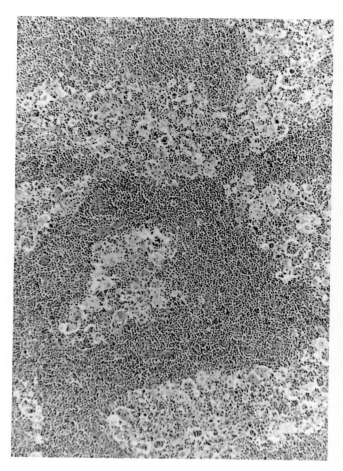

Fig. 20-23. Sinus histiocytosis with massive lymphadenopathy. An exquisitely sinusoidal pattern is seen at low magnification.

diagnosis of sinus histiocytosis with massive lymphadenopathy in a lymph node also includes sinusoidal involvement by metastatic carcinoma, malignant melanoma, and sinusoidal malignant lymphoma. Careful attention to the cytologic features of the proliferating cells and differing immunohistochemical profiles will distinguish sinus histiocytosis with massive lymphadenopathy from the malignant tumors.

Whipple's Disease

Whipple's disease is a bacterial infection involving the small intestine caused by *Tropheryma whippeli*.[150] Typically, Whipple's disease is seen in adult men who have symptoms of malabsorption.[151] Regional lymph nodes are frequently involved and peripheral lymphadenopathy may be seen in approximately one-half of cases. Microscopically, the lymph node sinuses are dilated and filled with enlarged histiocytes and large round empty spaces. The cytoplasm of the histiocytes contains copious amounts of diastase-resistant PAS-positive rod-shaped forms that correspond to the causative bacillus.[151–153] The vacuoles are formed by loss of lipid materials during tissue processing. These features are similar to lymphadenopathy due to the

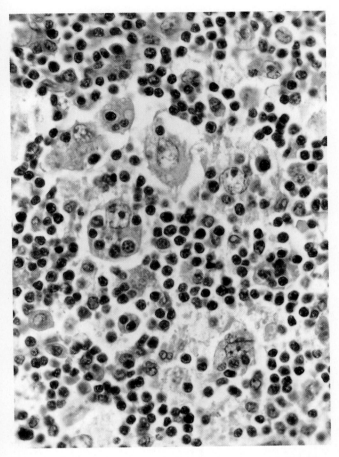

Fig. 20-24. Sinus histiocytosis with massive lymphadenopathy. Histiocytic cells with a vesicular nucleus and abundant cytoplasm exhibiting lymphophagocytosis characteristic of this disease.

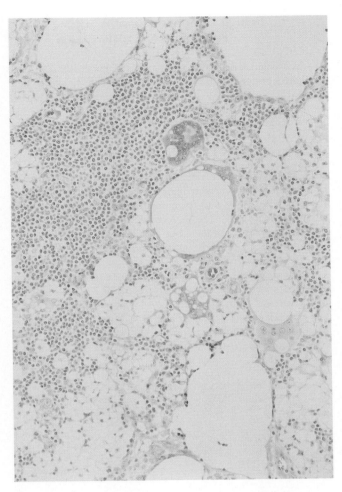

Fig. 20-25. Silicone lymphadenopathy. Large spaces lined by attenuated foreign body giant cells and numerous foamy macrophages are present.

deposition of exogenous lipid substances. *Mycobacterium avium-intracellulare* infection of the lymph node, which may be seen in patients with AIDS, may be mistaken for Whipple's disease involving the lymph node, because the histiocytes of both entities contain PAS-positive material. An acid-fast stain reveals that histiocytes are stuffed with acid-fast bacilla in the mycobacterial infection, allowing easy distinction from Whipple's disease, which is acid-fast negative.

Lymphadenopathy Due to Deposition of Exogenous Lipids

Exogenous lipid substances may be deposited in lymph nodes and be responsible for lymphadenopathy in several settings, including lymphangiography dye and silicone, polyvinylpyrrolidone (PVP), and prosthetic materials. Lymphangiography dye is an oily base that reaches the lymph nodes via the lymphatics. The material collects in the sinuses, and a foreign body giant cell reaction ensues.[154] During routine tissue processing, the injected medium dissolves, leaving behind sinuses with large empty vacuoles up to 100 μm in diameter. Silicone lym-

phadenopathy usually involves lymph nodes draining the site of silicone implants, usually from breast or joints. The histologic findings resemble lymphangiography changes, but since the process has usually been around for a longer period, there are usually more foamy histiocytes[155] (Fig. 20-25). Silicone is usually not completely removed during processing, so that refractile, nonbirefringent material can often be demonstrated in the spaces.

The deposition of exogenous lipids in lymph nodes must be distinguished from endogenous lipid deposition. *Lipogranulomatosis* refers to the reaction in lymph node (or spleen) to any lipid material arising from such endogenous sources as hematomas, tumors, cholesterol deposits, xanthomatous lesions, fat embolism, and fat necrosis.[156] Lymph nodes in the porta hepatis and celiac axis are most frequently involved. The lipid accumulation manifests as vacuolization of sinus histiocytes, eventually with the formation of small lipid granulomas with multinucleate giant cells. The vacuoles are much smaller than those seen with lymphangiography effect or silicone.

Benign Lymphadenopathy with Prominent Necrosis

Any benign lymphadenopathy or lymphadenitis may have focal areas of necrosis, including both primary follicular or paracortical hyperplasias.[157] However, in some diseases, extensive necrosis is the primary or most characteristic finding. The lymph node necrosis may be complete or subtotal.

Complete Lymph Node Necrosis

Complete lymph node necrosis is seen within two main settings. In the first, there is liquefactive necrosis, consisting of karyorrhectic debris and fragments of neutrophils, often with abscess formation.[157] This is more commonly seen at autopsy than in surgical specimens, but may be seen in the setting of AIDS, either due to fungi such as histoplasmosis or a wide variety of bacteria.

In the second type of complete necrosis, coagulative necrosis is seen as a result of vascular compromise (Fig. 20-26). The areas of necrosis often show ghosts of lymphoid cells, and generally lack inflammatory cells. The rim of the lymph node may be partially viable, whereas the perinodal soft tissue usually contains granulation tissue, and there may be venous thrombosis.

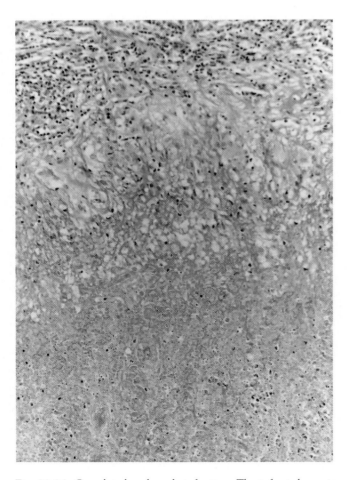

Fig. 20-26. Complete lymph node infarction. The infarcted area is rimmed by granulation tissue.

The most important cause of coagulative necrosis is malignant lymphoma, usually a non-Hodgkin's lymphoma of diffuse large cell type.[158] Occasionally, the lymphoma may be identified in a rim of viable lymph node parenchyma. More often, immunostains will identify a diffuse infiltrate of ghosts of B cells in the infarcted area, as the membrane antigens remain viable for a time after the cells have histologically undergone complete necrosis.[159] Rebiopsy, either immediately or within 6 months, will often reveal more definitive evidence of malignant lymphoma.

Kikuchi's Histiocytic Necrotizing Lymphadenitis

Histiocytic necrotizing lymphadenitis (of Kikuchi and Fujimoto) is a self-limiting, well defined clinicopathologic disorder of unknown etiology that most commonly affects young Asian women, although both sexes and all ages and ethnic groups may be afflicted.[160–164] Patients usually present with isolated cervical or posterior cervical lymphadenopathy, which may be tender to palpation. Lymphadenopathy of several months' duration is the only symptom in most patients. However, reported symptomatology may also include a mild fever associated with upper respiratory symptoms, and constitutional symptoms. The prognosis for the large majority of patients with histiocytic necrotizing lymphadenitis is excellent, with spontaneous resolution of the disease usually occurring within 1 to 4 months.

Microscopically, the lymph node architecture is only partially effaced, and the uninvolved lymphoid tissue is usually normal, with dormant nonhyperplastic follicles. Scattered throughout the paracortex and, less often, the cortex, are discrete foci of large deposits of eosinophilic amorphous material, abundant karyorrhectic debris, and viable cells (Fig. 20-27). The latter consist of histiocytes that exhibit phagocytosis and occasionally contain foamy cytoplasm, reactive immunoblasts, and plasmacytoid monocytes. The absence of intact neutrophils, plasma cells, and eosinophils in the areas of extensive necrosis is a very useful diagnostic feature. Immediately adjacent to the well circumscribed necrotic areas, one generally sees a proliferation of reactive immunoblasts. The sinuses may be focally distended by monocytoid B lymphocytes, but this is not a usual finding. The lymph node capsule may be thickened adjacent to the necrotic foci.

Immunohistochemical studies show a predominance of T cells and macrophages within involved areas of the lymph node. In lesions detected and biopsied early, helper/inducer T cells may predominate, whereas the majority of biopsies taken late after presentation appear to contain cytotoxic/suppressor T cells. There is some evidence that the karyorrhectic debris may be derived from T lineage-associated plasmacytoid cells.[165]

Eliciting the characteristic clinical history of histiocytic necrotizing lymphadenitis is extremely useful in distinguishing it from non-Hodgkin's lymphoma. The abundant karyorrhectic debris and sheets of macrophages seen in histiocytic necrotizing lymphadenitis may impart a superficial appearance of a high grade lymphoma. However, one must keep in mind that the only lymphomas to have a large amount of karyorrhexis are Burkitt's type and large cell immunoblastic lymphoma. The monotonous and malignant cells of these lymphomas are not present in lymph nodes with histiocytic necrotizing lymphadenitis. In node-based non-Hodgkin's lymphoma, the in-

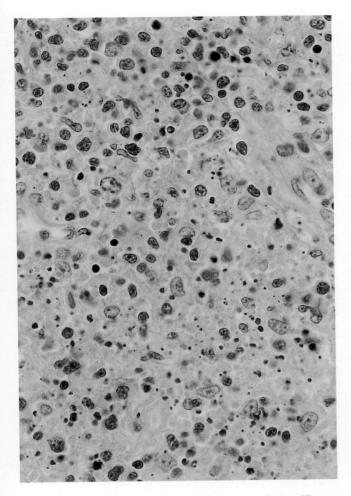

Fig. 20-27. Kikuchi's histiocytic necrotizing lymphadenitis. There is abundant necrosis with karyorrhectic debris and histiocytes with twisted nuclei.

farcted areas are generally rimmed by granulation tissue, and may contain the "ghosts" of the malignant cells. The differential diagnosis of histiocytic necrotizing lymphadenitis also includes Hodgkin's disease and lymph nodes with manifestations of infectious agents such as *Yersinia* enterocolitis or the cat-scratch organism, because they all are associated with stellate areas of necrosis (stellate microabscesses). In the latter entities, the presence of neutrophils in and around the necrotic foci allow easy separation from histiocytic necrotizing lymphadenitis. The differentiation of histiocytic necrotizing lymphadenitis from systemic lupus erythematosis and Kawasaki disease is discussed below.

Systemic Lupus Erythematosis Lymphadenopathy

Lymph nodes involved by systemic lupus erythematosus share morphologic features with lymph nodes involved by histiocytic necrotizing lymphadenitis, particularly the presence of discrete necrotic foci and eosinophilic deposits.[166] Histologic features that favor systemic lupus erythematosis are the presence of basophilic necrotic material that is often deposited in vessel walls

and sometimes forms hematoxyphilic bodies, and the presence of more than occasional plasma cells. However, distinguishing between histiocytic necrotizing lymphadenitis and lupus may be impossible on a purely morphologic basis, so clinical investigation should be undertaken. Some investigators hypothesize that histiocytic necrotizing lymphadenitis represents a self-limited autoimmune condition resembling systemic lupus erythematosis.

Kawasaki Disease Lymphadenopathy

Kawasaki disease (mucocutaneous lymph node syndrome) is an acute febrile disease of uncertain etiology, usually occurring in young children.[167] Five of the following six clinical criteria must be present to establish the diagnosis: fever, congestion of the conjunctiva, oral mucous membrane lesions, distal extremity lesions, polymorphous exanthem, and acute cervical adenopathy. The disease may be life threatening when coronary arteritis is present. Lymph node biopsies from patients with Kawasaki disease show necrotizing lesions, with fibrin, karyorrhectic debris, and neutrophils in association with the areas of necrosis[168] (Fig. 20-28). In addition, fibrin thrombi in

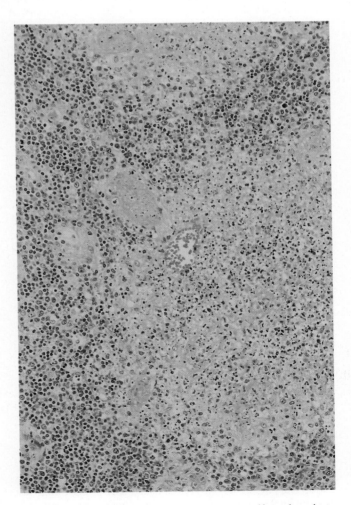

Fig. 20-28. Kawasaki disease. There are numerous fibrin thrombi in small vessels in and adjacent to areas of necrosis.

small vessels is usually a prominent feature, and an arteritis with fibrinoid necrosis may be present. Fibrin thrombi may also occur in thrombocytopenic purpura and rickettsial infection. Histiocytic necrotizing lymphadenitis may have fibrin thrombi, but they are not usually a prominent feature; the presence of neutrophils should also suggest Kawasaki disease.

Granulomatous Disorders

Noninfectious Granulomatous Lymphadenopathy

Granulomatous lymphadenopathy may be noninfectious or infectious. Noninfectious causes of granulomatous lymphadenopathy include berylliosis, Hodgkin's disease and non-Hodgkin's lymphomas, lymph nodes draining neoplasms, lymph nodes draining Crohn's disease, and sarcoidosis.[169,170] Granulomas may be found in the lymph nodes of Hodgkin's disease and non-Hodgkin's disease under two circumstances. First, they may be seen in conjunction with involvement of the lymph node by neoplasm. In Hodgkin's disease, the granulomas may be so numerous as to easily obscure the Reed-Sternberg cells and variants. The phenomenon is less common in non-Hodgkin's lymphomas, but has been reported in a variety of types, including Burkitt's lymphoma.[171] Similar to Hodgkin's disease, some cases have such an exuberant granulomatous response that the lymphoma may be obscured.[172] Second, non-caseating granulomas may seen in uninvolved lymph nodes in patients with Hodgkin's disease, non-Hodgkin's lymphomas, as well as carcinoma and other neoplasms. In Hodgkin's disease, the presence of noncaseating granulomas may be associated with a slightly better prognosis within a given stage.[173]

Sarcoidosis

Despite long-standing intensive research, the etiology of sarcoidosis is still not known. Sarcoidosis is a systemic disease of unknown etiology that affects adults most commonly between the ages of 20 and 40.[170] The male/female ratio is 2:1, and blacks are affected approximately 10 times more frequently than whites. Multiorgan involvement is the rule, particularly lymph nodes, lungs, eyes, and skin. Mediastinal and hilar lymph nodes are most frequently involved, but there may be generalized lymphadenopathy. The lymph node architecture is partially or wholly replaced by well formed noncaseating granulomas. The granulomas contain numerous epithelioid histiocytes, Langhans type multinucleate giant cells, and scattered lymphocytes. Occasional granulomas may show central foci of fibrinoid necrosis, but foci of classic caseating necrosis should be absent. Birefringent crystals (3 to 10 mm) of calcium oxalate are common and should not be mistaken for foreign body material. In addition, Schaumann bodies (large concentrically laminated basophil bodies consisting of protein containing calcium carbonate and iron), asteroid bodies (acidophilic star-shaped inclusions), and Hamazaki-Wesenberg bodies (PAS-positive intracellular and extracellular inclusions that represent giant lysosomes) may also be present, but have no diagnostic significance. Supporting laboratory data such as a positive skin test (Kveim test) and an elevated serum angiotensin-converting en-

zyme level may support the diagnosis, but are not specific to sarcoidosis.

The differential diagnosis of sarcoidosis includes infectious granulomatous lymphadenitis as well as all of the other causes of noninfectious granulomatous lymphadenitis. Special stains for organisms are generally not of use unless some necrosis is present. However, appropriate cultures for acid-fast, fungal, and bacterial organisms should be performed on any case in which an infectious etiology is being considered.

Infectious Granulomatous Lymphadenitis

Two types of infectious granulomatous lymphadenitis have been recently delineated. In the classic type, as exemplified by tuberculosis, nonsuppurative, hypersensitivity type granulomas are found.[174] Immunohistochemical studies demonstrate a predominance of histiocytes with lesser numbers of T cells and dendritic cells. Small, round mantle B cells are found at the periphery of the granulomas, but no B cells are present within the granulomas. In the second type, as exemplified by cat-scratch disease, suppurative granulomas containing numerous neutrophils and monocytoid B cells are found.[175] Immunohistochemical studies also demonstrate a predominance of histiocytes, but show variable number of B cells either at the periphery or in the center of suppurative granulomas in addition to T cells and dendritic cells. It has been suggested that the monocytoid B cells are recruited by the development of a T independent, macrophage-mediated immune response against antigens. Furthermore, the monocytoid B cells may have a role in the recruitment of neutrophils and in the development of the necrosis. Alternatively, the presence of aggregates of monocytoid B cells may be the primary event, followed by necrosis and infiltration by neutrophils, followed finally by the formation of granulomatous inflammation at the periphery.

Tuberculosis, once thought to be under control, has undergone a dramatic resurgence in the number of cases, due to complacency and the growing number of drug-resistant strains. Involvement of lymph nodes is usually accompanied by pulmonary involvement, but lymphadenopathy, usually cervical, accounts for about 40 percent of nonrespiratory infections. Tuberculous lymphadenopathy may be histologically indistinguishable from sarcoidosis, although the former usually contains caseating granulomas or areas of caseation with a rim of granulomatous reaction. When necrosis is prominent, there is sometimes a draining sinus to the skin. Organisms are most easily demonstrated by PCR or appropriate culture. When organisms are demonstrable by acid-fast stains, it is usually in the necrotic areas.

Atypical mycobacterial infections are an even more common cause of isolated granulomatous lymphadenitis than tuberculosis. Again, cervical lymph nodes are most commonly involved. The histologic changes may be similar to tuberculosis or may show less granulomatous changes and a greater degree of acute inflammation with abscess formation.[176] In immunocompromised patients such as AIDS patients, different features may be seen. There is often foamy histiocytic infiltration beginning in the superficial paracortex and extending to involve the entire parenchyma. An acid-fast stain reveals tremendous numbers of acid-fast bacilli in the histiocytes. Alternatively, there may be a more spindled proliferation of fibroblasts and histiocytes mimicking inflammatory pseudotumor.[48] Special stains demonstrate the presence of numerous bacilli within the spindled histiocytes.

A variety of histologic appearances may also be seen in *lepromatous lymphadenitis*, depending on the status of the patient's immunity. In patients with relatively intact cellular immunity, the tuberculoid form of leprosy is seen. Generally, lymph nodes are uninvolved by leprosy but may be enlarged due to reactive paracortical hyperplasia. In patients with borderline leprosy, numerous noncaseating granulomas are found in the paracortex; acid-fast organisms may or may not be identified by Fite stains. In patients with defective cellular immunity, the lepromatous form of leprosy is seen. In this form, generalized lymphadenopathy is often present. There are numerous foamy macrophages containing numerous organisms present in the paracortical areas, and there may also be reactive follicular hyperplasia with abundant plasma cells. The macrophages may coalesce into syncytial clumps and giant cells may be seen, but true granulomas are not present.

Fungal infections seldom present initially in lymph nodes but rather usually involve lymph nodes as part of a systemic fungal infection. A wide variety of fungi may cause lymphadenitis, but histoplasmosis most commonly causes isolated lymphadenitis. Histologically, a granulomatous reaction is usually seen, although one may also see acute inflammation with abscess formation. Organisms are most easily demonstrated by appropriate fungal cultures although fungal organisms may often be demonstrated by PAS, Gridley, or Grocott methenamine silver stain.

Pneumocystis carinii is a protozoal organism that is seen most commonly in patients with AIDS. Lymph nodes are rarely involved, but cases of lymphadenitis with granulomatous lesions containing the organism have been reported.[177]

Cat-Scratch Lymphadenitis

Cat-scratch disease is the most common cause of suppurative granulomas in lymph nodes.[178] It is a benign infectious illness caused by a bacterium introduced through the skin following a scratch by a cat or, less commonly, by a dog. A skin lesion may or may not be present. This is followed in several weeks by regional lymphadenopathy, usually in the axillary, inguinal, or cervical regions. The disease usually affects children and young adults, with an equal male/female ratio. It has been demonstrated that cat-scratch disease is caused by a bacterium,[179] but the exact causative organism is still somewhat controversial. Many investigators believe that a majority of cases is caused by *Rochalimaea henselae*, but a minority of cases may be caused by *Afipia felis*.[180,181] In occasional cases, both organisms have been identified, and in rare cases, neither organism has been identified.

Lymph nodes initially show florid reactive follicular hyperplasia with a monocytoid B cell proliferation in the sinuses and paracortical areas.[182] Subsequently, there are small suppurative granulomas located adjacent to or within the monocytoid B cells composed of histiocytes with central aggregates of neutrophils (Figs. 20-29 and 20-30). In the final stages, there are discrete stellate microabscesses composed of neutrophils and necrotic or fibrinoid material, with a rim of palisading epithe-

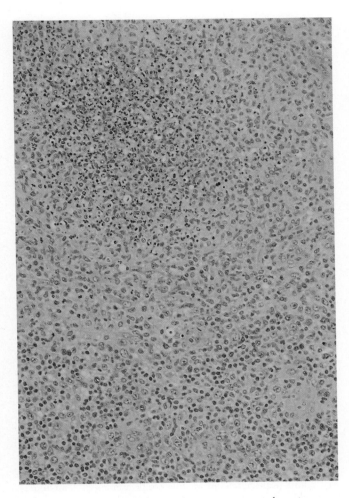

Fig. 20-29. Cat-scratch disease. A suppurative granuloma is seen.

lioid histiocytes. Langhans type giant cells are generally not frequent, but numerous mature plasma cells and occasional immunoblasts may be present at the periphery of some of the granulomas and in the paracortical areas. The lymph node capsule is often fibrotic or acutely inflamed. Warthin-Starry silver impregnation stain performed at a pH of 3.8 to 4.0 may show delicate pleomorphic bacilli; the Gram stain is usually negative.[179] The bacilli are commonly observed in the walls of capillaries, in macrophages lining sinuses or near germinal centers, and in areas of necrosis; they may occur singly, in chains, or in clumps.

The differential diagnosis includes the other bacterial causes of suppurative granulomatous lymphadenitis discussed below as well as some of the fungal and mycobacterial organisms discussed previously. Usually the clinical setting can differentiate among the different infectious possibilities. In questionable cases, an indirect fluorescent-antibody test is available and serology, culture, and PCR tests may also be used to specifically identify the organism. The differential diagnosis also includes causes of nonsuppurative granulomatous lymphadenitis; these can be distinguished histologically by the usual absence of stellate microabscesses, the absence of large numbers of B cells (in-

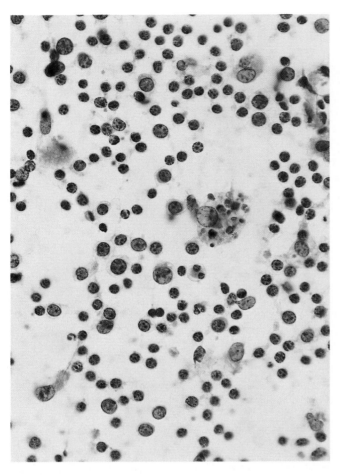

Fig. 20-30. Cat-scratch disease, fine needle aspiration. A mixture of lymphoid cells, with scattered tingible body macrophages and neutrophils, is seen.

cluding monocytoid B cells), and the more frequent occurrence of Langhans giant cells in the latter. Hodgkin's disease, in particular the syncytial variant of nodular sclerosing type, can also be difficult to distinguish from cat-scratch disease. Close examination of the cells at the edge of the necrosis will disclose numerous Reed-Sternberg cells and variants in this type of Hodgkin's disease.

Lymphogranuloma Venereum Lymphadenitis

Lymphogranuloma venereum is a sexually transmitted disease caused by *Chlamydia*.[183] It almost always affects inguinal lymph nodes. Because this lesion often presents at a later stage, there is often more matting of adjacent nodes than typically seen in cat-scratch disease. Histologically, the changes are very similar to that seen in cat-scratch disease. However, early lesions are less often seen, and at the time of biopsy, there are usually multiple stellate abscesses within the nodal parenchyma, sometimes with coalescence and often with extension outside the fibrotic capsule into the adjacent perinodal soft tissues. Giemsa staining may show inclusion bodies. The diagnosis can be confirmed by serologic testing.

Yersinial Lymphadenitis

Yersinial lymphadenitis is caused by the bacteria *Yersinia enterocolitica* or *pseudotuberculosis*.[184] It usually occurs in children or young adults who present with symptoms of acute appendicitis. However, laparoscopy reveals a grossly normal appendix, but markedly enlarged mesenteric lymph nodes draining the ileocecal region. Histologically, the lymph nodes initially show florid reactive hyperplasia. Later, there are suppurative granulomas identical to those seen in cat-scratch disease. However, the suppurative granulomas may commonly involve the germinal centers. Gram-negative acid-fast diplobacilli may be identified in the lesions. Similar changes may be noted in the appendix when it is removed.

ANGIOIMMUNOBLASTIC LYMPHADENOPATHY

Angioimmunoblastic lymphadenopathy with dysproteinemia (AILD) (immunoblastic lymphadenopathy) is an uncommon disorder of uncertain nature that has characteristic clinicopathologic features.[185–187] It generally occurs in the elderly, with a male/female ratio of about 2:1. Patients usually present with generalized lymphadenopathy, hepatosplenomegaly, and a skin rash. This is usually accompanied by severe constitutional symptoms, such as fever, night sweats, and malaise. Laboratory studies usually reveal hypergammaglobulinemia and an autoimmune hemolytic anemia. The clinical behavior is unpredictable with some patients having an indolent course and others having a rapidly progressive one. Response to therapy, including chemotherapy and steroids, is also unpredictable. Many patients succumb to severe infections. Others may eventually develop definitive evidence of a peripheral T cell lymphoma, usually AILD-like T cell lymphoma.[188–190] A minority of patients may develop a B cell lymphoma, usually an EBV-associated immunoblastic lymphoma.

Because so many patients with AILD develop AILD-like T cell lymphoma and because it is often difficult to distinguish between AILD and AILD-like T cell lymphoma, many hematopathologists now believe that AILD represents a peripheral T cell lymphoma from the outset.[9] Other hematopathologists still believe that it may be a reactive or preneoplastic disorder, which has a propensity to progress to lymphoma.[191]

Histologically, the lymph node is usually normal in size or mildly enlarged. Sinuses are often still patent, and the capsule is usually intact. However, there is usually diffuse effacement of architecture, although small regressed lymphoid follicles may still be present (Fig. 20-31). The lymph node parenchyma has the appearance of lymphoid depletion with intense vascular proliferation, and occasionally there are intercellular deposits of a PAS-positive amorphous substance. At high magnification, one sees a mixture of small and large lymphoid cells, including immunoblasts, plasma cells, eosinophils, and scattered epithelioid histiocytes.

Immunohistochemical studies show a marked predominance of T cells, usually of helper phenotype, with few B cells.[192] Aberrant T cell phenotypes are not found. Molecular studies

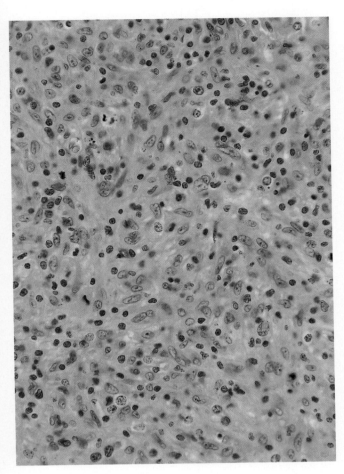

Fig. 20-31. Angioimmunoblastic lymphadenopathy. There is lymphoid depletion with marked hypervascularity. A mixture of lymphoid cells is seen, without striking atypia.

show a germline configuration for the antigen receptor genes or light bands on analyses of the immunoglobulin or beta-T cell receptor genes, consistent with the presence of small monoclonal populations of lymphoid cells.[192–194] Cytogenetic studies may show small clonal populations with cytogenetic abnormalities.[195]

The most important and most difficult entity in the differential diagnosis is AILD-like T cell lymphoma (which is a nonissue for those who feel these represent the same disease). The presence of clusters and small sheets of atypical lymphoid cells often containing clear cytoplasm, particularly around blood vessels, should raise suspicion that progression to AILD-like lymphoma has occurred. The presence of an aberrant T cell phenotype on frozen section immunohistochemical studies or the demonstration of sizeable monoclonal populations by gene rearrangement or cytogenetic studies would indicate AILD-like T cell lymphoma. For this reason, these studies should probably be performed in most cases in which the diagnosis of AILD vs. AILD-like lymphoma is being considered, unless aggressive treatment is not a clinical option.

CLASSIC HODGKIN'S DISEASE

Hodgkin's disease is a neoplastic proliferation of Reed-Sternberg cells and variants (Hodgkin's cells). Lukes and Butler[196] recognized six categories of Hodgkin's disease, including nodular and diffuse lymphocytic and histiocytic (L&H), nodular sclerosis, mixed cellularity, diffuse fibrosis, and reticular.[196] In the subsequent Rye modification, the categories of nodular and diffuse L&H were combined into a new category of lymphocyte predominance, whereas diffuse fibrosis and reticular was combined into lymphocyte depletion.[197] In recent years, it has been recognized that the L&H forms of Hodgkin's probably represent a distinctive clinicopathologic entity separate from the rest of Hodgkin's disease.[198] Therefore, this section covers "classic" Hodgkin's disease; a subsequent section discusses the L&H forms.

Hodgkin's disease accounts for about 15 percent of all cases of malignant lymphoma, with about 8,000 new cases per year.[199] The overall male/female ratio is 1.5:1, although the male predominance is not seen in cases of nodular sclerosis.[200] In the United States, there is a peak of incidence in young adults with a second slow rise of incidence in older adults. About 40 to 50 percent of cases have been associated with EBV in the neoplastic cells, although a clear etiologic role has not yet been identified.[201,202] Cases of mixed cellularity and lymphocyte depletion, particularly occurring in children or older adults, are most likely to be associated with EBV. There may be a genetic component to Hodgkin's disease, particularly in cases of nodular sclerosis occurring in young adulthood.[203] Some other environmental/genetic factors that have been implicated include higher social class, employment in wood-related industries, and certain HLA types.[204–208] Patients with Hodgkin's disease usually present with slowly growing, enlarged lymph nodes, most often in the cervical or axillary regions, or a mediastinal mass.[209] Low neck or mediastinal presentations are particularly common in females with nodular sclerosis. About one-quarter of patients have constitutional symptoms (so-called B symptoms), including unexplained fever (>38°C) during the previous months, recurrent drenching night sweats during the previous month, and unexplained weight loss (>10 percent of body weight) during the previous 6 months. Pruritis or pain after alcohol ingestion may also occur. Laboratory studies can usually document a deficiency in cellular immunity.

Hodgkin's disease spreads in a predictable fashion, usually from one contiguous lymph node group to another; therefore staging is generally of great use in determining the optimal treatment.[209] The Cotswolds staging classification, a minor modification of the Ann Arbor classification, is outlined in Table 20-6.[210,211] Clinical staging includes history, physical examination, plain chest radiograph, and computed tomography of chest and abdomen.[212] Additional studies that are commonly performed in many institutions include lymphangiography, magnetic resonance imaging, and gallium scanning. Routine pathologic staging procedures include bilateral bone marrow biopsies. Staging laparotomy is no longer routinely performed in many institutions due to long-term increase in the risk of acute leukemia and infections,[212] but still may be performed when detection of disease might alter therapy.

Table 20-6. The Cotswolds Staging Classification of Hodgkin's Disease

Classification	Description
Stage I	Involvement of a single lymph node region or lymphoid structure
Stage II	Involvement of two or more lymph node regions on the same side of the diaphragm (the mediastinum is considered a single site, whereas hilar lymph nodes are considered bilaterally
Stage III	Involvement of lymph node regions or structures on both sides of the diaphragm
Stage III-1	With or without involvement of splenic hilar, celiac, or portal nodes
Stage III-2	With involvement of para-aortic, iliac, and mesenteric nodes
Stage IV	Involvement of one or more extranodal sites in addition to a site for which the designation "E" has been used
Designations applicable to any disease stage	
A	No symptoms
B	Fever (temperature >38°C), drenching night sweats, unexplained loss of >10% of body weight within the preceding 6 months
X	Bulky disease (a widening of the mediastinum by more than one-third or the presence of a nodal mass with a maximal dimension >10 cm)
E	Involvement of a single extranodal site that is contiguous or proximal to the known nodal site
CS	Clinical stage
PS	Pathologic stage (as determined by laparotomy)

(Data from Lister et al.[210,211])

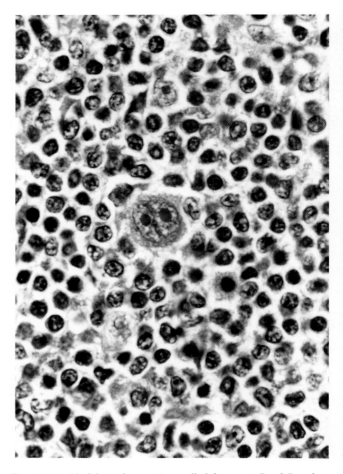

Fig. 20-32. Hodgkin's disease. A so-called diagnostic Reed-Sternberg cell is present.

Histopathologic Diagnosis

The diagnosis of Hodgkin's disease is established by the definitive identification of Reed-Sternberg cells and variants (Hodgkin's cells) (Figs. 20-32 to 20-34). Their identification is facilitated by recognition of the characteristic cellular milieu in which these cells are usually found. Thus, attention to both the atypical cells as well as the background cells is important to the histologic diagnosis of Hodgkin's disease. Reed and Sternberg described the classic Reed-Sternberg cell as a large cell with multilobed nucleus, often "owl's-eye" with two mirror-image nuclei, each containing a single large inclusion-like eosinophilic nucleolus; the cytoplasm is abundant and eosinophilic (Fig. 20-32). Mononuclear variants are similar to the classic Reed-Sternberg cells, but have a single nucleus and large eosinophilic nucleoli (Fig. 20-33). Formalin-fixed cases of nodular sclerosis contain many lacunar cells, which are mononuclear cells with abundant, often clear cytoplasm, and relatively less conspicuous nucleoli (Fig. 20-34). In all types of classic Hodgkin's disease, one can see apoptotic Hodgkin's cells

("mummified" cells), with degenerated nuclei and shrunken, highly eosinophilic cytoplasm. Although most hematopathologists require the presence of at least one classic Reed-Sternberg cell to establish a definitive diagnosis of Hodgkin's disease, we disagree and merely require that one is confident in the identification of Hodgkin's cells, either by histopathologic examination or by confirmation with immunohistochemical stains. At the time of surgery, touch or scrape preparations may be more useful than the actual frozen section for the recognition of Hodgkin's cells.

Hodgkin's cells generally comprise less than 1 percent of the cellular elements of the involved tissue. The background cells usually consist of varying numbers of small, round lymphocytes, histiocytes, eosinophils, neutrophils, plasma cells, and fibroblasts. Occasional immunoblasts may be present, but a spectrum of lymphoid size and atypia should raise consideration of diagnoses other than Hodgkin's disease. The histiocytes may be epithelioid in appearance, and occasionally well formed granulomas may be found. On rare occasions, foamy histiocytes may predominate. Eosinophils may vary in number from few to many, with the formation of eosinophilic abscesses. Neutrophils are usually not abundant in number, and tend to be most

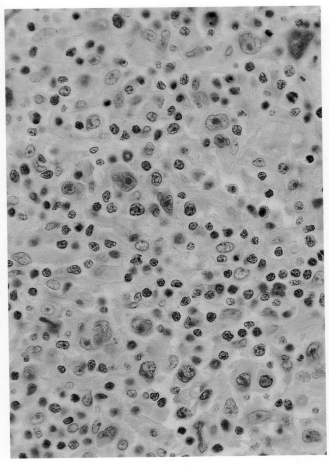

Fig. 20-33. Hodgkin's disease, mixed cellularity type. Several mononuclear Hodgkin's cells are present. Note also the background cells, including small round lymphocytes, histiocytes, eosinophils, and plasma cells.

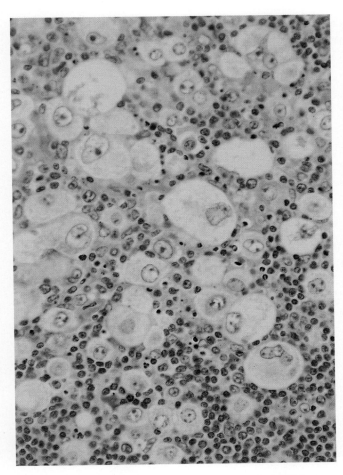

Fig. 20-34. Hodgkin's disease, nodular sclerosing type. Many lacunar cells are seen.

often found in patients with "B" symptoms. Plasma cells are usually scattered throughout the tissue, and when found in sheets should raise doubt about the diagnosis of Hodgkin's disease. Fibroblasts are usually few in number, but may occasionally be so numerous as to simulate a sarcoma such as malignant fibrous histiocytoma.

As discussed above, the Rye classification of Hodgkin's disease recognizes nodular sclerosis, lymphocyte predominance, mixed cellularity, and lymphocyte depletion types.[196] In the REAL classification, a provisional entity of lymphocyte-rich classic Hodgkin's disease is included to recognize those cases of lymphocyte predominance that are not of the L&H type.[9] Nodular sclerosis is the most frequently diagnosed subtype of Hodgkin's disease, comprising about 50 to 70 percent of cases in Western populations, and is defined by the presence of at least focal fibrous bands[196] (Fig. 20-35). These bands usually extend from a thickened capsule to separate the lymphoid parenchyma into nodules, but may be extremely focal, with the remainder of the lymph node showing diffuse effacement, or rarely, an interfollicular pattern of infiltration. The bands are

composed of dense collagen with interspersed small lymphocytes and usually incorporate blood vessels radiating from the capsule. The nodules are usually composed of lacunar cells, which may be few in number or quite numerous, the latter termed the *syncytial variant* of nodular sclerosis[213] (Fig. 20-36) Eosinophils are generally abundant.

The British National Lymphoma Investigation group has subdivided cases of nodular sclerosis into two grades that, in some series, have prognostic value.[214–217] Cases are classified as grade II if (1) more than 25 percent of the nodules show reticular or pleomorphic lymphocyte depletion; (2) greater than 80 percent of the nodules show fibrohistiocytic lymphocyte depletion; or (3) more than 25 percent of the nodules contain numerous bizarre and highly anaplastic-appearing Hodgkin's cells with lymphocyte depletion.[215] All other cases are classified as grade I.

Lymphocyte-rich classic Hodgkin's disease, mixed cellularity, and lymphocyte depletion represent a spectrum of the remainder of cases not of nodular sclerosis subtype. Generally, diffuse effacement of architecture is present, although a vague nodularity is characteristic at low magnification. In rare cases, however, an interfollicular pattern of involvement is present[62]; even more rarely, Hodgkin's disease may have a follicular pat-

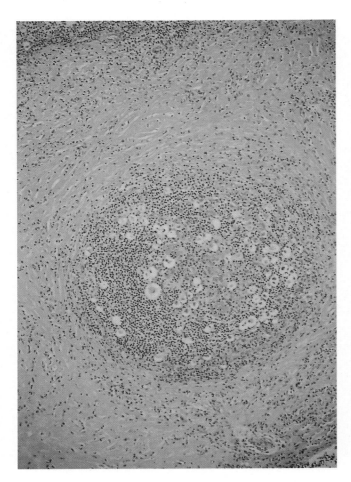

Fig. 20-35. Hodgkin's disease, nodular sclerosing type. A nodule is delineated by broad fibrous bands.

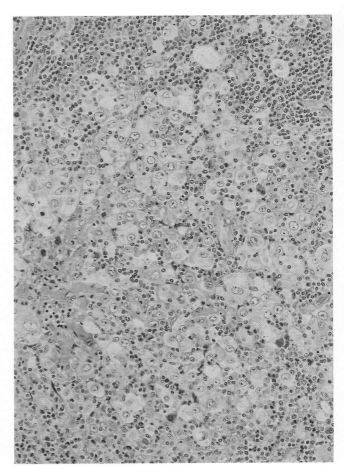

Fig. 20-36. Hodgkin's disease, nodular sclerosing type, syncytial type. Sheets of lacunar cells are seen, adjacent to an area of necrosis.

tern.[218] The capsule is usually intact, without extension of the lymphoid proliferation into the surrounding soft tissues. Varying amounts of interstitial fibrosis may be seen, particularly in lymphocyte depletion in which individual cells are often surrounded by thin wisps of collagen. The presence of any discrete, thick bands would exclude any of these subtypes and warrant classification as nodular sclerosis. There are no quantitative cutoffs between lymphocyte rich classic Hodgkin's disease, mixed cellularity, and lymphocyte depletion, although in practice, almost all cases not of nodular sclerosing type represent mixed cellularity.

Determination of the subtype of Hodgkin's disease is best made on the initial biopsy, and preferably in a lymph node. Recurrences of Hodgkin's disease in untreated sites usually resemble the initial specimen, but recurrences of Hodgkin's in treated sites generally show an increase in the number and atypia of the Hodgkin's cells.[219] Hodgkin's disease at autopsy may show a striking degree of Hodgkin's cell proliferation and atypia.[220] Biopsies performed in successfully treated cases of Hodgkin's often show hypocellular or acellular fibrous scars. These scars may present as mass-occupying lesions that necessitate biopsy to rule out residual or recurrent disease.

Fine Needle Aspiration Cytopathology

Fine needle aspiration biopsy may be a means of diagnosing and staging Hodgkin's disease; in one study, the accuracy for diagnosing Hodgkin's disease was over 90 percent.[221] On low magnification, the aspirate smears usually show a dispersed population of lymphoid cells in which scattered large cells are evident (Fig. 20-37). At high magnification, these latter cells have bilobed or polylobated nuclei with prominent nucleoli and moderately abundant cytoplasm. Immunohistochemical studies may be helpful for confirmation. Fine needle aspiration studies are of less use in subclassifying Hodgkin's disease, although one study reported an accuracy of 58 percent.[221] Fine needle aspiration may be of great use in the diagnosis of recurrence of Hodgkin's disease, as Hodgkin's cells are sometimes more easily identified in this instance.

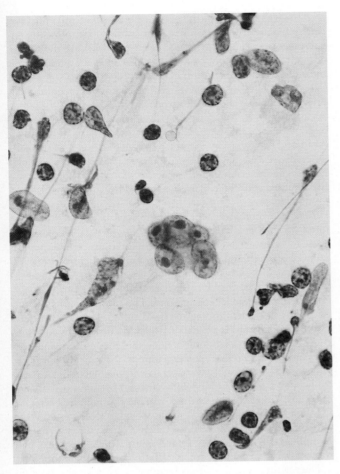

Fig. 20-37. Hodgkin's disease, fine needle aspiration. Hodgkin's cells are usually easily appreciated in smear preparations.

Table 20-7. Paraffin Section Immunophenotype of Hodgkin's Cells vs. L&H Cells

	Hodgkin's Cells (%)	L&H Cells (%)
CD45	10	90
CD30	90	40
CD15	90	10[a]
CD20	25	90
CD3	5	0
CD43	5	0
EMA	0	40

Abbreviation: EMA, epithelial membrane antigen; L&H, lymphocytic and histiocytic.

[a] Without neuraminidase predigestion.

Adjunctive Studies

Immunohistochemical studies have become an important adjunct to the diagnosis of Hodgkin's disease.[222] Paraffin section studies are better than frozen sections for the assessment of Hodgkin's cells, because morphology is much better preserved. Flow cytometry studies in Hodgkin's disease are not generally of use, and may even be misleading. Typically, the latter merely demonstrate a polyclonal population of B cells and a mixture of helper and suppressor T cells; the phenotype of the Hodgkin's cells is not demonstrated, even with attempts to gate on the large cell population, due to the infrequency of these cells. In paraffin sections, Hodgkin's cells have a characteristic phenotype: CD45−, CD30+, CD15+, CD20−, CD3−, CD43− (Table 20-7 and Fig. 20-38).[2,20,21,223,224] However, as Table 20-7 indicates, exceptions are seen with all stains, particularly with CD20, and therefore one needs to assess the overall staining pattern. In addition to case-to-case variation, the phenotype may vary from biopsy to biopsy, a factor to consider when eval-

uating possible recurrences.[225] Cases of EBV-associated Hodgkin's disease will show positivity for the EBV latent membrane protein.[201]

Molecular studies are not generally of practical use in Hodgkin's disease.[226] Southern blotting studies usually demonstrate a germline configuration for the immunoglobulin and beta-T cell receptor genes, although some cases, particularly those that have large numbers of Hodgkin's cells, have demonstrated clonal rearrangements (most often of the immunoglobulin genes).[227] Similarly, highly sensitive PCR studies have identified small monoclonal immunoglobulin gene rearrangements, particularly in cases expressing B lineage antigens such as CD20.[228] Cytogenetic studies are generally not useful in the routine diagnosis of Hodgkin's disease, due to the scarcity of Hodgkin's cells and their slow growth in cell culture. Successful studies usually show complex hyperdiploid karyotypes without consistent structural abnormalities.[229] EBV EBER in situ hybridization is a reliable test to identify this virus in EBV-associated cases.[230]

Despite years of investigation, the cell of origin of Hodgkin's disease has not been definitively established; however, a lymphoid origin is favored by most investigators. Lymphoid antigens, particularly B lineage antigens, can be identified in many cases when an extensive battery of paraffin and frozen section studies is performed, and the immunoglobulin-associated heterodimer has been identified in Reed-Sternberg cells.[231,232] In addition, the presence of clonal lymphoid antigen receptor genes in some cases strongly supports a lymphoid origin. However, other possibilities are still considered by some investigators, particularly a follicular dendritic cell lineage.[233] Although *bcl-2* gene rearrangements have been identified in Hodgkin's tissues by PCR,[234] it is likely that they derived from the reactive population and not the Reed-Sternberg cells.[226] Although one group has identified the t(2;5),[235] a translocation typically found in T cell/null cell anaplastic large cell lymphoma, other studies have not confirmed this finding.[236,237]

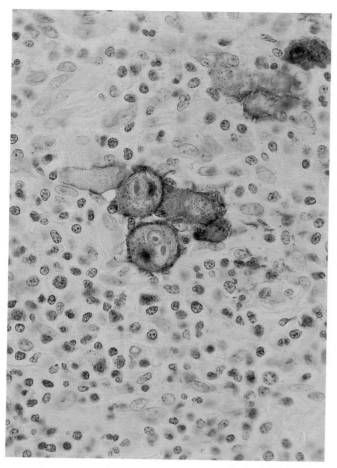

Fig. 20-38. Hodgkin's disease, CD15 stain. Membrane and paranuclear staining of Hodgkin's cells is present.

The nature of the accompanying infiltrate in Hodgkin's disease has also been the focus of intense interest. It is likely that much of the reactive lymphoid infiltrate represents an immune response to the neoplastic element. However, it has been demonstrated that Hodgkin's cells express a wide range of cytokines, including various interleukins, tumor necrosis factor, and transforming growth factor-β.[238] Production of one or more of these factors may explain some of the characteristic features of individual cases. For example, the production of interleukin-5 has been correlated with tissue and blood eosinophilia.[239]

Differential Diagnosis

The differential diagnosis of Hodgkin's disease is wide and includes carcinoma, malignant melanoma, germ cell tumor, sarcoma, reactive lymphoid hyperplasia, and malignant lymphoma. Cases of nodular sclerosing Hodgkin's disease with numerous Reed-Sternberg cells (the syncytial variant) can easily be misdiagnosed as a carcinoma, malignant melanoma, or a germ cell tumor. The localization of the neoplastic cells adja-

cent to areas of necrosis, the presence of admixed inflammatory cells particularly eosinophils, and subtotal lymph node involvement may suggest the possibility of Hodgkin's disease. In difficult cases, immunohistochemical studies may be of great use, with the demonstration of keratin positivity in carcinoma, S-100 positivity in malignant melanoma, and placental alkaline phosphatase and/or keratin positivity in germ cell tumors. As mentioned above, Hodgkin's disease may sometimes be confused with sarcoma, particularly in cases with an exuberant fibroblastic proliferation. Attention should be given to the cells possessing cytologic atypia. In sarcomas, the spindle cell elements will show significant atypia, while in Hodgkin's disease the spindled cells have bland nuclei and the atypical cells have rounded features.

Reactive immunoblastic proliferations may be easily confused with Hodgkin's disease, particularly interfollicular variants. In reactive immunoblastic proliferations, numerous immunoblasts with large nuclei and prominent nucleoli are found in expanded paracortical areas; occasionally, architectural effacement may be present. Cells resembling diagnostic Reed-Sternberg cells may even be found. The immunoblasts tend to be evenly dispersed in reactive conditions, whereas clustering of the atypical cells is typical of Hodgkin's disease. In addition, there is usually a background of numerous plasma cells and lymphoplasmacytoid cells in reactive immunoblastic proliferations, whereas only scattered plasma cells without lymphoplasmacytoid cells are found in Hodgkin's disease. Immunohistochemical studies may be of great use, as reactive immunoblasts are usually CD45+ and CD15−, while Hodgkin's cells are CD45− and CD15+; both are usually CD30+. In addition, the immunoblasts as well as the lymphoplasmacytic elements may show polyclonal staining for cytoplasmic immunoglobulins.

Necrotizing granulomatous lymphadenitis may also be difficult to distinguish from Hodgkin's disease, which may show patchy areas of necrosis. In these cases, it is important to examine the areas adjacent to the necrosis. In Hodgkin's disease, Hodgkin's cells will almost always be found adjacent to the necrosis, while in necrotizing granulomatous lymphadenitis, the lining cells will be bland histiocytes, often with epithelioid features.

Non-Hodgkin's lymphoma may be even more difficult to distinguish from Hodgkin's disease. Cases of small lymphocytic lymphoma may be confused with cases of lymphocyte-rich classic Hodgkin's disease. Large cells with prominent nucleoli are typically found as part of the proliferating element in small lymphocytic lymphoma; attention should be given to the background proliferation of small, regular lymphoid cells and the lack of eosinophils and other inflammatory elements. Immunohistochemical studies demonstrate a predominant B cell proliferation, often with coexpression of CD43, in small lymphocytic lymphoma, and a predominant T cell proliferation in Hodgkin's disease.

Rare cases of small lymphocytic lymphoma may have Reed-Sternberg-like cells or even true Reed-Sternberg cells.[240] The biology of these cases has yet to be fully clarified, but they may represent true composite lymphoma, as some of these patients, particularly those in which the atypical cells have the typical immunophenotype of Hodgkin's cells, eventually developed disseminated Hodgkin's disease. Most of these cases may be identified by EBV in situ hybridization, as the Reed-Sternberg-like cells (and not the small lymphocytes) are EBV positive in almost all cases.

Peripheral T cell lymphoma may be easily mistaken for Hodgkin's disease, because both diseases commonly feature a mixed proliferation of cells with an inflammatory component including eosinophils, histiocytes (including epithelioid histiocytes), and plasma cells. A range of cytologic atypia is usually found in peripheral T cell lymphoma, with atypical small, medium, and large-sized cells. Immunohistochemical studies will demonstrate a T cell prominence in both neoplasms, and CD30+ and even CD15+ cells may be present in both. The identification of CD45 and T lineage or T-associated antigens such as CD3 and CD43 on the atypical cells favors peripheral T cell lymphoma. Frozen section immunohistochemical studies will demonstrate an aberrant T cell phenotype in the majority of cases of peripheral T cell lymphoma. Occasionally, gene rearrangement studies may be necessary; the identification of a sizeable monoclonal beta-T cell receptor gene rearrangement would favor T cell lymphoma over Hodgkin's disease. T cell-rich B cell lymphoma may be difficult to distinguish from cases of lymphocyte-rich or mixed cellularity Hodgkin's disease, as the neoplastic B cells in T cell-rich lymphoma may very closely simulate Hodgkin's cells. Hodgkin's disease may also be confused with large B cell lymphoma, particularly in cases in which the Hodgkin's cells form sheets, such as in the syncytial variant of nodular sclerosis Hodgkin's disease. Large cell B cell lymphoma may show significant amounts of sclerosis, particularly in the mediastinum, the site where the syncytial variant of nodular sclerosis most commonly occurs. The demonstration of CD45 negativity and CD15 positivity strongly favors Hodgkin's disease over these B cell lymphomas; one must keep in mind that CD20 is positive in 10 to 20 percent of cases of Hodgkin's disease. Rarely, Hodgkin's disease and B cell lymphoma may coexist in the same patient, either simultaneously in the same site (composite lymphoma), or simultaneously at different sites (discordant lymphoma).[241] Non-Hodgkin's lymphomas may arise in patients successfully treated for Hodgkin's disease,[242] and conversely, Hodgkin's disease may occur in patients with a history of non-Hodgkin's lymphoma.[243]

Finally, anaplastic large cell lymphoma may be extremely difficult to distinguish from Hodgkin's disease, because both neoplasms contain a proliferation of large, highly atypical cells with prominent nucleoli. Clinical features may be of use, as anaplastic large cell lymphoma frequently involves the skin, an infrequent site of occurrence of Hodgkin's disease, and is more common in children. A preferential localization to sinuses would favor anaplastic large cell lymphoma over Hodgkin's disease, because Hodgkin's disease usually does not involve sinuses until there is extensive involvement of the paracortical region. The presence of abundant neutrophils and plasma cells would also favor anaplastic large cell lymphoma over Hodgkin's disease, which usually has more numerous eosinophils. Both neoplasms are CD30+, and CD45 may be negative in up to one-third of cases of anaplastic large cell lymphoma.[20] The expression of epithelial membrane antigen or T lineage-associated antigens such as CD43 would favor anaplastic large cell lymphoma, and the expression of CD15+ would favor Hodgkin's disease, although some cases of anaplastic large cell lymphoma may also be CD15+. Molecular studies may be helpful, as the presence of a sizeable monoclonal beta-T cell receptor gene rearrangement or the demonstration of a t(2;5) would strongly favor anaplastic large cell lymphoma. Some investigators believe there is a biologic overlap between anaplastic large cell lymphoma and Hodgkin's disease, referring to these cases as Hodgkin's-like anaplastic large cell lymphoma.[9,244] Some of these transitional cases seem to behave as Hodgkin's disease, whereas others may require aggressive therapy such as is given for high grade non-Hodgkin's lymphomas.[245]

L&H LYMPHOCYTE PREDOMINANCE HODGKIN'S DISEASE

As discussed above, Lukes and Butler[196] recognized nodular and diffuse L&H categories of Hodgkin's disease.[196] In the last two decades, a plethora of evidence has established that the L&H variants of Hodgkin's disease represent a clinicopathologic entity distinct from classic Hodgkin's disease.[198] L&H lymphocyte predominance is defined as a proliferation of L&H cells, cells morphologically and immunologically distinct from the Reed-Sternberg cells and variants found in classic Hodgkin's disease. It is also known as nodular paragranuloma in the European literature.[76] It is not clear whether L&H lymphocyte predominance is a neoplastic or a reactive proliferation, although most of the current evidence supports the former possibility.

L&H lymphocyte predominance comprises approximately 4 percent of cases of Hodgkin's disease.[246] There is a male/female ratio of about 2.5:1, and the disease occurs in all age groups, with a median age of about 35 years.[247,248] It is not associated with EBV,[249] and there are no known predisposing factors, although rare patients have a history of progressive transformation of germinal centers.[76,77] Patients usually present with isolated lymphadenopathy of greater than 3 months' duration, usually involving cervical, axillary, or inguinal lymph nodes.[247,248] About one-half of patients present in Ann Arbor stage I, and "B" symptoms are uncommon. Liver and spleen involvement occur in about 10 to 15 percent of cases, but bone marrow and other visceral organ involvement is very uncommon. In one study of nodular L&H lymphocyte predominance, the disease tended to recur independently of time and treatment, suggesting a clinical course distinct from classic Hodgkin's disease,[250] although not all other studies have confirmed this finding. The optimal treatment of L&H lymphocyte predominance is still not clear.[251] The overall prognosis is excellent and similar to that of the general population, particularly in patients with low stage disease. Patients with stage III disease with splenic involvement and stage IV disease have only about a 60 percent survival, with death usually occurring within the first year.[248]

At low magnification, L&H lymphocyte predominance usually shows a nodular architecture, with the nodules larger than the follicles of follicular lymphoma (Fig. 20-39). Occasionally, the nodules are highlighted by a rim of epithelioid histiocytes. Often, there is a rim of uninvolved lymph node that may show reactive follicular hyperplasia or progressive transformation of

Fig. 20-39. Lymphocytic and histiocytic lymphocyte predominance Hodgkin's disease. At low magnification, large nodules are almost always present.

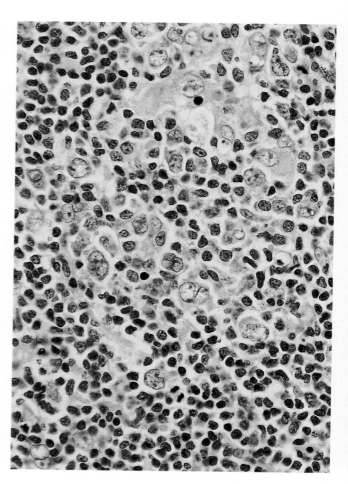

Fig. 20-40. Lymphocytic and histiocytic (L&H) lymphocyte predominance Hodgkin's disease. Several L&H cells are seen, including a polylobated one in the center.

germinal centers. The nodules are composed of numerous small, round lymphocytes and scattered epithelioid histiocytes and L&H cells. L&H cells are large cells with large nuclei and scant cytoplasm (Fig. 20-40). The nuclear outlines are usually highly irregular ("popcorn" or "elephant foot" cells), but may be round. The chromatin is usually vesicular. There are one to several moderately sized nucleoli that are usually less eosinophilic and smaller in size than in the Reed-Sternberg cells of classic Hodgkin's disease. Although rare cells closely resembling classic Reed-Sternberg cells may be found, these are not a requisite for the diagnosis. The internodular areas are usually compressed, and are composed of small, round lymphocytes and scattered plasma cells. Eosinophils are generally sparse in both the nodular and internodular areas.

In a minority of cases, diffuse effacement of architecture is present, without the formation of nodules. Occasionally, both a nodular and diffuse pattern is present in the same node. More commonly, a nodular appearance is seen in one biopsy, while a subsequent biopsy shows diffuse effacement.

L&H cells show a B lineage immunophenotype distinct from the Reed-Sternberg cells of classic Hodgkin's disease. The cells are typically CD45+ and CD20+, CD15–, and CD30 and epithelial membrane antigen positive or negative.[222,252–255] J chain, a protein associated with immunoglobulin synthesis, has been found in the cytoplasm of L&H cells,[256] but the expression of immunoglobulins is controversial. In some studies, a polyclonal staining pattern is seen,[255] in other studies no expression is seen,[248,252,256,257] while in one study kappa light chain restriction was found in most cases.[258] Most of the small lymphocytes in the nodules are polyclonal B lymphocytes, although there are also significant numbers of T cells.[255] Many of these T cells express the natural killer (NK) marker CD57, and a ring of CD57+ cells may sometimes be found around the L&H cells.[259] A network of dendritic reticulum cells is found in the nodules.[260]

The true nature of the L&H cells is still not clear. Immunophenotyping studies have indicated that they are of B lineage, but whether they are polyclonal or monoclonal has not been resolved. As mentioned above, the results of immunoglobulin protein studies have been controversial. The results of in situ hybridization studies for immunoglobulin mRNA have been equally confusing and have paralleled the immunohistochemical studies, with some studies demonstrating a lack of immunoglobulin mRNA,[257] other studies demonstrating a polyclonal pattern, and still other studies finding monotypic kappa mRNA restriction.[249] One recent PCR study employing single cell dissection has found a polyclonal pattern of light chain mRNA expression.[261]

Differential Diagnosis

The differential diagnosis of L&H lymphocyte predominance is wide and includes progressive transformation of germinal centers, classic Hodgkin's disease, and non-Hodgkin's lymphoma, including follicular lymphoma, T cell-rich/histiocyte-rich B cell lymphoma, and diffuse large cell lymphoma. Progressive transformation generally does not show the effacement of architecture seen in L&H lymphocyte predominance; rather, the progressively transformed germinal centers are found in the context of reactive follicular hyperplasia.[77] However, the most important differentiating feature is the presence of L&H cells in L&H lymphocyte predominance and their absence in progressive transformation. Immunostains for CD20 may be very useful in highlighting the L&H cells, although it must be remembered that CD20+ immunoblasts may be present in progressive transformation. Stains for epithelial membrane antigen are positive in a subset of cases of L&H lymphocyte predominance but always negative in immunoblasts.[222] In addition, CD57 staining of small lymphocytes in L&H lymphocyte predominance may also be helpful, particularly when there is ringing of CD57+ cells around the L&H cells.[259]

Lymphocyte rich cases of classic Hodgkin's disease may be difficult to distinguish from L&H lymphocyte predominance, particularly diffuse variants of L&H lymphocyte predominance. It is likely that both were included in the Rye category of lymphocyte predominance Hodgkin's disease. Although a distinctly nodular architecture would favor L&H lymphocyte predominance, the crucial difference rests in the character of the large atypical cells, L&H cells vs. other Hodgkin's cells. L&H cells tend to have more delicate and more irregular nuclear membranes and less prominent nucleoli than classic Hodgkin's cells. In difficult cases, immunohistochemical studies may be of great use (Table 20-7).

Follicular lymphoma, particularly the floral variant, may be difficult to distinguish from nodular forms of L&H lymphocyte predominance.[262] The nodules in L&H lymphocyte predominance are almost always larger than seen in follicular lymphoma, and there is usually not the compression between adjacent follicles seen in the latter. Cytologically, L&H lymphocyte predominance does not contain the small and large cleaved cells that compose the neoplastic element of follicular lymphoma. The distinction between T cell-rich/histiocyte-rich B cell lymphoma and L&H lymphocyte predominance may be extremely difficult. A significant degree of nodularity would favor L&H lymphocyte predominance, whereas clustering of the large atypical cells into small sheets of cells would favor B cell lymphoma. Immunohistochemical studies may not be helpful, since the phenotypes, B lineage with possible expression of epithelial membrane antigens, may be identical. In fact, some have speculated that histiocyte-rich B cell lymphoma and diffuse L&H lymphocyte predominance represent the same disease, al-

though it is stated that the histiocytes are epithelioid and nonepithelioid in L&H lymphocyte predominance, but nonepithelioid in histiocyte-rich B cell lymphoma.[263]

Some cases of L&H lymphocyte predominance contain large numbers of L&H cells, raising consideration of large cell lymphoma, a complication that has been reported in about 5 percent of cases.[264] We diagnose large cell transformation when sheets of large cells are present in the internodular areas. The large cell lymphomas complicating L&H lymphocyte predominance are usually (but not always) of B lineage, and lack EBV or *bcl-2* gene rearrangements.[265] In one recent study, PCR studies demonstrated that the same B cell clone was found in the B cell lymphoma and in the preceding specimen that showed L&H lymphocyte predominance.[266]

NON-HODGKIN'S LYMPHOMA

Non-Hodgkin's lymphoma is defined by what it is not, that is, it includes all neoplasms of lymphoid origin other than Hodgkin's disease. It occurs five times more frequently than Hodgkin's disease, with about 40,000 new cases each year, and has been increasing by a rate of 3 to 4 percent per year.[199,267] Some of the increase is due to the increase in number of HIV-associated cases.[268] Environmental exposures, such as exposure to hair dyes, herbicides, and organic chemicals, may account for an additional part of the increase.[269–271] A subset of cases is associated with human T cell leukemia virus (HTLV)-1,[272] and other subsets of cases are associated with EBV.[201] Non-Hodgkin's lymphoma occurs in both children and adults, with an overall male/female ratio of 1.3:1. Although more common in adults, it accounts for a relatively high percentage of cancer occurring in children.

Non-Hodgkin's lymphoma usually presents as painless, localized or generalized enlargement of lymph nodes with or without hepatosplenomegaly. However, it may present as a tonsillar, mediastinal, or abdominal mass, or as localized or generalized lesions involving every organ or organ system. "B" symptoms may occur, but are less commonly seen than in Hodgkin's disease. The signs and symptoms may occur acutely or may have been present for a long period of time, occasionally years. Although progression does not occur in as orderly a fashion as in Hodgkin's disease, the Ann Arbor system has still been used for the staging of non-Hodgkin's lymphoma.[273]

Non-Hodgkin's lymphomas represent a heterogeneous mixture of neoplasms of different cell lineages frozen at different stages of development. Eighty to 90 percent represent B lineage neoplasms, most often related to cells of the germinal center.[274] Other B cell lymphomas may be related to cells of the B cell mantle or marginal zone or B cell populations native to extranodal tissues. A minority of cases represent T lineage neoplasms, including neoplasms of immature (thymic) as well as mature T cell phenotype (post-thymic or peripheral). Some cases may be of NK cell lineage or indeterminate lineage, the latter usually referred to as null cell type. Some investigators include neoplasms of true histiocytic lineage among the malignant lymphomas, because of clinical and morphologic similarities.

In general, non-Hodgkin's lymphomas are monoclonal pro-

Table 20-8. Non-Hodgkin's Lymphomas and Frequency of Monoclonal Gene Rearrangements

	Ig Heavy (%)	Ig Light (%)	T-Beta (%)
Most B cell lymphomas	100	100	5–10
B lymphoblastic	100	40	20–30
Peripheral T cell lymphoma	5–10	<1	90
T lymphoblastic	20–30	1	90

Abbreviation: Ig, immunoglobulin.
(Modified from Weiss et al,[511] with permission.)

liferations.[11] Thus, B cell lymphomas expressing immunoglobulin will generally show only one of the light chains, so-called light chain restriction. Monoclonal immunoglobulin gene rearrangements are usually detectable, and aberrant clonal rearrangements of the beta-T cell receptor gene are also detectable in a minority of cases, particularly in the immature lymphoblastic neoplasms (Table 20-8). There is no good marker for monoclonality analogous to analysis of light chains for T cell lymphomas, although many T cell lymphomas may show aberrant loss of one or more T lineage antigens.[275] Monoclonal beta-T cell receptor gene rearrangements are found in most, but not all, T cell lymphomas, and similar to B cell lymphomas, aberrant monoclonal immunoglobulin heavy chain gene rearrangements are also detectable in a minority of cases, again particularly in the immature lymphoblastic neoplasms. Many types of non-Hodgkin's lymphomas are associated with characteristic cytogenetic abnormalities, usually balanced translocations (Table 20-9). Typically, a cellular oncogene is translocated to adjacent to one of the antigen receptor genes.

The classification of non-Hodgkin's lymphoma has been an extremely controversial issue over the past several decades. Classifications have been proposed that have been based primarily on morphologic, immunologic, ontogenic (developmental), or molecular genetic features. Summarizing thousands of papers in the literature, it is safe to conclude that there is still no one uniformly accepted classification of non-Hodgkin's lymphoma. Currently, most cases of non-Hodgkin's lymphoma in the United States are classified using the Working Formulation,[276] whereas most cases in Europe are classified using the Updated Kiel classification of 1988.[277] The Working Formulation was devised in 1982 as a means of translation between six different classifications, but has come to be used as an independent classification[276] (Table 20-10). It is most closely related to the previous Rappaport classification,[56] being morphologically based. It recognizes 10 major categories of lymphoma, organized into three histologic grades: low grade, with a median survival of 6.0 years; intermediate grade, with a median survival of 3.5 years; and high grade, with a median survival of 1.4 years. The Updated Kiel classification is a combined immunologic and cytologic classification recognizing several cytologic types of B and T cell lymphoma, organized into low and high grade[277] (Table 20-11). Recently, a new proposal has come from the International Lymphoma Study Group, termed the Revised European-American Lymphoma (REAL) classification[9] (Table 20-12). This system recognizes about 25 separate categories of lymphoma thought to represent well established (or provisional) clinicopathologic entities as defined by combined morphologic, immunologic, ontogenic, and molecular genetic features.

Complicating the difficulty in classification is the recognition that a minority of lymphomas may have different histologic appearances in different sites; these lymphomas are termed *discordant lymphomas*. Rarely, lymphomas may have two or more distinctly different histologic appearances at the same site (including coexisting non-Hodgkin's lymphoma and Hodgkin's disease); these lymphomas are termed *composite lymphoma*.[278] In addition, it is not uncommon for a low grade lymphoma to transform over time to a lymphoma of higher grade. Finally, some lymphomas show close overlap with leukemic counterparts, and it is likely that both represent the same biologic entity with different clinical manifestations.

Fine needle aspiration biopsy has been used for the primary diagnosis of non-Hodgkin's lymphoma, but there are limitations due to the difficulties involved in both the diagnosis as well as classification. The key to the recognition of most non-Hodgkin's lymphomas on fine needle aspiration is the identifi-

Table 20-9. Common Chromosomal Translocations Found in Non-Hodgkin's Lymphomas

Translocation	Lymphoma	Antigen Receptor Gene	Oncogene
t(11;14)(q13;q32)	Mantle cell	IgH	*PRAD1/cyclin/CCND1/bcl-1*
t(14;18)(q32;q21)	Follicular; some diffuse large cell	IgH	*bcl-2*
t(3;v)(q27;v)	Diffuse large cell lymphoma	Variable	*bcl-6/laz-3*
t(2;5)(p23;q35)	Anaplastic large cell lymphoma	Not involved (*npm* gene)	*alk*
t(8;14)(q24;q32)	Burkitt's; some diffuse large cell	IgH	*c-myc*
t(2;8)(2p12;q24)	Burkitt's; some diffuse large cell	Kappa	*c-myc*
t(8;22)(q24;q11)	Burkitt's; some diffuse large cell	Lambda	*c-myc*

(Modified from Weiss et al,[511] with permission.)

Table 20-10. Working Formulation of Non-Hodgkin's Lymphomas for Clinical Usage

Low grade
  A. Small lymphocytic
          Consistent with CLL; plasmacytoid
  B. Follicular predominantly small cleaved cell
          Diffuse areas, sclerosis
  C. Follicular mixed small cleaved and large cell
          Diffuse areas, sclerosis

Intermediate grade
  D. Follicular predominantly large cell
          Diffuse areas, sclerosis
  E. Diffuse small cleaved cell
          Sclerosis
  F. Diffuse mixed, small and large cell
          Sclerosis, epithelioid cell component
  G. Diffuse large cell
          Cleaved cell, noncleaved cell, sclerosis

High grade
  H. Large cell, immunoblastic
          Plasmacytoid, clear cell, polymorphous, epithelioid cell
          component
  I. Lymphoblastic
          Convoluted, nonconvoluted
  J. Small noncleaved cell
          Burkitt's, follicular areas

Miscellaneous
          Composite, mycosis fungoides, histiocytic, extramedullary plasmacytoma, unclassifiable, other

(Modified from Non-Hodgkin's Lymphoma Pathologic Classification Project,[276] with permission.)

Table 20-11. Updated Kiel Classification of Non-Hodgkin's Lymphomas

B cell	T cell
Low grade	
Lymphocytic—chronic lymphocytic and prolymphocytic leukemia; hairy cell leukemia	Lymphocytic chronic lymphocytic, and prolymphocytic leukemia
Lymphoplasmacytic/cytoid	Lymphoepithelioid
Plasmacytic	Angioimmunoblastic
Centroblastic/centrocytic	T zone
Centrocytic	Pleomorphic, small cell
High Grade	
Centroblastic	Pleomorphic, medium and large cell
Immunoblastic	Immunoblastic
Large cell anaplastic	Large cell anaplastic
Burkitt's lymphoma	
Lymphoblastic	Lymphoblastic
Rare types	Rare types

(From Stansfeld et al,[277] with permission.)

Table 20-12. List of Lymphoid Neoplasms Recognized by the International Lymphoma Study Group

B cell neoplasms
  I. Precursor B cell neoplasm: B precursor lymphoblastic leukemia/lymphoma
  II. Peripheral B cell neoplasms
    1. B cell chronic lymphocytic leukemia/prolymphocytic leukemia/small lymphocytic lymphoma
    2. Lymphoplasmacytoid lymphoma/immunocytoma
    3. Mantle cell lymphoma
    4. Follicle center lymphoma, follicular
       Provisional cytologic grades: I (small cell), II (mixed small and large cell), III (large cell)
       Provisional subtype: diffuse, predominantly small cell type
    5. Marginal zone B cell lymphoma
       Extranodal (MALT type ± monocytoid B cells)
       Provisional category: nodal (± monocytoid B cells)
    6. Provisional category: splenic marginal zone lymphoma (± villous lymphocytes)
    7. Hairy cell leukemia
    8. Plasmacytoma/plasma cell myeloma
    9. Diffuse large B cell lymphoma
       Subtype: primary mediastinal (thymic) B cell lymphoma
    10. Burkitt's lymphoma
    11. Provisional category: high grade B cell lymphoma, Burkitt's-like

T cell and putative NK cell neoplasms
  I. Precursor T cell neoplasm: T precursor lymphoblastic lymphoma/leukemia
  II. Peripheral T cell and NK cell neoplasms
    1. T cell chronic lymphocytic leukemia/prolymphocytic leukemia
    2. Large granular lymphocyte leukemia (LGL)
    3. Mycosis fungoides/Sézary's syndrome
    4. Peripheral T cell lymphoma, unspecified
       Provisional cytologic categories: subtypes: medium-sized cell, mixed medium and large cell, large cell, lymphoepithelioid cell
       Provisional subtype: hepatosplenic gamma/delta T cell lymphoma
       Provisional subtype: subcutaneous panniculitic T cell lymphoma
    5. Angioimmunoblastic T cell lymphoma (AILD)
    6. Angiocentric lymphoma
    7. Intestinal T cell lymphoma (± enteropathy associated)
    8. Adult T cell lymphoma/leukemia (ATL/L)
    9. Anaplastic large cell lymphoma (ALCL), CD30 +, T and null cell types
    10. Provisional subtype: anaplastic large cell lymphoma, Hodgkin's-like

Hodgkin's disease
  I. Lymphocyte predominance
  II. Nodular sclerosis
  III. Mixed cellularity
  IV. Lymphocyte depletion
  V. Provisional entity: lymphocyte-rich classic Hodgkin's disease

(From Harris et al,[9] with permission.)

Table 20-13. International Prognostic Index
for Aggressive Lymphomas

Risk factors	
Age >60 years	
Stage III or IV	
Number of extranodal sites of disease >1	
Performance status ≤2	
Serum lactate dehydrogenase level greater than normal	
Low risk (73% 5 year survival)	0 or 1 of above risk factors
Low intermediate risk (51% 5 year survival)	2 of above risk factors
High intermediate risk (43% 5 year survival)	3 of above risk factors
High risk (26% 5 year survival)	4 or 5 of above risk factors

(Data from The International Non-Hodgkin's Lymphoma Prognostic Factors Project.[285])

cation of a monotonous lymphoid cell population. The monotony is reflected not so much in the nuclear size, but in the essentially uniform cell-to-cell appearance of the chromatin pattern. Lymphomas composed of a heterogeneous mixture of neoplastic cells (e.g., peripheral T cell lymphoma) may be very difficult to recognize by fine needle aspiration, unless highly bizarre or pleomorphic cells are identified. The efficacy of fine needle aspiration biopsy in the primary diagnosis of non-Hodgkin's lymphoma can be dramatically improved when supplemented with immunohistochemical and molecular studies. Precise classification may still be quite difficult to perform; however, the distinction between low grade and high grade lymphomas can usually be made. In one series, about 90 percent of non-Hodgkin's lymphomas were correctly diagnosed, with the correct assignment of grade in virtually all cases.[279] The specific diagnosis of low grade lymphomas is more difficult to make than with high grade lymphomas. Fine needle aspiration biopsy is more easily applied to the staging of non-Hodgkin's lymphoma, allowing easy, widespread sampling of different sites. It may also be used to diagnose recurrent or residual disease, or to identify large cell transformation in a patient with a history of low grade lymphoma.

Recently, there has been intense interest in better defining prognostic factors in non-Hodgkin's lymphoma. In addition to histologic grade and stage, clinical factors such as age, sex, Karnofsky performance index, number of nodal and extranodal sites of disease, size of tumor, and beta-2-microglobulin and lactate dehydrogenase levels have been found to affect prognosis.[280–284] Recently, an International Prognostic Index has been developed for aggressive non-Hodgkin's lymphoma patients, based on age, stage, number of extranodal sites of disease, performance status, and serum lactate dehydrogenase levels[285] (Table 20-13). This index may also be applicable to other types of non-Hodgkin's lymphoma.[286] In addition, a variety of immunobiologic factors may be of importance in determining prognosis, including proliferative rate, cytotoxic T cell response, loss of molecules of immune recognition, loss of cell ad-

hesion antigens, gain of drug resistance molecules, acquisition of aneuploidy, gain of specific oncogenes, or loss of specific tumor suppressor genes.[286–289]

Follicular Lymphoma

Follicular lymphoma is defined as a neoplasm of B cell derivation showing some component of follicular architecture. In the Working Formulation, it is divided into small cleaved, mixed small cleaved and large cell, and predominantly large cell categories.[276] The small cleaved and mixed variants are of low grade, whereas the large cell variant is of intermediate grade. In the REAL classification, follicular lymphoma is a specific clinicopathologic entity called "follicle center lymphoma, follicular," with three provisional cytologic grades: small cell, mixed small and large cell, and large cell.[9]

In the United States, follicular lymphoma is a relatively common type of non-Hodgkin's lymphoma, representing about 40 percent of cases. The mean age of occurrence is 55 years, with only rare cases reported in childhood, and few under the age of 40.[290] Roughly equal numbers of cases occur in males and females. Patients usually present with one or several enlarged lymph nodes, often of long duration. However, the vast majority of cases are already in stage IV, with bone marrow, liver, and spleen involvement common. Involvement of peripheral blood also occurs frequently, either at presentation or during the course of disease.

Follicular lymphoma is usually an indolent lymphoma, with occasional spontaneous regressions, slow progression, and numerous relapses occurring over time seemingly independent of treatment.[291,292] Because of this, most cases of follicular lymphoma are not treated aggressively, although the large cell variant is often treated with standard anthracyclin-based chemotherapy with curative intent.[286] In about 40 to 50 percent of cases, transformation to a diffuse large cell lymphoma occurs. With this event, survival is usually less than 1 year, although some patients undergo remissions with aggressive chemotherapy.

The hallmark of follicular lymphoma is the presence of a true follicular architecture, at least focally within the tumor (Fig. 20-41). In most cases, the follicles are evenly dispersed throughout the entire lymph node parenchyma, often with extension into the perinodal adipose tissue. In some cases, there are areas of follicular and diffuse effacement of architecture (most often seen in the large cell type). The presence of diffuse areas may adversely affect prognosis, particularly in the mixed and large cell variants.[286, 293] For example, we consider follicular mixed small cleaved and large cell lymphomas to be of intermediate grade if over 75 percent of the tumor area has diffuse architecture. Occasionally, the follicular areas may only be focally appreciated; usually the remainder of the lymph node shows diffuse effacement of architecture, although rarely there is normal architecture. In the latter case, adjacent lymph nodes may show a greater degree of involvement. The follicles are classically round and relatively homogeneously sized; occasionally, however, the follicles are highly irregular, with varied size and shape. The mantles are usually absent, but when present, are a thin rim or of normal thickness. Rarely, small mantle cells larger than small, mature lymphocytes and have relatively condensed chromatin without prominent nucleoli. The most distinctive feature are the highly irregular nuclear outlines, which are contorted and twisted. Large cleaved cells are similar cells with nuclei about two to three times the size of small cleaved cells. Large noncleaved cells are slightly larger in size and have rounded nuclear outlines, a vesicular chromatin pattern, and one to several moderately sized nucleoli, often apposed to the nuclear membrane. A moderate amount of amphophilic or slightly basophilic cytoplasm is typically present.

Cases are usually classified as predominantly small cleaved when there are greater than 75 percent small cleaved cells or less than five large noncleaved cells per high power field (× 10 eyepiece and × 40 objective).[35,296, 297] Cases are usually classified as mixed small cleaved and large cells type when there are between 25 and 50 percent large cells or between 5 and 15 large cells per high power field. Cases are usually classified as predominantly large cell type when there are greater than 50 percent large cells or greater than 15 large cells per high power field. In practice, the distinction is often arbitrary, perhaps at

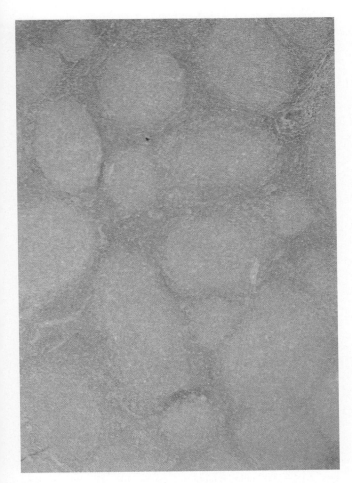

Fig. 20-41. Follicular lymphoma. Numerous follicles are present, with only a small amount of intervening interfollicular areas.

may invaginate between and separate small clusters of follicular lymphoma cells, expanding the neoplastic follicles in the process; these unusual cases have been termed the *floral variant of follicular lymphoma*.[262,294] In most cases, the interfollicular regions are compressed, and often there is a back-to-back arrangement of the follicles. In some cases, the follicles coalesce into one another. However, in some cases the interfollicular areas may be of normal size, and the follicles clearly distinct. In rare cases, the marginal zones (the areas just outside of the mantle zone) may be expanded by a proliferation of monocytoid cells forming a pale collar around the neoplastic follicles; in these cases, the proliferating monocytoid cells are part of the lymphomatous process.[295] Sclerosis is common in follicular lymphoma, and usually consists of broad collagenous bands. Deposition of an amorphous extracellular material may be found within the follicles, but is not specific for neoplastic follicles.

The cytologic features are as important as the architectural features in establishing a morphologic diagnosis of follicular lymphoma. The cells in the follicles are varying mixtures of small cleaved cells, large cleaved cells, and large noncleaved cells (Figs. 20-42 and 20-43). Small cleaved cells are slightly

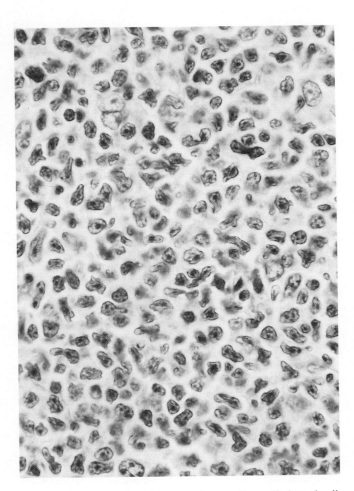

Fig. 20-42. Follicular lymphoma, predominantly small cleaved cell type. Most of the cells are small and have contorted nuclear outlines, but occasional larger cells are also present.

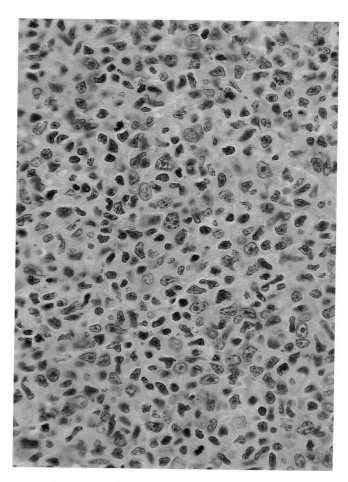

Fig. 20-43. Follicular lymphoma, mixed small cleaved cell and large cell type. A mixture of atypical cells is seen. Both large cleaved and large noncleaved cells are present.

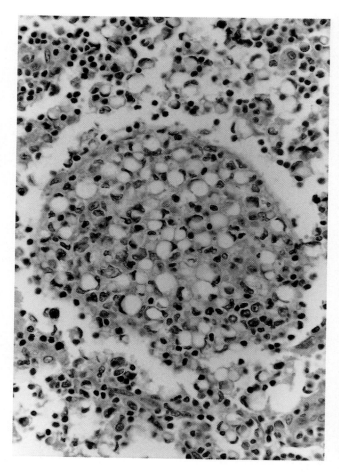

Fig. 20-44. Follicular lymphoma, signet ring cell type. Striking cytoplasmic vacuolization is seen in this unusual variant of follicular lymphoma.

least partially explaining the poor reproducibility among even experienced hematopathologists. Approximately two-thirds of cases of follicular lymphoma are predominantly small cleaved cell type, about 25 percent of cases are diagnosed as mixed small cleaved and large cell type, and about 10 percent are classified as predominantly large cell type. Tingible body macrophages are rare in follicular lymphoma of predominantly small cleaved and mixed cell types, but may be a feature of the large cell type. Similarly, the mitotic rate is usually low in the small cleaved and mixed cell types, but may be brisk in the large cell type.

Rarely, there may be other cytologic variants of follicular lymphoma. These include the presence of clear or eosinophilic cytoplasmic inclusions, the so-called signet ring cell variant of follicular lymphoma[298] (Fig. 20-44). In addition, the cells may rarely have small round nuclei (termed *follicular small lymphocytic lymphoma*),[299] cerebriform nuclei reminiscent of the cells of mycosis fungoides,[300] multilobated nuclei,[301] plasmacytoid nuclear and cytoplasmic features,[302] immunoblastic features,[303] and blastic nuclei resembling the nuclei of lymphoblastic leukemia.[304]

Fine needle aspiration biopsy smears of follicular lymphoma

often show vague nodular aggregates, imparting a nodular pattern at low magnification. Small cleaved cells appear as small hyperchromatic cells with a wrinkled or indented nuclear outline (Fig. 20-45). Large cells typically have rounded or cleaved vesicular nuclei with irregularly thick and thin nuclear membranes. The recognition of the mixed cell type may be extremely difficult cytologically, but immunohistochemical and molecular studies may be helpful in establishing a diagnosis of follicular lymphoma.

Immunohistochemical studies demonstrate that all follicular lymphomas are of B lineage, expressing multiple B lineage antigens in both paraffin and frozen sections (Table 20-14). Approximately 90 percent express surface immunoglobulins by flow cytometry/frozen section immunohistochemistry, usually IgM, and sometimes with a second isotype.[305] The large cell subtype is most likely to be immunoglobulin negative. Monotypic immunoglobulin may also be detected in paraffin sections in a significant proportion of cases, but this procedure is less dependable than frozen section studies. The bcl-2 oncoprotein is expressed by the neoplastic cells in about 80 to 90 percent of cases (Fig. 20-46); again, the large cell subtype is most likely to be bcl-2 protein negative.[306,307] The neoplastic cells express

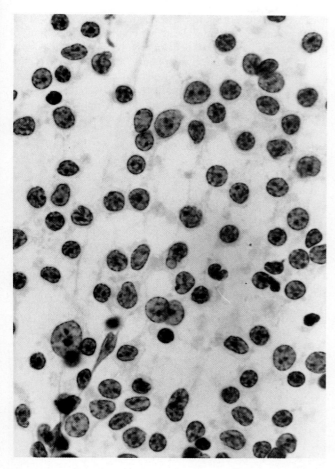

Fig. 20-45. Follicular lymphoma, fine needle aspiration. Many of the small lymphoid cells have irregular nuclear contours. This feature is often difficult to appreciate in smear preparations, unless the cells are carefully examined.

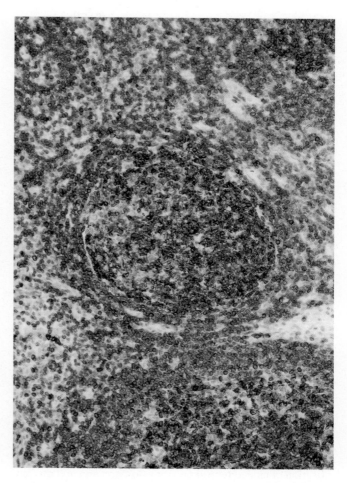

Fig. 20-46. Follicular lymphoma, bcl-2 stain. The follicles are strongly labeled for bcl-2, consistent with a follicular lymphoma.

CD10 in about 50 to 60 percent of cases, are usually negative for CD23, and are almost always negative for CD5. T lineage antibodies do not stain the neoplastic cells, but demonstrate a significant population of T cells within the neoplastic follicles. A subset of these T cells express the NK marker CD57. Stains such as CD35 demonstrate a rich network of follicular dendritic cells, similar to that seen in non-neoplastic follicles.

Clonal immunoglobulin heavy and light chain gene rearrangements are detectable in virtually all cases of follicular lymphoma. In addition, evidence of the t(14;18) can be found by a variety of techniques in about 90 percent of cases.[308–311]

Table 20-14. Summary of Immunophenotypes of Low to Intermediate Grade B Cell Lymphomas

	Follicular	SLL/CLL	Marginal	Lym-Plas	Mantle
Ig	90%	98%	98%	98%	98%
Heavy	IgM,G	IgM ± IgD	IgM,D,A	IgM	IgM + IgD
K/L	2:1	2:1	2:1	2:1	1:1
CD20	100%	98%	98%	98%	99%
CD43	2%	85%	50%	60%	60%
CD5	1%	90%	10%	25%	80%
CD10	60%	10%	10%	10%	25%
CD23	5%	90%	15%	30%	15%

Abbreviations: SLL/CLL, small lymphocytic lymphoma/chronic lymphocytic leukemia; Lym-Plas, lymphoplasmacytic; Ig, immunoglobulin; heavy, common heavy chain(s); K, kappa; L, lambda.

The t(14;18) at the molecular level involves translocation of the *bcl-2* gene on chromosome 18 into the immunoglobulin heavy chain gene, leading to its deregulation and overexpression.[312] Evidence of the t(14;18) can also be detected by sensitive molecular techniques in a high proportion of peripheral blood and bone marrow specimens from these patients, consistent with the disseminated nature of the disease.[313] The presence of other cytogenetic abnormalities, such as abnormalities involving chromosome regions 1p21-22, 6q23-26, and the short arm of chromosome 17 may be associated with adverse prognosis.[314] Mutations of the tumor suppressor gene p53 have been identified in a subset of cases of large cell transformation.[315,316]

The differential diagnosis of follicular lymphoma vs. reactive follicular hyperplasia has already been discussed in the section on reactive follicular hyperplasia. The differential diagnosis with nodular L&H lymphocyte predominance Hodgkin's disease has already been discussed in the section on that disease. Follicular lymphoma may also be confused with mantle cell lymphoma and marginal cell lymphoma. Mantle cell lymphoma may have nodular variants in which the germinal centers as well as the mantle zone regions become replaced by neoplastic mantle cells. Cytologically, mantle cell lymphomas are characterized by a homogeneous population of small atypical cells without admixed large cleaved and noncleaved cells. Immunohistochemical studies may be very helpful, as the cells of mantle cell lymphoma often show aberrant coexpression of CD5 or CD43, very rare findings in follicular lymphoma. Marginal zone lymphomas may mimic follicular lymphoma by virtue of colonization of reactive germinal centers by neoplastic cells. The identification of typical areas of marginal zone lymphoma is helpful on low power magnification, and the identification of moderate to abundant pale cytoplasm and the lack of truly cleaved nuclei are helpful features on high power magnification. bcl-2 oncoprotein may be immunohistochemically positive in follicles colonized by marginal cell lymphoma, but evidence of a t(14;18) is lacking.

Small Lymphocytic Lymphoma

In the Working Formulation, the morphologic category of low grade lymphoma, small lymphocytic type probably included at least several clinicopathologic entities characterized by diffuse proliferation of relatively small lymphoid cells, including small lymphocytic lymphoma/chronic lymphocytic leukemia and marginal zone B cell lymphoma (particularly the extranodal variants), lymphoplasmacytic lymphoma/immunocytoma. Over the past decade, these entities have been more clearly delineated, and the REAL classification has now recognized these as separate categories of B cell lymphoma.[9] In this section, we have adopted the more limited REAL classification definition of small lymphocytic lymphoma as the lymph node equivalent of classic B cell chronic lymphocytic leukemia. One group has recommended designating cases as chronic lymphocytic leukemia if patients have greater than 5,000/mm³ circulating lymphocytes and greater than 30 percent lymphocytes in the marrow but the distinction is arbitrary.[317]

Small lymphocytic lymphoma is almost always seen in adults over age 40, with a peak in the seventh decade.[318,319] Most patients present with generalized lymphadenopathy. Many of these patients have or will develop involvement of the peripheral blood at some point in their course. Regardless of the clinical symptoms, the patients are usually in high stage at diagnosis, with frequent bone marrow, liver, and spleen involvement. Similar to low grade follicular lymphoma, the clinical course is indolent, with occasional spontaneous regressions, slow progression, and numerous relapses occurring over time seemingly independent of treatment. In about 10 to 20 percent of patients, transformation to large cell lymphoma occurs (Richter's syndrome).[320] As discussed above, rare cases may transform to a lymphoma with a Hodgkin's-like histologic appearance or even true Hodgkin's disease.[240,321]

At low magnification, diffuse effacement of lymph node architecture is usually seen, although occasionally germinal centers are still present.[322] There is often infiltration of the perinodal adipose tissues. In many cases, particularly cases associated with a peripheral blood lymphocytosis, pale areas can be discerned, representing proliferation centers (also called pseudofollicles)[323] (Fig. 20-47). The mitotic rate is generally low, but higher numbers may be found in the proliferation cen-

Fig. 20-47. Small lymphocytic lymphoma. Pale areas are present, termed *proliferation centers.*

ters. At high magnification, the predominant cell type is a small lymphocyte with condensed chromatin (Fig. 20-48). Although the cells are usually round, a mild degree of irregularity may be present.[9] Nucleoli are generally small, but may be moderate in size in some cases. Cytoplasm is generally scant, although some cases may have cells with somewhat plasmacytoid features. In addition to these small cells, a population of larger cells is always present. These cells may be medium sized, termed *prolymphocytes* or *paraimmunoblasts* or large sized, termed *immunoblasts*. Both have round nuclei with a vesicular chromatin pattern and medium- to large-sized nucleoli. It is the presence of these cells in aggregations that give rise to the proliferation centers appreciated at low magnification. Large numbers of other cells, including eosinophils, neutrophils, and histiocytes are not found. Rarely, paraimmunoblasts can predominate, termed the *paraimmunoblastic variant of small lymphocytic lymphoma*; these cases have a worse prognosis than other cases of small lymphocytic lymphoma, but still better than cases of de novo diffuse large cell lymphoma.[324] However, when immunoblasts predominate and form sheets, the prognosis is significantly worse, indicating transformation to a higher grade lymphoma. Fine needle aspiration biopsy smears show a

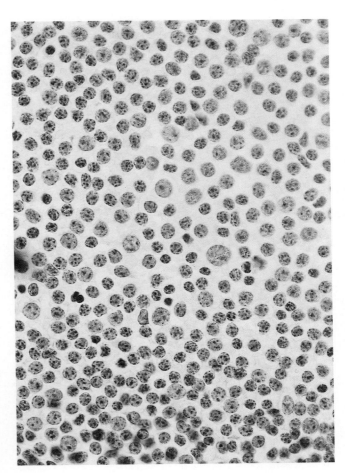

Fig. 20-49. Small lymphocytic lymphoma, fine needle aspiration. As in histologic sections, the cells consist mainly of small lymphocytes with round nuclear contours, with a minority population of larger cells with evident nucleoli.

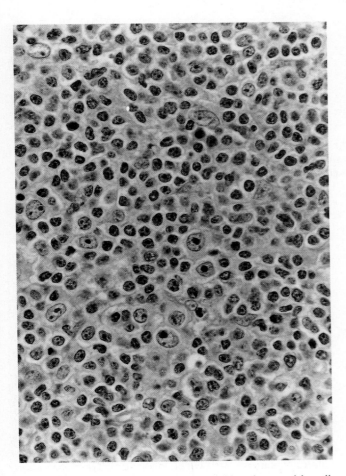

Fig. 20-48. Small lymphocytic lymphoma. Although most of the cells are small lymphocytes with round nuclear contours, a population of larger cells with prominent nucleoli are characteristic of this lymphoma.

preponderance of small lymphoid cells with round, regular nuclear membranes and clumped chromatin, with occasional admixed cells of similar size with an open chromatin pattern and a prominent nucleolus, representing prolymphocytes (Fig. 20-49).

By definition, small lymphocytic lymphoma is a neoplasm of B cell lineage, expressing CD20 in both paraffin and frozen sections (Table 20-14 and Fig. 20-50). Immunoglobulin expression with light chain restriction is seen in virtually all cases by flow cytometry/frozen section studies. Characteristically, both mu and delta heavy chains are present. Flow cytometry studies demonstrate that the level of immunoglobulin expression is typically low. When plasmacytoid features are seen histologically, immunoglobulin light chain restriction can also be demonstrated in paraffin sections. Aberrant expression of the paraffin T/myeloid marker CD43 is found in about 80 percent of cases (Fig. 20-50), and aberrant expression of the flow cytometry/frozen section T cell marker CD5 is found in about 80 to 90 percent of cases.[3,57,325] In contrast to most other low grade B cell lymphomas, CD23 is usually positive (in contrast to man-

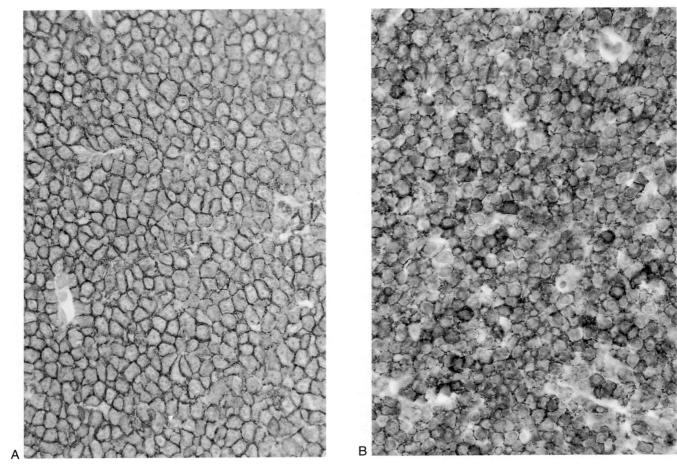

Fig. 20-50. Small lymphocytic lymphoma. (**A**) CD20 stain. Diffuse positivity is present, consistent with a B cell lymphoma. (**B**) CD43 stain. Diffuse positivity is also present, consistent with aberrant coexpression in a B cell lymphoma. The most strongly stained cells probably represent reactive T cells.

tle cell lymphoma), and CD10 is usually negative (in contrast to follicular lymphoma).[8,9,326] Monoclonal rearrangement of the immunoglobulin heavy and light chain genes is seen in virtually all cases. Trisomy of chromosome 12 is found in about one-third of cases.[327]

The differential diagnosis of small lymphocytic lymphoma is wide and includes reactive lymphoid proliferations, follicular lymphoma, and other low to intermediate grade diffuse small cell B cell lymphomas. Small lymphocytic lymphoma can usually be distinguished from reactive lymphoid proliferations by its monotonous cellular population. In difficult cases, paraffin section immunohistochemical stains are of great use, demonstrating a diffuse B cell infiltrate, most often with aberrant coexpression of CD43. In frozen sections, light chain restriction and aberrant CD5 expression is usually seen. If proliferation centers are prominent, one may mistake small lymphocytic lymphoma for follicular lymphoma. However, the proliferation centers are always more poorly defined than neoplastic follicles and lack small cleaved cells. They may contain follicular den-

dritic cells by immunohistochemistry, but the network is never as well developed as seen in follicular lymphoma. Small lymphocytic lymphoma may be very difficult to distinguish from other low to intermediate grade diffuse small cell B cell lymphomas. The presence of proliferation centers or CD23 positivity would favor small lymphocytic lymphoma over the other neoplasms. The presence of scattered larger cells also distinguishes small lymphocytic lymphoma from mantle cell lymphoma, whereas the identification of a t(11;14) would favor mantle cell lymphoma. The cells of marginal zone B cell lymphoma generally have more abundant cytoplasm than small lymphocytic lymphoma, and commonly have extranodal sites of involvement. Although small lymphocytic lymphoma may show somewhat plasmacytoid features, the presence of marked plasmacytic differentiation with Dutcher bodies and Russell bodies is more consistent with lymphoplasmacytic lymphoma. Clinically, patients with lymphoplasmacytic lymphoma often have large M protein spikes or even symptoms of Waldenström's macroglobulinemia.

Marginal Zone B Cell Lymphoma (Monocytoid B Cell Lymphoma/Lymphoma of Mucosal-Associated Lymphoma Tissues)

The normal marginal zone is the area just peripheral to the mantle zone of a secondary follicle. It is best seen in the spleen, and not easy to appreciate in normal lymph nodes outside of the abdominal region. Marginal zone B cell lymphoma is a low grade lymphoma theoretically showing differentiation similar to normal marginal zone B cells, cells that may differentiate into either monocytoid B cells or plasma cells. It encompasses the entity of monocytoid B cell lymphoma of the lymph node (nodal marginal zone B cell lymphoma) as well as extranodal marginal zone B cell lymphoma.[328–330] Extranodal marginal zone B cell lymphoma is also known as lymphoma of mucosa-associated lymphoid tissues (MALToma),[328,329,331] a term that may not be the most appropriate, because this lymphoma may occur in extranodal sites that are not usually thought of as mucosal associated. Many hematopathologists think that splenic marginal zone lymphoma, with or without villous lymphocytes, may represent a variant of marginal zone B cell lymphoma (see later section on splenic lymphomas).[9] In the Working Formulation, all variants of marginal zone B cell lymphoma were probably classified as low grade, small lymphocytic, with or without plasmacytoid differentiation.[276]

Nodal marginal zone B cell lymphoma is most often a disease of the elderly, with a median age of about 60; the male/female ratio is about 1:2.[332,333] Patients usually present with isolated or generalized lymphadenopathy. Bone marrow involvement occurs in 40 percent, splenomegaly in 20 percent, hepatomegaly in 15 percent, and involvement of the peripheral blood occurs in 5 percent. The presence of bone marrow or peripheral blood involvement adversely affects prognosis.[334] Nodal marginal zone B cell lymphoma is an indolent lymphoma, but transformation to large cell lymphoma occurs in about 10 percent and is another poor prognostic sign.[333] MALTomas typically occur in patients with a long history of autoimmune disease or antigenic stimulation, such as Sjögren's syndrome, Hashimoto's thyroiditis, or *Helicobacter* gastritis.[328,335,336] Many different extranodal organs may be affected, particularly the gastrointestinal tract, salivary glands, and conjunctiva.[328,329,335–337] Even organs without true mucosa, such as thyroid, soft tissue, and skin, may be affected. Patients with MALToma tend to have recurrences in other extranodal sites. If lymph nodes are involved, they tend to be regional nodes draining an area affected by MALToma.

At low magnification, involved lymph nodes may have partial or complete effacement of architecture.[128] Partial involvement preferentially affects the areas adjacent to the follicular mantle, the so-called marginal zone. In some cases, lymph nodes contain another lymphoma, usually follicular type.[333] At high magnification, the typical neoplastic monocytoid B cell has a small to medium-sized nucleus with round to slightly irregular nuclear outlines (Fig. 20-51). The chromatin is usually condensed and nucleoli are indistinct. A very characteristic feature is the presence of moderately abundant clear to pale cytoplasm. The cell membranes are often distinct and highlighted

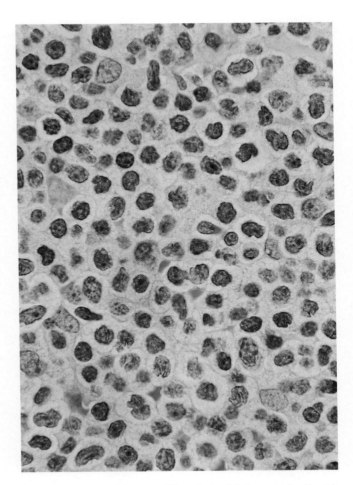

Fig. 20-51. Marginal zone B cell lymphoma. Medium-sized cells with small bland nuclei and abundant clear cytoplasm are present.

when two cells with clear or pale cytoplasm abut one another. Immunoblasts are often scattered among the monocytoid B cells. Lymphoid cells with plasmacytoid features, including Dutcher bodies, and mature plasma cells may also be present, either admixed with the other cells, or segregated apart, often next to the capsule or trabeculae. In some cases, one can see scattered neutrophils, similar to what may be seen in reactive monocytoid proliferations.

All marginal zone B cell lymphomas are of B lineage, and almost all cases express surface immunoglobulin (Table 20-14). About one-half of cases also express cytoplasmic immunoglobulin detectable in paraffin sections, particularly cases with plasmacytoid differentiation.[338] About one-half of cases show aberrant coexpression of CD43, a helpful feature also demonstrable in paraffin sections. CD5, CD10, and CD23 are usually negative. Monoclonal immunoglobulin heavy and light chain gene rearrangements are usually detectable, but *bcl-1* and *bcl-2* genes are germline. Trisomy 3 has been detected in a majority of cases of both nodal and extranodal cases, and numeric abnormalities of chromosomes 12 and 18 have also been found.[339,340]

The differential diagnosis of marginal zone B cell lymphoma includes the other low to intermediate grade B cell lymphomas. The cells of marginal zone B cell lymphoma generally have more abundant pale cytoplasm than the cells of small lymphocytic lymphoma, and proliferation centers are not seen. Coexpression of CD5 is usually seen in small lymphocytic lymphoma, but is present in only 10 percent of cases of marginal zone B cell lymphoma.[341] Marginal zone B cell lymphoma may be difficult to distinguish from lymphoplasmacytic lymphoma, because both may have areas with marked plasmacytoid differentiation, including Dutcher bodies. The presence of cells with more abundant pale cytoplasm would exclude lymphoplasmacytic lymphoma. Mantle cell lymphoma contains a more homogeneous population of cells and lacks large transformed cells, and the cells have a greater degree of nuclear irregularities. Coexpression of CD5 is usually seen, distinct from marginal zone B cell lymphoma.[341] Occasionally, marginal zone B cell lymphoma is difficult to distinguish from follicular lymphoma because the cells of marginal zone B cell lymphoma may colonize reactive germinal centers. Attention should be given to the cytologic features of cells, both within and outside the germinal centers. Truly small cleaved cells are absent within the germinal centers, whereas typical marginal zone B cells are found both within and outside the germinal centers. One must keep in mind, however, that true follicular lymphoma may also be found composite with marginal zone B cell lymphoma.[333] Marginal zone B cell lymphoma may be very difficult to histologically distinguish from lymph node involvement by hairy cell leukemia. However, the clinical circumstances are very different, as lymph node involvement by hairy cell leukemia never occurs without marked splenomegaly and obvious changes in the blood or bone marrow.

Lymphoplasmacytic Lymphoma

Lymphoplasmacytic lymphoma is a low grade lymphoma of small lymphocytes, plasma cells, and transitional forms between the two. It is called lymphoplasmacytoid lymphoma in the REAL classification, small lymphocytic with plasmacytoid differentiation in the Working Formulation, and lymphoplasmacytic immunocytoma in the Updated Kiel classification.[9,276,277] It is an uncommon lymphoma, comprising about 2 to 3 percent of non-Hodgkin's lymphomas in the United States. It is a disease of the elderly. Some patients present with symptoms of Waldenström's macroglobulinemia, with high amounts of a monoclonal serum paraprotein of IgM type, often with symptoms of hyperviscosity, whereas others present with symptoms resembling small lymphocytic lymphoma, with generalized lymphadenopathy with or without splenomegaly.[318] The clinical course is generally indolent, but transformation to large cell lymphoma, usually an immunoblastic lymphoma with plasmacytoid features, may occur in 5 to 10 percent of cases, and indicates a poor prognosis.

Histologically, there is diffuse architectural effacement. Proliferation centers are not present, but in occasional cases the germinal centers are still present. At high magnification, there is a mixed population of small lymphocytes, plasmacytoid lymphocytes, and plasma cells (Fig. 20-52). Scattered plasmacytoid

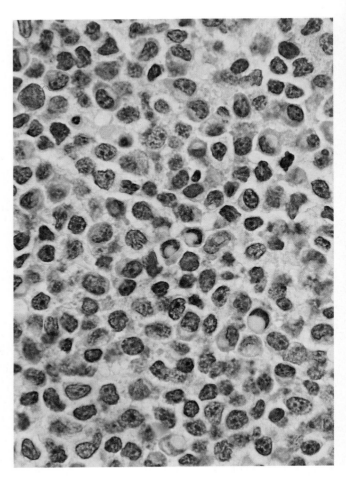

Fig. 20-52. Lymphoplasmacytic lymphoma. There is a range of lymphoplasmacytic differentiation. Note the numerous Dutcher bodies in this field.

immunoblasts are also often found. In occasional cases, numerous plasmacytoid immunoblasts may be present (polymorphous immunocytoma); these cases may be classified as diffuse mixed small and large cell with plasmacytoid differentiation in the Working Formulation, since they may be more aggressive. Dutcher bodies are usually frequently and easily identified, and Russell bodies may also be present. Scattered epithelioid histiocytes may be present, and occasionally marked infiltration may be seen, masking the lymphoma or simulating T cell lymphoma.[342] Mast cells may also be numerous.

The immunophenotypic hallmark of this lymphoma is the uniform presence of monotypic cytoplasmic and surface immunoglobulin of IgM type, usually easily demonstrated in paraffin sections (Table 20-14). As expected, these neoplasms usually express B lineage markers, and often show aberrant coexpression of CD43 in paraffin sections. The neoplastic cells usually do not stain for CD5, CD10, or CD23 in frozen sections or flow cytometric studies, but exceptions occur. Monoclonal gene rearrangement of the immunoglobulin heavy and light chain genes are detected in virtually all cases. A subset of cases may have a t(9;14) or a del(7)(32).[343,344]

The differential diagnosis of lymphoplasmacytic lymphoma includes reactive lymphoplasmacytic proliferations, other low to intermediate grade B cell lymphomas, Hodgkin's disease, and T cell lymphoma. The presence of more than rare numbers of Dutcher bodies would favor lymphoplasmacytic lymphoma over a reactive lymphoplasmacytic proliferation, but the distinction is perhaps most reliably accomplished by paraffin section staining for cytoplasmic immunoglobulin: polytypic in reactive proliferations and monotypic in lymphoplasmacytic lymphoma. All other low to intermediate grade B cell lymphomas may have lymphoplasmacytic differentiation. The diagnosis of lymphoplasmacytic differentiation is almost a diagnosis of exclusion—the lymphoma must lack evidence of other types of lymphomas. The presence of proliferation centers indicates a diagnosis of small lymphocytic lymphoma rather than lymphoplasmacytic lymphoma, despite the presence of lymphoplasmacytic features. Similarly, the presence of areas of neoplastic monocytoid B cells indicates a diagnosis of marginal zone B cell lymphoma. The presence of a homogeneous population of lymphoplasmacytoid cells with irregular nuclei favors mantle cell lymphoma, a diagnosis that may be supported by immunophenotypic studies demonstrating CD5 positivity. Even follicular lymphoma may rarely show lymphoplasmacytic features with numerous Dutcher bodies. Hodgkin's disease and peripheral T cell lymphoma may have scattered plasma cells and epithelioid histiocytes, which can simulate lymphoplasmacytic lymphoma. However, the plasma cells are polyclonal, and both neoplasms feature neoplastic elements (Reed-Sternberg cells in Hodgkin's disease and a spectrum of atypical lymphoid cells in peripheral T cell lymphoma) not present in lymphoplasmacytic lymphoma.

Mantle Cell Lymphoma

Mantle cell lymphoma is a lymphoma composed of neoplastic cells showing differentiation resembling mantle B cells.[61] It has many synonyms in the literature, including diffuse predominantly small cleaved cell (Working Formulation), centrocytic (Updated Kiel Classification), and intermediately differentiated lymphocytic lymphoma (modified Rappaport classification).[277,345] Most hematopathologists consider it to be an intermediate grade lymphoma because of its relatively poor overall survival. However, its clinical features are more similar to the low grade lymphomas in that there is no plateau in survival (patients are incurable) and relapses occur independently of time.[320,346,347]

Mantle cell lymphoma is relatively common, comprising approximately 10 percent of lymphomas in the United States. It occurs most commonly in elderly adults, and is rare in children. The male/female ratio is about 2:1. Patients frequently present in stage IV with generalized lymphadenopathy. Commonly involved sites include spleen, Waldeyer's ring, bone marrow, and peripheral blood. One interesting presentation is as multiple polypoid masses in the intestine (lymphomatous polyposis).[348] Transformation to large cell lymphoma is rare, if it occurs at all, but transformation to a "blastic" variant is not uncommon, and portends a poor prognosis.[8,346]

Architecturally, three patterns may be seen. Most often,

there is diffuse effacement of architecture. Occasionally, the neoplastic infiltrate replaces the mantle zone of reactive follicles, leaving naked germinal centers surrounded by thickened cuffs (Fig. 20-53); this mantle zone pattern may be a focal finding or may be present throughout the biopsy.[349] In a subset of cases, the germinal centers may also become replaced by the neoplastic infiltrate, leaving large nodules of mantle cell lymphoma. Cytologically, there is usually a highly monomorphic population of small- to medium-sized lymphocytes with condensed chromatin, inconspicuous nucleoli, and irregular nuclear outlines (Fig. 20-54). The nuclear irregularities are often marked, with abrupt deep indentations. In some cases, particularly those with suboptimal fixation, this may not be easily appreciated. Sometimes a cytoplasmic stain such as bcl-2 antibody may be helpful in demonstrating the irregular nuclear outlines to better advantage. It is important to stress that the neoplastic population is highly homogenous in almost all cases. In some cases, scattered large cells can be seen, usually present in small clusters; these cells may represent residual germinal center cells from follicles that have been completely overrun by tumor. In

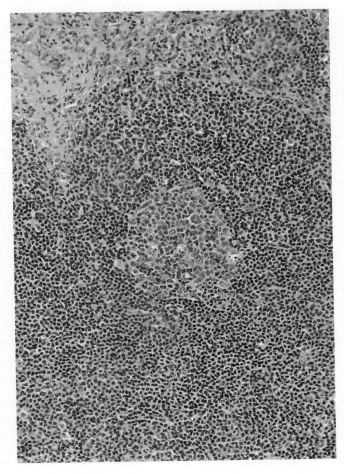

Fig. 20-53. Mantle cell lymphoma. A mantle zone architecture is present, with expanded mantle zones, around a small reactive germinal center.

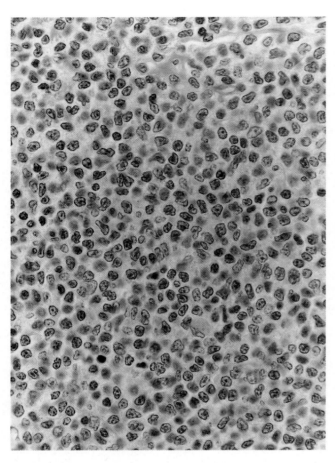

Fig. 20-54. Mantle cell lymphoma. A homogeneous population of small lymphoid cells with irregular nuclear contours is seen.

addition, scattered epithelioid histiocytes may be present, and can be helpful in suggesting the diagnosis. Fine needle aspiration biopsy smears of mantle cell lymphoma show small lymphoid cells with round and irregular nuclear contours. The chromatin pattern is usually less clumped or coarse than that seen in small lymphocytic or small cleaved cell lymphoma.[350]

Several variants of mantle cell lymphoma have been described. In the most common, the blastic (or lymphoblastoid) variant, some or most cells may have very fine chromatin, simulating lymphoblastic lymphoma.[346] These cases have a very high mitotic rate, and have a worse prognosis. In the centroblastic variant, the neoplastic cells are larger than usual and have more dispersed chromatin than ordinarily seen.[277,351] In the pleomorphic or anaplastic variant, the neoplastic cells are focally larger than usual, more hyperchromatic, and have prominent nuclear clefts.[277,351,352]

Mantle cell lymphoma is a B lineage lymphoma expressing monotypic surface immunoglobulin (Table 20-14). Interestingly, there is a slight predilection for lambda as opposed to kappa light chain restriction. Aberrant coexpression of the paraffin section marker CD43 is seen in about 60 percent of cases and aberrant coexpression of the frozen section marker

CD5 is seen in about 80 percent of cases. CD10 and CD23 are usually negative, but occasionally may be positive. There are paraffin section antibodies to cyclin D1 that stains the nuclei of the neoplastic cells of mantle cell lymphoma (see below).[353] Monoclonal rearrangements of the immunoglobulin heavy and light chain genes are present in virtually all cases. One-half to two-thirds of cases possess a t(11;14), involving juxtaposition of the *bcl-1* locus on the long arm of chromosome 11 with an immunoglobulin heavy chain gene enhancer sequence on chromosome 14.[354-359] The translocation results in deregulation and overexpression of the *PRAD1/cyclin D1* gene. This translocation can be detected by classic cytogenetics and Southern blotting, and the majority of the translocations can be detected by PCR. Overexpression of this gene can be detected in virtually all cases of mantle cell lymphoma by Northern blot analysis.[360]

The differential diagnosis of mantle cell lymphoma includes other diffuse low to intermediate grade B cell lymphomas. Small lymphocytic lymphoma may be very difficult to distinguish from mantle cell lymphoma, as the cells of the former may have somewhat irregular nuclear outlines, while the nuclei of the cells of the latter may appear round and regular. However, small lymphocytic lymphoma usually has proliferation centers at low magnification, and is composed of a mixture of cell types at high magnification, including scattered prolymphocytes and immunoblasts, whereas mantle cell lymphoma never has proliferation centers, and large cells with vesicular chromatin are not part of the neoplastic process (although occasionally residual non-neoplastic large cells may be present). Immunophenotypically, the cells of small lymphocytic lymphoma and mantle cell lymphoma may be quite similar with coexpression of both CD43 and CD5, but evidence of cyclin D1 overexpression or the t(11;14) would greatly favor mantle cell lymphoma. The homogeneous population of cells in mantle cell lymphoma also distinguishes it from the mixture of cells generally present in lymphoplasmacytic lymphoma and marginal zone B cell lymphoma. In addition, CD5 expression or evidence of cyclin D1 protein overexpression or the t(11;14) would strongly favor mantle cell lymphoma.

When mantle cell lymphoma has a mantle zone or nodular pattern, there may be confusion with follicular lymphoma. In the mantle zone pattern, the germinal centers are reactive and not neoplastic, and have the architectural and cytologic characteristics of reactive germinal centers. In the nodular pattern, the nodules are generally somewhat larger than the follicles of follicular lymphoma (because they encompass both the region of the germinal center and the mantle zone). In addition, the follicles of follicular lymphoma virtually always include at least some large cells, whereas the cells of mantle cell lymphoma are usually more homogeneous, without large cells.

The blastic variant of mantle cell lymphoma may be very difficult to distinguish from the cells of lymphoblastic lymphoma. A history of mantle cell lymphoma or the presence of areas of typical mantle cell lymphoma within the same specimen would favor mantle cell lymphoma. In addition, the cells of mantle cell lymphoma are terminal deoxynucleotidyl transferase (TdT) negative, whereas TDT is almost always positive in lymphoblastic malignant tumors.

Diffuse Mixed, Diffuse Large Cell, and Large Cell Immunoblastic Lymphomas of B Lineage

Diffuse mixed small and large, diffuse large cell, and large cell immunoblastic lymphomas of B cell lineage are diffuse aggressive lymphomas with a significant component of large lymphoid cells. They are included in three corresponding categories in the Working Formulation, the first two of intermediate grade and the third of high grade.[276] In the REAL classification, all three are combined into the entity of diffuse large B cell lymphoma.[9] These lymphomas correspond to centroblastic and B immunoblastic in the Updated Kiel classification.[277]

These lymphomas comprise about one-third of all non-Hodgkin's lymphomas, and occur in all age groups, with a median age at presentation of 55 years.[276] The male/female ratio is about 1.2:1. Most patients present with a single mass, either an enlarged lymph node (two-thirds of cases) or at an extranodal site (one-third of cases). Some patients have a history of a previous low grade lymphoma of B or T cell type. Follicular lymphoma, small lymphocytic lymphoma, marginal zone B cell lymphoma, lymphoplasmacytoid lymphoma, and mycosis fungoides all have a propensity for transformation to large cell lymphoma. Some patients have a history of immunodeficiency, either congenital, iatrogenic (including post-transplantation), or HIV-associated. There are no clear differences in survival between diffuse mixed, diffuse large cell, and large cell immunoblastic lymphomas of B lineage.[276,361] The International Prognostic Index for Aggressive Lymphomas was designed for large cell lymphoma, and works well to stratify patients into several prognostic groups.[285] These lymphomas are generally treated with multidrug chemotherapy, with response rates above 80 percent, and survival rates of about 60 percent.[362,363] Relapses generally occur early, with a plateau in survival seen after a few years. Large cell lymphoma arising in the mediastinum may have distinct clinicopathologic features, occurring in younger adults, with a male/female ratio of about 1:1.5.[364–368] Locally aggressive behavior may be problematic, but these neoplasms are responsive to aggressive therapies, and have overall survivals similar to other large cell lymphomas.[369]

By definition, these lymphomas have a diffuse architecture (Fig. 20-55), although focal follicular areas may be seen in a minority of cases as part of a residual follicular lymphoma component that has transformed. Similarly, in a subset of cases, areas of other low grade lymphomas may also be present, presumably also preceding the development of large cell lymphoma in these cases. Partial involvement of the lymph node may be seen, primarily involving the sinuses (sinusoidal large cell lymphoma) or the paracortical areas. A rare but distinctive variant is an exclusive or predominant intravascular component, found in soft tissue or extranodal sites (intravascular or angiotropic lymphoma)[370] (Fig. 20-56) Sclerosis occurs in up to one-half of cases, and may consist of broad bands surrounding large areas of tumor, a fine sclerosis enveloping single cells, or a compartmentalizing fibrosis enclosing clusters of cells, the latter particularly common in mediastinal large cell lymphoma[365] (Fig. 20-57).

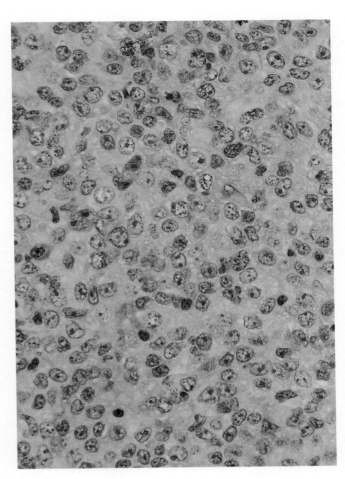

Fig. 20-55. Diffuse large cell B cell lymphoma. A mixture of large cleaved and large noncleaved cells is present.

All of these lymphomas have a significant component of large cells; in diffuse mixed small and large cell, the large cell component comprises between 25 percent and 50 to 75 percent of the elements, whereas in diffuse large cell and large cell immunoblastic lymphoma, greater than 50 to 75 percent of the cells are large (Fig. 20-55). The large cells have been divided into several types, including large cleaved and noncleaved cells (already described in the section on follicular lymphoma), multilobated large cells, and immunoblasts. Multilobated cells have greater than three lobes, and usually have a chromatin pattern intermediate between large cleaved and noncleaved cells. According to Lennert,[371] multilobated cells should be more than 10 to 20 percent for a case to be designated the multilobated variant. Immunoblasts have large nuclei with round contours, a vesicular chromatin pattern, and usually one prominent, centrally located nucleolus (Fig. 20-58). Cytoplasm is generally abundant and plasmacytoid or pale to clear. The large cells of mediastinal large cell lymphoma are often distinctive, with nuclei resembling large cleaved or noncleaved cells or multilobated cells and abundant clear to pale staining cytoplasm.[372] Despite the description of specific types of large cells, in many

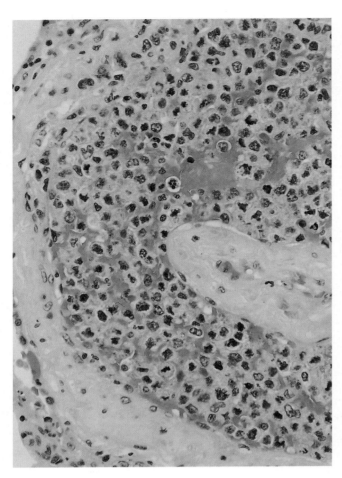

Fig. 20-56. Diffuse large cell B cell lymphoma, intravascular pattern. The small vessels of the lung are packed with large cell lymphoma cells in this case.

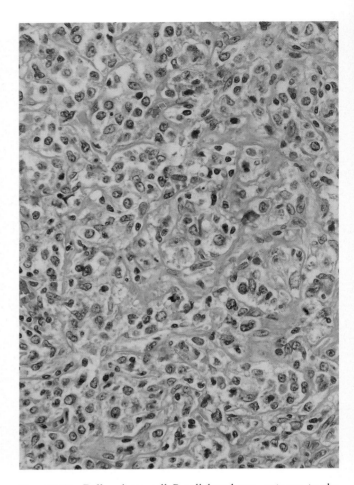

Fig. 20-57. Diffuse large cell B cell lymphoma, primary in the mediastinum. A compartmentalizing fibrosis is present, as is typical of large cell lymphomas primary in this site.

cases, the large cells defy categorization. Other admixed cells are always present, and are most frequent in diffuse mixed small and large cell lymphoma and least frequent in immunoblastic lymphoma. These cells may consist of small reactive T cells, atypical small B cells (not usually present, but when present, part of the neoplastic process), histiocytes, eosinophils, plasma cells, and, rarely, neutrophils.

Numerous histologic variants have been described. In T cell-rich B cell lymphoma, there is a predominant reactive component of small T cells, with only scattered large B cell lymphoma cells.[373–376] In histiocyte-rich B cell lymphoma, histiocytes predominate as the reactive component.[263] Rarely, large cell lymphomas may form a rosette-like structure (Fig. 20-59) or have myxoid or fibrillary stroma.[377,378] The neoplastic cells may be signet ring type (with either clear or eosinophilic inclusions); may have microvillous-like cytoplasmic projections; or, extremely rarely, may be spindled.[365,379,380]

Fine needle aspiration smears of diffuse large cell lymphoma usually show a dispersed population of cells with rounded or cleaved vesicular nuclei with irregularly thick and thin nuclear membranes, with one to multiple small nucleoli (Figs. 20-60).

Immunoblastic lymphoma usually has a single, more prominent nucleolus, and may have more abundant cytoplasm. The recognition of diffuse, mixed small and large cell lymphoma may be very difficult cytologically, and may require supportive immunohistochemical or molecular studies.

By definition, all of these large cell lymphomas are B lineage neoplasms, with virtually all positive for the B lineage marker CD20.[223] CD20 stains are particularly helpful in identifying the minority B cell component in T cell-rich B cell lymphoma (Fig. 20-61). Almost all large cell lymphomas are positive for CD45, with the exception of some cases of plasmacytoid immunoblastic lymphoma.[21] About two-thirds express surface immunoglobulin detectable in frozen sections or by flow cytometry,[381] and a subset express cytoplasmic immunoglobulin detectable in paraffin sections, particularly cases of plasmacytoid immunoblastic lymphoma. Aberrant coexpression of CD43 (paraffin sections) or CD5 (frozen sections) is found in about 20 percent and 5 percent of cases, respectively.[2,341] Virtually all cases have detectable immunoglobulin heavy or light chain gene rearrangement.[382] About 30 percent of cases have evidence of a t(14;18), particularly those cases with a history of follicular

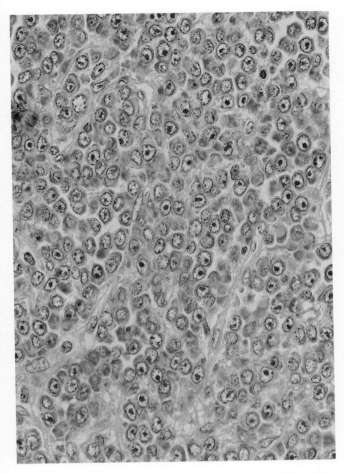

Fig. 20-58. Large cell immunoblastic lymphoma. The cells have large nuclei with a single centrally located prominent nucleolus. The cytoplasm is abundant and somewhat plasmacytoid.

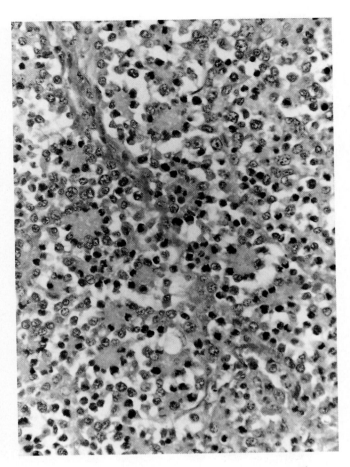

Fig. 20-59. Diffuse large cell B cell lymphoma, rosetting type. This rare variant of diffuse large cell B cell lymphoma closely simulates a small round blue cell tumor of childhood.

lymphoma.[309] *bcl-1* gene rearrangements are generally not found. Rearrangements involving *bcl-6 (laz-3)*, an oncogene on chromosome 3q27, is found in about 25 percent of cases, particularly cases presenting in extranodal sites.[383] The presence of a *bcl-6* rearrangement has been correlated with better overall survival as well as survival without disease progression. The prognostic significance of a t(14;18) in large cell lymphomas is still not clear, but its identification should suggest a search for history or coexistence of follicular lymphoma. A subset of cases may have evidence of *c-myc* rearrangements.

The differential diagnosis of the large cell lymphomas is very broad, and includes nonhematopoietic neoplasms, reactive lymphoid proliferations, other non-Hodgkin's lymphomas, classic Hodgkin's disease, and L&H lymphocyte predominance Hodgkin's disease (as discussed above). The differential diagnosis with true histiocytic tumor and extramedullary myeloid tumor will be discussed below. Reactive immunoblastic proliferations and Kikuchi's histiocytic necrotizing lymphadenitis are the reactive conditions most easily confused with diffuse large cell lymphoma. Clinical history is important, as a tonsillar lesion in a young adult with viral-like symptoms would raise

concern for infectious mononucleosis, whereas an enlarged cervical lymph node in an otherwise asymptomatic young female would raise concern for Kikuchi's disease. In reactive lymphoid proliferations, there is usually a greater maintenance of normal architecture, at least focally within the lymph node. In addition, reactive proliferations generally have a greater degree of cellular polymorphism, with immunohistochemical studies usually demonstrating a mixture of B and T cells (and usually a predominance of T cells). By contrast, B lineage large cell lymphomas generally have a more monomorphous appearance, with sheets of B lineage cells seen on immunohistochemical studies. Prominent exceptions include T cell-rich or histocyte-rich B cell lymphoma; however, these lymphomas generally lack a spectrum of B cell atypia, being composed of a mixture of small T cells (or histiocytes) and large B cells, without medium or small B cells.

Several different types of other non-Hodgkin's lymphomas can be confused with the large cell lymphomas, including the paraimmunoblastic variant of small lymphocytic lymphoma, and the centroblastic variant of mantle cell lymphoma. Features that differentiate large cell lymphoma from small non-

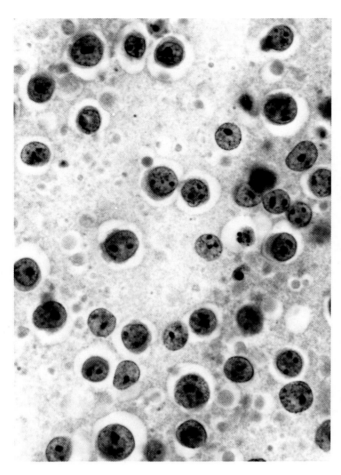

Fig. 20-60. Diffuse large cell B cell lymphoma, fine needle aspiration. A dispersed population of large atypical lymphoid cells is present.

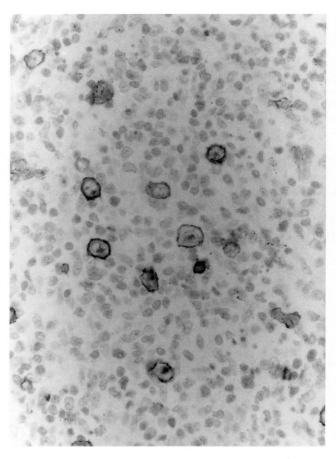

Fig. 20-61. T cell-rich B cell lymphoma, CD20 stain. This stain highlights the minority (but neoplastic) population of large B cells.

cleaved cell lymphoma and peripheral T cell lymphoma are discussed below. In the paraimmunoblastic variant of small lymphocytic lymphoma, there is often a prior history of small lymphocytic lymphoma/chronic lymphocytic leukemia. Morphologically, the cells are smaller, nucleoli generally less prominent, and the cytoplasm less abundant than the cells of large noncleaved or immunoblastic lymphoma. In the centroblastic variant of mantle cell lymphoma, the cells are also smaller than typical large cell lymphoma. However, the distinction may be morphologically very difficult to make and additional studies may be required. Immunohistochemical studies generally demonstrate CD5 positivity and molecular studies often demonstrate evidence of a t(11;14) in the centroblastic variant of mantle cell lymphoma.

Peripheral T Cell Lymphoma

Peripheral T cell lymphoma (post-thymic T cell lymphoma) is defined as a non-Hodgkin's lymphoma with a morphologic appearance and immunohistochemical profile consistent with mature T cells. It encompasses subsets of intermediate to high

grade lymphomas in the Working Formulation, including diffuse predominantly small cleaved, mixed small cleaved and large cell, and large cell lymphoma and large cell immunoblastic lymphoma.[276] In the REAL classification, it encompasses at least six categories of T cell lymphoma, with several provisional subtypes and several more cytologic categories.[9] In the Updated Kiel classification, peripheral T cell lymphoma encompasses at least eight categories of T cell lymphoma.[277] Several clinicopathologic entities are included within the broad definition of peripheral T cell lymphoma, including mycosis fungoides and adult T cell leukemia/lymphoma. Some hematopathologists include T lineage cases of anaplastic large cell lymphoma within the definition of peripheral T cell lymphoma, but this entity is discussed in a separate section in this chapter.

Peripheral T cell lymphoma is uncommon, accounting for about 10 percent of cases of diffuse non-Hodgkin's lymphoma. It occurs in all ages, but particularly the elderly, with a median age around 60.[384–386] The male/female ratio is about 1.5:1. Patients usually present with generalized lymphadenopathy, and often have a history of autoimmune disease. Approximately two-thirds of patients have stage III or IV disease, often with involvement of extranodal organs such as skin, spleen, and liver. "B" symptoms are common, and patients are often anemic. The clinical course is variable, with some patients following a rapid course to death, whereas some patients have indolent disease. Peripheral T cell lymphoma is usually treated similarly to B lineage large cell lymphoma with aggressive multidrug chemotherapy.[387] Although the issue is still highly controversial, it appears that patients with peripheral T cell lymphoma have a worse prognosis than equivalent patients with B cell lymphoma, particularly if treatment is suboptimal.[388]

Peripheral T cell lymphomas show focal or diffuse effacement of architecture. Focal involvement usually affects the paracortical areas, sparing the follicles (T-zone pattern). Vascularity is often markedly increased, with prominent high endothelial venules. Characteristically, the neoplastic population is composed of a spectrum of atypical cells with nuclei of varying shapes and sizes from small to large (Fig. 20-62). The small cells generally have highly irregular nuclei with condensed chromatin, whereas the large cells may have round or irregular nuclei, condensed or vesicular chromatin, and generally have prominent nucleoli. Cytoplasm may be scant or abundant, often pale or clear. Also characteristic is the presence of an exuberant host infiltrate, including small round lymphocytes, epithelioid and nonepithelioid histiocytes, eosinophils,

neutrophils, and plasma cells. Rarely, hemophagocytosis is seen in benign histiocytes, either within the neoplasm or at distant sites. In theory, the morphologic features of peripheral T cell lymphoma are distinctive, but the histologic differentiation between B and T cell lymphomas is extremely difficult in practice.[389] The fine needle aspiration biopsy diagnosis of peripheral T cell lymphoma may be extremely difficult, because a mixed population is usually seen. The identification of highly bizarre or anaplastic cells would favor a diagnosis of lymphoma. Immunohistochemical or molecular studies are helpful in confirming a diagnosis of lymphoma, and are essential for the recognition of T cell lineage.

Approximately 90 percent of peripheral T cell lymphomas express CD45.[21] By definition, these lymphomas express one or more definitive T cell antigens in the absence of B antigen expression. In paraffin sections, the T-associated antigens CD3, CD45RO, and CD43 are expressed in about 80 to 90 percent of cases (Fig. 20-63), whereas the B-associated antigen CD20 is always negative.[2,21] In frozen sections, peripheral T cell lymphomas often express an aberrant T cell phenotype with aberrant loss of one or more of the pan-T markers CD5, CD7, CD3, or CD2.[275,390] A helper (CD4+, CD8−) phenotype is usually

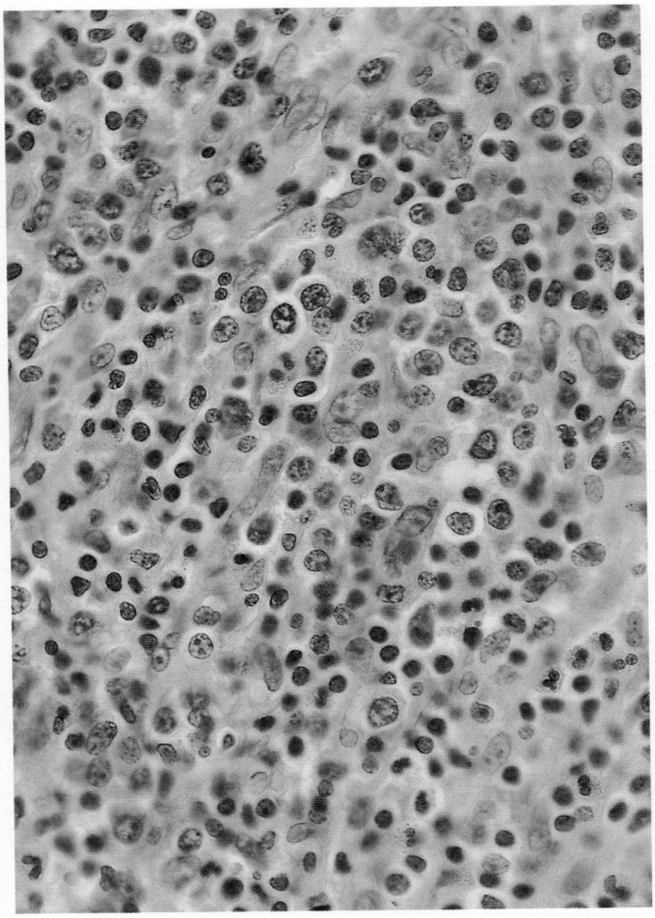

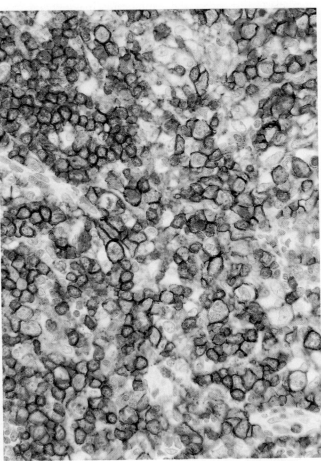

Fig. 20-62. Peripheral T cell lymphoma. A spectrum of lymphoid atypia is present in a mixed inflammatory background.

Fig. 20-63. Peripheral T cell lymphoma, CD45RO stain. The atypical lymphoid cells are labeled with this T lineage marker. The CD20 stain was negative.

seen but a suppressor/cytotoxic (CD4−, CD8+) or aberrant phenotype may also be present. A subset of T cell lymphomas expresses CD56, the neural cell adhesion molecule (N-CAM); these cases have a predilection for involvement of unusual extranodal sites.[391, 392]

About 80 to 90 percent of cases of peripheral T cell lymphoma have detectable beta-T cell receptor gene rearrangements. Approximately 10 to 15 percent lack detectable beta-T cell receptor gene rearrangements.[393] These are generally cases that have aberrant loss of multiple pan-T cell antigens and often expression of one or more markers of NK cell differentiation; thus their true lineage is in doubt.

The differential diagnosis of peripheral T cell lymphoma includes reactive paracortical proliferations, Hodgkin's disease (discussed in the section on Hodgkin's disease), and B cell lymphoma. The distinction of benign paracortical hyperplasia from peripheral T cell lymphoma may be extremely difficult, requiring immunohistochemical studies to demonstrate an aberrant T cell immunophenotype or molecular studies to demonstrate a monoclonal T cell population. Histologically, paracortical hyperplasia generally shows a mottled appearance at low magnification, because there is a mixed population of discrete cell types, including small lymphocytes, immunoblasts, histiocytes, and granulocytes. In peripheral T cell lymphoma, there is a usually a more continuous spectrum of atypia, from small to large lymphoid cells. Peripheral T cell lymphoma is more likely to show complete effacement of architecture, but an exclusive paracortical (T-zone) distribution may occur. However, the intervening follicles are usually atrophic in lymphoma, whereas they are usually highly hyperplastic in a reactive proliferation.

As mentioned above, the histologic distinction between B and T cell lymphoma is very difficult, even for experienced hematopathologists. A diffuse proliferation of atypical lymphoid cells, the presence of a spectrum of lymphoid atypia, the presence of more than occasional eosinophils, or a paracortical distribution should all raise the possibility of a T cell lymphoma. Nonetheless, any histologic suspicions should always be confirmed by immunohistochemical or molecular studies. The presence of CD3+ atypical cells is a good indication of a T cell lymphoma, but staining for CD45RO or CD43 alone should not be used as definitive evidence for a T cell lymphoma, because both may stain some B cell lymphomas. However, positivity for CD45RO or CD43 in the absence of staining for the reliable B lineage markers CD20 and CD79a is strong presumptive evidence for T cell lymphoma.

Subtypes of Peripheral T Cell Lymphoma

Mycosis fungoides is a peripheral T cell lymphoma of CD4+ helper T cells arising in skin or rarely, another epithelial site.[35] It is an indolent disease, characterized by a neoplastic proliferation of small cerebriform cells. Patients with mycosis fungoides often have lymph node enlargement due to dermatopathic lymphadenitis, but lymph node involvement by mycosis fungoides may also commonly occur.[394] Lymph node involvement begins as very subtle infiltrates of atypical cells among the dendritic cells and macrophages within the areas of dermatopathic

change. The diagnosis of mycosis fungoides can generally be established histologically only when aggregates of cerebriform cells of 15 or more cells are found in the paracortical areas or when architectural effacement is present (Fig. 20-64). Transformation to large cell lymphoma may occur, and confers a poor prognosis.[395,396] Molecular studies to detect beta-T cell gene rearrangements are usually a more sensitive indicator of involvement by mycosis fungoides than light microscopy or immunohistochemistry in this setting.[397]

Adult T cell leukemia/lymphoma is a specific clinicopathologic variant caused by the human T cell leukemia virus (HTLV)-1.[398] The virus is endemic in southwestern Japan,[399] but can occur in other areas.[400] Patients usually present with widespread disease, including generalized lymphadenopathy. The patients are often hypercalcemic and characteristic atypical lymphoid cells with cloverleaf nuclei are usually seen in the peripheral blood. Less commonly, lymphomatous, chronic, and smoldering forms may occur.[401] Involved lymph nodes show histologic features similar to that described for peripheral T cell lymphoma, although marked pleomorphism can be seen.[272] Molecular studies show clonal integration of HTLV-1 in the tumor cells.

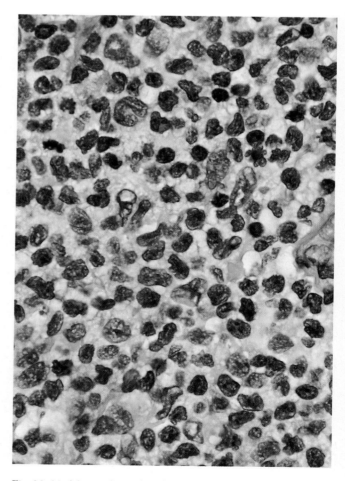

Fig. 20-64. Mycosis fungoides. Sheets of atypical small lymphoid cells are present in this case.

Lymphoepithelioid T cell lymphoma (Lennert's lymphoma) is not so much a specific clinicopathologic entity as it is a peripheral T cell lymphoma with distinctive histologic features. The characteristic finding is the presence of numerous epithelioid histiocytes throughout the lymph node, as single cells or small clusters, but not forming discrete granulomas[402] (Fig. 20-65). The neoplastic component may be overshadowed by the epithelioid histiocytes unless the biopsy is carefully examined. One should keep in mind that lymphoplasmacytic lymphoma may occasionally have extensive infiltrates of epithelioid histiocytes. The absence of well formed granulomas and necrosis makes granulomatous lymphadenitis an unlikely diagnosis.

Angioimmunoblastic lymphadenopathy (AILD)-like T cell lymphoma is a peripheral T cell lymphoma with clinical and histologic features similar to AILD.[189,403] As discussed in the section on AILD, some hematopathologists consider all cases of AILD to represent AILD-like lymphoma ab initio, whereas other hematopathologists still regard AILD as a possible polyclonal or preneoplastic T cell disorder. Lymphoma should be suspected when there are clusters and small sheets of atypical lymphoid cells (Fig. 20-66), particularly around vessels, and should be diagnosed when there are large sheets of atypical lymphoid cells,

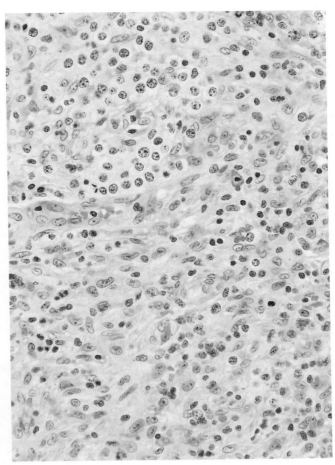

Fig. 20-66. Angioimmunoblastic lymphadenopathy-like peripheral T cell lymphoma. Although the overall features resemble angioimmunoblastic lymphadenopathy, there are small sheets of atypical cells with clear cytoplasm.

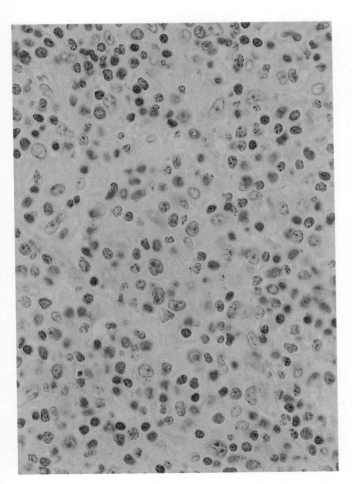

Fig. 20-65. Lymphoepithelioid T cell (Lennert's) lymphoma. The sheets of epithelioid histiocytes masked the tumor cell population.

immunohistochemical evidence of an aberrant T cell immunophenotype, or molecular evidence of a sizeable (>1 to 5 percent) monoclonal T cell population.[192]

Angiocentric T cell lymphoma is found in extranodal sites such as the upper respiratory tract, particularly the nose.[404–407] A subset of cases of lymphomatoid granulomatosis may also represent angiocentric T cell lymphoma. It is more common in Asian populations but occurs sporadically in the United States. There is a very strong association with EBV.[404–406] Histologically, there is an angiocentric and angiodestructive atypical infiltrate in the wall of blood vessels, usually leading to extensive necrosis of the surrounding tissues. Many of these cases lack multiple T cell antigens and beta-T cell receptor gene rearrangements, but express the NK-associated antigen CD56, raising a question as to whether they are NK rather than T cell lineage; however, they generally lack other markers of NK cell lineage.

Hepatosplenic T cell lymphoma is a rare lymphoma of gamma/delta T cells, as opposed to the usual alpha/beta T cells.[408] Patients present with hepatosplenomegaly, and histologic involvement of the splenic red pulp and the hepatic sinusoids is seen. The tumor cells exhibit an aberrant T cell phenotype and have detectable rearrangements of the delta- and gamma-T cell receptor gene, whereas the beta-T cell receptor gene is germline. The neoplasm is discussed further in the section on lymphomas in the spleen.

Intestinal T cell lymphoma (ulcerative jejunitis) is a rare lymphoma derived from the intestinal intraepithelial T cells.[409,410] It usually occurs in patients with a history of celiac sprue. Patients often present with an acute abdomen, and ulcers are often found in the jejunum. The base of the ulcer contains an infiltrate of atypical lymphoid cells, and atypical cells are often found in the adjacent nonulcerated mucosa. An aberrant T cell phenotype is usually present, along with expression of CD103, a marker of normal mucosal-associated T lymphocytes.[411]

Anaplastic Large Cell Lymphoma

Anaplastic large cell lymphoma is a neoplasm of anaplastic lymphoid cells that virtually always expresses the CD30+ antigen.[412,413] There is no true equivalent in the Working Formulation, but cases are best classified as high grade, immunoblastic, polymorphous type.[276] Both B cell and T cell types of large cell anaplastic lymphoma are recognized in the Updated Kiel classification,[277] but the REAL classification only recognizes T and null cell types.[9] Any lymphomas with morphologic features of anaplastic large cell lymphoma but of B lineage phenotype should be included within the category of diffuse large B cell lymphoma in that classification.

Anaplastic large cell lymphoma comprises less than 5 percent of all non-Hodgkin's lymphomas, but about 10 percent of the lymphomas in the pediatric age group.[414,415] There are three main presentations. Most often, there is a lymphomatous presentation, with involvement of lymph nodes or a variety of extranodal sites, including the gastrointestinal tract or soft tissue.[416] This presentation has a bimodal age distribution, with one peak in children, and the second in the fifth decade. The clinical course in these cases is aggressive, similar to other large cell non-Hodgkin's lymphomas, and with a similar response to multidrug chemotherapy. In the second type of presentation, which occurs primarily in adults, there are one to multiple skin papules and nodules without extracutaneous involvement, similar to lymphomatoid papulosis; in fact, there is probably a clinical, histologic, and biologic continuum between this type of anaplastic large cell lymphoma and lymphomatoid papulosis.[417–419] The disease is very indolent, does not require systemic therapy, and waxes and wanes over time, although systemic dissemination may occur eventually, heralding a more aggressive course. In the third type of presentation, patients with a history of another type of lymphoma, including both non-Hodgkin's lymphoma or Hodgkin's disease, transform to anaplastic large cell lymphoma; the prognosis in these cases is usually poor.[420]

Involved lymph nodes may show complete effacement of architecture, but partial involvement is more common. Characteristically, there is preferential infiltration of the sinuses (Fig. 20-67), although extension to the paracortical regions is very common. Often, there is capsular fibrosis, with focal extension

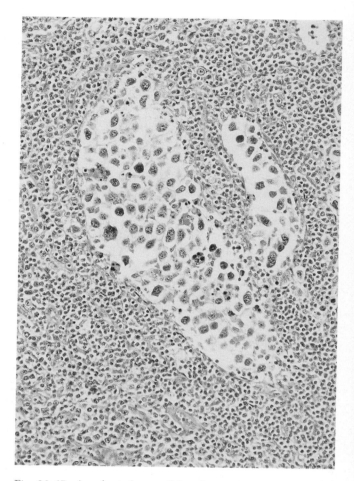

Fig. 20-67. Anaplastic large cell lymphoma. A striking sinusoidal pattern of infiltration is seen.

into the lymph node parenchyma. The mitotic rate is high, and a starry sky pattern may be present. Cytologically, two main variants have been recognized.[421,422] In the more common pleomorphic type, there are numerous highly anaplastic cells, often with multilobation or multinucleation (Fig. 20-68). Cells with doughnut-shaped nuclei and Reed-Sternberg-like cells can be identified. In the monomorphic type, the tumor cells appear monotonous. They generally have large round to oval nuclei, without multinucleation, and fairly abundant basophilic cytoplasm without a paranuclear hof. In some cases, features intermediate between the pleomorphic and monomorphic types are seen. Usually accompanying the neoplastic population are a mixed population of host reactive cells, including small lymphocytes, histiocytes, plasma cells, eosinophils, and neutrophils. Occasionally, histiocytes may be very abundant (lymphohistiocytic T cell lymphoma).[423]

Several other less common variants of anaplastic large cell lymphoma have been recognized. These include a small cell variant, in which the predominant cell is a small lymphoid cell with highly irregular nuclear outlines, with scattered anaplastic large cells present singly or in small groups.[424] The relationship to anaplastic large cell is inferred by the characteristic im-

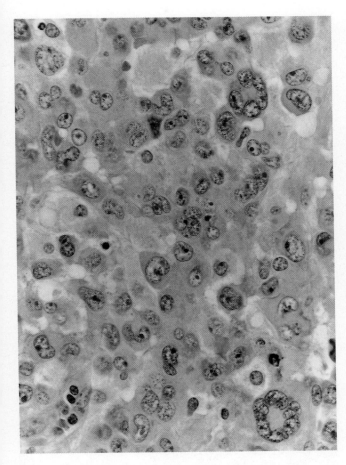

Fig. 20-68. Anaplastic large cell lymphoma. Large pleomorphic cells are seen, including two "doughnut" cells.

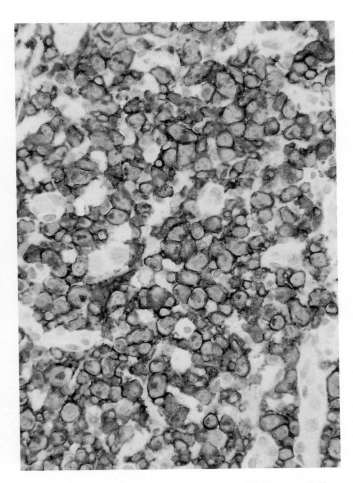

Fig. 20-69. Anaplastic large cell lymphoma, CD30 stain. Diffuse strong reactivity is seen on the tumor cell membranes.

munohistochemical profile (see below) as well as progression in some cases to typical anaplastic large cell lymphoma. Other variants include cases with a sarcomatoid pattern,[425] and a Hodgkin's-like variant, featuring Reed-Sternberg-like cells.[245] The Hodgkin's-like variant is particularly common in the mediastinum, and may actually represent an anaplastic variant of nodular sclerosing Hodgkin's disease.

The immunohistochemical hallmark of anaplastic large cell lymphoma is the almost universal expression of CD30[412,413] (Fig. 20-69). Typically, all or virtually all of the neoplastic cells are positive. This is in contrast to CD30 expression when it occurs in most other non-Hodgkin's lymphomas, in which the staining is usually focal. CD45 is positive in only two-thirds of cases, the lowest rate of positivity of any of the major categories of non-Hodgkin's lymphoma.[21] Most cases are of T lineage, expressing CD43, CD3, and CD45RO, and showing aberrant T cell phenotypes in frozen section studies.[412,413] A significant minority are of null cell lineage, although CD43 is still usually positive. If B lineage cases are accepted within the definition of anaplastic large cell lymphoma, about 20 percent are positive for B cell antigens. Epithelial membrane antigen is usually positive in systemic cases,[426] whereas the cutaneous lymphocyte

antigen HECA-452 is usually positive in the cutaneous cases.[418] Occasional cases may be CD15+,[427] and rare cases may be keratin positive.[428]

About three-fourths of cases have detectable monoclonal gene rearrangements of the beta-T cell receptor gene. If B lineage cases are accepted within the definition of anaplastic large cell lymphoma, those cases usually have detectable immunoglobulin gene rearrangements.[429,430] A significant minority of cases do not have detectable gene rearrangements of either the beta-T cell receptor gene or the immunoglobulin heavy or light chain genes. About one-half to two-thirds of cases of systemic anaplastic large cell lymphomas possess a t(2;5), involving the *alk* gene on chromosome 2p23 and the *npm* gene on chromosome 5q35.[431–434] The incidence of this translocation is higher in neoplasms from children than from adults, in systemic cases compared to cutaneous cases, and in T cell or null cell cases compared to B cell cases. The alk-npm gene product may be detected by paraffin section immunohistochemistry.[435]

The differential diagnosis of anaplastic large cell lymphoma includes metastatic carcinoma and malignant melanomas (covered in the section on metastatic neoplasms), classic Hodgkin's disease (covered in the section on Hodgkin's disease), other large cell lymphomas, and malignant histiocytosis. Anaplastic large cell lymphoma is distinguished from other large cell lymphomas by the combination of its characteristic anaplastic histologic appearance and diffuse positivity for CD30. Most non-Hodgkin's lymphomas usually show negative or focal staining for CD30, with only occasional cases exhibiting diffuse positivity. As discussed above, many hematopathologists exclude a diagnosis of anaplastic large cell lymphoma in any B lineage neoplasm. The specificity of t(2;5) for anaplastic large cell lymphoma is currently being studied; preliminary data suggest that it is characteristic of anaplastic large cell lymphoma, but may occasionally be identified in other large cell lymphomas.

Malignant histiocytosis was described as a sinusoidal carcinoma of histiocytic derivation, but many of the cases previously diagnosed as malignant histiocytosis have been found to be anaplastic large cell lymphoma when studied using modern techniques.[436] Complete immunophenotyping should be performed in any case suspected to be of histiocytic derivation to rule out the possibility of an anaplastic large cell lymphoma.

Lymphoblastic Lymphoma

Lymphoblastic lymphoma is a neoplasm of cells frozen at the level of immature lymphoid cells, either T lineage thymocytes or immature B lineage bone marrow lymphoid cells. It is a category of high grade lymphoma in the Working Formulation.[276] In the Updated Kiel classification, it is separated into B and T cell types.[277] In the REAL classification, it is also separated into B and T cell types and called precursor lymphoblastic lymphoma/leukemia.[9] This was done to indicate that the cells of lymphoblastic lymphoma are equivalent to the neoplastic cells of acute lymphoblastic leukemia. When greater than 10 percent circulating blasts are found in the peripheral blood or greater than 25 percent bone marrow involvement is seen, many clinicians prefer using the designation acute lymphoblastic leukemia, but the cutoff between the two is arbitrary.[437,438]

Lymphoblastic lymphoma has a median age of incidence of 17 years and a male/female ratio of 2:1.[276,437–440] Accounting for about one-third of non-Hodgkin's lymphomas in childhood, it nonetheless occurs in all age groups. Patients usually present with a symptomatic mediastinal mass, often associated with pleural or pericardial effusions, or supradiaphragmatic lymphadenopathy. Mediastinal presentation is a strong predictor for a T cell phenotype, although rare cases of B lineage mediastinal lymphoblastic lymphoma have been reported. Skin involvement is relatively common in cases of B lineage.[441] Lymphoblastic lymphoma shows rapid progression, often with involvement of the peripheral blood and bone marrow, central nervous system, and gonads. It responds well to multidrug chemotherapeutic regimens similar or identical to those given for acute lymphoblastic leukemia. Adverse prognostic factors include high stage, involvement of the central nervous system, and a high serum lactate dehydrogenase.[437]

Histologically, lymphoblastic lymphoma shows diffuse effacement of normal nodal architecture. In fact, lymphoblastic lymphoma often effaces the entire lymph node structure, with capsular destruction and extensive infiltration of the adjacent

soft tissues. In the soft tissues and in the adventitia of blood vessels, single file cell infiltration is often seen. The mitotic rate is generally high and a starry sky pattern may be focally present. It is a monomorphous lymphoma, composed of a uniform population of small to medium-sized cells (Fig. 20-70). These cells have a very fine chromatin pattern with inconspicuous nucleoli and only a small amount of cytoplasm. In many cases, the nuclear outlines are highly irregular and convoluted (convoluted variant), whereas in other cases the nuclear outlines appear rounded or oval (nonconvoluted variant). In about 10 percent of cases, the cells may be slightly larger than usual, and may possess larger nuclei that may contain one or two small but distinct nucleoli.[442] There are usually very few host cells, although occasional cases may have scattered plasma cells or eosinophils. Fine needle aspiration smears of lymphoblastic lymphoma show a monomorphous population of medium-sized lymphoid cells with a very fine chromatin pattern and very inconspicuous nucleoli (Fig. 20-71). The cytologic appearance is identical to acute lymphoblastic leukemia in bone marrow aspirate or peripheral blood smears.

Virtually all lymphoblastic lymphomas express Tdt, a marker that can be applied in frozen and paraffin sections.[443,444] CD45

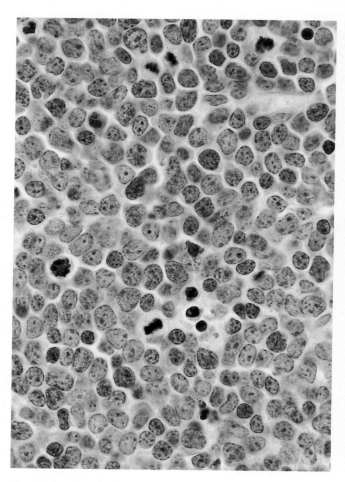

Fig. 20-70. Lymphoblastic lymphoma. A diffuse proliferation of medium-sized cells with a fine chromatin pattern is present. Note the high mitotic rate.

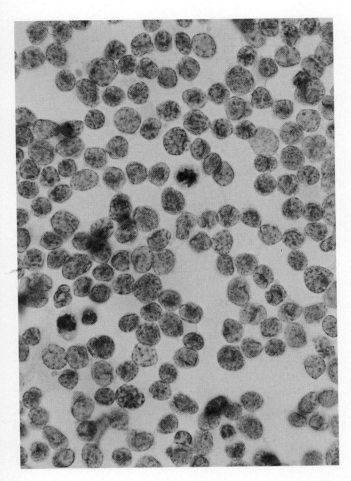

Fig. 20-71. Lymphoblastic lymphoma, fine needle aspiration. The nuclei have a very fine chromatin pattern without discernible nucleoli. Several mitotic figures are present in this field.

is positive in about 80 percent of cases, a rate of positivity lower than all non-Hodgkin's lymphoma except anaplastic large cell lymphoma.[21] About 85 percent of lymphoblastic lymphomas are T lineage neoplasms, almost always expressing CD43 and cytoplasmic or surface CD3.[445,446] These cases express phenotypes consistent with the different stages of intrathymic T cell maturation[447] (Table 20-15). About 20 percent of these cases may also show strong positivity for the NK markers CD16 and CD57; in one study, these latter cases occurred more often in

females and had a more aggressive course.[448,449] About 15 percent of cases of lymphoblastic lymphoma are of B lineage.[446,450] Due to their immaturity, only about one-half of cases express CD20, but all B lineage cases will stain for the B lineage markers CD19 (frozen) or CD79a (paraffin) and the CALLA antigen CD10.[451,452] Surface immunoglobulin is only rarely positive,[453] and cytoplasmic immunoglobulin may be positive (pre-B) or negative (pre-pre-B). About 90 percent of T lineage lymphoblastic lymphomas have detectable monoclonal beta-T cell receptor gene rearrangements; in addition, immunoglobulin heavy chain gene rearrangements may be present in about 25 percent of cases.[454,455] Virtually all B lineage lymphoblastic lymphomas have detectable monoclonal immunoglobulin heavy chain gene rearrangements, but light chain gene rearrangements are detectable in only about 40 percent of cases. Similar to the presence of immunoglobulin heavy chain gene rearrangements in T lineage lymphoblastic lymphoma, beta-T cell receptor gene rearrangements may be present in 25 percent of cases of B lineage lymphoblastic lymphoma.[454,456] Other molecular findings in lymphoblastic neoplasms are discussed in Chapter 21.

The differential diagnosis of lymphoblastic lymphoma includes other types of non-Hodgkin's lymphoma, extramedullary myeloid tumor, thymoma, and small cell undifferentiated carcinoma. TdT is an extremely useful marker in the differential diagnosis of lymphoblastic lymphoma vs. other non-Hodgkin's lymphomas, as it is positive in virtually all cases of lymphoblastic lymphoma, but negative in all other types of non-Hodgkin's lymphoma.[443] Morphologically, lymphoblastic lymphoma can be easily confused with small noncleaved cell lymphoma and the blastic variant of mantle cell lymphoma. The cells of lymphoblastic lymphoma have a finer chromatin pattern than those of small noncleaved cell lymphoma, whereas the latter have more distinct nucleoli and a greater amount of cytoplasm that tends to square off on adjacent cells. The blastic variant of mantle cell lymphoma may be morphologically indistinguishable from lymphoblastic lymphoma. Areas of more typical mantle cell lymphoma or a past history of that lymphoma can be helpful, but immunohistochemical studies may be necessary. Besides TdT, lineage determination may be of use, because most cases of lymphoblastic lymphoma are of T lineage.

Lymphoblastic lymphoma may also be very difficult to distinguish from an extramedullary myeloid tumor, because both can show single file pattern of infiltration in fibrous tissue, and both feature a fine chromatin pattern. The presence of eosinophils or cells with more than scant cytoplasm should suggest the diagnosis of extramedullary myeloid tumor. Occasional

Table 20-15. Stages of T Cell Maturation

Prethymic	CD7+	CD2−	cCD3±						
Stage I	CD7+	CD2+	cCD3+	CD1−	CD4−	CD8+			
Stage II	CD7+	CD2+	cCD3+	CD1+	CD4−	CD8−	or	CD4+	CD8+
Stage III	CD7+	CD2+	sCD3+	CD1−	CD4+	CD8−	or	CD4−	CD8+

Abbreviations: c, cytoplasmic; s, surface.

cases of extramedullary myeloid tumor may be TdT positive. Myeloperoxidase is a relatively sensitive marker for extramedullary myeloid tumor, but rare cases may be negative. Bone marrow examination should be recommended in any questionable cases. The proliferating thymocytes of thymoma may have close morphologic and immunohistochemical similarities to the cells of lymphoblastic lymphoma.[457] Attention should be given to the presence of the epithelial cells of thymoma, which are scattered larger cells with vesicular chromatin. Confirmation can be obtained using keratin stains, which demonstrate a network of epithelial cells throughout thymoma, keeping in mind that occasional residual thymic epithelial cells can be seen in mediastinal masses of lymphoblastic lymphoma. The confusion between the thymocytes of thymoma and the cells of lymphoblastic lymphoma can be greatest when examining flow cytometric data, which may demonstrate an immature thymic phenotype in thymoma and not detect the epithelial population. Finally, small cell undifferentiated carcinoma can be confused with lymphoblastic lymphoma, particularly in suboptimal preparations. Immunohistochemical studies including keratin should be performed in any questionable case.

Small Noncleaved Cell Lymphoma

Small noncleaved cell lymphoma is a high grade lymphoma in the Working Formulation, consisting of Burkitt's and non-Burkitt's subtypes.[276] In the REAL classification, Burkitt's lymphoma is recognized as an entity, whereas high grade B cell lymphoma, Burkitt-like is recognized as a provisional entity.[9] In the Updated Kiel classification, only Burkitt's lymphoma is recognized.[277] The neoplastic cells of small noncleaved lymphoma are biologically equivalent to the French-American British (FAB)-L3 cells of acute lymphoblastic leukemia.

There are two clinical forms of small noncleaved cell lymphoma: endemic and sporadic. The endemic form, which occurs in equatorial Africa, affects children (particularly males) who present with jaw tumors or other extranodal masses.[458] Sporadic small noncleaved cell lymphoma has peaks of incidence in both childhood and adults, with abdominal presentations most common.[459–462] There are not marked clinical differences between the Burkitt's and non-Burkitt's subtypes, although the non-Burkitt's subtype may present in an older population and have a higher incidence of peripheral lymphadenopathy. Small noncleaved cell lymphoma is an extremely aggressive lymphoma treated primarily by multidrug chemotherapy, although there may be a role for bone marrow transplantation.[463,464] Survival rates are now in the range of 80 percent; relapses, if they occur, usually manifest in the first year. There are not marked differences in survival between the Burkitt's and non-Burkitt's subtype.[463,465]

At low magnification, small noncleaved cell lymphoma usually shows diffuse effacement of architecture, although rare cases show focal involvement of germinal centers.[466] A striking finding is the presence of a starry sky pattern, imparted by a high mitotic rate, numerous apoptotic cells, and evenly dispersed tingible body macrophages (Fig. 20-72); this pattern is invariably present in the Burkitt's subtype and almost always present in the non-Burkitt's subtype. At high magnification,

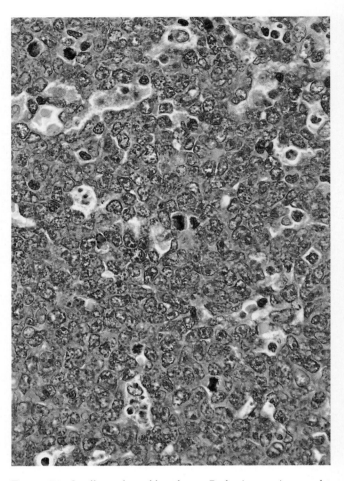

Fig. 20-72. Small noncleaved lymphoma, Burkitt's type. A starry sky pattern is present. The tumor cells are very homogeneous.

Burkitt's lymphoma is composed of a very homogeneous population of medium-sized cells with round nuclei, a vesicular chromatin pattern, several moderately sized nucleoli, and a moderate rim of basophilic cytoplasm that tends to square off as it abuts adjacent cells (Fig. 20-72). In the non-Burkitt's subtype, more cell-size heterogeneity is seen, and nucleoli tend to be fewer in number, but more prominent (Fig. 20-73). Fine needle aspirate smears of small noncleaved lymphoma, Burkitt's type, show a homogeneous population of medium-sized cells with round nuclei, a coarsely reticulated chromatin pattern, and several nucleoli. The cytoplasm is relatively abundant, basophilic, and usually shows small vacuoles on air-dried smears. The non-Burkitt's type contains similarly sized rounded nuclei with a finer chromatin pattern and usually one conspicuous nucleolus.

All cases of small noncleaved cell lymphoma are B lineage neoplasms, almost always expressing monotypic immunoglobulins. Aberrant coexpression of CD43 is seen in a significant subset of cases. In frozen sections, CD10 is usually positive in the Burkitt's subtype, but CD5 and CD23 are negative. Virtually all cases have detectable immunoglobulin heavy and light chain gene rearrangements. In addition, virtually all Burkitt's cases have a translocation involving the c-myc gene on chromosome

proliferative index may be helpful, with the highest rates present in small noncleaved cell lymphoma.

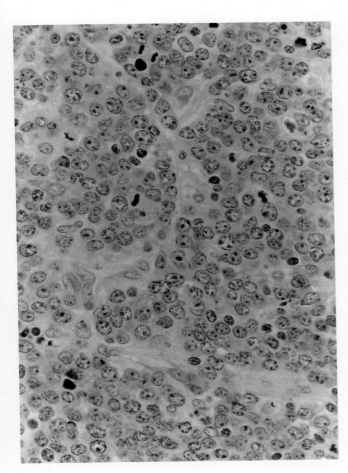

Fig. 20-73. Small noncleaved lymphoma, non-Burkitt's type. The mitotic rate is very high. Although the cells are somewhat monomorphous, some variability is present.

8—either a t(8;14) involving the immunoglobulin heavy chain gene, found in 85 percent of cases, a t(2;8) involving the kappa gene, found in 10 percent of cases, or a t(8;22) involving the lambda gene, found in 5 percent of cases.[467,468] Many of the translocations are not easily detected by Southern blotting due to heterogeneity of the breakpoints at the molecular level.

The differential diagnosis of small noncleaved cell lymphoma includes lymphoblastic lymphoma, discussed in the previous section, and the large cell lymphomas, particularly large cell immunoblastic lymphoma. Small noncleaved cell lymphoma is generally more homogeneous than large cell lymphoma, lacking host cells other than histiocytes, and more consistently has a starry sky appearance. Although one would expect that size could be used as a criterion in the discrimination between small noncleaved cell lymphoma and the large cell lymphomas, in practice there is a gradation of nuclear sizes for each, without distinct differences in many cases. In our opinion, there is occasionally not a clear distinction between some cases of the non-Burkitt's subtype of small noncleaved cell lymphoma and some cases of large cell immunoblastic lymphoma. In questionable cases, Ki-67 (mib-1) stains to assess the

LYMPHOPROLIFERATIONS IN IMMUNODEFICIENT INDIVIDUALS

Patients with immunodeficiencies are at increased risk of lymphoproliferative disorders, most often EBV-associated non-Hodgkin's lymphomas. The incidence and specific types of lymphoproliferative disorders vary with the specific type of immunodeficiency. The primary immunodeficiencies most often associated with lymphoproliferative disorders are X-linked lymphoproliferative syndrome, ataxia-telangiectasia, common variable immunodeficiency, Wiskott-Aldrich syndrome, and severe combined immunodeficiency.[469] About 65 percent of patients with X-linked lymphoproliferative syndrome, 15 percent of patients with Wiskott-Aldrich syndrome, and 5 percent of patients with common variable immunodeficiency syndrome develop on intermediate to high grade diffuse non-Hodgkin's lymphoma that is usually extranodal. Patients with common variable immunodeficiency more often have lymphadenopathy that reveals chronic granulomatous inflammation, reactive hyperplasia, or atypical lymphoid hyperplasia.[470] About 10 percent of patients with ataxia-telangiectasia and 3 percent of patients with severe combined immunodeficiency develop lymphoid neoplasia, including both non-Hodgkin's lymphoma and Hodgkin's disease. The non-Hodgkin's lymphomas in ataxia-telangiectasia reflect the lymphomas occurring in the normal population, while those in severe combined immunodeficiency are usually intermediate to high grade and arise in multiple extranodal sites. The cases of Hodgkin's disease are usually of mixed cellularity or lymphocyte depletion types.

Secondary immunodeficiencies associated with lymphoproliferative disorders include HIV infection and iatrogenic causes, usually as a result of immunosuppression after organ transplantation, but occasionally after treatment for a collagen vascular disease. The benign lymphadenopathies associated with HIV infection have already been discussed. About 3 percent of HIV-infected patients develop non-Hodgkin's lymphoma, roughly accounting for about 10 percent of cases of non-Hodgkin's lymphoma currently diagnosed in the United States.[268] These lymphomas are usually B lineage, either of small noncleaved cell, diffuse large cell, or large cell immunoblastic type. The small noncleaved cell type usually occurs in patients at an early stage of HIV infection and involves lymph nodes, whereas the large cell immunoblastic lymphomas tend to occur in patients who already have a diagnosis of AIDS and involve extranodal sites. The molecular lesions also differ between the small noncleaved cell and large cell immunoblastic cases.[471] HIV-infected patients occasionally develop other types of malignant lymphoma, including Hodgkin's disease and T cell lymphomas.[472]

Patients who are receiving immunosuppression after organ transplantation are at greatly increased risk of the development of post-transplantation lymphoproliferative disorders, with the specific risk dependent on age, the type of organ transplant, and the drug regimen used. These lesions have recently been classified into several types: plasmacytic hyperplasia, polymorphous B cell hyperlasia, polymorphic B cell lymphoma, immunoblastic lymphoma, and multiple myeloma.[473] In plasmacytic hyperplasia, there is expansion of the paracortical areas by a predominant population of plasmacytoid lymphocytes and plasma cells; plasmacytoid immunoblasts may be present but are few in number. Follicles may be hyperplastic, show regression, or be absent. In the polymorphic lesions, the entire range of B lymphocyte forms is seen, including small lymphocytes, plasma cells, small lymphoplasmacytoid forms, plasmacytoid immunoblasts, and small and large cleaved and noncleaved lymphoid cells (Fig. 20-74). In both polymorphic hyperplasia and lymphoma, marked disturbance of underlying architecture is usually seen. Polymorphic B cell lymphoma is diagnosed when there is significant atypia, with atypical immunoblasts. As this classification implies, most of the frank non-Hodgkin's lymphomas that occur in this setting are large cell immunoblastic, but small noncleaved and diffuse large cell (not otherwise specified) lymphomas also occur. Molecular studies demonstrate that almost all the polymorphic B cell lesions and all of the monomorphic lesions harbor monoclonal B cell populations

and are almost all EBV associated.[473] The monomorphic lymphomas have additional genetic mutations that apparently confer a more neoplastic phenotype. Rarely, post-thymic T cell lymphoma, low grade non-Hodgkin's lymphoma, and Hodgkin's disease have also been reported in transplant recipients.

Patients with collagen vascular disease who are treated with methotrexate are also at increased risk of malignant lymphomas, including both non-Hodgkin's lymphoma and Hodgkin's disease.[474] Some of these lymphomas have undergone regression upon withdrawal of the methotrexate.

OTHER NEOPLASMS

Langerhans Cell Histiocytosis (Histiocytosis X)

Langerhans cell histiocytosis, also known as histiocytosis X and Langerhans cell granulomatosis, historically includes three main and sometimes overlapping clinical syndromes: unifocal disease (solitary eosinophilic granuloma), multifocal unisystem disease (Hand-Schüller-Christian syndrome), and multifocal multisystem disease (Letterer-Siwe syndrome).[475] Lymph nodes may be the site of unifocal disease or multifocal unisystem disease, or as part of multifocal multisystem disease. Patients with isolated lymph node involvement (usually cervical or inguinal region) are most often children or young adults who are typically afebrile and may have painful lymphadenopathy.[476,477]

Langerhans cell histiocytosis may be diagnosed in lymph nodes draining the site of disease, in multisystem disease, in isolated disease (as a primary site), or rarely, adjacent to a focus of malignant lymphoma.[476,478,479] The morphologic features of involved lymph nodes in disseminated and localized forms of Langerhans cell histiocytosis are virtually identical. Affected lymph nodes may be small and show focal involvement of the sinuses. Dermatopathic changes may be seen in the paracortex, resulting in slight lymph node enlargement. The lymph node architecture is almost always intact. However, in advanced cases, one may see partial or complete architectural effacement by a proliferation of Langerhans cells in the sinusoids, which often causes marked sinus distention and may extend into the perinodal tissues.

The histologic appearance of Langerhans cell histiocytosis lesions may vary greatly, but one always sees varying degrees of a sinusoidal proliferation of Langerhans cells in the appropriate cellular background (Fig. 20-75). Langerhans cells are mononuclear, approximately 12 to 15 μm in diameter, and have a moderate amount of eosinophilic cytoplasm, (Fig. 20-76). The Langerhans cell has a characteristic folded or grooved nucleus ("coffee-bean" appearance), with small inconspicuous nucleoli. The nuclei appear bland, but slight cytologic atypia may be seen. Mitotic activity varies widely from lesion to lesion, but is generally low. The Langerhans cells are accompanied by mononuclear and multinucleated histiocytes, eosinophils, neutrophils, and small lymphocytes; plasma cells are rare or absent. Clusters of eosinophils may be associated with necrosis, form-

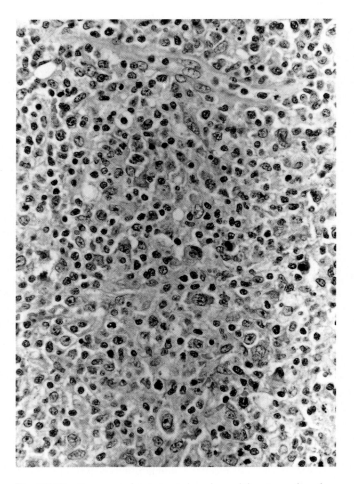

Fig. 20-74. Post-transplantation lymphoproliferative disorder, polymorphous hyperplasia type. A mixed population of lymphoid cells is seen, without striking atypia.

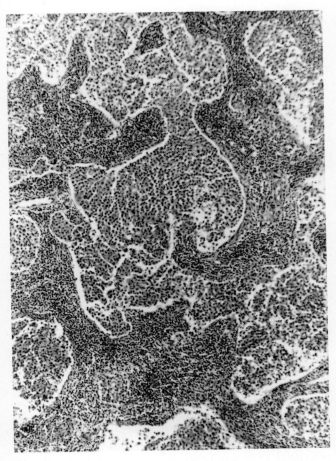

Fig. 20-75. Langerhans cell histiocytosis. A sinusoidal pattern of infiltration is present.

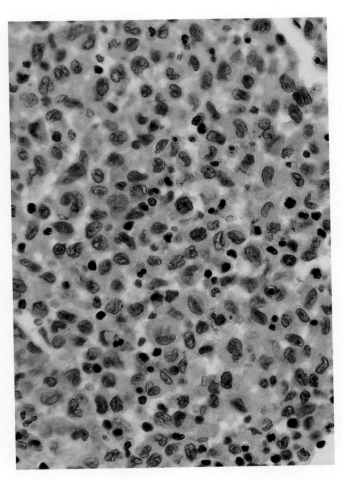

Fig. 20-76. Langerhans cell histiocytosis. Langerhans cells, with their characteristic grooved nuclei, are seen admixed with eosinophils.

ing so-called eosinophilic microabscesses. Rare cases may contain Langerhans cells with unequivocally malignant cytologic features, and have been called malignant histiocytosis X or malignant Langerhans cell histiocytosis.[480]

By immunohistochemistry, neoplastic Langerhans cells virtually always express S-100 protein, and a portion of the neoplastic cells express CD68 and antiplacental alkaline phosphatase.[481–483] Importantly, Langerhans cells stain for CD1, which is of great diagnostic utility, because CD1 expression is limited to reactive and neoplastic Langerhans cells, immature thymocytes, and T lineage lymphoblastic neoplasms. Other histiocytic and dendritic cells lack CD1 expression.[484] Ultrastructurally, one should see characteristic Birbeck granules, which are racket-shaped organelles approximately 200 to 400 nm long, 33 nm wide, with an osmiophilic core and a double outer sheath.[485] By studying the patterns of X-chromosome inactivation in the X-linked human androgen-receptor gene, researchers have demonstrated that Langerhans cell histiocytosis is a monoclonal proliferation.[486] Molecular hybridization studies show a germline configuration for the immunoglobulin heavy chain and alpha-, beta-, and gamma-T cell receptor genes.[487]

Lymph node involvement by Langerhans cell histiocytosis should be distinguished from other diseases that involve the sinuses, including reactive sinus hyperplasia, sinus histiocytosis with massive lymphadenopathy, metastatic neoplasms, and sinusoidal malignant lymphoma. The characteristic Langerhans cells and abundant eosinophils of Langerhans cell histiocytosis are not features of benign sinusoidal hyperplasia. The rounded nuclei with vesicular chromatin and prominent nucleoli, and the abundant cytoplasm of sinus histiocytosis with massive lymphadenopathy cells differ from the folded, grooved nuclei of Langerhans cell histiocytosis. Also, in contrast to Langerhans cell histiocytosis, sinus histiocytosis with massive lymphadenopathy lymph nodes shows phagocytosis and high numbers of plasma cells and lacks eosinophils. The malignant cytology of cells of metastatic malignancies and sinusoidal malignant lymphoma differs from that of Langerhans cell histiocytosis. Large numbers of Langerhans cells are present in the paracortical region of lymph nodes with dermatopathic lymphadenitis, and not the sinuses, as is the case in Langerhans cell histiocytosis. In dermatopathic lymphadenopathy, the proliferating cells are accompanied by numerous melanin-containing histiocytes and interdigitating reticulum cells.[119]

Dendritic Cell Neoplasms

Dendritic cell neoplasms are rare tumors with lineage consistent with follicular dendritic cells or interdigitating dendritic cells.[35,488–491] Follicular dendritic cell tumors have a tendency to recur, either locally or at multiple sites, although the prognosis has generally been good. Interdigitating cell tumors are more aggressive, with approximately one-half of patients dying of their disease.

Follicular dendritic tumors are neoplasms composed of spindled cells containing oval to spindled nuclei with bland nuclear features (Fig. 20-77). Admixed small lymphocytes are often found, between the tumor cells and in perivascular spaces. By electron microscopy, long cytoplasmic processes are evident, connecting to one another by numerous desmosomes. *Interdigitating dendritic tumors* may closely resemble follicular dendritic tumors, or they may more closely resemble lymphoma. Electron microscopy of interdigitating dendritic tumors reveals interdigitating cell processes without well formed desmosomes. Immunohistochemical studies are important in establishing the diagnosis of these tumors. Follicular dendritic tumors may be positive or negative for CD45 or S-100 protein, but are typically positive for the follicular dendritic markers CD21 and

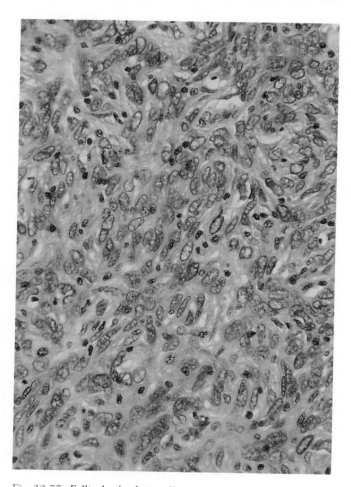

Fig. 20-77. Follicular dendritic cell tumor. A spindle cell proliferation is seen. Note the admixed small lymphocytes.

CD35, antigens detectable in paraffin sections. They are also positive for CD68. Interdigitating tumors are usually positive for CD45, S-100 protein, and CD68. Both tumors are negative for B and T lineage antigens.

The differential diagnosis of dendritic cell neoplasms includes any spindled lesion occurring in lymph nodes. In particular, thymomas may appear similar to these tumors, but thymomas rarely occur in lymph nodes, and are keratin positive. The differentiation between follicular dendritic tumors and interdigitating dendritic tumors essentially rests on immunohistochemical data.

True Histiocytic Lymphoma/ Malignant Histiocytosis

True histiocytic lymphoma and malignant histiocytosis are terms for a rare neoplasm in which the malignant cells demonstrate lineage consistent with histiocytes.[492,493] Historically, the diagnosis of malignant histiocytosis was made when the morphologic and cytochemical features of the tumor cells were considered those of histiocytes. Unfortunately, neither the appearance nor the cytochemical studies were unique to the neoplasm. With the use of more recently available study techniques that have high specificity, the majority of cases of malignant histiocytosis studied in earlier reports are now known to be lymphoid in origin.[436,494–497] We prefer to use the term true histiocytic lymphoma for the neoplasms that remain in the category of histiocytic tumors after a lymphoid origin has been excluded, because the term malignant histiocytosis has been misused in the past.

True histiocytic lymphoma accounts for approximately 0.5 percent of all hematolymphoid neoplasms and occurs most commonly in adults.[498] The lymph nodes are a commonly involved site; other extranodal sites of involvement have been reported.[499] Patients generally present with fever, fatigue, and weakness, and may have weight loss, lymphadenopathy, skin lesions, or splenomegaly. Laboratory tests are usually unremarkable.

Involved lymph nodes may be partially or completely effaced by a proliferation of cytologically malignant cells that resemble histiocytes (Fig. 20-78). The malignant cells vary in size and have a large, eccentrically placed, oval nucleus with a prominent irregular nucleolus and abundant eosinophilic cytoplasm. Multinucleated tumor cells with bizarre nuclei and multiple nucleoli and hemophagocytosing tumor cells may also be present. Mitotic activity is quite brisk. Because the tumor cells of true histiocytic lymphoma have no unique morphologic characteristics, immunophenotypic and molecular studies are essential for diagnosis.

One must have strong immunologic evidence of histiocytic lineage, accompanied by absence of specific T and B lineage markers, and molecular evidence of a germline configuration for the T cell receptor and immunoglobulin genes.[3,429,495] By paraffin section immunohistochemistry, the tumor cells of true histiocytic lymphoma should express CD68 and they should not stain with CD30, any B lineage or T lineage-specific antibodies, S-100, any of the antikeratin antibodies, or HMB 45.[492,498,499] Frozen section immunohistochemical studies should show reactivity of the malignant cells with CD45 and multiple histiocytic markers.[492]

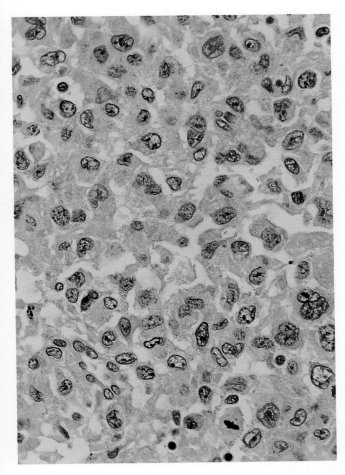

Fig. 20-78. True histiocytic tumor. This case was proved to be a true histiocytic lymphoma after a large panel of immunohistochemical and molecular studies. The cells have pleomorphic nuclei and abundant cytoplasm.

The differential diagnosis of true histiocytic lymphoma includes anaplastic large cell lymphoma, B cell sinusoidal large cell lymphoma, anaplastic carcinomas showing hemophago-cytosis, malignant lymphomas associated with benign erythro-phagocytosis, follicular dendritic cell neoplasms, hepatosplenic T cell lymphoma, infection-associated hemophagocytic syndrome, storage diseases such as Gaucher's disease and Nie-mann-Pick disease, and familial hemophagocytic lymphohistio-cytosis. The strict morphologic, phenotypic, and molecular criteria of true histiocytic lymphoma, along with clinical presentation, help separate true histiocytic lymphoma from the other cancers listed above.[139,500,501]

Myeloid Leukemia

When myeloid leukemia involves extramedullary sites, it is known as granulocytic sarcoma, extramedullary myeloid tumor, or chloroma.[502] Lymph node involvement by granulocytic sarcoma has several modes of presentation.[503,504] It may occur in patients with known acute myeloid leukemia. It may be seen as the first sign of blastic transformation in a patient with known chronic myeloid leukemia, other myeloproliferative disorder, or myelodysplastic syndrome. Finally, it may occur in a patient with no known history of leukemia.

The granulocytic sarcoma cells may involve the sinusoidal, interfollicular, or perinodal spaces of a lymph node or diffusely efface the normal lymph node architecture. Sheets of monotonous malignant cells are often accompanied by eosinophilic myelocytes (Fig. 20-79). The malignant cells have intermediately sized round or lobated nuclei, with fine delicate or vesicular chromatin and small to prominent nucleoli. The cytoplasm is scant or moderate, and may contain granules. The tumor usually has a high mitotic rate, and a starry sky pattern may be seen, owing to interspersed tingible body macrophages. Touch imprints or frozen sections, if available, can be examined cytochemically for myeloperoxidase or Sudan Black B.[502] In tissues, the Leder stain (chloroacetate esterase reaction) will be positive in approximately 75 percent of cases, but the number of positive blasts can be very low. Immunohistochemistry is extremely useful, with antimyeloperoxidase, CD43, CD68, and antilysozyme; each positive in a high percentage of cases.[505]

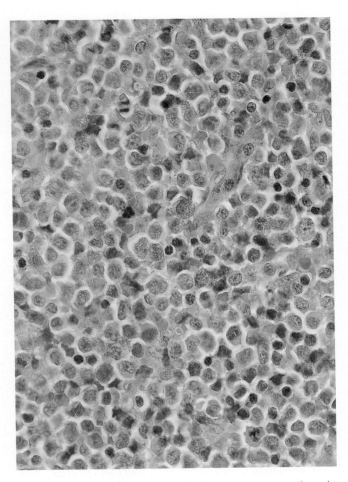

Fig. 20-79. Extramedullary myeloid tumor. A relatively monomorphous population of cells with a fine chromatin pattern is seen. Note the occasional myelocytes.

Flow cytometric expression of CD34, CD33, CD13, and c-kit is also seen.

When one sees an immature proliferation of cells in a lymph node from a patient with known myeloid leukemia, myeloproliferative disorder, or myelodysplastic syndrome, one may make the diagnosis of granulocytic sarcoma more easily than when granulocytic sarcoma in a lymph node is the initial presentation of a myeloid malignancy. Granulocytic sarcoma may be histologically confused with non-Hodgkin's lymphoma, particularly lymphoblastic or large cell subtypes. The larger size and more prominent nucleoli of myeloid cells compared to lymphoblasts and the finer chromatin pattern compared to cells of large cell lymphoma help distinguish between these entities. Identifying myelocytes or cytoplasmic granules also favors a myeloid process. Cytochemical and immunohistochemical studies are extremely useful in the differential diagnosis.

Plasmacytoid T cell lymphoma, also known as plasmacytoid monocytic lymphoma, is closely related to myeloid leukemia[506] and may involve lymph nodes. Immunohistochemical studies show a characteristic phenotype for plasmacytoid monocytic cells: reactivity for histiocytic markers, often with aberrant coexpression of CD5.

Miscellaneous Neoplasms

Hairy cell leukemia may involve the lymph nodes, but rarely without concomitant involvement of the bone marrow and spleen.[507] The outer cortex of the lymph node is preferentially involved, and the morphology and immunologic profile are the same as those of hairy cell leukemia involving other sites. Regional lymph nodes near a site of solitary plasmacytoma may be involved by plasmacytoma.[508] *Primary plasmacytoma* of lymph node is extremely rare. Rare cases of plasmacytoma of lymph node are associated with amloidosis.[509] Lymph nodes may rarely be involved in cases of *systemic mastocytosis*.[510] The mast cell infiltrate is found predominantly in the medullary cords and perivascular areas and is composed of bland cells, with small, or indented nuclei, fine chromatin, and a moderate of pale cytoplasm. Eosinophils and sclerosis typically accompany the mast cell clusters. Giemsa, chloracetate esterase, and toluidine blue stains are used to identify mast cell granules.

THE SPLEEN

Outside of the United States, fine needle aspiration of the spleen is used with some frequency and with excellent results. This procedure has been accurately used to diagnose metastatic disease, splenic involvement by malignant lymphoma, and primary splenic tumors, as well as infectious diseases, with very little morbidity.[512–516] Ultrasound guided core biopsies of the spleen have also been reported to give excellent results.[517] Despite these reports, these techniques are infrequently used in the United States, presumably due to the concern of excessive hemorrhage from the procedures. Thus, the splenectomy specimen remains as the only sample from this organ to be evaluated by most surgical pathologists.

A wide range of clinical events may result in a patient undergoing a splenectomy. Although a spleen removed due to traumatic injury, either preoperatively or intraoperatively, generally offers little difficulty to the surgical pathologist, most other causes for splenectomy are diagnostically challenging. A variety of reactive, metabolic, autoimmune, and neoplastic processes can result in splenic enlargement,[518] and the clinical indication for splenectomy must be adequately communicated to the pathologist examining the specimen. Although splenic enlargement is often related to a systemic disease process, the splenectomy specimen may be the first opportunity for diagnosis. Adequate sampling, fixation, and processing are all vital to identify many of these disease processes, which may be histologically subtle.

Whenever possible, the spleen should be examined, weighed, and sectioned prior to fixation. One centimeter thick sections can be easily made through a fresh specimen, although thinner sectioning may be desired when the splenectomy is performed as a staging procedure. Each breadloafed section should be carefully examined and accentuations of the white pulp should be sampled. The sections submitted for tissue processing and microscopic examination should be thin (2 mm or less in thickness) and adequately fixed prior to processing. We routinely fix one specimen in B5 and place the remaining sections in formalin. If B5 is not available, formalin fixation alone is generally adequate. The tissue, however, must be fixed adequately in the formalin and should be fixed overnight prior to processing, if the specimen is received late in the day. The number of required sections will vary greatly by the clinical indication for the procedure. Touch preparations of the fresh spleen should also be made for Wright-Giemsa staining. The cut surface of the spleen should be dried with towels to reduce the amount of blood prior to making the impressions. The touch preparations should be made from areas that include areas of accentuated white pulp, if present. Additional unstained slides can be made for possible immunocytochemical studies, although we generally prefer to perform phenotypic studies on paraffin sections and less frequently on frozen tissue.

Additional tissue may also be collected from the fresh specimen. A portion of tissue should be snap frozen if there is any possibility of a hematopoietic neoplasm. This tissue should be stored for possible frozen section immunohistochemical studies or gene rearrangement studies. Also, if available, fresh tissue should be collected for flow cytometric immunophenotyping if an hematopoietic neoplasm is in the differential diagnosis.

We find H&E stained sections to be adequate for evaluation of most spleen sections, although others have advocated the routine use of silver stains and the PAS stain. Reticulin staining and iron stains may be useful in selected cases.

Normal Histology

The normal anatomy and histology of the spleen are described in more detail elsewhere.[519,520] The simplest approach to spleen histology is to divide the cellular constituents into the white and red pulp. The red pulp is the largest of the two components and is involved in the filtering function of the spleen. It is primarily composed of the open sinuses lined by flattened endothelium and is surrounded by the splenic cords (of Billroth). The lymphoid component of the normal red pulp is minimal, with only rare scattered lymphocytes and plasma cells identified by immunohistochemical studies. The white pulp contains the major lymphoid component of the spleen, with a fairly high proportion of B lymphocytes. The malpighian corpuscles vary in their appearance with age, with prominent germinal center formation present in children and in antigenically stimulated adults (Fig. 20-80). Adults that are not antigenically stimulated have more involuted white pulp without germinal center formation.

In the child, three distinct white pulp zones of lymphocytes are seen. The central germinal center and surrounding mantle zone are B cell regions that are similar to the primary follicle of the lymph node. A third distinct lymphocyte zone is also normally present in the splenic white pulp. This splenic marginal zone is composed predominantly of B lymphocytes with slightly more open nuclear chromatin than the mantle zone cells and with moderately abundant, clear cytoplasm. These cells are morphologically similar to the monocytoid B lymphocytes seen in some reactive lymph nodes. The region analogous to the normal splenic marginal zone, however, is not present routinely in lymph nodes. T lymphocytes are scattered within the germinal centers, similar to lymph node follicles, as well as admixed around white pulp follicles with the marginal zone cells. In addition, periarterial lymphatic sheaths without follicle formation and small red pulp arterioles are surrounded by T lymphocytes.

Splenosis and Accessory Spleen

Splenosis is the term for autotransplantation of the spleen following surgery or trauma that results in multiple small, dark red nodules attached to the abdominal mesentery.[521,522] Microscopically, most cases show a diffuse red pulp proliferation, although lymphoid nodules with or without germinal centers (white pulp elements) may be seen. The capsule of splenosis is often thinner than the usual splenic capsule. Accessory spleens are present in 16 to 19 percent of individuals and may have similar morphologic features to a nodule of splenosis with both red and white pulp elements.[518,523] Most accessory spleens are solitary, in contrast to the multiple nodules usually found with splenosis.[518,523] The distinction between these two processes may not be possible solely on morphologic grounds, and may depend on the clinical and operative findings.

Splenic Rupture

Examination of the ruptured spleen following major trauma is of value primarily to document the gross pathologic findings. Microscopic examination of the spleen when it is ruptured in relation to minor or no trauma is important because this unusual occurrence is usually related to an underlying disease process involving the spleen. A variety of infectious disease processes are associated with splenic rupture; most notable of these are infectious mononucleosis and malaria. In addition, patients with splenic involvement by lymphoma, acute leukemia, or metastatic malignant tumors may rarely present with spontaneous splenic rupture.[524] Splenic rupture may be the initial manifestation of the disease process in these patients.

Infectious Diseases

Splenomegaly may be caused by a variety of infectious diseases. *Splenic abscesses* are rare, but may be treated by splenectomy.[525,526] They may be single or multiple, and may occur following trauma, in patients with bacterial endocarditis (especially intravenous drug users), or in patients with sepsis.[525,527] The abscess is usually well circumscribed with a fibrous wall and may be accompanied by white pulp hyperplasia of the surrounding splenic tissue. Bacterial and fungal cultures should be taken in all cases, because many different organisms have been implicated in abscess formation.[528] Rarely, patients with splenic abscess have presented with splenic rupture.[525]

More than one-half of patients with *infectious mononucleosis* have associated splenomegaly. Although many different infectious diseases are associated with an increased risk of rupture, only recurrent malaria infection is associated with more splenic

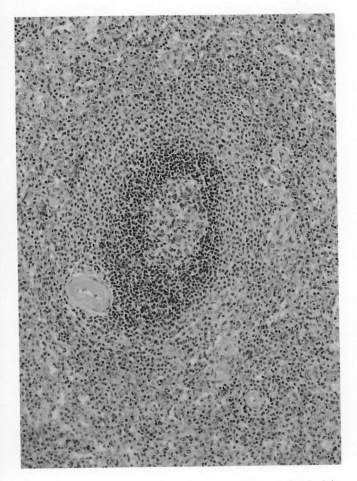

Fig. 20-80. Splenic white pulp in an antigenically stimulated adult. Note the central germinal center, the surrounding, darkly stained mantle zone, and the outer more pale staining splenic marginal zone.

ruptures than EBV infection.[529] Most cases of splenic rupture in infectious mononucleosis are associated with trauma, often minor, although rare cases of spontaneous rupture have been documented.[530,531] The morphologic features of infectious mononucleosis in the spleen may be confused with malignant lymphoma. The white pulp may be expanded or depleted with a wide spectrum of cell types (Fig. 20-81) ranging from small lymphocytes and plasma cells to plasmacytoid immunoblasts and cells simulating Reed-Sternberg cells. Such cells may also be seen in increased numbers in the red pulp cords and are generally of T lineage with a suppressor cell phenotype. Areas of individual cell necrosis may be present as well as larger areas of necrosis. Epithelioid granulomas may also be seen. The striking polymorphism of the cellular infiltrate is helpful for excluding a malignant process. In addition, discrete nodules as typically seen in Hodgkin's disease are not usually present in infectious mononucleosis.

Infection-associated, *familial*, and *secondary hemophagocytoses* (Fig. 20-82) also frequently result in splenomegaly and are often associated with EBV infection, although other infectious agents may cause identical findings.[132,532] Two morphologic patterns may be seen with the infection-associated and the fa-

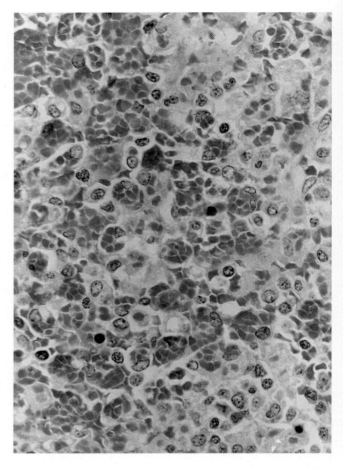

Fig. 20-82. Infection-associated hemophagocytosis showing marked erythrophagocytosis within the splenic red pulp.

milial disorders. The most common is one of white pulp atrophy, which is usually accompanied by lymphocyte depletion of lymph nodes. A second pattern of white pulp expansion with cellular polymorphism is similar to that seen in infectious mononucleosis. Both patterns also exhibit a marked expansion of the red pulp by histiocytes showing marked hemophagocytosis.[532] Secondary hemophagocytosis occurs in patients with T cell lymphomas,[532,533] and evidence of hemophagocytosis may be present in organs that are not involved by lymphoma. Many of these T cell lymphomas are EBV related, and admixed pleomorphic large lymphoid cells may be seen within the splenic red pulp along with the non-neoplastic hemophagocytic histiocytes.

Granulomas are commonly seen in the spleen and may be associated with infectious diseases as well as with malignant tumors. Tuberculosis, fungal diseases, infectious mononucleosis, and brucellosis, among others, all may cause extensive necrotizing granuloma formation in the spleen, similar to those seen in lymph nodes. Granulomas of the spleen, however, are not always infection related and may also be seen in patients with Hodgkin's disease, non-Hodgkin's lymphomas, sarcoidosis, chronic uremia, and selective IgA deficiency.[534] In Hodgkin's

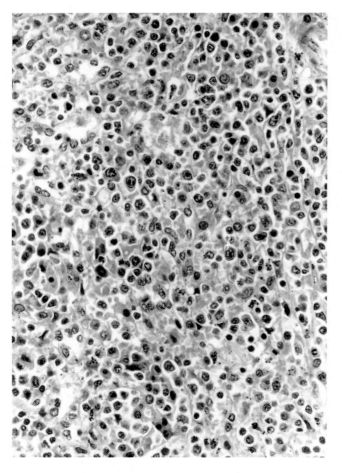

Fig. 20-81. Infectious mononucleosis involving the spleen showing a spectrum of lymphocytes, including plasmacytoid immunoblasts.

disease, granulomas may be present in an otherwise uninvolved spleen and care must be taken to not over interpret such granulomas as representing disease involvement. The presence of epithelioid granulomas in Hodgkin's disease has been reported to be a favorable prognostic sign.[173,535] Lipogranulomas (follicular lipidosis or mineral oil lipidosis) of the spleen are common in North America, present in approximately one-half of autopsy specimens, while virtually nonexistent in other geographic areas.[536,537] This difference is presumed to be due to differences in dietary intake or food packaging. Aggregates of vacuolated histiocytes are present surrounded by lymphocytes and plasma cells. They differ from lymphangiography-associated changes by the lack of epithelioid, foreign body type histiocytes that are commonly seen in tissues following the radiographic procedure.

Splenic-Gonadal Fusion

Splenic-gonadal fusion is a congenital disorder that primarily affects males, almost always involving the left testicle. Putschar and Manion[538] described two forms. *Continuous* splenic-gonadal fusion has a direct cord-like attachment of splenic and fibrous tissue between the gonad and the spleen, whereas the *discontinuous* type represents a fusion between an accessory spleen and the gonad. A subset of cases are associated with congenital defects of the extremities and mandible.

Metabolic Diseases

A variety of congenital enzyme deficiencies cause the red pulp accumulation of histiocytes in the spleen with resultant splenomegaly.[519,539] The lysosomal storage diseases are the major group that result in splenomegaly. These disorders generally present in infants and children, although adults are affected by some of these storage diseases, such as type 1 Gaucher's disease. The enlarged spleen generally demonstrates a firm mottled to homogeneous cut surface. The red pulp cords are expanded by large aggregates of histiocytes with abundant cytoplasm. The morphologic detail of the histiocytes is best visualized on touch imprints where the tissue-paper character of the Gaucher cell cytoplasm (Fig. 20-83) can more easily be distinguished from the multivacuolated cytoplasm seen with Niemann-Pick disease. Heavily vacuolated balloon cells may be seen both with the gangliosidoses, including Tay-Sach's disease, and the mucopolysaccharidoses, including Hunter's and Hurler's syndromes. Less descript foamy-appearing histiocytes are seen in several disorders, including Fabry's disease, Wolman's disease, and von Gierke's disease, whereas ceroid-containing histiocytes (seablue histiocytes) with granular cytoplasm may be seen in familial Hermansky-Pudlak syndrome. The presence of ceroid histiocytes, however, is nonspecific and they may be seen in other storage diseases as well as in chronic myelogenous leukemia, red blood cell disorders, and autoimmune disorders.[8]

Tangier's disease (familial high density protein lipoprotein deficiency) may also result in splenomegaly. The red pulp histiocytes seen in these patients contain intracytoplasmic lipid droplets as well as identifiable cholesterol crystals.[539]

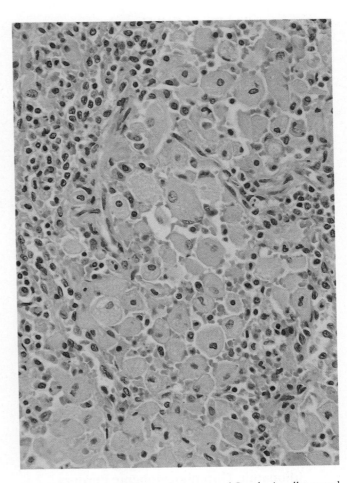

Fig. 20-83. Gaucher's disease. Aggregates of Gaucher's cells expand the splenic red pulp.

The wide morphologic overlap in these diseases makes a definite diagnosis difficult by H&E alone, and differences in cytochemical staining patterns may be useful to differentiate some of these processes. Gaucher's cells and ceroid histiocytes contain strongly diastase-resistant, PAS-positive material, in comparison to the cells of Neimann-Pick disease, which are only weakly PAS positive. In addition, Neimann-Pick cells contain neutral fat that can be demonstrated in unfixed tissue with an oil red O or other fat stain. In addition to being PAS positive, ceroid histiocytes are positive for acid fast stains. Specific ultrastructural changes are also described for certain storage diseases, and fresh tissue might be collected for electron microscopy in certain cases. This requires communication between the clinician and pathologist prior to examination and fixation of the specimen. Biochemical evaluation to determine the enzymatic defect is essential for the precise classification of the various storage diseases. Many of the genes involved in these disorders have now been cloned, and molecular studies will continue to gain diagnostic importance in these diseases as well. The pathologist must correlate the molecular and enzymatic ancillary test results with the morphologic findings to properly diagnose these cases.

Red Blood Cell Disorders

Splenomegaly may result from abnormalities of red blood cells. Hereditary spherocytosis is probably the best example of this phenomenon. The red cells in this usually autosomal dominant disorder have abnormalities of the surface protein spectrin or other related proteins. These defects result in a loss of red cell pliability, which is needed for the cells to pass through the cords of Billroth into the splenic sinuses. The sequestration of red blood cells that subsequently occurs results in splenomegaly and anemia. The initial diagnosis is generally made prior to surgery, and splenectomy for this disease is a therapeutic procedure. The morphologic features consist of an expanded red pulp with red blood cell engorgement of the cords and relatively clear sinuses.

Sickle cell anemia is another disorder of red blood cells that the surgical pathologist may encounter. Although autosplenectomy frequently occurs in late childhood, splenomegaly is more common in infants and young children with sickle cell anemia. Again, the loss of pliability of the sickled red blood cells within the spleen leads to splenic sequestration and splenomegaly. The morphologic features of such a spleen are similar to those of hereditary spherocytosis, with engorged cords and fairly clear sinuses. With good histologic preservation, sickled red blood cells can be identified within the cords. Other less common red blood cell disorders, including hemoglobin C disease and hemoglobin SC disease, may also result in splenomegaly with similar features. Both alpha and beta thalassemia are also associated with progressive splenomegaly, although such spleens are not commonly received as surgical pathology specimens.

Idiopathic Thrombocytopenic Purpura

The surgical pathologist frequently receives splenectomy specimens for idiopathic thrombocytopenic purpura (ITP). The diagnosis is usually well established prior to surgery. Gross examination of these specimens is often only remarkable for slight accentuation of the white pulp. The most common microscopic findings are white pulp hyperplasia with secondary follicle formation and focal red pulp lymphoplasmacytic aggregates. In addition, phagocytosed platelets and extramedullary hematopoiesis may be seen in the red pulp. Foamy, lipid-laden macrophages are also commonly present, presumably containing the degenerated by-products of phagocytosed platelets.[540,541] The plasmacytosis and white pulp hyperplasia, which is also seen with Felty's syndrome,[542] may be absent in ITP patients treated with corticosteroids prior to splenectomy. The platelet-filled red pulp foamy macrophages, however, are usually still present after steroid therapy.[543] The microscopic examination of the spleen in these cases is most important to exclude other causes of hypersplenism, particularly splenic involvement by malignant lymphoma or chronic lymphocytic leukemia. The morphologic features of these disorders will be described subsequently.

Rarely, multiple myeloma will involve the spleen with aggregates of red pulp plasma cells, morphologically mimicking ITP. The clinical presentation of these two disorders is usually quite different and can aid in this differential diagnosis. If necessary, immunohistochemical studies on paraffin sections will usually identify a monotypic plasma cell population in multiple myeloma in contrast to the polytypic plasma cells of ITP.

Cysts

Cysts of the spleen are found in less than 1 percent of splenectomy specimens.[544] These rare lesions most frequently occur in young adults in the third decade, but may be seen at any age, and a male predominance has been reported. An abdominal mass is the most common presenting symptom, although abdominal pain and other gastrointestinal tract disturbances may be present or the patient may be asymptomatic. In one large series,[545] the average size of splenic cysts was 10 cm.

Fairly elaborate classification systems have been proposed for the different cyst types[56,544,546,547]; however, we prefer the simple classification[545] of primary (or true) cysts and secondary (or false) cysts (Table 20-16). Most cysts of either type are unilocular. Primary cysts have a firm but slightly roughened to trabecular internal surface that has been likened to the endocardial surface of the heart. The cyst wall is composed of thick fibrous tissue that is at least partially surfaced by mesothelium or squamous epithelium, or a mixture of both (Fig. 20-84). Subdivision of these cysts based on the type of lining probably does not accurately reflect a difference in pathogenesis.[548] Primary cysts may be parasitic or nonparasitic. There are geographic differences in the frequency of primary parasitic (echinococcal) cysts. Garvin and King[545] found parasitic cysts to represent less than 2 percent of all splenic cysts accessioned at the Armed Forces Institute of Pathology. The nonparasitic, primary cysts are felt to arise from congenital inclusions.

Secondary cysts are approximately four times as common as primary cysts and are frequently associated with a history of significant trauma. Their gross appearance is similar to the primary cyst, except the lining is generally smoother. Microscopically, the cyst wall is composed of dense fibrous tissue without any epithelial lining; approximately 25 percent of cases will have areas of calcification within the cyst wall. Iron may be demonstrated within the cyst wall, probably reflecting previous hemorrhage related to trauma. Because the major difference in the two cyst types is based on the presence or absence of cyst lining cells, multiple sections of the cyst wall should be submitted to identify the possibly incomplete epithelial lining of primary cysts.

Table 20-16. Splenic Cysts

Type	Characteristic Features
Primary (true) cyst	
Parasitic	Entirely or partially epithelial lined, parasite scolices identified
Nonparasitic	Entirely or partially epithelial lined, no scolices identified
Secondary (false) cyst	No epithelial lining identified on examination of multiple histologic sections, ± calcification

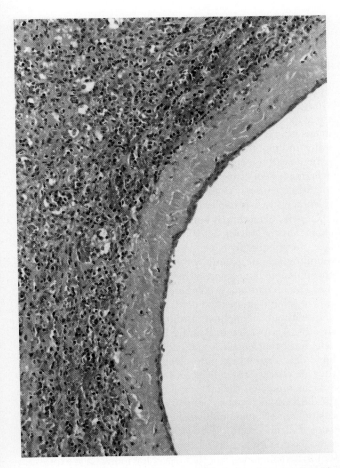

Fig. 20-84. Primary or true splenic cyst. Note that the cyst is lined by a thin layer of flattened epithelium.

Benign Tumors and Proliferations

Vascular and Lymphatic Proliferations

Hemangiomas are the most common primary tumors of the spleen. Similar to splenic cysts, these lesions are seen most often in young adults.[545] They are often asymptomatic, but may present as abdominal masses, with abdominal discomfort or hypersplenism. The spleen is usually only slightly enlarged (300 to 400 g) with an average size of the lesion reported as 5 to 8 cm.[545] The lesion generally has a cystic and bloody gross appearance. The morphologic features are similar to hemangiomas at other sites and usually have a cavernous component. Hemangiomas may undergo infarction with resultant fibrosis and possible cystic change.

Peliosis of the spleen is a rare, diffuse vascular proliferation, primarily of adults, which is infrequently associated with splenomegaly. It is usually an incidental finding, although rare cases have been associated with splenic rupture.[549,550] Although it is usually found in conjunction with peliosis of the liver, approximately 17 percent of cases of peliosis involve only the spleen.[551] Peliosis of the spleen is most often associated with anabolic steroid use, malignancy, tuberculosis, and aplas-

tic anemia. The process is usually evident grossly with diffuse, dilated vascular spaces of up to 1 mm.[551,552] Microscopically, round to oval blood-filled spaces are lined by a single layer of cells without cordal fibrosis (Fig. 20-85).

Patients with *lymphangiomas* may be asymptomatic or present with abdominal pain. The cystic nature of the gross lesions may suggest a primary or secondary cyst in some cases, and 10 percent of cystic spleen lesions described by Fowler[546] were thought to be lymphangiomas. Smaller lymphangiomas may be less cystic in appearance and multiple splenic lymphangiomas may also occur.[553] These proliferations are most often found in children and young adults and have a reported predilection for a subcapsular location,[545] compared to hemangiomas that occur in no specific splenic location. Microscopically, the lesions consist of a single layer of endothelium surrounding the variably sized cystic spaces containing proteinaceous material. The lining cells reportedly immunoreact for factor VIII-related antigen as well as CD31, while negative for CD68; however, we have found solitary "lymphangiomas" to actually represent keratin-positive primary mesothelial cysts.[553a] *Lymphangiomatosis* is a rare condition associated with lymphangiomas of multiple sites, including the spleen as well as other organs, including bone.[554]

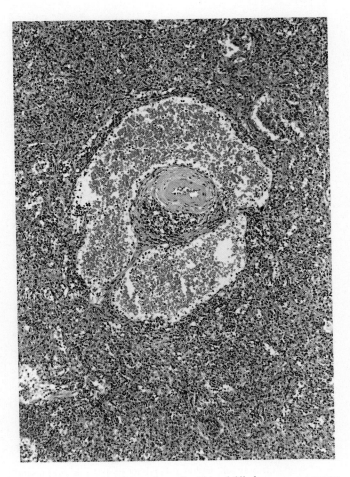

Fig. 20-85. Peliosis of the spleen. Oval blood-filled spaces are present throughout the splenic parenchyma.

Littoral cell angioma (LCA) of the spleen is an endothelial-lined proliferation of the spleen that differs both morphologically and immunohistochemically from hemangiomas and lymphangiomas. The tumor may occur at any age. Patients most commonly presented with splenomegaly in the report of Falk et al,[555] although the tumors in this series varied greatly in size, from 0.2 to 9 cm. LCAs are grossly nodular dark spongy lesions that are frequently multiple and may be cystic. Microscopically, they contain tall endothelial cells with small nucleoli, a low mitotic rate, and no nuclear pleomorphism, although the cells may be large with abundant cytoplasm and enlarged nuclei (Fig. 20-86). The endothelial cells commonly form papillary projections that are often accompanied by endothelial cell sloughing into the lumina of the lesion. The intraluminal cells may show evidence of hemophagocytosis. LCA may be confused with other benign vascular lesions or with angiosarcoma, although mitoses are not increased and nuclear atypia is not prominent. Immunohistochemically, the lining cells of LCA stain for factor VIII-related antigen as well as for CD31 and CD68.[555,556] The expression of CD68 presumably reflects a pattern of dual differentiation in this lesion of both vascular and histiocytic

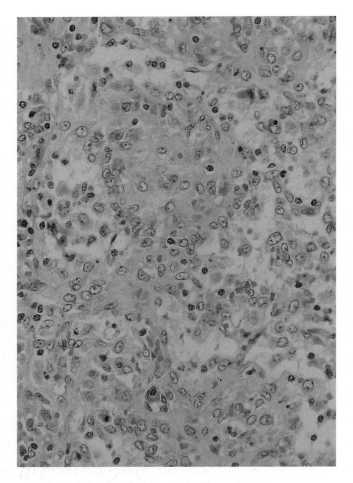

Fig. 20-86. Littoral cell angioma. Papillary projections are present with sloughing of endothelial cells into the lumina. Although there is enlargement of the endothelial cells, no nuclear atypia is seen.

origin. The expression of CD68 is a useful feature in excluding other vascular lesions.

Hamartoma

Splenic hamartoma, also termed *splenoma* or "spleen in spleen" syndrome, is a rare, generally asymptomatic lesion with only three such lesions found in almost 200,000 surgical spleen specimens in one series.[557] Because most lesions are incidental autopsy findings, they have been found most commonly in elderly patients with no apparent sex predilection. Hamartomas, however, may occur at any age, and may be seen in spleens removed for other causes. In addition, rare cases may present with splenomegaly, hypersplenism, or splenic rupture.[558,559]

Grossly, hamartomas appear well circumscribed and have a characteristic bulging cut surface. Other than the bulging surface, they frequently have a similar gross appearance to the surrounding splenic parenchyma. Microscopically, they are not encapsulated, but compress the surrounding normal splenic tissue. The hamartoma is composed of a homogeneous proliferation of splenic sinuses and cords similar to the surrounding red pulp without malpighian corpuscles or periarterial lymphoid sheaths. An increase in B and T lymphocytes as well as plasma cells has been seen in some cases.[560] Although some reports have described white pulp elements within hamartomas,[561] they are characteristically absent.

Hemangioma is the major splenic tumor to be considered in the differential diagnosis of hamartoma. Because both have vascular channels, immunohistochemical study may be of limited value. Falk and Stutte,[560] however, have reported an absence of follicular dendritic cells in hamartoma while these cells are present in hemangioma. Another report has found CD8 expression by the endothelial cells of a splenic hamartoma but not in an hemangioma.[562] Morphologically, the absence of a cavernous component associated with the vascular channels is the most helpful finding in excluding hemangioma.

Inflammatory Pseudotumor

Inflammatory pseudotumor of the spleen is now well described[563–565] and may be seen in a wide age range, from young adulthood to the elderly. The patients may be asymptomatic or may present with abdominal pain or an abdominal mass. Some patients present with anemia, weight loss, malaise, and fever, suggestive of an infectious disease. The lesions may or may not be associated with splenomegaly and are usually solitary, although occasional multifocal lesions are seen. Inflammatory pseudotumors are characteristically well circumscribed, but not encapsulated, with a white or yellow cut surface that may contain areas of necrosis (Fig. 20-87). They can vary greatly in size, from 1.5 to over 12 cm. Microscopically, they are composed of an admixture of cells. Lymphocytes and plasma cells are present at least focally, and foci of neutrophils and occasional eosinophils may also be present. Clusters of histiocytes, often foamy, are present in some tumors. Fibrosis, sclerosis, plump spindled cells and often vascular proliferation are other characteristic features of these tumors (Fig. 20-88). Foci of necrosis are present in some cases. Although the etiology of most cases of inflammatory pseudotumor at any site is not known, at least

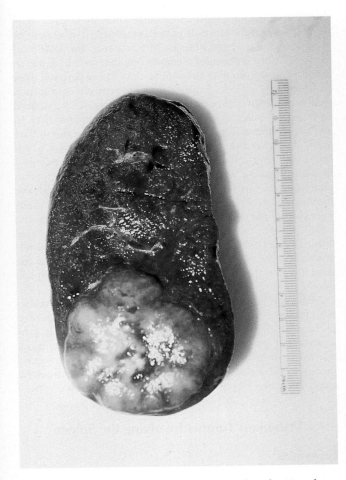

Fig. 20-87. Inflammatory pseudotumor of the spleen forming a large, well circumscribed nodule, simulating a malignant neoplasm.

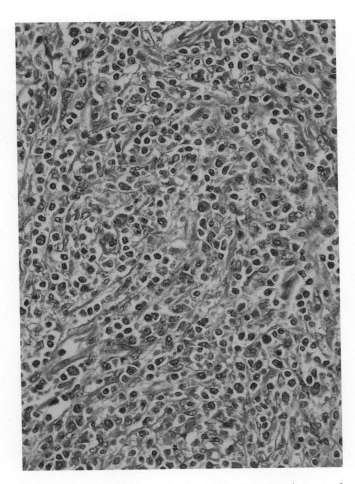

Fig. 20-88. Inflammatory pseudotumor of the spleen. An admixture of stromal cells, lymphocytes, and plasma cells is present.

some contain evidence of the EBV.[566] In particular, the spindled cells of some splenic inflammatory pseudotumors have been shown to contain this virus.

The gross appearance of these tumors may simulate a metastatic lesion, and the morphologic features may superficially mimic those of Hodgkin's disease. The lack of identifiable Reed-Sternberg cells or their mononuclear variants excludes such a neoplastic process.

Localized Reactive Lymphoid Hyperplasia

Small localized hyperplastic foci of the spleen have been reported, usually in spleens of normal weight, which may grossly mimic malignant tumors.[567] Similar to inflammatory pseudotumors, these foci are well circumscribed, but are not encapsulated. They are smaller than inflammatory pseudotumors, usually 0.1 to 1.0 cm, and contain prominent reactive follicular hyperplasia. Some cases may have accompanying sclerosis and a plasma cell infiltrate. The surrounding splenic white pulp in these cases frequently shows evidence of reactive hyperplasia. These lesions offer a similar differential diagnosis to inflammatory pseudotumors, and caution must be used in diagnosing lo-

calized reactive lymphoid hyperplasia in the setting of Hodgkin's disease. In these cases, it is advisable to examine multiple tissue levels for the presence of neoplastic cells.

The relationship between these lesions and inflammatory pseudotumor is not clear because there is some overlap in the morphologic features of the two proliferations in the spleen. Small size and the presence of abundant lymphoid hyperplasia would favor a diagnosis of localized reactive lymphoid hyperplasia.

Systemic Mast Cell Disease

Systemic mast cell disease, or mastocytosis, is a rare multiorgan proliferation of mast cells that may be subclassified into benign and malignant categories. Patients with malignant mastocytosis have an associated malignant tumor, usually a myeloproliferative disorder or myelodysplasia, and usually do not have the cutaneous involvement seen in benign mast cell disease. Over two-thirds of patients with systemic mast cell disease have splenomegaly,[568] and a splenectomy specimen may be the first diagnostic specimen received in such a patient. The spleen may vary widely in weight, from a normal weight to over 2,000 g.[510,568] The largest spleens are seen in patients with malignant mastocytosis, although pathologic examination of the spleen alone cannot conclusively distinguish between the benign and malignant forms of mast cell disease. The splenic capsule usually shows fibrous thickening, and the cut surface demonstrates an expanded red pulp without prominent white pulp. In spleens of near normal weight, no other gross lesions may be identifiable. One to two millimeter nodules may be identified throughout the cut surface in the more enlarged specimens.

Microscopically, the grossly identified nodules represent multiple areas of fibrosis, usually radiating from blood vessels, or nodular collections of mast cells. The mast cells have central, dark staining, round to irregular nuclei and abundant, often clear cytoplasm or they may have a more spindled cell appearance admixed with a surrounding fibrous stroma (Fig. 20-89). Only rarely, more typical mast cells with basophilic or granular cytoplasm may be present, and eosinophils are more obvious than the mast cells in many cases. Despite the pattern, the fibrous areas of the spleen are almost pathognomonic of mast cell

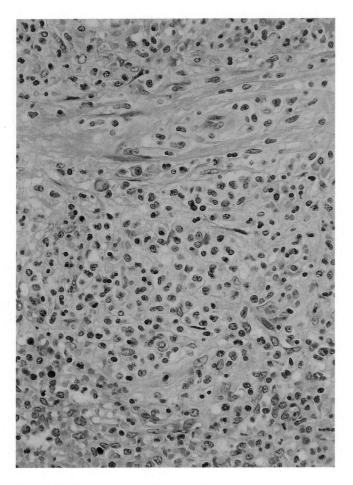

Fig. 20-89. Systemic mast cell disease of the spleen. An aggregate of mast cells with abundant clear cytoplasm is present with adjacent fibrosis.

disease, forming multiple areas of stellate fibrosis. Both a diffuse red pulp and focal white pulp pattern of splenic involvement by mastocytosis have been described[568]; however, the multifocal fibrotic pattern is the most common one that we see. These fibrous areas are often so prominent that the underlying mast cells are easily missed. Identification of the pattern of fibrosis as well as the scattered eosinophils should increase the surgical pathologist's index of suspicion of a mast cell proliferation. In addition to the multiple aggregates of mast cells or the stellate areas of fibrosis, the splenic red pulp may be expanded in patients with mast cell disorders. Extramedullary hematopoiesis is frequently present. Mast cells are generally positive for chloracetate esterase, Giemsa, and toluidine blue stains, although the demonstration of neoplastic mast cells with cytochemical stains is frequently pH dependent.[569] Mast cells may also express the CD43, CD45, and CD68 antigens.[570] Although all of these antigens can be detected in paraffin sections, they are also relatively nonspecific and we find the H&E findings to be the most useful in the diagnosis of splenic involvement by mast cell disease.

Malignant mast cell disease is associated with several malignant tumors.[571] In the spleen, these patients may have acute or chronic myeloproliferative disorders or myelodysplastic syndromes that infiltrate the splenic red pulp. Careful attention, therefore, must be placed on the identification of a second process in these patients. Solid tumors, in organs other than the spleen, may also be present in patients with mast cell disease.

Malignant Tumors Involving the Spleen

Leukemias

Acute leukemias may secondarily involve the spleen with resultant splenomegaly. Both acute myeloid and lymphoblastic leukemia predominantly involve the splenic red pulp. Blast cells are identifiable in both the splenic cords and sinuses as a relatively monotonous cell composition with fine nuclear chromatin and a high mitotic rate. Lymphoblasts may be difficult to distinguish from small lymphocytes if the cytologic details are not well preserved. Paraffin section immunohistochemistry may be helpful in determining the lineage of the cellular infiltrate as well as confirming the immature nature of lymphoid cells. Myeloperoxidase staining will identify the majority of cells of myeloid derivation. Precursor-B lymphoblasts may be identified by staining for both the B cell antigen CD79a and TdT. CD3 antigen and TdT expression may be detected in many cases of acute lymphoblastic leukemia of T lineage. An even more detailed phenotypic analysis may be performed if fresh tissue is submitted for flow cytometric evaluation.

The chronic myeloproliferative disorders all generally cause splenomegaly to varying degrees. Splenectomy may be performed for some of these disorders, most notably for *myelosclerosis with myeloid metaplasia* (agnogenic myeloid metaplasia).[572] In myelosclerosis with myeloid metaplasia, the spleen is almost always significantly enlarged, averaging approximately 2,000 g.[573,574] The splenic capsule is often thickened with patchy fibrosis, and the spleen has a homogeneous red to brown cut surface with indistinct malpighian corpuscles. Areas of infarction may be present, especially in the larger spleens. Gross nodules corresponding to areas of hematopoiesis are occasionally seen. Microscopically, the white pulp is decreased or absent with little or no germinal center formation. The red pulp is congested with prominent areas of extramedullary hematopoiesis present in both the cords and sinuses, but primarily within the splenic cords (Fig. 20-90). Of the maturing hematopoietic elements, the megakaryocytes are the most morphologically striking, showing dysplastic features with smaller cells and pleomorphic nuclei as well as the presence of immature megakaryocytes.[574,575] Fibrosis of the red pulp cords may be prominent, especially in the larger spleens. The etiology of this fibrosis appears to differ from the bone marrow fibrosis seen in these patients and does not appear to be related to the megakaryocyte proliferation. Instead, the spleen fibrosis appears to be secondary to splenic congestion, similar to the red pulp fibrosis found in patients with portal hypertension. Additional cases may demonstrate a red pulp plasmacytosis, and others may contain areas of hemorrhage and scarring. The morphologic findings of the spleen in myelosclerosis with myeloid metaplasia are not pathognomonic and similar findings may be found in the other chronic myeloproliferative disorders, especially chronic myelogenous leukemia. Correlation with clinical, cytogenetic, peripheral blood, and bone marrow findings are all essential for the proper classification of these disorders.

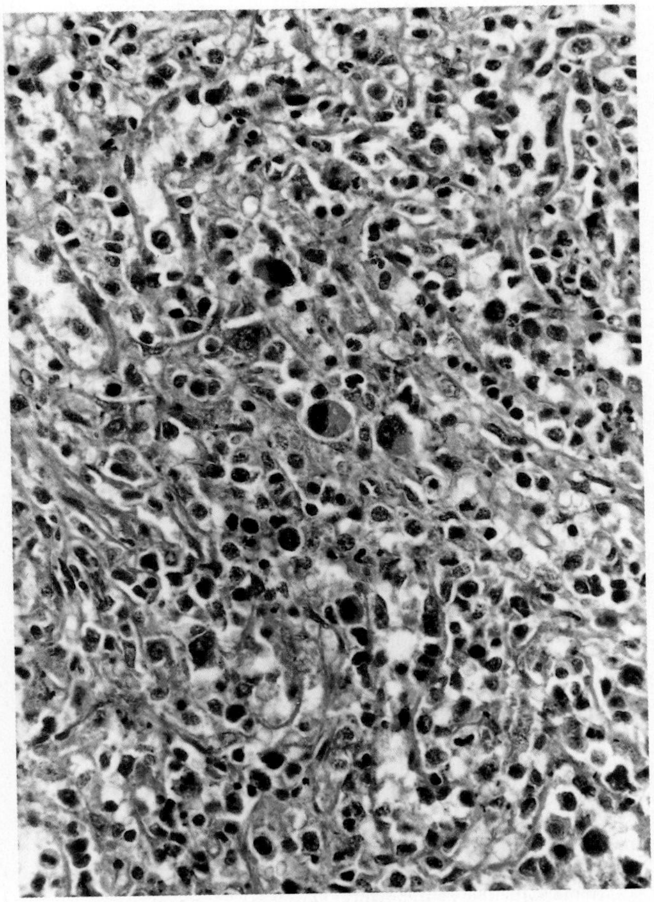

In *chronic myelogenous leukemia*, the red pulp infiltrate of the spleen may show more numerous maturing myeloid cells and a lesser degree of extramedullary hematopoiesis than seen in myelosclerosis with myeloid metaplasia. Varying numbers of blast cells may also be present, and blast crisis of chronic myelogenous leukemia may present with a rapidly enlarging spleen. In *essential thrombocythemia*, the spleen may be small and atrophic or enlarged.[56] When enlarged, the red pulp is congested and contains numerous platelet-filled histiocytes. Occasional megakaryocytes may be present, but other evidence of extramedullary hematopoiesis is not prominent. In *polycythemia vera*, there are two different patterns of splenomegaly.[576] In the erythrocytotic phase of polycythemia vera, the white pulp is decreased and there is marked congestion of the red pulp by red blood cells. This congestion is presumably secondary to the elevated red blood cell mass in these patients. Extramedullary hematopoiesis is minimal, and the average splenic weight is 800 to 900 g. In the spent phase of polycythemia vera, the spleen is even larger, averaging over 2,000 g. Marked extramedullary hematopoiesis is present in the splenic cords and sinuses with all three bone marrow cells lines evident. Immature precursor cells become more evident as the spleen enlarges.

The chronic lymphoid leukemias also frequently involve the spleen. *Chronic lymphocytic leukemia* and *prolymphocytic leukemia* primarily involve the splenic white pulp with secondary involvement of the red pulp. This distribution is discussed in more detail below with small lymphocytic lymphoma. *Hairy cell leukemia* is a rare chronic lymphoid leukemia of B lineage that frequently presents in elderly patients with pancytopenia and splenomegaly.[507] The spleen in this disorder is massively enlarged, usually over 1,000 g, although splenic involvement by hairy cell leukemia without splenomegaly has been reported.[577] The spleen has a homogeneous cut surface with diminished malpighian bodies. Unlike the majority of chronic lymphoproliferative disorders of B lineage, hairy cell leukemia primarily involves the splenic red pulp. A diffuse red pulp proliferation, with or without residual white pulp follicles, is present, and is composed of small, relatively homogeneous lymphoid cells with ovoid nuclei and abundant clear to pink staining cytoplasm (Fig. 20-91). Dilated, blood-filled sinuses, also known as red cell lakes, may be present, but are not pathognomonic. Paraffin section immunohistochemistry for CD20 may be useful to identify the marked increase of B lineage cells within the red pulp. In addition, the cells are characteristically DBA.44 positive. Frozen section or flow cytometric immunophenotyping will identify a monoclonal B cell population that is CD5– and CD10–, while commonly expressing CD11c, CD25, and CD103. Imprint preparations will more clearly demonstrate the cytologic features of the tumor cells than can be appreciated on H&E sections. The cells have slightly indented nuclei with abundant cytoplasm and irregular (hairy) cytoplasmic borders. Cytochemical studies may be performed on imprint preparations to demonstrate the characteristic tartrate-resistant acid phosphatase positivity of the hairy cells.

Large granular lymphocytosis is a T cell or NK cell proliferation that is associated with neutropenia and an increased risk

Fig. 20-90. Myelosclerosis with myeloid metaplasia. Extramedullary hematopoiesis is present in the splenic red pulp. Megakaryocytes are the cell type most easily identified.

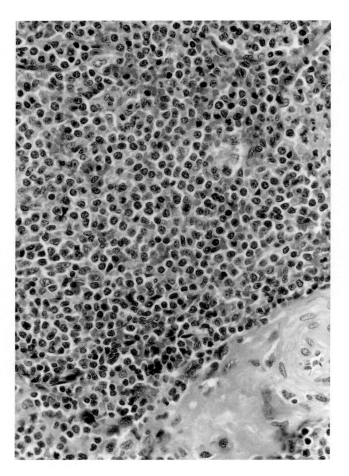

Fig. 20-91. Hairy cell leukemia. A monotonous population of small lymphoid cells with moderately abundant cytoplasm diffusely replacs the splenic red pulp.

fections. Splenectomy has been reported to reduce the degree of neutropenia in these patients.[578] Grossly the spleen is enlarged, weighing from 450 to 1,650 g with no gross lesions.[578,579] Microscopically, the white pulp may be expanded, but uninvolved by the neoplastic proliferation while the red pulp is expanded by the tumor cells. On H&E sections, the infiltrate has the appearance of small lymphocytes and may be confused with hairy cell leukemia. Well fixed sections, however, will show that the cells lack the abundant clear cytoplasm of hairy cells. Imprint preparations show the characteristic large cytoplasmic granules that are associated with the NK/T cell phenotype of this proliferation. Immunohistochemical studies will also exclude a B cell proliferation such as hairy cell leukemia. The large granular lymphocytes are often CD3+ or mark for the less specific, T lineage-associated antigen CD43. Many cases also express CD57 (Leu 7), which can also be detected by paraffin section immunohistochemistry. Frozen section or flow cytometric immunophenotyping may identify additional T lineage antigens or the NK cell-associated antigens CD16 or CD56. Correlation with the peripheral blood and clinical findings are helpful in the differential diagnosis with other T cell proliferations, especially hepatosplenic T cell lymphoma.

Malignant Lymphoma Secondarily Involving the Spleen

Malignant lymphoma of the spleen usually represents secondary involvement. Any of the malignant lymphomas previously described can secondarily involve the spleen with morphologic features similar to lymph node involvement. A great deal has been written concerning the pattern of splenic involvement by various malignant tumors, especially lymphoma.[580–583a] Traditionally, malignant lymphomas of B lineage and chronic lymphocytic leukemia are described as involving primarily the white pulp whereas acute leukemias, chronic myeloproliferative disorders, histiocytic malignant tumors, and T cell lymphomas reportedly primarily involve the splenic red pulp. These generalizations hold true for the leukemias, but are fairly inconsistent for the malignant lymphomas. Immunophenotyping studies demonstrate that some T lineage neoplasms involve the white pulp primarily and many B lineage lymphomas may primarily involve the red pulp.

Table 20-17 shows the overlap of pattern of splenic lymphomas. Most low grade B cell lymphomas diffusely involve the splenic white pulp and often cause gross accentuation of the malpighian bodies. The spleen may be massively enlarged in these patients. In chronic lymphocytic leukemia and small lymphocytic lymphoma, the markedly expanded white pulp nodules fuse to form large dumbbell-shaped aggregates of tumor. In addition, small lymphoid cells of B lineage spill over into the surrounding red pulp (Fig. 20-92). This secondary red pulp infiltration is a helpful feature in distinguishing reactive white pulp hyperplasia from splenic lymphoma because this differential diagnosis may be problematic in patients that undergo

Table 20-17. Common Patterns of Splenic Involvement by Hematopoietic Malignant Tumors

Predominantly white pulp disease
  Chronic lymphocytic leukemia/small lymphocytic lymphoma
  Prolymphocytic leukemia
  Follicular center lymphoma[a]
  Mantle cell lymphoma
  Splenic marginal zone lymphoma/marginal zone B cell lymphoma
  Lymphoplasmacytic lymphoma[a]
  Early involvement by B lineage large cell and immunoblastic lymphoma[a]

Predominantly red pulp disease
  Acute myeloid leukemia
  Acute lymphoblastic leukemia/lymphoblastic lymphoma
  Chronic myeloproliferative disorders
  Hairy cell leukemia
  Lymphoplasmacytic lymphoma[a]
  Hepatosplenic T cell lymphoma
  Large granular lymphocytosis
  Some T cell lymphomas[a]
  Rare B lineage large cell lymphomas[a]

Predominantly nodular disease
  Most large cell and immunoblastic lymphomas, B or T lineage[a]
  Some follicular center lymphomas[a]
  Hodgkin's disease

[a] More than one pattern may be seen with these tumor types.

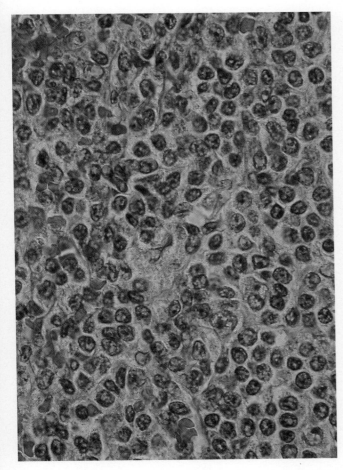

Fig. 20-92. Small lymphocytic lymphoma/chronic lymphocytic leukemia. Small lymphocytes with scattered larger prolymphocytes expand the splenic white pulp and secondarily infiltrate the red pulp. This red pulp involvement, demonstrated in the figure, is a helpful clue in the diagnosis of splenic involvement by lymphoma.

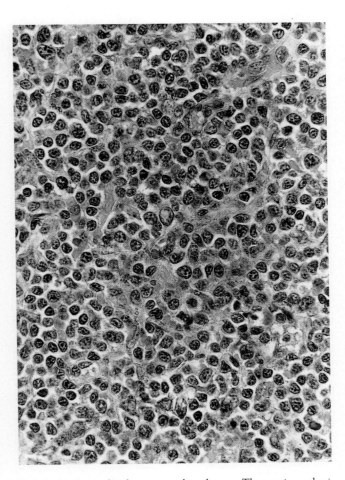

Fig. 20-93. Lymphoplasmacytic lymphoma. The entire splenic parenchyma may be replaced by plasmacytoid cells. The identification of intranuclear inclusions (Dutcher bodies) is a useful diagnostic feature.

splenectomy for presumed ITP that is actually related to low grade lymphoma. Early involvement of the spleen by lymphoma may be morphologically similar to the expanded white pulp of an ITP patient and immunohistochemical studies are useful to demonstrate an abnormal increase in red pulp B lymphocytes in involved spleens. Prolymphocytoid transformation of small lymphocytic lymphoma and prolymphocytic leukemia may show a zone of transformed cells at the periphery of the expanded white pulp, adjacent to the red pulp.[584]

Lymphoplasmacytic lymphomas may have the white pulp pattern of small lymphocytic lymphomas or may diffusely infiltrate the splenic red pulp (Fig. 20-93). The frequent presence of intranuclear inclusions, or Dutcher bodies, is helpful in distinguishing this type of lymphoma from leukemic infiltrates, including hairy cell leukemia. Monotypic light chain expression of the plasmacytoid cells is often identifiable with paraffin section immunohistochemistry in these cases.

Mantle cell lymphoma of the spleen shows a similar pattern of splenic involvement to small lymphocytic lymphoma, but

does not contain the larger prolymphocytes seen in small lymphocytic lymphoma (Fig. 20-94). Clusters of epithelioid histiocytes may be present in cases of mantle cell lymphoma and may obscure the neoplastic infiltrate in rare cases.

Follicular lymphomas also primarily involve the splenic white pulp. They generally involve the central portion of the malpighian body with surrounding residual non lymphomatous white pulp elements. With extensive splenic involvement, follicular nodules may become evident within a markedly expanded white pulp nodule.

Large cell and immunoblastic lymphomas of either T or B lineage frequently form tumor nodules that are grossly apparent. Such nodules are presumably overgrowths of the white pulp. These firm tan-white nodules are grossly similar to splenic involvement by metastatic carcinoma or Hodgkin's disease (Fig. 20-95). Some T cell lymphomas will not form nodules and will primarily involve the splenic red pulp. Many such cases in the past were considered examples of malignant histiocytosis. Rarely, large cell lymphomas of B lineage will primarily involve the splenic red pulp (Fig. 20-96), and immunohistochemical studies may be necessary to differentiate these tumors from T

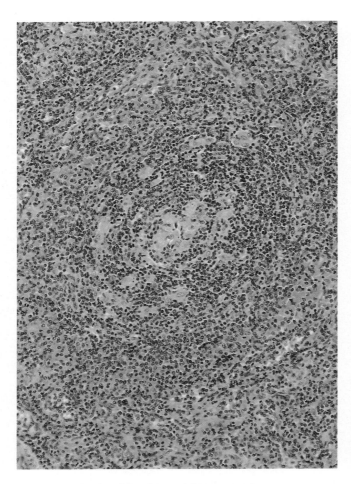

Fig. 20-94. Mantle cell lymphoma. A distinct mantle zone pattern may not be obvious in all cases. The lack of prolymphocytes is useful in distinguishing this lymphoma type from small lymphocytic lymphoma.

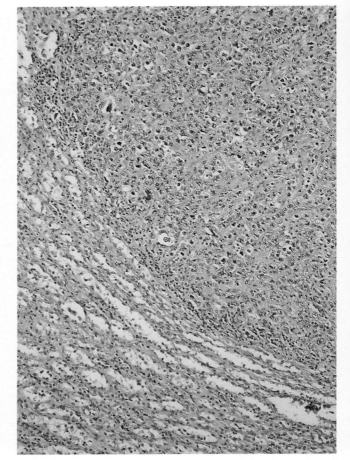

Fig. 20-95. Large cell lymphoma forming a large tumor aggregate within the spleen.

cell lymphomas or leukemic infiltrates. These case have also been interpreted as variants of angiotropic B cell lymphoma. Because of the great variability in the pattern of splenic involvement by malignant lymphoma, it is ill advised to presume lineage of a process without immunophenotypic studies.

Hodgkin's disease characteristically forms grossly obvious tumor nodules that are similar to the nodules of large cell lymphoma and metastatic carcinoma (Fig. 20-97). Very early involvement of the spleen by Hodgkin's disease may only demonstrate a small tan-white nodule and may grossly mimic an area of accentuated white pulp. The spleen should be carefully examined for such minute nodules in any patient with a history of Hodgkin's disease. As discussed previously, however, the presence of granulomatous inflammation is not sufficient for a diagnosis of splenic involvement by Hodgkin's disease. Reed-Sternberg cells or their mononuclear variants must be identified for such a diagnosis. Nodular lymphocyte predominance Hodgkin's disease only rarely involves extranodal sites, but when present, it also generally forms tumor nodules in the spleen.[585]

Primary Splenic Lymphomas

Any type of malignant lymphoma may on rare occasion present as a primary splenic lymphoma,[583a, 586–588] although most cases that present with splenomegaly have evidence of disease elsewhere at the time of splenectomy. For this reason, it is not clear if these cases actually represent primary splenic lymphomas and some authors have used the term malignant lymphoma with prominent splenomegaly rather than primary splenic lymphoma.[589] Three more recently described disorders appear to be unique to the spleen and are discussed in more detail.

Splenic Marginal Zone Lymphoma

Splenic marginal zone lymphoma appears to be a unique form of B cell lymphoma that was primarily believed to arise from the marginal zone of the splenic white pulp.[590–593] The tumor is apparently distinct from nodal "marginal zone" lymphomas such as low grade B cell lymphoma of mucosa-associated lymphoid tissue and monocytoid B cell lymphoma,[9] although primary splenic monocytoid B cell lymphoma and splenic marginal zone

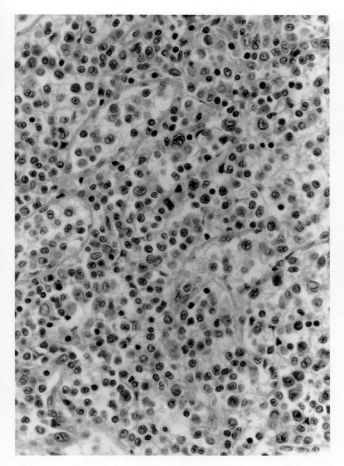

Fig. 20-96. Large cell lymphoma primarily involving the splenic red pulp. This relatively unusual pattern of splenic involvement by large cell lymphoma can easily be mistaken for splenic involvement by acute leukemia.

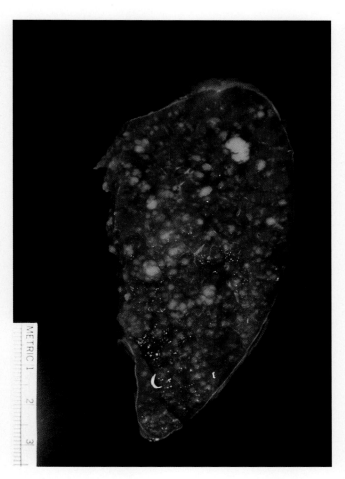

Fig. 20-97. Hodgkin's disease. A similar gross pattern of splenic involvement may be seen with large cell lymphoma.

lymphoma probably represent the same disease process. This entity was originally described by Neiman et al[590] in 1979 as a malignant lymphoma that simulated hairy cell leukemia.

In most cases, the spleen is massively enlarged, weighing 1,000 g or more. Rarely, involved spleens are normal in weight or only slightly enlarged, apparently representing an early phase of the disease.[594] The cut splenic surface of the cases with splenomegaly show a miliary pattern similar to the gross pattern of involvement by other low grade lymphomas. On microscopic examination, the white pulp is markedly expanded. This expansion is due to an increase in cells in the marginal zone of the spleen as well as the smaller lymphocytes of the central white pulp (Fig. 20-98). The marginal zone lymphoma cells are small to medium-sized lymphocytes with moderately abundant cytoplasm and little to no nuclear pleomorphism. In addition to the expanded marginal zones, aggregates of lymphoma cells form small nodules within the splenic red pulp. The neoplastic B cells are characteristically CD20+, CD5–, and usually CD43–.

The differential diagnosis of splenic marginal zone lymphoma includes hairy cell leukemia and reactive marginal zone cell hyperplasia. The diffuse red pulp involvement of hairy cell leukemia, sparing the residual white pulp, is not seen in marginal zone lymphoma. In addition, the neoplastic marginal zone cells differ from hairy cells by being tartrate-resistant acid phosphatase negative and usually negative for the antigens CD11c and CD103. An expanded marginal zone may also be seen in reactive conditions and in follicular lymphomas involving the spleen and care must be taken not to overdiagnosis marginal zone lymphoma in these cases. The lack of a red pulp component is helpful in suggesting a reactive process. Immunophenotyping or molecular studies for clonality are useful for this differential diagnosis, especially in cases that are not accompanied by massive splenic enlargement.

Splenic Lymphoma with Circulating Villous Lymphocytes

Splenic lymphoma with circulating villous lymphocytes (SLVL) is a rare clinicopathologic disorder that is most common in elderly males and is characterized by splenomegaly, a mild lymphocytosis, and circulating lymphocytes with unipolar villous cytoplasmic projections.[595] Clinically, the disorder is most likely to mimic hairy cell leukemia; however, the gross ap-

T lymphocytes. Although the majority of normal circulating T lymphocytes are alpha/beta T cells, approximately 4 percent of T cells carry the gamma/delta T cell antigen receptor. In the normal spleen, these gamma/delta cells are over-represented, accounting for approximately 17 percent of all splenic T lymphocytes, and are localized to the splenic red pulp.[607]

Patients with hepatosplenic T cell lymphoma are usually adolescents or young men who present with hepatosplenomegaly and no adenopathy. The patients may also have anemia and/or thrombocytopenia and subtle bone marrow involvement by disease at the time of diagnosis. Most do not have peripheral blood involvement by lymphoma, although one such case has been reported.[608] Grossly, the spleen is usually massively enlarged, often weighing several thousand grams, with a diffuse pattern of involvement. On microscopic examination, the red pulp cords and sinuses are extensively infiltrated by medium to large lymphoid cells with open nuclear chromatin and slightly irregular nuclear contours (Fig. 20-99). The cells may have moderately abundant cytoplasm, imparting a low power impression of splenic involvement by hairy cell leukemia. Rare cases of hepatosplenic T cell lymphoma are associated with prominent erythrophagocytosis, presumably

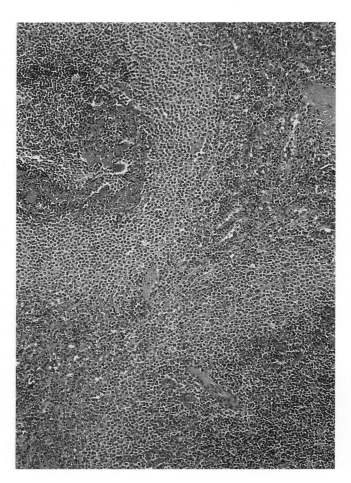

Fig. 20-98. Splenic marginal zone lymphoma. The marginal zone is expanded by cells with pale staining cytoplasm. Small aggregates of similar cells are usually also seen within the splenic red pulp.

pearance of the enlarged spleen in SLVL shows the miliary pattern more characteristic of a low grade lymphoma. Histologically, SLVL appears to represent a heterogeneous group of malignant lymphomas, although one report has suggested that SLVL and splenic marginal zone lymphoma are identical disease.[596] Other reports suggest that SLVL may encompass several lymphoma types.[595,597] As an example, t(11;14)(q13;q32), commonly seen in mantle cell lymphomas, is present in approximately 15 to 20 percent of cases of SLVL.[598] We favor the concept that a variety of malignant lymphomas can cause the syndrome of SLVL, and we prefer to classify the underlying splenic lymphoma based on the morphologic, immunologic, and molecular characteristics of the tumor. Therefore, we do not use the term "splenic lymphoma with circulating villous lymphocytes" diagnostically.

Hepatosplenic T Cell Lymphoma

This rare type of lymphoma is also known as hepatosplenic gamma/delta T cell lymphoma and probably includes cases originally described as erythrophagocytic T-gamma lymphoma.[408,599–606] It is a neoplastic proliferation of gamma/delta

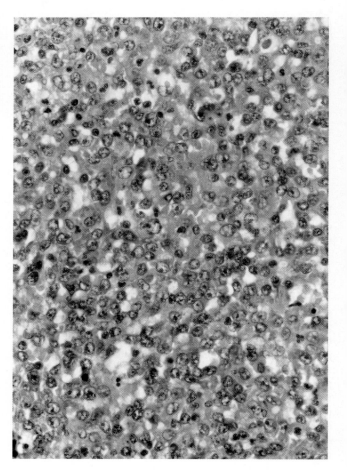

Fig. 20-99. Hepatosplenic T cell lymphoma. The splenic red pulp is expanded by a mixture of medium-sized and large lymphoid cells.

mimicking malignant histiocytosis, but this feature is not pronounced in most cases. Involvement of the hepatic sinuses by identical neoplastic T cells exists at the time of splenectomy.

Immunophenotyping easily excludes hairy cell leukemia from the differential diagnosis by the failure to identify evidence of B lineage. On paraffin sections, the neoplastic cells are usually positive for the T lineage and T lineage-associated antigens CD3, CD43, and CD45RO. Frozen section or flow cytometric immunophenotyping will identify the presence of additional T lineage associated antigens, and will often demonstrate loss of T cell antigen expression. The cells differ from alpha/beta T cells by being characteristically CD4– and CD8–. Some cases are reported to express NK cell-associated antigens, including CD16 and CD56, although this does not appear to be a constant finding in this type of lymphoma. The neoplastic cells fail to immunoreact with the beta-F1 antibody that detects the beta chain of alpha/beta T cells, whereas they generally react with the delta 1 antibody or other antibodies for the T cell delta or gamma chains. T cell receptor gamma chain gene rearrangements are detectable in these patients whereas beta chain rearrangements may or may not be detectable.

In addition to hairy cell leukemia, the morphologic findings of hepatosplenic T cell lymphoma overlap with splenic involvement by large granular lymphocytosis (LGL). A morphologic distinction between these two diseases may not be possible and the clinical setting must be considered. In LGL, the patients are older and frequently have an autoimmune disease. In addition, many LGL cases have CD57+ lymphocytes, an antigen that is not commonly expressed by hepatosplenic T cell lymphoma cells.

Although the delta and beta chain antibodies are not routinely available in many laboratories, the diagnosis of hepatosplenic T cell lymphoma can still be made. The identification of a T cell phenotype of the neoplastic cells in a diffuse red pulp pattern is generally sufficient for the diagnosis in the clinicopathologic setting of a young person with massive hepatosplenomegaly and no evidence of adenopathy.

Malignant Vascular Tumors

Angiosarcoma is the most common primary nonhematopoietic malignant tumor of the spleen.[545,609] In a series of 40 primary angiosarcomas of the spleen, Falk et al[610] found this tumor to occur at a median age of 59 years with no sex predilection. Unlike angiosarcoma of the liver, there is no apparent relationship between splenic tumors and exposure to arsenic, vinyl chloride, or Thorotrast. Most patients present with splenomegaly and abdominal pain and have a short survival, often dying within a year of diagnosis. Thirteen to 18 percent of patients will present with spontaneous splenic rupture and the disease is often associated with peripheral blood cytopenias and coagulation disorders.

Grossly, the spleen is enlarged, usually weighing over 500 g.[610] The cut splenic surface characteristically demonstrates multiple nodules, some of which may have a diffuse, infiltrating pattern or hemorrhagic cystic spaces. Areas of hemorrhage are present in over one-half of cases and approximately one-quarter of cases will have associated areas of infarction. Microscopically, angiosarcoma of the spleen may demonstrate great morphologic variation (Fig. 20-100). Solid areas of sarcomatous proliferation may be difficult to distinguish from malignant fibrous histiocytoma or fibrosarcoma on H&E stained sections alone. More vascular areas, however, are invariably present in other areas of the tumor, forming irregular vascular channels with atypical endothelial cells. Papillary and spindle cell patterns may also be seen. Hobnail cells with enlarged, atypical nuclei may be present, even in the absence of an obvious increase in mitotic figures. Immunohistochemical studies demonstrate vascular antigen expression in the tumor cells, which are characteristically factor VIII-related antigen and CD31 antigen positive.

Epithelioid hemangioendothelioma and epithelioid and spindle-cell hemangioendothelioma are low grade angiosarcomas that have abundant epithelioid cells and small signet ring-like vascular tumor cells. These tumors have a similar clinical presentation and gross appearance to high grade angiosarcomas, but several reports suggest a better survival than typical angiosarcomas of the spleen.[611,612]

The differential diagnosis of angiosarcoma includes both benign and malignant proliferations. Benign vascular proliferations, such as hemangiomas and peliosis, do not demonstrate

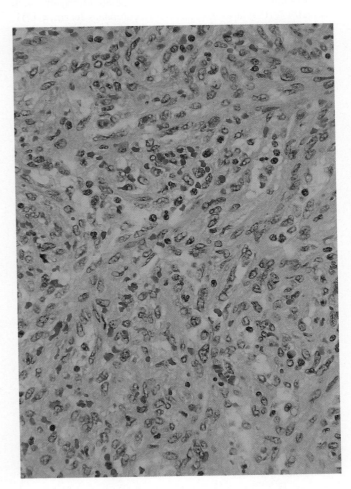

Fig. 20-100. Angiosarcoma of the spleen. Solid areas of spindled cells may mimic other types of sarcoma.

the nuclear atypia of angiosarcoma. In addition, the lack of an infiltrating gross and microscopic pattern into the surrounding red pulp is useful for the diagnosis of hemangioma. Littoral cell angiomas do have nuclear enlargement of lining cells, but not the nuclear atypia of angiosarcoma. A single case of *littoral cell angiosarcoma* has been reported[613] in which cytologic atypia was present as well as an infiltrating gross appearance and immunohistochemical evidence of both vascular and histiocytic antigen expression.

Kaposi's sarcoma may also rarely involve the spleen.[610,614] When present, Kaposi's sarcoma usually forms small tumor nodules without associated hemorrhage, in contrast to the more characteristic massive splenic involvement with hemorrhage of angiosarcoma. Numerous hyaline globules are also frequently present in Kaposi's sarcoma, as are areas of collagenous fibrosis. These features are uncommon in angiosarcoma.

The distinction of angiosarcoma from other sarcomas, especially malignant fibrous histiocytoma and fibrosarcoma, can be difficult in tumors that have extensive solid sarcomatous areas. Even when this pattern predominates, foci of irregular vascular channels lined by atypical tumor cells are usually present; therefore, extensive tumor sampling is essential. The immunohistochemical detection of vascular-associated antigens, such as factor VIII-related antigen, Ulex europaeus lectin, CD31, and CD34, is also helpful in excluding other types of sarcomas.

Other Sarcomas and Metastatic Tumors

Other primary sarcomas of the spleen are extremely rare, with reports of malignant fibrous histiocytoma, fibrosarcoma, and leiomyosarcoma primarily involving the spleen.[545,609] Careful sampling and immunohistochemical studies help to exclude an angiosarcoma mimicking one of these rare tumors.

Metastatic tumors involving the spleen are also quite rare and are usually discovered on autopsy. Solitary metastases may present with splenomegaly and may be treated with splenectomy.[615] Rare cases of splenic rupture have also been reported due to metastatic tumors.[616,617] In one autopsy series, one-third of patients with splenic metastases had no gross evidence of splenic tumor. When grossly seen, the majority of tumors formed large nodules, often with areas of necrosis. Lung and breast carcinomas are the most common primary tumors to metastasize to the spleen, although virtually any tumor may secondarily involve the spleen on rare occasions.[618]

REFERENCES

1. Pitts WC, Weiss LM: The role of fine needle aspiration biopsy in diagnosis and management of hematopoietic neoplasms. pp. 385–405. In Knowles DM (ed): Neoplastic Hematopathology. Williams & Wilkins, Baltimore, 1992
2. Arber DA, Weiss LM: CD43: a review. Appl Immunohistochem 1:88–96, 1993
3. Picker LJ, Weiss LM, Medeiros LJ, et al: Immunophenotypic criteria for the diagnosis of non-Hodgkin's lymphoma. Am J Pathol 128:181–201, 1987
4. Stein H, Lennert K, Feller AC, Mason DY: Immunohistological analysis of human lymphoma: correlation of histological and immunological categories. Adv Cancer Res 42:67–147, 1984
5. Braylan RC, Benson NA, Nourse VA: Cellular DNA of human neoplastic B-cells measured by flow cytometry. Cancer Res 44:5010–5016, 1984
6. Costa A, Mazzini G, Delbino G, Silvestra R: DNA content and kinetic characteristics of non-Hodgkin's lymphoma: determined by flow cytometry and autoradiography. Cytometry 2:185–188, 1981
7. Shackney SE, Skramstad KS, Cunningham RE, et al: Dual parameter flow cytometry studies in human lymphomas. J Clin Invest 66:1281–1294, 1980
8. Zukerberg LR, Medeiros LJ, Ferry JA, Harris NL: Diffuse low-grade B-cell lymphomas: four clinically distinct subtypes defined by a combination of morphologic and immunophenotypic features. Am J Clin Pathol 100:373–385, 1993
9. Harris NL, Jaffe ES, Stein H, et al: A revised European-American classification of lymphoid neoplasms. A proposal from the International Lymphoma Study Group. Blood 84:1361–1392, 1994
10. Weiss LM, Spagnolo DV: Assessment of clonality in lymphoid proliferations. Am J Pathol 142:1579–1582, 1993
11. Sklar J, Weiss LM: Application of antigen receptor gene rearrangements to the diagnosis and characterization of lymphoid neoplasms. Ann Rev Med 39:315–334, 1988
12. Cossman J, Aehnbauer B, Garrett C, et al: Gene rearrangements in the diagnosis of lymphoma/leukemia: guidelines for use based on a multiinstitutional study. Am J Clin Pathol 95:347–354, 1991
13. Cossman J, Uppenkamp M, Sundeen J, et al: Molecular genetics and the diagnosis of lymphoma. Arch Pathol Lab Med 134:117–127, 1988
14. Davis RE, Warnke RA, Dorfman RF, Cleary ML: Utility of molecular genetic analysis for the diagnosis of neoplasia in morphologically and immunophenotypically equivocal hematolymphoid lesions. Cancer 67:2890–2899, 1991
15. Hu E, Horning S, Flynn S, et al: Diagnosis of B cell lymphoma by analysis of immunoglobulin gene rearrangements in biopsy specimens obtained by fine needle aspiration. J Clin Oncol 4:278–283, 1986
16. Anastasi J: Interphase cytogenetic analysis in the diagnosis and study of neoplastic disorders. Am J Clin Pathol, suppl. 95:S22–S28, 1991
17. Aster JC, Kobayashi Y, Shiota M, et al: Detection of the t(14;18) at similar frequencies in hyperplastic lymphoid tissues from American and Japanese patients. Am J Pathol 141:291–299, 1992
18. Fisher ER, Gregorio RM, Redmond C, et al: Pathologic findings from the National Surgical Adjuvant Breast Project (Protocol No. 4). III The significance of extranodal extension of axillary metastasis. Am J Clin Pathol 65:439–444, 1976
19. Wells CA, Heryet A, Brochier J, et al: The immunocytochemical detection of axillary micrometastases in breast cancer. Br J Cancer 50:193–197, 1984
20. Chang KL, Arber DA, Weiss LM: CD30: a review. Appl Immunohistochem 1:244–255, 1993
21. Weiss LM, Arber DA, Chang KL: CD45: a review. Appl Immunohistochem 1:166–181, 1993
22. Weiss LM, Movahed LA, Butler AE, et al: Analysis of lymphoepithelioma and lymphoepithelioma-like carcinomas for Epstein-Barr viral genomes by in situ hybridization. Am J Surg Pathol 13:625–631, 1989
23. Robert NJ, Garnick MB, Frei E: Cancers of unknown origin: current approaches and future perspectives. Semin Oncol 9:526–531, 1983
24. Jesse RH, Perez CA, Fletcher G: Cervical lymph node metastasis; unknown primary cancer. Cancer 31:854–859, 1973
25. Copeland EM, McBride CM: Axillary metastasis from an unknown primary site. Ann Surg 178:25–27, 1973
26. Molinari R, Cantu G, Chiesa F, et al: A statistical approach to detection of the primary cancer based on the site of neck lymph node metastases. Tumori 63:267–282, 1977
27. Ryan JR, Ioachim HL, Marmer J, Loubeau JM: Acquired immune deficiency syndrome-related lymphadenopathies presenting in the salivary gland lymph nodes. Arch Otolaryngol 111:554–556, 1985

28. Holdsworth PJ, Hopkinson JM, Leveson SH: Benign axillary epithelial lymph node inclusions—a histological pitfall. Histopathology 13:226–228, 1988

29. Rosai J, Carcangiu ML, DeLellis RA: Tumors of the Thyroid Gland. Vol. 3. Armed Forces Institute of Pathology, Washington DC, 1992

30. Karp LA, Czernobilsky B: Glandular inclusions in pelvic and abdominal paraaortic lymph nodes, a study of autopsy and surgical material in males and females. Am J Clin Pathol 52:212–218, 1969

31. Clement PB: Pathology of endometriosis. Pathol Annu 1:245–295, 1990

32. Mills SE: Decidual and squamous metaplasia in abdomino-pelvic lymph nodes. Int J Gynecol Pathol 2:209–215, 1983

33. Bautista NC, Cohen S, Anders KH: Benign melanocytic nevus cells in axillary lymph nodes. A prospective incidence and immunohistochemical study with literature review. Am J Clin Pathol 102:102–108, 1994

34. Epstein JL, Erlandson RA, Rosen PP: Nodal blue nevi: a study of three cases. Am J Surg Pathol 8:907–915, 1984

35. Warnke RA, Weiss LM, Chan JKC, et al: Tumors of the Lymph Nodes and Spleen. Armed Forces Institute of Pathology, Washington DC, 1995

36. Chan JKC, Warnke RA, Dorfman RF: Vascular transformation of sinuses in lymph nodes: a study of its morphologic spectrum and distinction from Kaposi's sarcoma. Am J Surg Pathol 15:732–743, 1991

37. Cook PD, Czerniak B, Chan JKC, et al: Nodular spindle cell vascular transformation of lymph nodes: a benign process occurring predominantly in retroperitoneal lymph nodes draining carcinomas that can simulate Kaposi's sarcoma or metastatic tumor. Am J Surg Pathol 19:1010–1020, 1995

38. Chan JKC, Lewin KJ, Lombard CD, et al: The histopathology of bacillary angiomatosis of lymph nodes. Am J Surg Pathol 14:430–437, 1991

39. Finkbeiner WE, Egbert BM, Groundwater JR, Sagebiel RW: Kaposi's sarcoma in young homosexual men, a histopathologic study with particular reference to lymph node involvement. Arch Pathol Lab Med 106:261–264, 1982

40. Chang Y, Cesarman E, Pessin MS, et al: Identification of herpesvirus-like DNA sequences in AIDS-associated Kaposi's sarcoma. Science 266:1865–1869, 1994

41. Tsang WYW, Chan JKC, Dorfman RF, Rosai J: Vasoproliferative lesions of lymph nodes. Pathol Annu 29(Pt 1):63–133, 1994

42. Chan JK, Frizzera G, Fletcher CD, Rosai J: Primary vascular tumors of lymph nodes other than Kaposi's sarcoma: analysis of 39 cases and delineation of two new entities. Am J Surg Pathol 16:335–350, 1992

43. Chan JK, Tsang WY, Pau MY, et al: Lymphangiomyomatosis and angiomyolipoma: closely related entities characterized by hamartomatous proliferation of HMB-45-positive smooth muscle. Histopathology 22:445–455, 1993

44. Channer JL, Davies JD: Smooth muscle proliferation in the hilum of superficial lymph nodes. Virchows Arch [A] 406:261–270, 1985

45. Abell MR, Littler ER: Benign metastasizing uterine leiomyoma: multiple lymph node metastasis. Cancer 36:2206–2213, 1975

46. Davis RE, Warnke RA, Dorfman RF: Inflammatory pseudotumor of lymph nodes. Additional observations and evidence for an inflammatory etiology. Am J Surg Pathol 15:744–756, 1991

47. Perrone T, De Wolf-Peeters C, Frizzera G: Inflammatory pseudotumor of lymph nodes. A distinctive pattern of nodal reaction. Am J Surg Pathol 12:351–361, 1988

48. Chen KTK: Mycobacterial spindle cell pseudotumor of lymph nodes. Am J Surg Pathol 16:276–281, 1992

49. Fletcher CD, Stirling RW: Intranodal myofibroblastoma presenting in the submandibular region: evidence of a broader clinical and histological spectrum. Histopathology 16:287–293, 1990

50. Suster S, Rosai J: Intranodal hemorrhagic spindle cell tumor with "amianthoid" fibers. Report of six cases of a distinctive mesenchymal

51. neoplasm of the inguinal region that simulates Kaposi's sarcoma. Am J Surg Pathol 13:341–346, 1989

51. Weiss SW, Gnepp DR, Bratthauer GL: Palisaded myofibroblastoma. A benign mesenchymal tumor of lymph node. Am J Surg Pathol 13:341–346, 1989

52. Michaeli J, Niesvizky R, Siegel D, et al: Proteinaceous (angiocentric sclerosing) lymphadenopathy: a polyclonal stemic, nonamyloid deposition disorder. Blood 86:1159–1162, 1995

53. MacKenzie DH: Amyloidosis presenting as lymphadenopathy. BMJ 2:1449–1450, 1963

54. Ordi J, Grau JM, Junque A, et al: Secondary (AA) amyloidosis associated with Castleman's disease. Report of two cases and review of the literature. Am J Clin Pathol 100:393–397, 1993

55. Nathwani BN, Winberg CD, Diamond LW, et al: Morphologic criteria for the differentiation of follicular lymphoma from florid reactive follicular hyperplasia: a study of 80 cases. Cancer 48:1794–1806, 1981

56. Rappaport H: Tumors of the hematopoietic system. Series I, Armed Forces Institute of Pathology, Washington, DC, 1966

57. Ngan BY, Picker LJ, Medeiros LJ, Warnke RA: Immunophenotypic diagnosis of non-Hodgkin's lymphoma in paraffin sections. Co-expression of L60(Leu-22) and L26 antigens correlates with malignant histologic findings. Am J Clin Pathol 91:579–583, 1989

58. Wood BL, Bacchi MM, Bacchi CE, et al: Immunocytochemical differentiation of reactive hyperplasia from follicular lymphoma using monoclonal antibodies to cell surface and proliferation-related markers. Appl Immunohistochem 2:48–53, 1994

59. Utz GL, Swerdlow SH: Distinction of follicular hyperplasia from follicular lymphoma in B5-fixed tissues: comparison of MT2 and bcl-2 antibodies. Hum Pathol 24:1155–1158, 1993

60. Segal GH, Scott M, Jorgensen T, Braylan RC: Standard polymerase chain reaction analysis does not detect a t(14;18) in reactive lymphoid hyperplasia. Arch Pathol Lab Med 118:791–794, 1994

61. Banks PM, Chan J, Cleary ML, et al: Mantle cell lymphoma. A proposal for unification of morphologic, immunologic, and molecular data. Am J Surg Pathol 16:637–640, 1992

62. Doggett RS, Colby TV, Dorfman RF: Interfollicular Hodgkin's disease. Am J Med 78:22–28, 1983

63. Osborne BM, Butler JJ: Clinical implications of nodal reactive follicular hyperplasia in elderly patients with enlarged lymph nodes. Mod Pathol 4:24–30, 1991

64. Nosanchuk JS, Schnitzer B: Follicular hyperplasia in lymph nodes from patients with rheumatoid arthritis. Cancer 24:343–354, 1969

65. Kondratowicz GM, Symmons DP, Bacon PA, et al: Rheumatoid lymphadenopathy: a morphological and immunohistochemical study. J Clin Pathol 43:106–113, 1990

66. McCurley TJ, Collins D, Ball E, Collins RD: Nodal and extranodal lymphoproliferative disorders in Sjogren's syndrome: a clinical and immunopathologic study. Hum Pathol 21:482–492, 1990

67. Fishleder A, Tubbs R, Hesse B, Levine H: Uniform detection of immunoglobulin-gene rearrangement in benign lymphoepithelial lesions. N Engl J Med 316:1118–1121, 1987

68. Chan JKC, Hui PK, Ng CS, et al: Epithelioid hemangioma (angiolymphoid hyperplasia with eosinophilia) and Kimura's disease in Chinese. Histopathology 15:557–574, 1989

69. Hui PK, Chan JKC, Ng CS, et al: Lymphadenopathy in Kimura's disease. Am J Surg Pathol 13:177–186, 1989

70. Kuo TT, Shih LY, Chan HL: Kimura's disease. Involvement of regional lymph nodes and distinction from angiolymphoid hyperplasia with eosinophilia. Am J Surg Pathol 12:843–854, 1988

71. Dorfman RF, Remington JS: Value of lymph node biopsy in the diagnosis of toxoplasmosis. N Engl J Med 289:878–881, 1973

72. Stansfeld AG: The histologic diagnosis of toxoplasmic lymphadenitis. J Clin Pathol 14:565–573, 1961

73. Weiss LM, Chen YY, Berry GJ, et al: Infrequent detection of

Toxoplasma gondii genome in toxoplasmic lymphadenitis: a polymerase chain reaction study. Hum Pathol 23:154–158, 1992

74. Hartsock RJ, Halling LW, King FM: Luetic lymphadenitis: a clinical and histologic study of 20 cases. Am J Clin Pathol 53:304–314, 1970

75. Hansmann M-L, Fellbaum C, Hui PK, Moubayed P: Progressive transformation of germinal centers with and without association to Hodgkin's disease. Am J Clin Pathol 93:219–226, 1990

76. Poppema S, Kaiserling E, Lennert K: Hodgkin's disease with lymphocyte predominance, nodular type (nodular paragranuloma) and progressively transformed germinal centers: a cytohistologic study. Histopathology 3:295–308, 1979

77. Burns BF, Colby TV, Dorfman RF: Differential diagnostic features of nodular L&H Hodgkin's disease, including progressive transformation of germinal centers. Am J Surg Pathol 8:253–261, 1984

78. Osborne BM, Butler JJ: Clinical implications of progressive transformation of germinal centers. Am J Surg Pathol 8:725–733, 1984

79. Frizzera G: Castleman's disease and related disorders. Semin Diagn Pathol 5:346–364, 1988

80. Keller AR, Hochholzer L, Castleman B: Hyaline-vascular and plasma-cell types of giant lymph node hyperplasia of mediastinum and other locations. Cancer 29:670–683, 1972

81. Flendrig JA: Benign giant lymphoma: clinicopathologic correlation study. pp. 296–299. In Clark RL, Curnley RW (eds): The Year Book of Cancer. Year Book Medical, Chicago; 1970

82. Danon AD, Krishnan J, Frizzera G: Morpho-immunophenotypic diversity of Castleman's disease, hyaline-vascular type: with emphasis on a stroma-rich variant and a new pathogenetic hypothesis. Virchows Arch [A] 423:369–382, 1993

83. Madero S, Onate JM, Garzon A: Giant lymph node hyperplasia in an angiolipomatous mediastinal mass. Arch Pathol Lab Med 110:853–855, 1986

84. Gerald W, Kostianovsky M, Rosai J: Development of vascular neoplasia in Castleman's disease. Am J Surg Pathol 14:603–614, 1990

85. Chan JKC, Tsang WYW, Ng CS: Follicular dendritic cell tumor and vascular neoplasm complicating hyaline-vascular Castleman's disease. Am J Surg Pathol 18:517–525, 1994

86. Harris NL, Bhan AK: "Plasmacytoid T cells" in Castleman's disease: immunohistologic phenotype. Am J Surg Pathol 11:109–113, 1987

87. Soulier J, Grollet L, Oksenhendler E, et al: Molecular analysis of clonality in Castleman's disease. Blood 86:1131–1138, 1995

88. Kahn LB, Ranchod M, Stables DP, et al: Giant lymph node hyperplasia with haematological abnormalities. S Afr Med J 47:811–816, 1973

89. Beck JT, Hus SM, Wijdenes J, et al: Alleviation of systemic manifestations of Castleman's disease by monoclonal interleukin-6 antibody. N Engl J Med 330:602–605, 1994

90. Radaszkiewicz T, Hannsmann ML, Lennert K: Monoclonality and polyclonality of plasma cells in Castleman's disease of the plasma cell variant. Histopathology 14:11–24, 1989

91. Hsu SM, Waldron JA, Xie SS, Barlogie B: Expression of interleukin-6 in Castleman's disease. Hum Pathol 24:833–839, 1993

92. Frizzera G, Peterson BA, Bayrd ED, Goldman A: A systemic lymphoproliferative disorder with morphologic features of Castleman's disease: clinical findings and clinicopathologic correlations in 15 patients. J Clin Oncol 3:1202–1216, 1985

93. Weisenburger DD, Nathwani BN, Winberg CD, Rappaport H: Multicentric angiofollicular lymph node hyperplasia: a clinicopathologic study of 16 cases. Hum Pathol 16:162–172, 1985

94. Bitter MA, Komaiko W, Franklin WA: Giant lymph node hyperplasia with osteoblastic bone lesions and the POEMS (Takatsuki's) syndrome. Cancer 56:188–194, 1985

95. Frizzera G, Massarelli G, Banks PM, Rosai J: A systemic lymphoproliferative disorder with morphologic features of Castleman's disease: pathological findings in 15 patients. Am J Surg Pathol 7:211–231, 1983

96. Hanson CA, Frizzera G, Patton DF, et al: Clonal rearrangement for immunoglobulin and T-cell receptor genes in systemic Castleman's disease: association with Epstein-Barr virus. Am J Pathol 131:84–91, 1988

97. Soulier J, Grollet L, Oksenhendler E, et al: Kaposi's sarcoma-associated herpesvirus-like DNA sequences in multicentric Castleman's disease. Blood 86:1276–1280, 1995

98. Centers for Disease Control and Prevention: Persistent, generalized lymphadenopathy among homosexual males. MMWR 31:249–251, 1982

99. Chadburn A, Metroka C, Mouradian J: Progressive lymph node histology and its prognostic value in patients with acquired immunodeficiency syndrome and AIDS-related complex. Hum Pathol 20:579–587, 1989

100. Brynes RK, Chan WC, Spira TJ, et al: Value of lymph node biopsy in unexplained lymphadenopathy in homosexual men. JAMA 250:1313–1317, 1983

101. Ioachim HL, Cronin W, Roy M, Maya M: Persistent lymphadenopathies in people at high risk for HIV infection. Clinicopathologic correlations and long-term follow-up in 79 cases. Am J Clin Pathol 93:208–218, 1990

102. Pileri S, Rivano MT, Raise E, et al: The value of lymph node biopsy in patients with acquired immunodeficiency syndrome (AIDS) and the AIDS-related complex (ARC): a morphological and immunohistochemical study of 90 cases. Histopathology 10:1107–1129, 1986

103. Burns BF, Wood GS, Dorfman RF: The varied histopathology of lymphadenopathy in the homosexual male. Am J Surg Pathol 9:287–297, 1985

104. Biberfeld P, Chayt KJ, Marselle LM, et al: HTLV-III expression in infected lymph nodes and relevance to pathogenesis of lymphadenopathy. Am J Pathol 125:436–442, 1986

105. Wood GS, Garcia CF, Dorfman RF, Warnke RA: The immunohistology of follicle lysis in lymph node biopsies from homosexual men. Blood 66:1092–1097, 1985

106. Childs CC, Parham DM, Berard CW: Infectious mononucleosis: the spectrum of morphologic changes simulating lymphoma in lymph nodes and tonsils. Am J Clin Pathol 53:304–314, 1987

107. Strickler JG, Fedeli F, Hurwitz CA, et al: Infectious mononucleosis in lymphoid tissue. Histopathology, in situ hybridization, and differential diagnosis. Arch Pathol Lab Med 117:269–278, 1993

108. Shin SS, Berry GJ, Weiss LM: Infectious mononucleosis: diagnosis by in situ hybridization in two cases with atypical features. Am J Surg Pathol 15:625–631, 1991

109. Vago JF, Titman WE, Swerdlow SH: CMV-associated lymphadenopathy in the "normal" host: a histopathologic and immunophenotypic description, abstracted. Lab Invest 60:100A, 1989

110. Younes M, Podesta A, Helie M, Buckley P: Infection of T but not B lymphocytes by cytomegalovirus in lymph nodes. An immunophenotypic study. Am J Surg Pathol 15:75–80, 1991

111. Rushin JM, Riordan GP, Heaton RB, et al: Cytomegalovirus-infected cells express Leu-M1 antigen: a possible source of diagnostic error. Am J Pathol 136:989–995, 1990

112. Tamaru J, Atsuo M, Horie H, et al: Herpes simplex lymphadenitis. Report of two cases with review of the literature. Am J Surg Pathol 14:571–577, 1990

113. Gaffey MJ, Ben-Ezra J, Weiss LM: Herpes simplex lymphadenitis. Am J Clin Pathol 95:709–714, 1991

114. Gams RA, Neal JA, Conrad FG: Hydantoin-induced pseudolymphoma. Ann Intern Med 69:557–568, 1968

115. Saltzstein SL, Ackerman LV: Lymphadenopathy induced by anticonvulsant drugs clinically and pathologically mimicking malignant lymphomas. Cancer 12:164–182, 1959

116. Abbondanzo SL, Irye NS, Frizzera G: Dilantin-associated lymphadenopathy: spectrum of histopathologic patterns. Am J Surg Pathol 19:675–686, 1995

117. Gould E, Porto R, Albores-Saavedra J, Ibe MJ: Dermatopathic lymphadenitis. The spectrum and significance of its morphologic features. Arch Pathol Lab Med 112:1145–1150, 1988

118. Burke JS, Colby TV: Dermatopathic lymphadenopathy. Comparison of cases associated and unassociated with mycosis fungoides. Am J Surg Pathol 5:343–352, 1981

119. Weiss LM, Beckstead JH, Warnke RA, Wood GS: Leu 6 expressing lymph node cells are dendritic cells and closely related to interdigitating cells. Hum Pathol 17:179–184, 1986

120. Rausch E, Kaiserling E, Goos M: Langerhans cells and interdigitating reticulum cells in the thymus-dependent region in human dermatopathic lymphadenitis. Virchows Arch B (Cell Pathol) 25:327–343, 1977

121. Albores-Saavedra J, Vuitch F, Delgado R, et al: Sinus histiocytosis of pelvic lymph nodes after hip replacement. A histiocytic proliferation induced by cobalt-chromium and titanium. Am J Surg Pathol 18:83–90, 1994

122. Black MM, Speer F: Sinus histiocytosis of lymph node in cancer. Surg Gynecol Obstet 106:163–175, 1958

123. Listinsky CM: Common reactive erythrophagocytosis in axillary lymph nodes. Hum Pathol 89:189–192, 1988

124. Gould E, Perez J, Albores-Saavedra J, Legaspi A: Signet ring cell sinus histiocytosis: a previously unrecognized histologic condition mimicking metastatic adenocarcinoma in lymph node. Am J Clin Pathol 92:509–512, 1989

125. Plank L, Hansmann ML, Fischer R: The cytological spectrum of the monocytoid B-cell reaction: recognition of its large cell type. Histopathology 23:425–431, 1993

126. Sheibani K, Fritz RM, Winberg CD, et al: "Monocytoid" cells in reactive follicular hyperplasia with and without multifocal histiocytic reactions: an immunohistochemical study of 21 cases including suspected cases of toxoplasmosis lymphadenitis. Am J Clin Pathol 81:453–458, 1984

127. Sohn CC, Sheibani K, Winberg CD, Rappaport H: Monocytoid B lymphocytes: their relation to the patterns of the acquired immuno-deficiency syndrome (AIDS) and AIDS-related lymphadenopathy. Hum Pathol 16:979–985, 1985

128. Nathwani BN, Mohrmann RS, Brynes RK, et al: Monocytoid B-cell lymphomas: an assessment of diagnostic criteria and a perspective on histogenesis. Hum Pathol 23:1061–1071, 1992

129. Risdall RJ, McKenna RW, Nesbitt ME, et al: Virus associated hemophagocytic syndrome. A benign histiocytic proliferation distinct from malignant histiocytosis. Cancer 44:993–1002, 1979

130. McKenna RW, Risdall RJ, Brunning RD: Virus associated hemophagocytic syndrome. Hum Pathol 12:395–398, 1981

131. Favara BE: Hemophagocytic lymphohistiocytosis: a hemophagocytic syndrome. Semin Diagn Pathol 9:63–74, 1992

132. Kikuta H, Sakiyama T, Matsumoto S, et al: Fatal Epstein-Barr virus-associated hemophagocytic syndrome. Blood 82:3259–3264, 1993

133. Chen R-L, Su I-J, Lin K-H, et al: Fulminant childhood hemo-phagocytic syndrome mimicking histiocytic medullary reticulosis. An atypical form of Epstein-Barr virus infection. Am J Clin Pathol 96:171–176, 1991

134. Farquhar JW, Claireaux AF: Familial hemophagocytic reticulosis. Arch Dis Child 27:519–525, 1952

135. Ladisch S, Holiman B, Poplack DG, Blaese RM: Immunodeficiency in familial erythrophagocytic lymphohistiocytosis. Lancet 1:581–583, 1978

136. Jaffe ES, Costa J, Fauci AS, et al: Malignant lymphoma and erythrophagocytosis simulating malignant histiocytosis. Am J Med 75:741–749, 1983

137. Falini B, Pileri S, DeSolas I, et al: Peripheral T-cell lymphoma associated with hemophagocytic syndrome. Blood 75:434–444, 1990

138. Wong KF, Chan JK: Reactive hemophagocytic syndrome—a clinico-

139. Chang C-S, Wang C-H, Su I-J, et al: Hematophagic histiocytosis: a clinicopathologic analysis of 23 cases with special reference to the association with peripheral T-cell lymphoma. J Formos Med Assoc 93:421–428, 1994

140. Rosai J, Dorfman RF: Sinus histiocytosis with massive lymphadenopathy: a newly recognized benign clinicopathologic entity. Arch Pathol 87:63–70, 1969

141. Rosai J, Dorfman RF: Sinus histiocytosis with massive lymphadenopathy: a pseudolymphomatous benign disorder. Analysis of 34 cases. Cancer 30:1174–1188, 1972

142. Foucar E, Rosai J, Dorfman RF: Sinus histiocytosis with massive lymphadenopathy (Rosai-Dorfman disease). Review of the entity. Semin Diagn Pathol 7:19, 1990

143. Leighton SEJ, Gallimore AP: Extranodal sinus histiocytosis with massive lymphadenopathy affecting the subglottis and trachea. Histopathology 24:393–394, 1994

144. Montgomery EA, Meis JM, Frizzera G: Rosai-Dorfman disease of soft tissue. Am J Surg Pathol 16:122–129, 1992

145. Komp DM: The treatment of sinus histiocytosis with massive lymphadenopathy (Rosai-Dorfman disease). Semin Diagn Pathol 7:83–86, 1990

146. Eisen RN, Buckley PJ, Rosai J: Immunophenotypic characterization of sinus histiocytosis with massive lymphadenopathy (Rosai-Dorfman disease). Semin Diagn Pathol 7:74–82, 1990

147. Naiem M, Gerdes J, Abdulaziz A, et al: Production of a monoclonal antibody reactive with human dendritic cells and its use in the immunohistological analysis of lymphoid tissue. J Clin Pathol 36:167–175, 1983

148. Parwaresch MR, Radzun HJ, Hansmann M-L, Peters K-P: Monoclonal antibody Ki-M4 specifically recognizes human dendritic cells (follicular dendritic cells) and their possible precursors in blood. Blood 62:585–590, 1983

149. Bonetti F, Chilosi M, Menestrina F, et al: Immunohistological analysis of Rosai-Dorfman histiocytosis. A disease of S-100+CD1– histiocytes. Virchows Arch [A] 411:129–135, 1987

150. Relman DA, Schmidt TM, McDermott RP, Falkow S: Identification of the uncultured bacillus of Whipple's disease. N Engl J Med 327:293–301, 1992

151. Fleming JL, Wiesner RH, Shorter RG: Whipple's disease: clinical, biochemical, and histopathologic features and assessment of treatment in 29 patients. Mayo Clin Proc 63:539–551, 1988

152. Schnitzer B: Reactive lymphoid hyperplasia. pp. 22–56. In Jaffe ES (ed): Surgical Pathology of the Lymph Nodes and Related Organs. Vol. 16. WB Saunders, Philadelphia, 1985

153. Sieracki JC, Fine G: Whipple's disease—observations on systemic involvement: II. Gross and histologic observations. Arch Pathol 67:81–93, 1959

154. Ravel R: Histopathology of lymph nodes after lymphangiography. Am J Clin Pathol 46:335–340, 1966

155. Truong LD, Cartwright J, Goodman D, Woznicki D: Silicone lymphadenopathy associated with augmentation mammoplasty: morphologic features of nine cases. Am J Surg Pathol 12:484–491, 1988

156. Warner NE, Friedman NB: Lipogranulomatous pseudosarcoid. Ann Intern Med 45:662–673, 1956

157. Strickler JG, Warnke RA, Weiss LM: Necrosis in lymph nodes. Pathol Annu 22 (Pt 2):253–282, 1987

158. Cleary KR, Osborne BM, Butler JJ: Lymph node infarction fore-shadowing malignant lymphoma. Am J Surg Pathol 6:435–442, 1982

159. Norton AJ, Ramsey AD, Isaacson PG: Antigen preservation in infarcted lymphoid tissue: a novel approach to the infarcted lymph node using monoclonal antibodies effective in routinely processed tissues. Am J Surg Pathol 12:759–767, 1988

160. Kikuchi M: Lymphadenitis showing focal reticulum cell hyperplasia

with nuclear debris and phagocytes: a clinico-pathological study (in Japanese). Nippon Ketsueki Gakkai Zasshi 35:379–380, 1972

161. Fujimoto Y, Kozima Y, Yamaguchi K: Cervical subacute necrotizing lymphadenitis. A new clinicopathologic entity. Naika 20:920–927, 1972

162. Pileri S, Kikuchi M, Helbron D, Lennert K: Histiocytic necrotizing lymphadenitis without granulocytic infiltration. Virchows Arch (Pathol Anat) 395:257–271, 1982

163. Dorfman RF, Berry GJ: Kikuchi's histiocytic necrotizing lymphadenitis: an analysis of 108 cases with emphasis on differential diagnosis. Semin Diagn Pathol 5:329–345, 1988

164. Chamulak GA, Brynes RK, Nathwani BN: Kikuchi-Fujimoto disease mimicking malignant lymphoma. Am J Surg Pathol 14:514–523, 1990

165. Feller AC, Lennert K, Stein H, et al: Immunohistology and aetiology of histiocytic necrotizing lymphadenitis: report of three instructive cases. Histopathology 7:825–829, 1983

166. Medeiros LJ, Kaynor B, Harris NL: Lupus lymphadenitis: report of a case with immunohistologic studies on frozen sections. Hum Pathol 20:295–299, 1989

167. Goldsmith RW, Gribetz D, Strauss L: Mucocutaneous lymph node syndrome (MLNS) in the continental United States. Pediatrics 57:431–435, 1976

168. Giesker DW, Pastuszak WT, Forouhar FA, et al: Lymph node biopsy for early diagnosis in Kawasaki disease. Am J Surg Pathol 6:493–501, 1982

169. Cook MG: The size and histological appearances of mesenteric lymph nodes in Crohn's disease. Gut 13:970–972, 1972

170. Bascom R, Johns CJ: The natural history and management of sarcoidosis. Adv Intern Med 31:213–241, 1986

171. Hollingsworth HC, Longo DL, Jaffe ES: Small noncleaved cell lymphoma associated with florid epithelioid granulomatous response: a clinicopathologic study of seven patients. Am J Surg Pathol 17:51–59, 1993

172. Braylan RC, Long JC, Jaffe ES, et al: Malignant lymphoma obscured by concomitant extensive epithelioid granulomas. Cancer 39:1146–1155, 1977

173. Sacks EL, Donaldson SS, Gordon J, Dorfman RF: Epithelioid granulomas associated with Hodgkin's disease: clinical correlations in 55 previously untreated patients. Cancer 41:562–567, 1978

174. van den Oord JJ, de Woolf-Peeters C, Facchetti F, Desmet VJ: Cellular composition of hypersensitivity-type granulomas. Immunohistochemical analysis of tuberculous and sarcoidal lymphadenitis. Hum Pathol 15:559–565, 1984

175. Facchetti F, Agostini C, Chilosi M, et al: Suppurative granulomatous lymphadenitis. Immunohistochemical evidence for a B-cell-associated granuloma. Am J Surg Pathol 16:955–961, 1992

176. Reid JD, Wolinsky E: Histopathology of lymphadenitis caused by atypical mycobacteria. Am Rev Respir Dis 99:8–12, 1969

177. Barnett RN, Hull JG, Vortel V: Pneumocystis carinii in lymph nodes and spleen. Arch Pathol Lab Med 88:175–180, 1969

178. Korbi S, Toccanier MF, Leyvraz G, et al: Use of silver staining (Dieterle's stain) in the diagnosis of cat scratch disease. Histopathology 10:1015–1021, 1986

179. Wear DJ, Margileth AM, Hadfield TL, et al: Cat-scratch disease: a bacterial infection. Science 221:1403–1404, 1983

180. Anderson B, Sims K, Regnery R, et al: Detection of Rochalimaea henselae DNA in specimens from cat scratch disease patients by PCR. J Clin Microbiol 32:942–948, 1994

181. Alkan S, Morgan MB, Sandin RL, et al: Dual role for Afipia felis and Rochalimaea henselae in cat-scratch disease, letter. Lancet 345:385, 1995

182. Naji AF, Carbonell F, Barker HJ: Cat scratch disease, a report of three new cases, review of the literature, and classification of the pathologic changes in the lymph nodes during various stages of the disease. Am J Clin Pathol 38:513–521, 1962

183. Walzer PD, Armstrong D: Lymphogranuloma venereum presenting as supraclavicular and inguinal lymphadenopathy. Sex Transm Dis 4:12–14, 1977

184. Schapers RFM, Reif R, Lennert K, Knapp W: Mesenteric lymphadenitis due to Yersinia enterocolitica. Virchows Arch A (Pathol Anat Histol) 390:127–138, 1981

185. Lukes RJ, Tindle BH: Immunoblastic lymphadenopathy: a hyperimmune entity resembling Hodgkin's disease. N Engl J Med 292:1–8, 1975

186. Frizzera G, Moran EM, Rappaport H: Angio-immunoblastic lymphadenopathy with dysproteinemia. Lancet 1:1070–1073, 1974

187. Frizzera G, Moran EM, Rappaport H: Angio-immunoblastic lymphadenopathy. Diagnosis and clinical course. Am J Med 59:803–818, 1975

188. Nathwani BN, Rappaport H, Moran EM, et al: Malignant lymphoma arising in angio-immunoblastic lymphadenopathy. Cancer 41:578–606, 1978

189. Shimoyama M, Minato K, Saito H, et al: Immunoblastic lymphadenopathy (IBL)-like T-cell lymphoma. Jpn Clin Oncol, suppl. 9:347–356, 1979

190. Watanabe S, Sato Y, Shimoyama M, et al: Immunoblastic lymphadenopathy, angioimmunoblastic lymphadenopathy, and IBL-like T-cell lymphoma. A spectrum of T-cell cell neoplasia. Cancer 58:2224–2232, 1986

191. Frizzera G, Kaneko Y, Sakurai M: Angioimmunoblastic lymphadenopathy and related disorders: a retrospective look in search of definitions. Leukemia 3:1–5, 1989

192. Weiss LM, Strickler JG, Dorfman RF, et al: Clonal T-cell populations in angioimmunoblastic lymphadenopathy and angioimmunoblastic lymphadenopathy-like lymphoma. Am J Pathol 122:392–397, 1986

193. Feller AC, Griesser H, Schilling CV, et al: Clonal gene rearrangement patterns correlate with immunophenotype and clinical parameters in patients with angioimmunoblastic lymphadenopathy. Am J Pathol 133:549–556, 1988

194. Lipford EH, Smith HR, Pittaluga S, et al: Clonality of angioimmunoblastic lymphadenopathy and implications for its evolution to malignant lymphoma. J Clin Invest 79:637–642, 1987

195. Schlegelberger B, Feller A, Godde W, Lennert K: Stepwise development of chromosomal abnormalities in angioimmunoblastic lymphadenopathy. Cancer Genet Cytogenet 50:15–29, 1990

196. Lukes RJ, Butler JJ: The pathology and nomenclature of Hodgkin's disease. Cancer Res 26:1063–1081, 1966

197. Lukes RJ, Craver LF, Hall TC, et al: Report of the nomenclature committee. Cancer Res 26:1311, 1966

198. Mason DY, Banks PM, Chan J, et al: Nodular lymphocyte predominance Hodgkin's disease: a distinct clinico-pathological entity. Am J Surg Pathol 18:528–530, 1994

199. Boring CC, Squires TS, Tong T: Cancer statistics, 1993. CA cancer J Clin 43:7–26, 1993

200. MacMahon B: Epidemiology of Hodgkin's disease. Cancer Res 26:1189–1200, 1966

201. Weiss LM, Chang KL: The association of the Epstein-Barr virus with hematolymphoid neoplasia. Adv Anat Pathol 3:1–15, 1996

202. Weiss LM, Chen Y-Y, Liu X-F, Shibata D: Epstein-Barr virus and Hodgkin's disease: a correlative in situ hybridization and polymerase chain reaction study. Am J Pathol 139:1259–1265, 1991

203. Mack TM, Cozen W, Shibata DK, et al: Concordance in identical twins suggests genetic susceptibility to young adult Hodgkin's disease. N Engl J Med 332:413–418, 1994

204. Prazak J, Hermanska Z: Study of HLA antigens in patients with Hodgkin's disease. Eur J Haematol 43:50–53, 1989

205. Gutensohn N, Cole P: Epidemiology of Hodgkin's disease in the young. Int J Cancer 19:595–604, 1977

206. Gutensohn N, Cole P: Epidemiology of Hodgkin's disease. Semin Oncol 7:92–102, 1980

207. Gutensohn N, Cole P: Childhood social environment and Hodgkin's disease. N Engl J Med 304:135–140, 1981

208. Grufferman S, Delzell E: Epidemiology of Hodgkin's disease. Epidemiol Rev 6:76–106, 1984

209. Kaplan HS: Hodgkin's Disease. Harvard University Press, Cambridge, MA, 1980

210. Lister TA, Crowther D, Sutcliffe SB, et al: Report of a committee convened to discuss the evaluation of staging of patients with Hodgkin's disease: Cotswolds meeting. J Clin Oncol 7:1630–1636, 1989

211. Lister TA, Crowther D: Staging for Hodgkin's disease. Sem Oncol 17:696–703, 1990

212. Urba WJ, Longo DL: Hodgkin's disease. N Engl J Med 326:678–687, 1992

213. Strickler JG, Michie SA, Warnke RA, Dorfman RF: The "syncytial variant" of nodular sclerosing Hodgkin's disease. Am J Surg Pathol 10:470–477, 1986

214. Ferry JA, Linggood RM, Convery KM, et al: Hodgkin's disease, nodular sclerosis type. Implications of histologic subclassification. Cancer 71:457–463, 1993

215. MacLennan KA, Bennett MJ, Tu A, et al: Relationship of histopathologic features to survival and relapse in nodular sclerosing Hodgkin's disease. Cancer 64:1686–1693, 1989

216. Georgii A, Fischer R, Hubner K, et al: Classification of Hodgkin's disease biopsies by a panel of four histopathologists. Report of 1,140 patients from the German National Trial. Leuk Lymphoma 9:365–370, 1993

217. Wijlhuizen TJ, Vrints LW, Jairam R, et al: Grades of nodular sclerosis (NSI-NSII) in Hodgkin's disease: are they of independent prognostic value? Cancer 63:1150–1153, 1989

218. Ashton-Key M, Thorpe PA, Allen JP, Isaacson PG: Follicular Hodgkin's disease. Am J Surg Pathol 19:1294–1299, 1995

219. Colby TV, Warnke RA: The histology of the initial relapse of Hodgkin's disease. Cancer 45:289–292, 1980

220. Colby TV, Hoppe RT, Warnke RA: Hodgkin's disease at autopsy: 1972–1977. Cancer 47:1852–1862, 1981

221. Das DK, Gupta SK, Datta BM, Sharma SC: Fine needle aspiration cytodiagnosis of Hodgkin's disease and its subtypes. I. Scope and limitations. Acta Cytol 34:329–336, 1989

222. Chittal SM, Caveriviere P, Schwarting R, et al: Monoclonal antibodies in the diagnosis of Hodgkin's disease. The search for a rational panel. Am J Surg Pathol 12:9–21, 1988

223. Chang KL, Arber DA, Weiss LM: CD20: a review. Appl Immunohistochem 4:1–15, 1996

224. Arber DA, Weiss LM: CD15: a review. Appl Immunohistochem 1:17–30, 1993

225. Chu W-S, Abbondanzo SL, Frizzera G: Inconsistency of the immunophenotype of Reed-Sternberg cells in simultaneous and consecutive specimens from the same patients. A paraffin section evaluation in 56 patients. Am J Pathol 141:11–17, 1992

226. Weiss LM, Chang KL: Molecular biologic studies of Hodgkin's disease. Semin Diagn Pathol 9:272–278, 1992

227. Weiss LM, Strickler JG, Hu E, et al: Immunoglobulin gene rearrangements in tissues involved by Hodgkin's disease. Hum Pathol 17:1006–1014, 1986

228. Tamaru J, Hummel M, Zemlin M, et al: Hodgkin's disease with a B-cell phenotype often shows a VDJ rearrangement and somatic mutations in the V$_H$ genes. Blood 84:708–715, 1994

229. Cabanillas F: A review and interpretation of cytogenetic abnormalities identified in Hodgkin's disease. Hematol Oncol 6:271–274, 1988

230. Chang KL, Chen Y-Y, Shibata D, Weiss LM: In situ hybridization methodology for the detection of EBV EBER-1 RNA in paraffin-embedded tissues, as applied to normal and neoplastic tissues. Diagn Mol Pathol 1:246–255, 1992

231. Schmid C, Pan L, Diss T, Isaacson PG: Expression of B-cell antigens by Hodgkin's and Reed-Sternberg cells. Am J Pathol 139:701–707, 1991

232. Kuzu I, Delsol G, Jones M, et al: Expression of the Ig-associated heterodimer (mb-1 and B29) in Hodgkin's disease. Histopathology 22:141–144, 1993

233. Delsol G, Meggetto F, Brousset P, et al: Relation of follicular dendritic reticulum cells to Reed-Sternberg cells of Hodgkin's disease with emphasis on the expression of CD21 antigen. Am J Pathol 142:1729–1738, 1993

234. Stetler-Stevenson M, Crush-Stanton S, Cossman J: Involvement of the bcl-2 gene in Hodgkin's disease. J Natl Cancer Inst 82:855–858, 1990

235. Orscheschek K, Mere H, Hell J, et al: Large-cell anaplastic lymphoma-specific translocation (t[2;5][p23;q35]) in Hodgkin's disease—indication of a common pathogenesis? Lancet 345:87–90, 1995

236. Weiss LM, Lopategui JR, Sun L-H, et al: Absence of the t(2;5) in Hodgkin's disease. Blood 85:2845–2847, 1995

237. Ladanyi M, Cavalchire G, Morris SW, et al: Reverse transcriptase polymerase chain reaction for the Ki-1 anaplastic large cell lymphoma-associated t(2;5) translocation in Hodgkin's disease. Am J Pathol 145:1296–1300, 1994

238. Hsu S-M, Waldron JW Jr, Hus P-L, Hough AJ Jr: Cytokines in malignant lymphomas: review and prospective evaluation. Hum Pathol 24:1040–1057, 1993

239. Samoszuk M, Nansen L: Detection of interleukin-5 messenger RNA in Reed-Sternberg cells of Hodgkin's disease with eosinophilia. Blood 75:13–16, 1990

240. Momose H, Jaffe ES, Shin SS, et al: Chronic lymphocytic leukemia/small lymphocytic lymphoma with Reed-Sternberg-like cells and possible transformation to Hodgkin's disease. Mediation by Epstein-Barr virus. Am J Surg Pathol 16:859–867, 1992

241. Gonzalez CL, Medeiros LJ, Jaffe ES: Composite lymphoma. A clinicopathologic analysis of nine patients with Hodgkin's disease and B-cell non-Hodgkin's lymphoma. Am J Clin Pathol 96:81–89, 1991

242. Zarate-Osorno A, Medeiros LJ, Longo DL, Jaffe ES: Non-Hodgkin's lymphomas arising in patients successfully treated for Hodgkin's disease. A clinical, histologic, and immunophenotypic study of 14 cases. Am J Surg Pathol 16:885–895, 1992

243. Zarate-Osorno A, Medeiros LJ, Kingma DW, et al: Hodgkin's disease following non-Hodgkin's lymphoma. A clinicopathologic and immunophenotypic study of nine cases. Am J Surg Pathol 17:123–132, 1993

244. Rosso R, Paulli M, Magrini U, et al: Anaplastic large cell lymphoma, CD30/Ki-1 positive, expressing the CD15/Leu-M1 antigen. Immunohistochemical and morphological relationships to Hodgkin's disease. Virchows Arch [A] 416:229–235, 1990

245. Pileri S, Bocchia M, Baroni CD, et al: Anaplastic large cell lymphoma (CD30+/Ki-1+): results of a prospective clinicopathologic study of 69 cases. Br J Haematol 86:513–523, 1994

246. Lukes RJ, Butler JJ, Hicks EB: Natural history of Hodgkin's disease as related to its pathological picture. Cancer 19:317–344, 1966

247. Poppema S, Kaiserling E, Lennert K: Epidemiology of nodular paragranuloma (Hodgkin's disease with lymphocytic predominance, nodular). J Cancer Res Clin Oncol 95:57–63, 1979

248. Hansmann ML, Zwingers T, Boske A, et al: Clinical features of nodular paragranuloma (Hodgkin's disease, lymphocyte predominance type, nodular). J Cancer Res Clin Oncol 108:321–330, 1984

249. Stoler MH, Nichols GE, Symbula M, Weiss LM: Nodular L&H lymphocyte predominance Hodgkin's disease: evidence for a kappa light chain-restricted monotypic B cell neoplasm. Am J Pathol 146:812–818, 1995

250. Regula DP, Hoppe RT, Weiss LM: Nodular and diffuse types of lymphocyte predominance Hodgkin's disease. N Engl J Med 318:214–219, 1988

251. Borg-Grech A, Radford JA, Crowther D, et al: A comparative study of the nodular and diffuse variant of lymphocyte-predominant Hodgkin's disease. J Clin Oncol 7:1303–1309, 1989

252. Pinkus GS, Said JW: Hodgkin's disease, lymphocyte predominance type, nodular—a distinct entity? Unique staining profile of L&H variants of Reed-Sternberg cells defined by monoclonal antibodies to leukocyte common antigen, granulocyte specific antigen, and B-cell specific antigen. Am J Pathol 116:1–6, 1985

253. Pinkus GS, Said JW: Hodgkin's disease, lymphocyte predominance type, nodular—further evidence for a B cell derivation: L&H variants of Reed-Sternberg cells express L26, a pan B cell marker. Am J Pathol 133:211–217, 1988

254. Dorfman RF, Gatter KC, Pulford KAF, Mason DY: An evaluation of the utility of anti-granulocyte and anti-leukocyte monoclonal antibodies in the diagnosis of Hodgkin's disease. Am J Pathol 123:508–519, 1986

255. Timens W, Visser L, Poppema S: Nodular lymphocyte predominance type of Hodgkin's disease is a germinal center lymphoma. Lab Invest 54:457–461, 1986

256. Stein H, Hansmann ML, Lennert K, et al: Reed-Sternberg and Hodgkin cells in lymphocyte-predominant Hodgkin's disease of nodular subtype contain J chain. Am J Clin Pathol 86:292–297, 1986

257. Momose H, Chen Y-Y, Ben-Ezra J, Weiss LM: Nodular, lymphocyte predominant Hodgkin's disease: study of immunoglobulin light chain protein and mRNA expression. Hum Pathol 23:1115–1119, 1992

258. Schmid C, Sargent C, Isaacson PG: L and H cells of nodular lymphocyte predominant Hodgkin's disease show immunoglobulin light-chain restriction. Am J Pathol 139:1281–1289, 1991

259. Kamel OW, Gelb AB, Shibuya RB, Warnke RA: Leu7 (CD57) reactivity distinguishes nodular lymphocyte predominance Hodgkin's disease, T cell rich B cell lymphoma and follicular lymphoma. Am J Pathol 142:541–546, 1993

260. Alavaikko JF, Hansmann ML, Nebendahl C, et al: Follicular dendritic cells in Hodgkin's disease. Am J Clin Pathol 95:194–200, 1991

261. Delabie J, Tierens A, Wu G, et al: Lymphocyte predominance Hodgkin's disease: lineage and clonality determination using a single-cell assay. Blood 84:3291–3298, 1994

262. Goates JJ, Kamel OW, LeBrun DP, et al: Floral variant of follicular lymphoma. Immunological and molecular studies support a neoplastic process. Am J Surg Pathol 18:37–47, 1994

263. Delabie J, Vandenberghe E, Kennes C, et al: Histiocyte-rich B-cell lymphoma. A distinct clinicopathologic entity possibly related to lymphocyte predominant Hodgkin's disease, paragranuloma subtype. Am J Surg Pathol 16:37–48, 1992

264. Miettinen M, Franssila KO, Saxen E: Hodgkin's disease, lymphocytic predominance nodular: increased risk for subsequent non-Hodgkin's lymphomas. Cancer 51:2293–2300, 1983

265. Hansmann ML, Shibata D, Lorenzen J, et al: Incidence of Epstein-Barr virus, bcl-2 expression and chromosomal translocation t(14;18) in large cell lymphoma associated with paragranuloma (lymphocyte-predominant Hodgkin's disease). Hum Pathol 25:240–243, 1994

266. Wickert RS, Weisenburger DD, Tierens A, et al: Clonal relationship between lymphocyte predominance Hodgkin's disease and concurrent or subsequent large-cell lymphoma of B lineage. Blood 86:2312–2320, 1995

267. Devesa SS, Fears T: Non-Hodgkin's lymphoma time trends: United States and International Data. Cancer Res, suppl. 52:5432–5440, 1992

268. Gail MH, Pluda JM, Rabkin CS, et al: Projections of the incidence of non-Hodgkin's lymphoma related to acquired immunodeficiency syndrome. J Natl Cancer Inst 83:695–701, 1991

269. Scherr PA, Hutchison GB, Neiman RS: Non-Hodgkin's lymphoma and occupational exposure. Cancer Res, suppl. 52:5503–5509, 1992

270. Hoar SK, Blair A, Holmes FF, et al: Agricultural herbicide and risk of lymphoma and soft tissue sarcoma. JAMA 256:1141–1147, 1986

271. Cantor KP, Blair A, Everett G, et al: Hair dye use and risk of leukemia and lymphoma. Am J Public Health 78:570–571, 1988

272. Jaffe ES, Blattner WA, Blayney DW, et al: The pathologic spectrum of adult T-cell leukemia/lymphoma in the United States. Am J Surg Pathol 8:263–275, 1984

273. Rosenberg SA: Validity of the Ann Arbor Staging Classification for the non-Hodgkin's lymphomas. Cancer Treat Rep 61:1023–1027, 1977

274. Lukes RJ, Collins RD: Immunologic characterization of human malignant lymphomas. Cancer 34:1488–1503, 1974

275. Weiss LM, Crabtree GS, Rouse RV, Warnke RA: Morphologic and immunologic characterization of 50 peripheral T-cell lymphomas. Am J Pathol 118:316–324, 1985

276. Non-Hodgkin's Lymphoma Pathologic Classification Project: National Cancer Institute sponsored study of classifications of non-Hodgkin's lymphomas: summary and description of a Working Formulation for clinical usage. Cancer 49:2112–2135, 1982

277. Stansfeld AG, Diebold J, Kapanci Y, et al: Updated Kiel classification for lymphomas, letter. Lancet 1:292–293, 1988

278. Kim H, Hendrickson MR, Dorfman RF: Composite lymphoma. Cancer 40:959–976, 1977

279. Russell J, Skinner J, Orell S, Seshadri R: Fine needle aspiration cytology in the management of lymphoma. Aust NZ J Med 13:365–368, 1983

280. Velasquez WS, Jagannath S, Tucker SL, et al: Risk classification as the basis for clinical staging of diffuse large-cell lymphoma derived from 10-year survival data. Blood 74:551–557, 1989

281. Shipp MA, Yeap BY, Harrington DP, et al: The m-BACOD combination chemotherapy regimen in large-cell lymphoma: analysis of the completed trial and comparison with the M-BACOD regimen. J Clin Oncol 8:84–93, 1990

282. Hoskins PJ, Ng V, Spinelli JJ, et al: Prognostic variables in patients with diffuse large-cell lymphoma treated with MACOP-B. J Clin Oncol 9:220–226, 1991

283. Dixon DO, Neilan B, Jones SE, et al: Effect of age on therapeutic outcome in advanced diffuse histiocytic lymphoma: the Southwest Oncology Group experience. J Clin Oncol 4:295–305, 1986

284. Coiffier B, Gisselbrecht C, Vose JM, et al: Prognostic factors in aggressive malignant lymphomas: description and validation of a prognostic index that could identify patients requiring a more intensive therapy. J Clin Oncol 9:211–219, 1991

285. The International Non-Hodgkin's Lymphoma Prognostic Factors Project: A predictive model for aggressive non-Hodgkin's lymphoma. N Engl J Med 329:987–994, 1993

286. Bartlett NL, Rizeq M, Dorfman RF, et al: Follicular large-cell lymphoma: intermediate or low grade? J Clin Oncol 12:1349–1357, 1994

287. Grogan TM, Lippman SM, Spier CM, et al: Independent prognostic significance of a nuclear proliferation antigen in diffuse large cell lymphomas as determined by the monoclonal antibody Ki-67. Blood 71:1157–1160, 1988

288. Grogan TM, Spier CM, Richter LC, Rangel CS: Immunologic approaches to the classification of non-Hodgkin's lymphomas. pp. 31–148. In Bennett JM, Foon KA (eds): Immunologic Approaches to the Classification and Management of Lymphomas and Leukemias. Kluwer Academic, Boston 1988

289. Grogan TM: Immunobiologic correlates of prognosis in lymphoma. Semin Oncol 5:58–74, 1993

290. Pinto A, Hutchison RE, Grant LH, et al: Follicular lymphoma in pediatric patients. Mod Pathol 3:308–313, 1990

291. Horning SJ, Rosenberg SA: The natural history of initially untreated low grade non-Hodgkin's lymphomas. N Engl J Med 311:1471–1475, 1984

292. Rosenberg SA: The low-grade non-Hodgkin's lymphomas: challenges and opportunities. J Clin Oncol 3:299–310, 1985

293. Hu E, Weiss LM, Hoppe RT, Horning S: Follicular and diffuse mixed small cleaved and large cell lymphoma—a clinicopathologic study. J Clin Oncol 3:1183–1187, 1985

294. Osborne BM, Butler JJ: Follicular lymphoma mimicking progressive

transformation of germinal centers. Am J Clin Pathol 88:264–269, 1987

295. Slovak ML, Weiss LM, Nathwani BN, et al: Cytogenetic studies of composite lymphomas: monocytoid B-cell lymphoma and other non-Hodgkin's lymphomas. Hum Pathol 24:1086–1094, 1993

296. Harris NL, Ferry JA: Follicular lymphoma and related disorders (germinal center lymphomas). pp. 695–679. In Knowles DM (ed): Neoplastic Hematopathology. Williams & Wilkins, Baltimore, 1992

297. Mann RB, Berard CW: Criteria for the cytologic subclassification of follicular lymphomas: a proposed alternative method. Hematol Oncol 1:187–192, 1982

298. Kim H, Dorfman RF, Rappaport H: Signet-ring lymphoma: a rare morphologic and functional expression of nodular (follicular) lymphoma. Am J Surg Pathol 2:119–132, 1978

299. Chang KL, Arber DA, Shibata D, et al: Follicular small lymphocytic lymphoma: a rare but distinct clinicopathologic entity. Am J Surg Pathol 18:999–1009, 1994

300. Nathwani BN, Sheibani K, Winberg CD, et al: Neoplastic B cells with cerebriform nuclei in follicular lymphomas. Hum Pathol 16:173–180, 1985

301. van der Putte SC, Schuurman HJ, Rademakers LH, et al: Malignant lymphoma of follicular center cell with marked nuclear lobation. Virchows Arch [Cell Pathol] 46:93–107, 1984

302. Vago JF, Hurtubise PE, Redden-Borowski MN, et al: Follicular center-cell lymphoma with plasmacytic differentiation, monoclonal paraprotein, and peripheral blood involvement. Recapitulation of normal B-cell development. Am J Surg Pathol 9:764–770, 1985

303. Chan JK, Hui PK, Ng CS: Follicular immunoblastic lymphoma: neoplastic counterpart of the intrafollicular immunoblast? Pathology 22:103–105, 1990

304. Come SE, Jaffe ES, Andersen JC, et al: Non-Hodgkin's lymphomas in leukemic phase: clinicopathologic correlations. Am J Med 69:667–674, 1980

305. Warnke R, Levy R: The immunopathology of follicular lymphomas: a model of B-lymphocyte homing. N Engl J Med 298:481–486, 1978

306. Ngan B, Chen-Levy Z, Weiss LM, et al: Expression in non-Hodgkin's lymphoma of the bcl-2 protein associated with the t(14;18) chromosomal translocation. N Engl J Med 318:1638–1644, 1988

307. Pezzella F, Tse A, Cordell J, et al: Expression of the bcl-2 oncogene protein is not specific for the 14;18 chromosomal translocation. Am J Pathol 137:225–232, 1990

308. Yunis JJ, Oken MM, Kaplan ME, et al: Distinctive chromosomal abnormalities in histologic subtypes of non-Hodgkin's lymphoma. N Engl J Med 307:1231–1236, 1982

309. Weiss LM, Warnke RA, Sklar J, Cleary ML: Molecular analysis of the t(14;18) chromosomal translocation in malignant lymphomas. N Engl J Med 317:1185–1189, 1987

310. Yunis JJ, Mayer MG, Amesen MA: bcl-2 and other genomic alterations in the prognosis of large-cell lymphoma. N Engl J Med 320:1047–1054, 1989

311. Horsman DE, Gascoyne RD, Coupland RW, et al: Comparison of cytogenetic analysis, Southern analysis, and polymerase chain reaction for the detection of t(14;18) in follicular lymphoma. Am J Clin Pathol 103:472–478, 1995

312. Tsujimoto T, Cossman J, Jaffe E, Croce CM: Involvement of the bcl-2 gene in human follicular lymphoma. Science 288:1440–1443, 1985

313. Berinstein NL, Reis MD, Ngan BY, et al: Detection of occult lymphoma in peripheral blood and bone marrow of patients with untreated early-stage and advanced-stage follicular lymphoma. J Clin Oncol 11:1344–1352, 1993

314. Tilly H, Rossi A, Stamatoullas A, et al: Prognostic value of chromosomal abnormalities in follicular lymphoma. Blood 84:1043–1049, 1994

315. LoCoco F, Gaidano G, Louie DC, et al: p53 mutations are associated with histologic transformation of follicular lymphoma. Blood 92:2289–2295, 1994

316. Sander CA, Yano T, Clark HM, et al: p53 mutation is associated with progression in follicular lymphoma. Blood 82:1994–2004, 1993

317. Cheson BD, Bennett JM, Rai KR, et al: Guidelines for clinical protocols for chronic lymphocytic leukemia: recommendations of the National Cancer Institute-sponsored working group. Am J Hematol 29:152–163, 1988

318. Pangalis GA, Boussiotis VA, Kittas C: Malignant disorders of small lymphocytes. Small lymphocytic lymphoma, lymphoplasmacytic lymphoma, and chronic lymphocytic leukemia: their clinical and laboratory relationship. Am J Clin Pathol 99:402–408, 1993

319. Morrison WH, Hoppe RT, Weiss LM, et al: Small lymphocytic lymphoma. J Clin Oncol 7:598–606, 1989

320. Berger F, Felman P, Sonet A, et al: Nonfollicular small B-cell lymphomas: a heterogeneous group of patients with distinct clinical features and outcome. Blood 83:2829–2835, 1994

321. Brecher M, Banks PM: Hodgkin's disease variant of Richter's syndrome. Report of eight cases. Am J Clin Pathol 93:333–339, 1990

322. Ben-Ezra J, Burke JS, Swartz WG, et al: Small lymphocytic lymphoma: a clinicopathologic analysis of 268 cases. Blood 73:579–587, 1989

323. Dick FR, Maca RD: The lymph node in chronic lymphocytic leukemia. Cancer 41:283–292, 1978

324. Pugh WC, Manning JT, Butler JJ: Paraimmunoblastic variant of small lymphocytic lymphoma/leukemia. Am J Surg Pathol 12:907–917, 1988

325. Contos MJ, Kornstein MJ, Innes DJ, Ben-Ezra J: The utility of CD20 and CD43 in subclassification of low-grade B-cell lymphoma on paraffin sections. Mod Pathol 5:631–633, 1992

326. Dorfman DM, Pinkus GS: Distinction between small lymphocytic and mantle cell lymphoma by immunoreactivity for CD23. Mod Pathol 7:326–331, 1994

327. Knuutila S, Elonen E, Teerenhovi L, et al: Trisomy 12 in B cells of patients with B-cell chronic lymphocytic leukemia. N Engl J Med 314:865–869, 1986

328. Isaacson PG: Lymphomas of mucosa-associated lymphoid tissue (MALT). Histopathology 16:617–619, 1990

329. Isaacson PG, Wright DH: Malignant lymphoma of mucosa associated lymphoid tissue. A distinctive B cell lymphoma. Cancer 52:1410–1416, 1983

330. Sheibani K, Burke JS, Swartz WG, et al: Monocytoid B cell lymphoma. Clinicopathologic study of 21 cases of a unique type of low grade lymphoma. Cancer 62:1531–1538, 1988

331. Isaacson P, Spencer J: Malignant lymphoma of mucosa-associated lymphoid tissue. Histopathology 11:445–462, 1987

332. Shin SS, Sheibani K: Monocytoid B-cell lymphoma. Am J Clin Pathol 99:421–425, 1993

333. Ngan B-Y, Warnke R, Wilson M, et al: Monocytoid B-cell lymphoma: a study of 36 cases. Hum Pathol 22:409–421, 1991

334. Traweek ST, Sheibani K: Monocytoid B-cell lymphoma. The biologic and clinical implications of peripheral blood involvement. Am J Clin Pathol 97:591–598, 1992

335. Shin SS, Sheibani K, Fishleder A, et al: Monocytoid B-cell lymphoma in patients with Sjogren's syndrome: a clinicopathologic study of 13 patients. Hum Pathol 22:422–430, 1991

336. Parsonnet J, Hansen S, Rodriguez L, et al: Helicobacter pylori infection and gastric lymphoma. N Engl J Med 330:1267–1271, 1994

337. Pelstring RJ, Essell JH, Kurtin PJ, et al: Diversity of organ site involvement among malignant lymphomas of mucosa-associated tissues. Am J Clin Pathol 96:738–745, 1991

338. Chan JKC: Antibiotic-responsive gastric lymphoma? Adv Anat Pathol 1:33–37, 1994

339. Brynes RK, Almaguer PD, McCourty A, Nathwani BN: Numerical cytogenetic abnormalities of chromosomes 3, 7, and 12 in monocytoid B-cell lymphoma. Lab Invest 71:107A, 1995

340. Wotherspoon AC, Finn TM, Isaacson PG: Trisomy 3 in low-grade primary B-cell lymphomas of mucosa-associated lymphoid tissue (MALT). Blood 85:2000–2004, 1995

341. Arber DA, Weiss LM: CD5: a review. Appl Immunohistochem 3:1–22, 1995

342. Patsouris E, Noel H, Lennert K: Lymphoplasmacytic/lymphoplasmacytoid immunocytoma with a high content of epithelioid cells: histologic and immunohistochemical findings. Am J Surg Pathol 14:660–670, 1990

343. Offit K, Parsa NZ, Filippa D, et al: t(9;14)(p13;q32) denotes a subset of low-grade non-Hodgkin's lymphoma with plasmacytoid differentiation. Blood 80:2594–2599, 1992

344. Offit K, Louie DC, Parsa NZ, et al: del (7)(32) is associated with a subset of small lymphocytic lymphoma with plasmacytoid features. Blood 86:2365–2370, 1995

345. Weisenburger DD, Kim H, Rappaport H: Malignant lymphoma, intermediate lymphocytic type: a clinicopathologic study of 42 cases. Cancer 48:1415–1425, 1981

346. Lardelli P, Bookman MA, Sundeen J, et al: Lymphocytic lymphoma of intermediate differentiation. Morphologic and immunophenotypic spectrum and clinical correlations. Am J Surg Pathol 14:752–763, 1990

347. Fisher RI, Dahlberg S, Nathwani BN, et al: A clinical analysis of two indolent lymphoma entities: mantle cell lymphoma and marginal zone lymphoma (including the mucosa-associated lymphoid tissue and monocytoid B-cell categories): a Southwest Oncology Group study. Blood 85:1075–1082, 1995

348. O'Briain DS, Kennedy MJ, Daly PA, et al: Multiple lymphomatous polyposis of the gastrointestinal tract: a clinicopathologically distinctive form of non-Hodgkin's lymphoma of centrocytic type. Am J Surg Pathol 13:691–699, 1989

349. Weisenburger DD, Kim H, Rappaport H: Mantle zone lymphoma. A follicular variant of intermediate lymphocytic lymphoma. Cancer 49:1429–1438, 1982

350. Koo CH, Rappaport H, Sheibani K, et al: Imprint cytology of non-Hodgkin's lymphomas. Based on a study of 212 immunologically characterized cases. Hum Pathol, suppl. 20:1–137, 1989

351. Ott MM, Ott G, Kuse R, et al: The anaplastic variant of centrocytic lymphoma is marked by frequent rearrangements of the Bcl-1 gene and high proliferation indices. Histopathology 24:329–334, 1994

352. Lennert K: Malignant Lymphomas Other Than Hodgkin's Disease. Springer-Verlag, New York, 1978

353. Zukerberg LR, Yang W-I, Arnold A, Harris NL: Cyclin D1 expression in non-Hodgkin's lymphomas. Detection by immunohistochemistry. Am J Clin Pathol 103:756–760, 1995

354. Raffeld M, Jaffe ES: bcl-1, t(11;14), and mantle cell-derived lymphomas. Blood 78:259–263, 1991

355. Leroux D, Le Marc'hadour F, Gressin R, et al: Non-Hodgkin's lymphomas with t(11;14)(q13;q32): a subset of mantle zone/intermediate lymphocytic lymphoma? Br J Haematol 77:346–353, 1991

356. Williams ME, Swerdlow SH, Rosenberg CL, Arnold A: Chromosome 11 translocation breakpoints at the PRAD1/Cyclin D1 gene locus in centrocytic lymphoma. Leukemia 7:241–245, 1993

357. Rimokh R, Berger F, Delsol G, et al: Rearrangement and overexpression of the BCL-1/PRAD-1 gene in intermediate lymphocytic lymphomas and in t(11q13)-bearing leukemias. Blood 81:3063–3067, 1993

358. Rimokh R, Berger F, Cornillet P, et al: Break in the BCL1 locus is closely associated with intermediate lymphocytic lymphoma subtype. Genes Chromosom Cancer 2:223–226, 1990

359. Rimokh R, Berger F, Delsol G, et al: Detection of the chromosomal translocation t(11;14) by polymerase chain reaction in mantle cell lymphomas. Blood 83:1871–1875, 1994

360. Rosenberg CL, Wong E, Petty E, et al: Overexpression of PRAD1, a candidate BCL1 breakpoint region oncogene, in centrocytic lymphomas. Proc Natl Acad Sci USA 88:9638–9642, 1991

361. Kwak LW, Wilson M, Weiss LM, et al: Clinical significance of morphologic subdivision in diffuse large cell lymphoma. Cancer 68:1988–1993, 1991

362. Armitage JO: Treatment of non-Hodgkin's lymphoma. N Engl J Med 328:1023–1030, 1993

363. Urba WJ, Duffey PL, Longo DL: Treatment of patients with aggressive lymphomas: an overview. J Natl Cancer Inst Monogr 10:29–37, 1990

364. Addis BJ, Isaacson PG: Large cell lymphoma of the mediastinum: a B-cell tumour of probable thymic origin. Histopathology 10:379–390, 1986

365. Perrone T, Frizzera G, Rosai J: Mediastinal diffuse large-cell lymphoma with sclerosis: a clinicopathologic study of 60 cases. Am J Surg Pathol 10:176–191, 1986

366. Yousem SA, Weiss LM, Warnke RA: Primary mediastinal non-Hodgkin's lymphomas: a morphologic and immunologic study of 19 cases. Am J Clin Pathol 83:676–680, 1985

367. Davis RE, Dorfman RF, Warnke RA: Primary large cell lymphoma of the thymus: a diffuse B-cell neoplasm presenting as primary mediastinal lymphoma. Hum Pathol 21:1262–1268, 1990

368. Lamarre L, Jacobson JO, Aisenberg AC, Harris NL: Primary large cell lymphoma of the mediastinum. Am J Surg Pathol 13:730–739, 1989

369. Jacobson JO, Aisenberg AC, Lamarre L, et al: Mediastinal large cell lymphoma: an uncommon subset of adult lymphoma curable with combined modality therapy. Cancer 62:1893–1898, 1988

370. Sheibani K, Battifora H, Winberg CD, et al: Further evidence that "malignant angioendotheliomatosis" is an angiotropic large-cell lymphoma. N Engl J Med 314:943–948, 1986

371. Lennert K, Feller AC: Histopathology of non-Hodgkin's lymphomas (based on the updated Kiel Classification). Springer-Verlag, Berlin, 1992

372. Moller P, Lammler B, Erberlein-Gonska M: Primary mediastinal clear cell lymphoma of B-cell type. Virchows Arch 409:79–92, 1986

373. Macon WR, Williams ME, Greer JP, et al: T-cell-rich B-cell lymphomas. A clinicopathologic study of 19 cases. Am J Surg Pathol 16:351–363, 1992

374. Chittal SM, Brousset P, Voigt JJ, Delsol G: Large B-cell lymphoma rich in T-cells and simulating Hodgkin's disease. Histopathology 19:211–220, 1991

375. Ramsay AP, Smith WJ, Isaacson PG: T-cell-rich B-cell lymphoma. Am J Surg Pathol 12:433–443, 1988

376. Krishnan J, Wallberg K, Frizzera G: T-cell-rich large B-cell lymphoma. A study of 30 cases, supporting its histologic heterogeneity and lack of clinical distinctiveness. Am J Surg Pathol 18:455–465, 1994

377. Tsang WY, Chan JK, Tang SK, et al: Large cell lymphoma with fibrillary matrix. Histopathology 20:80–82, 1992

378. Tse CC, Chan JK, Yuen RW, Ng CS: Malignant lymphoma with myxoid stroma: a new pattern in need of recognition. Histopathology 18:31–35, 1991

379. Dardick I, Srinivasan R, Al-Jabi M: Signet ring cell variant of large cell lymphoma. Ultrastruct Pathol 5:195–200, 1983

380. Kinney MC, Glick AD, Stein H, Collins RD: Comparison of anaplastic large cell Ki-1 lymphomas and microvillous lymphomas in their immunologic and ultrastructural features. Am J Surg Pathol 14:1047–1060, 1990

381. Doggett RS, Wood GS, Horning S, et al: The immunologic characterization of 95 nodal and extranodal diffuse large cell lymphomas in 89 patients. Am J Pathol 115:245–252, 1984

382. Cleary ML, Trela MJ, Weiss LM, et al: Most null large-cell lymphomas are B cell neoplasms. Lab Invest 53:521–525, 1985

383. Offit K, Lo Coco F, Louie DC, et al: Rearrangement of the bcl-6 gene as a prognostic marker in diffuse large-cell lymphoma. N Engl J Med 331:74–80, 1994

384. Horning SJ, Weiss LM, Crabtree GS, Warnke RA: Clinical and phenotypic diversity of T cell lymphomas. Blood 67:1578–1582, 1986

385. Greer JP, York JC, Cousar JB, et al: Peripheral T-cell lymphoma: a clinicopathologic study of 42 cases. J Clin Oncol 2:788–798, 1984

386. Weis JW, Winter MW, Phyliky RL, Banks PM: Peripheral T-cell

lymphomas: histologic, immunohistologic, and clinical characterization. Mayo Clin Proc 61:411–426, 1986

387. Kwak LW, Wilson M, Weiss LM, et al: Similar outcome of treatment of B-cell and T-cell diffuse large-cell lymphomas: the Stanford experience. J Clin Oncol 9:1426–1431, 1991

388. Lippman SM, Miller TP, Spier CM, et al: The prognostic significance of the immunotype in diffuse large-cell lymphoma: a comparative study of the T-cell and B-cell phenotype. Blood 72:436–441, 1988

389. Jaffe ES, Strauchen JA, Berard CW: Predictability of immunologic phenotype by morphologic criteria in diffuse aggressive non-Hodgkin's lymphomas. Am J Clin Pathol 77:46–49, 1982

390. Borowitz M, Reichert TA, Brynes RK, et al: The phenotypic diversity of peripheral T-cell lymphomas. The Southeastern Cancer Study Group experience. Hum Pathol 17:567–574, 1986

391. Kern WF, Spier CM, Hanneman EH, et al: Neural cell adhesion molecule-positive peripheral T-cell lymphoma: a rare variant with a propensity for unusual sites of involvement. Blood 79:2432–2437, 1992

392. Wong KF, Chan JK, Ng CS, et al: CD56 (NKH1)-positive hematolymphoid malignancies: an aggressive neoplasm featuring frequent cutaneous/mucosal involvement, cytoplasmic azurophilic granules, and angiocentricity. Hum Pathol 23:798–804, 1992

393. Weiss LM, Picker LJ, Grogan TM, et al: Absence of clonal beta and gamma T-cell receptor gene rearrangements in a subset of peripheral T-cell lymphomas. Am J Pathol 130:436–443, 1988

394. Colby T, Burke J, Hoppe RT: Lymph node biopsy in mycosis fungoides. Cancer 47:351–359, 1981

395. Vonderheid EC, Diamond LW, Lai SM, et al: Lymph node histopathologic findings in cutaneous T-cell lymphoma. A prognostic classification system based on morphologic assessment. Am J Clin Pathol 97:121–129, 1992

396. Salhany KE, Cousar JB, Greer JP, et al: Transformation of cutaneous T cell lymphoma to large cell lymphoma. A clinicopathologic and immunologic study. Am J Pathol 132:265–277, 1988

397. Weiss LM, Hu E, Wood GS, et al: Clonal rearrangements of the T cell receptor gene in mycosis fungoides and dermatopathic lymphadenopathy. N Engl J Med 313:539–544, 1985

398. Bunn PA, Schecter GP, Jaffe E, et al: Clinical course of retrovirus-associated adult T-cell lymphoma in the United States. N Engl J Med 309:257–264, 1983

399. Tokunaga M, Sato E: Non-Hodgkin's lymphomas in a southern prefecture in Japan: an analysis of 715 cases. Cancer 46:1231–1239, 1980

400. Swerdlow SH, Habeshaw JA, Rohatiner AZS, et al: Caribbean T-cell lymphoma/leukemia. Cancer 54:687–696, 1984

401. Kikuchi M, Mitsui T, Takeshita M, et al: Virus associated adult T-cell leukemia (ATL) in Japan: clinical, histological and immunological studies. Hematol Oncol 4:67, 1986

402. Patsouris E, Noel H, Lennert K: Histological and immunohistological findings in lymphoepithelioid cell lymphoma (Lennert's lymphoma). Am J Surg Pathol 12:341–350, 1988

403. Nathwani BN, Rappaport H, Moran EM, et al: Malignant lymphoma arising in angioimmunoblastic lymphadenopathy. Cancer 41:578–606, 1978

404. Weiss LM, Arber DA, Strickler JG: Nasal T cell lymphoma. Ann Oncol suppl. 1, 5:39–42, 1994

405. Strickler JG, Meneses M, Habermann TM, et al: "Polymorphic reticulosis": a reappraisal. Hum Pathol 25:659–665, 1994

406. Arber DA, Weiss LM, Albujar PF, et al: Nasal lymphomas in Peru: high incidence of T-cell immunophenotype and Epstein-Barr virus infection. Am J Surg Pathol 17:659–665, 1993

407. Lipford EH, Margolich JB, Longo DL, et al: Angiocentric immunoproliferative lesions: a clinicopathologic spectrum of post-thymic T cell proliferations. Blood 5:1674–1681, 1988

408. Farcet JP, Gaulard P, Marolleau JP, et al: Hepatosplenic T-cell lymphoma: sinusal/sinusoidal localization af malignant cells expressing the T-cell receptor gd. Blood 75:2213–2219, 1990

409. Isaacson PG, Spencer J, Connolly CE, et al: Malignant histiocytosis of the intestine: a T-cell lymphoma. Lancet 2:688–691, 1985

410. Chott A, Dragosics B, Radaszkiewicz T: Peripheral T-cell lymphomas of the intestine. Am J Pathol 141:1361–1371, 1992

411. Spencer J, Cerf-Bensussan N, Jarry A, et al: Enteropathy-associated T-cell lymphoma is recognized by a monoclonal antibody (HML-1) that defines a membrane molecule on human mucosal lymphocytes. Am J Pathol 132:1–5, 1988

412. Kadin M, Sako D, Berliner N, et al: Childhood Ki-1 lymphoma presenting with skin lesions and peripheral lymphadenopathy. Blood 68:1042–1049, 1986

413. Stein H, Mason DY, Gerdes J, et al: The expression of the Hodgkin's disease associated antigen Ki-1 in reactive and neoplastic lymphoid tissue: evidence that Reed-Sternberg cells and histiocytic malignancies are derived from activated lymphoid cells. Blood 66:848–858, 1985

414. Sandlund JT, Pui CH, Santana VM, et al: Clinical features and treatment outcome for children with CD30+ large-cell non-Hodgkin's lymphoma. J Clin Oncol 12:895–898, 1994

415. Reiter A, Schrappe M, Tiemann M, et al: A successful treatment strategy for Ki-1 anaplastic large cell lymphoma of childhood. A prospective analysis of 62 patients enrolled in three consecutive BFM group studies. J Clin Oncol 12:899–908, 1994

416. Greer JP, Kinney MC, Collins RD, et al: Clinical features of 31 patients with Ki-1 anaplastic large-cell lymphoma. J Clin Oncol 9:539–547, 1991

417. Krishnan J, Tomaszewski MM, Kao GF: Primary cutaneous CD30+ anaplastic large cell lymphoma. Report of 27 cases. J Cutan Pathol 20:193–202, 1993

418. de Bruin PC, Beljaards RC, van Heerde P, et al: Differences in clinical behaviour and immunophenotype between primary cutaneous and primary nodal anaplastic large cell lymphoma of T-cell or null cell phenotype. Histopathology 23:127–135, 1993

419. Beljaards RC, Meijer CJLM, Scheffer E, et al: Prognostic significance of CD30 (Ki-1/Ber-H2) expression in primary cutaneous large-cell lymphomas of T-cell origin. A clinicopathologic and immunohistochemical study in 20 patients. Am J Pathol 135:1169–1178, 1989

420. Hansmann ML, Fellbaum C, Bohm A: Large cell anaplastic lymphoma: evaluation of immunophenotype of paraffin and frozen sections in comparison with ultrastructural features. Virchows Arch [A] 418:427–433, 1991

421. Chan JKC: Anaplastic large cell Ki-1 lymphoma. Delineation of two morphological types. Histopathology 15:11–34, 1989

422. Chott A, Kaserer K, Augustin I, et al: Ki-1 positive large cell lymphoma. A clinicopathologic study of 41 cases. Am J Surg Pathol 14:439–448, 1990

423. Pileri S, Falini B, Delsol G, et al: Lymphohistiocytic T-cell lymphoma (anaplastic large cell lymphoma CD30+/Ki-1+) with a high content of reactive histiocytes. Histopathology 16:383–391, 1990

424. Kinney M, Collins RD, Greer JP, et al: A small-cell-predominant variant of primary Ki-1 (CD30)+ T-cell lymphoma. Am J Surg Pathol 17:859–868, 1993

425. Chan JKC, Buchanan R, Fletcher CDM: Sarcomatoid variant of anaplastic large cell Ki-1 anaplastic large-cell lymphoma. J Clin Oncol 9:539–547, 1991

426. Delsol G, Al Saati T, Gatter KC, et al: Coexpression of epithelial membrane antigen (EMA), Ki-1, and interleukin-2 receptor by anaplastic large cell lymphomas. Diagnostic value in so-called malignant histiocytosis. Am J Pathol 130:59–70, 1988

427. Penny RJ, Blaustein JC, Longtine JA, Pinkus GS: Ki-1 positive large cell lymphomas, a heterogenous group of neoplasms. Morphologic, immunophenotypic, genotypic, and clinical features of 24 cases. Cancer 68:362–373, 1991

428. Frierson HF, Bellafiore FJ, Gaffey MJ, et al: Cytokeratin in anaplastic large cell lymphoma. Mod Pathol 7:317–321, 1994

429. Weiss LM, Picker LJ, Copenhaver CM, et al: Large-cell hemato-lymphoid neoplasms of uncertain lineage. Hum Pathol 19:967–973, 1988

430. O'Connor NTJ, Stein H, Falini B, et al: Genotypic analysis of large cell lymphomas which express the Ki-1 antigen. Histopathology 11:733–730, 1987

431. Benz-Lemoine E: Malignant histiocytosis: a specific t(2;5) (p23;q35) translocation? Review of the literature. Blood 72:1045–1047, 1988

432. Wellmann A, Otsuki T, Vogelbruch M, et al: Analysis of the t(2;5)(p23;q35) by RT-PCR in CD30+ anaplastic large cell lymphomas, in other non-Hodgkin's lymphomas of T-cell phenotype, and in Hodgkin's disease. Blood 86:2321–2328, 1995

433. Lopategui JR, Sun L-H, Chan JKC, et al: Low frequency association of the t(2;5)(p23;q35) chromosomal translocation with CD30+ lymphomas from American and Asian patients. A reverse transcriptase-polymerase chain reaction study. Am J Pathol 146:323–328, 1994

434. Lamant L, Meggetto F, AI Saati T, et al: High incidence of the t(2;5)(p23;q35) translocation in anaplastic large cell lymphoma and its lack of detection in Hodgkin's disease. Comparison of cytogenetic analysis, RT-PCR and P-80 immunostaining. Blood 87: 284–291, 1996

435. Shiota M, Nakamura S, Ichinohasama R, et al: Anaplastic large cell lymphomas expressing the novel chimeric protein p80NPM/ALK: a distinct clinicopathologic entity. Blood 86:1954–1960, 1995

436. Wilson MS, Weiss LM, Gatter KC, et al: Malignant histiocytosis: a reassessment of cases previously reported in 1975 based upon paraffin section immunophenotyping studies. Cancer 66:530–536, 1990

437. Coleman CN, Picozzi VJ, Cox RS, et al: Treatment of lymphoblastic lymphoma in adults. J Clin Oncol 4:1628–1637, 1986

438. Murphy SB: Current concepts in cancer. Childhood non-Hodgkin's lymphoma. N Engl J Med 299:1446–1448, 1978

439. Nathwani BN, Kim H, Rappaport H: Malignant lymphoma, lymphoblastic. Cancer 38:964–983, 1976

440. Nathwani BN, Diamond LW, Winberg CD, et al: Lymphoblastic lymphoma: a clinicopathologic study of 95 patients. Cancer 48:2347–2357, 1981

441. Sander CA, Medeiros LJ, Abruzzo LV, et al: Lymphoblastic lymphoma presenting in cutaneous sites: a clinicopathologic analysis of six cases. J Am Acad Dermatol 25:1023–1031, 1991

442. Griffith RC, Kelly DR, Nathwani BN, et al: A morphologic study of childhood lymphoma of the lymphoblastic type. The Pediatric Oncology Group experience. Cancer 59:1126–1131, 1987

443. Braziel RM, Keneklis T, Donlon JA, et al: Terminal deoxynucleotidyl transferase in non-Hodgkin's lymphoma. Am J Clin Pathol 80:655–659, 1983

444. Orazi A, Caggoretti G, John K, Neimen RS: Terminal deoxynucleotidyl transferase staining of malignant lymphomas in paraffin sections. Mod Pathol 1994:582–586, 1994

445. Weiss LM, Bindl JM, Picozzi VJ, et al: Lymphoblastic lymphoma: an immunophenotype study of 26 cases with comparison to T cell acute lymphoblastic leukemia. Blood 67:474–478, 1986

446. Cossman J, Chused TM, Fisher RI, et al: Diversity of immunological phenotypes of lymphoblastic lymphoma. Cancer Res 43:4486–4490, 1983

447. Bernard A, Boumsell L, Reinherz L, et al: Cell surface characterization of malignant T cells from lymphoblastic lymphoma using monoclonal antibodies: evidence for phenotypic differences between malignant T cells from patients with acute lymphoblastic leukemia and lymphoblastic lymphoma. Blood 57:1105–1110, 1981

448. Sheibani K, Winberg CD, Burke JS, et al: Lymphoblastic lymphoma expressing natural killer cell-associated antigens: a clinicopathologic study of six cases. Leuk Res 11:371–377, 1987

449. Sheibani K, Nathwani BN, Winberg CD: Antigenically defined

450. subgroups of lymphoblastic lymphoma: relationship to clinical presentation and biological behavior. Cancer 60:183–190, 1987

450. Weiss LM, Bindl JM, Picozzi VJ, et al: Lymphoblastic lymphoma: an immunophenotype study of 26 cases with comparison to T cell acute lymphoblastic leukemia. Blood 67:474–478, 1986

451. Mason DY, van Noesel C, Cordell JL, et al: The B29 and mb-1 polypeptides are differentially expressed during human B cell differentiation. Eur J Immunol 22:2753–2756, 1992

452. Mason D, Cordell J, Tse A, et al: The IgM-associated protein mb-1 as a marker of normal and neoplastic B-cells. J Immunol 147:2474–2482, 1991

453. Stroup R, Sheibani K, Misset JL, et al: Surface immunoglobulin-positive lymphoblastic lymphoma. A report of three cases. Cancer 65:2559–2563, 1990

454. Korsmeyer SJ, Arnold A, Bakhshi A, et al: Immunoglobulin gene rearrangement and cell surface antigen expression in acute lymphocytic leukemias of T-cell and B-cell precursor origins. J Clin Invest 71:301–313, 1983

455. Kitchingman GR, Robigatti U, Mauer AM, et al: Rearrangement of immunoglobulin heavy chain genes in T cell acute lymphoblastic leukemia. Blood 65:725–729, 1985

456. Felix CA, Poplack DG, Reaman GH: Characterization of immunoglobulin and T-cell receptor gene patterns in B-cell precursor acute lymphoblastic leukemia of childhood. J Clin Oncol 8:431–442, 1990

457. Rouse RV, Weiss LM: Human thymomas: evidence of immunologically defined normal and abnormal microenvironmental differentiation. Cell Immunol 111:94–106, 1988

458. Burkitt DP: A sarcoma involving the jaws in African children. Br J Surg 197:218–223, 1958

459. Grogan TM, Warnke RA, Kaplan HS: A comparative study of Burkitt's and non-Burkitt's "undifferentiated" malignant lymphoma: immunologic, cytochemical, ultrastructural, cytologic, histopathologic, clinical and cell culture features. Cancer 49:1817–1828, 1982

460. Levine AM, Pavlova Z, Pockros AW, et al: Small noncleaved follicular center cell (FCC) lymphoma: Burkitt and non-Burkitt variants in the United States. I. Clinical features. Cancer 52:1073–1079, 1983

461. Miliauskas JR, Berard CW, Young RC, et al: Undifferentiated non-Hodgkin's lymphomas (Burkitt's and non-Burkitt's types). The relevance of making this histologic distinction. Cancer 50:2115–2121, 1982

462. Aine R: Small non-cleaved follicular center cell lymphoma: clinicopathologic comparison of Burkitt and non-Burkitt variants in Finnish material. Eur J Cancer Clin Oncol 21:1179–1185, 1985

463. Bernstein JI, Coleman CN, Strickler JG, et al: Combined modality therapy for adults with small non-cleaved cell lymphoma (Burkitt's and non-Burkitt's types). J Clin Oncol 4:847–858, 1986

464. Magrath IT, Shiramizu B: Biology and treatment of small non-cleaved cell lymphoma. Oncology 3:41–53, 1989

465. Hutchison RE, Murphy S, Fairclough DL, et al: Diffuse small noncleaved cell lymphoma in children, Burkitt's versus non-Burkitt's types. Cancer 64:23–38, 1989

466. Mann RB, Jaffe ES, Braylan RC, et al: Non-endemic Burkitt's lymphoma. A B-cell tumor related to germinal centers. N Engl J Med 295:685–691, 1976

467. Magrath I: The pathogenesis of Burkitt's lymphoma. Adv Cancer Res 53:133–270, 1990

468. Leder P, Battey J, Lenoir G, et al: Translocations among antibody genes in human cancer. Science 222:765–771, 1983

469. Filipovich AH, Mathus A, Kamat D, Shapiro RS: Primary immunodeficiencies: genetic risk factors for lymphoma. Cancer Res suppl. 52:5465s–5467s, 1992

470. Sander CA, Medeiros LM, Weiss LM, et al: Lymphoproliferative lesions in patients with common variable immunodeficiency syndrome. Am J Surg Pathol 16:1170–1182, 1992

471. Ballerini P, Gaidano G, Gong JZ, et al: Multiple genetic lesions in AIDS-related non-Hodgkin lymphoma. Blood 81:166–176, 1993

472. Schoeppel SL, Hoppe RT, Dorfman RF, et al: Hodgkin's disease associated with individuals at risk for the acquired immune deficiency syndrome. Ann Intern Med 102:68–70, 1987

473. Knowles DN, Cesarman E, Chadburn A, et al: Correlative morphologic and molecular genetic analysis demonstrates three distinct categories of posttransplantation lymphoproliferative disorders. Blood 85:552–565, 1995

474. Kamel OW, van de Rijn M, LeBrun DP, et al: Lymphoproliferative lesions in patients with rheumatoid arthritis and dermatomyositis: frequency of Epstein-Barr virus and other features associated with immunosuppression. Hum Pathol 25:638–643, 1994

475. Lichtenstein L: Histiocytosis X: integration of eosinophilic granuloma of bone, Letterer-Siwe disease and Schüller-Christian disease as related manifestations of a single nosologic entity. Arch Pathol 56:84–102, 1953

476. Motoi M, Helbron D, Kaiserling E, Lennert K: Eosinophilic granuloma of lymph nodes: a variant of histiocytosis X. Histopathology 4:585–606, 1980

477. Williams JW, Dorfman RF: Lymphadenopathy as the initial manifestation of histiocytosis X. Am J Surg Pathol 3:405–421, 1979

478. Burns BF, Colby TV, Dorfman RF: Langerhans' cell granulomatosis (histiocytosis X) associated with malignant lymphomas. Am J Surg Pathol 7:529–533, 1983

479. Egeler RA, Neglia JP, Puccetti DM, et al: Association of Langerhans cell histiocytosis with malignant neoplasms. Cancer 71:865–873, 1993

480. Ben-Ezra J, Bailey A, Azumi N, et al: Malignant histiocytosis X. A distinct clinicopathologic entity. Cancer 68:1050–1060, 1991

481. Azumi N, Sheibani K, Swartz WG, et al: Antigenic phenotype of Langerhans cell histiocytosis. An immunohistochemical study demonstrating the value of LN-2, LN-3 and vimentin. Hum Pathol 19:1376–1382, 1988

482. Hage C, Willman CL, Favara BE, Isaacson PG: Langerhans' cell histiocytosis (histiocytosis X): immunophenotype and growth fraction. Hum Pathol 24:840–845, 1993

483. Ruco LP, Pulford KAF, Mason D: Expression of macrophage-associated antigens in tissues involved by Langerhans' cell histiocytosis (histiocytosis X). Am J Clin Pathol 92:273–279, 1989

484. Krenacs L, Tiszlavicz L, Krenacs T, Bournsell L: Immunohistochemical detection of CD1a antigen in formalin-fixed and paraffin-embedded tissue sections with monoclonal antibody O10. J Pathol 171:99–104, 1993

485. Mierau GW, Favara BE, Brenman JM: Electron microscopy in histiocytosis X. Ultrastruct Pathol 3:137–142, 1982

486. Willman CL, Busque L, Griffith BB, et al: Langerhans'-cell histiocytosis (histiocytosis X)—a clonal proliferative disease. N Engl J Med 331:154–160, 1994

487. Yu RC, Chu AC: Lack of T-cell receptor gene rearrangements in cells involved in Langerhans cell histiocytosis. Cancer 75:1162–1166, 1995

488. Monda L, Warnke R, Rosai J: A primary lymph node malignancy with features suggestive of dendritic reticulum cell differentiation. Am J Surg Pathol 122:562–572, 1986

489. Weiss LM, Berry GJ, Dorfman RF, et al: Spindle cell neoplasms of lymph nodes of probable reticulum cell lineage. True reticulum cell sarcoma? Am J Surg Pathol 14:405–414, 1990

490. Nakamura S, Hara K, Suchi T, et al: Interdigitating cell sarcoma. A morphologic, immunohistologic, and enzyme-histochemical study. Cancer 61:562–568, 1988

491. Vasef MA, Zaatari GS, Chan WC, et al: Dendritic cell tumors associated with low-grade B-cell malignancies. Report of three cases. Am J Clin Pathol 104:696–701, 1995

492. Hanson CA, Jaszcz W, Kersey JH, et al: True histiocytic lymphoma: histopathologic, immunophenotypic and genotypic analysis. Br J Haematol 73:187–198, 1989

493. Kamel OW, Gocke CD, Kell DL, et al: True histiocytic lymphoma: a study of 12 cases based on current definition. Leuk Lymphoma 18:81–86, 1995

494. Ornvold K, Carstensen H, Junge J, et al: Tumours classified as "malignant histiocytosis" in children are T-cell neoplasms. APMIS 100:558–566, 1992

495. Weiss LM, Trela MJ, Cleary M, et al: Frequent immunoglobulin and T cell receptor gene rearrangement in "histiocytic" neoplasms. Am J Pathol 121:369–373, 1985

496. Salter DM, Krajewski AS, Dewar AE: Immunophenotype analysis of malignant histiocytosis of the intestine. J Clin Pathol 39:8–15, 1986

497. Isaacson P, Wright DH, Jones DB: Malignant lymphoma of true histiocytic (monocyte-macrophage) origin. Cancer 51:80, 1983

498. Ralfkiaer E, Delsol G, O'Connor NTJ, et al: Malignant lymphomas of true histiocytic origin. A clinical, histological, immunophenotypic and genotypic study. J Pathol 160:9–17, 1990

499. Arai E, Su WPD, Roche PC, Li C-Y: Cutaneous histiocytic malignancy. Immunohistochemical re-examination of cases previously diagnosed as cutaneous "histiocytic lymphoma" and "malignant histiocytosis". J Cutan Pathol 20:115–120, 1993

500. Bucksy P, Favara B, Feller AC: Malignant histiocytosis and large cell anaplastic (Ki-1) lymphoma in childhood: guidelines for differential diagnosis—report of the Histiocyte Society. Med Ped Oncol 22:200–203, 1994

501. Okada Y, Nakanishi I, Nomura H, et al: Angiotropic B-cell lymphoma with hemophagocytic syndrome. Pathol Res Pract 190:718–727, 1994

502. Neiman RS, Barcos M, Berard C, et al: Granulocytic sarcoma: a clinicopathologic study of 61 biopsied cases. Cancer 48:1426–1437, 1981

503. Meis JM, Butler JJ, Osborne BM, Manning JT: Granulocytic sarcoma in nonleukemic patients. Cancer 58:2697–2709, 1986

504. Muller S, Sangster G, Crocker J, et al: An immunohistochemical and clinicopathological study of granulocytic sarcoma (chloroma). Hematol Oncol 4:101–112, 1986

505. Traweek ST, Arber DA, Rappaport H, Brynes RK: Extramedullary myeloid cell tumors. An immunohistochemical and morphologic study of 28 cases. Am J Surg Pathol 17:1011, 1993

506. Baddoura FK, Hanson C, Chan WC: Plasmacytoid monocytic proliferation associated with myeloproliferative disorders. Cancer 69:1457–1467, 1992

507. Chang KL, Stroup R, Weiss LM: Hairy cell leukemia. Current status. Am J Clin Pathol 97:719–738, 1992

508. Addis BJ, Isaacson P, Billings JA: Plasmacytosis of lymph nodes. Cancer 46:340–346, 1980

509. Kahn H, Strauchen JA, Gilbert HS, Fuchs A: Immunoglobulin-related amyloidosis presenting as recurrent isolated lymph node involvement. Arch Pathol Lab Med 115:948–950, 1991

510. Travis WD, Li CY: Pathology of the lymph node and spleen in systemic mast cell disease. Mod Pathol 1:4–14, 1988

511. Weiss LM, Chan WC, Schnitzer B: Lymph nodes. pp. 1115–1120. In Damjanov I, Linder J (eds): Anderson's Pathology. Mosby–Year Book, St. Louis, 1996

512. Suniluoto T, Päivänsalo M, Tikkakoski T, Apaja-Sarkkinen M: Ultrasound-guided aspiration cytology of the spleen. Acta Radiol 33:137–139, 1992

513. Zeppa P, Vetrani A, Luciano L, et al: Fine needle aspiration biopsy of the spleen. A useful procedure in the diagnosis of splenomegaly. Acta Cytol 38:299–309, 1994

514. Moriarty AT, Schwenk GR Jr, Chua G: Splenic fine needle aspiration biopsy in the diagnosis of lymphoreticular diseases. A report of four cases. Acta Cytol 37:191–196, 1993

515. Silvermann JF, Geisinger KM, Raab SS, Stanley MW: Fine needle aspiration biopsy of the spleen in the evaluation of neoplastic disorders. Acta Cytol 37:158–162, 1993

516. Haque I, Haque MZ, Krishnani N, et al: Fine needle aspiration cytology of the spleen in visceral leishmaniasis. Acta Cytol 37:73–76, 1993

517. Cavanna L, Civardi G, Fornari F, et al: Ultrasonically guided percutaneous splenic tissue core biopsy in patients with malignant lymphomas. Cancer 69:2932–2936, 1992

518. Eraklis AJ, Filler RM: Splenectomy in childhood: a review of 1413 cases. J Pediatr Surg 7:382–388, 1972

519. Wolf BC, Neiman RS, Bennington JL, (eds): Disorders of the Spleen. WB Saunders, Philadelphia, 1989

520. van Krieken JHJM, te Velde J: Spleen. p. 253. In Sternberg SS (ed): Histology for Pathologists. Lippincott-Raven, Philadelphia, 1992

521. Carr NJ, Turk EP: The histological features of splenosis. Histopathology 21:549–553, 1992

522. Fleming CR, Dickson ER, Harrison EG Jr: Splenosis: autotransplantation of splenic tissue. Am J Med 61:414–419, 1976

523. Wadham BM, Adams PB, Johnson MA: Incidence and location of accessory spleens. N Engl J Med 304:1111, 1981

524. Bauer TW, Haskins GE, Armitage JO: Splenic rupture in patients with hematologic malignancies. Cancer 48:2729–2733, 1981

525. Chun CH, Raff MJ, Contreras L, et al: Splenic abscess. Medicine 59:50–65, 1980

526. Paris S, Weiss SM, Ayers WH Jr, Clarke LE: Splenic abscess. Am Surg 60:358–361, 1994

527. Gadacz T, Way LW, Dunphy JE: Changing clinical spectrum of splenic abscess. Am J Surg 128:182–187, 1974

528. Chulay JD, Lankerani MR: Splenic abscess. Report of 10 cases and review of the literature. Am J Med 61:513–522, 1976

529. Smithe EB, Custer RP: Rupture of the spleen in infectious mononucleosis. A clinicopathologic report of seven cases. Blood 1:317–333, 1946

530. Rutkow IM: Rupture of the spleen in infectious mononucleosis. A critical review. Arch Surg 113:718–720, 1978

531. Farley DR, Zietlow SP, Bannon MP, Farnell MB: Spontaneous rupture of the spleen due to infectious mononucleosis. Mayo Clin Proc 67:846–853, 1992

532. Gaffey MJ, Frierson HF Jr, Medeiros LJ, Weiss LM: The relationship of Epstein-Barr virus to infection-related (sporadic) and familial hemophagocytic syndrome and secondary (lymphoma-related) hemophagocytosis: an in situ hybridization study. Hum Pathol 24:657–667, 1993

533. Su I, Hsu Y, Lin M, et al: Epstein-Barr virus-containing T-cell lymphoma presents with hemophagocytic syndrome mimicking malignant histiocytosis. Cancer 72:2019–2027, 1993

534. Neiman RS: Incidence and importance of splenic sarcoid-like granulomas. Arch Pathol Lab Med 101:518–521, 1977

535. O'Connell MJ, Schimpff SC, Kirschner RH, et al: Epithelioid granulomas in Hodgkin's disease. A favorable prognostic sign? JAMA 233:886–889, 1975

536. Cruickshank B: Follicular (mineral oil) lipidosis: I. Epidemiologic studies of involvement of the spleen. Hum Pathol 15:724–730, 1984

537. Cruickshank B, Thomas MJ: Mineral oil (follicular) lipidosis: II. Histologic studies of spleen, liver, lymph nodes, and bone marrow. Hum Pathol 15:731–737, 1984

538. Putschar WGJ, Manion WC: Splenic-gonadal fusion. Am J Pathol 32:15–33, 1956

539. Scriver CR, Beaudet AL, Sly WS, et al (eds): The Metabolic and Molecular Bases of Inherited Disease. 7th Ed. McGraw-Hill, New York, 1995

540. Salzstein SL: Phospholipid accumulation in histiocytes of splenic pulp associated with thrombocytopenic purpura. Blood 18:73–88, 1961

541. Firkin BG, Wright R, Miller S, Stokes E: Splenic macrophages in thrombocytopenia. Blood 33:240–245, 1969

542. Laszlo J, Jones R, Silberman HR, Banks PM: Splenectomy for Felty's syndrome. Clinicopathological study of 27 patients. Arch Intern Med 138:597–602, 1978

543. Hassan NMR, Neiman RS: The pathology of the spleen in steroid-treated immune thrombocytopenic purpura. Am J Clin Pathol 84:433–438, 1985

544. McClure RD, Altemeier WA: Cysts of the spleen. Ann Surg 116:98–102, 1942

545. Garvin DF, King FM: Cysts and nonlymphomatous tumors of the spleen. Pathol Annu 16:61–80, 1981

546. Fowler RH: Nonparasitic benign cystic tumors of the spleen. Int Abstr Surg 96:209–227, 1953

547. Fowler RH: Cystic tumors of the spleen. Int Abstr Surg 70:213–223, 1940

548. Bürrig K: Epithelial (true) splenic cysts. Pathogenesis of the mesothelial and so-called epidermoid cyst of the spleen. Am J Surg Pathol 12:275–281, 1988

549. Garcia RL, Khan MK, Berlin RB: Peliosis of the spleen with rupture. Hum Pathol 13:177–179, 1982

550. Kohr RM, Haendiges M, Taube RR: Peliosis of the spleen: a rare cause of spontaneous splenic rupture with surgical implications. Surg 59:197–199, 1993

551. Tada T, Wakabayashi T, Kishimoto H: Peliosis of the spleen. Am J Clin Pathol 79:708–713, 1983

552. Taxy JB: Peliosis: a morphologic curiosity becomes an iatrogenic problem. Hum Pathol 9:331–340, 1978

553. Chan KW, Saw D: Distinctive, multiple lymphangiomas of spleen. J Pathol 131:75–81, 1980

553a. Arber DA, Strickler JG, Weiss LM: Splenic mesothelial cysts mimicking lymphangiomas. Am J Surg Pathol (in press)

554. Ramani P, Shah A: Lymphangiomatosis. Histologic and immunohistochemical analysis of four cases. Am J Surg Pathol 17:329–335, 1993

555. Falk S, Stutte HJ, Frizzera G: Littoral cell angioma. A novel splenic vascular lesion demonstrating histiocytic differentiation. Am J Surg Pathol 15:1023–1033, 1991

556. Falk S: Immunodiescrepancy (IMDI). Am J Surg Pathol 18:428–429, 1994

557. Silverman ML, LiVolsi VA: Splenic hamartoma. Am J Clin Pathol 70:224–229, 1978

558. Morgenstern L, McCafferty L, Rosenberg J, Michel SL: Hamartomas of the spleen. Arch Surg 119:1291–1293, 1984

559. Beham A, Hermann W, Schmid C: Hamartoma of the spleen with haematological symptoms. Virchows Archiv A [Pathol Anat] 414:535–539, 1989

560. Falk S, Stutte HJ: Hamartomas of the spleen: a study of 20 biopsy cases. Histopathology 14:603–612, 1989

561. Steinberg JJ, Suhrland M, Valensi Q: The spleen in the spleen syndrome: the association of splenoma with hematopoietic and neoplastic disease—compendium of cases since 1864. J Surg Oncol 47:193–202, 1991

562. Zukerberg LR, Kaynor BL, Silverman ML, Harris NL: Splenic hamartoma and capillary hemangioma are distinct entities. Immunohistochemical analysis of CD8 expression by endothelial cells. Hum Pathol 22:1258–1261, 1991

563. Cotelingam JD, Jaffe ES: Inflammatory pseudotumor of the spleen. Am J Surg Pathol 8:375–380, 1984

564. Thomas RM, Jaffe ES, Zarate-Osorno A, Medeiros LJ: Inflammatory pseudotumor of the spleen. A clinicopathologic and immunophenotypic study of eight cases. Arch Pathol Lab Med 117:921–926, 1993

565. Sheahan K, Wolf BC, Neiman RS: Inflammatory pseudotumor of the spleen: a clinicopathologic study of three cases. Hum Pathol 19:1024–1029, 1988

566. Arber DA, Kamel OW, van de Rijn M, et al: Frequent presence of the Epstein-Barr virus in inflammatory pseudotumor. Hum Pathol 26:1093–1098, 1995

567. Burke JS, Osborne BM: Localized reactive lymphoid hyperplasia of the spleen simulating malignant lymphoma. A report of seven cases. Am J Surg Pathol 7:373–380, 1983

568. Horny H, Ruck MT, Kaiserling E: Spleen findings in generalized mastocytosis. A clinicopathologic study. Cancer 70:459–468, 1992

569. Klatt EC, Lukes RJ, Meyer PR: Benign and malignant mast cell proliferations. Diagnosis and separation using a pH-dependent toluidine blue stain in tissue section. Cancer 51:1119–1124, 1983

570. Horny H, Schaumburg-Lever G, Bolz S, et al: Use of monoclonal antibody KP1 for identifying normal and neoplastic human mast cells. J Clin Pathol 43:719–722, 1990

571. Travis WD, Li C, Bergstralh EJ: Solid and hematologic malignancies in 60 patients with systemic mast cell disease. Arch Pathol Lab Med 113:365–368, 1989

572. Barosi G, Ambrosetti A, Buratti A, et al: Splenectomy for patients with myelofibrosis with myeloid metaplasia: pretreatment variables and outcome prediction. Leukemia 7:200–206, 1993

573. Pitcock JA, Reinhard EH, Justus BW, Mendelsohn RS: A clinical and pathological study of seventy cases of myelofibrosis. Ann Intern Med 57:73–84, 1962

574. Falk S, Mix D, Stutte H: The spleen in osteomyelofibrosis. A morphologic and immunohistochemical study of 30 cases. Virchows Archiv A [Pathol Anat] 416:437–442, 1990

575. Theile J, Klein H, Falk S, et al: Splenic megakaryocytopoiesis in primary (idiopathic) osteomyelofibrosis. An immunohistochemical and morphometric study with comparison of corresponding bone marrow features. Acta Haematol 87:176–180, 1992

576. Wolf BC, Banks PM, Mann RB, Neiman RS: Splenic hematopoiesis in polycythemia vera. A morphologic and immunohistochemical study. Am J Clin Pathol 89:69–75, 1988

577. Burke JS, Sheibani K, Winberg CD, Rappaport H: Recognition of hairy cell leukemia in a spleen of normal weight. The contribution of immunohistologic studies. Am J Clin Pathol 87:276–281, 1987

578. Loughran TP Jr, Starkebaum G, Clark E, et al: Evaluation of splenectomy in large granular lymphocytic leukaemia. Br J Haematol 67:135–140, 1987

579. Griffiths DFR, Jasani B, Standen GR: Pathology of the spleen in large granular lymphocytic leukaemia. J Clin Pathol 42:885, 1989

580. van Krieken JHJM, Feller AC, te Velde J: The distribution of non-Hodgkin's lymphoma in the lymphoid compartments of the human spleen. Am J Surg Pathol 13:757–765, 1989

581. Butler JJ: Pathology of the spleen in benign and malignant conditions. Histopathology 7:453–474, 1983

582. Audouin J, Diebold J, Schvartz H, et al: Malignant lymphoplasmacytic lymphoma with prominent splenomegaly (primary lymphoma of the spleen). J Pathol 155:17–33, 1988

583. Burke JS: Surgical pathology of the spleen: an approach to the differential diagnosis of splenic lymphomas and leukemias. Part I. Diseases of the white pulp. Am J Surg Pathol 5:551–563, 1981

583a. Arber DA, Rappaport H. Weiss LM: Non-Hodgkin's lymphoproliferative disorders involving the spleen. Mod Pathol (in press)

584. Lampert I, Catovsky D, Marsh GW, et al: The histopathology of prolymphocytic leukaemia with particular reference to the spleen: a comparison with chronic lymphocytic leukaemia. Histopathology 4:3–19, 1980

585. Chang KL, Kamel OW, Arber DA, et al: Pathologic features of nodular lymphocyte predominance Hodgkin's disease in extranodal sites. Am J Surg Pathol 19:1313–1324, 1995

586. Falk S, Stutte HJ: Primary malignant lymphomas of the spleen. A morphologic and immunohistochemical analysis of 17 cases. Cancer 66:2612–2619, 1990

587. Spier CM, Kjeldsberg CR, Eyre HJ, Behm FG: Malignant lymphoma with primary presentation in the spleen. A study of 20 patients. Arch Pathol Lab Med 109:1076–1080, 1985

588. Kraemer BB, Osborne BM, Butler JJ: Primary splenic presentation of malignant lymphoma and related disorders. A study of 49 cases. Cancer 54:1606–1619, 1984

589. Narang S, Wolf BC, Neiman RS: Malignant lymphoma presenting with prominent splenomegaly. A clinicopathologic study with special reference to intermediate cell lymphoma. Cancer 55:1948–1957, 1985

590. Neiman RS, Sullivan AL, Jaffe R: Malignant lymphoma simulating leukemic reticuloendotheliosis. A clinicopathologic study of ten cases. Cancer 43:329–342, 1979

591. Schmid C, Kirkham N, Diss T, Isaacson PG: Splenic marginal zone cell lymphoma. Am J Surg Pathol 16:455–466, 1992

592. Mollejo M, Menárguez J, Lloret E, et al: Splenic marginal zone lymphoma: a distinctive type of low-grade B-cell lymphoma—a clinicopathological study of 13 cases. Am J Surg Pathol 19:1146–1157, 1995

593. Wu CD, Jackson CL, Medeiros LJ: Splenic marginal zone cell lymphoma: an immunophenotypic and molecular study of six cases. Am J Clin Pathol 105:277–285, 1996

594. Rosso R, Neiman RS, Paulli M, et al: Splenic marginal zone cell lymphoma: report of an indolent variant without massive splenomegaly presumably representing an early phase of the disease. Hum Pathol 26:39–46, 1995

595. Melo JV, Hegde U, Parreira A, et al: Splenic B cell lymphoma with circulating villous lymphocytes: differential diagnosis of B cell leukaemias with large spleens. J Clin Pathol 40:642–651, 1987

596. Isaacson PG, Matutes E, Burke M, Catovsky D: The histopathology of splenic lymphoma with villous lymphocytes. Blood 84:3828–3834, 1994

597. Imbing F, Kumar D, Kumar S, et al: Splenic lymphoma with circulating villous lymphocytes. J Clin Pathol 48:584–587, 1995

598. Jadayel D, Matutes E, Dyer MJS, et al: Splenic lymphoma with villous lymphocytes: analysis of BCL-1 rearrangements and expression of the cyclin D1 gene. Blood 83:3664–3671, 1994

599. Kadin ME, Kamoun M, Lamberg J: Erythrophagocytic Tγ lymphoma. A clinicopathologic entity resembling malignant histiocytosis. N Engl J Med 304:648–653, 1981

600. Gaulard P, Zafrani ES, Mavier P, et al: Peripheral T-cell lymphoma presenting as predominant liver disease: a report of three cases. Hepatology 6:864–868, 1986

601. Gaulard P, Bourquelot P, Kanavaros P, et al: Expression of the alpha/beta and gamma/delta T-cell receptors in 57 cases of peripheral T-cell lymphomas. Identification of a subset of γ/δ T-cell lymphomas. Am J Pathol 137:617–628, 1990

602. Sun T, Brody J, Susin M, et al: Extranodal T-cell lymphoma mimicking malignant histiocytosis. Am J Hematol 35:269–274, 1990

603. Krishnan J, Goodman Z, Frizzera G: Primary hepatic sinusoidal presentation of malignant T cell lymphoma, abstract ed. Mod Pathol 5:81a, 1992

604. Cooke CB, Greiner T, Raffeld M, et al: γ/δ T cell lymphoma: a distinct clinicopathologic entity, abstracted. Mod Pathol 7:106a, 1994

605. Salhany K, Kahn M, Kamoun M, et al: Hepatosplenic Tγδ cell lymphoma: an aggressive cytolytic peripheral T cell lymphoma presenting with severe neutropenia, abstracted. Mod Pathol 7:119a, 1994

606. Wong KF, Chan JKC, Matutes E, et al: Hepatosplenic γδ T-cell lymphoma. A distinct aggressive lymphoma type. Am J Surg Pathol 19:718–726, 1995

607. Bordessoule D, Gaulard P, Mason DY: Preferential localisation of human lymphocytes bearing γδ T cell receptors to the red pulp of the spleen. J Clin Pathol 43:461–464, 1990

608. Mastovich S, Ratech H, Ware RE, et al: Hepatosplenic T-cell lymphoma: an unusual case of a γδ T-cell lymphoma with blast-like terminal transformation. Hum Pathol 25:102–108, 1994

609. Wick MR, Smith SL, Scheithauer BW, Beart RW Jr: Primary nonlymphoreticular malignant neoplasms of the spleen. Am J Surg Pathol 6:229–242, 1982

610. Falk S, Krishnan J, Meis JM: Primary angiosarcoma of the spleen. A clinicopathologic study of 40 cases. Am J Surg Pathol 17:959–970, 1993

611. Suster S: Epithelioid and spindle-cell hemangioendothelioma of the

spleen. Report of a distinctive splenic vascular neoplasm of childhood. Am J Surg Pathol 16:785–792, 1992

612. Kaw YT, Duwaji MS, Kinsley RE, Esparza AR: Hemangioendothelioma of the spleen. Arch Pathol Lab Med 116:1079–1082, 1992

613. Rosso R, Paulli M, Gianelli U, et al: Littoral cell angiosarcoma of the spleen—case report with immunohistochemical and ultrastructural analysis. Am J Surg Pathol 19:1203–1208, 1995

614. Sarode VR, Datta BN, Savitri K, et al: Kaposi's sarcoma of the spleen with unusual clinical and histologic features. Arch Pathol Lab Med 115:1042–1044, 1991

21

Bone Marrow

Nora C. J. Sun

Bone marrow examination is a well established procedure in the study of hematologic disorders, in the workup of fever of unknown origin,[1] in the evaluation of other systemic diseases,[2–4] and for the staging of malignant lymphoma.[5,6] It is also used to monitor therapy and for the restaging of lymphohemopoietic neoplasia. Sections of bone biopsy provide added advantages of being able to evaluate bony architecture and marrow cellular distribution; to identify stromal disorders (such as marrow fibrosis or serous degeneration of the marrow) or bone disease (such as Paget's disease or osteoporosis); to detect infiltrative processes (such as granuloma, lymphoma, storage disease, or metastatic carcinoma); to follow the course of leukemias; and to supplement the information gained from the study of aspiration smears of the bone marrow. Bone marrow biopsy sections are particularly useful whenever there is a "dry tap" (an inability to aspirate bone marrow) regardless of whether it is caused by packed leukemic cells, bone marrow necrosis, or fibrosis.[7–13]

HANDLING AND PROCESSING OF SPECIMENS

The conventional approach to the study of bone marrow includes (1) a pertinent clinical history and physical examination, (2) complete blood cell and white cell differential counts, (3) sections of bone marrow aspiration (clot) and/or bone marrow biopsy, (4) smears of bone marrow aspirations or touch preparations of bone marrow biopsy, and (5) other tests.[14–16] Bilateral or multiple bone marrow biopsies have been advocated[3,17] in the staging of malignant lymphomas and in the search for other malignant tumors or granulomas. Serial sections or step sections may be required in some instances.

The choice of a site for bone marrow aspiration and/or biopsy depends on the age of the patient, the previous history of irradiation, the presence of local skin conditions, and the preference of the examiner. In general, anterior or posterior iliac crest is the choice for adults and anterior tibia is the choice for children. The density and content of hematopoietic elements, fat, and bony trabeculae vary in different parts of the bone. If care is taken to utilize different entry sites, either bone marrow aspiration or biopsy can be performed first. For that effect, a generous area of periosteum should be anesthetized. A Jamshidi biopsy needle is generally used.[7] Sometimes, two different needles may be used, one for aspiration and one for biopsy.[8] A bone biopsy should never be performed with a sternal puncture. A Salah or Klima marrow-puncture needle that has an adjustable

guard should be used for sternal puncture and bone marrow aspiration. A detailed description of bone marrow procedures is available in any major textbook of hematology and is not repeated here.

Proper selection of marrow particles for smears or electron microscopic study is an art learned by practice and experience. Some investigators advocate aspiration only, followed by concentration of particles for section preparation.[18] Others believe that sections of bone marrow biopsies have the added advantage of permitting the examination of the bony architecture to identify diseases affecting the bone and to study the distribution of hematopoietic elements and their relationship to bony trabeculae, and to study the effect of intramedullary disease on bone.[9,19] Touch preparations should be made from the bone biopsy, especially when there is a "dry tap." The air-dried smears and touch preparations may be used for Romanowsky's stain, special cytochemical stains, and immunohistochemical stain for the detection of cell antigens, such as terminal deoxynucleotidyl transferase (TdT). Cytologic study is most useful in classifying leukemia and myelodysplastic syndrome and in identifying dyspoiesis by examining the Romanowsky-stained smears. It is a valuable adjunct to the study of histologic sections. Extra slides may be fixed in acetone or alcohol for immunohistochemical stains by using a panel of monoclonal or polyclonal antibodies. The aspirated material should be submitted for flow cytometric study or cytogenetic analysis if the diagnosis of leukemia/lymphoma or myelodysplastic syndrome is suspected. The specimen should be placed in an anticoagulant with or without tissue culture media. The collected particles or the biopsy specimen may be submitted for electron microscopic study if such a study is indicated. The rest of the specimens are then fixed in Zenker's or B5 solutions. Specimens that have been well fixed in 10 percent buffered formalin and properly processed can also give satisfactory preparations for interpretation.

Decalcification of bone biopsy specimens frequently causes leaching of iron from the tissue, resulting in inaccurate assessment of body iron stores,[20] and it also interferes with histochemical and immunohistochemical stains.[9] Thus, these special studies are preferentially performed on smears or on bone marrow particle or clot sections. Routine stains for bone marrow examination include hematoxylin and eosin (H&E) and periodic acid-Schiff (PAS) stains. The latter highlights myeloid cells and megakaryocytes because these cells contain glycogen. Reticulin stain is particularly helpful in the study of myelofibrosis caused by a variety of diseases and for delineation of the marrow meshwork. The specific (naphthol AS-D

Table 21-1. Common Antibodies Used for Antigen Detection in Histologic Sections of Bone Marrow

Antibodies	Reactive Cells
HbA	Most of NRBCs and RBCs
HbF	Minority of NRBCs and RBCs
Glycophorin A	Most of NRBCs and RBCs
Myeloperoxidase	Granulocytes, including myeloblasts, some mono/histiocytes
Lysozyme	Granulocytes, mono/histiocytes
CD15 (Leu M1)	Most granulocytes and monocytes, some R-S cells
CD45 (leukocyte common antigen)	Lymphocytes, monocytes, and mast cells; some histiocytes, plasma cells, and polymorphonuclear leukocytes
CDw75 (LN1)	Germinal center B cells, NRBCs, peripheral B cells, some R-S cells
CD74 (LN2)	B cells in germinal center and mantle zone, interdigitating histiocytes, and R-S cells
HLA-DR (LN3)	HLA-DR antigen: B cells, mono/histiocytes, and activated T cells
CD20 (L26)	Most B cells
Immunoglobulin (heavy and light chains)	B immunoblasts and plasma cells; some large and small noncleaved follicular center cells
CD43 (Leu22)	T cell-associated antigen; early myeloid cells including myeloblasts in acute myeloid leukemia.
CD45RO (UCHL-1)	Thymocytes, activated T cells, and a proportion of resting T cells
Polyclonal CD3	Subsets of T cells
CD30 (BerH2)	Activated lymphoid cells and R-S cells
Vimentin	Endothelial cells, fibroblasts, fibrocytes
Ulex europaeus agglutinin (UEA)	Endothelial cells, mature and some immature megakaryocytes, some NRBCs
Factor VIII-related antigen	Megakaryocytes, platelets, endothelial cells

Abbreviations: NRBCs, nucleated red blood cells; R-S cells, Reed-Sternberg cells.

chloroacetate) esterase (Leder) stain may be used on formalin-fixed, paraffin-embedded sections and is a useful marker for neutrophils and tissue mast cells.[14] This stain is ineffective on tissues that were fixed in mercurial-based fixative.

Recent studies indicate that enzyme cytochemistry, immunocytochemistry, flow cytometry, DNA restriction enzyme analysis, and cytogenetic examinations are invaluable tools in classifying hematopoietic and lymphoreticular malignant tumors and in predicting the prognosis for these patients.[21–31] However, some of these techniques require special and expensive equipment and trained and experienced operators. If collaborative studies can be arranged, fresh specimens should be collected in tissue culture media for transportation. In most of the surgical pathology laboratories in daily practice, a panel of polyclonal and monoclonal antibodies may be applied to formalin-fixed or B5-fixed, paraffin-embedded sections by using an immunoperoxidase or an immunoalkaline phosphatase technique for identification and classification of hematologic disorders[21,32–38] (Table 21-1). In our laboratory, the immunoalkaline phosphatase method is preferred over immunoperoxidase to avoid the presence of endogenous peroxidase in most hematopoietic cells.

NORMAL BONE MARROW

The marrow is traversed by bony trabeculae, consists of vascular and hematopoietic compartments, and is organized about blood vessels. The vascular sinuses play an important role in many of the marrow's functions. The adventitial reticular cells of the vascular sinuses are capable of becoming voluminous, forming gelatinous or fat cells; if such change is extensive, the marrow may become grossly gelatinous or fatty. The proportion of fatty to hematopoietic marrow varies in different bones and in different age groups under normal conditions, although the relationship in a given age group and anatomic site is usually quite constant. Hartsock and associates,[39] on the basis of a study of bone marrow from the anterior iliac crest, concluded that the amount of hematopoietic tissue in the first decade was 80 percent, which diminished to about 50 percent at the age of 30 and remained relatively constant until the age of 70, at which time the mean value became 30 percent. Similar trends may be seen in bone marrow obtained from the ribs, sternum, and vertebrae. It is also important to remember that marrow cavities directly adjacent to cortical bone are frequently fatty in elderly individuals and are not representative of the cellularity in the rest of the marrow. Schmid and Isaacson[40] advocate that a bone biopsy should contain at least five well preserved marrow spaces before one considers it to be an adequate specimen. The reticular cells synthesize reticular (argentophilic, reticulin) fibers that, along with their cytoplasmic processes, extend into the hematopoietic compartments and form a meshwork on which hematopoietic cells rest.

The lymphohematopoietic elements include erythrocytes, granulocytes, megakaryocytes, lymphocytes, plasma cells, macrophages, mast cells, and their precursors. They are located in the marrow spaces in the extravascular compartments in a certain topographic distribution.[41] Erythropoietic islands and megakaryocytes are associated with the sinusoids in the central regions of the marrow cavities. Early myeloid precursors lie close to the endosteal surfaces and to the arterioles. As the myeloid cells mature, they are found in the central part of the marrow cavity. The myeloid/erythroid ratio is usually 3:1 or 4:1 but may range from 2:1 to 6:1 under physiologic conditions. This paradox of more myeloid elements in marrow despite more red cells in the peripheral blood is due to the much shorter life span of granulocytes (the time from myeloblast to death is 9 to 10 days, in comparison with the 120 day life span of a red cell). A marked derangement in myeloid/erythroid ratio indicates hematologic disorders. The histopathology of normal bone marrow has been reviewed recently.[42–44]

It is believed that a pluripotent stem cell gives rise to a series of progenitor cells for hematopoietic (erythrocytic, myeloid, and megakaryocytic) cells and to common lymphoid stem cells after a number of cell divisions and differentiation steps. These pluripotent stem cells possess the capacity of self-renewal and multilineate differentiation, whereas the progenitor cells (committed stem cells) are lineage committed. These cells may lack the self-renewal capabilities. A gradual decrease of CD34 expression with a concurrent increase in expression of the proliferation antigen CD38 is noted during the maturation of stem cells to progenitor cells. Stem cells express cell surface adhesion molecules (CAMs), which interact with specific structures (ligands) in the extracellular matrix produced by marrow stromal cells.[45] The interactions between CAMs and ligands facilitate the lodgement of stem cells in the marrow and permit the close cell to cell contacts that are required for cell proliferation and survival.[46] Adhesion receptor expression is a regulated process during hematopoietic maturation. The stromal cells consist of macrophages, fibroblasts, endothelial cells, fat cells, and reticular cells. These stromal cells and a microvascular network constitute the microenvironment that is essential for the growth and development of stem cells. The extracellular matrix is composed of a variety of substances, such as fibronectin (binds erythroid precursors), hemonectin (binds granulocytic precursors), laminin, collagen, and proteoglycans (acid mucopolysaccharides). Lymphohematopoietic growth factors (cytokines, glycoprotein hormones) regulate the proliferation and differentiation of lymphohemopoietic progenitor cells and functions of mature blood cells. They serve as either inducers or inhibitors of lymphohematopoiesis. They are produced by many cell types and usually affect more than one lineage. These cytokines are active at very low concentrations and generally act on the malignant counterpart of their normal target cells.

Most information about lymphohematopoietic regulators was obtained from in vitro culture system and animal studies. Some cytokines, such as stem cell factor (SCF), interleukin-1 (IL-1), IL-3, IL-6, IL-11, and granulocyte macrophage colony-stimulating factor (GM-CSF), are considered to be early acting growth factors. Others, such as macrophage colony-stimulating factor (M-CSF), granulocyte colony-stimulating factor (G-CSF), IL-5, erythropoietin (EPO), and thrombopoietin (TP) are considered to be lineage-specific hematopoietic growth factors. Other interleukins such as IL-2, IL-4, IL-7, IL-8, IL-9, and IL-10 also participate in the regulation of hematopoiesis. Although the precise pattern of colony formation stimulated by each purified regulator is quite distinctive, there is substantial overlap in function and synergism of these regulatory factors.[47] The availability of recombinant human hematopoietic growth factors provides the basis for clinical trials. They have been used to correct iatrogenic myelosuppression secondary to chemotherapy or radiotherapy, to stimulate hematopoiesis in primary bone marrow failure (such as aplastic anemia), and to activate effector cell functions in patients with leukocyte function disorders, acquired immunodeficiency syndrome (AIDS), or other toxic conditions. They have also been used as differentiation/maturation agents for the treatment of acute myelogenous leukemias and myelodysplastic syndromes. A detailed discussion of cytokines and their inhibitors is beyond the scope of this chapter.

Erythropoiesis

Islands of erythropoiesis are easily identified on histologic sections or smears. They are characterized by perfectly round nuclei, evenly distributed chromatin, and a moderate amount of cytoplasm, which is often intensely basophilic in proerythroblasts and basophilic normoblasts by the Giemsa stain and bright red with the methyl green pyronine stain. The more mature forms (polychromatophilic and orthochromatophilic normoblasts) have more condensed or pyknotic nuclei (Fig. 21-1). The former have a clear cytoplasm and the latter have eosinophilic cytoplasm with H&E stain as hemoglobinization of the cytoplasm becomes more evident. The nucleated red blood cells (NRBCs) may be easily differentiated from myeloid precursors by their PAS-negative cytoplasm (except in erythroleukemia and a few disease entities in which the cytoplasm of erythroblasts may contain PAS-positive granules or may be diffusely stained by the PAS method). Lymphocytes or lymphoid aggregates may at times be confused with NRBCs. However, foci of erythropoiesis usually contain a spectrum of NRBCs, indicating subsequent maturation, whereas small lymphocytes in lymphoid aggregates tend to be monomorphic. In addition, the nuclei of lymphoid cells are usually slightly irreg-

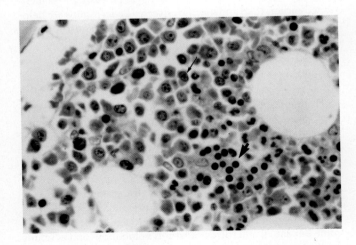

Fig. 21-1. Normal hematopoiesis. Islands of erythropoiesis are easily seen. The earlier erythroid precursors have round nuclei, prominent nucleoli, and fine chromatin (small arrows). As the cells mature, the nuclei become pyknotic and are surrounded by clear (hemoglobinized) cytoplasm (large arrow). (H&E stain, × 200.)

ular, the nuclear membranes are thickened, and the chromatin is more clumped. Plasma cells, blood vessels, transformed cells, and mast cells are often found in lymphoid aggregates. Erythropoiesis tends to be present in the vicinity of sinusoids. Hemosiderin-laden macrophages, which are found in the center of an erythroblastic island, may be easily identified by a Prussian blue (iron) stain. These macrophages are usually surrounded by a ring of erythroblasts.

Body iron stores are best assessed by an iron stain on the bone marrow smear or clot section. Although serum ferritin correlates well with the bone marrow iron stain under normal conditions, an increased serum ferritin concentration may be found in a variety of pathologic conditions unrelated to body iron stores.[48] Normally, iron is present in the histiocytes. A few (up to four) Prussian blue-positive (siderotic) granules may be normally seen in erythroid precursors (sideroblasts). Under pathologic conditions the NRBCs contain iron-laden mitochondria (sideromitochondria), which are distributed perinuclearly in humans, thus appearing as "ring sideroblasts" by iron stain. Sideroblastic anemia is defined as a refractory dyserythropoietic anemia with marked erythroid hyperplasia and an excess of iron and many ring sideroblasts in the marrow. It is a syndrome with diverse etiologies.

Myelopoiesis

The earlier myeloid precursors, myeloblasts and promyelocytes, have an oval vesicular nucleus, small but distinct nucleoli, and a moderate amount of eosinophilic cytoplasm (Fig. 21-2). Primary (azurophilic) granules are synthesized in the promyelocytes, which appear as purplish granules on Romanowsky-stained smears, but are usually unidentifiable on H&E stained sections. As the cells become more mature, the nuclear/cytoplasmic ratio decreases and specific (neutrophilic, basophilic, and eosinophilic) granules appear in the cytoplasm, which are synthesized by myelocytes. However, neutrophilic granules are often difficult to see on H&E-stained sections, and basophilic granules dissolve during tissue processing. As mentioned earlier, PAS and specific esterase (Leder) stains are helpful in recognizing neutrophilic granulocytes, and the Leder stain will highlight basophils and mast cells.

Megakaryopoiesis

The more primitive cells—megakaryoblasts and promegakaryocytes—are difficult to identify on H&E-stained sections, although they are readily recognizable on Romanowsky-stained smears. Their number is increased in acute megakaryocytic leukemia (M7), some chronic myeloproliferative disorders, and reactive conditions. Electron microscopic examination or specific monoclonal antibodies (such as glycoprotein IIB/IIIA or HP1-1D) are used to confirm their presence.[49,50] Following subsequent maturation, the cells are enlarged, the nuclei become lobulated, and the cytoplasm is voluminous and contains numerous granules on Romanowsky-stained smears or contains PAS-positive cytoplasm on histologic sections (Fig. 21-2). Margination of intensely PAS-positive granules may be seen on sections, which indicates platelet production. Occasionally

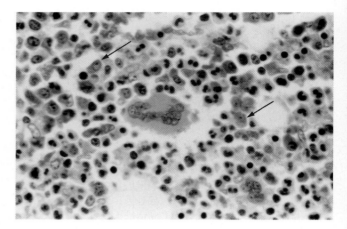

Fig. 21-2. Normal hematopoiesis. The earlier myeloid cells usually have an oval nucleus, lacy chromatin pattern, and one or more distinct nucleoli (arrows). Megakaryocytes are also present. (H&E stain, × 200.)

polymorphonuclear leukocytes or red cells are seen in the cytoplasm of megakaryocytes (emperipolesis).[51] Megakaryocytes are easily differentiated from osteoclasts. The latter are multinucleated cells in which each nucleus is identical, with an evenly distributed chromatin pattern and a small nucleolus. Osteoclasts are present along the bony trabeculae and are considered to be generated from the same hematopoietic stem cell as megakaryocytes. They are important in bony remodeling.[41]

Other Cells

Monocytes originate from the same stem cells as myeloblasts, but they are difficult to find in bone marrow sections that are in normal condition. *Histiocytes* with phagocytosis (phagocytes, macrophages), epithelioid cells, foamy cells, or other variations are seen in normal or pathologic conditions. *Lymphocytes* are present in an appreciable number in very young and very old individuals. Aggregates of lymphocytes in association with capillaries, histiocytes, plasma cells, and mast cells are seen in increased frequency in elderly individuals.[52] Very few *plasma cells* (<2 percent) are normally seen in the bone marrow[53]; they are usually scattered in the marrow cavity. A perivascular cuffing of plasma cells is seen in alcoholic liver disease, cirrhosis, collagen vascular disease, and other chronic conditions. *Osteoblasts*, cells that produce bone matrix, should be differentiated from plasma cells on bone marrow smears. These cells are often in clusters, with each cell containing one oval nucleus, evenly distributed smooth chromatin, and one small nucleolus. A hof is present away from the nucleus. Osteoblasts frequently line bony trabeculae in young children, as seen on sections. *Mast cells* lie adjacent to the endothelial cells of sinusoids, at the endosteal surface of the trabecular bone, and frequently at the edges of lymphoid nodules or aggregates. They are difficult to recognize in H&E-stained sections of bone marrow but are readily identifiable by PAS or Leder stains. Increased numbers of lymphocytes, plasma cells, and mast cells are frequently noted in hypoplastic or aplastic bone marrow.

PRACTICAL APPROACH TO BONE MARROW EXAMINATION

As stated earlier, knowledge of the clinical history, the peripheral blood cell count, the white cell differential count, and other important laboratory test results (such as serum and urine protein studies, serum levels of lactate dehydrogenase, iron) is

Table 21-2. Evaluation of the Bone Marrow Biopsy Sections: A Checklist

Quality of the specimen
    Satisfactory
    Inadequate
Bony architecture and content
    Evidence of remodeling
        Yes (increased, decreased)
        No
    Trabecular bone
        Normal
        Abnormal (osteoporosis, osteomalacia, osteosclerosis)
    Pagetoid change or other abnormalities
Marrow space
    Hematopoietic elements
        Cellularity (normal, increased, decreased)
        Fat/cell ratio
        Topographic distribution of hematopoiesis (normal or abnormal)
        Erythropoiesis and maturation sequence
        Granulopoiesis and maturation sequence
        Myeloid/erythroid ratio
        Megakaryopoiesis and maturation sequence
        Dyspoiesis (absent or involving which cell line)
        Marrow necrosis
    Stroma
        Fat
            Normal, increased, decreased
            Gelatinous degeneration
            Necrosis, edema, hemorrhage
        Blood vessels
            Normal
            Abnormal (vasculitis, arteriosclerosis, amyloid deposition, intravascular fibrin or platelet thrombi, vascular proliferation or tumor, dilation of sinuses, intrasinusoidal hematopoiesis)
    Reticulin meshwork
        Normal
        Abnormal (reticulin fibrosis or collagen fibrosis; focal or diffuse; collapsed reticulin meshwork)
    Other cells
        Histiocytes (phagocytes, foamy cells, epithelioid cells, giant cells, granulomas)
        Lymphocytes (small aggregates, nodules, follicles)
            Pattern of infiltration: focal or diffuse; interstitial, nodular, or paratrabecular
            Composition of infiltration: small, intermediate, or large cells
        Plasma cells
            Increased (perivascular, interstitial, focal, diffuse)
            Well differentiated, moderately well differentiated, or poorly differentiated
        Mast cells
        Foreign cells

essential prior to examination and interpretation of peripheral blood smears, bone marrow biopsy and clot sections, and bone marrow smears. Because this book is for surgical pathologists, a checklist for evaluation of bone marrow biopsy sections is given in Table 21-2.

A bone marrow report includes description, diagnosis, and comment. Needless to say, all pertinent findings should be described. A systemic approach is always helpful. For example, it can be started with the clinical history followed by examining the peripheral blood smear, bone marrow biopsy, bone marrow clot section, bone marrow smear and/or touch preparation, and the results of other special studies. One can also establish a routine while studying each of these preparations: for instance, the red cell series will be examined first and then the myeloid and megakaryocytic series and other cells in sequential order. It is important to know the patient's age (bony remodeling and cellularity), sex (especially in considering anemia), and ethnic background (for instance, hemoglobinopathy is common in certain ethnic groups). Sometimes a definitive diagnosis cannot be made; in this case a summation of pertinent findings is listed, followed by comments, which include a list of differential diagnoses and, frequently, suggestions for additional studies.

PATHOLOGY OF BONE MARROW

The pathology of bone marrow can be classified according to etiology (e.g., infectious disease, iron deficiency anemia), type of cell involved (e.g., red cell disorders, white cell disorders), and pathologic changes. I have chosen to discuss the marrow abnormalities according to the predominant pathologic changes in the following order: (1) cellularity, (2) fibrosis, (3) lymphocytic infiltrates, (4) granulomatous changes, (5) histiocytic proliferative disorders, (6) metastatic tumors, (7) bone marrow necrosis and infarction, and (8) vascular lesions in marrow.

Cellularity

The hematopoietic elements may become hypocellular or hypercellular in normal or pathologic conditions. A hypocellular bone marrow is often associated with peripheral cytopenia, whereas hypercellular bone marrow may be manifested as polycythemia, leukocytosis, thrombocytosis, or one or more cytopenias in the peripheral blood.

Normal or Hypocellular Bone Marrow

Hypocellular bone marrow is defined by a decrease in volume of hematopoietic elements in relation to fat, with the patient's age taken into consideration. The cellular components of a hypocellular marrow must be studied carefully, because the different cell series may not be affected to the same degree and because an increased number of blasts (acute leukemia) may be observed in hypocellular marrow (discussed below). Lymphocytes, plasma cells, histiocytes, and mast cells are usually quite prominent in such specimens. The common causes or clinical

Table 21-3. Common Causes or Clinical Conditions Associated with Hypocellular Bone Marrow

Normal aging process
Nutritional (anorexia nervosa)
Infectious (e.g., viral hepatitis or miliary tuberculosis)
Marrow toxicity (drugs, chemicals, or ionizing radiation)
Some leukemias
Some myelodysplastic syndromes
Paroxysmal nocturnal hemoglobinuria
Congenital (Fanconi's syndrome or constitutional hypoplastic anemia)
Idiopathic (aplastic anemia)

conditions associated with hypocellular bone marrow are listed in Table 21-3. Intramedullary hemorrhage following bone marrow aspiration should not be confused with hypocellular marrow. Likewise, the marrow cavities in the subcortical region are usually more hypoplastic (especially in old age) and should not be relied on for diagnosis. Selective hypoplasia in the iliac crest has also been observed in certain conditions, such as autoimmune states.[54] Growth factors, such as IL-3 (or multi-CSF), CSF or M-CSF, EPO, GM-CSF, and G-CSF may be selectively used to correct respective lineage hypoplasia.

Serous (Mucinous, Gelatinous) Degeneration of the Marrow

Serous degeneration of the marrow is characterized by multifocal gelatinous transformation of the nonhematopoietic marrow and is associated with malnutrition, emaciation, anorexia nervosa, and a variety of chronic disorders, including malignant disease, AIDS, tuberculosis, and chronic renal disease.[55–57] Microscopic examination reveals the fat cells to be decreased in size, with pink amorphous material in the interstitium (Fig. 21-3). They have a granular or fibrillary appearance on higher magnification and stain pale pink with the PAS stain (Fig.

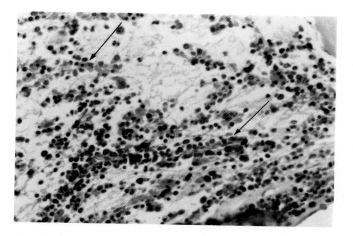

Fig. 21-3. Bone marrow biopsy from a patient with acquired immunodeficiency syndrome (AIDS). Note mucinous degeneration of fat (the fat cells become very small and poorly outlined). The plasma cells are markedly increased with perivascular cuffing (arrows). (H&E stain, × 100.)

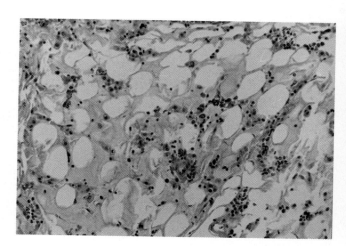

Fig. 21-4. Hypocellular bone marrow with gelatinous degeneration of fat cells. (H&E stain, × 70.)

21-4). Histochemical studies show that the extracellular substance consists primarily of hyaluronic acid[56] or a large amount of sulfated glycosaminoglycan in addition.[57] The adjacent marrow is usually hypoplastic, but the total amount of hematopoietic material is usually not decreased. Serous atrophy may be found in the adipose tissue in other parts of the body.

Aplastic Anemia

Aplastic anemia can be classified as constitutional (congenital or hereditary) or acquired and is usually characterized by peripheral blood pancytopenia and marrow panhypoplasia.[58] Isolated single cell-line deficiency may also occur. The congenital form is uncommon. The acquired form is frequently related to drugs, chemicals, ionizing radiation, or viral infections.[59] Sometimes the episode may be transient, and the marrow may recover after removal of the insulting agent(s). However, patients with aplastic anemia may develop myelodysplastic syndrome, paroxysmal nocturnal hemoglobinuria (PNH), or acute nonlymphocytic leukemia[60–62]; thus, it appears to be a stem cell defect. Bone marrow examination reveals moderately hypocellular (hypoplastic) or severely hypocellular (aplastic) marrow with an increased amount of adipose tissue (>75 percent of marrow space, age adjusted) with scattered lymphocytes, plasma cells, mast cells, and hemosiderin-laden macrophages. Small collections of erythroid, myeloid, or megakaryocytic precursors may be observed in hypoplastic anemia. There may be areas of normocellularity despite overall hypocellularity and lymphoid follicles may be prominent. Bone marrow transplantation is a treatment of choice in selected patients. The disease must be differentiated from other causes of pancytopenia, such as hypocellular acute leukemia, hypoplastic myelodysplastic syndrome, and hairy cell leukemia.

Pure Red Cell Aplasia

Pure red cell aplasia may be congenital (Diamond-Blackfan anemia) or acquired (associated with spindle cell thymoma or various types of malignancy, aplastic crisis in hemolytic anemia, drugs, or other causes).[63,64] Vacuolated erythroblasts are seen in chloramphenicol-associated aplasia, erythroleukemia, alcoholism (in which vacuolated myeloid precursors may also be present), and hyperosmolar coma. PAS-positive granules are usually demonstrated in erythroblasts of erythroleukemia. The marrow is normocellular or hypercellular.

Agranulocytosis

Agranulocytosis is a severe degree of neutropenia that is often drug related. Neutropenia may be caused by underproduction, excessive destruction, or abnormal distribution of neutrophils. Thus, although granulocytic hypoplasia in the bone marrow is always associated with neutropenia in the peripheral blood, not all neutropenias are associated with granulocytic hypoplasia in the marrow. Congenital abnormalities of granulopoiesis are rare. Some patients with autoimmune disorders or viral infections may have selective granulocytic hypoplasia.[65,66]

Megakaryocytic Hypoplasia

Isolated or selective megakaryocytic hypoplasia or aplasia is very rare,[67] although thrombocytopenia is not uncommon clinically. Several thrombocytopenias, such as immune thrombocytopenic purpura or thrombotic thrombocytopenic purpura, are associated with megakaryocytic hyperplasia. Refractory thrombocytopenia may be a manifestation of myelodysplastic syndrome.[68] Megakaryocytes may be quantitatively normal, increased, or decreased. However, dysmegakaryopoiesis is seen in all cases and dyspoiesis involving erythroid and/or granulocytic series is noted in some cases.[68]

Paroxysmal Nocturnal Hemoglobinuria

PNH is a stem cell disorder characterized by chronic hemolytic anemia associated with recurrent nocturnal exacerbations, neutropenia, and/or thrombocytopenia. The etiology of this acquired disorder is unknown. The clinical manifestations of pancytopenia and reticulocytosis are due to increased sensitivity of erythrocyte membranes to complement-mediated lysis. Sucrose hemolysis and Ham acid hemolysis tests are useful for the diagnosis. The marrow cellularity is quite variable.[63] However, a substantial number of patients with typical PNH show signs of bone marrow failure (pancytopenia, reduced bone marrow cellularity, and modest reticulocytosis in the face of very low hemoglobin). A number of biochemical defects have been detected in red blood cells (RBCs), neutrophils, monocytes, lymphocytes, and thrombocytes.[69] PNH may precede or follow the development of aplastic anemia. PNH has also been reported in association with acute leukemia and other myeloproliferative disorders.

Hypoplastic Acute Leukemia

Although acute leukemia is usually characterized by hypercellular bone marrow, some patients, mostly elderly men, may present with hypocellular marrow and other morphologic features indicative of acute leukemia (increased number of blasts, presence of Auer rods, dyserythropoiesis, and chromosomal abnormalities).[70,71] The diagnostic criteria consist of a hypocellular marrow (50 percent cellularity) and more than 30 percent primitive myeloid cells. Core biopsy of marrow is essential for an accurate diagnosis. The incidence of this form of acute leukemia was said to be 7.7 percent[71] to 10.7 percent.[70] Most of these patients had acute nonlymphocytic leukemia, and many of them responded to aggressive chemotherapy. However, a number of patients in both studies[70,71] do not fulfill the diagnostic criteria of acute leukemia as delineated by the French-American-British (FAB) cooperative group.[72–74] Gladson and Naeim[75] found that a history of alcohol abuse (30 percent), potential exposure to toxic chemicals (20 percent), second malignant tumors (20 percent), and aplastic anemia (25 percent) were common in this group of patients, and they also found that overall mortality was high, especially in patients undergoing chemotherapy. Antecedent myelodysplastic changes are found in one-third of cases and there is often a history of previous exposure to leukemogenic agents.[71,76] The pathogenesis of the hypocellularity is uncertain, but it appears that this condition is a true variant of acute leukemia. Hypoplastic myelodysplastic syndrome is discussed below.

"Preleukemic State" in Children

Transient pancytopenia has been occasionally noted preceding the onset of acute leukemia in children (2 percent).[77] These patients had peripheral pancytopenia and a hypocellular bone marrow aspirate. They responded rapidly to steroid therapy, but developed overt leukemia within 5 to 38 weeks of first presentation with features of marrow failure. Immunologic study revealed that blasts with acute lymphocytic leukemia (ALL) morphology possessed the phenotype of common ALL. This phenomenon has been described as a "preleukemic state" in the literature.[78] Although the terms *preleukemia* and *myelodysplastic syndrome* have been used interchangeably in the literature with regard to adult patients, and hypoplastic myelodysplastic syndrome has also been described in adults,[79] myelodyplastic syndromes are well defined entities and are discussed in detail in the section on myelodysplastic syndrome.

Postchemotherapy Bone Marrow Aplasia

Sequential evaluation of bone marrow changes following administration of chemotherapeutic agents for acute leukemias frequently reveals marrow necrosis and aplasia in the immediate post-therapy stage, with deposition of eosinophilic amorphous material in the interstitium, edema, and marked dilation of sinuses (Fig. 21-5). Erythroid cell regeneration usually appears first, followed by the megakaryocytic and granulocytic precursors in successfully treated patients. A similar process is observed in bone marrow necrosis of other etiologies (Fig. 21-6). Wittels[80] described two phases of marrow response to effective chemotherapy in acute leukemia: (1) cellular depletion characterized by progressive emptying of the initially packed marrow to leave an essentially vacant fibrillary reticulin stroma punctuated by dilated sinusoids containing fibrin; and (2) marrow reconstitution, during which the intertrabecular space is refilled by proliferation of hematopoietic cells and generation of fat cells, collagen, or bone. It should be emphasized that cytokine therapy will augment the chemotherapeutic effects on bone marrow. Special precaution should be taken when one interprets such a specimen (see below). In my experience, small clusters of leukemic cells are often scattered among a normocellular or hypocellular bone marrow in relapse of leukemia or in unsuccessfully treated patients with residual leukemic cells;

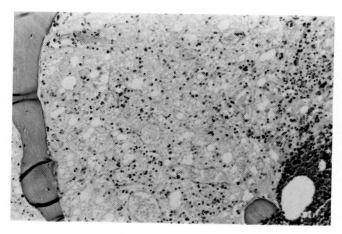

Fig. 21-5. Postchemotherapeutic effect. Note markedly hypocellular bone marrow, with edema and deposition of eosinophilic granular material in the interstitium and sinusoids. (H&E stain, × 40.)

thus, histologic section provides a better means for assessment than aspirated smears.

Bone Marrow Changes in Transplant Recipients

Bone marrow transplants have been widely used to treat patients with non-neoplastic and neoplastic diseases such as aplastic anemia, severe combined immunodeficiency, leukemias, and solid tumors, and have been received with considerable success. An examination of the recipient's bone marrow prior to bone marrow transplant should be carefully performed to confirm the clinical diagnosis and to serve as a baseline for future comparison. The bone marrow is usually markedly hypocellular during the first week after transplantation. Evidence of damaged marrow, such as necrosis, edema, and an increased number of histiocytes, especially foamy macrophages, scattered lymphocytes, and plasma cells is seen.

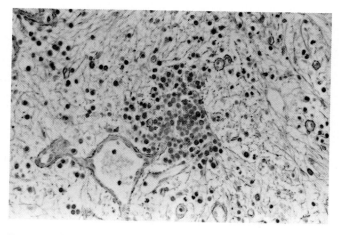

Fig. 21-6. Bone marrow biopsy from a patient who had SS disease (sickle cell anemia) in aplastic crisis. Note that the reticulin meshwork is maintained and enhanced, although the cellularity is markedly decreased. An island of erythropoiesis is seen in the center of the field. (Snook's reticulin stain, × 100.)

The engrafted bone marrow contains isolated, small clusters of erythroid and granulocytic cells at 1 to 3 weeks after transplantation. However, erythropoiesis is often in predominance and megakaryocytes are difficult to find. Both erythroid and granulocytic cells may show a moderate to marked left shift and dyspoietic changes are frequently seen. Between 4 and 8 weeks the marrow cellularity increases and blood counts rise progressively. Large hematopoietic islands containing mixed-lineage cell lines are evident. Dysplastic changes are minimal. Maturation proceeds normally. The rate of engraftment and return to normocellularity varies from patient to patient. It is usually achieved about 8 to 12 weeks following transplantation.

The first usual indication of graft rejection of an allogeneic bone marrow transplant is a decline in erythroid precursors. This is followed by the decrease of other hematopoietic elements and finally by marrow aplasia. Patients with graft-versus-host disease may have an increased number of lymphocytes, plasma cells, and eosinophils in their marrow. Lymphoid aggregates and granulomas have been found in some cases. Detection of relapse or residual acute leukemia in transplant recipients is difficult, because lymphocytosis is common in children and regenerated left-shifted myelopoiesis may be confused with myelogenous leukemic cells in adults. In addition, one should recognize the presence of hematogones, B lineage lymphoid precursor cells, in these patients. Hematogones are small to medium-sized lymphoid cells with a uniform or intermediate degree of chromatin condensation, nuclear irregularity, indistinct nucleoli, and scant agranular basophilic cytoplasm. An increased number of hematogones may be observed in regenerating bone marrow in children and in a variety of clinical conditions in adults.[81] It is best to follow these cases with serial bone marrow examination before reaching a conclusion.

Hypercellular Bone Marrow

Hypercellular bone marrow may be broadly classified as non-neoplastic or neoplastic hyperplasia (Table 21-4).

Non-Neoplastic Hyperplasia

Reactive hyperplasia is a compensatory mechanism responding to peripheral destruction or utilization of blood elements; the production and maturation of these elements are usually normal. Sometimes non-neoplastic hyperplasia may occur under nonphysiologic conditions, such as erythroid hyperplasia following ineffective hematopoiesis associated with megaloblastic anemia, or myeloid hyperplasia following cytokine (G-CSF) therapy.

Erythroid Hyperplasia. Erythroid hyperplasia may be normoblastic, megaloblastic, or megaloblastoid.

Normoblastic Hyperplasia. Normoblastic hyperplasia may be manifested as peripheral erythrocytosis or anemia. Erythrocytosis (secondary polycythemia) results from increased erythropoiesis due to increased production of erythropoietin. Chronic tissue hypoxia of various etiologies (such as living in high altitude or cardiopulmonary disease resulting in a right-to-left cardiac shunt) and hemoglobinopathy with increased oxy-

Table 21-4. Common Causes or Clinical Conditions Associated with Hypercellular Bone Marrow

Non-neoplastic conditions
  Newborn
  Compensatory increase in hematopoiesis
    Erythroid hyperplasia in hemoglobinopathies, hereditary red cell membrane defects, or enzymopathies, hemolytic anemia, pernicious anemia, hypoxia, and other conditions
    Leukemoid reaction to infections, drug reactions, neoplasia, or others
    Megakaryocytic hyperplasia in immune thrombocytopenic purpura
    Panhyperplasia in hypersplenism
  Congenital dyserythropoietic anemia
  Multilineage or single cell line hyperplasia following cytokine (growth factor) therapy
  Storage disorders, such as Gaucher's disease, Niemann-Pick disease, and others
Neoplastic conditions
  Leukemias, myelodysplastic syndromes, and chronic myeloproliferative disorders
  Chronic lymphoproliferative disorders and plasma cell dyscrasias
  Lymphomatous involvement
  Malignant histiocytosis and true histiocytic lymphoma
  Metastatic tumors

gen affinity are more common than inappropriate secretion of erythropoietin by a tumor (such as hypernephroma or cerebellar hemangioblastoma). The bone marrow shows erythroid hyperplasia without accompanying myeloid or megakaryocytic hyperplasia. Anemia of hereditary red cell abnormalities (red cell membrane defect, enzymopathy, or hemoglobinopathy) or of acquired disorders (nutritional deficiency anemia, hemolytic anemia, some forms of refractory anemias, or some forms of sideroblastic anemias) is often associated with erythroid hyperplasia. Erythroid hyperplasia also is observed a few days after acute massive hemorrhage or bleeding and in patients with congenital dyserythropoietic anemia.[82]

Hypochromic anemia, the most common form of anemia, is characterized by normocytic or microcytic, hypochromic red cell morphology. It includes a variety of clinical conditions (such as iron deficiency anemia, thalassemia, sideroblastic anemia, and anemia of chronic disease), all of which are related to impaired hemoglobin synthesis. Of the disease entities listed above, all but iron deficiency anemia are associated with iron overload.

A normal individual absorbs 5 to 10 percent of the total iron ingested, the rest being lost with sloughed mucosal cells of the small intestine. All body iron is combined (chelated) with one or another protein. For instance, plasma iron is transported bound to transferrin. By far the greatest amount of iron in the body is present within cells as heme iron (iron chelated to the porphyrin ring), which is then combined with globins and becomes hemoglobin (for oxygen transport), myoglobin (for oxygen storage), and cytochrome c (an enzyme responsible for oxygen activation in biologic oxidation).

Iron is stored equally as ferritin (ferric hydroxyphosphate micelles attached to apoferritin, a globulin) and hemosiderin (aggregates of ferritin particles) in the reticuloendothelial cells of the liver, spleen, and bone marrow and the parenchymal cells of the liver. Ferritin is finely dispersed within the cytoplasm, is water-soluble, and is invisible with the light microscope, although it is readily seen with the electron microscope. Hemosiderin is visible as yellow to brown granules on H&E-stained sections by light microscopy but is best demonstrated by the Prussian blue stain. Only intracellular granules should be considered in the evaluation of iron stores. The iron not utilized for the red cell pool is shifted to the stores. Prolonged intravascular hemolysis is associated with hemosiderinuria and depletion of iron stores. In extravascular hemolytic processes, including ineffective erythropoiesis (as in thalassemia), and also in patients who have received multiple blood transfusions for chronic anemias, increased hemosiderin is seen in the phagocytic histiocytes of the reticuloendothelial system (hemosiderosis). A subgroup of sideroblastic anemias is discussed in connection with myelodysplastic syndrome. Ring sideroblasts may be found in megaloblastic anemia, thalassemia, alcoholism, lead intoxication, drug reactions (to chloramphenicol or isoniazid), and in certain hereditary anemias.

Clinically, iron deficiency anemia may be divided into three stages: (1) iron depletion, (2) iron-deficient erythropoiesis, and (3) iron-deficient anemia. Although decreased levels of serum ferritin and marrow iron stores are noted in the earliest stage, it is not until the third stage that microcytic hypochromic anemia becomes evident.

Megaloblastic Hyperplasia. Megaloblastic anemia includes a group of disorders characterized by one or more peripheral cytopenias, oval macrocytosis, iron overload, and megaloblastic erythroid hyperplasia. It is commonly caused by a vitamin B_{12} or folate deficiency, resulting in impairment of DNA synthesis. A megaloblastic erythroid cell is larger than a corresponding normoblastic cell, with a high cytoplasmic/nuclear area ratio and an open, lacy chromatin pattern (dyssynchrony in nuclear and cytoplasmic maturation). Multinuclearity, nuclear fragments or Howell-Jolly bodies (dyserythropoiesis), and mitoses are seen. Megaloblastic change affects all dividing cells. Giant bands, monocytoid bands, hypersegmented neutrophils, and hyperlobulated megakaryocytes are all present. Ineffective erythropoiesis (premature death of erythroid cells during the maturation sequence in the marrow) is increased. Megaloblastic hyperplasia may be so florid as to be confused with acute leukemia (Fig. 21-7). Identification of intracytoplasmic HbA or HbF by an immunoperoxidase method may be helpful in recognizing that these immature cells are megaloblastic erythroblasts. Megaloblastic change is most evident on bone marrow smears, which also show dyspoiesis involving myeloid (giant bands, monocytoid bands, and hypersegmented neutrophils) and megakaryocytic (hyperlobulated forms) cells.

Pernicious anemia is a form of megaloblastic anemia, caused by atrophic gastritis with circulating antiparietal cell and/or intrinsic factor antibody in the blood, resulting in vitamin B_{12} deficiency. The most significant clinical manifestations are neurologic symptoms due to subacute combined degeneration of the spinal cord. It affects middle-aged or elderly women with a familial and racial disposition. A juvenile form has also been recognized.

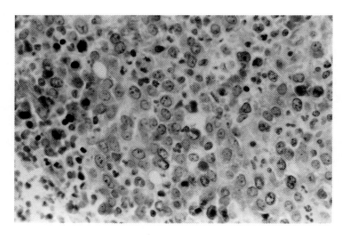

Fig. 21-7. Hypercellular bone marrow from a patient with megaloblastic anemia. Note marked erythroid hyperplasia, with cells characterized by a round or oval nucleus with smooth chromatin and multiple nucleoli. Compare these megaloblastic erythroblasts with normoblastic erythroblasts (Fig. 21-1) and myeloblasts (Fig. 21-2). Immunohistochemical stains may be used to distinguish erythroblasts from myeloblasts. Note that many immature cells are weakly stained by anti-hemoglobin A. (Immunoperoxidase stain, × 200.)

Megaloblastoid Hyperplasia. Megaloblastoid erythropoiesis displays morphologic features intermediate between those of megaloblastic and normoblastic erythropoiesis. It has been called "intermediate megaloblastic," "macronormoblastic," or "transitional megaloblastic" erythropoiesis. A megaloblastoid erythroid cell is larger than the corresponding erythrons of the normoblastic series, with evidence of dissociation in nuclear/cytoplasmic maturation. However, the chromatin pattern is punctate and clumping, and the chromatin strands are coarser than in megaloblastic maturation. Thus, there are more parachromatin spaces. Multinuclearity and nuclear fragmentation are common. Both megaloblastic and megaloblastoid erythropoiesis are dyserythropoietic, but the megaloblastoid change is more common clinically. It may be observed in acute and chronic myeloproliferative disorders (CMPDs), myelodysplastic syndrome (MDS), pregnancy, alcoholic liver disease, and in patients undergoing chemotherapy, especially those treated with antimetabolites. Lewis and Verwilghen[83] preferred to reserve the term *dyserythropoietic anemia* for congenital (and acquired primary) cases only.

Myeloid Hyperplasia. Myeloid hyperplasia with peripheral leukocytosis (in excess of 50×10^9 leukocytes/L) is often seen in leukemoid reaction. Leukemoid reaction may be elicited by bacterial (neutrophilic), viral (lymphoid), allergic (eosinophilic), or inflammatory diseases, necrosis, burns, drugs, toxins, and neoplasms. Reactive myeloid hyperplasia secondary to severe sepsis may occasionally be associated with leukopenia. Myeloid hyperplasia or granulocytic hyperplasia may display normal maturation with a marked increase in the myeloid/erythroid ratio. It can also exhibit a "shift to the left" (an increased number of the more immature granulocytic cells). The term *maturation arrest of the granulocytic series* is used to describe granulocytic hyperplasia with a shift to the left and very rare segmented neutrophils and bands. It may be associated with leukemia, or it may reflect granulocytic hyperplasia associated with an increased delivery of more mature granulocytes to the peripheral blood. Histologic differentiation between a leukemoid reaction and chronic granulocytic leukemia (CGL) in the marrow may not be possible, but the following guidelines may be helpful:

1. Granulocytic proliferation in CGL is most evident along the paratrabecular region, consisting of broad paratrabecular and perivascular seams of immature myeloid precursors and mature granulocytes in the central regions
2. Increased eosinophils and basophils are more commonly seen with CGL
3. Megakaryocytic hyperplasia with abnormal forms is common in CGL
4. Increased reticulin fibers are more frequently seen in CGL
5. The marrow fat cells are relatively well preserved in leukemoid reaction but not in CGL
6. The presence of Philadelphia chromosome [Ph:t(9;22)] and decreased leukocyte alkaline phosphatase score confirm the diagnosis of CGL

Hematologic Changes After Cytokine Therapy. Recombinant growth factors such as EPO, G-CSF, and GM-CSF have been used to treat patients with anemia or leukopenia (following chemotherapy for acute leukemia, lymphoma, or solid tumors or following human immunodeficiency virus [HIV] infections). These cytokines bind to specific surface receptors of lineage-specific progenitor cells and maturing cells and stimulate proliferation, differentiation, maturation, and activation of some mature cell functions. Elevation of neutrophil count to reach an absolute neutrophil count of greater than 0.5×10^9/L may be obtained 1 to 24 days (with an average of 5 to 6 days) after GM-CSF or G-CSF therapy.[84] The major findings in the blood are similar to those observed in a marked inflammatory reaction, with increased azurophilic granulation (toxic granules) and prominent Döhle bodies (some of which may be seen in the eosinophils) and left-shifted myeloid cells including myeloblasts.[84] Bone marrow examination at 2 to 4 days after cytokine therapy reveals marked myeloid hyperplasia with an increase in promyelocytes and myelocytes.[84,85] Both promyelocytes and myelocytes appear larger than normal. Even distribution of coarse azurophilic granules and a prominent perinuclear spherical area indicating the Golgi zone are characteristic findings of abnormal promyelocytes, whereas increased azurophilic granules and cytoplasmic basophilia are common features in myelocytes. It is at times difficult to differentiate a promyelocyte from a myelocyte. Bone marrow findings at 10 to 15 days after cytokine therapy include a normal myeloid/erythroid ratio, although toxic granules and Döhle bodies are still visible in myelocytes, metamyelocytes, and segmented neutrophils. The differential diagnosis for a leukemic patient status postchemotherapy includes residual leukemic cells (in the early stage of therapy) and infection. Close clinicopathologic correlations and sequential bone marrow examinations may lead to resolution of the problem.

Megakaryocytic Hyperplasia. Increased numbers of normal megakaryocytes with normal morphology are typically seen in immune thrombocytopenic purpura or other clinical conditions associated with increased destruction of platelets (thrombotic thrombocytopenic purpura, consumption coagulopathy, and so forth) or with peripheral thrombocytosis. Increased megakaryocytes with abnormal morphology are sometimes seen in AIDS, and are also characteristically found in some CMPDs, acute malignant myelosclerosis, and sometimes in acute leukemia (M7).

Neoplastic Hyperplasia

Included as forms of neoplastic hyperplasia are a group of acute leukemias, CMPDs, and MDS. Chronic lymphocytic leukemia and non-Hodgkin's lymphoma are discussed under the section on lymphocytic infiltrate. Hodgkin's disease and some non-Hodgkin's lymphomas in which granulomatous changes are constant features are discussed under granulomatous changes.

Acute Leukemia. Acute leukemia is defined as uncontrolled clonal proliferation of immature blood cells in the blood-forming organs, which chiefly affects the bone marrow and eventually replaces the normal hematopoietic cell lines, resulting in peripheral cytopenias. In clinical practice, acute leukemia is diagnosed when there are more than 30 percent of blasts in the bone marrow.[72,75]

The classification of acute leukemia is based on morphologic examination of Romanowsky-stained bone marrow smears, or touch preparations, supplemented by a few cytochemical stains.[14,86] According to the criteria proposed by the FAB Cooperative Group,[72–74,87] acute leukemias may be broadly classified into acute nonlymphocytic leukemia (ANLL) and acute lymphocytic leukemia (ALL) based on the presence (ANLL) or absence (ALL) of 3 percent or more blasts containing myeloperoxidase- or Sudan black B-positive granules. It should be emphasized, however, that immunologic study is important in classifying ALL, and that nonrandomized chromosomal changes are seen in specific types of acute leukemias.[88–95] It should also be pointed out that blasts in M7 (megakaryoblasts) do not contain myeloperoxidase- or Sudan black B-positive granules; therefore, other studies such as electron microscopy or

immunocytochemistry should be performed to confirm the diagnosis.[49,50,87,96] Likewise, the diagnosis for minimally differentiated acute leukemia (ANNL-M0) has to depend on immunophenotypic study.[97]

Acute Nonlymphocytic Leukemias. The FAB group now proposes to establish the percentage of erythroblasts as the first step in classifying ANLLs (Fig. 21-8). If erythroblasts comprise fewer than 50 percent of all nucleated bone marrow cells (ANC) and there are 30 percent or more blasts of ANC, then the leukemia may be classified as M1 to M5, and M7. If erythroblasts account for more than 50 percent of ANC and blasts represent 30 percent or more of nonerythroid cells (NEC), a diagnosis of erythroleukemia (M6) may be made. If erythroblasts account for more than 50 percent of ANC but blasts account for less than 30 percent of NEC, a diagnosis of MDS may be considered. The FAB classification of ANLLs is listed in Table 21-5.[74,87,95,97,98] The application of cytochemical and immunologic studies in the modified FAB classification is illustrated in Figure 21-9.

Most forms of ANLL exhibit a hypercellular marrow with few fat cells seen; however, hypocellular ANLL is not uncommon and has been discussed earlier (Fig. 21-10). Megakaryocytes and erythroid precursors are generally sparse, with the exception of M7 and M6, respectively. The blasts are usually large, with increased nuclear/cytoplasmic ratio, round to oval or folded nuclei, finely dispersed chromatin, and small but distinct nucleoli. Three types of blasts have been described. The type I blasts resemble myeloblasts without azurophilic granules. Type II blasts have identical features as type I blasts, but contain up to 20 delicate azurophilic granules in the cytoplasm. The type III blasts resemble type II blasts but have more than 20 fine azurophilic granules.[74,99] Type II and type III blasts should be differentiated from promyelocytes (see under MDS) (Fig. 21-11). Auer rods, which appear as eosinophilic rod-like structures, may be identified (Figs. 21-12 and 21-13). They are composed of primary granules and are positively stained by myeloperoxidase, PAS, and chloroacetate esterase (Leder) stains. They give a negative image with Sudan black B stain. A combination of chloroacetate esterase (CAE) stain and immunocytochemical stain for lysozyme (muramidase) or

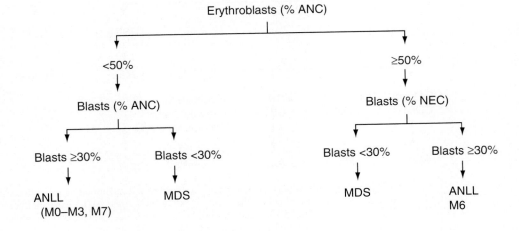

Fig. 21-8. Differentiation of acute nonlymphocytic leukemia (ANLL) from myelodysplastic syndrome (MDS) according to FAB classification. ANC, all nucleated cells; NEC, nonerythroid cells; Blasts, type I, type II, and type III myeloblasts. (Modified from Bennett et al,[74] with permission.)

Table 21-5. French-American-British (FAB) Classification of Acute Nonlymphocytic Leukemia

FAB Subtype	Morphologic and Other Characteristics	Frequency (%) Adults	Frequency (%) Children
M0	Acute myeloid leukemia, minimally differentiated (AML): ≥30% blasts; <3% blasts reactive for MPO, SBB, or NSE; blasts express CD13 and/or CD33, and may be TdT-positive	2–3	2
M1	Acute myeloblastic leukemia without maturation (AML): ≥30% blasts; ≥3% blasts reactive for MPO or SBB; blasts express CD13 and CD33; 3% may be Philadelphia chromosome-positive	20	13
M2	Acute myeloblastic leukemia with maturation (AML): ≥30% blasts; ≥3% blasts reactive for MPO or SBB; >10% promyelocytes and maturing myeloid cells; <20% monocytic cells; blasts express CD13, CD33, CD11, and CD15; 12% have t(8;21)	25–30	28
M3	Acute promyelocytic leukemia (APL): ≥30% blasts and abnormal promyelocytes; often contain bundles of Auer rods (faggot cells); hypergranular (M3) or microgranular (hypogranular, M3 variant [M3v]) forms; intense MPO and SBB reactivity; blasts express CD13, CD33, CD11, and CD15; most are HLA-DR negative; >90% have t(15;17)	10	6
M4	Acute myelomonocytic leukemia (AMMoL): ≥30% myeloblasts, monoblasts, and promonocytes; ≥20% abnormal monocytic cells in marrow (or ≥5 × 10⁹/L monocytic cells in blood) and ≥20% myeloblasts/promyelocytes in marrow; monocytic cells reactive for NSE; monocytic cells express CD14 and CD36; ≥5% abnormal eosinophils (containing single, unsegmented nucleus and large basophilic granules) may be seen in M4$_{EO}$ and associated with chromosome 16 abnormalities	20–25	19
M5	Acute monocytic leukemia (AMoL): ≥80% monocytic cells M5a: poorly differentiated [monoblasts ≥80% monocytic cells; NSE (+), MPO and SBB (−) or (±)] M5b: differentiated [monoblasts <80% of monocytic cells; NSE (+); MPO and SBB (±)]	10–15	21
M6	Acute erythroleukemia (AEL): ≥50% erythroblasts; myeloblasts, ≥30% of NEC; abnormal multinucleated erythroblasts are usually PAS positive and express glycophorin A and transferrin receptor	5	1
M7	Acute megakaryoblastic leukemia: ≥30% megakaryoblasts; blasts are reactive to platelet peroxidase by electron microscopy and express CD41 and CD61; myelofibrosis is common	<5	10

Abbreviations: MPO, myeloperoxidase; SBB, Sudan black B; NSE, nonspecific esterase; PAS, periodic acid-Schiff; TdT, terminal deoxynucleotidyl transferase; NEC, nonerythroid cells; CD, cluster designation; (+), positive; (±), weakly positive or few scattered positive granules; (−), negative. (Data from Pui[95] and Cline.[98])

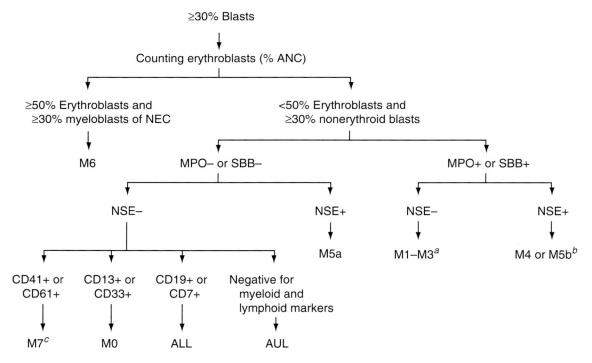

Fig. 21-9. Diagnosing acute leukemias based on cytochemical and immunologic studies. ANC, all nucleated cells; NEC, nonerythroid cells; ALL, acute lymphoid leukemia; AUL, acute undifferentiated leukemia; MPO, myeloperoxidase; SBB, Sudan black B; NSE, nonspecific esterase; ANAE, alpha-naphthyl acetate esterase. [a] M3 may stain moderately with NSE. [b] May be NSE-negative. [c] May be ANAE-positive. (Modified from Franzman and Bennett,[476] with permission.)

Fig. 21-10. Hypocellular acute leukemia of nonlymphocytic type (M1). Note that the vast majority of cells are immature with little differentiation. In comparison with megaloblasts in Fig. 21-7, these blasts have irregular nuclear contours and folded nuclei (H&E stain, × 400.)

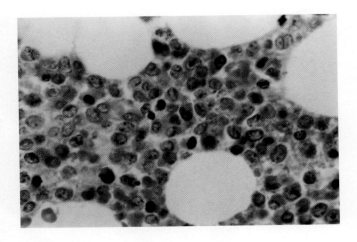

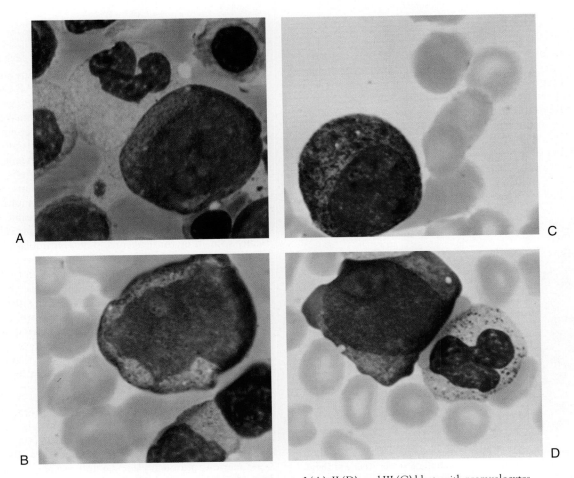

Fig. 21-11. **(A–D)** Composite picture to compare types I (A), II (D), and III (C) blasts with promyelocytes (B). See text for a description of each cell type. (Romanowsky stain, × 1,000.)

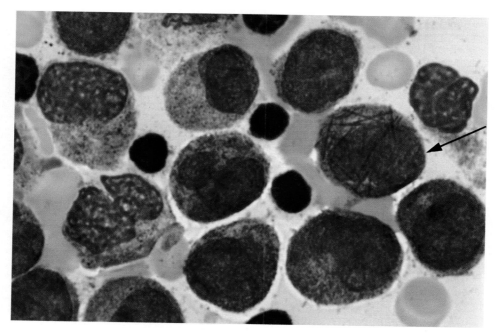

Fig. 21-12. Acute promyelocytic leukemia (M3, according to FAB classification). One of the leukemic cells contain bundles of Auer rods (Faggot cells) (arrow). Leukemic cells may contain one or multiple Auer rods in their cytoplasm. (Romanowsky stain, × 1,000.)

myeloperoxidase can differentiate a myelocytic component (positive with all three listed stains) from a monocytic component (negative with CAE stain). Maturing granulocytic cells may be seen interspersed among blasts, in contrast to ALL, in which CAE-positive maturing granulocytes are decreased and pushed aside to the periphery of the leukemic foci. Reticulin fibers are often slightly increased.

The incidence of various subgroups is somewhat different from report to report, and is different between adults and children (Table 21-5). However, children with Down's syndrome who have had transient myeloproliferative disorder as new-borns have a high incidence of developing M7.[100,101] A greater proportion of ANLLs secondary to chemotherapy and/or radiotherapy were unclassifiable according to the FAB classification in comparison with de novo ANLLs. Most subgroups of ANLLs that are associated with nonrandom chromosomal abnormalities are discussed below. The M5 and M4 subgroups are commonly associated with leukemic tissue infiltration.[102] M6 should be differentiated from megaloblastic anemia and acute myeloid leukemia (AML) with dyserythropoiesis. Although dyserythropoiesis is seen in all three conditions, vacuolated proerythroblasts and giant erythroblasts with multinucleation are only seen in erythroleukemia. Intracytoplasmic PAS-positive granules and PAS-positive cytoplasm are also characteristically seen in erythroleukemia. The erythroblasts in M6 are stained by nonspecific esterase or chloroacetate esterase.[86] In addition, a therapeutic trial of vitamin B_{12} and folic acid or blood transfusion often corrects the morphologic abnormalities in megaloblastic anemia and AML with dyserythropoiesis. It should be pointed out that PAS-positive normoblasts have been reported in thalassemia and in chronic renal disease, and vacuolated proerythroblasts are seen in a variety of clinical conditions, such as alcoholism, chloramphenicol therapy, copper deficiency, riboflavin deficiency, galactoflavin ingestion, and erythroleukemias.[86]

Extramedullary Myeloid Cell Tumors. The term *extramedullary myeloid cell tumors* (EMCT) was first introduced by Davey and associates[103] to designate malignant neoplasms of myeloid lineage that occur in a variety of anatomic sites other than the bone marrow, although *chloroma* and *granulocytic sarcoma* are better known synonyms for these neoplasms. The incidence of

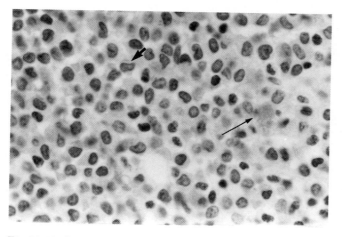

Fig. 21-13. Acute promyelocytic leukemia (M3). Bundles of Auer rods (small arrow) and leukemic cells containing a single Auer rod (large arrow) can be found. (H&E stain, × 400.)

EMCT from the hematology and/or surgical pathology file of one institute was 2.9 percent.[104] It may develop prior to, concurrently with, or following the onset of classic acute myeloid leukemia (AML). The tumor may occur anywhere in the body with peritoneum, soft tissue, bone, lymph node, nasal fossa, and skin as the most common sites.[105,106] Histopathologically, EMCT have been classified into (1) well differentiated, when numerous eosinophilic myelocytes are seen in any section of a given case, (2) poorly differentiated, when only occasional eosinophilic myelocytes can be found, and (3) blastic, if there is no evidence of granulocytic differentiation.[105] The neoplastic cells in EMCT often have oval or reniform nuclei with delicate nuclear membranes, a "dusty" or "salt-and-pepper" chromatin pattern, and multiple small but distinct nucleoli. Commonly used special stains include Leder stain and immunoperoxidase stain for lysozyme. Traweek and associates[107] found that 100 percent of their 28 cases were CD43+ (Leu22) and 75 percent were CD45+.[107] Roth and colleagues[108] concluded that CD43 (Leu22 or MT1), lysozyme, and myeloperoxidase were all very sensitive for these tumors. In nonleukemic patients and patients with CMPDs, the occurrence of granulocytic sarcoma was a harbinger of AML or blast crisis. However, if patients with EMCT were appropriately treated, they might undergo complete remission, and a few may be cured[104,106]; thus, accurate and timely diagnosis of EMCT is important.

Acute Malignant Myelosclerosis. Acute malignant myelosclerosis or acute myelofibrosis (AMF) is a rare but rapidly fatal disease, characterized by pancytopenia and minimal or no splenomegaly.[109,110] Teardrop cells, characteristically seen in AMM (agnogenic myeloid metaplasia or myelosclerosis with myeloid metaplasia), are rare in AMF, and there is little anisopoikilocytosis on the peripheral blood smear. The bone marrow examination often yields a "dry tap." Histologic examination of bone marrow biopsy specimens shows hypercellular bone marrow with replacement of normal hematopoieteic elements and fat by fibrous tissue (reticulin fibrosis) interspersed with sheets of blasts, dysplastic megakaryocytes, and residual dyspoietic hematopoietic cells. Cytogenetic studies support the concept that AMF is a primary malignant tumor of hematopoietic cells associated with secondary non-neoplastic fibrosis.[111,112] Chemotherapy is ineffective, but marrow transplantation may offer a cure.[113] Some patients terminate in acute leukemia.[114,115] Recent improvement in technology identified the blasts to be megakaryoblasts; thus, it indicated that these cases were variants of AML and should be classified as M7, according to FAB classifications.[49,116–118] However, Winfield and Polacarz[119] believed that megakaryoblastic leukemia (M7) and acute myelofibrosis were two different diseases because the blasts in M7 marked as megakaryocytic origin based on their positive reactivity with anti-factor VIII, whereas blasts in acute myelofibrosis are nonreactive to the same monoclonal antibody. They believed that acute myelofibrosis results from a proliferation of more primitive stem cells.

Acute Lymphocytic Leukemia. ALL is more common in children than in adults. The FAB group classifies this entity into three morphologic groups: L1, L2, and L3.[72] The L1 subgroup is characterized by a homogeneous population of small cells having up to twice the diameter of a small lymphocyte.

The nucleus is large and round, with occasional clefting or indentation. The amount of cytoplasm is scanty, with slight or moderate basophilia. The nucleoli are invisible or small and inconspicuous. L2 cells are large with considerable heterogeneity in size. Nuclear clefting, indentation, and folding are characteristic. Nucleoli are always present, and often large. The amount of cytoplasm varies but is often abundant. Cytoplasmic basophilia may be marked. L3 cells are large and characteristically homogeneous. The nucleus is oval to round and regular. The chromatin is finely stippled. One or more prominent vesicular nucleoli are seen in most cells. The cytoplasm is voluminous and intensely basophilic. Prominent cytoplasmic vacuolization is often present (Fig. 21-14).

L1 morphology has been associated with a better prognosis and is more common in children,[120] but it is nevertheless difficult to separate L1 from L2 at times. The FAB group has therefore modified its criteria and developed a score system for L1 and L2,[121] which is based on four features: (1) nuclear/cytoplasmic ratio, (2) presence, prominence, and frequency of nucleoli, (3) regularity of nuclear membrane outline, and (4) cell size. It has been stated that the overall concordance among observers is improved by using this score system.

With the exception of L3 (a B cell malignant tumor), there is no correlation between morphologic and immunologic classification.[86,121,122] L2, which is more common in adults, has to be differentiated from ANLL (M0 or M1). Scattered rare azurophilic granules may be seen in L2, but these granules do not react with myeloperoxidase. The FAB group claims that the presence of up to 3 percent peroxidase-positive blasts is still considered compatible with L2.[72]

L3 cells carry membrane surface immunoglobulin or intracytoplasmic immunoglobin (frequently IgM kappa) and are B cells. The vacuoles in blasts react with oil red O or Sudan IV (neutral lipid). Immunologic classification of ALL is given in Table 21-6.[95,122]

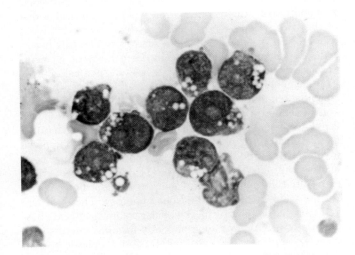

Fig. 21-14. Acute lymphocytic leukemia (L3, according to FAB classification). The nuclei of acute lymphocytic leukemia (L3) may be round to oval, the chromatin is evenly distributed, and each nucleus contains one or more prominent nucleoli. The cytoplasm is deeply basophilic and vacuolated. These vacuoles contain oil red O-positive but PAS-negative material. (Romanowsky stain, × 1,000.)

Table 21-6. Immunologic/Morphologic Classification
of Acute Lymphoblastic Leukemia

Immunologic Subtype	TdT	HLA-DR	CD19	CD10	Cμ	SIg	CD7	CD2	FAB Morphology
B Lineage									
Early B-precursor ALL	+	+	+	−	−	−			L1, L2
Common ALL	+	+	+	+	−	−			L1, L2
Pre-B ALL	+	+	+	+	+	−			L1
B-ALL	−	+	+	±	±	+			L3
T Lineage									
Early T-precursor ALL	+						+	−	L1, L2
T-ALL	+						+	+	L1, L2

Abbreviations: ALL, acute lymphoblastic leukemia; TdT, terminal deoxynucleotidyl transferase; Cμ, cytoplasmic IgM; SIg, membrane surface immunoglobulin; FAB morphology, French-American-British classification.

Terminal deoxynucleotidyl transferase (TdT) is a DNA polymerase, characteristically present in stem cells, pre-T cells, cortical thymocytes, and some pre-B cells. There are fewer than 2 percent TdT-positive cells in normal bone marrow. TdT positivity is found in 95 percent of patients with untreated ALL and in 30 to 60 percent of patients with CML in blast crisis.[86] In general, patients with common ALL and pre-B ALL have better prognosis than B- or T-ALL. Many early B-precursor ALLs simultaneously express early and/or late antigens that are not present on normal lymphoid cells.[88]

Unlike ANLL, in which tissue infiltration (granulocytic sarcoma, chloroma) is uncommon, ALL frequently presents with lymphadenopathy and/or hepatosplenomegaly with neoplastic infiltrate (lymphoma). These cases have been classified as lymphoma/leukemia. The L1 or L1/L2 ALL is frequently associated with lymphoblastic lymphoma (convoluted cell lymphoma), and the L3 is associated with Burkitt's lymphoma. Histologic examination of ALL in bone marrow is almost identical to that of the corresponding non-Hodgkin's lymphoma (NHL) in lymph nodes or other tissues. The marrow is markedly hypercellular with an absence of fat cells. Hematopoietic elements are markedly depleted. A few lymphocytes and plasma cells may be present, and mitoses may be numerous. Necrosis is not uncommon, but fibrosis is rarer than in ANLL.

Lymphoblastic lymphoma characteristically involves adolescent boys. These patients frequently present with a mediastinal mass and/or supradiaphragmatic lymphadenopathy. Extranodal involvement is not uncommon. Many patients also have bone marrow infiltrate. These patients tend to have a higher peripheral white cell count and blast count, with blasts displaying L1 (in the majority of cases) or L2 morphology. The blasts are TdT-positive, exhibiting focal globular paranuclear acid phosphatase positivity, and spontaneously forming rosettes with sheep erythrocytes (CD2 positivity). Most neoplastic cells in these cases express early T-precursor cell or T cell antigens; other lymphoblastic lymphomas may express pre-B cell antigens. Although they may initially respond to chemotherapy, remission duration is short, and testicular or central nervous system (CNS) relapse is common.[89–92]

The nonendemic (sporadic) Burkitt's lymphoma also affects young boys in their first two decades of life. Over 90 percent of the patients have abdominal disease, particularly in the terminal ileum. Other sites, including bone marrow, ovary, testis, pleura, CNS, and peripheral lymph nodes, may also be involved. When it becomes leukemic, leukemic blasts display L3 morphology. Rearrangement of c-myc oncogene is demonstrated in 80 percent of cases.[93–95]

Clonal Chromosomal Abnormalities. Nonrandom chromosomal changes have been frequently identified in subgroups of acute leukemias[95,98] (Tables 21-7 and 21-8). Molecular studies link these structural changes to genetic alterations. Although the mechanisms of leukemogenesis of the proto-oncogenes or tumor suppressor genes in leukemia and lymphomas are quite variable,[98] usually involving loss or gain of one or more entire chromosomes (hypodiploid or hyperdiploid) or long (q) or short (p) arms of a specific chromosome, other structural changes (translocations, inversion, or insertions) may also occur. One of the common abnormalities is that the protein prod-

Table 21-7. Common Nonrandom Chromosomal Abnormalities in Acute Nonlymphocytic Leukemias

Chromosomal Abnormalities	Genetic Alteration	FAB Classification
t(9;22) (q34;q11)	BCR-ABL fusion	M1
t(8;21) (q22;q22)	AML1-ETO fusion	M2
t(15;17) (q22;q11–12)	PML-RARA fusion	M3
inv(16) (p13;q22)	CBF-beta-MYH11 inversion	M4Eo (eosinophilia)
t(16;16) (p13;q22)	CBF-beta-MYH11 fusion	M4Eo (eosinophilia)
t(9;11) (p21–22;q23)	AF9-MLL fusion	M4, M5
t(6;9) (p23;q34)	DEK-CAN fusion	M2, M4 marrow basophilia
t(1;22) (p13;q13)	?	M7 (infancy)

(Data from Pui[95] and Cline.[98])

Table 21-8. Common Nonrandom Chromosomal Abnormalities in Acute Lymphoid Leukemias (ALL)

Chromosomal Abnormalities	Genetic Alteration	Immunologic Classification
t(1;19) (q23;p13.3)	E2A-PBX1 fusion	Pre-B ALL
t(9;22) (q34;q11)	BCR-ABL fusion	Predominant B lineage ALL
t(4;11) (q21;q23)	AF4-MLL fusion	CD10− B lineage ALL
t(8;14) (q24;q32.3)	MYC-IgH fusion	B-ALL (L3-Burkitt)
t(2;8) (p12;q24)	Kappa-MYC fusion	B-ALL (L3-Burkitt)
t(8;22) (q24;q11)	MYC-lambda fusion	B-ALL (L3-Burkitt)
t(11;14) (p13;q11)	TTG2-TCR alpha/delta fusion	T-ALL
t(8;14) (q24;q11)	MYC-TCR alpha/delta fusion	T-ALL
t(1;14) (p32;q11)	SCL(tal-1)-TCR alpha/delta fusion	T-ALL
t(7;9) (q35;p13)	TCR-beta-tal-2 fusion	T-ALL

(Data from Pui[95] and Cline.[98])

ucts of these genes bind to specific DNA sequences near target genes and enhance the synthesis of messenger RNA (activating transcription).[98,123] These recurring (or nonrandom) chromosomal changes correlate with a particular subgroup of acute leukemias with characteristic morphologic and clinical findings. They provide important information regarding response to therapy and overall prognosis.

t(8;21) (q22;q22). This chromosomal abnormality is the single most common structural rearrangement seen in ANLL and is most often associated with M2 morphology with large prominent Auer rods or pseudo-Chédiak-Higashi anomaly.[124] The marrow frequently has increased number of eosinophils. It commonly affects young males. Extramedullary myeloid cell tumor may be the initial clinical presentation. It is associated with most favorable prognosis.

t(15;17) (q22;q11). Almost all patients with M3 ANLL will have t(15;17) whether by cytogenetic study or molecular analysis (polymerase chain reaction [PCR] or fluorescent in situ hybridization [FISH]).[125] Both hypergranular promyelocytic leukemia (M3) and microgranular promyelocytic leukemia (M3V) will have this t(15;17). Disseminated intravascular coagulation (DIC) may be the initial presenting sign or soon develops after the initiation of conventional therapy. The leukemic cells can be induced to differentiate into mature granulocytes following exposure to differentiating agents such as all-trans-retinoic acid. However, hyperleukocytosis develops because of a rapid increase in the number of mature leukemic cells in the blood. A *retinoic acid syndrome* may occur in some patients. These patients have hyperleukocytosis, fever, and respiratory failure. Pleural and pericardial effusions and peripheral edema may also develop. Early introduction of cytotoxic

chemotherapy prevents onset of this syndrome. If remission is attained, these patients tend to have a long remission duration and survival compared to other forms of ANLL. Heparin should be given once the diagnosis of M3 is made.

Inv (16) (p13q22). A subgroup of ANLL M4 that is characterized by bone marrow eosinophilia with atypical eosinophilic precursors is associated with rearrangement of chromosome 16p13q22.[126] In this type of leukemia (M4Eo), 5 percent or more of the nonerythroid bone marrow cells have a mixture of eosinophilic and basophilic granules. These cells are positive for chloroacetate esterase and PAS (coarse granules). This M4Eo subtype has a higher frequency of CNS involvement, but has a more favorable prognosis and a higher remission rate than the M4 subtype in general.

t(9;22) (q34;q11). The Philadelphia chromosome may be seen in de novo ANLL. When seen, it is most often associated with the FAB M1 subtype. It is also seen in 5 percent of children and 20 to 30 percent of adults with ALL. Most ALL cells have a breakpoint within the *bcr* gene that differs from the breakpoint in chronic myelocytic leukemia (CML). The protein product of the fusion gene on chromosome 22 is smaller (p185) than that in CML (p210), but it also has abnormally modulated tyrosine kinase activity.[98] Philadelphia chromosome-positive ALL usually has FAB L2 morphology but may occasionally be L1. Most of these cases have immature B cell phenotype. Patients with Philadelphia chromosome-positive ALL appear to respond to induction chemotherapy but have significantly shorter remission durations and survival compared with patients without this translocation.[95]

t(1;19) (q23;p13). This chromosomal abnormality occurs quite frequently (25 percent) in pre-B and less commonly (1 percent) in early B-precursor ALL. It is the most common translocation in childhood ALL. An association of pre-B-immunophenotype with t(1;19) denotes poor prognosis (with increased leukocyte count) and requires intensified chemotherapy. Pre-B-ALL without t(1;19) and early B-precursor ALL with t(1;19) are not associated with a poor prognosis.[95]

t(4;11) (q21;q23). Approximately 5 percent of all children and 70 percent of infants with ALL have 11q23 rearrangements, primarily the t(4,11) (q21;q23).[95] This chromosomal abnormality is associated with markedly elevated leukocyte count, splenomegaly, and a very poor prognosis.[127,128] Most cases have an early B-precursor phenotype, usually CD10−. However, many have either features of myeloid leukemias or of mixed phenotype leukemias defined by cytochemical, immunophenotypic, or ultrastructural studies. Undifferentiated and, rarely, T cell or B cell ALL with t(4;11) have been reported. Rearrangements involving 11q23 are the most frequent cytogenetic abnormalities in ANLL M5, especially in infants.[95] Coagulation disorders and CNS leukemia are characteristics for this type of leukemia.[95] The 11q23 breakpoints are molecularly identical in both ALL and ANLL, suggesting that the involved gene, MLL, has an important regulatory role in both differentiation pathways.[129]

t(8;14) (q24;q32.3). Reciprocal translocations involving c-*myc* oncogene (8q24) with an immunoglobulin gene, FAB L3

Table 21-9. Prognostic Factors in ANLL

Favorable	Intermediate	Unfavorable
Normal karyotype	t(15;17) (q22;q11)	Old age (>60 yr)
t(8;21) (q22;q22)	Abnormal 11q23	Complex chromosomal abnormalities
Rearrangement of 16q22		−7/7q− or −5/5q− t(9;22) (q34;q11) Abnormal 3q p53 mutation Decreased Rb protein Deletion of p16(9q21)

morphology, and B cell phenotype (SIg+) are found in 1 to 3 percent of cases of ALL. Less common translocations involving light chain genes [t(2;8), and t(8;22)] have also been reported. Many of these patients may also have a malignant lymphoma (high grade, small noncleaved, Burkitt's type) of the small bowel (terminal ileum). They are often designated as having leukemia/lymphoma. There is a high rate of CNS involvement. The prognosis is poor.

t(11;14) (p13;q11). This chromosomal abnormality is the most common form seen in T-ALL. In this condition, the T cell receptor (TCR) alpha/delta on chromosome 14q11 is spliced to a proto-oncogene and then serves as the driving force in dysregulated oncogene expression. The leukemic cells often express mature T cell antigens. The presence of t(11;14) is often correlated with a poor prognosis.[130]

Prognostic Factors in Acute Leukemias. As discussed above, certain nonrandomized chromosomal abnormalities have been associated with a better or worse clinical course. Currently, about 70 to 80 percent of ALL and about 50 percent of ANLL in children are curable.[131] The results are not nearly as dramatic as in adults.[132] The differing prognosis in adults and children has been attributed to differences in disease biology and in treatment tolerance. Tables 21-9 and 21-10 list the favorable and unfavorable prognostic factors in ANLL and ALL, respectively. With powerful tools such as PCR amplification, and flow cytometry combined with FISH, minimal residual dis-

Table 21-10. Prognostic Factors in ALL

Favorable	Unfavorable
FAB L1 morphology	Age <1 and >9 yr
CD10 expression	High WBC count (>50 × 10⁹/L)
Hyperdiploid (>50 chromosomes)	B or T cell phenotype
	Myeloid coexpression
Normal karyotype	Hypodiploid (<46 chromosomes)
del (6) (q15;q21)	t(9;22) (q34;q11)
	Rearrangement of 8q24 (c-myc)
	Rearrangement of 11q23 (MLL)
	t(4;11) (q21;q23)

ease may be detected with these molecular biologic techniques beyond the recognition by light microscopy. Although the presence of minimal residual disease in ALL and ANLL M3 appears to be associated with a high risk of relapse,[133,134] the detection of minimal residual disease does not foretell relapse.[135,136] It is obvious that more large cooperative studies are needed in this area.

Acute Mixed Leukemia. By using a multiparameter approach, mixed-lineage antigen expression has been detected in as many as 22 percent of cases of ALL[137,138] and 60 percent of cases of AML.[137,139,140] However, the incidences of these cases may be considerably decreased if one uses the expression of two or more markers of the opposite lineage as diagnostic criteria (6 percent of patients with ALL and 17 percent of those with AML). This lineage infidelity or lineage promiscuity is also common in adult ALL, and the myeloid antigen-positive ALL in adults is associated with a poor prognosis.[30] The prognostic significance in childhood mixed phenotype ALL is still inconclusive.[95] This type of leukemia frequently appears as FAB-L2 morphology in children. There is an increased incidence of chromosomal translocations involving 11q23, 14q32, or t(9;22) in mixed phenotype ALL. Clinically, mixed (hybrid) leukemias may be classified as biphenotypic leukemia (the individual leukemic blasts express both myeloid and lymphoid antigens), bilineal leukemia (in which the leukemic cells are heterogeneous and display either lymphoid or myeloid antigens but they originate from the same neoplastic clone), or biclonal leukemia (in which the heterogeneous leukemic cells are derived from two separate clones). Biphenotypic leukemia is probably the most common.

Myeloproliferative Disorders. The term *myeloproliferative syndrome* was introduced by Dameshek[141] to include a heterogeneous group of disorders characterized by simultaneous proliferation of any or all cell lines originating from the marrow during the course of the disease.

Chronic myeloproliferative disorders (CMPDs) are clonal disorders of the hemopoietic stem cells, characterized by excessive proliferation of one or more hemopoietic cell lines with relatively normal differentiation and effective hematopoiesis, resulting in an increase in the quantities of one or more hematopoietic elements (cytosis) in the peripheral blood. CMPDs consist of four well defined clinical entities: polycythemia vera (PV), idiopathic thrombocythemia (IT), chronic myeloid leukemia (CML), and agnogenic myeloid metaplasia (AMM, or idiopathic myelofibrosis [myelofibrosis/osteomyelosclerosis]). Histologic recognition and classification of CMPDs depend on (1) the predominant proliferative cell line, (2) the degree of its differentiation, and (3) the fibrotic reaction. It should be emphasized that subgroups of CMPDs often overlap. PV, AMM, and CML may evolve to acute leukemia. Chronic myelomonocytic leukemia (CMML) and juvenile CML share the characteristics of myeloproliferative disorder and myelodysplastic syndrome (MDS), and are discussed under MDS.

Polycythemia Vera. PV is a slowly progressive myeloproliferative disorder characterized by an absolute erythrocytosis, hypervolemia, and panhyperplasia of the bone marrow[142] (Fig.

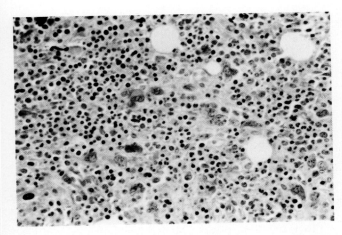

Fig. 21-15. Spent phase of polycythemia vera. Panhyperplasia of marrow is noted with aggregates of megakaryocytes. (H&E stain, × 100.)

21-15). Megakaryocytic hyperplasia may be striking, with abnormal forms present (variably sized and shaped nuclei and variable cytoplasmic density). In addition, they frequently cluster together. Increased reticulin fibers may be demonstrated by special stains. Irregularly dilated and expanded sinusoids are seen, some of which contain islands of nucleated red cells and megakaryocytes. Occasionally, bilinear hyperplasia consisting of erythrocytic and megakaryocytic lines only or erythrocytic and granulocytic lines only may be seen. Occasionally, patients with PV will have a normocellular marrow.[143] Even in those, close observation will reveal clustering of enlarged and atypical megakaryocytes. It appears that those patients with marked megakaryocytic hyperplasia on bone marrow biopsies tend to develop myelofibrosis.[144] The laboratory abnormalities include an increase in the red cell mass; mild to moderate leukocytosis with neutrophilia, eosinophilia, and basophilia; and thrombocytosis. The leukocyte alkaline phosphatase (LAP) score is typically increased. Absent iron stores are characteristic, which may be due to increased consumption in response to erythroid hyperplasia or may be secondary to repeated phlebotomies. The diagnostic criteria have been established by the Polycythemia Study Group and were essentially based on the red blood cell mass, arterial blood oxygen saturation, and splenomegaly, and some other laboratory tests.[145] Among those patients who lived more than 8 years, about 10 to 25 percent developed postpolycythemic myeloid metaplasia[146] and another 5 to 10 percent developed AML.[147,148] The incidence of acute leukemia was higher in patients who developed a myeloid metaplasia phase as compared to those who did not develop myeloid metaplasia. The onset of the disease in patient under 40 years of age appears to be associated with a more grave illness.[149] Chromosomal abnormalities have been demonstrated in 25 to 50 percent of patients. The most common abnormalities included +8, +9, and 20q−.[150,151] Patients who have abnormal clones at diagnosis appear to have a shorter survival than those patients who do not have them. In addition, abnormal clones emerge with progression of the disease. The differential diagnosis includes (1) secondary erythrocytosis (in which megakaryocytes are normal in number and in morphology, with preservation of fat cells and

reticulin structure); (2) CML (in which the erythroid precursors are usually decreased in number and in addition, the LAP score is decreased and Philadelphia chromosome is demonstrated in most cases); and (3) AMM. This cannot be differentiated from postpolycythemic myeloid metaplasia.[146]

Idiopathic Thrombocythemia. Idiopathic (or essential) thrombocythemia (IT) is characterized by a sustained increase in the platelet count at a level of $1,000 \times 10^9$ L or higher. Bone marrow cellularity is variable, but there is definite hyperplasia of megakaryocytes. These cells frequently form clusters of polymorphic cells of variable size and shape, which contain polymorphic nuclei. Megakaryocytes are found not only at the walls of the sinusoids but also projecting into their lumina. Progression into myelofibrosis is seen.[152–154] Bartl and associates[144] suggest that the presence of clustered polymorphic megakaryocytes may represent a more aggressive stage of the disease.[144] These investigators also believe that a falling platelet count signals the transition either to the immature (promegakaryocytic) subtype or to myelofibrosis.

The differential diagnosis includes other subgroups of CMPDs and reactive thrombocytosis associated with inflammatory conditions, neoplasms, and postsplenectomy.[155] However, the platelet counts in these reactive thrombocytoses may not reach such a magnitude as in IT. Furthermore, the morphologies of megakaryocytes are usually normal. The differential diagnosis from other CMPDs is difficult. The criteria for diagnosis proposed by the Polycythemia Vera Study Group should be followed.[156]

Chronic Myeloid Leukemia. CML is a clonal disorder due to malignant transformation of a primitive cell probably involving the pluripotent hemolymphopoietic stem cell. The Philadelphia chromosome, originally described as shortening of the long arm of chromosome 22[157] and its fusion protein product, is identified in more than 95 percent of CML, 20 percent of adult ALL, and 5 percent of adult ANLL, as well as 5 percent of childhood ALL.[95,98] This marker chromosome Philadelphia has been found in erythroid, granulocytic, monocytic, and megakaryocytic lineages, as well as in B and T cells from patients with CML.[158,159] The Philadelphia chromosome translocation activates the cellular Abelson (c-abl) proto-oncogene on chromosome 9q34 by joining 3′ abl coding sequences with the regulatory and 5′ coding sequences of the "breakpoint cluster region" (bcr) gene on chromosome 22q11. The fusion proteins abl-bcr of CML, ALL, and AML have increased tyrosine kinase activity and show a transforming potential in vitro and in animal models. The shorter p185 or p190 protein is associated almost exclusively with ALL and AML, whereas the protein 210 is present in both chronic phase and blast crisis of CML and also in 50 percent of Philadelphia chromosome-positive ALL.[160] It is of note that the transforming ability of p190 is greater than that of p210 in vitro. Additional chromosomal abnormalities are often identified in CML in blast crisis.

CML is primarily a disease of middle-aged adults, but may occur at any age, including infancy. The most common symptoms relate to anemia, splenomegaly, and an increased metabolic rate. The leukocyte count is usually in excess of 50×10^9/L. Signs of leukostasis may be seen in those with excessive leukocytosis. Neutrophilia with left shift, eosinophilia, basophilia, and thrombocytosis are common findings. The neutrophil alkaline phosphatase (LAP) level is decreased in most patients unless the patient has concurrent infection, in which case the LAP level may be normal or even elevated. The bone marrow is extremely hypercellular with marked granulocytic hyperplasia evidenced by broad paratrabecular and perivascular seams of immature myeloid precursors and mature granulocytes in the central regions of marrow cavity. Although granulopoiesis appears to be normal in maturation, there is a marked increase in eosinophils and basophils. Mast cells are usually normal. Erythropoiesis is appreciably decreased, with a myeloid/erythroid ratio of 15:1 to 20:1 (Fig. 21-16). The number of megakaryocytes varies even within different marrow spaces in a single biopsy; they frequently display abnormal morphology (dyspoietic features). Histiocytes containing crystalloid structures (Gaucher-like cells) are seen. Reticulin fibers may be increased.

As stated earlier, a marker chromosome, the Philadelphia chromosome, is demonstrated in 95 percent of cases. Molecular studies of Philadelphia chromosome-negative CML reveal that approximately one-half of these patients have genetic mutation characteristics of the Philadelphia chromosome; reassessment of other Philadelphia chromosome-negative CML has resulted in the reclassification of all but a few as some disorders other than CML (such as CMML [MDS]).[161,162] Rarely, a Philadelphia chromosome-positive clone may disappear during the course of the disease, or patients who are Philadelphia chromosome negative at presentation become positive after a varying period of time. There is no morphologic difference between Philadelphia chromosome-positive and Philadelphia chromosome-negative CML.[144] Bartl and associates[144] divided CML into two main groups. First was the unilinear granulocytic-type (45 percent) with a striking proliferation of granulopoiesis. Neutrophilic CML was the most common type, but eosinophilic and basophilic variants were also encountered. Second was the bilinear granulocytic/megakaryocytic type (55 percent) with concomitant cytologic and topographic alterations of megakaryopoiesis. These investigators found that 69 percent of the unilinear granulocytic type transform into blast crisis, whereas 70 percent of bilinear granulocytic/megakaryocytic type evolve into myelofibrosis/osteomyelosclerosis.

Some CML patients will develop progressive marrow failure with increasing anemia and thrombocytopenia. These patients may also have increasing myelofibrosis, basophilia in excess of 20 percent, karyotypic evolution, and an increase in blasts (but <30 percent). It appears that these patients have undergone a transformation of CML from a chronic phase to an accelerated phase.[163] The bone marrow examination may show an increase in immature cells involving myeloid, monocytic, megakaryocytic, and erythroid series. These cells often display marked dyspoiesis, and may be circulating in the peripheral blood. An increase in eosinophils may also be noted. The duration for this accelerated phase is unpredictable. Progression to a blast phase may occur.

Blastic transformation of CML is generally defined as 30 percent or more blasts in the blood or bone marrow smears or a focus of blasts in a marrow biopsy or extramedullary site. The blasts may show myeloid (most common), lymphoid, megakaryocytic, or mixed[164] differentiation morphologically and immunophenotypically. The histopathology of the bone marrow may be indistinguishable from that of acute leukemias, except that an increase of eosinophils and basophils is more common in CML in blast crisis than in acute leukemias.

Agnogenic Myeloid Metaplasia. AMM or chronic idiopathic myelofibrosis is a clonal disorder of hematopoietic cells with reactive fibrosis. It is characterized by marked poikilocytosis with dacrocytes and a leukoerythroblastic blood picture, panmyelosis, bone marrow fibrosis, and extramedullary hematopoiesis. The patients usually present with symptoms of anemia, hepatosplenomegaly, and hyperuricemia. Atypical, large and hypogranular platelets and abnormal megakaryocyte nuclei are circulating in the blood. Blasts may be present in the blood. A basophilia is also noted. Radiographic evidence of osteosclerosis has been reported in 30 to 70 percent of patients. Bone marrow aspiration is usually unsuccessful (dry tap). Bone biopsy is necessary for diagnosis. The following histologic patterns have been described[165]:

1. Panhyperplasia: the marrow is hypercellular with effacement of normal architecture and compartmentalization of hematopoiesis. Aggregates of dysplastic megakaryocytes are frequently surrounded by reticulin fibers. The sinusoids are irregular in shape, often dilated, with sclerosis of sinusoidal walls. Intrasinusoidal hematopoiesis is evident
2. Myeloid atrophy and fibrosis: alternating areas of fibrosis and hematopoiesis are seen. All hematopoietic cell lines are usually present but megakaryocytes predominate
3. Myelofibrosis and osteosclerosis: this is characterized by replacement of the marrow cavity with broad, irregular, twisted trabeculae (without the regular lamellar appearance) and fibrotic marrow. Normal hematopoietic elements are markedly decreased. The hematopoietic cells present are primarily megakaryocytes

These different patterns may be found simultaneously in different parts of the skeleton or even of the same section. However, as the disease progresses, reticulin fibrosis is often replaced with collagen fibrosis (Fig. 21-17). The topic of myelofibrosis

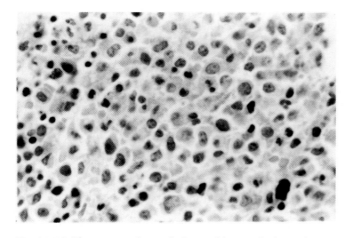

Fig. 21-16. Chronic granulocytic leukemia. Note marked granulocytic hyperplasia with a predominance of myelocytes and metamyelocytes. Only a few nucleated red cells and one megakaryocyte are identified. (H&E stain, × 250.)

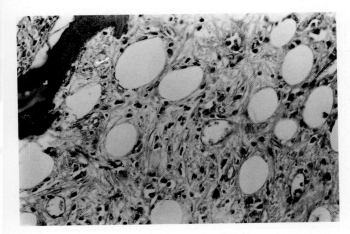

Fig. 21-17. Fibrotic bone marrow with marked decrease in hematopoietic elements. Snook's reticulin stain does not show increased reticulin. Trichrome stain displays increased collagen fibers. (Snook's reticulin stain, × 100.)

has been recently reviewed by several groups.[166–168]

The pathogenesis of the reticulin and collagen myelofibrosis in the myeloproliferative disorders is not clear. Two basic pathogenetic mechanisms have been proposed: (1) chronic inflammatory reaction, possibly mediated by circulating immune complexes[169] and by the presence of plasma cells, mast cells, and lymphoid nodules—all known to have the capabilities to produce various growth factors; (2) the release of fibroblast-stimulating growth factors derived from megakaryocytes and platelets (platelet-derived growth factor [PDGF]) and of a collagenase-inhibiting factor (platelet factor 4) by the disintegrating megakaryocytes and platelets. These cytokines induce fibroblast proliferation and production of collagen (subtypes I, II, and IV).[170,171]

The differential diagnosis includes secondary myelofibrosis following other CMPDs, metastatic tumors, leukemia, Hodgkin's disease, and non-Hodgkin's lymphoma. Myelofibrosis may occur in response to other stimuli, such as toxins, drugs, radiotherapy, and bone disease.[172]

Fibrosis of the bone marrow is discussed further in a later section. Please refer to standard hematology textbooks for other uncommon CMPDs.

Myelodysplastic Syndrome. Preleukemia syndromes, myelodysplastic syndromes (MDSs), hematopoietic dysplasias, and dysmyelopoietic syndromes are some of the terms used to describe a group of clinically well recognized, heterogeneous acquired clonal stem cell disorders characterized by qualitative and quantitative changes within one or more hematopoietic cell lines. These disorders are refractory to treatment; most patients die of complications of bone marrow dysfunction or hematopoietic neoplasia. About 15 to 25 percent of the patients having the disease finally develop acute leukemia. MDSs occur as primary diseases or therapy-related disorders. Therapy-related MDSs occur in patients who have been exposed to chemotherapy and radiotherapy.[173,174] Most of the following discussions are referred to primary MDS. Therapy-related MDSs are difficult to classify and carry with them a worse prognosis.

The affected patients are usually in their sixth or seventh decade, with an insidious onset and slowly progressive course. Cytopenias with refractory anemia and dyspoiesis of marrow cell lines are pertinent laboratory findings. The morphologic, biochemical, and functional changes of the hematopoietic cell lines have been well described.[175] The term *preleukemia syndromes* should not be used to designate any congenital or hereditary disorders known to be associated with an increased incidence of acute leukemia, or to designate those well defined myeloproliferative disorders in which the terminal event is often acute leukemia.

The qualitative abnormalities involving hematopoiesis seen in MDSs are listed in Table 21-11. The FAB Cooperative Group subclassifies the MDSs into five groups[73]: (1) refractory anemia (RA); (2) RA with ring sideroblasts (RARS); (3) RA with excess of blasts (RAEB); (4) chronic myelomonocytic leukemia (CMML); and (5) RAEB in transformation (RAEB-T). The characteristics of the various subtypes are listed in Table 21-12. The FAB states that, when the percentage of blasts present in the bone marrow is 30 percent or more, a diagnosis of acute leukemia is made. The number of blasts present in the bone marrow of patients with MDS can range from normal to less than 30 percent (Fig. 21-8). Recognition of these subtypes may be difficult in a core biopsy specimen.[119,176] It

Table 21-11. Morphologic Abnormalities Seen in MDS

Peripheral blood
    Anemia with oval macrocytosis; dimorphic red cell population; anisopoikilocytosis; reticulocytopenia
    Less common finding include leukoerythroblastic picture and the following:
        Neutropenia or neutrophilia with qualitative granulopathy: Pelger-Huet-like anomaly, hypersegmented neutrophils, coarse granulation, abnormal granulation (pseudo-Chédiak-Higashi), degranulation, abnormally small or large forms, mirror image of segmented nucleus or band nucleus, "doughnut nucleus" or other nuclear abnormalities
        Thrombocytopenia with bizarre platelet size and shape, abnormal granulations
        Monocytosis or atypical monocytoid cells
        Circulating blasts (type I, type II, or type III blasts)
Bone marrow
    Erythroid hyperplasia or hypoplasia with megaloblastoid changes: dyssynchrony in nuclear/cytoplasmic maturation, multinucleation, nuclear lobulation, nuclear fragmentation, gigantic erythroblasts with abnormal nuclei, karyorrhexis, impaired hemoglobinization, ± ring sideroblasts, maturation arrest
    Myeloid hyperplasia or hypoplasia with dyspoiesis described above; abnormal granulation (pseudo-Chédiak-Higashi anomaly); abnormal eosinophils with dimorphic (containing both eosinophilic and basophilic) granules; ring or rodent nuclei (doughnut-shaped nuclei); increased number of type I, II, and III blasts (but less than 30%); abnormal localization of immature precursors (ALIP)
    Megakaryocytic hyperplasia with dyspoiesis: micromegakaryocytes, polynucleated megakaryocytes, large mononucleated megakaryocytes, megakaryocytes with odd-numbered lobes; degranulated, abnormally granulated, or vacuolated cytoplasm
    Increased monoblasts, promonocytes, and monocytes with dyspoiesis, reactive with naphthol-ASD-chloroacetate esterase

Table 21-12. Comparison of Morphologic Features in Subgroups of Myelodysplastic Syndrome
According to FAB Classification

| Subgroup | Blasts (%) | | Marrow Cellularity | Dyspoiesis Seen in Bone Marrow | | | |
	PB	BM		Erythroid	Myeloid	Megakaryocytic	Other
RA	<1	<5	Hyper-, normo-, or hypo-	Yes	No	No	—
RARS	<1	<5	Same as above	Yes	Some	Some	≥15% Ring sideroblasts
RAEB	<5	5–20	Same as above	Yes	Yes	Some	No Auer rods
CMML	<5	<20	Hypercellular	Some	Yes	Variable	Absolute monocytosis, and ≥20% monocytic cells in marrow
RAEB-T	>5	20–29	Hypercellular	Yes	Yes	Some	Auer rods may be present

should be noted that not all patients who have dysplastic changes, especially megaloblastoid erythropoiesis, have MDS. The demonstration of a clonal chromosomal abnormality in a patient with a suspected MDS lends strong support to the diagnosis. A normal karyotype, however, does not exclude the diagnosis. Further, FAB classification only includes major subgroups of MDS.[68,177–179]

The cellularity of marrow may be variable, although hypercellular marrow is most common. All hematopoietic cell lines may exhibit dysplastic changes, with increased precursors. In addition, the normal topographic distribution of erythropoiesis, myelopoiesis, and megakaryopoiesis may be disrupted. Tricot and associates[176] noted that clustered myeloblasts may be present in the central part of the marrow prior to the increased blast count by aspiration.[176] These investigators observed that patients with this abnormal localization of immature precursors had a more rapid progression to acute leukemia than patients with MDS without this abnormal pattern. Abnormal localization of immature precursors (ALIP) is defined as the presence of three or more myeloblasts or promyelocytes clustering centrally in the marrow. There must be more than three ALIPs per section before they can be considered to be of diagnostic importance.[176,180] It should be pointed out that ALIP is not specific for MDS. Similar changes may be observed in regenerating marrows in patients who were treated for acute leukemias. It is also seen in patients with AIDS with dyspoiesis. Further, it is important to recognize that aggregates of immature erythroid and megakaryocytic cells, as demonstrated by immunohistochemistry, may also mimic the appearance of an ALIP (pseudo-ALIP).[181] The core biopsy is very useful for the detection of reticulin fibrosis, for the accurate diagnosis of the rare hypoplastic variant of MDS, and for the identification of a uniform population of monolobulated micromegakaryocytes in 5q– syndrome.[79,179,182,183] Riccardi et al[184] found that a hypocellular bone marrow appeared to be a favorable prognostic factor in MDS. Patients with refractory cytopenias, especially those with a hypocellular bone marrow, may respond to androgens.[184]

The FAB classification is based on the presence of dyspoietic features with quantification of the erythrocytic precursors and the number of type I and type II blasts in the bone marrow smears (Fig. 21-8). A type I blast is a primitive cell without granules but with a basophilic cytoplasm. It usually contains two or more prominent centrally placed nucleoli with an uncondensed fine nuclear chromatin pattern. A type II blast is slightly larger with a lower nuclear/cytoplasmic ratio than a type I blast and contains a few azurophilic (primary) granules. The nucleus is centrally positioned with one or multiple prominent nucleoli. The chromatin remains fine and uncondensed. Type II blasts must be distinguished from normal promyelocytes. The latter have an eccentrically placed nucleus, lower nuclear/cytoplasmic ratio than the blasts, clumped or condensed nuclear chromatin, a single large nucleolus, and a slightly basophilic cytoplasm containing a prominent Golgi zone and a moderate number of azurophilic granules. A type III blast has also been described by the FAB group.[99] This blast resembles type II blasts but contains numerous azurophilic granules (more than 20). A prominent nucleolus may be present (Fig. 21-11). The diagnosis of MDS is usually based on complete blood cell count and morphology of peripheral blood smear and bone marrow examination. The qualitative abnormalities (dyspoiesis) are listed in Table 21-11. The changes in RA and RARS are relatively mild, and they may require the presence of clonal chromosomal abnormalities to support the diagnosis. RAEB and RAEB-T must be differentiated from ANLL-M6, and the diagnostic criteria set by the FAB group should be closely adhered to (Fig. 21-8).

Chronic Myelomonocytic Leukemia. CMML possesses MDS and CMPD characteristics. These patients present with peripheral blood monocytosis (>1 × 10⁹/L), normocellular or hypercellular bone marrow accompanied by dysgranulopoiesis, dyserythropoiesis, or dysmegakaryopoiesis. The percentage of blasts is less than 5 in the peripheral blood and less than 20 in the bone marrow, with absent Auer rods. Although erythropoiesis and megakaryopoiesis may be ineffective, granulopoiesis is usually effective and often associated with extreme leukocytosis. Splenomegaly and hepatomegaly are common. About 20 to 30 percent of CMML patients transform to ANLL, most commonly M2 or M4. Chromosomal abnormalities are found in 30 to 50 percent of patients and there are no specific clonal abnormalities that can differentiate CMML from other

MDSs.[185–187] CMML should be differentiated from Philiadelphia chromosome-negative CML in adults.[162] In general, patients who have suffered from CML tend to be younger and have a higher white cell count with basophilia but no monocytosis; no dysplastic changes are seen in bone marrow cells, and the patients usually have a better prognosis.

Recently, the FAB group has redefined CML and CMML. They called the classic form of CML (Ph+ or Ph–, but BCR+ CML) chronic granulocytic leukemia (CGL), chronic phase. They then used several parameters to compare CGL, atypical CML, and CMML. They found that the percentage of basophils, the percentage of immature granulocytes, and percentage of erythroid precursors in the marrow were useful indicators for differentiating the above disease categories. CGLs were characterized by an elevated basophil count and an increased number of immature granulocytes. The atypical CMLs had an increased number of immature granulocytes but they had granulocyte dysplasia as well. The CMMLs characteristically had increased monocytes and increased bone marrow erythroid precursors.[188] Patients with CMML do not have the Philadelphia chromosome, but they have –7/7q–, –5/5q–, +8, 20q–, and other complex chromosomal abnormalities.

5q– Syndrome: The 5q– syndrome is a distinct hematologic disorder, occurring principally in elderly women, characterized by macrocytic, therapy-resistant anemia with normal or elevated platelet count, erythroid hypoplasia, and unilobulated megakaryocytes in the bone marrow[183,189] (Fig. 21-18). The clinical course is usually mild, with infrequent progression to acute leukemia, at which time additional chromosomal abnormalities are often identified.

Other manifestations of MDS include isolated refractory thrombocytopenia[68] and myelodysplastic syndromes with bone marrow fibrosis.[178,179] The latter should be differentiated from malignant myelosclerosis and AMM as described above.

Cytogenetic Abnormalities. Cytogenetic abnormalities are common in MDS, their incidence ranging from 20 to 90 percent of cases in the literature.[190] Most studies report that the bone marrows of 40 to 60 percent of patients contain nonrandom chromosomal abnormalities, the most common of which affect chromosomes 5 and 7.[26] It appears that the incidence of chromosomal abnormalities varies with the subgroups of MDS. Jacobs and associates[191] reported that chromosomal abnormalities were found in 29 percent of patients with RA, 13 percent with RARS, 89 percent with RAEB, 80 percent with RAEB-T, and 20 percent with CMML. A new entity, 5q– anomaly, has been described.[183,189] It appears that patients who have monosomy 7 tend to have a markedly shortened survival, although patients with multiple chromosomal abnormalities in a marrow clone have a high chance of developing acute leukemia or other complications of hemopoietic dysfunction.[192]

Prognostic Factors. As stated earlier, the presence or absence of chromosomal abnormalities and specific changes of chromosomes not only correlates to the progression of MDS to acute leukemia (42 percent of patients with an abnormal karyotype transformed to ANLL in comparison with 10 percent of those with an initially normal karyotype[191]) but also to overall survival. Aul et al[193] introduced a new scoring system that appears to correlate with clinical outcome. This system is based on the following parameters: (1) bone marrow blasts 5 percent

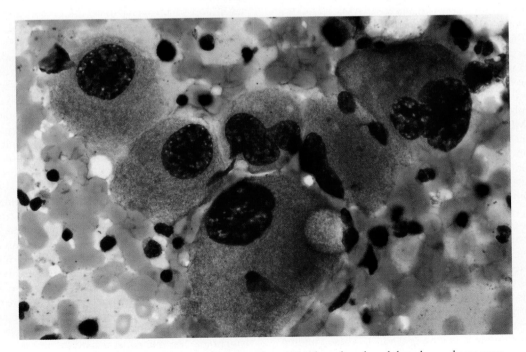

Fig. 21-18. 5q-syndrome. Note an aggregate of mononucleated or hypolobated megakaryocytes. (Romanowsky stain, × 400.)

or more, (2) LDH greater than 200 v/L, (3) hemoglobin 9 g/dl or less, and (4) platelets 100×10^9/L or less. Each parameter is assigned one score. As a function of their total score, patients were divided into three risk groups (group A score 0; group B score 1–2; group C score 3–4). The cumulative survival 2 years after diagnosis in their studied group was 91 percent in group A, 52 percent in group B, and 9 percent in group C. The actual risk of transformation to ANLL at 2 years was 0, 19, and 54 percent, respectively.

Therapy-Related MDS and ANLL. Therapy-related MDS and ANLL occur in individuals previously treated with cytotoxic agents and radiotherapy.[173,174,194–197] The majority of cases are characterized by panmyelosis, which makes precise classification difficult according to the FAB diagnostic criteria.[198] In most cases, the patients were treated with alkylating agents and radiotherapy, often associated with abnormalities of chromosomes 5 and 7. These cases usually have RAEB, or evolving ANLL, M2, M4, or M6 subtypes. In epipodophyllotoxin-associated MDS or ANLL, abnormalities of 11q23 and a monocytic component (such as CMML or M4 and M5) are frequently seen. Orazi and associates[198] found that the presence of ALIP, marrow fibrosis, and augmented CD34 expression in bone marrow biopsies are ominous prognostic factors. Therapy-related MDS generally has a more aggressive clinical course than primary MDS.

Preleukemia and Myelodysplastic Syndromes in Children. Since the FAB Cooperative Group subclassified MDS, the term preleukemia has been almost abandoned because not all patients with MDS will develop acute leukemia. Saarinen and Wegelius[199] reviewed 24 cases in the literature and added 4 of their own cases who all evolved into overt acute leukemia within a period ranging from 2 to 42 months. These authors separated the cases into a pre-ALL and a pre-AML group. It is interesting to note the differences: (1) the pre-ALLs occur most commonly in the 1 to 6 year age group with a female predominance, whereas the AMLs occur at extreme age groups (<1 year and >10 years) with a male predominance; (2) the bone marrows show true hypoplasia without any morphologic changes involving hematopoietic cells in pre-ALLs, whereas the marrows are hyperplastic with dyspoiesis involving one or more cell lines in pre-AMLs; (3) no specific chromosomal abnormalities are detected in pre-ALLs, whereas missing group C chromosome is found in 50 percent of pre-AML cases. Therefore, it appears that MDS occur in the pre-AML group only. Passmore and associates[200] collected data on 68 children (only one of whom had therapy-related MDS) who had the diagnosis of MDS at their own institute. They found that the FAB system of classification was applicable to all cases except three who had eosinophilia. Nineteen of the patients had other clinical abnormalities (e.g., Shwachman's syndrome, familial platelet storage pool defects, and neurofibromatosis) or a family history of MDS. In addition to the FAB classification, these investigators identified two other groups: (1) juvenile CML is defined as a child who had CMML with an elevated fetal hemoglobin (HbF >10 percent), and who did not have monosomy 7; and (2) infantile monosomy 7 syndrome (IMO7). These children were under 4 years of age at presentation with any type of MDS and monosomy 7. Both groups were associated with poor prog-

nosis because they either did not respond or responded poorly to chemotherapy.

Therapy-related MDS or ANLLs are extremely uncommon in pediatric patients.[201] Most of the children had a prior diagnosis of Hodgkin's disease, non-Hodgkin's lymphoma, or neuroblastoma. Unlike the primary MDS in pediatric patients who often had abnormalities involving chromosome 7 (monosomy 7), 8(+8), 21(+21), or 5, the therapy-related MDS and ANLL showed t(9;11), t(8;21) with or without del 16(q22), complete loss of chromosome 7, and 11q23 abnormality. The treatment responses of patients with therapy-related leukemia have been extremely poor.[201]

Fibrosis

Fibrosis of the bone marrow, or myelofibrosis, may be primary (idiopathic) or secondary. The peripheral blood in both chronic idiopathic myelofibrosis (agnogenic myeloid metaplasia [AMM]) and secondary myelofibrosis is characterized by a leukoerythroblastic picture (presence of immature myeloid and erythroid series in the peripheral blood, accompanied by giant and bizarre thrombocytes) with circulating teardrop erythrocytes. The number of circulating nucleated RBCs is often excessive compared with the degree of anemia. Reticulocytosis is not seen in most cases. This peripheral blood picture is specific for myelophthisic anemia (a normocytic, normochromic anemia with leukoerythroblastosis due to replacement of normal bone marrow by nonmarrow elements). The bone marrow shows reticulin (demonstrated by silver impregnated reticulin stain) fibrosis in the early stage, and collagen fibrosis later. However, both reticulin and collagen fibers consist of type I, III, IV, and V collagen with a predominance of the type III collagen and its precursor molecule procollagen III.[202] An increased level of procollagen III aminoterminal fragments is detected in the serum of patients with primary and secondary myelofibrosis. In addition, fibronectin, a product of both fibroblasts and endothelial cells, is extensively deposited in the myelofibrotic marrow. Likewise, laminin and collagen IV proteins, which are synthesized by endothelial and epithelial cells, are found exclusively in vascular basement membrane.[203] It has been postulated that megakaryocytes and platelets, as well as their degraded products in the macrophages, produce platelet-derived growth factor (PDGF), transforming growth factor-beta (TGF-beta), endothelial cell growth factor (ECGF), and platelet factor 4 (PF4).[204] TGF-beta and PDGF are mitogenic to fibroblasts and therefore stimulate collagen type I and III synthesis. The breakdown and removal of the collagen is mediated by monocytes, macrophages, and granulocytes that contain collagenase. PF4 can inhibit collagenase. The imbalance between collagen synthesis and degradation could be responsible for an accumulation of fibers in the mesenchymal compartment of the bone marrow. Clusterings of megakaryocytes with abnormal morphology are usually seen in primary myelofibrosis and myelofibrosis associated with CMPDs. Other changes, such as metastatic tumor or malignant lymphoma, are related to secondary fibrosis. Clinical conditions that are associated with marrow fibrosis are listed in Table 21-13.[202,205,206]

Table 21-13. Clinical Conditions Associated with Bone Marrow Fibrosis

Hematopoietic disorders
    Primary idiopathic myelofibrosis
        Acute malignant sclerosis
        Chronic idiopathic myelofibrosis (AMM)
    Chronic myeloproliferative disorders
        Postpolycythemic myelofiboris
        Transitional myeloproliferative disorder
        Chronic myeloid leukemia
        Idiopathic thrombocythemia
    Acute leukemias
    Chronic lymphocytic leukemia, hairy cell leukemia, adult T cell leukemia/lymphoma, Waldenström's macroglobulinemia, and multiple myeloma
    Malignant lymphomas
    Myelodysplastic syndrome
    Aplastic anemia
    Malignant histiocytosis
    Paroxysmal nocturnal hemoglobinuria
    Mast cell disease
    Gray platelet syndrome
Metastatic tumors
Inflammatory and reparative processes
    Autoimmune diseases
    Granulomatous diseases
    Osteomyelitis
    Previous bone marrow biopsy site
    Following bone marrow necrosis or infarction
    Following bone marrow radiation
    Exposure to toxins, such as thorium dioxide
Storage diseases
Metabolic disorders
    Renal osteodystrophy
    Osteopetrosis
    Vitamin D deficiency
    Hypoparathyroidism
    Hyperparathyroidism
Paget's disease

Primary Myelofibrosis

The clinical presentation of primary myelofibrosis may be acute or chronic. Acute myelosclerosis is uncommon, and morphologic change in peripheral blood is often minimal. Chronic myelofibrosis, or agnogenic myeloid metaplasia, is a form of CMPD. Both entities have been discussed earlier.[109–115,165–168]

Secondary Myelofibrosis

Secondary myelofibrosis may be caused by chemicals, radiation exposure, occlusive vascular disease, metastatic carcinomas, leukemias, and malignant lymphomas. It is also common in CMPDs, such as chronic myelogenous leukemia or polycythemia vera. Focal myelofibrosis may be seen in areas of inflammatory reaction to an infectious agent (such as tuberculosis) or sarcoidosis, or in areas adjacent to bone marrow necrosis and fracture of bone.[202,205] The hematopoietic elements are normal or decreased in most of these disorders (with the exception of fibrosis associated with CMPDs and leukemias), and the morphology of megakaryocytes is normal. The primary cause of fibrosis (such as metastatic carcinoma) may be identified on the same bone marrow section or on deeper sections. It is interesting to note that bone marrow fibrosis in childhood ALL is associated with common ALL antigen (CALLA-positive [CD10+]) and B cell markers.[207] Islam et al[208] found that at least some increase in fiber content is present in 35 percent of the patients with ANLL at presentation.[208] There is no correlation between subgroups of FAB classification and the presence or absence or degree of marrow fibrosis. Bone marrow fibrosis regresses after effective chemotherapy. They conclude that an increase in marrow fiber content at diagnosis does not affect hematopoietic regeneration after treatment and achievement of complete remission.

Primary osseous, renal, or endocrine diseases, such as osteitis fibrosa cystica, fibrous dysplasia, and osteopetrosis, are also associated with marrow fibrosis and osteosclerosis. Microcystic resorption of bone, marrow fibrosis, and increased osteoclastic activity are seen in the recently recognized and studied adult T cell leukemia/lymphoma (discussed below).

Lymphocytic Infiltration

Lymphocytic infiltrates may be broadly separated into (1) benign lymphocytic infiltrate, which may be physiologic (in young children) or reactive (infectious lymphocytosis, infectious mononucleosis, tuberculosis); and (2) malignant lymphoproliferative disorders, including chronic lymphocytic leukemia (CLL) and related disorders, bone marrow involvement by non-Hodgkin's lymphoma (NHL) with or without leukemic picture, and multiple myeloma and related disorders. Hodgkin's disease and some NHLs in which granulomatous change is a part of the pathology are discussed in the section on granuloma.

Non-Neoplastic Lymphocytic Infiltration

Lymphocytes, a normal component of the bone marrow, may constitute up to 50 percent of all nucleated cells in marrow in a child 1 month to 1 year old and about 20 percent of all nucleated cells from 1 year old and onward. Lymphoid nodules or lymphoid aggregates are a relatively common finding in routine bone marrow examination; their reported incidence varies from 1 to 9 percent in antemortem specimens and from 21 to 62 percent in autopsy material. Prevalences of 17.9 and 47 percent, respectively, were cited in two large series.[52,209] These nodules are more commonly seen in older women and are frequently present around the blood vessels, associated with plasmacytosis and lipid granulomas. They are composed of small lymphocytes, a few plasma cells, histiocytes, and occasionally eosinophils and mast cells, organized around a capillary or arteriole within a reticulin fiber network. Rywlin and associates[52] divided lymphoid nodules into lymphoid infiltrates and lymphoid follicles, which measured from 0.08 to 0.6 mm in greatest dimension. These authors defined nodular lymphoid hyperplasia (NLH) of the bone marrow as present when (1) four or more normal lymphoid nodules are seen in any low power (80 mm²) field or (2) a lymphoid nodule exceeds 0.6 mm in greatest dimension. The nodules in NLH may consist of both lymphoid follicles or lymphoid infiltrates, although the former type is more common. Some patients have associated infectious or autoimmune disorders; other may be immunodeficient. Identification of lymphoid nodules or NLH in a patient with a history of lymphoma of small lymphocytes often creates diagnostic difficulty. Irregularity, asymmetry, great variability in size and shape, tendency to fragmentation of the nodules, and abnormal cytology with increased number of large "blastic" lymphocytes are criteria for malignant lymphoma. Table 21-14 lists some of the parameters that can be used to differentiate benign from malignant lymphoid lesions.

Recently, immunohistochemical stains have been used to further delineate benign from malignant lesions. Horny and associates[210] used antibodies to CD45RO (UCHL-1) and beta-F_1 for identifying T cells and antibody to CD20 (L26) for B cells to study the number of T and B cells in normal bone marrow or other conditions. They found that normal bone marrow contained seven T cells and one to five B cells, however, both T and B cell numbers were increased in reactive conditions (T cells from 7 to 11 and B cells from 1.5 to 3). Both T and B cells were decreased in number in neoplastic conditions, such as AML, CML, and carcinomas. A significant increase in T or B cells was only seen in their respective chronic lymphocytic leukemias. Bluth and colleagues[211] found three patterns of staining using anti-CD20 to study small cell lymphoid aggregates in paraffin-embedded marrow particle preparations: (1) homogeneous, (2) mixed, and (3) focally homogeneous. The homogeneous pattern was usually associated with B cell neoplasia, whereas mixed and focally homogeneous were commonly seen in reactive conditions. Sangster and co-workers[212] using the immunogold-silver technique demonstrated the presence of surface immunoglobulin in paraffin sections. However, this method has not been commonly adopted in the routine histologic laboratory. It appears that morphologically benign lymphoid aggregates should not be ignored in iliac crest biopsy specimens from patients who do not have a lymphoproliferative disorder (LPD), because Faulkner-Jones et al[213] found that 37 percent of such patients eventually developed confirmed or suspected LPD.

Lymphoproliferative Disorders

Acute lymphocytic leukemia has been discussed earlier. The FAB Cooperative Group proposed the following classifications for the chronic B and T lymphoid leukemias: the B-LPD includes CLL, PLL (prolymphocytic leukemia), HCL (hairy cell leukemia), SLVL (splenic lymphoma with villous lymphocytes), leukemic phase of NHL, Waldenström's macroglobulinemia (WMG), and plasma cell leukemia. The T-LPD includes CLL, PLL, adult T cell leukemia/lymphoma (ATLL), and Sézary's syndrome.[214] Many of these entities are discussed in the chapter on malignant lymphoma (see Ch. 20).

Chronic Lymphocytic Leukemia and Related Disorders
Chronic Lymphocytic Leukemia. CLL is a disease of elderly men. It is the most common form of leukemia in Western countries.[215,216] The clinical presentations are variable, but the general criterion for the diagnosis of CLL is a sustained and absolute lymphocytosis in peripheral blood and bone marrow that is not attributable to any other cause. Minimum requirements for a diagnosis of CLL include sustained mature-appearing lymphocytosis of greater than 10×10^9/L in peripheral blood and bone marrow lymphocytosis of at least 30 percent in bone marrow aspirates.[215] The National Cancer Institute-sponsored working group[217] on CLL recommends an absolute lymphocyte count threshold value of more than 5×10^9/L. However, other investigators consider that the diagnosis of CLL may be made if B cell monoclonality is demonstrated in a proper clinical setting regardless of the absolute lymphocyte count,[218] because most cases (>95 percent) of CLLs in Western countries are B-CLL. In typical cases of B-CLL, the neoplastic lymphocytes are small with a narrow rim of basophilic cytoplasm, and the nuclear chromatin is dense and nucleoli are not visible. However, some morphologic variation is seen from patient to patient. Two CLL mixed cell types have been described: (1) a spectrum of small to large lymphocytes with occasional (<10 percent) prolymphocytes, and (2) a mixture of small lymphocytes and prolymphocytes (>10 percent to <55 percent) designated CLL/PL.[214]

Immunologic study shows that most of the neoplastic small lymphocytes possess weak monoclonal surface immunoglobu-

Table 21-14. Comparison of Benign (Reactive) Lymphocytic Infiltrates and Malignant Lymphocytic Lesions (Leukemia or Lymphoma) in Bone Marrow Sections

Benign	Malignant
Randomly distributed	Frequently paratrabecular or around a large sinus
Small, well circumscribed	Large, irregularly shaped, with ill-defined borders
Polymorphic, consisting of small lymphocytes, plasma cells, transformed lymphocytes, immunoblasts, and histiocytes; often organized around a capillary or blood vessel, within a delicate network of reticulin fibers	Usually monomorphic; cytology of neoplastic infiltrate depends on the type of malignant cells involved (cytologic atypia common)
Germinal centers may be present	Germinal centers are absent
A mixture of T and B cells by immunohistochemical study	Most commonly B cells with atypical morphology. Aberrant T cell phenotypes in T cell LPD

Abbreviation: LPD, lymphoproliferative disorder.

lins (SIgM and SIgD) on their cell membrane, and they also carry weak complement and Fc receptors as well as receptors for mouse erythrocytes. In addition, CLL cells express the following antigens: CD19, CD20, CD24, HLA-DR, CD5, CD23, and CD43. "Deviation" from the typical CLL phenotype is seen in cases of CLL with mixed cell types, in which strong expression of SIg and reactivity with FMC7/CD22 may be seen.[214] In addition, CD5– CLL and CLL with expression of myelomonocytic markers (such as CD11c and CD13) have been described.[219–221]

A clinical staging system for CLL was introduced by Rai and colleagues[222] to assess the tumor burden. Later, Binet and associates[223] proposed a new system consisting of three stages. Both staging systems are based on the degree of peripheral lymphocytosis, thrombocytopenia, anemia, and the presence of organomegaly (liver, spleen, cervical, axillary, and inguinal lymph nodes). For instance, Rai's "Stage 0" is defined by lymphocytosis alone; "stage I," lymphocytosis and lymphadenopathy; "stage II," lymphocytosis, spleen or liver enlargement, or both; "stage III," lymphocytosis and anemia (hemoglobin <11 g/dl); "stage IV," lymphocytosis and thrombocytopenia (platelet count $<100 \times 10^{12}$/L). The Rai classification has now been condensed to three stages that differ with respect to survival: good prognosis (equivalent to original Rai stage 0); intermediate prognosis (Rai stage I or II); and poor prognosis (Rai stage III or IV).[215,216,218] Several recent studies indicate that clinical stages, bone marrow histopathologic findings, blood lymphocyte counts, lymphocyte doubling time, and cytogenetic abnormalities are good predictors of survival.[215,216,218]

Histopathologic findings in the bone marrow that were capable of predicting prognosis in patients with CLL were first noted by Rozman and associates.[224] These authors described four different histologic patterns: (1) interstitial lymphoid infiltration without displacement of fat cells (Fig. 21-19); (2) nodular (abnormal lymphoid nodule without interstitial infiltration) (Fig. 21-20); (3) mixed (combination of interstitial and nodular patterns); and (4) diffuse (replacement of both hematopoietic cells and fat cells by lymphoid infiltration). The difference between normal and neoplastic nodules has been described earlier. Cytologically the neoplastic lymphocytes are small and contain round or slightly irregular nuclei, clumped chromatin, and an indiscernible amount of cytoplasm. A small nucleolus may be observed in some cells. Some intermediate lymphocytes may also be present. These transformed lymphocytes resemble those seen in proliferation centers in lymph nodes from patients with CLL. The reticulin framework is moderately accentuated in most cases. The pattern of bone marrow histology (diffuse or nondiffuse) in B-CLL patients has been proved to be one of the best prognostic parameters.[225] The diffuse pattern of bone marrow histology is considered the best criterion for initiation of therapy in these patients.[226] Pangalis and associates[227] also observed that bone marrow involvement in patients with malignant lymphoma of small lymphocytes always displayed nodular patterns even though these patients had advanced disease.

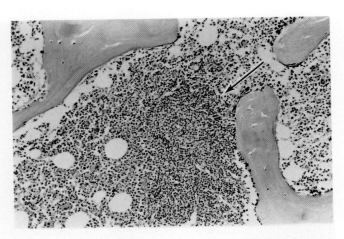

Fig. 21-20. Nodular infiltrate of CLL. This pattern of CLL infiltrate (arrow) is difficult to differentiate from benign lymphoid nodules. Immunohistochemical stains or flow cytometric studies are necessary for a definitive diagnosis. (H&E stain, × 40.)

Cytogenetic analysis by karyotyping of in vitro stimulated lymphocytes in B-CLL revealed clonal chromosomal changes in 218 out of 391 patients (56 percent) studied.[228] The most common abnormalities were trisomy 12 (31 percent) and structural abnormalities of chromosome 13 (23 percent), which frequently involved the site of the retinoblastoma gene, and of chromosome 14 (19 percent). The incidence of trisomy 12 increases when a FISH technique is used.[229,230] Several reports indicate an association of trisomy 12 with atypical CLL[229–231] and a worse prognosis. Patients with a normal karyotype had a median overall survival of more than 15 years, in contrast to 7.7 years for patients with clonal changes; patients with single abnormalities did significantly better than those with complex karyotypes; patients with abnormalities involving chromosome 14q had poorer survival than those with aberrations of chromosome 13q.[228] Among patients with single abnormalities, those with trisomy 12 alone had poorer survival than patients with single aberrations of chromosome 13q.[228] The bcl-1 gene (11q13) rearrangement has been occasionally demonstrated in patients with B-CLL and has been associated with atypical morphology and surface expression of CD11b,[232] although this genetic abnormality is frequently seen in mantle cell lym-

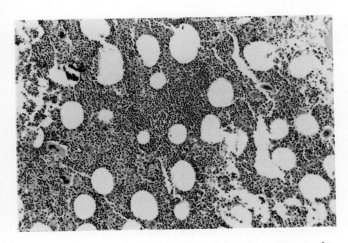

Fig. 21-19. Interstitial infiltration in CLL. Note monomorphic leukemic infiltrate interspersed by hematopoietic cells. (H&E stain, × 40.)

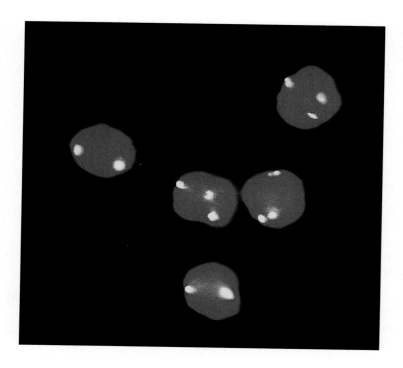

Fig. 21-21. Mixed CLL/PLL. Three of the five leukemic cells have trisomy 12. (Fluorescence in situ hybridization, ×, 1,000.) (Courtesy of Russell Brynes.[249])

phomas.[233–235] Cyclin D_2 mRNA was found to be overexpressed in 29 of 34 B-CLL cases and in all cases of lymphoplasmacytic lymphoma.[236] It is interesting to note that the human cyclin D_2 gene ($CCND_2$) has been mapped to chromosome 12p13 and trisomy 12 is the most common chromosomal change in B-CLL and immunocytomas[236] (Fig. 21-21). Translocation t(14;18) (q32.3;q21.3) was detected cytogenetically in three cases of B-CLL. In addition, t(2;18) (p11;q21.3) or t(18;22) (q21.3;q11) have been detected cytogentically in two cases of B-CLL.[237] It should be pointed out that translocation involving the bcl-2 locus at 18q21.3 is observed in about 80 percent of cases of follicular B cell NHLs.[238]

Differential Diagnosis. The differential diagnosis includes a variety of chronic B cell leukemias, such as prolymphocytic leukemia (PLL), hairy cell leukemia (HCL), splenic lymphoma with villous lymphocytes (SLVL), and leukemic phase of mantle cell lymphoma (MCL) and follicular center cell lymphoma, small cleaved cell (FCC, SC). The immunophenotypic characteristics of these entities are listed in Table 21-15.

Transformation of CLL. In most cases of CLL there is clinical and morphologic evolution to an aggressive phase of the disease. There may be an abrupt increase in absolute lymphocytes with appearance of many prolymphocytes in the blood or bone marrow, accompanied by enlarging lymph nodes and spleen (prolymphocytoid transformation). Other cases may be manifested by systemic symptoms, a rapid increase in lymphadenopathy, or extranodal involvement (Richter's syndrome).

Prolymphocytoid transformation may represent an accelerated phase of CLL in which the disease undergoes an insidious, although aggressive, change in character, with increasing refractoriness to treatment.[239] These patients not only have a previous history of CLL but also have a double population of lymphocytes (prolymphocytes and "mature" small lymphocytes) that retain most of the marker characteristics of B-CLL. The prolymphocytes are large cells with moderately abundant cytoplasm and a round or oval nucleus containing condensed nuclear chromatin and a large centrally located nucleolus. Bone marrow examination shows marked hypercellularity with replacement of normal marrow by a mixed infiltrate of small lymphocytes and prolymphocytes. Melo and associates[240–243] have recently studied the relationship of CLL and prolymphocytic leukemia in detail. They divided chronic lymphocytic leukemia and prolymphocytic leukemia into three groups: (1) typical CLL group (prolymphocytes <10 percent); (2) CLL/PL group (prolymphocytes 11 to 55 percent); and (3) PLL (prolymphocytes >55 percent). Patients who fall into the second group were found to have intermediate features between CLL and PLL. The degree of splenomegaly was disproportionate to the lymph node enlargement. This group includes at least two types of CLL, one with increased proportions of prolymphocytes but otherwise typical disease, and another in prolymphocytoid transformation.[240] The third group have clinical and laboratory features characteristic of PLL. The percentage of prolymphocytes is defined as the proportion of prolymphocytes among the peripheral blood lymphoid population.[240] It was found that absolute prolymphocyte count and spleen size carry with them prognostic significance.[243] Prolymphocytoid transformation should be differentiated from Galton's prolymphocytic leukemia.[244]

Richter's syndrome is characterized by fever, weight loss, localized lymphadenopathy, dysglobulinemia, and a pleomorphic malignant lymphoma occurring terminally in patients with a previous history of CLL.[245–248] Immunohistopathologic study has revealed that the malignant lymphoma was a B cell immunoblastic sarcoma in most instances. The incidence ranges

Table 21-15. Comparison of Chronic Lymphoproliferative Disorders of B Cell Origin

Markers	CLL/SLL	PLL	MCL	FCC/SCC	MZL	HCL	SLVL	PCL
SIg	Weak	+	+	+	+	+	+	−
CIg	−	−/+	−	−	−/+	+/−	+/−	+
Pan B	+	+	+	+	+	+	+	−
CD10	−	−/+	−/+	+/−	−	−/+	−/+	−/+
CD23	+	−	−/+	−/+	−	−	−/+	−
CD5	+	−/+	+	−	−	−	−/+	−
CD43	+	+	+	−	−/+	−	−	−/+
CD11c	−/+	−	−	−	−/+	+	+/−	−
CD25	−/+	−	−	−	−	+	−/+	−
FMC7/CD22	−/+	+	+	+	+/−	+	+	?
CD38	−	−	−	−/+	−	−/+	−/+	+
bcl-1 (R)	−/+	−	+/−	−	−	−	−/+	−/+
bcl-2 (R)	−	−	−	+	−	−	−	−

Abbreviations: CLL/SLL, chronic lymphocytic leukemia/small lymphocytic lymphoma; PLL, prolymphocytic leukemia; MCL, mantle cell lymphoma; FCC/SCC, follicular center cell lymphoma, small cleaved cell; MZL, marginal zone lymphoma, including monocytoid B cell lymphoma; HCL, hairy cell leukemia; SLVL, splenic lymphoma with villous lymphocytes; PCL, plasma cell leukemia; (R), rearrangement; SIg, membrane surface immunoglobulin; CIg, cytoplasmic immunoglobulin.

from 1 to 10 percent of CLL patients with most reports indicating 3 percent. Thirty-three percent of 39 cases studied presented with extranodal involvement.[248] The median interval between diagnosis of CLL and large cell lymphoma (Richter's syndrome) was 48 months.[248] Clonality analysis suggested that Richter's syndrome was most commonly a true transformational event in one study,[248] but it was found to be an acquired abnormality in another report.[249] Transformation of CLL to other types of malignant lymphomas has also been described.[250–252] A similar evolution has been reported in other lymphoproliferative disorders of small B cell type, including multiple myeloma.[253]

T-CLL is uncommon, accounting for about 2 percent of CLL in Western countries. In most cases, the cells are large granular lymphocytes (LGLs).[254–256] These cells are large and have an oval, round, or slightly folded nucleus, and an abundant amount of pale blue cytoplasm containing fine or coarse azurophilic granules. A diagnosis of T-CLL may be made if T lymphocytosis of greater than 5×10^9/L persists for over 6 months and consists of a relatively uniform population of lymphocytes.[214] LGLs comprise 10 to 15 percent of normal blood mononuclear cells and may be of either CD3−(NK cells) or CD3+ (T cell) lineage. T-LGL leukemia is defined as a clonal proliferation of CD3+ LGL and is found in 80 percent of cases with LGL leukemia. Most of these cases run a chronic clinical course and have a CD3+, CD4−, CD8+, CD16+, CD56−, CD57+, and often HLA-DR+ phenotype. Rarely, T-LGL leukemia may be CD4+, or CD4+CD8+. TCR alpha/beta or gamma/delta gene rearrangement is often demonstrated. NK-LGL leukemia results from a clonal proliferation of CD3− LGL. They are usually CD3−, CD4−, CD8−, CD16+, CD56+, and CD57−. Nonrandom chromosomal abnormalities may be demonstrated in NK-LGL leukemia, although TCR rearrange-

ment is lacking.[257–259] Patients with T-LGL leukemia frequently present with severe neutropenia, anemia, or red cell aplasia. Recurrent infections, rheumatoid arthritis, and other autoimmune phenomena (such as autoantibodies) have also been observed. Hepatosplenomegaly is common; lymphadenopathy and cutaneous lesions are unusual. Patients with NK-LGL leukemia are younger, more often have systemic B symptoms, and have more massive hepatosplenomegaly. Lymphadenopathy and gastrointestinal involvement are frequently seen. The bone marrow cellularity is variable. Lymphocytic infiltration also varies and frequently occurs in an interstitial pattern, but it may be diffuse. Cytologically, the neoplastic cells may be indistinguishable from those of B-CLL. T-CLL should be differentiated from reactive lymphocytosis, which is self-limiting and rarely exceeds 5×10^9/L, and Sézary's syndrome, which is characterized by generalized erythroderma, pruritus, peripheral lymphadenopathy, hepatomegaly, and the presence of Sézary cells in the skin and peripheral blood. Sézary cells usually express T helper cell markers.[260]

Prolymphocytic Leukemia of Galton. Prolymphocytic leukemia (PLL), as defined by Galton and associates,[244] is an uncommon variant of CLL. Patients with PLL are often elderly men, with massive splenomegaly, absent or minimal lymphadenopathy, striking lymphocytosis (average lymphocyte count 355×10^9/L), resistance to conventional therapy for CLL, and a poor prognosis.[244,261] Histologically, PLL may be differentiated from CLL by the characteristic cytology of the neoplastic cells (a larger cell than CLL, with an immature-appearing round nucleus containing one prominent nucleolus and an abundant amount of cytoplasm).[262] A minor population of small lymphocytes with clumped chromatin is commonly present. Phenotypically the neoplastic cells marked as B cells in the majority of cases, but T-PLLs have been reported.[263,264] Histologic examination shows a nodular, interstitial, mixed or diffuse pattern. Some of the nodules are paratrabecular in location.

Matutes and associates[264] collected data on 78 cases of T-prolymphocytic leukemia. The median age for this group of patients was 69 years, with a male/female ratio of 1.33:1. Seventy-three percent of these patients presented with splenomegaly. Lymphadenopathy (53 percent) and hepatomegaly (40 percent) were also common, and skin lesions were seen in 27 percent of patients. Most patients had leukocytosis (>100 × 10⁹/L) with circulating prolymphocytes (containing a large prominent nucleolus). A small prolymphocyte variant was described (19 percent of cases). The neoplastic cells expressed mature T cell phenotype with CD4+, CD8– being the most common subset. The expression of CD7 was a consistent finding, in contrast to ATLL, LGL leukemia, and Sézary's syndromes, in which CD7 was often negative. Chromosomal abnormalities involving 14q11 [inv(14) (q11;q32)], trisomy 8, and occasional cases with t(11;14) (q13;q32) have been reported. The clinical course was progressive with a median survival of 7.5 months.

Hairy Cell Leukemia. HCL is a chronic lymphoproliferative disorder, primarily affecting middle-aged men with a median age of 50 years at the onset of the disease. The neoplastic cell is a mononuclear cell of intermediate to large size. The eccentrically located nucleus often contain lacy chromatin and a small and inconspicuous nucleolus. The light blue cytoplasm displays typical fine filamentous ("hairy") projections on peripheral blood smear. Hairy cells generally express pan B cell antigens CD20 and CD10. They are also positive for PCA-1, CD11c, CD22, and CD25[265] (Fig. 21-22) (Table 21-15). Rare cases of T cell HCL have been reported.[265–267] Some of these cases have been linked with HTLV-II,[268] a retrovirus that infects humans. The leukemic cells are characteristically stained with acid phosphatase (multiple paranuclear granules), and this positive reaction is resistant to tartaric acid inhibition.[269] One or more ribosome-lamellar complexes may be demonstrated intracytoplasmically by electron microscopy.[270] However, none of these characteristics are pathognomonic, and hairy cell leukemia may simulate a variety of myeloid and lymphoid proliferative disorders.[265,271,272]

In a typical case the disease is characterized by an insidious onset, marked splenomegaly, pancytopenia, and circulating hairy cells. Although peripheral lymphadenopathy is usually minimal, significantly enlarged mediastinal, retroperitoneal, and abdominal lymph nodes were seen in 15 of 22 patients in one series.[273] The bone marrow aspiration often yields a dry tap. The marrow cellularity is variable in biopsy specimens. The neoplastic infiltrate may be focal, patchy, or diffuse and is composed of uniform mononuclear cells with a distinct cell membrane, giving a "mosaic" pattern or a "honeycomb" or "sponge" appearance (Fig. 21-23). The nucleus may be round, ovoid, indented, or coffee-bean in shape, surrounded by a "halo" of pale cytoplasm imparting a "fried egg" feature; the nuclear chromatin is finely stippled, and the nucleolus is indistinct (Fig. 21-24). Mitoses and nuclear pleomorphism are usually absent. This loose network of monomorphic cells is in contrast to the

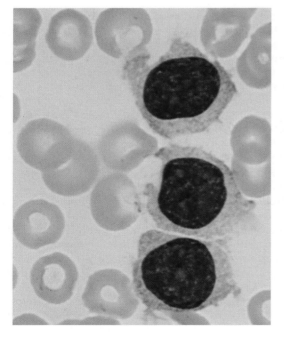
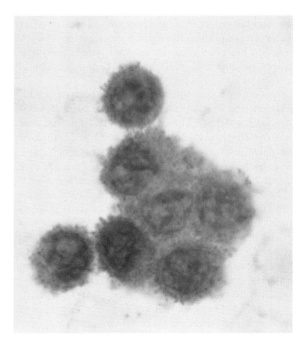

Fig. 21-22. Hairy cell leukemia. This composite picture depicts circulating hairy cells in the blood. Note the typical nuclear chromatin and hairy cytoplasmic projection. Leukemic cells express CD11c. (Romanowsky stain and immunoalkaline phosphatase stain, × 1,000.)

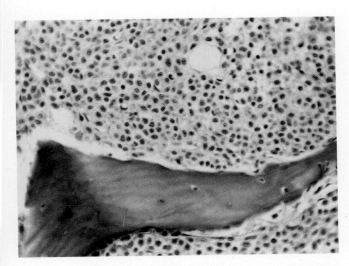

Fig. 21-23. Hairy cell leukemia (HCL). Diffuse infiltrate of bone marrow by HCL. Each leukemic cell has clear cytoplasm. (H&E stain, × 100.)

tightly packed, paratrabecular arrangement of lymphomatous involvement of the marrow. Increased reticulin fibers are seen in the infiltrated areas.

The changes in the spleen are characteristic.[265,274,275] It is usually moderately to massively enlarged and appears congested on gross examination. Microscopically, the red pulp cords and sinuses are infiltrated by the neoplastic hairy cells, whereas the white pulp appears atrophic or totally replaced by the tumor.

Nonrandomized chromosomal abnormalities have been reported in more than 50 percent of cases with HCL.[276] Clonal aberrations in chromosome 5 manifested as trisomy 5, pericentric inversions, or interstitial deletions involving band 5q13 have been demonstrated in 12 of 30 patients (40 percent).[276] Other important findings include pericentric inversions and deletions of chromosome 2, and structural abnormalities of band 1q42.[276]

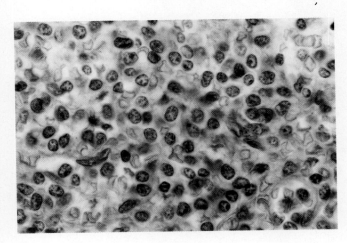

Fig. 21-24. Hairy cell leukemia (HCL). Higher magnification reveals round, oval, or coffee bean-shaped nuclei, evenly distributed chromatin, and indistinct nucleoli typical of HCL. (H&E stain, × 400).

Several variants of hairy cell leukemia (HCL-V) have been described.[265] One such variant is characterized by splenomegaly, moderate anemia, and thrombocytopenia with leukocytosis-containing neoplastic lymphoid cells.[277] Monocytopenia, which is common in typical HCL, is absent in these patients with HCL-V. The tartrate-resistant acid phosphatase reaction is negative. The leukemic cells from a majority of patients express CD19, CD20, CD22, FMC-7, HLA-DR, and CD11c; they are negative for CD25 and HC-2. Bone marrow examinations show interstitial infiltration by neoplastic cells, which often contain condensed chromatin and visible nucleoli, and are packed together surrounded by a moderate amount of reticulin.

The differential diagnosis includes splenic lymphoma with villous lymphocytes, monocytoid B cell lymphoma (marginal zone lymphoma),[274,275,278] follicular center cell lymphoma, chronic lymphocytic leukemia, prolymphocytic leukemia, and mast cell disease. These entities are discussed elsewhere in this text.

Splenic Lymphoma with Villous Lymphocytes. SLVL is a low grade B cell lymphoma that primarily afflicts elderly men or women with a median age of 66 years and a mean of 70 years.[275,278] These patients present with anemia, thrombocytopenia, leukocytosis with circulating neoplastic cells, monoclonal gammopathy, and splenomegaly.[279] The circulating cells are slightly larger than a small lymphocyte, have a round or oval nucleus containing condensed nuclear chromatin and a small nucleolus, and exhibit short and thin cytoplasmic villi. Sometimes the cytoplasmic projections are localized to one pole or two opposite poles of the cell. The nuclear/cytoplasmic ratio is higher than in hairy cells of HCL and HCL-V. A few cells showing lymphoplasmacytic features are often present. The histopathology of the spleen shows infiltration of white pulp in a marginal zone pattern or complete replacement of follicles in the white pulp. The bone marrow is not infiltrated in half of the cases; in others there is moderate to pronounced diffuse or nodular infiltration.[214] The results of phenotypic and genotypic studies in these cases are listed in Table 21-15.

Sézary's Syndrome. Sézary's syndrome is characterized by generalized erythroderma, pruritis, peripheral lymphadenopathy, hepatomegaly, and the presence of Sézary (Lutzner) cells in the skin and peripheral blood.[260] Lutzner and associates[280] proposed the term cutaneous T cell lymphoma to include both the Sézary's syndrome and mycosis fungoides (MF). The neoplastic cells of both diseases possess similar morphologic findings (cerebriform nuclei), express T cell (helper cell) markers (CD2+, CD3+, CD4+, and CD5+; TdT-negative, HLA-DR-negative, and CD7−), and have a predilection for the skin. Circulating atypical lymphoid (Sézary) cells are classically present in Sézary's syndrome but much rarer in MF. Two cell types have been recognized.[281,282] The large cells range from 12 to 25 μm in diameter and characteristically have a cerebriform nucleus. The cytoplasm is clear to slightly basophilic and may contain vacuoles. The small cells vary from 8 to 11 μm in diameter and may resemble the normal small lymphocytes. However, they contain a moderate amount of vacuolated, basophilic cytoplasm. These vacuoles are PAS-positive and form a "necklace" around the nucleus. Histopathologic examination of bone marrow biopsy samples reveals limited involvement.[260,281,283] The cellularity is usually normal. The hematopoietic elements are not decreased, although the neoplastic cells may infiltrate in the interstitium or form small aggregates. It has been said that the interstitial pattern of marrow involvement is associated with circulating neoplastic cells in the blood whereas the nodular pattern is not associated with peripheral blood involvement.[283] These cells have a very high nuclear/cytoplasmic ratio and contain a hyperchromatic nucleus with irregular nuclear contour. Nuclear indentation or convolution may be appreciated under oil immersion with fine adjustment.

Adult T Cell Leukemia/Lymphoma. ATLL or subacute leukemia of Japan is linked to human T cell leukemia virus.[284] This disorder was first described by Japanese investigators and was found in an endemic area in southwest Japan.[285] Later, it was reported from the West Indies and Africa and in blacks in the southeastern United States.[284,286,287] Patients with ATLL characteristically present with subacute leukemia, hypercalcemia, lytic lesions in bones, generalized lymphadenopathy, hepatosplenomegaly, and cutaneous lesions. Although the disease has an insidious or subacute onset, it frequently runs an aggressive course, leading to death in a few months to a year. The malignant cell is a small to intermediate T cell, with a markedly irregular ("knobby") nucleus (Fig. 21-25). Polymorphism is characteristic of ATLL. These cells frequently mark as T helper/inducer cells (CD2+, CD3+, CD4+, CD5+, and CD25+; and TdT-negative, CD7−, and CD8−), but they generally do not have detectable helper function. Neoplastic cells in some cases may function as suppressor/cytotoxic T cells. Variation in the clinical manifestations has been described.[288]

Bone marrow biopsies show microcystic resorption with focal fibrosis and increased osteoclastic activity in some patients. Of those patients who had lymphomatous involvement in the marrow, the degree of marrow replacement was not prominent. The infiltrate is patchy or interstitial but not paratrabecular. Some patients who had circulating leukemic cells did not have evidence of bone marrow involvement.[284] Histopathology of involved lymph nodes exhibits a spectrum of morphology, and there is no correlation between clinical course and histologic type.[284,289,290]

Bone Marrow Involvement in Non-Hodgkin's Lymphoma

Bone marrow involvement is quite common in NHL. However, the incidence varies among different series of studies, different histologic types, and different methods of obtaining the specimens. As a rule, histologic examination of a bone marrow clot section or biopsy specimen is better than that of Wright-Giemsa-stained bone marrow smears,[13] bilateral bone marrow biopsy is better than unilateral biopsy,[17] and open bone marrow biopsy is better than needle biopsy.[6] However, bilateral needle biopsies are adequate for staging purposes.[291] Bone marrow involvement was found in 89 percent of multiple myeloma, 64 percent of non-Hodgkin's lymphoma, and 8 percent of Hodgkin's disease by Bartl and associates[292] after studying 3,229 patients with lymphoproliferative disorder. Schmid and Isaacson[40] found a similar prevalence: 90 percent (141 of 157 patients) of multiple myeloma, 64 percent (311 of 490) of low grade non-Hodgkin's lymphoma; 15 percent (30 of 199) of high grade non-Hodgkin's lymphoma, and 9 percent of Hodgkin's disease involved bone marrow. The clinical symptoms vary with the type of NHL. The classifications of malignant lymphomas and their clinical, histologic, immunophenotypic, and

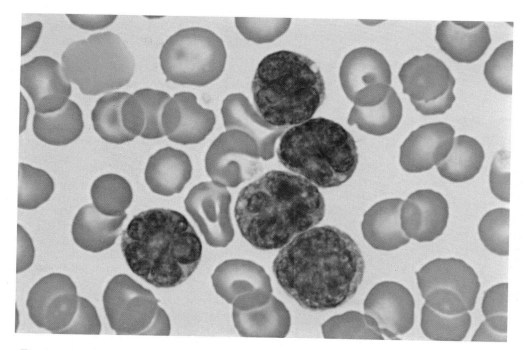

Fig. 21-25. Adult T cell leukemia lymphoma. Note the "flower-like" or "knobby" nuclei that are characteristic of this type of leukemic cell. (Romanowsky stain, × 100.)

genotypic characteristics are discussed in detail in Chapter 20. The terminologies used in the International Working Formulation are applied in this chapter for discussion.[293] Whenever it is necessary, terms used in the Revised European-American Classification (REAL) of lymphoid neoplasms are employed.[278]

Bone marrow involvement is more frequently seen in patients with lymphomas of small lymphocytes (low grade) than in those with large cell lymphomas, high grade NHLs, and peripheral T cell lymphoma[292,294,295] although lymphocytic lymphomas of small lymphocytic cells and small cleaved cells often have a more indolent clinical course. The initial histologic diagnosis of malignant lymphoma was established by bone marrow biopsy in 36 percent of the positive cases in one series.[296] Bone marrow examination frequently changes clinical staging from a more localized form of disease to a disseminated form (stage IV). A positive bone marrow examination is frequently obtained in patients with a normal complete blood cell count and without evidence of a leukoerythroblastic picture. The absolute blood lymphocyte count is considered to be an important diagnostic criterion in differentiating malignant lymphomas from leukemic infiltration of the bone marrow; that is, when the blood lymphocyte count is 10×10^9/L or greater, lymphocytic leukemia is the preferred diagnosis.[214]

Histopathologic examination of a bone marrow biopsy reveals the following patterns: (1) interstitial, (2) nodular, (3) paratrabecular, or (4) packed marrow.[296] Combinations of one or more of the above patterns are also observed. The neoplastic lymphocytes are seen infiltrating between fat cells and replacing normal hematopoietic elements in the interstitial pattern. The focal or nodular involvement in small cleaved follicular center cell (FCC) lymphoma is characterized by a paratrabecular distribution (Fig. 21-26). The pattern of infiltration is unre-

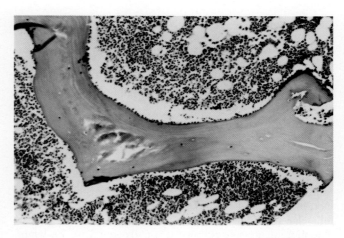

Fig. 21-26. Paratrabecular infiltrate of intermediate grade malignant lymphoma with small cleaved cells. (H&E stain, × 40.)

lated to the histologic finding of follicular or diffuse small cleaved cell lymphoma in the lymph node biopsy. On the contrary, bone marrow involvement in small lymphocytic lymphomas is usually randomly focal, whereas small noncleaved cell and lymphoblastic lymphomas generally display an interstitial or diffuse pattern of infiltration.[297–299] Cytologically, lymphomatous infiltration in the marrow generally shows morphologic features similar to those observed in lymph node biopsies from the same patients. Extensive blood involvement was noted most frequently in small cleaved FCC lymphomas, and the term *lymphosarcoma cell leukemia* has been used widely in the literature[86] (Fig. 21-27). Lymphosarcoma cell leukemia,

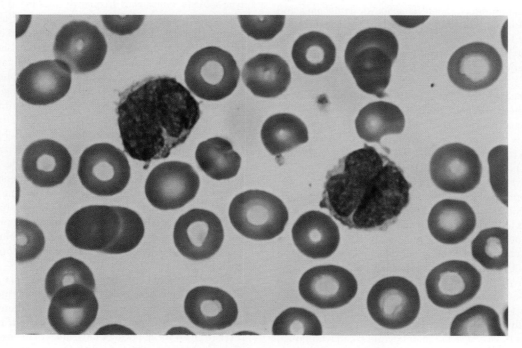

Fig. 21-27. Leukemic phase of non-Hodgkin's lymphoma. Note that neoplastic lymphocytes have deeply clefted or indented nuclei and clumped chromatin. (Romanowsky stain, ×, 1,000.)

however, is a confusing term and may have different meanings to different people, as it may describe (1) a variant of CLL, (2) a leukemic phase of poorly differentiated lymphocytic lymphoma, or (3) a leukemic phase of any non-Hodgkin's lymphoma. Strictly speaking, the term should be reserved for the leukemic phase of small cleaved FCC lymphoma (poorly differentiated lymphocytic lymphoma).

Morphologic Discordance Between the Lymph Node and Bone Marrow. When comparative histologic examinations of malignant lymphomas in lymph node and bone marrow were made, a discordance between these two anatomic sites is noted in 22 to 60 percent of cases.[300,301] Divergent histology is common in large cell lymphomas (including immunoblastic), and follicular and diffuse, mixed small and large cell types.[301–303] The more aggressive subtype is usually found in the lymph node. The typical discordant pattern shows large cell or immunoblastic in the lymph node, but mixed small and large cell, small cleaved cell or small lymphocytic histology in the bone marrow.[301–303] Of the lymphomas that were immunophenotyped and had bone marrow involvement, 52 percent of the B cell lymphomas and 38 percent of the T cell lymphomas showed discordant histology between lymph node and bone marrow.[303]

Isolated bone marrow non-Hodgkin's lymphoma without systemic involvement is relatively rare.[304] Three of the four cases reported by Ponzoni and Li[304] were T cell lymphoma. They may create diagnostic difficulty. Bone marrow examination is important in pathologic staging of clinical stage I and II disease and in following patients with advanced disease for response to therapy. Its significance for patients with advanced clinical stages is uncertain.[305]

Low Grade Lymphomas. *Small lymphocytic lymphoma* and chronic lymphocytic leukemia are nearly identical disorders with neoplastic lymphocytes displaying the same morphologic, immunophenotypic, and genotypic findings.[226,227] Lymphomatous involvement of the marrow is seen in 80 to 90 percent of cases.[291,299]

Lymphoplasmacytoid lymphoma is an uncommon low grade lymphoma, although bone marrow involvement is seen in 85 percent of cases at the time of initial diagnosis.[292] The pattern of infiltration is nodular or interstitial/nodular. The subtype, Waldenström's macroglobulinemia (WMG), is discussed under the heading of plasma cell dyscrasia.

Mantle cell lymphoma (mantle zone lymphoma, centrocytic lymphoma, intermediate lymphocytic lymphoma, or small cleaved cell follicular center cell lymphoma in the Working Formulation) is a disease of elderly men, characterized by lymphadenopathy and liver and bone marrow involvement.[306] It is believed to be a low grade B cell lymphoma of follicular mantle cell in origin, although a blastic variant has been described.[306] The immunologic and genotypic findings are presented in Table 21-15. Bone marrow involvement has been observed in 65 to 82 percent of cases.[307,308] The pattern of involvement is usually randomly focal or interstitial.

Marginal zone B cell lymphoma (monocytoid B cell lymphoma, low grade B cell lymphoma of MALT type)[278] is a low grade lymphoma, and primarily involves lymph nodes or extranodal sites (MALT).[309–311] Splenomegaly, bone marrow involve-

ment, and leukemic conversion are uncommon. An incidence of 2 percent is cited in one report,[311] 38 percent in another,[310] and 49 percent in a more recent report.[312]

Follicular center cell lymphoma: Approximately 50 to 60 percent of the follicular lymphomas of predominantly small cleaved cell and follicular mixed small cleaved and large cell lymphomas involves bone marrow.[297,299] These types of lesions frequently display a focal and paratrabecular pattern (Fig. 21-27). The neoplastic cells usually consist of a predominance of small cleaved cells regardless of the lymph node histology. A high incidence of discordant histologic types between the bone marrow and the lymph node has been observed in this group of lymphomas and was discussed earlier.

Intermediate Grade Lymphomas. *Diffuse small cleaved cell lymphomas,* many of which are mantle cell lymphomas, have been reported to involve the bone marrow in approximately 65 to 82 percent of cases.[307,308]

Diffuse mixed small and large cell and *diffuse large cell lymphomas* include a morphologic spectrum of B and T cell lymphomas. The overall incidence of marrow involvement for this group varies from 30 to 56 percent.[297,299] A discordant histology between lymph node and bone marrow is observed in this morphologic category and is more common in B cell lymphomas.[301–303] However, the diagnostic difficulty of bone marrow involvement usually occurs in the peripheral T cell lymphomas. Because these neoplasms often consist of a mixed cellular infiltrate including histiocytes and pose a differential diagnosis with Hodgkin's disease, this entity is discussed under granulomatous changes in this chapter.

High Grade Lymphomas. Among the high grade lymphomas, *lymphoblastic lymphomas* frequently involve the bone marrow (50 to 60 percent of cases).[297,299] Tura and associates[295] reported that 18 of their 43 patients (42 percent) with lymphoblastic lymphoma showed circulating blasts. The lymphoma cells in approximately 70 percent of cases express a T cell immunophenotype (convoluted cell lymphoma) and in 30 percent of cases type as pre-B cells. The histologic and cytologic features of lymphoblastic lymphoma are identical to those of acute lymphocytic leukemia (L1 or rarely L2 morphology according to FAB classification).[88–92] If lymphoblasts constitute more than 25 percent of all nucleated cells in the marrow, a diagnosis of acute lymphocytic leukemia is made. The pattern of infiltration in the marrow is nearly always interstitial or diffuse. A "starry-sky pattern" may be observed in some cases, which is due to the presence of tingible body macrophages. The neoplastic cells range from the size of a small lymphocyte to three or four times larger than a small lymphocyte. Nuclear irregularity, fine chromatin pattern, and a high mitotic rate are frequently observed.[313]

The L3 type of acute lymphocytic leukemia is the counterpart of *small noncleaved cell lymphoma.* Bone marrow involvement and leukemic presentation vary in different studies, occurring in 5 to 57 percent.[72,299] The pattern may be diffuse, interstitial, or focal. Focal or large areas of necrosis may be seen. The size of the neoplastic nucleus approximates that of a histiocyte. The nuclei are round or oval with coarse but evenly distributed chromatin and two to four small, distinct nucleoli. The neoplastic cells have a moderate amount of vacuolated py-roninophilic cytoplasm. Mitotic figures are numerous.

Immunoblastic lymphomas seldom involve the bone marrow with the exception of some T immunoblastic lymphomas (polymorphous and epithelioid cell component), which are now classified as peripheral T cell lymphomas and are discussed under the section on granulomatous changes. Immunoblastic lymphoma of clear cell type may be either B or T cell in origin.[314] More than two-thirds of T cell immunoblastic lymphoma, clear cell variant, present with stage III/IV disease clinically.

It is not clear whether *Ki-1(+) anaplastic large cell lymphoma* is classified as an immunoblastic lymphoma or some other large cell lymphoma. However, 17 percent of 42 patients with anaplastic large cell lymphoma were found to have bone marrow involvement at diagnosis by morphologic examination.[315] However, occult malignant cells were detected in 23 percent of the patients with negative bone marrow biopsy on routine histology after immunohistochemical stains using CD30 and epithelial membrane antigen as markers.[315] It should be pointed out that some anaplastic large cell lymphomas resemble Hodgkin's disease. The lower percentage of positive cases on routine morphologic examination compared to immunohistochemical study was explained by the authors as follows: (1) the scarcity of neoplastic cells that were scattered among hematopoietic cells; (2) the difficulty of distinguishing malignant cells from immature hematopoietic elements; and (3) the absence of alteration of the reticulin network.[315]

Multiple Myeloma and Related Diseases

The plasma cell is an end cell of B cell lineage, and a small number of plasma cells are normally present in the marrow. Plasmacytic disorders may also be divided into non-neoplastic and neoplastic diseases. A mixed proliferation of lymphocytes and plasma cells is sometimes seen.

Non-Neoplastic Plasma Cell Disorders. *Reactive Plasmacytosis.* Reactive plasmacytosis is a common feature of several clinical disorders, including carcinomatosis, chronic granulomatous infections, hepatic diseases, and autoimmune disorders. The prevalence of plasmacytosis (defined as 2 percent or more of plasma cells in the differential count of the bone marrow cells) was found to be 29 percent in a series of consecutive studies of 1,000 bone marrow aspirates.[53] The morphology of plasma cells is often mature, and they cluster around (cuffing) the blood vessels on histologic sections (Fig. 21-3). Reactive plasmacytosis should be differentiated from plasma cell myeloma.

Monoclonal Gammopathy of Undetermined Significance. Bone marrow examination in patients with monoclonal gammopathy of undetermined significance (MGUS) often reveals normal marrow, although a mild or moderate degree of plasmacytosis may be observed. These patients lack other clinical and/or laboratory findings seen in multiple myeloma, Waldenström's macroglobulinemia, heavy chain disease, or other lymphoproliferative disorders. Plasma cells usually constitute less than 10 percent of all nucleated cells in marrow and they are normal in morphology. In addition, plasma cells are usually evenly distributed or concentrated around the blood vessels. However, continuous follow-up should be undertaken because progression to a malignant lymphoplasmacytic disorder is observed in a minority of patients.[316]

Neoplastic Proliferation of Plasma Cells. Neoplastic proliferation of plasma cells may be classified as (1) diagnostic, (2) prognostic, and (3) therapeutic.[317] It is the diagnostic classification that is discussed here: (1) solitary myeloma of bone, (2) extramedullary plasmacytoma, (3) myelomatosis (smoldering myeloma, indolent myeloma, non-secretory myeloma, light chain myeloma, and others), and (4) plasma cell leukemia.

Solitary Myeloma of Bone. Solitary myeloma of bone is a localized plasma cell tumor characterized by a bone marrow plasmacytosis in excess of 15 percent and a single symptomatic area of bony destruction without evidence of other lytic lesions or bone marrow plasmacytosis in other areas. It commonly involves the spine, pelvis, and femur. Anemia, azotemia, or hypercalcemia are absent. Serum immunoglobulin concentrations are usually within normal limits. These patients are often younger than patients with classic multiple myeloma.[318–320] About 5 percent of patients with multiple myeloma initially present with a solitary plasmacytoma. The usual course is progression to multiple myeloma within 2 to 10 years.

Extramedullary Plasmacytoma. Solitary extramedullary plasmacytomas often involve the mucous membranes or soft tissue of the upper respiratory tract.[318,320] They seldomly evolve to multiple myeloma.

Multiple Myeloma. Multiple myeloma (plasma cell myeloma) is a neoplastic proliferation of plasma cells in the bone marrow, which accounts for slightly more than 10 percent of hematologic malignant tumors. The disease commonly affects elderly men. The usual presentation includes bone pain, anemia, renal insufficiency, and hypercalcemia. Multiple osteolytic lesions or diffuse osteoporosis, clonal proliferation of plasma cells in the bone marrow, serum monoclonal paraprotein (M protein), and/or Bence-Jones proteinuria are frequent laboratory findings.[321–323] Several subtypes, such as localized myeloma, indolent myeloma, smoldering myeloma, nonsecretory myeloma, light chain myeloma, and multiple myeloma with osteosclerotic lesions have been described.[323]

The histologic pattern of myelomatous involvement of the bone marrow is variable, ranging from nodular or patchy to diffuse. In most instances solid sheets of plasma cells infiltrate the fat and replace the normal elements of the marrow; occasionally an "interstitial" pattern may be observed, with preservation of fat cells but with replacement of the normal hematopoietic elements. The cytology of myeloma cells may be poorly differentiated, resembling an immunoblastic lymphoma of B cells (Fig. 21-28), or may be well differentiated, displaying characteristics of normal plasma cells with little cellular pleomorphism or atypism.[324,325] A multivariate linear regression analysis of survival data revealed that morphologic classification of mature, immature, and plasmablastic correlated with survival time.[324] Bartl and associates[325] also demonstrated that the quantity of plasma cell burden and the degree of neoplastic cell

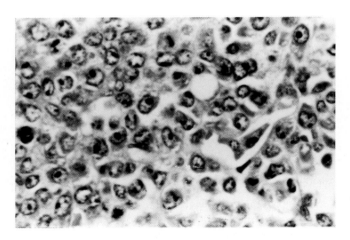

Fig. 21-28. Anaplastic myeloma with plasma cell leukemia. Note that neoplastic cells have large vesicular nuclei and one or two prominent nucleoli, with basophilic cytoplasm. (H&E stain, × 400.)

differentiation were useful criteria for histologic staging of multiple myeloma, which in turn might be used to guide the therapeutic modalities.

There is no agreement on the minimum percentage of plasma cells in the marrow smear that is necessary to make a diagnosis of myeloma. Reactive plasmacytosis of up to 20 percent of all the marrow cells may be observed in rheumatoid arthritis, chronic liver disease, Hodgkin's disease, carcinomatosis, AIDS, and occasionally in immunoreactions to drugs or collagen vascular disease. Binucleated, trinucleated, or tetranucleated mature-appearing plasma cells, and plasma cells with intranuclear and intracytoplasmic inclusions, may all be observed in reactive states as well as in multiple myeloma. Documentation of monoclonality by immunohistochemical technique is useful to distinguish a reactive from a neoplastic plasma cell proliferation.[326] In addition, pleomorphism, multinuclearity, prominent nucleoli, and nucleocytoplasmic asynchronism are helpful hints pointing to a malignant tumor. Kyle[322] suggested that minimal criteria for the diagnosis of multiple myeloma included the presence of at least 10 percent abnormal plasma cells in the bone marrow or histologic proof of a plasmacytoma, the usual clinical features of multiple myeloma, and at least one of the following abnormalities: monoclonal serum protein (usually greater than 3 g/dl), monoclonal protein in the urine, or osteolytic lesions.

Recent studies indicate several markers may be useful to differentiate benign from malignant plasmacytosis. Harada et al[327] found that normal plasma cells express CD19+CD56–, whereas mature myeloma plasma cells were CD19–CD56+. Both CD19+CD56– and CD19– CD56+ plasma cells were found in MGUS. Kawano and colleagues[328] believed that one could use VLA-5, one of the integrin adhesion molecules, to differentiate immature, proliferative myeloma cells (VLA-5–) and mature myeloma cells (VLA-5+). San Miguel and co-workers,[329] using a DNA/CD38 double-staining technique and flow cytometry in which plasma cells can be clearly discriminated from residual bone marrow cells based on their CD38 expression, found that the number of S-phase plasma cells was the most important in-

dependent prognostic factor.[329] Kyle[330] in a recent editorial pointed out that in spite of numerous efforts, better prognostic factors are needed for multiple myeloma. Nonrandom chromosomal abnormalities may be demonstrated in 46 percent of patients with evaluable karyotype.[331] It is not surprising that chromosome 14q32 translocation is the most common abnormality,[332] because it involves the heavy chain immunoglobulin gene.

Smoldering Myeloma. Smoldering myeloma was defined by Kyle and Greipp[333] as a lesion occurring in a group of asymptomatic patients who had 10 percent or more plasma cells in the bone marrow and an M protein peak of at least 3 g/dl in the serum and who remained stable without specific therapy for 5 or more years. These investigators advocated no specific therapy for these patients. These cases resemble MGUS clinically.[316]

Indolent Myeloma. Indolent myeloma was defined as the presence of a monoclonal IgG spike greater than 2.5 g/dl or an IgA peak greater than 1.0 g/dl and by a bone marrow plasmacytosis of greater than 15 percent.[320] All patients were asymptomatic. These patients had an intermediate survival rate between the rate for solitary myeloma of bone and that for overt myeloma.

Nonsecretory Myeloma. This variant of multiple myeloma is rare (5 percent) and requires immunohistochemical stains or electron microscopic examination to demonstrate that the cells are immunoglobulin-secreting cells. These individuals may present with typical or atypical clinical features of myeloma. M protein cannot be detected in serum or urine. Despite bone marrow plasmacytosis greater than 20 percent and radiologic bone lesions, these patients have significantly longer median survival time than patients with M proteins.[334]

Light Chain Myeloma. The reported incidence of multiple myeloma associated with only monoclonal light chains varies from 9 to 26 percent in the literature.[321,335,336] These patients usually have atypical presentations, such as "idiopathic" renal failure, "solitary" tumor of the bone, primary amyloidosis, or leukemia. Serum protein study often reveals hypogammaglobulinemia and an absence of monoclonal spike. Urine protein electrophoresis may reveal an M protein. They usually run a more aggressive clinical course with a short survival.[335,336]

Multiple Myeloma with Osteosclerotic Lesions. Osteosclerotic lesions may appear as the only skeletal manifestation of multiple myeloma in occasional patients; in others, both osteosclerotic and osteolytic lesions coexist. Driedger and Pruzanski collected data on 68 such patients. They and others found that this group of patients appears to be younger than the general group with multiple myeloma, and that peripheral neuropathy, organomegaly due to extraosseous myelomatous infiltration, endocrinopathy, monoclonal gammopathy, and skin lesions (POEMS) are common.[337–339] The monoclonal protein level is quantitatively low and usually consists of lambda light chain coupled with IgG or IgA. On radiographic examination the lesions should be differentiated from metastatic carcinoma or myelofibrosis and myeloid metaplasia.

Plasma Cell Leukemia. Plasma cell leukemia is defined as a number of plasma cells in the blood that is greater than 20 percent of total leukocytes or an absolute plasma cell count exceeding 2.0×10^9/L.[340,341] The bone marrow is hypercellular and is diffusely infiltrated by neoplastic plasma cells. The cytologic characteristics of the neoplastic plasma cells vary from small, mature plasma cells resembling plasmacytoid lymphocytes to those resembling pleomorphic blastic cells. The neoplastic cells may secrete IgG, light chains, IgA, or IgE. Plasma cell leukemia is uncommon. It may occur as a terminal event of multiple myeloma or may be the initial presentation in some patients with IgD or IgE myeloma. Patients with plasma cell leukemia are younger, have more aggressive disease, poorer response to therapy, and a significantly shorter survival time than patients with more typical myeloma.

Bone destruction is the usual manifestation of multiple myeloma, frequently demonstrated by radiology and histology. Pathologic fractures are common. Occasionally, myeloma may be associated with osteosclerotic lesions, as mentioned above. Bone marrow biopsy is also useful for the study of primary amyloidosis.[342]

Primary Amyloidosis. Primary amyloidosis is considered to be a clonal plasma cell proliferative disorder resulting in deposition of amyloid protein in the walls of blood vessels and interstitium of visceral organs. Amyloid protein seems to be homogeneous and amorphous by light microscopy, and is stained positively by Congo red, producing apple-green birefringence when viewed with polarized light. The amorphous, hyaline-like substance consists of rigid, nonbranching, aggregated fibrils 7.5 to 10 nm wide and of indefinite length. The fibrils consist of the N-terminal amino acid residues of the variable portion of a monoclonal light chain.[343] Primary amyloidosis may be divided into (1) primary amyloid, and (2) primary amyloid associated with multiple myeloma. However, both disorders are plasma cell proliferative processes with much overlap. Of the 474 cases of primary amyloidosis studied at the Mayo Clinic, 16 percent had monoclonal gammopathy of undetermied significance, 15 percent had multiple myeloma, 3 percent had smoldering multiple myeloma, 1 percent had macroglobulinemia, and 0.5 percent had solitary plasmacytoma of bone at the time of diagnosis of primary amyloidosis.[343]

Although bone marrow aspiration and biopsy should be performed in all cases that are suspected of having primary amyloidosis, histologic sections or aspiration smears of the marrow range from having no identifiable pathologic changes to extensive replacement of the hematopoietic elements by amyloid or overt myeloma. Kyle and Gertz[343] reported that 56 percent of their patients showed positive stain for amyloid in the bone marrow biopsy, and virtually all patients have an M protein in the serum or urine or a monoclonal population of plasma cells in the marrow.[343]

Waldenström's Macroglobulinemia. Waldenström's macroglobulinemia (WMG) is a neoplastic clonal proliferation of B lymphocytes that secrete monoclonal IgM.[344–346] Clinically, these patients have hyperviscosity syndrome and resemble those having malignant lymphoma, with generalized lym-

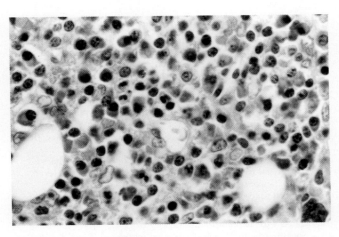

Fig. 21-29. Waldenström's macroglobulinemia. A mixed infiltrate of plasma cells, plasmacytoid lymphocytes, and lymphocytes is present. (H&E stain, × 250.)

phadenopathy and splenomegaly. The bone marrow may be partially or largely replaced by lymphocytes, plasmacytoid lymphocytes (or lymphocytoid plasma cells), and plasma cells (Fig. 21-29). Intranuclear or intracytoplasmic PAS-positive inclusions (Dutcher bodies) may be identified. These inclusions are usually composed of M protein.

Heavy Chain Diseases. Heavy chain diseases consist of a group of lymphoproliferative disorders characterized by the production of monoclonal defective immunoglobulins (i.e., composed of incomplete heavy chains with light chain deletions).[347] *Gamma heavy chain disease* has more of the features of a malignant lymphoma than of multiple myeloma.[348] The bone marrow, lymph nodes, and spleen are infiltrated by lymphoplasmacytic cells or plasma cells.[349,350] *Alpha chain disease* predominantly involves the gastrointestinal tract and mesenteric lymph nodes, although there is also a respiratory variant. These cases are also more like a malignant lymphoma.[351] The bone marrow is usually normal but alpha chain secreting plasma cells may be identified.[352] *Mu chain disease* is characterized by the presence of vacuolated plasma cells, small lymphocytes, and plasmacytoid lymphocytes in the bone marrow, with a prolonged antecedent history of CLL.[353] Serum protein study reveals hypogammaglobulinemia with the presence of a mu chain. Light chain (kappa) may be detected in the urine.

Granulomatous Changes and Granuloma-Like Lesions

A granuloma is defined as a host chronic inflammatory reaction with a predominance of cells of the macrophage series admixed with inflammatory cells, such as lymphocytes and plasma cells, with or without eosinophils. Giant cells of Langhans type or foreign body type may be present. A granulomatous reaction may be elicited by a wide variety of stimuli mediated by immunologic or chemical mechanisms, but the etiology may be difficult to establish from a tissue examination alone. A list of possible causes that may produce a granulomatous response in

Table 21-16. Possible Causes of Granulomatous Lesions in the Marrow

Nonspecific: lipid granuloma

Infectious
  Mycobacteria: tuberculosis, leprosy, and atypical mycobacteria
  Fungi: coccidioidomycosis, histoplasmosis, cryptococcosis, and others
  Viruses: infectious mononucleosis, cytomegalovirus, hepatitis B virus, and others
  Bacteria: typhoid fever, brucellosis, tularemia, and others
  Rickettsial disease: Q fever, Rocky Mountain spotted fever
  Spirochetes: syphilis (secondary stage)
  Others: toxoplasmosis, leishmaniasis, *Pneumocystis carinii*, mycoplasma pneumonia

Associated with neoplastic disorders
  Specific lesion: Hodgkin's disease, peripheral T cell lymphoma, eosinophilic granuloma, Hand-Schüller-Christian disease, Letterer-Siwe disease, and others
  Nonspecific lesion: sarcoid-like granuloma associated with Hodgkin's disease, non-Hodgkin's lymphoma including mycosis fungoides, multiple myeloma, acute lymphocytic leukemia, and carcinomatosis

Lesions resembling granuloma: systemic mastocytosis including eosinophilic fibrohistiocytic lesion of the bone marrow, metastatic carcinoma

Miscellaneous: Sarcoidosis, angioimmunoblastic lymphadenopathy, foreign body granuloma, drug reactions, allergic/autoimmune disorders, and others

Unknown

(Modified from Sun,[354] with permission.)

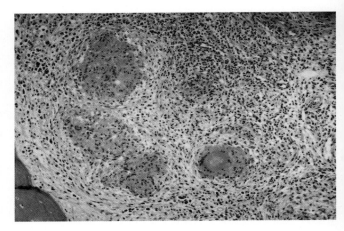

Fig. 21-30. Noncaseating granulomas of the marrow with marrow fibrosis and chronic inflammatory cell infiltrate. Langhans giant cells are seen. The patient was later found to have sarcoidosis. (H&E stain, × 40.)

the bone marrow is presented in Table 21-16.[354,355] The reason for including some lymphoproliferative disorders under the heading of "granulomatous changes" is to emphasize that histiocytic proliferation and granuloma formation are integral features of their pathology. Mast cell disease produces lesions simulating granulomas and is also discussed here. Unifocal or multifocal eosinophilic granulomas are discussed under histiocytic proliferative disorders.

A granulomatous lesion may be classified as proliferative, necrotic, or suppurative. The latter two types are most commonly seen in infectious disease as a form of systemic reaction. Proliferative granuloma is characterized by a focal aggregation of epithelioid cells with or without Langhans giant cells and may be seen in a variety of conditions, including sarcoidosis, infectious mononucleosis, tuberculosis, Hodgkin's disease, NHL, multiple myeloma, liver disease, and drug reactions (Fig. 21-30). It has been speculated that proliferative or epithelioid granuloma may be a manifestation of host immune response to overload of antigens or of defective lymphocyte-macrophage function[356]; others have demonstrated nonimmune mechanisms for granuloma formation.[357] A large study disclosed that the most common cause of granulomatous lesions in bone marrow is infection (38 percent), followed by carcinoma (21 percent), drug reaction (12 percent), allergic or autoimmune disease (9 percent), and sarcoidosis (7 percent).[355] However, the etiology of granulomatous disease in marrow was unknown in

13 percent of patients in the same study. It should be pointed out that bone marrow granuloma is considered to be an uncommon finding with an incidence of 0.5 to 1.23 percent in the pre-AIDS era[355] but granulomatous change in bone marrow is very common now in HIV-infected patients, ranging from 13 to 24 percent in the literature.[358,359] A variety of microorganisms may be identified by special stains or bone marrow cultures, including *Pneumocystis carinii*.[360]

Benign Nonhematologic Conditions

Infectious Granulomata and Acquired Immunodeficiency Syndrome

The morphology of the granuloma in some infectious diseases is quite characteristic and is similar to that in other parts of the body. Microorganisms may be demonstrated on H&E-stained or special-stained sections. Serial sections or step sections are sometimes needed to localize the granuloma or to identify the Reed-Sternberg cells in the case of Hodgkin's disease. A "doughnut" granuloma, which is characterized by a central empty space surrounded by polymorphonuclear leukocytes, epithelioid cells, and/or eosinophils, has been observed in Q fever[361] (Fig. 21-31). Similar lesions have been described in typhoid fever and Hodgkin's disease.[354]

Acquired immunodeficiency syndrome (AIDS) is an infectious disease caused by a retrovirus, human immunodeficiency virus (HIV). Most patients develop one or more cytopenias during the course of the disease.[358,359,362–365] Bone marrow examinations often reveal normal or decreased fat cells, with hematopoietic elements occupying the rest of the marrow spaces (normocellular or hypercellular bone marrow). Serous or mucinous degeneration of fat cells may be observed in the late stage of the disease, and the density of hematopoietic cells is often decreased, with deposition of eosinophilic granular or fibrillar material in the interstitium. This material may or may not be stained by PAS and is usually unstained by reticulin. It is similar to that observed in patients after radiation or chemotherapy and may represent disintegrated cellular ele-

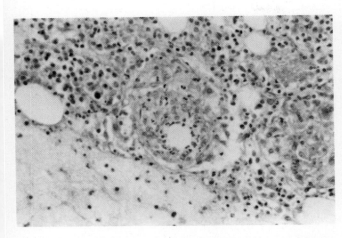

Fig. 21-31. "Doughnut" granuloma is characterized by a central clear space surrounded by a rim of polymorphonuclear leukocytes, fibrinoid material, and epithelioid cells. Epithelioid cells are also seen in the right side of the photomicrograph. The material is taken from a patient with Q fever. (H&E stain, × 100.)

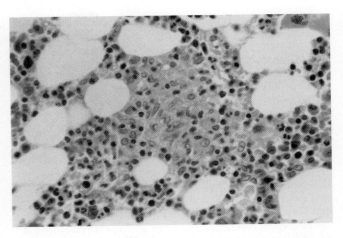

Fig. 21-32. Epithelioid granuloma from a patient with AIDS and disseminated histoplasmosis. *Histoplasma capsulatum* was demonstrated by PAS and methenamine silver stains. (H&E stain, × 160.)

ments. Mehta and associates[57] found that the gelatinous material in AIDS patients was composed exclusively of glycosaminoglycans. They hypothesized that the damaged microenvironment leads to failure of hematopoiesis in some of these patients. The myeloid/erythroid ratio is usually increased, with a normal or increased number of megakaryocytes. Dyserythropoiesis is common, observed in 69 to 100 percent of cases.[358,363] However, true myelodysplastic syndrome and acute leukemia are uncommon. Marrow plasma cells and lymphocytes (including immunoblasts and transformed lymphocytes) are increased, with cuffing of plasma cells around the blood vessels. Lymphocytic aggregates were identified in 35 percent of biopsied specimens.[358] Lymphoid infiltrates may also be present. Increased iron stores are usually demonstrable by Prussian blue stain, and focal increase in reticulin fibers is also noted with the reticulin stain.

Granulomas (usually small, epithelioid, and without necrosis) may be present (Fig. 21-32), and special stains are required to demonstrate the microorganisms within them. It should be pointed out that the methenamine silver stain appears to be superior to PAS in demonstrating fungi on bone marrow biopsy. As a matter of fact, special stains for mycobacteria and fungi should be routinely used in bone marrow specimens from these patients. One of the studies, however, indicates that bone marrow cultures give a higher yield for the identification of microorganisms in comparison to special stains.[366] Another study demonstrated intracytoplasmic negatively stained linear inclusions within histiocytes in bone marrow aspiration smears as clues for mycobacterial infection.[367] Foamy cells in the marrow of these patients should alert the observers to the possibility of *M. avium-intracellulare* infection (Fig. 21-33). None of these findings are pathognomonic for AIDS. However, a decreased number of fat cells with low density hematopoietic elements interspersed by eosinophilic granular or fibrillary material in a young man should alert the observer to the possibility of AIDS or AIDS-related complex.

The mechanism of peripheral cytopenias in an AIDS patient with normal or hypercellular marrow is unclear. Hypotheses include (1) peripheral destruction secondary to hypersplenism; (2) immune complex mediated autoimmune phenomenon; (3) drug reactions to trimethoprim-sulfamethoxazole for presumed *Pneumocystis* pneumonia; (4) stimulation of the reticuloendothelial system due to multiple viral infections; (5) damaged microenvironment; and (6) primary infection of hematopoietic stem cells by HIV. It is most likely that several factors are contributing to the pancytopenia.[359]

An increased incidence of non-Hodgkin's lymphoma and Hodgkin's disease in AIDS patients has been well recognized.[368–371] These lesions also involve bone marrows. Lymphoreticular malignant tumors were found in 18 of 216 HIV-infected patients (8 percent).[358] Although the occurrence of

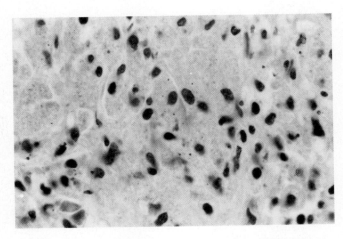

Fig. 21-33. Foamy histiocytes from a patient with AIDS. Note that the cytoplasm contains granular or linear structures. Fite-Faraco stain revealed clumps of acid-fast microorganisms in the cytoplasm of the foamy cells. (H&E stain, × 250.)

Kaposi's sarcoma is common in HIV-infected homosexual men, its involvement of the bone marrow is very unusual.[358,372]

Lipid Granuloma

Lipid granuloma is a relatively common finding in elderly patients and patients with diabetes mellitus.[373] The morphology is similar to that found in the liver or spleen. Lipid granuloma consists of a collection of macrophages containing vacuoles of various sizes, which are, however, always smaller than the single vacuole in normal fat cells. Plasma cells, lymphocytes, and sometimes eosinophils and mast cells are all seen in the lipid granuloma. Microcysts lined by compressed histiocytes and multinucleated giant cells may also be present. Lipid granulomas associated with hyperlipidemia often contain foam cells and Touton type giant cells. Foamy cells may be seen in a variety of clinical conditions[354] (Table 21-17 and Figs. 21-33 and 21-34). It is important to differentiate the nonspecific lesion of lipid granuloma from other granulomatous lesions.

Granulomatous Changes Associated with Hematologic Disorders

Lymphomas or lymphoma-like lesions may contain granulomas or display granulomatous changes.[354] These include Hodgkin's disease, peripheral T cell lymphoma, and angioimmunoblastic lymphadenopathy. Other lesions, such as eosinophilic fibrohistiocytic lesion of the bone marrow, systemic mastocytosis, and Langerhans cell histiocytosis, may produce lesions simulating granulomas. Langerhans cell histiocytosis is discussed under histiocytic proliferative disorders. The diagnostic criteria for these lesions in the bone marrow are the same as those in other parts of the body.

Hodgkin's Disease

Hodgkin's disease is a lymphoreticular malignant disease characterized by a neoplastic proliferation of malignant cells (Reed-Sternberg cells) associated with an impaired host immune response.[374] Identification of the classic Reed-Sternberg cell is necessary for the diagnosis of Hodgkin's disease, although the

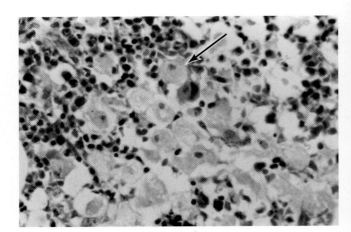

Fig. 21-34. Foamy histiocytes from a patient with Gaucher's disease. Note crystalloid structures in the cytoplasm (arrow). (H&E stain, × 160.)

mere presence of such a cell is not sufficient for this diagnosis. A classic Reed-Sternberg cell has a lobulated nucleus or is multinucleated. Each lobe or individual nucleus contains a large, homogeneous, eosinophilic, inclusion-like nucleolus, which often reaches the size of a red cell or the nucleus of a small lymphocyte. The cytoplasm contains a large quantity of ribonucleic acid and is strongly pyroninophilic when stained by methyl green pyronine. Several types of Reed-Sternberg variants have been described and are very useful in the subclassification of the disease.

The nature of Reed-Sternberg cells is not completely understood. However, they are known to be reactive with monoclonal or polyclonal antibodies directed against the following antigens: CD15, CD20, CDw75, CD74, HLA-DR, peanut agglutinin, CD30, CD45, and both lambda and kappa light chains.[375]

Bone marrow involvement is not uncommon in certain subtypes of Hodgkin's disease, although the overall frequency of bone marrow involvement reported in the literature ranges from 5 to 22 percent.[5,376–378] Bartl and associates[379] noted that bone marrow involvement was found in 10 percent of untreated and 25 percent of treated patients with Hodgkin's disease. The most frequent type of Hodgkin's disease involving bone marrow is the diffuse fibrosis of the lymphocytic depletion type, with a reported incidence varying from 40 to 79 percent.[380–382] Bone marrow involvement also occurs in patients with other types of Hodgkin's disease. It is more commonly seen in older men who have constitutional symptoms and advanced clinical stages.[379] It appears that bone marrow involvement does not have an adverse effect on the patient's response to treatment, ability to achieve complete remission, or overall prognosis.[377,378] Furthermore, marrow fibrosis due to increased collagen or reticulin in the pretreatment specimens was found to have completely disappeared in many patients, with a reversion to normal marrow, after therapy.[378] Peripheral complete blood cell counts generally appear to be unreliable indicators of bone marrow involvement.

The histopathologic diagnosis of Hodgkin's disease of the

Table 21-17. Clinical Conditions with Foamy Cells in the Marrow

Common conditions
   Lipophages associated with alcoholic liver disease or diabetes mellitus
   Fat necrosis secondary to bony fracture, infarction, pancreatitis, and status postchemotherapy for acute leukemias and other malignant tumors
Less common conditions
   Infections: such as leprosy, Whipple's disease, M. avium-intracellulare, leishmaniasis, histoplasmosis, and others
   Metastatic tumors: metastatic renal cell carcinoma and others
   Storage diseases: Niemann-Pick disease, Gaucher's disease, Fabry's disease, Farber's disease, Wolman's disease, some mucopolysaccharidoses, mucolipidoses, glycogen storage disease, and others
   Langerhans cell histiocytosis: eosinophilic granuloma, Hand-Schüller-Christian disease, and others

(Adapted from Sun,[354] with permission.)

marrow is not difficult to make when the normal marrow architecture is disrupted and is focally or diffusely replaced by a polymorphic cellular infiltrate consisting of lymphocytes, plasma cells, eosinophils, histiocytes, and classic Reed-Sternberg cells, especially when the diagnosis of Hodgkin's disease has been previously established by lymph node biopsy (Fig. 21-35). The general rule of thumb is that if a tissue diagnosis has not been established by a previous lymph node biopsy, the criteria should be more rigid, and diagnostic or classic Reed-Sternberg cells must be identified in the lesion; otherwise, polyploid cells that contain at least one huge nucleolus or Reed-Sternberg variants in a proper cellular background are adequate for the diagnosis of Hodgkin's disease involving the marrow[383,384] (Figs. 21-36 and 21-37). The frequency of Hodgkin's disease involvement of marrow apparently depends on the size or volume of the specimen, the method of examination, and the histologic type (i.e., an open biopsy is better than a bilateral needle biopsy, a histologic examination is superior to an aspiration smear, and patients with diffuse fibrosis and mixed cellularity have a higher prevalence of marrow involvement). It is not advisable to subclassify Hodgkin's disease based on bone marrow biopsy alone. Osseous changes may also be noted in the area adjacent to the lesion. Massive intramedullary phagocytosis, an uncommon phenomenon in Hodgkin's disease, has been reported in two cases.[385] Hodgkin's disease should be differentiated from peripheral T cell lymphoma, angioimmunoblastic lymphadenopathy, and anaplastic large cell lymphoma. Immunohistochemical stain and molecular genetic analysis can usually assist in reaching a definitive diagnosis.

Sarcoid-like granulomas may be found in the bone marrow of patients with Hodgkin's disease[386,387] and should not be confused with the specific lesions of this disease. It has been said, however, that survival and relapse-free survival are significantly more favorable for those patients who have noncaseating granulomas in the material obtained at initial staging procedures than for those who do not.[387] Benign lymphoid aggregates are also occasionally seen in involved or uninvolved marrow from patients with Hodgkin's disease.

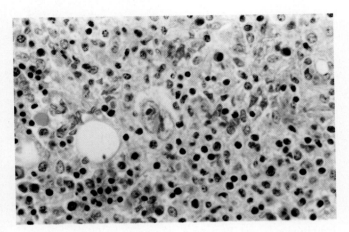

Fig. 21-36. Hodgkin's disease. A binucleate giant cell is seen in the center of this photomicrograph. Note that the size of the nucleolus reaches that of a small lymphocyte. The morphology is that of a Reed-Sternberg cell. Note also polymorphic cellular background. (H&E stain, × 250.)

Angioimmunoblastic (Immunoblastic) Lymphadenopathy

Angioimmunoblastic lymphadenopathy is a distinct clinicopathologic entity characterized by an acute clinical onset with fever, sweats, weight loss, and generalized lymphadenopathy. Skin rash, pruritus, hepatosplenomegaly, hypergammaglobulinemia, and Coombs-positive hemolytic anemia are other common features. A history of hypersensitivity reaction to drugs or other substances immediately preceding the onset of symptoms may be obtained in some patients. The disease is generally considered to be an abnormal immune response involving a deficiency of T cell regulatory function or an exaggeration of lymphocyte transformation of the B cell system.[388–390]

Bone marrow involvement occurred in approximately 40 to 70 percent of patients who underwent bone marrow examina-

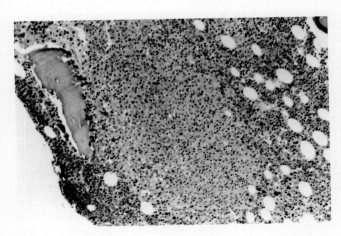

Fig. 21-35. Hodgkin's disease. A solitary lesion is seen in the marrow. This pattern of infiltrate is common for Hodgkin's disease, peripheral T cell lymphoma, and other randomly focal lesions. (H&E stain, × 40.)

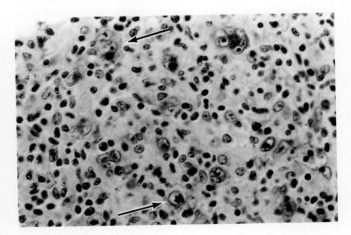

Fig. 21-37. Hodgkin's disease (same case as Fig. 21-36). Paranuclear, membranous and diffuse intracytoplasmic stain with CD15 (Leu M1) (arrows) is demonstrated in the Reed-Sternberg cells and their variants by an immunoperoxidase method. (Immunoperoxidase stain with DAB as chromogen, × 160.)

tion.[388,391] The lesions are usually hypocellular, focal, and rarely paratrabecular in distribution. Diffuse infiltration with replacement of normal hematopoietic elements has been described.[392] Cells with fibroblast-like spindle-shaped nuclei are often prominent. In addition, lymphocytes, transformed lymphocytes, immunoblasts, histiocytes, plasma cells, and eosinophils are present in the lesion. Increased numbers of reticulin fibers that arrange in a whorled pattern are frequently demonstrated. Proliferation and arborization of small blood vessels with deposition of eosinophilic amorphous material in the interstitium are present. The involvement of bone marrow did not correlate with the clinical course and prognosis in one study,[391] but was associated with unfavorable outcome in another.[392] The lesion should be differentiated from Hodgkin's disease, granulomas in other disorders, and peripheral T cell lymphomas.[392–394] Transformation to malignant lymphomas has been described.[392,395]

Peripheral T Cell Lymphoma

Peripheral T cell lymphoma (PTCL) is a neoplastic disorder of post-thymic ("mature") T cells, exclusive of T-CLL, T-PLL, large granular lymphocytosis/leukemia, cutaneous T cell lymphoma, and anaplastic large cell lymphoma. It chiefly affects elderly men and is characterized by constitutional symptoms at presentation, disseminated disease at diagnosis, histopathologic diversity, and an aggressive clinical course. In the International Working Formulation, PTCL is included in the diffuse small cleaved cell, diffuse mixed small and large cell, diffuse large cell, and immunoblastic lymphomas.[293] In the REAL classification, PTCL includes (1) PTCL, unspecified, and (2) PTCL, specific variants (angioimmunoblastic T cell lymphoma, angiocentric lymphoma, intestinal T cell lymphoma, and adult T cell lymphoma/leukemia).[278] All these tumors are relatively uncommon in Western countries. Bone marrow involvement has been described in 11 to 80 percent of the cases.[396–402] Sometimes, lymphomatous involvement of the marrow in an asymptomatic patient with peripheral cytopenia is the first evidence of the disease.[400] The frequency of bone marrow involvement is related to histologic subtype of PTCL, that is, patients with small cell histologic type had a significantly higher incidence of marrow infiltration and circulating lymphoma cells than patients with mixed or large cell/immunoblastic type.[396,398]

The pattern of infiltration may be diffuse or randomly focal[396,402] (Fig. 21-35). In the mixed and large cell/immunoblastic types, the lesions are usually composed of a spectrum of lymphoid cells with variable size and configuration among a heterogeneous population of eosinophils, plasma cells, neutrophils, histiocytes, epithelioid histiocytes, and capillaries. Prominent vascularity and reticulin fibrosis are often observed. The epithelioid cells are often found in clusters and may impart a granulomatous appearance. Most of the large lymphocytes and immunoblasts show prominent nuclear irregularity, multilobation, and multinucleation. Some immunoblasts have large eosinophilic nucleoli, resembling Reed-Sternberg cells or their variants. Unlike follicular center cell lymphomas, in which discordant morphology between lymph node and marrow may occur in 20 to 40 percent of cases, the histopathology of PTCL in the bone marrow corresponds to that observed in the lymph nodes.[396] The differential diagnosis includes polymorphous reactive lymphoid lesions, angioimmunoblastic lymphadenopathy, Hodgkin's disease, and systemic mastocytosis. Immunohistochemical studies may be helpful in reaching a correct diagnosis.[401,402] The small cell variant of PTCL resembles T-CLL or T-PLL. Hanson and associates[396] found that there was no apparent correlation between the presence or absence of bone marrow involvement at diagnosis and median survival.

Some patients with PTCL initially present as abnormal myelopoiesis, ranging from a picture resembling myelodysplastic syndrome to myeloproliferative disorder.[403] Lymphomatous involvement of the marrow was found in follow-up specimens.[403] Other investigators report that patients with PTCL may present a picture that mimics malignant histiocytosis.[404,405] They have an acute onset of illness, characterized by high fever, weight loss, prominent hepatosplenomegaly, slight or no lymphadenopathy, and profound pancytopenia. All these patients are immunocompetent, however, and run a rapidly downhill course and die shortly. The major pathologic finding is the infiltration of the spleen, liver, and bone marrow by neoplastic T cells, accompanied by striking hemophagocytosis by benign-appearing histiocytes. It was found later that these cases are associated with Epstein-Barr virus infection.[406]

Mast Cell Disease

Mast cells are normally found in the bone marrow, skin, lungs, and mucosa and submucosa of other organs. *Reactive mastocytosis* may be observed in a variety of hematopoietic or lymphoreticular disorders, chronic liver disease, chronic renal disease, and osteoporosis. Mast cell disease may be classified as (1) localized mastocytosis, (2) urticaria pigmentosa, and (3) systemic mast cell disease (SMCD).[407] *Urticaria pigmentosa* of children and infants is usually limited to the skin and frequently regresses at puberty. However, urticaria pigmentosa in adults usually develops into systemic mastocytosis (SMCD). A pathologic increase of mast cells in extracutaneous tissues that is not attributable to a reactive process is the diagnostic criterion for SMCD. *Systemic mastocytosis* may be manifested clinically in two ways: (1) an infiltrative process characterized by osteoporosis or osteosclerosis, hepatosplenomegaly, lymphadenopathy, and/or mast cell infiltration in the skin (urticaria pigmentosa), bone marrow, gastrointestinal tract, heart, and lungs, and (2) pharmacologic effects secondary to release of chemicals following degranulation of mast cells. These are characterized by flushing, pounding headache, bronchospasm, hypotension, diarrhea, rhinorrhea, urticaria, palpitation, dyspnea, peptic ulcer, and gastrointestinal bleeding. Various combinations and clinical syndromes are seen.[408]

Travis and associates[409,410] classified SMCD into (1) indolent SMCD, (2) SMCD with associated hematologic disorders, (3) mast cell leukemia, and (4) aggressive SMCD (nonleukemic) based on clinical manifestations and outcomes. Urticaria pigmentosa is common in indolent SMCD, but uncommon in other groups of patients, whereas patients with other groups of SMCD have constitutional symptoms and hepatosplenomegaly. Bone marrow involvement is seen in all groups.[409] Histopathologic examination of bone marrow biopsy shows patchy or focal infiltration of spindle-shaped mast cells, usually in perivascular or paratrabecular regions, with concomitant fibrosis and osteosclerosis in the vast majority of cases with SMCD. An increased number of eosinophils, lymphocytes, and histiocytes is noted within the lesion or at the periphery. These foci often exhibit a granulomatous appearance and are sharply demarcated from the adjacent tissue. The differential diagnosis includes granulomatous disease, Hodgkin's disease, angioimmunoblastic lymphadenopathy, and eosinophilic fibrohistiocytic lesion. It was later recognized that this eosinophilic fibrohistiocytic lesion of the bone marrow represents a form of mast cell lesion.[411–413]

Horny and associates[414] described three types of histopathologic patterns based on their study of 38 bone marrow biopsies: type 1 (focal mast cell lesions, normal hematopoiesis, and fat cell content in adjacent areas), type 2 (focal mast cell lesions, hypercellular bone marrow with markedly increased granulocytopoiesis or increased blast cells), and type 3 (diffuse mast cell infiltrates with replacement of normal hematopoiesis). Patients with type 2 findings frequently had associated myeloproliferative disorders. Patients with type 3 lesions were found to have mast cell leukemias. Both groups of patients had poor prognosis.[414] Indeed, 33 percent (22 of 66) of patients with SMCD studied by Travis and associates[415] were found to have associated hematologic disorders. Patients with hematologic disorders were different from other SMCD patients in that they were older and more likely to be anemic and to have constitutional symptoms. The associated hematologic disorders included myelodysplastic syndrome (10 patients), myeloproliferative disorders (5), acute nonlymphocytic leukemia (3), and chronic neutropenia (1). Chromosomal abnormalities that were characteristics of neoplastic myeloid disorders were found in 4 patients. The clinical course of these patients was usually determined by the hematologic disorder rather than SMCD.[415]

Diffuse marrow infiltration is seen in patients with mast cell leukemia. These patients have at least 10 percent atypical mast cells circulating in the peripheral blood.[410] The diagnosis of mast cell leukemia may be difficult because it may resemble basophilic leukemia, acute promyelocytic leukemia, or a blastic variant of hairy cell leukemia.[409] The nuclei of many of the atypical mast cells are indented, multilobated, and multinucleated.[409,414] Neoplastic mast cells are strongly positive for acid phosphatase and tartrate-resistant acid phosphatase, naphthol-ASD chloroacetate esterase, aminocaproate esterase, and Giemsa or toluidine blue stain.[409,414] They are negative for peroxidase, alpha-naphthyl butyrate esterase, and alkaline phosphatase.[409,414] Immunohistochemical staining shows mast cells expressing vimentin, leukocyte common antigen (CD45), lysozyme, alpha-1-antitrypsin, and alpha-1-antichymotrypsin, but they are negative for CD45RO (UCHL-1), CD45RA (MB1), CD57 (Leu7), CD11 (OKM1), Ki-B3, KL-1, desmin, S-100 protein, factor VIII-related antigen, and chromogranin A.[409,416] These histochemical and immunohistochemical stains are useful for the identification of mast cells in mast cell disease.

Histiocytic Proliferative Disorders

The concept and understanding of histiocytic proliferative disorders have progressed in the last 10 years with the availability of many monoclonal antibodies, molecular biologic techniques, and cytogenetic analysis. Histiocytes, originating from bone marrow CD34+ stem cells, may be divided into two functionally different systems: (1) antigen-presenting cells, and (2) antigen-processing cells. The former include Langerhans cells, interdigitating reticulum cells (IRC), and dendritic reticulum cells (DRC). The latter consist of monocytes and histiocytes in various organs (such as alveolar macrophages in the lung, Küpffer cells in the liver, cordal macrophages in the spleen, microglial cells in the brain, and osteoclasts in the bone).[417,418] The term *mononuclear phagocyte and immunoregulatory effector (M-PIRE) system* has been proposed to replace the old term reticuloendothelial system.[418]

Common to all these antigen-presenting cells (or immune accessory cells) is the surface antigen expression of HLA-DR, class I or II histocompatibility antigens, CD45, Fc receptors for IgG, S-100 protein, CD1, and DRC. Some of them are also positive for ATPase and acid phosphatase. The Langerhans cells contain Birbeck granules (intracytoplasmic structures that are rod or tennis racquet-shaped organelles with a central zipper-like striation) by electron microscopic examination. The antigen-processing cells (monocytes-phagocytes) express HLA-DR, CD45, CD11, CD25, CD4, CD68, MAC387, CD11b, CD11c, CD14, and CD15, with variable expression of CD13 and CD33. They are also positive for lysozyme, acid phosphatase, and alpha-naphthyl esterase, and react with alpha-1-antitrypsin and alpha-1-antichymotrypsin antibodies. They contain secondary lysozymes (phagosomes) and lysosomes on electron microscopic examination.[417,418]

Several classifications have been proposed for the histiocytic proliferative disorders.[417–419] Those that involve bone marrow include reactive histiocytic proliferations, storage diseases and hemophagocytic syndromes, acute monocytic leukemia, chronic myelomonocytic leukemia, malignant 5q35 histiocytosis, malignant histiocytosis, and Langerhans cell histiocytosis.[417]

Reactive Histiocytic Proliferation

Reactive histiocytic proliferation is usually transient and is caused by an infectious process or increased cell death. Granulomatous lesions described above are examples of histiocytic reaction. Storage diseases and hemophagocytic syndromes are other forms of reactive histiocytic proliferations.

Storage Diseases

This group of diseases is usually caused by an enzyme defect in a normal degradative or catabolic pathway that leads to intracellular accumulation of biologic products in the histiocytes. It is important to recognize that enzymatically normal macrophages can sometimes be overwhelmed by excessive tissue breakdown, such as in chronic hemolytic anemia, chronic myelogenous leukemia, or idiopathic thrombocytopenic purpura, resulting in the appearance of the cells found in the storage diseases.[420,421] However, storage cells are much fewer in number in these conditions in comparison to those seen in genetic disorders. In addition, the underlying hematologic disorders often coexist.

Gaucher's disease is the most common storage disease and is most likely to be diagnosed by bone marrow examination.

Gaucher cells are large histiocytes, 20 to 100 μm in diameter, with one or more small, often eccentrically placed nuclei and a characteristic "reticular," "striated," "fibrillary" or "wrinkled tissue paper" appearance of the cytoplasm (Fig. 21-34). They are usually present in aggregates or sheets, focally or completely replacing the normal marrow. Characteristic storage cells can also be found in other metabolic disorders such as Niemann-Pick disease and sea-blue histiocyte syndrome. The histiocytes in Niemann-Pick disease are also large with a single, small nucleus, and an abundant vacuolated cytoplasm. The sea-blue histiocytes measure up to 20 μm in diameter and are filled with sea-blue granules.

Hemophagocytic Syndromes

Hemophagocytic syndrome (HPS) is characterized by marked systemic hemophagocytosis, associated with fever, hepatosplenomegaly, cytopenia, abnormal liver function tests, and coagulopathy. An infectious etiology can be detected in most cases.[422–429] A familial form (familial hemophagocytic syndrome) has also been described.[430,431] Finally, hemophagocytosis may be observed in a variety of malignant disorders in which either malignant cells phagocytize hematopoietic cells or there is hemophagocytosis by benign histiocytes as a manifestation of underlying malignant diseases (Figs. 21-38 and 21-39).[404–406,432–439] It should be noted that hemophagocytosis by itself is not diagnostic of any disease. It indicates a stimulated (activated) reticuloendothelial system and may be observed in a variety of clinical conditions as described above. The pathogenesis is unclear, but they are probably related to defects in the immune system.

Infection-associated HPS is a systemic disorder characterized by widespread reactive proliferation of phagocytic histiocytes in response to a variety of infections. The incriminating agents include viruses (e.g., EBV, CMV, and herpes simplex virus), bacteria (brucella, salmonella, mycobacteria), fungi (candida, actinomyces, histoplasma), protozoa (leishmania, babesia), and mycoplasma. The bone marrow shows cellular destruction with deposition of eosinophilic granular material and a decrease in density of cells. Both erythropoiesis and myelopoiesis are decreased. Megakaryopoiesis may be normal or increased. Histiocytes phagocytizing red cells, nucleated red cells, leukocytes, and platelets are diffusely scattered throughout the marrow. These histiocytes have a slightly oval nucleus, minimally condensed chromatin, and indistinct nucleoli. The voluminous cytoplasm contains hematopoietic cells or their degradation products or vacuoles. Lymphocytes and plasma cells may be increased in number. Lymphoid aggregates and granulomas are uncommon findings.

Infection-associated HPS must be differentiated from *malignant HPS*. The latter includes a variety of hematopoietic or nonhematopoietic malignant tumors in which phagocytic cells may be benign histiocytes or malignant cells. The most common malignant tumor that manifests HPS is peripheral T cell lymphoma.[404–406,439] These T cell lymphomas are often associated with EBV infection and clinically resemble malignant histiocytosis.[406,440] Patients with EBV-associated T cell lymphoma often present with fever, hepatosplenomegaly, cutaneous or mucosal lesions, and jaundice. Pancytopenia, hyperbilirubinemia, markedly elevated LDH, mild liver dysfunction, coagulopathy, and hypertriglyceridemia are common laboratory findings. Histopathologic study shows compart-

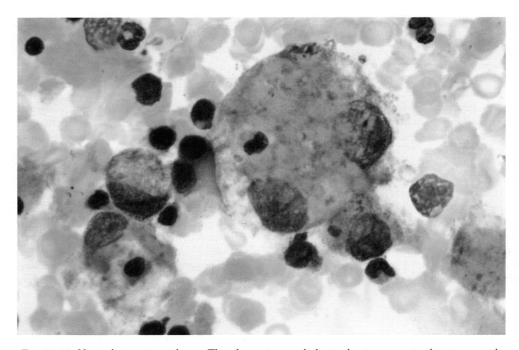

Fig. 21-38. Hemophagocytic syndrome. This photomicrograph depicts benign-appearing histiocytes with phagocytized red blood cells, white blood cells, even platelets. This particular patient had EBV-associated T cell lymphoma with marked hemophagocytosis in the marrow. (Romanowsky stain, × 600.)

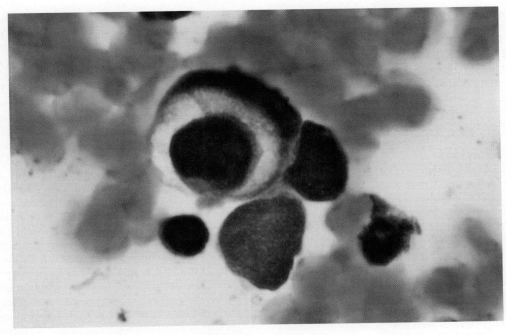

Fig. 21-39. Oat cell carcinoma with metastasis to the marrow. Note the close resemblance of carcinoma cells to lymphoblasts. However, the carcinoma cells are cohesive. One of the neoplastic cells engulfs another neoplastic cell. (Romanowsky stain, ×, 1,000.)

mentalization and segregation of malignant lymphoma and HPS. The erythrophagocytic cells appear to be benign, and lack atypia. Hemophagocytosis is found in the red pulp of the spleen, sinusoids of the liver, lymph node sinuses, and bone marrow. Cytologically malignant T lymphoma cells are present in the white pulp of the spleen, portal triads of the liver, and various other organs, such as lymph nodes, lungs, skin, and kidneys. Diagnosis is often delayed, and prognosis is poor. Malignant histiocytosis is discussed later.

Familial erythrophagocytic lymphohistiocytosis is an autosomal recessive disorder affecting very young children. These patients present with fever, failure to thrive, hepatosplenomegaly, pancytopenia, hepatic dysfunction, bleeding diathesis, and neurologic manifestations. Hypertriglyceridemia, hypofibrinogenemia, and hyperbilirubinemia are common.[431] It is difficult to differentiate from infection-associated HPS.

Malignant Histiocytic Proliferative Disorders

Neoplastic histiocytic proliferation includes clonal proliferation of antigen-presenting cells (which are very uncommon with the exception of Langerhans cell histiocytosis and are discussed in Ch. 20), and antigen-processing cells (monocytes-phagocytes).

Acute Monocytic Leukemia and Chronic Myelomonocytic Leukemia

These disorders were discussed earlier. *Malignant 5q35 histiocytosis* of children, described by Nezelof and colleagues,[441] is such an uncommon disorder that it is not clear whether these pa-

tients have malignant histiocytosis or Ki-1 positive anaplastic large cell lymphoma.

Malignant Histiocytosis

Malignant histiocytosis is a systemic malignant tumor of histiocytes affecting the entire reticuloendothelial system at presentation. It occurs in patients of all ages. Fever, weight loss, generalized lymphadenopathy and hepatosplenomegaly are common. Some patients may also have skin lesions that form nodular or ulcerated tumors based in the subcutaneous fat.[434] Peripheral cytopenia involving one or more of the three major blood cell lines and circulating atypical histiocytes have been reported.[434] The bone marrow may be focally or diffusely involved by the neoplastic cells. These cells are large and have a round or irregular nucleus, one or more prominent eosinophilic nucleoli, and an abundant lightly eosinophilic cytoplasm. These cells are cytologically malignant and may or may not display phagocytosis. However, reactive phagocytic histiocytes may be intermixed with the malignant histiocytes. In the aspirate smear, the malignant cells may be up to 50 μm in diameter with increased nuclear/cytoplasmic ratio. The nucleus is large with irregular contour, containing reticular chromatin and large prominent nucleoli. The cytoplasm is deeply basophilic and vacuolated. Phagocytosis may or may not be observed in the malignant histiocytes. Immunohistochemical and cytochemical studies are essential to demonstrate the histiocytic (phagocytic) nature of the neoplastic cells. When the lesion consists of "well differentiated" or "reactive" histiocytes, with or without hemophagocytosis, caution should be exercised to rule out infection-associated HPS.

Malignant histiocytosis may overlap with true histiocytic lymphoma (when the disease is localized), and acute monocytic leukemia.[442,443] It should be pointed out that some cases that were diagnosed as malignant histiocytosis or histiocytic medullary reticulosis are currently classified as infection-associated HPS or a variety of non-Hodgkin's lymphoma including PTCL and Ki-1 positive anaplastic large cell lymphoma.[425,440,444–446] True histiocytic lymphomas are very uncommon[435,447,448] and they seldom involve bone marrow.

Langerhans Cell Histiocytosis

The term *Langerhans cell histiocytosis* (LCH) is currently used to replace the term *histiocytosis X* that was proposed by Lichtenstein in 1953.[449] LCH can be divided into unifocal or multifocal *eosinophilic granuloma* (the latter has also been referred to as *Hand-Schüller-Christian disease* when the classic triad of calvarial lesions, exophthalmos, and diabetes insipidus is present), and disseminated LCH (progressive LCH or *Letterer-Siwe disease*). The clinical presentation of LCH is variable depending on the type of the disease, the age of the patient, and the organ involved. However, all LCH are caused by proliferation of Langerhans histiocytes that express CD1 antigen and S-100 protein, and contain Birbeck granules. In addition, they also express CD11c and CD14, which are not present in the normal Langerhans cells but are associated with phagocytic histiocytes.[449] They are also vimentin positive, CD74 (LN2)+, HLA-DR (LN3)+, CD4+, CD15+, but CD30– and CD45–.[450]

Unifocal eosinophilic granuloma, the most common form of LCH, seldomly involves the iliac crest, although bone marrow involvement may be seen in multifocal eosinophilic granuloma. Both entities are characterized by chronicity and granulomatous-like lesions with or without necrosis. The Langerhans cells have an indented or grooved nucleus that contains delicate chromatin and inconspicuous nucleoli ("coffee-bean"-like nuclei). The cytoplasm is eosinophilic.[451] Multinucleated giant cells, plasma cells, eosinophils, lymphocytes, neutrophils, and foamy histiocytes may be identified (Fig. 21-40).

Letterer-Siwe disease is commonly seen in children with visceral and hematopoietic involvement. Massive lymphadenopathy, hepatosplenomegaly, characteristic scaly brown-red eczematoid or seborrheic cutaneous eruptions, and numerous osseous defects of the skull, ribs, and femur are common findings. Other organs involved may include thymus, bone marrow, kidney, gastrointestinal tract, muscle, lungs, and pituitary.[417] The proliferating cells in the bony and visceral lesions have the morphologic and phenotypic characteristics of Langerhans cells. The bone marrow may be focally or diffusely involved by the polymorphic infiltrate described above. It should be noted that there is poor correlation between histologic appearance of the lesions and clinical behavior of the disease.[452]

LCH has long been considered a reactive proliferative condition, perhaps resulting from an immunoregulatory defect.[442] However, a recent report provides strong evidence that all forms of Langerhans cell histiocytoses are clonal.[453] It is possible that unifocal eosinophilic granuloma represents an early lesion. Its relationship to other LCH is similar to the relationship of monoclonal gammopathy of undetermined significance to multiple myeloma.

Metastatic Tumors

The frequency of metastatic carcinoma in bone marrow from all patients who have had marrow examinations has varied

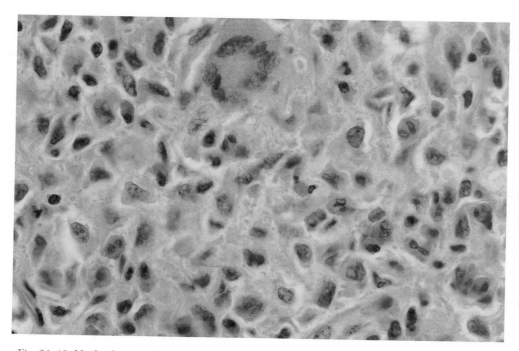

Fig. 21-40. Unifocal eosinophilic granuloma. Note the mixed infiltration of Langerhans cell histiocytes and eosinophils. A multinuclated Langerhans histiocyte is also present. (H&E stain, × 600.)

from 1 to 2.7 percent.[2,454,455] A routine bone marrow examination of patients with nonhematopoietic malignant tumors revealed metastatic carcinoma in 9.1 percent.[456] Metastasis was most frequent in patients with neuroblastoma (48 percent), Ewing's sarcoma (36 percent), oat cell carcinoma (21 percent), prostatic carcinoma (20 percent), and breast carcinoma (20 percent).[456] The frequency of positive bone marrow pathology in patients suspected of having or showing evidence of metastatic carcinomas was even higher (37 to 44 percent).[17,457] The incidence of metastatic lesions in bone marrow varies from series to series, depending on the purpose of the study, the histopathologic type of tumor, the stage of the disease, and the method of bone marrow examination.[458] Generally, both biopsy and aspiration should be performed when evaluating metastatic disease of the marrow.[459] Although trephine biopsy appears to be superior to aspiration smear because of frequently associated fibrosis and necrosis, these two methods complement each other.[460]

The most common metastatic tumors in bone marrows are carcinomas of the lung, breast, and prostate in adults, and neuroblastomas in children. Metastatic tumor may be focally and diffusely infiltrating in the marrow and associated with necrosis,[461] fibrosis,[462] increased osteoblastic activity (most notably in carcinomas of the prostate and breast but also in other tumors), osteoclastic activity (as in metastatic oat cell carcinoma of the lung or metastatic carcinoma of the colon), or a combination of both (most common form of bone reaction) (Figs. 21-41 and 21-42). Oat cell carcinoma and neuroblastoma may produce a picture simulating malignant lymphoma, but metastatic tumor cells are often larger than lymphoma cells, the neoplastic cells are more coherent than lymphoma cells, and immunohistochemical technique or electron microscopic study can differentiate these entities in a majority of difficult cases. The surrounding hematopoietic elements may show dyspoiesis and hypercellularity. In addition, increased numbers of plasma cells, eosinophils, and lymphocytes are seen. It is interesting to note that bone marrow necrosis in children with malignant disease does not appear to confer a poor prognosis,[463] and bone

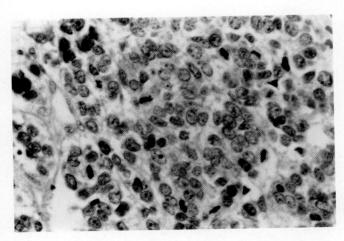

Fig. 21-41. Metastatic undifferentiated small cell (oat cell) carcinoma. Note the cohesion of neoplastic cells, with numerous mitoses. (H&E stain, × 200.)

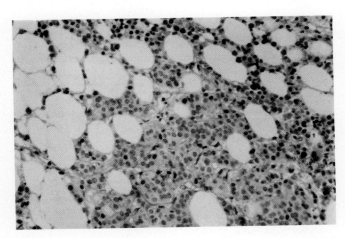

Fig. 21-42. Metastatic breast carcinoma. Islands of well differentiated adenocarcinoma are illustrated. Compare these cells with normal erythropoietic islands. (H&E stain, × 100.)

marrow fibrosis associated with metastatic tumor often regresses after successful treatment for malignant disease.[460]

Although the bone marrow aspiration smears are often of poor quality, isolated clusters of metastatic tumor are often found at the periphery of the smear. The neoplastic cells usually form coherent three-dimensional structures, with a great variability in nuclear size, shape, and staining characteristics. The nuclear/cytoplasmic ratio is variable, depending on the type of primary tumor; nevertheless, these tumor cells are usually two to five times larger than the hematopoietic cells. Nuclear molding at the cell border is often visible. The nuclear chromatin is usually hyperchromatic with irregular condensation or smudged appearance. The volume of cytoplasm is also variable. It may be deeply basophilic and contain vacuoles. Rosette-like structures may be seen in metastatic neuroblastoma.

The peripheral blood findings range from mild anemia to leukoerythroblastic picture to carcinocythemia.[458,464] It appears that leukoerythroblastic reaction is correlated with metastatic carcinoma[459]; carcinocythemia indicates a terminal event and ominous prognosis.[464]

Recent research effort has been concentrated on the detection of micrometastases in patients with breast cancer. Detection is important in identifying early recurrence, in detecting hormonal receptors in patients who have not had the determination done on the primary tumor, and in the practice of autologous marrow transplants.[460] However, these highly technical procedures are currently available in major centers only.

Bone Marrow Necrosis and Infarction

Bone marrow necrosis is very uncommon, with a prevalence ranging from 0.15 to 7 percent,[463,465,466] although another retrospective study revealed that approximately one-third of 368 bone marrow biopsy specimens displayed focal necrosis and degenerative changes.[467] The most commonly associated clinical conditions are sickle cell disease, myeloproliferative disorders, acute leukemia, malignant lymphoma, and metastatic carcino-

Table 21-18. Clinical Conditions Associated with Bone Marrow Necrosis

Benign	Malignant
Caisson disease	Leukemia, acute or chronic
Sickle cell anemia and sickle trait	Malignant lymphoma
	Multiple myeloma
Systemic lupus erythematosus	Myeloproliferative disorders
Disseminated intravascular coagulation	Malignant histiocytosis
Severe bacterial infections and septicemia	Metastatic carcinoma
	Status postchemotherapy or radiotherapy
Tuberculosis and mycotic disease	
Bacterial endocarditis	
Eclampsia	
Alcohol abuse	
Chronic renal failure	

(Modified from Mehta et al,[470] with permission.)

mas. Bone marrow necrosis may also occur in patients with sepsis, vasculitis, or disseminated intravascular coagulation[463,465,467-471] (Table 21-18). The frequency of bone marrow necrosis in an autopsy series may be as high as 15 percent among patients who died of acute leukemias. A serious and even fatal complication is fat or bone marrow embolization.

Bone marrow necrosis is often a diffuse process affecting multiple foci. Frequently, the necrotic marrow is unaspirable, resulting in a "dry tap" or very scant material for diagnosis. Histopathologic examination may reveal a spectrum of morphologies ranging from total necrosis and infarction to individual cell necrosis (Fig. 21-43). In foci of bone marrow necrosis, the fatty and hematopoietic marrow are replaced by granular eosinophilic debris. Ghost cells and cells with poorly defined

cytoplasmic borders and pyknotic nuclei may be identified. It is important to identify the underlying disease, such as acute leukemia or metastatic carcinoma. Deep sections or step sections may be needed to search for viable cells or tissues. Occasionally, repeated biopsy is indicated.

Fat necrosis of bone marrow is identical with that seen in other adipose tissues. The causes include fracture of bone and infarction. During the healing process, lipophages (foamy cells) and lipid granulomas are seen.

The pathogenesis of bone marrow necrosis is unclear. It may be due to vascular obstruction caused by tumor emboli or by extrinsic compression by rapidly dividing neoplastic cells. Bone marrow necrosis may also occur after induction therapy in leukemias or malignant lymphomas.[469,472] Rapid lysis of tumor cells following effective chemotherapy may be the underlying cause for some cases. The prognosis of bone marrow necrosis associated with a malignant neoplasm is still controversial. Although some investigators believe that bone marrow necrosis in these patients is an ominous finding,[469,470] other researchers, particularly those who deal with children with acute lymphocytic leukemia and neuroblastoma, indicate a more optimistic picture.[463]

Vascular Lesions in Marrow

Vascular lesions, either localized in the marrow[372] or systemic (whenever a pathologic process affects the blood vessels, such as arteriosclerosis, thrombosis, vasculitis, thrombotic thrombocytopenic purpura, systemic lupus erythematosus, Kaposi's sarcoma or amyloidosis), may be diagnosed on histologic sections of bone marrow.[343,358,365,473,474] Cholesterol emboli can be recognized with ease and may be a manifestation of a multisystem illness.[475] Kaposi's sarcoma is very uncommon in the bone marrow even in this era of the worldwide endemic spread of AIDS, only two instances having been reported[358,372] (Fig. 21-44). The lesion should be differentiated from a variety of disorders associated with primary or secondary myelofibrosis and vascular proliferation.

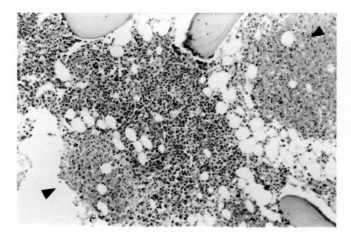

Fig. 21-43. Malignant lymphoma with bone marrow necrosis. Foci of eosinophic granular material admixed with pyknotic nuclei and cellular debris are seen in the upper and lower corners (arrowheads), of this specimen from a patient with malignant lymphoma. (H&E stain, × 40.)

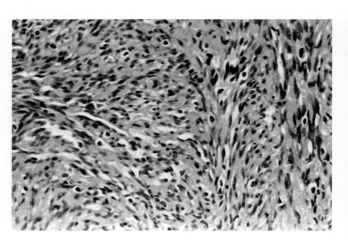

Fig. 21-44. Kaposi's sarcoma of bone marrow. Note the interlacing spindle cells, which form slits and spaces. Mitotic figures are seen. (H&E stain, × 100.) (Courtesy of Dr. Richard Conran and associates.)

REFERENCES

1. Petersdorf RG, Beeson PB: Fever of un-explained origin: Report on 100 cases. Medicine (Baltimore) 40:1–30, 1961
2. Contreras E, Ellis LD, Lee RE: Value of the bone marrow biopsy in the diagnosis of metastatic carcinoma. Cancer 29:778–783, 1972
3. Ellman L: Bone marrow biopsy in the evaluation of lymphoma, carcinoma and granulomatous disorders. Am J Med 60:1–7, 1976
4. Pease GL: Granulomatous lesions in bone marrow. Blood 11:720–734, 1956
5. O'Carroll DI, McKenna RW, Brunning RD: Bone marrow manifestations of Hodgkin's disease. Cancer 38:1717–1728, 1976
6. Rosenberg SA: Bone marrow involvement in the non-Hodgkins lymphomata. Br J Cancer, suppl. II, 31:261–264, 1975
7. Jamshidi K, Swaim WR: Bone marrow biopsy with unaltered architecture: a new biopsy device. J Lab Clin Med 77:335–342, 1971
8. Islam A: A new bone marrow biopsy needle with core securing device. J Clin Pathol 35:359–364, 1982
9. Westerman MP: Bone marrow needle biopsy: an evaluation and critique. Semin Hematol 18:293–300, 1981
10. Rywlin AM: Histopathology of the Bone Marrow. pp. 1–13. Little, Brown, Boston, 1976
11. Brynes RK, McKenna RW, Sundberg RD: Bone marrow aspiration and trephine biopsy. An approach to a thorough study. Am J Clin Pathol 70:753–759, 1978
12. Gruppo RA, Lampkin BC, Granger S: Bone marrow cellularity determination: comparison of the biopsy, aspirate and buffy coat. Blood 49:29–31, 1977
13. Liao KT: The superiority of histologic sections of aspirated bone marrow in malignant lymphomas: a review of 1,124 examinations. Cancer 27:618–628, 1971
14. Sun NCJ: Hematology: An Atlas and Diagnostic guide. pp. 23–49. WB Saunders, Philadelphia, 1983
15. Bain NT, Pickett JP: Glycol methacrylate for routine, special stains, histochemistry, enzyme histochemistry and immunohisto-chemistry. A simplified method for surgical biopsy tissue. J Histotechnol 2:125–130, 1979
16. Beckstead JH, Bainton DF: Enzyme histochemistry on bone marrow biopsies: reactions useful in the differential diagnosis of leukemia and lymphoma applied to 2-micron plastic sections. Blood 55:386–394, 1980
17. Brunning RD, Bloomfield CD, McKenna RW, et al: Bilateral trephine bone marrow biopsies in lymphoma and other neoplastic diseases. Ann Intern Med 82:365–366, 1975
18. Lukes RJ, Tindle BH: An approach to bone marrow evaluation by pathologists. pp. 86–92. In Nordmann M, Merten R, Lommel H (eds): Anatomic and Clinical Pathology Proceedings. American Elsevier, New York, 1973
19. Gruber HE, Stauffer ME, Thompson ER, et al: Diagnosis of bone disease by core biopsies. Semin Hematol 18:258–278, 1981
20. Fong TP, Okafor LA, Thomas W Jr, et al: Stainable iron in aspirated and needle-biopsy specimens of marrow: a source of error. Am J Hematol 2:47–51, 1977
21. Van der Valk P, Mullink P, Huijgens PC, et al: Immunohistochemistry in bone marrow diagnosis. Value of a panel of monoclonal antibodies on routinely processed bone marrow biopsies. Am J Surg Pathol 13:97–106, 1989
22. Hanson CA, Abaza M, Sheldons S, et al: Acute biphenotypic leukemia: immunophenotypic and cytogenetic analysis. Br J Haematol 84:49–60, 1993
23. Cossman J, Zehnbauer B, Garrett CT, et al: Gene rearrangements in the diagnosis of lymphoma/leukemia: guidelines for use based on a multi-institutional study. Am J Clin Pathol 95:347–354, 1991
24. Parker JW: Flow cytometry in the diagnosis in hematologic diseases. Ann Clin Lab Sci 16:427–442, 1986
25. Christensson B, Tribukait E, Linder I-L, et al: Cell proliferation and DNA content in non-Hodgkin's lymphoma: flow cytometry in relation to lymphoma classification. Cancer 58:1295–1304, 1986
26. Bitter MA, LeBeau MM, Rowley JD, et al: Associations between morphology, karyotype, and clinical features in myeloid leukemias. Hum Pathol 18:211–225, 1987
27. Sandberg AA: The chromosomes in human leukemia. Semin Hematol 23:201–217, 1986
28. Foon KA, Gale RP, Todd RF III: Recent advances in the immunologic classification of leukemia. Semin Hematol 23:257–283, 1986
29. Fend F, Gscwwentner A, Gredler E, et al: Detection of monoclonal B-cell populations in decalcified, plastic-embedded bone marrow biopsies with the polymerase chain reaction. Am J Clin Pathol 102:850–855, 1994
30. Sobol RE, Mick R, Royston I, et al: Clinical importance of myeloid antigen expression in adult acute lymphoblastic leukemia. N Engl J Med 316:1111–1117, 1987
31. Taubenberger JK, Cole DE, Raffeld M, et al: Immunophenotypic analysis of acute lymphoblastic leukemia using routinely processed bone marrow specimens. Arch Pathol Lab Med 115:338–342, 1991
32. Pinkus GS, Said JW: Intracellular hemoglobin—a specific marker for erythroid cells in paraffin sections. Am J Pathol 102:308–313, 1981
33. Ishii T, Takami T, Yuasa H, et al: Two distinct antigen systems in human B lymphocytes: identification of cell surface and intracellular antigens using monoclonal antibodies. Clin Exp Immunol 58:183–192, 1984
34. Kubic VL, Brunning RD: Immunohistochemical evaluation of neoplasms in bone marrow biopsies using monoclonal antibodies reactive in paraffin-embedded tissue. Mod Pathol 2:618–629, 1989
35. Motoi M, Stein H, Lennert K: Demonstration of lysozyme, alpha 1-antichymotrypsin, alpha 1-antitrypsin, albumin, and transferin with immunoperoxidase method of lymph node cells. Virchows Arch [B] 35:73–82, 1980
36. Ordonez NG: Comparison of Ulex Europaeus I lectin and factor VIII-related antigen in vascular lesions. Arch Pathol Lab Med 108:129–132, 1984
37. Kurtin PJ, Pinkus GS: Leukocyte common antigen—a diagnostic discriminant between hematopoietic and non-hematopoietic neoplasms in paraffin sections using monoclonal antibodies: correlation with immunologic studies and ultrastructural localization. Hum Pathol 16:353–365, 1985
38. Linder J, Ye Y, Harrington DS, et al: Monoclonal antibodies marking T lymphocytes in paraffin-embedded tissue. Am J Pathol 127:1–8, 1987
39. Hartsock RJ, Smith EB, Petty CS: Normal variations with aging of the amount of hematopoietic tissue in bone marrow from the anterior iliac crest. A study made from 177 cases of sudden death examined by necropsy. Am J Clin Pathol 43:326–331, 1965
40. Schmid C, Isaacson PG: Bone marrow trephine biopsy in lymphoproliferative disease. J Clin Pathol 45:745–750, 1992
41. Frisch B, Lewis SM, Burkhardt R, et al: Biopsy Pathology of Bone and Bone Marrow. pp. 18–46. Lippincott-Raven, Philadelphia, 1985
42. Wilkins BS: Histology of normal haemopoiesis: bone marrow histology I. J Clin Pathol 45:645–649, 1992
43. Brown DC, Gafter KC: The bone marrow trephine biopsy: a review of normal histology, Histopathology 22:411–422, 1993
44. Gulati GL, Ashton JK, Hyun BH: Structure and function of the bone marrow and hematopoiesis. Hematol Oncol Clin North Am 2:495–511, 1988
45. Liesveld JL, Winslow J, Kempski MC, et al: Adhesive interactions of normal and leukemic human CD34+ myeloid progenitors: role of marrow stromal fibroblast and cytomatrix components. Exp Hematol 19:63–70, 1991
46. Clark BR, Gallagher JT, Dexter M: Cell adhesion in the stromal regulation of hematopoiesis. Baillieres Clin Haematol 5:619–652, 1992

47. Metcalf D: Hematopoietic regulators: redundancy or subtlety?, review. Blood 82:3515–3523, 1993

48. Brittenham GM, Danish EH, Harris JW: Assessment of bone marrow and body iron stores: old techniques and new technologies. Semin Hematol 18:194–221, 1981

49. Huang B-J, Li C-Y, Nichols WL, et al: Acute leukemia with megakaryocytic differentiation: a study of 12 cases identified immunocytochemically. Blood 64:427–439, 1984

50. Ruiz-Arguelles GJ, Marin-Lopez A, Lobato-Mendizabal E, et al: Acute megakaryoblastic leukemia: a prospective study of its identification and treatment. Br J Haematol 62:55–63, 1986

51. Larsen TE: Emperipolesis of granular leukocytes within megakaryocytes in human hematopoietic bone marrow. Am J Clin Pathol 53:485–489, 1970

52. Rywlin AM, Ortega RS, Dominguez CJ: Lymphoid nodules of the bone marrow: normal and abnormal. Blood 43:389–400, 1974

53. Hyun BH, Kwa D, Gabaldon H, et al: Reactive plasmacytic lesions of the bone marrow. Am J Clin Pathol 65:921–928, 1976

54. Farrant A, Rodham J, Cordier A, et al: Selective hypoplasia of pelvic bone marrow. Scand J Haematol 25:12–18, 1980

55. Seaman JP, Kjeldsberg CR, Linker A: Gelatinous transformation of the bone marrow. Hum Pathol 9:685–692, 1978

56. Amrein PC, Friedman R, Kosinsku K, et al: Hematologic changes in anorexia nervosa. JAMA 241:2190–2191, 1979

57. Mehta K, Gascon P, Robboy S: The gelatinous bone marrow (serous atrophy) in patients with acquired immunodeficiency syndrome. Evidence of excess sulfated glycosaminoglycan. Arch Pathol Lab Med 116:504–508, 1992

58. Alter BP, Potter NU, Li FP: Classification and aetiology of the aplastic anemia. Clin Haematol 7:431–465, 1978

59. The International Agranulocytosis and Aplastic Anemia Study: Risks of agranulocytosis and aplastic anemia—a first report of their relation to drug use with special reference to analgesics. JAMA 256:1749–1757, 1986

60. Narayanan MN, Geary CG, Freemont AJ, et al: Long term follow-up of aplastic anemia. Br J Haematol 86:837–843, 1994

61. De Planque MM, Kluin-Nelemans HC, Van Krieken HJM, et al: Evolution of acquired severe aplastic anemia to myelodysplasia and subsequent leukemia in adults. Br J Haematol 70:55–62, 1988

62. Socie G, Henry-Amar M, Bacigalupo A, et al: Malignant tumors occurring after treatment of aplastic anemia. N Engl J Med 329:1152–1157, 1993

63. Diamond LK, Blackfan KD: Hypoplastic anemia. Am J Dis Child 56:464–467, 1938

64. Slater WM, Schultz MJ, Armentrout SA: Remission of pure red cell aplasia associated with nonthymic malignancy. Cancer 44:1879–1881, 1979

65. Levitt LJ, Ries CA, Greenberg PL: Pure white cell aplasia. Antibody mediated autoimmune inhibition of granulopoiesis. N Engl J Med 308:1141–1146, 1983

66. Carmel R: An unusual case of autoimmune agranulocytosis with total absence of myeloid precursors. Am J Clin Pathol 79:611–615, 1983

67. Stoll DB, Blum S, Pasquale D, et al: Thrombocytopenia and decreased megakaryocytes. Evaluation and prognosis. Ann Intern Med 94:170–175, 1981

68. Menke DM, Colon-Otero G, Cockerill KJ, et al: Refractory thrombocytopenia: a myelodysplastic syndrome that may mimic immune thrombocytopenic purpura. Am J Clin Pathol 98:502–510, 1992

69. Rotoli B, Luzatto L: Paroxysmal nocturnal hemoglobinuria. Semin Hematol 26:201–207, 1989

70. Howe RB, Bloomfield CD, McKenna RW: Hypocellular acute leukemia. Am J Med 72:391–395, 1982

71. Needleman S, Burns CP, Dick FR, et al: Hypoplastic acute leukemia. Cancer 48:1410–1414, 1981

72. Bennett JM, Catovsky D, Daniel M-T et al: Proposals for the classification of the acute leukemias. Br J Haematol 33:451–458, 1976

73. Bennett JM, Catovsky D, Daniel MT, et al: Proposals for the classification of the myelodysplastic syndrome. Br J Haematol 51:189–199, 1982

74. Bennett JM, Catovsky D, Daniel M-T, et al: Proposed revised criteria for the classification of acute myeloid leukemia: a report of the French-American-British Cooperative Group. Ann Intern Med 103:626–629, 1985

75. Gladson CL, Naeim F: Hypocellular bone marrow with increased blasts. Am J Hematol 21:15–22, 1986

76. Berdeaux DH, Glasser L, Serokmann R, et al: Hypoplastic acute leukemia: review of 70 cases with multivariate regression analysis. Hematol Oncol 4:291–305, 1986

77. Breatnach F, Chessells JM, Greaves MF: The aplastic presentation of childhood leukemia: a feature of common ALL. Br J Haematol 49:387–393, 1981

78. Sills RH, Stockman JA III: Preleukemic states in children with acute lymphoblastic leukemia. Cancer 48:110–112, 1981

79. Nand S, Godwin JE: Hypoplastic myelodysplastic syndrome. Cancer 62:958–964, 1988

80. Wittels B: Bone marrow biopsy change following chemotherapy for acute leukemia. Am J Surg Pathol 4:135–142, 1980

81. Davis RE, Longacre TA, Cornbleet J: Hematogones in the bone marrow of adults. Immunophenotypic features, clinical settings, and differential diagnosis. Am J Clin Pathol 102:202–211, 1994

82. Sun NCJ: Hematology: An Atlas and Diagnostic Guide. pp. 74–122. WB Saunders, Philadelphia, 1983

83. Lewis SM, Verwilghen RL: Dyserythropoiesis and dyserythropoietic anemias. Prog Hematol 8:99–129, 1973

84. Schmitz LA, McClure JS, Litz CE, et al: Morphologic and quantitative changes in blood and marrow cells following growth factor therapy. Am J Clin Pathol 101:67–75, 1994

85. Harris AC, Todd WM, Hackney H et al: Bone marrow changes associated with recombinant granulocyte-macrophage and granulocyte colony-stimulating factors. Discrimination of granulocytic regeneration. Arch Pathol Lab Med 118:624–629, 1994

86. Sun NCJ: Hematology: An atlas and Diagnostic Guide. pp. 173–185, 228–258, 288–322. WB Saunders, Philadelphia, 1983

87. Bennett JM, Catovsky D, Daniel M-T, et al: Criteria for the diagnosis of acute leukemia of megakaryocyte lineage (M7). A report of the French-American-British Cooperative Group. Ann Intern Med 103:460–462, 1985

88. Hurwitz CA, Loken MR, Graham ML, et al: Asynchronous antigen expression in B lineage acute lymphoblastic leukemia. Blood 72:299–307, 1988

89. Picozzi VJ, Coleman CN: Lymphoblastic lymphoma. Semin Oncol 17:96–103, 1990

90. Weiss LM, Bindl JM, Picozzi VJ, et al: Lymphoblastic lymphoma: an immunophenotype study of 26 cases with comparison to T-cell acute lymphoblastic leukemia. Blood 67:474–478, 1986

91. Sander C, Jaffe ES, Gebhardt FC, et al: Mediastinal lymphoblastic lymphoma with an immature B-cell immunophenotype. Am J Surg Pathol 16:300–305, 1992

92. Pui CH, Behm FG, Singh B, et al: Heterogeneity of presenting features and their relation to treatment outcome in 120 children with T-cell acute lymphoblastic leukemia. Blood 75:174–179, 1990

93. Pavlova Z, Parker JW, Taylor CR, et al: Small non-cleaved follicular center cell lymphoma; Burkitt's and non-Burkitt's variants in the U.S. II. Pathologic and immunologic features. Cancer 59:1892–1902, 1987

94. Hutchinson RE, Murphy SB, Fairclough DL et al: Diffuse small noncleaved cell lymphoma in children, Burkitt's versus non-Burkitt's type. Results from the Pediatric Oncology Group and St. Jude Children's Research Hospital. Cancer 64:23–28, 1989

95. Pui C-H: Childhood leukemias, review. N Engl J Med 332:1618–1630, 1995

96. Sun NCJ: Diagnosing leukemias with granulated leukemic cells (excluding eosinophilic leukemia) editorial. Mayo Clin Proc 62:1059–1061, 1987

97. Bennett JM, Catovsky D, Daniel M-T, et al: Proposal for the recognition of minimally differentiated acute myeloid leukemia (AML-MO). Br J Haematol 78:325–329, 1991

98. Cline MJ: The molecular basis of leukemia, review. N Engl J Med 330:328–336, 1994

99. Goasguen J-E, Bennett JM, Cox C, et al: Prognostic implication and characterization of the blast cell population in the myelodysplastic syndrome. Leuk Res 15:1159–1165, 1991

100. Zipursky A, Poon A, Doyle J: Leukemia in Down syndrome: a review. Pediatr Hematol Oncol 9:139–149, 1992

101. Kojima S, Matsuyama T, Sato T, et al: Down's syndrome and acute leukemia in children: an analysis of phenotype by use of monoclonal antibodies and electron microscopic platelet peroxidase reaction. Blood 76:2348–2353, 1990

102. Shaw MT: Monocytic leukemias. Hum Pathol 11:215–227, 1980

103. Davey FR, Olson S, Kurec AS, et al: The immunophenotyping of extramedullary myeloid cell tumors in paraffin-embedded tissue sections. Am J Surg Pathol 12:699–707, 1988

104. Krause JR: Granulocytic sarcoma preceding acute leukemia. A report of six cases. Cancer 44:1017–1021, 1979

105. Neiman RS, Barcos M, Berard C, et al: Granulocytic sarcoma: a clinicopathologic study of 61 biopsies cases. Cancer 48:1426–1437, 1981

106. Meis JM, Butler JJ, Osborne BM, et al: Granulocytic sarcoma in non-leukemic patients. Cancer 58:2697–2709, 1986

107. Traweek ST, Arber DA, Rappaport H, et al: Extramedullary myeloid cell tumor: an immunohistochemical and morphologic study of 28 cases. Am J Surg Pathol 17:1011–1019, 1993

108. Roth MJ, Medeiros LJ, Elenitoba-Johnson K, et al: Extramedullary myeloid cell tumors: an immunohistochemical study of 29 cases using routinely fixed and processed paraffin-embedded tissue sections. Arch Pathol Lab Med 119:790–798, 1995

109. Lewis SM, Szur L: Malignant myelosclerosis. BMJ 2:472–477, 1963

110. Bearman RM, Pangalis GA, Rappaport H: Acute (malignant) myelosclerosis. Cancer 43:279–293, 1979

111. Shah I, Mayeda K, Koppitch F, et al: Karyotypic polymorphism in acute myelofibrosis. Blood 60:841–844, 1982

112. Clare N, Elson D, Manhoff L: Case report: cytogenetic studies of peripheral myeloblasts and bone marrow fibroblasts in acute myelofibrosis. Am J Clin Pathol 77:762–766, 1982

113. Rozman C, Granena A, Hernandez-Nieto M, et al: Bone marrow transplantation for acute myelofibrosis. Lancet 1:618, 1982

114. Puckett JB, Cooper MR: Acute myelofibrosis evolving into acute myeloblastic leukemia. Ann Intern Med 94:545–546, 1981

115. Tada T, Nitta M, Kishimoto H: Acute myelofibrosis terminating in erythroleukemic state. Am J Clin Pathol 78:102–104, 1982

116. Truong LD, Saleem A, Schwartz MR: Acute myelofibrosis. A report of four cases and review of the literature. Medicine (Baltimore) 63:182–187, 1984

117. Cuneo A, Mecucci C, Kerim S, et al: Multiple stem cell involvement in megakaryoblastic leukemia. Cytologic and cytogenetic evidence in 15 patients. Blood 74:1781–1790, 1989

118. Hirt A, Leuthy AR, Mueller B, et al: Acute megakaryoblastic leukemia in children identified by immunological marker studies. Am J Pediatr Hematol Oncol 12:27–33, 1990

119. Winfield DA, Polacarz SV: Bone marrow histology 3: value of bone marrow core biopsy in acute leukemia, myelodysplastic syndromes, and chronic myeloid leukaemia. J Clin Pathol 45:855–859, 1992

120. Miller DR, Krailo M, Bleyer WA, et al: Prognostic implications of blast cell morphology in childhood acute lymphoblastic leukemia: a report from the Children's Cancer study Group. Cancer Treat Rep 69:1211–1221, 1985

121. Bennett JM, Catovsky D, Daniel MT, et al: The morphological classification of acute lymphoblastic leukemia: concordance among observers and clinical correlations. Br J Haematol 47:553–561, 1981

122. Pui C-H, Behm FG, Crist WM: Clinical and biologic relevance of immunologic marker studies in childhood acute lymphoblastic leukemia, review. Blood 82:343–362, 1993

123. Nichols J, Nimer SD: Transcription factors, translocations, and leukemia, review. Blood 80:2953–2963, 1992

124. Rowley JD, Testa JR: Chromosome abnormalities in malignant hematologic disease. Adv Cancer Res 36:103–148, 1982

125. Larson RA, Kondo K, Vardiman JW, et al: Evidence for a 15;17 translocation in every patient with acute promyelocytic leukemia. Am J Med 76:827–841, 1984

126. LeBeau MM, Diaz MO, Karin M, et al: Metallothionein gene cluster is split by chromosome 16 rearrangements in myelomonocytic leukemia. Nature 313:709–711, 1985

127. Katz F, Malcolm S, Gibbons B, et al: Cellular and molecular studies on infant null acute lymphoblastic leukemia. Blood 71:1438–1447, 1988

128. Pui C-H, Frankel LS, Carroll AJ, et al: Clinical characteristics and treatment outcome of childhood acute lymphoblastic leukemia with the t(4;11) (q21;q23): a collaborative study of 40 cases. Blood 77:440–447, 1991

129. Hunger SP, Tkachuk DC, Amylon MD, et al: HRX involvement in de novo and secondary leukemias with diverse chromosome 11q23 abnormalities. Blood 81:3197–3203, 1993

130. Pui C-H, Crist WM, Look AT: Biology and clinical significance of cytogenetic abnormalities in childhood acute lymphoblastic leukemia. Blood 76:1449–1463, 1990

131. Gaynon PS: Acute leukemia in children. Curr Opin Hematol 2:240–246, 1995

132. Crump M, Keating A: Acute leukemia in adults. Curr Opin Hematol 2:247–254, 1995

133. Brisco MJ, Condon J, Hughes E, et al: Outcome prediction in childhood acute lymphoblastic leukemia by molecular quantitation of residual disease at the end of induction. Lancet 343:196–200, 1994

134. Miller WH, Levine K, DeBlasio A, et al: Detection of minimal residual disease in acute promyelocytic leukemia by a reverse transcription polymerase chain reaction assay for the PML/RAR alpha mRNA. Blood 82:1687–1693, 1993

135. Maruyama F, Stass SA, Estey EH, et al: Detection of AML1/ETO fusion transcript as a tool for diagnosing t(8;21) positive acute myelogenous leukemia. Leukemia 8:40–45, 1994

136. Hubert J, Cayuela JM, Daniel MT, et al: Detection of minimal residual disease in acute myelomonocytic leukemia with abnormal marrow eosinophils by vested polymerase chain reaction with allele specific amplification. Blood 84:2291–2296, 1994

137. Pui C-H, Raimondi SC, Head DR, et al: Characterization of childhood acute leukemia with multiple myeloid and lymphoid markers at diagnosis and at relapse. Blood 78:1327–1337, 1991

138. Fink F-M, Koller U, Mayer H, et al: Prognostic significance of myeloid-associated antigen expression on blast cells in children with acute lymphoblastic leukemia. Med Pediatr Oncol 21:340–346, 1993

139. Smith FO, Lampkin BC, Versteeg C, et al: Expression of lymphoid-associated cell surface antigens by childhood acute myeloid leukemia cell lacks prognostic significance. Blood 79:2415–2422, 1992

140. Kuerbitz SJ, Civin CI, Krischer JP, et al: Expression of myeloid associated and lymphoid-associated cell surface antigens in acute myeloid leukemia of childhood. A Pediatric Oncology Group Study. J Clin Oncol 10:1419–1429, 1992

141. Dameshek W: Some speculations on the myeloproliferative syndromes. Blood 6:372–375, 1951

142. Anger B, Haug U, Seidler R, et al: Polycythemia vera. A clinical study of 141 patients. Blut 59:493–500, 1989

143. Ellis JT, Peterson P: The bone marrow in polycythemia vera. Pathol Annu 14:383–403, 1979

144. Bartl R, Frisch B, Wilmanns W: Potential of bone marrow biopsy in chronic myeloproliferative disorders (MPD). Eur J Haematol 50:41–52, 1993

145. Berlin NI: Polycythemia. I. Diagnosis and classification of the polycythemias. Semin Hematol 12:339–351, 1975

146. Silverstein MN: Postpolycythemia myeloid metaplasia. Arch Intern Med 134:113–117, 1974

147. Ellis JT, Peterson P, Geller SA, et al: Studies of the bone marrow in polycythemia vera and the evolution of myelofibrosis and secondary hematologic malignancies. Semin Hematol 23:144–155, 1986

148. Landaw SA: Acute leukemia in polycythemia vera. Semin Hematol 23:156–165, 1986

149. Najean Y, Mugnier P, Dresch C, et al: Polycythemia vera in young people: an analysis of 58 cases diagnosed before 40 years. Br J Haematol 67:285–291, 1987

150. Berger R, Bernheim A, Le Coniat M, et al: Chromosome studies in polycythemia vera patients. Cancer Genet Cytogenet 12:217–223, 1984

151. Diez-Martin JL, Graham DL, Petitt RM, et al: Chromosome studies in 104 patients with polycythemia vera. Mayo Clin Proc 66:287–299, 1991

152. Bellucci S, Janvier M, Tobelem G, et al: Essential thrombocythemias: clinical evolutionary and biological data. Cancer 58:2440–2447, 1986

153. Adams JA, Barrett AJ, Beard J, et al: Primary polycythemia, essential thrombocythemia and myelofibrosis—three facets of a single disease process? Acta Haematol 79:33–37, 1988

154. Fenaux P, Simon M, Caulier MT, et al: Clinical course of essential thrombocythemia in 147 cases. Cancer 66:549–556, 1990

155. Mitus AJ, Schafer AI: Thrombocytosis and thrombocythemia. Hematol Oncol Clin North Am 4:157–178, 1990

156. Murphy S, Iland H, Rosenthal D, et al: Essential thrombocythemia: an interim report from the polycythemia vera study group. Semin Hematol 23:177–182, 1986

157. Nowell PC, Hungerford DA: Chromosome studies in human leukemia. II. Chronic granulocytic leukemia. J Natl Cancer Inst 27:1013–1021, 1961

158. Martin PJ, Najfeld V, Hansen JA, et al: Involvement of the B-lymphoid system in chronic myelogenous leukemia. Nature 287:49–50, 1980

159. Sun T, Susin M, Koduru P, et al: Extramedullary blast crisis in chronic myelogenous leukemia: demonstration of T-cell lineage and Philadelphia chromosome in a paraspinal tumor. Cancer 68:605–610, 1991

160. Gorska-Flipot I, Norman C, Addy L, et al: Molecular pathology of chronic myelogenous leukemia. Tumor Biol, suppl. 111:25–43, 1990

161. Carabasi MH: Chronic myelogenous leukemia. Cancer Invest 11:408–419, 1993

162. Travis LB, Pierre RV, DeWald GW: Ph negative chronic granulocytic leukemia: a nonentity. Am J Clin Pathol 85:186–193, 1986

163. Kantarjian HM, Deisseroth A, Kurzrock R, et al: Chronic myelogenous leukemia: a concise update. Blood 82:691–703, 1993

164. Korostoff NR, Sun NCJ, Okun DB: Atypical blast crisis in chronic myelogenous leukemia. JAMA 245:1245–1246, 1981

165. Ward HP, Block MH: The natural history of agnogenic myeloid metaplasia (AMM) and a critical evaluation of its relationship with the myeloproliferative syndrome. Medicine (Baltimore) 50:357–420, 1971

166. Varki A, Lottenberg R, Griffith R, et al: The syndrome of idiopathic myelofibrosis. A clinicopathologic review with emphasis on the prognostic variables predicting survival. Medicine (Baltimore) 62:353–371, 1983

167. Visani G, Fineli C, Castelli V, et al: Myelofibrosis with myeloid metaplasia: clinical and haematological parameters predicting survival in a series of 133 patients. Br J Haematol 75:4–9, 1990

168. Weinstein IM: Idiopathic myelofibrosis: historical review, diagnosis and management. Blood Rev 5:98–104, 1991

169. Hasselbalch H, Nielsen H, Berild D, et al: Circulating immune complexes in myelofibrosis. Scand J Haematol 34:177–180, 1985.

170. Reilly JT: Pathogenesis of idiopathic myelofibrosis: role of growth factors. J Clin Pathol 45:461–464, 1992

171. Fava RA, Casey TT, Wicox J, et al: Synthesis of transforming growth factor-β1 by megakaryocytes and its localization to megakaryocyte and platelet alpha-granules. Blood 76:1946–1955, 1990

172. Frisch B, Bartl R: Histology of myelofibrosis and osteomyelosclerosis. pp. 51–86. In Lewis SM (ed): Myelofibrosis. Marcel Dekker, New York, 1985

173. Stone RM: Myelodysplastic syndrome after autologous transplantation for lymphoma: the price of progress. Blood 83:3437–3440, 1994

174. Rosenbloom B, Schreck R, Koeffler HP: Therapy-related myelodysplastic syndrome. Hematol Oncol Clin North Am 6:707–722, 1992

175. Sun NCJ: Hematology: An Atlas and Diagnostic Guide. pp. 140–157. WB Saunders, Philadelphia, 1983

176. Tricot G, De Wolf-Peeters C, Hendrickx B, et al: Bone marrow histology in myelodysplastic syndromes. I. Histologic findings in myelodysplastic syndromes and comparison with bone marrow smears. Br J Haematol 57:423–430, 1984

177. Kempmeyer P, Anastasi J, Vardiman JW: Issues in the pathology of the myelodysplastic syndrome. Hematol Oncol Clin North Am 6:501–522, 1992

178. Verhoef GEG, de Wolf-Peeters C, Ferrant A, et al: Myelodysplastic syndrome with bone marrow fibrosis: a myelodysplastic disorder with proliferative features. Ann Hematol 63:235–241, 1991

179. Lambertenghi-Deliliers G, Orazi A, Luksch R, Annaloro C: Myelodysplastic syndrome with increased marrow fibrosis: a distinct clinico-pathological entity. Br J Haematol 78:161–166, 1991

180. Tricot G, De Wolf-Peeters C, Vlietinck R, et al: Bone marrow histology in myelodysplastic syndromes. II. Prognostic value of abnormal localization of immature precursors in MDS. Br J Heaematol 58:217–225, 1984

181. Mangi MH, Mufti GJ: Primary myelodysplastic syndromes: diagnostic and prognostic significance of immunohistochemical assessment of bone marrow biopsies. Blood 79:198–205, 1992

182. Tuzuner N, Cox C, Rowe JM, et al: Hypocellular myelodysplastic syndrome (MDS): new proposals. Br J Haematol 91:612–617, 1995

183. Boultwood J, Lewis S, Wainscoat JS: The 5q– syndrome, review. Blood 84:3253–3260, 1994

184. Riccardi A, Geordano M, Girino M, et al: Refractory cytopenias: clinical course according to bone marrow cytology and cellularity. Blut 54:153–163, 1987

185. Fenaux P, Jouet JP, Zandecki M, et al: Chronic and subacute myelomonocytic leukemia in the adult: a report of 60 cases with special reference to prognostic factors. Br J Haematol 65:101–106, 1987

186. Tefferi A, Hoagland HC, Therneau TM, et al: Chronic myelomonocytic leukemia: natural history and prognostic determinants. Mayo Clin Proc 64:1246–1254, 1989

187. Kantarjian HM, Keating MJ, Walters RS, et al: Clinical and prognostic features of Philadelphia chromosome-negative chronic myelogenous leukemia. Cancer 58:2023–2030, 1986

188. Bennett JM, Catovsky D, Daniel MT, et al: The chronic myeloid leukaemias: guidelines for distinguishing chronic granulocytic, atypical chronic myeloid, and chronic myelomonocytic leukaemia. Proposals by the French-British Cooperative Leukaemia Group. Br J Haematol 87:746–754, 1994

189. van den Berghe: The 5q– syndrome. Scand J Haematol 36:78–81, 1986

190. Koeffler HP: Myelodysplastic syndromes (preleukemia). Semin Hematol 23:284–299, 1986

191. Jacobs RH, Cornbleet MA, Vardiman JW, et al: Prognostic implications of morphology and karyotype in primary myelodysplastic syndromes. Blood 67:1765–1772, 1986

192. Nowell PC, Besa EC, Stelmach T, et al: Chromosome studies in

preleukemic states. V. Prognostic significance of single versus multiple abnormalities. Cancer 58:2571–2575, 1986

193. Aul C, Gattermann N, Heyll A, et al: Primary myelodysplastic syndromes: analysis of prognostic factors in 235 patients and proposals for an improved scoring system. Leukemia 6:52–59, 1992

194. Kantarjian HM, Keating MJ: Therapy-related leukemia and myelodysplastic syndrome. Semin Oncol 14:435–443, 1987

195. Le Beau MM, Albain KS, Larson RA, et al: Clinical and cytogenetic correlations in 63 patients with therapy-related myelodysplastic syndrome and acute non-lymphocytic leukemia: further incidence for characteristic abnormalities of chromosomes no. 5 and 7. J Clin Oncol 4:325–345, 1986

196. Whitlock JA, Greer JP, Lukens JN: Epipodophyllo-toxin-related leukemia. Identification of a new subset of secondary leukemia. Cancer 68:600–604, 1991

197. Winick NJ, McKenna RW, Shuster JJ, et al: Secondary acute myeloid leukemia in children with acute lymphoblastic leukemia treated with etaposide. J Clin Oncol 11:209–217, 1993

198. Orazi A, Cattoretti G, Soligo D, et al: Therapy-related myelodysplastic syndromes: FAB classification, bone marrow histology, and immunohistology in the prognostic assessment. Leukemia 6:838–847, 1993

199. Saarinen UM, Wegelius R: Preleukemic syndrome in children. Report of four cases and review of literature. Am J Pediatr Hematol Oncol 6:137–145, 1984

200. Passmore SJ, Hann IM, Stiller CA, et al: Pediatric myelodysplasia: a study of 68 children and a new prognostic scoring system. Blood 85:1742–1750, 1995

201. Pui C-H, Hancock ML, Raimondi SC, et al: Myeloid neoplasia in children treated for solid tumours. Lancet 336:417–421, 1990

202. Smith RE, Chelmowski MK, Szabo EJ: Myelofibrosis: a concise review of clinical and pathological features and treatment. Am J Hematol 29:174–180, 1988

203. Reilly JT, Nash JRG, Mackie MJ, McVerry BA: Endothelial cell proliferation in myelofibrosis. Br J Haematol 60:625–630, 1985

204. Thiele J, Braeckel C, Wagner S, et al: Macrophages in normal human bone marrow and chronic myeloproliferative disorders: an immunohistochemical and morphometric study by a new monoclonal antibody (PG-M$_1$) on trephine biopsies. Virchows Arch A Pathol Anat 421:33–39, 1992

205. McCarthy DM: Fibrosis of the bone marrow: content and causes. Br J Haematol 59:1–7, 1985

206. Hasselbalch H: Idiopathic myelofibrosis: a clinical study of 80 patients. Am J Hematol 34:291—300, 1990

207. Wallis JP, Reid MM: Bone marrow fibrosis in childhood acute lymphoblastic leukaemia. J Clin Pathol 42:1253–1254, 1989

208. Islam A, Catovsky D, Goldman JM, et al: Bone marrow fiber content in acute myeloid leukaemia before an after treatment. J Clin Pathol 37:1259–1263, 1984

209. Maeda K, Hyun BH, Rebuck JW: Lymphoid follicles in bone marrow aspirates. Am J Clin Pathol 67:41–48, 1977

210. Horny H-P, Wehrmann M, Griesser H, et al: Investigation of bone marrow lymphocyte subsets in normal, reactive, and neoplastic states using paraffin-embedded biopsy specimens. Am J Clin Pathol 99:142–149, 1993

211. Bluth RF, Casey TT, McCurley TL: Differentiation of reactive from neoplastic small cell lymphoid aggregates in paraffin-embedded marrow particle preparations using L-26 (CD20) and UCHL-1 (CD45RO) monoclonal antibodies. Am J Clin Pathol 99:150–156, 1993

212. Sangster G, Crocker J, Nar P, et al: Benign and malignant (B-cell) focal lymphoid aggregates in bone marrow trephines shown by means of an immunogold-silver technique. J Clin Pathol 39:453–457, 1986

213. Faulkner-Jones BE, Howie AJ, Boughton BJ, Franklin IM: Lymphoid aggregates in bone marrow: study of eventual outcome. J Clin Pathol 41:768–775, 1988

214. Bennett JM, Catovsky D, Daniel M-T, et al: Proposals for the classification of chronic (mature) B and T lymphoid leukemias. J Clin Pathol 42:567–584, 1989

215. Dighiero G, Travade P, Chevret S, et al: B-cell chronic lymphocytic leukemia: present status and future directions, review. Blood 78:1901–1914, 1991

216. Rozman C, Montserrat E: Chronic lymphocytic leukemia, review. N Engl J Med 333:1052–1057, 1995

217. Cheson BD, Bennett JM, Rai KR, et al: Guidelines for clinical protocols for chronic lymphocytic leukemia: recommendations of the National Cancer Institute-sponsored working group. Am J Hematol 29:152–163, 1988

218. Tefferi A, Phyliky RL: A clinical update on chronic lymphocytic leukemia. I. Diagnosis and prognosis. Mayo Clin Proc 67:349–353, 1992

219. Geisler CH, Larson JK, Hansen NE, et al: Prognostic importance of flow cytometric immunophenotyping of 540 consecutive patients with B-cell chronic lymphocytic leukemia. Blood 78:1795–1802, 1991

220. Wormsley SB, Baird SM, Gadol N, et al: Characteristics of CD11c+CD5+ chronic B-cell leukemias and the identification of noval peripheral blood B-cell subsets with chronic lymphoid leukemia immunophenotypes. Blood 76:123–130, 1990

221. Ikematsu W, Ikematsu H, Okamura S, et al: Surface phenotype and Ig heavy-chain gene usage in chronic B-cell leukemias: expression of myelomonocytic surface markers in CD5– chronic B-cell leukemia. Blood 83:2602–2610, 1994

222. Rai KR, Sawitsky A, Cronkite EP, et al: Clinical staging of chronic lymphocytic leukemia. Blood 46:219–234, 1975

223. Binet J, Auquier A, Dighiero G, et al: A new prognostic classification of chronic lymphocytic leukemia derived from a multivariate analysis. Cancer 48:198–206, 1981

224. Rozman C, Hernandez-Nieto L, Montserrat E, et al: Prognostic significance of bone-marrow patterns in chronic lymphocytic leukemia. Br J Haematol 47:529–537, 1981

225. Rozman C, Montserrat E, Rodriguez-Fernandez JM, et al: Bone marrow histologic pattern—the best single prognostic parameter in chronic lymphocytic leukemia: a multivariate survival analysis of 329 cases. Blood 64:642–648, 1984

226. Pangalis GA, Roussou PA, Kittas C, et al: B-chronic lymphocytic leukemia. Prognostic implication of bone marrow histology in 120 patients: experience from a single hematology unit. Cancer 59:767–771, 1987

227. Pangalis GA, Roussou PA, Kittas C, et al: Patterns of bone marrow involvement in chronic lymphocytic leukemia and small lymphocytic (well differentiated) non-Hodgkin's lymphoma. Its clinical significance in relation to their differential diagnosis and prognosis. Cancer 54:702–708, 1984

228. Juliusson G, Oscier DH, Fitchett M, et al: Prognostic subgroups in B-cell chronic lymphocytic leukemia defined by specific chromosomal abnormalities. N Engl J Med 323:720–724, 1990

229. Criel A, Wlodarska I, Meeus P, et al: Trisomy 12 is uncommon in typical chronic lymphocytic leukemias. Br J Haematol 87:523–528, 1994

230. Escudier SM, Pereira-Leahy JM, Drach JW, et al: Fluorescence in situ hybridization and cytogenetic studies of trisomy 12 in chronic lymphocytic leukemia. Blood 81:2702–2707, 1993

231. Que TH, Marco JG, Ellis J, et al: Trisomy 12 in chronic lymphocytic leukemia detected by fluorescence in situ hybridization: analysis by stage, immunophenotype, and morphology. Blood 82:571–575, 1993

232. Newman RA, Peterson B, Davey FR, et al: Phenotypic markers and bcl-1 gene rearrangements in B-cell chronic lymphocytic leukemia: a cancer and leukemia group B study. Blood 82:1239–1246, 1993

233. Bosch F, Jares P, Campo E, et al: PRAD-1/cyclin D1 gene overexpression in chronic lymphoproliferative disorders: A highly specific marker of mantle cell lymphoma. Blood 84:2726–2732, 1994

234. Rimokh R, Berger F, Delsol G, et al: Rearrangement and overexpression of the bcl-1/prad-1 gene in intermediate lymphocytic lymphomas and in t(11q13)-bearing leukemia. Blood 81:3063–3067, 1993

235. Zukerberg LR, Yang W-O, Arnold A, et al: Cyclin D1 expression in non-Hodgkin's lymphomas. Detection by immunohistochemistry. Am J Clin Pathol 103:756–760, 1995

236. Delmer A, Ajchenbaum-Cymbalista F, Tang R, et al: Overexpression of cyclin D2 in chronic B-cell malignancies. Blood 85:2870–2876, 1995

237. Dyer MJ, Zani VJ, Lu WZ, et al: Bcl2 translocations in leukemias of mature B cells. Blood 83:3682–3688, 1994

238. Korsmeyer SJ: Bcl-2 initiates a new category of oncogenes. Regulators of cell death. Blood 80:879–886, 1992

239. Enno A, Catovsky D, O'Brien M, et al: "Prolymphocytoid" transformation of chronic lymphocytic leukemia. Br J Haematol 41:9–18, 1979

240. Melo JV, Catovsky D, Galton DAG: The relationship between chronic lymphocytic leukaemia and prolymphocytic leukemia. I. Clinical and laboratory features of 300 patients and characterizations of an intermediate group. Br J Haematol 63:377–387, 1986

241. Melo JV, Catovsky D, Galton DAG: The relationship between chronic lymphocytic leukaemia and prolymphocytic leukaemia. II. Patterns of evolution of "prolymphocytoid" transformation. Br J Haematol 64:77–86, 1986

242. Melo JV, Wardle J, Chetty M, et al: The relationship between chronic lymphocytic leukaemia and prolymphocytic leukaemia. III. Evaluation of cell size by morphology and volume measurements. Br J Haematol 64:469–478, 1986

243. Melo JV, Catovsky D, Gregory WM, et al: The relationship between chronic lymphocytic leukaemia and prolymphocytic leukaemia. IV. Analysis of survival and prognostic features. Br J Haematol 65:23–29, 1987

244. Galton DAG, Goldman JM, Wiltshaw E, et al: Prolymphocytic leukemia. Br J Haematol 27:7–23, 1974

245. Richter MN: Generalized reticular cell sarcoma of lymph nodes associated with lymphocytic leukemia. Am J Pathol 4:285–292, 1928

246. Armitage JO, Dick FR, Corder MP: Diffuse histiocytic lymphoma complicating chronic lymphocytic leukemia. Cancer 41:422–427, 1978

247. Foucar K, Rydell RE: Richter's syndrome in chronic lymphocytic leukemia. Cancer 46:118–134, 1980

248. Robertson LE, Pugh W, O'Brien S, et al: Richter's syndrome: a report on 39 patients. J Clin Oncol 11:1985–1989, 1993

249. Brynes RK, McCourty A, Sun NCJ, et al: Trisomy 12 in Richter's transformation of chronic lymphocytic leukemia. Am J Clin Pathol 104:199–203, 1995

250. Pistoia V, Roncella C, Di Celle PF, et al: Emergence of a B-cell lymphoblastic lymphoma in a patient with B-cell chronic lymphocytic leukemia: evidence for the single-cell origin of the two tumors. Blood 78:797–804, 1991

251. Brecher M, Banks PM: Hodgkin's disease variant of Richter's syndrome. Report of eight cases. Am J Clin Pathol 93:333–339, 1990

252. Lee A, Skelly ME, Kingma DW, Medeiros LJ: B-cell chronic lymphocytic leukemia followed by high grade T-cell lymphoma. An unusual variant of Richter's syndrome. Am J Clin Pathol 103:348–352, 1995

253. Sun NCJ, Fishkin BG, Nies KM, et al: Lymphoplasmacytic myeloma. An immunological, immunohistochemical and electron microscopic study. Cancer 43:2268–2278, 1979

254. Brouet JC, Flandrin G, Sasportes M, et al: Chronic lymphocytic leukemia of T-cell origin. Immunologic and clinical evaluation in eleven patients. Lancet 2:890–893, 1975

255. Newland AC, Catovsky D, Linch D, et al: Chronic T cell lymphocytosis. A review of 21 cases. Br J Haematol 58:433–446, 1984

256. Loughran TP Jr, Kadin ME, Starkbaum G, et al: Leukemia of large granular lymphocytes: association with clonal chromosomal abnormalities and autoimmune neutropenia, thrombocytopenia, and hemolytic anemia. Ann Intern Med 102:169–175, 1985

257. Taniwaki M, Tagawa S, Nishigaki H, et al: Chromosomal abnormalities define clonal proliferation in CD3-large granular lymphocyte leukemia. Am J Hematol 33:32–38, 1990

258. Loughran TP, Starkebaum G, Aprile JA: Rearrangement and expression of T-cell receptor genes in large granular lymphocyte leukemia. Blood 71:822–824, 1988

259. Imamura N, Kusunoki Y, Kawa-ha K, et al: Aggressive natural killer cell leukaemia/lymphoma: report of few cases and review of the literature. Br J Haematol 75:49–59, 1990

260. Sun, NCJ: Hematology: An Atlas and Diagnostic Guide. pp. 323–347. WB Saunders, Philadelphia, 1983

261. Bearman RM, Pangalis GA, Rappaport H: Prolymphocytic leukemia. Clinical, histopathological and cytochemical observations. Cancer 42:2360–2372, 1978

262. Stone RM: Prolymphocytic leukemia. Hematol Oncol Clin North Am 4:457–471, 1990

263. Catovsky D, Galletto J, Okos A, et al: Prolymphocytic leukemia of B and T cell type. Lancet 2:232–234, 1973

264. Matutes E, Brito-Babapulle V, Swansbury J, et al: Clinical and laboratory features of 78 cases of T-prolymphocytic leukemia. Blood 78:3269–3274, 1991

265. Chang KL, Stroup R, Weiss LM: Hairy cell leukemia. Current status. Am J Clin Pathol 97:719–738, 1992

266. Saxon A, Stevens RH, Golde DW: T-lymphocyte variant of hairy cell leukemia. Ann Intern Med 88:323–326, 1978

267. Demeter J, Poloczi K, Foldi J, et al: Immunological and molecular biological identification of a true case of T-hairy cell leukemia. Eur Haematol 43:339–345, 1989

268. Kalyanaraman VS, Sarngadharan MG, Robert-Guroff M, et al: A new subtype of human T-cell leukemia virus (HTLV-II) associated with a T-cell variant of hairy cell leukemia. Science 218:571–573, 1982

269. Yam LT, Li CY, Lam KW: Tartrate-resistant acid phosphatase isoenzyme in the reticulum cells of leukemic reticuloendotheliosis. N Engl J Med 284:357–360, 1971

270. Katayama I, Li CY, Yam LT: Ultrastructural characteristics of the "hairy cells" of leukemic reticuloendotheliosis. Am J Pathol 67:361–370, 1972

271. Sun NCJ: Hematology: An Atlas and Diagnostic Guide. pp. 348–370. WB Saunders, Philadelphia, 1983

272. Burke JS, Rappaport H: The differential diagnosis of hairy cell leukemia in bone marrow and spleen. Semin Oncol 11:334–346, 1984

273. Vardiman JW, Colomb HM: Autopsy findings in hairy cell leukemia. Semin Oncol 11:370–380, 1984

274. Neiman RS, Sullivan AL, Jaffe R: Malignant lymphoma simulating leukemic reticuloendotheliosis. A clinicopathologic study of ten cases. Cancer 43:329–342, 1979

275. Isaacson PG, Matutes E, Burke M, et al: The histopathology of splenic lymphoma with villous lymphocytes. Blood 84:3828–3834, 1994

276. Haglund U, Juliusson G, Stellan B, et al: Hairy cell leukemia is characterized by clonal chromosome abnormalities clustered to specific regions. Blood 83:2637–2645, 1994

277. Sainati L, Matutes E, Mulligan S, et al: A variant form of hairy cell leukemia resistant to α-interferon: clinical and phenotypic characteristics of 17 patients. Blood 76:157–162, 1990

278. Harris NL, Jaffe ES, Stein H, et al: A revised European-American classification of lymphoid neoplasms: a proposal from the international lymphoma study group. Blood 84:1361–1392, 1994

279. Melo JV, Robinson DSF, Gregory C, et al: Splenic B cell lymphoma with "villous" lymphocytes in the peripheral blood: a disorder distinct from hairy cell leukemia. Leukemia 1:294–299, 1987

280. Lutzner M, Edelson R, Schein P, et al: Cutaneous T-cell lymphoma: the Sézary syndrome, mycosis fungoides, and related disorders. Ann Intern Med 83:534–552, 1975

281. Edelson RL, Lutzner MA, Kirkpatrick CH, et al: Morphologic and functional properties of the atypical T lymphocytes of the Sézary syndrome. Mayo Clin Proc 49:558–566, 1974

282. Flandrin G, Brouet JC: The Sézary cell: cytologic, cytochemical, and immunologic studies. Mayo Clin Proc 49:575–583, 1974

283. Salhany KE, Greer JP, Cousar JP, et al: Marrow involvement in cutaneous T-cell lymphoma. A clinicopathologic study of 60 cases. Am J Clin Pathol 92:747–754, 1989

284. Broder S (moderator): T-cell lymphoproliferative syndrome associated with human T-cell leukemia/lymphoma virus. Ann Intern Med 100:543–557, 1984

285. Uchiyama T, Yodoi J, Sagawa K, et al: Adult T-cell leukemia: clinical and hematologic features of 16 cases. Blood 50:481–492, 1977

286. Catovsky D, Greaves MF, Rose M, et al: Adult T-cell lymphoma-leukaemia in blacks from the West Indies. Lancet 1:639–643, 1982

287. Blayney DW, Jaffe ES, Blattner WA, et al: The human T-cell leukemia/lymphoma virus associated with American adult T-cell leukemia/lymphoma. Blood 62:401–405, 1983

288. Kawano F, Yamaguchi K, Nishimura H, et al: Variation in the clinical courses of adult T-cell leukemia. Cancer 55:851–856, 1985

289. Jaffe ES, Blattner WA, Blayney DW, et al: The pathologic spectrum of adult T-cell leukemia/lymphoma in the U.S. Am J Surg Pathol 8:263–275, 1984

290. Tajima K: The T and B-cell malignancy study group and co-authors. The 4th nationwide study of adult T-cell leukemia/lymphoma (ATL) in Japan estimates of risk of ATL and its geographical and clinical features. Int J Cancer 45:237–243, 1990

291. Juneja SK, Wolf MM, Cooper IA: Value of bilateral bone marrow biopsy specimens in non-Hodgkin's lymphoma. J Clin Pathol 43:630–632, 1990

292. Bartl R, Frisch B, Burkhardt R, et al: Lymphoproliferations in the bone marrow: identification and evolution, classification and staging. J Clin Pathol 37:233–254, 1984

293. National Cancer Institute Sponsored Study of Classifications of Non-Hodgkin's Lymphoma: Summary and description of a working formulation for clinical usage. The non-Hodgkin's lymphoma Pathology Classification Project. Cancer 49:2112–2135, 1982

294. Chabner BA, Fisher RI, Young RC, et al: Staging of non-Hodgkin's lymphoma. Semin Oncol 7:285–291, 1980

295. Tura S, Mazza P, Lauria F, et al: Non-Hodgkin's lymphomas in leukemic phase: incidence, prognosis and therapeutic implications. Scand J Haematol 35:123–131, 1985

296. Bartl R, Frisch B, Burkhardt R, et al: Assessment of bone marrow histology in the malignant lymphomas (non-Hodgkin's): correlation with clinical factors for diagnosis, prognosis, classification and staging. Br J Haematol 51:511–530, 1982

297. Lai HS, Tien HF, Hsieh HC, et al: Bone marrow involvement in non-Hodgkin's lymphoma. J Formos Med Assoc 88:114–121, 1989

298. McKenna RW, Hernandez JA: Bone marrow in malignant lymphoma. Hematol Oncol Clin 2:617–635, 1988

299. Foucar K, McKenna RW, Frizzera G, Brunning RD: Bone marrow and blood involvement by lymphoma in relationship to the Lukes-Collins classifications. Cancer 49:888–897, 1982

300. Bartl R, Hansmann M-L, Frisch B, et al: Comparative histology of malignant lymphomas in lymph node and bone marrow. Br J Haematol 69:229–237, 1988

301. Fisher DE, Jacobson JO, Ault KA, et al: Diffuse large cell lymphoma with discordant bone marrow histology. Clinical features and biological implications. Cancer 64:1879–1887, 1989

302. Robertson LE, Redman JR, Butler JJ, et al: Discordant bone marrow involvement in diffuse large-cell lymphoma: a distinct clinical-pathologic entity associated with a continuous risk of relapse. J Clin Oncol 9:236–242, 1991

303. Conlan MG, Bast M, Armitage JO, et al: Bone marrow involvement by non-Hodgkin's lymphoma: the clinical significance of morphologic discordance between the lymph node and bone marrow. J Clin Oncol 8:1163–1172, 1990

304. Ponzoni M, Li C-Y: Isolated bone marrow non-Hodgkin's lymphoma: a clinicopathologic study. Mayo Clin Proc 69:37–43, 1994

305. Bennett JM, Cain KC, Glick JH, et al: The significance of bone marrow involvement in non-Hodgkin's lymphoma: the Eastern Cooperative Oncology Group experience. J Clin Oncol 4:1462–1469, 1986

306. Weisenburger DD, Chan WC: Lymphomas of follicles. Mantle cell and follicular center cell lymphoma, review. Am J Clin Pathol 99:409–420, 1993

307. Weisenburger DD, Duggan MJ, Perry DA, et al: Non-Hodgkin's lymphoma of mantle zone origin. Pathol Annu 26:139–158, 1991

308. Berger F, Felman P, Sonet A, et al: Nonfollicular small B-cell lymphomas: a heterogeneous group of patients with distinct clinical features and outcome. Blood 83:2829–2835, 1994

309. Sheibani K, Burke J, Swartz W, et al: Monocytoid B-cell lymphoma: clinicopathologic study of 21 cases of a unique type of low grade lymphoma. Cancer 62:1531–1538, 1988

310. Nathwani BN, Mohrmann RL, Brynes RK, et al: Monocytoid B-cell lymphomas: an assessment of diagnostic criteria and a perspective on histogenesis. Hum Pathol 23:1061–1071, 1992

311. Traweek ST, Sheibani K: Monocytoid B-cell lymphoma. The biologic and clinical implications of peripheral blood involvement. Am J Clin Pathol 97:591–598, 1992

312. Fisher RI, Dahlberg S, Nathwani BN, et al: A clinical analysis of two indolent lymphoma entities: mantle cell lymphoma and marginal zone lymphoma (including the mucosa-associated lymphoid tissue and monocytoid B-cell subcategories): a Southwest Oncology Group Study. Blood 85:1075–1082, 1995

313. Nathwani BN, Kim H, Rappaport H: Malignant lymphoma, lymphoblastic. Cancer 38:964–983, 1976

314. Nakamine H, Masih AS, Strobach RS: Immunoblastic lymphoma with abundant clear cytoplasm. A comparative study of B-and T-cell types. Am J Clin Pathol 96:177–183, 1991

315. Fraga M, Brousset P, Schlaifer D, et al: Bone marrow involvement in anaplastic large cell lymphoma. Immunohistochemical detection of minimal disease and its prognostic significance. Am J Clin Pathol 103:82–89, 1995

316. Kyle RA: Monoclonal gammopathy of undetermined significance and smoldering myeloma. Eur J Haematol, suppl. 51:70–75, 1989

317. Hansen OP, Galton AG: Classification and prognostic variables in myelomatosis. Scand J Haematol 35:10–19, 1985

318. Wiltshaw E: The natural history of extramedullary plasmacytoma and its relation to solitary myeloma of bone and myelomatosis. Medicine 55:217–238, 1976

319. Dimopoulos MA, Moulopoulos A, Delasalle K, Alexanian R: Solitary plasmacytoma of bone and asymptomatic multiple myeloma. Hematol Oncol Clin North Am 6:359–369, 1992

320. Alexanian R: Localized and indolent myeloma. Blood 56:521–525, 1980

321. Kyle RA: Multiple myeloma. Review of 869 cases. Mayo Clin Proc 50:29–40, 1975

322. Kyle RA: Diagnostic criteria of multiple myeloma. Hematol Oncol Clin North Am 6:347–358, 1992

323. Sun NCJ: Hematology: An Atlas and Diagnostic Guide. pp. 259–287. WB Saunders, Philadelphia, 1983

324. Carter A, Hocherman I, Linn S, et al: Prognostic significance of plasma cell morphology in multiple myeloma. Cancer 60:1060–1065, 1987

325. Bartl R, Frisch B, Fateh-Moghadam A, et al: Histologic classification and staging of multiple myeloma. A retrospective and prospective study of 674 cases. Am J Clin Pathol 87:342–355, 1987

326. Wolf BC, Brady K, O'Murchadha MT, et al: An evaluation of immunohistologic stains for immunoglobulin light chains in bone marrow biopsies in benign and malignant plasma cell proliferations. Am J Clin Pathol 94:742–746, 1990

327. Harada H, Kawano MM, Huang N, et al: Phenotypic difference of normal plasma cells from mature myeloma cells. Blood 81:2658–2663, 1993

328. Kawano MM, Huang N, Harada H, et al: Identification of immature and mature myeloma cells in the bone marrow of human myelomas. Blood 82:564–570, 1993

329. San Miguel JF, Garcia-Sanz R, Gonzalez M, et al: A new staging system for multiple myeloma based on the number of S-phase plasma cells. Blood 85:448–455, 1995

330. Kyle RA: Why better prognostic factors for multiple myeloma are needed. Blood 83:1713–1716, 1994

331. Gould J, Alexander R, Goodacre A, et al: Plasma cell karyotype in multiple myeloma. Blood 71:453–456, 1988

332. Taniwaki M, Nishida K, Takashima T, et al: Nonrandom chromosomal rearrangements of 14q32.3 and 19p13.3 and preferential deletion of 1 p in 21 patients with multiple myeloma and plasma cell leukemia. Blood 84:2283–2290, 1994

333. Kyle RA, Greipp PR: Smoldering multiple myeloma. N Engl J Med 302:1347–1349, 1980

334. Dreicer R, Alexanian R: Nonsecretory multiple myeloma. Am J Hematol 13:313–318, 1982

335. Stone MJ, Frenkel EP: The clinical spectrum of light chain myeloma. A study of 35 patients with special reference to the occurrence of amyloidosis. Am J Med 58:601–619, 1975

336. Shustik C, Bergsagel DE, Pruzanski W: κ and λ light chain disease: survival rates and clinical manifestations. Blood 48:41–51, 1976

337. Driedger H, Pruzanski W: Plasma cell neoplasia with osteosclerotic lesions. A study of five cases and a review of the literature. Arch Intern Med 139:892–896, 1979

338. Bardwick PA, Zvaifler NJ, Gill GN, et al: Plasma cell dyscrasia with polyneuropathy, organomegaly, endocrinopathy, M protein and skin changes: the POEMS syndrome. Report on two cases and review of the literature. Medicine 59:311–322, 1980

339. Miralles GD, O'Fallon JR, Talley NJ: Plasma cell dyscrasia with polyneuropathy. The spectrum of POEMS syndrome. N Engl J Med 327:1919–1923, 1992

340. Kosmo MA, Gale RP: Plasma cell leukemia. Semin Hematol 24:202–208, 1987

341. Noel P, Kyle RA: Plasma cell leukemia: an evolution of response to therapy. Am J Med 83:1062–1068, 1987

342. Wolf BC, Kumar A, Vera JC, et al: Bone marrow morphology and immunology in systemic amyloidosis. Am J Clin Pathol 86:84–88, 1986

343. Kyle RA, Gertz MA: Primary systemic amyloidosis: clinical and laboratory features in 474 cases. Semin Hematol 32:45–59, 1995

344. Harris NL, Bhan AK: B cell neoplasms of the lymphocytic, lymphoplasmacytoid and plasma cell types: immunohistologic analysis and clinical correlation. Hum Pathol 16:829–837, 1985

345. Kyle RA, Garton KP: The spectrum of IgM monoclonal gammopathy of 430 cases. Mayo Clin Proc 62:719–731, 1987

346. Feiner HD, Rizk CC, Finfer MD, et al: IgM monoclonal gammopathy/Waldenstrom's macroglobulinemia: a morphological and immunophenotypic study of the bone marrow. Mod Pathol 3:348–356, 1990

347. Seligmann M, Mihaesco E, Preudhomme JL, et al: Heavy chain diseases: current findings and concepts. Immunol Rev 48:145–167, 1979

348. Bloch KJ, Lee L, Mills JA, et al: Gamma heavy chain disease—an expanding clinical and laboratory spectrum. Am J Med 55:61–70, 1973

349. Kyle RA, Greipp PR, Banks PM: The diverse picture of gamma heavy chain disease: report of seven cases and review of literature. Mayo Clin Proc 59:439–451, 1981

350. Fermand JP, Brouet JC, Danon F, et al: Gamma heavy chain "disease": heterogeneity of the clinicopathologic features. Report of 16 cases and review of the literature. Medicine (Baltimore) 68:321–335, 1989

351. Seligmann M: Immunochemical, clinical and pathological features of α-chain disease. Arch Intern Med 135:78–82, 1975

352. Price SK: Immunoproliferative small intestinal disease: a study of 13 cases with alpha heavy-chain disease. Histopathology 17:7–17, 1990

353. Franklin EC: Mu-chain disease. Arch Intern Med 135:71–72, 1975

354. Sun NCJ: Hematology: An Atlas and Diagnostic Guide. pp. 398–425. WB Saunders, Philadelphia, 1983

355. Bodem CR, Hamory BH, Taylor HM, Kleopfer L: Granulomatous bone marrow disease. A review of the literature and clinicopathologic analysis of 58 cases. Medicine (Baltimore) 62:372–383, 1983

356. Choe JK, Hyun BH, Salazar GH, et al: Epithelioid granulomas of the bone marrow in non-Hodgkin's lymphoproliferative malignancies. Am J Clin Pathol 80:19–24, 1983

357. Jagadha V, Andavolu RH, Huang CT: Granulomatous inflammation in the acquired immune deficiency syndrome. Am J Clin Pathol 84:598–602, 1985

358. Karcher DS, Frost AR: The bone marrow in human immunodeficiency virus (HIV)-related disease. Morphology and clinical correlation. Am J Clin Pathol 95:63–71, 1991

359. Sun NCJ, Shapshak P, Lachant NA, et al: Bone marrow examination in patients with AIDS and AIDS-related complex (ARC). Morphologic and in situ hybridization studies. Am J Clin Pathol 92:589–594, 1989

360. Heyman MR, Rasmussen P: Pneumocystis carinii involvement of bone marrow in acquired immunodeficiency syndrome. Am J Clin Pathol 87:780–783, 1987

361. Okun DB, Sun NCJ, Tanaka KR: Bone marrow granulomas in Q fever. Am J Clin Pathol 71:117–121, 1979

362. Castella A, Croxson TS, Mildvan D, et al: The bone marrow in AIDS: a histologic, hematologic, and microbiologic study. Am J Clin Pathol 84:425–432, 1985

363. Schneider DR, Picker LJ: Myelodysplasia in the acquired immune deficiency syndrome. Am J Clin Pathol 84:144–152, 1985

364. Stricker RB: Hemostatic abnormalities in HIV disease. Hematol Oncol Clin North Am 5:249–265, 1991

365. Yospur LS, Sun NCJ, Figueroa P, Niihara Y: Concurrent thrombotic thrombocytopenic purpura and immune thrombocytopenic purpura in an HIV positive patient: a case report and a review of the literature. Am J Hematol 50:73–78, 1996

366. Farhi DC, Mason UG III, Horsburgh CR: The bone marrow in disseminated Mycobacterium avium-intracellulare infection. Am J Clin Pathol 83:463–468, 1985

367. Godwin JH, Stopeck A, Chang VT, et al: Mycobacteremia in acquired immune deficiency syndrome. Rapid diagnosis based on inclusions in the peripheral blood smear. Am J Clin Pathol 95:369–375, 1991

368. Levine AM: AIDS-related lymphoma review. Blood 80:1–12, 1992

369. Knowles DM, Chamulak GA, Subar M, et al: Lymphoid neoplasia associated with the acquired immunodeficiency syndrome (AIDS): the New York University Medical Center experience with 105 patients (1981–1986). Ann Intern Med 108:744–753, 1988

370. Ziegler JL, Beckstead JA, Volberding PA, et al: Non-Hodgkin's lymphoma in 90 homosexual men. Relation to generalized lymphadenopathy and the acquired immune deficiency syndrome (AIDS). N Engl J Med 311:565–570, 1984

371. Prior E, Goldberg AF, Conjalka MS, et al: Hodgkin's disease in homosexual man. An AIDS-related phenomenon? Am J Med 81:1085–1088, 1986.

372. Conran RM, Granger E, Reddy VB: Kaposi's sarcoma of the bone marrow. Arch Pathol Lab Med 110:1083–1085, 1986

373. Rywlin AM, Ortega R: Lipid granulomas of the bone marrow. Am J Clin Pathol 57:457–462, 1972

374. Kaplan HS: Hodgkin's disease: biology, treatment, prognosis review. Blood 57:813–822, 1981

375. Hsu S-M, Yang K, Jaffe ES: Phenotypic expression of Hodgkin's and Reed-Sternberg cells in Hodgkin's disease. Am J Pathol 118:209–217, 1985

376. Webb DI, Urogy G, Silver RT: Importance of bone marrow biopsy in the clinical staging of Hodgkin's disease. Cancer 26:313–317, 1970

377. Rosenberg SA: Hodgkin's disease of the bone marrow. Cancer Res 31:1733–1736, 1971

378. Myers CE, Chabner BA, De Vita VT, et al: Bone marrow involvement in Hodgkin's disease: pathology and response to MOPP chemotherapy. Blood 44:197–204, 1974

379. Bartl R, Frisch B, Burkhardt R, et al: Assessment of bone marrow histology in Hodgkin's disease. Correlation with clinical factors. Br J Haematol 51:345–360, 1982

380. Kinney NC, Greer JP, Stein RS, et al: Lymphocyte-depletion Hodgkin's disease. Histopathologic diagnosis of marrow involvement. Am J Surg Pathol 10:219–226, 1986

381. Bearman RM, Pangalis GA, Rappaport H: Hodgkin's disease, lymphocytic depletion type. A clinicopathologic study of 39 patients. Cancer 41:293–302, 1978

382. Neiman RS, Rosen PJ, Lukes RJ: Lymphocyte depletion Hodgkin's disease: a clinicopathologic entity. N Engl J Med 288:751–754, 1973

383. Lukes RJ: Criteria for involvement of lymph node, bone marrow, spleen and liver in Hodgkin's disease. Cancer Res 31:1755–1767, 1971

384. Rappaport H, Berard CW, Butler JJ, et al: Report of the committee on histopathological criteria contributing to staging of Hodgkin's disease. Cancer Res 31:1864–1865, 1971

385. Korman LY, Smith JR, Landaw SA, Davey FR: Hodgkin's disease: intramedullary phagocytosis with pancytopenia. Ann Intern Med 91:60–61, 1979

386. Kadin ME, Donaldson SS, Dorfman RF: Isolated granulomas in Hodgkin's disease. N Engl J Med 283:859–861, 1970

387. Sacks EL, Donaldson SS, Gordon J, Dorfman RF: Epithelioid granulomas associated with Hodgkin's disease: clinical correlations in 55 previously untreated patients. Cancer 41:562–567, 1978

388. Lukes RJ, Tindle BH: Immunoblastic lymphadenopathy. A hyperimmune entity resembling Hodgkin's disease. N Engl J Med 292:1–8, 1975

389. Frizzera G, Moran EM, Rappaport H: Angioimmunoblastic lymphadenopathy: diagnosis and clinical course. Am J Med 59:803–818, 1975

390. Neiman RS, Dervan P, Haudenschild C, Jaffe R: Angioimmunoblastic lymphadenopathy: an ultrastructural and immunologic study with review of the literature. Cancer 41:507–518, 1978

391. Pangalis GA, Moran EM, Rappaport H: Blood and bone marrow findings in angioimmunoblastic lymphadenopathy. Blood 51:71–83, 1978

392. Schnaidt U, Vykoupil KF, Thiele J, Georgii A: Angioimmunoblastic lymphadenopathy. Histopathology of bone marrow involvement. Virchows Arch A Pathol Anat Histol 389:369–380, 1980

393. Kaneko Y, Naseki N, Sakurai M, et al: Characteristic karyotypic pattern in T-cell lymphoproliferative disorders with reactive angioimmunoblastic lymphadenopathy with dysproteinemia-type features. Blood 72:413–421, 1988

394. Frizzera G, Kaneko Y, Sakurai M: Angioimmunoblastic lymphadenopathy and related disorders: a retrospective look in search of definitions. Leukemia 3:1–5, 1989

395. Nathwani BN, Rappaport H, Moran EM, Pangalis GA, Kim H: Malignant lymphoma arising in angioimmunoblastic lymphadenopathy. Cancer 41:578–606, 1978

396. Hanson CA, Brunning RD, Gajl-Peczalska KJ, et al: Bone marrow manifestations of peripheral T-cell lymphoma. A study of 30 cases. Am J Clin Pathol 86:449–460, 1986

397. Horning SJ, Weiss LM, Crabtree GS, et al: Clinical and phenotypic diversity of T-cell lymphomas. Blood 67:1578–1582, 1986

398. Armitage JO, Greer JP, Levine AM, et al: Peripheral T-cell lymphoma. Cancer 63:158–163, 1989

399. Caulet S, Delmer A, Audouin J, et al: Histopathological study of bone marrow biopsies in 30 cases of T-cell lymphoma with clinical, biological and survival correlations. Hematol Oncol 8:155–168, 1990

400. White DM, Smith AG, Whitehouse JMA, Smith JL: Peripheral T-cell lymphoma: value of bone marrow trephine immunophenotyping. J Clin Pathol 42:403–408, 1989

401. Gaulard P, Kanavaros P, Farcet J-P, et al: Bone marrow histologic and immunohistochemical findings in peripheral T-cell lymphoma: a study of 38 cases. Hum Pathol 22:331–338, 1991

402. Chott A, Augustin I, Wrba F, et al: Peripheral T-cell lymphomas: a clinicopathologic study of 75 cases. Hum Pathol 21:1117–1125, 1990

403. Auger MJ, Nash JRG, Mackie MJ: Marrow involvement with T-cell lymphoma initially presenting as abnormal myelopoiesis. J Clin Pathol 39:134–137, 1986

404. Jaffe ES, Costa J, Fauci AS, et al: Malignant lymphoma and erythrophagocytosis simulating malignant histiocytosis. Am J Med 75:741–749, 1983

405. Falini B, Pileri S, De Solas I, et al: Peripheral T-cell lymphoma associated with hemophagocytic syndrome. Blood 75:434–444, 1990

406. Su I-J, Hsieh HC: Clinicopathological spectrum of Epstein-Barr virus-associated T-cell malignancies. Leukemia Lymphoma 7:47–53, 1992

407. Lichtman MA: Basophilopenia, basophilia, and mastocytosis. pp. 852–858. In Beutler E, Lichtman MA, Coller BS, Kipps TJ (eds): William's Hematology. 5th Ed. McGraw-Hill, New York, 1995

408. Lennert K, Parwaresch MR: Mast cells and mast cell neoplasia: a review. Histopathology 3:349–365, 1979

409. Travis WD, Li C-Y, Hoagland HC, et al: Mast cell leukemia: report of a case and review of the literature. Mayo Clin Proc 61:957–966, 1986

410. Travis WD, Li C-Y, Bergstralh EJ, et al: Systemic mast cell disease. Analysis of 58 cases and literature review. Medicine (Baltimore) 67:345–368, 1988

411. Rywlin AM, Hoffman EP, Ortega RS: Eosinophilic fibrohistiocytic lesion of bone marrow: a distinct new morphologic finding, probably related to drug hypersensitivity. Blood 40:464–472, 1972

412. Te Velde J, Vismans FJFE, Leenheers-Binnendijk L, et al: The eosinophilic fibrohistiocytic lesion of the bone marrow: a mastocellular lesion in bone disease. Virchows Arch [Pathol Anat] 377:277–235, 1978

413. Rwylin AM: Mastocytic eosinophilic fibrohistiocytic lesion of the bone marrow. Histopathology 24:1–4, 1982

414. Horny H-P, Parwaresch MR, Lennert K: Bone marrow findings in systemic mastocytosis. Hum Pathol 16:808–814, 1985

415. Travis WD, Li C-Y, Yam LT, et al: Significance of systemic mast cell disease with associated hematologic disorders. Cancer 62:965–972, 1988

416. Horny HP, Kaiserling E: Lymphoid cells and tissue mast cells of bone marrow lesions in systemic mastocytosis: a histological and immunohistological study. Br J Haematol 69:449–455, 1988

417. Cline MJ: Histiocytes and histiocytosis, review. Blood 84:2840–2853, 1994

418. Foucar K, Foucar E: The mononuclear phagocyte and immunoregulatory effector (M-PIRE) system. Evolving concepts. Semin Diagn Pathol 7:4–18, 1990

419. The Writing Group of the Histiocytic Society: Histiocytosis syndromes in children. Lancet 1:208–209, 1987

420. Sawitsky A, Rosner F, Chodsky S: The sea-blue histiocyte syndrome, a review: genetic and biochemical studies. Semin Hematol 9:285–297, 1972

421. Dosik H, Rosner F, Sawitsky A: Acquired lipidosis: Gaucher-like cells

and "blue cells" in chronic granulocytic leukemia. Semin Hematol 9:309–316, 1972

422. Matzner Y, Behar A, Beeri E, et al: Systemic leishmaniasis mimicking malignant histiocytosis. Cancer 43:398–402, 1979

423. Risdall RJ, Brunning RD, Hernandez JI, et al: Bacteria-associated hemophagocytic syndrome. Cancer 54:2968–2972, 1984

424. Auerbach M, Haubenstock A, Soloman G: Systemic babesiosis. Another cause of the hemophagocytic syndrome. Am J Med 80:301–303, 1986

425. Chen R-L, Su I-J, Lin K-H, et al: Fulminant childhood hemophagocytic syndrome mimicking histiocytic medullary reticulosis. An atypical form of Epstein-Barr virus infection. Am J Clin Pathol 96:171–176, 1991

426. Risdall RJ, McKenna RW, Nesbit ME, et al: Virus-associated hemophagocytic syndrome: a benign histiocytic proliferation distinct from malignant histiocytosis. Cancer 44:993–1002, 1979

427. Mroczek EC, Weisenburger DD, Grierson L, et al: Fatal infectious mononucleosis and virus-associated hemophagocytic syndrome. Arch Pathol Lab Med 111:530–535, 1987

428. Reiner AP, Spivak JL: Hematophagic histiocytosis. A report of 23 new patients and a review of the literature. Medicine 67:369–388, 1988

429. Campo E, Condom E, Miro M-J, et al: Tuberculosis-associated hemophagocytic syndrome. A systemic process. Cancer 58:2640–2645, 1986

430. Wieczorek R, Greco MA, McCarthy K, et al: Familial erythrophagocytic lymphohistiocytosis: immunophenotypic, immunohistochemical, and ultrastructural demonstration of the relation to sinus histiocytes. Hum Pathol 17:55–63, 1986

431. Favara BE: Hemophagocytic lymphohistiocytosis: a hemophagocytic syndrome. Semin Diagn Pathol 9:63–74, 1992

432. James JP, Stass SS, Peterson V, et al: Abnormalities of bone marrow simulating histiocytic medullary reticulosis in a patient with gastric carcinomas. Am J Clin Pathol 71:600–602, 1979

433. Monoharan A, Catovsky D, Lampert I, et al: Histiocytic medullary reticulosis complicating chronic lymphocytic leukemia: malignant or reactive: Scand J Haematol 26:5–13, 1981

434. Ducatman BS, Wick MR, Morgan TW, et al: Malignant histiocytosis: a clinical, histologic, and immunohistochemical study of 20 cases. Hum Pathol 15:368–377, 1984

435. Ven der Valk P, Meijer CJLM, Willemze R, et al: Histiocytic sarcoma (true histiocytic lymphoma): a clinicopathologic study of 20 cases. Histopathology 8:105–123, 1984

436. Colon-Otero G, Li C-Y, Dewald GW, et al: Erthrophagocytic acute lymphocytic leukemia with B-cell markers and with a 20q– chromosome abnormality. Mayo Clin Proc 59:678–682, 1984

437. Falini B, Bucciarelli E, Grigani F, et al: Erythrophagocytosis by undifferentiated lung carcinoma cells. Cancer 46:1140–1145, 1980

438. Fitchen JH, Lee S: Phagocytic myeloma cells. Am J Clin Pathol 71:722–723, 1979

439. Kadin ME, Kamoun M, Lamberg J: Erythrophagocytic T-gamma lymphoma: a clinicopathologic entity resembling malignant histiocytosis. N Engl J Med 304:648–653, 1981

440. Su I-J, Hsu Y-H, Lin M-T, et al: Epstein-Barr virus containing T-cell lymphoma presents with hemophagocytic syndrome mimicking malignant histiocytosis. Cancer 72:2019–2027, 1993

441. Nezelof C, Barbey S, Gogusev J, et al: Malignant histiocytosis in childhood: a distinctive CD30-positive clinicopathological entity associated with a chromosomal translocation involving 5q35. Semin Diagn Pathol 9:75–89, 1992

442. Gonzalez CL, Jaffe ES: The histiocytoses: clinical presentation and differential diagnosis. Oncology 4:47–60, 1990

443. Ben-Ezra JM, Choo CH: Langerhans' cell histiocytosis and malignancies of the M-PIRE system, review. Am J Clin Pathol 99:464–471, 1993

444. Wilson MS, Weiss LM, Gatter KC, et al: Malignant histiocytosis. A reassessment of cases previously reported in 1975 based on paraffin section immunophenotyping studies. Cancer 66:530–536, 1990

445. Kadin ME, Sako D, Berliner N, et al: Childhood Ki-1 lymphoma presenting with skin lesions and peripheral lymphadenopathy. Blood 68:1042–1049, 1986

446. Kaneko Y, Frizzera G, Edamura S, et al: A noval translocation t(2;5) (p23;q35) in childhood phagocytic large T-cell lymphoma mimicking malignant histiocytosis. Blood 73:806–813, 1989

447. Weiss LM, Trela MJ, Cleary ML: Frequent immunoglobulin and T-cell receptor rearrangement in "histiocytic" neoplasms. Am J Pathol 121:369–373, 1985

448. Hanson CA, Jaszcz W, Kersey JH, et al: True histiocytic lymphoma: histopathologic, immunophenotypic and genotypic analysis. Br J Haematol 73:187–198, 1989

449. Lichentein L: Histiocytosis X: integration of eosinophilic granuloma of bone. "Letterer-Siwe disease" and "Schuller-Christian disease" as related manifestations of a single nosologic entity. Arch Pathol 56:84–102, 1953

450. McMillan EM, Humphrey GB, Stoneking L, et al: Analysis of histiocytosis X infiltrates with monoclonal antibodies directed against cells of histiocytic, lymphoid, and myeloid lineage. Clin Immunol Immunopathol 3:295–301, 1986

451. Dehner LP: Morphologic findings in the histiocytic syndromes. Semin Oncol 18:3–7, 1991

452. Ben-Ezra J, Bailey A, Azumi N, et al: Malignant histiocytosis X. A distinct clinicopathologic entity. Cancer 68:1050–1060, 1991

453. Willman CL, Busque L, Griffity B, et al: Langerhans'-cell histiocytosis [histiocytosis X]—a clonal proliferative disease. N Engl J Med 331:154–160, 1994

454. Savage RA, Hoffman GC, Shaker K: Diagnostic problems involved in detection of metastatic neoplasms by bone marrow aspirate compared with needle biopsy. Am J Clin Pathol 70:623–627, 1978

455. Pittman G, Tung KSK, Hoffman GC: Metastatic cells in bone marrow: study of 83 cases. Cleve Clin Q 38:55–64, 1971

456. Anner RM, Drewinko B: Frequency and significance of bone marrow involvement by metastatic solid tumors. Cancer 39:1337–1344, 1977

457. Leland J, MacPherson B: Hematologic findings in cases of mammary cancer metastatic to bone marrow. Am J Clin Pathol 71:31–35, 1979

458. Sun NCJ: Hematology: An Atlas and Diagnostic Guide. pp. 158–172. WB Saunders, Philadelphia, 1983

459. Bearden JD, Ratkin GA, Coltman CA: Comparison of the diagnostic value of bone marrow biopsy and bone marrow aspiration in neoplastic disease. J Clin Pathol 27:738–740, 1974

460. Papac RJ: Bone marrow metastases, review. Cancer 74:2403–2413, 1994

461. Colvin BT, Revell PA, Ibbotson RM, et al: Necrosis of bone marrow and bone in malignant disease. Clin Oncol 6:265–272, 1980

462. Rubins JM: The role of myelofibrosis in malignant leukoerythroblastosis. Cancer 51:308–311, 1983

463. Pui C-H, Stass S, Green A: Bone marrow necrosis in children with malignant disease. Cancer 56:1522–1525, 1985

464. Gallivan MVE, Lokich JJ: Carcinocythemia (carcinoma cell leukemia). Report of two cases with English literature review. Cancer 53:1100–1102, 1984

465. Hansen PV, Andersen J, Mygind H: Bone marrow necrosis: report of a case and a brief review of the literature. Acta Med Scand 214:331–336, 1983

466. Kiraly JF III, Wheby MS: Bone marrow necrosis. Am J Med 60:361–368, 1976

467. Cowan JD, Rubin RN, Kies MS, et al: Bone marrow necrosis. Cancer 46:2168–2171, 1980

468. Vesteby A, Jensen OM: Aseptic bone/bone marrow necrosis in leukaemia. Scand J Haematol 35:354–357, 1985

469. Cassileth PA, Brooks JSJ: The prognostic significance of

myelonecrosis after induction therapy in acute leukemia. Cancer 60:2363–2365, 1987

470. Mehta K, Pawel BR, Gadol C: Bone marrow necrosis in leukemic phase follicular lymphoma. Arch Pathol Lab Med 115:89–92, 1991

471. Brown CH: Bone marrow necrosis in a study of seventy cases. Johns Hopkins Med J 131:189–203, 1972

472. Dann EJ, Gillis S, Polliack A, et al: Tumor lysis syndrome following treatment with 2-chlorodeoxyadenosine for refractory chronic lymphocytic leukemia. N Engl J Med 329:1547–1548, 1993

473. Krause JR: Value of bone marrow biopsy in the diagnosis of amyloidosis. South Med J 70:1072–74, 1977

474. Kwaan HC: Clinicopathologic features of thrombotic thrombocytopenic purpura. Semin Hematol 24:71–81, 1987

475. Pierce JR, Wren MV, Cousar JB: Cholesterol embolism: diagnosis antemortem by bone marrow biopsy. Ann Intern Med 89:937–938, 1978

476. Franzman C, Bennett JM: Classification of acute leukemias. Contemp Oncol 2:46–54, 1992

22

Non-Neoplastic Diseases of Bones and Joints

Peter G. Bullough

This chapter discusses both the special problems that relate to the interpretation of bone lesions and, briefly, the more common orthopedic diseases that may come across the surgical pathologist's desk.

METHODS OF EXAMINATION

A major problem in dealing with bone specimens is the preparation of reasonable histologic sections. In many laboratories bone tissue is either overdecalcified or the acid is inadequately removed; in both cases poor staining results. In our laboratory, after sectioning of the bone into slices 3 to 5 mm thick and adequate fixation with buffered formalin, decalcification is achieved with 5 percent nitric acid. The volume of acid should be at least 10 times that of the tissue, and because the acid is neutralized as the calcium is removed from the tissue, the acid must be changed twice a day. To ensure access of the acid to the tissue, gentle agitation is provided by means of a shaker. By using this technique, most bones are decalcified in 1 or 2 days. After decalcification adequate washing is essential; otherwise good differentiation of the hematoxylin and eosin (H&E) stain is not possible. We have found that better sections of bone are obtained after vacuum embedding. This is very simply arranged and well worth the effort involved.

Gross

Bone specimens received by the surgical pathologist often consist only of fragments, the anatomic site of which cannot be recognized. By contrast, when a larger piece of bone is submitted, anatomic landmarks should be carefully sought. Large specimens should be cut into parallel slices 4 or 5 mm thick with a band saw, so the interior appearance of the bone may be examined.

On occasion, the color of the bone may be particularly helpful; for example, necrotic bone is an opaque yellow, in contrast to the rather translucent and pink appearance of living bone. A generalized or localized increase in porosity or sclerosis should be sought. When multiple pieces are received, the pieces chosen for embedding should be preferably those that appear to show the most departure from normal.

A particularly useful adjunct to gross examination is the preparation of radiographs of the surgical specimens with low voltage x-rays (Faxitron x-ray machine) and industrial film (Kodalith Ortho film, type 3). These radiographs not only help in choosing the areas to section but also are frequently helpful in the interpretation of histologic material, for example, in bone-forming tumors, finding a nidus in osteoid osteoma, or defining an infarct (Fig. 22-1). Because bone and cartilage are somewhat translucent, it is frequently difficult to get acceptable black and white photographs. This problem can be overcome by using a monochromatic short wave light source, such as ultraviolet.[1]

Microscopic

The histologist uses various staining techniques to demonstrate the components of the matrix.

The collagen may be demonstrated by a trichrome stain or van Gieson's stain and also by the use of polarized light. This latter technique is particularly useful because it not only clearly shows the collagen fibers but also allows us to determine the orientation of the collagen and to study the microarchitecture of the tissue.[2,3]

The proteoglycans can be demonstrated by the use of safranin O or alcian blue stains and less specifically by toluidine blue and periodic acid-Schiff (PAS) stains.[4]

Mineral components can only be demonstrated in undemineralized tissue. It is possible, by embedding the tissue in plastic and using specially hardened knives, to cut histologic sections that still contain the minerals within the bone matrix. The mineral may be stained by two techniques: alizarin red, which will stain the calcium components of the hydroxyapatite, and the von Kossa method, which will stain the phosphate component. The distribution of mineral in the tissue may also be studied by the technique of microradiology.[5] By using low kilovoltage x-rays from an x-ray tube with a very fine focal spot, radiographs are made from thin slices of bone, which have been cut with a diamond saw at approximately 100 mm. Undecalcified sections are particularly important in the assessment of metabolic disturbances.

An essential component in interpretation of bone and joint histology is careful correlation with the clinical radiographs and history.

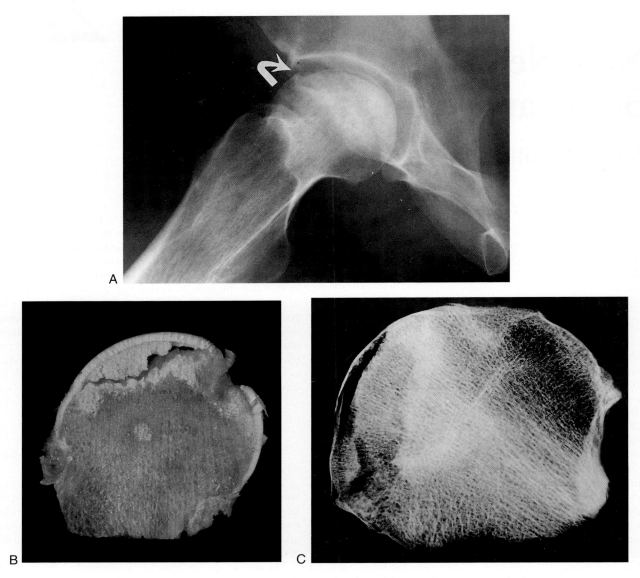

Fig. 22-1. **(A)** Radiograph of the hip of a young person with sickle cell disease. There is segmental infarction of the superior portion of the femoral head recognized radiologically by the presence of a small step-fracture at the lateral margin of the femoral head (arrow) and a radiolucent crescent on the superior surface of the femoral head just beneath the articular surface. **(B)** Photograph of a frontal section through a femoral head resected because of pain. The infarcted area is clearly differentiated from the surrounding bone by its opaque yellow-white appearance. At the margin of the infarct there is hyperemia, and there is a fracture extending from the articular surface through the infarcted bone. **(C)** Radiograph of the specimen shown in Fig. B demonstrates that the margin of the infarct is sclerotic. This sclerosis is the result of reparative bone formation. (See also Figs. 22-9 and 22-10.)

BONES AND BONE TISSUE

Bones

Bone structure[6,7] may be briefly summarized as follows. Each bone has a delimiting shell or cortex, which varies in thickness from bone to bone and from area to area within a given bone. The interior of a bone is occupied by a varying amount of porous, cancellous bone tissue. The proportion of cortical to cancellous bone reflects the mechanical requirements of the bone as a whole. In the spaces between the plates and rods of cancellous bone are blood vessels, nerve fibers, fat, and hematopoietic tissue. In the adult most of the hematopoietic tissue is confined to the axial skeleton (spine, pelvis, and shoulder girdles). However, occasionally hematopoietic tissue may be seen in the femoral head or humeral head. By contrast, in the infant the entire skeleton contains hematopoietic tissue. During growth the hematopoietic tissue in the appendicular skeleton (arms and legs) is slowly replaced by fat advancing proximally until the adult state is reached.

Except for the insertion of the tendons and the articular ends of the bone, the cortex is covered by a thin layer of dense fibrous tissue, the periosteum. The periosteal layer adjacent to the bone, the cambium layer, has bone-forming potential. This potential becomes apparent after trauma and infection and in association with certain tumors. In the child the periosteum is only loosely attached to the underlying bone, whereas in the adult it is firmly attached; this accounts for the more extensive periosteal reaction seen in children as compared with adults.

The terms *epiphysis, metaphysis,* and *diaphysis* are used to designate regions of bones. The epiphysis is the portion of the bone that lies between the joint and the site of the growth plate; the metaphysis is the region of bone adjacent to the growing side of the growth plate; and the diaphysis is the portion of the bone between the growth plates.

Bone Tissue

In studying and interpreting bone connective tissues,[8,9] it is important to realize that unlike parenchymal organs, the bulk of which is formed of cells, the bulk of connective tissue is made up largely of an extracellular matrix, and the cells represent only a small percentage of the tissue bulk. Bone, cartilage, and fibrous connective tissues differ not only grossly and microscopically but also in their mechanical properties. This variation reflects the variable composition of their extracellular matrices; for example, tendons, whose function is to resist tension, are formed mainly of well oriented parallel bundles of collagen. By contrast, cartilage and bone, which are subject to compression, have in addition to collagen either large molecules of proteoglycan (cartilage) or hydroxyapatite crystals (bone). These substances, restrained by the collagen running between them, resist compressive forces and provide rigidity to the tissue.

Microscopic examination reveals two possible appearances of bone tissue. In lamellar bone, the type found normally, the collagen is in sheets of parallel fibers, stacked one upon another, giving rise in cross-section to a striped appearance, which can be heightened by polarized light. The bone cells (osteocytes) are widely separated from each other, and the osteocytic lacunae are flattened (Fig. 22-2).

In the fetus and in conditions in which the metabolism of the skeleton is accelerated, such as fracture repair, periosteal reactions, parathyroid dysfunction, and tumors, the collagen is arranged haphazardly, again made more apparent by examination with polarized light. The osteocytes are more closely packed together, and the lacunae are larger and rounder than those seen in lamellar bone. This type of bone is called woven bone, fiber bone, or immature bone (Fig. 22-3). (It is incorrect to refer to this type of bone as osteoid, as is often done.)

Recognition of these two types of bone tissue is very important to the surgical pathologist in the interpretation of bone disease.

It is also important to look for other alterations in the intercellular matrix resulting from trauma or metabolic disturbances such as disruption of the collagen fibers, with or without repair, metaplastic changes in the type of matrix being produced, microcystic changes, and so on; here again examination with polarized light is extremely helpful.

Bone Cells

The skeleton is not merely an inanimate structure serving a mechanical need; it is composed of living, constantly changing tissue involved in both skeletal homeostasis, with the capability of growth and repair, and mineral homeostasis. These processes are effected through the bone cells, which include the osteoblasts, the osteocytes, and the osteoclasts.[8,9]

Osteoblasts

Osteoblasts are the cells responsible for the synthesis of bone matrix. They form a continuous covering over the bone tissue, and at any particular time they may be either actively forming bone or inactive. The active cells are plump and crowded along the bone surface, whereas inactive osteoblasts are flat and inconspicuous. In those areas where bone is actively being made, the cells lie on a thin, smooth layer of unmineralized bone matrix called osteoid. The junction between the mineralized bone and the unmineralized osteoid at the surface is often marked in H&E-stained sections by a basophilic line indicating the mineralization front.

Osteocytes

Osteoblasts, when incorporated into the bone after the process of matrix formation, are called osteocytes. The osteocytes are connected with one another and also with the surface of the bone by an intricate network of canals, the osteocytic canaliculi. Through these canaliculi cytoplasmic processes extend from osteocyte to osteocyte and also to the osteoblasts on the surface, making tight junctions with one another. The elaborate structure of the osteocytic network strongly suggests a metabolic function, probably for mineral homeostasis.

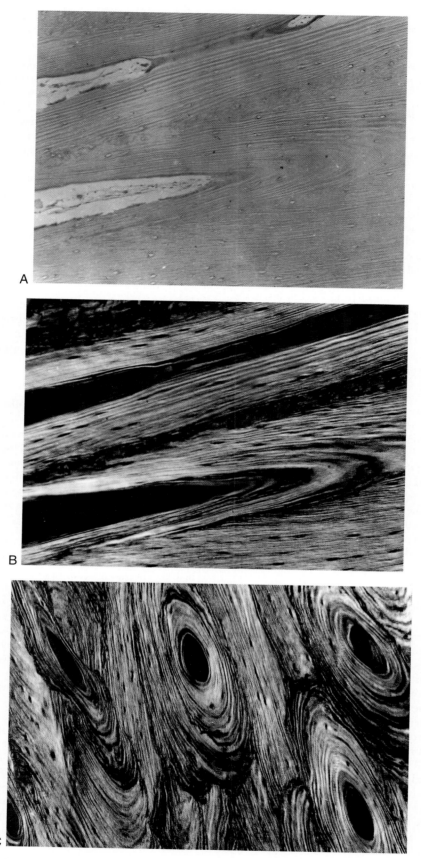

Fig. 22-2. **(A)** Photomicrograph of lamellar bone. Note the distribution of the osteocytes in the orientation of the lamellae. **(B)** Same field as in Fig. A but examined under polarized light. **(C)** Cortical bone in transverse section to demonstrate the osteons. (Polarized light microscopy.)

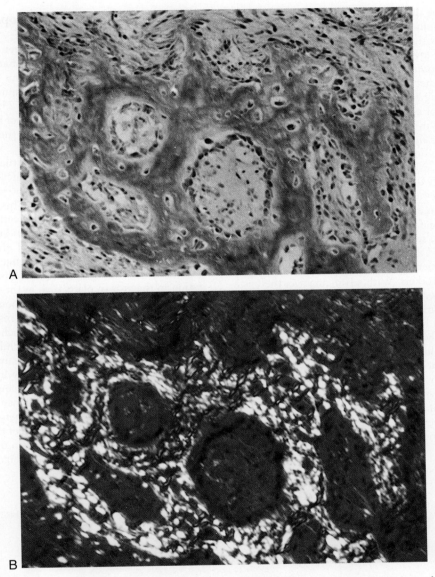

Fig. 22-3. Photomicrograph of a section taken from fracture callus to demonstrate the appearance of woven bone. Note the irregularity of the bone trabeculae that are being formed, the prominent osteoblasts and osteocytes, and the collagen fibers arranged in a basketweave pattern. **(A)** Transmitted light. **(B)** Polarized light. (H&E.)

Osteoclasts

Those portions of the bone surface undergoing resorption have an irregular, gnawed-out appearance. Covering this irregular surface are mononuclear and sometimes multinucleate osteoclasts. By electron microscopy these cells are seen to have ruffled borders on the surface facing the bone, numerous cytoplasmic vesicles, lysosomal bodies, and mitochondria, but unlike osteoblasts, little endoplasmic reticulum. In sections of normal bone, multinucleate osteoclasts are rarely seen, although irregular resorbing surfaces are apparent over about 7 to 20 percent of the total bone surface. The absence of multinucleate osteoclasts from normal bone may simply reflect the fact that giant

cells are obvious only when resorption is proceeding at an extraordinary or pathologic rate.

Bone Physiology

As already indicated, the bones have two quite different basic functions: (1) mechanical, providing for movement and protection, and (2) maintenance of the "milieu interieur," especially with respect to plasma calcium, phosphorus, and magnesium. As a consequence, the bone and bone tissue are a compromise in both form and structure.

The formation and resorption of bone continue throughout

life, and in normal bone these processes are more or less in balance. Microscopic examination will often show one surface of a trabeculum to be smooth with a layer of active osteoblasts, while the other shows irregular resorption (Fig. 22-4). In this way, spatial reorganization of the cancellous and cortical bone to accommodate the mechanical requirements is constantly taking place. Resorbing surfaces that have become inactive later become the site for active bone deposition, and evidence of this process is seen in the form of cement lines (reversal lines), dense basophilic lines separating distinct areas of bone matrix. The chemical composition of the cement line is not known, but examination by polarized light will show that no collagen fibers cross it.[10] In processes in which there is accelerated remodeling of bone (e.g., Paget's disease), the cement lines may become very prominent (Fig. 22-5).

The density of the bone in healthy people depends on several factors, including race, sex, and occupation. On the whole, blacks have heavier and denser bones than whites, men have denser bones than women, and manual workers have denser bones than sedentary workers. With advancing age, there is a steady loss of bone tissue, which occurs in everyone but is more likely to give rise to clinical problems (e.g., osteoporosis) in a white woman than in a black man, because the white woman starts with so much less bone.[11] (Osteoporosis is a clinical term, which indicates an absolute loss of bone tissue sufficient to lead to fracture, whereas osteopenia indicates a decrease in bone mass and is often used by radiologists to indicate a decrease in radiodensity. Although such a decrease in radiodensity may be due to osteoporosis, it may also result from a decrease in the amount of mineralized bone tissue, as in rickets or osteomalacia because it is only the mineralized bone that is visualized on a radiograph.)

Skeletal Development

Developmental disease is rarely seen by the surgical pathologist, with the exception of certain hamartomatous malformations, such as bone islands or fibrous dysplasia, and developmental aberrations, such as the common osteochondroma, all of which are described in Chapter 23. However, the surgical pathologist should know the basics of bone growth and development because they are helpful to the understanding of bone disease in general.

Most bones are preformed in a cartilage model, which, in the course of development, undergoes calcification followed by vascular invasion and the laying down of osseous tissue on the remnants of calcified cartilage matrix. This process is known as endochondral ossification. The viable cartilage continues to grow and subsequently calcifies, thus providing for the growth of the skeletal elements. During most of childhood the principal source of cartilage growth and subsequent endochondral ossification is found in the growth plate. Disturbances in cell maturation in the growth plate, such as those that occur in achondroplasia and may also occur in hormonal disturbances such as hypothyroidism or hypopituitarism, result in decreased cartilage proliferation and decreased endochondral ossification, the ultimate effect being dwarfing of the child. Hyperpituitarism results in giantism and in adult acromegaly because of stimulation of cartilage growth and subsequently increased endochondral ossification. (Interpretation of the changes in the growth plate require familiarity with the appearance of the normal growth plate at the various stages of growth up to adolescence, and such considerations are outside the scope of this chapter.)

The bone that is first laid down on the calcified cartilage is referred to as the primary spongiosa (Fig. 22-6). This mixture of

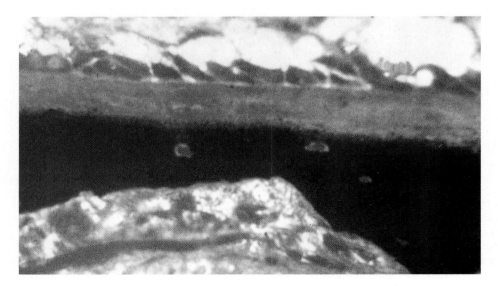

Fig. 22-4. Photomicrograph of an individual trabeculum from a patient with a metabolic disturbance, showing on the upper surface bone formation with active osteoblasts and on the lower surface the irregular gnawed-out appearance of resorption. This section of undecalcified bone was stained by the von Kossa stain. Mineralized bone is black, whereas the unmineralized osteoid is a smooth gray zone between the osteoblastic cell layer on the surface and the fully mineralized bone beneath.

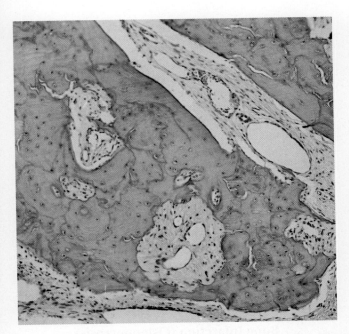

Fig. 22-5. Photomicrograph of a section taken from pagetoid bone. The cement lines are seen as irregular wavy gray lines coursing through the matrix of the bone. In many areas clefts are seen in the region of these lines. These clefts represent a cracking artifact at the time of sectioning. They indicate the ease with which this bone will fracture. The marrow spaces are fibrotic, and large dilated vessels are present.

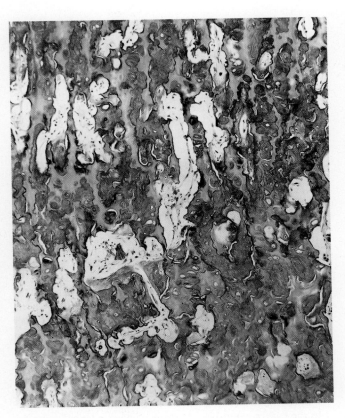

Fig. 22-7. Photomicrograph of a section of the cancellous bone from a patient with osteopetrosis. Note the increased amount of bone, the loss of the normal trabecular architecture, and the residual calcified cartilage within the bone. In this condition the osteoclasts, although present, do not appear to resorb the bone.

bone and calcified cartilage is remodeled by osteoclastic activity and eventually the bone trabeculae are formed only of bone tissue, referred to as the secondary spongiosa. A rare disease results from a failure of the normal remodeling of primary to secondary spongiosa. In this condition, osteopetrosis,[12] most of the skeletal tissue is formed of primary spongiosa. This bone is extremely dense, and pieces of bone from osteopetrotic subjects will be found to be unduly heavy and difficult to decalcify and section (Fig. 22-7).

SKELETAL DISEASE

The clinical symptoms of disease in the skeletal tissues, whether we are speaking of bones or joints, are most likely to result from mechanical failure.

Fracture Healing

A broken bone results from either a violent force or significant weakening (pathologic fracture). The latter may occur because of either a localized replacement by tumor or a general-

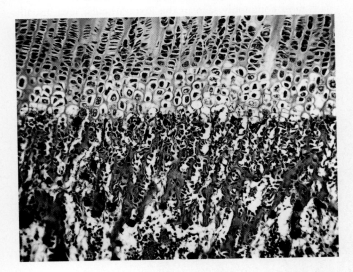

Fig. 22-6. Photomicrograph of the growth plate in a 2-month-old pig. In the upper part of the photograph one can see the columnar arrangement of the hypertrophic zone of the growth plate, which then goes into the degenerative and calcified zone of the growth plate. The calcified zone is invaded by capillaries, which deposit the first bone onto the surface of calcified cartilage matrix. The bone trabeculae of the metaphysis are therefore characterized by a central core of calcified cartilage and a thin layer of bone matrix on the surface. This bone is called the *primary spongiosa*.

ized disturbance (e.g., senile osteoporosis, osteomalacia, Paget's disease, osteogenesis imperfecta).

The reparative response[13] depends on the site of injury and the bone involved; in general, it corresponds to the richness of the vascular bed. For example, a fracture through the midshaft of the tibia in a poorly vascularized area is notorious for both delayed healing and nonunion.[14]

A fracture inevitably results in some degree of necrosis. We tend to speak of bone necrosis, but only cells can necrose. The extracellular matrix is nonviable to begin with. However, the extracellular matrix may undergo enzymatic degradation. An example of this is the so-called hyalinization of the collagen. In favorable circumstances, the necrosis of the cellular elements (i.e., bone cells and bone marrow cells) extends for only a short distance on each side of the fracture line, but, depending on local factors, large fragments may become necrotic and significantly interfere with the healing process. In the process of bone healing the necrotic bone will be resorbed by osteoclasts.

The periosteum is an extremely important source of repair tissue (callus) following fracture. At the time of the initial injury the periosteum may be elevated from the underlying bone by hemorrhage, and the osteogenic cells of the cambium layer may rapidly become activated and begin to lay down woven bone. This immature subperiosteal bone eventually bridges the fracture site and renders the fractured bone stable. In the medullary cavity, the osteoblasts lining the trabeculae on either side of the fracture site also become very active and lay down new bone on the existing bone trabeculae.

In the face of extensive soft tissue damage, a large amount of callus may be seen in the surrounding soft tissues. This takes the form of irregular trabeculae of woven bone, and in fractures that are particularly unstable, this extraosseous callus may be quite immature and contain a high proportion of cellular cartilage, giving rise to a pseudosarcomatous appearance (Fig. 22-8).

After stabilization of the fracture, remodeling takes place, with restoration to an anatomic state similar to that present before fracture. Stabilization of the fracture usually takes place in 4 to 8 weeks, but anatomic restitution takes many months or even years. Because the callus serves to immobilize the fracture, it should be obvious that the amount of callus is in general proportional to the stability of the fracture, and therefore, in a fracture that has been immobilized surgically by internal fixation, little or no callus may form.

It is important for the surgical pathologist to know that fracture can occur in a bone without the patient being aware of it. These fractures classically occur in healthy young athletic adults and are termed *stress fractures*; they are common in the metatarsals and tibia. In such a case the patient may complain of pain and swelling over a bone, and radiographs may show localized exuberant new bone. Biopsy will show a very proliferative osseous and cartilaginous tissue, which because of its deranged pattern and cellularity may be mistaken for osteogenic sarcoma (Fig. 22-8). Obviously, this is a most important differential diagnosis and requires careful correlation of the clinical history, radiographs, and pathologic findings.

Bone Infarction (Osteonecrosis)

Localized bone and bone marrow death (osteonecrosis)[15] is a common complication of osteomyelitis and conditions in which the bone marrow is replaced by massive cellular infiltrates, such as Gaucher's disease, lymphoma, or primary or metastatic tumor. Osteonecrosis may also occur as a result of the "bends" in deep sea divers or hemoglobinopathies such as sickle cell disease and is frequently seen in association with cortisone therapy and alcoholism. In clinical practice, osteonecrosis is most commonly seen in the juxta-articular area, usually the hip, and gives rise to articular symptoms, as described below.

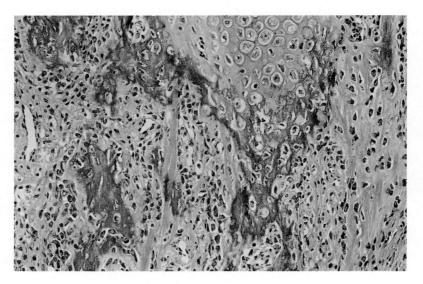

Fig. 22-8. Photomicrograph of a section taken from a fracture approximately 10 days old. The irregularity of the bone and cartilage being formed, together with the crowded and varying appearance of the stromal cells, imparts a pseudosarcomatous appearance.

Grossly, dead bone is generally yellow and chalky in appearance (Fig. 22-1B). The recognition of dead bone microscopically is not difficult: the marrow cells are necrotic and ghostlike, the walls of the fat cells break down to form irregular fat cysts, and sometimes calcification of the fat occurs. The bone matrix is usually palely stained and the osteocytic lacunae enlarged and empty. As occurs with infarcts in other organs, the necrotic tissue is invaded at its margins by granulation tissue, removed, and replaced by scar. However, in the case of bone, the scar tissue is organized as osseous tissue (Fig. 22-9).

In revascularized bone, the bone marrow space is filled with fibrous granulation tissue, and it is common to see a layer of new living bone being deposited on a core of dead bone tissue, a process that is often referred to as "creeping substitution" (Fig. 22-10).

Clinically, infarction is usually seen adjacent to a joint, particularly the femoral head, although it may occur in other joints. In the femoral head it commonly complicates fracture[16] but is also frequently seen without fracture, in which case there is frequently a clinical history of either cortisone therapy or alcoholism. In alcoholics and following corticosteroid therapy the systemic nature of the disease is apparent by the presence of multiple bone infarcts in almost 50 percent of the patients.

The radiologic features of infarction of the femoral head are increased bone density and a change in joint contour. The increased density is the result of reparative new bone and trabecular thickening at the edge of the infarct. The change in the contour of the articular surface is due to a failure of repair and central collapse of the infarcted area with the overlying articular cartilage.

Gross examination of the femoral head resected because of early stage osteonecrosis is likely to reveal fairly intact articular cartilage, although there will probably be wrinkling of the surface marking the edge of the necrotic area (Fig. 22-1). On vertical sectioning, the infarcted zone exhibits a characteristic bright yellow, opaque appearance. At its margin there is a hyperemic zone or a band of fibrous scar tissue. In the later stages of the disease, the articular cartilage becomes detached over the infarcted area, the underlying bone gradually fragments and

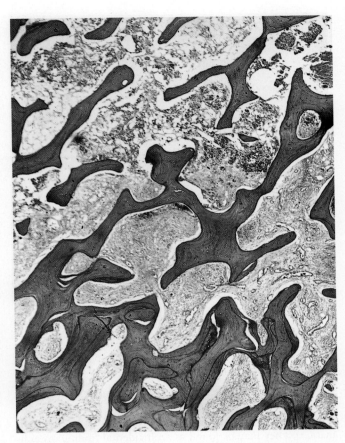

Fig. 22-10. Photomicrograph of area outlined in Fig. 22-9. In the upper part, the fatty marrow is necrotic. The amorphous granular material seen within the fat is calcium soap. In this area the bone trabeculae have an abnormal outline, but a close view would show that the osteocytic lacunae are empty. In the lower part of the picture, a layer of new bone is seen covering the original bone trabeculae. This is evidence of healing and is known as creeping substitution. The bone marrow in this area is hyperemic and, together with the new bone formation, represents the repairing margin of the infarct.

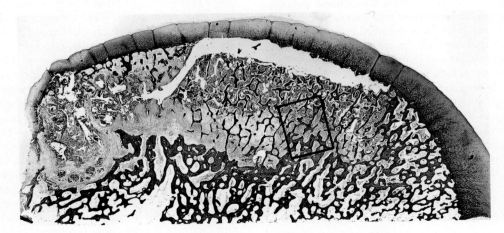

Fig. 22-9. Photomicrograph of a histologic preparation of the specimen shown in Fig. 22-1. An enlarged view of the outlined area is shown in Fig. 22-10.

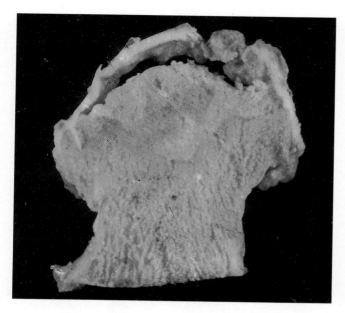

Fig. 22-11. Photograph of a coronal section through the femoral head of a patient with more advanced osteonecrosis than that shown in Fig. 22-1. The articular cartilage is almost entirely detached. Once the cartilage detaches, the necrotic bone beneath will rapidly be eroded away, and secondary osteoarthritis will ensue.

erodes, and secondary osteoarthritis ensues (Fig. 22-11). Infarcts in the shafts of long bones are likely to be asymptomatic.[17] They may be found as an incidental finding on radiographic films, in which case they are frequently misinterpreted as tumors, particularly cartilaginous tumors. There have been several reports of sarcomas, usually malignant fibrous histiocytoma, developing as a complication of long-standing infarcts in long bones.[18]

Heterotopic Calcification and Bone Formation

The distinction between calcification in soft tissue and ossification in soft tissue is an important one. Extensive calcification of soft tissue may result from disturbed calcium metabolism, as in hyperparathyroidism, metastatic carcinoma, myeloma, and hypervitaminosis D, or may complicate systemic connective tissue diseases such as scleroderma. Localized diffuse calcification may be seen in fat necrosis, old tuberculous cavities, phlebolithiasis, or synovioma (Fig. 22-12).

The most common sites of heterotopic bone are in calcified laryngeal or tracheal cartilage and in the media of calcified arteries. In these situations bone is formed by vascular invasion of calcified tissue, similar to endochondral ossification of the growth plate (see above). However, any tissue that has calcified may later ossify.

Myositis Ossificans

Two entirely separate conditions are included under the diagnosis of myositis ossificans. The first is a congenital progressive

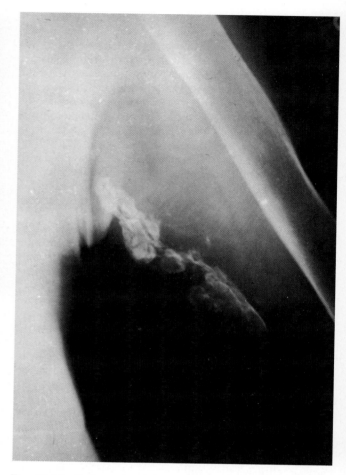

Fig. 22-12. Radiograph of the upper arm of a 50-year-old man complaining of a swelling on the inner aspect of the left arm. A heavily calcified mass is apparent, which following removal, was found to be a calcified lipoma.

disease in which groups of tendons and muscle, usually around major joints, become progressively ossified, producing severe functional disability.[19] Microscopic examination will reveal poorly organized bone, both lamellar and woven, and dense fibrous scar tissue. Occasionally, one may observe islands of poorly formed cartilage.

The second condition is myositis ossificans circumscripta, in which the patient usually has a lump in a muscle, which has been present for some weeks and may have been somewhat painful.[20] A history of trauma can usually be elicited but is often of a trivial nature and occasionally may be absent. A radiograph taken soon after the onset of symptoms may not show an opacity, but within 1 or 2 weeks a poorly defined shadow will appear, and over the following weeks the periphery will become increasingly well delineated from the surrounding soft tissue.

On gross examination, a focus of myositis ossificans circumscripta present for a few months shows a shell of bony tissue with a more or less soft red-brown central area. It is usually 2 to 5 cm in diameter and adherent to the surrounding muscle.

Microscopic examination reveals, in the central part of the

lesion, an irregular mass of active mesenchymal cells with foci of interstitial microhemorrhage that are rarely extensive (Fig. 22-13A). Occasionally, hemosiderin-filled macrophages and degenerative muscle fibers are encountered. The whole lesion is intensely vascular, the vessels being dilated channels lined by endothelium but without any formed media or adventitia. At some distance from the center of the lesion, depending on the age of the lesion in question, one finds small foci of osteoid production and, rarely, even cartilage production; this tissue may be disorganized and hypercellular. As one approaches the periphery there are more and more clearly defined trabeculae (Fig. 22-13B). The bone is usually of the primitive woven type with large, round, and crowded osteocytes; however, in cases of long standing the bone is mature and has a lamellar pattern.

Histologically it may be difficult to differentiate a focus of myositis, especially in its acute and active stage, from a sarcoma. A careful correlation of the clinical and radiographic findings is therefore essential. An important distinction that must be emphasized is that whereas myositis ossificans is most mature at its periphery and least mature at its center (Fig. 22-13C), the opposite is true of osteosarcoma. Post-traumatic reactive lesions similar to myositis ossificans are sometimes seen on the small bones of the hand where they are often referred to as reactive periostitis.

Metabolic Disease

Skeletal disease secondary to disturbed metabolism can be considered under three headings of disturbance or disease, which are discussed below.

Disturbances in the Formation or Breakdown of the Matrix Components

Skeletal disease due to matrix component disturbances may involve the collagen, proteoglycan, or mineral components of the matrix.

Collagen

An abnormality in collagen synthesis may result from an inborn error such as occurs with osteogenesis imperfecta or the Ehlers-Danlos syndrome (diseases characterized histologically by severe osteoporosis, often a hypercellular immature bone tissue, and deficient fibrous connective tissue throughout the body)[21] or from extrinsic disturbances such as vitamin C deficiency and lathyrism, in which the intracellular formation of the collagen molecule is disturbed.

Proteoglycan

Most disturbances of proteoglycan metabolism are the result of overproduction of one or another type of glycosaminoglycan (mucopolysaccharide), most commonly dermatan sulfate and heparan sulfate. Accumulation of glycosaminoglycan occurs within the reticuloendothelial cells of many organs, and this may or may not be associated with excess excretion in the urine of these substances. These disorders, which are collectively known as the mucopolysaccharidoses, may exhibit marked skeletal abnormalities.[22] One of these diseases, Morquio's disease, probably specifically involves a defect in the proteoglycan metabolism of cartilage.

Minerals

Disturbances in the mineral component of the matrix may result from inborn errors in metabolism in which there is either a relative absence or excess of the enzyme alkaline phosphatase. Hypophosphatasemia[23] is characterized by an extremely osteopenic skeleton, which radiologically mimics rickets. Microscopically the bone tissue is disorganized and poorly mineralized, with an excess of unmineralized osteoid tissue. Hyperphosphatasemia,[24] by contrast, results in a dense and irregularly formed skeleton. Histologically the bone tissue resembles that of Paget's disease. Hyperphosphatasemia is often referred to as juvenile Paget's disease.

A number of metallic elements may also deposit in the bone, resulting in interference with the normal process of mineralization. These include lead, iron, and aluminum. Aluminum toxicity has recently been recognized as a major complication of the administration of phosphate bindings in the management of renal dialysis patients. Not only does aluminum result in an encephalopathy, eventually leading to an irreversible psychosis, but it also deposits at the mineralization fronts in the bone, effectively blocking further mineralization and leading to an osteomalacia-like picture. In undecalcified sections the aluminum in the bone can be demonstrated by using the aurintricarboxylic acid stain, which stains the aluminum red.[25] Fluoride in excessive amounts, either endemic or iatrogenic, results in increased bone formation, the matrix of the newly formed bone showing a patchy and abnormal mineralization.[26]

Osteoporosis

Osteoporosis is a decrease in mass of normally mineralized bone, which often leads to fracture. It results in thinning of the bone cortices and in thin, widely spaced trabeculae in the cancellous bone (Fig. 22-14). It is the result of a relative decrease in osteoblastic (bone-forming) activity as compared with osteoclastic (bone-resorbing) activity, usually with an increase in osteoclastic activity.

Osteoporosis may be localized or generalized. Localized osteoporosis occurs after immobilization, for example, in a plaster cast. It may also be seen in the region of a joint associated with localized pain and hyperemia (Sudeck's atrophy). This type of localized patchy osteoporosis occasionally seems to involve several joints, usually in the lower limbs, in a transient fashion—so-called idiopathic transient osteoporosis.[27] In one form of localized osteoporosis, disappearing bone disease, the bone may eventually entirely disappear on the radiograph.[28] In all these forms of localized osteoporosis, no specific microscopic appearance other than the obvious loss of bone tissue and some increase in osteoclastic activity, has been identified, although it has been suggested that there is an increased vascularity of the bone.

Clinical osteoporosis as a result of age is most common in white women for the reasons discussed earlier. It may also occur in a severe form after menopause, presumably as a result of endocrine imbalance, and it also complicates hypercortisonism.

Proper evaluation of osteoporosis, as of the other metabolic

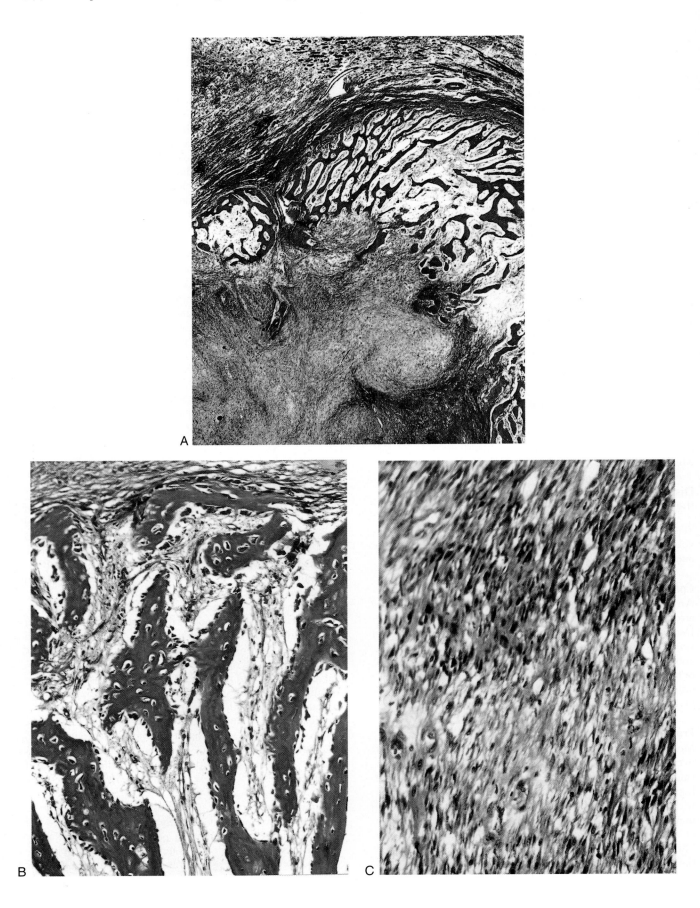

A

B   C

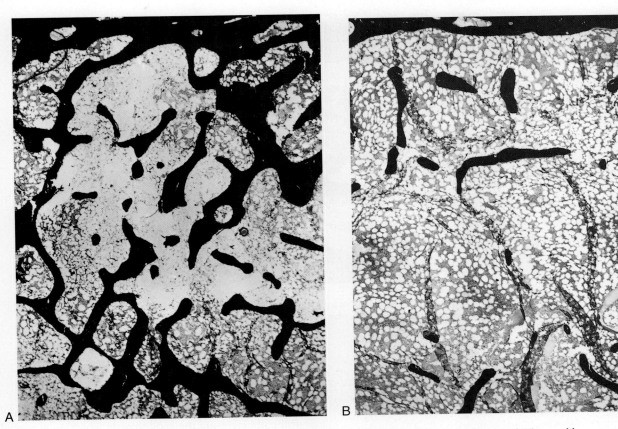

Fig. 22-14. **(A)** Photomicrograph of a core biopsy specimen of the iliac crest in a normal 35-year-old woman. Note that for the most part the trabeculae are connected with one another and to the cortex, a portion of which is seen in the upper part of the picture. Compare this appearance with that in **(B)** which is from an osteoporotic 65-year-old woman. In Fig. B not only are the trabeculae much thinner and sparser, but they are not connected with one another or with the cortical bone at the surface.

disturbances of bone, requires quantitative histology; the parameters to measure are the percentage of tissue occupied by bone tissue as opposed to marrow, and the percentage of the bone surface that is actively laying down bone or that is actually resorbing bone as compared with the inactive surfaces. (For a full discussion, see Rasmussen and Bordier.[29]) Clinical history and thorough biochemical studies are essential to determine etiology and treatment.

Disturbances in Calcium Homeostasis

Disturbances in calcium homeostasis result in osteitis fibrosa (hyperparathyroidism) and/or osteomalacia (rickets).

Hyperparathyroidism

Hyperparathyroidism may be either primary, due to a functioning adenoma, primary hyperplasia, or, rarely, a carcinoma of the parathyroid glands[30] or secondary, due to renal disease.[31] With the advent of renal dialysis the latter form of disease (secondary hyperparathyroidism) has become much more frequent. In hyperparathyroid bone disease the characteristic microscopic change is localized osteoclastic resorption of the bone tissue, which characteristically and frequently shows a dissecting pattern (Fig. 22-15). Associated with the foci of osteoclastic resorption, localized fibrosis of the marrow adjacent to the bone is seen. (The localization of the fibrosis against the bone trabeculae distinguishes this type of fibrosis from that seen in

Fig. 22-13. **(A)** Photomicrograph showing a portion of a specimen of myositis ossificans circumscripta. In the upper part of the photograph, there is scar tissue with compressed muscle fibers. The lesion itself shows trabecular bone at the periphery and at the center a cellular tissue. **(B)** Photomicrograph showing detail of periphery of lesion shown in Fig. A. Note the trabeculae of woven bone with crowded osteocytes and prominent osteoblasts on the surface of the trabeculae. Between the trabeculae there is innocuous fibrous tissue. **(C)** Photomicrograph showing detail of center of lesion in Fig. A. Note the crowded spindle cells, which give a pseudosarcomatous appearance to the lesion.

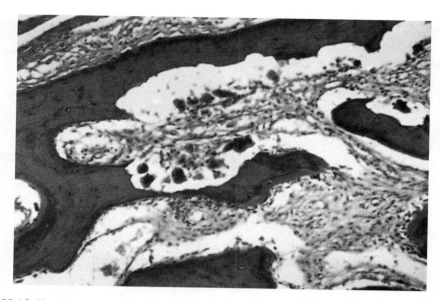

Fig. 22-15. Photomicrograph of section taken from a patient with hyperparathyroidism. Note the way the resorbing surfaces dissect into the bone trabeculae, resulting in a tunneling effect characteristic of hyperparathyroidism.

myelofibrosis.) The increased bone resorption results in a secondary increase in bone deposition, and the result is an increased turnover rate that is generalized throughout the skeleton, although it is more apparent in sections of cancellous bone than in sections of dense cortical bone.

Occasionally, the proliferation of osteoclasts and fibrous tissue is associated with hemorrhage and a giant cell reaction. This results in the so-called brown tumor of hyperparathyroidism, which may be confused with a giant cell tumor. This error may be avoided by careful correlation of the microscopic appearance with the clinical chemistry findings and radiographs.

Osteomalacia

Although childhood rickets is now an uncommon condition, this is not the case with adult rickets, or osteomalacia. Osteomalacia may result from malabsorption syndrome, after intestinal surgery or poor diet, or from a disturbance in vitamin D metabolism.[32] One current cause of disturbance in vitamin D metabolism is treatment with anticonvulsive drugs such as diphenylhydantoin (Dilantin). However, whatever the cause of the disturbance in vitamin D metabolism or calcium absorption, the effects are similar. The bone that is laid down fails to be calcified. As a result the osteoblasts tend to be overactive, laying down even more bone, which in turn remains unmineralized. It is not possible to appreciate the extent of unmineralized bone tissue unless undecalcified sections are prepared (Fig. 22-16). When this is done, most of the bone trabeculae are covered by a prominent layer of unmineralized bone or osteoid, and this can be best appreciated by the use of the von Kossa stain. In osteomalacia not only is upward of 40 percent of the bone unmineralized, but it will also be apparent that the mineralization front is very irregular and fuzzy in appearance.

Disease Resulting From Deposition of Abnormal Extrinsic Metabolic Products

The last group of metabolic disturbances commonly seen by the surgical pathologist are the conditions in which an abnormal extrinsic metabolic product is deposited in the skeleton. Such conditions include the so-called lipid histiocytoses (Gaucher's, Niemann-Pick, and Tay-Sachs diseases), ochronosis,[33] cystinosis, and oxalosis,[34] but the two most common diseases are calcium pyrophosphate dihydrate crystal deposition disease and gout.

Calcium Pyrophosphate Dihydrate Deposition Disease (Pseudogout)

Calcium pyrophosphate dihydrate is a chalky white material often found in the synovial membrane, articular cartilage, and/or fibrocartilaginous menisci of elderly people, and it does not usually result in clinically significant disease.[35] However, some cases of inflammatory joint disease and secondary osteoarthritis may be the result of deposition of calcium pyrophosphate, and occasional patients are seen who develop clinically significant pseudogout before the age of 35. These individuals have an autosomal dominant pattern of inheritance.

The histologic appearance of these deposits, as well as the clinical presentation in some cases, is similar enough to that of gout to have given rise to the term *pseudogout* to describe the clinical syndrome. In histologic sections the material is usually crystalline, the crystals being small and rectangular and exhibiting a weak positive birefringence. On occasion, noncrystalline deposits that do not polarize may also be seen. These crystalline deposits are sometimes surrounded by giant cells and occasional histiocytes and chronic inflammatory cells (Fig. 22-17).

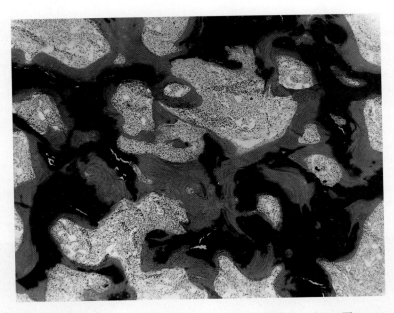

Fig. 22-16. Photomicrograph of a section taken from a patient with osteomalacia. The section has been prepared from undecalcified bone and stained by the von Kossa method. The area stained black represents mineralized bone. On the surface, there is a thick layer of nonmineralized bone matrix (osteoid). This osteoid seam, which is characteristic of osteomalacia, cannot be appreciated on decalcified sections.

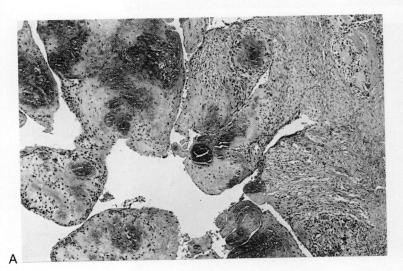

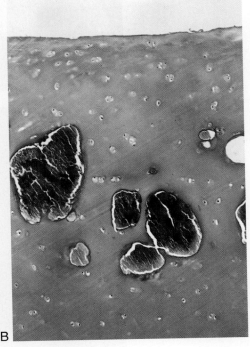

Fig. 22-17. (A) Photomicrograph of a section of synovium taken from a patient with calcium pyrophosphate dihydrate deposition disease. The deposits of calcium pyrophosphate are often crystalline and surrounded in some areas by histiocytes, giant cells, and a mild chronic inflammatory infiltrate. (B) Photomicrograph of section of articular cartilage from the same case demonstrated in Fig. A. Large irregular noncrystalline deposits of calcified material are present. Undecalcified frozen section stained by the von Kossa method.

Gout

Gout[36] results from the precipitation of monosodium urate monohydrate in the synovial fluid and other tissues after prolonged hyperuricemia. It is most commonly seen in the kidney and the large joints, especially the first metatarsophalangeal joint. There are three stages of involvement to the joint by gout: (1) acute gouty synovitis; (2) the deposition of sodium urate in the form of chalky concretions or tophi in the synovium, bone, bursae, and subcutaneous tissues; and (3) chronic gouty arthritis. In patients with acute gouty arthritis, the synovial fluid invariably contains crystals that are usually needle-shaped and when examined with polarized light demonstrate strong negative birefringence. The crystals may be free in the synovial fluid or may be engulfed within polymorphonuclear leukocytes. The ingested crystals result in the release of lysosomal enzymes, which in turn perpetuate the acute inflammatory reaction. After a number of years, chalky deposits of sodium urate, known as tophi, may develop in the articular and periarticular tissues. These deposits are surrounded by chronic inflammatory cells, foreign body giant cells, and dense fibrous scar. Destruction of the bone and capsular tissues results in chronic arthritis with disabling deformities (Fig. 22-18).

Gaucher's Disease

Gaucher's disease[37] is a lipid histiocytosis resulting from an accumulation of glycocerebrosides within the histiocytes of the reticuloendothelial system, particularly in bones and spleen. It is mostly seen in Ashkenazic Jews and is transmitted as an au-

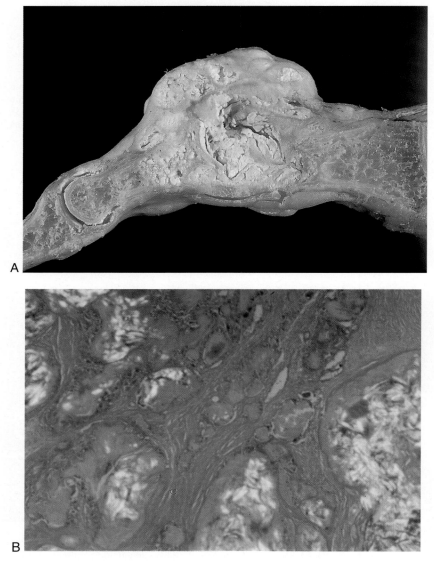

Fig. 22-18. **(A)** Photograph of a sagittal section through a metatarsophalangeal joint affected by tophaceous gout. **(B)** Photomicrograph of the sodium urate deposits with surrounding giant cell, histiocytic, and fibroblastic response in a case of tophaceous gout. As seen in this photograph the urate crystals are refractile when examined with polarized light.

tosomal recessive trait. The bone marrow shows more or less replacement by sheets of large pale cells, with a distinctive crumpled appearance to the cytoplasm. Because the disease is inherited, the bone marrow replacement may result in developmental deformities in the more rapidly growing parts of the skeleton, that is, the lower end of the femur, the upper tibia, and the upper end of the humerus. This takes the form of widening of the metaphyseal portion of bone, resulting in a deformity known as the "Erlenmeyer flask deformity." Radiographically, the affected bones are frequently osteoporotic and may show a lytic or soap bubble appearance. The extending mass of lipid-laden histiocytes may interfere with the blood supply to the bone and cause infarction. Unilateral or bilateral avascular necrosis of the femoral head is a common complication of Gaucher's disease and may be the presenting clinical sign. Because of the relative ischemia of the affected bone, biopsy is attended by a high incidence of secondary infection.

Paget's Disease

Paget's disease[38] is a localized disturbance in bone cell activity, the cause of which is unknown, although recently there have been reports of viral inclusions in the osteoclasts.[39] It is a fairly common disease, occurring in about 4 percent of the northern European male population over the age of 40. However, in most instances the disease is not clinically significant, usually being confined to only one vertebral body or one other focus in the skeleton. Generalized clinical Paget's disease is much less common.

The microscopic appearance of Paget's disease is variable and depends on the state of activity. In active disease, the histologic appearance is difficult to distinguish from that of hyperparathyroidism (Fig. 22-19). There is very active osteoclastic resorp-

tion and, associated with this, increased osteoblastic activity. These changes result in an increased number of reversal lines (cement lines), which are apparent even in the early or active stage of the disease. The marrow spaces are fibrosed, but the dissecting type of resorption, which typifies hyperparathyroidism, is not usually seen. In the later, quiescent stages of the disease, the bone becomes very dense, and the previous overactivity is represented by multiple cement lines, giving rise to the descriptive mosaic appearance (Fig. 22-5). The bone marrow will be noted to have many dilated vascular channels, which is consistent with the clinical observation that these patients frequently have a high output type of failure. In a small percentage of patients sarcoma may develop[40] (see Ch. 23).

Infection

Before the advent of antibiotics, infection[41,42] was among the most common indications for inpatient treatment in orthopedic hospitals, and in developing countries bone infection is still the most common cause of bone and joint disease. In the United States, however, it is now rare and for this reason may give rise to problems in differential diagnosis.

Infection of the bones and joints may result from either hematogenous spread or direct implantation. In the latter case, the infection usually complicates either a compound fracture or surgery, nowadays particularly prosthetic replacement of joints.

Hematogenous osteomyelitis is most commonly seen in children and is usually due to *Staphylococcus aureus* infection. Bacteremia alone is probably not sufficient to cause osteomyelitis, and generally a history of trauma will be elicited from the patient, the trauma presumably giving rise to local blood stasis or thrombosis, thereby providing a site for bacterial growth. Infection is most commonly seen in children in the metaphyseal re-

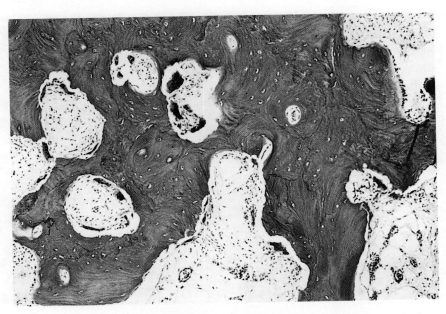

Fig. 22-19. Photomicrograph of a section taken from a patient with active Paget's disease. At the surface of the bone there is considerable osteoclastic activity. Some of these osteoclasts have many nuclei. Giant osteoclasts tend to be characteristic of Paget's disease. In other areas, abundant osteoblastic activity can be discerned.

gion of long bones and particularly around the knee joint. Usually, the patient has a high fever, pain, and local tenderness, and during the first week or so of the disease radiographs will not show any bony change. (Nowadays, because patients with fever are frequently treated with antibiotics without further diagnosis, osteomyelitis in children may present as a chronic problem.)

In adults, hematogenous osteomyelitis is less common. When it is seen, it is more common in the vertebral column. It has been described recently as occurring in heroin addicts and may also complicate urinary tract infection, presumably via Batson's plexus. An unusual form of osteomyelitis is the multiple bony involvement seen in patients with sickle cell disease, in which the causative organism is often *Salmonella*.

In osteomyelitis, the inflammatory exudate usually results in widespread bone and bone marrow necrosis. This results from the increased pressure within the closed cavity of the cancellous bone, which rapidly leads to vascular occlusion. The inflammatory exudate tracks through the haversian systems of the cortex to elevate the overlying periosteum, which in turn is activated to form a sleeve of new bone (the involucrum) around the necrotic infected bone (the sequestrum) beneath. This classic sequence is aborted by the use of adequate antibiotic therapy. However, unless the disease is treated with adequate doses of antibiotics, it may become chronic and in this case is likely to continue for many years with recurrent episodes of local infection, which may be accompanied by sinus formation. Rare long-term complications of osteomyelitis include secondary amyloidosis and the formation of squamous cell carcinoma in the sinus tract.[43]

Occasional adult patients with hematogenous osteomyelitis may present without significant systemic signs. As likely as not,

the radiologic diagnosis on these patients will be that of a tumor, possibly a malignant round cell tumor. A biopsy specimen revealing small, round inflammatory cells may also be misinterpreted by the pathologist as a round cell tumor, and on occasion this differential diagnosis may be problematic. In this regard it also should be noted that occasional children with Ewing's tumor may have an elevated temperature, increased sedimentation rate, and leukocytosis.

Granulomatous infection is usually due to *Mycobacterium tuberculosis*, but occasionally to blastomycosis, cryptococcosis, coccidioidomycosis, or sporotrichosis; rarely, it results from sarcoidosis. These infections are most commonly seen either in the spine or in the large joints (the hip and the knee). Histologically, typical granulomas with giant cells, epithelioid cells, and chronic inflammatory cells are seen. Organisms may be difficult to demonstrate in bony tissue. Often, granulomatous infection, because of its rarity, is not suspected clinically, and the diagnosis does not become apparent until the pathologist has examined the tissue. For this reason cultures may not have been taken, and the causative organism may be difficult to establish.

The Histiocytoses

The histiocytoses are characterized by the proliferation of histiocytes in the bone and/or soft tissues.[44] Depending on the presentation, they have been classified as eosinophilic granuloma, Hand-Schüller-Christian disease, or Letterer-Siwe disease. Nowadays these lesions are usually all included under the rubric of eosinophilic granuloma or Langerhans granulomatosis.

In the skeleton, eosinophilic granuloma is usually unifocal but occasionally may be multifocal. Most patients are under age 10. It may occur anywhere in any bones, but the most common

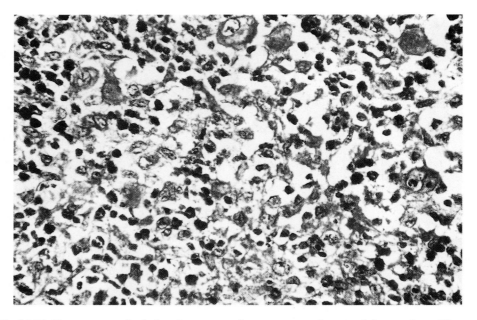

Fig. 22-20. Photomicrograph of a histologic section from a patient with eosinophilic granuloma. There is a background of pale-staining histiocytic cells with abundant loose cytoplasm, which vary considerably in size and shape. The small dark cells are mostly eosinophils, but there are a few plasma cells and lymphocytes present. This microscopic appearance can be confused on occasion with Hodgkin's disease or with infection.

sites are the skull, the shafts of the long bones (particularly the femur and tibia), and the ilium. The patient usually has localized aching pain and, less commonly, a low grade fever and an elevated erythrocyte sedimentation rate. In radiographs the lesions are osteolytic and generally round to oval, but they may show considerable periosteal reaction and a ragged appearance suggestive of a malignant tumor. Involvement of the vertebral body frequently leads to collapse and flattening (so-called Calve's disease). On gross examination, the curetted material is usually scant and pinkish gray. Microscopic examination will reveal masses of histiocytes (Langerhans cells) and focal or diffuse collections of eosinophils (Fig. 22-20). On electron microscopic examination, the Langerhans cell displays characteristic racket-shaped inclusion bodies in the cytoplasm (Birbeck granules). Occasionally, lymphocytes and plasma cells may also be present. During the healing phase, scar tissue and lipid-laden macrophages may become predominant.

Overdecalcification of the tissue may result in the eosinophilic granules not being apparent, and the lesion may be mistaken for osteomyelitis. The numerous histiocytes, occasionally with large nuclei and even occasionally binucleate forms, can lead to the erroneous impression of Hodgkin's disease.

The term *Hand-Schüller-Christian syndrome*, which originally referred to a classic triad of skull defects, exophthalmos, and diabetes insipidus, is now used to include instances of more chronic evolution, occurring generally in children older than 3 years, with multiple cranial and other bony lesions and sometimes involvement of other systems or with one of the other classic symptoms (exophthalmos or diabetes insipidus). However, the complete triad has been rarely noted in the reported cases.

Letterer-Siwe disease is a rare condition affecting infants less than 2 years of age and is characterized by an acute onset of hepatosplenomegaly, lymphadenopathy, and sometimes bone lesions. In the past, this has been considered a form of histiocytosis, but Lieberman et al[44] have suggested that the cases can be separated into two groups. In one group anaplastic histiocytes predominate, and this lesion would appear to be a form of malignant lymphoma. In the other group the histiocytes have a benign cytology, and this lesion may well be an infantile form of multifocal eosinophilic granuloma.

JOINT TISSUES

The joints[45] provide for motion and stability. These functions are achieved through the anatomy of the joint—its shape and the cartilage and bone of which it is made—and through the neuromuscular control of the joint. Dysfunction of the joint, which is generally called arthritis, occurs because of an alteration in the anatomy or its neuromuscular control. Obviously, such changes may result from congenital disease, metabolic disturbances, infection, or mechanical trauma.

The diarthrodial joints are composed of the articulating cartilages, synovial membrane, bone ends, and surrounding ligaments, tendons, and muscles.[46] Disease may begin in any of these structures, but by the time it comes to the attention of a physician, most or all of them are involved.

The synovial membrane, which lines the inner surface of the joint capsule and all other intra-articular structures with the exception of the articular cartilage, is composed of a smooth moist intimal layer and either a fibrous or a fatty subsynovial (or subintimal) supportive or backing layer. Microscopic examination shows at the surface a layer of closely packed cells with elliptical nuclei and abundant cytoplasm.

The articular cartilage is largely composed of collagen, proteoglycan, and water, and it distributes the load through the joint onto the underlying subchondral bone. To achieve this, the collagen fibers are distributed in a very precise way, as is the proteoglycan.[9] The cells on the surface of the cartilage are flat with their long axes parallel to the surface. The cells that are lower down in the cartilage are rounded and lie in well defined lacunae. Other forms of cartilage in the body (epiphyseal cartilage, fibrocartilage, and elastic cartilage) do not function in the same way as articular cartilage and therefore have a different chemical composition and a different organization of the extracellular matrix.[47]

JOINT DISEASE

The most important therapeutic advance since the 1960s has been the development of artificial articulations to replace joints affected by various disease. On most orthopedic services, endoprosthetic replacements probably account for about one-third of all operations. For the surgical pathologist this means a considerable increase in the amount of orthopedically related tissue to be studied and reported on.

The most common pathologic diagnoses made in patients having total hip replacement in our experience are osteoarthritis (about 65 percent), avascular necrosis (about 20 percent), and rheumatoid arthritis (about 15 percent). (It should be emphasized that these diagnoses are not completely objective and that end-stage hip disease, like end-stage kidney disease or end-stage liver disease, looks very much the same regardless of its etiology.)

The arthritides that are the result of metabolic disturbances and infection are referred to earlier and are not further discussed here.

Osteoarthritis

Osteoarthritis[48] (degenerative joint disease, osteoarthrosis) is generally regarded as a noninflammatory condition that begins as a disruption of the bearing surfaces of the articular cartilage and ends with disintegration of the mechanical joint. In about one-fifth of the cases, an antecedent condition causally related to the osteoarthritis is evident to the clinician. These conditions include Perthes disease, slipped epiphysis, previous infection, and osteonecrosis.

A patient with clinical osteoarthritis usually complains of pain and disability. Movement of the affected joint may be very limited. Examination of a joint removed at surgery or autopsy shows the most obvious features of an osteoarthritic joint to be a change in the shape of the articular surfaces and damage of the cartilage. In the weight-bearing areas of a joint, the cartilage may be entirely absent, and the exposed subchondral bone has a dense polished appearance like marble (eburnation) (Fig. 22-21). In these areas of absent cartilage, the bone trabeculae are markedly thickened (sclerotic), and, adjacent to the surface in the subchondral bone there may be cystic defects filled by loose fibromyxoid tissue or sometimes by a thick fluid. In the eburnated areas the superficial bone may be necrotic, presumably from the excessive pressure. In some specimens the weight-bearing surface may be covered by few or many tufts of fibrocartilage, and this seems to be a reparative phenomenon. In the areas of the joint that are not weight bearing and around the margins, there are bony and cartilaginous overgrowths (osteophytes or exostoses), which on the medial and inferior aspect of the femoral head may be in the form of large, flat plaques of bone and cartilage.

The cartilage that remains on the joint surface may have many clefts in its substance, most, but by no means all, being vertical in disposition. The cartilage cells may show considerable proliferation, with the formation of prominent cell nests (Fig. 22-22). Generally, basophilic staining of the matrix with hematoxylin stain will be found to be diminished. The synovial membrane shows some villous proliferation and mild hyperplasia of the intima. There may be a mild chronic inflammation (Fig. 22-23). Small osteochondral loose bodies are not unusual both in the synovium and also free in the joint. In Charcot joints, which are very severe examples of osteoarthritis, the synovium is generally full of bone and cartilage fragments, and there are many loose bodies.

On the basis of anatomic features, Nichols and Richardson[49]

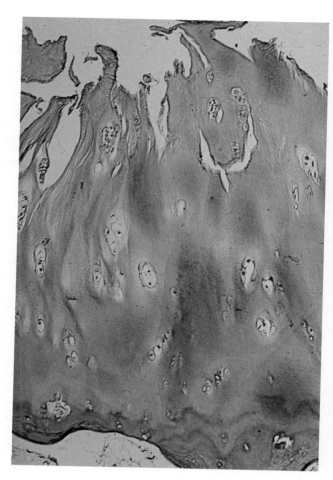

Fig. 22-22. Photomicrograph of a section of fibrillated cartilage from a patient with osteoarthritis. Note the proliferating nests of chondrocytes particularly evident toward the surface.

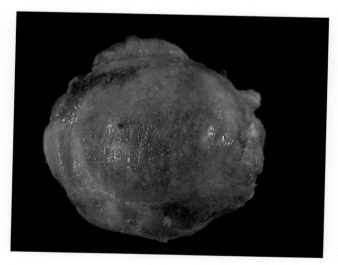

Fig. 22-21. Photograph of a femoral head removed from a patient with osteoarthritis of the hip joint. The superior articular surface has a shiny appearance where the articular cartilage has been worn away and the underlying bone exposed and polished. The cartilage that remains around the periphery is irregular and roughened.

in 1909 distinguished the two forms of chronic arthritis that we would call, respectively, inflammatory arthritis and degenerative arthritis—most of the former comprising the clinical syndrome of rheumatoid arthritis and the latter that of osteoarthritis.

How well are we able to distinguish rheumatoid arthritis and osteoarthritis of the hip using histopathologic criteria? This is a summary of my own experience:

1. Histologically, there is more inflammation in association with the clinical diagnosis of rheumatoid arthritis than with the clinical diagnosis of degenerative joint disease. However, there is considerable overlap, and in about 40 percent of the cases no clear distinction can be made on the basis of the inflammatory infiltrate.
2. Pannus, a fibrous or inflammatory covering of the cartilage, often regarded as a hallmark of rheumatoid arthritis, is not uncommon in osteoarthritis.
3. The principal difference rests in the production of osteophytes

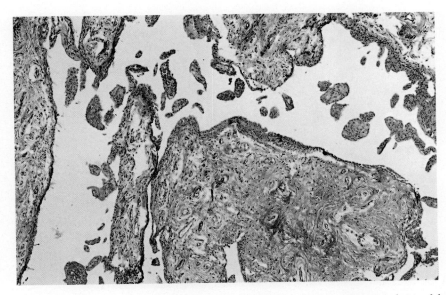

Fig. 22-23. Photomicrograph of a section of synovium taken from a patient with osteoarthritis of the hip joint. The synovial membrane is hypertrophied, hyperplastic, and thrown up into a fine villous structure. In the subsynovial tissue there is a mild chronic inflammatory infiltrate.

and dense sclerosis in the bony joint surfaces of osteoarthritis versus the destructive and nonproductive qualities of rheumatoid arthritis.

Salvati et al[50] reported on the specific activity of cathepsin D in synovial membrane and a histologic quantification of inflammation on synovial tissue obtained from 36 patients undergoing total hip replacement. Among patients with degenerative hip disease, two groups could be identified. In the first, which accounted for 20 percent of the cases, there were high enzyme levels and high histologic scores. In the rest low enzyme levels were accompanied by low histologic scores. It would seem, therefore, that there are a significant number of patients who have an inflammatory arthritis by all pathologic criteria even though clinically they have been diagnosed as having osteoarthritis.

Some patients with osteoarthritis have a spontaneous tendency to improve symptomatically and radiologically.[51] This may be explained by the histologic finding that in advanced stages of disease, eburnated areas tend to resurface with fibrocartilage. It suggests that osteoarthritis is not necessarily a progressive and continually degenerative process, but rather that there are two opposing processes occurring in a joint, namely breakdown and repair.

Rheumatoid Arthritis

Rheumatoid arthritis[52] is a chronic systemic disease frequently involving peripheral joints, two to three times more common in females, and characterized by spontaneous remission and exacerbation.[53] Of all affected patients, 70 to 80 percent have histocompatibility antigen Dw4, which implies a strong hereditary component.[54]

Clinically, the acutely affected joint is hot, swollen, and tender. The synovial effusion is milky and turbid and contains 20,000 to 50,000 inflammatory cells, about 50 percent of which are polymorphonuclear leukocytes (compared with septic arthritis, in which the count is in excess of 100,000 with 75 percent polymorphonuclear leukocytes). No causative organism has been identified.

The principal morphologic feature of rheumatoid disease is joint destruction. Unlike osteoarthritis, there is little reparative activity, and osteophytes and new bone formation are not prominent.

The earliest histologic finding (Fig. 22-24) is a nonsuppurative chronic inflammation of the synovium characterized by:

1. Hypertrophy and hyperplasia of the synovial cells, resulting in a papillary and villous pattern at the surface of the synovium
2. An infiltrate of lymphocytes and plasma cells, the latter often containing eosinophilic inclusions (Russell bodies, evidence of gamma globulin production); neutrophils are common in the synovial exudate but much less so in the synovial membrane
3. Lymphoid follicles (Allison-Ghormley bodies)
4. Fibrinous exudation both at the surface of the synovium and within the synovial tissue

Although these histologic changes are very typical of rheumatoid arthritis, similar changes may also be seen in patients with systemic lupus erythematosus, psoriasis, Lyme disease and other inflammatory arthritides. For this reason a definitive diagnosis of rheumatoid arthritis cannot be made on histologic examination of the synovium alone.

The hypertrophied, inflamed synovium often extends over the articular surface (pannus) and destroys the underlying cartilage by enzymatic degradation of the matrix (Fig. 22-25). The end result of this inflammatory destruction of the articular sur-

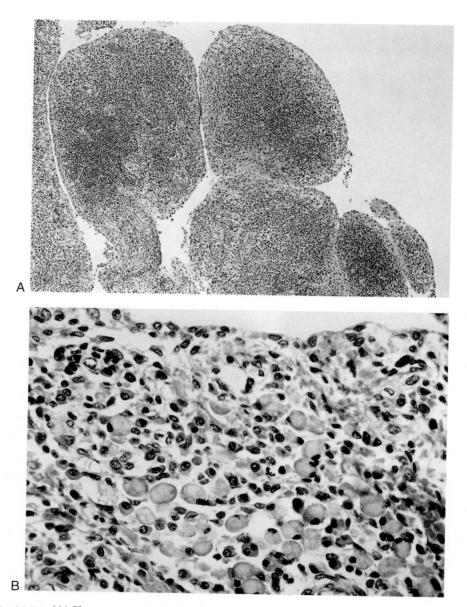

Fig. 22-24. **(A)** Photomicrograph of a histologic section of synovium from a patient with rheumatoid arthritis. There is prominent villous proliferation, with a heavy subsynovial inflammatory infiltrate and marked hyperplasia of the synovial lining cells. **(B)** High power view of this synovium showing the plasma cell and lymphocyte infiltrate. Many of the plasma cells contain cytoplasmic inclusions (Russell bodies).

faces may be fusion of the joint (ankylosis), either by fibrous granulation tissue or by bone. (Note: ankylosis is not a feature of osteoarthritis.)

As well as destroying the cartilaginous surfaces of the joint, the rheumatoid synovium may invade the bone at the articular margin, the joint capsule, and other periarticular supportive tissues, resulting in marked instability of the joint and, frequently, subluxation or complete dislocation. Extra-articular synovitis may lead to carpal tunnel syndrome in which there is compression of the median nerve, or trigger finger, and on occasion these clinical syndromes may be heralds of rheumatoid arthritis.

One histologic feature that is not usually commented on is considerable chronic inflammation and lymphoid follicle formation in the subchondral bone. In some cases this inflammatory tissue may destroy the articular cartilage from below.

Radiographs of affected joints will usually show osteopenia of the juxta-articular bone ends. This may be due to either inflammation of the subchondral bone or hyperemia secondary to inflammation of the synovium.

About 25 percent of patients with rheumatoid arthritis have subcutaneous nodules, most commonly over the extensor surfaces of the elbow and forearm. The nodules may also occur in synovial membrane and in the gastrointestinal tract, lung, and

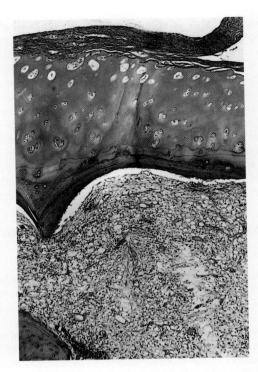

Fig. 22-25. Photomicrograph of a section of the articular surface of a joint involved by rheumatoid arthritis. Covering the articular cartilage is a layer of inflamed synovium (pannus). Underlying the pannus the chondrocytic lacunae are markedly enlarged. A heavy inflammatory infiltrate is also seen in the subchondral bone.

heart. The nodules may be present before any other sign of rheumatoid disease. The rheumatoid nodule is characterized histologically by an irregular shape and a central zone of necrotic fibrinoid material surrounded by histiocytes and some chronic inflammatory cells. The long axes of these histiocytes are frequently radially disposed or palisaded. Generalized vasculitis is much more common in patients with rheumatoid nodules, which is is consistent with the belief that the nodules result from vascular damage[55] (Fig. 22-26).

Although the ultimate cause of rheumatoid disease is unknown, there are two important contributory factors: an immunologic reaction and increased degradative enzymes. Patients with rheumatoid arthritis have a number of immunoglobulins in their serum and synovial fluid, most commonly IgM. These immunoglobulins are known as rheumatoid factors and, as can be demonstrated by immunofluorescence, are made by plasma cells in the synovium and lymphoid system. They can be seen microscopically in H&E-stained sections, both intracellularly and extracellularly as dense homogeneous eosinophilic globules (Russell bodies).

As already noted, in the late stages of rheumatoid arthritis the affected joint may show very little in the way of inflammation and may be anatomically indistinguishable from osteoarthritis.

Traumatic and Hemorrhagic Arthropathy

Severe acute or chronic trauma to a joint that results in bleeding into the joint frequently results in hemosiderotic synovitis and sometimes even green-black discoloration of the articular cartilage. As an end result, secondary osteoarthritis is not uncommon.

Hemorrhage into a joint space, resulting in a hot, painful, and swollen joint, is one of the commonly observed clinical complications of hemophilia or other bleeding diatheses. These bloody joint effusions can be precipitated by even minor trauma and typically involve the knees, elbows, and ankles. Chronic, bloody effusions into the joint spaces may lead to a destructive arthropathy characterized on radiographic studies by a narrow

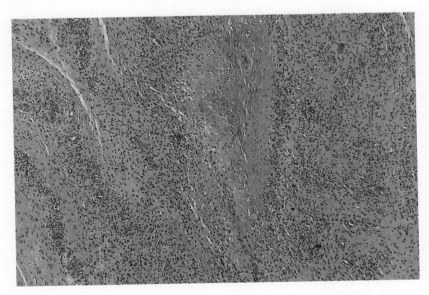

Fig. 22-26. Photomicrograph of a portion of a rheumatoid nodule. Note the geographic central fibrinoid necrosis with the surrounding palisaded histiocytes with fibrosis and chronic inflammation.

joint space, cartilage destruction, bone erosion, multiple juxta-articular cysts, and, if the lesion has progressed over a long period, osteophytes. Radiographs may also reveal a peculiar juxtaepiphyseal osteoporosis. On the basis of gross examination of the hemosiderotic synovium of hemophilia and other forms of chronic bleeding into the joint, the differential diagnosis includes rheumatoid arthritis and pigmented villonodular synovitis. However, microscopic examination of the synovium in hemophilia-related destructive joint disease does not reveal the striking lymphoplasmacytic infiltrate that characterizes rheumatoid arthritis, nor is there the nodular proliferation of mononuclear and giant cells characteristic of pigmented villonodular synovitis.

Cytopathology of Synovial Fluid

Normal synovial fluid, a dialysate of plasma to which hyaluronic acid produced by the "B" cells of the synovial lining is added, is viscous, pale yellow, and clear. Even in large joints the volume is small.

Examination of synovial fluid is extremely helpful in the diagnosis of arthritis for determining both the cause and severity of the disease. Whatever the cause of arthritis, the synovial fluid is altered (Table 22-1).

In cases of inflammatory arthritis, there is an increased volume of synovial fluid with large numbers of neutrophils in the fluid and some free synovial cells. The amount of hyaluronic acid is markedly diminished and this leads to a typical decrease in viscosity. However, in degenerate forms of arthritis, the amount of hyaluronic acid is increased, resulting in an extremely viscous fluid.

An important diagnostic procedure for the clinical diagnosis of crystal synovitis is examination of synovial fluid for crystals and identification of these crystals by polarized light microscopy. This examination requires a polarizing microscope with a compensating first-order red filter. With the red filter in position, the crystals in the synovial fluid should be aligned so that their long axis is parallel to the line that is drawn on the compensating filter, which is the axis of slow vibration.

Sodium urate crystals are usually needle-shaped and exhibit strong negative birefringence; that is, they appear bright yellow when aligned parallel with the line on the compensating filter. Calcium pyrophosphate dihydrate crystals are usually rhomboidal and they exhibit weakly positive birefringence (i.e., when their long axis is aligned with the line on the compensating filter, they appear blue and much less bright than urate crystals).

Synovitis and Other Tissue Responses to Implanted Artificial Joints

A small percentage of total joint replacements fail either because of mechanical loosening or breakage, or, less commonly, because of infection. In these cases the prosthesis is usually removed.[56]

In patients who have had a prosthesis in which metal articulates on metal, it is not uncommon to see a distinct gray-black discoloration at the synovial surface.[56] Microscopic examination of removed tissue shows irregular metal fragments measuring between 1 and 3 mm, mostly within histiocytes. The metallic nature of these particles has been confirmed by various techniques.[57]

Wear particles from the plastic, polyethylene components of artificial joints are only visible when the tissue is examined by polarized light. Mostly, they are intracellular and thread-like and measure about 1 mm across and 4 to 10 mm in length. A severe histiocytic response in the synovium is frequently ob-

Table 22-1. Examination of Synovial Fluid

	Condition			
	Normal	Noninflammatory	Chronic Inflammatory	Septic
Clinical example		Osteoarthritis	Rheumatoid arthritis	Bacterial infection
Cartilage debris	0	+	0	0
Volume (ml) (knee)	<3.5	>3.5	>3.5	>3.5
Color	Clear	Clear yellow	Opalescent yellow	Turbid yellow to green
Viscosity	High	High	Low	Low
White blood cells/mm³	200	200–2,000	2,000–100,000	>100,000
Polymorphonuclear leukocytes (%)	<25	<25	50% or more	90% or more
Culture	Negative	Negative	Negative	Positive
Mucin clot	Firm	Firm	Friable	Friable
Fibrin clot	None	Small	Large	Large
Glucose (% blood glucose)	~50–100	~50–100	~20–75	~1–5
Total protein		Equal to normal joint	Elevated	Elevated

(From Paget and Bullough,[66] with permission.)

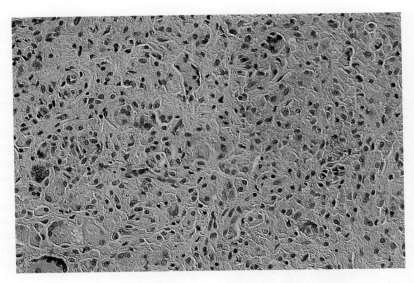

Fig. 22-27. Photomicrograph of a histologic section taken from the synovium of a patient with a failed total knee replacement. There is a marked histiocytic and giant cell reactive process. Irregular fragments of plastic can be demonstrated in these giant cells by polarized light. Proliferative synovium such as this may result in periarticular erosion of the bone.

served, and foreign body giant cells are common. Occasionally, the fragments of polyethylene result in a tumor-like mass developing in the joint capsular tissue, and occasionally erosion of the periarticular bone has been observed (Fig. 22-27).

Both the polyethylene and the metallic components of the artificial joint are usually keyed to the underlying bone by an interposed layer of methyl methacrylate cement.

Abraded particles of cement produce in the capsular tissues a foreign body giant cell reaction. Often the particles are fairly small (10 to 30 mm), in which case they are surrounded by recognizable giant cells. Sometimes the pieces are very large (≥ 100 mm), and in this case histologic sections reveal large irregular spaces surrounded by flattened giant cells (Fig. 22-28). In the routine preparation of histologic sections, any cement in the tissue will be dissolved out by the solvents used in the processing, and microscopic examination will reveal only spaces where the cement was. However, it usually leaves behind a marker in the form of the insoluble barium sulfate that is put into the cement to render it radiopaque.

In all the removed prostheses we have examined, wear debris from one or all of these three sources was present histologically. This debris may be found also in draining lymph nodes. The long-term effects on the body are not known.

Pigmented Villonodular Synovitis and Tenosynovitis

Pigmented villonodular synovitis and tenosynovitis[58] is characterized by a nodular or diffuse proliferation of mononuclear cells, resembling synoviocytes, in the synovium of a tendon sheath or a joint. Frequently, these cells coalesce to form multinucleate giant cells, and for this reason the lesion is some-

times called a giant cell tumor of tendon sheath. In addition to the mononuclear histiocytic type cells, one may also see some admixed chronic inflammatory cells (Fig. 22-29). A varying degree of collagen will be observed in the lesion; this may be minimal in amount or may be so extensive as to obliterate most of the cellular elements. The more cellular the tumor, the more likely one is to see mitotic figures and occasional bizarre cells.

Although grossly these lesions most often show some brown-

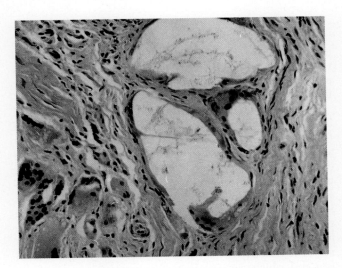

Fig. 22-28. Photomicrograph of a section of synovial tissue taken from a patient with a failed knee prosthesis. The large irregular spaces surrounded by flattened giant cells originally contained methyl methacrylate cement, dissolved out during processing. The finely granular material seen in these spaces is barium sulfate, which is used as a clinical radiopaque marker.

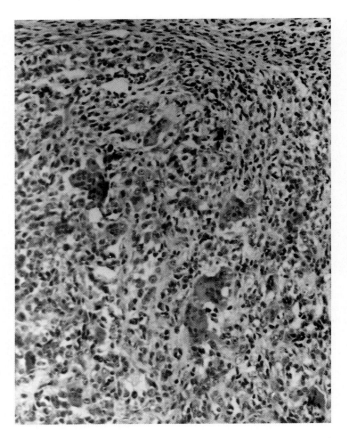

Fig. 22-29. Photomicrograph of a section taken from a patient with pigmented villonodular synovitis. The tissue is composed of sheets of mononuclear cells, some of which are forming multinucleate giant cells. An admixture of chronic inflammatory cells is also present.

tan staining, despite the name pigmented villonodular synovitis hemosiderin pigment is not abundant microscopically. It is probably an incidental finding secondary to hemorrhage rather than an etiologic factor.

This lesion is most commonly seen in the fingers, where it has been called by various names, including giant cell tumor of tendon sheath, benign synovioma, and fibroxanthoma. It usually occurs in the flexor tendon sheath and is rarely seen on the extensor surface of the finger. In most instances of major joint involvement, it is the knee that is involved, although occasionally one may see involvement of the hip or other joints. It is grossly nodular and slow growing. In rare instances, multiple sites may be involved in the form of multiple nodules or a diffuse involvement of the synovium. In the latter case total removal may be impossible. Often the bone underlying the lesion is eroded, which may give rise to the erroneous impression on a radiograph that one is dealing with an osseous tumor that has broken out of the bone into the soft tissue. In such a case, multiple giant cells could lead to the incorrect diagnosis of a giant cell tumor of bone.

Although most patients with pigmented villonodular syn-

ovitis are middle-aged at the time the disease manifests, it may occur at any age. There is a high rate of local recurrence after surgery, particularly when the lesion involves a large joint.

Synovial Chondromatosis

Foci of metaplastic cartilage within the synovial tissues are not an uncommon finding in patients with various types of underlying arthritis, and often the cartilaginous nodules in the synovium may become detached and grow independently within the synovial fluid, where they may attain very large sizes.[59] In most instances, synovial chondromatosis is secondary to some underlying joint condition, and frequently one can find at the centers of the loose bodies small fragments of bone or necrotic articular cartilage or fibrin that acted as seeds on which the cartilaginous loose body grew, rather like pearl formation inside an oyster. When such a loose body is sectioned, one will find evenly spaced chondrocytes of uniform size, although the cartilage will be excessively cellular (Fig. 22-30). When the cartilage nodules are in the form of loose bodies, they will undergo recurrent calcification as they get larger, leaving rings of calcium rather like the rings in a tree trunk. If the cartilage nodule is within the synovial membrane, then it may become invaded by blood vessels and endochondral ossification may occur.

Primary chondromatosis, by contrast, is a very uncommon disease and is not preceded by any recognizable underlying arthritis. Histologically, the lesions in primary synovial chondromatosis or chondrometaplasia are much more bizarre. The chondrocytes are cloned into very cellular atypical nests of chondrocytes, calcification occurs in a haphazard and diffuse manner, and the lesional tissue could easily be mistaken for chondrosarcoma (Fig. 22-31). After excision, the rate of recurrence is high. The lesions may occur both in large joints and also in the synovial sheaths of tendons, particularly in the fingers.

Torn Meniscus

A very common orthopedic lesion that frequently follows trauma is a tear of one or another of the menisci of the knee.[60] The tear is usually in the posterior horn and usually runs for some distance within the substance of the meniscus before turning medially to extend onto the medial edge, consequently giving rise to a tag or on occasion a "bucket handle" type of tear. If these lesions have been present for a long time, the edges become very rounded, and occasionally a tag of the posterior meniscus may become detached into the joint, giving rise to a fibrocartilaginous loose body. Histologically, the meniscus is formed of a relatively avascular, highly collagenized tissue, in which the blood vessels are confined to the outer third. Cystic degeneration with mucoid-filled microcysts is fairly common. Occasionally, large cysts may form, particularly in the lateral meniscus.

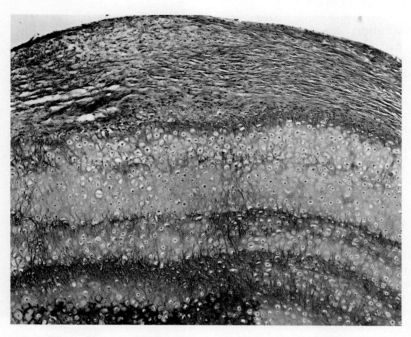

Fig. 22-30. Photomicrograph of a loose body that formed secondary to a detached portion of the articular surface of a knee. The proliferating cartilage is very cellular but with regularly spaced chondrocytes. Concentric rings of calcification are apparent. Compare this photograph with Fig. 22-31.

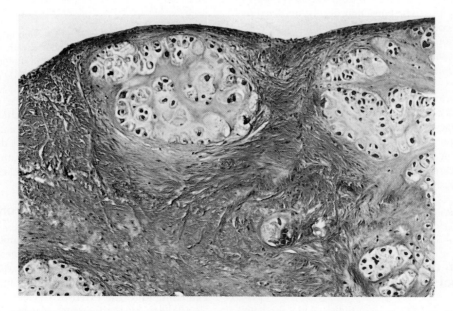

Fig. 22-31. Photomicrograph of a section taken from the synovium of a patient with primary synovial chondromatosis. The islands of cartilage, which form metaplastically within the synovium, are very irregular. The chondrocytes are crowded and vary considerably in size and shape.

MISCELLANEOUS DISEASES OF CONNECTIVE TISSUE

Ganglion

A ganglion is a fibrous walled cyst filled by clear mucinous fluid and usually without a recognizable cyst lining. Ganglia occur in the soft tissues, usually around the hands and feet, and particularly on the extensor surfaces near joints. They may arise as herniations of the synovium or from mucinous degeneration within dense fibrous connective tissue, possibly secondary to trauma. On occasion, they may erode the adjacent bone and even become totally intraosseous; the most common site for such an intraosseous ganglion is the medial malleolus of the tibia.[61]

Bursitis

Acute or chronic bursitis is clinically characterized by pain, redness, and/or swelling of one of the many synovium-lined bursae that lie between muscles, tendons, and bone prominences, especially around the joints. Bursitis is usually caused by chronic trauma. It often occurs in the shoulders of professional athletes and in the prepatellar and infrapatellar bursae of those who frequently kneel. Bursitis is sometimes observed as a complication of rheumatoid arthritis or infection. In cases of rheumatoid arthritis, a cyst may occur particularly in the popliteal area (where it is known as a Baker's cyst) and may extend far into the calf. In the past, bursitis from infection was frequently due to tuberculosis. The bursa may also be involved in other conditions that commonly affect the synovial membrane (e.g., gout, synovial chondromatosis, or pigmented villonodular synovitis). Sometimes extensive calcification may complicate a chronically inflamed bursa, which renders it visible on radiologic examination.

On gross examination of an inflamed bursa, the wall of the bursal sac is usually markedly thickened and the lining often appears injected and shaggy owing to fibrinous exudation into the cavity. The microscopic findings depend on the etiology, and the various disease that might affect the synovium, including infection, should be carefully sought. However, in most cases that are post-traumatic in origin, scarring and chronic inflammation predominate.

Treatment depends on the etiology and the extent of the lesion.

Trigger Finger, de Quervain's Disease, and Carpal Tunnel Syndrome

In both trigger finger and de Quervain's disease,[62] a thickening of the tendon sheath gives rise to clinical problems with movement of the tendon through the sheath. In carpal tunnel syndrome[62] there is compression of the median nerve by thickening of the tissue forming the transverse carpal ligament. These conditions may precede or accompany some systemic disease of the connective tissues such as rheumatoid arthritis. His-

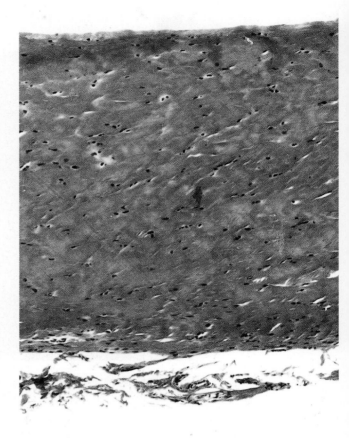

Fig. 22-32. Photomicrograph of a section taken from a patient with a trigger finger. The wall of the tendon sheath, which is normally a very delicate structure, shows a localized thickening by densely collagenized tissue with cells resembling cartilage cells (i.e., fibrocartilage).

tologic examination of the resected thickened tendon sheath will generally show a rather clear-cut cartilaginous or fibrocartilaginous metaplasia of the otherwise delicate tendon sheath (Fig. 22-32). In some cases of carpal tunnel syndrome, amyloid deposits have been recognized as the causative agent.[63]

Morton's Neuroma

Morton's neuroma[64] is a lesion characterized by thickening of the interdigital nerve as it runs between the third and fourth metatarsal heads. Clinically, the patient, who is usually a woman, experiences sharp shooting pains in the sole of the foot extending onto the extensor surface. The resected specimen usually includes the neurovascular bundle and the bifurcation to the third and fourth toe. Just proximal to the bifurcation a fusiform thickening of the neurovascular bundle can usually be observed. Histologic sections will generally show two characteristic features: (1) an occlusion of the digital artery, and (2) extensive fibrosis both around and within the nerve, giving rise to a marked depletion of axons within the digital nerve (Fig.

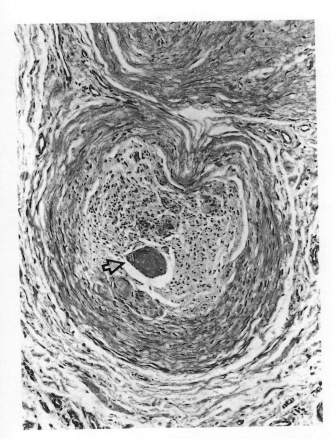

Fig. 22-33. Photomicrograph of a histologic section taken from a patient with Morton's neuroma. The nerve bundles show considerable fibrous proliferation and collagen deposition in the perineurium, as well as within the endoneurium. There is a marked diminution in the number of axons present, and on occasion focal deposits of homogeneous pink material (Renaut bodies, arrow).

22-33). The term neuroma is a misnomer, because there is no evidence in the vast majority of cases of either a traumatic type of neuroma or a neurilemoma.

Prolapsed Intervertebral Disc

Curettage of prolapsed intervertebral disc tissue[65] is an operation commonly undertaken by either the orthopedic surgeon or the neurosurgeon. It usually provides multiple gelatinous pieces of tissue, which on histologic examination will be seen to be composed of portions of fibrous tissue, fibrocartilage, and cartilaginous tissue, the latter with a considerable amount of myxoid material in the matrix. Often, the chondrocytes are necrotic, but in other areas the chondrocytes may be seen to be proliferating, and large clones of cells may be observed. Just as cartilage loose in the joint may give rise to cartilage proliferation, growth, and loose bodies, it is entirely possible that prolapsed intervertebral disc tissue may also, when removed from the constraints of the annulus fibrosa, undergo cellular proliferation and growth and result in secondary nerve root compression.

ACKNOWLEDGMENT

I am extremely grateful to Dr. E. DiCarlo for his help in the preparation of this chapter.

REFERENCES

1. Drury DJ, Bullough PG: Improved photographic reproduction of bone and cartilage specimens using ultraviolet illumination. Med Biol Illus 20:57–58, 1970
2. Bullough PG, Goodfellow J: The significance of the fine structure of articular cartilage. J Bone Joint Surg 50:852–857, 1968
3. Minns RJ, Steven FS: The collagen fibril organization in human articular cartilage. J Anat 123:437–457, 1977
4. Scott JE: The histochemistry of cartilage proteoglycans in light and electron microscopy. pp. 19–32. In Ali SY, Elves MW, Leaback DH (eds): Normal and Osteoarthrotic Articular Cartilage. Institute of Orthopaedics (University of London), London, 1974
5. Jowsey J: The Bone Biopsy. Plenum Medical, New York, 1977
6. Enlow DH: Principles of Bone Remodeling. An Account of Postnatal Growth and Remodeling Processes in Long Bones and the Mandible. Charles C Thomas, Springfield, IL, 1963
7. Jaffe HL: Metabolic, Degenerative and Inflammatory Disease of Bones and Joints. Lea & Febiger, Philadelphia, 1972
8. Bourne GH (ed): The Biochemistry and Physiology of Bone. Vols. 1–4. Academic Press, Orlando, FL, 1971–1976
9. Cormack DH: Bone. Ch. 12. In: Ham's Histology. 9th Ed. Lippincott-Raven, Philadelphia, 1987
10. Sokoloff L: Note on the histology of cement lines. p. 135. In Kenedi RM (ed): Perspectives in Biomedical Engineering. MacMillan, London, 1973
11. Avioli LV: Senile and postmenopausal osteoporosis. Adv Intern Med 21:391–415, 1976
12. Johnston CC, Lavy N, Lord T, et al: Osteopetrosis: a clinical, genetic, metabolic and morphologic study of the dominantly inherited, benign form. Medicine (Baltimore) 47:149–167, 1968
13. Ham AW, Harris WR: Repair and transplantation of bone. Ch. 10. In Bourne GH (ed): Biochemistry and Physiology of Bone. 2nd Ed. Academic Press, Orlando, FL, 1971
14. Cruess R, Dumont J: Healing of bone, tendon and ligament. p. 97. In Rockwood CA Jr, Green DP (eds): Fractures. Lippincott-Raven, Philadelphia, 1975
15. Davidson JK: Aseptic Necrosis of Bone. American Elsevier, New York, 1976
16. Catto M: A histological study of avascular necrosis of the femoral head after transcervical fracture. J Bone Joint Surg Br 47:749–776, 1965
17. Bullough PG, Kambolis CP, Marcove RC, et al: Bone infarctions not associated with caisson disease. J Bone Joint Surg Am 47:477–491, 1965
18. Mirra JM, Bullough PG, Marcove RC, et al: Malignant fibrous histiocytoma and osteosarcoma in association with bone infarcts: report of four cases, two in caisson workers. J Bone Joint Surg Am 56:932–940, 1974
19. Smith R, Russell RGG, Woods CG: Myositis ossificans progressiva. J Bone Joint Surg Br 58:48–57, 1976
20. Paterson DC: Myositis ossificans circumscripta. J Bone Joint Surg Br 52:296–301, 1970
21. Trelstad RL, Rubin D, Gross J: Osteogenesis imperfecta congenita: evidence for a generalized molecular disorder of collagen. Lab Invest 36:501–508, 1977
22. McKusick VA, Neufeld EF, Kelly TE: The mucopolysaccharide storage diseases. p. 1282. In Stanbury JB, Wyngaarden JB, Frederickson DS (eds):

The Metabolic Basis of Inherited Disease. 4th Ed. McGraw-Hill, New York, 1978

23. Teitelbaum SL, Rosenberg EM, Bates M, et al: The effects of phosphate and vitamin D therapy on osteopenic, hypophosphatemic osteomalacia of childhood. Clin Orthop 116:38–47, 1976

24. Whalen JP, Horwith M, Krook L, et al: Calcitonin treatment in hereditary bone dysplasia with hyperphosphatasemia: a radiographic and histologic study of bone. AJR 129:29–35, 1977

25. Malluche HH, Faugere MC, Smith AJ, Friedler RM: Aluminum intoxication of bone in renal failure—fact or fiction? Kidney Int, suppl. 18:570–573, 1986

26. Epker BN: A quantitative histologic study of the effects of fluoride on resorption and formation in animal and human bone. Clin Orthop 49:77–87, 1966

27. Langloh ND, Hunder GG, Riggs LB, et al: Transient painful osteoporosis of the lower extremities. J Bone Joint Surg Am 55:1188–1196, 1973

28. Bullough PG: Massive osteolysis. NY State J Med 71:2267–2278, 1971

29. Rasmussen H, Bordier P: The Physiological and Cellular Basis of Metabolic Bone Disease. Williams & Wilkins, Baltimore, 1974

30. Wilde CD, Jaworski ZF, Villaneuva AR, et al: Quantitative histological measurements of bone turnover in primary hyperparathyroidism. Calcif Tissue Res 12:137–142, 1973

31. Teitelbaum SL, Bullough PG: The pathophysiology of bone and joint disease. Am J Pathol 96:283–354, 1979

32. DeLuca HF: Recent advances in our understanding of the vitamin D endocrine system. J Lab Clin Med 87:7–26, 1976

33. O'Brien WM, Banfield WG, Sokoloff L: Studies on the pathogenesis of ochronotic arthropathy. Arthritis Rheum 4:137–152, 1961

34. Kinnett JG, Bullough PG: Identification of calcium oxalate deposits in bone by electron diffraction. Arch Pathol Lab Med 100:656–659, 1976

35. McCarty DJ (ed): Conference on pseudogout and pyrophosphate metabolism. Arthritis Rheum 19:275–285, 1976

36. Wyngaarden JB, Holmes EW: Clinical gout and the pathogenesis of hyperuricemia. p. 1193. In McCarty DG (ed): Arthritis and Allied Conditions, a Textbook of Rheumatology. 9th Ed. Lea & Febiger, Philadelphia, 1979

37. Brady RO: Glucosyl ceramide lipidosis (Gaucher's disease). p. 731. In Stanbury JB, Wyngaarden JB, Fredrickson DS (eds): Metabolic Basis of Inherited Disease. 4th Ed. McGraw-Hill, New York, 1978

38. Barry H: Paget's Disease of Bone. Williams & Wilkins, Baltimore, 1969

39. Rebel A, Malkain K, Basel M, et al: Osteoclast ultrastructure in Paget's disease. Calcif Tissue Res 20:187–199, 1976 ·

40. Price CHG, Goldie W: Paget's sarcoma of bone. A study of 80 cases. J Bone Joint Surg Br 51:205–224, 1969

41. Kelly PJ, Fitzgerald RH (eds): Symposium on infections in orthopedics. Orthop Clin North Am 6:915–1144, 1975

42. Miller J (ed): Bone infections symposium. Clin Orthop 96:2–344, 1973

43. Spjut HJ, Dorfman HD, Fechner RE, et al: Tumors of bone and cartilage. p. 387. In: Atlas of Tumor Pathology, Series 2. Fasc. 5. Armed Forces Institute of Pathology, Washington, DC, 1970

44. Lieberman PH, Jones CR, Dargeon HWK, et al: A reappraisal of eosinophilic granuloma of bone, Hand-Schüller-Christian syndrome and Letterer-Siwe syndrome. Medicine (Baltimore) 48:375–400, 1969

45. Cormack DJ: Joints. Ch. 13. In: Ham's Histology. 9th Ed. Lippincott-Raven, Philadelphia, 1987

46. Hamerman D, Rosenberg LC, Schubert M: Diarthrodial joints revisited. J Bone Joint Surg Am 52:725–774, 1970

47. Muir IHM: Biochemistry. p. 145. In Freeman MAR (ed): Adult Articular Cartilage. 2nd Ed. Pittman Medical, Kent, 1979

48. Meisel AD, Bullough PG: Atlas of Osteoarthritis. Lea & Febiger, Philadelphia, 1984

49. Nichols EH, Richardson FL: Arthritis deformans. J Med Res 21:149–221, 1909

50. Salvati EA, Granda JL, Mirra J, et al: Clinical, enzymatic and histologic study of synovium in coxarthrosis. Int Orthop 1:39–42, 1977

51. Perry GH, Smith JG, Whiteside CG: Spontaneous recovery of the joint space in degenerative hip disease. Ann Rheum Dis 31:440–448, 1972

52. Sokoloff L: Pathology of rheumatoid arthritis and allied disorders. p. 429. In McCarty DJ (ed): Arthritis and Allied Conditions, a Textbook of Rheumatology. 9th Ed. Lea & Febiger, Philadelphia, 1979

53. Schumacher HR, Klippel JH, Koopman WJ (eds): Primer on the Rheumatic Diseases. 10th Ed. Arthritis Foundation, Atlanta, 1993

54. Winchester RJ: B Lymphocyte alloantigens, cellular expression, and disease significance with special reference to rheumatoid arthritis. Arthritis Rheum 20:S159–163, 1977

55. Sokoloff L: Pathophysiology of peripheral blood vessels in collagen diseases. In Orbison JL, Smith DE (eds): The Peripheral Blood Vessels. Williams & Wilkins, Baltimore, 1963

56. DiCarlo EF, Bullough PG: The biologic responses to orthopedic implants and their wear debris. Clin Mater 9:235–260, 1992

57. Semlitsch M, Willert HG: Gewebsveranderungen im Bereiche metallischer Huftgelenke; mikroanalytische Untersuchungen mittels Spektralphotometrie, Elektronemikroscopie und der Elektronen-strahlmikrosonde. VI Internat Symp fur Mikrochemie, Vol C, p. 70, 1970

58. Byers PD, Cotton RE, Deacon OW, et al: The diagnosis and treatment of pigmented villonodular synovitis. J Bone Joint Surg Br 50:290–305, 1968

59. Villacin AB, Brigham LN, Bullough PG: Primary and secondary synovial chondrometaplasia. Hum Pathol 10:439–451, 1979

60. Smillie IS: Surgical pathology of the menisci. In: Injuries of the Knee Joint. Churchill Livingstone, Edinburgh, 1978

61. Kambolis C, Bullough PG, Jaffe HL: Ganglionic cystic defects of bone. J Bone Joint Surg Am 55:496–505, 1973

62. Phalen GS: The carpal-tunnel syndrome. J Bone Joint Surg Am 48:211–228, 1966

63. Massachusetts General Hospital: Case records. Weekly clinico-pathological exercises. Case 10. N Engl J Med 286:534–539, 1972

64. Asbury AK, Johnson PC: Morton's neuroma. p. 204. In: Pathology of Peripheral Nerve. WB Saunders, Philadelphia, 1978

65. Schmorl G: The displacement of intervertebral disc tissue in the human spine. p. 158. In Junghanns H (ed): Besemann EF (trans-ed): Health and Disease. 5th German Ed., 2nd American Ed. Grune & Stratton, Orlando, FL, 1971

66. Paget S, Bullough PG: Synovivm and synovial fluid. pp. 18–22. In Owen R, Goodfellow JW, Bullough PG (eds): Scientific Foundation of Orthopaedics and Traumatology. WB Saunders, Philadelphia, 1980

23

Neoplasms and Tumor-Like Lesions of Bone

Alberto G. Ayala

Jae Y. Ro

Lisa A. Teot

Harlan J. Spjut

CLINICAL AND RADIOGRAPHIC CONSIDERATIONS

Neoplasms of bone are often a diagnostic problem because they are uncommon and represent a rather small part of the diagnostic experience of most pathologists. Even so, the pathologist may enhance the diagnosis of neoplasms of bone with knowledge of their clinical presentation, biologic behavior, and radiologic features. In addition, close cooperation with an orthopedic surgeon and a radiologist is essential for arriving at an accurate diagnosis.[1-5] Admittedly, the clinical manifestation of most neoplasms of bone is rather nonspecific in that the patient has pain, tenderness, or swelling of the affected part. Nevertheless, if the pathologist is aware of a few pieces of clinical information, such as the location of the lesion, its radiologic features, and the age of the patient, reasonable differential diagnostic possibilities can be considered. For example, it is distinctly uncommon for giant cell tumors to occur before the age of 15 years. Thus, a pathologist insisting on a diagnosis of giant cell tumor in a child aged 10 or 11 years must give strong consideration to some other lesion that contains many multinucleated giant cells. By contrast, chondrosarcomas are most likely to occur after the age of 20 years, whereas a Ewing's sarcoma is common before age 20. Similar observations can be applied to localization in a long bone. For example, a giant cell tumor is epiphyseal and metaphyseal in location; thus, when having to diagnose a lesion that histologically contains numerous multinucleated giant cells but has no epiphyseal component on radiographs, one must strongly consider other lesions. The same holds true for chondroblastomas, which are recognized to be epiphyseal lesions, but commonly have a metaphyseal component. Osteosarcomas of the long bones are likely to be metaphyseal, whereas Ewing's sarcoma or malignant lymphoma may involve the diaphysis or the metaphysis, or both. The latter three tumors are unlikely to be epiphyseal only. Thus, if the pathologist takes care to review the clinical and radiologic

information, the differential diagnosis of neoplasms of bone can be more practical.

Radiologic findings are one of the most important parameters in the diagnosis of bone tumors. Plain radiographs remain the most valuable tool with which to diagnose a bone tumor. Computed tomography (CT) and magnetic resonance imaging (MRI) are also integral parts of the examination of a patient with a bone tumor; whereas in some instances they can provide diagnostic clues (such as the demonstration of the nidus with CT scan), these procedures usually provide information that is more valuable in the management of the lesion (extent of involvement in the bone and soft tissue) than in the diagnosis. Radionucleide scans often detect the lesion but are not specific; however, in some instances, such as in osteoid osteoma and stress fractures, radionucleide scans are very valuable in demonstrating the site of the disease.

The radiologic features often represent the only opportunity that the pathologist has of seeing the tumor intact because many benign lesions are curetted, depriving the pathologist of an intact lesion. In effect, radiologic findings represent the gross findings for many neoplasms as far as the pathologist is concerned. Therefore, the pathologist must be familiar with radiologic features of neoplasms and lesions that simulate neoplasms of bone to be able to interpret histologic material properly. Obviously, detailed interpretation of the radiographs must be done by a radiologist, with whom the pathologist should have a consultative working relationship. Some tumors, such as nonossifying fibroma, osteoid osteoma, and some cartilaginous lesions, are almost specifically diagnosable by their radiologic features.

In the same light, an understanding of the anatomic and histologic features of bone is essential in the diagnosis of skeletal tumors. Awareness of the epiphysis, the growth plate, the metaphysis, and the diaphysis is important in regard to differential diagnosis of neoplasms of long bones. It is of interest to remember that ossification centers in the pelvis and vertebrae serve as sites of tumors that are generally considered to arise from an epiphysis (e.g., chondroblastoma and giant cell tumor).

BONE TUMOR BIOPSY

Once a radiologic diagnosis of a bone tumor has been made, a biopsy should be considered. There are two types of biopsies: closed and open. Closed biopsies refer to the application of a needle to obtain cells for cytologic examination or a core of tissue for histologic examination. Open biopsies may be incisional or excisional. Included in these is the common practice of the curettage biopsy. The type of biopsy depends on the radiologic interpretation of the bone lesion. As a general rule, if a malignant lesion is suspected, the biopsy should be made by the surgeon who will be involved in the management of the patient's disease, especially if a limb-sparing procedure is contemplated. The site, size, and type of the biopsy have to be perfectly planned in relation to the ultimate surgical procedure so that the latter, whether a major amputation or a limb salvage procedure, is not marred by a poorly placed incision that will require additional surgery. The old custom of performing a biopsy before referring the patient to a major institution is discouraged because an improper biopsy may handicap any attempt at limb salvage.

Not all bone lesions need to be biopsied; for example, it may not be necessary to do a biopsy on a lesion entirely characteristic of a nonossifying fibroma that is found incidental to radiographic examination of the limb for other reasons. The same might be said for lesions characteristic of fibrous dysplasia. However, if it is not possible to suggest a specific radiologic diagnosis, or if the findings strongly point to a malignant lesion, a biopsy is needed. It should be kept in mind that some malignant tumors may appear to be benign and that benign lesions such as osteomyelitis or eosinophilic granuloma may mimic malignant lesions.

After the need for biopsy has been determined, the site where the biopsy material is to be taken from becomes important. Radiographic features are of great importance in this decision; areas on radiographs that show disease progression and active destruction should be chosen because these sites should contain diagnosable rather than reactive tissue. Densely sclerotic sites may not be diagnostic because they may consist of bone or of calcified necrotic tissue. Tumors such as parosteal osteosarcomas are uniformly dense, leaving little choice as to biopsy site. Many malignant bone tumors frequently have an extracortical component that is an ideal site for biopsy and from which to retrieve tissue for frozen section examination.

The type of biopsy must be considered. For lesions that are benign and have radiographic features strongly suggestive of tumors, such as chondroblastoma, osteoid osteoma, aneurysmal bone cyst, enchondroma, and fibrous dysplasia, the biopsy may be a fine needle aspiration (FNA), a core, an excision, or a curettage; the latter two also serve as definitive treatments. Skeletal location leads to modification of the biopsy technique; for example, an aneurysmal bone cyst of a vertebra is not likely to be excised, whereas one of the fibula may be resected en bloc. Incisional biopsy should be considered for large lesions that might require a major surgical procedure for their extirpation (e.g., chondrosarcoma of the upper end of the femur or of the pelvic bones). If incisional biopsy is decided, a deep wedge is suggested to avoid the possibility of only including the reactive tissues around an expanding neoplasm. Reactive tissues have been mistaken for neoplasm by both surgeons and pathologists. Thus, in nearly all instances, we advise the orthopedic surgeon to obtain tissue for frozen section examination from the material removed at biopsy. It is not always possible to select tissue that can be cut on frozen section, but in most cases, small particles of tissue free of bone or containing osteoid can be submitted for frozen section. Even though a specific diagnosis may not be made or the surgeon may not be willing to accept the diagnosis, the frozen section serves the purpose of demonstrating that lesional tissue has been obtained. This is important to avoid a second biopsy, should only reactive tissue be included in the biopsy material.

PROCESSING OF BIOPSY SPECIMENS

We have had considerable experience with needle biopsies in the diagnosis of bone neoplasms.[6,7] The site for needle biopsy is carefully determined after thorough radiographic examination of the lesion. Usually, an FNA is done initially and the material is submitted for immediate cytologic interpretation. If the material is diagnostic (e.g., as it would be for metastatic carcinoma or eosinophilic granuloma) no additional tissue is obtained. If the material is not diagnostic, a core of tissue is obtained that can be used for frozen section examination if necessary. In most cases, a specific diagnosis can be made from needle biopsy specimens.[6,7] The needle biopsy has the advantage of usually not requiring general anesthesia, thus saving the patient the risk (however minor) and the expense of an operating room. We are conservative in the interpretation of needle biopsy specimens. If a diagnosis cannot be made or is equivocal, open biopsy is done. The liquid material obtained from cystic lesions should be routinely submitted for cytologic examination.

Regardless of the type of biopsy, tissue should be saved for electron microscopic examination. In most cases, examination with the electron microscope is not necessary for a diagnosis, but occasionally it is an important part of the diagnosis. This is particularly true of undifferentiated malignant tumors such as Ewing's sarcoma, malignant lymphomas, and metastatic tumors such as neuroblastoma and undifferentiated carcinoma.

As with any surgical specimen, proper fixation, appropriate choice of tissue selection, and thickness of blocks are keys to obtaining adequate histologic sections. In addition, when bone or calcific areas are present, decalcification must be done. Many solutions are available for decalcification, all of which serve the purpose well. The pathologist must be careful that the tissues are not over-decalcified because this will distort the osseous and soft tissue components. Decalcified tissues seem to take up eosin rather avidly; thus, during the staining process, allowing more time for hematoxylin stain and less for eosin stain is advisable.

PROCESSING OF RESECTION AND AMPUTATION SPECIMENS

Intact, locally excised lesions and amputation specimens deserve special attention. In addition to adequate descriptions and measurements, radiologic examination of the intact and sliced specimen may be useful. The radiologic studies may also reveal areas that may be of interest for histologic examination. For smaller specimens, slicing may be done with a sharp hand saw or a power band saw. Amputation specimens may be examined in two ways.[8] In the first, the specimen may be deep frozen and then cut sagittally or crosswise using a hand saw or a power band saw with the soft tissues left intact. This has the advantage of maintaining the relations of the soft tissues (particularly the muscles and neurovascular bundles) to the neoplasm. It has the disadvantage that freezing artifact may appear in the subsequent histologic examinations. To circumvent freezing artifacts, it is suggested that blocks of the tumor be removed before the specimen is frozen. This ordinarily does not distort the specimen greatly because the biopsy site is usually present.[8]

For the second method of dissection, the soft tissues are removed after careful notation of their relationship to the tumor: the specimen can be either fixed or cut fresh with a hand saw or a power band saw. After fixation of the slices, the blocks are selected. It may be desirable to indicate the site of the blocks diagrammatically in the event that careful radiologic and gross correlations are to be undertaken (Fig. 23-1). With amputation specimens, it is desirable to obtain marrow specimens proximal to the tumor to determine whether intramedullary sites of the neoplasm were undetected on radiographs. In addition, the amputation site should be examined histologically for the possibility of spread to this area. If there is transection of a bone rather than disarticulation, the proximal end of the bone is curetted by the orthopedic surgeon at the time of the amputation and submitted as a separate specimen; frozen section may be done. If the amputation specimen includes lymph node-bearing areas, the nodes, of course, should be isolated and examined. In all instances, photographic documentation of the specimen is helpful.

CLASSIFICATION OF BONE TUMORS

The classification of tumors of bone is and has been based on histologic patterns and on tissue or cell of origin, which, in turn, have generally correlated with the biologic behavior of the tumor.[9] Although this type of classification is not ideal, it serves the purpose of grouping lesions according to histologic patterns, enabling a means of communication among physicians who treat patients and those who report in medical journals.

We have modified the system of the World Health Organization classification[10] as follows:

I. Bone-forming tumors
  A. Benign
    1. Osteoma
    2. Osteoid osteoma
    3. Osteoblastoma
  B. Indeterminate
    1. Aggressive osteoblastoma
  C. Malignant
    1. Conventional osteosarcoma (osteogenic sarcoma)
    2. Parosteal osteosarcoma (juxtacortical osteosarcoma)

Fig. 23-1. Hemisection of a femoral osteosarcoma showing the blocks to be submitted for sectioning. A film of the specimen is on the left.

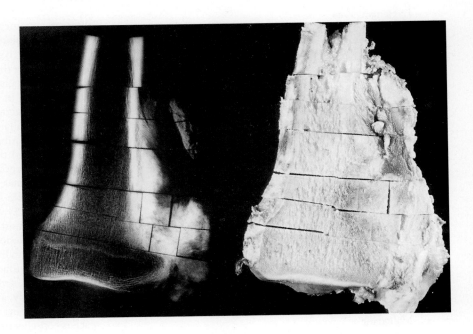

3. Periosteal osteosarcoma

4. High grade osteosarcoma on the surface

5. Intraosseous well differentiated osteosarcoma

6. Osteosarcoma of the jaws

7. Rare osteosarcomas: intracortical, arising in Paget's disease, irradiated bone, or bone infarct

II. Cartilage-forming tumors

A. Benign

1. Osteochondroma (osteocartilaginous exostosis)

2. Chondroma (enchondroma)

3. Chondroblastoma

4. Chondromyxoid fibroma

5. Periosteal chondroma

B. Malignant

1. Chondrosarcoma

2. Mesenchymal chondrosarcoma

3. Dedifferentiated chondrosarcoma

4. Clear cell chondrosarcoma

5. Extraosseous chondrosarcoma

6. Extraskeletal myxoid chondrosarcoma

III. Giant cell tumor

IV. Marrow tumors

1. Ewing's sarcoma-peripheral neuroectodermal tumor (PNET)

2. Malignant lymphoma

3. Myeloma

4. Mastocytosis

V. Vascular tumors

A. Benign

1. Hemangioma

2. Skeletal angiomatosis

3. Massive osteolysis (Gorham's disease)

4. Lymphangioma

5. Glomus tumor (glomangioma)

B. Intermediate or indeterminate

1. Epithelioid/histiocytoid hemangioendothelioma

2. Hemangiopericytoma

C. Malignant

1. Angiosarcoma (high grade angiosarcoma)

VI. Connective tissue lesions

A. Benign

1. Metaphyseal fibrous defect/nonossifying fibroma

2. Fibrous histiocytoma, atypical fibrous histiocytoma, and fibroxanthoma

B. Indeterminate or intermediate

1. Desmoplastic fibroma

C. Malignant

1. Fibrosarcoma

2. Malignant fibrous histiocytoma

D. Other tumors

1. Chest wall mesenchymal hamartoma

2. Lipoma

3. Liposarcoma

4. Malignant mesenchymoma

5. Leiomyosarcoma

VII. Other tumors

1. Chordoma and parachordoma

2. Adamantinoma of long bones

3. Neurogenic tumors (neurilemoma and neurofibroma)

VIII. Tumor-like lesions

1. Solitary bone cyst (simple or unicameral bone cyst)

2. Aneurysmal bone cyst

3. Juxta-articular bone cyst (intraosseous ganglion)

4. Eosinophilic granuloma

5. Fibro-osseous lesions (fibrous dysplasia/ossifying fibroma and osteofibrous dysplasia)

6. Localized myositis ossificans

7. Brown tumor of hyperparathyroidism

IX. Metastatic malignant neoplasms

BONE-FORMING TUMORS

Benign Tumors

Osteoma

Osteomas are uncommon bony lesions that are predominantly found in the paranasal sinuses, particularly the frontal sinus.[11] They may be seen at any age and are usually solitary. Solitary or multiple lesions that occur in the skull and mandible are also reported in association with Gardner's syndrome.[12] Osteomas are uncommon in bones other than those of the paranasal sinuses, but extracranial osteomas have been described that involve the medullary cavity or the surface of a bone.[1,13] Dahlin and Unni[1] described two osteomas (one in the tibia and the other in the rib) that involved extracranial bones. Bertoni et al[13] recently reported on 14 patients who had extracranial parosteal osteomas, 13 involving the long bones and 1 the clavicle. The 8 males and 6 females ranged in age from 21 to 66 years (median, 43 years; average, 45 years). The femur and the tibia were the most commonly affected bones.

Grossly, the lesion is rock hard and nodular, correlating with the radiologic findings of a radiodense, somewhat lobulated lesion. The cut surface of an osteoma demonstrates bone that is dense and hard, similar to normal cortical bone.

Histologically, the lesion consists of cortical bone with haversian systems and broad bony trabeculae. The marrow space is consequently sparse. Osteoblasts are usually inconspicuous. Osteoma probably does not have a malignant counterpart.

The surface lesions most likely to be confused with osteoma are bony spurs, osteochondroma, and parosteal osteosarcoma. The bony spur is radiologically not as dense as the osteoma, nor is it lobular in pattern. The same holds true for osteochondromas, which generally involve the metaphysis of long bones and have a pedicle that melds with the cortex. Histologically, a bony spur is likely to exhibit osteoblastic activity and does not have the extreme thickness of the bony trabeculae seen in osteoma. Osteochondromas are identified by a cartilaginous cap, but in the absence of such a cap, islands of cartilage may be found in the bony trabeculae. The trabeculae are not as broad or dense as those of an osteoma. Parosteal osteoma shows the same histologic features as its medullary counterpart, including the haversian system. Parosteal osteoma differs from parosteal osteosarcoma in that on radiographs it appears as a dense solid bone lesion without areas of radiolucency and has smooth lobulated surfaces; histologically it does not contain a spindle cell stroma.

Osteoma requires no treatment unless it is symptomatic. A simple excision should be curative.

Osteoid Osteoma

Osteoid osteoma is a benign neoplasm, accounting for about 12 percent of all benign bone tumors.[1] It occurs predominantly in males. Most cases (85 percent) occur in people between the ages of 5 and 24 years and rarely in those younger than 5 years or older than 50 years. Osteoid osteoma is most commonly seen in the metadiaphyseal portion of long bones, particularly the tibia and femur, although a wide variety of skeletal locations have been described. This is a lesion that may be diagnosed quite readily by its radiographic features and often by its clinical features.[14]

The classic clinical presentation is pain in the affected part (e.g., the thigh) that is usually more severe during the night and can be relieved by aspirin. However, this clinical presentation represents the minority of patients who have an osteoid osteoma. Osteoid osteoma of the vertebra may produce pain that

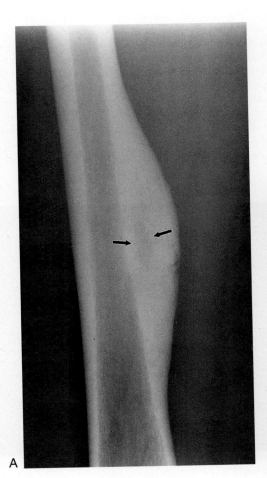 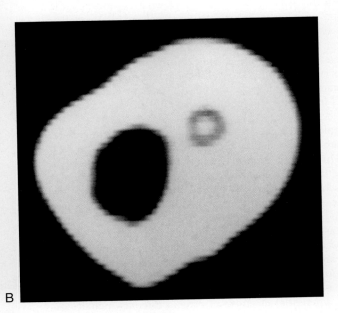

Fig. 23-2. **(A)** Anteroposterior and lateral views of an osteoid osteoma of the femur. It is cortical in location and has resulted in bony sclerosis. Arrows indicate the nidus. **(B)** Computed tomography demonstrates the nidus surrounded by the thickened reactive cortical bone.

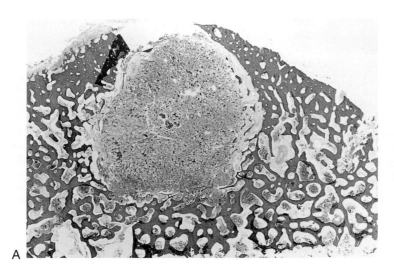
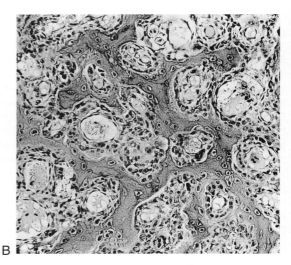

Fig. 23-3. **(A)** Whole-mount section of an osteoid osteoma. The nidus seems to lie loosely in the surrounding sclerotic bone. **(B)** Osteoid osteoma. Irregular partially mineralized bone, abundant osteoblasts, and numerous small blood vessels comprise the nidus.

simulates intervertebral disc disease.[15] Scoliosis may sometimes be due to osteoid osteoma, which is said to be the most common cause of painful scoliosis in children.[16] Osteoid osteoma located near an articular surface, particularly the hip, may be associated with the early onset of degenerative disease.[17]

Radiologically, osteoid osteoma may occupy the medullary cavity, the cortex, or the surface of the bone, but the most common presentation is in the cortex. On plain films one sees a zone of bony sclerosis, particularly if the osteoid osteoma involves the cortex of a long bone. Within the zone of sclerosis a radiolucency represents the nidus (Fig. 23-2). The amount of sclerosis surrounding the nidus is somewhat dependent on its location, with less seen in nidi of periosteal and intramedullary locations. An abscess of bone may exhibit a similar radiologic picture.

Grossly, the nidus is hyperemic, round, and surrounded by a zone of sclerotic bone. The nidus usually measures 1 cm or less in diameter. Radiologic studies of the gross specimen may be helpful in locating the nidus, should it be inconspicuous (Fig. 23-2).

Histologically, poorly oriented bony trabeculae are present; some are heavily calcified and others show little or no calcification. The irregular arrangement of the bony trabeculae serves to set the nidus off from the surrounding medullary or compact bone, which may be nearly normal. Osteoblasts lining the trabeculae of the nidus are abundant. Although large, they are uniform and show no nuclear pleomorphism (Fig. 23-3). Osteoclasts occur quite frequently and are of normal configuration. The intertrabecular stroma is loose areolar tissue that is highly vascular. There are no inflammatory cells, but nerve fibers have been demonstrated in the nidus.[18] Further confirmation of the nerve fibers has been found using S-100 protein immunostaining.[19]

The differential diagnosis of osteoid osteoma includes osteomyelitis, osteoblastoma, and osteosarcoma. Bone abscesses may simulate osteoid osteoma radiologically but not histologi-

cally. Osteoblastoma has an identical histologic pattern to that of osteoid osteoma and is therefore indistinguishable. The lesion is distinguished from osteoid osteoma on the basis of size, with the nidus of osteoblastoma exceeding 2 cm in greatest dimension. On radiographs, osteoblastoma shows considerably less bony sclerosis than does osteoid osteoma. Osteoid osteoma is only a problem (in relation to a diagnosis of osteosarcoma) when the nidus is curetted and the pathologist is unaware of the radiologic or clinical findings. Attention to the radiologic findings will alleviate any possibility of mistaking these two lesions.

Complete removal of the nidus is the treatment of choice. A

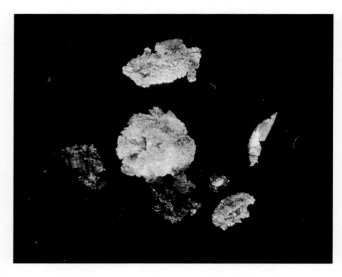

Fig. 23-4. Ultraviolet light examination of nidus. The nidus shows a golden yellow color on ultraviolet light examination. The patient received tetracycline 2 days before excision of the nidus.

simple technique to detect the nidus during surgery is to give the patient tetracycline 1 or 2 days before surgery.[20] Tetracycline binds to osteoid and can be detected by ultraviolet light. The resected specimen is examined in a dark room under the ultraviolet light; the nidus fluoresces, with a yellow-golden granular appearance (Fig. 23-4). Other techniques to detect the nidus employ radionucleides. The patient is given a dose of radioactive technetium, which localizes in the nidus. During surgery the radiation emitted by the radionucleide in the nidus is measured with a Geiger counter. When there is no longer any radioactivity in the surgical bed, the nidus has been removed.

If the nidus is not completely removed, symptoms may persist or recur.[21] It is possible that some "recurrences" are due to multicentric nidi.[22] Evidence also shows that they may regress occasionally.[18] Apparently no malignant counterpart of osteoid osteoma exists.

Osteoblastoma

Osteoblastoma accounts for about 1 to 4 percent of all primary bone neoplasms and has a significant male predominance (3:1).[1,23] The age range is 5 to 78 years, with the second and third decades of life representing the years of most common occurrence.[24]

Osteoblastoma is usually localized to long bones and the vertebrae and is less likely to provoke the outstanding bony sclerosis typical of osteoid osteoma.[18,25] Radiologically, it is a lucent defect surrounded by a narrow zone of bony sclerosis. At times, the sclerosis may be as marked as that of osteoid osteoma. Osteoblastomas are 2 cm or more (possibly as large as 10 cm) in diameter. Because radiographically the lesion may be large and radiolucent, it may be mistaken for a more serious lesion, such as osteosarcoma. Grossly, the tumor is hyperemic and often loosely attached to the surrounding bone. The cut surfaces are red to red-brown, somewhat nodular, and gritty, with the grittiness correlating with bone.

Histologically, it is similar to, if not indistinguishable from, osteoid osteoma (Fig. 23-5). It has been stated that the bony trabeculae of osteoblastoma are slightly wider than those of osteoid osteoma and that there is less irregularity in their arrangement. The major histologic problem of osteoblastoma is its differentiation from osteosarcoma and aggressive osteoblastoma. Conventional osteosarcoma is not a diagnostic problem because it contains a malignant spindle, fibroblastic, or cartilaginous stroma that produces osteoid. A diagnostic problem arises in tumors that have been termed osteoblastoma-like osteosarcomas, which are osteoblastic, show a relatively bland stroma, and may have a cartilaginous component.[26] The presence of cartilage in an osteoid-producing lesion should alert the pathologist to consider a diagnosis of osteosarcoma. Although some osteoblastomas have been reported to contain cartilage, most of them do not.[27] The presence of malignant cartilage places the lesion in the osteosarcoma category.

Equally difficult to determine is the distinction between benign osteoblastoma and aggressive (epithelioid) osteoblastoma.[24,28] In the latter lesion, the osteoblasts are large, epithelioid, and often arranged in clusters; they have abundant cytoplasm and their nuclei show a fine nuclear chromatin pat-

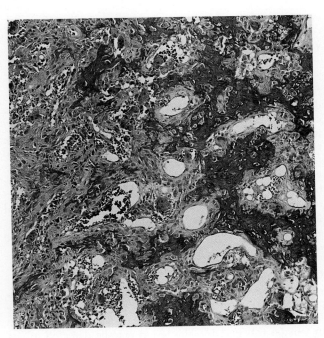

Fig. 23-5. Osteoblastoma. The similarity with osteoid osteoma is apparent. At higher magnification osteoblasts and osteoclasts are readily seen.

tern, often with a large prominent nucleolus. Mitotic activity may be present. The bony trabeculae, although similar to osteoblastoma, are larger and thicker and often display pagetoid cement lines. If these findings are present, then one should consider the possibility of aggressive osteoblastoma or osteosarcoma. In contrast to osteoid osteoma, a few acceptable cases of osteosarcoma that arose either in association with or from an osteoblastoma have been reported, but this is a rare occurrence.[28]

The management for osteoblastoma is curettage with bone packing. The local relapse rate is about 15 percent, even with incomplete curettage.[29] A second curettage is almost always curative. Excision may be attempted if feasible.

Aggressive (Epithelioid) Osteoblastoma

Aggressive (epithelioid) osteoblastoma is so designated partly on the basis of its clinical behavior and partly on the basis of its histologic features. Histologically, this tumor is not always easily defined, but Dorfman and Weiss[30] pointed out the feature of plump epithelioid osteoblasts that is helpful in distinguishing aggressive osteoblastoma from other osteoblastic tumors. In addition, it has been noted that the clinical behavior of these lesions is aggressive: recurrences are common, often with extension into adjacent tissues, and may be massive. Differentiation of this lesion from osteosarcoma is difficult and sometimes impossible.[30] Hence, some authorities believe it should be considered as a variant of osteosarcoma. At the University of Texas M.D. Anderson Cancer Center, aggressive osteoblastoma is considered a locally aggressive malignant tumor and is treated with the same protocol utilized for osteosarcoma.

Malignant Tumors

Osteosarcoma

Several different malignant bone-producing tumors are identified under the term osteosarcoma. These lesions have the production of malignant osteoid, bone, and/or cartilage as their common denominator, and each has a distinct natural behavior. Until recently we have utilized the classification of osteosarcoma proposed by Dahlin and Unni[1]; however, Raymond et al[8] proposed another classification that incorporates new developments and reorganizes existing concepts. In this classification, four major groups are considered: (1) conventional osteosarcoma, (2) osteosarcoma arising in special clinical settings, (3) osteosarcoma defined by histologic parameters, and (4) osteosarcoma arising on the surface of a bone (Table 23-1).

Conventional Osteosarcoma

Conventional osteosarcoma is the most common and most important of the osteosarcomas. It has a peak occurrence in the second decade of life and occurs more frequently in males than in females (about 2:1). The lesion may be detected in any decade of life but is rare in children younger than 5 years and less frequently arises de novo in adults.[1,31] When diagnosed in an adult, predisposing factors should be sought such as Paget's disease of bone, previous irradiation, bone infarct, or history of fibrous dysplasia.[1–4]

Osteosarcoma most frequently involves the metaphysis of the long bones, with the distal end of the femur, proximal tibia, and proximal humerus being the most common sites of involvement. However, osteosarcoma has also been described in almost all skeletal sites.[1–4]

Generally, the signs and symptoms of osteosarcoma are nonspecific. Pain is frequently present (which usually awakens the patient at night) and/or swelling in the affected part, commonly near the knee. Depending on the size of the mass, the swelling may be slight or marked. At times there may be heat and redness of the overlying skin. Often, there is a history of recent trauma, a factor that calls the attention of the patient to a preexisting lesion. Laboratory data are often noncontributory, although a few patients may have an elevated level of alkaline phosphatase.

The major prebiopsy diagnostic procedure is the radiologic study. A careful radiologic examination is important because it is often the first indication of whether the lesion in question is benign or malignant and it also reveals the probability of the lesion being an osteosarcoma. On plain films the tumor may be predominantly blastic, predominantly lytic, or a combination of both (Fig. 23-6). The metaphysis of a long bone is the preferred site of involvement, with tumor reaching the cartilage of growth. The latter serves as a temporary barrier, but not infrequently the tumor breaks through and invades the epiphysis. The cortex may be permeated or destroyed by tumor. A Cod-

Table 23-1. Osteosarcoma Classification

Conventional
    Osteoblastic
    Chondroblastic
    Fibroblastic

Clinical variants
    Osteosarcoma of the jaws
    Postradiation osteosarcoma
    Osteosarcoma in Paget's disease of bone
    Multifocal osteosarcoma
    Osteosarcoma arising in benign conditions

Morphologic variants
    Intraosseous well differentiated osteosarcoma
    Osteosarcoma resembling osteoblastoma
    Telangiectatic osteosarcoma
    Small cell osteosarcoma
    ? Dedifferentiated chondrosarcoma
    ? Malignant fibrous histiocytoma

Surface variants
    Parosteal osteosarcoma
    Dedifferentiated parosteal osteosarcoma
    Periosteal osteosarcoma
    High grade surface osteosarcoma

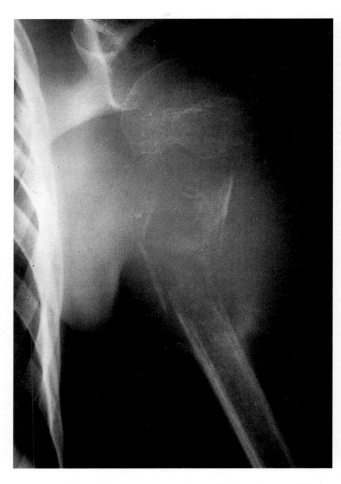

Fig. 23-6. Humeral osteosarcoma with a pathologic fracture. The lesion permeates the humerus and destroys cortex. The extraosseous component is evident.

man's triangle—a reactive elevation of the periosteum—is often present. Typically, the extraskeletal component is predominantly made up of unmineralized osteoid, which makes it amenable for biopsy.

CT[32,33] and MRI[34,35] provide information about the extent of the lesion and its relation to adjacent anatomic structures. In particular, MRI is very valuable in the evaluation of the extent of the tumor into the marrow, information vital to the planning of limb-sparing surgery. Radionuclide scintigraphy is also complementary to other imaging techniques. Although not specific, it can identify the primary tumor as well as any skip metastases (areas of tumor discontinuous from the primary tumor in the same bone).[36] Chest imaging with plain films and CT should be done to exclude metastases to the lungs. Arteriography is no longer utilized routinely unless the patient receives intra-arterial chemotherapy. In such cases arteriography is extremely valuable in the evaluation of the tumor's response to chemotherapy.[37]

Either incisional or needle biopsy will provide satisfactory tissue in a suspected osteosarcoma. However, a biopsy should not be done indiscriminately because contamination of the soft

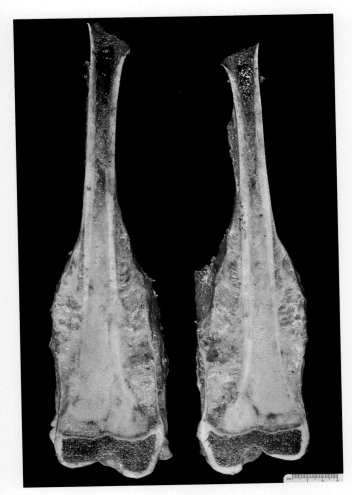

Fig. 23-7. Hemisection of an osteosarcoma of the femur. The tumor involves the distal diaphysis and the metaphysis reaching the growth plate. A significant extraosseous component is also present.

tissues, along with a poorly placed incision, may handicap a limb-salvage procedure.[6,7] In our hands, a needle core biopsy often yields satisfactory results in that an osteosarcoma can be identified.[6,7] FNA may also be sufficient for the diagnosis of osteosarcoma.[38] Should there be any question about the diagnosis, an incisional biopsy is recommended.[6,7,38] If an incisional biopsy is performed, then we recommend that a frozen section examination be done on a portion of the specimen to determine with certainty that lesional tissue has been obtained. Our practice is also to save a fragment of tissue for electron microscopic study, should it be needed, and we save tissue for flow cytometric analysis. In addition to determining the adequacy of the biopsied tissue, the frozen section examination will yield a specific diagnosis of osteosarcoma in most cases and enable an immediate amputation, should it be advisable. However many treatment protocols for osteosarcoma presently call for preoperative administration of chemotherapeutic agents followed by delayed amputation or resection. Thus, a specific diagnosis of osteosarcoma from a frozen section may not be critical and should not be attempted if the pathologist is not familiar with the appearance of this tumor on frozen section.

The gross features of an osteosarcoma are somewhat varied, but there is destruction of the cortex and replacement of the medullary cavity by tumor that varies from gray-white to brown-red (Fig. 23-7). The firmness is also variable. Evidence of necrosis is frequent. If a cartilaginous element is dominant, the lesion will have a shiny gray appearance. Osteosarcomas are often hypervascular, and extensive areas of hemorrhagic necrosis and even cystic alteration may be present. If this is a dominant pattern, then the tumor is probably a telangiectatic osteosarcoma. Periosteal reaction may be identified, with evidence of bone production and spiculation. Destruction and permeation of the cortex lead to an extraosseous component of the osteosarcoma. If the growth plate has not closed, it serves as a barrier to the advancement of the osteosarcoma into the epiphysis. However, not uncommonly, osteosarcoma penetrates the growth plate and even the articular cartilage. The interface of tumor and medullary bone is often quite distinct but may show slight sclerosis or evidence of fibrosis; tumor permeation may be subtle.

Conventional osteosarcoma is composed of malignant, undifferentiated stroma that produces osteoid, bone, and cartilage (Fig. 23-8). Osteoblasts with pleomorphic, often bizarre, nuclei and frequent mitoses are associated with the neoplastic osteoid and bone. The osteocytes show similar cytologic features. In addition to these components, cytologically malignant cartilage and a stroma often resembling that of a fibrosarcoma or malignant fibrous histiocytoma may be seen in osteosarcoma. Foci of necrosis are common. In some osteosarcomas with abundant osteoid, the pattern of the osteoid is complex (filigreed) and is itself suggestive of osteosarcoma. At times, the osteoid is sparse and requires many blocks or step sections to identify neoplastic osteoid. It is not always easy to be certain of the presence of osteoid; special stains are not helpful. Only the rimming of the spicule by neoplastic osteoblasts serves to identify osteoid.

Conventional osteosarcoma is subclassified on the basis of the dominant tissue identified: osteoblastic, chondroblastic, or fibroblastic.[1-4] In the latter two, even though malignant carti-

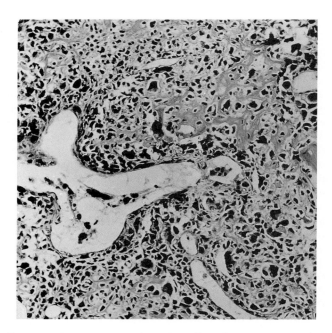

Fig. 23-8. Osteosarcoma with cytologically malignant stroma producing lace-like deposition of osteoid.

lage or a malignant fibrous stroma is dominant, malignant osteoid and bone are identifiable somewhere in the sections. Although the malignant osteoid or bone is a minor element, the tumor is still designated as an osteosarcoma rather than a chondrosarcoma or fibrosarcoma. Whether this subclassification will remain pertinent in the prognosis in relation to chemotherapy remains to be determined.

Morphologic Variants of Osteosarcoma

Morphologic variants of osteosarcoma include essentially three subgroups: high grade lesions, low grade lesions, and lesions that share some features with osteosarcoma.[8]

High Grade Lesions: Telangiectatic and Small Cell Osteosarcoma. The first group is represented by telangiectatic osteosarcoma[39,40] and small cell osteosarcoma.[41-44] The definition of telangiectatic osteosarcoma includes radiologic findings of a totally lytic destructive lesion of the affected bone (Fig. 23-9). Grossly, these tumors are hemorrhagic, destructive, and often partly cystic; because they contain large vascular channels (Fig. 23-10A), they may be mistaken for aneurysmal bone cysts. Histologically, they show a proliferation of anaplastic spindle cells with little or no osteoid (Fig. 23-10B); however, with ample sampling, malignant osteoid will be identified. Such histologic changes distinguish these tumors from aneurysmal bone cysts. As with other tumors of bone, the radiologic features are an important aid in this regard. Similar to telangiectatic osteosarcoma, small cell osteosarcoma occurs in the same age group and bone location as conventional osteosarcoma. Radiologically, most small cell osteosarcomas are mixed blastic and lytic, but occasionally a lesion may be entirely lytic. Histologically, small

cell osteosarcoma is composed of small round cells that can form three patterns: Ewing's-like, lymphoma-like, or spindle cells. Although these patterns simulate the histology of nonosteosarcoma entities, all cases show evidence of osteoid formation histologically or radiologically.[41-44]

Low Grade Osteosarcomas. Osteosarcomas that resembles osteoblastomas[26] and well differentiated medullary osteosarcomas[45-47] are low grade osteosarcomas.[45] The former lesion has histologic features that closely mimic osteoblastoma, except that the neoplastic cells are more atypical and have some mitotic activity and the matrix is more complex.[24,26] Well differentiated medullary osteosarcoma is more likely to be mistaken for a benign neoplasm or tumor-like lesion of bone than for a malignant one. In the reported cases, the most frequent benign diagnosis made from a biopsy specimen was fibrous dysplasia, which indicates the well differentiated pattern of the lesion. Histologically, it is the medullary counterpart of parosteal osteosarcoma.[45-47] In contrast to telangiectatic osteosarcoma, which is particularly aggressive, well differentiated medullary osteosarcoma behaves in a rather indolent fashion and has a low rate of metastasis to distant sites.[45-47]

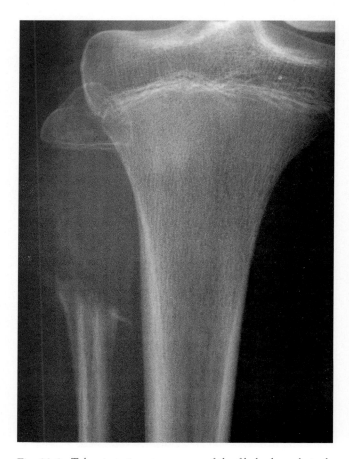

Fig. 23-9. Telangiectatic osteosarcoma of the fibula shows lytic destruction of the metaphysis. At the lower end of the tumor, Codman's triangle represents periosteal reaction to tumor.

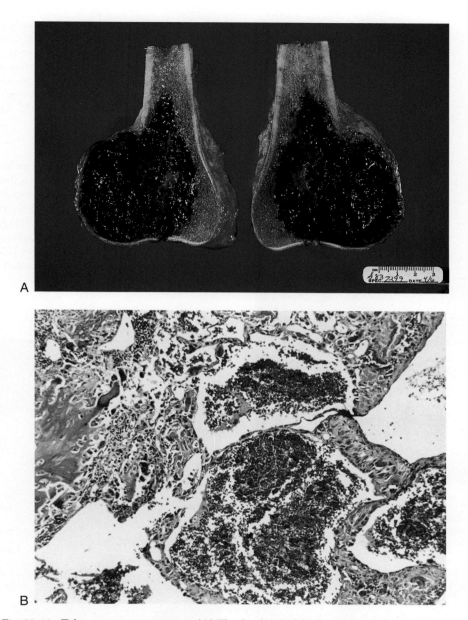

Fig. 23-10. Telangiectatic osteosarcoma. **(A)** The distal end of the femur shows a hemorrhagic destructive mass involving the metaphysis-epiphysis of the bone. **(B)** Histologically, telangiectatic osteosarcoma shows large vascular spaces resembling an aneurysmal bone cyst but differs from it because it contains a highly malignant cellular stroma.

Surface Osteosarcomas. Surface osteosarcomas include parosteal osteosarcoma,[48,49] dedifferentiated parosteal osteosarcoma,[50] periosteal osteosarcoma,[51,52] and high grade surface osteosarcoma.[53] High grade osteosarcoma on the surface is identical in morphology to conventional (medullary) osteosarcoma.[53,54] It is extremely rare and behaves like conventional osteosarcoma.

Parosteal Osteosarcoma. Parosteal osteosarcoma is a low grade osteosarcoma that occurs predominantly at the posterior distal end of the femur but may develop in other locations and

is more common in females.[1–5] It affects patients in the third through fifth decades of life. Radiologically, the lesion may be small, but if it remains undiagnosed for many years, it may become large in bulk. It is not unusual to see a tumor arising from the cortex of a bone showing extension around the entire shaft (Fig. 23-11).

Grossly parosteal osteosarcoma grows from the cortical surface and has a broad base (Fig. 23-12). The cut surface is made up of dense bone and should not have areas of soft tumor tissue. If these are present, they should be sampled because they may harbor an area or areas of dedifferentiation. This lesion should

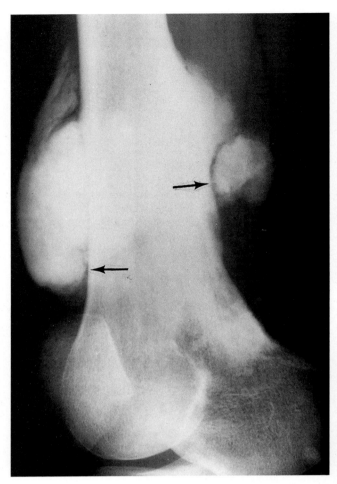

Fig. 23-11. Lobular radiodensity of parosteal osteosarcoma. Note linear zone of radiolucency, fairly characteristic of parosteal osteosarcoma (arrows). The lesion was recurrent in a 30-year-old woman.

Periosteal Osteosarcoma. Periosteal osteosarcoma also arises on the surface of a bone (Fig. 23-14A) but, unlike parosteal osteosarcoma, occurs in a younger age group. The prognosis is similar to or better than that of conventional osteosarcoma, but worse than that of parosteal osteosarcoma. Histologically, it is composed of a proliferation of malignant chondroblastic tissue and minimal osteoid formation[51,52] (Fig. 23-14B & C).

Clinical Variants

The clinical variants of osteosarcoma include those associated with Paget's disease, infarct of bone, or irradiation, and those arising in fibrous dysplasia.[1-4] Histologically, osteosarcomas arising in these situations are similar to conventional osteosarcoma. Other variants include osteosarcoma of the jaws,[56] multifocal osteosarcoma,[57] osteosarcoma, malignant fibrous histiocytoma type,[58] epithelioid types,[59,60] intracortical osteosarcoma,[61] and osteosarcoma associated with other benign conditions.[1-4,62,63]

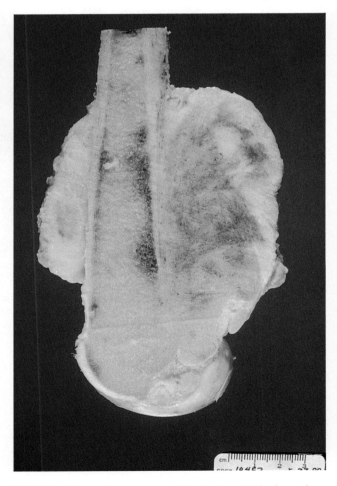

Fig. 23-12. Parosteal osteosarcoma. The distal end of the femur shows a large solid mass arising from the surface of the bone. Note that the cortex and medullary cavity are intact.

not have an intramedullary portion, although a relatively minor component may be allowed in large lesions.[55]

Histologically, parosteal osteosarcoma has well differentiated bone and stroma that may vary little from normal bone.[48,49] The bony trabeculae may be poorly oriented or may have a parallel arrangement; they may be thin or broad, but osteoblasts are not prominent. The stroma is fibrous and at least focally hypercellular (Fig. 23-13). Not infrequently rare mitoses are found. Cartilage may be present and rarely may form a cap. These tumors are often mistaken histologically for fibrous dysplasia and, because of the cartilage, for osteochondroma. Occasionally, areas characteristic of conventional osteosarcoma may be present. When they occur, the tumor has dedifferentiated toward a high grade tumor. Radiologically, the presence of large lytic areas (usually vascular on angiographs), in a parosteal osteosarcoma suggests dedifferentiation. Dedifferentiated parosteal osteosarcoma is more aggressive than parosteal osteosarcoma and is treated like conventional osteosarcoma.[50,53,54]

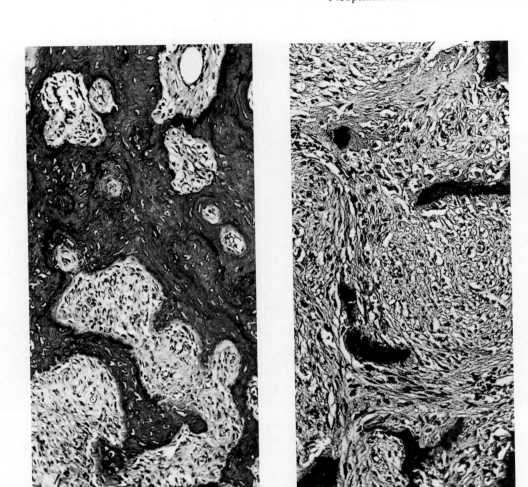

Fig. 23-13. **(A & B)** Parosteal osteosarcoma shows mature but irregularly shaped bony spicules and a slightly hypercellular stroma.

Osteosarcoma of the jaws shows a slight predilection for males in the third and fourth decades of life.[1–4,56] The infrastructure of the maxilla and the body of the mandible are the most common sites of involvement, and the chondroblastic variant is the most common histologic type. Radical surgery is the management of choice for this type of osteosarcoma. Systemic metastases occur in about 35 percent of cases.[56]

Therapy

Primary chemotherapy, whether before or after surgery, has become the standard treatment for conventional osteosarcoma. Some protocols involve preoperative chemotherapy administered either systemically or intra-arterially; whether the patient is treated surgically or receives preoperative chemotherapy initially, all patients receive postoperative chemotherapy.

Before the advent of chemotherapy, the 5 year survival rate for patients with osteosarcoma was at best 20 percent.[64] Since the institution of the various treatment protocols, the prognosis has dramatically improved.[65–68] The 5 year survival rate for patients with osteosarcoma is now 65 to 80 percent.[65–68] Tumor necrosis resulting from chemotherapy has been found to be an excellent prognostic factor in patients treated with intra-arterial infusion of cisplatin and systemic doxorubicin.[8] When tumor necrosis, as determined by detailed histologic examination, is in excess of 90 percent, a long-term survival rate of 80 to 90 percent is expected. On the other hand, tumor necrosis of less than 90 percent is associated with a poor prognosis and a long-term survival rate of 10 to 40 percent.[8,65,66,69]

Conventional osteosarcoma frequently metastasizes to the lungs, and massive metastases are the cause of death. Metastases to other visceral organs and bones are less common, but metastases to regional lymph nodes occur in approximately 5 percent of patients. Parosteal and intraosseous well differentiated osteosarcomas have an excellent disease-free survival rate of more than 90 percent, provided all the tumor tissue is ablated with clear margins. Incomplete surgery usually leads to recurrences. Dedifferentiation in either of these tumors, however, hampers survival. These patients require chemotherapy. The expected survival rate for patients with periosteal osteosarcoma is roughly 50 percent. Telangiectatic osteosarcoma is highly re-

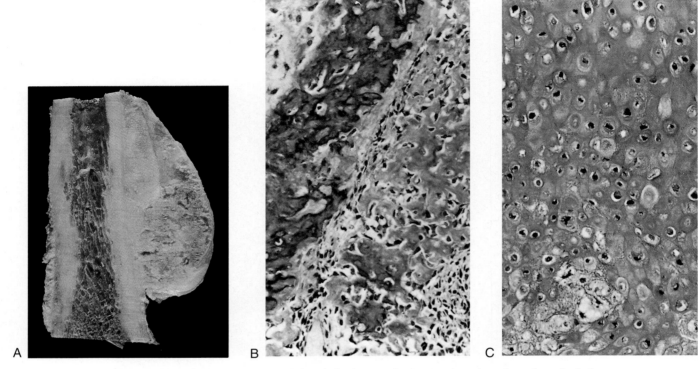

Fig. 23-14. Periosteal osteosarcoma. **(A)** Grossly, there is a large mass arising from the surface of a shaft of the femur. Note cartilaginoid appearance of this tumor. **(B & C)** Histologically, periosteal osteosarcoma shows different patterns of malignant osteoid and cartilage.

sponsive to chemotherapy and consequently the 5 survival rate is in the range of 68 percent.[69,70]

Cytopathology of Bone-Forming Tumors

A variety of bone tumors produce osteoid and its mineralized end product, woven bone. By contrast, lamellar bone is seen only in osteoma and enostosis (bone islands). Osteoid is the unmineralized matrix produced by osteoblasts and consists predominantly of type I collagen, with a minor component of noncollagenous proteins and growth factors. Due to biochemical and staining similarities, osteoid may be difficult or impossible to distinguish from acellular or relatively hypocellular fragments of dense, fibroblastic collagen; however, this distinction is important diagnostically. Fibroblastic collagen has a distinctly fibrillar, longitudinal arrangement. By contrast, osteoid forms irregular, amorphous masses that have a hard, waxy quality. Osteoid appears bright magenta in air-dried, Romanowsky-stained preparations, and green-blue in wet-fixed, Papanicolaou-stained smears.[71] Osteoblasts, which may be benign or malignant, become entrapped in the matrix, creating a lacy, interwoven pattern (Fig. 23-15).

Benign Tumors

Osteoma

Osteomas are poor candidates for FNA. Due to the cortical bone that comprises these lesions, attempts to penetrate osteomas with standard 22 to 25 gauge needles may result in bent or broken tips, and aspirates are unlikely to yield diagnostic material.

Osteoid Osteoma

To our knowledge, diagnosis of osteoid osteoma by FNA has not been reported. Preoperatively, the diagnosis is usually apparent from the radiographic or clinical findings (or both); this feature, combined with the characteristic intracortical location and extensive peripheral sclerosis, makes aspiration of these lesions unlikely.[14]

In the intraoperative setting, smears or touch preparations of the nidus may be useful for distinguishing osteoid osteoma from a bone abscess when the latter cannot be excluded from the preoperative differential diagnosis.[72] Cytologically, osteoid osteomas are composed of plump osteoblasts, osteoclasts, and rare, bland spindle cells in a bloody background. In our experience, bony trabeculae, with and/or without osteoblastic rim-

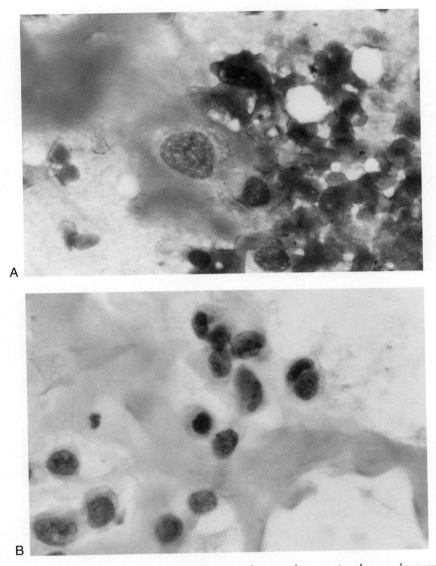

Fig. 23-15. Osteosarcoma. **(A)** An air-dried, Romanowsky-stained preparation shows a pleomorphic tumor cell entrapped in bright magenta osteoid matrix. **(B)** A Papanicolaou-stained smear from the same case demonstrates the green-blue appearance of the osteoid matrix.

ming, are present and may be numerous in smears, but are absent from touch preparations. Inflammatory cells and necrotic debris, which are the hallmarks of bone abscesses, are not seen in osteoid osteoma.

Osteoblastoma

In contrast to osteoid osteoma, osteoblastoma is usually bordered by a narrow rim of bony sclerosis and thus may be more accessible to sampling by FNA. Aspirates yield variably cellular smears composed of a polymorphous population of benign mesencyhmal elements, including osteoblasts, osteoclasts, and spindle cells. The osteoblasts are typically hypertrophic and have round nuclei with evenly dispersed chromatin and a single, round, often prominent nucleolus. Osteoblasts are individually dispersed, as well as arrayed in rows rimming fragments of

osteoid and/or partially mineralized bony trabeculae.[71-73] Irregular fragments of fibrovascular stroma, as well as individually dispersed, benign spindle cells of fibroblastic and endothelial origin, are also present. The background is usually bloody, reflecting the richly vascular nature of osteoblastoma.

Malignant Tumors

Osteosarcoma

FNA is increasingly utilized in the initial pathologic evaluation of osteosarcomas. Due to cortical destruction or extraosseous extension, or both, these tumors are often readily accessible to either direct or image-guided FNA.[74] Although osteoid may be scarce or absent, the sarcomatous nature of the lesion is usually obvious in the aspirate smears. The cytologic findings, in con-

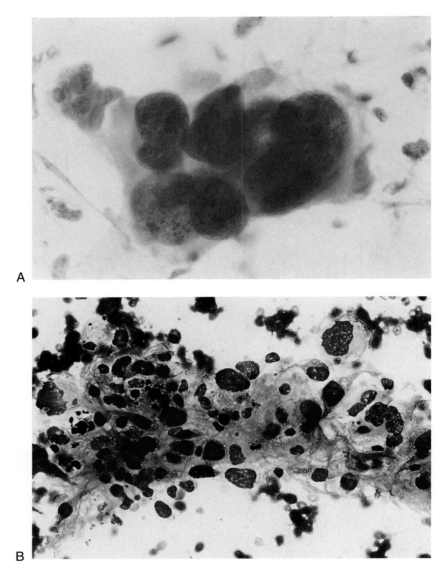

Fig. 23-16. Osteosarcoma. **(A)** FNA material of an osteosarcoma demonstrates a cluster of large pleomorphic cells with obvious variation in nuclear size and shape. **(B)** An air-dried, Romanowsky-stained preparation demonstrates a cluster of malignant cells with anisocytosis and nuclear pleomorphism.

cert with the clinical and radiographic features, allow the pathologist to render either a specific diagnosis or a narrow differential diagnosis.[75] Accuracy rates for the diagnosis of osteosarcomas on FNA have been reported to be between 80 and 90 percent in experienced hands, with the main problem being inconclusive aspirates with inadequate material.[76–78]

Conventional Osteosarcoma

Osteosarcoma has a spectrum of cytologic appearances, reflecting the histologic variability of these tumors.[77] FNA of conventional osteosarcoma yields variably cellular smears, depending on the amount of matrix within the area sampled. Aspirates are composed of varying proportions of malignant spindle cells

(Fig. 23-16A) and bizarre, multinucleated tumor giant cells.[77,78] The former are characterized by considerable anisocytosis, nuclear pleomorphism, and increased nuclear/cytoplasmic ratios. The enlarged nuclei have irregular contours, coarsely clumped chromatin, and prominent, irregular nucleoli (Fig. 23-16B). Mitotic figures, including abnormal forms, are evident and may be abundant. Variable numbers of round or polygonal malignant osteoblasts are also present. The malignant cells occur singly, in irregular aggregates, and in association with osteoid or other matrix (Fig. 23-17).

The amount of osteoid in the aspirates varies considerably. It may be abundant, but more often is scant and focal. In our experience, osteoid may be reliably distinguished from dense col-

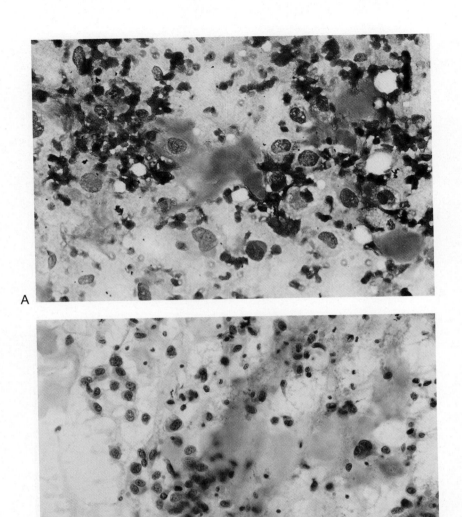

Fig. 23-17. Osteosarcoma. **(A)** Osteoid matrix associated with single malignant cells is readily apparent in this air-dried, Romanowsky-stained preparation. **(B)** A Papanicolaou-stained smear shows malignant cells arrayed singly or in small aggregates in close association with osteoid.

lagen in air-dried, Romanowsky-stained smears by the amorphous, lace-like quality of the former and the presence of entrapped or adjacent malignant cells reminiscent of osteoblasts (Figs. 23-15A and 23-17A). When these features are absent, osteoid may be difficult or impossible to distinguish from dense collagen.

Malignant chondroid and fibrous matrices are also present in aspirates from chondroblastic and fibroblastic variants of osteosarcoma, respectively (Fig. 23-18). These matrices may dominate the smears, and in the absence of convincing osteoid, cytologic distinction from chondrosarcoma and fibrosarcoma or malignant fibrous histiocytoma may be difficult or impossible. Because the treatments for osteosarcoma and chondrosarcoma

are significantly different, distinction between these two entities preoperatively is essential. The clinical context is often helpful in distinguishing chondroblastic osteosarcoma from chondrosarcoma; however, either core or open biopsy must be performed when a definitive cytologic diagnosis cannot be rendered. By contrast, preoperative distinction among osteosarcoma, fibrosarcoma, and malignant fibrous histiocytoma may not be necessary, as these entities may be treated with similar protocols in some cases.

Telangiectatic Osteosarcoma

Telangiectatic osteosarcoma is a high grade, intramedullary tumor with prominent intralesional blood lakes and scant evi-

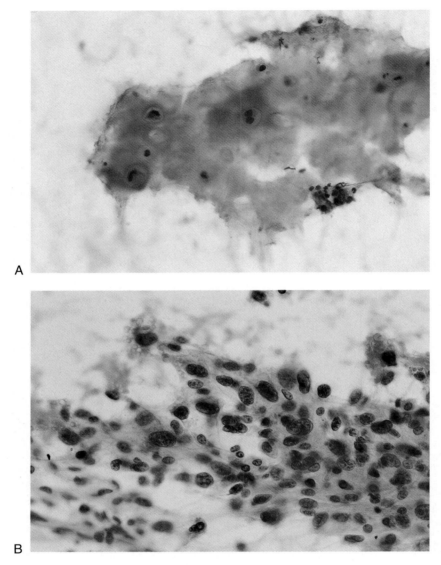

Fig. 23-18. **(A)** A Papanicolaou-stained smear from a chondroblastic osteosarcoma demonstrates neoplastic chondroid matrix. **(B)** A Papanicolaou-stained smear from a high grade osteosarcoma shows a fibrosarcoma-like area.

dence of osteoid formation. FNA of these tumors yields variably cellular smears composed of anaplastic cells that are individually dispersed and arrayed in irregular clusters. Blood and variable amounts of necrotic debris comprise the background. Osteoid is exceedingly scant or absent. Due to the hemorrhagic, cystic, and necrotic nature of these tumors, FNA is more likely to yield diagnostic material than core biopsy.[75]

Small Cell Osteosarcoma

The cytologic features of the small cell variant differ considerably from those of other types of osteosarcoma. Aspirates are composed of small, round or ovoid cells with scant cytoplasm, oval to elongate nuclei with finely dispersed or clumped chromatin, and very high nuclear/cytoplasmic ratios. Nuclear pleo-

morphism is present, but not marked. Cells occur singly and in cohesive fragments.

CARTILAGINOUS TUMORS

Interpretation of cartilaginous tumors of the skeleton presents some of the most difficult histologic problems related to neoplasms of bone. The proper histologic interpretation of cartilaginous tumors must include, in addition to adequate biopsy specimens and well prepared slides, the clinical data, the age of the patient, the location of the tumor, its size, and a review of the radiographs.[1–5]

Osteochondroma

Osteochondromas are the most common of the benign neoplasms of bone, representing approximately 35.8 to 45 percent of benign tumors.[1,5] Most are discovered in patients younger than 21 years, but they may be observed at almost any age. Generally, osteochondromas cease to grow at puberty, but those that keep growing after puberty should be viewed with suspicion for malignant transformation. There is a male predominance of 1.3:1, and tumors may be solitary or multiple. Multiple osteochondromatosis is a hereditary autosomal-dominant disease that is similar in presentation and histology to solitary osteochondroma.[79,80]

On radiographs, an osteochondroma is a bony projection that seems to be an extension of the cortex. Often, the lesion has a readily visible pedicle topped by a lobular radiodense mass. The density varies with the amount of cartilage and with the degree of calcification of the cartilaginous component (Fig. 23-19). At the base of the osteochondroma, there is a continuation or sweeping up of the cortex into the pedicle of the osteochondroma. This feature serves to distinguish it from other lesions such as the parosteal osteosarcoma and localized myositis ossificans and bizarre osteochondroma of Nora.

Grossly, the anatomy of osteochondromas corresponds well to the radiologic appearance (Fig. 23-20). They are cartilaginous-capped bony projections, often from the metaphyseal end of a tubular bone. The pedicle is bony, cortical, and cancellous, and the head consists of a combination of cartilage and bone. The cartilaginous cap varies to some degree in thickness, re-

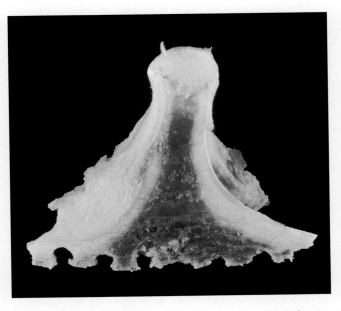

Fig. 23-20. Osteochondroma. A roughly triangular lesion showing the cartilaginous cap at the tip of the exostosis. Note that the medullary cavity has been carried out into the body of the lesion.

lated to the age of the patient; the younger the patient the thicker the cap may be. It may measure from 1 mm to 1 cm or more. The cartilaginous surfaces are shiny, lobulated, and gray-white and resemble hyaline cartilage.

Histologically, the cartilage is hyaline, which retains a normal organization of the chondrocytes. Typically, the chondrocytes form parallel columns, with the most active growth toward the outer surface and endochondral ossification toward the medullary cavity, which resembles an epiphyseal plate. The nuclei of the chondrocytes tend to be small and irregular. Occasionally, one may encounter slightly enlarged nuclei. Even in mature osteochondromas small islands of cartilage may be retained in the bony trabeculae.

Sometimes it is difficult to distinguish large osteochondromas (6 cm or larger in greatest dimension) from a well differentiated peripheral chondrosarcoma. In such cases, radiologic features, including the dimensions of the lesion, are helpful in arriving at a proper interpretation (those larger than 6 cm should be viewed with suspicion for chondrosarcoma). Many blocks must be taken of the cartilaginous component and must be studied for nuclear atypia, enlarged nuclei, and binucleate cells. Because of the gross configuration of an osteochondroma, it is frequently considered that the peripheral type of chondrosarcomas arise from osteochondromas, but this is difficult to prove. However, it is accepted that patients who have multiple hereditary exostoses have a higher risk of developing chondrosarcoma from one of their lesions.[1-4]

Osteochondromas that are asymptomatic and solitary require no treatment, but those that become painful or have a protruding unsightly mass are treated by excision. For patients who have multiple osteochondromas, it is impractical to excise each lesion. Thus, excision is reserved for those lesions that apparently increase in size or otherwise become symptomatic.

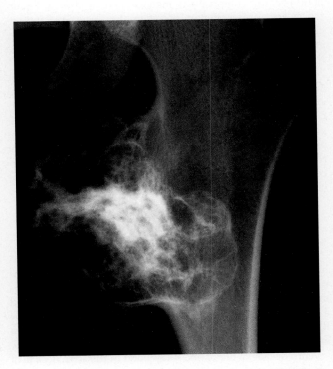

Fig. 23-19. Broad-based osteochondroma of the upper end of the femur. It is shown en face with the lobular nature and ossification evident. The sweep of the cortex into the pedicle is also seen at the top.

A relatively common lesion, *subungual exostosis*, is a proliferative process that affects the tips of the fingers or toes; it is most likely related to trauma and has also been referred to as traumatic osteochondroma. Histologically, this lesion shows a cellular cartilaginous proliferation, often with nuclear atypia and mitotic activity, and an osseous formation that resembles a malignant tumor. The subungual location suggests this lesion.[81,82]

Another rare surface lesion is *bizarre parosteal osteochondroma of the hands and feet*.[83,84] It most commonly arises from the surface of the phalanges but may occur in the long bones. Although it simulates an osteochondroma, the contents of the medullary cavity are not pulled into the protruding mass as occurs in ordinary osteochondroma. This lesion may recur.[83,84]

Enchondroma

Enchondroma (chondroma) is a benign hyaline cartilaginous tumor that arises in the medullary cavity of a bone. Although enchondroma has been described in almost any bone, tubular or flat, it is best to consider those occurring in the long bones as different entities because they are often difficult, if not impossible, to differentiate from low grade chondrosarcoma. Therefore, in this discussion, the term *enchondroma* is restricted to those lesions that occur in the hands or feet.

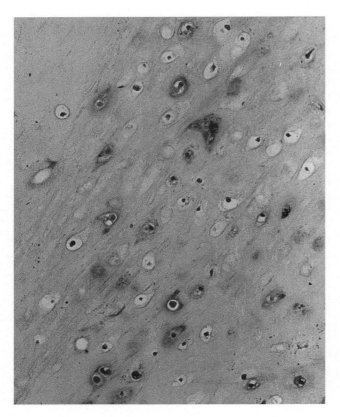

Fig. 23-21. Hyaline cartilage from a phalangeal chondroma. The cells are in lacunae, and most of the nuclei are small and dark.

Enchondroma occurs in all ages, but most often before the fourth decade of life, and has an almost equal predominance in males and females. It is the most common tumor of the small bones of the hands and feet, involving, in order of frequency, the phalanges of the fingers, the metacarpal bones, the phalanges of the toes, and the metatarsal bone.[85] Enchondroma is usually asymptomatic, but it may occasionally cause pain, mass, or fractures.

Radiologically, enchondromas of the bones of the hands are radiolucent and have a multilobular appearance with some slight deformity of the bone and thinning of the cortex. At times, evidence of calcification is noted. This calcification may be semilunar or circular in contour, reflecting the lobular nature of the tumor, and has a fluffy radiodense appearance. Enchondromas may be large, involving the entire length of the small tubular bone, and their somewhat lobular appearance will result in scalloping of the internal cortical surface.

Grossly, enchondromas usually arise in the metaphyseal region of the bone, extend to the remainder of the bone, and often expand the medullary cavity. The tumor tissue is a gray shiny cartilage with white or yellow-white areas that represent calcification. Enchondromas resected intact may show scalloping of the inner cortex.

Histologically, the neoplastic cartilage maintains, to some extent, the normal hyaline cartilage pattern of the chondrocytes (Fig. 23-21). In many specimens, there may be evidence of mucoid degeneration of the matrix and nuclear abnormalities that raise the possibility of a tumor. Even though the small enchondromas may have histologic alterations that suggest malignancy, they should be considered benign. Curettage and bone packing comprise the management of choice. Recurrences are not uncommon, but even after recurrence, an enchondroma should still be treated conservatively because progression to a malignant state seldom occurs. Local amputation should be the last resort.

Enchondromas may occur as multiple lesions and may cause deformity of the affected bones. A person who has multiple enchondromas (Ollier's disease) has a high risk of chondrosarcoma.[1–5] Maffucci's disease is another entity made up of multiple enchondromas, but in this disease the enchondromatosis is associated with soft tissue angiomas and a high susceptibility for the development of malignant tumors, including chondrosarcoma, vascular sarcoma, fibrosarcoma, and other malignancies.[2,86]

Chondromyxoid Fibroma

Chondromyxoid fibroma is a benign bone tumor that combines connective tissue and chondroid and myxoid components. It is rare, accounting for less than 0.5 percent of all primary benign bone tumors.[1] A slight predominance in males and a wide age range are seen, but the lesion is most commonly found in patients younger than 40 years, with a peak occurrence at 20 years.[1–5,87–89] A second peak has been described in the seventh decade of life in one study[87] and in the sixth decade of life in another.[88]

The patients often seek medical aid because of pain and swelling over the affected part. This pain may be of several

Fig. 23-22. Chondromyxoid fibroma. The distal end of the femur demonstrates a predominantly metaphyseal lesion with well delimited borders. The cut surface of the lesion is light pink and glistening, typical of a cartilaginous lesion. Compare with adjacent film.

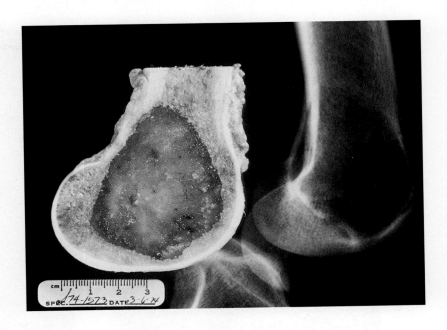

weeks' or months' duration. Sometimes a patient may seek medical aid because of a pathologic fracture through the lesion.

The lesion is most commonly found in metaphyses of the tubular bones, especially the proximal tibia and distal femur; it is uncommon in the flat bones.[87] Forty-two percent are found in the long bones, 25 percent in the flat bones, 20 percent in the small tubular bones, 8 percent in the spine, and 5 percent in the ribs.[88]

Radiologically, chondromyxoid fibroma is metaphyseal, eccentrically located, well circumscribed, and radiolucent and appears to be multilobulated.[90] The margins show a thin rim of bony sclerosis, but there may be destruction of the cortex. In some lesions, bony sclerosis may dominate much of the pattern. In the smaller bones, the bony contours will be deformed.

Excised specimens are grossly lobulated, solid, somewhat firm, and gray-white with tan areas (Fig. 23-22). The tumor has a cartilaginous texture but usually lacks the sliminess that one might expect from the myxoid component. The cortex is often expanded and may be eroded. The periosteum serves to confine the tumor.

The microscopic pattern reflects the gross pattern in that a lobular outline is often maintained by thin fibrous trabeculae traversing the lesion. Chondromyxoid fibromas are quite varied, being predominantly myxoid with small chondroid areas intermingled with fibrous or collagenized zones. The lobules are outlined by peripheral accumulations of spindled, chondroblastic, and occasionally multinucleated giant cells. From the periphery toward the center of the lobules (Fig. 23-23A), decreasing cellularity is seen. In the central areas, the myxoid features are identified by the elongation of cytoplasmic processes that give a stellate pattern to many cells (Fig. 23-23B). At the periphery of the lobule the cells are larger than those of the center, and the nuclei are commonly reniform with nuclear grooves and an often eccentric situation. Ultrastructurally, the stellate cells have irregular cell processes, scalloping of the cell membrane, and often abundant cytoplasmic fib-

rils.[91,92] Calcifications have been reported in 14 percent in one study[88] and 27 percent in another.[89] Determination of the cartilaginous origin is based on the histologic characteristics, including the presence of mixed chondroblastic and chondromyxoid fibromatous components, similarity of histochemical reactions to those of normal cartilage, and a positive reaction for S-100 protein, a marker that stains cartilage.[93]

These lesions are best treated by resection in expendable bones, en bloc resection when possible, or curettage, particularly when the tumor is located in bones near a joint or in bone for which function must be preserved. The risk of local recurrence is estimated to be approximately 25 percent.[87–89,94] For all practical purposes, the lesion is benign, with only rare cases recorded that presumably have undergone a malignant transformation.[89] These cases are open to question as one may wonder whether the original diagnosis of chondromyxoid fibroma was correct. In other words, the lesion may have been a chondrosarcoma originally.

Chondroblastoma

Chondroblastoma is an uncommon benign neoplasm of bone that accounts for 1 percent of all benign bone tumors.[1] It is seen most commonly in males in the second decade of life.[1]

Clinically, chondroblastoma causes pain near or in the affected joint. Often the pain seems more severe than would be expected from the size of the lesion and is due to irritation of the synovial membrane. Evidence of swelling may be present, including effusion of the joint, but this is not especially common; pathologic fractures are infrequent. Chondroblastoma is a cartilaginous tumor with a predilection for an epiphyseal location in long bones and a preference for the upper end of the humerus and tibia and the lower end of the femur. Flat bones such as the sternum, ribs, and pelvis are rarely involved.[95,96]

Radiologically, a chondroblastoma should be suspected in

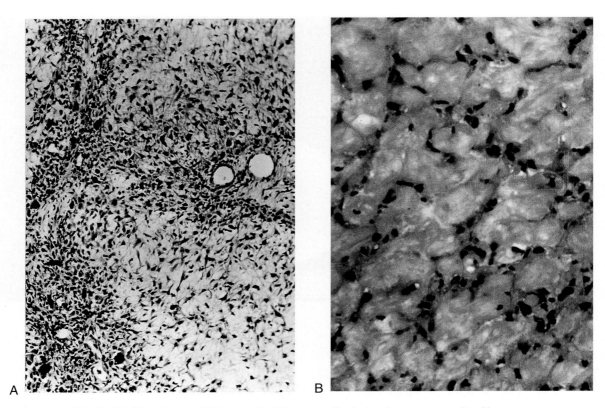

Fig. 23-23. Chondromyxoid fibroma. (A) Microscopically the lobular pattern is outlined by a congregation of cells with few cells in the center. (B) The center of the lobule shows spindle stellate cells over a myxoid background.

any teenager who has a radiolucent lesion that involves the epiphyseal end of a long bone (Fig. 23-24). Chondroblastomas are often multilobar, with a well defined sclerotic margins. They may be small, measuring 1 or 2 cm in greatest dimension, or so large as to involve the entire epiphyseal-metaphyseal portion of a long bone. The large lesions may destroy the cortex and may alter the gross form of the bone. Some chondroblastomas are lightly to heavily calcified. Because of the calcification and a high number of giant cells, chondroblastomas originally were named calcifying epiphyseal giant cell tumors.

Grossly, the intact lesions are well demarcated from the surrounding bone. They may be ovoid to rounded and have a lobular pattern, as do most cartilaginous tumors. The cut surfaces are shiny gray to blue-gray and gray-yellow and suggest cartilage. Calcium deposits are seen as white to yellow-white material. If considerable calcium is present, the cut surfaces are gritty. Occasionally, a chondroblastoma is partially cystic, and rare lesions may be predominantly cystic. In the latter situation, a small nubbin of chondroblastoma may persist on one wall of the cyst.

Histologically, chondroblastoma is often richly cellular and therefore is mistaken for a malignant tumor, especially chondrosarcoma.[97,98] Multinucleated giant cells may be common, and thus the pathologist may diagnose giant cell tumor. However, the basic cell of the lesion has a round to oval eccentric nucleus that has a bean or reniform shape or shows nuclear grooves (Fig. 23-25). The cell boundaries are often quite distinct, and the cytoplasm varies from acidophilic to almost colorless. Variations of this cell are seen, even to the extent of being spindled. Mitotic activity has been described in 77 percent of the chondroblastomas; they range from 1 to 3 mitoses/10 high power fields (hpf). The cells of chondroblastoma stain with the S-100 protein.[99,100] Small amounts of chondroid material may be identified, and in some lesions it may be a major component. Calcification is frequently seen in undecalcified sections. The typical pattern of calcification is the outlining of individual chondroblasts to form a delicate network that has been termed chicken-wire calcification. Fibrosis, cystic alteration, and secondary aneurysmal bone cyst formation may be found in chondroblastomas. Electron microscopic studies have demonstrated that the basic cell of this lesion is compatible with that of a chondroblast.[96] Cartilage is present in 95 percent of these tumors and appears as small areas of pink amorphous material that often resembles osteoid.

Chondroblastoma may occur in the cranial bones, but it presents definite clinical differences: the patients are older (generally over 30 years), chondroid differentiation is not always clearly seen, and the tumor has a high incidence of recurrence.[101] Most chondroblastomas are treated by curettage. The recurrence rate is about 16 percent,[4] but it may be as high as 40 percent.[96] Cranial chondroblastoma, by contrast, has a 50 percent recurrence rate after curettage.

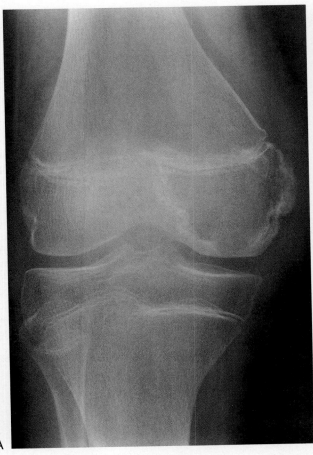
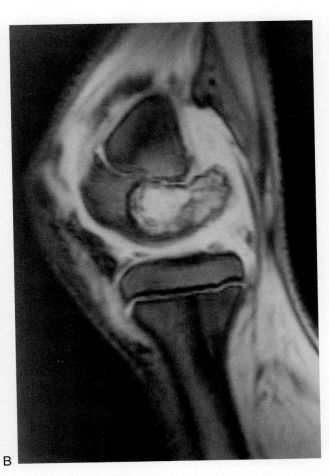

Fig. 23-24. Chondroblastoma of the distal femur. **(A)** This radiograph demonstrates a radiolucent lesion in the epiphysis surrounded by sclerotic margins. Note the open growth plate. **(B)** Magnetic resonance image of the same patient's lesion demonstrates it as a white area. The margins appear as the thick black area around the lesion.

Chondroblastoma is generally considered a benign tumor, but individual cases of pulmonary metastases have been reported.[102] The pulmonary metastases maintain the histologic appearance of the primary benign chondroblastoma. Most of the metastases developed after multiple attempts to resect the primary chondroblastoma; hence, it is possible that the metastases were the result of the surgical procedures. At any rate, the risk of malignant transformation of benign chondroblastoma is small.[103]

Periosteal Chondroma

A periosteal chondroma is a benign cartilaginous tumor that apparently arises from the periosteum.[1–4,104] It is more common in males than in females (ratio about 2:1), and the peak incidence is in the second and third decades of life, although it may be seen in subsequent decades.[105] It may present with mild pain or as an asymptomatic mass or may be discovered incidentally on radiologic studies done for other reasons.[106] The metaphyseal area of the proximal humerus, phalanges of the hand, dis-

tal femur, proximal tibia, and proximal femur have been cited as the most common sites of occurrence of this lesion.[105]

Radiologically, the lesion is shown to erode the underlying cortical bone to form a cup-shaped or saucer-like alteration of the cortex. The surrounding cortical bone becomes sclerotized. The lesion usually contains some matrix calcifications typical of cartilage, and its periphery is well delimited by the elevated periosteum, which may be calcified (Fig. 23-26). Grossly, periosteal chondroma is a well circumscribed lesion confined to the cortex, with its outer surface being covered by periosteum (Fig. 23-27). The margins are well demarcated from the surrounding cortex, and the cut surfaces demonstrate a somewhat lobular cartilaginous tumor that is blue-gray to gray-white with evidence of calcification.

Histologically, the lesion is composed of hyaline cartilaginous cells ranging from cells that contain small dark pyknotic nuclei to cells that show larger nuclei with a fine nuclear chromatin pattern and an occasional nucleolus. When the larger cells predominate, the possibility of a chondrosarcoma arises, but such atypia is not diagnostic of malignancy. It has been demonstrated that these lesions do not metastasize, despite atypical histologic

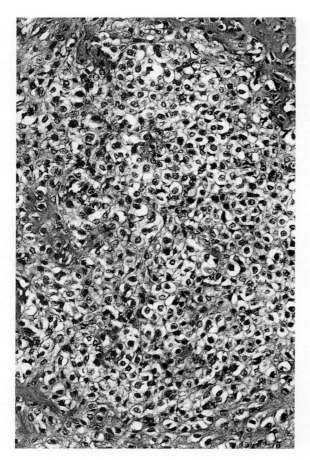

Fig. 23-25. Cellular pattern of a chondroblastoma. The chondroblasts are rounded, with almost colorless cytoplasm. The cell outlines are frequently distinct.

findings. Periosteal chondrosarcoma may mimic periosteal chondroma radiologically and histologically. The former is more aggressive radiologically; histologically, it often invades the soft tissues.[106] Therapy is curettage or en bloc excision; local recurrence of about 3.5 percent has been reported.[103,104]

Chondrosarcoma

Chondrosarcoma is the second most common primary malignant tumor of bone, osteosarcoma being the most common.[5] In contrast to osteosarcoma, chondrosarcoma occurs at a later age, more frequently in the fourth through sixth decades of life.[1–5,107] It is found predominantly in males.[1–5] Chondrosarcoma may occur at any site in the skeleton but has a preference for the pelvis and upper ends of the femur, humerus, and scapula.[1–4] Most patients with chondrosarcoma will seek medical aid because of a mass or swelling at the site of the lesion. Discomfort or pain are frequently associated.

Radiologically and grossly, chondrosarcoma may be divided into two types: a peripheral type that arises from the surface of a bone and grows into the surrounding tissue and a central type that arises in the medullary cavity of the bone.[1–5] Radiologically, the peripheral form is quite characteristic and is often

specifically diagnosable. It is a cauliflower-shaped mass that varies in its degree of calcification (Fig. 23-28). The shape is due to its lobulation, and calcification around and within the lobules account for the semilunar and ring-shaped calcifications that are quite specific for both benign and malignant cartilaginous tumors. With proper imaging studies the attachment of the chondrosarcomatous mass to the underlying bone can often be seen and aids in planning the surgical procedure.

Central chondrosarcomas have radiologic features that indicate the cartilaginous nature of the lesion (Fig. 23-29A). These are characterized by the presence of small fluffy calcifications often described as popcorn, ringlet-like, annular, punctate, stippled, or small ill-defined radiodense calcifications. Although this radiologic pattern identifies cartilage, it does not discriminate benign from malignant lesions. The lesion may be heavily calcified and may mimic an infarct of bone. Different degrees of cortical erosion are present, and if the cortex is penetrated, this would be an important sign of underlying chondrosarcoma. At times an extraosseous component may be large and may mask the origin of the lesion as a central chondrosarcoma.

Grossly, chondrosarcoma is a lobular mass of cartilage that on cut surface is shiny gray to gray-white (Fig. 23-29). Variable amounts of bone and calcified matrix may be visible. The central chondrosarcomas reside in the medullary cavity of bone, causing varied changes

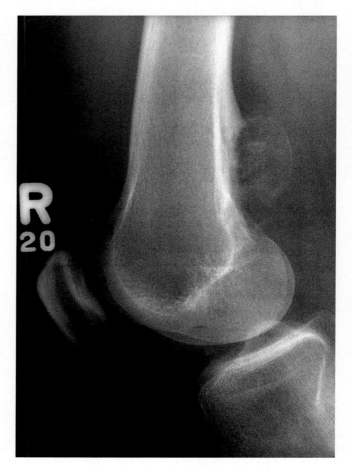

Fig. 23-26. Periosteal chondroma. The distal femur exhibits a rounded well delimited radiolucent lesion arising from the surface of the bone.

Fig. 23-27. Periosteal chondroma. Whole-mount section of the lesion includes a rim of normal cortex and the surrounding periosteum. The tumor is made up of hyaline cartilage.

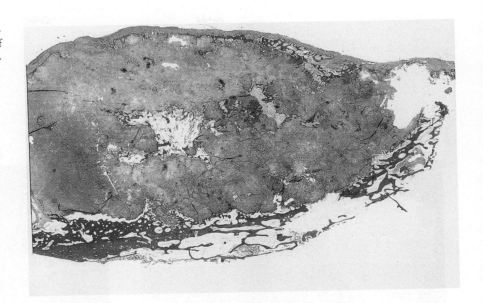

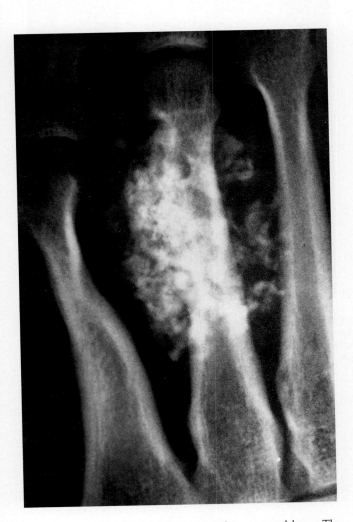

Fig. 23-28. Peripheral chondrosarcoma of a metatarsal bone. The fluffy calcification and the ring forms of calcification are prominent.

that include scalloping of the endosteum, remodeling (enlargement) of the medullary cavity, and various degrees of cortical disruption. The margins may be infiltrative, isolating fragments of cancellous bones. Yellow-white to white areas of calcium deposition may be seen and palpated throughout the lesion. Chondrosarcomas are variable in size, with peripheral chondrosarcomas generally measuring more than 5 cm in greatest dimension and occasionally exceeding 20 or 25 cm. Central chondrosarcomas likewise vary in size, measuring up to 8 or 10 cm, and may involve the entire shaft of the bone. They are often elongated because of their location within the medullary cavity. Surface chondrosarcomas usually have a broad base and a lobulated cartilaginoid appearance (Fig. 23-29B). They often trap or invade skeletal muscle as they grow out.

Histologically, the diagnosis of chondrosarcoma may be difficult, particularly when the well differentiated lesions are in question. In such cases, the hyaline cartilage of the tumor closely resembles normal cartilage. The histologic examination is important and requires that many blocks be taken. Among the slides, the pathologist should search for nuclear changes that comprise binucleated cells and enlarged nuclei of the chondrocytes. If these are found, then, with the proper radiologic and gross features, one can diagnose well differentiated chondrosarcoma.

Grading

Chondrosarcomas have been graded according to the degree of nuclear alteration[108] (Fig. 23-30). Evans et al[108] have proposed the following system. Grade 1 lesions are characterized by a marked preponderance of small, densely staining nuclei, absence of cellular areas, and lack of mitoses. Grade 2 tumors are cellular lesions in which evidence of malignancy is more easily found. The nuclei are medium sized and occasionally large, with visible intranuclear detail, and cellular areas are evident at the periphery of the lobule. Rarely, one may find mitoses; when present, fewer than 2 mitoses/10 hpf should be seen. We have recently modified our grading system by dividing the grade 2 category into grades 2a and 2b lesions.[109] Grade 2b lesions are as described above. Grade 2a lesions are cellular tumors that retain the lacunar pattern; the cells are larger than the nucleus of a mature lymphocyte and the nuclei demonstrate a fine nuclear

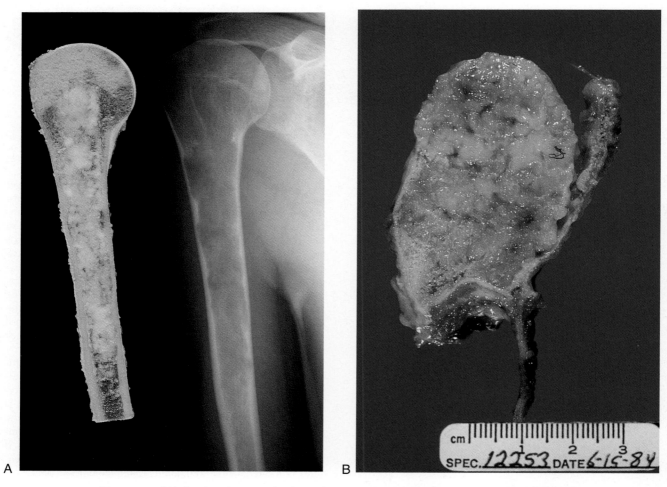

Fig. 23-29. **(A)** Combined gross and radiographic appearance of chondrosarcoma of the humerus. The tumor involves predominantly the shaft of the humerus and produces scalloping of the endosteal surface, best seen in the radiograph. **(B)** Surface chondrosarcoma of the scapula. The lesion shows a glistening white cut surface and a prominent multilobular pattern.

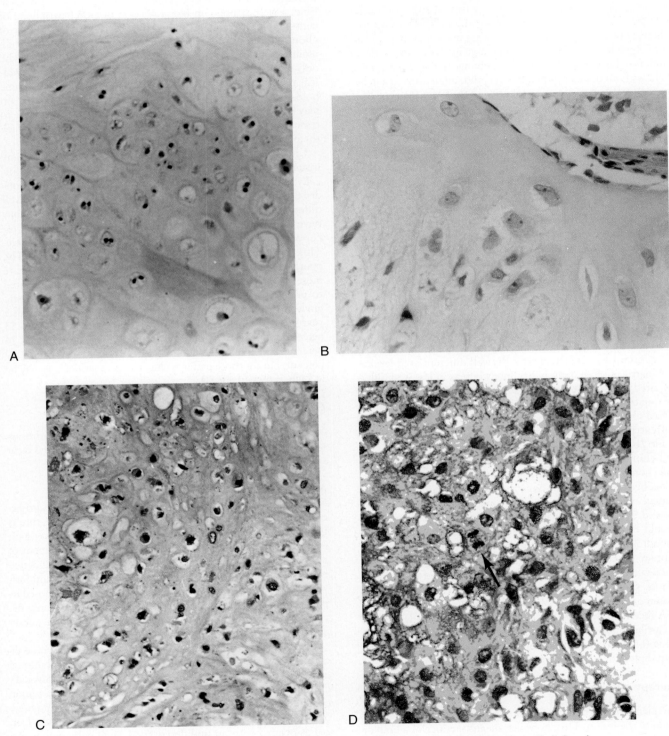

Fig. 23-30. Chondrosarcoma. (A) Grade 1 lesions consist of hyaline cartilage cells with small, dark and pyknotic nuclei. Grade 1 lesions fit the clinical concept of enchondroma. (B) Grade 2a lesions show larger nuclei than grade 1; some may have fine nuclear chromatin pattern and are more cellular than grade 1 lesions. (C) Grade 2b lesions show definitive nuclear atypia and very rare mitoses. (D) Grade 3 lesions exhibiting nuclear anaplasia contain more than 2 mitoses/10 high power fields (see mitotic figure at arrow).

chromatin pattern, often with a prominent nucleolus. Mitoses do not occur but large bizarre cells with karyorrhectic nuclei may be seen in this grade. However, the presence of myxoid change of the matrix with cells showing nuclear atypia is a feature of grade 2b tumors. Myxoid change may occur in grade 2a tumors but is usually a degenerative change or is associated with cells without nuclear atypia. It is very difficult to distinguish degenerative change versus neoplastic but the presence of nuclear atypia should help to place the lesion into grade 2b category. Histologically, grade 3 tumors are obviously malignant with cellular areas that contain 2 or more mitoses/10 hpf.[108]

Grading is related to survival. Grade 1 lesions may behave indolently or may be locally aggressive with only the potential for recurrence but not for metastases. Grade 1 tumors may fit into the so-called enchondroma of long bones, but to make this diagnosis, the lesion has to be in the medullary cavity of the long bone without evidence of remodeling, endosteal scalloping, or pain related to the lesion. We prefer to diagnose these lesions as hyaline cartilage tumors (grade 1) with potential for local recurrence but not for metastasis. This way the message for a lesion that may be only locally aggressive is conveyed. Grade 2a lesions also have a low aggressive behavior; they may recur but do not metastasize. Grade 2b lesions have the potential to metastasize but do so less commonly than do grade 3 lesions.[109]

In addition to grading on the basis of nuclear morphology, it is important to note the matrix. In well differentiated lesions, the matrix is often densely hyaline, whereas in less well differentiated lesions, one is more likely to find mucoid alterations of the matrix that give the tumor a less dense appearance. As stated above, the presence of a single focus of myxoid matrix with atypical cartilaginous cells upgrades a grade 2a tumor to a grade 2b tumor. The histologic findings of peripheral and central chondrosarcomas are similar. One may find bone within the chondrosarcomas, but this is not an indication of osteosarcoma because it does not have the cytologic features of malignancy, even though it is part of the neoplasm. Should bone or osteoid be found with features of malignancy, then the lesion should be classified as a chondroblastic osteosarcoma. Most chondrosarcomas fall into grades 1 and 2; approximately 20 percent are poorly differentiated grade 3 tumors.[108–110] In general, the recurrences and metastases reflect the grade of the original lesion. Occasionally, after repeated recurrences, the chondrosarcoma may take on a higher degree of malignancy.

A recent study on p53 expression and DNA ploidy analysis of cartilaginous tumors has demonstrated that aneuploid, high grade (grade 3) chondrosarcomas contain higher levels of p53 than diploid, low grade, or benign cartilaginous lesions.[111]

Therapy and Recurrence

The ideal form of therapy for chondrosarcoma is complete ablation of the lesion. This, however, means sacrifice of a limb or even greater portion of the body in many instances. Recognizing that the major problem is local recurrence for well differentiated lesions (grades 1 and 2a), one should consider procedures that will preserve the function of a part or a limb. Thus, grades 1 and 2a lesions are amenable to curettage with cement packing of the cavity. Some investigators may freeze the surgical bed

with liquid nitrogen before cementation. If curettage is not feasible, a well planned en bloc resection of either peripheral or central chondrosarcomas should be undertaken. In the case of chondrosarcomas localized to the bony pelvis, an internal, modified, or classic hemipelvectomy may be considered the only means of tumor ablation; for many smaller lesions, less radical procedures can be accomplished with success. The same holds true for central chondrosarcomas, in which amputation may be necessary to ablate the lesion. However, it is possible to resect portions of the femur or tibia, for example, and replace them with a prosthesis or bone graft.

Chondrosarcomas are slowly evolving tumors that in many instances have been present for years before becoming clinically apparent. This is reflected in the behavior of the chondrosarcomas after therapy because a major problem with well differentiated lesions is local recurrence.[108] Some patients may have multiple excisions over a number of years before the recurrences become so massive as to make resection impossible. This is commonly seen in low grade lesions of the pelvis. The poorly differentiated chondrosarcomas (grades 2b and 3) are more aggressive and more likely to metastasize. Factors related to prognosis include tumor location, tumor size, histologic grade, and DNA content of the chondrocytes.[112] The overall 5 year survival rate for patients with chondrosarcoma is 28 to 53 percent; for those who accept treatment, it may be as high as 76 percent. Likewise, the overall 10 year survival rate is nearly 39 percent, but for those patients who accept treatment, it may be as high as 69 percent.[113]

Chondrosarcoma Variants

Variants of chondrosarcoma are mesenchymal chondrosarcoma,[114–117] dedifferentiated chondrosarcoma,[118–122] and clear cell chondrosarcoma.[123–126]

Mesenchymal Chondrosarcoma

Mesenchymal chondrosarcoma resembles ordinary chondrosarcoma both radiologically and grossly. An interesting feature is that about one-third of the cases arise in nonskeletal sites such as the meninges or thigh. It accounts for less than 1 percent of all primary malignant neoplasms of bone.[1] The peak incidence is in the second decade of life; this tumor is rare in children younger than 10 years. Most cases (80 percent) are diagnosed in patients younger than 40 years.[2] The sites more commonly involved include the lower extremities (31 percent), the pelvic girdle (17 percent), and the cranial bones (14 percent).[3]

Radiologically, this tumor shows features similar to those of conventional chondrosarcoma. Grossly, evidence of lobules of cartilage may be present, but generally one finds a partially calcified or ossified mass with a light tan or hemorrhagic tumor component in soft tissue. Histologically, the tumor is composed of islands of hyaline cartilage usually of low grade (grade 1 or 2a) associated with an undifferentiated small cell component (Fig. 23-31). A hemangiopericytomatous pattern is commonly seen, as well as some degree of endochondral ossification.

The management of choice is complete ablation of the tumor and chemotherapy. These tumors, however, have a high risk of local recurrence and seem to metastasize more widely than do other chondrosarcomas to unusual sites such as liver, lymph

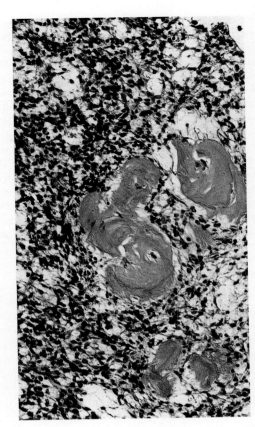

Fig. 23-31. Mesenchymal chondrosarcoma. Islands of cartilage in an undifferentiated stroma.

nodes, kidneys, and brain. The lungs are the most common site of metastases. Although survival may be prolonged, the long-term survival rate is poor, reported as 27 percent at 10 years.[114–117]

Dedifferentiated Chondrosarcoma

Dedifferentiated chondrosarcoma is the cartilaginous tumor with the worst prognosis of any chondrosarcoma.[118–120] It accounts for about 11 percent of all chondrosarcomas and has an equal sex distribution.[118] Most cases are diagnosed in the sixth or subsequent decades of life, and pain is the most common initial symptom. In some cases, there may have been a history of a long indolent enchondroma. This tumor is believed to represent a dedifferentiation of a benign, low grade hyaline cartilage tumor to a high grade sarcoma. Another theory postulates that the high grade component derives from a different cell line and not from that of a low grade cartilage tumor.[120,121] The pelvis and the femur are the most common locations of this tumor, followed by the proximal humerus, distal femur, and ribs.[118]

Radiographically, the tumor may simulate a central chondrosarcoma, but a lytic component is often present associated with considerable expansion and destruction that indicates a malignant state. Grossly, the cartilaginous portion may be identified, but the undifferentiated portion may be dominant and

may suggest a sarcoma other than a chondrosarcoma (Fig. 23-32). Histologically, the tumor is identifiable by portions of well differentiated chondrosarcoma associated with a component that may have characteristics of malignant fibrous histiocytoma, osteosarcoma, rhabdomyosarcoma, or anaplastic sarcoma[118,121] (Fig. 23-33).

The expression of p53, a tumor suppressor gene, was found by Simms and collaborators[122] to be consistently positive in the high grade sarcomatous component of the dedifferentiated chondrosarcoma but negative in the low grade cartilaginous component. In this study the authors also found that proliferative activity measured by Ki-67 and proliferating cell nuclear antigen was also increased in the high grade sarcomatous components of these tumors.

Current management is a combination of radical surgery and chemotherapy. The prognosis is poor, with most patients (about 90 percent) dying within 5 years.[118–120]

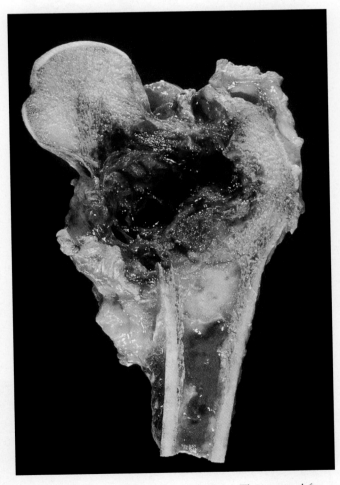

Fig. 23-32. Dedifferentiated chondrosarcoma. The proximal femur displays a large hemorrhagic mass involving the neck and greater trochanter of the femur with an associated pathologic fracture. In the upper diaphysis note a nodule of white glistening cartilaginous tissue representing the low grade hyaline cartilage tumor.

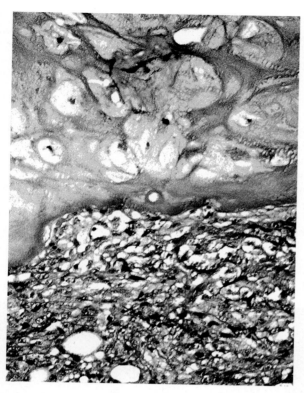

Fig. 23-33. Well differentiated chondrosarcoma in the upper half of the field and undifferentiated sarcoma in the lower half.

Clear Cell Chondrosarcoma

The clear cell type is the rarest, accounting for about 2 percent of all chondrosarcomas. It is also the least malignant.[123-126] Most patients affected with this tumor are in the third and fourth decades of life, but it has been reported in patients in the second through ninth decades. Pain and a mass, usually present for several months or years, are the most common complaints.

Clear cell chondrosarcoma varies radiologically from ordinary chondrosarcoma in that it usually involves the epiphysis of a long bone, thus simulating a chondroblastoma.[123] Calcification in this tumor is not as common as in ordinary chondrosar-

coma; in fact, a lytic lesion is the most common finding. It frequently expands a bone and may break through the cortex, particularly in long-standing processes.

Grossly, it is not always recognized as cartilaginous because some clear cell chondrosarcomas are cystic and have been mistaken for aneurysmal bone cysts. Histologically, the tumor is made up of large cells that have colorless to faintly acidophilic to densely acidophilic cytoplasm[123-126] (Fig. 23-34). In some lesions, the more conventional form of well differentiated chondrosarcoma may be seen. Endochondral ossification is commonly seen, as is aneurysmal bone cyst formation. The radiologic involvement of an epiphyseal end of bone and the cartilaginous nature of the lesion have suggested the possibility that clear cell chondrosarcomas are related to chondroblastoma, but this theory has not been proved.[1-4] Surgical resection or en bloc excision, if feasible, is the management of choice. The 5 year survival rate is 85 percent.[123-126]

Extraosseous Chondrosarcoma

Another form is the extraosseous chondrosarcoma. This lesion apparently arises in the soft tissues and is radiologically, grossly, and histologically similar to conventional chondrosarcoma. To date, data on the biologic behavior of the lesion are sparse. Extraskeletal myxoid chondrosarcoma is similar but has myxoid areas that in themselves may be mistaken for carcinoma.[127,128] This tumor is slow to grow but has a tendency toward local recurrence and late metastases.[127,128]

Cytopathology of Cartilaginous Tumors

FNA is gaining acceptance as a primary modality for the pathologic diagnosis of cartilaginous tumors of the skeleton.[129-131] Nonetheless, these lesions remain a major source of diagnostic difficulty in cytologic, as well as histologic, specimens.[132,133] Significant overlap exists in the morphologic features of benign and malignant lesions, and in addition, considerable morphologic variation is often present within a single tumor. In most cases, it is possible to differentiate low grade lesions with minimal risk of metastasis (i.e., chondromas and grades 1 and 2a chondrosarcomas) from high grade lesions with significant risk of metastasis (i.e., grades 2b and 3 chondrosarcomas) in cytologic specimens, and it is this distinction that is

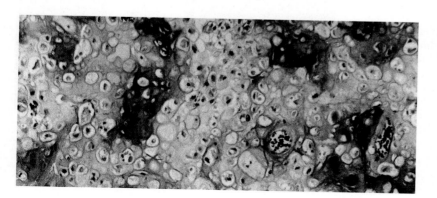

Fig. 23-34. Clear cell chondrosarcoma. Large cells and nuclear aberrations are apparent. Note enchondral ossification.

Fig. 23-35. Chondrosarcoma. This Papanicolaou-stained smear contains abundant, sheet-like fragments of metachromatic chondroid.

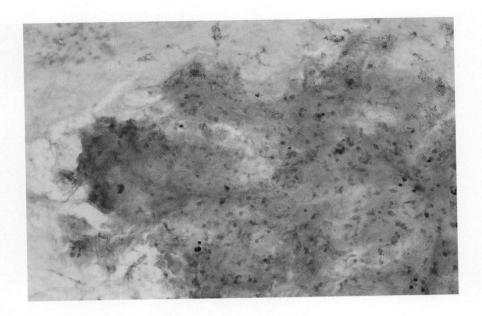

most relevant clinically.[132,133] As with histologic specimens, FNA of cartilaginous tumors must be interpreted in the context of the clinical data and radiographic findings. When different patterns of growth are present within the same lesion, the radiographic studies may also guide the selection of the most appropriate site for FNA. Heavily calcified areas are more likely to be composed of benign or low grade chondrosarcomatous elements, whereas purely lytic foci usually represent high grade or dedifferentiated tumor.

Cartilaginous tumors are characterized by the presence of benign or malignant chondroid matrix. Like osteoid, chondroid is intensely metachromatic but, in contrast to osteoid, often occurs in large, sheet-like fragments or clumps (Fig. 23-35). It may appear opaque or may have a fibrillar or filmy quality.[130,134] The fragments often have relatively well defined borders and may be acellular or have variable numbers of benign or malignant cells embedded in the stroma (Fig. 23-36).

Enchondroma

FNA biopsy of enchondroma yields paucicellular smears dominated by benign cartilaginous matrix that has a filmy or granular quality and appears bright magenta to purple in air-dried, Romanowsky-stained smears and blue-green to blue-gray in Papanicolaou-stained preparations.[134] Fragments of matrix may have a lobulated appearance that recapitulates the histologic pattern. Embedded in the matrix, usually within lacunar spaces, are variable numbers of uniform, round or ovoid chondrocytes that have small, round, dark nuclei without apparent nucleoli. Binucleated cells are rare, and multinucleated forms and mitotic figures are absent. Within the lacunae, cells occur singly, as doublets, or occasionally in clusters. Individually dispersed chondrocytes may also be identified. Foci of calcification within the matrix are often evident (Fig. 23-37).

The previously described features apply to enchondromas arising in sites other than the hands and feet. In the latter two sites, hypercellularity and cytologic atypia are common and,

unless the location is considered, may lead to a false positive diagnosis of low grade chondrosarcoma (Fig. 23-38). Regardless of site, the presence of significant myxoid degeneration or necrosis, or both, should arouse suspicion of malignant change. Table 23-2 summarizes the features that help to distinguish enchondroma from low grade chondrosarcoma.

Chondromyxoid Fibroma

FNA of chondromyxoid fibroma yields mildly to moderately cellular smears in which fragments of chondromyxoid matrix are admixed with stellate, spindled, and round cells.[135–137] The stellate and spindled cells appear to float in the chondromyxoid matrix and also occur as individually dispersed elements.[135] These cells are moderately pleomorphic, with variably shaped nuclei and finely clumped to dark chromatin. Binucleated and multinucleated forms may be found. In addition, variable numbers of uniform, small, round to ovoid cells are also present, either singly or in small clusters. These cells are morphologically similar or identical to chondroblasts and have dense, well defined cytoplasm and round to ovoid nuclei with pale, finely dispersed chromatin.[137] Nuclear grooves or convolutions are often present. Mitotic figures are absent. The chondromyxoid matrix is magenta or pale purple in air-dried, Romanowsky-stained smears or pale blue-green or gray-blue in Papanicolaou-stained preparations and has a watery or filmy quality.[135–137]

Chondroblastoma

FNA biopsy of chondroblastoma yields variably cellular smears composed of small, mononuclear cells arranged singly and in clusters, osteoclast-like giant cells, and fragments of chondroid matrix[138] (Fig. 23-39A). The mononuclear cells have dense cytoplasm with distinct borders, and eccentric, round to oval nuclei with finely dispersed chromatin and absent or inconspicuous nucleoli.[137,139–141] Longitudinal nuclear grooves or convolutions are characteristic (Fig. 23-39B). Fragments of

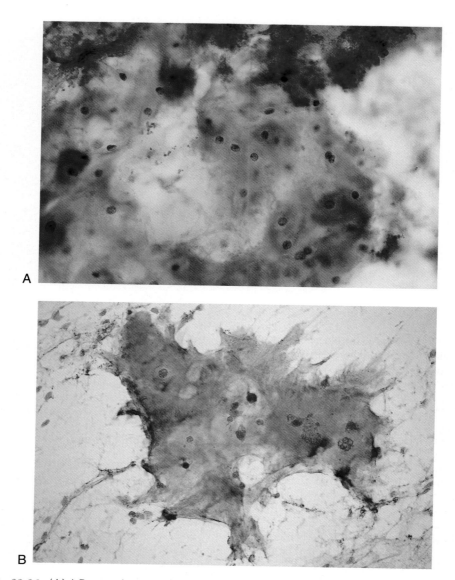

Fig. 23-36. **(A)** A Papanicolaou-stained smear from a digital enchondroma shows a well defined fragment of chondroid matrix with uniform cells embedded within lacunar spaces. **(B)** Chondrosarcoma. Malignant cells are embedded in chondroid matrix, which has irregular, frayed edges.

chondroid matrix are typically small, have an amorphous or fibrillar quality, and may be calcified. Cellular aggregates in which matrix, with or without calcification, surrounds individual mononuclear cells in a chicken-wire pattern may be present and are virtually diagnostic of chondroblastoma. Particularly in the absence of calcification, chicken-wire chondroid is best appreciated in air-dried, Romanowsky-stained smears.

The differential diagnosis of chondroblastoma includes giant cell tumor of bone. In the latter, nuclei lack longitudinal grooves and are essentially identical in the mononuclear stromal cells and multinucleated giant cells. Although chondroid is absent from giant cell tumor of bone, it is often inconspicuous or lacking in smears from chondroblastoma.

Chondrosarcoma

FNA of chondrosarcoma yields variably cellular smears composed of malignant chondrocytes that occur singly, in small clusters, and embedded within chondroid matrix[129–131] (Fig. 23-40). In low grade chondrosarcomas, the neoplastic cells are round, oval, or polygonal and have abundant vacuolated or granular cytoplasm and relatively uniform, round to oval nuclei with evenly dispersed, fine to coarse chromatin[142,143] (Fig. 23-41). Nucleoli may be absent; when present, they are small, round, and regular. Binucleated forms may occur. Within the matrix, cells occur singly, as doublets, or in small clusters and tend to fill the lacunar spaces. The chondroid matrix typically

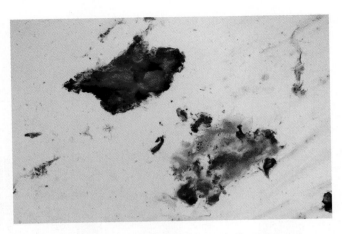

Fig. 23-37. Enchondroma. Large foci of calcification are present within the cartilaginous matrix.

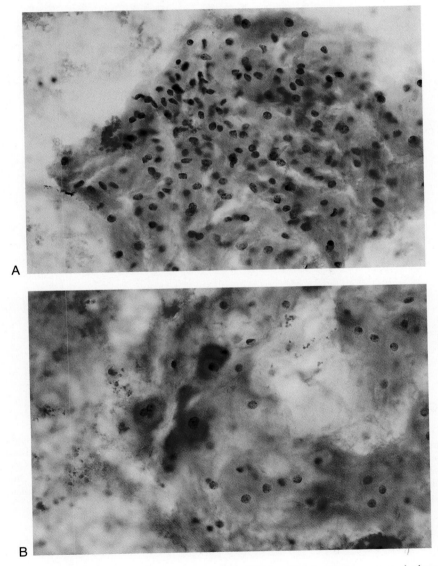

Fig. 23-38. **(A & B)** Papanicolaou-stained smears of a digital enchondroma demonstrate the hypercellularity and cytologic atypia that may be seen in these lesions. Careful attention to the skeletal location, as well as the clinical and radiographic features of these lesions, is essential for avoiding a false positive diagnosis of low grade chondrosarcoma.

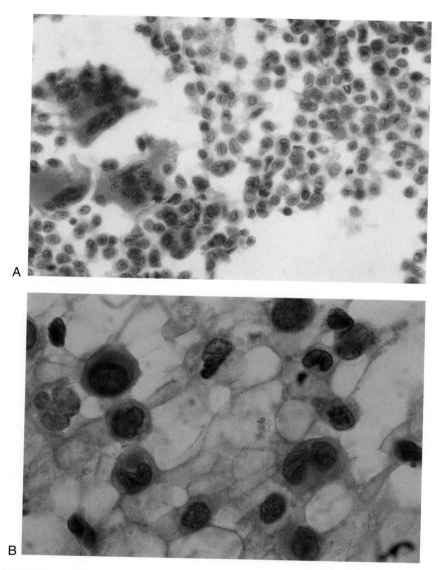

Fig. 23-39. Chondroblastoma. **(A)** In this highly cellular Papanicolaou-stained smear, single and clustered mononuclear cells are interspersed with osteoclast-like giant cells. The mononuclear cells have distinct cell borders, round to oval nuclei, and finely dispersed chromatin. Characteristic longitudinal grooves are easily identified. (Courtesy of Terri Johnson, M.D., Henry Ford Hospital, Detroit, MI.) **(B)** On FNA the cells of this tumor exhibit reniform-, horse shoe-, or kidney-shaped nuclei that on perpendicular position appear to have nuclear grooves.

Table 23-2. Useful Features for Distinguishing Enchondroma From Low Grade Chondrosarcoma

Feature	Enchondroma (EC)	Low Grade Chondrosarcoma (LCS)
Binucleated cells	Occasional (EC < LCS)	Occasional to frequent (LCS > EC)
Cellular morphology	Small, bland cells Do not fill lacunar space Atypia absent or minimal except in digital EC	Larger, "plump" cells Tend to fill lacunae Mild atypia
Nuclear morphology	Small, round nuclei Dark, pyknotic-appearing nuclei, chromatin detail absent	Larger, round nuclei ± Evenly dispersed open chromatin ± Small nucleoli
Pattern of growth	Well circumscribed Usually surrounded by a rim of trabecular bone Lobulated architecture	Infiltrative Invades/surrounds host bone Erodes and destroys cortex Architecture less organized
Skeletal location	Small bones of hands and feet, long bones, especially femur and humerus	Pelvis, axial skeleton, proximal long bones
Clinical history	Painless, usually asymptomatic Most often discovered incidentally or after pathologic fracture	Usually painful (± night or rest pain)

has a dense or opaque amorphous appearance. Occasional foci of myxoid degeneration may be present, imparting a fibrillar or stringy quality to the matrix (Fig. 23-42).

Low grade chondrosarcomas are extremely difficult or impossible to distinguish from enchondromas on the basis of cytologic features alone. However, correlation of the cytologic findings with the clinical and radiographic data may allow accurate diagnosis of these lesions[133,144] (Table 23-2). In most cases, a diagnosis such as "low grade cartilaginous neoplasm: low grade chondrosarcoma versus enchondroma" provides sufficient information for the clinician to plan appropriate therapy. Clinically, a more important problem is underdiagnosis of a high grade lesion due to sampling error.[75] Close communication among the radiologist, pathologist, and orthopedic surgeon should ensure that aspirates are obtained from the most worrisome areas; the importance of such communication cannot be overemphasized.

In contrast to low grade lesions, high grade chondrosarcomas are characterized by obvious cellular and nuclear atypia.[130] Nuclei are enlarged and hyperchromatic, with irregular contours and prominent, often irregular nucleoli. In grade 3 lesions, anaplastic cells are the predominant cell type. Mitotic figures, including abnormal forms, are present; and myxoid degeneration or necrosis, or both, are usually evident. In grade 3 lesions, chondroid matrix may be scant.

Mesenchymal Chondrosarcoma

FNA of mesenchymal chondrosarcoma yields highly cellular smears dominated by small, round cells arrayed singly and in loosely cohesive aggregates[143,145] (Fig. 23-43). These cells have scant or moderate amounts of granular cytoplasm, distinct cytoplasmic borders, and central, round to oval nuclei with coarsely granular chromatin and small nucleoli. The nuclear membranes are smooth and thickened, and longitudinal nuclear grooves may be present. A chondroid component indistinguishable from low grade chondrosarcoma is usually present but may be extremely scant or absent, making distinction from other small round cell tumors difficult.[139] Immunocytochemistry performed on smears, cytospin preparations, or a cell block may be used to clarify the diagnosis. Cells in mesenchymal chondrosarcoma are immunoreactive for vimentin and S-100 protein but negative for markers of lymphoid, neuroendocrine, and plasmacytic differentiation.[146]

Dedifferentiated Chondrosarcoma

The cytologic appearance of dedifferentiated chondrosarcoma depends in large part on where the lesion is sampled. Thus smears may be composed of only high grade, noncartilaginous sarcoma (Fig. 23-44) or only low grade chondrosarcoma (Fig. 23-45), or both.[147] Clearly, definitive diagnosis requires both noncartilaginous and cartilaginous elements. The cytologic features of high grade fibrosarcoma, malignant fibrous histiocytoma, and osteosarcoma are described elsewhere in this chapter. When present, the chondrosarcomatous component has features as described above.

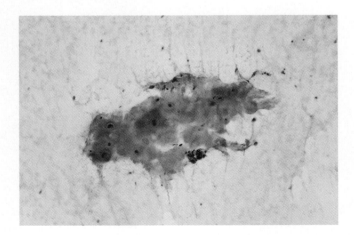

Fig. 23-40. Chondrosarcoma. A Papanicolaou-stained smear shows a fragment of chondroid matrix with embedded tumor cells.

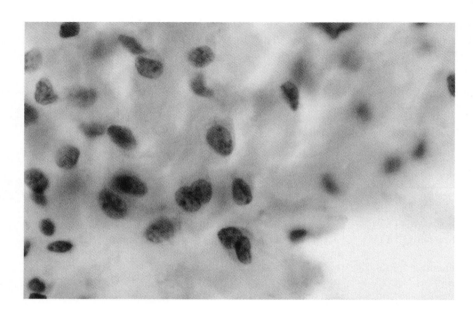

Fig. 23-41. Low grade chondrosarcoma. Neoplastic cells in this Papanicolaou-stained smear have granular cytoplasm and round to oval nuclei with coarse chromatin and small nucleoli.

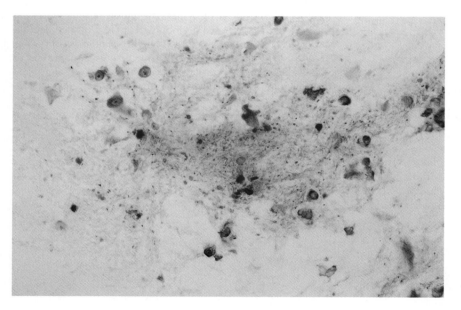

Fig. 23-42. Low grade chondrosarcoma. A Papanicolaou-stained preparation shows an area of myxoid degeneration that imparts a fibrillar or stringy quality to the matrix.

Fig. 23-43. Mesenchymal chondrosarcoma. This highly cellular, air-dried, Romanowsky-stained preparation is composed almost entirely of small round cells arrayed singly and in loosely cohesive aggregates. Without additional information, it would be difficult to distinguish this tumor from other small round blue cell tumors.

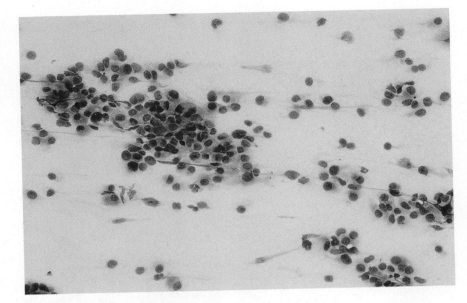

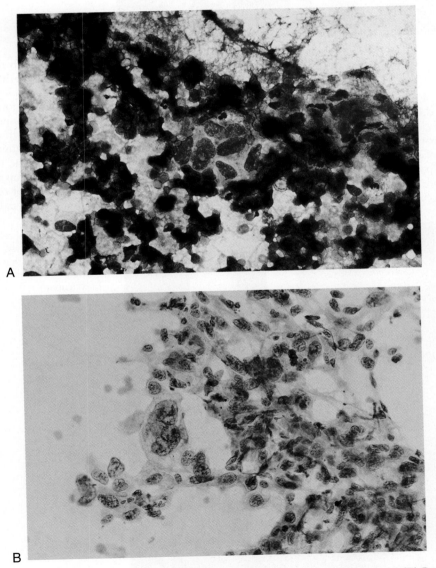

A

B

Fig. 23-44. Dedifferentiated chondrosarcoma. **(A)** Air-dried, Romanowsky-stained and **(B)** Papanicolaou-stained smears show the high grade sarcomatous component of this tumor.

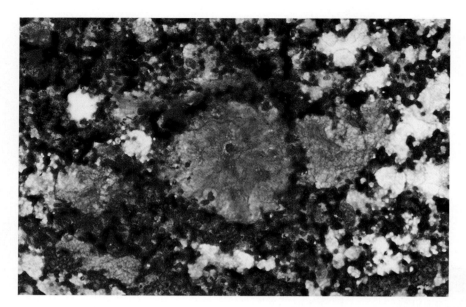

Fig. 23-45. Dedifferentiated chondrosarcoma. An air-dried, Romanowsky-stained preparation from the case illustrated in Fig. 23-44 demonstrates the chondroid component of the lesion.

GIANT CELL TUMOR

Giant cell tumor is a neoplasm that develops from mesenchymal cells with differentiation toward fibroblast-like stroma, multinucleated giant cells, and a mixture of other cells, predominantly inflammatory. It is a tumor of bone that can be suspected on the basis of its radiologic and clinical features.[1-4] It rarely occurs in the pediatric age group or after the age of 50.[1,148] The peak incidence is within the third and fourth decades of life, and it occurs more frequently in females than in males.[1-4] Giant cell tumor has been reported as occurring in most bones, with a predominance in the distal end of the femur and in the proximal end of the tibia.[1,149] Only rarely has giant cell tumor occurred in the skull[150] or in multiple sites.[151] Thus giant cell tumor should be strongly suspected in a patient in late adolescence or in the third or fourth decade of life who has swelling around the knee and indicative radiologic findings.

Radiologically, the characteristic giant cell tumor has a metaphyseal and an epiphyseal component. Without an epiphyseal component, the lesion is not readily diagnosable. The features of the lesion are those of a radiolucent expanding le-

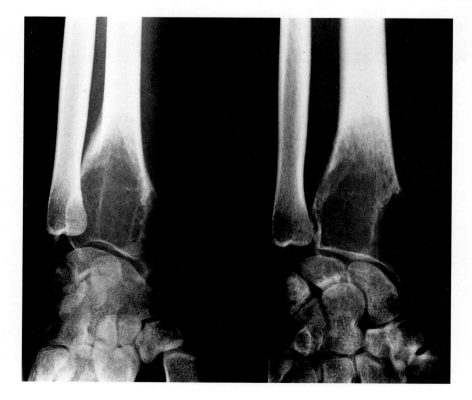

Fig. 23-46. Giant cell tumor of the radius. The epiphysis-metaphysis of the bone is expanded by a lytic process that characteristically reaches the subchondral area of the bone. Note ill-defined margins at the junction of the tumor with the medullary cavity.

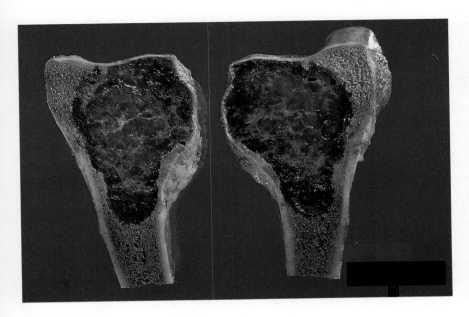

Fig. 23-47. Giant cell tumor of the distal end of the femur. Characteristically this tumor involves subchondral bone and is predominantly epiphyseal in location with extension into the metaphysis. The cut surface demonstrates a red-brown discoloration, reflecting the vasculature of the tumor.

sion, typically with indistinct margins. Sclerotic margins are not a feature of this tumor, but at times there may be focal sclerosis. The cortex becomes attenuated and almost imperceptible. In the large tubular bones, the entire width of the bone may be involved. In the small tubular bones, the entire bone may be involved and in effect may be destroyed. A very important radiologic feature is extension of the tumor until it abuts the articular cartilage (Fig. 23-46). At times, the giant cell tumor will penetrate the cortex and have an extraosseous component. Nonepiphyseal origin of giant cell tumor is rarely seen. In the series of Fain et al,[152] 14 of 1,682 cases of giant cell tumor of the bone presented with a nonepiphyseal origin; 10 were metaphyseal, 2 were metadiaphyseal, and 2 were diaphyseal.

Grossly, giant cell tumors are gray-white to gray-red to red-brown and are well circumscribed; as would be expected from the radiologic findings, they extend to and abut the articular cartilage (Fig. 23-47). They are often hemorrhagic (sometimes predominantly) and may be partly cystic. Occasionally areas of fibrosis are present, which may be extensive. Because of the presence of lipid-laden histiocytes, which in some cases may be numerous, yellow areas may be distinguished.

Histologically, giant cell tumor is identifiable by myriad multinucleated giant cells that are usually dispersed throughout the tumor (Fig. 23-48) except in areas of degeneration or fibrosis. The intervening stroma is somewhat variable, being composed of rounded to spindle-shaped cells; often the rounded cells predominate. Foamy macrophages, scattered inflammatory cells such as lymphocytes and plasma cells, and hemosiderin are often present. Giant cell tumors have been graded histologically, but recent studies indicate that the grade does not necessarily correspond to the aggressiveness. For this reason, a tendency exists among pathologists to discard grading. The degree of aggressiveness displayed by giant cell tumors on radiographs more closely relates to its behavior than does histologic grading.[153] Electron microscopic studies suggest that the basic cell of giant cell tumor is the mononuclear stromal cell.[154,155] These may be of fibroblastic or perhaps histiocytic origin.

The multinucleated giant cells are considered to be the result of the fusion of stromal cells, which is borne out by immunohistochemical studies indicating that the multinucleated giant cell originates from mononuclear phagocytes.[156] Thus, alpha-1-antitrypsin and alpha-1-antichymotrypsin have been found in both stromal and giant cells. S-100 protein may occasionally stain the stromal cells, a fact to be remembered when trying to rule out a chondroblastoma.[157]

Metastases from giant cell tumors are identical to the primary lesion. For the most part, metastases from giant cell tumors have occurred only after surgical intervention, with the impli-

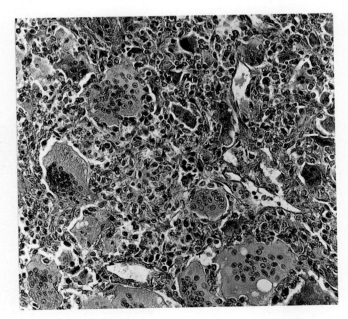

Fig. 23-48. Giant cell tumor. Histologically, many large multinucleated giant cells are seen over a rounded to spindle cell vascular stroma.

cation that they are iatrogenic. Metastases are overwhelmingly to the lungs.

Differential Diagnosis

Histologically, giant cell tumor presents a wide range of differential diagnostic possibilities, as almost any disease of bone may exhibit multinucleate giant cells. However, the knowledge that the lesion is in the epiphysis-metaphysis of a long bone in a skeletally mature individual narrows the differential diagnosis. Chondroblastoma, an epiphyseal lesion, may have a significant number of giant cells, but the presence of cartilage and chondroblasts helps to make this distinction. In difficult cases immunostaining with S-100 protein may demonstrate the cartilaginous nature of the lesion. The radiologic features of chondroblastoma should also help to rule out this lesion. Giant cell tumor may contain a significant component of aneurysmal bone cyst and, in fact, in a biopsy, all the tissue may be represented by the aneurysmal bone cyst component. However, aneurysmal bone cyst is a metaphyseal lesion. Hence the importance of knowing the radiologic features of both giant cell tumor and aneurysmal bone cyst.

Other tumors contain giant cells, but each has its own clinicoradiologic features. These lesions, including fibrous cortical defect/nonossifying fibroma and brown tumor of hyperparathyroidism, are described later in this chapter.

Giant cell reparative granuloma, now believed to be the solid variant of aneurysmal bone cyst (see aneurysmal bone cyst discussion), occurs mainly in the jaws but has been described in other bones, particularly of the hands and feet.[158,159] Histologically, it may be indistinguishable from a giant cell tumor. Usually it has fewer and smaller multinucleated giant cells and considerably more stroma, which is more likely to be fibrous. The giant cells have a tendency to congregate around areas of hemorrhage, in contrast to the usual more diffuse distribution seen in giant cell tumors. In addition, there may be evidence of bone production, although osteoid and cartilage may also be found in the genuine giant cell tumor. Multinucleated giant cells will be found in a wide variety of lesions, including chronic osteomyelitis, Paget's disease of bone, eosinophilic granuloma, healing fracture, benign chondroblastoma, osteosarcoma, and nodular tenosynovitis or pigmented villonodular synovitis that invades bone. If close attention is paid to the pathologic, clinical, and radiologic findings, the pathologist is not likely to mistake these lesions for a genuine giant cell tumor.

Treatment and Natural History

The ideal form of therapy for a giant cell tumor is ablation of the lesion. This is accomplished in an "expendable" bone such as the fibula. The current management of giant cell tumor is curettage and cement packing with methylmetacrylate.[160]

The local recurrence rate with curettage and bone packing has been high, exceeding 50 percent,[153] but with curettage and cementation this rate has been reduced to about 30 to 35 percent.[160] Cryosurgery after the curettage and before cementation is also being utilized in some centers.[161]

An aneuploid pattern has been described in giant cell tumor. Sara et al[162] found that 16 of 60 cases of giant cell tumor presented an aneuploid pattern, but none of these cases behaved any differently than tumors with a diploid pattern.

Malignant giant cell tumors, which are also termed dedifferentiated giant cell tumor,[163] may arise from nontreated benign giant cell tumors, but most patients have had previous surgical treatment with added irradiation.[164] To confirm this transformation, one should endeavor to demonstrate histologically benign areas in an otherwise malignant tumor. Malignant giant cell tumors are rare and occur at a slightly older age than does

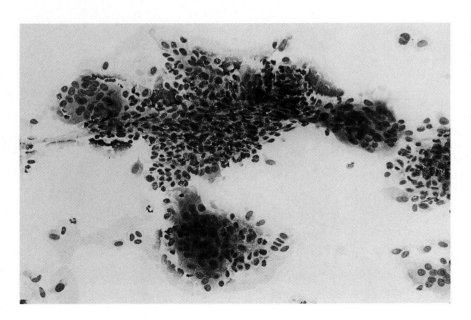

Fig. 23-49. Giant cell tumor. This air-dried, Romanowsky-stained smear is highly cellular and contains cohesive sheets and clusters of stromal cells with interspersed giant cells.

Fig. 23-50. Giant cell tumor. Mononuclear stromal cells have a syncytial appearance and are intimately admixed with multinucleated giant cells in this cellular aggregate. Nuclei are essentially the same in both cell types.

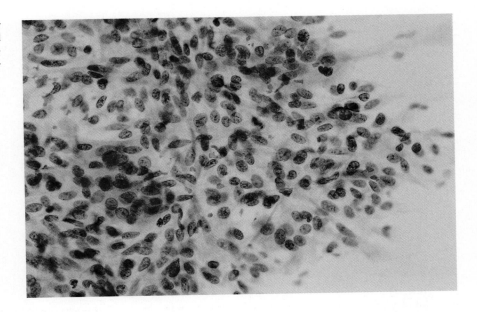

the usual giant cell tumor. They are most commonly seen at the distal end of the femur or at the proximal end of the tibia. Radiologically, evidence of a malignant lesion is widespread destruction of bone, appearing diffusely radiolucent. Most malignant giant cell tumors are fibrosarcomas or malignant fibrous histiocytomas, and a few are osteosarcomas. Survival is poor, with a death rate of 68 percent.[164]

Cytopathology of Giant Cell Tumor

FNA of giant cell tumor yields moderately or highly cellular smears composed of a biphasic population of multinucleated osteoclast-like giant cells and mononuclear stromal cells arrayed in cohesive sheets, in clusters, and singly[165,166] (Fig. 23-49). Within the cellular aggregates, giant cells are fairly evenly dispersed and intimately admixed with mononuclear stromal cells. The latter are plump, spindled cells with scant to moderate cytoplasm, which has a syncytial appearance in clustered cells[165] (Fig. 23-50). Nuclei are round to oval, with smooth contours, finely granular chromatin, and regular, round to oval nucleoli. Mitotic figures are uncommon. The osteoclast-like giant cells contain few to greater than 50 nuclei, which are morphologically identical to those in the mononuclear stromal cells and are randomly distributed throughout the cytoplasm.[165–167] The latter feature is a hallmark of giant cell tumor and, combined with the clinical and radiographic features, helps to distinguish it from other lesions with a prominent giant cell component, such as chondroblastoma, aneurysmal bone cyst, and brown tumor of hyperparathyroidism. The cytologic features of these lesions are described elsewhere in this chapter.

MARROW TUMORS

Ewing's Sarcoma and Peripheral Neuroectodermal Tumor

Ewing's sarcoma, which accounts for approximately 5 to 6 percent of all malignant bone tumors, is basically an undifferentiated malignant small cell neoplasm that arises in bone and soft tissue and has a poor prognosis.[1–4] Recent studies indicate that Ewing's sarcoma is a spectrum of several small cell tumors (including classic Ewing's sarcoma, atypical Ewing's sarcoma, and peripheral neuroectodermal tumor) that are linked by the constant chromosomal translocation t(11;22) (q24;q12).[2–4,168–170] The finding of neural markers (neuron-specific enolase, Leu-7 [HNK-1], neurofilament 200 kd, and S-100 protein) in Ewing's sarcoma and in peripheral neuroectodermal tumor also supports the concept that these lesions are closely related and are most likely primitive neuroectodermal tumors differing only in the extent of neuroectodermal phenotype and morphologic differentiation.[171]

Almost all skeletal sites have been the source of Ewing's sarcoma. The femur, humerus, and tibia are the most common locations of Ewing's sarcoma of the long bones, and the ilium and ribs are the most frequently involved flat bones.[1–5] Ewing's sarcoma is mainly a disease of childhood and adolescence; at least 80 percent of the lesions occur before the age of 30 years, and most occur between the ages of 10 and 20 years.[1–5,172,173] Females are less frequently affected than males.[1,5] Interestingly, Ewing's sarcoma has a strong racial predilection for white persons, and blacks are rarely affected.[1–4,172,173] Most patients complain of pain and swelling in the area of the tumor. The

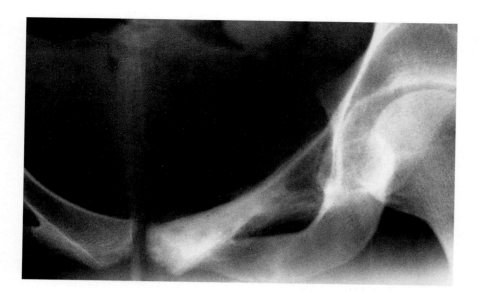

Fig. 23-51. Ewing's sarcoma of the pubis and ischium with sclerotic and lytic areas.

function of adjacent joints may be altered. Fever, anemia, elevated sedimentation rates, and occasionally leukocytosis may be present. Pathologic fractures are infrequent.

Radiologically, Ewing's sarcoma has a variety of patterns. It may cause considerable sclerosis or may be radiolucent with sclerotic areas (Fig. 23-51). Often it expands and deforms the bone to some degree. Ewing's sarcoma provokes considerable periosteal reaction (immature) in most cases. It is a permeative lesion and thus has indistinct boundaries. The periosteal layering (onion-skin effect) is said to be characteristic, but not necessarily specific, for Ewing's sarcoma. Although the radiologic features are not specific, they nearly always suggest a malignant tumor. A young person with a radiologically malignant lesion of a flat bone has a strong possibility of Ewing's sarcoma. A periosteal origin[174] has been described as well as origin in the soft tissue.[175]

CT and MRI techniques provide invaluable information regarding the extent of tumor in soft tissue and marrow. Intact gross specimens are rarely available for examination (Fig. 23-52). Usually, only a biopsy is done of the tumor, and the surgeon encounters a soft, somewhat hemorrhagic, gray-pink to gray-red tissue that resembles lymphoid tissue. In those few specimens that are resected, evidence exists of permeation by the sarcoma of the medullary cavity, with extension through the cortex into the surrounding soft tissues. The cut surfaces are homogeneous and gray-white to pink-gray; the softness and homogeneity, aside from the areas of necrosis, correlate with the rich cellularity of Ewing's sarcoma.

Histologically, Ewing's sarcoma exhibits a highly cellular, rather monotonous pattern of round to ovoid nuclei.[1–4] The cell boundaries are often indistinct, and the cytoplasm appears to be somewhat scanty. Necrosis is often present. The stroma is ordinarily scant but vascular. The tumor nuclei are fairly uniform in size, shape, and stainability and have little pleomorphism (Fig. 23-53A). The chromatin is usually not dense, but occasionally cellular foci are present in which the nuclear chro-

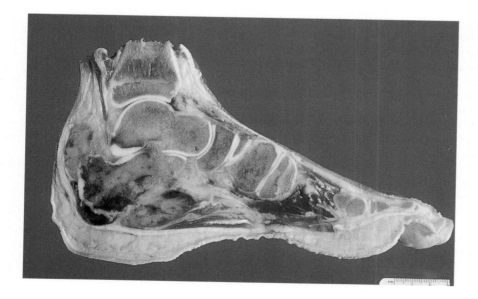

Fig. 23-52. The calcaneus shows massive replacement by a fish-flesh-like tumor that extends into the pre-achilles tendon area.

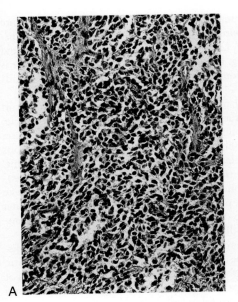
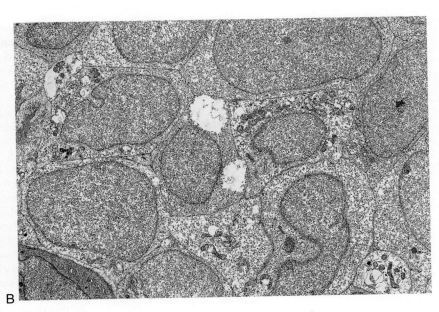

Fig. 23-53. **(A)** The uniform cellularity of Ewing's sarcoma is apparent. The nuclei are quite uniform in size and shape, and cytoplasmic boundaries are indistinct. **(B)** Ewing's sarcoma, ultrastructure. The cells show round to oval nuclei with smooth contours. The chromatin is evenly and finely dispersed, and there are rare small nucleoli. The cytoplasm contains no significant number of organelles. In the center, there is a cell showing two irregular electron-lucent areas, which represent glycogen. The cytoplasmic membranes show occasional junctions. ($\times$ 4,900.)

matin is dense, representing perhaps a second cell population. Possibly the cells with increased nuclear density represent degenerating cells. Nucleoli are present but are generally small and inconspicuous. Atypical (large cell) Ewing's sarcoma differs from classic Ewing's sarcoma in that it shows nuclear pleomorphism, lacks glycogen, has an increased number of mitoses (2/hpf), and has evidence of vascular transformation.[176,177] A reticulin stain demonstrates sparse fibers that are seldom related to individual cells. Approximately 80 percent of Ewing's sarcomas will show intracytoplasmic glycogen (periodic acid-Schiff reaction with and without diastase). By contrast, intracytoplasmic glycogen is rarely if ever found in the cytoplasm of malignant lymphomas and only on rare occasions is it found in the cytoplasm of neuroblastomas. The presence of glycogen or its absence does not mean that the tumor is or is not a Ewing's sarcoma. The stain should be considered an aid in the diagnosis. Material that is positive for periodic acid-Schiff may be seen in the cytoplasm of leukocytes, but this material is diastase resistant.

Immunohistochemical studies have shown that the Ewing's sarcoma complex reacts with several markers, including neuron-specific enolase, neuroblastoma cell surface antigen, neuron cell surface antigen, and neurofilament.[178–180] S-100 protein and keratin have also been found to be present in some of the cells of Ewing's sarcoma, but they are not constant findings. These markers are unfortunately nonspecific. A cell surface antigen, MIC2 (HBA71), is also expressed in the Ewing's complex of small cell tumors but does not discriminate between Ewing's sarcoma and peripheral neuroectodermal tumor.[180–184] This marker has also been described in other small cell neoplasms. Riopel and collaborators[185] found that 37 of 40 (93 per-

cent) lymphoblastic lymphomas and 4 of 20 large cell lymphomas showed strong immunoreactivity for this marker; in addition, all T cell acute lymphocytic leukemias also demonstrated immunoreactivity.[185] A recent study also noted its presence in synovial sarcoma.[186] Therefore, caution should be taken in the interpretation of this marker as it is not restricted to the Ewing's/peripheral neuroectodermal tumor complex.

Electron microscopically the cells of Ewing's sarcoma have a few cytoplasmic organelles and round to ovoid nuclei[187,188] (Fig. 23-53B). A few tight junctions and cytoplasmic filaments may be seen. An important feature is the presence of glycogen granules in the cytoplasm, correlating with the histologic finding of positivity for periodic acid-Schiff.

Peripheral neuroectodermal tumor differs from classic Ewing's sarcoma in that the primitive cells contain neural processes and neurosecretory granules. In our opinion ultrastructural examination is the only reliable method to establish a diagnosis of peripheral neuroectodermal tumor. Although a number of neural markers stain the small cells of this small cell tumor complex, they are not reliable. Askin and collaborators[189] have reported a small cell tumor that occurs in the chest wall. This lesion is often referred to as *Askin's tumor* and represents a Ewing's sarcoma/peripheral neuroectodermal tumor spectrum.[189,190] Metastases from Ewing's-peripheral neuroectodermal tumor may be widespread. Although anywhere from 40 to 75 percent of patients will have involvement of other bones, the lungs are usually the first metastatic site. Metastases to lymph nodes and other viscera are infrequent.[191]

At the moment, the treatment of Ewing's sarcoma is dominated by chemotherapy followed by surgical ablation of the involved bone (if feasible) or radiotherapy, or both. Because of the high incidence of sarcomas developing after a combination of chemotherapy and radiotherapy, a shift toward less radiotherapy appears to be occurring. The prognosis of Ewing's sarcomas has improved with the institution of a multidisciplinary treatment approach. The expected 5 year survival rate before chemotherapy was 0 to 10 percent, in contrast with the current 5 year disease-free survival rate of 60 percent and the 5 year survival rate of 65 percent obtained with modern therapy.[192,193]

Malignant Lymphoma of Bone

Primary lymphoma of bone is uncommon, making up approximately 4 percent of primary malignant bone tumors. It arises in most bones, predominantly those of the lower extremities and the flat bones. It occurs predominantly in males, with a ratio of 2:1 to 3:2.[194–199] In contrast to Ewing's sarcoma, malignant lymphoma of bone usually occurs after the second decade of life, and 50 percent of the patients are older than 40 years. Thus, it is an uncommon tumor in the pediatric age group.[1–4]

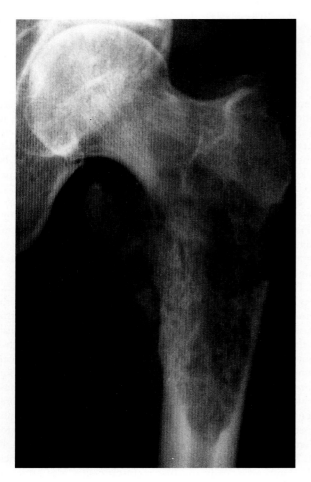

Fig. 23-54. Malignant lymphoma of the upper end of the femur in a 50-year-old woman. The tumor is permeative and destructive of the cancellous and cortical bone.

As with most malignant bone tumors, pain and swelling are common complaints. The pain becomes more severe and distressing at night. Local tenderness and heat may be associated with the swelling, but, in contrast to Ewing's sarcoma, fever is uncommon. Laboratory examinations are generally unrewarding.

Radiologically, malignant lymphoma of bone is frequently an extensively destructive lesion of the medulla and cortex (Fig. 23-54). Even though destruction is usually a prominent feature, areas of patchy sclerosis may exist, and (rarely) some lesions may be mostly sclerotic. Periosteal reaction, although present, is not as noteworthy as that seen in Ewing's sarcoma. An extraosseous component is common, but some lesions do not have one. In the older patient, the findings of a primary lymphoma may mimic those of metastatic carcinoma, an important consideration in the differential diagnosis.[1–4]

The gross features of primary lymphoma of bone are not distinctive. It may be difficult to distinguish them from metastatic carcinoma, Ewing's sarcoma, or some other primary sarcoma of bone. The findings correspond well with the radiologic findings in that there is destruction and permeation of the marrow cavity, erosion and penetration of the cortex, and nearly always an extraosseous component. Necrosis and hemorrhage into the tumor are frequent. The cut surfaces are homogeneous, vary from light red to pink-gray, and, because of their homogeneity and friability, suggest rich cellularity. Aside from the location of the lesion in bone, the gross features are similar to those of a malignant lymphoma of a lymph node.

Histologically and cytologically, primary malignant lymphomas of bone resemble those of lymph nodes (see Ch. 20). The most common type is the large cell lymphoma of B cell lineage.[200] The cells have indistinct cell boundaries with faintly acidophilic or basophilic cytoplasm. The nuclei are approximately the same size as those of a Ewing's sarcoma, but the nucleus is often indented, and nucleoli are commonly prominent. Most primary lymphomas of bone are made up of large cells or have a mixed cell population. Lymphomas composed of large cleaved cells have a better prognosis than those containing large noncleaved cells.[197–199] Aside from the lymphomatous component, quantities of a fibrous stroma are varied, and the lesions are often notably vascular. Areas of necrosis and hemorrhage and occasionally granulomatous lesions may be seen. Hodgkin's disease of bone has rarely been reported.

Immunohistochemistry is very valuable for confirming the diagnosis of lymphoma and characterizing the cell lineage. Leukocytic common antigen is a useful marker for all lymphoid lesions. CD20 (L26), a pan-B cell marker, is also extremely helpful.[200,201] T cell markers may be utilized but only after the B cell markers have been found to be negative. T cell lymphoma and anaplastic Ki-1 lymphomas are uncommon in bone.[200] Electron microscopic examination is also helpful in distinguishing this tumor from other round cell tumors of bone.

Primary malignant lymphoma of bone in all likelihood will be indistinguishable from secondary lymphomatous involvement of bone. Thus, it is important in diagnosing skeletal lymphoma that the clinician be alerted to the possibility that the lesion may be secondary. Only careful clinical and hematologic evaluation and follow-up will firmly establish the diagnosis of a primary lymphoma of bone. Metastases to visceral organs and other bones are common; metastases to regional lymph nodes occur in approximately one-fifth of the cases. Widespread metastases may occur.

The treatment of primary lymphoma of bone has been irradiation. The 5 year survival rate is between 40 and 45 percent, and the 10 year survival rate is close to 35 percent. Chemotherapy followed by radiotherapy has been recently advocated. Bacci et al[202] have reported an 88 percent disease-free survival rate during an average follow up of 87 months.

Plasma Cell Myeloma

Plasma cell myeloma is a neoplastic proliferation of plasma cells that presents as a clinically localized osseous lesion or as part of a systemic disease. Skeletal involvement is almost universal; therefore, myeloma is one of the most common malignant tumors involving bone. Within the wide age range, myeloma occurs most commonly in persons older than 40 years. The male/female ratio is approximately 2:1.[1] The clinical manifestations of myeloma are many and are often related to the overproduction of immunoglobulins. Pathologic fractures are frequent and are often the presenting complaint of otherwise asymptomatic patients. The laboratory data, which are important in the diagnosis and evaluation of patients with myeloma, are described in Chapter 21.

Radiologically, myeloma is commonly a destructive bone lesion; only occasionally is it sclerotic. The manifestations in the skeleton vary from site to site. Skull lesions often have well circumscribed, punched-out, lucent areas, whereas in the long bones or pelvis, myeloma may appear as a purely radiolucent area with maintenance of the contours of the bone. Myeloma may be a multiloculated lesion. The most common sites of involvement are the vertebral column, ribs, skull, pelvis, and long bones.

Grossly, myeloma is red-gray, soft, and fairly homogeneous. Cancellous bone shows destruction, as does the cortex, if involved. It is difficult to distinguish myeloma from other cellular lesions, such as lymphoma or some metastases. Myeloma might present as diffuse involvement of an area of bone or as a multinodular lesion that has the same features described above.

Solitary myeloma is a localized lesion without evidence of systemic disease. Males are affected in 70 percent of cases and pain is a common symptom. Any bone may be affected, but one-third of the cases occur in the spine. To accept a case as a solitary myeloma, the following criteria are required: a solitary bone lesion; negative skeletal survey; absence of plasma cell infiltrates in random marrow biopsies; lack of anemia, hypercalcemia, or renal involvement; and a proliferation of monoclonal plasma cells.[203]

The histologic features of myeloma cells are described in Chapter 21. Differentiation of myeloma varies from cases in which the plasma cells appear normal (Fig. 23-55) to those in which the plasma cells are poorly differentiated and histologically may mimic a plasmacytoid high grade lymphoma or an undifferentiated carcinoma. If these three cannot be distinguished by careful histologic examination, immunopathologic proce-

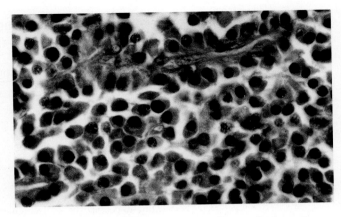

Fig. 23-55. Well differentiated plasma cells in multiple myeloma.

dures will be helpful. Monoclonality of the cells with either kappa or lambda light chain immunoglobulins would support a diagnosis of myeloma versus one of a reactive or inflammatory process. If this fails, electron microscopic studies may serve as the means by which histologic confirmation of myeloma can be made.

Nearly all (85 percent) solitary plasmacytomas of the skeleton will eventually disseminate. The presence of both nuclear immaturity and nucleoli has been cited as the best indicator to predict the development of multiple myeloma in cases of solitary tumors.[204] Considering the patient's age and the radiologic findings of a malignant tumor, the major differential diagnostic possibility is metastatic carcinoma. This is stated to highlight the importance of myeloma in the differential diagnosis of destructive bone lesions in adults. Irradiation remains the treatment of choice for localized myelomas. For those that are disseminated, a combination of chemotherapy and radiation will serve to prolong life.[205] With chemotherapy the average survival has been remarkably improved.[205] Aside from the complications of dissemination, patients with myeloma die of infections, cardiopulmonary disease, uremia, and hemorrhage.

Mastocytosis

Mastocytosis is mentioned merely as a means of differential diagnosis in regard to its radiologic and histologic findings. About 15 percent of the patients with mastocytosis will have radiologic changes in the skeleton.[5] A presumptive diagnosis can be made from the bony abnormalities when the typical skin lesions are present and are confirmed by histologic examination. It is rare for a patient to have skeletal involvement without the dermal lesions. Radiologically, the lesion may appear to be permeative and occasionally sclerotic; in a child it may be mistaken for a Ewing's sarcoma. However, the lesions are often multiple and extensive. Histologically, mastocytosis may closely mimic a malignant lymphoma or histiocytosis. The granules may be demonstrated with Wright and Giemsa stains. Electron microscopic studies will demonstrate the classic features of mastocytes.

Table 23-3. Useful Features for Distinguishing Between Small Round Cell Tumors of Bone

Features	ES/PNET	Lymphoma	Plasma Cell Myeloma	Mesenchymal Chondrosarcoma
Cytoplasm	ES: scant, indistinct borders PNET: ± wispy extensions	Scant to moderate	Moderate to abundant	Scant, distinct borders
Cytoplasmic glycogen (PAS + diastase digestible)	Usually prominent	Absent	Absent Cells may be PAS ± diastase resistant	Rare
Nuclear features	Oval to round ES: evenly dispersed chromatin PNET: fine to coarse chromatin, ± small nucleoli	Irregular contours; coarse or vesicular chromatin; nucleoli usually prominent	Round; clumped "clock-faced" chromatin; ± nucleoli; ± binucleated forms	Oval to spindled shaped; fine to coarse chromatin; ± nucleoli
Matrix	Absent	Absent	Absent	Focal chondroid (may be scant)
ICC	ES: + vimentin, MIC2[a] PNET: +vimentin, NSE, PGP 9.5, chromogranin, MIC2, synaptophysin; (−) LCA	+ LCA B cell: + CD20, CD79, LN2 T cell: + CD43, UCHL1	(−) LCA; + EMA; + kappa or lambda (light chain restriction)	+ vimentin, ± S-100 protein
Pattern	ES: single cells PNET: single cells, clusters, and pseudorosettes	Single cells; lymphoglandular bodies	Single cells	Single cells
Age range	10–20 yr	Broad	40–60 yr	10–40 yr
Extraosseous mass	Usually prominent	Usually prominent	Usually absent	Common

Abbreviations: ES/PNET, Ewing's sarcoma/peripheral neuroectodermal tumor; PAS, periodic acid-Schiff; NSE, neuron-specific enolase; PGP 9.5, protein gene product 9.5; LCA, leukocyte common antigen; EMA, epithelial membrane antigen; ICC, immunocytochemistry.
[a] MIC2 (HBA71) can be positive in other small cell malignant tumors.

Cytopathology of Marrow Tumors

A distinctive group of malignant neoplasms of bone are the so-called small round blue cell tumors. These include Ewing's sarcoma, peripheral neuroectodermal tumor, primary malignant lymphoma, plasmacytoma/multiple myeloma, mesenchymal chondrosarcoma, and small cell osteosarcoma. Metastatic lesions such as neuroblastoma, rhabdomyosarcoma, and small cell undifferentiated carcinoma should also be considered in the differential diagnosis of small round blue cell tumors of bone.

Because each of these tumors is composed of a relatively monomorphous population of small, round cells with scant cytoplasm and hyperchromatic nuclei, distinction between these neoplasms may be difficult or impossible without ancillary studies. The principle exceptions are small cell osteosarcoma and mesenchymal chondrosarcoma, in which the presence of the appropriate matrix allows accurate diagnosis. In most cases of small round blue cell tumors involving bone, the use of ancillary studies including special stains, immunocytochemistry, flow cytometry, cytogenetics, and/or electron microscopy permits a definitive diagnosis. The importance of immediate, on-site assessment of the FNA in the diagnosis of these tumors cannot be overstated, as it allows collection of additional material for appropriate ancillary studies and often obviates the need for a more invasive diagnostic biopsy. Features that help to distinguish some of the more common small round blue cell tumors of bone are summarized in Table 23-3.

Ewing's Sarcoma and Peripheral Neuroectodermal Tumor

Due to the cortical destruction and extraosseous extension that characterize these neoplasms, Ewing's sarcoma and peripheral neuroectodermal tumor are often readily accessible to FNA.[206] Aspirates are highly cellular and contain individually dispersed and loosely clustered cells[207] (Fig. 23-56). In addition, larger aggregates and pseudorosettes are usually present in peripheral neuroectodermal tumor.[208] Ewing's sarcoma consists of relatively uniform, small, round to ovoid cells with scant cytoplasm and indistinct cellular borders[204] (Fig. 23-57). In air-dried, Romanowsky-stained smears, the cytoplasm often appears vacuolated due to abundant glycogen.[207] Nuclei are round to ovoid and have finely granular, evenly dispersed chromatin and inconspicuous nucleoli. Although mitotic figures are present, they are usually few in number. Naked nuclei and DNA streaks (crush artifact) are common. Necrosis is usually present but is not a dominant feature. In peripheral neuroectodermal tumor, the cells may be more pleomorphic than those comprising Ewing's sarcoma.[208] Cytoplasmic projections may be apparent in

Fig. 23-56. Ewing's sarcoma. This highly cellular Papanicolaou-stained smear demonstrates a dispersed monomorphous population of primitive small round blue cells.

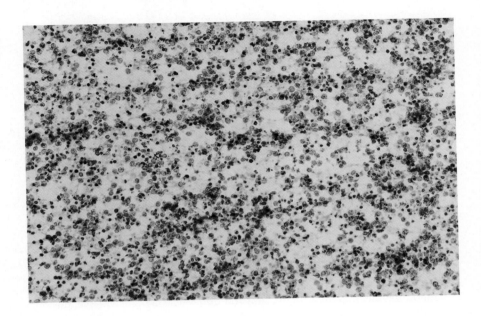

Fig. 23-57. Ewing's sarcoma. This Papanicolaou-stained smear shows cells having round to oval nuclei with finely granular evenly dispersed chromatin and inconspicuous nucleoli. Numerous naked nuclei and necrotic nuclear debris are evident.

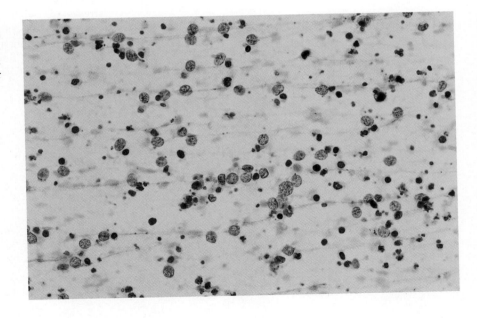

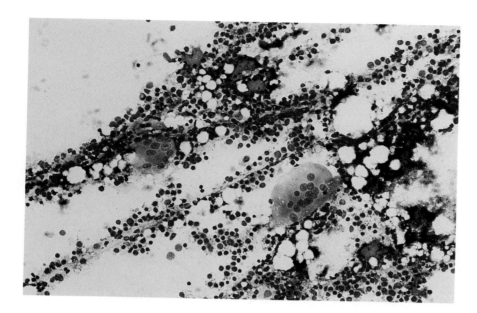

Fig. 23-58. Lymphoma. An air-dried, Romanowsky-stained smear from a primary lymphoma of bone shows a monomorphic population of malignant cells with interspersed osteoclasts.

some cells. Nuclei are round to ovoid and have irregular membranes, clumped chromatin, and small nucleoli. Necrosis is often more prominent than in Ewing's sarcoma. Considerable overlap exists in the cytologic features of Ewing's sarcoma and peripheral neuroectodermal tumor, and the differences between theses entities may be quite subtle. In some cases, ancillary studies may be needed to distinguish these entities with certainty[210] (Table 23-3).

Malignant Lymphoma of Bone

Malignant lymphoma of bone frequently presents with a large extraosseous component that is readily accessible to FNA. The cytologic features resemble those of lymphomas arising in other sites (see Ch. 20). Aspirates yield highly cellular smears composed of a relatively monotonous or (in mixed lymphomas) biphasic population of cells that occur singly and in loosely cohesive, pseudoepithelial clusters[211,212] (Fig. 23-58). Due to cytoplasmic fragility, the background usually contains numerous lymphoglandular bodies that are best appreciated in air-dried, Romanowsky-stained smears (Fig. 23-59). In addition, DNA streaks are usually evident. Necrosis is variably present. In many cases, the lymphoid origin of the malignant cells is readily apparent; in such cases, additional cytologic material should be obtained for flow cytometry and immunocytochemistry. When the cell of origin is less certain, as in anaplastic large cell

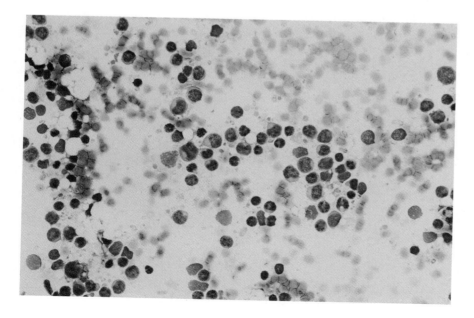

Fig. 23-59. Lymphoma. Lymphoglandular bodies are evident in this air-dried, Romanowsky-stained smear.

Fig. 23-60. Plasma cell myeloma. An air-dried, Romanowsky-stained preparation demonstrates typical cytologic features of malignant plasma cells.

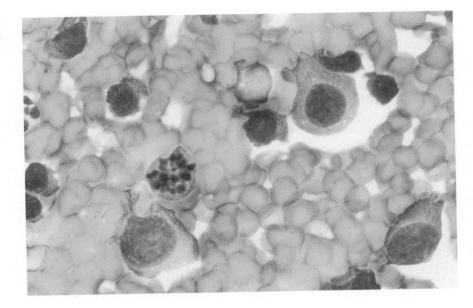

lymphomas, material should also be obtained for electron microscopy and, if possible, cytogenetics and molecular studies.

Plasma Cell Myeloma

Diagnosis of myeloma is usually based on laboratory data and bone marrow biopsy, combined with the appropriate clinical features. FNA is most likely to be performed on solitary myelomas that may mimic a variety of primary and metastatic bone lesions, or to confirm the identity of a new lesion in a patient with known myeloma. Aspirates are highly cellular and consist of individually dispersed neoplastic plasma cells that may vary from essentially normal to anaplastic[213,214] (Fig. 23-60). Immunocytochemistry may be useful for confirming the monoclonal nature of the proliferation and/or differentiating these lesions from plasmacytoid lymphoma or anaplastic carcinoma.

TUMORS OF VASCULAR ORIGIN

Hemangioma

Hemangiomas or vascular malformations are common skeletal lesions, particularly of the vertebral bodies, but those associated with symptoms such as mass, pain, or pathologic fracture are uncommon.[215] Among those that are clinically significant, there is a slight predominance in the female. Hemangiomas are seen in different age groups, with a peak in the third through seventh decades of life.

Radiologically, the lesions are usually solitary and may mimic other neoplasms. They are frequently well circumscribed and radiolucent, but they may produce considerable bony sclerosis with a so-called sunburst pattern (Fig. 23-61). At times hemangiomas may cause sclerotic streaking and linear radiolucency that mimic osteomyelitis or a malignant lesion such as lymphoma or Ewing's sarcoma. The most common sites of he-

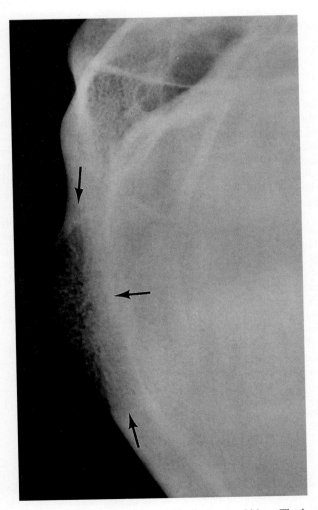

Fig. 23-61. Hemangioma of the skull of a 2-year-old boy. The bony defect and the spiculation are evident.

mangiomas are the skull, ribs, long bones, vertebra, mandible, and facial bones.[5]

Grossly, hemangiomas are blue-red to dark red. The cut surfaces may have a spongy appearance owing to the bony trabeculation. The histologic pattern of most hemangiomas of bone is that of a cavernous hemangioma. Capillary hemangiomas are rare. The treatment varies with the location of the lesion, but generally surgical excision is recommended. For inaccessible lesions, radiotherapy may be effective in relieving symptoms.

Lymphangioma

Lymphangioma is a rare lesion of bone that has histologic features similar to lymphangiomas of skin and soft tissue.[216] Whether lymphatics exist within the medullary portion of bone has been questioned, but lymphangiographic studies in patients with lymphedema have confirmed the presence of intraosseous lymphatic channels. Radiologically, the lesions, being similar to hemangioma, are often well outlined and have a soap bubble appearance. Although rare, the reported examples of lymphangioma have all involved multiple bones.[216] The histologic features are similar to those of lymphangioma occurring in more common sites.

Skeletal Angiomatosis

Skeletal angiomatosis is characterized by multicentric vascular tumors of the skeleton. The lesion is chiefly discovered in children and has a predominance in males.[217] Approximately 50 percent of patients have associated angiomas in skin, soft tissue, and visceral sites. Usually, medical aid is sought because the skeletal lesions have led to vertebral compression and neurologic symptoms. Involvement of all bones has been reported; the most common sites are the skull, ribs, pelvis, scapula, humerus, tibia, and femur.

Radiologically, the lesion is characterized by multiple bubbly defects of the skeleton, often associated with bony sclerosis. The multiplicity of lesions is the key to the radiologic diagnosis. The gross examination of intact specimens is similar to that of hemangiomas. In most cases, only a biopsy specimen is submitted, and it is not particularly characteristic of any lesion. Histologically, skeletal angiomatosis is similar to localized hemangiomas. The lesions are generally combinations of cavernous and capillary formations.

For patients with lesions confined to the skeleton, the prognosis is good; in most instances the lesions tend to stabilize, but progression may occur. Patients with skeletal and visceral lesions may die because the disease may be complicated by heart failure, hemolytic anemia, microangiopathic anemia, and thrombocytopenia.[217]

Massive Osteolysis

Massive osteolysis is a rare, destructive lesion of bone also known as disappearing bone disease or Gorham's disease.[218] It affects young people, usually under the age of 30 years, and is widely destructive of one or more bones.[219] This results in pathologic fractures and sometimes death, particularly if bones of the thorax or vertebrae (or both) are involved. Radiologically, the lesions may resemble hemangiomas, but they may often show destruction of a bone to the point where the bone or bones are imperceptible. Histologically, the lesion is angiomatous. Thus, the disease is defined by its clinical manifestation, its radiologic features, and, to a lesser degree, the histologic findings. A possible variant of massive osteolysis has similar clinical features; histologically, however, it is *not vascular* but exhibits extensive bone resorption with abundant osteoclasts.[220]

Glomus Tumor

Glomus tumor is a benign lesion that commonly occurs in the medullary cavity of a distal phalanx and is typically painful. It affects females more frequently than males and occurs most commonly between 20 and 40 years of age.[1-4] Histologically glomus tumor consists of round monotonous cells associated with vascular structures. Not uncommonly the cells of glomus tumor appear to be arising from the wall of a thick vessel, and they react to smooth muscle actin. Excision of the lesion is the management of choice.

Low Grade Malignant Vascular Tumors

Because of the numerous terms applied to low and high grade vascular lesions, significant confusion on this subject has developed. Early investigators knew that two types of malignant vascular tumors existed, those with a low grade behavior and those with a high grade behavior.[221-224] Unfortunately the terms hemangioendothelioma, hemangiosarcoma, and angiosarcoma were utilized interchangeably. Rosai et al[225] have clarified much of the confusion. Epithelioid/histiocytoid vascular tumors range from small, well differentiated, benign lesions to the cellular tumors that may be confused with other malignant tumors.[226,227] The common denominator of all these lesions is the presence of numerous vessels lined by large plump epithelioid/histiocytoid endothelial cells.[225,226,228]

In this discussion these benign, low grade, vascular tumors are referred to simply as *epithelioid/histiocytoid hemangioendotheliomas*. They vary from the small benign lesions that are similar to angiolymphoid hyperplasia of the skin[229] to the cellular tumors that have been termed epithelioid hemangioendotheliomas.[226,227] The latter lesion simulates carcinoma or sarcoma because the endothelial cells are so numerous and closely packed that they obliterate the lumina of the vessels and produce the appearance of a solid tumor. Furthermore, myxoid stroma may be a component of these lesions, which further compounds the histologic picture.[226,227]

These lesions may be solitary or multicentric. They occur from the second through the sixth decades of life with about equal frequency but are definitively uncommon in people younger than 10 years of age.[230,231] They affect more males than females and may involve any bone. Several bones of an extremity may be involved in multicentric cases, but development of lesions beyond the extremity is unlikely. In the multi-

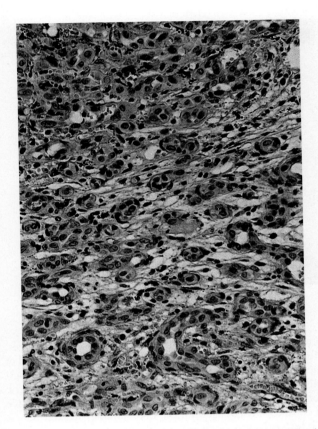

Fig. 23-62. Epithelioid/histiocytoid hemangioendothelioma. This lesion is characterized by the presence of numerous vascular channels lined by large plump epithelioid/histiocytoid cells.

centric cases there is no predilection for any specific part of the anatomy of the bone. In solitary lesions the metaphysis-epiphysis is more likely to be involved than is the diaphysis.

Radiologically, single lesions appear as lytic change, often with sclerotic borders. Macroscopically, the curetted or excised lesions are hemorrhagic and gritty on palpation.

Histologically, these lesions show vascular cords, sometimes anastomosing, that are lined by plump endothelial cells (Fig. 23-62). On cross-section, a cord may present a lumen or may be totally obliterated. Inflammatory cells are nearly always present; of these, eosinophils are a common companion, but lymphocytes and plasma cells may also be found. Reactive bone formation may also be present. Mitotic activity ranges from 2 to 10 mitoses/10 hpf. The solid lesions may be difficult to diagnose and some may be confused with carcinoma, chondrosarcoma, chondromyxoid fibroma, chordoma, or other neoplasms. In these cases endothelial markers are helpful in establishing the correct diagnosis. Factor VIII, Ulex europaeus agglutinin-1, and CD31 are commonly utilized.

Management of solitary lesions should be curettage with bone or cement packing. The tumor may recur, but usually several years after the initial treatment. Multicentric lesions are difficult to control conservatively and may require a major surgical procedure.

Angiosarcoma

High grade vascular tumors or angiosarcomas of the skeleton are rare lesions that may be seen at almost any age but are more common in adults.[1–4,232] There does not appear to be a skeletal site of predilection because they are seen in both flat and long bones. The clinical manifestation is not specific, usually being that of pain or swelling of the affected part, or both. Laboratory findings are not contributory. Radiologically, angiosarcomas are ordinarily radiolucent, appearing as areas of destruction; they may appear well circumscribed or permeative. Often they have a soap bubble appearance (Fig. 23-63). Periosteal reaction may or may not be present.

Grossly, the tumors are bloody, dark red to blue-red, and soft and may appear to be spongy (Fig. 23-64). Evidence of bony destruction and permeation of the cortical and medullary bone is often present. Histologically, the major feature to seek is enlarged cytologically malignant endothelial cells (Fig. 23-65). These are identified by enlarged nuclei with chromatin clumping and large nucleoli. In addition to the cytologic changes, the configuration of the vessels suggests an angiosarcoma (i.e., the vessels are varied in size and shape, often with irregular ramifications and anastomoses). Angiosarcomas may metastasize widely, with the most common sites being lungs, brain, liver, pleura, and occasionally lymph nodes. Treatment has generally been local excision, amputation, irradiation, or a combination

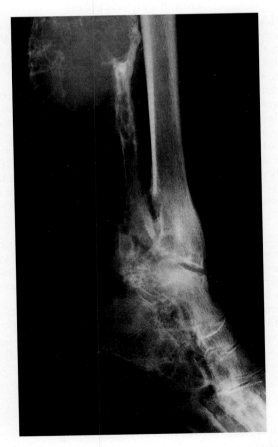

Fig. 23-63. Angiosarcoma of the fibula in a 65-year-old woman. Note the enlarged multiloculated mass and multiple lucent areas elsewhere in the fibula, tibia, and bones of the foot.

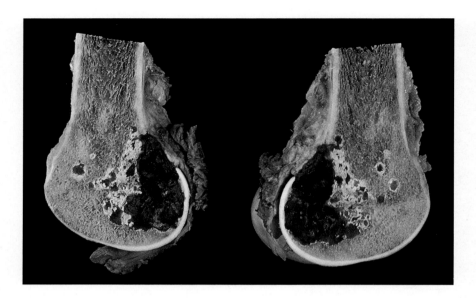

Fig. 23-64. High grade angiosarcoma. The distal femur shows a large epiphyseal-metaphyseal hemorrhagic mass focally destroying the cortex. Note satellite nodules.

of these modalities. Occasional survivors who have been treated by irradiation only have been reported.[1-4]

Hemangiopericytoma

Hemangiopericytoma is an extremely rare lesion of the skeleton that accounts for 0.1 percent of all primary malignant bone tumors. The age at presentation ranges from 10 to 80 years, with a peak incidence in the fourth and fifth decades of life; hemangiopericytoma affects both sexes equally.[2]

Histologically, hemangiopericytoma presents the same pattern in bone as it does in the soft tissues.[2,233] A grading system has been applied to these lesions. Grade 1 lesions show bland nuclear features and less than 1 mitosis/10 hpf. Grade 2 lesions show more nuclear atypism and from 1 to 5 mitoses/10 hpf. Grade 3 lesions have definite nuclear anaplasia and more than 6 mitoses/10 hpf. Although lesions of all grades have the potential to metastasize, metastases from grade 1 lesions are uncommon; they occur in 50 percent of grade 2 lesions and in 75 percent of grade 3 lesions.[2,234]

Cytopathology of Vascular Tumors

FNA of benign intraosseous vascular lesions is not recommended. In most cases, the diagnosis can be made or strongly suggested based on the clinical presentation and radiographic features. When surgical therapy is indicated, a preoperative pathologic diagnosis is not usually required.

Intraosseous malignant vascular tumors are exceedingly rare, and their diagnosis by FNA has only rarely been reported.[235,236] The cytologic features of these lesions resemble those of malignant vascular lesions arising in the soft tissue (see Ch. 18).

CONNECTIVE TISSUE LESIONS

Benign Fibrous Lesions

Metaphyseal Fibrous Defect/Nonossifying Fibroma

Nonossifying fibroma and its companion, fibrous cortical defect, are common bone lesions found in an estimated 50 per-

cent of children who have radiographs taken of their knees. Fibrous cortical defect has a predilection for the distal end of the femur, apparently arising in the periosteum. Radiologically, it causes what appears to be a scooped-out defect of the cortex.[5,237] Histologically, it is densely fibrous with evidence of considerable collagenization. Like nonossifying fibroma, it tends to involute. Nonossifying fibroma is intimately related

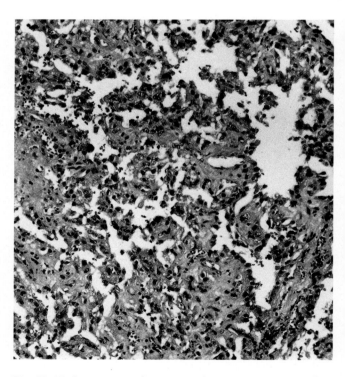

Fig. 23-65. Intricate vascular pattern of an angiosarcoma. Papillary structures lined by anaplastic endothelial cells are present.

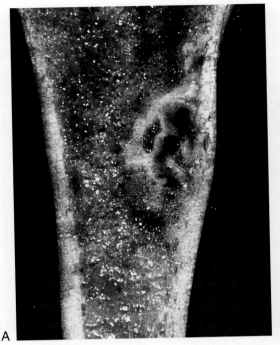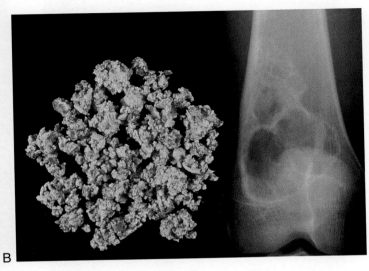

Fig. 23-66. **(A)** Nonossifying fibroma. The lobular pattern and sclerotized margins are identical to the radiologic picture. (Courtesy of S. Saltzstein, M.D., San Diego, CA.) **(B)** Combined specimen and radiograph of a nonossifying fibroma. The specimen curettage shows the yellow-brown appearance typical of a nonossifying fibroma. The color denotes the high lipid content of the cells of this lesion.

to fibrous cortical defect; the only difference, if any, is perhaps its larger size. Most patients are asymptomatic, and if symptoms appear, they usually follow those of a pathologic fracture. The most common sites are the metaphyses of the lower end of the femur and upper end of the tibia.[5] Distal ends of the tibia and fibula are also fairly common sites of occurrence.

Nonossifying fibroma is readily diagnosable from radiographs[1–4]; the lesion is well circumscribed, eccentric, and usually radiolucent. The margins are sclerotic and exhibit a lobular pattern. The cortex may be thin. As the lesion matures, it becomes increasingly sclerotic, as it has been demonstrated that the nonossifying fibroma heals by bony sclerosis.

Grossly, the lesion is usually seen as curettings, and these fragments of tissue vary from light brown to dark brown with yellow areas. Occasionally, an intact nonossifying fibroma is seen in conjunction with an amputation (Fig. 23-66A). These lesions correlate perfectly with radiologic findings (i.e., there is sclerosis of the margins of an eccentrically located metaphyseal lesion that on the cut surface is yellow-brown to brown) (Fig. 23-66B).

Histologically, the lesion has the pattern of a fibrous histiocytoma (i.e., the spindled stroma has a storiform pattern) (Fig. 23-67A). In contrast to a genuine giant cell tumor, the multinucleated giant cells, although present, are scattered and may be clustered. Hemosiderin and numerous foamy histiocytes are frequently identified (Fig. 23-67B). Specimens from patients in late adolescence or their early twenties may show evidence of bone

formation. In the immature and in those with nontraumatized nonossifying fibroma, bone and osteoid are not seen. Histologically, nonossifying fibroma and fibrous cortical defect are identical and are generally considered to be the same lesion, except that fibrous cortical defect is smaller and more likely to be confined to the cortex. Bosch et al[237] suggested that a histochemical difference existed between the two. Basically, the lesion is self-limiting, and a major reason for surgical intervention is danger of fracture in large lesions or lesions that continue to grow.[238,239]

Fibrous Histiocytoma and Atypical Fibrous Histiocytoma

When fibrous tumors that exhibit the same morphologic characteristics as nonossifying fibroma occur in a site different from the usual location for nonossifying fibroma, they are referred to as fibrous histiocytoma, including atypical fibrous histiocytoma.[240,241] The reason for a different terminology is that they do not involute with time and may recur. Wold[241] described the Mayo Clinic's experience with 38 cases of fibrous histiocytoma and atypical fibrous histiocytoma. The age distribution is wide, with a slight peak in the fourth decade of life, and the pelvis and femur are the two most common locations.

Radiologically, this lesion is found in the metaphyseal-epiphyseal area of a long bone and presents a radiolucent appearance. This lesion may have a peripheral sclerotic rim of dense bone tissue. Other cases are purely lytic and may be similar to the radiologic aspects of a giant cell tumor of bone. Morpho-

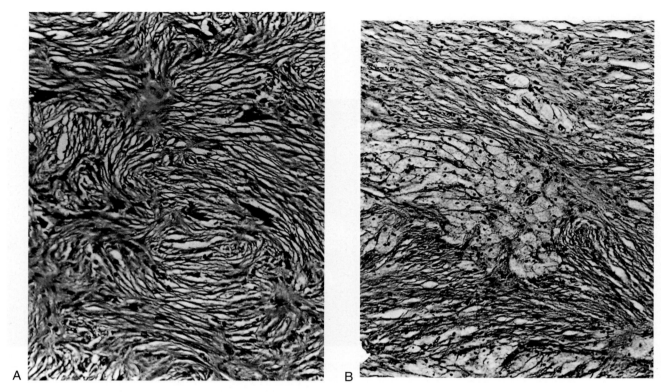

Fig. 23-67. Nonossifying fibroma. **(A)** Fibrous stroma with storiform pattern. **(B)** Note clusters of foamy histiocytes and scattered multinucleated cells.

logically, the lesion is not different from nonossifying fibroma. When some degree of nuclear atypia exists, as well as an increased number of mitoses, atypical fibrous histiocytoma has been diagnosed. Management should be conservative, with curettage and bone or possibly cement packing. Close follow-up is suggested because of possible recurrences.

Xanthoma/Fibroxanthoma

Xanthoma/fibroxanthoma is an extremely rare lesion; some authors deny its existence because they believe it is a degenerative change that replaces a pre-existing benign bone lesion. However, Bertoni et al[242] reported a pure fibroxanthoma that was not associated with any prior benign bone tumors. Histologically, this lesion contains a proliferation of histiocytic cells with marked xanthomatous change. Curettage should be curative. Partial xanthomatous change may be seen in several benign bone lesions, including giant cell tumor of bone, nonossifying fibroma, and fibrous dysplasia.[1-4]

Fibrous Lesions with Indeterminate/Intermediate Biologic Behavior

Desmoplastic Fibroma

Desmoplastic fibroma, an uncommon benign tumor of bone, is formed by fibrous tissue and collagen. It accounts for less than 0.1 percent of bone tumors, and most patients are younger than

40 years.[2,243] The mandible is the most common site of occurrence, followed by the metaphysis of the long bones (femur, tibia, and humerus).[2]

Radiologically, desmoplastic fibroma is radiolucent, and thus may be mistaken for a malignancy or for lesions such as aneurysmal bone cyst, solitary bone cyst, or chondromyxoid fibroma. Occasionally a pathologic fracture may occur through the tumor.

Grossly, desmoplastic fibroma shows the hard rubbery consistency of fibrous lesions, and its cut surface demonstrates white-tan discoloration, with prominent fibrous cords or bands traversing the tumor (Fig. 23-68).

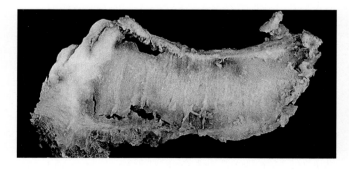

Fig. 23-68. Desmoplastic fibroma of pubic bone. There is fibrous replacement of the cancellous bone.

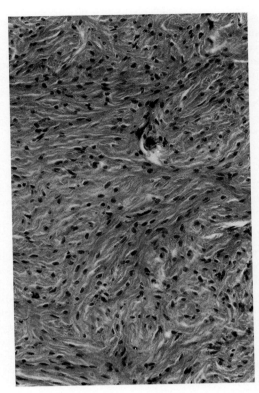

Fig. 23-69. Desmoplastic fibroma. The mature fibrous nature of the lesion can be seen.

Histologically, desmoplastic fibroma is similar to desmoid tumor of the soft tissue (Fig. 23-69). Ultrastructurally, myofibroblasts are common and are mixed with fibroblasts and primitive mesenchymal cells.[244] When the lesion occurs in the jaws, especially in children, it appears to be more aggressive than it is in the long bones, extending into the adjacent soft tissue and recurring multiple times.[245,246]

Management of desmoplastic fibroma is surgical. However, in lesions arising in the jaw bones, preoperative chemotherapy has given excellent tumor reduction results, allowing a conservative and less disfiguring surgical resection.[241]

The term periosteal desmoid, a synonym for fibrous cortical defect, is frequently used in radiologic jargon, but we discourage its use as a pathologic term because it may imply a true desmoid tumor of periosteal or soft tissue origin.

Malignant Tumors

Fibrosarcoma and Malignant Fibrous Histiocytoma

Fibrosarcoma is a rare primary malignant tumor of bone that apparently arises from fibrous elements and histologically resembles fibrosarcoma of the soft tissues[247–249] (Fig. 23-70). Much of what is known about fibrosarcoma comes from the older literature and possibly such information may no longer be valid. Since the recognition of malignant fibrous histiocytoma as an

entity that occurs in both soft tissue and bone, the diagnosis of fibrosarcoma has faded. In a study from the Mayo Clinic on malignant fibrous histiocytoma of bone, many of the tumors were obtained from the pool of tumors originally interpreted to be fibrosarcomas.[250] Therefore, it is reasonable to assume that most high grade spindle cell sarcomas that were previously interpreted to be fibrosarcomas are presently recognized as malignant fibrous histiocytomas. The term fibrosarcoma, however, is still useful for the well differentiated fibrous tumor that shows spindle cells with the typical herring-bone arrangement. Malignant fibrous histiocytoma, a common malignant tumor of soft tissue, also arises primarily in bone. Although recently described, it is not a new lesion but was formerly, as stated above, included among other tumors of bone such as fibrosarcomas and osteosarcomas.[250]

The lesion predominates in males and has a wide age range, with most patients being in the third decade of life and older.[250–252] Patients often have pain in the affected part and a slowly enlarging mass. Symptoms may have been present for a short period or for several months to 1 or 2 years. Pathologic fractures are apparently rare. Malignant fibrous histiocytoma has a wide skeletal distribution, but about 75 percent arise in the lower extremities and pelvis.[253] Occasionally malignant fibrous histiocytoma has been noted to occur in the jaws. This lesion may arise secondary to irradiation, infarcts of bone, and fibrous dysplasia.[253–256]

Radiologically, malignant fibrous histiocytoma is permeative and generally an osteolytic lesion.[251] Occasionally there may be dense mottling and slight sclerosis at the margin of the lesion

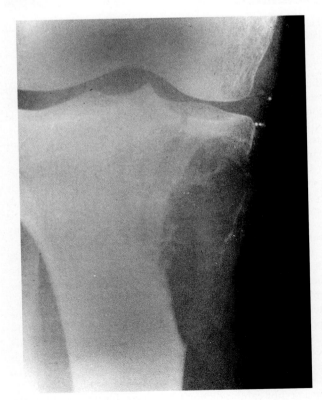

Fig. 23-70. Fibrosarcoma of the tibia. The inner margin is fairly distinct.

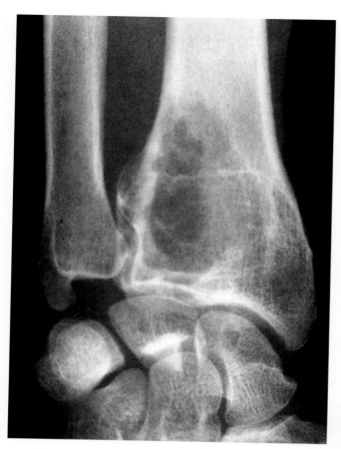

Fig. 23-71. Malignant fibrous histiocytoma of the distal radius, simulating a giant cell tumor.

broblastic or histiocytic derivations.[252] Malignant fibrous histiocytoma frequently metastasizes to other bones, to the lungs, and occasionally to the lymph nodes.[250]

Management of this lesion includes a combination of chemotherapy, surgery, and irradiation. Survival from treatment of malignant fibrous histiocytoma is somewhat variable, but as many as one-third of patients may survive beyond 5 years. Of the malignant fibrous histiocytoma variants, the angiomatoid may rarely occur in bone also.

Rare Connective Tissue Tumors

Other rare lesions of bone include chest wall mesenchymal hamartoma,[257] lipoma,[258] liposarcoma,[259] leiomyosarcoma,[260,261] and fibrocartilaginous mesenchymoma.[262,263]

Chest Wall Mesenchymal Hamartoma

Chest wall mesenchymal hamartoma presents dramatic clinical, radiologic, and pathologic findings.[257] It occurs in newborn babies, who present with severe respiratory symptoms or a palpable chest wall mass, or both. Radiologically, the chest wall exhibits a large mass arising in the ribs or chest wall and often involves more than one rib; it may opacify the hemithorax and may cause a shift of the mediastinum. Grossly, this lesion is well circumscribed and at times pseudoencapsulated; its cut surface shows multiple cystic cavities, solid areas, and occasionally visible bone and cartilage (Fig. 23-74A). Histologically, there is aneurysmal

(Fig. 23-71). There is destruction of the cortex, and periosteal reaction is frequent, although not always present. A soft tissue component may be identified. Radiologically, the features add up to those of a malignant disease, and the differential diagnosis would include osteosarcoma, fibrosarcoma, and malignant lymphoma.

Grossly, malignant fibrous histiocytoma is a fairly well circumscribed tumor because of its consistency and color (Fig. 23-72). It destroys the medullary portion of bone and often extends beyond the confines of the bone. The cut surfaces are yellow to gray-white and tan or brown, often with focal necrosis. Bony trabeculae may be identified in the tumor.

Histologically, malignant fibrous histiocytoma has features identical to those of the same neoplasm arising in the soft tissues (Fig. 23-73) (see also Ch. 18). The storiform pattern of the stroma is present, but not in all fields. Pleomorphism of the nuclei is common, and foamy cells may be present that have the appearance of Touton giant cells. Bizarre mitotic figures, clusters of foamy cells, and a sprinkling of inflammatory cells are frequent. Special stains are not helpful in the diagnosis of this lesion, but stains for lipids will be positive. Huvos et al[253] noted that different histologic variants of malignant fibrous histiocytoma do not exhibit different behaviors. Electron microscopic studies suggest a variety of origins for this lesion, including fi-

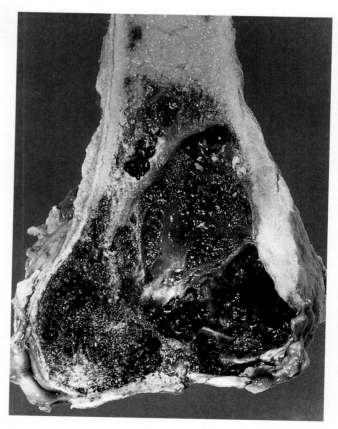

Fig. 23-72. Malignant fibrous histiocytoma of the distal femur. The tumor is partly cystic and hemorrhagic.

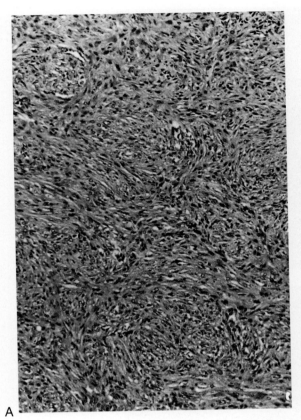
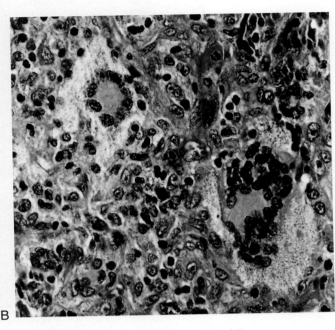

Fig. 23-73. Malignant fibrous histiocytoma. **(A)** Storiform fibroblastic pattern. **(B)** Histiocytes and Touton giant cells.

bone cyst formation, which accounts for the grossly visible cysts. The solid areas contain cartilaginous tissue in different stages of maturation (Fig. 23-74B): there may be mature hyaline cartilage tissue, immature cartilage, and areas resembling chondroblastoma, including the chicken-wire type of calcification. The presence of immature cartilage, including ossification, led some authors to consider this lesion a chondrosarcoma. Despite the alarming features, the lesion behaves in a benign fashion.[257] Management may be conservative if the lesion is asymptomatic, or surgical intervention may be required.

Lipoma, Liposarcoma, and Leiomyosarcoma

Lipoma manifests as a radiolucent defect of bone and is histologically identical to lipomas of the soft tissues.[258] The importance of this lesion lies mainly in the differential diagnosis from findings on radiographs in regard to radiolucent defects of bone. Liposarcoma[259] and leiomyosarcoma[260,261] manifest radiologically as malignant lesions without specific changes to suggest the underlying tumor. All these lesions are histologically identical to their counterparts in soft tissue.

Fibrocartilaginous Mesenchymoma

Fibrocartilaginous mesenchymoma is a rare tumor of bone that was described by Dahlin et al[262] in 1984. It occurs between the ages of 9 and 25 years and is slightly more common in females

than in males. The metaphysis of the long bones is the site of occurrence; the most commonly involved bone is the fibula, followed by the humerus and tibia.[263]

Radiologically, the lesion is radiolucent and abuts the metaphysis but may extend to the epiphysis in patients in whom the metaphysis is already closed. The cortex may be scalloped or may be destroyed, and focal calcifications may be seen. Histologically, three components are present: spindle cells, cartilage, and bone. The spindle cell component is made up of closely packed bundles of slender spindle cells that have rare or no mitoses. The characteristic feature of this lesion is the presence of islands of hyaline cartilage that resemble the physis. These cartilaginous islands are present throughout the lesion. The bone component is variable and in some areas resembles the bone formation of fibrous dysplasia.[262,263]

With curettage, recurrences are common, but metastatic disease has not been reported.[261,262]

Malignant Mesenchymoma

Malignant mesenchymoma requires the presence of two totally different sarcomas. This is a very rare type of sarcoma and one must be careful in making this diagnosis. For instance, dedifferentiated chondrosarcoma may contain a mixture of sarco-

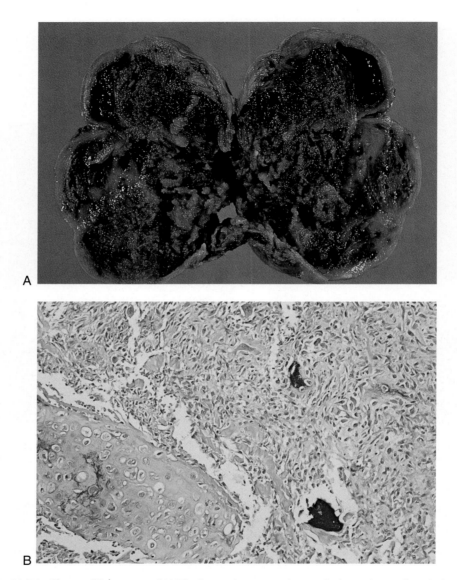

Fig. 23-74. Chest wall hamartoma. (A) This bisected specimen shows a thick pseudocapsule and a brown hemorrhagic appearance. (B) Histologically, there are components of cartilage, osteoid and bone, and giant cells.

mas, such as chondrosarcoma, osteosarcoma, malignant fibrous histiocytoma, and rhabdomyosarcoma, but these characteristics do not place the lesion in question in the malignant mesenchymoma category.

OTHER TUMORS

Chordoma

Chordoma, a lesion derived from the notochord, represents about 4 percent of the primary malignant bone tumors.[1] Males are affected more commonly than females and it is very rare in chil-

dren; the peak incidence is in the sixth decade of life.[1-4] The sacrococcygeal region accounts for 50 percent of cases, and the spheno-occipital region or base of the skull accounts for 37 percent of cases. The remainder of cases reported occur, in descending order of frequency, in the cervical, thoracic, and lumbar spine.[2]

The symptomatology depends on the site of involvement. Pain is a common complaint in sacrococcygeal lesions, and as the tumor grows additional symptoms related to compression and destruction of nerve roots, bone, and viscera develop. Elevated intracranial pressure or cranial nerve symptoms (or both) may develop in lesions in the base of the skull.

Radiologically, lesions at the base of the skull show a radio-

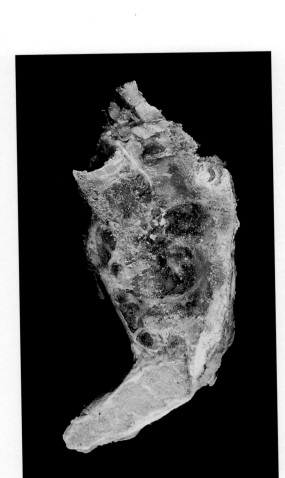

Fig. 23-75. Chordoma. This vertical section of the sacrum shows a large intra- and extraosseous mass that has a lobulated appearance. Note the myxoid characteristics of the lesion.

lucency usually situated in the clivus. In the sacrum the radiolucency may be difficult to visualize on plain films, but CT and MRI scans should demonstrate both the lesion and its extension. Although chordoma produces no matrix, one may find calcifications that represent residual destroyed bone tissue or dystrophic calcification.[264]

On gross examination of resected sacral chordomas, the tumors may be well circumscribed, but more often they are ill defined at the margins. The cut surface shows a gray-white sometimes glistening appearance with a slimy consistency because of the mucoid content (Fig. 23-75). Focal necrosis is usually evident.

Histologically, evidence of lobulation is revealed on low power examination. The chordoma cells are arranged in cords that form a trabecular arrangement but that may grow as solid sheets (Fig. 23-76). A myxoid background is nearly always present and when it is disposed around single or double cells may give the appearance of a myxoid cartilaginous tumor. The individual cells are large, sometimes polygonal and other times round, and contain abundant cytoplasm. Vacuolization is present and usually is multiple. When multiple vacuolization occurs in large cells, these have been termed physaliferous cells

because of the resemblance to jellyfish. Chordomas contain glycogen[265] and express cytokeratin, epithelial membrane antigen, vimentin, and S-100 protein.[266,267] Chordomas of the skull may contain hyaline cartilage, in which case they are referred as to chondroid chordomas.[268–271] Controversy exists about whether there is true cartilage or not.[264,269] This variant is slow growing and indolent.[269–271]

The management of chordomas is surgical. However, because of their location in the sacrum, spine, or skull, resection with wide margins is nearly impossible to conduct. Local recurrences and invasion of adjacent tissues are common; distant metastases usually develop late in the course of the disease.

The term *dedifferentiated chordoma* has been applied to chordomas when they develop a high grade spindle cell sarcoma component, usually malignant fibrous histiocytoma. This variant has a poor prognosis because distant metastases are likely to occur rapidly.[272–274]

Parachordoma

Parachordoma is a rare, slow-growing tumor that has potential for recurrence. It shares histologic features with chordoma and extraskeletal myxoid chondrosarcoma.[275,276] This tumor arises in soft tissues near or on the surface or cortex of a bone. Unlike chordoma, it has an indolent behavior.

Adamantinoma of Long Bones

Adamantinoma of the long bones is a rare lesion of the skeleton of unknown histogenesis.[277–279] The name derives from its histologic resemblance to adamantinoma of the jaw bones. Considerable discussion is found in the literature about its histogenesis; a vascular or epithelial origin is most prominently mentioned. Histologically, most of these tumors display areas with a vascular appearance and, in many, areas of epithelial differentiation. Ultrastructurally, support has been advanced for both histogenetic theories. Immunohistochemical studies confirm an epithelial component but do not add to the understanding of the histogenesis of adamantinoma.[280,281] Nevertheless, adamantinoma represents a distinct tumor of the skeleton.

The lesion occurs in young adults and is slightly more common in males than in females.[277–279] Clinical manifestations are not specific, but often a mass or slight discomfort is present over the lesion. Approximately 90 percent of adamantinomas occur in the tibia. Only occasionally have adamantinomas been reported in the femur and in the long bones of the upper extremity. Occasionally, multiple adamantinomas may occur in the same patient.

Radiologically, the lesion is fairly distinct, particularly if the tibia is involved. It presents with sharply outlined margins and signs of trabeculation that impart a lobulated or bubbly effect to the tumor. Multiple, small, lucent zones may be seen in the vicinity of a larger mass. Sclerosis of the cortex around the tumor is often present.[277]

Grossly, adamantinoma is well circumscribed with adjacent bony sclerosis. The cut surfaces are often shiny gray-white (Fig. 23-77). Multiple separate foci of gray-white tissue may be seen or, in some lesions, broad areas of fibrous tissue, which correspond histologically to sites that resemble fibrous dysplasia.

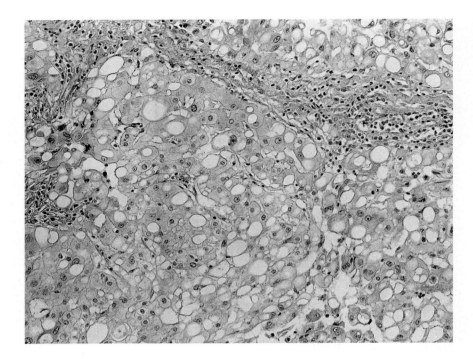

Fig. 23-76. Chordoma. Microscopically there are large cells with abundant cytoplasmic vacuolization.

Histologically, adamantinomas exhibit a variable pattern.[277,278] Strands of small dark cells may be embedded in fibrous tissue, spaces may resemble blood vessels (Fig. 23-78A), and other sites may have an epithelial appearance (Fig. 23-78B). Keratin expression is found in the epithelial cells of adamantinoma.[282] In fact, the epithelial areas occasionally show evidence of keratinization. In some of the epithelial areas, there is reticulation of the cells, which imparts an appearance similar to that of adamantinoma of the jaws. Campanacci et al[283] classified the histologic patterns into four types: spindle, basaloid, squamous, and trabecular. Apparently these have no prognostic implications but do help to simplify diagnostic difficulties. In some areas, the epithelial components and those that appear to be vascular may be large enough to present as small cysts. The stroma between the more cellular elements is fibrous and has no malignant features. On occasion, the stroma may predominate, giving a fibrous dysplasia-like appearance.

The term *differentiated (regressing) adamantinoma* has been used to describe tibial lesions that would otherwise be classified as osteofibrous dysplasia of Campanacci.[284] These lesions show a fibro-osseous proliferation identical to, if not the same as, osteofibrous dysplasia of Campanacci, but some of the spindle cells react to the cytokeratin antibody. The authors believe that this lesion is a form of regressing adamantinoma. Of the cases reported, none has shown progression to typical adamantinoma, and some authors believe that these lesions should be considered osteofibrous dysplasia.[285]

Histologically, a prominent differential diagnostic problem with adamantinoma is metastatic carcinoma, most commonly metastatic squamous or transitional cell carcinoma. In addition, primary angiosarcoma must be ruled out. Attention to the variety of patterns frequently present in the adamantinoma will help solve the histologic dilemma. If the radiograms are studied in concert with the histologic features, the proper diagnosis can usually be made.

Adamantinomas are malignant, even though they have a slow evolution. The management of choice is en bloc excision of the lesion, but extensive lesions may necessitate an amputation. Patients may survive for a number of years with adamantinoma, even though it is recurrent. Metastasis to the lung occurs, usually many years after the initial surgery. In a series of 85 patients reported by Keeney et al,[286] the average time that elapsed from resection of the primary tumor to metastatic disease to the lung was 8.2 years.

Neurogenic Tumors

Schwannoma (neurilemoma) arises from the nerve sheath and is rarely primary in bone. Radiologically, it is a radiolucent area that has benign but not distinctive characteristics. Most intraosseous Schwannomas have occurred in the mandible, with others in the femur, humerus, small bones of the hand, scapula, sacrum, and maxilla.[1] Grossly, the few that have been removed intact show features similar to those of the same neoplasm occurring in soft tissue (i.e., cystic degeneration of a well defined, gray-white to gray-yellow nodule). Histologically, the lesion is also identical to schwannoma in the soft tissues. Treatment of these lesions is curettage or en bloc excision, where feasible.

Among the patients with *neurofibromatosis* are many who have skeletal involvement and deformities. One of the common skeletal deformities is kyphoscoliosis, which occurs in 10 to 41 percent of patients with neurofibromatosis.[287] Any part of

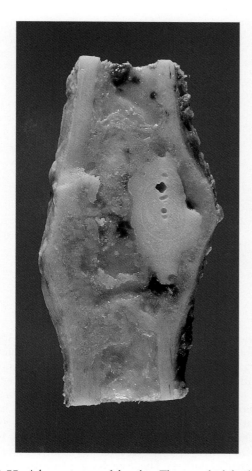

Fig. 23-77. Adamantinoma of the tibia. This is a tibial diaphysis exhibiting a white-tan tumor involving the medullary cavity and breaking through the cortex. A cement plug is present at the site of the previous biopsy site.

the vertebral column may be involved, with the thoracic spine being the most common site. Other bony lesions include localized overgrowth (a form of focal giantism that may involve any part of the skeleton), bowing deformity of the long bones, pseudoarthrosis, and erosive lesions resulting from neurofibroma.[288] The latter often have sclerotic zones on radiographs and may appear as grooves or subperiosteal blisters. Neurofibromas are not necessarily seen in the lesions described above. Several, such as kyphoscoliosis, are considered to be dysplastic change of bone related to neurofibromatosis.

A rare neurogenic lesion is *ganglioneuroma*, which presents as a radiolucent defect in bone. Histologically, the lesion has features identical to ganglioneuroma occurring in extraosseous sites[289] (see Ch. 59).

Cytopathology of Connective Tissue Lesions

Benign Fibrous Lesions

Metaphyseal Fibrous Defect/Nonossifying Fibroma
Due to its virtually diagnostic radiographic appearance and tendency to involute, nonossifying fibroma is rarely aspirated. When surgical intervention is indicated, usually due to impending fracture or atypical clinical or radiographic features, FNA may be used to confirm the diagnosis preoperatively. Aspirates vary from paucicellular to moderately cellular and are composed of variable numbers of bland spindle cells, multinucleated giant cells, foamy histiocytes, and hemosiderin-laden macrophages. Cells are arrayed in cohesive sheets and clusters and as individually dispersed elements. In some fragments, the spindle cells may have a recognizable storiform pattern. The cytologic features of nonossifying fibroma overlap considerably with those of aneurysmal bone cyst, giant cell reparative granuloma, and, to a lesser extent, giant cell tumor of bone.[290] In

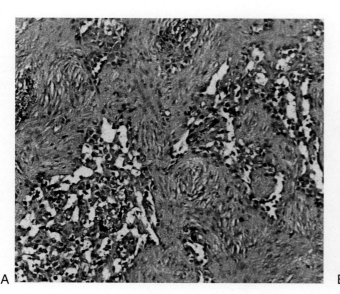

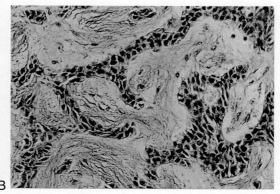

Fig. 23-78. **(A)** Adamantinoma with a vascular appearance. **(B)** Adamantinoma exhibiting an epithelial appearance.

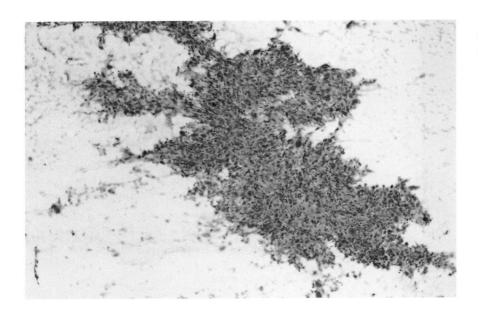

Fig. 23-79. Malignant fibrous histiocytoma of bone. A Papanicolaou-stained preparation shows an irregular aggregate of pleomorphic spindle cells arrayed in a vaguely storiform pattern.

the presence of atypical radiographic features, it may be difficult or impossible to render a specific cytologic diagnosis, although the benign nature of the lesion is usually readily apparent. Both microscopic and overt pathologic fractures may occur in nonossifying fibromas. Unless the cytologic findings are correlated with clinical and radiographic data, the presence of early fracture callus in an aspirate may lead to a false positive diagnosis of sarcoma.

Malignant Tumors

Fibrosarcoma and Malignant Fibrous Histiocytoma

The cytologic features of intraosseous fibrosarcoma and malignant fibrous histiocytoma are essentially identical to those of their counterparts arising in the soft tissues (see Ch. 18). The

cytologic appearance is variable, reflecting the broad spectrum of differentiation observed in these lesions.[291–293] Aspirates are variably cellular, depending on the amount of collagenous matrix, with cells arrayed singly and in irregular sheets and clusters. In low grade fibrosarcoma, smears are composed of spindle cells with oval to elongate nuclei, finely to coarsely granular chromatin, and one or more, often irregular nucleoli. Nuclear enlargement, pleomorphism, and hyperchromasia may be minimal. Mitotic figures, including abnormal forms, are present but may be few in number. The distinction between low grade fibrosarcoma and benign fibrous lesions may be difficult or impossible solely on cytologic grounds. By contrast, the malignant nature of high grade fibrosarcoma and malignant fibrous histiocytoma is readily apparent. Smears are highly cellular and contain obviously malignant spindle cells with marked nuclear

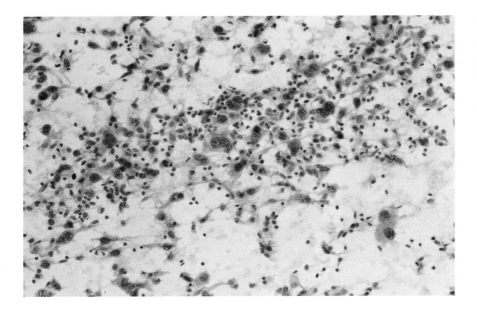

Fig. 23-80. Malignant fibrous histiocytoma of bone. In this Papanicolaou-stained preparation, bizarre tumor cells as well as smaller malignant spindle cells are arrayed in loosely cohesive clusters and singly.

pleomorphism and hyperchromasia (Fig. 23-79). Mitoses, including abnormal forms, are often abundant. In malignant fibrous histiocytoma, variable numbers of histiocytoid cells, multinucleated cells, and bizarre tumor giant cells are also present (Fig. 23-80). A storiform pattern may be apparent in some of the tissue fragments. As discussed in a previous section, malignant fibrous histiocytoma may be difficult or impossible to differentiate from high grade osteosarcoma.

Other Tumors

Chordoma

FNA of chordoma yields cellular smears in which cells are arranged singly and in small clusters. Cells are large, with abundant bubbly cytoplasm, distinct cytoplasmic borders, and one or two large, round nuclei with evenly dispersed chromatin and round nuclei.[294–296] Smaller, epithelioid cells may also be present. The background contains abundant, intensely metachromatic, myxoid matrix that forms a delicate network surrounding individual cells. Cytologically, chordoma may be difficult to distinguish from myxoid chondrosarcoma. In the latter, cells are typically smaller, and the delicate pattern of interlacing matrix is absent. Immunocytochemistry may help to distinguish these entities: both tumors express S-100 protein, but, in contradistinction to chondrosarcoma, chordoma is immunoreactive for cytokeratin and epithelial membrane antigen. When only wet-fixed, Papanicolaou-stained smears are available, the matrix may be not be appreciated, and the possibility of a metastatic clear cell carcinoma may be entertained.

Adamantinoma

FNA of adamantinoma yields moderately to highly cellular smears with cells arrayed singly and in sheets and clusters. The cellular composition may be triphasic, biphasic, or monomorphous.[297–299] The three types of cells include (1) small, round cells with indistinct cytoplasm, hyperchromatic nuclei, and absent or inconspicuous nucleoli (basaloid cells); (2) polygonal cells with large round nuclei, vesicular chromatin, and one or more prominent nucleoli; and (3) spindle cells with scant cytoplasm, oval nuclei, finely dispersed chromatin, and micronucleoli. Clusters of basaloid cells may show peripheral pallisading. Mitotic figures may be scarce or frequent. Necrosis is absent. The cytologic differential diagnosis includes metastatic carcinoma and epithelioid hemangioendothelioma. The latter may be distinguished from adamantinoma using immunocytochemical stains: epithelioid hemangioendothelioma is immunoreactive for factor VIII-related antigen, CD31, and Ulex europaeus agglutinin, but negative for cytokeratin, whereas the opposite pattern of reactivity is seen in adamantinoma. Differentiation between adamantinoma and metastatic carcinoma requires clinical, radiographic, and/or histologic information, as immunocytochemistry is not helpful for distinguishing these entities.

Neurogenic Tumors

To our knowledge, FNA of neurogenic tumors arising in bone has not been reported. Nonetheless, it seems reasonable to assume that, if an intraosseous neurogenic tumor were to be encountered in an FNA, the cytologic features would resemble those of its counterpart arising in soft tissues (see Chs. 18 and 59).

TUMOR-LIKE LESIONS

Solitary Bone Cyst

A solitary bone cyst is a benign, often unicameral, fluid-containing lesion of unknown etiology. Approximately three-fourths are located in the upper end of the humerus or the upper end of the femur and frequently lie near to or abut the epiphyseal plate. Solitary bone cyst is seen most commonly in children and adolescents but may occur in people as old as 72 years. A male predominance is seen, with the male/female ratio being approximately 3:1.[5] Clinically, solitary bone cysts are often asymptomatic, being diagnosed only as a result of a pathologic fracture. Uncommonly, patients have pain or swelling caused by the lesion. Solitary bone cysts involving flat bones are usually asymptomatic.

Radiologically, solitary bone cysts are radiolucent and, unless complicated by fracture or previous treatment, do not deform the contours of the bone. Characteristically, in a young person, the lesion is cone shaped and abuts the epiphyseal growth plate (Fig. 23-81). The cortex is attenuated although intact. The cyst may appear to be loculated because of bony trabeculation of the wall. The boundaries of the lesion are often fairly distinct because they are slightly sclerotized. The cysts that abut the

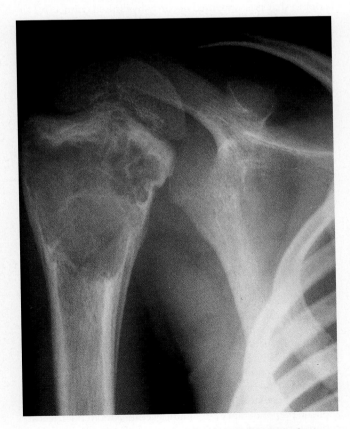

Fig. 23-81. Simple cyst of the upper end of the humerus of a 4-year-old boy. The cyst abuts on the epiphyseal growth plate. Mature periosteal reaction is seen on the medial humeral surface reflecting previous trauma.

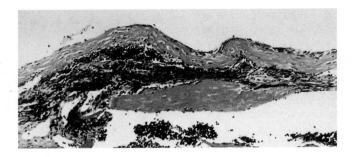

Fig. 23-82. Solitary bone cyst. Lining consists of a collagenous membrane.

growth plate are known as active cysts, and those that have "grown" away are inactive cysts.

Grossly, the contents shine through a thin cortex and impart a blue discoloration. The fluid in an uncomplicated cyst is clear yellow and sometimes blood tinged. It may be bloody if fracture has occurred previously. Examination of fluid indicates that it is similar to serum. The solitary bone cysts are usually composed of one compartment with bony trabeculation. The lining membrane may be thickened.

Histologically, the lining membrane is somewhat nondescript in that it is composed of partly hyalinized connective tissue (Fig. 23–82). Evidence of osteoid formation and vascular proliferation may be present. A cementum-like bony formation has been described in some of these lesions.[300] In lesions complicated by trauma, areas of inflammation and multinucleated giant cells as well as evidence of fracture repair may be seen. Because of the latter, the curettings from a cyst may be mistaken for fibrous dysplasia or giant cell tumor. Therefore, review of the radiographs by the pathologist is important.

The current management for solitary bone cysts is the instillation of steroids (methylprednisolone acetate) into the cystic cavity.[301,302] The healing rate is about 70 percent in contrast with the 53 percent healing rate after curettage.[303]

Aneurysmal Bone Cyst

Aneurysmal bone cyst is a benign expansile lesion of bone. Its pathogenesis is somewhat controversial, but it may arise de novo or may be secondary to a pre-existing benign lesion such as chondroblastoma, fibrous dysplasia, or giant cell tumor.[1,5] Some question has always existed on whether aneurysmal bone cyst represents a neoplasm or a reaction to injury. The importance of aneurysmal bone cyst lies in the fact that it occurs in the metaphysis of the long bones in patients younger than 20 years, paralleling the site and clinical presentation of conventional osteosarcoma.

Aneurysmal bone cyst may occur at any age but is most common in the pediatric and adolescent age groups, seemingly with a female preponderance.[1,304] Pain, swelling, and tenderness are common signs and symptoms. Because many of the lesions are located near the distal end of the femur and the proximal end of the tibia, limitation of motion of the nearby joint may be associated. A number of aneurysmal bone cysts may involve the vertebrae, particularly the posterior elements; in their expansion, they may impinge on nerves, causing pain and paresthesias.

Radiologically, aneurysmal bone cyst is an expansile lesion that in long bones is often eccentric (Fig. 23-83). However, it may be widely destructive and may simulate a malignant tumor, particularly osteosarcoma. Many aneurysmal bone cysts have a bubbly appearance on radiographs that correlates with the multicystic features seen grossly. Some aneurysmal bone cysts are centrally located and do not cause the typical blow-out pattern seen on radiographs. Those located near the end of long bones may be mistaken for osteosarcomas. The long bones of the limbs (distal end of femur and proximal tibia) are the most common sites. Approximately 10 percent of aneurysmal bone cysts involve the vertebral column; a few involve the flat bones.[1,5,304,305]

The gross features of intact specimens are those of a spongy, bloody, somewhat lobulated mass (Fig. 23-84). The cortex is often attenuated or destroyed. On the outer surfaces, the periosteum is intact and thickened. The cut surfaces are dark red to brown, with multiple cystic spaces of varied sizes containing

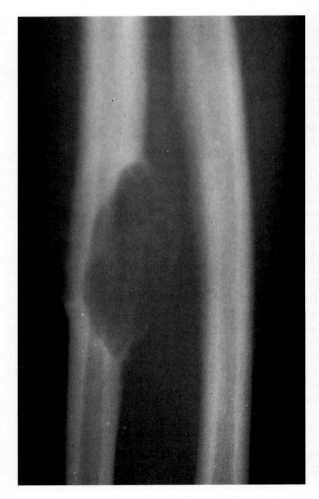

Fig. 23-83. Aneurysmal bone cyst in a 20-year-old woman. Eccentric, expansile, lucent lesion of the midshaft of the ulna. The borders are well defined.

blood and clotted blood. In some lesions, solid fibrous areas may be seen.

Histologically, aneurysmal bone cysts are composed of blood-filled spaces with walls formed by fibrous tissue and, in many instances, osteoid and bone (Fig. 23-85A). In some areas, the walls of the blood spaces may be lined by multinucleated giant cells (Fig. 23-85B), but there is no evidence of an endothelial lining. Some aneurysmal bone cysts may be almost totally composed of a solid component, an observation that has given origin to the term *solid aneurysmal bone cyst*[306,307]; in the past the solid aneurysmal bone cyst was classified under giant cell reparative granuloma. In some of the cellular areas, the stroma may be spindled and may raise the possibility of a malignant neoplasm; in other areas, multinucleated giant cells may be abundant, raising the consideration of a giant cell tumor. Osteoid formation suggests osteosarcoma (Fig. 23-85C). To rule out other lesions, as mentioned earlier, one must pay careful attention to the radiologic features, and numerous blocks of the lesion should be taken to determine whether the aneurysmal bone cyst is actually part of a giant cell tumor or whether, for example, one is examining an aneurysmal component of malignant fibrous histiocytoma or osteosarcoma. In the case of either of the latter two lesions, the stroma should have histologically malignant characteristics, and in the case of an osteosarcoma, histologically malignant osteoid and bone should be identifiable.

FNA characteristically yields bloody, paucicellular smears. Cellular elements include variable numbers of osteoclast-like giant cells, as well as benign spindle cells consistent with fibroblasts and myofibroblasts[290] (Fig. 23-86). In some cases, osteoblasts and osteoid are also noted. Mitotic figures may be present in the spindle cells, particularly in rapidly growing lesions, but abnormal forms are absent. The cytologic differential diagnosis includes giant cell tumor, chondroblastoma, brown tumor of hyperparathyroidism, and possibly osteosarcoma. In contrast to aneurysmal bone cysts, osteosarcomas usually yield cellular smears and contain frankly malignant spindle cells. Similarly, aspirates from chondroblastomas are usually cellular and contain numerous chondroblasts with longitudinal nuclear grooves that are not present in aneurysmal bone cysts. Distinction among aneurysmal bone cyst, giant cell tumor, and brown tumor may be difficult or impossible solely on cytologic grounds, although the benign nature of the lesion is usually apparent.

Surgical removal of the aneurysmal bone cyst by curettage and bone packing is the management of choice, but en bloc resection may be done in expendable bones such as the fibula. Recurrence, particularly with curettage, has been reported in as many as one-third of patients.[364,365]

Intraosseous Ganglion

Intraosseous ganglion is a cystic benign lesion of bone that radiologically is well defined and osteolytic. The lesion should be considered as a possibility for any well defined radiolucent lesion seen near a joint. Most of the patients are adolescents or adults, with an almost equal number being male and female. Intraosseous ganglion is most commonly seen at the ends of long tubular bones, but it has been described in flat and small bones and in a periosteal location.[308]

Grossly, the lesions have characteristics similar to those of ganglion of the soft tissues. They have a fibrous wall and contain a thick viscous fluid. Histologically, the wall is fibrous, with evidence of collagenization. Only occasionally may synovial tissue be identified. The lining may be similar to that of a solitary bone cyst, but the fluid is viscid rather than watery as in solitary cysts. Because intraosseous ganglion occurs at distal ends of long bones, a chondroblastoma may be considered in the radiologic differential diagnosis. Those that are metaphyseal and eccentric raise the possibility of nonossifying fibroma, chondromyxoid fibroma, or aneurysmal bone cyst.[309] Cysts associated with degenerative joint disease are similar in histology to ganglion cysts, but they are associated with changes on the

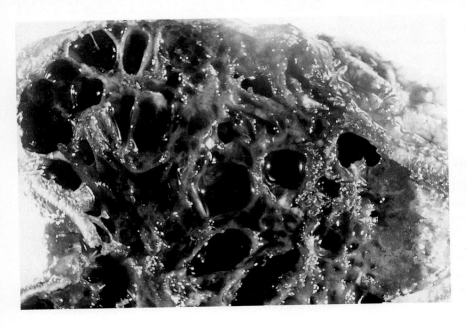

Fig. 23-84. Multicystic hemorrhagic cut surface of an aneurysmal bone cyst.

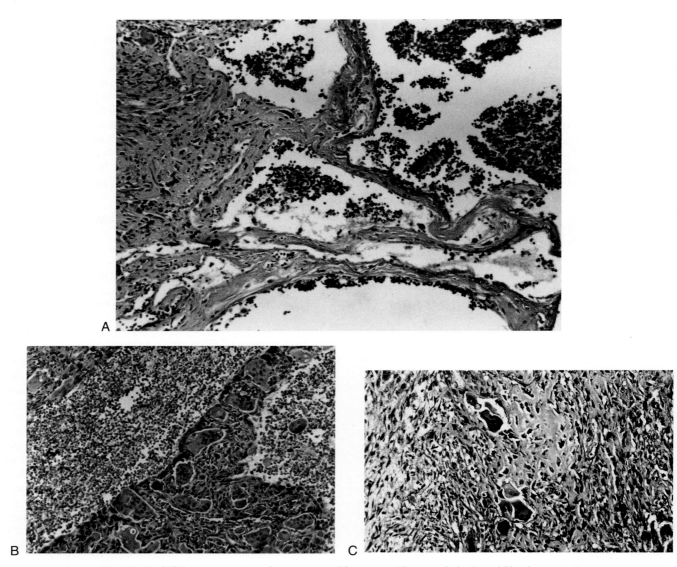

Fig. 23-85. **(A)** Low power view of an aneurysmal bone cyst. The irregularly shaped blood spaces are formed by fibrous tissue and osteoid. **(B)** Aneurysmal bone cyst. Blood spaces are partly lined by multinucleated cells. The trabeculae are formed by a cellular stroma in which many multinucleate cells are seen. **(C)** Osteoid and multinucleate cells in a solid area of an aneurysmal bone cyst.

articular surface, and a communication between the surface and the underlying cyst is invariably present.

Eosinophilic Granuloma

Eosinophilic granuloma of bone is the solitary form of Langerhans cell histiocytosis, formerly known as histiocytosis X.[310] Letterer-Siwe disease, the acute form, and Hand-Schüller-Christian disease, the chronic form, are not discussed here, but all three have as a common denominator the presence of the Langerhans histiocyte. Langerhans cell histiocytosis has been considered a non-neoplastic process, but clonality of the cells has been recently demonstrated, strongly supporting a neoplastic origin.[311,312]

Eosinophilic granuloma is a benign solitary or multicentric lesion that affects children and young adults and is slightly more common in females than in males.[2–4] About 50 percent of cases occur in the first decade of life, but rare cases may occur in the fourth decade. In a recent review of Langerhans cell histiocytosis of bone by Kilpatrick et al[313] (including cases with solitary, multiple bone, and extraosseous involvement), children under 17 years of age disclosed an age range of 2 months to 16 years, with a mean of 6.4 years and a median of 5 years. For adults the age range was from 17 years to 71 years, with a mean of 34 years and a median of 32 years. In this study the skull was the most commonly involved bone, followed by the femur, jaw, pelvis, and spine in children and the skull, ribs, jaw, femur, and pelvis in adults.[313] The usual symptom is pain in the

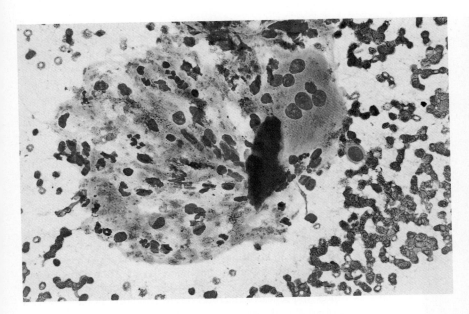

Fig. 23-86. Aneurysmal bone cyst. This air-dried, Romanowsky-stained preparation is composed of occasional spindle cells, inflammatory cells, and giant cells in a bloody background. A fragment of reactive bone was also present.

affected region, but limping may be the initial complaint if the lesion is located in the lower extremity. Localized swelling is another symptom.

Radiologically, eosinophilic granuloma demonstrates a lytic lesion in the medullary cavity of the bone or in the cortex; a periosteal reaction that may be laminated is commonly found. This picture is similar to that produced by small cell neoplasms, especially Ewing's sarcoma and malignant lymphoma. MRI findings are nonspecific and may also simulate malignancy.[314]

Histologically, eosinophilic granuloma consists of a proliferation of Langerhans histiocytes admixed with a variable eosinophilic and chronic inflammatory cell infiltrate. The histiocytes are positive for S-100 protein and for peanut agglutinin and ultrastructurally contain Birbeck granules. These rod-shaped granules contain a central stria similar to a zipper and have a tennis-racket-shaped end.

Eosinophilic granuloma yields moderately to highly cellular smears containing a polymorphous population of individually dispersed cells, including Langerhans histiocytes, eosinophils, osteoclast-like giant cells, lymphocytes, and plasma cells[315,316] (Fig. 23-87A). The Langerhans cells have abundant cytoplasm and eccentric, oval to reniform nuclei with pale, evenly dispersed chromatin and inconspicuous nuclei[317] (Fig. 23-87B). Nuclear folds or grooves are characteristic and help to distinguish these cells from ordinary macrophages. Definitive diagnosis usually requires ancillary studies, including immunocytochemistry or electron microscopy (or both), to confirm the identity of the Langerhans histiocytes.[315] In contrast to ordi-

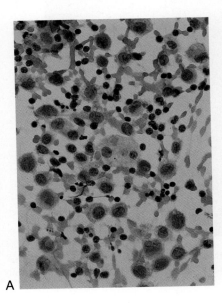
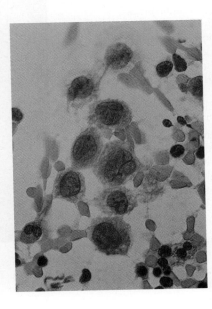

A   B

Fig. 23-87. Eosinophilic granuloma. (A) This highly cellular smear contains a polymorphous population of Langerhans histiocytes, eosinophils, lymphocytes, plasma cells, and osteoclast-like giant cells. (B) Langerhans histiocytes have abundant cytoplasm and oval to reniform nuclei with a characteristic nuclear groove that distinguishes them from ordinary macrophages. (Courtesy of Terri Johnson, M.D., Henry Ford Hospital, Detroit, MI.)

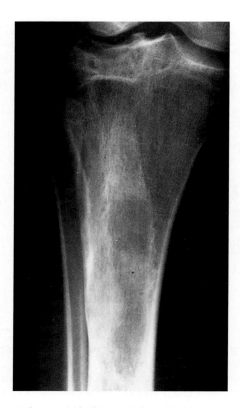

Fig. 23-88. Admixture of sclerotic and lucent areas in tibial fibrous dysplasia. The boundaries of the lesion are vague. There is little deformity of the tibia.

nary macrophages, Langerhans histiocytes are immunoreactive for S-100 protein and negative for lysozyme, alpha-1-antitrypsin, and CD68.

The usual clinicoradiologic differential diagnosis includes small cell tumor and osteomyelitis. Histologically and cytologically, the main differential diagnosis is with acute and chronic osteomyelitis. Both of these lesions may contain the same types of cells, but osteomyelitis shows polymorphonuclear leukocytes, which are rarely seen in eosinophilic granuloma. The presence of numerous plasma cells would also favor a diagnosis of osteomyelitis. In difficult cases, staining with S-100 protein may help to solve the problem.

The current treatment for eosinophilic granuloma is the instillation of methylprednisolone in the lesion.[316,318] Curettage and radiation are other options for its management.[313,318]

Kilpatrick et al[313] concluded that the prognosis of patients with osseous involvement alone was excellent. Ninety-five percent were disease free (162 of 171 patients), and no patient died of isolated skeletal disease. The management of these patients *did not* include intralesional injection of methylprednisolone.

Fibro-osseous Lesions

Two fibro-osseous lesions affect the skeleton: fibrous dysplasia and osteofibrous dysplasia of Campanacci.[319,320] In the discussion of fibrous dysplasia, we also include lesions that have been variously named ossifying fibroma, cemento-ossifying fi-

broma, and psammomatoid ossifying fibroma, which commonly affects the jaw bones. The above terminology is rife with confusion, as a lesion of the tibia and fibula, now known as osteofibrous dysplasia of Campanacci,[320,321] has also been termed ossifying fibroma.[322]

Fibrous Dysplasia

Fibrous dysplasia is a benign fibro-osseous lesion of bone that may be monostotic or polyostotic. About one-third of patients will have polyostotic involvement.[1-4] Polyostotic fibrous dysplasia is more likely to be symptomatic and to present with bone pain or bone deformities. It is much more common in females than in males; girls may present with precocious menarche. The triad of polyostotic dysplasia (typically unilateral), skin discoloration (café-au-lait spots), and endocrine dysfunction (precocious puberty) constitutes Albright's syndrome. Other manifestations such as hyperthyroidism, hypophosphatemia, and hearing loss may occur.[323] The monostotic form is usually asymptomatic, coming to the attention of the patient because of the presence of a mass or pathologic fracture. Fractures and repeated fractures occur frequently in patients with polyostotic disease. The lesion may involve almost any bone, with the skull, ribs, femur, and tibia being common sites.[319] The polyostotic form is more likely to be associated with focal skin pigmentation than is monostotic fibrous dysplasia.

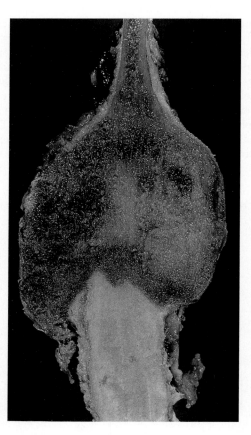

Fig. 23-89. Hemisection of fibrous dysplasia of a rib at the costochondral junction. The rib is enlarged, and the lesion gives the impression of grittiness.

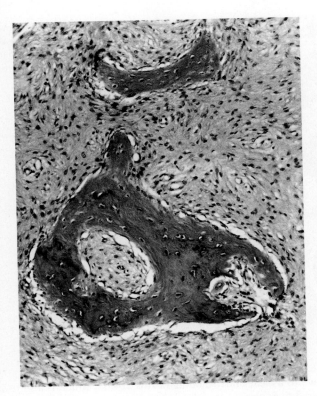

Fig. 23-90. Fibrous dysplasia. Oddly shaped bony trabeculae are evident.

Radiologically, fibrous dysplasia exhibits a variety of alterations[324] (Fig. 23-88). Typically, it is a fairly well circumscribed lesion that expands a bone. The lesion is faintly osteosclerotic, imparting the so-called ground-glass appearance. Some may appear cystic. At times, the lesion may be dominated by osteosclerosis, and in patients with polyostotic fibrous dysplasia, bony deformities are fairly frequent and may be severe (shepherd's crook deformity).

Grossly, the cut surface imparts a gritty sensation to palpation (Fig. 23-89). The surfaces are gray-white to yellow-white to light brown. Occasionally, fibrous dysplasia exhibits microcysts or is mainly cystic. The margins are not clearly defined, with the lesion appearing to blend with the surrounding bone.[1]

Histologically, fibrous dysplasia is composed of bony trabeculae and a fibrous stroma, which mingle intimately. The bony trabeculae often form numerous bizarre shapes such as "O's" and "C's" (Fig. 23-90). The bone in most portions of the specimen will be woven or immature, readily demonstrable by polarized light. Osteoblasts around the bony trabeculae are not present unless a previous fracture has occurred. The stroma varies in cellularity and is fibrous. Quite commonly, the stroma has foci that resemble a fibrous histiocytoma. In some areas, vascularity may be prominent; occasionally, clusters of multinucleate giant cells are seen. A hyaline cartilage component has also been described that at times may predominate over the fibrous component.[325] Secondary aneurysmal bone cyst formation may also occur.[326]

FNA biopsy yields paucicellular smears composed of bland spindle cells arrayed in irregular, cohesive fragments and singly. The spindle cells have scant, indistinct cytoplasm and oval or elongate nuclei with smooth contours, finely granular chromatin, and inconspicuous nucleoli. Mitotic figures are rare or absent. Short, curved fragments from trabeculae of osteoid or woven bone may also be present.[297]

Treatment of monostotic fibrous dysplasia is excision or curettage, depending on the location of the lesion. In most instances, this is successful, although recurrence may be observed after curettage. The recurrences usually maintain the histologic pattern of the original lesion. In polyostotic fibrous dysplasia, orthopedic correction may be required because of bony deformities, and some lesions may have to be resected because of symptoms caused by compression (i.e., large rib lesions compressing the lungs).

A rare complication of either polyostotic or monostotic fibrous dysplasia is transformation into a malignant tumor.[327,328] In a recent study from the Mayo Clinic, the authors found 28 cases of malignancy occurring in 1,122 patients who had fibrous dysplasia.[328] Nineteen occurred in patients with monostotic fibrous dysplasia and nine in cases of polyostotic disease. In order of frequency the histologic type were osteosarcoma in 19 cases, fibrosarcoma in 5, chondrosarcoma in 3, and malignant fibrous histiocytoma in 1. The craniofacial bones were commonly affected (13 cases), followed by the proximal femur (7 cases) and humerus, tibia, pelvis, tibia, and scapula (1 case each). The prognosis of these patients was reported to be poor.[328]

Cemento-ossifying fibroma, a lesion commonly seen in the paranasal sinuses, is also referred to as ossifying fibroma, cementifying fibroma, juvenile active ossifying fibroma, psammomatoid (juvenile) ossifying fibroma of the orbit, and aggressive psammomatoid ossifying fibroma of the sinonasal region.[329–332] This fibroma comprises a group of fibro-osseous lesions characterized by the presence of bone and fibrous stroma. Unlike fibrous dysplasia, the major bony component is in the form of small, round bone formations called ossicles, cementicles, or psammomatoid formations (Fig. 23-91), hence the different terms. These ossicles show no osteoblastic rimming and may be found admixed with larger bony trabeculae. The stroma also differs from the stroma of fibrous dysplasia in that it is more cellular; thus the background is made up of closely packed small spindle cells that may have rare mitoses.

Recent studies have demonstrated that this lesion represents one end of the spectrum of fibrous dysplasia. Sissons et al[333] and Voytek et al[334] have demonstrated that some cases of typical fibrous dysplasia may contain areas of cemento-ossifying fibroma and that some cases of typical cemento-ossifying fibroma may contain areas of fibrous dysplasia. Furthermore, these combined lesions have been seen in areas other than the paranasal sinuses.

Cemento-ossifying fibromas were previously thought to have a worse prognosis than fibrous dysplasia, but Voytek et al[334] found no difference in clinical behavior.

Osteofibrous Dysplasia

A fibro-osseous lesion of the long bones, formerly termed ossifying fibroma of the long bones[322] or intracortical fibrous dysplasia,[2] is now called osteofibrous dysplasia. Campanacci[320,321]

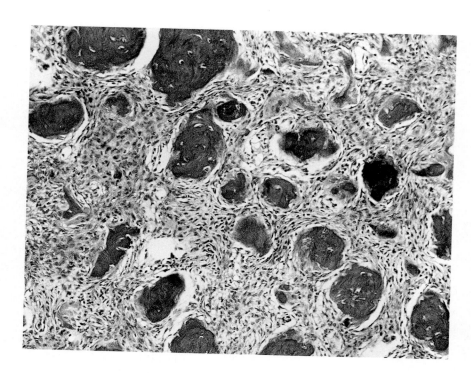

Fig. 23-91. Cemento-ossifying fibroma. In this lesion there are numerous small ossified areas (cementicles; ossicles) and a fibrous cellular stroma.

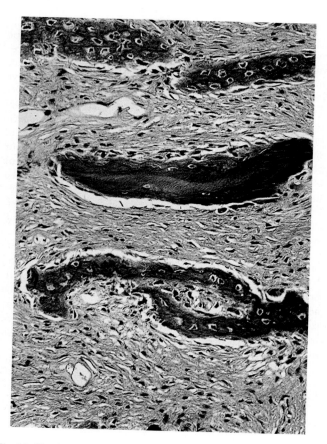

Fig. 23-92. Osteofibrous dysplasia. Note the fairly orderly orientation of bony trabeculae. The stroma is only moderately cellular, and osteoblasts are associated with the bony trabeculae.

gave us a clear understanding of this disease, which is also referred to as osteofibrous dysplasia of Campanacci. A disease of children aged 5 to 10 years, it progresses slowly to involution after skeletal maturity. It is slightly more common in boys than in girls, affecting the tibia predominantly and less commonly the fibula.

Radiographically the cortex of the shaft of the tibia demonstrates a single lucent area (sometimes multiple areas) surrounded by bony sclerosis. The anterior cortex of the tibia is the preferred site of involvement, and the medullary cavity is rarely involved. As the disease progresses, an anterior bowing of the tibia usually develops. Most specimens are the product of a curettage. The fragments have a tough fibrous-gritty consistency reflecting the bony and fibrous contents.

Microscopically the predominant finding is the presence of a fibrous and bony proliferation. The fibrous tissue is variably cellular and produces some fibers or bundles of collagen. The bone spicules show osteoid or bone both with and without osteoblastic activity (Fig. 23-92).

The differential diagnosis is with fibrous dysplasia and adamantinoma. Fibrous dysplasia is usually ruled out on a radiologic basis. Histologically these lesions are different in that osteofibrous dysplasia shows a combination of bony spicules with and without osteoblastic activity whereas fibrous dysplasia does not. Classic adamantinoma may have a significant fibrous component. As a general rule, adamantinoma occurs in older patients, and histologically the lesion should have definitive evidence of an epithelial component. As discussed in the section on adamantinoma, the cells of osteofibrous dysplasia may react to cytokeratin markers. When such a reaction to keratin is found, the lesion has been referred to as regressing adamantinoma.[284] In a recent report on such cases, no patients have developed classic adamantinoma.[285]

The management of this lesion is conservative as the lesion heals spontaneously. However, reconstructive procedures or fixing of fractures may have to be done. Patients who have undergone surgical procedures before puberty usually develop recurrences.

Localized Myositis Ossificans

Localized myositis ossificans (heterotopic bone and cartilage formation) is mentioned briefly because it enters into the differential diagnoses for extraskeletal osteosarcoma, parosteal osteosarcoma, periosteal osteosarcoma, and osteochondroma (see Ch. 22 for further discussion). Localized myositis ossificans may be localized entirely in the soft tissues, but when it is juxtacortical or periosteal, it raises questions in the differential diagnosis.[5] The lesion is not always associated with a known incident of trauma, but when it is and a series of films are available, its development and maturation are most helpful in ruling out malignant neoplasms. An osteosarcoma, for example, would not be expected to mature. A juxtacortical localized myositis ossificans may be quite difficult to distinguish on radiographs from parosteal osteosarcoma. The latter is usually lobulated, whereas localized myositis ossificans ordinarily has a smooth outline.

Histologically, the problems are evident by the names pseudomalignant and pseudosarcomatous that have been applied to localized myositis ossificans.[335,336] With a deep wedge or excisional biopsy of a developing lesion of localized myositis

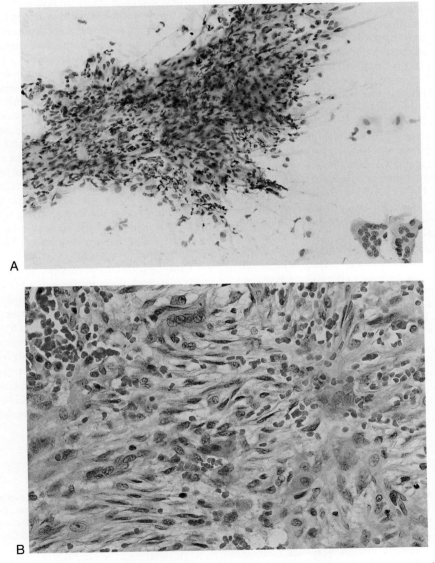

A

B

Fig. 23-93. Brown tumor of hyperparathyroidism. **(A)** This moderately cellular smear is composed of benign spindle cells with numerous osteoclast-like giant cells and hemosiderin pigment. **(B)** A section from the cell block demonstrates loose vibrovascular stroma with admixed giant cells, hemosiderin, and blood.

ossificans, it can be seen that the interior is highly proliferative and, taken in itself, appears to be malignant. However, toward the periphery of the lesion, maturation of bone and stroma is seen, which is most helpful in interpreting these reactive lesions. Because cartilage may be present, osteochondroma or chondrosarcoma have been mistakenly considered in the differential diagnosis. All in all, the zoning phenomenon—maturation from interior to periphery of the mass—is an important key to the correct diagnosis. Small biopsy specimens, however, are easily misinterpreted as being from some other lesion. As with skeletal neoplasms, radiologic studies are an integral part in the proper interpretation of localized myositis ossificans and the tumors that it simulates.[5]

Brown Tumor of Hyperparathyroidism

Two complications of hyperparathyroidism occur in bone: brown tumor, when a mass develops in a bone, and osteitis fibrosa cystica, when no mass is present.[1–5,337] A brown tumor may affect any bone and any part of a bone and usually presents a radiolucent aspect on plain radiographs. It may be solitary or multiple. Typical radiologic signs of hyperparathyroidism include subperiosteal resorption in the bones of the hands and generalized osteopenia. Rarely osteitis fibrosa cystica may simulate metastatic disease.[337]

Histologically a brown tumor displays a proliferation of osteoclastic type giant cells over a fibrous stroma rich in hemosiderin. From the histologic point of view, brown tumor may be difficult to distinguish from a giant cell tumor of bone. The differences, however, should be looked for in the site of presentation of the bone lesion. Giant cell tumor is a lesion that involves the epiphyseal-metaphyseal aspect of the bone and invariably reaches the subarticular cartilage. Typical radiologic changes in the hands also help to establish the diagnosis of hyperparathyroidism. The level of calcium in serum demonstrating hypercalcemia should give the clue to the correct diagnosis.

Brown tumor of hyperparathyroidism yields moderately cellular smears composed of benign spindle cells and osteoclastlike giant cells that occur singly or within irregular fragments of loose fibrous stroma[338,339] (Fig. 23-93). Hemosiderin is often abundant, and the background may be bloody. As discussed in previous sections, these lesions may be difficult or impossible to distinguish from giant cell tumor and aneurysmal bone cyst on cytologic grounds.

METASTATIC AND SECONDARILY INVASIVE TUMORS

In the differential diagnosis of bone neoplasms, secondary involvement should be given at least a passing thought, or prime consideration in certain situations. Benign or malignant extraosseous tumors may invade adjacent bone. Examples of benign lesions that may secondarily involve bone are nodular tenosynovitis, pigmented villonodular synovitis, glomus tumors, epidermal cysts, and fibromatoses. Soft tissue sarcomas may invade bone. In some of the lesions, such as pigmented vil-

lonodular synovitis, bony destruction seen on radiographs may be extensive enough to suggest malignancy. Many of the lesions, both benign and malignant, cause alterations that are at least suggestive of an extraosseous lesion. Radiologically, the bone is often saucerized, probably the result of long-continued pressure. The defect is smooth and not necessarily indicative of malignancy. By contrast, carcinoma invading bone (e.g., gingival carcinoma invading the mandible) is destructive and generally interpreted as malignant.

Metastatic tumors to the bone are more common than primary bone lesions in adults and elderly patients. Metastatic carcinoma is the most common malignant tumor to involve bone. When encountering a lesion of bone that is radiologically malignant in a person older than 40 years, one should first rule out the possibility of a metastasis. Plasma cell myeloma must also receive top consideration in the same circumstances.

Radiologically, most metastases are destructive (radiolucent); some exhibit both bone destruction and bone formation, and others are predominantly productive of bone. Purely lytic metastases are usually from renal, thyroid, and gastrointestinal carcinomas, as well as melanomas. Combined lytic and blastic metastases together or in different bones stem from breast and lung adenocarcinomas and, less commonly, gastrointestinal carcinomas. Purely or predominantly blastic metastases are generally produced by metastatic prostatic carcinoma, carcinoid tumor, and, less commonly, breast and pancreatic carcinomas. Mucinous carcinomas not infrequently develop calcifications that may simulate a malignant cartilaginous tumor.[340]

Aside from radiologic and radionucleide studies, marrow aspirations and biopsies from the iliac crest have been an aid in the diagnosis of metastases. The latter yield cancer cells, even though a lesion is not demonstrable at the aspiration site.[341] FNA will yield diagnostic material from metastatic lesions, particularly those that are destructive. This procedure may forestall the need for open biopsy.

Patients with known cancer and adults who incur what appear to be pathologic fractures should have tissue submitted for pathologic examination if open fixation is carried out. In fact, a biopsy should be done of any fracture site, particularly in an elderly person, if open reduction and fixation are required.

Treatment of bony metastases incorporates all modalities. Satisfactory response may occur with irradiation, chemotherapy, or hormonal manipulation. For the patient with cancer who develops a pathologic fracture, internal fixation has proved successful in reducing pain and re-establishing function. The latter is important to facilitate mobilization.[342]

REFERENCES

1. Dahlin DC, Unni K: Bone Tumors. General Aspects and Data on 8,542 Cases. 3rd Ed. Charles C Thomas, Springfield, IL, 1986
2. Fechner RE, Mills SE: Tumors of Bones and Joints. Atlas of Tumor Pathology. Series 3, Fascicle 8. Armed Forces Institute of Pathology, Washington, DC, 1993
3. Huvos AG: Bone Tumors: Diagnosis, Treatment, and Prognosis. 2nd Ed. WB Saunders, Philadelphia, 1991
4. Mirra J, Picci P, Gold RH: Bone Tumors: Clinical, Radiologic, and Pathologic Correlations. Lea & Febiger, Philadelphia, 1989

5. Spjut HJ, Dorfman HD, Fechner RE: Tumors of Bone and Cartilage. Atlas of Tumor Pathology. Second Series. Armed Forces Institute of Pathology, Washington, DC, 1970

6. Ayala AG, Zornoza J: Primary bone tumors: percutaneous needle biopsy. Radiologic-pathologic study of 222 biopsies. Radiology 149:675–679, 1983

7. Ayala AG, Raymond AK, Ro JY, et al: Needle biopsy of primary bone lesions. Pathol Annu 24:219–251, 1989

8. Raymond AK, Chawla SP, Carrasco CH, et al: Osteosarcoma chemotherapy effect: a prognostic factor. Semin Diagn Pathol 4:212–236, 1987

9. Spjut HJ: Histologic classification of primary tumors of bone. p. 57. In: Management of Primary Bone and Soft Tissue Tumors. Year Book Medical, Chicago, 1977

10. Skyjacks F, Cessans HA, Sabin LH: The World Health Organization's Histologic Classification of Bone Tumors. A commentary on the second edition. Cancer 75:1208–1214, 1995

11. Children J: Osteoma of sinuses, frontal and sphenoid bone: report of fifteen cases. Arch Otolaryngol 30:63–72, 1939

12. Jarvinen HJ, Peltokallio P, Landtman M, Wolf J: Gardner's stigmas in patients with familial adenomatosis coli. Br J Surg 69:718–721, 1982

13. Bertoni F, Unni K, Beabout JA, Sim FH: Parosteal osteoma of the skull and face. Cancer 75:2466–2473, 1995

14. Swee RG, McLeod RA, Beabout JW: Osteoid osteoma. Detection, diagnosis, and localization. Radiology 130:117–123, 1979

15. Mehta MH, Murray RO: Scoliosis provoked by painful vertebral lesions. Skeletal Radiol 1:223–230, 1977

16. Pettine KA, Klassen RA: Osteoid-osteoma and osteoblastoma of the spine. J Bone Joint Surg [Am] 68:354–361, 1986

17. Norman A, Abdelwahab IF, Buyon J, Matzkin E: Osteoid osteoma of the hip stimulating an early onset of osteoarthritis. Radiology 158:417–420, 1986

18. Byers PD: Solitary benign osteoblastic lesions of bone. Cancer 22:43–57, 1968

19. Hasegawa T, Hirose T, Sakamoto H, et al: Mechanism of pain in osteoid osteomas: an immunohistochemical study. Histopathology 22:487–491, 1993

20. Ayala AG, Murray JA, Erling MA, Raymond AK: Osteoid osteoma: intraoperative tetracycline-fluorescence demonstration of the nidus. J Bone Joint Surg [Am] 68:747–751, 1986

21. Sim FH, Dahlin DC, Beabout JW: Osteoid-osteoma: diagnostic problems. J Bone Joint Surg [Am] 57:154–166, 1975

22. Glynn JJ, Lichtenstein L: Osteoid-osteoma with multicentric nidus: a report of two cases. J Bone Joint Surg [Am] 55:855–858, 1973

23. Lucas DR, Unni K, McLeod RA, et al: Osteoblastoma: clinicopathologic study of 306 cases. Hum Pathol 25:117–134, 1994

24. Marsh BW, Bonfiglio M, Brady LP, Enneking WF: Benign osteoblastoma: range of manifestations. J Bone Joint Surg [Am] 57:1–9, 1975

25. Boriani S, Capanna R, Donati D, et al: Osteoblastoma of the spine. Clin Orthop 278:37–45, 1992

26. Bertoni F, Unni K, McLeod RA, Dahlin DC: Osteosarcoma resembling osteoblastoma. Cancer 55:416–426, 1985

27. Bertoni F, Unni K, Lucas DR, McLeod RA: Osteoblastoma with cartilaginous matrix: an unusual morphologic presentation in 18 cases. Am J Surg Pathol 17:69–74, 1993

28. Skyjacks F, Lemos C: Malignant osteoblastoma. J Bone Joint Surg [Br] 58:202–211, 1976

29. Kroon HM, Schurmans J: Osteoblastoma: clinical and radiologic findings in 98 new cases. Radiology 175:783–790, 1990

30. Dorfman HD, Weiss SW: Borderline osteoblastic tumors: problems in the differential diagnosis of aggressive osteoblastoma and low-grade osteosarcoma. Semin Diagn Pathol 1:215–234, 1984

31. Uribe-Botero G, Russell WO, Sutow WW, Martin RG: Primary osteosarcoma of bone: a clinicopathologic investigation of 243 cases, with necropsy studies in 54. Am J Clin Pathol 67:427–435, 1977

32. Heller M, Jend HH, Bucheler E, et al: The role of CT in diagnosis and follow-up of osteosarcoma. J Cancer Res Clin Oncol, suppl. 106:43–48, 1983

33. Shirkhoda A, Jaffe N, Wallace S, et al: Computed tomography of osteosarcoma after intraarterial chemotherapy. Am J Radiol 144:95–99, 1985

34. O'Flanagan SJ, Stack JP, McGee HMJ, Dervan P: Imaging of intramedullary tumor spread in osteosarcoma: a comparison of techniques. J Bone Joint Surg [Br] 73:998–1001, 1991

35. Boyko OB, Cory DA, Cohen MD, et al: MR imaging of osteogenic and Ewing's sarcoma. Am J Radiol 148:317–322, 1987

36. Knop J, Montz R: Bone scintigraphy in patients with osteogenic sarcoma: study group COSS 80. J Cancer Res Clin Oncol, suppl. 106:49–50, 1983

37. Carrasco CH, Charnsangavej C, Raymond AK, Richli WR: Osteosarcoma: angiographic assessment of response to preoperative chemotherapy. Radiology 170:839–842, 1989

38. White VA, Fanning CV, Ayala AG, et al: Osteosarcoma and the role of the fine needle aspiration: a study of 51 cases. Cancer 62:1238–1246, 1988

39. Matsuno T, Unni K, McLeod RA, Dahlin DC: Telangiectatic osteogenic sarcoma. Cancer 38:2538–2547, 1976

40. Farr GH, Huvos AG, Marcove RC, et al: Telangiectatic osteogenic sarcoma. A review of twenty-eight cases. Cancer 34:1150–1158, 1974

41. Sim FH, Unni K, Beabout JW, Dahlin DC: Osteosarcoma with small cells simulating Ewing's tumor. J Bone Joint Surg [Am] 61:207–215, 1979

42. Ayala AG, Ro JY, Raymond AK, et al: Small cell osteosarcoma: clinicopathologic study of 27 cases. Cancer 64:2162–2173, 1989

43. Ayala AG, Ro JY, Papadopoulos NK, et al: Small cell osteosarcoma. In Humphrey GB (ed): Osteosarcoma in Adolescents and Young Adults. Kluwer Academic, Boston, 1993

44. Devaney R, Vinh TN, Sweet D: Small cell osteosarcoma of bone: an immunohistochemical study with differential diagnostic considerations. Hum Pathol 24:1211–1225, 1993

45. Unni K, Dahlin DC, McLeod RA, Pritchard DJ: Intraosseous well differentiated osteosarcoma. Cancer 40:1337–1347, 1977

46. Kurt AM, Unni K, McLeod DJ: Low-grade intraosseous osteosarcoma. Cancer 65:1418–1428, 1990

47. Bertoni F, Bacchini P, Babbri N, et al: Osteosarcoma: low-grade intraosseous-type osteosarcoma, histologically resembling parosteal osteosarcoma, fibrous dysplasia, and desmoplastic fibroma. Cancer 71:338–345, 1993

48. Unni K, Dahlin DC, Beabout JW, Ivins JC: Parosteal osteogenic sarcoma. Cancer 37:2466–2475, 1976

49. Heul RO van der, Ronnen JR von: Juxtacortical osteosarcomas: diagnosis, differential diagnosis, treatment, and an analysis of eighty cases. J Bone Joint Surg [Am] 49:415–439, 1967

50. Raymond AK, Ayala AG, Kirsch HC, et al: Parosteal osteosarcoma vs dedifferentiated: preoperative identification, abstracted. Lab Invest 54:53A, 1986

51. Unni K, Dahlin DC, Beabout JW: Periosteal osteogenic sarcoma. Cancer 37:2476–2485, 1976

52. Spjut HJ, Ayala AG, de Santos LA, Murray JA: Periosteal osteosarcoma. p. 79. In: Management of Primary Bone and Soft Tissue Tumors. Year Book Medical, Chicago, 1977

53. Raymond AK: Surface osteosarcoma. Clin Orthop 270:140–148, 1991

54. Wold LE, Unni K, Beabout JW, Prichard DJ: High-grade surface osteosarcoma. Am J Surg Pathol 8:181–186, 1984

55. Picci P, Campanacci M, Bacci G, et al: Medullary involvement in parosteal osteosarcoma. A case report. J Bone Joint Surg [Am] 69:131–136, 1987

56. Goepfert H, Raymond AK, Spires JR, et al: Osteosarcoma of the head and neck. Cancer Bull 42:347–354, 1990

57. Parham DM, Pratt CB, Parvey LS, et al: Childhood multifocal osteosarcoma: clinicopathologic and radiologic correlates. Cancer 55:2653–2658, 1985

58. Ballance WA, mendelsohn G, Carter JR, et al: Osteogenic sarcoma: malignant fibrous histiocytoma type. Cancer 62:763–771, 1988

59. Hasegawa T, Shibata T, Hirose T, et al: Osteosarcoma with epithelioid features: an immunohistochemical study. Arch Pathol Lab Med 117:295–298, 1993

60. Kramer K, Hicks DG, Palis J, et al: Epithelioid osteosarcoma of bone: immunohistochemical evidence suggesting divergent epithelial and mesenchymal differentiation in a primary osseous neoplasm. Cancer 71:2977–2982, 1993

61. Kyriakos M, Gilula LA, Becich MJ, Schoenecker PL: Intracortical osteosarcoma. Clin Orthop 279:269–280, 1992

62. Torres FX, Kyriakos M: Bone infarct-associated osteosarcoma. Cancer 70:2418–2430, 1992

63. Resnick CS, Aisner SC, Young JWR, Levine A: Case report 767: osteosarcoma arising in bone infarct. Skeletal Radiol 22:58–61, 1993

64. Taylor WF, Ivins JC, Dahlin DC, et al: Trends and variability in survival from osteosarcoma. Mayo Clin Proc 53:695–700, 1978

65. Benjamin RS, Chawla SP, Carrasco HC, et al: Preoperative chemotherapy for osteosarcoma with intravenous Adriamycin and intra-arterial cis-platinum. Ann Oncol, suppl. 3:3–6, 1992

66. Hudson M, Jaffe MR, Jaffe N, et al: Pediatric osteosarcoma: therapeutic strategies, results, and prognostic factors derived from a 10 year experience: J Clin Oncol 8:1988–1997, 1990

67. Bacci G, Picci P, Ferrari S, et al: Primary chemotherapy and delayed surgery for nonmetastatic osteosarcoma of the extremities: results in 164 patients preoperatively treated with high dose methotrexate followed by cisplatin and doxorubicin. Cancer 72:3227–3238, 1993

68. Link MP, Goorin AM, Horowitz M, et al: Adjuvant chemotherapy of high grade osteosarcoma of the extremity: updated results of the multi-institutional osteosarcoma study. Clin Orthop 270:8–14, 1991

69. Picci P, Bacci G, Campanacci M, et al: Histologic evaluation of necrosis in osteosarcoma induced by chemotherapy: regional mapping of viable and nonviable tumor. Cancer 56:1515–1521, 1985

70. Rosen G, Huvos AG, Marcove R, Niremberg A: Telangiectatic osteogenic sarcoma. Improved survival with combination chemotherapy. Clin Orthop 207:164–173, 1986

71. Walaas L, Kindblom LG: Light and electron microscopic examination of fine-needle aspirates in the preoperative diagnosis of osteogenic tumors: a study of 21 osteosarcomas and two osteoblastomas. Diagn Cytopathol 6:27–38, 1990

72. Wilkerson JA, Crowell WT: Intraoperative cytology of osseous lesions. Diagn Cytopathol 2:5–12, 1986

73. Mondal A, Misra DK: CT-guided needle aspiration cytology (FNAC) of 112 vertebral lesions. Indian J Pathol Microbiol 37:255–261, 1994

74. Logan PM, Connell DG, O'Connell JX, et al: Image-guided percutaneous biopsy of musculoskeletal tumors: an algorithm for selection of specific biopsy techniques. Am J Radiol 166:137–141, 1996

75. Ayala AG, Ro JY, Fanning CV, et al: Core needle biopsy and fine-needle aspiration in the diagnosis of bone and soft-tissue lesions. Hematol Oncol Clin North Am 9:632–651, 1995

76. Kreicbergs A, Bauer HCF, Brosjö O, et al: Cytologic diagnosis of bone tumors. J Bone Joint Surg [Br] 78:258–263, 1996

77. Bhatia A, Ashokraj G: Cytologic diversity of osteosarcoma. Indian J Cancer 29:56–60, 1992

78. White VA, Fanning CV, Ayala AG, et al: Osteosarcoma and the role of fine-needle aspiration. Cancer 62:1238–1246, 1988

79. Peterson HA: Multiple hereditary osteochondromata. Clin Orthop 239:222–230, 1989

80. Shapiro F, Simon S, Glimcher MJ: Hereditary multiple exostoses: anthropometric, roentgenographic, and clinical aspects. J Bone Joint Surg [Am] 61:815–824, 1979

81. Evison G, Price CHG: Subungual exostosis. Br J Radiol 39:451–455, 1966

82. Miller-Breslow A, Dorfman HD: Dupuytren's (subungual) exostosis. Am J Surg Pathol 12:368–378, 1988

83. Nora F, Dahlin DC, Beabout JW: Bizarre parosteal osteochondromatous proliferations of the hands and feet. Am J Surg Pathol 7:245–250, 1983

84. Meneses MF, Unni K, Swee RG: Bizarre parosteal osteochondromatous proliferation of bone (Nora's lesion). Am J Surg Pathol 17:691–697, 1993

85. Perlman MD, Gild ML, Schor AD: Enchondroma: a case report and literature review. J Foot Surg 27:556–569, 1988

86. Sun TC, Swee RG, Shives TC, Unni K: Chondrosarcoma in Maffucci's syndrome. J Bone Joint Surg [Am] 67:1214–1219, 1985

87. Gherlinzoni F, Rock M, Picci P: Chondromyxoid fibroma. The experience at the Istituto Orthopedico Rizzoli. J Bone Joint Surg [Am] 65:198–204, 1983

88. Zillmer DA, Dorfman HD: Chondromyxoid fibroma of bone: thirty six cases of clinicopathologic correlation. Hum Pathol 20:952–964, 1989

89. Rahimi A, Beabout JW, Ivins JC, Dahlin DC: Chondromyxoid fibroma: a clinicopathologic study of 76 cases. Cancer 30:726–736, 1972

90. Wilson AJ, Kyriakos M, Ackerman LV: Chondromyxoid fibroma: radiographic appearance in 38 cases and in a review of the literature. Radiology 179:513–518, 1991

91. Steiner GC: Ultrastructure of benign cartilaginous tumors of intraosseous origin. Hum Pathol 10:71–86, 1979

92. Ushigome S, Takakuwa T, Shinagawa T, et al: Chondromyxoid fibroma of bone: an electron microscopic observation. Acta Pathol Jpn 32:113–122, 1984

93. Bleiweiss IJ, Klein MJ: Chondromyxoid fibroma: report of six cases with immunohistochemical studies. Mod Pathol 3:664–666, 1990

94. Troncoso A, Ro JY, Edeiken J, et al: Case report 798: recurrent chondromyxoid fibroma in connective tissue. Skeletal Radiol 22:445–448, 1993

95. Bloem JL, Mulder JD: Chondroblastoma: a clinical and radiological study of 104 cases. Skeletal Radiol 14:1–9, 1985

96. Huvos AG, Marcove RC, Erlandson RA, Mike V: Chondroblastoma of bone. A clinicopathologic and electron microscopic study. Cancer 29:760–771, 1972

97. Springfield DS, Capanna R, Gherlinzoni F, et al: Chondroblastoma. A review of seventy cases. J Bone Joint Surg [Am] 67:748–755, 1985

98. Kurt AM, Unni K, Sim FH, McLeod RA: Chondroblastoma of bone. Hum Pathol 20:965–976, 1989

99. Weiss APC, Dorfman HD: S-100 protein in human cartilage lesions. J Bone Joint Surg [Am] 68:521–526, 1986

100. Breches ME, Simon MA: Chondroblastoma: an immunohistochemical study. Hum Pathol 19:1043–1047, 1988

101. Bertoni F, Unni K, Beabout JW, et al: Chondroblastoma of the skull and facial bones. Am J Clin Pathol 88:1–9, 1987

102. Reyes CV, Kathuria S: Recurrent and aggressive chondroblastoma of the pelvis with late malignant neoplastic changes. Am J Surg Pathol 3:449–455, 1979

103. Kyriakos M, Land VJ, Penning L, Parker SG: Metastatic chondroblastoma. Cancer 55:1770–1789, 1985

104. Fornasier VL, McGonigal D: Periosteal chondroma. Clin Orthop 124:233–236, 1977

105. Boriani S, Bachinni P, Bertoni F, Campanacci M: Periosteal chondroma: a review of twenty cases. J Bone Joint Surg [Am] 65:205–212, 1983

106. Nojima T, Unni K, McLeod RA, Pritchard DJ: Periosteal chondroma and periosteal chondrosarcoma. Am J Surg Pathol 9:666–677, 1985

107. Huvos AG, Marcove RC: Chondrosarcoma in the young: a clinicopathologic analysis of 79 patients younger than 21 years of age. Am J Surg Pathol 11:930–942, 1987

108. Evans HL, Ayala AG, Romsdahl MM: Prognostic factors in chon-

drosarcoma of bone: a clinicopathologic analysis with emphasis on histologic grading. Cancer 40:818–831, 1977

109. Ayala AG, Ro JY, Han W, et al: Chondrosarcoma: a clinicopathologic study of 173 cases with a minimal 5 years follow-up, abstract #3. Lab Invest 64:2A, 1991

110. Gitelis S, Bertoni F, Picci P, Campanacci M: Chondrosarcoma of bone. The experience at the Istituto Ortopedico Rizzoli. J Bone Joint Surg [Am] 63:1248–1257, 1981

111. Coughlan B, Feliz A, Ishida T, et al: p53 expression and DNA ploidy of cartilage lesions. Hum Pathol 26:620–624, 1995

112. Kreicbergs A, Boquist L, Borssen B, Larsson SE: Prognostic factors in chondrosarcoma. Cancer 50:577–583, 1982

113. Spjut HJ: Cartilaginous malignant tumors arising in the skeleton. p. 921. In: Seventh National Cancer Conference Proceedings. American Cancer Society, New York, 1973

114. Nakashima Y, Unni K, Shives CT, et al: Mesenchymal chondrosarcoma of bone and soft tissue. A review of 111 cases. Cancer 57:2444–2453, 1986

115. Shapeero LG, Vanel D, Couanet D, et al: Extraskeletal mesenchymal chondrosarcoma. Radiology 186:819–826, 1993

116. Swanson PE, Lillemoe TJ, Manivel JC, Wick MR: Mesenchymal chondrosarcoma: an immunohistochemical study. Arch Pathol Lab Med 114:943–948, 1990

117. Jacobs JL, Merriam JC, Chadburn A, et al: Mesenchymal chondrosarcoma of the orbit; report of three new cases and review of the literature. Cancer 73:399–345, 1994

118. Frassica FI, Unni K, Beabout JW, Sim FH: Dedifferentiated chondrosarcoma: a report of the clinicopathologic features and treatment of seventy-eight cases. J Bone Joint Surg [Am] 68:1197–1205, 1986

119. Campanacci M, Bertoni F, Capanna R: Dedifferentiated chondrosarcomas. Ital J Orthop Traumatol 3:331–341, 1979

120. Johnson S, Tetu B, Ayala AG, Chawla SP: Chondrosarcoma with additional mesenchymal component (dedifferentiated chondrosarcoma). I. A. clinicopathologic study of 26 cases. Cancer 58:278–286, 1986

121. Tetu B, Ordonez NG, Ayala AG, Mackay B: Chondrosarcoma with additional mesenchymal component (dedifferentiated chondrosarcoma). II. An immunohistochemical and electron microscopic study. Cancer 58:287–298, 1986

122. Simms WW, Ordonez NG, Johnston D, et al: p53 expression in dedifferentiated chondrosarcoma. Cancer 76:23–237, 1995

123. Unni K, Dahlin DC, Beabout JW, Sim FH: Chondrosarcoma: clear-cell variant: a report of sixteen cases. J Bone Joint Surg [Am] 58:676–683, 1976

124. Bjornsson J, Unni K, Dahlin DC, et al: Clear cell chondrosarcoma of bone: observations in 47 cases. Am J Surg Pathol 8:223–230, 1984

125. Wang LT, Liu TC: Clear cell chondrosarcoma of bone: a report of three cases with immunohistochemical and affinity histochemical observations. Pathol Res Pract 189:411–415, 1993

126. Present D, Bacchini P, Pgnatti G, et al: Clear cell chondrosarcoma of bone. A report of 8 cases. Skeletal Radiol 20:187–191, 1991

127. Luger AM, Ansbacher L, Farrell C, et al: Extraskeletal myxoid chondrosarcoma. Skeletal Radiol 6:291–?7, 1981

128. Saleh G, Evans HL, Ro JY, Ayala AG: Extraskeletal myxoid Chondrosarcoma: a clinicopathologic study of ten patients with long-term follow-up. Cancer 70:2827–2830, 1992

129. Kumar RV, Hazarika D, Mathews T, et al: Fine needle aspiration biopsy cytology of chondrosarcoma. Indian J Pathol Microbiol 36:436–441, 1993

130. Tunc M, Ekinci C: Chondrosarcoma diagnosed by fine needle aspiration cytology. Acta Cytol 40:283–288, 1996

131. Abdul-Karim FW, Wasman JK, Pitlik D: Needle aspiration cytology of chondrosarcoma. Acta Cytol 37:655–660, 1993

132. Mirra JM, et al: A new histologic approach to the differentiation of enchondroma and chondrosarcoma of the bones. A clinicopathologic analysis of 51 cases. Clin Orthop 201:214–237, 1985

133. Schiller AL: Diagnosis of borderline cartilage lesions of bone. Semin Diagn Pathol 2:45–62, 1985

134. Walaas L, Kindblom LG, Gunterberg B, Bergh P: Light and electron microscopic examination of fine-needle aspirates in the preoperative diagnosis of cartilaginous tumors. Diagn Cytopathol 6:396–408, 1990

135. Gupta S, Dev G, Marya S: Chondromyxoid fibroma: a fine-needle aspiration diagnosis. Diagn Cytopathol 9:63–65, 1993

136. Layfield LJ, Ferreiro JA: Fine-needle aspiration cytology of chondromyxoid fibroma: a case report. Diagn Cytopathol 4:148–151, 1988

137. Hazarika D, Kumar RV, Rao CR, et al: Fine needle aspiration cytology of chondroblastoma and chondromyxoid fibroma: a report of two cases. Acta Cytol 38:592–596, 1994

138. Fanning CV, Sneige NS, Carrasco CH, et al: Fine needle aspiration cytology of chondroblastoma of bone. Cancer 65:1847–1863, 1990

139. Pohar-Marinsek Z, et al: Chondroblastoma in fine needle aspirates. Acta Cytol 36:367–370, 1992

140. Hicks DG, Krasinskas AM, Sickel JZ, et al: Chondroblastoma: in situ hybridization and immunocytochemical evidence supporting a cartilaginous origin. Int J Surg Pathol 1:155–162, 1994

141. Fanning CV, Sneige NS, Carrasco CH, et al: Fine needle aspiration cytology of chondroblastoma of bone. Cancer 65:1847–1863, 1990

142. Olszewski W, Woyke S, Musiatowicz B: Fine needle aspiration biopsy cytology of chondrosarcoma. Acta Cytol 27:345–349, 1983

143. Kumar RV, Rao CR, Hazarika D, et al: Aspiration biopsy cytology of primary bone lesions. Acta Cytol 37:83–89, 1993

144. Sanerkin NG: The diagnosis and grading of chondrosarcoma of bone: a combined cytologic and histologic approach. Cancer 45:582–594, 1980

145. Doria MI, Wang HH, Chinoy MJ: Retroperitoneal mesenchymal chondrosarcoma: report of a case diagnosed by fine needle aspiration cytology. Acta Cytol 34:529–532, 1990

146. Swanson PE, Lillemoe TJ, Manivel JC, et al: Mesenchymal chondrosarcoma: an immunohistochemical study. Arch Pathol Lab Med 114:943, 1990

147. Dee S, et al: Pleomorphic ("dedifferentiated") chondrosarcoma: report of a case initially examined by fine needle aspiration biopsy. Acta Cytol 35:467–471, 1991

148. Schutte HE, Taconis WK: Giant cell tumor in children and adolescents. Skeletal Radiol 22:173–176, 1993

149. Goldenberg RR, Campbell CJ, Bonfiglio M: Giant-cell tumor of bone: an analysis of two hundred and eighteen cases. J Bone Joint Surg [Am] 52:619–664, 1970

150. Bertoni F, Unni K, Beabout JW, Ebersold MJ: Giant cell tumor of the skull. Cancer 70:1124–1132, 1992

151. Singson R, Feldman F: Multiple (multicentric) giant cell tumors of bone. Skeletal Radiol 9:276–281, 1983

152. Fain JS, Unni K, Beabout JW, Rock MG: Nonepiphyseal giant cell tumor of the long bones: clinical, radiologic, and pathologic study. Cancer 71:3514–3519, 1993

153. Campanacci M, Baldini N, Boriani S, Sudanese A: Giant-cell tumor of bone. J Bone Joint Surg [Am] 69:106–114, 1987

154. Hanaoka H, Friedman B, Mack RP: Ultrastructure and histogenesis of giant-cell tumor of bone. Cancer 25:1408–1423, 1970

155. Steiner GC, Ghosh L, Dorfman HD: Ultrastructure of giant cell tumors of bone. Hum Pathol 3:569–586, 1972

156. Brecher ME, Franklin WA, Simon MA: Immunohistochemical study of mononuclear phagocyte antigens in giant cell tumor of bone. Am J Pathol 125:252–257, 1986

157. Regezi JA, Zarbo RJ, Lloyd RV: Muramidase, alpha-1-antitrypsin, alpha-1-antichymotrypsin, and S-100 protein immunoreactivity in giant cell lesions. Cancer 59:64–68, 1987

158. Picci P, Baldini N, Sudanese A: Giant cell reparative granuloma and other giant cell lesions of the bones of the hands and feet. Skeletal Radiol 15:415–421, 1986

159. Lorenzo JC, Dorfman HD: Giant cell reparative granuloma of short

tubular bones of the hands and feet. Am J Surg Pathol 4:551–563, 1980

160. Pearson BM, Ekelund L, Lovdahl R, Gunterberg B: Favourable results of acrylic cementation for giant cell tumors. Acta Orthop Scand 55:209–214, 1984

161. Marcove RR, Weis LD, Vaghalwalla MR, Pearson R: Cryosurgery in the treatment of giant cell tumors of bone: a report of 52 consecutive cases. Clin Orthop 134:275–289, 1978

162. Sara AS, Ayala AG, El-Naggar A, et al: Giant cell tumor of bone: a clinicopathologic and DNA flow cytometric analysis. Cancer 66:2186–2190, 1990

163. Meis JM, Dorfman HD, Nathanson D, et al: Primary malignant giant cell tumor of bone: "dedifferentiated" giant cell tumor. Mod Pathol 2:541–546, 1988

164. Rock MG, Sim FH, Unni K, et al: Secondary malignant giant-cell tumor of bone: clinicopathologic assessment of nineteen patients. J Bone Joint Surg [Am] 69:1073–1079, 1986

165. Sneige N, Ayala AG, Carrasco CH, et al: Giant cell tumor of bone: a cytologic study of 24 cases. Diagn Cytopathol 1:111–117, 1985

166. Vetrani A, Fulciniti F, Boschi R, et al: Fine needle aspiration biopsy diagnosis of giant-cell tumor of bone: an experience with nine cases. Acta Cytol 34:863–867, 1990

167. van Hoeven KH, Kellogg K, Bavaria JE: Pulmonary metastasis from histologically benign giant cell tumor of bone. Report of a case diagnosed by fine needle aspiration cytology. Acta Cytol 38:401–404, 1994

168. Turc-Carel C, Philip T, Berger MP, et al: Chromosome study of Ewing's sarcoma (ES) cell lines: consistency of a reciprocal translocation t(11;22) (q24;q12). Cancer Genet Cytogenet 12:1–19, 1984

169. Turc-Carel C, Aurias A, Mugneret F, et al: Chromosomes in Ewing's sarcoma. I. An evaluation of 85 cases of remarkable consistency of t(11;22) (q24;q12). Cancer Genet Cytogenet 32:229–238, 1988

170. Whang-Peng J, Triche TJ, Knutsen T, et al: Chromosome translocation in peripheral neuroepithelioma. N Engl J Med 311:584–585, 1984

171. Navarro S, Cavazzana AO, Llombart-Bosch A, Triche TJ: Comparison of Ewing's sarcoma of bone and peripheral neuroepithelioma. An immunocytochemical and ultrastructural analysis of two primitive neuroectodermal neoplasms. Arch Pathol Lab Med 118:608–615, 1994

172. Maygarden SJ, Askin FB, Siegal SP, et al: Ewing's sarcoma of bone in infants and toddlers: a clinicopathologic report from the Intergroup Ewing's study. Cancer 71:2109–2118, 1993

173. Wilkins RM, Pritchard DJ, Burgeret EO Jr, Unni K: Ewing's sarcoma of bone: experience with 140 patients. Cancer 58:2551–2555, 1986

174. Bator SM, Bauer TW, Marks KE, Norris DG: Periosteal Ewing's sarcoma. 58:1781–1784, 1986

175. Llombart-Bosch A, Carda C, Peydro-Olaya A, et al: Soft tissue Ewing's sarcoma: characterization in established cultures and xenografts with evidence of neuroectodermal phenotype. Cancer 66:2589–2601, 1990

176. Nascimiento AG, Unni K, Pritchard DJ, Cooper KL: A clinicopathologic study of 20 cases of large-cell (atypical) Ewing's sarcoma of bone. Am J Surg Pathol 4:29–36, 1980

177. Hartman KR, Triche TJ, Kinsella TJ, Miser JS: Prognostic value of histopathology in Ewing's sarcoma. Cancer 67:163–171, 1991

178. Ushigome S, Shimoda T, Takaki K, et al: Immunocytochemical and ultrastructural studies of the histogenesis of Ewing's sarcoma and putatively related tumors. Cancer 64:52–62, 1989

179. Moll R, Lee I, Gould VE, et al: Immunocytochemical analysis of Ewing's tumors: pattern of expression of intermediate filaments and desmosomal proteins indicate cell type heterogeneity and pluripotential differentiation. Am J Pathol 127:288–304, 1987

180. Cavazzana AO, Miser JS, Jefferson J, Triche TH: Experimental evidence for a neural origin of Ewing's sarcoma of bone. Am J Pathol 127:507–518, 1987

181. Felliner EJ, Garin-Chesa P, Glasser DB, et al: Comparison of cell surface antigen HBA71 (p30/32^{MIC2}), neuron-specific enolase, and vimentin in the immunohistochemical analysis of Ewing's sarcoma of bone. Am J Surg Pathol 16:746–755, 1992

182. Fellinger EJ, Garin-Chesa P, Triche TJ, et al: Immunohistochemical analysis of Ewing's sarcoma cell surface antigen p30/32^{MIC2}. Am J Pathol 139:317–325, 1991

183. Fellinger EJ, Garin-Chesa P, Su SL, et al: Biochemical and genetic characterization of HBA71 Ewing's sarcoma cell surface antigen. Cancer Res 51:336–340, 1991

184. Perlman EJ, Dickman PS, Askin FB, et al: Ewing's sarcoma—routine diagnostic utilization of MIC2 analysis: a Pediatric Oncology Group/Children's Cancer Group Intergroup Study. Hum Pathol 25:304–307, 1994

185. Riopel M, Dickman PS, Link MP, Perlman EJ: MIC2 analysis in pediatric lymphomas and leukemias. Hum Pathol 25:396–399, 1994

186. Dei Tos AP, Wadden C, Calonje E, et al: Immunohistochemical demonstration of glycoprotein p30/32^{MIC2} in synovial sarcoma. A potential cause of diagnostic confusion. Appl Immunohistochem 3:168–173, 1995

187. Mahoney JP, Alexander RW: Ewing's sarcoma. A light and electron microscopic study of 21 cases. Am J Surg Pathol 2:283, 1978

188. Mawad JK, Mackay B, Raymond AK, Ayala AG: Electron microscopy in the diagnosis of small round cell tumors. Ultrastruct Pathol 18:263–268, 1994

189. Askin FB, Rosai J, Sibley RK, et al: Malignant small cell tumor of the thoracopulmonary region in childhood: a distinctive clinicopathologic entity of uncertain histogenesis. Cancer 43:2438–2451, 1979

190. Dehner LP: Primitive neuroectodermal tumor and Ewing's sarcoma. Am J Surg Pathol 17:1–13, 1993

191. Telles NC, Rabson AS, Pomeroy TC: Ewing's sarcoma: an autopsy study. Cancer 41:2321–2329, 1978

192. Sutow WW: Chemotherapy of Ewing's sarcoma. p. 97. In Jaffe N (ed): Bone Tumors in Children. PSG Publishing, Littleton, MA, 1979

193. Nesbitt ME, Gehan EA, Burgert EO, et al: Multimodal therapy for the management of primary, nonmetastatic Ewing's sarcoma of bone: a long-term follow-up of the First Intergroup study. J Clin Oncol 8:1664–1674, 1990

194. Shoji H, Miller TR: Primary reticulum cell sarcoma of bone: significance of clinical features upon the prognosis. Cancer 28:1234–1244, 1971

195. Boston HC Jr, Dahlin DC, Ivins JC, Cupps RE: Malignant lymphoma (so-called reticulum cell sarcoma) of bone. Cancer 34:1131–1137, 1974

196. Ostrowski ML, Unni K, Banks PM, et al: Malignant lymphoma of bone. Cancer 58:2646–2655, 1986

197. Clayton F, Butler JJ, Ayala AG, et al: Non-Hodgkin's lymphoma in bone: pathologic and radiologic features with clinical correlates. Cancer 60:2494–2501, 1987

198. Dosoretz DE, Raymond AK, Murphy GF, et al: Primary lymphoma of bone: the relationship of morphologic diversity to clinical behavior. Cancer 50:1009–1014, 1982

199. Baar J, Burkes RL, Bell R, et al: Primary non-Hodgkin's lymphoma of bone: a clinicopathologic study. Cancer 73:1194–1199, 1994

200. Pettit CK, Zukerber LR, Gray MH, et al: Primary lymphoma of bone: a B-cell neoplasm with a high frequency of multilobated cells. Am J Surg Pathol 14:329–334, 1990

201. Linder J, Ye Y, Armitage JO, Weisenburger DD: Monoclonal antibodies on paraffin-embedded tissues. Mod Pathol 1:29–34, 1988

202. Bacci G, Jaffe N, Emiliani E, et al: Therapy for primary non-Hodgkin's lymphoma of bone and a comparison of results with Ewing's sarcoma. Ten years' experience at the Instituto Ortopedico Rizzoli. Cancer 57:1468–1472, 1986

203. Dimopoulos MA, Moulopoulos A, Delasalle K, Alexanian R: Solitary plasmacytoma of bone and asymptomatic multiple myeloma. Hematol Oncol Clin North Am 6:359–369, 1992

204. Meis JM, Butler JJ, Osborne BM, Ordonez NG: Solitary plasmacytomas of bone and extramedullary plasmacytomas: a clinicopathologic and immunohistochemical study. Cancer 59:1475–1485, 1987

205. Kyle RA, Elveback LR: Management and prognosis of multiple myeloma. Mayo Clin Proc 51:751–760, 1976

206. Schaller RT, Schaller JF, Buschmann C, Kiviat N: The usefulness of percutaneous fine-needle aspiration biopsy in infants and children. J Pediatr Surg 18:398–405, 1983

207. Akhtar M, Ali MA, Sabbah R, et al: Fine-needle aspiration biopsy diagnosis of round cell malignant tumors of childhood: a combined light and electron microscopic approach. Cancer 55:1805–1817, 1985

208. Silverman JF, Berns LA, Holbrook CT, et al: Biopsy of small round cell tumors of childhood: cytomorphologic features and the role of ancillary studies. Diagn Cytol 10:245–255, 1994

209. Akhtar M, Ali MA, Sabbah R: Aspiration cytology of Ewing's sarcoma: light and electron microscopic correlations. Cancer: 56:2051–2060, 1985

210. Åkerman M, Alvegård T, Eliiasson J, et al: A case of Ewing's sarcoma diagnosed by fine needle aspiration: light microscopy, electron microscopy and chromosomal analysis. Acta Orthop Scand 59:589–592, 1988

211. Nieman TH, Thomas PA: Primary lymphoma of bone: diagnosis by fine-needle aspiration biopsy in a pediatric patient. Diagn Cytol 12:165–167, 1995

212. Ascoli V, Facciolo F, Nardi F: Cytodiagnosis of a primary non-Hodgkin's lymphoma of bone. Diagn Cytol 11:168–173, 1994

213. Cooper GL, Shaffer DW, Raval HB: Fine-needle aspiration biopsy of multiple myeloma in a patient with renal-cell carcinoma: a case report. Diagn Cytol 9:551–554, 1993

214. Gutmann EJ: Granulomatous inflammation related to amyloid deposition in a focus of multiple myeloma. Report of a case with diagnosis by fine needle aspiration biopsy. Acta Cytol 39:793–797, 1995

215. Baker ND, Klein MJ, Greenspan A, Neuwirth M: Symptomatic vertebral hemangiomas: a report of four cases. Skeletal Radiol 15:458–463, 1986

216. Falkmer S, Tilling G: Primary lymphangioma of bone. Acta Orthop Scand 26:99–110, 1956

217. Gutierrez RM, Spjut HJ: Skeletal angiomatosis: report of three cases and review of the literature. Clin Orthop 85:82–97, 1972

218. Gorham LW, Stout AP: Massive osteolysis (acute spontaneous absorption of bone, phantom bone, disappearing bone): its relation to hemangiomatosis. J Bone Joint Surg [Am] 37:985–1004, 1955

219. Halliday DR, Dahlin DC, Pugh DG, Young HH: Massive osteolysis and angiomatosis. Radiology 82:637–644, 1964

220. Pastakia B, Horvath K, Lack EE: Seventeen year follow-up and autopsy findings in a case of massive osteolysis. Skeletal Radiol 16:291–297, 1987

221. Stout AP: Hemangioendothelioma: a tumor of blood vessels featuring vascular endothelial cells. Ann Surg 118:445–464, 1943

222. Hartman WH, Stewart FW: Hemangioendothelioma of bone: unusual tumor characterized by indolent course. Cancer 15:846–854, 1962

223. Otis J, Hutter RVP, Foote FW, et al: Hemangioendothelioma of bone. Surg Gynecol Obstet 127:295–305, 1968

224. Dorfman HD, Steiner GC, Jaffe HL: Vascular tumors of bone. Hum Pathol 2:253–276, 1971

225. Rosai J, Gold J, Landy R: The histiocytoid hemangiomas: a unifying concept embracing several previously described entities of skin, soft tissue, large vessels, bone and heart. Hum Pathol 10:707–730, 1979

226. Tsuneyoshi M, Dorfman HD, Bauer TW: Epithelioid hemangioendothelioma of bone: a clinicopathologic, ultrastructural, and immunohistochemical study. Am J Surg Pathol 10:754–764, 1986

227. Weiss SW, Enzinger FW: Epithelioid hemangioendothelioma: a vascular tumor often mistaken for carcinoma. Cancer 50:970–981, 1982

228. O'Connell JX, Kattapuram SV, Mankin HJ, et al: Epithelioid hemangioma of bone: a tumor often mistaken for low-grade angiosarcoma or malignant hemangioendothelioma. Am J Surg Pathol 17:610–617, 1993

229. Castro C, Winkelmann RK: Angiolymphoid hyperplasia with eosinophilia in the skin. Cancer 34:1696–1705, 1974

230. Bollinger BK, Laskin WB, Knight CB: Epithelioid hemangioendothelioma with multiple site involvement. Cancer 73:610–615, 1994

231. Campanacci M, Boriani S, Giunti A: Hemangioendothelioma of bone: a study of 29 cases. Cancer 46:804–814, 1980

232. Wold LE, Unni K, Beabout JW, et al: Hemangioendothelial sarcoma of bone. Am J Surg Pathol 6:59–70, 1982

233. Wold LE, Unni K, Cooper KL, et al: Hemangipericytoma of bone. Am J Surg Pathol 6:53–58, 1982

234. Tang JSH, Gold RH, Mirra JM, Eckardt J: Hemangiopericytoma of bone. Cancer 62:848–859, 1988

235. Khiyami A, Green LK, Gyorkey Flandon G: Primary angiosarcoma of the cuboidal bone: a case report. Diagn Cytol 7:520–523, 1991

236. Jayaram G, Kapoor R, Saha MM: Hemangioendothelioma. Cytologic appearances in two cases presenting with multiple soft tissue and bone lesions. Acta Cytol 31:497–501, 1987

237. Bosch AL, Olaya AP, Fernandez AL: Non-ossifying fibroma of bone. A histochemical and ultrastructural characterization. Virchows Arch A Pathol Anat Histopathol 362:13–21, 1974

238. Caffey J: On fibrous defects in cortical walls of growing tubular bones: their radiologic appearance, structure, prevalence, natural course, and diagnostic significance. Adv Pediatr 7:13–51, 1955

239. Drennan DB, Maylahn DJ, Fahey JJ: Fractures through large non-ossifying fibromas. Clin Orthop 103:82–88, 1974

240. Bertoni F, Calderoni P, Bacchini P, et al: Benign fibrous histiocytoma of bone. J Bone Joint Surg [Am] 68:1225–1230, 1986

241. Wold LE: Fibrous histiocytic tumors of bone. In Unni K (ed): Bone tumors. Churchill Livingstone, New York, 1988

242. Bertoni F, Unni K, McLeod RA, Sim FH: Xanthoma of bone. Am J Clin Pathol 90:377–384, 1988

243. Specchiulli F, Florio U: Desmoplastic fibroma of bone: a study of three cases. Ital J Orthop Traumatol 2:141–150, 1976

244. Lagacé R, Delage C, Bouchard HL, Seemayer TA: Desmoplastic fibroma of bone. An ultrastructural study. Am J Surg Pathol 3:423–430, 1979

245. Inwards CY, Unni K, Beabout JW, Sim FH: Desmoplastic fibroma of bone. Cancer 68:1978–1983, 1991

246. Ayala AG, Ro JY, Goepfert H, et al: Desmoid fibromatosis: a clinicopathologic study of 25 children. Semin Diagn Pathol 3:138–150, 1986

247. Campanacci M, Olmi R: Fibrosarcoma of bone. A study of 114 cases. Ital J Orthop Traumatol 3:199–206, 1977

248. Taconis WK, van Rijssel TG: Fibrosarcoma of long bones. A study of the significance of areas of malignant fibrous histiocytoma. J Bone Joint Surg [Br] 67:111–116, 1985

249. Taconis WK, van Rijssel TG: Fibrosarcoma of the jaws. Skeletal Radiol 15:10–13, 1986

250. Dahlin DC, Unni K, Matsuno T: Malignant fibrous histiocytoma of bone—fact or fancy? Cancer 39:1508–1516, 1977

251. Feldman F, Lattes R: Primary malignant fibrous histiocytoma (fibrous xanthoma) of bone. Skeletal Radiol 1:145–160, 1977

252. McCarthy EF, Matsuno T, Dorfman HD: Malignant fibrous histiocytoma of bone: a study of 35 cases. Hum Pathol 10:57–70, 1979

253. Huvos AG, Heilweil M, Bretski SS: The pathology of malignant fibrous histiocytoma of bone: a study of 130 patients. Am J Surg Pathol 9:853–871, 1985

254. Abrahams TG, Hull M: Malignant fibrous histiocytoma (MFH) arising in an infarct of bone. Skeletal Radiol 15:578–583, 1986

255. Little DC, McCarty SW: Malignant fibrous histiocytoma of bone: the experience of the New South Whales Bone Tumor Registry. Aust NZ J Surg 63:346–351, 1993

256. Yokoyama R, Tsuneyoshi N, Enjoji M, et al: Prognostic factors of ma-

lignant fibrous histiocytoma of bone: a clinical and histopathologic analysis of 34 cases. Cancer 72:1902–1908, 1993

257. Ayala AG, Ro JY, Bolio-Solis A, et al: Mesenchymal hamartoma of the chest wall in infants and children: a clinicopathologic study of five patients. Skeletal Radiol 22:469–476, 1993

258. Moorefield WG, Urbaniak JR, Gonzalvo AA: Intramedullary lipoma of the distal femur. South Med J 69:1210–1211, 1976

259. Larsson SE, Lorentzon R, Boquist L: Primary liposarcoma of bone. Acta Orthop Scand 46:869–876, 1975

260. Myers JL, Arocho J, Bernreuter W, et al: Leiomyosarcoma of bone: a clinicopathologic, immunohistochemical, and ultrastructural study of five cases. Cancer 67:1051–1056, 1991

261. Fornasier VL, Paley D: Leiomyosarcoma in bone: primary or secondary? A case report and review of the literature. Skeletal Radiol 10:147–153, 1983

262. Dahlin DC, Bertoni F, Beabout JW, Campanacci M: Fibrocartilaginous mesenchymoma with low grade malignancy. Skeletal Radiol 12:263–269, 1984

263. Bulychova IV, Unni K, Bertoni F, Beabout JW: Fibrocartilaginous mesenchymoma of bone. Am J Surg Pathol 18:830–836, 1993

264. Pinto RS, Lin JP, Firooznia H, Lefleur RS: The osseous and angiographic features of vertebral chordomas. Neuroradiology 9:231–241, 1975

265. Uhrenholt L, Stimpel H: Histochemistry of sacrococcygeal chordoma. Acta Pathol Microbiol Scand 93:203–204, 1985

266. Meis JM, Giraldo AA: Chordoma: an immunohistochemical study of 20 cases. Arch Pathol Lab Med 112:553–556, 1988

267. Abenoza P, Sibley RK: Chordoma: an immunohistochemical study. Hum Pathol 17:744–747, 1986

268. Wojno KD, Aruban RH, Garlin-Chesa P, Huvos AG: Chondroid chordomas and low grade chondrosarcomas of the craniospinal axis. Am J Surg Pathol 16:1144–1152, 1992

269. Jeffrey PB, Biava CG, Davis RL: Chondroid chordoma. A hyalinized chordoma without cartilaginous differentiation. Am J Clin Pathol 103:271–279, 1995

270. Heffelfinger MJ, Dahlin DC, MacCarty CS, Beabout JW: Chordomas and cartilaginous tumors at the base of the skull. Cancer 32:410–420, 1973

271. Rosenberg AE, Brown GA, Bhan AK, Lee JM: Chondroid chordoma: a variant of chordoma: a morphologic and immunohistochemical study. Am J Clin Pathol 101:36–41, 1994

272. Meis JM, Raymond AK, Evans HL, et al: "Dedifferentiated" chordoma: a clinicopathologic and immunohistochemical study of three cases. Am J Surg Pathol 11:516–525, 1987

273. Hruban RH, Traganos F, Reuter VE, Huvos AG: Chordomas with malignant spindle cell components. Am J Pathol 137:435–447, 1990

274. Fleming GF, Heimann PS, Stephens JK, et al: Dedifferentiated chordoma: response to aggressive chemotherapy in two cases. Cancer 72:714–718, 1993

275. Dabska M: Parachordoma. A new clinicopathologic entity. Cancer 40:1586–1592, 1977

276. Shin HJ, Mackay B, Ichinose H, et al: Parachordoma. Ultrastruct Pathol 18:249–256, 1994

277. Weiss SW, Dorfman HD: Adamantinoma of long bone: an analysis of nine cases with emphasis on metastasizing lesions and fibrous dysplasia-like changes. Hum Pathol 8:141, 1977

278. Moon NF: Adamantinoma of the appendicular skeleton—a statistical review of reported cases and inclusion of 10 new cases. Clin Orthop 43:189–213, 1965

279. Moon NF, Mori H: Adamantinoma of the appendicular skeleton—updated. Clin Orthop 204:215–237, 1986

280. Perez-Atayde AR, Kozakewich HP, Vawter GF: Adamantinoma of the tibia. An ultrastructural and immunohistochemical study. Cancer 55:1015–1023, 1985

281. Eisenstein W, Pitcock JA: Adamantinoma of the tibia: an eccrine carcinoma. Arch Pathol Lab Med 108:246–250, 1984

282. Hazelbag HM, Fleuren GC, Broeck LJCM, et al: Adamantinoma of the long bones: keratin subclass immunoreactivity pattern with reference to its histogenesis. Am J Surg Pathol 17:1225–1233, 1993

283. Campanacci M, Giunti A, Bertoni F, et al: Adamantinoma of the long bones. Am J Surg Pathol 5:533–542, 1981

284. Czerniak B, Rojas-Corona RR, Dorfman HD: Morphologic diversity of long bone adamantinomas: the concept of differentiated (regressing) adamantinoma and its relationship to osteofibrous dysplasia. Cancer 64:2319–2334, 1989

285. Sweet DE, Tuyethoa NV, Devaney K: Cortical osteofibrous dysplasia of long bone and its relationship to adamantinoma: a clinicopathologic study of 30 cases. Am J Surg Pathol 16:282–290, 1992

286. Keeney GL, Unni K, Beabout JW, Pritchard DJ: Adamantinoma of long bones: a clinicopathologic study of 85 cases. Cancer 64:730–737, 1989

287. Winter RB, Moe J, Bradford DS, et al: Spine deformity in neurofibromatosis. A review of one hundred and two patients. J Bone Joint Surg [Am] 61:677–694, 1977

288. Holt JF: Neurofibromatosis in children. AJR 130:615–639, 1978

289. Wilber MC, Woodcock JA: Ganglioneuromata in bone: report of a case. J Bone Joint Surg [Am] 39:1385–1388, 1957

290. Vergel De Dios AM, Bond JR, Shives TC, et al: Aneurysmal bone cyst: a clinicopathologic study of 238 cases. Cancer 69:2921–2931, 1992

291. Kannan V, von Ruden D: Malignant fibrous histiocytoma of bone: initial diagnosis by aspiration biopsy cytology. Diagn Cytopathol 4:262–264, 1988

292. Silverman JF, Lannin DL, Larkin EW, et al: Fine-needle aspiration cytology of postirradiation sarcomas, including angiosarcoma with imunocytochemical confirmation. Diagn Cytol 5:275–281, 1989

293. Nanda M, Rao ES, Behera KC, et al: Fine needle aspiration cytology (FNAC) in malignant bone tumors. Indian J Pathol Microbiol 37:247–253, 1994

294. Walaas L, Kindblom LG: Fine-needle aspiration biopsy in the preoperative diagnosis of chordoma: a study of 17 cases with application of electron microscopic, histochemical, and immunocytochemical examination. Hum Pathol 22:22–28, 1991

295. Nijhawan VS, Rajwanshi A, Das A, et al: Fine-needle aspiration cytology of sacrococcygeal chordoma. Diagn Cytopathol 5:404–407, 1989

296. Finley JL, Silverman JF, Dabbs DJ, et al: Chordoma: diagnosis by fine-needle aspiration biopsy with histologic, immunocytochemical and ultrastructural confirmation. Diagn Cytopathol 2:330–337, 1986

297. Laucirica R, Mody D, MacLeay L, et al: Adamantinoma. A case report with aspiration cytology and differential diagnostic and immunohistochemical considerations. Acta Cytol 36:951–956, 1992

298. Galera-Davidson H, Fernandez-Rodriquez A, Torres-Olivera FJ, et al: Cytologic diagnosis of a case of recurrent adamantinoma. Acta Cytol 33:635–638, 1989

299. Hales MS, Ferrell LD: Fine-needle aspiration biopsy of tibial adamantimoma: a case report. Diagn Cytopathol 4:67–70, 1988

300. Adler CP: Tumour-like lesions in the femur with cementum-like material. Does "cementoma" of long bone exist? Skeletal Radiol 14:26–37, 1985

301. Scaglietti O, Bartolozzi P: The effects of methylprednisolone acetate in the treatment of bone cysts: results of three years follow-up. J Bone Joint Surg [Br] 61:200–204, 1979

302. Scaglietti O, Marchetti PG, Bartolozzi P: Final results obtained in the treatment of bone cysts with methylprednisolone acetate (Depomedrol) and a discussion of results achieved in other bone lesions. Clin Orthop 165:33–42, 1982

303. Farber JM, Stanton RP: Treatment options in unicameral bone cysts. Orthopedics 13:25–32, 1990

304. Ruiter DJ, van Rijssel TG, van der Velde EA: Aneurysmal bone cysts. A clinicopathological study of 105 cases. Cancer 39:2231–2239, 1977

305. Vergel de Dios AM, Bond JR, Shives TC, et al: Aneurysmal bone cyst: a clinicopathologic study of 238 cases. Cáncer 69:2921–2931, 1992

306. Oda Y, Tsuneyoshi M, Shinohara N: "Solid" variant of aneurysmal bone cyst (extragnathic giant cell reparative granuloma) in the axial skeleton and long bones: a study of its morphologic spectrum and distinction from allied giant cell lesions. Cancer 70:2642–2649, 1992

307. Bertoni F, Bacchini P, Capanna R, et al: Solid variant of aneurysmal bone cyst. Cancer 71:729–734, 1993

308. McCarthy EF, Matz F, Steiner GC, Dorfman HD: Periosteal ganglion: a cause of cervical bone erosion. Skeletal Radiol 10:243–246, 1983

309. Yaghmai I, Foster WC: Case report 404. Intraosseous ganglion of the distal end of the ulna with a pathological fracture. Skeletal Radiol 16:153–156, 1987

310. Lichtenstein L, Jaffe HL: Eosinophilic granuloma of bone, with report of case. Am J Pathol 16:595–604, 1940

311. Yu RC, Chu C, Buluwela L, Chu AC: Clonal proliferation of Langerhans cells in Langerhans' cell histiocytosis. Lancet 343:767–768, 1994

312. Williams CL, Busque L, Griffith BB, et al: Langerhans' cell histiocytosis (histiocytosis X): a clonal proliferative disease. N Engl J Med 331:154–160, 1994

313. Kilpatrick SE, Wenger DE, Gilchrist GS, et al: Langerhans' cell histiocytosis (histiocytosis X) of bone. A clinicopathologic analysis of 261 pediatric and adult cases. Cancer 76:2471–2484, 1995

314. Beltran J, Aparisi F, Bonmati LM, et al: Eosinophilic granuloma: MRI manifestations. Skeletal Radiol 22:157–161, 1993

315. Katz RL, Silva AG, de Santos L, Lukeman JM: Diagnosis of eosinophilic granuloma of bone by cytology, histology, and electron microscopy of transcutaneous bone-aspiration biopsy. J Bone Joint Surg [Am] 62:1284–1290, 1980

316. Shabb N, Fanning CV, Carrasco CH, et al: Diagnosis of eosinophilic granuloma of bone by fine-needle aspiration with concurrent institution of therapy: a cytologic, histologic, clinical, and radiologic study of 27 cases. Diagn Cytopathol 9:3–12, 1993

317. Elsheikh T, Silverman JF, Wakely PE, et al: Fine-needle aspiration cytology of Langerhans' cell histiocytosis (eosinophilic granuloma) of bone in children. Diagn Cytopathol 7:261–266, 1991

318. Nauert C, Zornoza J, Ayala AG, Harle TS: Eosinophilic granuloma of bone: diagnosis and management. Skeletal Radiol 10:227–235, 1983

319. Dehner LP: Fibro-osseous lesions of bone. p. 209. In Ackerman LV, Spjut HJ (eds): Bones and Joints. International Academy of Pathology Monograph. Williams & Wilkins, Baltimore, 1976

320. Campanacci M: Osteofibrous dysplasia of long bones. A new clinical entity. Ital J Orthop Traumatol 2:221–237, 1976

321. Campanacci M, Laus M: Osteofibrous dysplasia of the tibia and fibula. J Bone Joint Surg [Am] 63:367–375, 1981

322. Kempson R: Ossifying fibroma of the long bones. A light and electron microscopic study. Arch Pathol 82:218–233, 1968

323. Lee PA, Van Dop C, Migeon CJ: McCune-Albright syndrome. Long-term follow-up. JAMA 256:2980–2984, 1986

324. Ishida T, Dorfman HD: Massive chondroid differentiation in fibrous dysplasia of bone (fibrocartilaginous dysplasia). Am J Surg Pathol 17:924–930, 1993

325. Wojno KJ, McCarty EF: Fibro-osseous lesions of the face and skull with aneurysmal bone cyst formation. Skeletal Radiol 23:15–18, 1994

326. Kransdorf MJ, Moser RP, Gilkey FW: Fibrous dysplasia. Radiographics 10:519–537, 1990

327. Halawa M, Aziz AA: Chondrosarcoma in fibrous dysplasia of the pelvis. J Bone Joint Surg [Br] 66:760–764, 1984

328. Ruggieri P, Sim FH, Bond JR, Unni K: Malignancies in fibrous dysplasia. Cancer 73:1411–1424, 1994

329. Johnson LC, Yousefi M, Vinh TN, et al: Juvenile active ossifying fibroma. Its nature, dynamics and origin. Acta Otolaryngol, suppl. 488:3–40, 1991

330. Margo CE, Ragsdale BD, Perman KI, et al: Psammomatoid (juvenile) ossifying fibroma of the orbit. Ophthalmology 92:150–159, 1985

331. Hamer JE, Scofield HH, Cornyn J: Benign fibro-osseous jaw lesions of peripheral origin. Cancer 22:861–878, 1968

332. Wenig BM, Vinh TN, Smirniotopoulos JG, et al: Aggressive psammomatoid ossifying fibromas of the sinonasal region. A clinicopathologic study of a distinct group of fibro-osseous lesions. Cancer 76:1155–1165, 1995

333. Sissons HA, Steiner GC, Dorfman HD: Calcified spherules in fibro-osseous lesions of bone. Arch Pathol Lab Med 17:284–290, 1993

334. Voytek TM, Ro JY, Edeiken J, Ayala AG: Fibrous dysplasia and cemento-ossifying fibroma: a histologic spectrum. Am J Surg Pathol 19:775–781, 1995

335. Lagier R, Cox JN: Pseudomalignant myositis ossificans: a pathological study of eight cases. Hum Pathol 6:653–665, 1975

336. Dahl I, Angervall L: Pseudosarcomatous proliferative lesions of soft tissue with or without bone formation. Acta Pathol Microbiol Immunol Scand [A] 85:577–589, 1977

337. Bassler T, Wong ET, Brymes RK: Osteitis fibrosa cystica simulating metastatic tumor: an almost forgotten relationship. Am J Clin Pathol 100:697–700, 1993

338. Gupta RK, Voss DM, McHutchinson AG, Hatfield PJ: Osteitis fibrosa cystica (brown tumor) in a patient with renal transplantation. Report of a case with aspiration cytodiagnosis. Acta Cytol 36:555–558, 1992

339. Watson CW, Unger P, Kaneko M, Gabrilove JL: Fine needle aspiration of osteitis fibrosa cystica. Diagn Cytopathol 1:157–160, 1985

340. Ribalta T, Shannon RL, Ro JY, et al: Bone metastasis from urachal carcinoma simulating chondrosarcoma. Case report 645. Skeletal Radiol 19:616–619, 1990

341. Savage RA, Hoffman GC, Shaker K: Diagnostic problems involved in detection of metastatic neoplasms by bone-marrow aspirate compared with needle biopsy. Am J Clin Pathol 70:623–627, 1978

342. Vaughn PB, Brindley HH: Pathologic fractures of long bones. South Med J 72:788–794, 1979

24

Skeletal Muscle

Umberto De Girolami
Alan H. Beggs

The proper evaluation of a muscle biopsy requires the joint assessment of the patient's medical history, physical examination, laboratory values, electromyogram (EMG)/nerve conduction (NCV) studies, together with the morphologic and biochemical data derived from study of the muscle tissue itself. In this chapter we present the following topics in turn: a short account of muscle biopsy indications and techniques, a summary of the characteristics of normal skeletal muscle, a review of the structural manifestations of some of the basic reactions of muscle tissue to injury, and a discussion of the major categories of skeletal muscle diseases, including their salient clinical features, morphologic findings, and current understanding of their pathogenesis. The reader interested in an extensive discussion of these topics will be rewarded by finding several fine treatises on the subject.[1-4]

SKELETAL MUSCLE BIOPSY INDICATIONS AND TECHNIQUES

Often, the clinician who decides on a muscle biopsy is not the person who performs the surgical procedure. Communication between the two physicians is therefore essential so that the appropriate muscle site is selected based on clinical assessment, EMG/NCV values, or radiologic data. Prior notification of the pathology laboratory is also needed so that preparations for the proper handling of the biopsy specimen can be made beforehand. It is important to note that the muscle chosen for biopsy should be one that is moderately affected as determined by the physical findings and EMG studies, because clinically uninvolved muscles are less likely to show histopathologic abnormalities, and severely affected muscle may only demonstrate end-stage changes (Fig. 24-1). Sites of previous biopsy, EMG needle implantation, intramuscular injection, or prior trauma should be avoided by the surgeon because the inflammatory and reactive changes that attend these procedures will invariably confuse the interpretation of the biopsy. The biopsy should be taken from the belly of the muscle because at the tendinous insertion, the collagenous connective tissue, the variability in the cross-sectional diameter of the fibers, and the increased number of internalized nuclei within the fibers that is typically seen at the polar ends of the muscle fiber, could be misinterpreted as abnormal tissue (Fig. 24-2). Finally, the biopsy should be per-

formed by someone who is well versed in muscle biopsy technique.

In most instances, to allow for a complete analysis, we prefer an open biopsy of the muscle obtaining two separate specimens: an unclamped and a clamped sample. The specimens are processed as follows: (1) The first specimen is removed in situ on a muscle biopsy clamp to avoid contraction artifacts (hypercontraction bands of Nageotte[5]) (Fig. 24-3) and processed for light and electron microscopy. A portion of this specimen is placed in a fixative favorable for light microscopy (e.g., buffered formalin), embedded in paraffin and processed for cross-and longitudinal sections, stained with hematoxylin and eosin (H&E) at three levels and special stains as needed. The other portion of this specimen is fixed in glutaraldehyde, embedded in plastic, cross-and longitudinal sections are cut as semithin sections, stained with toluidine blue or other suitable stain, examined with the light microscope, and then selected regions are processed for electron microscopic study. (2) The second specimen, the unclamped muscle, is retained unfixed and wrapped in a saline-moistened gauze for transfer to the pathology laboratory. There, one portion of it is snap-frozen in isopentane cooled by liquid nitrogen mounted in a suitable embedding medium on a chuck that will allow for cryostat sections. The essence of the procedure is to drop the temperature of the specimen from room temperature to below freezing as quickly as possible, causing the water to freeze in situ, thereby preventing nidus formation of ice crystals that would disrupt the shape of the fiber (Fig. 24-4). Frozen sections are then processed with a battery of histochemical reactions and other special stains. The battery of histochemical reactions and special stains employed will vary somewhat from one laboratory to another; we routinely perform (H&E), modified Gomori trichrome, nicotinamide adenine dinucleotide-tetrazolium reductase (NADH-TR), periodic acid-Schiff (PAS) with and without diastase, oil red O, acid phosphatase, and adenosine triphosphatase (ATPase) performed at pH 4.3, 4.6, and 9.4. In selected instances (e.g., inflammatory myopathies) frozen sections can also be processed with a battery of reactions that bring out immunoglobulin deposits. Immunoperoxidase methods for the demonstration of abnormalities in the dystrophinopathic and nondystrophinopathic muscular dystrophies are becoming available in many specialized laboratories. Computer-assisted morphometric studies, performed on transverse frozen sections prepared with the ATPase reaction and compared with age-

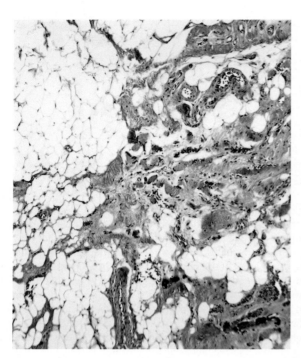

Fig. 24-1. End-stage neuromuscular disease. Most of the muscle has been replaced by fibroadipose tissue. The few remaining fibers are surrounded by collagen fibers. This pattern may be the end result of many neuromuscular diseases, either neuropathic or myopathic. (Courtesy of the Armed Forces Institute of Pathology.)

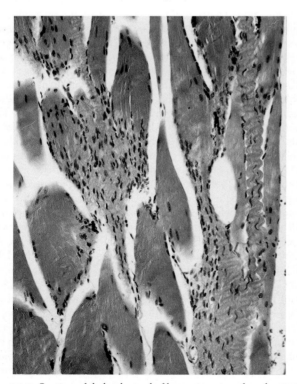

Fig. 24-2. Section of skeletal muscle fibers at a point of tendon insertion. Note the extensive fibrous tissue surrounding some of the fibers and the numerous internal nuclei. These changes may be mistaken for pathologic alterations. (Courtesy of the Armed Forces Institute of Pathology.)

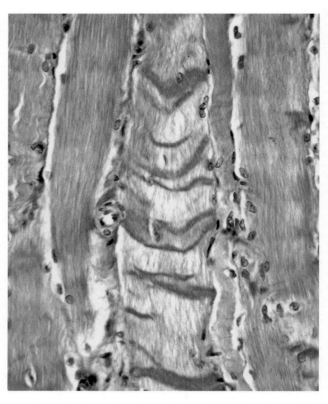

Fig. 24-3. Contraction artifact. Note the alternating dark (overly contracted) bands and pale areas. The myofibrils have been physically disrupted and have contracted into dense regions in the fiber. This artifact precludes meaningful evaluation of the architecture of the fiber and can be prevented by isometric fixation.

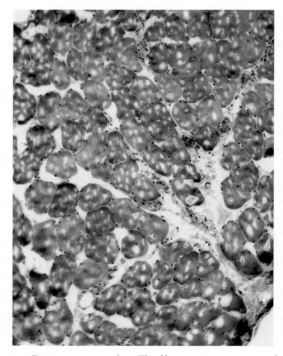

Fig. 24-4. Frozen section artifact. The fibers contain numerous "holes" caused by the development of large ice crystals due to slow freezing. (Courtesy of the Armed Forces Institute of Pathology.)

matched controls, are especially useful in the evaluation of muscle biopsies in pediatric patients. The second portion of the unclamped specimen is frozen directly in liquid nitrogen for specialized biochemical and molecular biologic studies. Frozen tissues may be stored in a deep freeze at – 70°C for extended periods and may yield important information as new molecular genetic methods become available.

NORMAL MUSCLE

Histology (Light and Electron Microscopy)

The earliest cell recognized as committed to develop into skeletal muscle is the myoblast, a proliferating cell containing intracytoplasmic myosin and actin filaments. Myoblasts soon acquire the capacity to fuse with one another forming primary myotubes, multinucleate cells with a roughly cylindrical configuration. As sarcomere structure develops peripherally, the nuclei are initially arranged internally about a myofibril-free zone. (Fig. 24-5). There is no further development until the muscle fiber becomes innervated by the terminus of a lower motor neuron. By the time the myotube is ready for innervation, the sarcolemma contains abundant, diffuse receptor protein for the neurotransmitter acetylcholine (ACh). This is the nicotinic acetylcholine receptor (AChR), and its presence seems necessary for the process of innervation. When the tip of the nerve fiber comes in contact with the muscle fiber, establishing

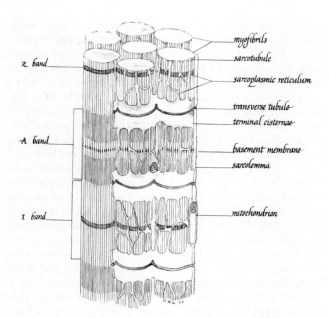

Fig. 24-6. Diagram of a portion of a skeletal muscle fiber. Note the arrangement of the sarcoplasmic reticulum and mitochondria (the membranous organelles) that surround the myofibrils. This network stains red with the modified Gomori trichrome stain, blue with Harris hematoxylin, and dark blue with the NADH-TR technique. The transverse tubular network, a continuation of the sarcolemma, is closely related to the dilated portion (cistern) of the sarcoplasmic reticulum. When isometrically fixed, the bands of the individual myofibrils are in register giving the entire muscle fiber its striated pattern.

a motor endplate, the receptor proteins become concentrated at the myoneural junction and disappear from the surface of the fiber elsewhere. It is possibly the disappearance of these extrajunctional receptors that prevents innervation of a fiber by more than one nerve terminal. Once innervated, the nuclei move to the periphery and the interior becomes packed with regular arrays of myofibrils as the myotube becomes a mature myofiber.

Mature striated muscle is composed of groups of fasciculi of longitudinally oriented muscle cells (fibers) (Fig. 24-6 and 24-7). Individual fibers run the length of the muscle from origin to insertion. Human myofibers vary considerably in length and diameter, depending on the position and function of the muscle, age, skill, and the state of exercise (e.g., extrinsic eye muscles 17.5 to 20 mm, gluteus 87.5 mm in diameter). Males tend to have larger fibers than females. The cross-sectional shape of the adult muscle fiber is polygonal. Infant and fetal muscles and extrinsic eye muscle outlines are rounder. Muscle fibers are multinucleated cells bounded by a cell membrane (sarcolemma) and a basement membrane (basal lamina). The cell membrane is smooth and of even density (300 to 400 nm). The basement membrane overlies the sarcolemma and is separated from it by a space ranging from 1,000 to 3,000 nm. Variability in thickness and regularity of this membrane and redundancy or reduplication of it are quite commonly seen both normally (e.g., contracted fiber) and in disease. The familiar striations of skeletal muscle, seen as alternating dark and light regions with phase contrast, polarized light, or interference mi-

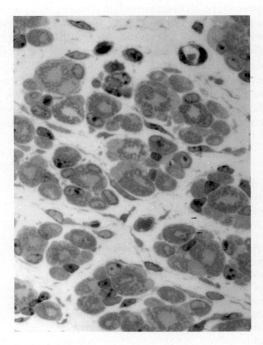

Fig. 24-5. Myotubes. Cross-section of developing skeletal muscle (mouse). Many of the fibers are at the myotube stage and are characterized by a pale homogeneous central zone or a single, central nucleus. The latter is relatively large and vesicular. The myofibrils are arranged around the periphery. (Courtesy of the Armed Forces Institute of Pathology.)

croscopy, are imparted by repeating units of interlaced, longitudinally directed, thin myofilaments and thick, dark myofilaments. The dark regions do not permit light to pass through them and are referred to as *anisotropic*, whereas the light regions do and are *isotropic*. The anisotropic region or A band is composed of myosin filaments alternating with actin filaments, whereas the isotropic region or I band contains only actin filaments. A narrow dark band, the Z disc (primarily alpha-actinin), bisects the I band and a narrow region of intermediate density, the H zone, composed of myosin filaments, bisects the A band (Figs. 24-7 and 24-8). A sarcomere is the distance between two Z discs; a myofibril is a longitudinally oriented cord of sarcomeres that runs the length of a fiber. The number of myofibrils in each fiber will vary considerably with the size of the fiber but on average runs in the hundreds. Each myofibril is 0.5 to 1.0 mm thick and separated from its neighbors by a loop of the T system, smooth endoplasmic (sarcoplasmic) reticulum, mitochondria, fat globules, and intervening unstructured myoglobin-containing cytoplasm. The T system is an invagination of the sarcolemmal membrane into the interior of the cell. In longitudinal sections it appears as a round or oval space bordered by a thick membrane. The T system runs parallel to the Z discs and is often seen beside the I band. It is accompanied by two cisterns of endoplasmic (sarcoplasmic) reticulum on either side. The profile of a centrally placed T tubule flanked by the two cisterns of sarcoplasmic reticulum is called a *triad*. The muscle fiber nuclei are in close proximity to the plasma membrane and separated from the underlying sarcomeres by mitochondria, fat globules, glycogen granules, smooth endoplasmic reticulum, and the Golgi apparatus. The nuclei are slender oval structures positioned beneath the sarcolemma and spaced about 10 to 50 mm apart. The chromatin is finely distributed and nucleoli are relatively inconspicuous except during active regeneration. Internalized nuclei are estimated to occur in no more than about 3 percent of normal adult fibers. Satellite cells, a reserve muscle cell population active in regeneration, occupy a position between the basement and plasma membranes and comprise about 4 to 10 percent of the nuclei seen in a biopsy specimen.

The Motor Unit, Muscle Fiber Types, and Histochemical Staining Methods

The functional unit of the neuromuscular system is the motor unit. Each motor unit consists of (1) a neuron located in the anterior horn of the spinal cord, or motor nucleus in the brain stem; (2) the axon of that neuron leaving the cord or stem, traversing the subarachnoid space, continuing on as the peripheral portion of the spinal or cranial nerve, terminating at the motor endplate, and (3) the muscle fibers it innervates. The number of muscle fibers within a motor unit (i.e., those innervated by the axon of a single motor neuron) vary from a few to many hundreds. Muscles with highly refined movements, like the extrinsic muscles of the eye, have a high neuron/muscle fiber ratio (1:10); those with relatively coarse and stereotyped movements, like the calf muscles, have a much lower ratio (1:2,000). These autonomous units can be called on to fire with increasing voluntary effort, thus explaining the gradation of power of a particular muscle.

The muscle fibers of any given motor unit can be identified by selected histochemical methods (see below) as belonging to either one of two prototypes: type 1 ("slow twitch") or type 2 ("fast twitch") myofibers. The type 1 fiber is concerned mainly with slow, sustained contractions and a slow twitch speed and is fatigue resistant. This type of fiber derives most of its energy from breakdown of lipid. Type 1 fibers are mitochondria- and oxidative enzyme-rich and glycogen- and glycolytic enzyme-poor. The type 2B fiber is concerned mainly with strong, short duration contractions; this type of fiber has a fast twitch speed, fatigues easily, and derives most of its energy from glycogen breakdown. Type 2B fibers are rich in glycolytic but poor in oxidative enzymes. A third fiber type (type 2A) shares characteristics with both type 1 and type 2B fibers. This fast twitch fiber is relatively fatigue resistant; it is well endowed with both glycolytic and oxidative enzyme systems. A fourth fiber type (2C) is believed to represent undifferentiated fibers and is seen in fetal tissue. These functional properties are listed in Table 24-1.

Although in some animals, entire muscles are composed of one or another fiber type, in the most commonly biopsied hu-

Fig. 24-7. **(A)** Diagram of a sarcomere. The Z disc is the most dense band and apparently is a continuation of the actin filaments. It bisects the lighter (isotropic) I band, which is mainly composed of actin filaments arranged in a hexagonal array. The dark A band (anisotropic) is composed of overlapping actin and myosin filaments, the latter situated within the hexagonal space formed by the former. In the central region of the A band, where there are no overlapping filaments, there is a lighter zone (H zone). In the center of the H zone, the myosin filaments are thickened, and there is apparent intermolecular bridging, which is a thin dark line called the M line. A sarcomere, the functional and structural unit of the myofibril, extends from one Z disc to the next. **(B)** Model of the molecular organization of the actin-dystrophin-dystroglycan-laminin axis. Dystrophin is drawn as a monomer with its amino terminus bound to cytoskeletal F-actin and its carboxy-terminus associated with membrane-bound dystroglycan. All known members of the dystroglycan, sarcoglycan, and syntrophin complexes are indicated although it is not proven that they all associate simultaneously with the same dystrophin molecule. The sarcoglycan complex copurifies with dystroglycan and dystrophin. When dystrophin is absent, dystroglycan is present, but the sarcoglycans are reduced or missing, suggesting that they may interact directly with dystrophin. The 25 kd species associates less tightly with the sarcoglycans and has not yet been named. Not all syntrophins may be present simultaneously in the same complex and both syntrophins and dystroglycan are found in tissues lacking dystrophin, suggesting that they also interact with other cytoskeletal elements. (Fig. B, data from Campbell,[46] Ozawa et al,[47] Worton,[48] and Ann and Kunkel.[49])

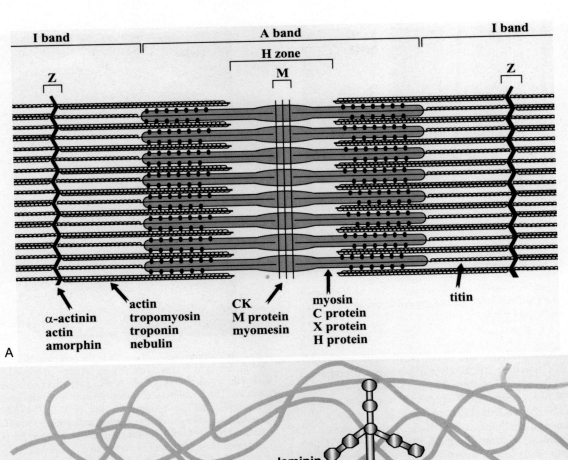

A

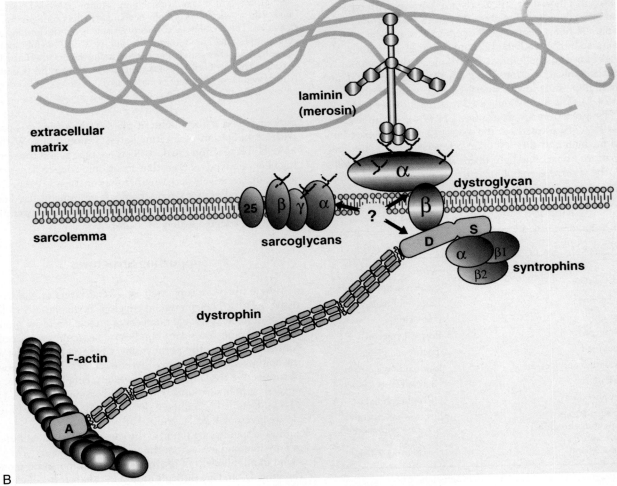

B

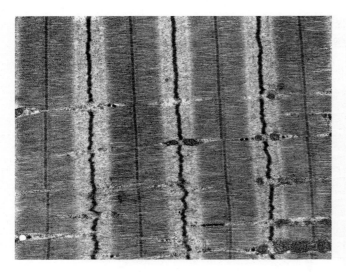

Fig. 24-8. Electron micrograph of a longitudinal section of skeletal muscle. Note the parallel arrangement of the myofibrils, so that the Z discs (dark) and A and I bands are in register.

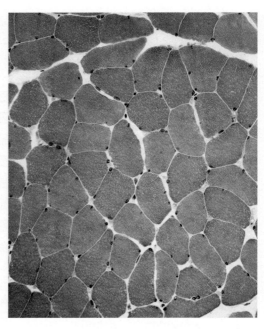

Fig. 24-9. Normal muscle fibers. Note the complete absence of shrinkage artifact, which is unavoidable in paraffin-embedded tissue. This makes the assessment of atrophy or changes in fiber configuration more accurate. The endomysial connective tissue is not discernible. Nuclei are peripheral. The intermyofibrillar network (membranous organelles), which is barely perceptible, stains blue with Harris hematoxylin. The myofibrils are pink. (Frozen section, H&E.) (Courtesy of the Armed Forces Institute of Pathology.)

man muscles both oxidative and glycolytic fibers are randomly distributed in a mosaic or "checkerboard" pattern, with types 1, 2A, and 2B each comprising about 30 percent of the total number of muscle fibers. Figure 24-9 demonstrates normal muscle fibers stained by the H&E method and Figure 24-10 with the alkaline ATPase histochemical technique. Other commonly used histochemical reactions bring out the fiber types and are extremely important in the interpretation of muscle biopsies (Table 24-2). The most widely used method for fiber typing is the ATPase reaction run at alkaline pH (9.4); in the reverse ATPase (RATPase) method, the sections are preincubated in an acid medium and this results in a reversal of the checkerboard pattern or dark and light fibers. If the preincubation is at pH 4.3, the reversal is complete, with the type 1 fibers staining

dark and type 2 fibers light; at pH 4.6, the reversal is partial, with a population of intermediate-staining fibers. With the NADH-TR reaction the dark fibers are type 1, and the remaining fibers are type 2. Fibers that are atrophic due to denervation are often excessively dark whether they are type 1 or type 2. Recently, procedures for typing the fibers in formalin-fixed paraffin-embedded tissue have been devised and these newer methods may be adopted widely in the future.[6]

Supporting Structures

Muscle fibers are supported by several layers of connective tissue sheaths. The epimysium envelops single muscles or large groups of fibers. Variable numbers of muscle fibers are grouped in primary and secondary bundles or fasciculi, enveloped by connective tissue, the perimysium, which is contiguous with the epimysium. The endomysium consists of a delicate network of connective tissue fibers, blood vessels, lymphatic tissue, and nerves, which surrounds the individual muscle fibers (Fig. 24-11). Detailed accounts of the microvascular supply of muscle are given by Kakulas and Adams.[4]

Muscle spindles are found at the edge of a fasciculus or on the perimysium and away from the tendinous insertions. They are found in all muscles but are more numerous in certain muscles (lumbricals) and are difficult to find in others (eye). Each limb muscle might contain as many as 100 of these structures, al-

Table 24-1. Muscle Fiber Types

Type I (37%)	Type II (63%)
Red	White
Sustained action	Sudden action
Weight-bearing	Purposeful motion
Slow twitch	Fast twitch
Soleus (pigeon)	Pectoral (pigeon)
Trichrome: red	Trichrome: green
High oxidative enzymes	Low oxidative enzymes
Low ATPase	High ATPase
Low phosphorylase	High phosphorylase
Electron microscopy	Electron microscopy
Many mitochondria	Few mitochondria
Abundant fat	Little fat
Wide Z band	Narrow Z band

Abbreviation: ATPase, adenosine triphosphatase.

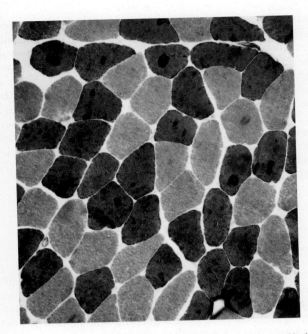

Fig. 24-10. Normal muscle fibers. The alkaline myosin myofibrillar ATPase stain is the basis for classifying fiber types. There is a crisp distinction between the dark (type 2) and light (type 1) fibers. This distinction is maintained even in advanced pathologic states of the fiber. The stain, done at an alkaline pH of 9.4, is deposited on the myofibrillar component of the fibers, in contrast to the NADH-TR reaction product, which is deposited on the membranous organelles. (Frozen section, ATPase.) (Courtesy of the Armed Forces Institute of Pathology.)

though not necessarily evenly distributed throughout the muscle. Spindles are fusiform structures varying in length from 0.5 to 3.0 mm. They are oriented parallel to the direction of the muscle fibers and attach at the poles to the aponeuroses and connective tissue sheaths surrounding the muscle fasciculi. The

Table 24-2. Histochemical Staining of Muscle Fibers

| | Fiber Type | | |
Stain	I	IIA	IIB
H&E	+ +	+	+
Trichrome	+ + +	+ +	+ +
ATPase, pH 9.4	+	+ + +	+ + +
ATPase, pH 4.6	+ + +	0	+ +
ATPase, pH 4.3	+ + +	0	0
NADH-TR	+ + +	+ +	+
Oil red O	+ +	+	+
PAS	+	+ + +	+ +
Phosphorylase	+	+ + +	+ + +

Abbreviations: H&E, hematoxylin and eosin; ATPase, adenosine triphosphatase; NADH-TR, nicotinamide adenine dinucleotide-tetrazolium reductase; PAS, periodic acid-Schiff.

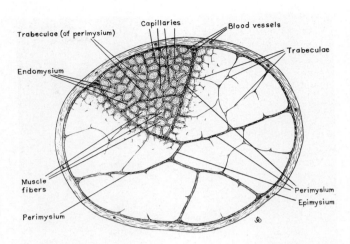

Fig. 24-11. Schematic diagram of the connective tissue sheaths of muscle.

normal muscle spindle has a very distinctive histologic appearance (Fig. 24-12). It is a rounded structure in cross section varying in diameter from 200 to 1,000 mm. The spindle contains easily distinguishable elements: a capsule, intrafusal muscle fibers, nerve fibers, specialized nerve endings, and blood vessels. The intrafusal fibers contained within the capsule (between 4 and 16) are structurally similar but not identical to fibers outside the spindle (extrafusal fibers). The intrafusal fibers are either nuclear bag fibers (20 to 30 mm in diameter) or nuclear chain fibers (4 to 8 mm in diameter). Both fibers are generally round in cross section and have unique histochemical reactions. The larger of the two, the nuclear bag fibers, contains a collection of nuclei at the equatorial zone of the fiber. Nuclear chain fibers have a row of internalized nuclei extending the length of the fiber. The muscle spindle capsule is a highly spe-

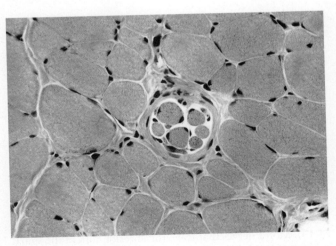

Fig. 24-12. Normal muscle spindle. Note the prominent multilayered capsule. Six intrafusal fibers are well visualized. The extrafusal fibers show some variability in size. The biopsy specimen was taken from an 11-year-old girl with neurogenic muscular atrophy. (Frozen section, H&E.)

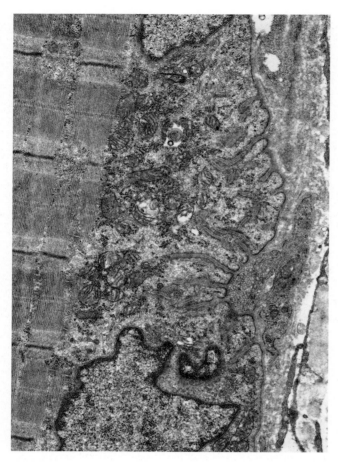

Fig. 24-13. Normal motor endplate (rat) (electron micrograph). Note the infolding of the sarcoplasmic membrane and the adjacent axon terminal with synaptic vesicles and mitochondria. (Courtesy of Dr. Richard Evans, Chief Medical Examiner, Commonwealth of Massachusetts.)

cialized structure containing several collagenous layers with intervening tight junctions that prevent the entrance of tracer substances applied to the surface of the spindle. The motor nerve supply is via the fusimotor system of efferents, and the afferent sensory fibers take origin from the primary (flower-spray) and secondary (annulospiral) endings. The function of spindles is sensory, responding to stretch in muscles and thus maintaining muscle tone.

The junction of nerve and muscle (motor endplate, neuromuscular junction [NMJ]) is difficult to recognize in ordinary H&E-stained paraffin-embedded sections. It generally appears as an aggregate of nuclei and nerve fibers on the surface of the muscle fiber. Special techniques utilizing intravital dyes, metallic impregnation, histo-/immunohistochemical reactions, or electron microscopy are required for their identification (Fig. 24-13). Motor nerves that leave the anterior horn of the spinal cord en route to skeletal muscles penetrate the connective tissue sheaths and subdivide into many branches until a single nerve fiber makes contact with a single muscle fiber. Occasionally, the same nerve fiber can be shown to give off two motor endplates to adjoining fibers. The myelin sheath of the motor

nerve fiber terminates in a series of folds, and beyond this point, for a distance of about 100 to 500 mm, the axon is covered only by a connective tissue sheath, which is then continuous with the endomysium. At the site of the motor end plate on the surface of the muscle fiber, the nerve splits in an elaborate terminal arborization to make synaptic contact with the muscle. Each of the terminal branches has an expansion that lies in a relatively elevated portion of the muscle fiber, in which the surface membrane thickens into a series of folds. The end portion of the axon—the axon terminal—contains synaptic vesicles and mitochondria. The space of the synaptic cleft is about 70 nm wide and is filled with fine granular material.

MOLECULAR STRUCTURE AND FUNCTION OF MUSCLE

Skeletal muscle is a highly organized and complex tissue with specialized molecular machinery for receipt of an excitatory stimulus from nerve, transmission of that stimulus to the contractile apparatus, and contraction and relaxation. The brief discussion that follows outlines the molecular basis for these functions with particular attention paid to components whose dysfunction results in some of the pathology described later in this chapter. A detailed treatment of these topics can be found in Engel and Franzini-Armstrong.[3]

Ion Channels and the Control of Excitation and Contraction

When a motor neuron fires, the action potential depolarizes the presynaptic nerve terminal causing voltage-dependent calcium channels to open allowing calcium to enter. In response, synaptic vesicles fuse with the presynaptic membrane releasing their ACh into the synaptic cleft. The ACh is bound by AChR on the muscle membrane causing them to open allowing sodium influx and potassium efflux. The sodium current predominates leading to depolarization of the muscle fiber creating an endplate potential. If threshold is reached, an action potential is produced, propagated along the myofiber membrane and down the T tubules, eventually transferring to the sarcomeric reticulum. One unique property of the sarcoplasmic reticulum is its ability to accumulate calcium and maintain very low intracellular concentrations of this ion. The wave of depolarization spreading down the T tubules alters calcium permeability in the sarcoplasmic reticulum, resulting in calcium release into the myofilamentous milieu. Contraction occurs and is followed a few milliseconds later by relaxation and ATP-dependent calcium reuptake by the sarcoplasmic reticulum. Several membrane-spanning ion channels are essential to the control of myofibrillar ion levels in the resting state and during depolarization.[7] There are at least four types of potassium channels in skeletal muscle with diverse roles.[8] Inward rectifiers modulate inward potassium current as the membrane potential changes relative to the potassium equilibrium potential and likely play a significant role in helping maintain the resting potential.[7,9] Voltage-dependent delayed rectifiers in surface membranes and T tubules are responsible for repolarization after the action potential by creating an outward potassium current.[8] There are also calcium-activated potassium channels that may regulate calcium entry or contribute to spike repolarization.[10] Finally, ATP-dependent potassium channels are blocked by high levels of ATP and may open during exercise, reducing excitability and forcing the muscle to rest.[11]

Chloride conductance is particularly high in skeletal muscle.[12,13] In fact, there are multiple types of chloride channels that together are responsible for 65 to 85 percent of the resting membrane conductance and help stabilize the transmembrane potential at resting values. Defects in this system result in hyperexcitability and myotonia as described later in this chapter. Transmission of an action potential along the muscle membrane and down the T tubules is primarily propagated by the rapid kinetics of voltage-dependent sodium channels.[14] Active channels create an inward sodium current depolarizing the membrane and opening more channels. This positive feedback loop, combined with fast activation kinetics, produces the rapid upstroke of an action potential and synchronizes calcium release from the sarcoplasmic reticulum. Defects in the adult muscle sodium channel alpha-subunit gene are responsible for several of the channelopathies discussed below. Excitation-contraction coupling at the T tubule/sarcoplasmic reticulum junctions (i.e., triads) is largely the role of dihydropyridine-sensitive calcium channels in the T tubules, which interact with ryanodine receptors in the sarcoplasmic reticulum.[15–17] The skeletal muscle L-type voltage-dependent calcium channel is a pentamer with alpha-1, alpha-2, beta, gamma, and delta subunits.[18] The alpha-1 subunit is the central component and contains binding sites for dihydropyridine, verapamil, and diltiazem. These dihydropyridine receptors are thought to function as voltage sensors for the transmission of the excitatory stimulus to the ryanodine receptor, which in turn releases calcium from the sarcoplasmic reticulum to the myofibrillar milieu.[19] The ryanodine receptor is a large protein of 564 k that forms an elaborate tetrameric structure in the junctional face membrane of the sarcoplasmic reticulum.[20] Repolarization of the myofiber membrane and T tubules results in closing of the ryanodine receptors. However, reuptake of calcium is an energy-dependent process mediated by a magnesium-calciumactivated ATPase, which hydrolyzes one molecule of ATP in the active transport of two calcium ions.[17] Mutations in the dihydropyridine-sensitive calcium channel and the ryanodine receptor are responsible for several of the channelopathies as well as central core disease (see below).

Myofibrillar Apparatus

Much is understood about the molecular structure and function of the myofibrillar apparatus. It has been known since 1954 that muscle contracts because the actin filaments slide between the myosin filaments. A number of other associated structural and regulatory proteins are present at the sarcomere to maintain the ordered myofibrillar array and coordinate contraction (Fig. 24-7). Myosin is a large hexameric structural protein that also has enzymatic activity (ATPase). The C-terminal halves of two heavy chains (MHC) are alpha-helical and twist around

each other to form a 155 nm long tail.[21–23] The N-termini form two globular heads in association with two light chain (MLC) polypeptides each. The tails are capable of self-association while the heads bind actin and contain ATPase activity. The myosin-containing thick filaments (in the A bands) interdigitate with thin filaments, which are made up of a double-strand helix of globular actin monomers (e.g., F actin).

Tropomyosin and troponin are two regulatory molecules closely associated with F actin. At rest, tropomyosin, which is a two-stranded, alpha-helical, coiled coil molecule, lies along the actin filament in a potential myosin-binding site, sterically inhibiting myosin-actin interactions. Troponin is a calcium-binding complex of three subunits, TN-I (inhibitory), TN-T (tropomyosin-binding), and TN-C (calcium-binding).[24] When muscle is stimulated, the intracellular concentration of calcium increases to a critical level and TN-C binds calcium releasing the inhibitory effect of TN-I. Tropomyosin moves into the groove between actin helices, and myosin binding sites are unmasked. Myosin heads then bind ATP, form cross bridges with actin, rotate (causing filament sliding and muscle shortening), and detach, releasing adenosine diphosphate (ADP) and phosphate. Although its function is well known, Z line structure is only poorly understood. Alpha-actinin, a 105 kd actin binding and cross-linking protein, is certainly the primary constituent where it is believed to anchor the overlapping ends of thin filaments through strong interactions with actin and nebulin.[25–27] Amorphin,[28] actin,[29] and desmin[30] are also components. Desmin and vimentin,[30–32] intermediate filaments, are present between adjacent Z lines where they are believed to link Z lines of adjacent myofibrils together helping maintain the lateral register of sarcomeres. Titin and nebulin are two extremely large structural proteins that may confer elasticity and maintain the ordered sarcomeric structure.[33] Titin (sometimes known as connectin) is an enormous (approximately 3,000 kd) elongated peptide that stretches from the Z line to the M line.[34–36] The I band portion is elastic and helps maintain the position of the thick filaments equidistant between Z lines. The A band portion is inelastic when bound with myosin and is considered an integral part of the thick filaments. At over 600 kd in size, nebulin also ranks as one of the largest known proteins. Nebulin has binding sites for both actin and alpha-actinin and is anchored at the Z lines where it may form a defined template for actin polymerization, thus regulating the length of thin filaments in skeletal muscle.[37]

The thick filaments contain a number of other proteins whose functions are less well defined. These include C, X, and H proteins,[38,39] which are detectable as stripes superimposed on the A bands. The M line also contains several additional peptides including creatine kinase,[40,41] M protein,[42,43] and myomesin.[44] The creatine kinase is important for resynthesizing ATP[45]; its release from injured muscle provides the basis for an important diagnostic test of muscle integrity. Although the structure and function of proteins of the myofibrillar apparatus is relatively well understood, their role in contributing to neuromuscular disease is less clear. An alpha-tropomyosin mutation was recently shown to cause one form of nemaline myopathy (see below) and mutations of cardiac-specific isoforms of MHC, troponin T, alpha-tropomyosin, and C protein have been implicated in inherited cardiomyopathies (see Ch. 31).

Membrane Cytoskeleton and the Extracellular Matrix

In mononuclear cells, the cytoskeleton functions to establish and maintain cell shape and control cell movement. Actin filaments, microtubules, and intermediate filaments (e.g., vimentin, cytokeratin, desmin, neurofilaments, and glial fibrillary acidic protein) make up the major classes of structural components, each with an attendant group of associated structural and regulatory partners. The membrane cytoskeleton serves to link the intracellular networks with transmembrane complexes that, in turn, provide direct connections with the extracellular matrix and extracellular contacts. If skeletal muscle is extracted with nonionic detergents and high concentrations of potassium-iodide, the membrane and contractile elements are removed leaving behind an insoluble skeleton of intermediate filaments. The primary constituent is desmin although vimentin may also be present.[32] The desmin distribution is circumferential around the Z lines, potentially serving to connect adjacent sarcomeres. Where Z lines abut the plasma membrane, desmin connections can be seen linking these two structures.

In skeletal muscle, the membrane cytoskeleton plays a critical role in maintenance of myofiber flexibility and integrity. In addition, transmembrane protein complexes provide important links between the intracellular force-generating myofibrillar apparatus and the extracellular matrix (Fig. 24-7). Indeed, when various components of this actin-dystrophin-dystroglycan/sarcoglycan-merosin axis are absent, the muscle undergoes dystrophic changes such as those seen in the dystrophinopathies, limb girdle dystrophies, and congenital muscular dystrophies[46–48] (see below). In mature myofibers, much of the cytoplasmic space is taken up with the contractile apparatus containing muscle-specific alpha-actin, but cytoskeletal actin isoforms are found in the subplasmalemmal network where they are associated with spectrin, dystrophin, and vinculin. Dystrophin is a 427 kd rod-shaped cytoskeletal protein with sequence similarities to the spectrins and alpha-actinin.[49,50] It is present in a subsarcolemmal network where the actin-binding amino-terminal domain creates a direct link with cytoskeletal actin.[51] The central rod domain contains 24 triple alpha-helical repeats that likely confer size and flexibility to the molecule. The carboxy terminus encodes two domains, D and S,[47] with which the dystroglycans, the syntrophins, and dystrobrevin interact. The syntrophin complex is a triplet of subsarcolemmal 59 kd proteins (alpha-, beta-1, and beta-2) whose functions are currently unknown.[52] The dystroglycans[53,54] are composed of two glycopeptides, alpha and beta, derived from the same gene. Beta-dystroglycan (43DAG) is a 43 kd transmembrane protein. Its cytoplasmic side is associated with dystrophin, whereas the extracellular side binds to alpha-dystroglycan (156DAG). Alpha-dystroglycan in turn binds the laminin alpha-2 chain or merosin,[55] thus completing the link between the intracellular cytoskeleton and the extracellular matrix. Dystrobrevin (AO) is a 94 kd dystrophin-related protein that copurifies with the syntrophins.[47,56] Also associated with beta-dystroglycan is the sarcoglycan complex composed of the transmembrane glycoproteins alpha-sarcoglycan (adhalin, 50DAG, A2, or SL50), beta-sarcoglycan (43DAG or A3b), gamma-sarcoglycan (35DAG or A4), and delta-sarcoglycan. This complex copurifies with the dystroglycans although the exact interactions are not known.[47] Finally, a 25 kd transmembrane protein, 25DAP or A5, also copurifies with the glycoprotein complex but its specific interactions and function are currently unknown.[47]

Costameres are sites on the myofiber plasma membrane where sarcomeric actin is anchored via the Z lines. Confocal immunofluorescence studies have demonstrated a costameric localization for dystrophin,[57] suggesting that the dystrophin complex may participate in linking the contractile apparatus to the extracellular matrix via these specialized structures. It remains to be seen if the syntrophins, sarcoglycans, and dystrobrevin have other structural and/or enzymatic activities. Additional associated proteins are likely to be identified in the future.

GENERAL REACTIONS OF SKELETAL MUSCLE

The general reactions of skeletal muscle to injury are discussed in detail in the monographs by Dubowitz,[2] Engel and Franzini-Armstrong,[3] and Kakulas and Adams.[4]

Atrophy and Hypertrophy

The term *atrophy* as applied to a muscle fiber refers to a reaction of the fiber characterized by a reduction in its girth. This may follow an abnormality involving its innervation (i.e., neurogenic atrophy) or may be the consequence of a primary disease of the muscle fiber itself. The most commonly encountered type of atrophy is neurogenic. Muscle fiber atrophy can also be observed as a result of immobilization, malnutrition, compression, aging, vascular insufficiency, and other mechanisms. Atrophic fibers are smaller than normal because the cytoplasmic contractile proteins are greatly reduced but the integrity of the cell and the cell membrane is preserved; as the cytoplasmic content is diminished, nuclei tend to pile up or line up in a chain. On transverse section the fiber may assume a roughly triangular (angulated) shape where the angles taper off acutely, sometimes partially encircling neighboring normal fibers and conforming to their shape.

In experimental animals, within the first 3 weeks following nerve section, there is about a two-thirds reduction of the average cross-sectional area of the fiber. In the same period of time, the decrease in volume is less pronounced with immobilization (bed confinement, bone fracture, and splinting, experimental tenotomy, upper motor neuron paralysis). The first fibers to atrophy in the early phases of immobilization and denervation are those fibers involved mainly in phasic movements (type 2B fibers histochemically). With the electron microscope one can observe a reduction in the number of myofibrils beginning at the periphery of the fiber. The nuclei are unremarkable, and sarcotubular profiles and mitochondria increase in density. The sarcolemma remains intact but there is duplication and thickening of the basal lamina. In chronic conditions the normal sarcomeric organization is eventually unrecognizable and all that remains are aggregates of haphazardly oriented "units" composed of thickened Z lines from which emanate filaments of variable thickness interspersed with loose myofilaments. Cell death and ingrowth of connective/adipose tissue ensues in the terminal stages. This histologic picture is referred to as *end-stage* muscle injury and marks the terminal phase of muscle disease be it neuropathic or myopathic. The distribution of atrophic fibers in relation to normal ones, and the histochemical characteristics of the affected fibers are important considerations in evaluating muscle atrophy due to denervation (see below). Muscle fiber atrophy can also occur in myopathic injury both in hereditary myopathies and in inflammatory myopathies; here the fibers are smaller than normal but retain either a polygonal or rounded contour.

Hypertrophied fibers are larger than normal, although well proportioned in terms of shape and constituent organelles (Fig. 24-14). They may develop as a consequence of excessive work demands or as a consequence of faulty reinnervation. Work hypertrophy of muscle is the basis for increase in muscle bulk in some athletes. The volumetric enlargement of the fiber is due to an increase in the number of myofibrils. The stimulus for this work-induced hypertrophy is presumably neurogenic, as repetitive firing of motor units induces the muscle to do more work. Experimental studies on compensatory hypertrophy induced by tenotomizing the synergist of a muscle have demonstrated vol-umetric fiber enlargement following denervation of the synergist. In pathologic states hypertrophy of muscle fibers occurs in both myopathies (e.g., dystrophinopathies) or following denervation (e.g., spinal muscular atrophy).

Especially in children, precise assessment of the extent and significance of variability of muscle size, whether atrophy or hypertrophy, requires computer-assisted morphometric study with matched controls (for a given age, sex, muscle).

Necrosis and Regeneration

An important category of myocyte injury deals with those changes associated with destruction of segments of the fiber and regeneration or death and phagocytosis of the cell in its entirety (Fig. 24-15). The early phases of this type of injury can be distinguished histologically from the cellular atrophies just described. The severity of the insult and the efficacy of the regenerative response will determine the potential for functional restoration of the muscle. As in other tissues, the major stumbling blocks in the accurate identification of acute injury are the difficulties in distinguishing surgical, postmortem, or preparative artifact from disease. Indeed, the borderline between very acute injury and artifact may be blurred. Muscle fibers may be destroyed massively as can be seen in instances of extensive trauma, ischemia, exposure to toxic chemicals, radiation injury, or invasion by microorganisms. By contrast, there are other circumstances wherein muscle fibers may be affected to a very slight extent, focally or segmentally. Segmental necrosis is found in myopathies due to vascular immunologic factors. The affected fiber shows focal loss of cross-striations for a relatively short segment along the length of a fiber where the nor-

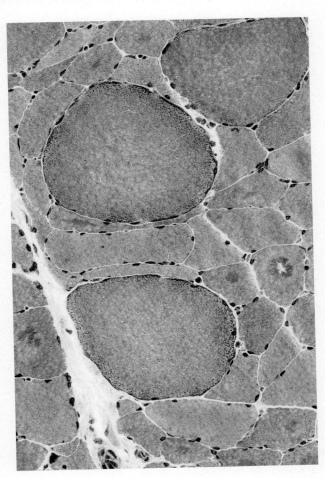

Fig. 24-14. Hypertrophy. Note the presence of three very large fibers. (Frozen section, MGT.)

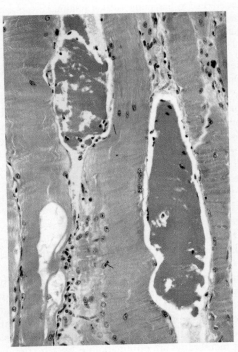

Fig. 24-15. Degeneration. Two fibers demonstrate hyaline degeneration, vacuolization, and fragmentation. (Paraffin section, H&E.)

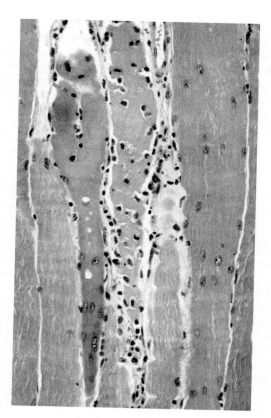

Fig. 24-16. Regenerating and degenerating muscle fibers. Note two abnormal fibers in the center of the field. The right one is a degenerating fiber characterized by fragmentation and disintegration of the sarcoplasm and invasion by macrophages. The left one is a regenerating fiber characterized by basophilic (darker staining) cytoplasm and large internalized nuclei with prominent nucleoli. The biopsy was taken from a patient with polymyositis. (Paraffin section, H&E.)

mal fiber is replaced by a smudge of hyalinized, somewhat darker-staining material. There may be bulging of the cell at this site or irregular shrinkage of its diameter. The subsarcolemmal myofibrils are damaged preferentially and the sarcolemma may rupture, resulting in extrusion of portions of the sarcoplasm. At the same time, neighboring nuclei become pyknotic or disappear. Eventually, phagocytes are seen within the necrotic segments and regeneration follows.

The regenerating portion of the fiber has a number of distinctive features (Fig. 24-16). As visualized on H&E the cytoplasm is light blue and the affected portion of the fiber is somewhat narrower than normal, the cross-striations are not apparent, and there is an increase in the size of the nuclei, which also appear larger, vesiculated, and more numerous and contain one or more large nucleoli. Fibers sometimes take on the appearance of multinucleated cells or giant cells. Fusion between basophilic regenerating fibers and normal fibers is not infrequent. Ultrastructurally, regeneration can be recognized by the demonstration of large nuclei and nucleoli, sometimes occupying an internal position within the fiber. The plasma and basement membranes are unremarkable, and the number of organelles is not different from normal, except perhaps for an increased number of free ribosomes. The most striking cellular al-

terations in regeneration are found in the contractile system. There may be large areas of the fiber in which the filaments are poorly organized into myofibrils, although these may be oriented in parallel. The phenomenon of "fiber splitting," which describes the light microscopic appearance of a muscle fiber in cross-section that shows one or more lengthwise "cracks," is seen especially in muscular dystrophy often in the context of fiber regeneration.[58]

MUSCLE DISEASES

The classification of muscle diseases followed below is presented in Table 24-3.

Neurogenic Atrophy

The term *neurogenic atrophy* refers to those morphologic changes occurring in muscle that result from interruption of its normal innervation (i.e., denervation). These changes can be a reflection of disease involving the lower motor neuron anywhere along its course, ranging from abnormalities affecting the

Table 24-3. Classification of Muscle Diseases

Neurogenic atrophy
Muscular dystrophy
    Dystrophinopathies
        Duchenne muscular dystrophy
        Becker muscular dystrophy
    Nondystrophinopathies
        Facioscapulohumeral muscular dystrophy
        Limb-girdle syndromes
        Emery-Dreifuss muscular dystrophy
        Congenital muscular dystrophy (and Fukuyama type)
        Myotonic dystrophy
        Extraocular muscle-specific dystrophy
Inflammatory myopathy
    Idiopathic polymyositis or dermatomyositis
    Inclusion body myositis
    Granulomatous myositis
    Infectious myositis
Ischemia
Trauma
Congenital myopathy
    Central core disease
    Nemaline myopathy
    Centronuclear (myotubular) myopathy
    Congenital fiber type disproportion
    Other congenital myopathies
Glycogenoses
Endocrine myopathy
Mitochondrial myopathy
Lipid myopathy
Channelopathy
Toxic myopathy
Disorders of the neuromuscular junction

anterior horn cell, such as amyotrophic lateral sclerosis (ALS) or poliomyelitis, to disorders of the axonal processes, as observed in anterior root disease and peripheral neuropathy.

Clinical and Pathologic Manifestations

Clinically, muscles damaged by neurogenic disease are weaker and thinner than normal. Deep tendon reflexes gradually diminish as the disease progresses. In general, neurogenic atrophy tends to involve the distal musculature before the proximal, in contrast to many of the myopathic disorders, such as polymyositis or muscular dystrophy, in which the proximal muscles are more severely affected early in the course of the disease. The histologic appearance of denervated muscle although distinctive, generally does not allow for discrimination between the many denervating diseases. For example, denervation atrophy observed in a muscle biopsy from a patient with ALS cannot reliably be distinguished from that seen in a peripheral neuropathy. Correlation of the histopathologic changes observed in the muscle with the clinical and laboratory findings is therefore necessary so as to put the morphologic changes in proper perspective.

Myofiber Atrophy

The principal morphologic response of the muscle to denervation is atrophy of individual myofibers. The involved fibers become progressively smaller and assume a characteristic angular, sharply contoured shape (Fig. 24-17). These configurational changes are thought to be largely the result of distortion of the atrophic fibers by the surrounding normal fibers. As fiber atrophy progresses, the amount of cytoplasm shrinks to the point where only small aggregates or clumps of pyknotic nuclei are

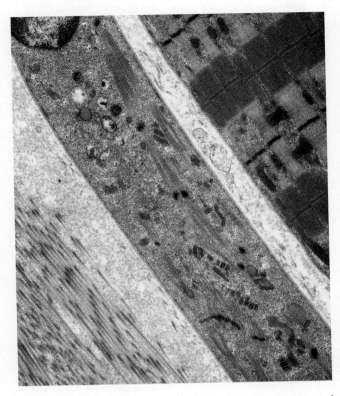

Fig. 24-18. Denervation atrophy. An atrophic fiber is next to a normal fiber. Note the loss of normal sarcomere structure. Disorganized myofibrils and organelles are present in the cytoplasm. The sarcolemmal and basement membranes are intact.

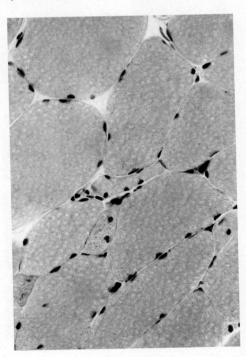

Fig. 24-17. Denervation atrophy. Note the two small angulated fibers in the center of the field. (Frozen section, H&E.)

visible by light microscopy. On electron microscopy, denervated fibers show loss of myofibrils beginning at the periphery of the fiber (Fig. 24-18). With time, there is gradual dissolution of both thick and thin myofilaments and smearing of the Z lines. The sarcolemma becomes wrinkled and the basement membrane is thrown into redundant folds. In the early stages of denervation, when only a few anterior horn cells or axons may be involved by disease, the atrophic fibers are distributed more or less randomly throughout the muscle. With progression of the disease, the atrophic fibers tend to cluster in small groups— "group atrophy" (Fig. 24-19). With histochemical staining using the myofibrillar ATPase reactions, the angular atrophic fibers are both type 1 and type 2 (Fig. 24-20). Another characteristic histochemical feature of denervation is that, with an oxidative enzyme stain such as NADH-TR or the nonspecific esterase reaction, virtually all the atrophic fibers tend to stain quite darkly regardless of their fiber type (Fig. 24-21).

Reinnervation

Denervated fibers acquire the ability to synthesize extrajunctional ACh receptor along the sarcoplasmic membrane, analogous to the myotube stage of embryonic muscle. Coincident with this, adjacent intramuscular nerve twigs are stimulated to initiate collateral sprouting. By this process, previously dener-

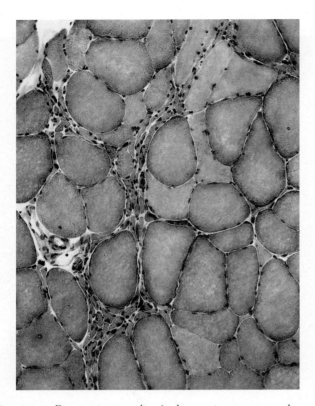

Fig. 24-19. Denervation atrophy. As denervation progresses, the angular fibers appear in groups. There are pyknotic nuclear clumps among them, and many of the surrounding fibers have undergone hypertrophy. Some of the latter have internal nuclei. (Frozen section, H&E.) (Courtesy of the Armed Forces Institute of Pathology.)

vated fibers may become reinnervated. The reinnervated muscle fibers, however, will assume the fiber type of their new innervation. This will eventually lead to loss of the normal random histochemical checkerboard pattern, with the formation of small or large groups of contiguous fibers having the same histochemical fiber type. The process is referred to as fiber type grouping and is virtually pathognomonic of reinnervation, hence denervation (Fig. 24-22). At least 15 or more contiguous fibers of the same histochemical type should be present for the recognition of definitive fiber type grouping. Also, ideally, groups composed of both major types should be seen, so that type grouping due to reinnervation may be distinguished from fiber type predominance. In some chronic, slowly progressive denervating conditions (e.g., spinal muscular atrophy) or in patients who have suffered an acute episode of injury to the motor neurons in the remote past (e.g., in old poliomyelitis), reinnervation keeps close pace with denervation, resulting in a muscle that may appear essentially normal on H&E-stained sections. It follows that fiber type grouping (thus reinnervation) can only be reliably detected with histochemical techniques. If the denervating process is relentlessly progressive, the pace of denervation will exceed that of reinnervation, leading to atrophy of the enlarged previously reinnervated motor units with resultant type-specific group atrophy. This entire process is depicted schematically in Figure 24-23.

Target Fibers

Another morphologic change that may be observed in approximately 30 to 40 percent of cases of denervation is the target fiber.[59] This change affects predominantly type 1 fibers, and is best recognized in frozen sections stained for an oxidative enzyme such as NADH-TR. The affected fibers show a central area of diminished or absent enzyme activity surrounded by a narrow intermediate zone of increased activity, which is in turn surrounded by normally stained sarcoplasm. The combined effect of these zones of variable oxidative enzyme staining results in a characteristic bullseye appearance (Fig. 24-24). On electron microscopy, the target fiber shows a central area of clearing of membranous organelles including mitochondria, surrounded by a ring of condensed sarcoplasmic reticulum and mitochondria. In the central zone, the myofibrils may be preserved initially but will eventually degenerate. When the latter occurs, the target fiber may then be recognized by light microscopy with other staining methods (H&E, Masson trichrome, ATPase). Target fibers are generally considered to be a manifestation of neurogenic disease. Sometimes muscle fibers may be observed that have an appearance similar to that of target fibers but that lack the intermediate zone of increased oxidative enzymatic activity. These are known as *targetoid fibers*. Targetoid fibers can also be seen in denervation but they are not specific for neurogenic disease.

Myopathic Changes

In some long-standing denervative disorders, such as Charcot-Marie-Tooth disease, spinal muscular atrophy, and radicu-

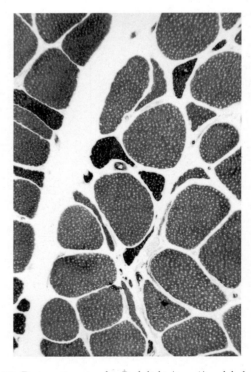

Fig. 24-20. Denervation atrophy. Both light (type 1) and dark (type 2) small angulated fibers are seen randomly dispersed throughout the field. (Frozen section, ATPase pH 9.4.)

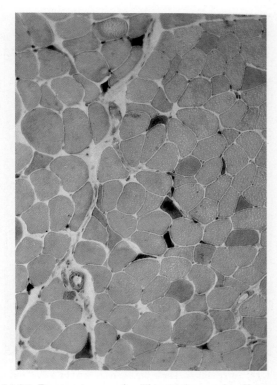

Fig. 24-21. Denervation atrophy. The angular atrophic fibers are excessively stained, a feature suggestive of denervation atrophy. The small, dark, oval structures are pyknotic nuclear clumps, representing a late stage of atrophy. Pyknotic nuclear clumps are the end stage of fiber atrophy due to many causes and are not specific for denervation. (Frozen section, esterase.) (Courtesy of the Armed Forces Institute of Pathology.)

lopathies, the affected muscles may show, in addition to the typical histologic features of neurogenic atrophy, changes that may be described as myopathic in nature, such as increased numbers of internal nuclei, fiber splitting, focal necrosis, regeneration, and mild interstitial inflammation.[60] These so-called secondary myopathic changes may be reflected clinically by the presence of mild elevations of serum creatine kinase (CK).

Hereditary Spinal Muscular Atrophies

An important group of denervation atrophies that have a somewhat different range of morphologic abnormalities from the rest of the denervation atrophies are the hereditary spinal muscular atrophies (SMA).[61] These include the acute form Werdnig-Hoffmann disease (SMA 1), the intermediate form or chronic Werdnig-Hoffmann (SMA 2), and Kugelberg-Welander disease (SMA 3).

Clinical Presentation

The clinical presentation of the most severe type of SMA 1 is that of a child who presents soon after birth with hypotonia, generalized weakness, and respiratory difficulties or alternately, the infant may be normal at birth but by 3 to 6 months of age develops increasing feeding difficulties and fails to develop the

expected motor milestones. On physical examination the legs are flexed at the knee ("frog leg" position) and the arms are externally rotated, abducted, and flexed at the elbow. The extraocular muscles are not affected but the muscles of deglutition and respiration often are involved. Sensory function is preserved. Death occurs by 2 to 3 years of age, due to respiratory failure and pulmonary infection. SMA 2 begins between 6 and 18 months of age. Although the child never gains the ability to bear weight on the legs or walk unaided, independent sitting is achieved. The disease is generally slowly progressive with the development of skeletal deformities and joint contractures. The cause of death is respiratory insufficiency.

In SMA 3 the clinical course is very slowly progressive with onset of proximal weakness of the legs and then of the shoulders and arms between 5 and 15 years of age after independent ambulation has been achieved. The typical muscle biopsy findings of SMA 1, and to a large extent SMA 2, consist of panfascicular atrophy of some muscle fibers groups and hypertrophy of others, sometimes with intermixing of bundles of hypertrophic and atrophic fibers (Figs. 24-25 and 24-26). The atrophic fibers are of both fiber types whereas the hypertrophic ones are largely type 1 fibers; in some cases fiber typing is weak and it is not easy to discriminate the two fiber types. The abnormally small or large fibers retain a rounded contour and internalized nuclei or

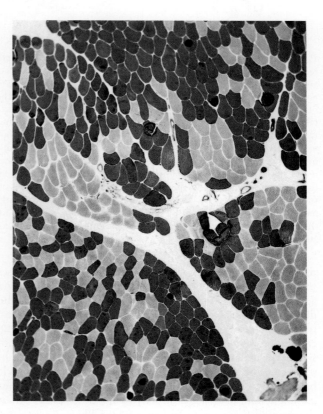

Fig. 24-22. Type grouping. Note the loss of the normal checkerboard pattern. Groups of contiguous fibers are of the same histochemical type. This may be the only sign of a neuropathic process and represents reinnervation. (Frozen section, ATPase.) (Courtesy of the Armed Forces Institute of Pathology.)

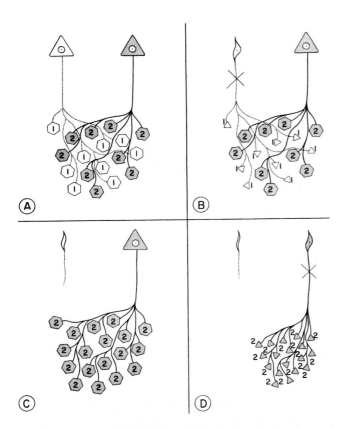

Fig. 24-23. Schematic illustration of the process of denervation and reinnervation. **(A)** Normal. The light motor unit is composed of the anterior horn cell, nerve fibers, and the randomly distributed hexagonal muscle fibers labeled 1. The dark motor unit comprises the muscle fibers labeled 2. This accounts for the normal checkerboard pattern. **(B)** Random fiber atrophy. The muscle fibers of the light motor unit (triangles) have become atrophic because of interruption of their normal innervation. **(C)** Fiber type grouping. Through collateral sprouting, the previously denervated muscle fibers of the light motor unit are reinnervated by the dark motor unit. The atrophic fibers have regained their normal proportions but now have the histochemical properties of the dark motor unit. **(D)** Type-specific group atrophy. As the dark motor unit becomes affected by disease, all the fibers belonging to that unit (including those previously reinnervated) undergo atrophy.

myopathic changes are not observed. As the disease progresses there is replacement of damaged muscle cells with fibrous and adipose tissue. In the early stages of the disease it may be quite difficult to make the diagnosis histologically in spite of clinical neurologic impairment. Furthermore, there is remarkably little correlation between the degree of clinical severity and prognosis and the extent of muscle atrophy in an individual case.[60] In some cases of the Kugelberg-Welander syndrome the muscle biopsy shows random fiber or group atrophy that is indistinguishable from neurogenic atrophy of any other cause; others show rounded atrophic and hypertrophic fibers, internalized nuclei, and increased endomysial connective tissue.

Mode of Inherited Transmission
SMA is an autosomal recessive disease with an incidence of 1 in 200,000 live births with a carrier frequency of 1 in 60 to 80.

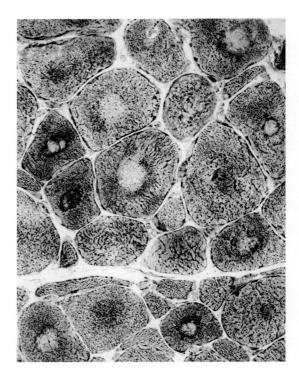

Fig. 24-24. Target fibers. These are characterized by a clearing of the membranous organelles from the central portion of the fibers. The NADH-TR stain will show the structure most consistently. They are characteristic of denervation and occur in type 1 fibers. (Frozen section, NADH-TR.) (Courtesy of the Armed Forces Institute of Pathology.)

Carriers are phenotypically normal. In some countries with a high rate of consanguinity, the disease incidence is at least 40-fold greater. In 1990 the genetic abnormality responsible for SMA was localized to chromosome 5q11.2-13.3. The genes for all three types of childhood SMA are linked to the same locus in a number of studies, indicating phenotypic heterogeneity with genetic homogeneity similar to that observed in Duchenne/Becker muscular dystrophy.[63] Analysis of 5q-linked SMA families supports the view that, with certain exceptions, there is little intrafamilial phenotypic variability. If the index patient satisfies the diagnostic criteria noted above, over 90 percent of all SMA families currently appear to be linked to chromosome 5q markers; the proportion of SMA 1 families linked to 5q11.2-13.1 is higher and may approach 100 percent. The probable SMA-determining gene (termed the *survival motor neuron* [SMN] gene) has been identified. Mutation analysis of SMN in 229 patients with 5q SMA (types 1,2 and 3)[64] revealed homozygous deletions in 226, while the other 3 had one deleted allele and one allele with a point mutation or other small mutation Simple polymerase chain reaction (PCR) tests are now available for identification of SMN gene deletions, allowing rapid confirmation of the diagnosis.[65,66] The function of the gene product is not yet known, but it is expressed in a wide variety of tissues, including spinal cord. No phenotype-genotype correlation between the gene defect and the type of SMA was detected, although deletions of contiguous segments of DNA appeared to be more frequent in type 1 than in type 2 pa-

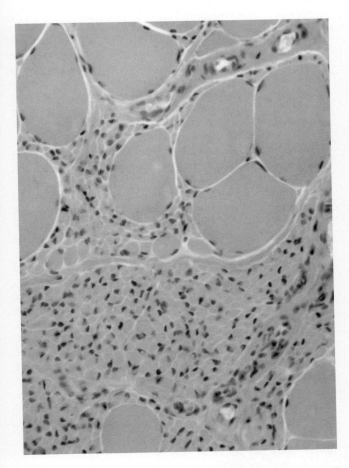

Fig. 24-25. Werdnig-Hoffmann disease. There are groups of small, rounded atrophic fibers; normal-sized fibers; and clusters of fibers that are markedly hypertrophied. (Frozen section, H&E.) (Courtesy of Dr. T.W. Smith, University of Massachusetts Medical School, Worcester, MA.)

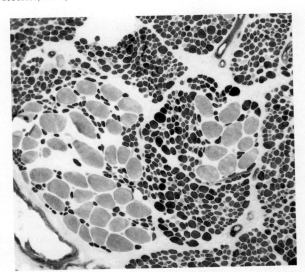

Fig. 24-26. Werdnig-Hoffmann disease. The normal and atrophic fibers are types 1 and 2. The hypertrophied fibers are characteristically type 1. (Frozen section, ATPase.) (Courtesy of the Armed Forces Institute of Pathology.)

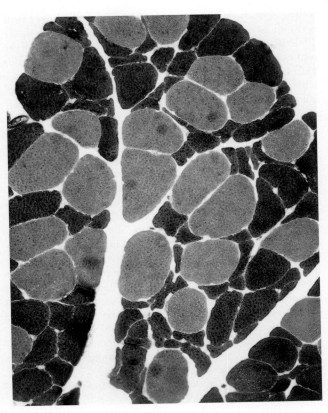

Fig. 24-27. Type 2 atrophy. Note that the type 1 fibers are not atrophic, and that all the small angular fibers are type 2. The atrophic fibers are not excessively dark with the NADH-TR and esterase reactions. This pattern, without histochemical studies, is often mistaken for denervation. (Frozen section, ATPase pH 9.4.) (Courtesy of the Armed Forces Institute of Pathology.)

tients. The SMN gene region is unstable and contains a number of other genes and it remains to be seen if any of these contribute to the pathology of SMA.

Diagnosis

The diagnosis of early neurogenic atrophy requires the demonstration of both type 1 and type 2 atrophy. Atrophy of type 2B is nonspecific and commonly seen in muscle biopsies (Fig. 24-27); it tends to be associated with long-term immobilization or steroid treatment.

Muscular Dystrophy

Muscular dystrophy is a generic term that refers to a large category of hereditary diseases of muscle, often beginning in childhood, with a variable rate of progression, clinical picture, and molecular genetic mechanisms of injury.[48]

Dystrophinopathies

The dystrophinopathies include cases of Duchenne muscular dystrophy (DMD) and Becker muscular dystrophy (BMD) as well as individuals with atypical mild forms of BMD.[67–69] DMD is the more common of the two conditions, occurring in 1 of 3,500 live male births; approximately one-third of cases represent new mutations. This X-linked condition was described by Duchenne and others.[70–73] There have been rare reports of DMD in girls with Turner or Turner mosaic syndromes or X-autosomal translocations. The disorder becomes clinically manifest by the age of 5, progressing relentlessly until death in the early 20s.[74] Boys with DMD are normal at birth and early motor milestones are met on time. Walking, however, is often delayed and the first indications of muscle weakness are clumsiness and inability to keep up with peers. Weakness begins in the pelvic girdle muscles and then extends to the shoulder girdle. Pseudohypertrophy of the calf muscles is an important clinical finding (Fig. 24-28A). The abnormally large muscle bulk is caused initially by an increase in the size of the muscle fibers and then, as the muscle atrophies, by an increase in fat and connective tissue. Myocardial involvement is common, often presenting as a dilated cardiomyopathy. Serum enzyme levels indicative of muscle destruction (e.g., CK) are always extremely elevated during the first decade of life but may decline to the normal range as muscle bulk diminishes in the later stages of the disease. Death results from respiratory insufficiency, pulmonary infection, and/or cardiac decompensation. Many patients have an associated static encephalopathy manifest as mild to moderate mental retardation.[75]

BMD has a lower incidence (1 of 30,000 male births), gener-ally presents later in childhood, and has a more protracted and/or variable course than does DMD.[76] Most affected boys run well as children and generally remain ambulatory until the second to fourth decade. One hallmark of family histories is that affected males never pass the disease to their sons, although their daughters are carriers and may pass the disease to their grandsons. The histopathologic alterations in DMD are distinctive and generally typify the muscle changes in the dystrophies as a group. Abnormalities include (1) variability in range in the cross-sectional fiber diameter (due to the presence of both small and giant fibers) and fiber splitting (Fig. 24-28B); (2) internalization of subsarcolemmal nuclei (beyond the normal range of 3 to 5 percent); (3) degeneration, necrosis, and phagocytosis of muscle fibers (Fig. 24-29A); (4) regeneration of muscle fibers; and (5) proliferation of endomysial connective tissue. One additional feature, which is said to be especially characteristic of Duchenne dystrophy, is the presence of enlarged, rounded, hyaline fibers that have lost their normal cross-striations ("hyaline fibers," "hypercontracted fibers"). Muscle spindles are relatively preserved until the end.[77] Fiber typing utilizing histochemical stains shows either type 1 fiber predominance or, more often, no alterations in the proportion and distribution of fiber types. Fibers sometimes cannot be typed. Immunohistochemistry with antibodies directed against the dystrophin protein (rod domain, carboxyl terminus, and amino terminus) fails to demonstrate immunoreactivity in the subsarcolemmal region of muscle fibers from patients with

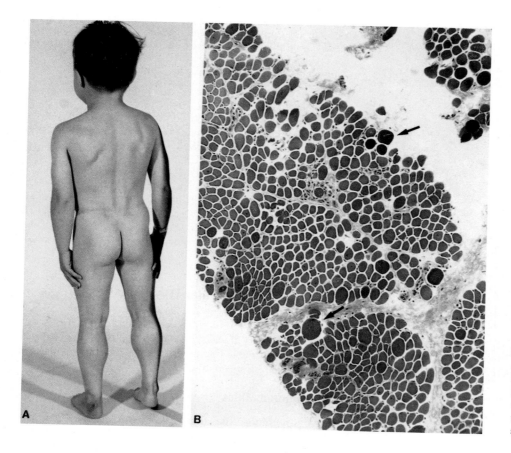

Fig. 24-28. (A) Duchenne muscular dystrophy. Note enlargement (pseudohypertrophy) of the calf muscles. (B) Duchenne muscular dystrophy. Note variation in fiber size and enlarged round hyaline fibers (arrows). (Frozen section, H&E.)

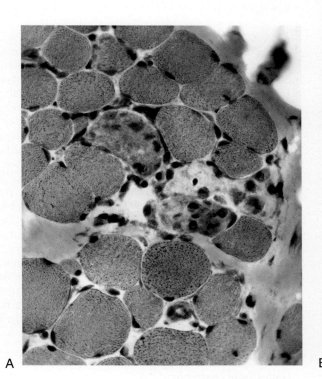

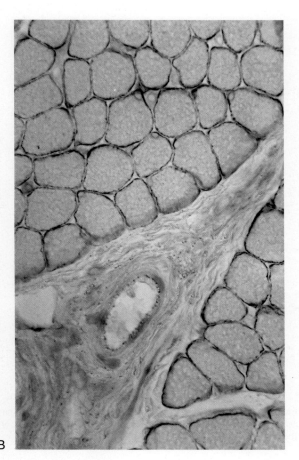

Fig. 24-29. Duchenne muscular dystrophy: **(A)** Several fibers are degenerating and undergoing phagocytosis. There is beginning endomysial fibrosis. (Frozen section, MGT.) (Courtesy of the Armed Forces Institute of Pathology.) **(B)** Normal muscle showing dystrophin immunoreactivity indicated as dark outline of sarcolemma; immunoreactivity is absent in Duchenne muscular dystrophy. (Frozen section dystrophin immunoperoxidase.)

DMD (Fig. 24-29B). Electron microscopic study shows muscle fibers in various stages of degeneration and regeneration but is generally of little diagnostic value (Fig. 24-30). In later stages of the disorder, the muscles eventually become almost totally replaced by adipose and connective tissue. At this point, the histologic picture is indistinguishable from the end stage of other severe myopathies, such as polymyositis, or neurogenic atrophy. Cardiac involvement, which may lead to arrhythmias and occasionally to congestive heart failure, consists of nonspecific interstitial fibrosis, more prominent in the epimyocardial portion of the left ventricle.[78]

In BMD the muscle biopsy findings observed in routine preparations are similar, although often less severe than those seen in DMD. The large hyalinized fibers seen in DMD are infrequent.[79] Later in the course, signs of chronic myopathy, such as fiber splitting and endomysial fibrosis supervene. Bradley and co-authors[80] have described modest neurogenic changes, such as angulated atrophic fibers, nuclear clumps, and mild fiber type grouping. Histochemical staining generally shows better fiber type differentiation; type 2B fibers, which may not be demonstrable in DMD, are usually not deficient in BMD. Immunohistochemical staining with antibodies directed to dystrophin (especially those against the carboxyl terminus) reveals patchy positivity in the subsarcolemmal region; however, Western blot analysis of dystrophin is a more sensitive test.[67]

Recent research developments have elucidated the genetic and biochemical basis of DMD/BMD, establishing the allelic nature of the two disorders.[46,50,81–84] The responsible gene is located on the Xp21 region of the X chromosome and spans more than 2 million base pairs. It includes more than 79 exons and encodes the 427 kd protein dystrophin.[49] It is the large size of the DMD/BMD gene that accounts for the high rate of spontaneous mutation. The dystrophin protein represents 0.01 percent of skeletal muscle protein but it comprises fully 2 percent of total sarcolemmal protein.[85] Its tissue distribution (skeletal, smooth and cardiac muscle, and brain) correlates well with the known clinical features of DMD/BMD. Most (65 to 75 percent) affected DMD/BMD boys have demonstrable mutations (deletions or duplications) of one or more exons. Mutations that disrupt the translational reading frame or the promoter result in an

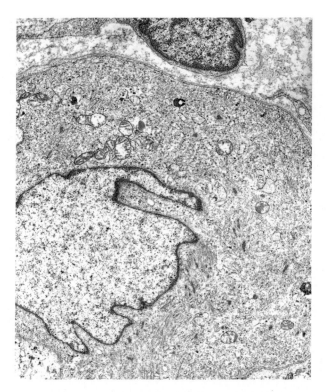

Fig. 24-30. Duchenne muscular dystrophy (electron micrograph). Dystrophic fiber showing complete dissolution of the normal myofibrillar structure. The basement membrane and sarcolemmal membranes of this fiber are intact.

absent or truncated and presumable unstable protein correlating with the severe DMD phenotype. By contrast, mutations that do not disrupt the translational reading frame or the promoters yield a lower molecular weight and semifunctional dystrophin, correlating with the less severe BMD phenotype. The dystrophin test (dystrophin immunoblotting) provides definitive biochemical diagnosis.[50] In addition, dystrophin testing permits prediction of the severity of the phenotype in early or preclinical cases (i.e., the relative absence of dystrophin predicts the severe DMD course), whereas dystrophin of abnormal size/quantity predicts the more benign BMD. Dystrophin immunohistochemistry of muscle tissue is a useful means of carrier detection (for the purpose of genetic counseling or establishing the diagnosis of manifest carrier) for a woman whose family does not have a demonstrable deletion recognized by direct DNA analysis or a pedigree suitable for restriction fragment length polymorphism (RFLP) analysis. Because of lyonization (inactivation of one or the two X chromosomes in females) DMD/BMD carriers may have a mosaic pattern of dystrophin immunoreactivity, that is, dystrophin-positive muscle fibers (expressing the normal X chromosome) are intermixed with dystrophin-negative fibers (expressing the dystrophin-deficient X chromosome). However, up to two-thirds of carrier females may have normal dystrophin immunohistochemistry due to preferential survival of dystrophin-positive myofibers, so that genetic analysis is required for confirmation. Genetic testing for deletions is easily accomplished by PCR.[86]

Nondystrophinopathies

The nondystrophinopathies include facioscapulohumeral (FSH) muscular dystrophy, the limb-girdle syndromes, Emery-Dreifuss muscular dystrophy (EDMD), the congenital muscular dystrophies, and extraocular muscle-specific dystrophy.

Facioscapulohumeral Muscular Dystrophy

FSH dystrophy was originally described as a distinct entity by Landouzy and Dejerine,[87,88] and is inherited as an autosomal dominant trait in the vast majority of cases. The age of onset is variable, but the more typical cases begin in the second or third decade. The muscles of the face (orbicularis oculi, zygomaticus, orbicularis oris), neck, and shoulder girdle are the first to be affected, and subsequently the disease may spread to the pelvic girdle. The disorder, much milder than DMD, is insidious in onset and the clinical course is slowly progressive. Patients may remain ambulatory even at advanced stages of illness. Cardiac involvement is observed infrequently. The histologic findings on muscle biopsy are not specific, although most observers agree that the most common findings are variation in fiber size, with both markedly hypertrophied and severely atrophic, sometimes angular fibers, and relatively few degenerating/regenerating myofibers. In some pedigrees the muscle biopsy may show an unusually prominent focal interstitial mononuclear inflammatory response.[89] Most families segregate an FSH gene on 4q35,[90] although there is some evidence for genetic heterogeneity of FSH.[91] The gene product has not been identified; however, prenatal diagnosis for 4q35-linked families is available by RFLP analysis.

Limb-Girdle Dystrophy

Limb-girdle dystrophy (LGMD) is a heterogeneous group of disorders that may be inherited as an autosomal recessive, autosomal dominant, or sporadic trait.[92] The onset of the disease as well as its prognosis are extremely variable including the childhood-onset forms previously called "severe childhood autosomal recessive muscular dystrophy" or SCARMD. Classically, LGMD usually begins in the second or third decade of life, involving either the pelvic or shoulder girdle muscles with spread to others after a variable period. Cardiac involvement and pseudohypertrophy are rare. The disorder is generally slowly progressive, and patients may remain ambulatory for 20 or more years. The muscle biopsy is typically dystrophic, exhibiting marked variation in fiber size with many extremely large fibers, pronounced fiber splitting, and many internalized nuclei. Degenerative and regenerative changes are also seen. Some LGMDs are really misdiagnosed sporadic BMD or manifesting carriers of DMD/BMD. Current nomenclature is in flux as the molecular genetics of this heterogeneous group is currently being elucidated.[48,93] Dominant forms of LGMD are type 1, whereas recessive forms are type 2. LGMD1A has been mapped to chromosome 5q.[94] There are currently at least seven recessive forms (LGMD2A-G). LGMD2A maps to 15q15.1-q21.1 and is due to mutations of the proteolytic enzyme calpain 3.[95] The LGMD2B gene is on chromosome 2q[96] and may be allelic with Miyoshi myopathy.[97] LGMD types 2C, D, E, and F are due to mutations in each of four sarcoglycans (gamma, alpha, beta, and delta, respectively) in the dystrophin-associated glycoprotein complex.[98–101,284] Finally,

LGMD2G currently represents any LGMD not linked to the above loci; however, this is likely a heterogeneous group.

Emery-Dreifuss Muscular Dystrophy

EDMD is an X-linked recessive muscular dystrophy characterized by slowly progressive weakness, early contractures, and cardiomyopathy, and was first described in detail in a large kindred from Virginia by Emery and Dreifuss.[102] The disease begins in early childhood initially with humeral and peroneal muscle weakness and atrophy and later with involvement of the muscles of the pelvic girdle. Toe walking is often the initial symptom. The eventual appearance of cardiopathy (initially first-degree atrioventricular block) and contractures at the elbow, posterior neck, and heels is typical. The CK elevation is mild. Female carriers may be found to have subtle clinical manifestations of the disease. Muscle biopsy studies have shown variation in fiber size, atrophic rounded type 1 fibers, scattered regenerating fibers, internalized nuclei, and some endomysial connective tissue proliferation.[103–105] The EDMD gene is located on the long arm of the X chromosome in band Xq2842. It has been recently reported that this locus encodes emerin, a serine-rich protein in skeletal and cardiac muscle with some structural similarities to membrane-bound proteins involved in vesicular transport in the secretory pathway.[106]

The scapuloperoneal syndrome (SPS) is a clinically, genetically, and pathologically heterogeneous disorder characterized by mild weakness of the scapular muscle and foot extensors. Accompanying features can include contractures of the elbow and cardiomyopathy. The age of onset is quite variable and the disease generally runs a very slowly progressive course. Many cases of X-linked SPS (or humeroperoneal neuromuscular disease)[107] are now known to be EDMD and Emery has proposed that the term SPS be reserved for autosomal dominant cases that may be either myopathic or neuropathic.[108]

Congenital Muscular Dystrophies

The designation *congenital muscular dystrophy* (CMD) includes a number of hereditary neuromuscular diseases characterized by some degree of hypotonia and muscle wasting evident at birth or in early infancy. Cases can be subclassified on the basis of magnetic resonance imaging (MRI) abnormalities and ocular and cognitive deficits. The clinical course is quite variable; some patients have progressive weakness, others improve with time.[109] Although there has been considerable variability from case to case, the histologic changes observed in skeletal muscle are similar in kind, if not in degree, to those seen in the muscular dystrophies that occur at an older age. Endomysial fibrosis has been especially striking. Fukuyama congenital muscular dystrophy (FCMD),[110] muscle-eye-brain (MEB or Santavuori's) disease, and WalkerWarburg syndrome all present with CMD, mental retardation, and ocular abnormalities.[109,111,112] FCMD is an autosomal recessive form endemic to Japan characterized by polymicrogyria and profound mental retardation. The genetic locus has been identified on chromosome 9q31-33.[113] Although there is controversy over the distinction between FCMD, MEB, and the Walker-Warburg syndrome,[114] European cases of MEB are genetically distinct.[115] CMD without clinical central nervous system (CNS) involvement can be sub-

divided into cases with abnormal white matter changes on MRI, and those with normal MRI findings. These patients generally present with contractures, weakness, and hypotonia at birth. Immunohistochemical and molecular studies of muscle biopsies from most MRI-abnormal cases reveal an absence of merosin, a muscle-specific laminin,[116,117] and merosin gene mutations on chromosome 6q have been identified in many of these cases.[118] These patients often have elevated serum CK levels. Merosin-normal cases may be clinically milder and likely represent a heterogeneous group of diseases.

Myotonic Dystrophy

Myotonic dystrophy (Steinert's disease[119]) is a not uncommon autosomal dominant multisystem disorder characterized primarily by weakness and myotonia. The disease begins in late childhood with gait difficulty secondary to weakness of foot dorsiflexors, then progressing to weakness of the hand intrinsic muscles and wrist extensors. Atrophy of muscles of the face (hatchet face) and ptosis ensue. Myotonia, or sustained involuntary contraction of a group of muscles, can be demonstrated in the tongue and thenar eminence upon percussion, vigorous contraction, or exposure to cold.

The disease tends to increase in severity and to come on at a younger age in succeeding generations (anticipation phenomenon). The diagnosis can usually be confirmed by EMG, which shows characteristic myotonic discharges (the so-called dive-bomber effect). To a large extent, the skeletal muscles may show many of the typical features of a dystrophy, although necrosis, regeneration, and fibrosis are generally not seen. In addition, there is a striking increase in the number of internal nuclei (Fig. 24-31). On longitudinal sections, these may form

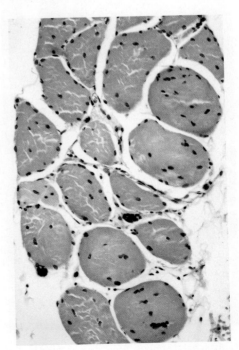

Fig. 24-31. Myotonic dystrophy. Note the striking increase in numbers of internalized nuclei and variation in fiber size. (Paraffin section, H&E.)

conspicuous chains. Another well recognized feature of myotonic dystrophy is the presence of ring fibers (Ringbinden, striated annulets). This is an abnormality of the muscle fiber in which there is a circumferential wrapping of a strip of the diseased fiber around itself (Fig. 24-32). On cross-section, the abnormal fiber has a rim of sarcoplasm in which the myofibrils can be seen running tangentially in relation to the longitudinally oriented fibrils in the center of the fiber.[120] The ring fiber may be associated with an irregular mass of sarcoplasm (sarcoplasmic mass) extending outward from the ring. These sarcoplasmic masses stain blue with H&E, red with Gomori trichrome, and intensely blue with the NADH histochemical reaction. Ultrastructurally, ring fibers show the subsarcolemmal myofilaments running perpendicular to the length of the fiber and sarcoplasmic masses appear as foci devoid of organized sarcoplasm and contain glycogen, mitochondria, ribosomes, and dense bodies (Fig. 24-33).

The relation of the ring fiber to myotonia is not understood. Both the ring fiber and the sarcoplasmic masses may be seen in neuromuscular disorders other than myotonic dystrophy. Histochemical techniques have demonstrated a relative atrophy of type 1 fibers in some cases early in the course of the disease (Fig. 24-34). A congenital form of myotonic dystrophy has been described in the neonate. Clinically, infants have severe hypotonia, facial diplegia, and respiratory difficulty. Pathologically the muscle may be normal or show atrophy of either type 1 or II fibers. Some fibers may be extremely small with internalized nuclei. Histochemical fiber type differentiation may be impaired.

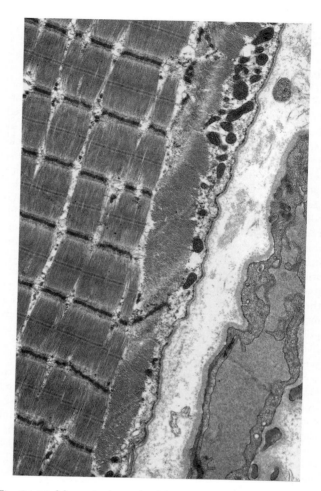

Fig. 24-33. Myotonic dystrophy (electron micrograph). Ring fiber with disorganized myofibrils running perpendicular to the length of the fiber beneath the sarcolemma.

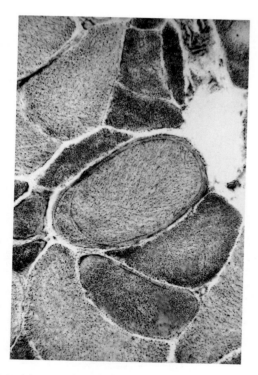

Fig. 24-32. Myotonic dystrophy. Ring fibers. A fiber in the center of the field demonstrates a thin circumferential strip of myofibrils running at right angles to the myofibrils in the rest of the fiber. (Frozen section, NADH-TR.)

Smooth and cardiac muscle involvement is common in autopsy studies and is characterized histologically by fibrous replacement. In a study of four patients with myotonic dystrophy and mental retardation, a disorder of cortical lamination was demonstrated at postmortem examination.[121] In congenital and infantile myotonic dystrophy the muscle may be normal or show atrophy of either type 1 or 2 fibers.[122,123] Some fibers may be extremely small with internalized nuclei. Recent molecular genetic research has not only identified the underlying molecular lesion but has also provided an explanation for the phenomenon of "anticipation.[124] The mutation event is expansion of a trinucleotide (CTG) repeat in the untranslated region of a protein kinase gene on chromosome 19. The length of the sequence correlates with the phenotype: normal individuals have from 5 to 30 copies whereas mildly (classically) affected patients have between 50 and 500. The severe congenital cases are associated with expansions of greater that 1,000 CTG repeats and are almost exclusively the result of maternal inheritance of a mutant myotonic dystrophy allele.[125] A recent report describes three patients from two families with myotonic dys-

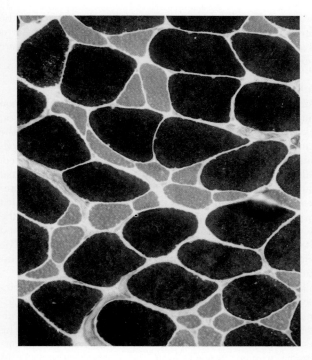

Fig. 24-34. Myotonic dystrophy. The type 1 fibers (light) are small and angulated, whereas the type 2 fibers (dark) are relatively unaffected. (Frozen section, ATPase pH 9.4.) (Courtesy of the Armed Forces Institute of Pathology.)

trophy who did not show an abnormal expansion of CTG trinucleotide repeats within the myotonic dystrophy gene.[126]

Extraocular Muscle-Specific Dystrophies

A number of entirely separate neuromuscular diseases preferentially involve the extraocular muscles (EOMs). However, it is noteworthy that many disorders of limb muscle (e.g., DMD/BMD, LGMD, CMD, FSH) tend to spare the EOMs. Similarly, disorders of EOMs are often associated with minimal limb muscle dysfunction. EOM pathology may be a primary feature of myasthenia gravis and the mitochondrial myopathies, but as these diseases represent dysfunction at a systemic level and often involve other muscles and/or organs, they are discussed later in this chapter. Much of the specificity of EOM-specific diseases can probably be attributable to the highly specialized structure and function of these muscles.[127] EOMs are designed to accomplish a variety of complex and finely controlled rapid movements without becoming fatigued. Relative to limb and trunk muscles, they have a unique embryonic origin, are smaller, rounder and more variable in size than mature limb muscle fibers, and have a more substantial epimysium. EOMs also display a unique constellation of fiber types, some of which contain EOM-specific isoforms of contractile proteins. EOM has a very high innervation ratio including some multiply innervated fibers and there may even be differences between EOM and limb muscle AChRs.

Clinically, EOM dysfunction presents as ptosis and external ophthalmoplegia. Often, it may be difficult to determine if the

underlying defect is at the level of the brain stem, the innervating cranial nerve(s), the neuromuscular junction, or the muscle itself. Because of their unique biology, their response to disease is not typical of that seen in other muscles. Indeed, normal EOM appears myopathic by the standards applied to limb muscle. Denervation of EOM may result in inflammatory, degenerative, and regenerative changes, responses more typical of myopathy than neurogenic insult in limb muscle.

Oculopharyngeal muscular dystrophy (OPMD) is typically a disease of late onset characterized by progressive ptosis and weakness of extraocular muscles, associated with difficulty in swallowing.[128] Weakness of the face, jaw, and limb muscles may occur later in the course of the disease. The largest affected communities have been of French-Canadian origin, but several kindreds from Europe, Latin America, and Japan have also been recognized. The mode of inheritance is most often autosomal dominant; sporadic and autosomal recessive cases are on record and onset in childhood has been described.[129] Skeletal muscles show myopathic changes, including variation in fiber size, internalized nuclei, and increased endomysial connective tissue. There may also be scattered type 1 angular fibers. In addition rimmed vacuoles are a characteristic feature (Fig. 24-35). The structure of the vacuoles is best demonstrated with the modified

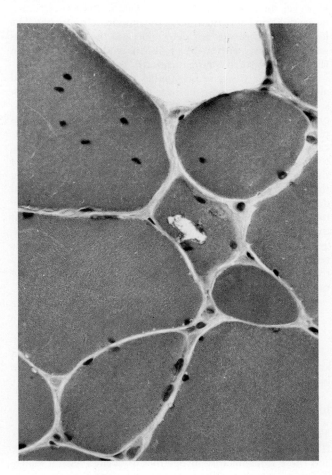

Fig. 24-35. Oculopharyngeal dystrophy. Note variability in fiber size and internalized nuclei. The fiber in the center of the field contains a rimmed vacuole. (Frozen section, H&E.)

Gomori trichrome reaction on frozen sections. Single or multiple intracytoplasmic vacuoles are typically found in type 1 fibers, which contain granular material that stains red and are lined by a rim of darker material. Ultrastructural studies have demonstrated membranous debris and disruption or the sarcomeric structure within the vacuole and intranuclear unbranched filaments, which measure 7 to 9 μm in diameter,[130,131] but are demonstrable only after an assiduous search. An OPMD gene has recently been mapped to 114q11.2-q13 by linkage analysis in a group of French-Canadian kindreds.[132]

Congenital fibrosis of the extraocular muscles (CFEOM), also referred to as "ocular congenital fibrosis syndrome,"[133] "hereditary congenital external ophthalmoplegia,"[134] or "congenital familial external ophthalmoplegia with co-contractures,"[135] presents with nonprogressive ptosis and external ophthalmoplegia.[136] Defining features include autosomal dominant inheritance with complete penetrance and bilateral involvement with the globes fixed in a downward gaze. Pathologically, the EOMs are reported to be fibrotic, although in some cases this may reflect sampling of the normal connective tissue at the tendinous insertion. Postmortem study of one recent case revealed histologically normal-appearing superior oblique, inferior oblique, inferior, medial, and lateral recti. However there was absence of the superior division of cranial nerve three and abnormalities of the muscles it innervates. The levator palpebrae was not detectable and the superior rectus was diminutive with areas of fibrosis and fatty infiltration (Engle EC, personal communication).

Genetic analysis of seven families with CFEOM as defined above has mapped the gene near the centromere of chromosome 12 and shown that this is a genetically homogenous disorder.[137,138] Given that it is presently unclear what role fibrosis plays in this disease, it may be preferable to refer to this genetically homogenous disorder as *autosomal dominant congenital external ophthalmoplegia* (ADCEO).[138] Congenital ptosis is one of the most common congenital neuromuscular disorders affecting the EOMs. Cases of isolated ptosis can be sporadic or autosomal dominant with reduced penetrance and some patients may have unilateral or bilateral involvement.[139,140] It is unclear if this is a primary myopathy of the levator palpebrae or a neurogenic disorder involving the third cranial nerve. The levator is reported as fibrotic or absent and other structures innervated by the third nerve (e.g., pupil and ciliary muscle) are apparently normal.

Inflammatory Myopathies

Inflammatory myopathies, either idiopathic or due to a known infectious agent, represent about 25 percent of muscle biopsy cases.[141]

Idiopathic Myopathies

The idiopathic inflammatory myopathies include polymyositis (PM), dermatomyositis (DM) (childhood DM and adult DM), and those inflammatory myopathies associated with a malignant tumor and/or collagen vascular disease. Inclusion body myositis (IBM) is a special category. In general, these disorders are characterized by subacute, progressive proximal muscle weakness. The distal musculature tends to be affected in the later stages except in IBM, where early distal involvement is common. In all types, muscles innervated by cranial nerves are rarely affected.[141–143]

Polymyositis and Dermatomyositis

Polymyositis often begins insidiously with asymmetric proximal muscle weakness variably associated with pain in the arms or, less often, leg muscles (e.g., difficulty climbing stairs, raising the arms for combing or grooming). Dysphagia occurs in about one-third of cases and weakness of neck flexors is commonly noted. Adult dermatomyositis is characterized by progressive proximal muscle weakness with erythematous skin lesions that may precede, coincide with, or follow the weakness and is accompanied by subungual telangiectases. The facial skin rash begins in the face (periorbital, malar, perioral regions) anterior neck and chest regions, as well as the extensor surfaces of the joints. The skin lesions progress to scaling, brown discoloration, and induration.

In both PM and DM, electrocardiographic abnormalities have been described. In different series around the world the incidence of associated malignant tumors in middle-aged or elderly patients ranges between about 10 to over 40 percent. The detection of the neoplasm (in women, ovarian and breast carcinoma; in men, stomach, lung, and intestinal carcinoma; in Chinese, nasopharyngeal carcinoma) may precede or follow the onset of neurologic symptoms. Both PM and adult DM may be associated with well defined collagen vascular diseases such as rheumatoid arthritis, scleroderma, polyarteritis nodosa, Sjögren's syndrome, lupus erythematosus, and mixed connective tissue disease. Laboratory studies show that the CK is elevated, and the EMG discloses short, polyphasic potentials with fibrillations, positive waves, and pseudomyotonic bursts. Radionuclide and MRI studies have been used recently to identify involved regions and to aid in directing the site for needle biopsy.

The typical clinical picture of childhood DM consists of erythematous malar violaceous, heliotrope rash, also involving the skin over the extensor surfaces of the joints, and muscle weakness of insidious onset relentlessly progressing over a period or weeks or months. In many cases other associated manifestations include subcutaneous calcifications, gastrointestinal bleeding, and respiratory insufficiency.[144] A rare, congenital form of inflammatory myopathy, clinically similar to CMD, has also been reported.[145] Inflammatory cells are found in some 75 percent of patients. In large series, 10 to 20 percent of patients will show no evidence of inflammation.

The muscle biopsy findings in PM and DM share a number of important similarities, although there are also significant differences between the two conditions. The typical findings are those of an inflammatory myopathy (i.e., changes reflecting acute segmental necrosis of muscle, manifest by smudging and eosinophilia of the cytoplasm and myophagocytosis by invading macrophages (Fig. 24-36). Along with these destructive changes there is often concomitant regeneration of muscle fibers, sometimes seen adjacent to the regions of myophagocytosis. The extent and distribution of the chronic mononuclear inflammatory cell infiltrates will vary somewhat in the two conditions. In PM inflammatory cells are present in the endomysium between and among muscle fibers (Fig. 24-37), whereas in

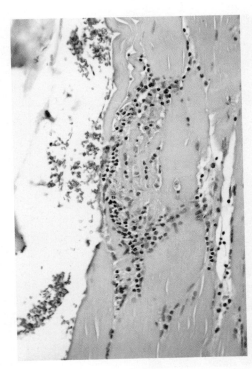

Fig. 24-36. Polymyositis. The muscle fiber in the center of the field is undergoing segmental necrosis, with focal destruction of the sarcoplasm and invasion by phagocytic inflammatory cells. (Paraffin section, H&E.)

suggests previous sensitization to muscle fiber surface-associated antigens, but no target antigen has yet been identified. Viral infection has long been suspected to be the inciting factor that triggers the immune response but there is little evidence for this hypothesis in spite of active search over many years.[152,153] The possible contribution of the humoral immune system in the development of the disease is unresolved at this time. In patients with PM, immunoglobulin deposits have been visualized by immunofluorescence within the walls of small intramuscular blood vessels, but these observations have not been consistent or specific, and therefore such examinations have largely been abandoned as a useful adjunct to diagnosis. Similarly, the diagnostic utility of localizing the membrane attack complex (MAC) to necrotic fibers[154] in PM and DM is questionable. In adult DM, humoral immunity appears to play an important part. The inflammatory infiltrate is composed mainly of B cells and helper T cells, although macrophages and cytotoxic/suppressor T cells are also present. In support of the notion that DM is an immune-mediated vasculopathy is the observation that the complement system has been found to be deposited, bound, and activated to completion within the intramuscular microvasculature of patients with childhood DM (to a lesser extent in adult DM). Ultrastructural and morphomet-

DM (both childhood and adult types) they tend to be angiocentric. An important structural characteristic of DM (rare in PM) is the tendency for fibers at the periphery of the fascicle to appear smaller than normal (so-called perifascicular atrophy) (Fig. 24-38A). These small fibers are either rounded or somewhat angulated; they are often basophilic, perhaps regenerating. On ultrastructural examination in both adult and childhood DM characteristic undulating tubulo reticular inclusions may be demonstrable in the cytoplasm of capillary endothelial cells and pericytes[146] (Fig. 24-38B).

In PM or DM associated with neoplasia there are no distinctive muscle biopsy features. In PM associated with a collagen vascular disease, the pathology most closely resembles that seen in DM. In congenital inflammatory myopathy the muscle biopsy shows perivascular/interstitial chronic inflammatory cell infiltrates with degenerating and regenerating fibers.[145] End-stage inflammatory myopathy is characterized by extensive fibro adipose replacement of muscle fibers with little inflammatory reaction. Mechanisms of fiber damage in these diseases have yet to be completely defined, but there is much evidence to implicate immunologic factors. In PM a cell-mediated immunopathogenesis of the muscle fiber destruction is suggested by the available evidence. The predominant inflammatory cells have been demonstrated to be T cells (about 70 percent) and macrophages. The T cells are mostly cytotoxic/suppressor CD8+ and some CD4+ cells.[147–150] MHC-I expression is demonstrable on and in affected fibers.[151] The focal invasion and destruction of muscle fibers by T cells and macrophages

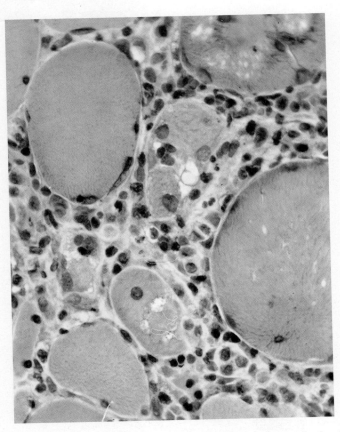

Fig. 24-37. Polymyositis. Note degenerating fibers and extensive interstitial infiltrate of mononuclear inflammatory cells. The cluster of nuclei within the oval fiber in the center are probably phagocytes. (Frozen section, H&E.) (Courtesy of the Armed Forces Institute of Pathology.)

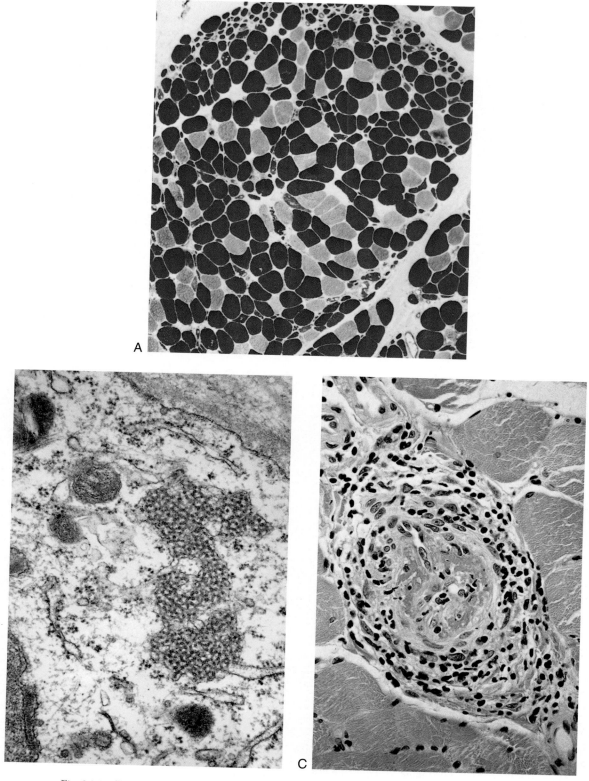

Fig. 24-38. Dermatomyositis. **(A)** The atrophy and degeneration selectively involve the periphery of the fascicle. The pattern is frequently present in childhood dermatomyositis and is less often present in the adult form. (Frozen section, ATPase.) (Courtesy of AFIP.) **(B)** Tubuloreticular inclusion in cytoplasm of endothelial cell (electron micrograph). **(C)** Necrotizing vasculitis involving skeletal muscle. (Courtesy of Dr. Jeffrey Joseph, Beth Israel Hospital, Boston, MA.)

ric studies evidencing capillary lesions early in the course of the disease have also been published.[155,156] In childhood DM, microcirculatory abnormalities and necrosis and thrombosis of capillaries, small arteries, and venules has been found especially in those vessels at the periphery of muscle fascicles, presumably accounting for the perifascicular atrophy.[157–159] In PM associated with the collagen vascular disease scleroderma, an immunologic response mediated by T cells appears to be directed against a connective tissue or vascular element, and not against the muscle fiber.

Vasculitis affecting skeletal muscle can be seen in polyarteritis nodosa (PAN), in the Churg-Strauss syndrome (allergic granulomatosis/angiitis), secondary to connective tissue disease (as in rheumatoid arthritis, Sjögren's syndrome, systemic lupus erythematosus), in Wegener's granulomatosis, in Behçet's syndrome, and in nonsystemic vasculitis. These diseases are discussed in detail elsewhere in this text. From the perspective of muscle pathology it is worth mentioning a few points that are of importance in the interpretation of the muscle biopsy. PAN is characterized by an inflammatory and necrotizing angiopathy that focally affects the walls of small muscular-walled arteries of a diameter of 100 to 250 mm. Muscle biopsy may be diagnostic in the acute phase where there may be necrosis of all components of the vessel wall, often with fibrin deposition within the necrotic remnants (fibrinoid necrosis), and infiltration of the diseased region with inflammatory cells, mainly polymorphonuclear neutrophils (Fig. 24-38C). Later stages are characterized by a mononuclear inflammatory reaction with lymphocytes and macrophages and fibroblastic proliferation, collagen deposition, and narrowing of the lumen. The disease tends to affect the vessel walls in a focal or segmental manner, such that the lesions on gross inspection present the appearance of nodules along the course of the vessel. The rare subvariety of PAN known as the Churg-Strauss syndrome has some additional features that have led to its being separately designated. The disorder appears on a background of asthma and is accompanied by blood eosinophils; many eosinophils accompany the acute vasculitic lesion and there is a tendency for granulomas to form in later stages of the process. In a small group of cases, a necrotizing vasculitis is found in skeletal muscles in the absence of any indications of systemic disease or involvement of other organs.

Inclusion Body Myositis
In 1971 Yunis and Samaha[160] introduced the term *inclusion body myositis* for a specific type of inflammatory myopathy; an earlier report also described the structural abnormality.[161] In the following 25 years many subsequent case studies and review articles have expanded and further clarified the distinctive features of this disease.[141–143,162–165] Clinically IBM can be separated from PM and DM because the disorder comes on in a somewhat older, particularly male, patient population, skin manifestations are not a feature of the illness, the distribution of the weakness tends to be both distal and proximal, and the course of the illness is perhaps more protracted. The CK levels are either in the normal range or mildly elevated, although ordinarily not above levels that are commonly seen in PM and DM. EMG findings are, for the most part, myopathic. The disease appears to be refractory to corticosteroid treatment and other therapeutic measures that are utilized for PM and DM.

An association with connective tissue diseases has been noted in a minority of cases and some familial cases are on record.

The histopathologic findings on muscle biopsy include sparse, or entirely absent, interstitial chronic inflammatory cell infiltrates of lymphocytes (largely CD8+ T cells surround the non-necrotic fibers) and macrophages, and rarely, myophagocytosis and regenerating fibers. The characteristic rimmed vacuoles are best demonstrable on frozen sections with the modified Gomori trichrome stain, although they can also be seen well on H&E preparations (they are ordinarily not well seen on paraffin-embedded sections) (Fig. 24-39). These are single or multiple rounded defects within the muscle fibers that are either empty or filled with red granular debris and are outlined by a rim of darkly staining material. Angular fibers, and sometimes grouping of atrophic fibers, are also frequent. Ultrastructurally the vacuoles contain non-membrane-bound whorls and skeins of "myeloid" membranous debris and dissolution of the myofibrillar architecture. There may also be twisted tubofilament 15 to 18 nm wide structures scattered in the disrupted cytoplasm or within neighboring nuclei (Fig. 24-39); the beta-amyloid fragment (A-beta) of the beta-amyloid precursor protein (beta-APP) has been colocalized to the filaments in both sporadic and familial cases.[166,167] The filamentous inclusions do not appear to be specific for IBM.[168] Recent observations have also reported the presence of other proteins and mRNA localized to the vacuoles including ubiquitin, prion proteins, apolipoprotein E (APO-E), hyperphosphorylated tau, and AChR proteins.[169,170] Muscle biopsies from patients with IBM, as in PM/DM, have been studied carefully for evidence of paramyxovirus infection but, although studies have successfully demonstrated the presence of virus in some affected individuals,[171,172] such evidence is lacking in most others.[163,165,173]

Granulomatous Myositis
Occasional patients with classic PM may have foci of granulomatous infiltrate in the muscle biopsy specimen. In these cases a search for microorganisms (e.g., parasites, tubercle bacilli, and fungi) may establish the diagnosis. A non specific epithelioid giant cell reaction in skeletal muscle may occur in a number of other conditions, including neoplasia, myasthenia gravis, rheumatologic disorders (including rheumatoid arthritis), and related connective tissue diseases, and may also be found idiopathically (i.e., in the absence of any known systemic illness)[174–176] (Fig. 24-40). In many patients with sarcoidosis there is extension of the disease into skeletal muscle.[177] Clinically, most patients with sarcoidosis are asymptomatic as regards signs and symptoms of muscle involvement but a minority have proximal muscle weakness, myalgia, and cramps.[178] Peripheral nerve involvement may lead to neurogenic atrophy. The muscle biopsy in sarcoid myositis shows relatively little active muscle fiber destruction; the granulomatous infiltrate is noncaseating, contains epithelioid histiocytes with relatively few lymphocytes, and extends into the perivascular connective tissue.[179]

Eosinophilic infiltration of inflamed muscle is a characteristic of parasitic infection. It can, in addition, be a feature of a number of rare and poorly understood conditions.[180] Reference has been made above to the toxic eosinophilia myalgia syndrome associated with contaminated L-tryptophan. Polymyositis in the setting of eosinophilia in affected tissues and/or

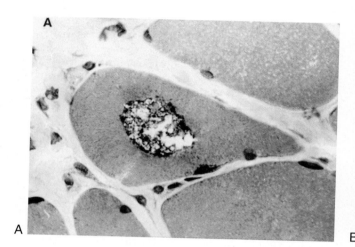
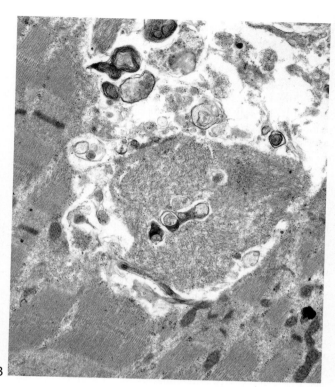

Fig. 24-39. **(A)** Inclusion body myositis. A characteristic feature is the presence of vacuoles containing basophilic granules (rimmed vacuoles) within muscle fibers. (Frozen section, H&E.) **(B)** Inclusion body myositis. Electron microscopy discloses disruption of the sarcomere and accumulation of abnormal filaments within the cytoplasm.

in the peripheral blood is characteristic of the hypereosoinophilic syndrome; some of these cases have been described under the term *eosinophilic polymyositis*. In Schulman's syndrome (diffuse fasciitis with eosinophilia), a clinical syndrome with scleroderma-like manifestations, hypergammaglobulinemia, and hypereosinophilia, there are eosinophilic inflammatory infiltrates in fascia and skeletal muscle.

Infectious Myopathies

Infectious agents including bacteria, viruses, and parasites can cause an inflammatory myopathy.

Pyogenic (bacterial) myositis is uncommon in the developed world except for occasional cases of gas gangrene associated with *Clostridium welchii*, usually the result of complicated mechanical trauma or postoperative wound infection. In the tropics, patients may present with multiple acute muscle abscesses, which are most often due to staphylococci. Pathologically, the affected muscle initially shows acute interstitial edema, followed by a pleomorphic inflammatory infiltrate consisting first of lymphocytes and then of neutrophils. At this stage, the muscle fibers show necrosis, phagocytosis, and regeneration.[181,182]

Acute viral myositis affects children and adults. Most cases are caused by the influenza virus and the enteroviruses (Coxsackie and Echo groups). The usual clinical syndrome is myalgia occurring in the setting of an acute febrile illness. The patient develops tender and swollen muscles as well as muscle weakness. Serum CK is elevated and there may be myoglobinuria as well as an abnormal EMG. When performed, the muscle biopsy discloses scattered muscle fiber necrosis, regeneration, and interstitial inflammatory reaction. Other less frequent pathogens include hepatitis B, herpes simplex, and the Epstein-Barr virus.[180] Human T cell leukemia/lymphoma-1 (HTLV-1), which is known to cause neurologic manifestations related to a myelopathy, can cause a mild inflammatory myopathy.[183,184]

A variety of parasitic infections may involve muscle. The most common is trichinosis, which results from ingesting the larvae of the nematode *Trichinella spiralis* in uncooked pork. After maturation of the ingested larvae in the human bowel, fertilized females penetrate the mucosa and deposit large numbers of embryos, which enter venules and lymphatics. These larvae then widely disseminate throughout the body, including the skeletal muscles. During the invasive stage, the affected individual will experience systemic symptoms accompanied by eosinophilia and variable muscle pain and weakness. Biopsy of an affected muscle shows the presence of encysted larvae, variable inflammation, degeneration and phagocytosis of muscle fibers, and focal connective tissue proliferation. In time, the larvae will die and frequently become calcified (Fig. 24-41). Other parasitic infections that may occasionally involve skeletal muscle include cysticercosis (*Taenia solium*) and hydatid disease (*Echinococcus*). Infection of skeletal muscle by *Toxoplasma gondii* occurs now most often in patients with systemic immunosuppression and especially in cases of acquired immuno deficiency disease (AIDS).[185]

Lyme disease, which is caused by infection with *Borrelia burgdorferi*, is often associated with muscle pain and weakness. Peripheral neuropathy demonstrable on clinical, NCV, and biopsy examinations is the most common cause of the muscle weakness. Muscle biopsy studies have shown minimal and nonspecific changes consisting primarily of scattered interstitial inflammatory cell infiltrates. Neurogenic atrophy may also occur. Rarely, the spirochete has been demonstrated within the skeletal muscle of patients with Lyme disease, but it is uncertain whether the clinical myalgia is due to a direct effect of the organism.[180,186]

Opportunistic viral (e.g., cytomegalovirus), parasitic (e.g., toxoplasmosis), and fungal (e.g., candidasis) infections have been recorded in many biopsy and autopsy studies of patients with AIDS.[187–189] The toxic myopathy associated with AZT (zidovudine) treatment in these patients is discussed below. In addition, an idiopathic polymyositis-like syndrome, which does not seem to be directly related to the virus, also occurs.[190] In some cases there is immunohistochemical and molecular evidence of human immunodeficiency virus (HIV) viral infection

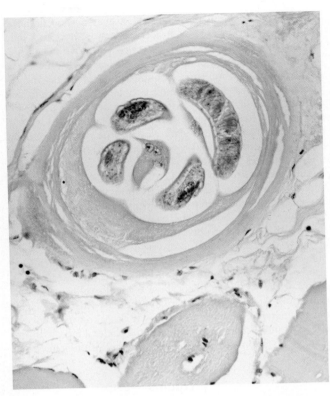

Fig. 24-41. Trichinosis. An encysted organism is present in the center of the field. A scanty endomysial inflammatory infiltrate is present. The presence of eosinophils or granulomas in the infiltrate should prompt a search for such organisms. (Paraffin section, H&E.) (Courtesy of Dr. T.W. Smith, University of Massachusetts Medical School, Worcester, MA.)

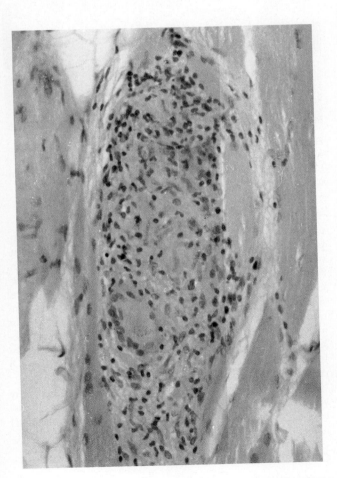

Fig. 24-40. Sarcoid myopathy. A granuloma containing a Langhans-type giant cell separates the muscle fibers. (Paraffin section, H&E.)

as well as hemosiderin deposits within macrophages invading skeletal muscle.[191,192]

Other inflammatory disorders

Under the generic term *inflammatory pseudotumor* are included a number of inflammatory disorders of muscle characterized by selective regional involvement of specific muscle groups. These encompass reported cases of focal myositis, proliferative myositis, nodular fasciitis, and myositis ossificans. The principal histopathologic features are variation in fiber size with interstitial and fascial chronic inflammation.[193] Myositis ossificans is a skeletal muscle lesion characterized by deposition of trabeculae of woven bone about a focus of chronically inflamed and fibrotic muscle. These histologic findings have been described in seemingly disparate entities, including hereditary disorders (fibrodysplasia ossificans progressiva), post-traumatic or ischemic injury to muscle, neoplastic-like lesions, and end-stage muscle disease.

Ischemia

Skeletal muscle is relatively resistant to ischemic injury because of its rich blood supply with many collateral branches.

Varying degrees of ischemic damage, however, may occur in the following conditions: (1) occlusion of a major artery to a limb by a thromboembolus; (2) severe arteriosclerosis with occlusion of multiple small peripheral arteries and veins (e.g., diabetes); (3) thrombosis of multiple intramuscular vessels, as in polyarteritis nodosa; (4) Volkmann's ischemic contracture (a rare complication of fractures; attributed to arterial spasm); (5) swelling and hemorrhage of certain muscles enclosed in rigid compartments, with secondary compromise of their vascular supply (e.g., anterior tibial syndrome); and (6) trauma. The histologic changes in the early stages consist of fragmentation of muscle fibers with focal loss of cross-striations. The fibers then become eosinophilic, acquiring a hyaline or waxy appearance. The nuclei become pyknotic and eventually disappear. The interstitium becomes edematous, separating individual fibers, and shows infiltration by polymorphonuclear leukocytes. After about 48 to 72 hours, there is invasion of macrophages, which phagocytize the dead muscle fibers. About this time, there is also beginning proliferation of fibroblasts in the endomysium. Many of the surviving fibers show marked swelling and vacuolization. At the edge of the infarct there is evidence of vigorous regenerative activity. Relatively little is known about the effects of more chronic ischemia on the skeletal muscle in humans (e.g., chronic arteriosclerotic vascular insufficiency).

Trauma

Skeletal muscle may be traumatized through application of an external force, in which case the amount of damage is related to the degree of the force, fracture of adjacent bones, and damage to blood vessels. Muscle may also be damaged secondary to violent exertion. This may be the result of herniation of the muscle through a tear in the covering fascia, or through actual rupture of the muscle itself. Histologic examination of the injured muscle shows rupture of many muscle fibers, with tearing of their sarcolemmal sheaths. Adjacent fibers may show myopathic changes. These changes are often accompanied by interstitial edema and hemorrhage. The cellular reaction ranges from predominantly neutrophilic in the early stages to mononuclear later on, with phagocytosis of dead fibers and evidence of regenerative activity. Associated ischemic changes secondary to vascular damage are common. If the parallel arrangement of the endomysial tubes is disrupted, this may lead to marked fibrous tissue proliferation. Primary hemorrhage into skeletal muscle may be secondary to trauma, thrombosis of intramuscular veins (due to severe infection), or hemorrhagic diathesis (anticoagulants, thrombotic thrombocytopenic purpura).

Congenital Myopathies

The congenital myopathies constitute a group of disorders defined largely on the basis of the morphologic appearance of the muscle. Most of these conditions share clinical features, including onset in early life, nonprogressive or slowly progressive course, proximal or generalized muscle weakness, and hypotonia.[194–196] Individuals affected at birth or in early infancy may

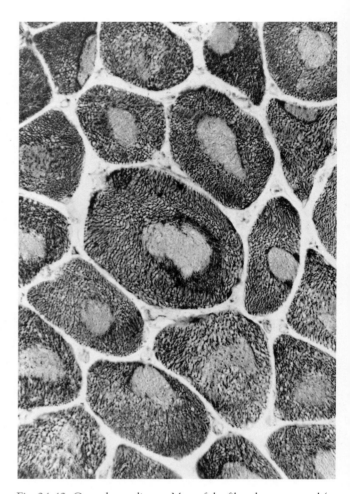

Fig. 24-42. Central core disease. Most of the fibers have a central (or sometimes eccentric) area of pallor. The cores occur only in type 1 fibers, and the ATPase stain usually shows a marked type 1 predominance. (Frozen section, NADH-TR.)

present as floppy babies. A genetic predisposition is usually apparent, although the mode of inheritance is variable. Some patients may have associated dysmorphic skeletal abnormalities. Serum muscle enzymes are usually normal or only slightly elevated, and the EMG shows myopathic features. Because of the similarities in the clinical presentation of these disorders, accurate diagnosis depends on study of the muscle biopsy. This must always include the use of histochemical and electron microscopic techniques, since many of the characteristic morphologic features cannot be reliably identified on conventional paraffin-embedded material.

Only the better defined categories of congenital myopathy are discussed in some detail; these include (1) central core disease, (2) nemaline myopathy, (3) centronuclear (myotubular) myopathy, and (4) congenital fiber type disproportion.

Central Core Disease

Central core disease was the first of the morphologically distinct congenital myopathies to be described.[194] Shy and Magee in 1956[196] described five patients within three generations of a family who manifested hypotonia and weakness. The disorder may be inherited as an autosomal dominant trait or may occur sporadically. Typically, the disease is characterized by hypotonia and nonprogressive weakness involving proximal more than distal musculature. Skeletal deformities, most commonly congenital dislocation of the hip and kyphoscoliosis, may be present. On occasion, histologic features of central core disease have been seen in adult patients who are nearly asymptomatic. Histologic examination of the muscle reveals a virtually pathognomonic picture. Many fibers show a central (or sometimes eccentric) area of pallor best recognized in frozen sections stained with an oxidative enzyme reaction such as NADH-TR (Fig. 24-42). On H&E- and trichrome-stained sections, the cores appear slightly pale, having the same color as, but appearing more homogeneous than, the surrounding sarcoplasm. The cores also show decreased glycolytic enzyme activity, as evidenced by reduced staining on the PAS and myophosphorylase reactions. On longitudinal sections,the cores extend the entire length of the fibers. Cores are only found in type 1 fibers, and most cases show a striking type 1 fiber predominance. On electron microscopy, the cores usually show some disruption of the sarcomeric pattern with degeneration of myofilaments and Z lines and diminution or loss of mitochondria, sarcoplasmic reticulum, and glycogen (Fig. 24-43). Most, if not all cases of autosomal dominant central core disease are due to missense mutations of the ryanodine (sarcoplasmic reticulum calcium release channel) receptor gene on chromosome 19.[197–199] Mutations of this gene are also associated with the malignant hyperthermia trait; the latter susceptibility is well documented in patients with central core disease. Interestingly, Fananapazir et al[200] have recently reported histologically typical central cores in soleus biopsies from patients with hypertrophic cardiomyopathy due to mutation of the beta-myosin heavy chain gene, although these findings remain to be replicated.

Nemaline Myopathy

Nemaline myopathy was first described in 1963 by two independent groups of investigators.[194,201–203] The disorder can present in infancy as well as in later life. Usually the clinical course in infancy is nonprogressive despite the presence of weakness, hypotonia, and delayed motor development. The weakness tends to involve the proximal limb muscles most severely and can also affect the facial and bulbar musculature. Skeletal abnormalities such as narrow face, high arched palate, kyphoscoliosis, and clubbed feet may be present. The mode of inheritance is variable. The pathologic hallmark of this disorder is the nemaline or rod body. Rod bodies are best visualized in frozen sections stained by the modified trichrome method, appearing as aggregates of red-purple granular or bacilliform structures, 2 to 7 mm in length, which tend to accumulate in the subsarcolemmal regions of the muscle (Fig. 24-44). They are difficult to detect in paraffin-embedded sections stained with H&E but can be seen with phosphotungstic acid hematoxylin (PTAH) stain. Nemaline rods are not stained by the oxidative enzyme or ATPase reactions. They occur predominantly in type 1 fibers. A variable degree of type 1 fiber predominance may be present. The number of fibers containing rod bodies, as well as the number of rods present in a given muscle fiber, can vary considerably from case to case. On electron microscopy, nemaline rods appear as moderately electron dense, lattice-like structures with periodic lines oriented parallel and perpendicular to the long axis (Fig. 24-45). They closely resemble normal Z lines and can often be observed in continuity with them. The "free" ends of the rod bodies appear to be continuous with the thin myofilaments. Biochemical studies have shown that the major component of the nemaline bodies is alpha-actinin, which is also the principal protein component of Z lines. Rod bodies are not specific for nemaline myopathy, as they may be occasionally observed in other hereditary myopathies, in inflammatory myopathies, following tenotomy, and in toxic myopathies (see zidovudine myopathy later in this chapter). Molecular analysis is incomplete. One large Australian family with autosomal dominant inheritance of mildly progressive weakness presenting in adolescence has been shown to carry a mutation in the tropomyosin gene TPM3 on chromosome 1.[204,205] Northern European cases with autosomal recessive inheritance have been shown to be genetically distinct, [206] and this second genetic locus was recently mapped to chromosome 2.[207] The etiology of sporadic cases also remains to be determined.

Centronuclear (Myotubular) Myopathy

Centronuclear (myotubular) myopathy was first described by Spiro and colleagues[208] in 1966 and given the name myotubular myopathy because of the resemblance of the affected muscle

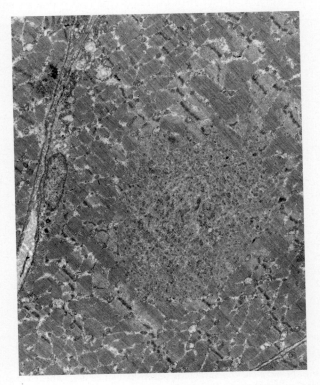

Fig. 24-43 Central core disease (electron micrograph). The core consists of degenerated myofibrils and loss of formed membranous organelles. (Courtesy of the Armed Forces Institute of Pathology.)

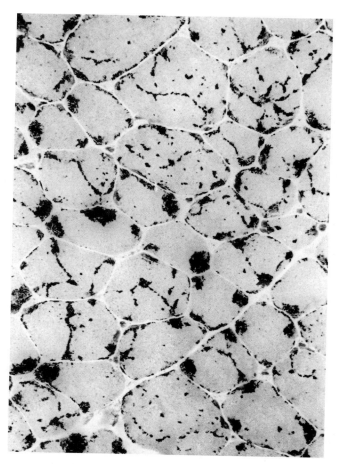

Fig. 24-44. Nemaline myopathy. The nemaline (rod) bodies are visualized as aggregates of red-purple granular or bacilliform structures located predominantly in the subsarcolemmal regions of the fibers. The rod bodies are found mainly in type 1 fibers, and there is often a type 1 predominance. (Frozen section, MGT.)

fibers to fetal myotubes. Shortly thereafter, another group of investigators introduced the term *centronuclear myopathy* for this group of disorders. The designation "type 1 fiber hypotrophy and central nuclei"[209] has also been used. All these terms remain in current usage and there is speculation that there may be fundamental differences between the prototypes. Several clinical variants with different modes of inheritance are recognized. The most common form, inherited as an autosomal recessive trait, presents in infancy or early childhood and clinically shows prominent involvement of extraocular and facial muscles in addition to hypotonia and slowly progressive limb muscle weakness. Other less common variants include a severe X-linked recessive form characterized by marked hypotonia and respiratory distress and milder, often later-onset autosomal dominant and sporadic forms.[194,210]

The characteristic pathologic feature of this group of disorders is the presence of a centrally located nucleus in most of the muscle fibers (Fig. 24-46A). In some pedigrees (especially the X-linked cases) the central nuclei are surrounded by a clear perinuclear halo that lacks ATPase activity. Ultrastructurally the

perinuclear region is devoid of myofibrils and may show increased numbers of mitochondria and glycogen (Fig. 24-46B). The central nuclei are usually confined to type 1 fibers but can occur in both types. Usually there is a predominance of type 1 fibers, and these fibers are often smaller than usual. On transverse sections, the central nuclei can be seen to occupy a variable number of fibers, ranging from 25 to 90 percent H&E, trichrome, and NADH-TR staining may reveal radial striations of affected fibers on cross-section. Central nuclei are also found in the extraocular muscles.[211] There are conflicting reports of an abnormality (persistence) of desmin and vimentin.[212–215] Current molecular genetic studies indicate that the gene for the X-linked form of myotubular myopathy is on Xq28; however, additional genetic linkage studies are needed to examine the possibility of genetic heterogeneity.[216,217] The molecular basis of the milder autosomal dominant or recessive phenotypes has not been established.

Congenital Fiber Type Disproportion

Patients with the muscle biopsy findings characteristic of congenital fiber type disproportion develop symptoms in early infancy with hypotonia, proximal muscle weakness, and delayed motor development. Approximately one-half of affected persons have skeletal abnormalities, including congenital hip dislocation, joint contractures, foot deformities, high arched palate, and kyphoscoliosis. Respiratory difficulties may be present. The mode of inheritance is unclear and there is concern that the condition may not be a discrete nosologic entity. The muscle biopsy characteristically shows type 1 fibers that are uni-

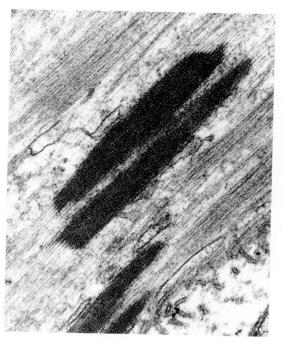

Fig. 24-45. Nemaline myopathy (electron micrograph). The red granular structures seen by light microscopy correspond to these electron-dense rod-shaped masses that seem to arise from the Z disc. (Courtesy of the Armed Forces Institute of Pathology.)

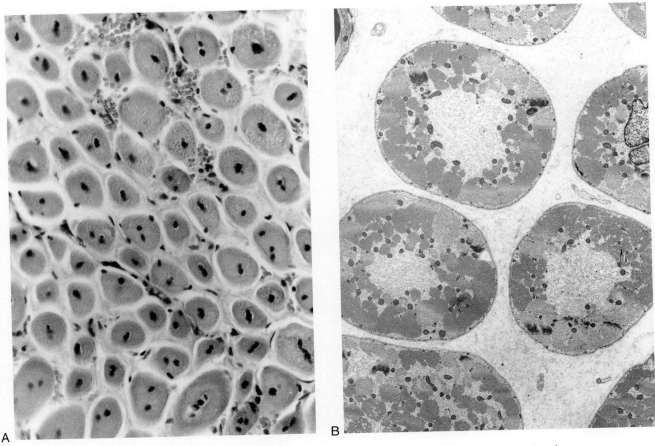

Fig. 24-46. Centronuclear myopathy. **(A)** Most of the muscle fibers contain a centrally located nucleu. (Paraffin section, H&E.) **(B)** Many fibers have central area devoid of contractile filaments (electron micrograph).

formly smaller than type 2 fibers by 12 percent or more (Figs. 24-47 and 24-48). This size disparity is well illustrated in histograms showing two distinct peaks. The type 2 fibers are of normal size or slightly hypertrophied. Type 1 fiber predominance is often present. There is some uncertainty about whether this disease is a distinct disorder. Genetic studies have indicated considerable heterogeneity; some pedigrees have shown autosomal dominant and others autosomal recessive inheritance.

Other Congenital Myopathies

A number of other poorly understood myopathies have been included with the congenital myopathies and defined in isolated case reports primarily on the basis of the demonstration of characteristic histochemical and/or ultrastructural features. These include multicore disease, fingerprint body myopathy, reducing body myopathy, sarcotubular myopathy, myopathy with tubular aggregates, familial myopathy with probable lysis of myofibrils in type 1 fibers, trilaminar fiber myopathy, cap disease, zebra body myopathy, cytoplasmic or spheroid body myopathy, and desmin storage myopathies.[194] The nosologic status of these entities is tenuous and their molecular basis is unknown.

Glycogen Storage Diseases (Glycogenoses)

In the course of intracellular digestion, glycogen is hydrolyzed within lysosomes by acid maltase. When this process fails to take place, glycogen, accumulating within lysosomal vacuoles, leads to muscle fiber damage, the clinical consequence of which is painless, progressive muscle weakness. Glycogen in the cytosol is a major fuel for glycolytic, fast twitch, type 2A and 2B fibers. As it is metabolized anaerobically to pyruvate and lactate, ATP is generated. Abnormalities in glycolytic enzymes lead to glycogen accumulation in the sarcoplasm, reduced lactate production, reduced formation of ATP, and impairment in muscle fiber metabolism, leading to rhabdomyolysis. Thus, clinical manifestations include myalgia (aches, cramps, and pains), fatigue, and myoglobinuria.[3,218]

Acid Maltase Deficiency (Pompe's Disease)

In 1963, Hers[219] discovered that a deficiency of acid maltase (alpha-1,4-glucosidase) caused a rapidly fatal disorder of infancy characterized by accumulation of glycogen in skeletal muscle, heart, and nervous system (Figs. 24-49 and 24-50). Elucidation of the enzyme defect led to the recognition of milder, later-onset forms. The mechanisms of muscle fiber injury in acid maltase deficiency (AMD) are thought to involve both the excessive storage of undergraded lysosomal material, which compromises vital cellular structures, and increased lysosomal activity. Both the severe and more benign forms are inherited as autosomal recessive traits. Acid maltase deficiency is due to alterations of the gene on chromosome 17.[220] The infantile form (Pompe's disease) is first noted at about 1 month of age, with severe hypotonia, weakness, and heart failure. There is enlargement of the heart, liver, and tongue. Death occurs by 2 years of age from cardiac and respiratory failure. The childhood form has a later onset. There is a delay in reaching motor milestones, followed by progressive weakness of proximal limb and trunk muscles. The liver and tongue may be enlarged but cardiomegaly is rare. Death occurs before the end of the second decade from respiratory insufficiency. In the adult form symptoms begin in the third or fourth decade, with slowly progressive weakness and wasting of proximal limb and trunk muscles, with sparing of bulbar musculature. Respiratory muscle weakness may occur and rarely results in death from ventilatory failure. The heart and liver are not affected. The adult variant can present as a limb girdle dystrophy, polymyositis, or spinal muscular atrophy. CK is elevated in most patients. The EMG discloses myopathic motor unit potentials, fibrillations, positive sharp waves, bizarre high frequency discharges, and true myotonic bursts. Occasionally, reduced recruitment with long duration, high amplitude motor unit potentials suggests a neurogenic component.

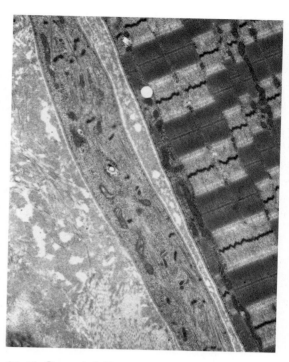

Fig. 24-48. Congenital fiber type disproportion (electron micrograph). A small fiber is present next to a normal fiber. The ultrastructural appearance of the small fiber is similar to that in neurogenic atrophy.

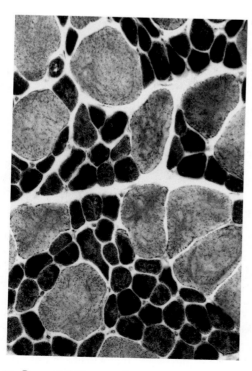

Fig. 24-47. Congenital fiber type disproportion. Note the two populations of fibers. The small (dark) fibers are exclusively type 1. (Frozen section, NADH-TR.)

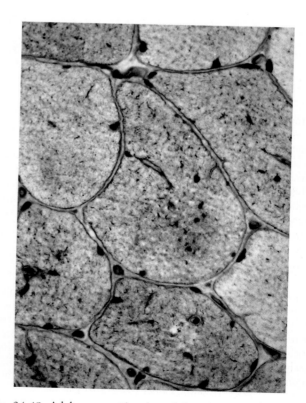

Fig. 24-49. Adult-onset acid maltase deficiency. The muscle fibers contain scattered coarse granules of PAS-positive (and diastase-sensitive) material. (Frozen section, PAS.) (Courtesy of the Armed Forces Institute of Pathology.)

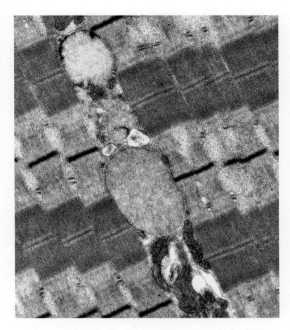

Fig. 24-50. Adult-onset acid maltase deficiency (electron micrograph). Same biopsy as Fig. 24-49. Distended membrane-bound sacs are filled with glycogen granules. (Courtesy of the Armed Forces Institute of Pathology.)

Of all the glycogenoses, AMD has the most distinct morphologic pattern. Because acid maltase is a lysosomal enzyme, a deficiency or absence of this enzyme leads to the accumulation of glycogen within lysosomes. It is therefore the only glycogenosis in which one finds packets of membrane-bound glycogen. There is a massive accumulation of granules and vacuoles of varying size filled with diastase-sensitive, PAS-positive material (Fig. 24-51). In spite of the marked devastation of the muscle fiber and the replacement of its contents with membrane-bound glycogen, there is little in the way of regenerative activity. Many fibers show almost complete dissolution of the myofibrillar content, but without apparent activation of the satellite cells or evidence of a reparative process. Indeed, the satellite cells themselves can be shown to contain membrane-bound glycogen. Electron microscopy shows clusters of glycogen granules free in the cytoplasm, in membranous sacs, and in autophagic vacuoles with other cytoplasmic products (Fig. 24-52). In adult cases, the glycogen-containing vacuoles may be few and small, making identification of the disease difficult. The histology of clinically unaffected muscles may be normal, and even in biopsies from weakened muscles, abnormalities may be slight. Most vacuoles contain PAS-positive granules that are removed by diastase and show high acid phosphatase activity.

Phosphorylase Deficiency (McArdle's Disease)

Phosphorylase deficiency was the first hereditary myopathy in which a specific enzyme defect was identified. In 1951, McArdle[221] described a 30-year-old man with a history of cramps and exercise intolerance since childhood. He postulated that the disorder was caused by a defect in glycogen breakdown. Later, it

was shown that skeletal muscle phosphorylase was absent and muscle glycogen increased.[222,223] In most cases, the disease is inherited as an autosomal recessive trait, although autosomal dominant transmission has been reported. The disease is caused by a deficiency of myophosphorylase, which is restricted to skeletal muscle. The clinical manifestations of the disease are well defined. Males outnumber females by a ratio of 3:1. In childhood, there is easy fatigability and mild weakness. Later, vigorous activity is accompanied by painful cramps in the exercising muscles. In about one-half of patients, muscle necrosis and myoglobinuria occur. Renal failure, a life-threatening complication of myoglobinuria, occurs in 8 percent of patients.

Patients learn to avoid sudden bursts of activity and prefer less intense but sustained exercise such as walking. Many patients experience a prominent second wind phenomenon attributable to mobilization of fatty acids and increased muscle blood flow that occurs with exercise. Between attacks, patients are well and can lead reasonably normal lives. Mild, permanent weakness is present in 20 percent of patients. Rarely, the disease presents with weakness and wasting in adult life without exercise intolerance, suggesting an acquired late-onset myopathy. In patients suspected of having the disease, ischemic forearm exercise should be performed under standard conditions. The peak level of venous lactate occurs within 3 to 5 minutes after

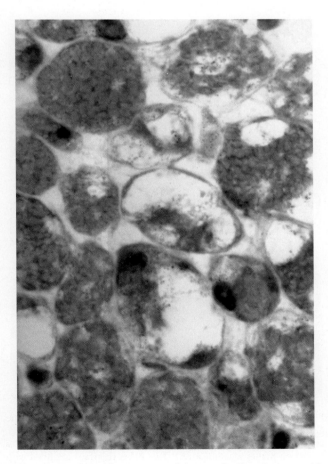

Fig. 24-51. Pompe's disease. Most of the muscle fibers have variably sized granules and vacuoles that, with appropriate stains, can be shown to contain glycogen. (Frozen section, H&E.)

exercise in normal subjects, reaching three to five times the resting pre-exercise level. Because patients with McArdle's disease are unable to break down glycogen, venous lactate fails to rise. Reduced lactate production, however, is not specific for McArdle's disease and is seen with other defects of the glycolytic pathway. The CK is elevated in most patients at rest and the EMG is abnormal in almost one-half of patients, showing myopathic potentials especially in patients with permanent weakness. The biopsy specimen may be structurally normal, except for the complete absence of phosphorylase activity. Often, however, in addition to a negative phosphorylase stain there are subsarcolemmal vacuoles that are filled with glycogen (Fig. 24-53). Biopsies often also show scattered necrotic and regenerating fibers, especially prominent if the patient has had a recent episode of myoglobinuria. Ultrastructural studies demonstrate that the glycogen granules are not membrane bound (Fig. 24-54). The gene that encodes for the enzyme was initially localized to the long arm of chromosome 11,[224] and recent advances in the molecular biology of the disease are summarized by DiMauro and Tsujino.[225] Isoenzymes under separate genetic control are present in other tissues. Multiple genetic mutations have been demonstrated in McArdle's disease, but the most common mutation is the substitution of thymine for cytosine at codon 49.[225,226]

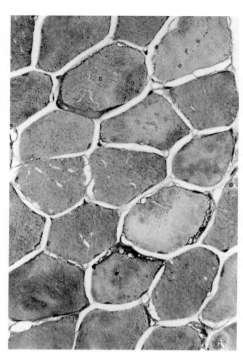

Fig. 24-53. McArdle's disease. Note subsarcolemmal collections of PAS-positive (darkly staining) material. (Frozen section, PAS.)

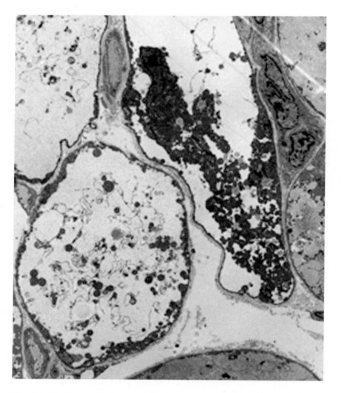

Fig. 24-52. Pompe's disease (electron micrograph). Several fibers are almost empty, with remnants of membranes, scattered mitochondria, and a few membrane-bound vesicles that contain glycogen granules (based on higher magnification). Two fibers (bottom) are filled with glycogen, much of which is membrane bound. Very few myofibrils are visible. (Courtesy of the Armed Forces Institute of Pathology.)

Phosphofructokinase Deficiency

In 1965, Tarui and colleagues [227] described three siblings with a clinical picture identical to McArdle's disease. Phosphofructokinase (PFK), the glycolytic enzyme that catalyzes the conversion of fructose 6-phosphate to fructose 1,6-diphosphate, was absent in these patients' muscles. Tarui et al also noted that their patients had a mild hemolytic anemia and found that red blood cell PFK activity was reduced by 50 percent. The M (muscle) subunit of the enzyme is present in muscle and red blood cells; red blood cells also have the L (liver) subunit. Genetic transmission of the syndrome is autosomal recessive. The gene encoding the M subunit of PFK is on chromosome 1[228] and multiple different mutations have been identified.[229] The muscle biopsy findings are identical to those of McArdle's disease except that, unlike phosphorylase deficiency, hyaline polysacharide inclusions (Lafora body-like by light and electron microscopy) have been found in some cases.[230] This polysaccharide stains with PAS but is not digested by salivary diastase. The accumulated material is similar to that found in patients who have brancher enzyme deficiency. In patients with PFK deficiency, there is absence of PFK activity as determined by histochemical or quantitative biochemical techniques.

Debrancher Enzyme Deficiency

Debrancher enzyme deficiency is an autosomal recessive disease that begins in infancy with hepatomegaly, growth retardation, fasting hypoglycemia, and cirrhosis. The enzyme defect has

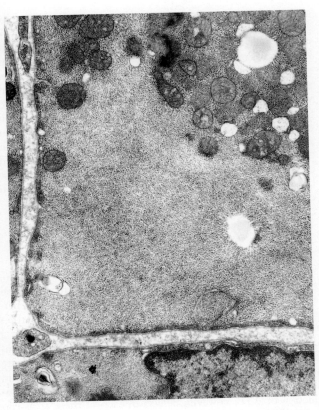

Fig. 24-54. McArdle's disease (electron micrograph). The subsarcolemmal vacuoles contain non-membrane-bound glycogen. This is not specific and can be seen in other glycogenoses or in diseases not related to glycogenosis. (Courtesy of the Armed Forces Institute of Pathology.)

been demonstrated in muscle, liver, leukocytes, and red blood cells. In the absence of debrancher enzyme activity, phosphorylase may hydrolyze the 1,4-glycosidic linkages to the point of branching. The resultant glycogen molecule has an excess number of exposed 1,6-glycosidic linkages and is referred to as *limit dextrin*. Myopathy is sometimes difficult to recognize in very ill infants, but it is not unusual to find hypotonia, lethargy, or delayed motor milestones. The disease has also been recognized as a cause of slowly progressive weakness in adult life. Unlike McArdle's disease and PFKD, cramps and myoglobinuria are not seen. The venous lactate level does not rise during ischemic exercise. Serum CK may be markedly elevated. The EMG shows myopathic features or a mixture of myopathic and neurogenic patterns. The muscle biopsy shows a severe vacuolar myopathy with subsarcolemmal and intramyofibrillar coarse, PAS-positive vacuoles that are digested by diastase. Ultrastructural studies show findings similar to those seen in McArdle's disease (i.e., pools of non-membrane-bound glycogen). The debrancher enzyme locus has been assigned to chromosome 1p21. The pathogenesis of the muscle weakness is obscure. There is a concomitant peripheral neuropathy, with glycogen accumulations in Schwann cells, which may contribute to the neurologic disability.

Other Glycogenoses

Other rarer glycogenoses, recently reviewed by DiMauro and Tsujino,[225] include deficiencies of phosphoglycerate kinase (chromosome Xq13), phosphoglycerate mutase (chromosome 7), and lactate dehydrogenase (chromosome 11, subunit M; chromosome 12, subunit H). The enzyme defects in all three diseases may produce muscle pain, weakness, and, when exercise persists in the face of myalgia, myoglobinuria. None of these enzyme defects produces a complete block of the glycolytic pathway, and thus severe glycogen accumulation does not occur. Brancher enzyme deficiency is a rapidly progressive autosomal recessive lethal disease of childhood with prominent liver dysfunction; hypotonia has been observed in some patients. Muscle biopsy studies have shown intensely PAS-positive intracytoplasmic deposits that are incompletely digestible with diastase. In these cases and in variants thereof, ultrastructural studies have shown Lafora-like bodies, while the glycogen granules appear normal; similar structures are also found in the central and peripheral nervous system.[231]

Endocrine Myopathies

Many of the generalized endocrine disorders can be associated with a myopathy.[232] In most cases, evidence of muscle involvement may even be subclinical, revealed only by special studies (e.g., serum enzymes, EMG, muscle biopsy) performed in the course of evaluation of the endocrine disorder. However, in some instances (e.g., thyrotoxicosis), the muscle symptoms may be a prominent, often presenting feature of the endocrine disorder. Most of these myopathies are readily reversed after correction of the underlying endocrine disturbance. As a general rule, the histologic changes present in the muscle tend to be mild and nonspecific, sometimes even in the face of severe muscle weakness and wasting. The endocrinopathies most consistently associated with myopathic features include hyperthyroidism, hypothyroidism, hyperparathyroidism, hyperadrenalism (Cushing's disease), hypoadrenalism (Addison's disease), and acromegaly. These are briefly discussed below.

Hyperthyroidism

Four different neuromuscular disorders may be seen in hyperthyroidism: thyrotoxic myopathy, myasthenia gravis, thyrotoxic periodic paralysis, and exophthalmic ophthalmoplegia. A chronic myopathy manifested largely by generalized proximal muscle weakness is a commonly observed finding in hyperthyroidism. It may at times precede other signs of thyrotoxicosis. The EMG may show myopathic abnormalities in about 90 percent of cases of hyperthyroidism. Nevertheless, light microscopic examination of the muscle may show essentially no abnormality or only mild myofiber atrophy. Other relatively minor histologic changes reported have included interstitial edema, single fiber necrosis, glycogen depletion, increased subsarcolemmal nuclei, and fatty infiltration. Ultrastructural abnormalities that have been described include papillary projections on the muscle fiber surface, various mitochondrial abnormalities, focal myofibrillar degeneration, tubular aggregates, and subsarcolemmal glycogen deposits. Neither the light microscopic nor the ultrastructural changes are specific for thyrotoxicosis.

Hypothyroidism

Patients with hypothyroidism often have a myopathy characterized by proximal weakness, slowed movements and reflexes, stiffness, myalgias, and less commonly cramps and/or muscle enlargement. Serum CK is usually elevated. Muscle biopsy specimens usually show nonspecific myopathic changes such as fiber atrophy (most often involving type 2 fibers), increased internal nuclei, glycogen accumulation, ring fibers, and endomysial fibrosis. Ultrastructural changes may include mitochondrial abnormalities, myofibrillar degeneration, glycogen accumulation, dilated sarcoplasmic reticulum, T tubule proliferation, lipoid granules, and autophagic vacuoles. Basophilic degeneration has been described in long-standing cases of hypothyroidism. None of the light or electron microscopic changes appears sufficient to explain the cause of the weakness in these patients.

Hyperparathyroidism

Both primary and secondary hyperparathyroidism may be associated with a myopathy. Clinically, this affects mainly proximal muscles, often with associated pain and fatigability, waddling gait, and hyperreflexia. The histologic changes seen in muscle biopsies from these patients are often surprisingly mild and have included nonspecific fiber atrophy, type 2 fiber atrophy, and focal vacuolar and degenerative changes.

Hyperadrenalism (Cushing's Disease)

Patients with Cushing's disease frequently have a myopathy characterized by proximal muscle weakness and wasting affecting especially the lower extremities. A myopathy can also be seen in association with exogenous corticosteroid therapy. The most consistent and characteristic histologic change observed in muscle biopsies in both conditions is selective atrophy of type 2 fibers. Sometimes this may involve more specifically the type 2B fibers. Occasionally type 1 fibers may show excess lipid deposition. Electron microscopy may show an apparent increase in glycogen within type 2 fibers. Other light microscopic and ultrastructural changes have been described but appear to be much less common and not as well documented.

Hypoadrenalism (Addison's Disease)

A myopathy characterized by severe generalized muscle weakness, cramping, and fatigue may occur in 25 to 50 percent of patients with adrenal insufficiency, regardless of its etiology. Serum muscle enzymes and EMG are usually normal. The muscle biopsy usually appears normal, except perhaps for some glycogen depletion.

Acromegaly

Proximal muscle weakness and diminished exercise tolerance may be present in about 50 percent of patients with acromegaly.[233] The muscle weakness may be insidious in onset, slowly progressive, and associated with some diminution in muscle bulk. Serum CK levels may be slightly elevated. The EMG shows myopathic changes in about 50 percent of patients with acromegaly. Histologic examination of muscle biopsy specimens has shown single fiber necrosis, nuclear enlargement with prominent nucleoli, proliferation and hypertrophy of satellite cells, increased glycogen, lipofuscin accumulation, and, rarely, mononuclear inflammatory infiltrates.[234] Hypertrophy of type 1 and/or type 2 fibers has also been described. Electron microscopic studies have noted excessive accumulation of glycogen and lipofuscin, myofibrillar degeneration, capillary basement membrane thickening, and increased satellite cells.[235]

Mitochondrial Myopathies

The mitochondrial encephalomyopathies are a set of heterogeneous disorders with many clinical manifestations, a wide variety of molecular pathogenic mechanisms, and variable patterns of inheritance. In the mitochondrial myopathies myopathic symptoms and signs arise as a consequence of a demonstrable abnormality in mitochondrial function. The underlying mechanism of disease may be due to defective substrate utilization, oxidative phosphorylation, or respiratory chain function. In each case, the common end point is deficient production of ATP; however, defects in each of these areas can have different patterns of pathology. Abnormal substrate utilization occurs in carnitine palmitoyltransferase (CPT) and carnitine deficiencies as well as disorders of pyruvate metabolism. Morphologic alterations of mitochondria are lacking in these diseases. By contrast, defects in oxidative phosphorylation or respiratory chain function are associated with characteristic histopathologic findings.

The presence of ragged-red fibers (Fig. 24-55) in muscle biopsy is a defining criterion in these diseases.[236] These are abnormally contoured fibers with an irregular/frayed outline best demonstrable on transverse frozen sections of muscle. When a modified Gomori trichrome reaction is run on the specimen the ragged-red fibers stain intensely red. The red staining is due to the presence of coarse granules that may be patchily dispersed throughout the cell, bulge out from the surface, form a crescent beneath the sarcolemma, or overwhelm the entire fiber. The involved fibers are often smaller than normal and are randomly distributed throughout the biopsy. They may be suspected on H&E sections when pale basophilic subsarcolemmal aggregates are noted; they are also well demonstrated with oxidative enzyme histochemical reactions. Electron microscopy is useful for delineating the abnormal mitochondria in cases where the light microscopic features are clear-cut or it is sometimes the diagnostic procedure when the light microscopic findings are ambiguous.

Ultrastructural features of ragged-red fibers include abnormally numerous subsarcolemmal intermyofibrillar mitochondria. The mitochondria and their crista structure are also often misshapen and there are characteristic intramitochondrial paracrystalline "parking lot" inclusions (Fig. 24-56). In addition other inclusions may be seen such as spiral/cylindrical structures, dense bodies, excessive accumulations of glycogen, and abnormal lipid deposits. Mitochondria are unique subcellular organelles in having their own genome that encodes genes for a small proportion of mitochondrial proteins. These include 13 components of the respiratory chain, a number of transfer RNAs, and two ribosomal RNAs. Because a fertilized zygote receives mitochondria from only the ovum, mutations are passed on only through the maternal lineage. All offspring likely inherit mutant mitochondria, but each cell contains a random mixture of mutant and normal mitochondria and cells receiving low proportions of mutant organelles may not express the defect (i.e., the threshold effect). Furthermore, some tissues are more dependent on oxidative metabolism, and thus, more likely to express a defect in mitochondrial function. These en-

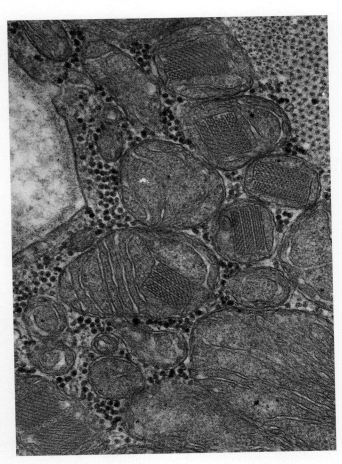

Fig. 24-56. Ragged-red fiber (electron micrograph). The granular deposits seen by light microscopy consist of pleomorphic abnormal mitochondria, some of which have paracrystalline structures. (Courtesy of the Armed Forces Institute of Pathology.)

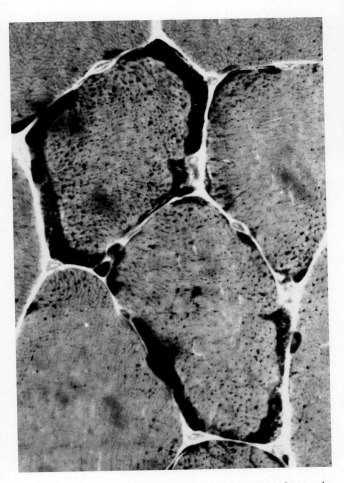

Fig. 24-55. Ragged-red fibers. The fibers have a red-purple granular-reticular network, often with prominent subsarcolemmal deposits. This material stains positively with the NADH-TR and succinic dehydrogenase reactions, indicating that it represents mitochondria. (Frozen section, MGT.)

ergy-dependent tissues include the CNS, skeletal and cardiac muscle (EOMs in particular), and kidney and liver. Because most mitochondrial proteins are encoded by the nuclear genome, autosomal dominant or recessive inheritance is also possible. Mitochondrial disorders with maternal inheritance and a myopathic component include MERRF (myoclonus epilepsy and ragged-red fibers), MELAS (mitochondrial encephalomyopathy, lactic acidosis, and stroke-like episodes), and NARP (developmental delay, retinitis pigmentosa, dementia, seizures, ataxia, proximal neurogenic muscle weakness, and sensory neuropathy). KSS/CPEO (Kearns-Sayre syndrome/chronic progressive external ophthalmoplegia) is also caused by mitochondrial mutations but is inherited as a sporadic trait.

MERRF is characterized by myoclonic seizures, mitochondrial myopathy, and cerebellar ataxia and can be slowly progressive or rapidly fatal. Muscle biopsy reveals ragged-red fibers and numerous cytochrome oxidase-negative fibers. The causative mutation in most cases is an A to G transition at nucleotide 8344 in the mitochondrial tRNA^{Lys} gene.[237] Because the tRNA^{Lys} is probably essential for proper synthesis of all mitochondrially encoded proteins, biochemical defects may be found in any of respiratory chain complexes I, II, III, and IV. The primary clinical presentation in MELAS is of a severe, progressive encephalomyopathy with stroke-like episodes. Up to 10 percent of patients may also have progressive external ophthalmoplegia (PEO). Most patients have a lactic acidosis and muscle biopsy reveals ragged-red fibers. Like MERRF, MELAS is due to a specific point mutation at nucleotide 3243 in the mitochondrial tRNA^{LEU} gene resulting in abnormalities of several respiratory chain complexes.[238] NARP is a clinically variable syndrome of developmental delay, retinitis pigmentosa, dementia, seizures, ataxia, proximal neurogenic muscle weakness, and sensory neuropathy.[239] Muscle biopsy is nonspecific, revealing neurogenic changes and no ragged-red fibers. Electron microscopy shows small subsarcolemmal accumulations of mitochondria, some of which had abnormal cristae, but there are no paracrystalline inclusions. A mitochondrial point mutation at position 8993 changes a leucine to arginine in subunit 6 of the mitochondrial H$^+$-ATPase. The clinical variability correlates to some degree with the amount of mutant mitochondrial DNA in the patients.

The Kearns-Sayre syndrome (KSS) is a sporadic neurologic disorder characterized clinically by onset in the second decade, PEO, pigmentary retinal degeneration, and heart block and pathologically by the finding of ragged-red fibers and cytochrome oxidase-negative fibers. Additional clinical manifestations include ataxia, hearing loss, dementia, endocrinologic disturbances, and peripheral neuropathy. The characteristic mutations are deletions, or occasionally duplications, of the mitochondrial DNA.[240] So-called incomplete KSS presents with PEO and some, but not all, of the other features of KSS. Similar deletions in incomplete KSS demonstrate the identity of this syndrome with KSS. At the mild end of the spectrum are cases of isolated PEO with proximal limb weakness and ragged-red fibers. Up to 50 percent of these patients may also have deletions of their mitochondrial DNA.[241] Two autosomally inherited defects involving mitochondrial DNA are known. Patients with the multiple deletion syndrome present with PEO, weakness of proximal limb and respiratory muscles, cataracts, and hearing loss.[242] Patients have a lactic acidosis and ragged-red fibers on muscle biopsy and biochemical studies reveal defective oxidative phosphorylation. Southern blot analysis of mitochondrial DNA from affected tissues reveals a heterogeneous population of molecules with different deletions originating in the D loop. The disease follows autosomal dominant inheritance and linkage studies have mapped the defective gene to chromosome 10q.[243] Depletion of mitochondrial DNA is a quantitative defect that presents variably as a myopathy, liver, and/or renal dysfunction.[244] Lactic acidosis and ragged-red fibers are seen, as are abnormalities of the respiratory chain. The degree of clinical severity in a given organ correlates with reductions in amount of mitochondrial DNA but the numbers of mitochondria are increased, implying that many contain no

DNA. There is no evidence for maternal inheritance and the disorder seems to be autosomal recessive.

Lipid Myopathies

Fatty acids are the major fuel for muscle at rest, in the fasting state, and during prolonged, low intensity aerobic exercise. They are mobilized from fat deposits and oxidized in muscle mitochondria. Short chain fatty acids penetrate the mitochondrial membrane with ease, but long chain fatty acids (palmitic and oleic) are impermeable unless combined with carnitine, which facilitates their transport to intramitochondrial sites. Inside the muscle fiber, fatty acids are activated to fatty acyl-CoA derivatives. On the outer mitochondrial membrane, these are joined to carnitine by carnitine palmitoyltransferase I (CPT I) to form a permeable derivative, fatty acylcarnitine, which moves across the mitochondrial membrane into the mitochondria. There, CPT II catalyzes the reverse reaction, with the formation of fatty acyl-CoA, which can then undergo oxidation. Two main categories of disordered muscle lipid metabolism have been identified: (1) carnitine deficiency, characterized by progressive weakness and excessive muscle fiber lipid storage; and (2) CPT deficiency, causing recurrent muscle pain and myoglobinuria with little muscle fiber lipid accumulation.

Carnitine Deficiency

Carnitine deficiency was first described in 1972 by Engel and Siekert[245] who reported the case of a 19-year-old woman with lifelong mild generalized weakness that rapidly progressed, rendering her bed-fast and in need of respiratory support. Muscle biopsy disclosed excessive lipid accumulation, especially in type 1 fibers. Since that description, additional familial cases have been further described that fall into two seemingly distinct groups. In the myopathic form there is a progressive weakness, most marked in proximal and trunk muscles, generally beginning in childhood. Rarely, there is rapid worsening associated with respiratory failure; heart involvement may give rise to cardiomyopathy. The serum CK is moderately increased in most patients and the EMG shows myopathic changes. The muscle biopsy shows intrafiber lipid droplets, most marked in type 1 fibers (Fig. 24-57). There is less lipid accumulation in the fibers with reduced oxidative capacity (the type 2A and type 2B fibers). Ultrastructurally (Fig. 24-58), droplets are not membrane bound and accumulate in parallel rows between myofibrils or beneath the sarcolemma. The systemic form was first described by Karpati et al,[246] who described an 11-year-old boy with lifelong clumsiness, thin muscles, and a short history of generalized weakness. At ages 3 and 9 he had episodes of unexplained liver failure with hepatic encephalopathy, but recovery was good. The muscle biopsy showed lipid accumulation in most type 1 fibers, and carnitine was virtually absent from muscle and reduced by 80 to 90 percent in liver and plasma. In additional cases that have been reported, the onset is generally in childhood and the main clinical features are progressive weak-

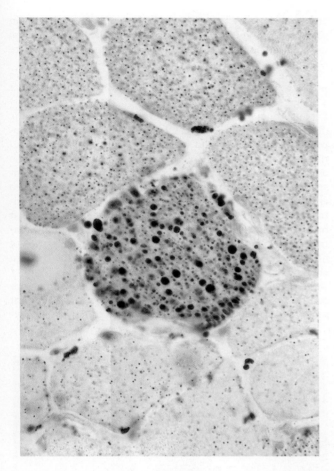

Fig. 24-57. Lipid storage myopathy. The muscle fiber in the center contains an excessive number of coarse lipid globules. (Frozen section, oil red O.)

ness and recurrent hepatic encephalopathy with metabolic acidosis. Death from respiratory failure has occurred before the age of 20 in most cases.[247] The molecular genetics of carnitine deficiency is not completely understood at present.

Carnitine Palmitoyltransferase Deficiency

Carnitine palmitoyltransferase (CPT) deficiency, first described by DiMauro and Melis-DiMauro[248] and further characterized clinically in subsequent reports, is a disease that begins in childhood. The major clinical feature is myoglobinuria associated with muscle pain provoked by prolonged exercise, fasting, or both. The frequency of myoglobinuria appears to be much higher in CPT deficiency than in McArdle's disease or other glycolytic defects. Between attacks, patients are well and there is no permanent weakness. The muscle biopsy is usually normal unless there has been a previous episode of myoglobinuria, in which case scattered necrotic and regenerating fibers are found. Lipid content is either normal or mildly increased. CPT deficiency shows a striking male predominance and is probably transmitted as an autosomal recessive trait. This CPT-

deficient myopathy is now known to result from CPT II gene mutations on chromosome 1p32.[249,250]

Channelopathies

The channelopathies are a large group of primarily inherited myopathies characterized by abnormalities in ion-channel structure/and function and include the periodic paralyses, paramyotonia congenita, myotonia congenita (Thomsen's disease, and Becker's myotonia) and malignant hyperthermia.

Periodic Paralysis

Periodic paralysis constitutes a group of disorders that share in common the clinical feature of attacks of paralysis with associated flaccidity, and a tendency to remit and relapse. Three forms of the disorder are recognized, classified according to the level of serum potassium present during an attack. All three variants are usually inherited as autosomal dominant traits, although they can also occur sporadically. The hypokalemic variant is the most common form of periodic paralysis. It is more common in males and usually has its onset between the ages of 20 and 35. The disorder is characterized by the appearance of sudden attacks of generalized muscle paralysis with relative sparing of the external ocular and respiratory muscles. The attacks usually occur at night and are precipitated by prior strenuous exercise, a high carbohydrate meal, or exposure to cold.

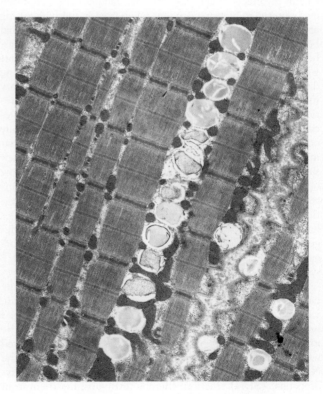

Fig. 24-58. Lipid storage myopathy (electron micrograph). Note subsarcolemmal and intermyofibrillar irregular electron-lucent lipid globules.

Serum potassium levels during an attack are low. Between attacks, patients are usually normal, although there may be some residual muscle weakness. The hyperkalemic variant usually begins in childhood and tends to affect both sexes equally. Unlike the hypokalemic variant, the attacks often occur during the daytime and are usually briefer but more frequent. There may be considerable variation in the extent and severity of weakness. Some patients may display myotonia, especially of face and hand muscles. Characteristically, there is a rise in serum potassium levels during an attack, although the elevation may at times be quite minimal. The attacks may be precipitated by exercise or exposure to cold, and can also be induced by the administration of potassium chloride. Normokalemic periodic paralysis shares many clinical features in common with the hyperkalemic variant. Serum potassium levels typically remain unchanged during an attack.

In addition to the primary periodic paralysis syndromes, secondary forms of both hypo- and hyperkalemic periodic paralysis may occur. Among the more common secondary hypokalemic forms are thyrotoxic periodic paralysis, periodic paralysis secondary to urinary or gastrointestinal potassium loss, and barium-induced periodic paralysis. Periodic paralysis due to hyperkalemia may be seen in patients with renal or adrenal failure. The pathologic findings in all forms of periodic paralysis are qualitatively similar but tend to be most pronounced in the hypokalemic variant. The principal light microscopic abnormality consists of the presence of variable numbers of vacuoles within myofibers[251] (Fig. 24-59). The vacuoles are more often encountered in biopsy specimens taken from individuals during an acute attack; the muscle may, in fact, appear fairly normal between episodes. The most conspicuous vacuolar changes, however, are seen in muscle biopsies obtained from patients who have a permanent myopathy resulting from long-standing disease with recurrent episodes of paralysis. The vacuoles vary in size but can be quite large, and they tend to occupy the interior rather than periphery of the fiber. Multiloculated vacuoles can also be seen. The vacuoles usually appear "empty" but may occasionally contain PAS-positive, diastase-digestible granular material and rarely calcium. In addition to the vacuoles, biopsies from patients with a permanent myopathy may also show other myopathic features including variation in fiber size, internal nuclei, fiber necrosis, moth-eaten fibers, and proliferation of connective tissue. Detailed electron microscopic studies have shown that the vacuoles arise from the proliferation, degeneration, and autophagic destruction of membranous organelles derived chiefly from the sarcoplasmic reticulum and T system tubules.

Another morphologic change often encountered in periodic paralysis, especially in the hyperkalemic and normokalemic variants, is the presence of tubular aggregates. In H&E-stained sections, they appear as basophilic deposits found in both the interior and periphery of muscle fibers. They stain intensely red with the modified trichrome method and dark blue with the NADH-TR reaction, but fail to stain with the succinic dehydrogenase (SDH) reaction, thereby distinguishing them from mitochondria (Fig. 24-60). They are found predominantly, but not exclusively, in type 2 fibers. Ultrastructurally, tubular aggregates consist of fascicular arrays of parallel double-walled tubules having a diameter of 60 to 90 nm (Fig. 24-61). On cross-section, they form a hexagonal profile. The tubules can sometimes be observed in continuity with the dilated terminal cisterns of the arcoplasmic reticulum, from which they are thought to be derived.

Paramyotonia Congenita

Paramyotonia congenita is an autosomal dominant myotonic disorder showing paradoxical myotonia (i.e., myotonia that appears during exercise and increases with continued exercise) that is especially severe after exposure to cold and involves the muscles of the face, neck, and distal upper extremities. The onset of the disease is in childhood and the clinical picture is also characterized by episodes of flaccid paresis that may be precipitated by exposure to cold.[252] The few muscle biopsy studies that have been reported describe minimal changes, including variation in fiber size, internalized nuclei, and poor differentiation of fiber types.[253] Different defects in the adult muscle sodium channel alpha-subunit gene (SSCN4A)[254] on chromosome 17 cause hyperkalemic periodic paralysis and paramyotonia congenita.[255] In hyperkalemic periodic paralysis, the mutant sodium channels fail to inactivate properly in response to hy-

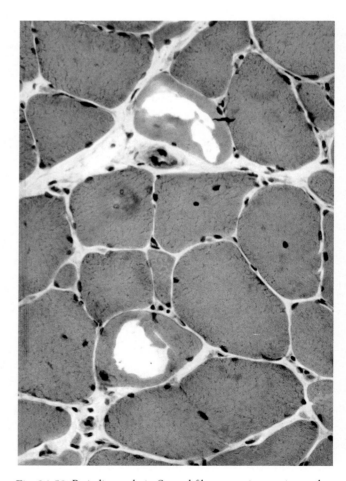

Fig. 24-59. Periodic paralysis. Several fibers contain prominent clear vacuoles. The muscle also shows variability in fiber size and internalized nuclei. (Frozen section, H&E.)

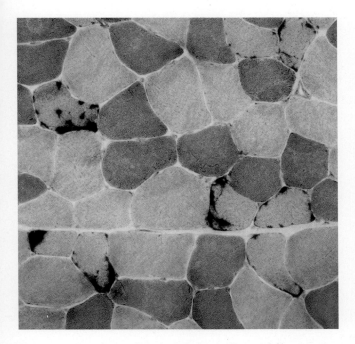

Fig. 24-60. Periodic paralysis, hyperkalemic. Scattered fibers contain large deposits of material that stains intensely with NADH-TR. These represent tubular aggregates. (Frozen section, NADH-TR.) (Courtesy of the Armed Forces Institute of Pathology.)

including internalized nuclei and variation in fiber size. One report describes a remarkable absence of type 2B fibers[259] whereas other cases have not shown this histochemical abnormality.[260] Both the dominant and recessive forms are channelopathies linked to the human skeletal muscle chloride channel gene (CLC-1) on chromosome 7 and a mutation has been identified in a family with the recessive Becker's form.[261] The muscle stiffness is a result of repetitive myofibrillar action potentials (myotonic runs). Chloride channels are responsible for most of the resting membrane conductance and defects likely lead to instability of the membrane potential and hence, hyperexcitability.

Malignant Hyperthermia

Malignant hyperthermia is a rare autosomal dominant clinical syndrome ordinarily occurring in previously asymptomatic individuals (children more often than adults) characterized by a dramatic hypermetabolic state (tachypnea, tachycardia, hypertension, and muscle spasm and later, rise in body temperature) triggered at the time of induction of general anesthesia (rarely, in the recovery period). The offending agents have mostly been halogenated inhaled anesthetic compounds and succinylcholine, but the attack may also be brought on in the absence of anesthesia, under stressful situations, or in individuals with other muscle diseases (CPT deficiency, central core disease, Duchenne/Becker dystrophy). In at least 50 percent of cases there is a previous history of uneventful anesthesia.

perkalemia following activity. The channels remain open, allowing excess sodium to enter the cell and enhancing membrane depolarization. This causes inactivation of the normal sodium channels encoded by the normal allele, and the membranes become inexcitable leading to paralysis. The abnormally high intracellular sodium levels lead to water uptake from the blood and a further rise in serum potassium, which enhances the severity of this cycle. Paramyotonia congenita may represent the first temperature-sensitive mutations identified in humans.[256] Cold-induced paramyotonia is due to persistent membrane depolarization presumably caused by abnormal sodium influx. By contrast, hypokalemic periodic paralysis is caused by mutations in the muscle dihydropyridine-sensitive calcium channel alpha-1 subunit (CACNL1A3) gene whose protein product participates in excitation-contraction coupling.[257] The pathogenesis of these mutations is presently unknown. There is evidence for further genetic heterogeneity in both hyper- and hypokalemic periodic paralyses.

Myotonia Congenita

Myotonia congenita presents in childhood with diffuse stiffness on initiation of motor activities (e.g., arising from a chair or starting to walk or run). Strength usually remains normal. The serum CK may be normal or up to three times normal and EMG studies show myotonic discharges. The autosomal dominant variant is referred to as Thomsen's disease[258] and it starts earlier in childhood than does the autosomal recessive form (Becker's myotonia). Muscle biopsy studies have shown minimal changes

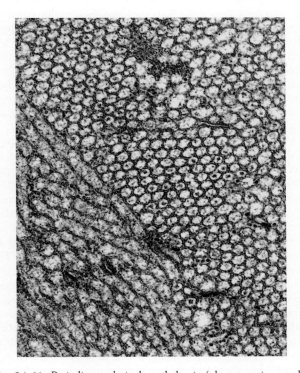

Fig. 24-61. Periodic paralysis, hyperkalemic (electron micrograph). Ultrastructure of tubular aggregate consisting of fascicular arrays of parallel double-walled tubules, 60 to 90 nm in diameter. (Courtesy of the Armed Forces Institute of Pathology.)

The only reliable method of diagnosis besides genetic analysis is the in vitro skeletal muscle biopsy contraction study, which is performed in very few centers around the world. The test is based on the observation that the skeletal muscle of affected individuals undergoes measurable halothane- or caffeine-potentiated contracture. A calcium uptake method applied to frozen sections is also used with unpredictable results. The muscle biopsy is structurally normal in most cases. The pathophysiology of the attack in the porcine model of malignant hyperthermia is that there is an anesthesia-generated loss of control of intracellular calcium because of a point mutation in the ryanodine receptor gene.[262,263] The frequency of a corresponding mutation in the chromosome 19 ryanodine receptor gene in humans is about 7 percent, but the genetic basis for most of the human cases is still not completely understood and there is evidence for several other loci on chromosomes 3,[264] 7,[265] and 17.[266] The chromosome 7 locus may be the voltage-dependent calcium channel alpha-2/delta subunit (CACNL2A).

Toxic Myopathies

Toxic drug-related myopathies have been reported with a wide variety of compounds.[267] Only those few that are associated with distinctive clinicopathologic syndromes are discussed briefly.

Alcoholics develop acute myopathic syndromes related to rhabdomyolysis (alcoholic myonecrosis) in the setting of alcohol withdrawal seizures. With obtundation and pressure exerted on dependent parts of the body they may also develop compartment syndromes. Histopathologic studies have shown multifocal acute fiber necrosis.[267] An acute painful myopathy may also develop associated with cramps, presumably related to impaired glycogen metabolism. There is no consensus on the existence of a chronic progressive myopathy directly related to the effects of the drug.[267] Other complicating factors include the effects on muscle related to alcoholism-associated electrolyte imbalances (e.g., hypokalemia), and nutritional or vitamin deficiencies.

Myopathy due to intoxication with the anti-inflammatory drug *colchicine* is relatively uncommon, but is now being reported more often, especially in a setting of progressive renal failure, as newer indications for the drug are being explored.[268] Muscle biopsy studies have shown a relatively distinctive toxic myopathy characterized by extensive monophasic individual fiber necrosis, vacuolization, prominent acid phosphatase activity in the necrotic fibers, and relatively little interstitial inflammation or endomysial connective tissue proliferation. The ultrastructural findings have also been fairly uniform consisting of multifocal subsarcolemmal or intermyofibrillar membranous whorls (myeloid bodies), dense bodies, and cytoplasmic degradation products[267,269] (Fig. 24-62). A very similar clinicopathologic picture has been observed with a variety of other drugs that contain a hydrophobic region and a primary or substituted amine group, which can bear a net positive charge. About 20 of these so-called *amphiphilic drugs* have now been recognized to give rise to myopathies, including chloroquine, imipramine, amiodarone, and perhexiline.[267,270,271] A related group of *cholesterol-lowering drugs*, including lovastatin (and

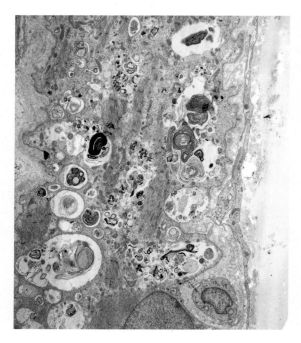

Fig. 24-62. Toxic myopathy (electron micrograph). Subsarcolemmal accumulation of membranous debris.

analogues), taken in isolation or in combination with gemfibrozil or cyclosporine, have also been reported to cause a toxic myopathy. These drugs inhibit cholesterol synthesis and presumably cause a toxic myonecrosis by damaging the cell membrane. The clinical syndrome, characterized by relatively abrupt onset of leg (greater than arm) weakness, sometimes associated with pain, and elevation of CK, is entirely reversible with discontinuation of the drug. Pathologic examination shows primarily muscle fiber necrosis and myophagocytosis with relatively little interstitial inflammation.[267,272]

Zidovudine (AZT) inhibits HIV reverse transcriptase and has been used extensively for the treatment of AIDS. Long-term administration of the drug has resulted in a previously unrecognized dose-related myopathy characterized by rapidly progressive proximal muscle weakness, myalgia, and elevated CK levels. Several muscle biopsy studies have shown a distinctive picture consisting of random muscle fiber necrosis and myophagocytosis with minimal inflammation and striking ragged-red fibers with ultrastructural abnormalities of mitochondria, cytoplasmic bodies, nemaline rods, and autophagic vacuoles.[273,274] With discontinuation of the drug the illness has been largely reversible after a few weeks.[275]

The *eosinophilia myalgia syndrome*, perhaps now only of historic interest, is a neuromyopathic symptom complex related to the ingestion of l-tryptophan (or a contaminant thereof apparently traced to a particular batch manufactured in Japan that was subsequently taken off the market) as health food/body building pills. This syndrome, first recognized 5 years ago, had considerable variability in severity ranging from a mild fasciitis with scleroderma-like dermatologic manifestations, myalgia, arthralgia, and hypereosinophilia to severe muscle weakness and respiratory insufficiency. Death from extreme emaciation occurred in a few cases. Histopathologic study of muscle and nerve has shown random fiber myophagocytosis, variable eosinophilia with fasciitis, and sometimes extreme proliferation of fibrous tissue in muscle and nerve.[267,276]

The neuromuscular syndrome of *chronic progressive distal weakness* that is seen in patients with end-stage renal disease is believed to be related to peripheral neuropathy rather than to a primary muscle disease. Light and electron microscopic studies have shown type 2 fiber atrophy, "moth-eaten" fibers, and calcium deposits.[277,278]

Unclassified

Myoadenylate deaminase deficiency (MAD) is a poorly understood condition characterized clinically by postexertional myalgias and cramps and histochemically/biochemically by the absence of myoadenylate deaminase reactivity in frozen sections of muscle and the biochemical demonstration of decreased myoadenylate deaminase activity in muscle tissue. No structural or ultrastructural abnormalities have been uncovered in this condition thus far. A responsible autosomal recessive trait has been postulated to be present in 1 to 2 percent of all individuals undergoing muscle biopsy. The gene has been localized to chromosome 1p13-p21 and several mutations have been identified.[279] There is no clear consensus on the relationship between the clinical condition and the enzymatic abnormality. The nosologic status of MAD is uncertain until more studies on affected individuals from different laboratories around the world become available.

Myasthenia Gravis and Other Disorders of the Neuromuscular Junction

Myasthenia gravis is an autoimmune disease that results from an antibody-mediated attack on the nicotinic AChR. The main clinical features of the illness are weakness and fatigability. The weakness has a special predilection for cranial nerve-innervated muscles. It affects all age groups but is especially common in young adult women and older men. Diplopia and ptosis are common presenting manifestations. Other early symptoms include dysphagia, dysarthria, difficulty in chewing, and difficulty in holding up the head. As the disease progresses, involvement of muscles of the shoulder and pelvic girdles as well as trunk muscles develops. In advanced cases and rarely, early in the course of the disease, respiratory muscles are affected. Laboratory studies disclose antibodies to AChR in 90 percent of patients. Repetitive nerve stimulation at low rates (2 Hz) is abnormal because of a decremental motor response. Ten to 15 percent of patients (especially the older men) will be found to have a thymoma. Muscle biopsy is usually normal. Patients who have been receiving corticosteroids may develop type 2 fiber atrophy.[280] Rarely, collections of lymphocytes (lymphorrhages) are seen. Electron microscopic studies of the muscle endplate region show a remarkably simplified postsynaptic region with degeneration of junctional folds (Fig. 24-63).

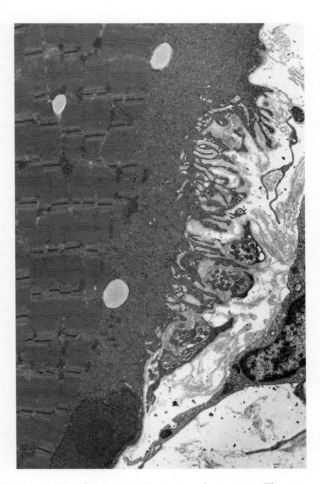

Fig. 24-63. Myasthenia gravis. Neuromuscular junction. The primary synaptic clefts are shallow and the secondary synaptic clefts are widened and shortened. The nerve terminals appear relatively normal.

When the myasthenic postsynaptic junction is stained for AChR, few are found on the terminal expansions of junctional folds, normally sites densely packed with AChR. Immunocytochemical studies show IgG, complement components C3 and C9, and the membrane attack complex all localized to the neuromuscular junction. This suggests that complement fixation and activation of the lytic phase of the complement reaction sequence occur in myasthenia gravis. The etiology of this disease is unknown, but much has been learned of its pathogenesis. First, there is complement-mediated lysis of the postsynaptic membrane, which causes loss of AChR. Second, autoantibodies bind to the AChR and result in accelerated degradation of receptor molecules. The first mechanism reduces membrane surface available for the insertion of new AChR. Third, autoantibodies may directly block the access of ACh to the receptor.

The *Lambert-Eaton myasthenic syndrome* (LEMS) usually develops as a paraneoplastic process, most commonly with small cell carcinoma of the lung (60 percent of cases), although it can be found in the absence of an underlying malignant tumor. Patients develop proximal muscle weakness along with evidence of autonomic dysfunction. No clinical improvement is found with the tensilon test and electrophysiologic studies show evidence of enhanced neurotransmission with repetitive stimulation. These clinical features allow this disorder to be separated from myasthenia gravis. The muscle biopsy is normal by light microscopy. Electron microscopic study has shown minimal or no abnormalities in the synaptic region.[281] Detailed electrophysiologic studies performed on muscle biopsies from patients with LEMS have shown that single vesicle content of ACh is normal and that the postsynaptic membrane is normally responsive to ACh, but that fewer vesicles are released in response to each presynaptic action potential. Although antibodies directed against the AChR are not present in these patients, their serum contains IgG species that allow passive transfer of LEMS-type electrophysiologic findings to animals. Recent studies have described a high frequency of P/Q-type calcium channel antibodies in patients with LEMS suggesting that these antibodies have a role in the pathogenesis of the presynaptic impairment of ACh releases in this disease.[282]

Other diseases of the neuromuscular transmission include inherited diseases largely of a nonimmunologic etiology. A number of syndromes have been described including both pre- and postsynaptic defects.[283] The typical presentation is that of an infant with ocular, bulbar, and respiratory weakness and associated generalized weakness that worsens with fatigue. The laboratory studies are unremarkable and the tensilon test is often negative. Muscle biopsy studies are often not performed in these children, but in the few reported instances when this was done, there have been no abnormalities noted by light microscopy, including enzyme histochemistry; abnormalities in the density of synaptic vesicle and in the junctional folds of the neuromuscular junction have been seen by electron microscopy.

ACKNOWLEDGMENTS

The authors acknowledge with pleasure all former collaborators who contributed to prior editions of this chapter: Drs. V. W. Armbrustmacher, D. Chad, and T. W. Smith.

REFERENCES

1. Carpenter S, Karpati G: Pathology of Skeletal Muscle. Churchill Livingstone, New York, 1984
2. Dubowitz V: Muscle Disorders in Childhood. 2nd Ed. Saunders/Baillière Tindall, Philadelphia/London, 1995
3. Engel AG, Franzini-Armstrong C (eds): Myology. Basic and Clinical. 2nd Ed. McGraw-Hill, New York, 1994
4. Kakulas BA, Adams RD: Diseases of Muscle. Pathological Foundations of Clinical Myology. 3rd Ed. Harper & Row, Philadelphia, 1985
5. Nageotte J: Sur la contraction extrême des muscles squelettiques chez les vertébrés. Zellforschung Mikroskopische Anatomie 26:603–624, 1937
6. Jay V, Becker LE: Fiber-type differentiation by myosin immunohistochemistry on paraffin-embedded skeletal muscle. A useful adjunct to fiber typing by the adenosine triphosphatase reaction. Arch Pathol Lab Med 118:917–918, 1994
7. Hille B: Ionic Channels of Excitable Membranes. Sinauer, Sunderland, 1992
8. Rudy B: Diversity and ubiquity of K channels. Neuroscience 25:729–749, 1988
9. Adrian RH: Rectification in muscle membrane. Prog Biophy Mol Bio 19:339–369, 1969
10. Latorre R, Oberhauser A, Labarca P, et al: Varieties of calcium-activated potassium channels. Ann Rev Physiol 51:385–399, 1989
11. Spruce AE, Standen NB, Stanfield PR: Studies of the unitary properties of adenosine-5′-triphosphate-regulated potassium channels of frog skeletal muscle. J Physiol 382:213–236, 1987
12. Bretag AH: Muscle chloride channels. Physiol Rev 67:618–724, 1987
13. Palade PT, Barchi RL: Characteristics of the chloride conductance in muscle fibers of the rat diaphragm. J Gen Physiol 69:325–342, 1977
14. Campbell DT, Hille B: Kinetic and pharmacological properties of the sodium channel of frog skeletal muscle. J Gen Physiol 67:309–323, 1976
15. Block BA, Imagawa T, Campbell KP, et al: Structural evidence for direct interaction between the molecular components of the transverse tubule/sarcoplasmic reticulum junction in skeletal muscle. J Cell Biol 107:2587–6000, 1988
16. Catterall WA: Excitation-contraction coupling in vertebrate skeletal muscle: a tale of two calcium channels. Cell 64:871–874, 1991
17. Fleischer S, Inui M: Biochemistry and biophysics of excitation-contraction coupling. Annu Rev Biophys Biophys Chem 18:333–364, 1989
18. Campbell KP, Leung AT, Sharp AH: The biochemistry and molecular biology of the dihydropyridine-sensitive calcium channel. Trends Neurosci 11:425–430, 1988
19. Rios E, Pizarro G: Voltage sensor of excitation-contraction coupling in skeletal muscle. Physiol Rev 71:849–908, 1991
20. Zorzato F, Fujii J, Otsu K, et al: Molecular cloning of cDNA encoding human and rabbit forms of the Ca^{2+} release channel (ryanodine receptor) of skeletal muscle sarcoplasmic reticulum. J Biol Chem 265:2244–2246, 1990
21. Craig R, Knight P: Myosin molecules, thick filaments and the actin-myosin complex. pp. 97–203. In Harris R (ed): Electron Microscopy of Proteins. Academic Press, San Diego, 1983
22. Elliott A, Offer G: Shape and flexibility of the myosin molecule. J Mol Biol 123:505–519, 1978
23. Lowey S, Cohen C: Studies on the structure of myosin. J Mol Biol 4:293–308, 1962
24. Weber A, Murray JM: Molecular control mechanisms in muscle contraction. Physiol Rev 53:612–673, 1973
25. Beggs AH, Byers TJ, Knoll JH, et al: Cloning and characterization of two human skeletal muscle α-actinin genes located on chromosomes 1 and 11. J Biol Chem 267:9281–9288, 1992
26. Blanchard A, Ohanian V, Critchley D: The structure and function of alpha-actinin. J Muscle Res Cell Motil 10:280–289, 1989
27. Nave R, Furst DO, Werber K: Interaction of alpha-actin and nebulin in vitro. FEBS Lett 269:163–164, 1990
28. Chowrashi PK, Pepe FA: The Z-band: 85,000-dalton amorphin and alpha-actinin and their relation to structure. J Cell Biol 94:565–573, 1982
29. Yamaguchi M, Izumimoto M, Robson RM, et al: Fine structure of wide and narrow vertebrate muscle Z-line. J Mol Biol 184:621–643, 1985
30. Tokuyasu KT, Dutton AH, Singer SJ: Immunoelectron microscopic studies of desmin (skeleton) localization and intermediate filament organization in chicken skeletal muscle. J Cell Biol 96:1727–1735, 1983
31. Goebel HH, Bornemann A: Desmin pathology in neuromuscular diseases. Virchows Arch 64:127–135, 1993
32. Granger BL, Lazarides E: Desmin and vimentin coexist at the periphery of the myofibril Z disc. Cell 18:1053–1063, 1979

33. Trinick J: Titin and nebulin: protein rulers in muscle? Trends Biochem Sci 19:405–409, 1994

34. Maruyama K, Kimura S, Ohashi K, et al: Connection, an elastic protein of muscle. Identification of "titin" with connectin. J Biochem (Tokyo) 89:701–709, 1981

35. Trinick J, Knight P, Whiting A: Purification and properties of native titin. J Mol Biol 180:331–356, 1984

36. Wang K, McClure J, Tu A: Titin: major myofibrillar components of striated muscle. Proc Nat Acad Sci USA 76:3698–3702, 1979

37. Kruger M, Wright J, Wang K: Nebulin as a length regulator of thin filaments of vertebrate skeletal muscles: correlation of thin filament length, nebulin size, and epitope profile. J Cell Biol 115:97–107, 1991

38. Bennett P, Craig R, Starr R, et al: Ultrastructural localization of C-protein, X-protein and H-protein in rabbit muscle. J Muscle Res Cell Motil 7:550–567, 1986

39. Offer G, Moos C, Starr R: A new protein of the thick filaments of vertebrate skeletal myofibrils. Extraction, purification and characterization. J Mol Biol 74:653–676, 1973

40. Turner DC, Willimann T, Eppenberger HM: A protein that binds specifically to M-line of skeletal muscle is identified as the muscle form of creatine kinase. Proc Nat Acad Sci USA 70:702–705, 1973

41. Wallimann T, Turner DC, Eppenberger HM: Localization of creatine kinase isoenzymes in myofibrils. I. Chicken skeletal muscle. J Cell Biol 75:297–317, 1977

42. Masaki T, Takaiti O: M-protein. J Biochem (Tokyo) 75:367–380, 1974

43. Trinick J, Lowey S: M-protein from chicken pectoralis muscle: isolation and characterization. J Mol Biol 113:343–368, 1977

44. Grove BK, Kurer V, Lehner C: A new 185,000 dalton skeletal muscle protein detected by antibodies. J Cell Biol 98:518–524, 1984

45. Wallimann T, Eppenberger HM: Localization and function of M-line bound creatine kinase: M-band model and creatine phosphate shuttle. Cell Muscle Motil 6:239–285, 1989

46. Campbell K: Three muscular dystrophies: loss of cytoskeleton-extracellular matrix linkage. Cell 80:675–679, 1995

47. Ozawa E, Yoshida M, Suzuki A, et al: Dystrophin-associated proteins in muscular dystrophy. Hum Mol Genet 4:1711–1716, 1995

48. Worton R: Muscular dystrophies; diseases of the dystrophin-glycoprotein complex. Science 270:755–756, 1995

49. Ahn AH, Kunkel LM: The structural and functional diversity of dystrophin. Nature Genet 3:283–291, 1993

50. Hoffman EP, Kunkel LM: Dystrophin abnormalities in Duchenne/Becker muscular dystrophy. Neuron 2:1019–1029, 1989

51. Hemmings L, Kuhlman PA, Critchley DR: Analysis of the actin-binding domain of alpha-actinin by mutagenesis and demonstration that dystrophy contains a functionally homologous domain. J Cell Biol 116:1369–1380, 1992

52. Suzuki A, Yoshida M, Hayashi K, et al: Molecular organization at the glycoprotein-complex-binding site of dystrophin: three dystrophin-associated proteins bind directly to the carboxy-terminal portion of dystrophin. Eur J Biochem 220:283–292, 1994

53. Campbell KP, Kahl SD: Association of dystrophin and an integral membrane glycoprotein. Nature 338:259–262, 1989

54. Yoshida M, Ozawa E: Glycoprotein complex anchoring dystrophin to sarcolemma. J Biochem 108:748–752, 1990

55. Ervasti JM, Campbell KP: A role for the dystrophin-glycoprotein complex as a transmembrane linker between laminin and actin. J Cell Biol 122:809–823, 1993

56. Sadoulet-Puccio HM, Khurana TS, Cohen JB, Kunkel LM: Cloning and characterization of the human homologue of a dystrophin related phosphoprotein found at the *Torpedo* electric organ post-synaptic membrane. Hum Molec Genet 5:489–496, 1996

57. Minetti C, Beltrame F, Marcenaro G, et al: Dystrophin at the plasma membrane of human muscle fibers shows a costameric localization. Neuromuscul Disord 2:99–109, 1992

58. Schwartz MS, Sargeant M, Swash M: Longitudinal fibre splitting in neurogenic muscular disorders—its relation to the pathogenesis of "myopathic" change. Brain 99:617–636, 1976

59. Kovarsky J, Schochet SS Jr, McCormick WF: The significance of target fibers: a clinicopathologic review of 100 patients with neurogenic atrophy. Am J Clin Pathol 59:790–797, 1973

60. Drachman DB, Murphy SR, Nigam MP, et al: "Myopathic" changes in chronically denervated muscle. Arch Neurol 16:14–24, 1967

61. Byers RK, Banker BQ: Infantile muscular atrophy. Arch Neurol 5:140–164, 1961

62. Munsat TL, Woods R, Fowler W, et al: Neurogenic muscular atrophy of infancy with prolonged survival. The variable course of Werdnig-Hoffmann disease. Brain 92:9–24, 1969

63. Gilliam TC, Brzustowicz LM: Molecular and genetic basis of the spinal muscular atrophies. pp. 883–887. In Rosenberg R, Prusiner S, DiMauro S, et al (eds): The Molecular and Genetic Basis of Neurologic Disease. Butterworths, Boston, 1993

64. Lefebvre S, Bürgien L, Reboullet S, et al: Identification and characterization of a spinal muscular atrophy-determining gene. Cell 80:155–165, 1995

65. Brahe C, Servidei S, Zappata S, et al: Genetic homogeneity between childhood-onset and adult-onset autosomal recessive spinal muscular atrophy. Lancet 346:741–742, 1995

66. Rodrigues NR, Owen N, Talbot K, et al: Deletions in the survival motor neuron gene on 5q13 in autosomal recessive spinal muscular atrophy. Hum Mol Genet 4:631–634, 1995

67. Beggs AH, Hoffman EP, Snyder JR, et al: Exploring the molecular basis for variability among patients with Becker muscular dystrophy: dystrophin gene and protein studies. Am J Hum Genet 49:54–67, 1991

68. Gospe SM Jr, Lazaro RP, Lava NS, et al: Familial X-linked myalgia and cramps: a nonprogressive myopathy associated with a deletion in the dystrophin gene. Neurology 10:1277–1280, 1989

69. Towbin JA, Hejtmancik JF, Brink P, et al: X-linked dilated cardiomyopathy. Molecular genetic evidence of linkage to the Duchenne muscular dystrophy (dystrophin) gene at the Xp21 locus. Circulation 87:1854–1865, 1993

70. Duchenne de Boulogne: De l'Électrisation localisée et de son Application à la Physiologie, à la Pathologie et à la Thérapeutique. Baillière, Paris, 1855

71. Duchenne de Boulogne: Recherches sur la paralysie musculaire pseudo-hypertrophique ou paralysie myo-sclérosique. Arch Gen Med 11:5–25, 179–209, 305–321, 421–443, 522–588, 868, 1868

72. Erb W: Ueber die "juvenile Form" der progressiven Muskelatrophie ihre Beziehungen zur sogenannten Pseudohypertrophie der Muskeln. Dtsch Archiv Klin Med 34:467–519, 1884

73. Erb W: Dystrophia muscularis progressiva. Klinische und pathologisch-anatomische Studien. Dtsche Zeitschrift Nervenheilkunde 1:13–94, 173–261, 1891

74. Brooke MH, Fenichel GM, Griggs RC, et al: Duchenne muscular dystrophy: patterns of clinical progression and effects of supportive therapy. Neurology 39:475–481, 1989

75. Marsh CG, Munsat TL: Evidence of early impairment of verbal intelligence in Duchenne muscular dystrophy. Arch Dis Child 49:118–122, 1974

76. Becker PE, Keiner F: Eine neue x-chromosomale Muskeldystrophie. Arch Psychiatr Nervenkrankheiten 193S:427–448, 1995

77. Cazzato G, Walton JN: The pathology of the muscle spindle. A study of biopsy material in various muscular and neuromuscular diseases. J Neurol Sci 7:15–70, 1968

78. Frankel KA, Rosser RJ: The pathology of the heart in progressive muscular dystrophy: epimyocardial fibrosis. Hum Pathol 7:375–386, 1976

79. Kaido M, Arahata K, Hoffman EP, et al: Muscle histology in Becker muscular dystrophy. Muscle Nerve 14:1067–1073, 1991

80. Bradley WG, Jones MZ, Fawcett PRW: Becker-type muscular dystrophy. Muscle Nerve 1:111–132, 1978

81. Engel AG, Yamamoto M, Fishbeck KH: Dystrophinopathies. pp. 1133–1185. In Engel AG, Franzini-Armstrong C (eds): Myology. Basic and Clinical. 2nd Ed. McGraw-Hill, New York, 1994

82. Harper P: The muscular dystrophies. pp. 2869–2902. In Scriver CR, Beaudet AL, Sly SS, Valle D (eds): The Metabolic Basis of Inherited Disease. 6th Ed. McGraw-Hill, New York, 1989

83. Padberg GW: The muscular dystrophies and dystrophin. Curr Opin Neurol 6:688–694, 1993

84. Specht L, Kunkel L: Duchenne and Becker muscular dystrophy. In Rosenberg R, Prusiner S, DiMauro S, et al (eds): The Molecular and Genetic Basis of Neurologic Disease. Butterworths, Boston, 1993

85. Ohlendieck K, Ervasti JM, Snook JB, et al: Dystrophin-glycoprotein complex is highly enriched in isolated skeletal muscle sarcolemma. J Cell Biol 112:135–148, 1991

86. Beggs AH: Multiplex PCR for the identification of dystrophin gene deletions. pp. 9.3.1–9.3.18. In Dracopoli NC, Haines JL, Korf BR (eds): Current Protocols in Human Genetics. John Wiley, New York, 1994

87. Landouzy L, Dejerine J: De la myopathie atrophique progressive (myopathie héréditaire débutant, dans l'enfance, par la face, sans altération du systéme nerveux). C R Hebdomadaires Séances Acad Sci 98:53–55, 1884

88. Landouzy L, Dejerine J: De la myopathie atrophique progressive. Myopathie sans neuropathie débutant d'ordinaire dans l' enfance, par la face. Rev Med 5:81–117, 253–266, 1885

89. Munsat TL, Piper D, Cancilla P, et al: Inflammatory myopathy with facioscapulohumeral distribution. Neurology 22:335–347, 1972

90. Sarfarazi M, Wijmenga C, Upadhyaya M, et al: Regional mapping of facioscapulohumeral muscular dystrophy gene on 4q35: combined analysis of an international consortium. Am J Hum Genet 51:396–403, 1992

91. Gilbert JR, Stajich JM, Wall S, et al: Evidence for heterogeneity in facioscapulohumeral muscular dystrophy (FSHD). Am J Hum Genet 53:401–408, 1993

92. Bushby KM: Diagnostic criteria for the limb-girdle muscular dystrophies: report of the ENMC Consortium on Limb-Girdle Dystrophies. Neuromuscul Disord 5:71–74, 1995

93. Bushby KMD, Beckmann JS: The limb-girdle muscular dystrophies—proposal for a new nomenclature. Neuromuscul Disord 5:337–343, 1995

94. Speer MC, Yamaoka LH, Gilchrist JH, et al: Confirmation of genetic heterogeneity in limb-girdle muscular dystrophy: linkage of an autosomal dominant form to chromosome 5q. Am J Hum Genet 50:1211–1217, 1992

95. Richard I, Broux O, Allamand V, et al: Mutations in the proteolytic enzyme calpain 3 cause limb-girdle muscular dystrophy type 2A. Cell 81:27–40, 1995

96. Bashir R, Strachan T, Keers S, et al: A gene for autosomal recessive limb-girdle muscular dystrophy maps to chromosome 2p. Hum Mol Genet 3:455–457, 1994

97. Bejaoui K, Hirabayashi K, Hentati F, et al: Linkage of Miyoshi myopathy (distal autosomal recessive muscular dystrophy) locus to chromosome 2p 12–14. Neurology 45:768–772, 1995

98. Bönnemann CG, Modi R, Noguchi S, et al: Beta-sarcoglycan (A3b) mutations cause autosomal recessive muscular dystrophy with loss of the sarcoglycan complex. Nature Genet 11:266–273, 1995

99. Lim LE, Duclos F, Broux O, et al: β-sarcoglycan: characterization and role in limb-girdle muscular dystrophy linked to 4q12. Nature Genet 11:257–265, 1995

100. Noguchi S, McNally EM, Ben Othmane K, et al: Mutations in the dystrophin-associated protein γ-sarcoglycan in chromosome 13 muscular dystrophy. Science 270:819–882, 1995

101. Roberds SL, Leturcq F, Allamand V, et al: Missense mutations in the adhalin gene linked to autosomal recessive muscular dystrophy. Cell 78:625–633, 1994

102. Emery AEH, Dreifuss FE: Unusual type of benign X-linked muscular dystrophy. J Neurol Neurosurg Psychiatry 29:338–342, 1966

103. Case Records of the Massachusetts General Hospital: case 34–1992. N Engl J Med 327:549–557, 1992

104. Merlini L, Granata C, Dominici P, et al: Emery-Dreifuss muscular dystrophy: report of five cases in a family and review of the literature. Muscle Nerve 9:481–485, 1986

105. Rowland LP, Fetell M, Olarte M, et al: Emery-Dreifuss muscular dystrophy. Ann Neurol 5:111–117, 1979

106. Bione S, Maestrini E, Rivella S, et al: Identification of a novel X-linked gene responsible for Emery Dreifuss muscular dystrophy. Nature Genet 8:323–327, 1994

107. Thomas PK, Calne DB, Elliot CF: X-linked scapuloperoneal syndrome. J Neurol Neurosurg Psychiatry 35:208–215, 1972

108. Emery AE: Emery-Dreifuss syndrome. J Med Genet 26:637–641, 1989

109. Banker BQ: The congenital muscular dystrophies. pp. 1275–1289. In Engel AG, Franzinini-Armstrong C (eds): Myology. Basic and Clinical. 2nd Ed. McGraw-Hill, New York, 1994

110. Fukuyama Y, Osawa M, Suzuki H: Congenital progressive muscular dystrophy of the Fukuyama type—clinical, genetic and pathological considerations. Brain Dev 3:1–29, 1981

111. Gordon N: Muscle and brain disease: an update. Child Care Health Dev 20:278–287, 1994

112. Lenard HG: Congenital muscular dystrophies—problems of classification. Acta Paediatr Jpn 33:256–260, 1991

113. Toda T, Segawa M, Nomura Y, et al: Localization of a gene for Fukuyama type congenital muscular dystrophy to chromosome 9q31–33. Nature Genet 5:283–286, 1993

114. Yoshioka M, Kuroki S: Clinical spectrum and genetic studies of Fukuyama congenital muscular dystrophy. Am J Med Genet 53:245–250, 1994

115. Ranta S, Pihko H, Santavuori P, et al: Muscle-eye-brain disease and Fukuyama type congenital muscular dystrophy are not allelic. Neuromuscl Disord 5:221–225, 1995

116. Tomé FMS, Evangelista T, Leclerc A, et al: Congenital muscular dystrophy with merosin deficiency. C R Acade Sci III 317:351–357, 1994

117. Yamada H, Tomé FMS, Higuchi I, et al: Laminin abnormality in severe childhood autosomal recessive muscular dystrophy. Lab Invest 72:715–722, 1995

118. Helbling-Leclerc A, Zhang X, Topaloglu H, et al: Mutations in the laminin α-2-chain (LAMA2) cause merosin-deficient congenital muscular dystrophy. Nature Genet 11:216–218, 1995

119. Steinert H: Über das klinische and anatomische Bild des Muskelschwunds der Myotoniker. Dtsche Z Nervenheilkunde 37:58–104, 1909

120. Schotland DL, Spiro D, Carmel P: Ultrastructural studies of ring fibers in human muscle disease. J Neuropathol Exp Neur 25:431–442, 1966

121. Rosman NP, Rebeiz JJ: The cerebral defect and myopathy in myotonic dystrophy. A comparative clinicopathological study. Neurology 17:1106–1112, 1967

122. Argov Z, Gardner Medwin D, Johnson NA, et al: Congenital myotonic dystrophy. Fiber type abnormalities in two cases. Arch Neurol 37:693–696, 1980

123. Karpati G, Carpenter S, Watters GV, et al: Infantile myotonic dystrophy. Histochemical and electron microscopic features in skeletal muscle. Neurology 23:1066–1076, 1973

124. Brook JD, McCurrach ME, Harley HG, et al: Molecular basis of myotonic dystrophy; expansion of a trinucleotide (CTG) repeat at the 3′ end of a transcript encoding a protein kinase family member. Cell 68:799–808, 1992

125. Harley HG, Rundle SA, MacMillan JC, et al: Size of the unstable CTG-repeat in relation to phenotype and parental transmission in myotonic dystrophy. Am J Hum Genet 52:1164–1174, 1993

126. Thornton CA, Griggs RC, Moxley RT: Myotonic dystrophy with no trinucleotide repeat expansion. Ann Neurol 35:269–272, 1994

127. Porter J, Baker R, Ragusa R, et al: Extraocular muscles: basic and clinical aspects of structure and function. Surv Ophthalmol 39:451–484, 1995

128. Victor M, Hayes R, Adams RD: Oculopharyngeal muscular dystrophy. A familial disease of late life characterized by dysphagia and progressive ptosis of the eyelids. N Engl J Med 267:1267–1272, 1962

129. Lacomis D, Kupsky WJ, Kuban KK, et al: Childhood onset oculopharyngeal muscular dystrophy. Pediatr Neurol 7:382–384, 1991

130. Smith TW, Chad D: Intranuclear inclusions in oculopharyngeal dystrophy. Muscle Nerve 7:339–340, 1984

131. Tomé FMS, Fardeau M: Nuclear inclusions in oculopharyngeal dystrophy. Acta Neuropathol 49:85–87, 1980

132. Brais B, Xie Y-G, Sanson M, et al: The oculopharyngeal muscular dystrophy locus maps to the region of the cardiac α and β myosin heavy chain genes on chromosome 14q11.2-q13. Hum Mol Genet 4:429–434, 1995

133. Nemet P, Godel V, Ron S, et al: Ocular congenital fibrosis syndrome. Metab Pediatr Syst Ophthalmol 8:172–174, 1985

134. Houtman WA, van Weerden TW, Robinson PH, et al: Hereditary congenital external ophthalmoplegia. Ophthalmologica 193:207–218, 1986

135. Cibis GW: Congenital familial external ophthalmoplegia with co-contraction. Ophthalmic Paediatr Geneti 3:163–168, 1984

136. Harley RD, Rodrigues MM, Crawford JS: Congenital fibrosis of the extraocular muscles. J Pediatr Ophthalmol Strabismus 6:346–358, 1978

137. Engle EC, Kunkel LM, Specht LA, et al: Mapping a gene for congenital fibrosis of the extraocular muscles to the centromeric region of chromosome 12. Nature Genet 7:69–73, 1994

138. Engle EC, Marondel I, Houtman WA, et al: Congenital fibrosis of the extraocular muscles (autosomal dominant congenital external ophthalmoplegia): genetic homogeneity, linkage refinement, and physical mapping on chromosome 12. Am J Hum Genet 57:1086–1094. 1995

139. Briggs HH: Hereditary congenital ptosis with report of 64 cases conforming to the Mendelian rule of dominance. Am J Ophthalmol 2:408–417, 1919

140. Cohen MA: Congenital ptosis: a new pedigree and classification. Arch Ophthalmol 87:161–163, 1972

141. Heffner RR: Inflammatory myopathies. A review. J Neuropathol Exp Neurol 52:339–350, 1993

142. Carpenter S, Karpati G: The pathological diagnosis of specific inflammatory myopathies. Brain Pathol 2:13–19, 1992

143. Dalakas M: Polymyositis, dermatomyositis and inclusion body myositis. N Engl J Med 325:1487–1498, 1991

144. Banker BQ, Victor M: Dermatomyositis (systemic angiopathy) of childhood. Medicine 45:261–289, 1966

145. Shevell M, Rosenblatt B, Silver K, et al: Congenital inflammatory myopathy. Neurology 40:1111–1114, 1990

146. Jerusalem F, Rakusa M, G EA, et al: Morphometric analysis of skeletal muscle capillary ultrastructure in inflammatory myopathies. J Neurol Sci 23:391–402, 1974

147. Arahata K, Engel AG: Monoclonal antibody analysis of mononuclear cells in myopathies. I: Quantitation of subsets according to diagnosis and sites of accumulation and demonstration and counts of muscle fibers invaded by T cells. Ann Neurol 19:193–208, 1984

148. Arahata K, Engel AG: Monoclonal antibody analysis of mononuclear cells in myopathies. III: Immunoelectron microscopic aspects of cell-mediated muscle fiber injury. Ann Neurol 19:112–125, 1986

149. De Bleecker JL, Engel AG: Immunocytochemical study of CD45 T cell isoforms in inflammatory myopathies. Am J Pathol 146:1178–1187, 1995

150. Engel AG, Arahata K: Monoclonal antibody analysis of mononuclear cells in myopathies. II: Phenotypes of autoinvasive cells in polymyositis and inclusion body myositis. Ann Neurol 16:209–215, 1984

151. Emslie-Smith AM, Arahata K, Engel AG: Major histocompatibility complex class I antigen expression, immunolocalization of interferon subtypes, and T-cell-mediated cytoxicity in myopathies. Hum Pathol 20:224–231, 1989

152. Caulfield JB, Rebeiz J, Adams RD: Viral involvement of human muscle. J Pathol Bacteriol 96:232–234, 1968

153. Chou SM, Gutmann L: Picornavirus-like crystals in subacute polymyositis. Neurology 20:205–213, 1970

154. Kissel JT, Mendell JR, Rammohan KW: Microvascular deposition of complement membrane attack complex in dermatomyositis. N Engl J Medi 314:329–334, 1986

155. De Visser M, Emslie-Smith AM, Engel AG: Early ultrastructural alterations in adult dermatomyositis. Capillary abnormalities precede other structural changes in muscle. J Neurol Sci 94:181–192, 1989

156. Emslie-Smith AM, Engel AG: Microvascular changes in early advanced dermatomyositis: a quantitative study. Ann Neurol 27:343–356, 1990

157. Banker BQ: Dermatomyositis of childhood. Ultrastructural alterations of muscle and intramuscular blood vessels. J Neuropathol Exp Neurol 34:46–75, 1975

158. Carpenter S, Karpati G, Rothman S, et al: The childhood type of dermatomyositis. Neurology 26:952–962, 1976

159. Oshima Y, Becker LE, Armstrong DL: An electron microscopic study of childhood dermatomyositis. Acta Neuropathol 47:189–196, 1979

160. Yunis EJ, Samaha FJ: Inclusion body myositis. Lab Invest 25:240–248, 1971

161. Chou S-M: Myxovirus-like structures in a case of chronic polymyositis. Science 158:1453–1455, 1967

162. Carpenter S, Karpati G, Heller I, et al: Inclusion body myositis: a distinct variety of idiopathic inflammatory myopathy. Neurology 28:8–17, 1978

163. Griggs RC, Askanas V, DiMauro S, et al: Inclusion body myositis and myopathies. Neurology 38:705–713, 1995

164. Lotz BP, Engel AG, Nishino H, et al: Inclusion body myositis. Observations in 40 patients. Brain 112:727–747, 1989

165. Mikol J, Engel A: Inclusion body myositis. pp. 1384–1398. In Engel AG, Franzini-Armstrong C (eds): Myology. Basic and Clinical. 2nd Ed. McGraw-Hill, New York, 1994

166. Mendell JR, Sahenk Z, Gales T, et al: Amyloid filaments in inclusion body myositis. Novel findings provide insight into nature of filaments. Arch Neurol 48:1229–1234, 1991

167. Sivakumar K, Cervenáková L, Dalakas MC, et al: Exons 16 and 17 of the amyloid precursor protein gene in familial inclusion body myopathy. Ann Neurol 38:267–269, 1995

168. Figarella-Branger D, Pellissier J-F, Pouget J, et al: Myosites à inclusions et maladies neuromusculaires avec vacuoles bordées. Rev Neurol 148:281–290, 1992

169. Albrecht S, Bilbao JM: Ubiquitin expression in inclusion body myositis. An immunohistochemical study. Arch Pathol Lab Med 117–789, 1993

170. Garelepp MJ, Tabarias H, van Bockxmeer FM, et al: Apolipoprotein E ε4 in inclusion body myositis. Ann Neurol 38:957–959, 1995

171. Kallajoki M, Hyypiä T, Halonen P, et al: Inclusion body myositis and paramyxoviruses. Hum Pathol 22:29–32, 1991

172. Mikol J, Felten-Papaiconomou A, Ferchal F, et al: Inclusion-body myositis: clinicopathologic studies and isolation of an adenovirus type 2 from muscle biopsy specimen. Ann Neurol 11:576–581, 1982

173. Chou SM: Inclusion body myositis: a chronic persistent mumps myositis? Hum Pathol 17:765–777, 1986

174. Lynch PG, Bansal DV: Granulomatous polymyositis. J Neurol Sci 18:1–9, 1972

175. Michel D, Tommasi M, Rousset H, et al: Myosite granulomateuse au cours d'une collagénose (une observation) et d'un dysgerminome suprasellaire (une observation). Rev Neurol 135:3–14, 1979

176. Namba T, Brunner NG, Grob D: Idiopathic giant cell polymyositis. Report of a case and review of the syndrome. Arch Neurol 31:27–30, 1974

177. Wallace SL, Lattes R, Malia JP, et al: Muscle involvement in Boeck's sarcoid. Am J Med 26:497–511, 1958

178. Silverstein A, Sitlzbach L: Muscle involvement in sarcoidosis. Asymptomatic, myositis, and myopathy. Arch Neurol 21:235–241, 1969

179. Hewlett RH, Brownell B: Granulomatous myopathy: its relationship to sarcoidosis and polymyositis. J Neurol Neurosurg Psychiatry 38:1090–1099, 1975

180. Banker BQ: Other inflammatory myopathies. pp. 1461–1486. In Engel AG, Franzinini-Armstrong C (eds): Myology. Basic and Clinical. 2nd Ed. McGraw-Hill, New York, 1994

181. Felice K, De Girolami U, Chad D: Pyomyositis presenting as rapidly progressive generalized weakness. Neurology 41:944–945, 1991

182. Gibson RK, Rosenthal SJ, Lukert BP: Pyomyositis. Increasing recognition in temperate climates. Am J Med 77:768–772, 1984

183. Leon-Monzon M, Illa I, Dalakas MC: Polymyositis in patients infected with human T-cell leukemia virus type 1: the role of the virus in the cause of the disease. Ann Neurol 36:643–649, 1994

184. Smadja D, Bellance R, Cabre P, et al: Atteintes du système nerveux périphérique et du muscle squelettique au cours des paraplégies associées au virus HTL VI. Étude de 70 cas observés en Martinique. Rev Neurol 151:190–195, 1995

185. Gherardi R, Baudrimont M, Lionnet F, et al: Skeletal muscle toxoplasmosis in patients with acquired immunodeficiency syndrome: a clinical and pathological study. Ann Neurol 32:535–542, 1992

186. Reimers CD, de Koning J, Neubert U, et al: *Borrelia burgdorferi* myositis: a report of eight patients. J Neurol 240:278–283, 1993

187. Gabbai AA, Schmidt B, Castelo A, et al: Muscle biopsy in AIDS and ARC: analysis of 50 patients. Muscle Nerve 13:541–544, 1990

188. Gherardi RK: Skeletal muscle involvement in HIV-infected patients. Neuropathol Appl Neurobiol 20:232–237, 1994

189. Gray F (ed): Atlas of the Neuropathology of HIV Infection. Oxford University Press, Oxford, 1993

190. Gherardi RK, Florea-Strat A, Fromont G, et al: Cytokine expression in the muscle of HIV-infected patients: evidence for interleukin-1 α accumulation in mitochondria of AZT fibers. Ann Neurol 36:752–758, 1994

191. Chad DA, Smith TW, Blumenfeld A, et al: Human immunodeficiency virus (HIV)-associated myopathy: immunocytochemical identification of an HIV antigen (gp 41) in muscle macrophages. Ann Neurol 28:579–582, 1990

192. Leon-Monzon M, Lamperth L, Dalakas MC: Search for HIV proviral DNA and amplified sequences in the muscle biopsies of patients with HIV polymyositis. Muscle Nerve 16:408–413, 1993

193. Heffner RR, Armbrustmacher VW, Earle KM: Focal myositis. Cancer 40:301–306, 1977

194. Fardeau M, Tomé FMS: Congenital myopathies. pp. 1487–1532. In Engel AG, Franzini-Armstrong C (eds): Myology. Basic and Clinical. 2nd Ed. McGraw-Hill, New York, 1994

195. Greenfield JG, Cornman T, Shy GM: The prognostic value of the muscle biopsy in the "floppy infant." Brain 81:462–484, 1958

196. Shy GM, Magee KR: A new congenital non-progressive myopathy. Brain 79:610–621, 1956

197. Haan EA, Freemantle CJ, McCure JA, et al: Assignment of the gene for central core disease to chromosome 19. Hum Genet 86:187–190, 1990

198. Quane KA, Healy JMS, Keating KE, et al: Mutations in the ryanodine receptor gene in central core disease and malignant hyperthermia. Nature Genet 5:51–55, 1993

199. Zhang Y, Chen S, Khanna VK, et al: A mutation in the human ryanodine receptor gene associated with central core disease. Nature Genet 5:46–59, 1993

200. Fananapazir L, Dalakas MC, Cyran F, et al: Missense mutations in the beta-myosin heavy-chain gene cause central core disease in hypertrophic cardiomyopathy. Proc Natl Acad Sci USA 90:3993–3997, 1993

201. Brownell AKW, Gilbert JJ, Shaw Dt, et al: Adult onset nemaline myopathy. Neurology 28:1306–1309, 1978

202. Hopkins IJ, Lindsey JR, Ford FR: Nemaline myopathy. A long-term clinicopathologic study of affected mother and daughter. Brain 89:299–310, 1966

203. Shy GM, Engel WK, Somers JE, et al: Nemaline myopathy. A new congenital myopathy. Brain 86:793–810, 1963

204. Laing NG, Majda BT, Akkarri PA, et al: Assignment of a gene (NEM1) for autosomal dominant nemaline myopathy to chromosome 1. Am J Hum Genet 50:576–583, 1992

205. Laing NG, Wilton SD, Akkari PA, et al: A mutation of the α tropomyosin gene TPM3 associated with autosomal dominant nemaline myopathy. Nature Genet 9:75–79, 1995

206. Tahvanainen E, Beggs AH, Wallgren-Pettersson C: Exclusion of two candidate loci for autosomal recessive nemaline myopathy. J Med Genet 31:79–80, 1994

207. Wallgren-Pettersson C, Avela K, Marchand S, et al: A gene for autosomal recessive nemaline myopathy assigned to chromosome 2q by linkage analysis. Neuromuscul Disord 5:441–443, 1995

208. Spiro AJ, Shy GM, Gonatas NK: Myotubular myopathy. Persistence of fetal muscle in an adolescent boy. Arch Neurol 14:1–14, 1966

209. Engel WK, Gold GN, Karpati G: Type I fiber hypotrophy and central nuclei. A rare congenital muscle abnormality with a possible experimental model. Neurology 18:435–444, 1968

210. Wallgren-Pettersson C, Clarke A, Samson F, et al: The myotubular myopathies: differential diagnosis of the X-linked recessive, autosomal dominant, and autosomal recessive forms and present state of DNA studies. J Med Genet 32:673–679, 1995

211. Bergen BJ, Carry MP, Wilson WB, et al: Centronuclear myopathy: extraocular- and limb-muscle findings in an adult. Muscle Nerve 3:165–171, 1980

212. Ferrer X, Vital M, Coquet M, et al: Myopathie centronucléaire autosomique dominante. Rev Neurol 148:622–630, 1992

213. Figarella-Branger D, Calore EE, Boucraut J, et al: Expression of cell surface and cytoskeleton developmentally regulated proteins in adult centronuclear myopathies. J Neurol Sci 109:69–76, 1992

214. Misra AK, Menon NK, Mishra SK: Abnormal distribution of desmin and vimentin in myofibers in adult onset myotubular myopathy. Muscle Nerve 15:1246–1252, 1992

215. Sarnat H: Myotubular myopathy: arrest of morphogenesis of myofibers associated with persistence of fetal vimentin and desmin. Four cases compared with fetal and neonatal muscle. Can J Neurol Sci 17:109–123, 1990

216. Janssen EAM, Hensels GW, van Oost BA, et al: The gene for X-linked myotubular myopathy is located in a 8 Mb region at the border of Xq27.3 and Xq28. Neuromuscul Disord 4:455–461, 1994

217. Samson F, Mesnard L, Heimburger M, et al: Genetic linkage heterogeneity in myotubular myopathy. Am J Hum Genet 57:120–126, 1995

218. Scriver CR, Beaudet AL, Sly WS, et al: The Metabolic Basis of Inherited Disease. McGraw-Hill, New York, 1989

219. Hers HG: α-Glucosidase deficiency in generalized glycogen storage disease (Pompe's disease). Biochem J 86:11–16, 1963

220. Engel AG, Hirschhorn R: Acid maltase deficiency. pp. 1533–1553. In Engel AG, Franzini-Armstrong C (eds): Myology. 2nd Ed. McGraw-Hill, New York, 1994

221. McArdle B: Myopathy due to a defect in muscle glycogen breakdown. Clin Sci 10:14–35, 1951

222. Pearson CM, Rimer DG, Mommaerts WFHM: A metabolic myopathy due to absence of muscle phosphorylase. Am J Med 30:502–517, 1961

223. Schmid R, Mahler R: Chronic progressive myopathy with myoglobinuria: demonstration of a glycogenolytic defect in the muscle. J Clin Invest 38:2044–2058, 1959

224. Lebo RV, Gorin F, Fletterick RJ, et al: High-resolution chromosome sorting and DNA spot-blot analysis assign McArdle's syndrome to chromosome 11. Science 225:57–59, 1984

225. DiMauro S, Tsujino S: Nonlysosomal glycogenoses. pp. 1554–1576. In Engel AG, Franzini-Armstrong C (eds): Myology. Basic and Clinical. 2nd Ed. McGraw-Hill, New York, 1994

226. Tsujino S, Shanske S, DiMauro S: Molecular genetic heterogeneity of

myophosphorylase deficiency (McArdle's disease). N Engl J Med 329:241–245, 1993

227. Tarui S, Okuno G, Ikua Y, et al: Phosphofructokinase deficiency in skeletal muscle. A new type of glycogenosis. Biochem Biophys Res Commun 19:517–523, 1965

228. Vora S, Durham S, deMartinville B, et al: Assignment of the human gene for muscle-type phosphofructokinase (PFKM) to chromosome 1 (region cen-q32) using somatic cell hybrids and monoclonal anti-M antibody. Somat Cell Genet 8:95–104, 1982

229. Raben N, Sherman JB: Mutations in muscle phosphofructokinase gene. Hum Mutat 6:1–6, 1995

230. Hays AP, Hallett M, Delfs J, et al: Muscle phosphofructokinase deficiency: abnormal polysaccharide in a case of late-onset myopathy. Neurology 31:1077–1086, 1981

231. Herrick MK, Twiss JL, Vladutiu GD, et al: Concomitant branching enzyme and phosphorylase deficiencies. An unusual glycogenosis with extensive neuronal polyglucosan storage. J Neuropathol Exp Neurol 53:239–246, 1994

232. Kaminski HJ, Ruff RL: Endocrine myopathies (hyper- and hypofunction of the adrenal, thyroid, pituitary and parathyroid glands and iatrogenic corticosteroid myopathy). pp. 1726–1753. In Engel AG, Franzini-Armstrong C (eds): Myology. Basic and Clinical. 2nd Ed. McGraw-Hill, New York, 1994

233. Mastaglia FL, Barwick DD, Hall R: Myopathy in acromegaly. Lancet 2:907–909, 1970

234. Mastaglia FL: Pathological changes in skeletal muscle in acromegaly. Acta Neuropathol 24:273–286, 1973

235. Stern LZ, Payne CM, Hannapel LK: Acromegaly: histochemical and electron microscopic changes in deltoid and intercostal muscle. Neurology 24:589–593, 1974

236. Morgan-Hughes JA: Mitochondrial myopathies. pp. 1610–1660. In Engel AG, Franzinini-Armstrong C, (eds): Myology. Basic and Clinical. 2nd Ed. McGraw-Hill, New York, 1994

237. Shoffner JM, Lott MT, Lezza AMS, et al: Myoclonic epilepsy and ragged-red fiber disease (MERRF) is associated with a mitochondrial DNA tRNA^{Lys} mutation. Cell 61:931–937, 1990

238. Kobayashi Y, Momoi MY, Tominaga K, et al: A point mutation in the mitochondrial tRNA^{Leu}(UUR) gene in MELAS (mitochondrial myopathy, encephalopathy, lactic acidosis and stroke-like episodes). Biochem Biophys Res Commun 173:816–822, 1990

239. Holt IJ, Harding AE, Petty RKH, et al: A new mitochondrial disease associated with mitochondrial DNA heteroplasmy. Am J Hum Genet 46:428–433, 1990

240. Zeviani M, Moraes CT, DiMauro S, et al: Deletions of mitochondrial DNA in Kearns-Sayre syndrome. Neurology 38:1339–1346, 1988

241. Moraes CT, DiMauro S, Zeviani M, et al: Mitochondrial DNA deletions in progressive external ophthalmoplegia and Kearns-Sayre syndrome. N Engl J Med 320:1293–1299, 1989

242. Zeviani M, Servidei S, Gellera C, et al: An autosomal dominant disorder with multiple deletions of mitochondrial DNA starting at the D-loop region. Nature 339:309–311, 1989

243. Suomalainen A, Kaukonen J, Amati P, et al: An autosomal locus predisposing to deletions of mitochondrial DNA. Nature Genet 9:146–151, 1995

244. Moraes CT, Shanske S, Tritschler HJ, et al: mtDNA depletion with variable tissue expression: a novel genetic abnormality in mitochondrial disease. Am J Hum Genet 48:492–501, 1991

245. Engel AG, Siekert RG: Lipid storage myopathy responsive to prednisone. Arch Neurol 27:174–181, 1972

246. Karpati G, Carpenter S, Engel AG, et al: The syndrome of systemic carnitine deficiency. Neurology 25:16–24, 1975

247. Di Donato S: Disorders of lipid metabolism affecting skeletal muscle: carnitine deficiency syndromes, defects in the catabolic pathway, and chanarin disease. pp. 1587–1609. In Engel AG, Franzini-Armstrong C (eds): Myology. Basic and Clinical. 2nd Ed. McGraw-Hill, New York, 1994

248. DiMauro S, Melis-DiMauro PM: Muscle carnitine palmitoyltransferase deficiency and myoglobinuria. Science 182:929–931, 1973

249. Finocchiaro G, Taroni F, Rocchi M, et al: cDNA cloning, sequence analysis, and chromosomal localization of the gene for human carnitine palmitoyltransferase. Proc Natl Acad Sci USA 88:661–665, 1991

250. Taroni F, Verderio E, Dworzak F, et al: Identification of a common mutation in the carnitine palmitoyltransferase II gene in familial recurrent myoglobinuria patients. Nature Genet 4:314–320, 1993

251. Pearson CM: The periodic paralyses: differential features and pathological observations in permanent myopathic weakness. Brain 87:341–354, 1964

252. Eulenburg A: Ueber eine familiäre, durch 6 Generationen verfolgbare Form congenitaler Paramyotonie. Neurol Centralblatt 5:265–272, 1886

253. Thrush DC, Morris CJ, Salmon MV: Paramyotonia congenita; a clinical, histochemical and pathological study. Brain 95:537–552, 1972

254. George AL, Komisarof J, Kallen RG, et al: Primary structure of the adult human skeletal muscle voltage-dependent sodium channel. Ann Neurol 31:131–137, 1992

255. Lehmann-Horn F, Engel AG, Ricker K, et al: The periodic paralyses and paramyotonia congenita. pp. 1303–1334. In Engel AG, Franzini-Armstrong C (eds): Myology. Basic and Clinical. 2nd Ed. McGraw-Hill, New York, 1994

256. McClatchey AI, Van den Bergh P, Pericak-Vance MA, et al: Temperature-sensitive mutations in the III-IV cytoplasmic loop region of the skeletal muscle sodium channel gene in paramyotonia congenita. Cell 68:769–774, 1992

257. Ptacek LJ, Tawil R, Griggs RC, et al: Dihydropyridine receptor mutations cause hypokalemic periodic paralysis. Cell 77:863–868, 1994

258. Thomsen J: Tonische Krämpfe in willkürlich beweglichen Muskeln in Folge von ererbter psychischer Disposition (Ataxia muscularis?). Arch Psychiatrie Nervenkrankheiten 6:702–718, 1876

259. Crews J, Kaiser KK, Brooke MH: Muscle pathology of myotonia congenita. J Neurol Sci 28:449–457, 1976

260. Kuhn E, Feihn W, Seiler D, et al: The autosomal recessive (Becker) form of myotonia congenita. Muscle Nerve 2:109–117, 1979

261. Koch MC, Steinmeyer K, Ricker K, et al: The skeletal muscle chloride channel in dominant and recessive human myotonia. Science 257:797–800, 1992

262. Gronert GA: Malignant hyperthermia. pp. 1661–1678. In Engel AG, Franzini-Armstrong C (eds): Myology. Basic and Clinical. 2nd Ed. McGraw-Hill, New York, 1994

263. MacLennan DH, Phillips MS: The role of the skeletal muscle ryanodine receptor (RYR1) gene in malignant hyperthermia and central core disease. Soc Gen Physiol Ser 50:89–100, 1995

264. Sudbrak R, Procaccio V, Klausnitzer M, et al: Mapping of a further malignant hyperthermia susceptibility locus to chromosome 3q13.1. Am J Hum Genet 56:684–691, 1995

265. Iles DE, Lehmann-Horn F, Scherer SW, et al: Localization of the gene encoding the $\alpha 2/\delta$-subunits of the L-type voltage-dependent calcium channel to chromosome 7q and analysis of the segregation of flanking markers in malignant hyperthermia susceptible families. Hum Mol Genet 3:969–975, 1994

266. Olckers A, Meyers DA, Meyers S, et al: Adult muscle sodium channel α-subunit is a gene candidate for malignant hyperthermia susceptibility. Genomics 14:829–831, 1992

267. Victor M, Sieb JP: Myopathies due to drugs, toxins and nutritional deficiency. pp. 1697–1725. In Engel AG, Franzini-Armstrong C (eds): Myology. Basic and Clinical. 2nd Ed. McGraw-Hill, New York, 1994

268. Kuncl RW, Duncan G, Watson D, et al: Colchicine myopathy and neuropathy. N Engl J Med 316:1562–1568, 1987

269. Rutkove SB, De Girolami U, Preston DC, et al: Myotonia in colchicine myopathy. Muscle Nerve 19:870–875, 1996

270. Fardeau M, Tomé MS, Simon P: Muscle and nerve changes induced by perhexiline maleate in man and mice. Muscle Nerve 2:24–36, 1979

271. Hughes JT, Esiri M, Oxbury JM, et al: Chloroquine myopathy. Q J Med 40:85–93, 1971

272. Chucrallah A, De Girolami U, Freeman R, et al: Lovostatin/gemfibrozil myopathy: a clinical, histochemical, and ultrastructural study. Eur Neurol 32:293–296, 1992

273. Dalakas MC, Illa I, Pezeshkpour GH, et al: Mitochondrial myopathy caused by long-term zidovudine therapy. N Engl J Med 322:1098–1105, 1990

274. Mhiri C, Baudrimont M, Bonne G, et al: Zidovudine myopathy: a distinctive disorder associated with mitochondrial dysfunction. Ann Neurol 29:606–614, 1991

275. Chalmers AC, Greco CM, Miller RG: Prognosis in AZT myopathy. Neurology 41:1181–1184, 1991

276. Strongwater SL, Woda BA, Yood RA, et al: Eosinophilia myalgia syndrome associated with L-tryptophan ingestion: analysis of four patients and implications for differential diagnosis and pathogenesis. Arch Intern Med 150:2178–2186, 1990

277. Ahonen RE: Light microscopic study of striated muscle in uremia. Acta Neuropathol 49:51–55, 1980

278. Bundschu HD, Schlote W: Eleknronmikroskopische Untersuchungen der Skelettmuskulatur bei terminaler Niereninsuffizienz. J Neurol Sci 23:243–254, 1974

279. Morisaki T, Gross M, Morisaki H, et al: Molecular basis of AMP deaminase deficiency in skeletal muscle. Proc Nat Acad Sci USA 89:6457–6461, 1992

280. Brownell B, Oppenheimer DR, Spalding JMK: Neurogenic muscle atrophy in myasthenia gravis. J Neurol Neurosurg Psychiatry 35:311–322, 1972

281. Fukuhara N, Takamori M, Gutmann L, et al: Eaton-Lambert syndrome. Ultrastructural study of the motor end-plates. Arch Neurol 27:67–78, 1972

282. Lennon V, Kryzer T, Griesmann, et al: Calcium-channel antibodies in the Lambert-Eaton and other paraneoplastic syndromes. N Engl J Med 332:1467–1474, 1995

283. Engel AG: Myasthenic syndromes. pp. 1798–1835. In Engel AG, Franzini-Armstrong C (eds): Myology. Basic and Clinical. 2nd Ed. McGraw-Hill, New York, 1994

284. Nigro V, De Sá Moreira E, Piluso G, et al: Autosomal recessive limb-girdle muscular dystrophy, LGMD2F, is caused by a mutation in the δ-sarcoglycan gene. Nature Genet 14:195–196, 1996

Index

Page numbers followed by f indicate figures; those followed by t indicate tables.

1